Queen Elizabeth Hospital

UH00001331

D1422434

WO 660

WO 660

# LIVING DONOR ORGAN TRANSPLANTATION

# NOTICE

Medicine is an ever-changing science. As new research and clinical experience broaden our knowledge, changes in treatment and drug therapy are required. The authors and the publisher of this work have checked with sources believed to be reliable in their efforts to provide information that is complete and generally in accord with the standards accepted at the time of publication. However, in view of the possibility of human error or changes in medical sciences, neither the editors nor the publisher nor any other party who has been involved in the preparation or publication of this work warrants that the information contained herein is in every respect accurate or complete, and they disclaim all responsibility for any errors or omissions or for the results obtained from use of the information contained in this work. Readers are encouraged to confirm the information contained herein with other sources. For example and in particular, readers are advised to check the product information sheet included in the package of each drug they plan to administer to be certain that the information contained in this work is accurate and that changes have not been made in the recommended dose or in the contraindications for administration. This recommendation is of particular importance in connection with new or infrequently used drugs.

# LIVING DONOR ORGAN TRANSPLANTATION

*Editor*

## Rainer W.G. Gruessner, MD

Professor and Chairman, Department of Surgery, University of Arizona,
Tucson, Arizona

*Associate Editor*

## Enrico Benedetti, MD

Professor and Chairman, Department of Surgery, University of Illinois,
Chicago, Illinois

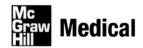

New York  Chicago  San Francisco  Lisbon  London  Madrid  Mexico City  Milan
New Delhi  San Juan  Seoul  Singapore  Sydney  Toronto

*The McGraw·Hill Companies*

**Living Donor Organ Transplantation**

Copyright © 2008 The **McGraw-Hill Companies**, Inc. All rights reserved.
Printed in the United States of America. Except as permitted under the
United States Copyright Act of 1976, no part of this publication may be reproduced or distributed in any form or by any means, or stored in a data base
or retrieval system, without the prior written permission of the publisher.

1 2 3 4 5 6 7 8 9 0   CCW CCW   0 9 8 7

ISBN 978-0-07-145549-7
MHID 0-07-145549-3

The editors were Marsha Loeb and Karen G. Edmonson.
The production supervisor was Catherine Saggese.
Project Management was provided by Aptara.
The cover designer was Aimee Nordin.
Courier Westford was printer and binder.
This book was set in ITC Galliard by Aptara.

This book is printed on acid-free paper.

**Library of Congress Cataloging-in-Publication Data**

Living donor organ transplantation / editor, Rainer W.G. Gruessner; associate
editor, Enrico Benedetti; color illustrations by Martin E. Finch.
     p. ; cm.
  ISBN–13: 978-0-07-145549-7 (alk. paper)
  ISBN–10: 0-07-145549-3 (alk. paper)
  1. Transplantation of organs, tissues, etc. 2. Donation of organs,
  tissues, etc. 3. Organ donors. I. Gruessner, Rainer W.G. II. Benedetti,
  E. (Enrico)
  [DNLM: 1. Organ Transplantation—methods. 2. Informed Consent.
  3. Living Donors—legislation & jurisprudence. 4. Tissue and Organ
  Procurement. 5. Transplantation Immunology. WO 660 L7845 2008]
RD129.5.L52 2008
617.9'54—dc22
         2007040358

# C O N T E N T S

v

                    *Angelika C. Gruessner, PhD*

C H A P T E R   22   **ISLET AUTOTRANSPLANTATION AFTER PANCREATECTOMY:**                               419
                    **HISTORY AND OUTCOMES**
                    *David E.R. Sutherland, MD, PhD, Takashi Kobayashi, MD, Bernhard J. Hering, MD,*
                    *Tun Jie, MD, Annelisa M. Carlson, MD*

C H A P T E R   23   **ISLET TRANSPLANTATION USING LIVING DONORS**                                     429
                    *Juliet Emamaullee, PhD, James Shapiro, MD, PhD*

**SECTION III   LIVER TRANSPLANTATION**

C H A P T E R   24   **PERSONAL REFLECTIONS AND HISTORY OF LIVING DONOR**                              438
                    **LIVER TRANSPLANTATION**
                    *Christoph E. Broelsch, MD, Silvio Nadalin, MD, Massimo Malagó, MD*

C H A P T E R   25   **REGIONAL VARIATIONS IN THE U.S. LIVING DONOR EXPERIENCE**                       442
                    *Mark Wang, MD, Irma Dixler, BSN, RN, Jonathan P. Fryer, MD*

C H A P T E R   26   **INSTITUTIONAL NEEDS FOR LIVING DONOR:**                                         448
                    **LIVER TRANSPLANTATION**
                    *Alan J. Koffron, MD, Michael Abecassis, MD*

C H A P T E R   27   **ROLE OF SPLIT LIVER TRANSPLANTATION FROM**                                      453
                    **DECEASED DONORS: LESSONS LEARNED**
                    *Andrew M. Cameron, MD, PhD, Hasan Yersiz, MD, Ronald W. Busuttil, MD, PhD*

C H A P T E R   28   **LIVER REGENERATION**                                                            459
                    *Jeroen de Jonge, MD, PhD, Kim M. Olthoff, MD*

C H A P T E R   29   **LIVING DONOR LIVER TRANSPLANTATION: THE DONOR**                                 468

                    29.1    **SELECTION AND WORKUP**                                                   468
                           *Abhinav Humar, MD, Cheryl Jacobs, MS, LICSW, Ann Kalis, RN*

                    29.2    **ANESTHESIOLOGIC CONSIDERATIONS**                                         475
                           *Suzanne Shamsolkottabi, MD, Kumar G. Belani, MBBS, MS*

                    29.3    **SURGICAL PROCEDURES**                                                    477

                           29.3.1a   **Adult Donor to Adult Recipient, Right Lobe**                    477
                                     *Giuliano Testa, MD, Massimo Malagó, MD, Enrico Benedetti, MD*

                           29.3.1b   **Adult Donor to Adult Recipient, Extended Right Lobe**           481
                                     *See Ching Chan, MD, MS, Chung Mau Lo, MD, MS*

                           29.3.1c   **Adult Donor to Adult Recipient, Left Lobe**                     484
                                     *Sander Florman, MD, Charles M. Miller, MD*

                           29.3.2    **Adult Donor to Pediatric Recipient**                            489
                                     *Thomas Heffron, MD, Todd Pillen, PA, Carlos Fasola, MD*

                           29.3.3    **Laparoscopic Donor Procedures for the Pediatric Recipient**     492
                                     *Kohei Ogawa, MD, Mikiko Ueda, MD, Koichi Tanaka, MD*

Color plates appear between pages 418 and 419.

# FOREWORD

## Living Donor Organ Transplantation

*By Joseph E. Murray, MD*

Alexis Carrel had received a Nobel Prize in 1912 "in recognition...of the transplantation of blood-vessels and organs." But neither he nor others who followed had studied their long-term function. The concept of "immunological rejection" was ten years in the future.

In 1943, George W. Thorn, MD, Physician-in-Chief of the Peter Bent Brigham (now Brigham/Women's) Hospital in Boston, initiated a program to study hypertension and renal disease. In 1948, Francis D. Moore, MD, new Surgeon-in-Chief, strongly supported the program.

Hemodialysis was first developed as a method to temporarily treat terminal uremia. At the same time, a series of experimental cadaveric thigh transplants was performed, under local anesthesia, with urine collected via an external ureterostomy. Results were published in 1952 by Drs. David Hume and John Merrill. Encouragingly, some of these thigh grafts had temporary function.

After returning to Boston in 1947 from three years of military service at Valley Forge Army Hospital in Pennsylvania, I enthusiastically joined the Transplant Team and replaced Dr. Hume as surgeon when he was recalled to the Navy during the Korean War. I continued performing occasional human thigh transplants, but my first laboratory protocol was to prove that a kidney graft without nerves and lymphatics could function permanently. Each experiment and human thigh transplant added to our knowledge. We were gradually filling the empty glass, drop by drop.

Progress in operating on patients with terminal uremia was steady. We had solid evidence in dogs that a transplanted kidney in the absence of immune rejection could function permanently for years. But no matter how experienced and confident in future success we were, all would have come to nothing without the selflessness of a young veteran of the Korean War. I am referring to Ronald Herrick, a healthy 23-year-old whose identical twin brother, Richard, was near death from chronic kidney disease.

In the hopes of saving his brother's life, Ronald agreed to serve as a living donor, to give his brother the one thing that he needed most: a new kidney. Because we knew that skin grafts between identical twins could function permanently, we believed the same would apply to kidney transplants.

Doctors are trained to "do no harm." The thought of performing an operation on a perfectly healthy person, not for his own benefit, was radical. The only benefit to Ronald was the possibility of saving the life of his brother Richard. That was all. Yet for Ronald, that was enough. On several occasions before the operation, our team met with the Herricks and their family, providing information about preparation, risk, and possible complications. The Herricks decided to put their trust in our hands.

Following the successful Herrick operation, surgeons, physicians, and scientists worldwide continued their transplantation research with renewed enthusiasm. It paved the way for doctors to transplant not only kidneys but also livers, hearts, lungs, pancreases, intestines, and other tissues and organs.

A half-century has followed since the first successful organ transplant. During this time, thousands of patients have survived transplants to lead healthy productive lives. It is appropriate to acknowledge the families and organ procurement agencies who have participated in the happiness of society. I also would like to acknowledge the far-sighted founders of medical schools and workshops that have allowed us to work so productively. Tom Starzl, the pioneer in liver and multiple cluster transplants, correctly summarized the role of the Brigham team on the 30th anniversary of the Herrick operation:

> "If gold medals...were awarded to institutions instead of individuals, the Peter Bent Brigham Hospital...would have qualified.... The qualities of leadership, creativity, courage, and unselfishness made the Peter Bent Brigham Hospital a unique world resource...."
>
> (Starzl TE. The Landmark Identical Twin Case. JAMA 251:2572, 1984)

*Joe Murray*

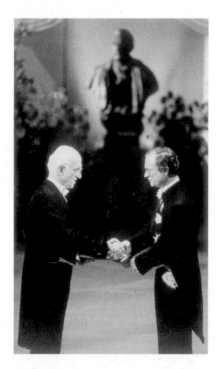

Joseph E. Murray receiving the Nobel prize from King Gustav IV of Sweden, in Stockholm, Sweden, December 10, 1990.

## Living Donor Organ Transplantation

*Rainer W.G. Gruessner, MD*
*University of Arizona, Tucson*

*Enrico Benedetti, MD*
*University of Illinois, Chicago*

The concept of living organ donation for transplantation is virtually unique in medicine, in that a healthy volunteer is exposed to the risk of surgery solely for the benefit of another individual. Because 2 individuals, a donor and a recipient, undergo a surgical procedure, living donor transplants have a potential mortality rate of 200%. The ethical, legal, medical, surgical, social, and psychological principles of this field have developed over time, yet it remains in evolution. This textbook summarizes merely our current understanding of solid organ transplants using living donors.

It has now been over half a century since the first successful kidney transplant between identical twins was performed by Dr. Joseph Murray in Boston on December 23, 1954. Since then, results of living (vs. deceased) donor kidney transplants have been more favorable. Consequently, and not surprisingly, in 2002, for the first time, more living than deceased donors were used for kidney transplants in the United States. A plethora of literature has been published demonstrating that living (vs. deceased) donor kidney transplants are associated not only with higher patient and graft survival rates, but also with lower immunologic and infectious complication rates and with the need for less immunosuppressive therapy.

The emergence of living donor liver transplants in the 1990s led to a decrease in the number of deaths on the liver waiting list. The number of pancreas and intestinal transplants using living donors, albeit in a fledgling state as compared with kidney and liver transplants, has also increased.

This textbook is a joint effort between the transplant divisions at the University of Minnesota, Minneapolis, and the University of Illinois, Chicago. Both have performed living donor transplants of all abdominal organs; 1 of these 2 institutions has also performed living donor islet and lung transplants. Since 2002, these 2 transplant divisions have jointly organized international conferences on living donor abdominal organ transplantation, held every other year. The 3 conferences held so far brought together distinguished scholars from Asia, Europe, and North America. The proceedings of the 2004 and 2006 conferences were published in the peer-reviewed literature, thereby sharing and advancing our knowledge in this field. It was, therefore, a logical step for our 2 transplant divisions to produce this textbook.

The goal of the editors was to assemble scholarly contributions from the most renowned experts in this field, including the very ones who pioneered the surgical aspects of living donor procedures. We are honored that Dr. Murray, in his foreword, described his early experience with living donor kidney transplants. We are also grateful to Dr. Francis Delmonico who, in his capacity as president of the United Network for Organ Sharing from June 25, 2005, through June 30, 2006, highlighted 2 state-of-the-art meetings on living donor transplantation that he had organized. The first meeting, held in Amsterdam in December 2004, focused on the care of living kidney donors; the second meeting, held in Vancouver in September 2005, focused on the care of living lung, liver, pancreas, and intestinal donors.

This textbook is dedicated to all living donors – they are our heroes because of their vision, their courage, and their trust in us to not place them unnecessarily in harm's way. We also want to remember those donors who, despite our best efforts, paid for their heroic effort with their lives; we are painfully aware that each individual donor death results in great grief on the part of their loved ones and the entire medical community.

This 4-part textbook is designed to provide an all-inclusive overview on living donor transplantation. Various procedural topics are touched on, from donor counseling and financial incentives to recipient workup and outcomes. Personal reflections of transplant pioneers offer historical background, while ample attention is also paid to future possibilities in this ever-changing field. Surgical and medical issues specific to living donor abdominal organ transplantation are discussed in detail, providing a wealth of information to both novices and experts.

The primary audience for this textbook includes transplant surgeons and physicians, along with researchers in related fields such as nephrology, hepatology, gastroenterology, endocrinology, pathology, immunology, radiology, and ethics. A definitive reference work, it will also be of interest to transplant fellows, residents, medical students, coordinators, nurses, and social workers, as well as hospital administrators and other medical professionals.

This textbook would not have been possible without the gracious assistance of many of our colleagues. We are indebted to Mary Knatterud, PhD, for her superb editing; to our secretaries, Lois Wolff, Barbara Bailey, and Ann Marie Papas, for their thoroughness; and to Lauren Rogers, Lul Seyum, and Kelsey Brandenburg for their assistance with the literature search. We also wish to express our appreciation to Martin Finch for his excellent art work. Finally, we are grateful to Karen Edmonson of the McGraw-Hill Companies for her continued support.

Rainer W.G. Gruessner, MD
University of Arizona, Tucson

Enrico Benedetti, MD
University of Illinois, Chicago

# DEDICATION

This book is dedicated to all living donors
for their vision and courage.

Michael Abecassis, MD, Professor, Department of Surgery, Division of Organ Transplantation, Northwestern University, Feinberg School of Medicine, Chicago, Illinois

Rita Alloway, PharmD, Research Professor of Medicine, Departments of Surgery and Internal Medicine, Divisions of Nephrology and Transplantation, University of Cincinnati, Cincinnati, Ohio

Estella M. Alonso, MD, Professor, Department of Pediatrics, Northwestern University Medical School, Director, Liver Transplantation, Children's Memorial Hospital, Chicago, Illinois

Bashar A. Aqel, MD, Assistant Professor, University of Minnesota, Division of Gastroenterology and Hepatology, Director, Hepatitis C Resource Center, Veterans Affairs Medical Center, Minneapolis, Minnesota

José G. Avila, MD, Research Instructor, Division of Transplantation, University of Illinois at Chicago, Chicago, Illinois

David Axelrod, MD, MBA, Assistant Professor, Department of Surgery, Dartmouth Medical School, Lebanon, New Hampshire

Rolf N. Barth, MD, Assistant Professor, Department of Surgery, University of Maryland School of Medicine, Baltimore, Maryland

Rodolfo R. Batarse, MD, Assistant Professor, Division of Nephrology, University of California San Diego, Center for Transplantation, San Diego, California

Scott Becher, Chief of Staff, Wisconsin State Capitol, Madison, Wisconsin

David S. Beebe, MD, Professor, Department of Anesthesiology, Director, Anesthesiology Residency Program, University of Minnesota Medical School, Minneapolis, Minnesota

Kumar G. Belani, MBBS, MS, Professor, Departments of Anesthesiology, Medicine, and Pediatrics, University of Minnesota, Minneapolis, Minnesota

Enrico Benedetti, MD, Professor, Department of Surgery, University of Illinois at Chicago, Chicago, Illinois

Peter Boros, MD, Associate Professor, Department of Surgery, Transplantation Institute, Mount Sinai School of Medicine, New York, New York

Ken Brayman, MD, PhD, Professor, Department of Surgery, University of Virginia, Charlottesville, Virginia

Christoph E. Broelsch, MD, Professor, Department of General Surgery and Transplantation, University Hospital of the Gerhard Mercator University Essen-Duisburg, Hufelandstr, Germany

Jonathan S. Bromberg, MD, Professor, Department of Surgery, Immunobiology and Gene and Cell Medicine, Transplantation Institute, Mount Sinai School of Medicine, New York, New York

Robert S. Brown Jr., MD, MPH, Associate Professor, Department of Surgery, Columbia University College of Physicians and Surgeons, Center for Liver Disease and Transplantation, New York-Presbyterian Hospital, New York, New York

Joseph Buell, MD, Professor, Department of Surgery, Division of Transplantation, University of Louisville, Louisville, Kentucky

Thomas Burroughs, PhD, Associate Professor, Department of Internal Medicine, Saint Louis University, Center for Outcomes Research, St. Louis, Missouri

Ronald W. Busuttil, MD, PhD, Professor, Department of Surgery, Division of Liver and Pancreas Transplantation, David Geffen School of Medicine, University of California, Los Angeles, California

Junchao Cai, MD, PhD, Terasaki Foundation Laboratory, Los Angeles, California

Clive O. Callender, MD, Professor, Department of Surgery, Howard University Transplant Center, Washington DC

Andrew M. Cameron, MD, PhD, Assistant Professor, Department of Surgery, Division of Transplantation, Johns Hopkins University School of Medicine, Baltimore, Maryland

Jeff Campsen, MD, Chief Surgical Resident, Division of Transplant Surgery, University of Colorado Health Sciences Center, Denver, Colorado

Annelisa M. Carlson, MD, Resident, Department of Surgery, Division of Transplantation, University of Minnesota, Minneapolis, Minnesota

Marilia Cascalho, MD, PhD, Assistant Professor, Departments of Surgery, Immunology, and Pediatrics, Mayo Clinic College of Medicine, Rochester, Minnesota

**Vincent Casingal, MD,** Assistant Professor, CMC Transplant Center, Charlotte, North Carolina

**J. Michael Cecka, PhD,** Director, Clinical Research, Department of Pathology, University of California, Los Angeles, California

**See Ching Chan, MD, MS,** Associate Consultant, Department of Surgery, Centre for the Study of Liver Disease, University of Hong Kong, Hong Kong, China

**Mark J. Cherry, PhD,** Associate Professor, Department of Philosophy, Saint Edward's University, Austin, Texas

**Laura L. Christensen, MS,** Biostatistician, Scientific Registry of Transplant Recipients, Ann Arbor, Michigan

**Erik N.K. Cressman. MD, PhD,** Assistant Professor, Department of Radiology, University of Minnesota Medical School, Minneapolis, Minnesota

**David C. Cronin II, MD, PhD,** Associate Professor, Department of Surgery, Yale University School of Medicine, New Haven, Connecticut

**John A. Daller, MD, PhD,** Director, Abdominal Organ Transplantation, Associate Professor, Surgery Temple University, Department of Surgery, 3322 N Broad Street, Philadelphia, Pennsylvania

**Phillip J. DeChristopher, MD, PhD,** Professor, Department of Pathology, Loyola University Medical Center, Maywood, Illinois

**Bernard de Hemptinne, MD, PhD,** Professor, General, Vascular, and Abdominal Surgery, Ghent University Hospital Medical School, Ghent, Belgium

**Jeron de Jonge, MD, PhD,** Assistant Professor, Department of Transplant and Gastrointestinal Surgery, Erasmus Medical Center, Rotterdam, The Netherlands

**Francis L. Delmonico, MD,** Professor, Department of Surgery, Harvard Medical School, Massachusetts General Hospital, Boston, Massachusetts

**Stefano DiDomenico, MD,** Research Fellow, Department of Surgery, University of Illinois, Chicago, Illinois

**Irma Dixler, BSN, RN,** Registered Nurse, Department of Surgery, Division of Transplantation, Northwestern University, Feinberg School of Medicine, Chicago, Illinois

**Ty Dunn, MD,** Assistant Professor, Department of Surgery, Division of Transplantation, University of Minnesota, Minneapolis, Minnesota

**Jean C. Emond, MD,** Professor, Department of Surgery, Columbia University, Transplantation Services, Center for Liver Disease and Transplantation, New York Presbyterian Hospital Center, New York, New York

**Bijan Eghtesad, MD,** Staff, Department of General Surgery and Liver Transplantation, Cleveland Clinic Foundation, Cleveland, Ohio

**Gunilla Einecke, MD,** Nephrology Fellow, Division of Nephrology, University of Alberta, Edmonton, Canada

**Juliet Emamaullee, PhD,** Post-doctoral Fellow, Shapiro Lab, University of Alberta, Edmonton, Canada

**Bo-Göran Ericzon, MD,** Professor, Division of Transplantation Surgery, Karolinska Institute, Karolinska University Hospital Huddinge, Stockholm, Sweden

**Sheung Tai Fan, MS, MD, PhD,** Professor, Department of Surgery, University of Hong Kong, Queen Mary Hospital, Hong Kong, China

**Carlos Fasola, MD,** Assistant Professor, Department of Surgery, Division of Transplantation, Emory Healthcare and Children's Healthcare of Atlanta, Atlanta, Georgia

**Ronald M. Ferguson, MD, PhD,** Professor, Department of Surgery, Division of Transplantation, Ohio State University, Columbus, Ohio

**Sander Florman, MD,** Associate Professor, Departments of Surgery and Pediatrics, Tulane University School of Medicine, Director, Liver Transplant, Tulane University Hospital and Clinic, New Orleans, Louisiana

**Christine A. Frederici, LCSW,** Licensed Clinical Social Worker, University of California Center for Transplantation, San Diego, California

**Jonathan P. Fryer, MD,** Associate Professor, Department of Surgery, Division of Transplantation, Northwestern University, Feinberg School of Medicine, Chicago, Illinois

**John J. Fung, MD, PhD,** Professor, Department of General Surgery, Director, Transplant Center, Cleveland Clinic Foundation, Cleveland, Ohio

**Hiroyuki Furukawa, MD,** Professor, Department of Surgery, Organ Transplantation, and Regenerative Medicine, Hokkaido University School of Medicine, Sapporo, Japan

**A. Osama Gaber, MD,** Professor, Department of Surgery, Methodist Hospital Physician Organization, Houston, Texas

**Carlos Galvani, MD,** Assistant Professor, Minimally Invasive Surgery Center, University of Illinois, Chicago, Illinois

**Antonio Gangemi, MD,** Research Fellow, University of Illinois, Chicago, Illinois

**Cathy Garvey, RN,** Transplant Coordinator, Department of Surgery, University of Minnesota, Minneapolis, Minnesota

**Roberto Gedaly, MD,** Assistant Professor, University of Kentucky, Transplant Center, Lexington, Kentucky

**Bernard Gert, PhD,** Professor, Department of Philosophy, Dartmouth College, Hanover, New Hampshire

**Ahad J. Ghods, MD,** Professor, Iran University of Medical Sciences, Director, Division of Nephrology and Transplantation, Hashemi Nejad Kidney Hospital, Tehran, Iran

**James M. Gloor, MD,** Associate Professor, Departments of Internal Medicine and Pediatrics, Mayo Clinic College of Medicine, Division of Nephrology, Mayo Clinic Transplant Center, Rochester, Minnesota

**David R. Grant, MD,** Professor, Department of Surgery, Multi-Organ Transplant, University of Toronto, Toronto, Ontario, Canada

**Thomas G. Gross, MD,** Associate Professor, Departments of Surgery, Pediatrics and Internal Medicine, Divisions of Nephrology and Transplantation, University of Cincinnati, Cincinnati, Ohio

**Angelika C. Gruessner, PhD,** Professor, Arizona Cancer Center, Tucson, Arizona

**Rainer W.G. Gruessner, MD,** Professor, Department of Surgery, University of Arizona, Tucson, Arizona

**Thomas Gutmann, PhD, MA,** Professor, Faculty of Law, Ludwig-Maximilians-University Munich, Muenchen, Germany

**Mehmet Haberal, MD,** Professor, Department of General Surgery, Transplantation and Burn Units, Baskent University, Ankara, Turkey

**Philip F. Halloran, MD, PhD,** Professor, Department of Medicine, Division of Nephrology, University of Alberta, Edmonton, Canada

**Thomas Heffron, MD,** Professor, Department of Surgery, Emory Healthcare and Children's Healthcare of Atlanta, Atlanta, Georgia

**Bernard Hering, MD, PhD,** Professor of Surgery, Diabetes Institute for Immunology and Transplantation, Division of Transplantation, University of Minnesota, Minneapolis, Minnesota

**Mark J. Holterman, MD, PhD,** Associate Professor, Department of Surgery, University of Illinois, Chicago, Illinois

**Santiago Horgan, MD,** Professor, Department of Surgery, University of California, San Diego, California

**Abhinav Humar, MD,** Professor, Department of Surgery, Division of Transplantation, University of Minnesota, Minneapolis, Minnesota

**Lawrence G. Hunsicker, MD,** Professor, Department of Medicine, Division of Nephrology, University of Iowa, Iowa City, Iowa

**Shin Hwang, MD, PhD,** Associate Professor, Department of Surgery, Hepato-Biliary Surgery and Liver Transplantation, University of Uisan College of Medicine, Asan Medical Center, Seoul, Korea

**Hassan N. Ibrahim, MD, MS,** Assistant Professor, Division of Renal Diseases and Hypertension, University of Minnesota, Minneapolis, Minnesota

**Cheryl Jacobs, MS, LICSW,** Clinical Transplant Social Worker, Department of Surgery, Living Donor Program, University of Minnesota, Minneapolis, Minnesota

**Jose Jessurun, MD,** Professor, Department of Pathology, University of Minnesota, Minneapolis, Minnesota

**Tun Jie, MD,** Medical Resident, Department of Surgery, Division of Transplantation, University of Minnesota, Minneapolis, Minnesota

**Micean Johnikin, MS,** Medical Student, Howard University, Washington DC

**Jeffrey Kahn, PhD, MPH,** Professor, Center for Bioethics, University of Minnesota, Minneapolis, Minnesota

**Fady Kaldas, MD,** Chief Surgical Resident, Department of Surgery, Division of Liver and Pancreas Transplantation, Northport VA Medical Center, Northport, New York

**Roberts S. Kalil, MD,** Assistant Professor, Department of Medicine, Division of Nephrology, University of Iowa, Iowa City, Iowa

**Ann Kalis, RN,** Transplant Nurse Coordinator, Department of Surgery, Division of Transplantation, University of Minnesota, Minneapolis, Minnesota

**Igal Kam, MD,** Professor, Division of Transplant Surgery, University of Colorado Health Sciences Center, Denver, Colorado

**Hideya Kamei, MD,** Clinical Transplant Fellow, Department of Transplantation Surgery, Nagoya University Hospital, Nagoya, Japan

**Andreas J. Karachristos, MD,** Transplant Fellow, Department of Surgery, Division of Nephrology Transplantation, University of Cincinnati, Cincinnati, Ohio

**Hamdi Karakayali, MD,** Associate Professor, Department of General Surgery, Baskent University, Ankara, Turkey

**David M. Kashmer, MD,** Transplantation Fellow, Department of Surgery, Abdominal Transplant, University of Virginia, Charlottesville, Virginia

**Bertram L. Kasiske, MD,** Professor, Department of Medicine, Hennepin County Medical Center, Minneapolis, Minnesota

**Avi Katz, MD,** Associate Professor, Department of Pediatrics, Division of Nephrology and Transplantation, University of Alabama, Birmingham, Alabama

**Dixon B. Kaufman, MD, PhD,** Professor, Department of Surgery, Feinberg School of Medicine, Northwestern University, Chicago, Illinois

**Anand K. Khakhar, MD,** Professor, Department of Surgery, Division of Transplantation, Columbia University Medical Center, Columbia University, New York, New York

**Mahmound El Khatib, MD,** Associate Professor, Departments of Surgery and Internal Medicine, Division of Nephrology and Transplantation, University of Cincinnati, Cincinnati, Ohio

**Dong-Sik Kim, MD,** Transplant Fellow, Department of Surgery, Division of Nephrology and Transplantation, University of Cincinnati, Cincinnati, Ohio

**Milan Kinkhabwala, MD,** Associate Professor, Department of Surgery, Columbia University, Center for Liver Disease and Transplantation, New York Presbyterian Hospital Center, New York, New York

**Tetsuya Kiuchi, MD, PhD,** Professor, Department of Transplantation Surgery, Nagoya University Hospital, Nagoya, Japan

**Goran B. Klintmalm, MD, PhD,** Professor, Chairman, Baylor Regional Transplant Institute, Dallas, Texas

**Stuart J. Knechtle, MD,** Professor, Department of Surgery, Division of Transplantation, University of Wisconsin, Madison, Wisconsin

**Takashi Kobayashi, MD,** Postdoctoral Associate, Department of Surgery, Division of Transplantation, University of Minnesota, Minneapolis, Minnesota

**Burak Kocak, MD,** Assistant Professor, Department of Urology, Ondokuz Mayis University School of Medicine, Samsun, Turkey

**Alan J. Koffron, MD,** Assistant Professor, Department of Surgery, Northwestern University, Feinberg School of Medicine, Chicago, Illinois

**Rohit Kohli, MBBS,** Fellow, Division of Pediatric Gastroenterology, Hepatology and Nutrition, Children's Memorial Hospital, Northwestern University Medical School, Chicago, Illinois

**Anil Kotru, MD,** Associate Professor, Department of Transplantation and Liver Surgery, Geisinger Medical Center, Danville, Pennsylvania

**Raul Koushik, MD,** Clinical Assistant Professor of Medicine University of Texas at San Antonio, Consultant in Nephrology, Hypertension and Transplant, San Antonio Kidney Disease Center, San Antonio, Texas

**Jerzy W. Kupiec-Weglinski, MD, PhD,** Professor, Department of Surgery, Pathology, and Laboratory Medicine, Division of Liver and Pancreas Transplantation, Dumont Transplant Center, University of California, Los Angeles, California

**John R. Lake, MD,** Professor, Department of Surgery, Division of Gastroenterology and Liver Transplantation, University of Minnesota, Minneapolis, Minnesota

**Walter G. Land, MD,** Professor, Baskent University, Anakara Turkey, Liaison Office Germany, Taufkirchen-Muenchen, Germany

**Dianne LaPointe Rudow, DrNP,** Assistant Professor, Columbia University, Senior Transplant Coordinator, Clinical Director, Living Donor Liver Transplantation, New York Presbyterian Hospital Center, New York, New York

**Marie Larsson, BSc,** Department of Transplantation Surgery, Karolinska University Hospital Huddinge, Stockholm, Sweden

**Jong Hoon Lee, MD, PhD,** Assistant Professor, Department of Surgery, Kwandong University College of Medicine, Division of Transplantation, Myongji Hospital, Goyang, South Korea

**SungGyu Lee, MD, PhD,** Professor, Department of Hepato-Biliary Surgery and Liver Transplantation, University of Ulsan College of Medicine, Director, Organ Transplantation Center, Asan Medical Center, Seoul, Korea

**Annette Lennerling, RN, MSc, PhD,** Department of Transplantation and Liver Surgery, Sahlgrenska University Hospital, Göteborg, Sweden

**Joseph R. Leventhal, MD, PhD,** Associate Professor, Department of Surgery, Northwestern Memorial Hospital, Division of Organ Transplantation, Chicago, Illinois

**David M. Levi, MD,** Associate Professor, Department of Surgery, University of Miami, Miller School of Medicine, Miami, Florida

**Chung Mau Lo, MD, MS,** Professor, Department of Surgery and Centre for the Study of Liver Disease, University of Hong Kong, Hong Kong, China

**Julian Losanoff, MD,** Transplant Fellow, University of Chicago Medical Center, Chicago, Illinois

**Fu Luan, MD,** Assistant Professor, Division of Nephrology, University of Michigan, Ann Arbor, Michigan

**Rose Luther-Campise, MD,** Assistant Professor, Department of Anesthesiology, University of Illinois, Chicago, Illinois

**M. Makuuchi, MD,** Professor, Department of Surgery, University of Tokyo, Tokyo, Japan

**Massimo Malagó, MD,** Professor, Department of General Surgery and Transplantation, University Hospital of the Gerhard Mercator University Essen-Duisburg, Hufelandstr, Germany

**Amadeo Marcos, MD,** Professor, University of Pittsburgh Medical Center, Thomas E. Starzl Transplantation Institute, Pittsburgh, Pennsylvania

**Arthur J. Matas, MD,** Professor, Department of Surgery, Division of Transplantation, University of Minnesota, Minneapolis, Minnesota

**Michael Mauer, MD,** Professor, Department of Pediatrics, University of Minnesota Medical School, Minneapolis, Minnesota

**Thomas R. McCune, MD,** Associate Professor, Department of Renal Transplantation, Eastern Virginia Medical School, Director, Renal Transplant Program, Sentara Norfolk General Hospital, Norfolk, Virginia

**Greg J. McKenna, MD,** Transplant Surgeon, Baylor Regional Transplant Institute, Dallas, Texas

**Herwig-Ulf Meier-Kriesche, MD,** Associate Professor, Department of Medicine, University of Florida, Gainesville, Florida

**J. Keith Melançon, MD,** Assistant Professor, Department of Surgery, Johns Hopkins University, School of Medicine, Baltimore, Maryland

**Patrice Miles,** Executive Director, National Minority Organ Tissue Transplant Education Program, Howard University, Washington, DC

**Charles M. Miller, MD,** Professor, Department of Surgery, Cleveland Clinic Lerner College of Medicine, Director, Liver Transplantation Program, Cleveland Clinic Foundation, Cleveland, Ohio

**J. Michael Millis, MD,** Professor, Department of Surgery, University of Chicago, Chicago, Illinois

**Robert A. Montgomery, MD, PhD,** Associate Professor, Department of Surgery, Johns Hopkins University School of Medicine, Baltimore, Maryland

**Joseph Murray, MD,** Professor Emeritus, Department of Surgery, Harvard Medical School, Massachusetts General Hospital, Wellesley, Massachusetts

**Silvio Nadalin, MD,** Assistant Professor, Department of General Surgery and Transplantation, University Hospital of the Gerhard Mercator University Essen-Duisburg, Hufelandstrasse, Germany

**John S. Najarian, MD,** Clinical Professor, Department of Surgery, Division of Transplantation, University of Minnesota, Minneapolis, Minnesota

**Seigo Nishida, MD, PhD,** Associate Professor, Department of Surgery, University of Miami, Miller School of Medicine, Miami, Florida

**José Oberholzer, MD,** Associate Professor, Department of Surgery, University of Illinois, Chicago, Illinois

**Kohei Ogawa, MD,** Assistant Professor, Department of Surgery, Division of Transplantation and Immunology, Kyoto University, Kyoto, Japan

**Brenda M. Ogle, PhD,** Assistant Professor, Transplantation Biology, Department of Physiology, Mayo Clinic College of Medicine, Rochester, Minnesota

**Yasuhiro Ogura, MD, PhD,** Assistant Professor, Department of Hepatobiliary, Pancreas, and Transplant Surgery, Kyoto University Hospital, Kyoto City, Kyoto, Japan

**Akinlolu O. Ojo, MD,** Professor, Division of Nephrology, University of Michigan, Ann Arbor, Michigan

**Michael Olausson, MD, PhD,** Professor, Department of Transplantation and Liver Surgery, Sahlgrenska University Hospital, Göteborg, Sweden

**Kim M. Olthoff, MD,** Associate Professor, Department of Surgery, Division of Transplant Surgery, University of Pennsylvania, School of Medicine, Liver Transplant Program, Philadelphia, Pennsylvania

**Stefan Pambuccian, MD,** Associate Professor, Department of Laboratory Medicine and Pathology, University of Minnesota, Minneapolis, Minnesota

**Fabrizio Panaro, MD,** Research Fellow, Division of Transplantation, University of Illinois, Chicago, Illinois

**Kiil Park, MD, PhD,** Professor, Department of Surgery, Kwandong University College of Medicine, Transplantation Center, Myongji Hospital, Goyang, South Korea

**Todd Pillen, PA,** Manager, Liver Transplantation, Emory Healthcare and Children's Healthcare of Atlanta, Atlanta, Georgia

**Jacques Pirenne, MD,** Professor, Department of Abdominal Transplant Surgery, University Hospitals, Leuven, Belgium

**Jeffrey L. Platt, MD,** Professor, Departments of Surgery, Immunology, and Pediatrics, Mayo Clinic College of Medicine Rochester, Minnesota

**Marleen Praet, MD, PhD,** Professor, Anatomy and Pathology, Ghent University Hospital Medical School, Ghent, Belgium

**Janet Radcliffe-Richards, BA, MA, Bphil,** Director, Centre for Biomedical Ethics and Philosophy of Medicine, Academic Center for Medical Education, London, United Kingdom

**Amer Rajab, MD,** Assistant Professor, Department of Surgery, Division of Transplantation, Ohio State University, Columbus, Ohio

**Lloyd E. Ratner, MD,** Professor, Department of Surgery, College of Physicians and Surgeons, Columbia University, New York, New York

**Mark E. Rosenberg, MD,** Professor, Department of Medicine, Division of Renal Diseases and Hypertension, University of Minnesota, Minneapolis, Minnesota

**Steven M. Rudich, MD,** Associate Professor, Departments of Surgery and Internal Medicine, Division of Nephrology and Transplantation, University of Cincinnati, Cincinnati, Ohio

**Mark W. Russo, MD, MPH,** Assistant Professor, Division of Gastroenterology and Hepatology, University of North Carolina, Chapel Hill, North Carolina

**David H. Sachs, MD,** Professor, Department of Surgery, Transplantation Biology Research Center, Harvard Medical School, Massachusetts General Hospital, Boston, Massachusetts

**Howard Sankary, MD,** Professor, Department of Surgery, University of Illinois, Chicago, Illinois

**Nancy Scheper-Hughes, PhD,** Professor, Department of Anthropology, Director, Organs Watch, University of California, Berkeley, California

**Tim Schmitt, MD,** Associate Professor, Department of Surgery, University of Virginia, Charlottesville, Virginia

**Mark A. Schnitzler, PhD,** Associate Professor, Department of Internal Medicine, Saint Louis University, Center for Outcomes Research, St. Louis

**Jesse D. Schold, MStat, MEd,** Assistant Instructor, Department of Medicine, University of Florida, Gainesville, Florida

**Elizabeth R. Seaquist, MD,** Professor, Department of Medicine, Division of Endocrinology and Diabetes, Director, General Clinical Research Center, University of Minnesota, Minneapolis, Minnesota

**Shimul A. Shah, MD,** Clinical Fellow, Department of Surgery, Multi-Organ Transplantation, University of Toronto, Toronto, ON Canada

**Suzanne Shamsolkottabi, MD,** Assistant Professor, Department of Anesthesiology, University of Minnesota, Minneapolis, Minnesota

**James Shapiro, MD, PhD,** Director, Clinical Islet Transplant Program, Research Transplantation, Edmonton, Alberta, Canada

**Thomas Shaw-Stiffel, MD,** Associate Professor, Department of Kidney, Pancreas, and Liver Transplantation, University of Pittsburgh Medical Center, Thomas E. Starzl Transplantation Institute, Pittsburgh, Pennsylvania

**Surendra Shenoy, MD, PhD,** Associate Professor, Department of Surgery, Section of Transplantation, Washington University School of Medicine, Barnes Jewish Hospital, St. Louis, Missouri

**Hosein Shokouh-Amiri, MD,** Professor, Department of Surgery, Louisiana Shreveport University, Living Related Liver Transplant Program, Shreveport, Louisiana

**Roshan Shrestha, MD,** Professor, University of North Carolina, Division of Gastroenterology and Hepatology, Center for Liver Diseases and Transplantation, Chapel Hill, North Carolina

**Sunil Shroff, MD, FRCS,** Professor, Department of Urology, Sri Ramachandra Medical College and Research Institute, Porur, Chennai, India

**Mark Siegler, MD,** Professor, Department of Medicine and Surgery, University of Chicago, Director, MacLean Center for Clinical Medical Ethics, Chicago, Illinois

**Aaron J. Simon, MHA, CHE,** Assistant Hospital Director, University of Illinois, Chicago, Illinois

**Hans W. Sollinger, MD, PhD,** Professor, Department of Surgery, Division of Transplantation, University of Wisconsin, Madison, Wisconsin

**Aaron Spital, MD,** Professor, Mount Sinai School of Medicine, Department of Nephrology, Elmhurst Hospital Center, Elmhurst, New York

**Jean-Paul Squifflet, MD, PhD,** Professor, Department of Abdominal Surgery and Transplantation, University of Liege, Liege, Belgium

**Mark D. Stegall, MD,** Professor, Department of Surgery, Division of Transplantation, Mayo Clinic College of Medicine, Rochester, Minnesota

**Robert W. Steiner, MD,** Professor, Division of Nephrology, University of California, Center for Transplantation, San Diego, California

**Peter G. Stock, MD, PhD,** Professor, Department of Surgery, University of California, San Francisco, California

**Mark L. Sturdevant, MD,** Assistant Professor, Department of Surgery, Recanati/Miller Transplantation Institute, Mount Sinai Medical Center, Mount Sinai College of Medicine, New York, New York

**B. Subbarao, MD, FRCS,** Professor, Department of Urology, Sri Ramachandra Medical College and Research Institute, Consultant Nephrologist, Apollo Hospitals, Chennai, India

**Yasuhiko Sugawara, MD,** Associate Professor, Department of Surgery, University of Tokyo, Tokyo, Japan

**David E. R. Sutherland, MD, PhD,** Professor of Surgery, Diabetes Institute for Immunology and Transplantation, Division of Transplantation, University of Minnesota Minneapolis, Minnesota

**Steven K. Takemoto, PhD,** Associate Professor, Department of Internal Medicine, Saint Louis University, Center for Outcomes Research, St. Louis, Missouri

**Henkie P. Tan, MD, PhD,** Associate Professor, Department of Kidney, Pancreas, and Liver Transplantation, University of Pittsburgh Medical Center, Thomas E. Starzl Transplantation Institute, Pittsburgh, Pennsylvania

**Kazunari Tanabe, MD, PhD,** Associate Professor, Department of Urology, Tokyo Women's Medical University, Professor, Graduate School of Medicine, Department of Urology, Tokyo Women's Medical University, Tokyo, Japan

**Koichi Tanaka, MD,** Professor, Department of Surgery, Division of Transplantation and Immunology, Kyoto University, Kyoto, Japan

**Sarah Taranto, BA,** SAS Analyst, United Network for Organ Sharing, Richmond, Virginia

**Abel E. Tello, Jr. MD,** Renal Fellow, Division of Renal Diseases and Hypertension, University of Minnesota, Minneapolis, Minnesota

**Paul Terasaki, PhD,** Professor of Surgery Emeritus, Terasaki Foundation Laboratory, Los Angeles, California

**Giuliano Testa, MD,** Associate Professor, Department of Surgery, University of Chicago, Chicago, Illinois

**Amit D. Tevar, MD,** Assistant Professor, Departments of Surgery and Internal Medicine, Divisions of Nephrology and Transplantation, University of Cincinnati, Cincinnati, Ohio

**Nicholas L. Tilney, MD,** Professor, Department of Surgery, Brigham and Women's Hospital and Harvard Medical School, Boston, Massachusetts

**Satoru Todo, MD,** Professor, Department of Surgery, Hokkaido University School of Medicine, Sapporo, Japan

**Alexander Horacio Toledo, MD,** Fellow, Division of Transplantation, Department of Surgery, Northwestern University, Northwestern Memorial Hospital, Chicago, Illinois

**Luis H. Toledo-Pereyra, MD,** Professor, Department of Surgery, Michigan State University, East Lansing; Borgess Research Institute, Western Michigan University, Kalamazoo Center for Medical Studies, Kalamazoo, Michigan

**Kusum Tom, MD,** Assistant Professor, Department of Kidney, Pancreas, and Liver Transplantation, University of Pittsburgh Medical Center, Thomas E. Starzl Transplantation Institute, Pittsburgh, Pennsylvania

**Roberto Troisi, MD, PhD,** Professor, Department of Hepato-Biliary and Liver Transplantation, Ghent University Hospital Medical School, Ghent, Belgium

**Christoph Troppmann, MD,** Professor, Department of Surgery, Division of Transplantation, University of California, Davis Medical Center, Sacramento, California

**James F. Trotter, MD,** Associate Professor, Department of Medicine, Division of Transplant Surgery, University of Colorado Health Sciences Center, Denver, Colorado

**Sei-ichiro Tsuchihashi, MD, PhD,** Department of Surgery, Division of Liver and Pancreas Transplantation, Dumont-UCLA Transplant Center, Los Angeles, California

**Stefan G. Tullius, MD,** Associate Professor, Department of Surgery, Brigham and Women's Hospital and Harvard Medical School, Boston, Massachusetts

**Andreas G. Tzakis, MD, PhD,** Professor, Department of Surgery, University of Miami, Miller School of Medicine, Division of Transplantation, Miami, Florida

**Mikiko Ueda, MD,** Assistant Professor, Department of Surgery, Division of Transplantation and Immunology, Kyoto University, Kyoto, Japan

**Anatolie Usatii, MD,** Department of Surgery, Division of Transplantation, Sioux Valley Hospital, Sioux Falls, South Dakota

**Prashanth Vallabhajosyula, MD,** Research Fellow, Department of Surgery, Transplantation Biology Research Center, Harvard Medical School, Massachusetts General Hospital, Boston, Massachusetts

**Raghu Varadrajan, MD,** Transplant Fellow, Department of Surgery, College of Physicians and Surgeons, Columbia University, New York, New York

**Santiago R. Vera, MD,** Professor, Department of Surgery and Liver Transplantation, Methodist University Transplant Institute and the University of Tennessee Health Sciences Center, Memphis, Tennessee

**W. Ben Vernon, MD,** Director, Centura Transplant Services, Porter Adventist Hospital, Denver, Colorado

**Jonas Wadström, MD, PhD,** Associate Professor, Department of Surgery, University Hospital, Uppsala, Sweden

**Mark Wang, MD,** Medical Student, Department of Surgery, Division of Transplantation, Northwestern University, Feinberg School of Medicine, Chicago, Illinois

**Gregor Warnecke, MD,** Professor, Department of Cardiovascular and Thoracic Surgery, Hannover Medical School, Hannover, Germany

**Daniel S. Warren, PhD,** Assistant Professor, Department of Surgery, Johns Hopkins University School of Medicine, Baltimore, Maryland

**Peter F. Whitington, MD,** Professor, Department of Pediatrics and Transplantation, Northwestern University Medical School, Division of Gastroenterology, Hepatology, and Nutrition, Children's Memorial Hospital, Chicago, Illinois

**Steve Wieckert,** State Representative, Policy Advisor, Wisconsin State Capitol, Madison, Wisconsin

**Henryk F. Wilczek, MD, PhD,** Associate Professor, Department of Transplantation Surgery, Karolinska University Hospital Huddinge, Stockholm, Sweden

**Charles Winans, MD,** Staff, General Surgery and Liver Transplantation, Cleveland Clinic Foundation, Cleveland, Ohio

**Kathryn J. Wood, DPhil,** Professor, Department of Surgery, University of Oxford, John Radcliffe Hospital, Oxford, U.K.

**E. Steve Woodle, MD,** Professor, Departments of Surgery and Internal Medicine, Division of Nephrology and Transplantation, University of Cincinnati, Cincinnati, Ohio

**Kenneth J. Woodside, MD,** Clinical Lecturer Division of Transplantation Department of Surgery University of Michigan Health System, Ann Arbor, Michigan

**Kazuhiko Yamada, MD, PhD,** Associate Professor, Department of Surgery, Transplantation Biology Research Center, Harvard Medical School, Massachusetts General Hospital, Boston, Massachusetts

**Hasan Yersiz, MD,** Associate Professor, Division of Liver and Pancreas Transplantation, David Geffen School of Medicine, University of California, Los Angeles, California

**Andrea A. Zachary, PhD,** Professor, Immunogenetics Laboratory, Johns Hopkins University School of Medicine, Baltimore, Maryland

**Nan Zhang, PhD,** Research Associate, Departments of Gene and Cell Medicine, Transplantation Institute, Mount Sinai School of Medicine, New York, New York

# The Amsterdam and Vancouver Conferences on Living Organ Donation

*Francis L. Delmonico, MD*
*Professor of Surgery*
*Harvard Medical School*
*Massachusetts General Hospital*

The current practice of organ transplantation has extended beyond what the pioneers considered possible or even acceptable. In many countries around the world, living individuals have become the sole source of organs for transplantation. If one analyzes these organ transplantation practices geographically and from a socioeconomic perspective, there is virtually no deceased organ transplantation in countries where resources do not enable a diagnosis of brain death. Further, in these same countries, there are no policies for the recovery of organs after the determination of death by cardiorespiratory criteria. Hospitals may not be equipped to provide the extended end-of-life care in the intensive care unit that would make such a determination of brain death possible.

In China, executed prisoners provide organs for transplantation: there are virtually no other donor sources to accommodate the estimated 6,000 transplants now performed in China each year. In other Asian countries such as Japan, the concept of death determined by neurologic criteria has not been widely accepted, necessitating the living individual to be the source of transplantable organs.

These developments are not indicative of a practice of transplantation that some of our predecessors intended. In his memoirs, Dr. Thomas Starzl writes: "a donor death had occurred at one of the premier centers. Although I was one of the first to use the expedient of living kidney donation and never had a donor die, I was shaken by the report of these discussions (donor death). The concept of living donation seemed less and less acceptable … and in 1972, I stopped using kidneys from any live donors. Obtaining organs from people who are dead was the alternative."

In 1991, the World Health Organization (WHO) issued guiding principles of transplantation to assert emphatically that "organs for transplantation should be removed preferably from the bodies of deceased persons." Adult living persons were considered acceptable, but only when genetically related to the recipient. Nevertheless, the current demand for organs has taken us far beyond these WHO guiding principles. WHO has now revised its policy to support spouses and friends who donate their kidneys to loved ones.

These revisions were necessary given the current success of unrelated living donor kidney transplants; however, the appreciation of the transplant community for an altruistic donation has seemingly now turned to an expectation that there is an unlimited source of living donors to meet the demand. The burden and possibility of the success of organ transplant are now regularly placed upon the willingness of a well human being to provide at least one of these organs for transplantation: a kidney, a lobe of a lung, a segment of the liver, or a portion of the pancreas or intestine. The widespread practice of living organ transplantation despite the attendant risks is clearly counter to what historically had been a medical dictum to do no harm. Thus, the Forums in Amsterdam and Vancouver were conceived and developed because of these emerging hazards for those who are being called upon to donate an organ (1, 2, 3).

The goal of these Forums was to present timely and definitive statements regarding the responsibility of the transplant community to care for the living organ donor. The person who consents to be a living organ donor should be informed of the risks; willing to donate, free of coercion; and medically and psychosocially suitable to be a donor. The ethics of a continuing practice of living donor transplantation demands an international recognition that prioritizes the sustained well-being of the donor and not the restored health of the intended recipient.

In Amsterdam, Forum participants agreed that prior to donation, the living kidney donor must receive a complete medical and psychosocial evaluation, give appropriate informed consent, and be capable of understanding the information presented in that process to make a voluntary decision. Forum participants also discussed the evaluation of current medical issues not uncommonly identified in a potential donor, such as donor hypertension, dyslipidemia, malignancy, and a history of metabolic or infectious diseases such as renal lithiasis, tuberculosis, or hepatitis.

At the Vancouver Forum, 4 organ-specific work groups were assembled: lung, liver, pancreas, and intestine. Each organ work group addressed the following topics: the evaluation of the potential living donor; the criteria of living donor medical suitability; operative events, donor morbidity, and mortality; and responsibility and duration of donor follow-up.

The Vancouver Forum participants acknowledged the heroism of those living volunteers who have provided a lifesaving organ for a transplant recipient, because the reported rate of complications was high, ranging from 20% to 60%, with a donor mortality after right lobe hepatectomy of 0.4%. The death of a living donor is a tragedy of immeasurable proportion that brings an ethical dimension distinct from the complications that might be experienced in a recipient. The Vancouver Forum also provided an opportunity for the Ethics Committee of the Transplantation Society to address issues of informed consent, living donor selection, donor autonomy and satisfaction, and procedural safeguards.

We remain in a time of medical history that necessitates clinical decisions in circumstances contrary to the principles that are at the core of every physician: to harm no one in the pursuit of helping another. The content of this book is a recording of that dilemma. Its authors recommend practices that require the best of medical judgment. The lives of the potential donors are dependent upon that judgment.

Even as these decisions are currently made with no other immediate options, this book also reveals the obvious conflict inherent in placing individuals who are otherwise well at medical risk. That practice, although understandable now, must not be the final testimony for the future. The science and medicine of transplantation must find alternatives that free the well living individual from the necessity to be an organ donor.

1. The consensus statement of the Amsterdam Forum on the Care of the Live Kidney Donor. Transplantation. 2004 Aug 27; 78(4): 491-2.
2. A report of the Amsterdam Forum on the Care of the Live Kidney Donor: data and medical guidelines. Transplantation. 2005 Mar 27; 79(6 Suppl): S53-66.
3. A report of the Vancouver Forum on the Care of the Live Organ Donor: Lung, liver, pancreas, and intestine: data and medical guidelines. Transplantation. 2006 May 27; 81: 1373-85.

PART I

# GENERAL ASPECTS OF LIVING DONOR ORGAN TRANSPLANTATION

# CHAPTER 1

# INTRODUCTION AND RATIONALE

*Rainer W.G. Gruessner, MD, Sarah Taranto, BA, Angelika C. Gruessner, PhD*

Why should organ donation from living donors (LDs) be promoted and healthy individuals place their health and life at stake? Can we justify placing LDs in harm's way? What is the current status of living donation, and what are the risks for the donors? What safeguards and incentives should be implemented?

Solid organ transplantation owes its very existence to LDs.[1] In the mid-1950s, a kidney transplant was immunologically successful only if the kidney was procured from a healthy twin donor: because of this specific relationship, the immunologic barrier that exists between human leukocyte antigen (HLA) and non-identical human beings could be overcome. With the advent of potent immunosuppressive therapy and, in particular, with the introduction of mono- and polyclonal antibodies for induction and calcineurin inhibitors for maintenance therapy, transplants from deceased donors (DDs) became immunologically successful and routine.

Nowadays, continued use of LDs is essential to transplant prospective candidates early and to avoid long waiting times associated with high morbidity and mortality rates. In fact, since the first successful kidney transplant (between identical twins) in 1954 by Joseph Murray,[2] the number of LD kidney transplants has continuously increased (Figure 1). In the United States, in 2001, 2002, and 2003, there were more kidney LDs than kidney DDs. The

initiation of the "Donation and Transplantation Breakthrough Collaborative" (sponsored by the Department of Health and Human Services with key national leaders and practitioners from the transplantation and hospital communities) in April 2003 has increased awareness of organ donation, in particular for DDs.[3] As a result, since 2004, the number of kidney DDs has again surpassed the number of kidney LDs.

According to the United Network for Organ Sharing (UNOS), from January 1 through December 31, 2005, the total number of donors from whom organs were recovered was 14,489. Of those, 7,593 were DDs and 6,896 were LDs. In the same year (2005), the total numbers of abdominal transplants performed in the United States were as follows: 16,476 kidney transplants alone, 6,444 liver transplants, 903 combined pancreas and kidney transplants, 541 pancreas transplants alone, and 178 intestinal transplants (see Table 1, which also includes the number of thoracic transplants).

Of all abdominal organ transplants, kidney transplants used the most LDs in 2005: a total of 6,563 LD kidney transplants took place, representing 39.8% of all kidney transplants that year. In contrast, in 2005, LDs were used significantly less frequently for liver transplants (323 LD liver transplants, 5% of all such transplants that year; Figure 2), pancreas transplants (2 LD pancreas transplants, 0.1%), and intestinal transplants (7 LD intestinal transplants, 3.9%; Table 1). Thus, in 2005, a total of 6,895 LDs were used for abdominal organ transplants (only 1 LD lung transplant was reported to UNOS that year).

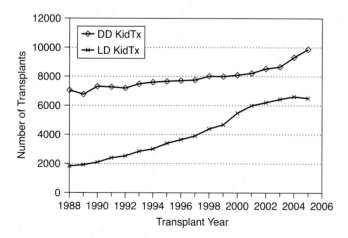

**FIGURE 1**

Living vs Deceased Kidney Transplants in the United States (UNOS data, January 1, 1988, to December 31, 2005). LD = living donor; DD = deceased donor; Kid = kidney; Tx = transplant.

**TABLE 1**

### NUMBER AND TYPE OF TRANSPLANTS PERFORMED IN 2005 (JANUARY 1 TO DECEMBER 31)

| Type of Transplant | No. of DD + LD Transplants | No. of LD Transplants Only |
| --- | --- | --- |
| Kidney (alone) transplants | 16,476 | 6,563 |
| Kidney–pancreas transplants | 903 | 1 |
| Pancreas (alone) transplants | 541 | 1 |
| Liver transplants | 6,444 | 323 |
| Intestine transplants | 178 | 7 |
| Heart transplants | 2,125 | — |
| Heart–lung transplants | 35 | — |
| Lung transplants | 1,406 | 1 |
| Total | 28,110 | 6,896 |

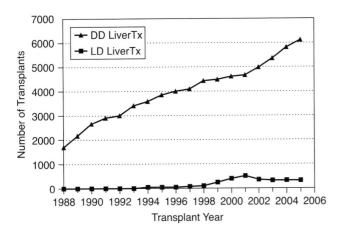

**FIGURE 2**

Living vs Deceased Donor Liver Transplants in the United States (UNOS data, January 1, 1988, to December 31, 2005). LD = living donor; DD = deceased donor; Tx = transplant.

Of the 245 U.S. kidney[9] transplant programs that performed at least 1 kidney transplant in 2005, 238 (97%) used LDs; of the 122 liver transplant programs, 45 (37%); of the 118 combined pancreas and kidney transplant programs, 1 (1%); of the 88 pancreas transplant alone programs, 1 (1%); and of the 20 intestinal transplant programs, 3 (15%).

Given these numbers, it is evident that the use of LDs for kidney transplants has a significant impact on the treatment of end-stage renal disease in the United States—in 2005 alone, 40% of all kidney transplants and 97% of all kidney transplant programs used LDs. The impact of LDs on liver, pancreas, and intestinal transplantation has been less pronounced. The main reason is that the kidneys are paired organs, so kidney procurement does not require parenchymal dissection (as in liver or pancreas procurement) or reconstruction of organ integrity (as in intestinal procurement). Yet another reason is this well-documented fact: in kidney transplants the half-life of an LD (vs DD) graft is almost twice as long.[4] Similar analyses have not been done for extrarenal LD transplants because of the overall small numbers.

In addition, the morbidity and mortality risks associated with kidney donation are low: the risk of major complications is less than 5%. The mortality risk for kidney LDs has been estimated to be 1 in 8,000 to 10,000 (Chapter 15.7). In contrast, for liver LDs, depending on the type of resection, the risk of major complications is considerably higher; the mortality risk is estimated to be 1 in 900 for lateral segmentectomy and 1 in 500 for lobectomy (Chapter 29.5). Trotter et al. identified 19 liver donor deaths (and an additional donor in a chronic vegetative state); of those 19 deaths, 13 and the vegetative state were definitively, 2 were possibly, and 4 were unlikely related to donor surgery.[5] An overall mortality risk of 0.1% to 0.3% for liver LDs is definitely not insignificant. It is particularly troubling that these donor deaths occurred despite the fact that liver LDs are meticulously screened and healthy. For pancreas and intestinal LDs, the morbidity and mortality risks are more difficult to evaluate, because of the low numbers of such transplants. It is estimated that, so far, worldwide, the number of LD kidney transplants is over 250,000; LD liver transplants,

about 7,000; LD pancreas transplants, about 150; and LD intestinal transplants, about 45. To date (December 2006), no pancreas LD has died from procedure-related causes. However, given the lack of regenerative capacity of insulin-producing cells (in contrast to the adaptive hypertrophy of a liver or kidney), the risk of developing diabetes mellitus post-donation and requiring oral antidiabetic medications or insulin administration is about 3%.[6, 7] For intestinal LDs to date, the mortality rate is also 0%; if a standardized surgical technique is used, the morbidity risk (e.g., diarrhea, vitamin malabsorption) is minimal.[6, 8]

Unfortunately, for all types of solid organ LDs, the exact short- and long-term complication rates are unknown, because of the lack of a registry that specifically collects information on LDs.[9] Attempts are now being made in the United States to implement a national database for collecting long-term LD outcome data (i.e., morbidity and mortality, quality of life) and to require mandatory data submission to such a registry. But merely collecting LD data, whether through UNOS or, in Europe, through Eurotransplant, is not enough to protect the safety of LDs and to avoid organ trafficking (see Chapter 10). All countries that permit the use of LDs should be required to implement LD databases so that LD outcome can be compiled in a transparent and accountable fashion. Ideally, the World Health Organization (WHO) should oversee these databases in order to create a true international source for LD outcome data and for implementation of regulatory measures. The creation of an international LD database would also enable health professionals worldwide to accurately inform prospective LDs of their short- and long-term risks.

Without doubt, the use of LDs decreases transplant candidates' mortality rates on the DD waiting list. By the end of 2005 (December 31), the waiting list mortality for kidney-alone transplant candidates was 4.1% (Figure 3). For liver transplant candidates, the mortality rate was 6.2%, indicating that wider use of LDs could further decrease the mortality rate, as with kidney transplant candidates. Not surprisingly, for abdominal organ transplants that have used the fewest number of LDs, the mortality rates on the DD waiting list have been lower: for pancreas transplant candidates, 2.5%; for intestinal transplant candidates, 2.8%.

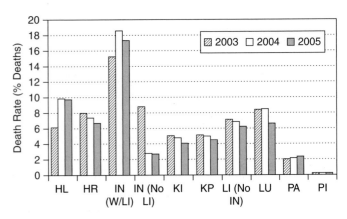

**FIGURE 3**

Waiting List Mortality Rates (percentage of deaths per patient waiting) in the United States (UNOS data, January 1, 2003, to December 31, 2005). HL = heart–lung; HR = heart; IN = intestine; KI = kidney; KP = kidney–pancreas; LI = liver; LU = lung; PA = pancreas; PI = pancreatic islets.

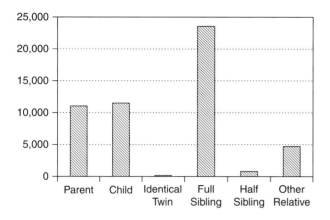

**FIGURE 4A**

Donor–Recipient Relationship in Kidney Transplantation: Biological Donors

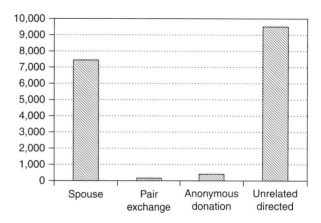

**FIGURE 4B**

Donor–Recipient Relationship in Kidney Transplantation: Nonbiological Donors

For transplant candidates who require both a kidney and a pancreas transplant, the mortality rate (4.5%) on the DD waiting list is slightly higher than that for kidney-alone transplant (4.1%) candidates. The mortality rate has been highest for combined intestine–liver transplant candidates: 17.3% of such candidates died while waiting, the majority being small children under the age of 2. For such children in need of a portion of the small bowel and a lateral segment of the liver, only a handful of LDs have been used. By expanding the LD pool in this category, the mortality rate on the waiting list can be further reduced. Overall, it is apparent that increased use of living unrelated donors, of altruistic donors, and of donor exchange programs (see Chapters 5, 16.6.1, and Figure 4) for all types of transplants can further decrease DD waiting list mortality.

The growing number of transplant candidates on the waiting list remains a concern—the proportional increase in the number of LD (and DD) transplants has not kept up with the proportional increase in listed candidates. As of September 15, 2006, a total of 67,723 candidates were waiting for a kidney transplant; 17,112, for a liver; 1,748, for a pancreas; 2,429, for a pancreas and a kidney; and 231, for an intestine (Table 2). This situation

can only be ameliorated if society as a whole is willing to accept nondirected or altruistic donation as a potential solution. One first step is to guarantee lifelong health insurance for all LDs. In addition, financial incentives for LDs may help bring about a steep increase in organ donation in the future. If financial incentives are considered, federal guidelines and laws as well as governmental oversight are required to avoid abuse of such a system (Chapter 8).

However, even with a possible increase in public willingness to donate for financial reasons, the major concern of such a program remains the same: the safety of LDs. Although we can certainly further minimize LD morbidity and mortality, we will not ever be able to completely eliminate the risks of donation. It takes courage and vision on the part of the LDs to accept these risks in order to end another human being's suffering. This book is dedicated to all living donors.

## References

1. Gaston RS, Eckhoff DE. Whiter living donors? *Am J Transplantation* 2004;4:2–3.
2. Murray JE, Merrill JP, Harrison JH. Renal homotransplantation in identical twins. *Surg Forum* 1955;6:432–436.
   http://www.organdonationnow.org
3. Cecka MJ. The OPTN/UNOS Renal Transplant Registry 2003. In: *Clinical Transplants 2003*. UCLA Immunogenetics Center, Los Angeles, CA; 2004:1–12.
4. Trotter JF, Adam R, Lo CM, Kenison J. Documented deaths of hepatic lobe donors for living donor liver transplantation. *Liver Transplant* 2006;12:1485–1488.
5. Barr ML, Belghiti J, Villamil FG, et al. A report of the Vancouver Forum on the care of the live organ donor: Lung, liver, pancreas, and intestine data and medical guidelines. *Transplantation* 2006;27:1373–1385.
6. Gruessner RW, Sutherland DE, Drangstveit MB, Bland BJ, Gruessner AC. Pancreas transplants from living donors: Short- and long-term outcome. *Transplant Proc* 2001;33:819–820.
7. Gruessner RWG, Sharp HL. Living-related intestinal transplantation: First report of a standardized surgical technique. *Transplantation* 1997;64:1605–1607.
8. Mulligan DC. A worldwide database for living donor liver transplantation is long overdue. *Liver Transplant* 2006;12:1443–1444.

**TABLE 2**

## OPTN NATIONAL PATIENT WAITING LIST FOR ORGAN TRANSPLANTS (AS OF SEPTEMBER 15, 2006)

| Type of Transplant | No. of Registration | No. of Patients Waiting |
| --- | --- | --- |
| Kidney transplant | 71,415 | 67,723 |
| Kidney–pancreas transplant | 2,487 | 2,429 |
| Pancreas transplant | 1,774 | 1,748 |
| Pancreas–islet transplant | 297 | 295 |
| Liver transplant | 17,574 | 17,112 |
| Intestine transplant | 232 | 231 |
| Heart transplant | 2,871 | 2,865 |
| Heart–lung transplant | 148 | 148 |
| Lung transplant | 2,918 | 2,897 |
| Total | 99,716 | 92,696 |

# CHAPTER 2

# CULTURAL DIFFERENCES IN LIVING ORGAN DONATION: A GLOBAL PERSPECTIVE

*Clive O. Callender, MD, Micean Johnikin, MS, Patrice Miles*

Organ donation is a deed, which across the globe can be looked at from every perspective imaginable. It has religious, moral, ethical, psychosocial, and linguistic ramifications. We believe in virtually all instances that humanistic goals are common to all: saving lives. The culture one finds oneself in, however, may well be the greatest determinant of the perspective one takes on this phenomenon. Our global analysis of the cultures of six of the seven continents and religious beliefs of these cultural perspectives of living donation are shared.

## INTRODUCTION

At first glance, organ donation seems a relatively simple deed; but as one looks deeply into this national and international act, the complexity of this gift is revealed. The roles of urban versus rural, developed versus developing countries, rich versus poor, and enslaved versus free are just some of the perspectives that our global journey depicts. Are these factors responsible for the apparent racial/ethnic differences, or are all of them cultural? What does cultural mean anyway? As we look at the earth we first recognize the large unpopulated oceanic and sea makeup. As we look at the populated earth there are seven large contiguous landmasses that constitute most of the dry land on the surface of the earth.[1] These landmasses are called continents and consist of Africa, Antarctica, Asia, Australia (Oceania), Europe, North America, and South America (Latin America). The Antarctica is uninhabitable and is excluded from our discussion.[2] We look at the other six landmasses and the people that live on each of the different continents and analyze their similarities and differences.[2,3] We quickly recognize that the cultural differences that make up these populations may be largely responsible for their varied behaviors. What are these factors? They include geographic location; climate, language, urban or rural setting, developed or developing countries, religious beliefs, moral or ethical beliefs; and ethnic, psychosocial, and cultural backgrounds. All of these factors must be considered as crucial to the perspectives taken on as personal an action as organ donation. *Culture* or *cultural differences* are terms that are commonly used in trying to understand human behavior from a global perspective. The *American College Dictionary* defines culture as the totality of socially transmitted behavior patterns, arts, beliefs, institutions, and all other products of human work and thoughts. In essence it means the "behavior that develops as a consequence of all exposures one encounters as one matures." With all of the possible ways of looking at the global perspectives of organ donation, in this chapter we decide to focus on the following: the six continents, their religions (including Islam [Muslim], Hinduism, Sikh, Confucianism, Buddhism, Christianity, and Judaism), the developed and developing countries, and altruistic and commercial

perspectives. The Middle East is in Asia but is discussed separately because of its unique religious and cultural differences.

This chapter shares the broad perspectives on how these differences and commonalities can help address the number one problem in transplantation: the worldwide shortage of donors. However, the primary focus is on the living donor perspective. Currently, living organ donation is only possible for kidney, liver, pancreas, small intestine, and lung transplantation.

## CONTINENTAL AND REGIONAL PERSPECTIVES

### Africa

Africa consists of 53 countries with a population of more than 800 million people.[1-3] We focus, for our discussions of the African continents cultural differences in organ donations, on the black Africans who are currently in Africa or have by virtue of the slave trade and the Diaspora emigrated to North and South America and Europe. Anthropologists have traced their emigration to the Caribbean, the United States, and the United Kingdom. Organ donation by those of African decent, in Africa and elsewhere, has been associated with a reluctance to become living or deceased organ donors. They have been exposed to very different cultural surroundings in North America, the Caribbean, the United Kingdom, and Africa. Interestingly, even though surrounded by different circumstances where those of African descent have landed, wherever they have landed, their reluctance to donate organs is similar.[4-8] In studies first conducted in the United States in the 1980s[5] and in the twenty-first century as well,[9-12] the reasons identified for reluctance to donate were: (1) lack of information, (2) religious myths and misperceptions, (3) distrust of health-care professionals, (4) fear of premature declaration of death, (5) racism, and (6) inequitable allocation systems. An analysis of the surveys and focus groups carried out in black African descendents located in the Caribbean, Africa, the United Kingdom, and South Africa[4-8] demonstrated commonalities, which suggest that although Africans or African descendants are raised in different regions, their complexion (blackness) may be the most indelible factor and even more influential than the Brutal Diaspora. Because culture is the totality of the person's exposures, one might have expected differences in the response of African descendants in the United States from those of African descendents elsewhere. This has not been the case! The barriers to increasing living organ donation in the United States have been overcome to a significant degree at the Washington Hospital Center and the North Carolinian groups.[13-14] The Coalition on Donation and the National Minority Organ Tissue Transplant Education Program (MOTTEP) have both launched African-American organ donation campaigns with different methodologies.[5,15] Conceptualized in 1991, the MOTTEP model has emphasized community education and empowerment by combining the grass-roots community education and empowerment campaign with mass media awareness campaigns. This dualistic strategy relied on community advisory groups developing their own unique strategic plans to identify and overcome the obstacles to minority organ donation in their localities. These successful campaigns were dependent on ethnically appropriate messengers (often transplant recipients, organ donors, or donor family members) delivering ethnically appropriate messages developed to increase organ donor rates and prevent the need for transplantation simultaneously.[5,16]

The Coalition on Donation began an awareness campaign in 1992 and initiated its African American Awareness Campaign in 2002.[15] Their campaigns are primarily donation awareness campaigns without the concentrated grass-roots community effort.

A look at the United Network for Organ Sharing (UNOS), African American living donation data between 1990 and 2000 reveal a dramatic increase in African American living donation rates from 22.4 organ donors per million in 1990 to 40.8 organ donors per million in 2000. We believe that the African American donation education efforts described previously contributed to this increase in African American living donation rates.

## Asia

Asia is the largest continent on the earth and the most populated consisting of 48 countries and independent islands.[1] Two out of every three people on earth are from this continent, which holds 3.9 billion people.[1–3] The 48 Asian countries all have very different cultures, beliefs, and languages. All of the main religions of the world began in Asia. The rich cultural and religious diversity of this region[1–3] is the reason we have considered the Middle East, which is part of Asia separately. The religious and cultural diversity of Asia makes it difficult to speak of the Asian perspective, as each of the different Asian countries has very critically different perspectives on many aspects of life and living donation.[17–32] One area where all of these religions and cultures agree is that there is no religious obstacle to living related and deceased organ donation and that saving a life is a noble deed. In general it seems best to characterize the different Asian perceptions separately (eg, the Philippines, the Vietnamese, the Cambodian, the Indonesian, the Korean, the Indian, the Japanese, the Chinese, the Pakistan, the Singapore). Because we know the transplant ideologies of less than half of the 48 countries that have transplant programs and make up Asia, any attempt to identify an Asian perspective could be labeled as "presumptuous." We discuss the transplant perspective of those Asian countries that are performing live organ transplants and share the known perspectives of some of these countries (see Table 2.1).

When speaking of the Asian perspective, it must be remembered that Asia consists of 3.9 billion of the 6.5 billion people in the world. One billion represent Indians and 1.3 billion are Chinese. Of the remaining 46 Asian countries, only 4 countries—Pakistan (162 million), Indonesia (241 million), Japan (121 million), and Bangladesh (141 million)—have populations that are in excess of 100 million people.[2,3]

Although successful living organ donation (kidney) began in the United States in 1954 and has flourished there ever since, kidney transplants in Asia were first performed in Korea and Japan in the 1960s.[18,21,23,25,28] Kidney donations in Pakistan have been taken to new heights, because of the absence of brain-death laws in this country. This has led to Pakistan moving aggressively into performing living kidney donations. They have made public awareness and education a priority and have shown their recognition of the donors' noble deed by providing job security and health insurance to the donors and free education to the donors' children. This was made possible by finance provided jointly by the Pakistani government and the community.[31] This model has applicability throughout the Asian continent and the world. The downside is that paid donations comprise 50% of all of their transplants.[32]

In Japan, kidney transplants have been in existence since 1964; and living liver transplants, since 1989. In Korea, kidney transplants began in 1969; and living liver transplants, in 1994. The total number of kidney transplants in Asian countries now exceeds 20,000 with excellent graft survival rates. No less non pareil has been their experience with living liver transplant programs with 600 living liver transplants performed in Korea and in excess of 1,500 living liver transplants in Japan without a single donor mortality and with donor morbidity rates of less than 10%.[18,23,28] The combination of the ever-widening donor recipient gap and the scarcity of deceased donor organs along with the unwillingness to accept deceased organ donation has been one of the hallmarks of the Asian continent.[20,21,25,28,30] For many reasons, the Chinese culture has been slow to accept many Western advances, most notably dialysis and transplantation.[20] Current donations are from deceased donors and next of kin donors in Hong Kong where this is the Law. In Singapore, Korea, Japan, Taiwan, Thailand, and other Asian countries, the legal obstacles to deceased organ donations are less problematic than the grass-roots notions and beliefs surrounding death and the bodies remaining intact after death, brain death, the buying and selling of organs, and the allocation of organs to needy recipients. What was most interesting in most of the Asian countries' transplant and donation surveys was the very high percentage of interviewees who had no religion or were not supportive of the importance of religious perspectives.[17,18,20,21,23–25,27–32] In the Hong Kong study, 59% had no religious beliefs[2,9]; in the Singapore study, 52% did not regard it as important to be a religious person;[27,30] and in the Korean study, 36% of those interviewed had no religious beliefs.[21] This was as surprising as was the similarity between the reasons given by the Asian donors for donating or not donating and the reasons given by the American/African American donors for not wanting to donate. This further substantiates the prejudice that people are people everywhere, and that they are distinctively products of their upbringing and culture. In the United States, Asian Americans[5] are the ethnic group associated with the longest graft survival rate after transplant of all organs and are among the fastest growing and the most diverse minorities in the United States. An effort to increase organ donation rates in the Filipino group in Hawaii was spectacularly successful.[33] This success was related to the availability of a transplant candidate program coordinator who was Filipino and who successfully received a kidney transplant. His role in increasing the Filipino organ donation rates from 5% to 20% over 5 years was a reminder that human interaction in all ethnic groups can overcome nearly all obstacles to donation.

## The Middle East

The Middle East[2,3] consists of 21 countries with a population of nearly 300 million people.[3] Transplantation in the Middle East has been practiced since the 1970s. Living related kidney transplants and most recently living liver transplants are performed there. The Middle East Society of Organ Transplantation (MESOT) has developed

**TABLE 2.1**
## A GLOBAL PERSPECTIVE OF LIVING ORGAN DONATION

| Continent | Country | Living Organs Currently Transplanted | Organ Procurement Organizations |
|---|---|---|---|
| Africa | Nigeria | Kidney | |
| | South Africa | Kidney, Liver | |
| Asia | China | Kidney | |
| | Hong Kong | Kidney | |
| | Korea | Kidney, Liver | Korean Network for Organ Sharing (KONOS) |
| | Taiwan | Kidney | |
| | India | Kidney | |
| | Japan | Kidney, Liver | |
| | Singapore | Kidney, Liver | Kidney Foundation of Singapore |
| | Phillipines | Kidney | |
| | Vietnam | Kidney, Liver | |
| | Thailand | Kidney | Organ Donation Centers Thai Red Cross Society (ODC) |
| Middle East | Egypt | Kidney, Liver | |
| | Iran | Kidney | Middle Eastern Society for Organ Transplantation (MESOT) |
| | Israel | Kidney | |
| | Pakistan | Kidney | MESOT |
| | Saudi Arabia | Kidney, Liver | Saudi Center for Organ Transplantation (SCOT) and MESOT |
| | Turkey | Kidney | MESOT |
| | Iraq | Kidney | MESOT |
| Australia (Oceania) | Australia | Kidney | Renal Transplant Advisory Committee |
| | New Zealand | Kidney, Liver | |
| Europe | Spain | Kidney, Liver | Euro Transplant |
| | Italy | Kidney, Liver | |
| | United Kingdom | Kidney, Liver, Lung | |
| North America | Canada | Kidney, liver, lung | Canadian Organ Replacement Register |
| | United States | Kidney, Liver, Lung, Pancreas, Small Intestine | United Organ Sharing Network (UNOS) |
| | Mexico | Kidney, Liver | Coordinating Center of Nuevo Leon, Mexico |
| | Cuba | Kidney, Liver | Investigociones Medico Quirargicas |
| South (Latin) America | Brazil | Kidney, Liver | |
| | Argentina | Kidney | |
| | Chile | Kidney | |
| | Venezuela | Kidney | VENEZ National Transplantation Organization |
| | Columbia | Kidney | |
| | Uruguay | Kidney, Liver | |
| | Peru | Kidney, Liver | |

with members of 29 countries and a population served of 600 million people.[34,35] MESOT membership consists of all of the Arab countries, Iran, Turkey, Pakistan, and the Central Asian countries. What is common to these members are organ transplantation programs, inadequate preventive medicine, poor health administrative infrastructure, poor awareness of the medical community and the public regarding transplantation and organ donation, poor governmental support of transplant, lack of effective health insurance, a lack of esprit de corps among transplant physicians, lack of planning for organ procurement, a large donor–recipient gap, and a long transplant waiting time.[35] Living organ donation is the most widely practiced type of donation, and deceased organ donors are scarce. There are three dominant distinctive models practiced in MESOT: the Saudi, Pakistan, and Iranian models. The Saudi Center for Organ Transplant (SCOT from 1985–present) is a model that presents a national organ procurement center: a governmental agency which supervises organ donation and transplant in Saudi Arabia.[34–36] The Pakistani model is a model that provides a partnership between the government and the community, which funds the management of End Stage Renal Disease (ESRD). This is a system in which 50% of living donors are paid, and the donors are also rewarded in many other ways. They recommend this for developing countries.[32,37] The Iranian model involves a partnership between the Government and the transplant society in which the living unrelated donors are paid to donate with careful oversight. Each of the 29 countries has the option of choosing the option best suited for its community. The Saudi model is best suited for these countries with the most resources, and the Pakistani and Iranian models are suited for those without religious, cultural, or ethical objectives to paid donation and the use of living unrelated donors which is banned by some of their religions. Previous public Middle Eastern surveys done in Saudi Arabia,[39] Turkey,[40] and Qatar leave many questions as to the likelihood of acceptance of the Iranian model or the Pakistani[41] model in their countries. Although the Pakistani model is more subject to modifications, that could make it acceptable in some of these countries. The fact that the Iranian model over the course of the last 10 years has eradicated the waiting list is a very powerful argument when patients are dying on the waiting list for organs that never come.[38]

## Australia (Oceania)

Australia (Oceania) is made up of seven states with a population of 20 million people. Geographic purists, however, consider Oceania the continent and consider it to consist of Australia (population 20 million), New Zealand (population 4 million), Papua New Guinea (population 5 million), Melanesia (population 7.4 million), and the 28 other countries or Islands whose total population comprises 32.75 million.[2,3] For our purposes we consider Australia and its transplant program as the continent. The native people of Australia, called Aborigines, live mainly in the outback and bush country. These lands make up 85% of the country of Australia. Data from the Australian and New Zealand Transplant Registries (their renal transplant advisory committee) demonstrate an increase in living donations from a low of 19% in 1994 to a high of 39% in 2001. This represents a doubling of living donors from 103 to 212 and a relative plateauing of deceased donors (337–328) during that 8-year period. The low deceased donors per million population (PMP), as low as 9 deceased donors PMP in 2003, is one of the lowest donor PMP rates by international standards.[42–45] Spain has the highest deceased donors PMP at 33.8, and Belgium is second with a 24.8 donors PMP. Australia has a growing dialysis population which has increased by 6% per annum over the past decade. Because kidney availability is decreasing with only 6.8% of people on dialysis receiving transplants in 2002, compared to 11.7% a decade ago, a relative transplant crisis exists (a shortage of kidneys for transplant). This has resulted in an increased number of altruistic-unrelated donors and to Australians[44,45] going overseas for overseas commercial sources for unrelated living donor kidneys.[44] The answer to why deceased donor rates are so low in Australia is thought to be the hospital retrieval systems, as there is perceived to be no lack of public support.[45]

## Europe

The European continent consists of 46 countries and 729 million people.[1–3] Many European countries work together for transplantation and have put together a group called "Euro transplant," which coordinates their transplant-related activities.[46,47] During the past 25 years, European transplant results have undergone steadfast improvement. Major efforts to increase organ donations have been launched in all European countries; Germany, France, Italy, and Scandinavian countries, for example, have initiated extensive national campaigns to increase donation rates. In addition to the public education and donor card initiatives of most European countries, Sweden, the Netherlands, Denmark, Belgium, and Austria have set up national registries that allow citizens to express their opinions about organ donation. Since 1986, the Belgium Registry allows registrations against donation; the Netherlands and Sweden register both for and against donations. Euro transplant data now show that countries with "opting-out" systems (Austria and Belgium) have higher donation rates than do countries with opting-in systems (Germany and the Netherlands).[46,47] The family refusal rates throughout European countries are approximately 30%. The European systems have identified the doctors' ability to approach the family as a very important factor influencing donation decisions and therefore have launched programs to train doctors to approach families regarding donations.[46–48] Family refusal rates have been lowered as a consequence, and such programs now exist in most European countries. In Europe, two other very effective influential donor programs have been the "Donor Action" programs that systematically facilitate hospital participation in organ donation and have increased donation rates by 50% in a single Hospital.[47] The second and most influential program in Europe and the world has been the Spanish Model, which has resulted in Spain being the only European country to raise donation rates continuously during the past 10 years.[47] The Spanish National Donation Agency (ONT) has hired individuals (physicians and other personnel) as transplant liaisons in their hospitals and ICUs. They participate in a standardized training program and have increased the number of organ donors exponentially. The public education campaigns alone have been unsuccessful, whereas the hospital efforts (Donor Action and the Spanish Model) have been spectacularly successful.[47]

Although many of the 46 European countries have large transplant centers,[47] only 21 of them have living related liver transplant programs. They perform these procedures with a 0.5% mortality rate and a 21% postoperative morbidity rate. The European Liver Transplant Registry (ELTR) is a rich resource for European liver transplant information and has accumulated data on all liver transplants since 1968.[46] These data report information for 124 transplant centers in 21 countries. Between 1991 and 2001, some 806 living donor transplants were performed in 46 centers from 15 European countries. Since 1968, more than 40,000 liver transplants have been performed in Europe and have been compiled by this research database (ELTR). More than 4,000 liver transplants are performed annually in Europe.[46] Eleven percent of these liver transplants performed annually are living related liver transplants[46] with a 1-year graft survival rate of 83%, which are the same as results for deceased donor transplants.

## North America

North America is made up of three large countries: Canada, Mexico, and the United States with a combined population of about 512 million people.[1–3]

Canada is the second largest nation in the world with a population of 32 million people.[1] In this country, kidney, heart, liver, pancreas, lung, and small bowel transplants are performed. Living kidney, liver, and lung transplant programs are very active. The Cadaver Organ Replacement Register is the data-reporting center for all Canadian cadaver transplant programs.[49] It has an organ transplant waiting list of more than 4,000 people. Over the past decade, living donor transplants rose nearly twofold from 124.9/1,000 transplants to 243.5/1,000 transplants. Living liver donor transplants were initially begun in Canada in 1993 and comprised 13% of all Canadian liver transplants. Lower donation rates plague Canada as its 13.5 donors PMP places it well below Spain's (32.5), but above Australia's (9.3 PMP).[49]

Mexico has a population of 106 million people.[1-3] In Mexico, kidney, liver, heart, and lung organ transplants are performed. Kidney transplants have been the most common solid organ transplanted in Mexico with 12,198 operations performed between 1963 and 2002. Since 1996, trimester reports from the 14 institutions licensed to perform organ tissue transplants have been reviewed by the Coordination Center of Nuevo Leon, Mexico.[50] Before 1996, virtually all organ transplants were from living donors. Living liver transplants were begun in Mexico in the year 2000. The first liver transplant was performed there in 1991, and since then, 23 liver transplants have been performed. The family referral rate for organ donation is 48% (8.4 deceased donors PMP). The experiences of Guadalajara and Nuevo Leon Mexico support the maintenance of the high percentage of living kidney donations while increasing the deceased donation rates.[50,51]

Cuba is the most populous of the Caribbean Islands with a population of 11.3 million,[1-3] and it has had a tremendous awakening recently of transplant activity since the creation in 1998 of the Centro de Investigaciones Medico Quirurgicas, the transplantation coordination office.[52] Although the original aim was to organize a system to support a liver transplant program, this office has changed the transplant donation process in the whole country. The deceased donor donation rates are now 71%. Between 1998 and 2002, 40 liver transplants were performed including a simultaneous liver–kidney transplant. During this period, 70 kidney transplants were performed: 29 from living related donors and 41 from deceased donor kidneys. This extraordinary result illustrates the role of transplant candidate programs and systems in developing as well as developed countries.[52]

The United States is the most populous country in North America (295 million).[1-3] The first successful human live donor kidney transplant was performed in 1954 (Dr. Joseph Murray). The first human liver transplant was performed here in 1963 (Dr. Thomas E. Starzl). Since that time, hundreds of thousands of organ transplants have been performed. Living donors are used for kidney, liver, pancreas, small intestine, and lung transplantation. Between 1954 and 1984, the U.S. Congress passed the National Organ Transplant Act, which defined the Federal Government as the Primary Administrator for organ allocation and transplantation oversight. A private contractor, the United Network for Organ Sharing (UNOS), was made responsible for data tracking, organ allocation, and recipient registration and would administer the Organ Procurement and Transplantation Network (OPTN).[53-55] This process coordinated virtually all aspects of organ transplants and also made paid organ donation illegal. This legislation was augmented in 2002 by the implementation of the "Final Rule," which put in place a new working system for liver allocation. A recent review of organ donation in the United States based on UNOS data between 1988 and 2002 demonstrated a 49% increase in deceased organ donations (6,082) and a 258% increase in living organ donations since 1988. The year 2001 represented the first year that there were more living donors than deceased donors.[53,54] This increase in donors was true for minority populations as well. In the minority population, donation rates for deceased donors during the same time period increased from 17% to 27% and for living donors from 24% to 30%. The percentage of living donors who were either spouses or unrelated to the recipient increased from 5% in 1998 to 27% in 2001, although Spain has the highest rate of organ donors per million in the world (33.4). The United States is third behind Belgium (24.6) with 22 donors per million.[2,3] It was inspired by former Secretary of Health, Tommy Thompson, to participate in a break through collaboration that is taking organ donation in the United States to a new high level.[56] This was necessitated by a transplant waiting list that had reached 89,000 by July 2005 and was creating an ever-increasing need for organ donors. This effort was desperately needed in order to prevent 16 people from dying daily, which this organ donor shortage had caused. Although this new collaborative effort is a hospital development system (not too dissimilar from the European Donor Action Model and the Spanish Model),[47] it is a system that is based on volunteerism, altruism, and using a system that is modeled for the success it has already achieved. Although this method is increasing deceased donation rates, it will also likely have a spillover effect on live donation rates as well.[56] No less vital to continuing the increases in living donation rates are successful public education programs like National MOTTEP.[5,16] These programs, when they are accompanied by serious studies of our public's concerns[56,57] about live donation and they follow the consensus recommendations made by the American consensus group (2000)[58] and the International Consensus Group (Amsterdam 2004),[59] augur well for ever-increasing living donation and deceased donation rates in the United States. The long-term success of living kidney donations and long-term analysis of living kidney donors followed for more than 2 decades has revealed low rates of kidney donor mortality of 0.01% and of < 5% morbidity rates.[60] A look at liver donors in Asia reveals no mortalities and a < 10% morbidity rate in Asia after the performance of over 2,400 donors. In Asia, they have now performed over 40,000 liver transplants.[61] In the United States since 1988 more than 51,000 liver transplants have been performed, but there is no liver registry, and the guestimate is that mortality rates range from 0.5% to 1% and morbidity rates from 20% to 60%. In the United States, as in Europe, 10% of liver transplants are living donor transplants.[60,61]

## South America

The continent of South America consists of 13 countries with a population of 379.5 million people. Although Central America is part of the North American continent,[1] many writings use the term *Latin American* in their discussions about organ donation and transplant. These writers lump Central America (Mexico and other countries) with South America under that terminology (Latin American). Therefore, there will be overlapping in the discussion of South America and their organ donation and transplant programs.

Central America and South America (Latin America) have carried out kidney transplants for more than 45 years (since 1958). Their transplant centers perform kidney, heart, liver, pancreas, and small bowel transplants.[50,51,63] The rate of organ donors PMP ranges from a low of 2 PMP per year to 12 PMP per year. The majority of kidney transplant donors are living related kidney donors.

The shortage of donors, however, has caused many countries to consider the use of living unrelated donors. Liver transplants in Latin America has reached the point where 1,100 liver transplants were performed in 2002, with Argentina, Brazil, and Chile being the most active liver transplant programs. Eighty percent of South American transplant programs perform liver transplants, whereas only one of six Central American transplant programs performs liver transplants.[51] In those countries performing liver transplants, living liver donation is used to help overcome the profound donor shortage for children with only three countries performing adult living liver donations.[51]

Latin American deceased donor donation rates in 2002 ranged from a high of 11.8 in Uruguay to a low of 4.5 donors PMP per year in Columbia; the range is from 2 donors PMP per year to 12 PMP per year, and patient and graft survival rates are 82% and 74%, respectively. Programs performing liver transplants are Brazil in 1968, Chile in 1969, Peru in 1973, Columbia in 1979, Mexico in 1985, Cuba in 1986, and Argentina in 1988. Most Latin American countries penalize organ traffic, have a transplant law that defines brain death criteria and living donor restrictions, and permit no economic benefit from donation. A few Latin American countries allow for presumed consent (Brazil and Columbia).[3] Family consent therefore is required for deceased donor usage, and family referral rates range from 30% to 55%.

Brazil is the largest and most populated country in South America (186 million people).[1-3] It is also the South American country where many attitude and practice surveys of the public, physicians, and academics have been carried out in order to find ways to increase their low organ donor rates.[64-67] These studies have been carried out in Porto Allegra[1], Sao Paulo[4], and Sao Jose do Rio Preto,[2] Brasilia.[1] Analysis of these well-carried-out studies teach us the following about Brazil. (1) Sixty-seven percent of their transplants were from living donors in 1989. (2) Blacks accounted for 24% of patients receiving transplants in 1989. (3) Graft survival for recipients of living related and non-living-related donors were not significantly different in 1989 (63% vs. 61%). (4) In 1998, there were only 7 deceased donors PMP from 2 PMP per year previously. (5) In 2000, 20% to 60% of the population were opposed to transplants. (6) Opinions about brain death were among the most important barriers to increasing transplants in 2000. (7) There is a positive correlation between education, social, and economic levels and willingness to donate. (8) Among those who did not agree with cerebral death as criteria for donation, 77% chose not to answer or justify their reasons. (9) Ninety percent of respondents did not agree to financial rewards for donation. (10) Sixty percent were in favor of first-come-first-serve for organ allocation except where children were concerned (a priority for children was approved (56%). (11) The physician in charge of the donors was preferred by 42% respondents to be the professional who should approach the donor family. (12) In 1999, 53% of organs transplanted were from living donors. (13) Reasons most commonly given for not agreeing to organ donation were lack of knowledge and information about cerebral death and more myths about the diagnosis of cerebral death (refusal to express thoughts about physician's definition of death or cerebral death). (14) Religious myths were not a significant barrier to donation. Finally, (15) Brazilians are supportive of donation and transplant.[65-67]

Brazilian legislation has explicitly prohibited organ commerce since 1988. The new Brazilian legislation of 1997 and 2001 stated that living unrelated donations could be accepted by careful case-by-case analysis by Judges; however, the laws seemed to enable the rich to exploit the poor and inadvertently predispose to organ commerce. The new law of 2001 (March 23) in article 9 enlarges the criteria for donation of organs between unrelated living people. Eighty percent of those interviewed felt that the law made possible the existence of rewarded donation, and 81% of them considered the requirement of judicial authorization an inefficient way of preventing organ commercialism.

In Venezuela, the new transplant coordination program has caused a sevenfold increase in organ donation and transplantation.[68] In Argentina, the third most populous South American country, a national education program on organ donation was introduced in grade schools and the education curriculum.[67] They propose that through education, younger generations will be able to erase ancestral behaviors for the welfare of current and future generations.[69]

## RELIGIOUS BELIEFS

*Culture* has also been previously defined as "behavior that develops as a consequence of all exposures one encounters as one matures." From a global perspective that includes in a very major way religious beliefs. The 12 major religions worldwide include (1) Christianity (1.9 billion [Catholics 1.05 billion of the 1.9 billion Christians]), (2) Islam (1.03 billion—Sunnites 83% of the Islams), (3) Hinduism (764 million), (4) Buddhism (338 million), (5) Chinese Folk religion (149 million), (6) New religions (128.9 million), (7) Tribal religions (99 million), (8) Sikhism (20 million), (9) Judaism (13.4 million), (10) Shamanism (11 million), (11) Confucianism (6.3 million), and (12) Bahaifaith (5.8 million).[2,3]

What is equally important to point out is that according to 1994 data, 1.1 billion humans have no religion (924 million) or are atheists (239 million). This is of the 5.6 billion people on earth (homo sapiens).[2,3]

It is significant to appreciate that to the true believers of all religions their religion is their complete code for living. The uniqueness and value of a human life is one of the important perspectives of virtually all major religions. This requires that all possible legal means be used to treat and save lives. Christianity is the religion that is associated with the largest number of people— 1.9 billion of which 1.05 billion are Catholics.[2,3] How important have the last three Papal decrees supporting transplantation and organ donation been in pointing Catholics and other Christians toward eliminating religious obstacles to donation and transplantation? This communication of support for transplantation and strong opposition to the commercialization of donation has been strongly supported by all of the major religions, and especially by the Islamic religion.

The way that the Islamic religion differs from the Christian religion is in the formal way it deals with special issues like transplantation, organ donation, and death. The Islam perspective identifies the Sharia, or the code on which Islamic laws are based. Fatwas are the opinions of important scholars giving the consensus of learned opinions. Fatwas regarding organ transplants are arrived at during Islamic conferences about religious matters not specifically mentioned in the Holy Quaran as in the sayings of the Prophet Muhammed and permits all types of transplants if the required conditions are fulfilled.[70] The Kingdom of Saudi Arabia is the most conservative Islamic country and plays a major role in formulating ethical Islamic Judicial views.

Between 1959 and 1998, there have been 18 fatwas dealing with transplantation. They have sanctioned live and cadaveric organ transplants; and skin, corneal, xenotransplantation;

and accept brain death criteria with and without heart death; and equated brain death with heart death in 1986. The Islam (Muslim) and Christian perspectives are identical as the Holy Quaran and the Bible; both emphasize altruism, selflessness, and helpfulness along with the value of the human being and the principle of Primun non nocere (first do no harm). Both prohibit human trafficking and organ commerce. The Islam religions' fatwas also prohibit unrelated living organ donation.[71] Both of these are violated in the Pakistani (97% Muslim) and Iranian (99% Muslim) models in which paid living unrelated donations are the rule rather than the exception.[70–73] There is no religious prohibition against organ transplantation or donation in the Sikh or Buddhist religions. Some Hindu commentators have proposed that Hindu donation is only acceptable if the desire to donate is expressed overtly before death. All other Asian religions do not prohibit organ donation. The Japanese Shinto religion is the one notable exception, for their Folk belief context considers injuring a dead body as a serious crime![74] Although religious beliefs are important for the maturation process of 80% of all Homo sapiens, it is rarely directly the reason for nondonation.

## COMMERICAL CONCERNS

*Commercial concerns commerce* is defined as the buying and selling of goods, especially on a large scale as between cities or nations (*American Heritage College Dictionary*). Has it come to this in renal transplantation? Have we come to the point where we speak of organs (kidneys) as commodities (something useful that can be turned into commercial or other advantages)? Is this not the antithesis of what most of the Islamic fatwas and Papal decrees were all about? Table 2.2 identifies the 15 countries in which commercial transplants and buying and selling of kidneys take place. Of the 15 countries, only 1 is nonreligious. China is atheist; the remainder are either Muslim (Islam) or Christian.

How did we get here, and how long has this been going on? Since 1978 in India, there have been more than 800 donors for paid kidney, living unrelated donation transplants; since 1990 in Pakistan, more than 50 kidney transplants per year have been performed; since 1992, in Iraq and Iran; and since 1993, in China.

Three of the strongest proponents for these practices are the Pakistani, Iran, and Israel transplant groups. Dr. Friedlaender of Israel, in his latest article of 2002,[75] puts it into the patient/physicians' perspective, which is that this is a practice that has been going on for the past 20 years. Patients who are now dying on the waiting list, know that others are receiving kidneys (paying in some circumstances as much as $200,000.00), getting off dialysis and having an improved quality of life, while at the same time their life is ebbing away from them as they wait for a kidney transplant that may not come in time. At first the transplant care that the paid donor recipients received was suboptimal, but as immunosuppressive management improved graft and patient survival rates and patient morbidity rates became more competitive as long as the deceased donor rate stayed low, the position of not allowing them to "buy a kidney" from a utilitarian perspective was becoming more paternalistic and less tenable.[76]

What are the basic problems that have stimulated the growth and development of commercial kidney transplant programs resulting in recipients acquiring kidneys from paid live nonrelated donors or from executed prisoners? They are contributed to by the prohibition of commercial kidney transplants by the legislation of most developed countries (including India where many of these transplants are still illegally performed). A. J. Ghods began a legalized state funded well-controlled paid living unrelated kidney donor program in Iran in 1988.[38] At that time there were (1) large numbers of dialysis patients who needed renal transplants, but had no potential living related donors; (2) the cadaver organ donation program had not been established and did not appear to be developed in the near future; and (3) by 1999 the renal transplant waiting list had been eliminated. In April 2000, legislation was passed in Iran supporting parliamentary acceptance for brain death and cadaver organ donation.[34,35,38,71]

By the end of 2001, a total of 12,607 renal transplants had been performed (2,614 living related donations, 9,839 living unrelated donations, 154 deceased donor renal transplants). More

**TABLE 2.2**

**CONTINENTS AND COUNTRIES WHERE PAID DONATION OCCURS**

| Continent | Country | Population | Major Religion (%) |
|---|---|---|---|
| Africa | South Africa | 49 million | Christian (86%) |
| Asia | China | 1.3 billion | Officially atheist |
| | India | 1 billion | Muslim (94%) |
| | Iran | 69 million | Muslim (99%) |
| | Iraq | 25.3 million | Muslim (97%) |
| | Lebanon | 3.7 million | Muslim (70%) |
| | Pakistan | 128 million | Muslim (97%) |
| | Philippines | 86 million | Catholic (83%) |
| | Turkey | 68.9 million | Muslim (99.8%) |
| Europe | Bulgaria | 7.5 million | Christian (85%) |
| | Estonia | 1.3 million | Christian |
| | Georgia | 4.9 million | Christian (75%) |
| | Romania | 22.3 million | Christian |
| | Russia | 143 million | Christian |
| South America | Brazil | 186 million | Catholic (80%) |

Based on data from references 2, 3, 44, 45, 75, 76.

than 78% of the renal transplants have been from paid living unrelated donations. The Dialysis and Transplant Patient Association (DATPA) funds the suitable living unrelated donations with financial incentives. The Government pays all renal transplant hospital expenses. After the renal transplant, each living unrelated donor receives a financial award from the Government and an arranged payment from the Dialysis and Transplant Patient Association. The renal transplant team receives no additional financial payments. The program is under close observation by the Iranian Society of Organ Transplantation regarding ethical issues. Foreigners are not allowed to undergo renal transplants from Iranian living unrelated donors. More than 50% of the living unrelated donors are from a poor socioeconomic background. A differing Islamic perspective on the Iranian Program is offered by Al-Khader[71] from Saudi Arabia who identifies (1) the low economic status and per-capita income in Muslim countries (a low of $100/year in Afghanistan to a high of $29,100/year in Qatar). Low renal transplant rates follow because of the expensive nature of transplants; (2) public attitude toward transplants—(a) a reluctance to accept living related donation (in Iran, but not believed to be present in other Muslim countries), (b) fear of body mutilation (a great Muslim fear), (c) a fear of premature declaration of brain death; (3) fatwas not being followed by laws in some Muslim countries (Pakistan, Egypt, Syria); and (4) that in Iran, the fatwa permitting transplants was based on the Quaranic verse, and if anyone saved a life it would be as if he or she saved the life of the whole people.

Quaran Chapter V, verse 35—"necessities allow prohibited matters—(iv) need is considered the same as necessity and (v) altruism and cooperation is paramount." Although Islam does not shun transplants from living unrelated donors; it states, however, that *paid donation is not permissible*[71]—one's body belongs to God and cannot be sold.

Other concerns Al-Khader has regarding the Iranian model are that 84% of the paid donors were from the poor class, and surveys of the donors paint a grim picture of the above encountered. Fifty-one percent of the donors expressed hatred toward their recipients, and 65% stated that promises given by the recipients prior to the surgery were never met. Eighty-three percent of paid donors were largely motivated by the financial incentive, and 76% of them feel that the practice should be banned.[71] Is the worse yet to come from this model?

After all is said and done, the religious models of Christianity and Islam have not prevented these commodifications of the human body. What does this say about the actual role of culture and religion when one has to make life or death decisions and when that life is your life?

## SUMMARY AND CONCLUSIONS

The shortage of organ donors across the earth is the number one problem in transplantation today. As a consequence of the donor shortage, transplant waiting lists are growing, and each day hundreds of people die waiting for an organ that does not come. The fight to live and survive may be the most primal urge of all. Among the most important factors that determine life or death if you have organ failure is where on the earth you are and whether you are rich or poor. Asians represent two thirds of the population and only one fourth of its wealth. This information must be factored into any conclusion we draw regarding the donor shortage and possible strategies we must employ to increase organ donations. On the face of it, better hospital systems, such as the Spanish Model (ONT), the Donor

Action Programs in Europe, The Break Through Collaborative in the United States; and Awareness Campaigns when combined with community education and empowering grass-roots efforts like the MOTTEP model of the United States; and the public-grade-school campaigns such as those employed in Argentina are likely to increase living donation rates.

The Saudi (SCOT), Pakistani, and Iranian models; the impact of Christianity; and the Papal decrees, along with the religious fatwas of the Muslims all in one way or another impact each of us in different parts of the globe based on our cultural upbringing: how different we are, yet how similar we are. When push comes to shove, however, it is the primal instinct of fighting for life that has the final say. How else can you explain that when 80% of the world, that is, 5 or 6 billion humans, is religious and two thirds are Islamic or Christian, that the one system that is most effective at eliminating the transplant waiting list is a program that highlights paid living unrelated donors. This is the case, even though Islamics and Christians alike recognize that this practice exploits the poor! On a less pessimistic note, the message that is loud and clear is that mankind is but mankind no matter where on the globe you find him or her. When we look at all the surveys no matter where they are on the earth, the factors that lead us to change our behaviors in our most sane moments are those that impact our cultural growth and development. While we mature on different parts of the globe, the fight for life, the fear of mutilation after death or in life, the premature declaration of death, religious myths and misperceptions, distrust of health providers, and lack of information and communication are common to us all and must be overcome in order for us to increase living donations, shorten transplant waiting lists, and save lives!

## References

1. "The Seven Continents." We Are the World. http://www.ri.net/schools/Central_Falls/v/218/index.html. Published July 1, 2005.
2. van der Heyden J.: "Global Statistics." GEOHIVE: Global Statistics. Geohive. http://www.geohive.com/. Published July 1, 2005.
3. "World Atlas of Maps Flags and Geography Facts." WorldAtlas.com. Woolwine—Moen Group. http://worldatlas.com/aatlas/world.htm. Published July 1, 2005.
4. Aghanwa HS, Akinsola A, Akinola DO, et al. Attitudes toward kidney donation. *JNMA* 2003;95:725–731.
5. Callender CO, Miles PA, Hall MB, et al. Blacks and whites and kidney transplantation: A disparity! But why and why won't it go away? *Transplant Rev* 2002;16(3):163–176.
6. Davis C, Randhawa G. "Don't know enough about it": Awareness and attitdes toward organ donation and transplantation among the black Caribbean and black African population in lambeth, southwark, and lewisham, United Kingdom. *Transplantation* 2004;78(3):420–425.
7. Modiba MC, Mzamane DV, Pantanowitz D, et al. Renal transplantation in black South Africans: The baragwanti experience. *Transplant Proc* 1989;21(1):2010–2011.
8. Mokotedi S, Modiba MC, Ndiovu Sr. Attitudes of black South Africans to living related kidney transplantation. *Transplant Procs* 2004;36:1896–1897.
9. Morgan SE, Cannon T: African americans' knowledge about organ donation: Closing the gap with more effective persuasive message strategies. *JNMA* 2003;95:1066–1071.
10. Rozon–Solomon M, Burrows L. 'Tis better to receive than to give: The relative failure of the African American community to provide organs for transplantation. *The Mount Sinai J Med* 1999;66(4):273–276.
11. Siminoff LA, Lawrence RH, Arnold RM. Comparison of black and white families' experiences and perceptions regarding organ donation requests. *Critical Care Med* 2003;31(1):146–151.

12. Terrell F, Mosley KL, Terrell AS, et al. The relationship between motivation to volunteer, gender, cultural mistrust, and willingness to donate organs among blacks. *JNMA* 2004;96(1):53–60.

13. Monet T, Pullen–Smith B, Haisch C, et al. Living renal donation in the African-American community. *Tranplant Proc* 1997;29(8): 3649–3650.

14. Trollinger J, Flores J, Corkill JK, et al. Increasing living kidney donation in African Americans. *Tranplant Proc* 1997;29(8):3748–3750.

15. Coalition on Donation, www.coalition@donatellife.net

16. Callender, CO; Maddox, GM; Miles, PV. In: David Satcher, MD, and Ruben J. Pamies, MD, eds. *Transplantation and Organ Donation: An Analysis of Ethnic Disparities: Multicultural Medicine and Health Disparities.* New York, McGraw–Hill; September 2005.

17. Bollinger RR, Cho W. Organ allocation for transplantation in the USA and Korea: The changing roles of equity and utility. *Yonsei Med J* 2004;45(6):1035–1042.

18. Cho W, Kim YS. Landmarks in clinical transplantation in korea. *Yonsei Med J* 2004;45(6):963–967.

19. de Villa VH, Lo CM, Chen CL. Ethics and rationale of living-donor liver transplantation in Asia. *Transplantation* 2003;75(3):S2–S5.

20. Ikels C. Kidney failure and transplantation in china. *Social Sci Med* 1997;44(9):1271–1283.

21. Ki JR, Elliot D, Hyde C. Korean health professionals' attitudes and knowledge toward organ donation and transplantation. *Intl J Nurs Studies* 2004;41:299–307.

22. Lee SH, Jeong JS, Ha HS, et al. Decision-related factors and attitudes toward donation in living related liver transplantation: Ten-year experience. *Transplant Proc* 2005;37:1081–1084.

23. Lo CM. Complications and long-term outcome of living liver donors: A survey of 1508 cases in five Asian centers. *Tranplantation* 2003;75(3):S12–S15.

24. Luvira U, Supaporn T. Role of patient support groups in the Thailand transplant program. *Transplant Proc* 2004;36:2004–2005.

25. Ota K. Strategies for increasing transplantation in Asia and prospects of organ sharing: The Japanese experience. *Transplant Proc* 1998;30:3650–3652

26. Randhawa G. An exploratory study examining the influence of religion on attitudes towards organ donation among the Asian population in Luton, UK. *Nephrol Dial Transplant* 1998;13:1949–1954.

27. Schmidt VH, Lim CH. Organ transplantation in Singapore: History, problems, and policies. *Social Sci Med* 2004;59:2173–2182.

28. Surman OS, Cosimi AB, Fukunishi I, et al. Some ethical and psychiatric aspects of right-lobe liver transplantation in the united states and japan. *Psychosomatics* 2002;43(5):347–353.

29. Yeung I, Kong SH, Lee J. Attitudes towards organ donation in hong kong. *Social Sci Med* 2000;50: 1643–1654.

30. Yew YW, Saw SM, Pan JCH, et al. Knowledge and beliefs on corneal donation in Singapore adults. *Brit J Ophthalmol* 2005;89:835–840.

31. Rizvi SA, Naqvi SA, Hashmi A, et al. Improving kidney and live donation rates in Asians: Living donation. *Transplant Proc* 2004;36: 1894–1895.

32. Rizvi SA, Naqvi SA, Hussain Z, et al. Renal transplantation in developing countries. *Kidney Int Suppl* 2003;83:S96–S100.

33. Personal Communication with Organ Donor Center of Hawaii/MOT-TEP of Hawaii, 2001.

34. Shaheen FA, Souquiyyeh MZ. Factors influencing organ donation and transplantation in the Middle East. *Transplant Proc* 2000;32: 645–646.

35. Shaheen FA, Souqiyyeh MZ, Abdullah A. Strategies and obstacles in an organ donation program in developing countries: Saudi Arabian experience. *Transplant Proc* 2000;32:1470–1472.

36. Al- Sebayel MI, Al- Enazi AM, Al- Sofayan MS, et al. Improving organ donation in central saudi arabia. *Saudi Med J* 2004;25(10): 1366–1368.

37. Rizvi SA, Naqvi SA. Our vision on organ donation in developing countries. *Transplant Proc* 2000;32:144–145.

38. Ghods, AJ. Should we have live unrelated donor renal transplantation in MESOT countries. *Transplant Proc* 2003;35; 2542–2544.

39. Sebayel MI, Khalaf H: Knowledge and attitude of intensivists toward organ donation in Riyadh, Saudi Arabia. *Transplant Proc* 36: 1883–1884.

40. Kececioglu N, Tuncer M, Sarikaya M. Detection of targets for organ donation in Turkey. *Transplant Proc* 1999;31:3373–3374.

41. El-Shoubaki H, Bener A. Public knowledge and attitudes toward organ donation and transplantation: A cross-cultural study. *Transplant Proc* 2005;37:1993–1997.

42. Hirsch N, Hailey, D, Martin C. The evolution of heart, lung and liver transplantation services in Australia. *Health Policy* 1995;34:6–71.

43. Chapman J, Russ, G. Geographic variance in access to renal transplantation in Australia. *Transplantation* 2003;76(9):1403–1406.

44. Kennedy SE, Shen Y, Charlesworth JA, et al. Outcome of overseas commercial kidney transplantation: An Australian perspective. *Med J Australia* 2005;182(5):224–227.

45. Matthew T, Faull R, Snelling P. The shortage of kidneys for transplantation in Australia. *Med J Australia* 2005;182(5):204–205.

46. Adam R, McMaster P, O'Grady JG, et al. Evolution of liver transplantation in Europe: report on the European liver transplant registry. *Liver* Transplant 2003; 9(12):1231–1243.

47. Schutt G. 25 Years of organ donation: European initiatives to increase organ donation. *Transplant Proc* 2002;34:2005–2006.

48. Gross T, Martinoli S, Spagnoli G. Attitudes and behavior of young European adults towards the donation of organs—A call for better information. *Am J Transplant* 1:74–81, 200.

49. McAlister VC, Badovinac K.: Transplantation in Canada: Report of the Canadian organ replacement register. *Transplant Proc* 2003;35:2428–2430.

50. Carbajal H, Cabriales H. Results from the organ and tissue transplant program in Nuevo Leon, Mexico, 1996 to 2001. *Transplant Proc* 2003;35:2851–2854.

51. Hepp J, Innocenti FA. Liver transplantation in latin America: Current status. *Transplant Proc* 2004;36:1667–1668.

52. Abdo A, Ugarte JC, Castellanos R, et al. The transplantation donation process in the Centro de Investigaciones Medico Quirurgicas de Cuba: 1999–2002. *Transplant Proc* 2003;35(5):1636–1637.

53. Ojo AO, Heinrichs D, Edmond JC, et al. Organ donation and utilization in the USA. *Am J Transplant* 2004;4(9):27–37.

54. Port FK, Dykstra DM, Merion RM, et al. Trends and results for organ donation and transplantation in the United States, 2004. *Am J Transplant* 2005;5(2):843–849.

55. Rosendale JD, Dean JR. Organ donation in the United States 1988–2001. *Clin Transplant* 2005;5(2):843–849.

56. Thompson, Tommy G, HHS Secretary, Organ Donation Break Through Collaborative: From Best Practice to Common Practice, April 2003–Present.

57. Boulware LE, Ratner LE, Sosa JA, et al. The general public's concerns about clinical risk in live kidney donation. *Am J Transplant* 2002; 2:186–193.

58. The Authors for the Live Organ Donor Consensus Group: Consensus statement on the live organ donor. *JAMA* 2000;284(22):2919–2926.

59. The Ethics Committee of the Transplantation Society: The consensus statement of the Amsterdam forum on the care of the live kidney donor. *Transplantation* 2004;78(4):491–492.

60. Dahlke MH, Popp FC, Eggert N, et al. Differences in attitude toward living and postmortal liver donation in the United States, Germany and Japan. *Psychosomatics* 2005;46(1):58–64.

61. Northup PG, Berg CL. Living donor liver transplantation: the historical and cultural basis of policy decisions and ongoing ethical questions. *Health Policy* 2005;72:175–185.

62. 2002 Annual Report The United States Organ Procurement and Transplantation Network and The Scientific Registry of Transplant Recipients. Transplant 1992–2001;76.

63. Garcia VD, Garcia CD, Santiago-Delphin EA. Organ transplants in Latin America. *Transplant Proc* 2003;35(5):1673–1674.

64. Passarinho LE; Goncalves MP, Garrafa V. Bioethical study of kidney transplantation in Brazil involving unrelated living donors: The inefficiency of law to prevent organ commercialism. *Rev Assoc Med Bras* Oct–Dec2003;49(4):382–388.

65. Brandao A, Fuchs S, Bartholomay E, et al. Organ donation in Porto Alegre, southern Brazil: Attitudes and practices of physicians working in intensive care units. *Transplant Proc* 1999;31:3073.

66. Duarte PS, Pericoco S, Miyazaki MCOS, et al. Brazilian's attitudes toward organ donation and transplantation. *Transplant Proc* 2002;34:458–459.

67. Roza BA, Schirmer J, Medina- Pestana JO. Academic community response to the brazilian legislation for organ donation. *Transplant Proc* 2002;34:447–448.

68. Milanes CL, Hernandez E, Gonzalez L, et al. Organ and tissue procurement system: A novel intervention to increase donation rates in Venezuela. *Progr Transplant* 2003 March 13;(1): 65–68.

69. Cantarovich F, Fagundes E, Biolcalti D, et al. School Education: A basis for positive attitudes toward organ donation. *Transplant Proc* 2000;32:55–56.

70. El–Shahat YI. Islamic viewpoint of organ transplantation. *Transplant Proc* 1999;31:3271–3274.

71. Al-Khader AA. The Iranian transplant programme: Comment from an Islamic perspective. *Nephrol Dial Transplant* 17:213–215.

72. Hayward C, Madill A. The meanings of organ donation: Muslims of Pakistani origin and white English nationals living in north England. *Social Sci Med* 2003;57:389–401.

73. Shaheen FA, Souquiyyeh MZ. Increasing organ donation rates from Muslim donors: Lesson from a successful model. *Transplant Proc* 2004;36:1878–1880.

74. Cooper ML, Taylor GJ. *SEOPF/UNOS, Organ and Tissue Donation: A Reference Guide for Clergy,* 4th ed. Richmond, VA; UNOS, 2000.

74. Friedlaender MM. The right to sell or buy a kidney: Are we failing our patients? *The Lancet* 2002;359:971–973.

76. Friedlaender MM. The role of commercial non–related living kidney transplants. *J Nephro* 2003;*J*16(7):S10–S15.

# CHAPTER 3

# ETHICAL AND LEGAL ISSUES

## 3.1 THE AMERICAN PERSPECTIVE

*David C. Cronin II, MD, PhD, Mark Siegler, MD*

The need for solid organ transplantation has rapidly expanded beyond the supply of available organ donors. Beginning with the first successful transplant performed in 1954, the number of registrants on the United Network for Organ Sharing (UNOS) waiting list now approaches 100,000.[1] In addition to the increasing number of registrants, the types of organs needed for transplantation have expanded beyond kidney transplants. Registrants now include individuals awaiting kidney, liver, lung, heart, pancreas, intestine, and multiorgan transplants. Unfortunately, the number of registrants who are successfully transplanted is limited by the availability of suitable donors with only 27,000 transplants performed in 2004.[2] These numbers, however, are not a complete representation of the crisis that exists in the field of transplantation. Because of the limited supply of organs, 9,204 registrants were removed from the transplant waiting list in 2004 because they died, were too sick to transplant or were medically unsuitable.[3] Many of the patients removed were listed for time-limited, live-saving organs (liver, heart, and lung) where medical therapies, such as dialysis, do not exist.

Various strategies have been employed to meet the continually increasing demand for organs and to narrow the disparity between the number of patients listed for transplantation and the number of transplants performed. One such strategy has been to expand the use of living organ donors from kidneys to include living donors of liver segments, lung lobes, and partial pancreas and small intestine grafts. It is noteworthy that in 2001, for the first time, the number of live donors exceeded the number of deceased donors as a source of organs for transplantation. Further, not only has the number of living donors and types of organs procured increased and expanded, but also there has been an expansion in acceptable relationships (or lack of relationship) between the recipient and the donor. The reasons that justified and compelled transplant surgeons to use living donors in the early experience of solid organ transplantation have fundamentally changed. Interestingly, much of this expansion has occurred without strict governmental or legal oversight. In distinction to the highly regulated and transparent system of deceased donor transplantation, much of the administration and control over living donation has been at the level of institutional and professional organizations. This chapter reviews the changes in the use of living donors in solid organ transplantation in the United States from the perspective of legal oversight and ethical justification.

### LEGAL OVERSIGHT*

From 1954 when the living organ donation was first used, the practice of living donor transplantation was conducted in very few centers, initially only between genetically identical twins and only for kidney transplantation. Further, use of living donors was performed with full disclosure within the medical community. In addition to demonstrating that transplantation is an acceptable therapy for the treatment of end-stage organ failure, use of living donors has undoubtedly saved many lives. As of January 20, 2006, more than 76,000 living donors have been used for transplant in the United States.[4] With the continued growth of the transplant waiting list and the relatively fixed supply of deceased donors the use and dependence on living donors has expanded. As with many surgical innovations and medical practices within the United States the practice of living donation is not specifically governed by federal legislation and is subjected to little state legislation. Recently, however, governmental legislation and regulations initially intended to govern deceased donor solid organ transplantation are now being applied to living donor transplantation.

In 1972, federal legislation mandated that patients suffering from end-stage renal disease be covered under Medicare. With this act, the treatment of end-stage renal failure with dialysis and transplantation was covered under a government-sponsored insurance program. Consequently the number of dialysis centers increased and the number of patients being maintained on dialysis increased. Improvements in immunosuppressive therapy, the acceptance of brain death, and the development of hypothermic storage techniques for organs expanded the source of donors from genetically identical living donors to include unrelated deceased donors for successful kidney transplantation. Transplantation proved to be the preferred treatment for end-stage renal failure and soon the number of kidney transplants performed rapidly outstripped the number of organs (from living and deceased donors) available for transplantation.

In 1984, in an effort to strengthen the nation's ability to provide organs for transplants, Congress passed the National Organ Transplant Act (NOTA).[5] This legislation brought the practice of organ donation and transplantation into public view and established a system for its regulation. NOTA provided for the following: (1) the appointment of a 25-member organ donation task force; (2) establishment and expansion of qualified organ procurement organizations (OPOs); (3) the authority for the Secretary of the Department

---

*Since this review was compiled and submitted, new federal legislation [2007] makes the OPTN responsible for developing policies governing the equitable allocation of living donor organs giving the OPTN/UNOS living donor committee new weight in protecting living donors and in standardizing the medical and administrative practices of living donation. The committee developed guidelines for the consent and medical evaluation of living donors, and teamed with the OPTN/UNOS membership and professional standards committee to create living kidney and liver program certification requirements.[5a]

of Health and Human Services to establish an Organ Procurement and Transplant Network (OPTN) by contract with a private, non-profit entity to coordinate the distribution of organs nationally and among regions and to maintain the registry of individuals needing organs; and (4) prohibition of organ purchases.

Under the authority of NOTA, the OPTN awarded the first operational contract to the UNOS in 1986. The intent of this organizational arrangement, OPTN being administered by UNOS, was to keep government bureaucracy out of the organ distribution system and, by membership rules, allow medical professionals involved in transplantation significant control.

Although the main focus of NOTA addressed the regulation of deceased donation and transplantation, there are some provisions that apply to live donation. First is the prohibition of commercial enterprise in organ transplantation specifically making the buying and selling of organs (deceased or living donors) illegal. Additionally, the Task Force on Transplantation produced a comprehensive report, which included recommendations to limit the use of live donors rather than supporting their expansion. Finally, all transplant centers (programs) receiving deceased donor organs within the United States must be members of UNOS and abide by all the policies, bylaws, and amendments.[6] The majority of UNOS policies specifically regulate the listing, organ allocation, and data reporting of solid organ transplantation using deceased donors. Nevertheless, patients who are listed with UNOS and subsequently receive a living donor transplantation are also included in the data-reporting obligations of the transplant center.

With the increased use of living donors, expansion of organs donated to include liver lobes and segments, increases in nondirected living donation, and concern for donor safety, the OPTN/UNOS Ad Hoc Living Donor Committee (2002) proposed guidelines for living donor and recipient evaluations. The committee developed guidelines for living kidney donor evaluation and living liver donor evaluation.[7, 8] Support for these guidelines was derived from the report to the New York State Transplant Council and New York Department of Health,[9] which established minimum criteria for living donor work-up which are independent of the requirement for data reporting. Recently, the OPTN/UNOS Board of Directors has begun a process of approval and certification of live donor kidney and liver programs and the Health Resources and Service Administration (HRSA), Department of Health and Human Services (HHS) has published a notice in the Federal Register to solicit comments on OPTN oversight and enforcement of living donor guidelines.[10] The intent of this action is to develop policies necessary and appropriate to promote the safety and efficacy of living donor transplantation for the donor and the recipient.

On a state level, New York became the first state to develop strict guidelines for living donor liver transplantation. In their report to the New York State Transplant Council and New York Department of Health, the New York State Committee on Quality Improvement in Living Liver Donation set forth the first set of guidelines governing the process of live donor liver transplantation for both donor and recipient.[9] Interestingly, the committee believed that despite the conditions that called this committee into formation, specifically the death of a donor, a moratorium on adult-to-adult live liver transplantation was not ethically acceptable due to the high mortality rate of patients on the waiting list for liver transplantation. The committee covered virtually all aspects of the process of adult-to-adult living donor liver transplantation and provided recommendations for donor and recipient evaluation and care, provision of informed consent, perioperative care and facility support, and discharge planning and donor follow-up. It is not surprising that this document has served as a model for the development of a national policy in living donor organ transplantation.

## ETHICAL JUSTIFICATION

*"Is it ever morally right and ethically acceptable to injure one person to help another?"*[11]

The answer to this question is as important today as it was when initially proposed at the time of the first successful living donor transplant performed in Boston on December 24, 1954. Since 1954, the use of living donors for solid organ transplantation has been a controversial practice.[12] As Dr. Moore's quote indicates, the fundamental moral tension is between saving the life of one person who otherwise would die while using and physically harming a second person, a healthy human being who volunteers to be a living donor. It might help to examine the fundamental ethical question in terms of the situation in which it was first raised in the 1950s and develop the justification for use of the living donor.

In 1954, the diagnosis of end-stage renal disease (ESRD) was uniformly fatal with no treatment available. Living donors, in the form of identical twins, were needed for the following reasons of the era: (1) the uniformly fatal outcome of ESRD; (2) the lack of understanding of immune rejection and immunosuppression; (3) extremely limited supply of deceased donor organs; and (4) inability to adequately preserve organs. In 1954, because of these reasons the use of living kidney donors was viewed as ethically acceptable, but just barely.

Despite these early justifications for the use of the living kidney donor many ethical issues still needed to be addressed. For example, use of the live donor violated the fundamental rule of medicine and surgery—*primum non nocere*. The removal of a kidney from a healthy volunteer donor unmistakably and unavoidably imparted significant surgical harm on the donor. In addition, the true morbidity and mortality of the donor operation and long-term effects were not known. It appeared that the human body was being used as a means to an end. Finally, the provision of informed consent was difficult if not impossible to obtain. The donor could not be fully protected from the potential pressures of coercion or exploitation in their "decision" to donate. This might be especially true if the intended recipient (as it was in most of the early transplants) was an identical twin.

What essentially appeared to be the justification for the use of living donors in the early years of transplantation was the net positive balance between recipient risk/benefit and donor risk/benefit. Clearly, the potential recipient of a kidney transplant would have the opportunity to postpone or escape death from kidney failure. The donor risk/benefit analysis was obvious with respect to risk: intentional surgical incision and removal of a healthy, functioning kidney. The complications associated with a major operation in the 1950s were not trivial. The long-term consequences of donor nephrectomy were not known. The benefit of living donation was more difficult to quantify in the 1950s than it is currently. Interestingly, the donor benefit appears to rest largely on the psychologic benefit derived from trying to improve or save the life of a loved one. Soon after the first few cases were performed, a Massachusetts court rendered the following opinion:

> … for identical twins, the loss of a kidney by the donor would be less devastating than the loss of an identical twin sibling. This operation is necessary for the continued good health and well-being of the donor and in performing the operation the surgeons are conferring a benefit upon the donor.

It appeared that the Massachusetts court almost mandated the use of the living donor for the benefit of the donor. This view, of psychological benefit for donors, seems to have held as donation has been extended to other family members in addition to identical twins.

Therefore, with the early use of live donors, the desperate case argument was sufficiently persuasive to override the moral problem of inflicting significant surgical harms to a consenting person to benefit someone else.

## CURRENT ETHICAL JUSTIFICATION

Many of the ethical justifications for using living donors have changed since 1954. For example, in the United States, we now have an improved and organized supply of deceased donor organs; further, we understand immune rejection and have developed excellent immunosuppressive medications; and, of course, we have excellent preservations solutions. But one central ethical justification remains as persuasive in 2007 as it was in 1954 and that is that the supply of organs needed to save lives remains insufficient. In fact, the gap is growing rapidly. This gap between the potential lives to be saved by using the living donor and actual lives currently being saved continues to be the strongest ethical justification for widespread use of living donors and for the expansion of living donors for organs other than kidney and of donors other than genetically or emotional related individuals. Every time there is an expansion of the use of living donors, the practice is always tested against the three central ethical criteria that pertain to living donors: (1) the risk/benefit to the donor and the recipient; (2) the absolute level of risk to the donor; and (3) the ability to obtain voluntary informed consent of donors. The remainder of this section examines the extension of living donation to organs other than kidney and extension of the practice beyond relatives and emotional related to include stranger donors.

## PEDIATRIC DONATION

Application of liver transplantation for pediatric patients with ESLD quickly revealed a dire clinical situation similar to that which existed at the beginning of living donor kidney transplantation. Within the pediatric population, the most frequent cause of ESLD is biliary atresia[13] with the majority of patients requiring liver transplantation before the age of 2.[14] Within this group of pediatric patients the death rate of patients listed and awaiting liver transplantation approached 30%.[15] The single most important variable responsible for this high mortality was the unavailability of a sufficient number of pediatric deceased donor grafts. With surgically innovative techniques such as reduced-size grafts[16] or split grafts the waiting list mortality diminished but was not eliminated.[15,17,18]

The continued need for life saving pediatric-size livers for transplantation prompted a few groups to attempt living donor liver transplantation. Two initial case reports, used the procedure to overcome the unavailability of deceased donor organs.[19,20] These initial reports prompted a team from the University of Chicago to define a model of research-ethics consultation to evaluate the clinical and ethical acceptability of the surgically innovative expansion in use of the living donor.[21] This group set forth an ethical framework for the introduction and investigation of innovative surgical therapies. The excellent results obtained in the initial study[22] and the improved results obtain from substantial modifications with the procedure[23–26] and recipient[27,28] and

donor selection[29] have resulted in over 2,000 adult-to-pediatric live donor liver transplants having been performed worldwide and its acceptance as standard procedure in pediatric liver transplantation.

Justification for the initiation of adult-to-pediatric living donor liver transplantation was similar to the initial situation in living donor kidney transplantation: there was an absolute need for the surgically innovative procedure; there was clear benefit to the recipients as demonstrated in diminished waiting list mortality and improved graft survival and patient survival after transplantation; the donors were primarily intimately related to the recipient (parents, uncles, aunts, grandparents, etc) and as such had a personal investment in (benefit from) saving the life of the recipient. And similar to the current justification of living donor kidney transplantation: the adult-to-pediatric living donor liver transplant procedure continues to provide life-saving recipient benefits oftentimes superior to those obtained with decease donors[23] and substantive donor benefit while limiting the donor risk to acceptable levels of morbidity and mortality.[30,31]

It is important to acknowledge the progression of ethical support and justification between the two procedures. In the initial series of living donor kidney transplantation, the experience was confined to a few highly experienced centers with continual exchange of results between centers and among the surgeons offering such a procedure. There was a life-saving need for the innovation and because of the immunologic requirements, the relationship between the donor and the recipient pair (identical twins) was very intimate and donor benefit apparent.

The development of pediatric living donor liver transplantation (PLDLT) addressed a similar life-saving need among pediatric patients in need of liver transplantation. The intimate relationship between the donor and recipient pair allowed for an easily recognized donor benefit. The restriction of the innovative procedure to one center and publication of results allowed for refinement of techniques before wide dissemination. It is important to note, however, that the expansion of the living donor into liver transplantation carried with it an increase in donor risk. Additionally, this was the first time that a surgically innovative procedure was introduced using the model of research-ethics consultation. Publication of the research protocol and discussion within the public and medical community before a single patient was enrolled into a prospective, Institutional Review Board (IRB)-approved protocol with immediate publication of the cohort results helped to establish what has become a clinically and ethically acceptable medical procedure.

## ADULT DONATION

The surgically innovative approach to liver transplantation using the living donor was expanded to an adult recipient in 1991 using a left lobe graft.[32] But it was not until 1997 when the next adult recipient was transplanted using an extended-right-lobe graft including the middle hepatic vein.[33] The method of introduction and application of this living donor procedure for adult recipients differed from the measured and ethically based model used for the pediatric recipients of a living donor graft.

Adult living donor liver transplantation (ALDLT) began as a series of case reports and small series published in peer-review journals.[33–36] Soon the procedure disseminated globally and was being applied in a variety of situations. This rapid expansion and dissemination of the ALDLT procedure left many critical components undefined. Despite more than 7 years of wide, global application, many of the critical areas in ALDLT are still in evolution.

Clearly, this procedure is associated with the highest rate of donor complication and mortality risk of any living donor operation currently performed.[37–39] Additionally, the technical aspects of the donor evaluation and surgical resection are still under development. Although more than 2,000 such operations have been performed, there is still controversy among programs and surgeons as to donor and recipient inclusion and exclusion criteria. Only recently has an NIH-sponsored multicenter study been initiated to answer some of the critical question associated with this procedure.[40]

With so many donor and recipient factors associated with the performance of ALDLT remaining undefined, ethical justification for the expansion of living donor liver transplantation to include adult recipients has been difficult at best. Clearly there is a need to perform more life-saving liver transplants. The waiting time for liver transplantation is continuing to increase as are the numbers of patients added to the list and the number of patients removed from the list because they died or were too sick to transplant. These recipients' needs do not, in themselves, justify the use of the living donor. In many ways the desperate situation in adult liver transplantation differs from living donor kidney and living donor pediatric liver transplant: (1) there is a supply of deceased donor grafts; (2) the allocation system for deceased donor liver transplantation favors the sickest patients (those with the highest mortality risk) first; (3) the dramatic improvements obtained in both patient and graft survival with living donor kidney and living donor pediatric liver transplantation are not readily apparent; (4) donor mortality and morbidity risk is greater with resection of a right or extended-right lobe; (5) a greater level of technical skill and institutional support is required to protect both recipients and donors.

The broad application of the ALDLT has failed to satisfactorily address the concept of double equipoise. The balancing of recipient benefits and risks with those of donor benefits and risks is difficult when the risks and benefits are being defined with the simultaneous execution of the procedure. Many of the complications experienced in both donors and recipients were a consequence of technical errors and a steep learning curve. Use of the living donor for a variety of recipient indications failed to define the most appropriate use and therefore failed to optimize the recipient benefit. Many other unknowns such as the minimal surgical skill required in performing the donor and recipient operations, institutional strength and capacity, how much hepatic mass is required for the recipient and how much is required to remain in the donor, and the long-term outcomes of donors and recipients are still in evolution. As such, the ability to provide sufficient information for informed consent and necessary protections for both donors and recipients is difficult.

## OTHER

With the advancement of surgical techniques, organs other than kidneys and liver lobes have been recovered from living donors for the purpose of transplantation. Fortunately, these transplants have been confined to relatively few centers that have demonstrated local expertise in the practice. Review of the UNOS database from 1988 to 2005 demonstrates a total of 28 intestinal, 70 pancreas, and 457 lung lobes have been recovered from live donors within the United States.[4] Ethical justification for many of these transplants is difficult to support at the present time for the following reasons. With respect to intestine and pancreas transplantation, the supply of life-saving deceased donor organs is not a limiting

factor as it was for the early kidney transplant and pediatric liver transplantation. Aside from some profound and unique immunologic benefit obtained from donation and transplant between identical twins, exposing the donor to the undefined short- and long-term risks of the procedure and variable recipient outcome does not appear warranted. Continued performance of such donations and transplants should be conducted under a strict research protocol. Donor safety and recipient benefit must be optimized and information gathered to provide a clear indication for the use of the living donor, the short-and long-term risks to the donors, and the appropriate recipient indications.

## SMALL INTESTINE

Isolated small bowel transplantation is a relatively infrequent procedure.[41] And although the number of candidates listed for isolated intestinal transplantation has continued to increase, the average time to transplantation has diminished.[42] In fact, despite the increase number of registrants, the mortality rate for those listed has not increased.[43] Further, registry data show no difference in graft survival or patient survival among recipients of a deceased donor or living donor small bowel transplant.[44] Therefore, use of living donors as a source for intestinal transplantation does not appear to be justified on the basis of an insufficient supply of deceased donor organs contributing to an increased death rate of patients on the waiting list or improved graft survival and patient survival in recipients of a living donor grafts.

The potential recipient benefits from a living donor small intestinal graft are obvious: decreased graft preservation time and ischemia; conversion of an urgent procedure to an elective procedure; elimination of waiting time; donor/recipient matching for graft size and human leukocyte antigen (HLA); pretransplant crossmatching; better preparation of the donor small intestinal graft; and the opportunity for immunomanipulation of the donor/recipient pair. Unfortunately, none of these potential benefits have been demonstrated to provide sufficient real benefit to offset the real risks experienced by the donor.

Donor risk associated with living donor small bowel transplantation is difficult to quantify secondary to the small number of cases performed and limited published information on donor outcomes. The risk associated with the donor evaluation is relatively minor and similar to the evaluation for living donor nephrectomy. The surgical risk should be viewed in three categories: (1) immediate risk associated with the surgical procedure; (2) risk associated with the removal of the intestine; and (3) long-term risk associated with the donation, both physical and psychological. The mortality risk associated with the surgery is probably equivalent to that associated with living donor nephrectomy, 0.03%. The potential morbidity (anastomotic breakdown or leak, enterocutaneous fistula, vascular trauma, wound infection, urinary tract infection, pneumonia, and incisional hernia) is similar to that of other healthy patients undergoing a small bowel resection. Except, this resection is performed to benefit the recipient and not the donor.

The risk associated with removal of the intestine is not trivial and can be serious. Living donor intestinal segments are based on a vascular pedicle and include a significant length of ileum. The actual length of the segment removed is dependent on the vascular arcade and the recipient's needs. Consequently, the potential morbidity experienced by the donor is variable. Depending on the length of intestinal segment removed, almost all donors experience diarrhea and fluid and electrolyte abnormalities, which require antimotility agents until intestinal adaptation occurs, which has been reported to take up to 2 years. Secondary to the removal of ileum, many donors are at risk for or develop weight loss and altered absorption of vitamin $B_{12}$. More serious complications include short bowel syndrome and the possible need for small bowel transplant in the donor.

Long-term risks include the development of adhesions in nearly all patients with the potential for bowel obstruction which may require further abdominal surgery, possible bowel resection, and an associated mortality risk of approximately 3%.[45–47]

The performance of living donor small bowel transplantation should be classified as experimental and only conducted under an IRB-approved protocol and in a fashion similar to that used for the introduction of PLDLT. There is insufficient data to adequately inform the donor about risk, and there is insufficient demonstration of benefit derived by the recipient of such a procedure. Further, the small numbers of deceased donor transplants performed, the continuous improvement in both graft and patient survival after transplant, and the wide variability in outcomes based on center volume further support the close regulation and oversight of this operation.[48]

## PANCREAS

Improvements in surgical techniques and immunosuppression protocols have contributed to the dramatic improvements in both graft and patient survival with simultaneous kidney–pancreas transplant and pancreas-after-kidney transplant in just 2 decades.[49,50] The earliest report using the living donor for pancreas transplantation occurred in 1980.[51] Since that time the operation has been expanded in magnitude from *just* a living donor pancreas to now include simultaneous kidney and pancreas transplantation from the same living donor and recently simultaneous kidney–pancreas transplantation using a living donor across a positive cross match.[52–54] Although donor mortality risk does not appear as high as that observed with living liver donation, the surgical morbidity is significant and the recipient benefit may be diminished by a technically more rigorous surgery which provides a smaller islet cell mass than standard deceased donor pancreas grafts. Despite an extensive and expanding donor evaluation, the incidence of morbidity is high.[54] The occurrence of general operative complications (splenectomy as high as 15%, pancreatitis, pseudocyst and fistula formation, intra-abdominal infection, and abscess and glucose dysregulation) may tip the balance against widespread utilization of living donor pancreas transplantation. Finally, because of the lack of regenerative ability of the pancreas and the increased risk of developing diabetes mellitus with age, donors should be followed for life. Currently, extensive donor follow-up is difficult and often not reimbursed under the current protocols. Donors themselves may be inconvenienced or not willing to submit to long-term follow-up especially if the recipient outcome is less than optimal.

Under specified conditions (genetically identical donor/recipient pair) use of the living donor may be acceptable. Additionally, if the surgical resection using laparoscopic techniques can safely deliver a segmental graft which does not expose the donor to insulin-deficient diabetes while providing a sufficient beta cell mass for successful islet transplantation, then the balance may tip in favor of a more widespread use of the living donor.[55]

## BEYOND LIVING *RELATED* DONORS

With current immunosuppression, the requirement for genetic identity between donor/recipient pair is no longer a prerequisite for successful transplantation. Immunological acceptable donors must only be blood-type compatible and cross-match negative. Even this requirement is being challenged.[56,57] Consequently, the *relatedness* of the donor/recipient pair has expanded to include: nonidentical family members, emotionally related donors, solicited donors, and directed and nondirected stranger donors. Although the donor risks associated with living donation are not different among the different types of recipient/donor relationships, donor benefit derived from such relationships likely is different.[58]

Emotionally related donors comprise individuals who have an intimate relationship with the intended recipient. These donors are usually a spouse, close friend, or significant other. The closeness of the relationship is readily apparent, and emotionally related donors are an increasing source of living donor organs.[59]

In situations where an acceptable living donation is prohibited due to blood-type incompatibility or a positive cross-match, a further extension of the living donor-to-recipient relationship has been undertaken: various forms of exchange programs.[60–62] Donor exchange programs seek to match donor/recipient pairs who have an incompatible blood type or cross-match with a complimentary donor/recipient pair in a similar situation. The donors and recipients of each pair are compatible across the pair. Due to the complexity of these exchanges and the large number of pairs required to realize meaningful benefit, many individual programs have combined within and across UNOS regions to improve the statistical likelihood of a successful exchange.

Historically, stranger or altruistic living donors have been deemed unacceptable based on poorly defined psychological grounds. Due to the increasing need for more donor organs, a few centers have begun to evaluate and accept stranger donors as a source of living donor organs.[62–64] These programs have subjected the potential donor to an extensive psychological evaluation before acceptance. Despite the high level of attrition among the potential donors, the increased utilization of program resources required for evaluation and the increased expense in running such a program, there appear to be individuals who sincerely and sanely wish to provide a charitable gift to their fellow man in the form of altruistic organ donation. Under current protocols, this process appears to be ethically justified and medically sound.[63] In fact, once psychiatric pathology has been excluded, these living donors potentially represent the only group of living donors among whom informed consent can be given freely, without exploitation or coercion.

Solicitation of living donors is not new in the field of organ transplantation. Prior to the passage of NOTA which resulted in a more organized distribution system for deceased donor organs, solicitation for living and deceased donor organs occurred in the media.[65] Recently, donor solicitation has become more organized and sophisticated with both donors and recipients aggressively defending the practice.

The current practice of donor solicitation is ethically troubling.[66,67] Defense of solicitation for both deceased donors and living donors has been justified as recipients taking their need for an organ into their own control and respect for donor autonomy. Although directed donation of deceased donor organs is legal,[68] advertising on billboards, in newspapers, and on the Internet can derail the current allocation scheme.[69] UNOS has matured into a system that fairly assigns a scarce resource, deceased donor organs, on the basis of medical need. When potential recipients seek to undermine the system for self-interest, organs become allocated for reasons other than medical benefit jeopardizing the justice and fairness of the system. It is unfortunate that organs are not readily available for all in need, but the practice of "cutting the line" should be discouraged if not prohibited.

Solicitation for living donors has matured into a well-organized and web-based enterprise. The most noteworthy is matchingdonors.com. This site allows recipients to post their needs and stories for potential donors to review and decide whether they might be willing donors. The potential problems with these sites are many. Web-based postings of patients in need and donors willing to donate do not provide equal access for all patients on the waiting list. The process is not transparent and is open for potential exploitation of donor and recipient alike. Claims that potential donors are well meaning and have good intentions and therefore should be allowed to donate are weakened when one realizes that their altruism can be implemented immediately by donating to the transplant waiting list at many transplant programs across the United States. They can volunteer to be a living organ donor in almost every region of the United States and donate to a program's waiting list or to the national waiting list. Their desire to "survey" the candidate pool and pick the individual who is worthy of their donation is suspect.

Financial incentives for organ donation both deceased and living are currently illegal.[5] However, reimbursement of donation-related expenses is being seriously considered as a way to eliminate financial disincentives associated with organ donation, for example, missed wages, lodging, travel expense, and compensation for pain and suffering associated with the donation process.[70] Additionally, many have argued that the living donor and their next-of-kin should be financially protected from the risk of organ donation by provision of term-life and disability insurance policies in case of death or serious complication arising from the donation process.

Ethical justification supporting the use of living donation rests heavily on the donor benefit derived from such a donation. As the relatedness of the donor/recipient pair become more extended and different, one of the basic tenets that justified the use of living donors, psychological benefit of the donor secondary to helping or saving the life of a loved one, becomes more difficult to

identify. Although the act and process of living organ donation is ethically justifiable and the numbers of living donors continue to increase, caution should be exercised as the transplant community and society expand the inclusion of individuals whose desires to donate and potential benefits derived from donation are different from the voluntary, altruistic basis on which living donation has been accepted.

## CONCLUSION

In little over 50 years, solid organ transplantation has become the preferred therapy for many forms of end organ failure. With improvements in immunosuppressive drugs, general medical care, and management of comorbid conditions, both graft and patient survival continue to lengthen. Consequently, the number of candidates added to the transplant list continues to increase. Unfortunately, the increased need for transplantation has not been paralleled by an equivalent increase in the number of organ donors resulting in patients dying without the opportunity for transplantation. Increases in the numbers of deceased donor organs have been modest, but the gains have occurred with use of expanded donor organs. Consequently, living donors have been used more frequently and supply organs other than kidneys for transplantation. In addition to expanding the number and type of organs used from living donors, the donor/recipient relationships have also expanded.

As expansion of the living donor continues, the double equipoise of the transplant which has always been implicit must now be explicit.[71] Merely extending the ethical arguments used to support the initial and current use of living kidney donors are probably not valid when applied to the current indications, relationships, organs used, and associated risks of donation (Table 3.1-1). Thus, the current system established to define the minimum criteria for allocation of deceased donor organs, certification and credentialing of institutions, and physicians performing deceased donor transplantation must now address the practice of living donation.

**TABLE 3.1-1**

**ETHICAL ACCEPTABILITY OF TRANSPLANT: THE BALANCE BETWEEN THE RISK (DONOR RISK) AND BENEFIT (POTENTIAL BENEFIT TO DONOR AND RECIPIENT) OF LIVING DONATION**

| Organ Donated | Recipient and Donor Relationship | | | | | |
|---|---|---|---|---|---|---|
| | G I | G R | E R | A D | S D | P D |
| Kidney—open nephrectomy | +* | + | + | + | ? | – |
| Kidney—laparoscopic nephrectomy | + | + | + | + | ? | – |
| Liver—left lateral segment | + | + | + | + | ? | – |
| Liver—right lobe | + | +/– | +/– | +/– | – | – |
| Liver—extended right lobe | + | +/– | +/– | +/– | – | – |
| Pancreas—segment | + | – | – | – | – | – |
| Pancreas—islets | + | – | – | – | – | – |
| Small intestine segment | + | – | – | – | – | – |

*Cells with a (+) have demonstrated recipient and donor benefit to balance the mortality/morbidity risk of the donation. Genetically identical donor/recipient pairs benefit from the availability of an organ and the added benefit of avoiding rejection without exposure to immunosuppressive drugs. Genetically related and emotionally related pairs share similar benefits of organ availability and use of a living donor (+). However, with increasing donor risk and unproven recipient benefits, the use of the living donor is more difficult to justify (+/–) or not appropriate (–). Use of solicited donors presents the transplant community with a potential donor benefit that is currently undefined (?).

GI: genetically identical, GR: genetically related, ER: emotionally related, AD: altruistic [stranger] donor, SD: solicited donor, PD: paid donor.

Many living donors decide to become donors before they present to the transplant center. Although the public sees living donation as possible therapy and assumes that if such a therapy is offered then it must be safe, acceptable, and ethically sound, it does not accept the most devastating complications associated with the practice. The practice of living donation must ensure donor safety and appropriate recipient outcomes as the practice extends to other organs and a variety of donor/recipient relationships. Despite the warning for greater self-regulation of the practice within the profession,[72] the potential for significant donor risk, and the devastating impact that a donor death can have on the transplant community, the New York State Department of Health defined the minimal criteria needed to undertake ALDLT in their state. Recently, OPTN/UNOS has begun a process to certify programs performing both kidney and liver living donor transplants.[7,8,67]

Although a formalized approach to help protect all parties and justify the ever-changing use of the living donor is warranted, in the last analysis, the decision must be between the surgeon and the living donor, and between them alone.[12]

## References

1. Current U.S. Waiting List Overall by Organ Based on OPTN data as of January 13, 2006.
2. U.S. Transplants Performed : January 1, 1988–October 31, 2005. Based on OPTN data as of January 13, 2006.
3. Removed from the Waiting List : January, 1995–October 31, 2005. Based on OPTN data as of January 13, 2006.
4. Donors Recovered in the U.S. by Donor Type January 1, 1988–October 31, 2005. Based on OPTN data as of January 20, 2006.
5. National Organ Transplant Act: Public Law 98-507. US Statut Large 1984;98:2339-48.
5a. Sokohl, K. keeping living donors safe. Living donor committee focuses on standardization. UNOS update. July-August 2007: 5.
6. UNOS Policy 1.0 Members Rights and Obligations. Accessed February, 2006.
7. Living liver donor evaluation and guidelines. Accessed February 2006
8. Living kidney donor evaluation guidelines.
9 http://www.health.state.ny.us/nysdoh/liver_donation/pgf/liver_donor_report_print.pdf. New York State Committee on Quality Improvement in Living Liver Donation. In: A Report to: New York State Transplant Council and New York State Department of Health; 2002.
10. Federal Register. In: 2006:3519–3520.
11. Moore F. Transplant. *The Give and Take of Tissue Transplantation*. New York: Simon and Schuster; 1972.
12. Starzl TE. Will live organ donations no longer be justified? *Hastings Cent Rep* 1985;15(2):5.
13. Burdelski M, Nolkemper D, Ganschow R, et al. Liver transplantation in children: Long-term outcome and quality of life. *Eur J Pediatr* 1999;158 Suppl 2:S34-42.
14. Amersi F, Farmer DG, Busuttil RW. Fifteen-year experience with adult and pediatric liver transplantation at the University of California, Los Angeles. *Clin Transpl* 1998:255–261.
15. Emond JC, Whitington PF, Thistlethwaite JR, Alonso EM, Broelsch CE. Reduced-size orthotopic liver transplantation: Use in the management of children with chronic liver disease. *Hepatology* 1989;10(5):867–872.
16. Bismuth H, Houssin D. Reduced-sized orthotopic liver graft in hepatic transplantation in children. *Surgery* 1984;95(3):367–370.
17. Broelsch CE, Emond JC, Thistlethwaite JR, Rouch DA, Whitington PF, Lichtor JL. Liver transplantation with reduced-size donor organs. *Transplantation* 1988;45(3):519–524.
18. Broelsch CE, Emond JC, Thistlethwaite JR, et al. Liver transplantation, including the concept of reduced-size liver transplants in children. *Ann Surg* 1988;208(4):410–420.

19. Raia S, Nery JR, Mies S. Liver transplantation from live donors. *Lancet* 1989;2(8661):497.
20. Strong RW, Lynch SV, Ong TH, Matsunami H, Koido Y, Balderson GA. Successful liver transplantation from a living donor to her son. *N Engl J Med* 1990;322(21):1505–1507.
21. Singer PA, Siegler M, Whitington PF, et al. Ethics of liver transplantation with living donors. *N Engl J Med* 1989;321(9):620–622.
22. Broelsch CE, Whitington PF, Emond JC, et al. Liver transplantation in children from living related donors. Surgical techniques and results. *Ann Surg* 1991;214(4):428–437.
23. Millis JM, Cronin DC, Brady LM, et al. Primary living-donor liver transplantation at the University of Chicago: technical aspects of the first 104 recipients. *Ann Surg* 2000;232(1):104–111.
24. Millis JM, Alonso EM, Piper JB, et al. Liver transplantation at the University of Chicago. *Clin Transpl* 1995:187–197.
25. Mori K, Nagata I, Yamagata S, et al. The introduction of microvascular surgery to hepatic artery reconstruction in living-donor liver transplantation—Its surgical advantages compared with conventional procedures. Transplantation 1992;54(2):263–268.
26. Furuta S, Ikegami T, Nakazawa Y, et al. Hepatic artery reconstruction in living donor liver transplantation from the microsurgeon's point of view. *Liver Transpl Surg* 1997;3(4):388–393.
27. Tanaka K, Uemoto S, Inomata Y, et al. Living-related liver transplantation for fulminant hepatic failure in children. *Transpl Int* 1994;7 Suppl 1:S108–S110.
28. Tanaka K, Uemoto S, Tokunaga Y, et al. Living related liver transplantation in children. *Am J Surg* 1994;168(1):41–48.
29. Hashimoto T, Suzuki T, Shimizu Y, et al. ABO-incompatible living related liver transplantation for fulminant hepatitis: Report of a successful pediatric case with long-term follow-up. *Transplant Proc* 1998;30(7):3510–3512.
30. Grewal HP, Thistlewaite JR, Jr., Loss GE, et al. Complications in 100 living-liver donors. *Ann Surg* 1998;228(2):214–219.
31. Yamaoka Y, Morimoto T, Inamoto T, et al. Safety of the donor in living-related liver transplantation—An analysis of 100 parental donors. *Transplantation* 1995;59(2):224–226.
32. Piper JB, Whitington PF, Woodle ES, et al. Pediatric liver transplantation at the University of Chicago Hospitals. *Clin Transpl* 1992:179–189.
33. Lo CM, Fan ST, Liu CL, et al. Adult-to-adult living donor liver transplantation using extended right lobe grafts. *Ann Surg* 1997;226(3):261–269.
34. Wachs ME, Bak TE, Karrer FM, et al. Adult living donor liver transplantation using a right hepatic lobe. *Transplantation* 1998;66(10):1313–1316.
35. Testa G, Malago M, Broelsch CE. Living-donor liver transplantation in adults. *Langenbecks Arch Surg* 1999;384(6):536–543.
36. Marcos A, Fisher RA, Ham JM, et al. Right lobe living donor liver transplantation. *Transplantation* 1999;68(6):798–803.
37. Pomfret EA, Pomposelli JJ, Lewis WD, et al. Live donor adult liver transplantation using right lobe grafts: donor evaluation and surgical outcome. *Arch Surg* 2001;136(4):425–433.
38. Brown RS, Jr., Russo MW, Lai M, et al. A survey of liver transplantation from living adult donors in the United States. *N Engl J Med* 2003;348(9):818–825.
39. Lo CM. Complications and long-term outcome of living liver donors: A survey of 1,508 cases in five Asian centers. Transplantation 2003;75(3 Suppl):S12–S15.
40. Adult to Adult Living Donor Liver Transplant Cohort Study (A2ALL). 2002.Published February 2006.
41. Table 10.4 Transplant Recipient Characteristics, 1995 to 2004 Intestine Recipients. OPTN/SRTR Annual Report, 2005. Published
42. Table 10.2 Time to Transplant, 1995 to 2004 New Intestine Waiting List Registrations. OPTN/SRTR Annual Report, 2005.
43. Table 10.3 Reported Deaths and Annual Death Rates Per 1,000 Patient-Years at Risk, 1995 to 2004 Intestine Waiting List. OPTN/SRTR Annual Report. Published 2005.
44. http://www.intestinaltransplant.org. The Intestinal Transplant Registry. Published 2003.

45. Bickell NA, Federman AD, Aufses JAH. Influence of Time on Risk of Bowel Resection in Complete Small Bowel Obstruction. *J Am College Surg* 2005;201(6):847–854.

46. Menzies D, Ellis H. Intestinal obstruction from adhesions—How big is the problem? *Ann R Coll Surg Engl* 1990;72(1):60–63.

47. Miller G, Boman J, Shrier I, Gordon PH. Etiology of small bowel obstruction. *Am J Surg* 2000;180(1):33–36.

48. Table 10.9 Unadjusted Graft Survival, Intestine Transplants Survival at 3 Months, 1 Year, 3 Years, and 5 Years. OPTN/SRTR Annual Report. Published 2005.

49. Demartines N, Schiesser M, Clavien PA. An evidence-based analysis of simultaneous pancreas-kidney and pancreas transplantation alone. *Am J Transplant* 2005;5(11):2688–2697.

50. Gruessner AC, Sutherland DE. Pancreas transplant outcomes for United States (US) and non-US cases as reported to the United Network for Organ Sharing (UNOS) and the International Pancreas Transplant Registry (IPTR) as of June 2004. *Clin Transplant* 2005;19(4):433–455.

51. Sutherland DE, Goetz FC, Najarian JS. Living-related donor segmental pancreatectomy for transplantation. *Transplant Proc* 1980;12(4 Suppl 2):19–25.

52. Benedetti E, Rastellini C, Sileri P, et al. Successful simultaneous pancreas-kidney transplantation from well-matched living-related donors. *Transplant Proc* 2001;33(1–2):1689.

53. Gruessner RW, Kandaswamy R, Denny R. Laparoscopic simultaneous nephrectomy and distal pancreatectomy from a live donor. *J Am Coll Surg* 2001;193(3):333–337.

54. Gruessner RW, Kendall DM, Drangstveit MB, Gruessner AC, Sutherland DE. Simultaneous pancreas-kidney transplantation from live donors. *Ann Surg* 1997;226(4):471–480 discussion 80-2.

55. Matsumoto S, Okitsu T, Iwanaga Y, et al. Insulin independence after living-donor distal pancreatectomy and islet allotransplantation. *Lancet* 2005;365(9471):1642–1644.

56. Warren DS, Zachary AA, Sonnenday CJ, et al. Successful renal transplantation across simultaneous ABO incompatible and positive cross-match barriers. *Am J Transplant* 2004;4(4):561–568.

57. Usuda M, Fujimori K, Koyamada N, et al. Successful use of anti-CD20 monoclonal antibody (rituximab) for ABO-incompatible living-related liver transplantation. *Transplantation* 2005;79(1):12–16.

58. Glannon W, Ross LF. Do genetic relationships create moral obligations in organ transplantation? *Camb Q Health Ethics* 2002;11(2):153–159.

59. Ross LF, Glannon W, Josephson MA, Thistlethwaite JR, Jr. Should all living donors be treated equally? *Transplantation* 2002;74(3):418–421; discussion 21-2.

60. Ross LF, Rubin DT, Siegler M, Josephson MA, Thistlethwaite JR, Jr., Woodle ES. Ethics of a paired-kidney-exchange program. *N Engl J Med* 1997;336(24):1752–1755.

61. Delmonico FL, Morrissey PE, Lipkowitz GS, et al. Donor kidney exchanges. *Am J Transplant* 2004;4(10):1628–1634.

62. Gilbert JC, Brigham L, Batty DS, Jr., Veatch RM. The nondirected living donor program: A model for cooperative donation, recovery and allocation of living donor kidneys. *Am J Transplant* 2005;5(1):167–174.

63. Adams PL, Cohen DJ, Danovitch GM, et al. The nondirected live-kidney donor: Ethical considerations and practice guidelines: A National Conference Report. *Transplantation* 2002;74(4):582–589.

64. Jacobs CL, Roman D, Garvey C, Kahn J, Matas AJ. Twenty-two nondirected kidney donors: an update on a single center's experience. *Am J Transplant* 2004;4(7):1110–1116.

65. Ross LF. Media appeals for directed altruistic living liver donations: Lessons from Camilo Sandoval Ewen. *Perspect Biol Med* 2002;45(3):329–337.

66. Steinbrook R. Public solicitation of organ donors. *N Engl J Med* 2005;353(5):441–444.

67. Delmonico FL, Graham WK. Direction of the Organ Procurement and Transplantation Network and United Network for Organ Sharing regarding the oversight of live donor transplantation and solicitation for organs. *Am J Transplant* 2006;6(1):37–40.

68. Undis DJ. LifeShares: Increasing organ supply through directed donation. *Am J Bioeth* 2005;5(4):22–24.

69. Appel JM, Fox MD. Organ solicitation on the Internet: every man for himself? *Hastings Cent Rep* 2005;35(3):14; discussion -5.

70. Delmonico FL, Arnold R, Scheper-Hughes N, Siminoff LA, Kahn J, Youngner SJ. Ethical incentives—not payment—for organ donation. *N Engl J Med* 2002;346(25):2002–2005.

71. Siegler M, Simmerling MC, Siegler JH, Cronin DC, 2nd ed. Recipient deaths during donor surgery: A new ethical problem in living donor liver transplantation (LDLT). *Liver Transpl* 2006;12(3):358–360.

72. Cronin DC, 2nd, Millis JM, Siegler M. Transplantation of liver grafts from living donors into adults—Too much, too soon. *N Engl J Med* 2001;344(21):1633–1637.

## 3.2    THE ASIAN PERSPECTIVE

### 3.2.1   East Asia

*Tetsuya Kiuchi, MD, PhD, Hideya Kamei, MD*

### INTRODUCTION

Details of medical practice in Asia are often outside of the information network in the English literature. Asia is known as an area where deceased donor (DD) organ transplantation is only poorly developed, yet the use of compensated living donor (LD) organs has evolved more rapidly than in Western countries. Furthermore, the longtime rumors of an organ trade or of organ retrieval from executed prisoners in limited areas of Asia have fueled skepticism about the ethical and psychosocial background, of the entire field of transplantation in Asia.

Collecting official transplant statistics in Asian countries is often difficult, given the frequent absence of registries. The ethical and psychosocial situation is even more difficult to analyze in terms of numerical data. In addition to our personal communications with transplant surgeons and physicians in East Asia, we herein describe the results of a questionnaire on LD liver transplants that we sent in April 2004 to 45 programs (44 hospitals) in Japan and to 23 programs in other East Asian areas (11 in mainland China, 1 in Hong Kong, 4 in Taiwan, and 7 in South Korea). The response rate was 100% for programs in Japan and 74% for other East Asian areas.

### STATISTICAL RESULTS

Table 3.2.1-1 shows the number of kidney and liver transplants in East Asia in 2003, with data from the United Network for Organ Sharing (UNOS) for comparison. Significant variations exist among East Asian countries. Proportionally, DD transplants are more commonly done in Hong Kong and Taiwan, as compared with other East Asian areas. In Japan, 96% of deceased DD kidneys are from controlled non-heart-beating donors. It is now well known that the vast majority of "DDs" in Mainland China are executed prisoners. Every year, a significant number of patients from Hong King and Taiwan visit Mainland China seeking a transplant; patients also come from Japan and South Korea. Professional brokers mediate such trips, in many cases. The organ transplantation law permitting organ retrieval from brain-dead donors—put into force in 1997 in Japan and in 2000 in South Korea—did not strongly stimulate DD transplants in either of these countries.

Regarding LD organ transplants, Japan performs the highest (absolute) number of both LD kidney and LD liver transplants in East Asia. However, the number per capita is higher in Hong Kong and South Korea. About three times more LD kidney transplants are done in South Korea than in Japan. The number of LD

**TABLE 3.2.1-1**

**NUMBER OF KIDNEY AND LIVER TRANSPLANTS BY DONOR SOURCE, IN EAST ASIA (2003)**

| Country or area | Mainland | Hong Kong China | Taiwan | South Korea | Japan | USA |
|---|---|---|---|---|---|---|
| Kidney transplants | | | | | | |
| DD* | 5470 | 44[†] | 164 | 124 | 138 | 8665 |
| (PMP)[b] | (4.2) | (6.8) | (7.3) | (2.6) | (1.1) | (29.8) |
| LD | 80 | 6 | 44 | 684 | 721 | 6468 |
| (PMP) | (0.06) | (0.9) | (1.9) | (14.2) | (5.6) | (22.2) |
| LD rate | 1.4% | 11.8% | 20.7% | 84.5% | 83.6% | 42.7% |
| | | | | | | |
| Liver transplants | | | | | | |
| DD | 1210[§] | 19 | 65 | 50 | 2 | 5350 |
| (PMP) | (0.9) | (2.8) | (2.9) | (1.0) | (0.02) | (18.3) |
| LD | 30 | 36 | 79 | 364 | 437[d] | 321 |
| (PMP) | (0.02) | (5.3) | (3.5) | (7.6) | (3.4) | (1.1) |
| LD rate | 2.2% | 65.4% | 54.7% | 88.4% | 99.4% | 5.7% |

*DD = deceased donor, LD = living donor
[†]decreased in 2003 due to SARS
[b]per million population
[§]increased twice in 2004
[d]increased by 25% to 30% in 2004

organ transplants is slowly increasing in Mainland China, which is still the least active LD transplant country in East Asia. It is notable that the number of LD kidney transplants per capita is much less in East Asia than in the United States.

In contrast, the number of LD liver transplants is extremely high in all East Asian countries except Mainland China. Liver transplant centers in East Asia outside Japan ($n = 17$) performed a total of 1,401 liver transplants in 2003 (1 to 500 transplants per center, median 50 transplants per center); of those, 447 were LD liver transplants (0 to 152 transplants per center, median 10 transplants per center). The cumulative number of LD liver transplants performed at these 17 centers was 1,927 transplants by the end of 2003 (1 to 673 transplants per center, median 40 transplants per center). In Japan, 437 liver transplants were reported in 2003 by 45 centers (0 to 95 transplants per center, median 4 transplants per center); of those, 435 were LD liver transplants (0 to 94 transplants per center, median 4 transplants per center). The cumulative number of LD liver transplants performed at those 45 centers was 2,667 by the end of 2003 (3 to 970 transplants per center, median 16 transplants per center).

The number of both LD and DD pancreas, islet, and small bowel transplants in East Asia remains very limited.

## ATTITUDE TOWARD LIVING DONOR ORGAN TRANSPLANTS

The most critical reason for the use of LDs in East Asia is the extreme scarcity of DD organs. Figure 3.2.1-1 summarizes some of the obstacles to DD organ transplants in East Asia.

In Japan and some other East Asian countries, the major obstacles to the use of DDs are "organizational problems" and "social indifference." This might be a surprising statement to some readers outside of Asia, but religion is not a key obstacle to DD organ transplants in East Asia. Buddhism and Shintoism (specific to Japan) are the leading religions in East Asia, followed by the minority religions Christianity and Islam. In parallel, Confucianism is a principle affecting the philosophy of most East Asians, although it is not a religion. The basic doctrines of all of these religions/philosophies are not against altruism or postmortem use of a part of the body for others. However, interpretation of the doctrines often varies by area; for example,

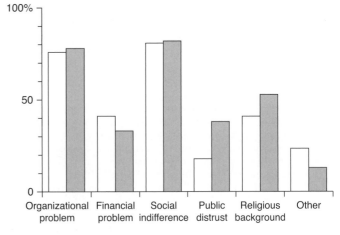

**FIGURE 3.2.1-1**

Obstacles to DD transplants in East Asia per April 2004 questionnaire. Multiple answers from 17 programs outside Japan (open column) and 45 programs in Japan (closed column) are shown. "Other" obstacles included cultural background, traditional ideas (outside Japan), government policy, indifference of medical personnel, family structure, culture to protect corpus, negative media coverage, and health insurance issues (in Japan).

some Buddhist temples in Japan object to the concept of brain death, in contrast to the attitude of the Catholic Church. Nonetheless, such religious restrictions are not strong among the young generation in Japan, although vague objections might spread even among those having no definite religion. In our April 2004 questionnaire, 43% of respondents in Japan and 65% of those in other East Asian countries said that their country's religious or cultural background helped create a positive attitude toward LD transplants.

Twice as many respondents in Japan as in other East Asian countries regarded "public distrust for medicine" as a significant obstacle to DD transplants—despite the increase in LD transplants. This paradoxical response seems to be based not only on personal experience but also, at least partly, on the negative impact of media coverage. The morbid details of the coverage of the first brain-dead donor organ transplant in Japan in 1998[2] sparked a debate on everything from journalistic ethics to medical transparency. Around the enactment of the Organ Transplant Law in 1997, the Japanese media introduced many negative campaigns against DD transplants.[3] The negative role of the media is also significant in other areas in East Asia.

## REGULATIONS AND TRENDS IN LIVING DONOR SELECTION

In East Asia, any organ trade or business seems to be extremely rare. The basic concept of pure altruism or voluntarism, without monetary or property reimbursement to LDs, is the ideal that is strived for. Of course, it is difficult to exclude motives of a sense of mission as a family member or some expectation of a nonmaterial exchange.

Legal regulations specific to LD selection do not exist in Japan, except for the law about physicians' practice in general. However, according to our questionnaire, three fourths of other East Asian programs do follow some legal regulations; perhaps they interpreted the term differently (Figure 3.2.1-2). The authority in Japan is primarily the relevant academic society, such as the local Transplantation Society or Liver Transplantation Society, whose guidelines are followed by the majority. But the regulatory role of such organizations, if any, seems to be low in other East Asian countries. In addition, at least 60% to 80% of programs have an institutional review board or an ethics committee regulating their practice.

All five areas (Japan, Mainland China, Hong Kong, Taiwan, South Korea) represented in our questionnaire have incomplete public insurance systems for LD transplants. The overall practice itself of LD transplants is not deeply affected by the lack or incompleteness of the insurance system. Yes, 60% of the programs in Japan and 57% of the programs in other countries said yes when asked if they had ever had a patient or a donor give up on a prospective LD liver transplant for economic reasons—clearly suggesting that better insurance coverage might make a difference. Our questionnaire also found that about half of the programs attach importance to self-regulation by the surgeon or physician.

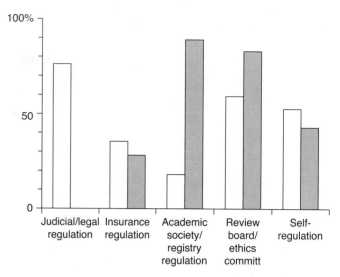

**FIGURE 3.2.1-2**

Factors regulating liver recipient and LD selection in East Asia, per April 2004 questionnaire. Multiple answers from 17 programs outside Japan (open column) and 45 programs in Japan (closed column) are shown.

Figure 3.2.1-3 shows the acceptable genetic or social relationship of potential LDs in liver programs in East Asia. In Japan, the acceptability of donor candidates clearly decreases in proportion to increased genetic or social distance. Programs in other East Asian areas generally accept a wider range of genetic or social relationships, including friends, lovers, and even Good Samaritans. In stark contrast to the United States, the acceptance of "nondirected living liver donation" has not yet been reported to the Japanese Registry.[4] Exchange (direct-swap or swap-around) and relay LD programs have achieved a success in some kidney programs in South Korea, but not in other East Asian areas.[5, 6]

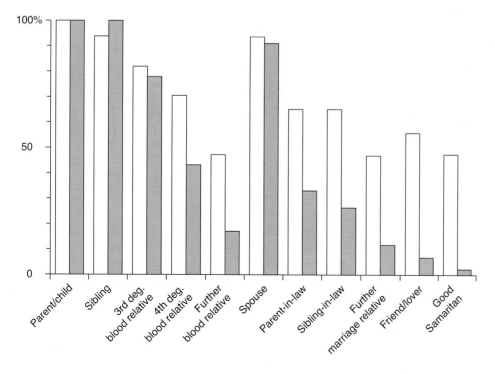

**FIGURE 3.2.1-3**

Acceptable genetic or social relationships between LD candidates and liver recipients in East Asia, per April 2004 questionnaire. Multiple answers from 17 programs outside Japan (open column) and 45 programs in Japan (closed column) are shown.

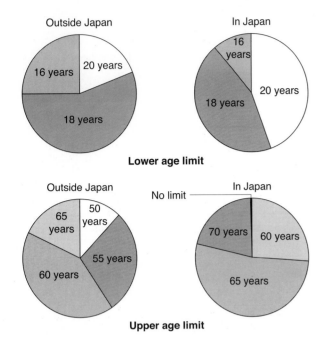

**FIGURE 3.2.1-4**

Acceptable age limit, both lower and upper, of LD candidates in liver programs in East Asia, per April 2004 questionnaire.

Figure 3.2.1-4 shows the acceptable age limit of potential LDs in liver programs in East Asia. The legal definition of an adult may differ by cultural background and by purpose (such as marriage, suffrage, property). The lower age limit for having an independent right to donate organs varies from 16 to 20 years old. In Japan, the acceptable age also varies by program, with liver programs more restrictive in their lower age limit. The upper age limit may reflect the recognition of risk to patients undergoing general anesthesia or a partial liver resection. A higher upper age limit may reflect more experience or less experience on the part of the program. Japanese programs are generally more radical in the acceptable upper age limit; on our questionnaire, many programs in Japan said that acceptance is not determined by age. We observed no relationship between acceptable LD age and program volume.

## LIVING DONOR ADVOCACY

A key concern is whether and how transplant programs try to protect LD candidates from coercion or interaction with their potential recipient and from psychosocial complications after donation. Our questionnaire found that only 59% of the LD liver programs in Japan and only 47% in other East Asian programs have an "independent" LD advocate, despite the New York State Committee guideline 1. The question of whether those responsible for a potential recipient can be completely neutral when evaluating the psychosocial and medical suitability of a potential LD is quite controversial. Not a few respondents seem to believe that their responsibility for the potential recipient does not interfere with their neutrality when they evaluate a potential LD.

Figure 3.2.1-5 shows the composition of the "independent" LD advocate teams in the liver programs in East Asia that have such teams. In Japan, the trend is to depend more on the physician and psychiatrist. Other East Asian programs seem to have a wider variety of composition on their teams. The role of the social worker and the ethicist, however, seems to be relatively small. Unfortunately, we have no information on the quality of LD advocates.

When we asked whether a program would shorten the period of reflection about a donor candidate according to the urgency of the recipient's status (eg, for someone in fulminant hepatic failure), 89% of the liver programs in Japan and 76% in other East Asian areas answered yes. Although this response may not necessarily reflect the quality of the donor advocate, it shows at least one aspect of the program's attitude. When we asked whether a program has allowed donation despite a suspicion of incompetence, hidden unwillingness, coercion, or psychological unfitness, but without an objective proof, 49% of the liver programs in Japan confessed yes—as compared with 0% of the other East Asian programs. Whether this clear contrast is due to an actual quality difference or merely to sensitivity to the question is unknown.

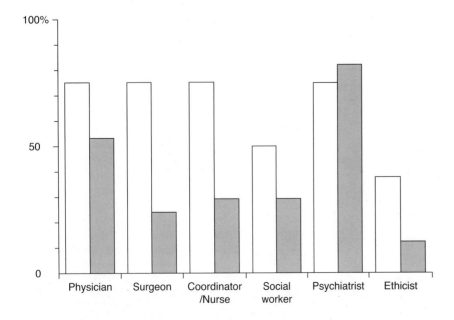

**FIGURE 3.2.1-5**

Composition of "independent" LD advocate teams in liver programs in East Asia, per April 2004 questionnaire. Multiple answers from 8 programs outside Japan (open column) and 18 programs in Japan (closed column) are shown.

## LIVING DONOR LD CARE

Removal of an organ or a part of an organ from healthy LDs for transplantation potentially bears not a few unfavorable, unanticipated sequelae. In addition to surgery-related or anesthesia-related complications in the acute phase, complications remaining or newly occurring in a distant chronic phase are within the range of the transplant program's responsibility.[7–9] The program should cover not only these physical sequelae but also any psychosocial consequences.[10–12]

Figure 3.2.1-6 shows the length of postdonation regular medical checkups and the presence of postdonation psychosocial care in liver programs in East Asia. Both in Japan and in other East Asian areas, most programs said that their scheduled follow-up ends within 6 to 12 months after the transplant. However, 16% in Japan and 6% in other East Asian areas do request LD medical checkups for 5 years or longer. A minority of programs have established postdonation psychosocial care programs; the incidence is higher outside Japan. However, 24% of the programs in Japan and 12% in other East Asian areas said they were aware of the necessity of lifelong coverage of LDs' psychosocial complications.

Apart from established psychosocial care programs, 44% of liver programs in Japan and 82% in other East Asian countries have a surveillance system for long-term quality of life in LDs, with more such systems under preparation (27% in Japan; 6%, other). Quality is again difficult to evaluate, but the methods of surveillance consisted of any or all of the following: (1) scheduled follow-up by a psychologist or psychiatrist (10% in Japan; 43%, other); (2) regular distribution of a survey (30% and 36%); and (3) regular phone calls by a coordinator or other staff (70% and 64%). These figures are similar to a report in the United States.[14]

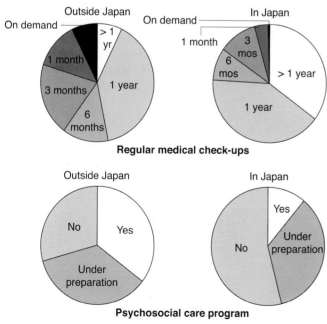

**Regular medical check-ups**

**Psychosocial care program**

**FIGURE 3.2.1-6**

Length of regular medical check-ups for LDs after donation (upper) and presence of psychosocial care program (lower) in liver programs in East Asia, per April 2004 questionnaire.

## SUMMARY

Given the extreme shortage of DD organs in East Asia, the rate of LD transplants is as high as 55% to 99% in East Asia (although the allocation system in Mainland China remains a confusing factor). Contrary to the common view outside Asia, religion is not a major factor interfering with postmortem organ donation. Instead, according to our April 2004 questionnaire results, most regard organizational problems and social indifference as the major obstacles to DD transplants. Distrust of medicine and negative media coverage also seem to discourage brain-dead organ donation in some areas of East Asia.

Despite these circumstances, as well as the suboptimal financial situation in East Asia, efforts to adhere to the ethical principles of LD transplants continue. Legal regulations, academic society guidelines, institutional review boards, and self-regulation play variable roles in East Asia. Although 85% of the LD liver programs in East Asia accept high-urgency recipients, most programs are aware of and try to reduce any psychosocial risks to LDs.

## ACKNOWLEDGMENTS

We are deeply indebted to the following institutes and contact persons who kindly responded to our questionnaire or to our inquiry.

Mainland, China: First Affiliated Hospital, Nanjing Medical University (Dr. Xuehao W), First Affiliated Hospital, Shanghai Jiaotong University (Dr. Zhihai P), First Hospital, Peking University (Drs. Long L/Liuming H), Liver Cancer Institute/ Shenzhen People Hospital (Dr. Xiaofang Y), People's Hospital, Peking University (Dr. Xisheng L), West China Hospital, Sichuan University (Dr. Lvnan Y), Xijing Hospital, Forth Military Medical University (Dr. Kefeng D), Zhongshan Hospital, Fudan University (Dr. Jia F).

Hong Kong, China: Queen Mary Hospital, Hong Kong University (Dr. Fan ST), Princess Margaret Hospital (Dr. Tong KL M).

Taiwan: Chang Gung Memorial Hospital, Kaohsiung (Dr. Chen CL), National Taiwan University (Dr. Lee PH).

South Korea: Asan Medical Center, Ulsan University (Dr. Lee SG), Catholic Medical Center, Catholic University (Dr. Kim DG), Kangdong Sacred Heart Hospital, Hallym University (Dr. Kim JS), Samsung Medical Center, SungKyunKwan University (Dr. Joh JW), Seoul National University (Drs. Suh KS/ Yi NJ/Ha J), Yonsei University (Dr. Kim SI).

Japan: Kyoto University (Dr. Takada Y), Tokyo University (Dr. Sugawara Y), Shinshu University (Dr. Hashikura Y), Kyusyu University (Dr. Soejima Y), Hokkaido University (Dr. Furukawa H), Tokyo Women's Medical University (Dr. Nakajima I), Tohoku University (Dr. Kawagishi N), Okayama University (Drs. Sadamori H/Yagi T), Keio University (Dr. Shimazu M),Nagoya City University (Dr. Hashimoto S), Jichi Medical University (Dr. Kawarazaki H), Kumamoto University (Dr. Inomata Y), Osaka University (Dr. Umeshita K), Niigata University (Dr. Satoh Y), Kanagawa Children's Medical Center (Dr. Murakami T), Hiroshima University (Dr. Ohdan H), Nagasaki University (Dr. Kabahara Y),

Kanazawa Medical University (Dr. Masuyama H), Matsunami General Hospital (Dr. Shimizu Y), Nihon University (Dr. Watanabe Y), Mie University (Dr. Mizuno S), Hyogo College of Medicine (Dr. Yamanaka J), Hirosaki University (Dr. Hakamada K), Yokohama City University (Dr. Sekido H), Gunma University (Drs. Kuwano H/Ohwada S), Tsukuba University (Dr. Fukunaga K), Osaka Medical College (Dr. Hayashi H), Fukushima Medical University (Dr. Saitoh T), Kanazawa University (Dr. Shimizu Y), Nippon Medical School (Dr. Akimaru K), Kobe University (Dr. Gu H), Chiba University (Dr. Miyauchi H), Ehime University (Drs. Nakamura T/Tohyama Y), Tokyo Medical University (Dr. Nagao T), Dokkyo University (Dr. Kubota K), Osaka City University (Dr. Hirohashi K), Kitasato University (Dr. Furuta.K), Nara Medical University (Dr. Nakajima S), Yamaguchi University (Dr. Oka M), National Okayama Medical Center (Dr. Akiyama T), Tokyo Medical and Dental University (Dr. Teramoto K), Kansai Medical University (Dr. Kaibori M), Kyoto Prefectural University of Medicine (Dr. Kaihara S), Nagoya University (Kiuchi.T).

We also deeply appreciate the excellent secretarial support of Ms. Kyoto Harada.

## References

1. Report by New York State Committee on Quality Improvement in Living Liver Donation. http://www.health.state.ny.us/nysdoh/liver_donation/pdf/liver_donor_report_web.pdf. Published December 2002.
2. Anonymous. Media coverage of first transplantation fuels public distrust Japan. *Lancet* 1999;354(July 17):229.
3. Kondo M, Nakano M, Miyazaki T, et al. *Reasons Why I Do Not Donate My Organs.* Tokyo: Yohsen-sha; 2000 (in Japanese).
4. Crowley-Matoka M, Switzer G. Non-directed living donation: A survey of current trends and practices. *Transplantation* 2005; 79:515.
5. Park K, Lee JH, Huh KH, et al. Exchange living-donor kidney transplantation: Diminution of donor organ shortage. *Transplant Proc* 2004;36:2429.
6. Park JH, Park JW, Koo YM, et al. Relay kidney transplantation in Korea: Legal, ethical and medical aspects. *Leg Med (Tokyo)* 2004;6:178.
7. Umeshita K, Fujiwara K, Kiyosawa K, et al. Operative morbidity of living liver donors in Japan. *Lancet* 2003;362(August 30):687.
8. Rizvi SA, Naqvi SA, Jawad F, et al. Living kidney donor follow-up in a dedicated clinic. *Transplantation* 2005;79:1247.
9. Beavers KL, Sandler RS, Fair JH, et al. The living donor experience: Donor health assessment and outcomes after living donor liver transplantation. *Liver Transplant* 2001;7:943.
10. Kim-Schluger L, Florman S, Schiano T, et al. Quality of life after lobectomy for adult liver transplantation. *Transplantation* 2002;73:1593.
11. Karliova M, Malago M, Valentin-Gamazo C, et al. Living-related liver transplantation from the view of the donor: a 1-year follow-up survey. *Transplantation* 2002;73:1799.
12. Walter M, Bronner E, Pascher A, et al. Psychosocial outcomes of living donors after living donor liver transplantation: a pilot study. *Clin Transplant* 2002;16:339.
13. Beavers KL, Cassara JE, Sherstha R. Practice patterns for long-term follow-up of adult-to-adult right lobectomy donors at US transplant centers. *Liver Transplant* 2003;9:645.

## 3.2.2   India

*B. Subbarao, MD, FRCS*

### INTRODUCTION

In India, a sovereign socialist secular democratic republic, the per capita income is U.S. $460 per year. Only 2.2% of the entire population (total per 2001 census, 1,028,612,328) earns above U.S. $1,000 a year; 29% lies below the poverty line, earning less than U.S. $100 a year. India is divided into various states based on the language spoken. The people elect the Indian parliament and legislative assemblies in the states once in 5 years. Subjects like defense, foreign affairs, and atomic energy come under the purview of the center; whereas health comes under both central and state governments, and any law relevant to health enacted in parliament needs to be endorsed by the state assembly with or without modification in order to make it a law. Of the total population, Hindus constitute 82%; Muslims, 12%; Christians, 2.3%; Sikhs, 2%; and others (including Buddhists, Jains, Parsis, and Jews), less than 2%. Hinduism has a large number of sects. Slightly more than 90% of Muslims are Sunni; the rest are Shi'a. The non-Hindu population is spread around the country. Large Muslim populations are found in the states of Uttar Pradesh, Bihar, Maharashtra, West Bengal, Andhra Pradesh, and Kerala; Muslims are a majority in Jammu and Kashmir. Christian populations are found in the northeastern states, as well as in the southern states of Kerala, Tamil Nadu, and Goa. Three small northeastern states have Christian majorities; Nagaland, Mizoram, and Meghalaya. The Sikhs are the majority population in the Punjab. Immigrants, primarily from Bangladesh, Sri Lanka, and Nepal, practice various religions. Health demographics in India have significantly changed over time, while remaining far below western standards (Table 3.2.2-1).

### LEGAL ISSUES

Transplantation in India began in the early 1970s, restricted mainly to teaching institutions and to well-equipped private institutions. With the introduction of cyclosporine in the 1980s, both graft and patient survival rates improved significantly, and transplantation was accepted as the best treatment for patients with end-stage renal disease (ESRD). Highly qualified clinicians in India, especially in cities like Vellore, Mumbai (formerly Bombay),

**TABLE 3.2.2-1**
### DEMOGRAPHIC CHANGES IN INDIA

| Indicator | 1951 | 1981 | 2000 |
|---|---|---|---|
| Life expectancy | 36.7 years | 54 years | 64.6 (RGI)[a] |
| Crude birth rate | 40.8% | 33.9 % (SRS) | 26.1% (SRS) |
| Crude death rate | 25% | 12.5% (SRS) | 8.7% (SRS) |
| IMR | 146 | 110 | 70 (SRS) |

[a]RGI, Registrar General of India; SRS, Sample Registration System; IMR, Infant Mortality Rate (per 1,000 births).
From NATIONAL HEALTH POLICY—2002 at http://mohfw.nic.in/np2002.htm

and Chennai (formerly Madras), made kidney transplantation successful in a short time span and lucrative for some hospitals. Given the availability of technical expertise, the lack of a clear legal framework, the lax enforcement of medical regulations, and a large impoverished and illiterate population willing to sell organs for a few hundred dollars, transplantation soon became a commercial trade. It was initially an internal Indian affair but soon trade became international, attracting customers from Southeast Asia, the Far and Middle East, Europe, Africa, and North America. In a matter of a few years, India became a kidney bazaar.[1]

Living donors (LDs) had been the only source of organs for transplantation in India before 1994. It was not legally permissible to use deceased donor (DD) organs until "The Transplantation of Human Organs Act" was passed in 1994 by the Indian parliament. The aim of the act was to curb commerce in transplantation by promoting DD transplantation, which was facilitated by accepting the concept of brain death and by laying down criteria for its diagnosis. The act became effective in February 1995 in the states of Goa, Himachal Pradesh, and Maharashtra; and in all Union Territories (Notification #S.O.80 [E]). However, some states, such as Bihar, Chattisgarh, and Jharkhand, have yet to adopt the act.

The act was stimulated by the innumerable scams involving removal of kidneys from poor people who were ill informed about the nature of surgery, for transplantation into patients who could afford to pay. The party that arranged the deal often got the best bargain in the transaction, be it a doctor, hospital staff, or a person who had donated a kidney earlier. Such scams involved almost all the regions of India. Some were sensational and rocked the Indian parliament and state assemblies.[2,3]

### The Transplantation of Human Organs Act

The act defines (1) "donor" as a person, not less than 18 years old, who voluntarily authorizes the removal of any of his or her human organs for therapeutic purposes; (2) "hospital" as a nursing home, clinic, medical center, or medical or teaching institution for therapeutic purposes; (3) "human organ" as a part of a human body consisting of a structured arrangement of tissues that, if wholly removed, cannot be replicated by the body; (4) "near relative" as a spouse, son, daughter, father, mother, brother, or sister; and (5) brainstem death by certain diagnostic criteria and procedures. The act regulates organ removal through an authorization committee; authorizes only certain hospitals to remove, store, and transplant organs through an appropriate body appointed by the state government; and empowers the government to investigate and punish people involved in the organ trade. The punishment includes 2 to 7 years of imprisonment and U.S. $250 to $500 in fines. Punishable under the act are people who (1) make or receive any payment for the supply of, or for an offer to supply, any human organ; (2) seek to find a person willing to supply for payment any human organ; (3) offer to supply any human organ for payment; (4) initiate or negotiate any arrangement involving payment for any human organ; (5) take part in the management or control of a body of persons, whether a society, firm, or company, whose activities include initiating or negotiating of any such arrangement; or (6) publish or distribute, or cause to be published or distributed, any advertisement inviting persons to supply for payment any human organ, offering to supply any human organ for payment, or indicating that the advertiser is willing to initiate or negotiate any such arrangement.

The major pitfall of the act is this provision: "no human organ removed from the body of a donor before his [or her] death shall be transplanted into a recipient unless the donor is a near relative of the recipient. If any donor authorizes the removal of any of his [or her] human organs before his [or her] death under subsection (1) of section 3 of The Transplantation of Human Organs Act, for transplantation into the body of such recipient, not being a near relative, as is specified by the donor by reason of affection or attachment towards the recipient or for any other special reasons, such human organ shall not be removed and transplanted without the prior approval of the Authorization Committee." This provision clearly put the onus on the Authorization Committee (appointed by the state government) to prove the relationship between the donor and the recipient and to ascertain true altruism, with no coercion or commerce involved. But what repeatedly occurred is that physicians, transplant surgeons, and hospitals colluded with the Authorization Committee. Many such cases have been brought to Indian courts; however, none of the offenders has been punished under the act so far, and every one of them is free on bail.

### ETHICAL ISSUES

Under the act, to give a valid consent, the donor must be competent to decide about donation. A transplant physician has the moral and legal duty to make sure that conditions favor the validity of the donor's consent, to make reasonable efforts to establish the donor's motives and reasons. In India, most transplants use living related or unrelated donors; a very small number of DD transplants have been done. We use the term *related* to mean either by blood or by marriage; *unrelated* means all other LD transplants.

Almost all unrelated donors are paid; such donors are typically uneducated, poor manual laborers, lured into the net by a middleman offering money that may amount to what they earn in a year. Unlike in developed countries, a huge difference in income between the poor and the rich exists and exploitation and coercion of poor and ill informed people is common. Donating organs for money has not improved their living standards; many studies by both international and national observers have confirmed this fact. One survey was conducted in February 2001 among 305 individuals who had sold a kidney in Chennai an average of 6 years earlier. The average amount received was U.S. $1,070, most of which was spent on debts, food, and clothing. Average family income declined by one third after nephrectomy (p < .001), the number of participants living below the poverty line increased, three fourths of the donors were still in debt at the time of the survey, and 86% reported deterioration in their health status after nephrectomy and said they would advise others not to sell a kidney.[4] This survey explodes the myth that the poor benefit substantially by donating their organs for financial gain. The findings also indicate that, if potential donors were better informed about their outcomes, they would be less likely to consider paid donation. A large number of the donors in the 2001 survey complained of ill health and inability to continue with hard labor.

Such frustration over the loss of steady income by poor and needy donors in India is in stark contrast to the feeling of well-being and the glow of contentment among altruistic, unpaid LDs, as observed in our programs, and in Western literature. Goyal et al, who reported the 2001 survey results, concluded that, in developing countries like India, potential donors need to be protected from exploitation; at a minimum, this might involve educating them about the likely outcomes of selling a kidney.[4]

The most pervasive argument against the commercial organ trade is that the poor are exploited to satisfy the needs of the rich. Extremely poor patients cannot be said to exercise autonomy when brokers who promise bright financial prospects lure them to donate their organs. In the case of poor relatives and domestic servants donating their organs out of "extreme affection and gratitude" (per the Authorization Committee) for their rich relative or employer, considerable coercion is likely: such donations are rarely voluntary. As for the utilitarian theory of the greatest good for the greatest number, only the recipient and the transplant team (not to mention the broker) benefit, whereas the donor is probably worse off than before.

The only way to increase the donor pool in India is for physicians and policymakers to encourage DD transplantation on a national scale. Importantly, we also need to work together to encourage lifestyle modification and to increase emphasis on primary prevention of common diseases like diabetes and hypertension that lead to kidney failure. Patients with ESRD deserve access to optimal treatment, but not if it entails exploitation of the poor. At least in India, paid organ donation slides down the slippery slope of exploitation and profiteering. Several ethicists in India defend the international ban on the outright selling of organs.

### Living Liver Donation

Liver transplantation was first attempted unsuccessfully in India in 1995 at the All India Institute of Medical Sciences, New Delhi. It was followed by more unsuccessful attempts there and in Chennai. The first successful DD liver transplant was carried out at Indraprasta Apollo Hospital, New Delhi, in 1998. About 60 LD liver transplants have been done in India so far, most at that hospital. The other major centers of LD liver transplantation are the Ganga Ram Hospital, New Delhi, and the Global Hospital, Hyderabad. A few of these LDs experienced significant morbidity; one died after surgery (personal communication). These hospitals have modern infrastructure and have been cleared by the appropriate state authority, yet it is more difficult to start a LD liver transplant program without acquiring sufficient experience in DD liver transplantation. The chief surgeons of these hospitals have acquired sufficient experience working overseas, but the rest of the team may still be in an early state of learning.

## RELIGIONS AND DONATION IN INDIA

### Hinduism

Although India is a land of many beliefs, Hinduism is the religion and way of life of 82% of the population. Hinduism has no founder, no creed, and no single source of authority. Many references support the concept of organ donation in Hindu scriptures. "Daan," the original word in Sanskrit for donation, means selfless giving. In the list of the ten Niyamas (virtuous acts), Daan comes third. Of all the things one can donate, the gift of one's own body is infinitely more praiseworthy. Hindus believe in transmigration of the soul, which results in incarnation. The law of Karma decides which way the soul will go in the next life; all people are part of a cycle of birth, death, and rebirth, a cycle that has no beginning and no end. The *Bhagavad-Gita*, the holy treatise of the Hindus, describes the mortal body and the immortal soul with this simple but profound metaphor: "As a person puts on new garments,

giving up the old ones, the soul similarly accepts new material bodies, giving up the old and useless ones." It is the strong belief of Hindus that good deeds done in this birth decide one's fate in the next birth. Moksha—the liberation from this cycle of birth, death, and rebirth—is the ultimate goal of a Hindu: Daan is one of the deeds that lead to this goal. Scientific and medical treatises (*Charaka,* and *Sushruta Samhita*) form an important part of the Vedas. Sage Charaka deals with internal medicine; Sage Sushruta, with organ and limb transplantation. Interestingly, there are a few mythological examples of organ donation and transplantation. Clearly, to an average Indian, the concept of transplantation is not new. The most famous mythological example is the story of Ganesha. In brief, the goddess Parvati ordered her son Vignesh to guard the door while she was having a bath. Shiva (her husband) came by to visit Parvati. He and Vignesh had not met before and did not recognize each other. Vignesh refused Shiva' entry to the house, and a fierce battle followed. Vignesh had been granted extraordinary power by his mother and was invincible. Shiva needed the help of another deity, Vishnu, to destroy Vignesh. Vishnu advised Shiva to trick Vignesh and beheaded him from behind. Parvati was furious and threatened to destroy the universe unless her son was brought back to life and made a God. Shiva was unable to find Vignesh's head and sent his henchmen to find the head of the first living creature that they found committing a crime against Mother Nature. They found a baby elephant sleeping with its head to the north (which in Hindu law, can disturb the peace of the universe). The elephant was slain and its head was brought to Shiva, who then successfully transplanted it onto Vignesh and brought him back to life. Vignesh was given eternal godhood and was thereafter called Ganesha. Thus, this mythological story represents the first example of a xenotransplant.

### Islam

Islam is the second most common (12%) religion in India. The majority of Muslims are Sunnis. Muslims are spread all over India, but in Jammu and Kashmir they represent the majority of the population. One of the basic aims of the Muslim faith is the saving of life. Allah greatly rewards those who save others from death: "Whosoever saves the life of one person it would be as if he saved the life of all mankind" (Holy Qur'an, chapter 5, verse 32). The issue of organ donation and transplantation has been discussed in various Fiqh seminars (Islamic jurisprudence). Most contemporary Islamic scholars base their views on the general and broad guidelines of Shariah (the code of Islamic law). The consensus is to permit organ donation, with some conditions.

The Second Fiqh Seminar, held in New Delhi in 1989, attracted more than 70 participants (jurists, intellectuals, and Ulama) from all parts of India, including many Islamic scholars. The following conclusions were arrived at unanimously: if an organ of a person stops functioning, and for the purpose of restarting its functioning, it becomes necessary to replace that organ, it is lawful to replace a part of a person's body with another part of the same person if necessity so demands. It is not permissible to sell one's organs. If a patient has reached ESRD, transplantation of human organ will be permissible to save his or her life. If a healthy person, in the opinion of medical experts, is sure that he or she can live with one kidney only, donating one kidney to an ailing relative is valid, if donation is necessary to save the relative's life and no other alternative is available: no price can be charged for the organ.

## Christianity

Only about 2.3% of India's population is Christian. Most of the original Apostles about 2,000 years ago worked in Europe to convert Europeans to Christianity. One Apostle, however, St. Judas Thomas, made his way to Kerala in southern India in 52 AD. He converted many locals, who were then called Syrian Christians. Most Indian Christians were converted by missionaries who arrived in India with European powers in the fifteenth century, beginning with the Portuguese, under the leadership of Vasco Da Gama, in southern India in 1498. The Portuguese were inspired by the Pope's order to baptize people to fight wars against the local Indian rulers. English missionaries started working in India much later, in 1660. Organ donation is morally and ethically acceptable to both Catholic and Protestant Christians. According to a survey in Delhi, more Christians (96.43%), as compared with Hindus (95.16%), were aware of organ donation; many of them were willing to be a donor after death.[5]

## Buddhism

Buddhism is the fourth largest religion in the world (after Christianity, Islam, and Hinduism). It was founded in northern India by Siddhartha Gauthama, called Buddha, in 535 BC. Buddhism expanded across Asia and initially evolved into largely independent forms: (1) Theravada (Hinayana) Buddhism, the dominant school in most of South East Asia since the thirteenth century, with establishments of monasteries in Sri Lanka, Thailand, Myanmar, Cambodia, and Laos; and (2) Mahayana Buddhism, the dominant school of Buddhism in China, Japan, Korea, Mongolia, and Tibet; a third school called Vajrayana was also established in Tibet. Nowadays, Buddhism has largely disappeared from India, its country of origin, except for refugees from Tibet and for a small number of converts from the lower castes of Hindus. Helping others is central to Buddhism, along with the belief that charity forms an integral part of a spiritual way of life. The *Sutra of Golden Light* (chapter 18) shows how Buddha gave his body to save a starving tigress and her cubs, which were later reborn as his disciples. For many Buddhists, organ donation is an extremely positive action. As long as it is truly the wish of the dying person, donation will not harm in any way the consciousness that is leaving the body. On the contrary, this final act of generosity accumulates good karma, according to *Sogyal Rinpoche—The Tibetan Book of Living & Dying*.

## Jainism

About 5,000,000 persons in India practice Jainism. Like Buddhism, it arose in the sixth century BC as a protest against the overdeveloped ritualism of Hinduism, particularly its sacrificial cults, and the authority of the Vedas. Of the 24 saits that originated the religion, the last one, Mahavira is an historical figure. He preached a rigid asceticism and solicitude as a means of escaping the cycle of birth and rebirth or the transmigration of souls. Mahavira organized a brotherhood of monks, who took vows of celibacy, nudity, self-mortification, and fasting. When a schism developed over the issue of nudity, Jains divided into Digambara (space clothed) and Svethambars (white clothed). Early Jainism, arising in North East India, quickly spread west,

particularly to Gujarat. As Jainism grew and prospered, reverence for Mahavira and other teacher passed into adoration. Modern Jains, eschewing any occupation that even remotely endangers animal life, are largely in commerce and finance; among them are many of India's most prominent industrialists and bankers as well as several important political leaders. Jains, known for philanthropy, contribute more than 50% of all eyes donated in India. They have no clear doctrine on organ donation, but their community accepts that donation is the supreme of all Daan (virtuous acts).

## Sikhism

Sikhism (founded over 500 years ago in Punjab, a northwest state of India) today has a following of over 20 million people worldwide and ranks as the world's fifth largest religion. Sikhism preaches a message of devotion and remembrance of God at all time, truthful living, and equality of mankind; and denounces superstitions and blind rituals. Sikhism is open to all through the teaching of its 10 Gurus enshrined in the Sikh Holy Book and Living Guru, Sri Guru Granth Sahib. The Sikh philosophy and teachings place great emphasis on the importance of giving and putting others before oneself: "Where self exists, there is no God. Where God exists, there is no self," (Guru Nanak, Guru Granth Sahib). Sikhism stresses the importance of performing noble deeds. There are many examples of selfless giving and sacrifice in Sikh teachings by the 10 Gurus and other Sikhs. They believe life after death is a continuous cycle but the physical body is not needed in this cycle—a person's soul is their real essence. The Sikh religion teaches that life continues after death in the soul, and not in the physical body. The last act of giving and helping others through organ donation is both consistent with and in the spirit of Sikh teachings.

## CONCLUSION

As long as economic inequality and the scarcity of DD organs persist in India, it is certain that commerce in transplantation will continue to flourish. To curb the organ trade, paid transplants must be completely abolished by amending the present Transplantation of Human Organs Act; stringent action must be taken against corrupt officials, doctors, and hospitals; and, simultaneously, DD transplants must be promoted. Religion, luckily, has not been a stumbling block to organ donation; most religions in India support organ donation.

## References

1. Menon P. Against organ trade. *Frontline* 2002;19(issue 10).
2. Ram V. Karnataka's unabating kidney trade. *Frontline* 2002;19(issue 07).
3. Gupta V, Singh N. Unholy Trade in the Holy City of Punjab. Kidney Transplant Racket in Amritsar, Punjab India, an interim report. Freeindiamedia.com
4. Goyal M, Mehta RL, Schneiderman LJ, et al. Economic and health consequences of selling a kidney in India. *JAMA* 2002;288:1589.
5. Mishra PH, Vij A, Sharma RK. A knowledge attitude and practice. Study of organ donation and its problems in the metropolitan city of Delhi. *JAHA* 2002;16:01.

### 3.2.3   The Near and Middle East

*Mehmet Haberal, MD, Hamdi Karakayali, MD*

## INRODUCTION

The Middle East Society for Organ Transplantation (MESOT), founded in Turkey in 1987, includes 29 countries from the Middle East, North Africa, and neighboring countries (total population, 635 million people).[1] The dialysis and kidney transplantation programs in these countries vary from nonexistent to large scale, correlating with the country's financial resources.

The annual per capita gross domestic product of MESOT countries ranges from $100 in Afghanistan to $29,100 in Qatar. In very low-income MESOT countries (eg, Afghanistan, Pakistan, Azerbaijan, Armenia, Turkmenistan, Yemen), health-care budgets are limited.[2] Dialysis and kidney transplant programs are small or nonexistent.

In low-income MESOT countries, the estimated annual number of new patients with end-stage renal disease (ESRD) is about 30,000; of these, 95% die each year because of lack of access to dialysis or kidney transplantation. Less than 5% are started on dialysis. Many also die because they cannot afford dialysis and cannot provide a living related donor (LRD) for a transplant.[3]

In low- to middle-income MESOT countries (eg, Egypt, Syria, Tunisia, Iraq, Lebanon, and Turkey), the estimated annual number of new patients with ESRD is about 30,000. Approximately 50% of the patients in these countries have access to dialysis. The kidney transplant programs are limited, and therefore many patients remain on dialysis permanently, which represents a great financial burden to the already-limited health-care systems.[2,3]

In high-income MESOT countries (eg, Bahrain, Kuwait, Qatar, Saudi Arabia) the estimated annual incidence of new patients with ESRD is 4,000. In these countries, although the dialysis facilities are adequate, transplantation remains limited. Health-care budgets in these countries cover all dialysis and transplantation expenses.[2,3]

Organs for transplantation come from three sources: deceased donors (DDs), whose families have consented to organ donation; LRDs, who are genetically related to the recipient (eg, parents, grandparents, brothers, sisters); and living unrelated donors (LURDs), who are genetically unrelated to the recipient but may be emotionally related (eg, spouse, in-law, adopted sibling, stepsister). LURDs who are not emotionally related may be altruistically motivated or may be compensated monetarily. Worldwide, kidney and liver transplants with living donors (LDs) have become ethically acceptable and common. Still, the shortage of donor organs remains a major obstacle for most MESOT countries, and this shortage can only be overcome by increasing the numbers of both LDs and DDs.[4,5] In MESOT countries, LDs are about 50% of the donor source of kidneys for transplantation.[6]

In many Middle Eastern countries, LURD renal transplant programs are in place and the number of transplants is growing. In these countries, the authorities that put the LURD programs into practice claim that they are financially advantageous, particularly in very-low-income countries where long-term dialysis is unavailable or limited. In low- and middle-income MESOT countries, LURD programs relieve the burden of dialysis expenses on health-care budgets. In high-income MESOT countries, LURD programs provide the treatment of choice for many patients with ESRD.

Some ethicists and transplantation authorities, particularly in Turkey and Saudi Arabia, oppose monetary compensation of LURDs.[7–10] Their solution has been to establish a Western model using DDs; however, many infrastructural deficiencies as well as strong cultural barriers have prevented any large-scale DD program from gaining a foothold. Another solution to the increasing organ demand is to increase awareness for LRD kidney transplants.[4,11,12]

The major arguments against compensation of LURDs are that such kidney donors would be poor and uneducated; that the donors would be exploited by middlemen and transplant teams; that only wealthy patients would be the recipients; that their medical care would be generally inadequate; that their use would inhibit DD and LRD transplants; and that sales would be uncontrolled.[7,13,14]

In the Asian countries of India and Pakistan, we can already see that use of LURDs may open the way to commercialism.[4,11,15] Recipients with enough resources come not only from within India and Pakistan but also from neighboring countries. There, the human kidney has become a marketable commodity. The debate for and against monetary compensation is sure to continue.

## LEGAL ISSUES AND COMMON PRACTICES

The MESOT countries, for the most part, have inadequate preventive medicine, incongruent health infrastructures, poor awareness by the medical community and the public of the importance of organ donation and transplantation, a high level of ethnicity, and poor government support of organ transplantation. In addition, they are plagued by a lack of collaboration among transplant physicians, a lack of coordination between organ procurement organizations and transplant centers, and a lack of effective health coverage.[11]

Patients seek a commercial transplant most of the time. The number of patients on waiting lists for organ transplants has increased with time, with an ever-increasing gap between the supply of and the demand for organs.[16] The number of kidney transplants in 2003, by MESOT country, is shown in Table 3.2.3-1.

Transplant activity in the MESOT region began as early as 1969, when a heart was transplanted in Turkey. The first LRD kidney transplant in Turkey was performed in November 1975 at Baskent University. This was followed by the first DD kidney transplant in October 1978 (the kidney was made available by Eurotransplant).[17] In the 1970s, sporadic kidney transplant programs were also started in other MESOT countries including Lebanon, Egypt, Jordan, Pakistan, Kuwait, Iran, and Kingdom of Saudi Arabia.[18] Other MESOT countries followed suit in the 1980s (Table 3.2.3-1). On June 3, 1979, the law on harvesting, storage, grafting, and transplantation of organs and tissues was enacted in Turkey (Table 3.2.3-2); one month later, the first local DD kidney transplant was performed.[9,10,19]

A Turkish law enacted in 1979 addressed ethical issues, such as the risks and benefits for both donor and recipient; the requirement of certified consent from the potential LD, or given by the DD before death or by the family after death; and brain death in potential DDs (Table 3.2.3-2).[20]

In 1986, Islamic theologians issued what became known as the Amman declaration, in which they clearly accepted brain death and the retrieval and transplantation of organs from LDs and DDs. After this declaration and similar ones, all countries in the Middle East (except for Egypt, Pakistan, and Iraq) passed laws that allowed DD transplants and regulated use of LDs. Several

TABLE 3.2.3-1

## KIDNEY TRANSPLANTS, BY MESOT COUNTRY (2003)

| Country | Population | Total No. of Tx | No./Year (2003) | Per Million/ Year |
|---|---|---|---|---|
| Algeria | 32,199,857 | 1200 | 42 | 1.3 |
| Bahrain | 676,461 | 280 | 12 | 17.7 |
| Cyprus | 773 | 520 | 22 | 28 |
| Egypt | 76,027,273 | 7000 | 380 | 5 |
| Iran | 68,753,499 | 16,810 | 1553 | 23 |
| Iraq | 25,257,859 | 3500 | 312 | 12.3 |
| Jordan | 5,450,418 | 1000 | 56 | 10.3 |
| Kingdom of Saudi Arabia | 25,607,367 | 6131 | 410 | 16.4 |
| Kuwait | 2,129,005 | 1146 | 97 | 45.6 |
| Lebanon | 3,774,670 | 941 | 70 | 19 |
| Libya | 5,596,976 | 680 | 45 | 8 |
| Morocco | 32,369,016 | 480 | 27 | 0.84 |
| Oman | 2,871,129 | 230 | 19 | 6.6 |
| Pakistan | 160,132,577 | 9000 | 2050 | 13 |
| Qatar | 779,559 | 230 | 14 | 18 |
| Sudan | 39,074,168 | 1150 | 50 | 1.3 |
| Syria | 17,970,525 | 630 | 102 | 6 |
| Tunisia | 9,977,049 | 535 | 29 | 3 |
| Turkey | 69,018,657 | 6686 | 605 | 8.7 |
| United Arab Emirates | 2,499,215 | 580 | 23 | 9.2 |
| Yemen | 19,743,645 | 288 | 19 | 1 |

MESOT countries also established laws and guidelines for transplant centers.[18]

In Iran, the Organ Transplantation and Brain Death Act was approved by the Parliament in 2000. According to this Act, which has similar properties with Turkish law, brain death must be diagnosed and certified by four physicians (one neurologist, one neurosurgeon, one medical specialist, and one anesthesiologist). Members of the team that diagnose and establish brain death must not be part of the transplant team. After confirming brain death, DD organs and tissues are used with consent of the deceased (ie, written will or signed donor card) or the next of kin. Despite support by religious leaders, some people do not offer permission for use of DDs.[21]

More than 78% of all kidney transplants in Iran have been from LURDs. According to the Iranian LURD kidney transplant program, the potential donor is referred to the Dialysis and Transplant Patient Association (DATPA) to match for a suitable LURD if the recipient has no LRD or the potential donor is not willing to donate. Those willing to volunteer as LURDs contact DATPA. All members of DATPA are patients with ESRD, and they receive no financial incentives for funding an LURD or for referring the patient and donor to a kidney transplant center. There is no role for a middleman or agency in this program. All kidney transplant centers are associated with university hospitals. The government pays all hospital expenses; each LURD receives an award from the government and most also receive a gift (or arranged payment) from the recipient. Transplant teams receive no incentives or government awards. The LURD program is under the close scrutiny of the Iranian Society of Organ Transplantation regarding ethical issues.[22] Foreigners are not allowed to undergo transplants using Iranian LURDs. Half of LURD recipients have been from a poor socioeconomic background.[23]

TABLE 3.2.3-2

## ARTICLES FROM TURKISH LAWS 2238 AND 2594 ON THE HARVESTING, STORAGE, GRAFTING, AND TRANSPLANTATION OF ORGANS AND TISSUES (JUNE 3, 1979)

Law No. 2238

**Article 3:** Buying and selling of organs and tissues against a monetary amount or another interest are forbidden.

**Article 6:** The consent for harvesting an organ must be obtained from a person/persons over 18 years of age and of sound mind verbally and in writing before at least two witnesses and approved by a physician.

**Article 7:** Physicians harvesting organs and tissues must:

   a) inform the donor about the risk involved, the medical, psychological, and domestic outcomes thereof in a suitable and detailed manner;

   b) inform the donor regarding the advantages the donor shall provide the recipient;

   c) refuse harvesting the organs and tissues of persons mentally and psychologically handicapped;

   d) investigate whether or not the donor is married, the spouse is aware of the donor's decision of donating his/her organs and tissues, and record the information;

   e) forbid and refuse the harvesting of organs and tissue donated for a monetary amount or any other interest than in the name of humanity;

   f) not reveal the donor's identity, with exception of blood and those who are related to the recipient by marriage or close personal relationships.

**Article 11:** Brain death must be medically established by 1 cardiologist, 1 neurologist, 1 neurosurgeon, and 1 anesthesiologist, according to the rules, methods, and practices equivalent to the level of science reached in the country.

Law No. 2594  AMENDMENT

**Article 1:** In results of any accident or natural death, provided that reason of death is not in any way related to the reason for organ harvesting and according to the conditions stated in Article 11, the suitable organs and tissues can be transplanted into persons whose lives depend upon this procedure without permission from the next of kin.

Egypt has an active LD transplant program. The LD ethical committee in Egypt consists of two top administrative officers, one judge, one senior surgeon, and one hepatologist (none involved in transplantation). This ethical committee sees every recipient and donor pair in order to document that both of them fully understand the risk–benefit relationship as explained by the transplant team. Informed consent is signed. In Egypt, use of DDs is still prohibited, forcing transplant candidates to seek this service abroad (which exacerbates organ scarcity in the Western hemisphere). Similarly, liver transplant candidates can only undergo liver transplants from LDs but not DDs.[24]

In Lebanon, all transplant costs are paid by the government (eg, Ministry of Health, national health insurance and securities, the army, municipalities, internal security, or police forces). The patient is the one who selects the center where the transplant is to be performed. The government has no hospital of its own. Most transplants use LURDs (60%) or LRDs (25.5%); DDs are used in 13.5%. The Ministry of Health must approve all transplants. No transplant is allowed between Lebanese and non-Lebanese. Residents of Lebanon (there are 1.5 million foreign workers) cannot donate their organs, even as DDs, except to nationals of their own country. Donors must sign a legal document with the government notary stating that the donation is of the person's own free will, with no peer pressure, and is given freely and for altruistic

**TABLE 3.2.3-3**

**LIVER, HEART, AND BONE MARROW TRANSPLANTS, BY MESOT COUNTRY**

| Country | Liver | Heart | Bone Marrow |
|---|---|---|---|
| Egypt | 200 | 5 | 1,700 |
| Iran | 131 | 78 | 3,120 |
| Kingdom of Saudi Arabia | 321 | 97 | 540 |
| Lebanon | 16 | 22 | 142 |
| Oman | 12 | 6 | 52 |
| Pakistan | 50 | 22 | 550 |
| Tunisia | 16 | 14 | 196 |
| Turkey | 703 | 132 | 2,882 |
| Total | 1,449 | 376 | 9,183 |

reasons. The document must be countersigned by a first-blood-line relative (i.e., father, mother, brother, spouse, child, uncle, or aunt). Patients from abroad can only use a donor of the same nationality, after documents similar to those used for Lebanese citizens are signed and witnessed by the embassy of the patient's country. Because of these rules, no tourist transplants occur in Lebanon.[18]

In the MESOT region, the first LRD segmental liver transplant was performed in March 1990 at Baskent University in Ankara, when a 10-month-old child received a mother's left lateral liver segments. One month later, a LRD liver transplant in an adult recipient (a father to his 22-year-old son) was successful. In 1992, again at Baskent University in Ankara, the first multiple-organ procurement from a living donor (a portion of liver and a kidney) was performed between a mother and her daughter.[25]

The declarations of Islamic authorities and the passage of laws paved the way to expand DD programs for liver, heart, pancreas, and lung transplants (see Table 3.2.3-3). Nonetheless, LD transplants are more common in MESOT countries (for kidney and partial liver transplant). DD transplants have great potential, but debate continues among the medical community regarding the concept of brain death. And the public is not fully aware of the importance of organ donation and transplantation.[8,11,26]

## ISLAMIC PHILOSOPHY AND ETHICS

Islam pays special attention to morality and ethics. The core of Islamic teaching is perfection of the ethical conduct of a human being. According to Islamic belief, each individual has a soul and a body. The human condition depends on the eternal soul. All humans are equally situated with respect to their spiritual perfection. God gave humans the basic knowledge of "good" and "bad," yet human acts are of value if done by informed freedom. Solutions to ethical problems are derived from Islamic principles and updated in the Holy Quran, which includes the traditions of the prophet of Islam and his successors (Sunna and Hadith), the consensus of scholars (Ijma), and wisdom (Aqul). According to religious sanctions (*fatwa*), vital organs (such as the heart) cannot

be donated before death. Donation of other organs is permitted but should not be harmful to the donor. Donor and recipient consent is necessary.[21]

All three forms of organ donation (use of DDs, LRDs, and LURDs) involve invasive procedures for both donor and recipient. Surgical transplantation of an organ (which is potentially beneficial to the recipient) seems acceptable ethically, because it is *beneficial* to the recipient (as long as the benefits of the surgery outweigh the risks). Ethically, it is similar to any other surgery performed on a human being. However, with regard to LDs, the principle of *nonmaleficence* (doing no harm) is breached because the surgery and the loss of a healthy organ or tissue carry risks for the donor.[6]

The fatwa permitting transplantation is based, among other things, on the Quranic verse "And if anyone saved a life, it would be as if he saved the life of the whole people" (Chapter V, Verse 35 [The verse number differs between 32 and 35 in different translations of the Holy Quran]) and on the two principles: "the necessities legitimize the prohibited" and "the greater detriment is warded off by the lesser detriment."[6] The benefit of transplantation should outweigh the harm caused by it in terms of risk to both donor and recipient. This demands that the potential success of transplant surgery be high.

In March 1980, the Supreme Board of Religious Affairs in Turkey stated that organ transplantation is lawful (Table 3.2.3-4). This was important. Although Turkey is a republic with a multiparty parliamentary democratic system like most Western democracies, almost 99.5% of the population is Muslim.[19] The first resolution of the Islamic council in Saudi Arabia (Senior Ulama Commission) about organ donation and transplantation was issued in 1982 (Table 3.2.3-5). It permitted tissue and organ transplantation from both LDs and DDs. This resolution marked a new era in organ transplantation in Saudi Arabia and led to formation of the Saudi Center of Organ Transplantation (SCOT).[27] SCOT led to DD liver transplant programs in Saudi Arabia and the first such DD transplant was performed in 1990.[28]

**TABLE 3.2.3-4**

**TURKISH SUPREME BOARD OF RELIGIOUS AFFAIRS DECISION DATED MARCH 6, 1980/396**

According to this decision, organ transplantation may only be performed under the following conditions:

1. Under necessity, that is, when a medical doctor, whose professional efficiency and integrity are respected, states that organ transplantation is the only way to save a patient's life or one of his vital organs.
2. When the medical doctor is of the prevailing opinion that organ transplantation is the only way to cure the disease.
3. When it is certain that the person, whose organ or tissue to be removed, is dead.
4. When the patient, who will receive a transplanted organ, gives his consent to the operation.

Only the person, to whom one donates on or his/her organs, oneself is responsible for all his/her good and evil deeds.

Chairman of the Supreme Board of Religious Affairs

**TABLE 3.2.3-5**

## PURPORT OF THE KINGDOM OF SAUDI ARABIA SENIOR ULAMA COMMISSION'S DECISION NO. 99 DATED 06-11-1402 H  (25-08-1982 G)[51]

The board unanimously resolved the permissibility to remove an organ, or a part thereof from a Muslim or Thimmi (non-Muslim) living person and graft it onto him, should the need arise, should there be no risk in the removal and should the transplantation seem likely successful. The board also resolved by the majority the following:

a) The permissibility to remove an organ or part thereof from a dead person for the benefit of a Muslim, should the need arise and cause no dissatisfaction and should the transplantation seem likely successful.

b) The permissibility for the living person to donate one of his organs or part thereof for the benefit of a Muslim in need thereof.  Scholars facilitated an early resolution about the view of Islam toward the issue of organ donation and transplantation.

---

## ARGUMENTS FOR AND AGAINST LURD TRANSPLANTS

Those who wish to ban paid donation through legislation, especially in developing countries, might do well to carefully study the case of India. In India, several thousand uncontrolled commercial kidney transplants were once performed in private backstreet clinics. Incomplete donor and recipient evaluations resulted in a high incidence of complications.[7,15] Many kidneys were sold by middlemen to wealthy patients. In the 1980s and 1990s, India was so criticized for allowing rampant commercialism that it responded in 1994 with a law that banned the sale of organs, recognized brain death, and facilitated use of DDs. However, the outcome was far from what was expected. The price of illegally transplanted kidneys in India increased sharply.[29,30] The law singularly failed. In 1998, the International Forum for Transplant Ethics concluded that organ trade should be regulated rather than banned.[31] Thus, some investigators proposed a strictly regulated and strongly ethics-based market in LD organs and tissues, in order to prevent illegal LURD transplants.[3,21,32]

Altruism and a sense of moral obligation have been reported to be the prime motivating factors in LRD kidney transplants. But gifted rewarding and exchange of money may occur even among LRDs.[14] Although most LRDs of kidneys cited love and affection as their prime motives, other factors such as financial dependence may play a significant role.[15]

LURD transplants can be motivated either by pure altruism or by real commercial interest.[6] In between, there is a zone that Daar et al.[33] the "grey area," subdivided into the realms of "compensated donation" and "donation with incentives." Most Muslims are guided by the example of the Prophet Mohammed who said, "If somebody confers on kindness (favor) to you, reward him." However, any reward is given after the kind act has been performed, so it should not be an advance part of the deal. Any agreement between donor and recipient (or a third party) to donate an organ that involves any the exchange of money (or its equivalent) should be considered as a *sale*, regardless of what it is called (eg, sale, reward, prize). Under the law of Islam, it is forbidden to sell oneself or any free person. The Prophet Mohammed said that Allah the Almighty says, "There are three

whose adversary I shall be on the Day of Resurrection: a man who has given his word by Me and has broken it; *a man who has sold a free man and has consumed the price;* and a man who has hired a workman, has exacted his due in full from him, and has not given him his wage." Islamic scholars clearly stated, centuries ago, that it is unlawful to sell a human being, and that such a sale is invalid. They stressed that what applies to the whole also applies to parts.

Another question that might arise is this: are LURD transplants permissible if they do not involve payment? One principle of Islamic law (Shariaa), "Closing the Door in the Face of Pretexts," means, "What is apparently permissible but leads *often* to what is not, is prohibited for that."[34] Among 32 Iranian LURDs interviewed by Bromand,[32] only one claimed that he had wanted to donate with true altruism; the other 31 donated for money. Nearly 95% of these LURDs had no follow-up. Zargooshi et al,[35] in a survey of 100 LURDs in Iran, gave a grim picture of abuse: he found that 51% of them expressed hate or anger toward their recipients, 65% stated that promises given by the recipient had not been met, 76% felt that the practice should be banned, and 97% were vendors. Zargooshi et al. concluded that the donor–recipient relationship is pathologic, with no similarity between LURDs emotionally related LRDs.

## PUBLIC AND FAMILY ATTITUDES TOWARD DD TRANSPLANTS

In general, regardless of whether the deceased is known to them, people in MESOT countries view the removal of organs from a body as a disrespectful act, further torture to the deceased, and disturbance of the soul. Separate from religious beliefs, Middle Eastern and mid-Asian countries have for centuries regarded and respected the dead as sacred. Famial refusal of DD transplants because of religious beliefs is a misconception; such refusal is not in line with the religious rulings of the three major religions practiced in MESOT countries.[36] For followers of Islam, Christianity, and Judaism, it is well known that no message prohibits use of organs and tissues in certain circumstances, provided there is no conflict of interest.[12,37–39] Religious beliefs are often simply an excuse for familial refusal of consent. People tend to stand by their traditional beliefs and superstitions more than religious teachings when faced with death and "matters unknown."[36]

Next to religious misconceptions, the most common reason for famial refusal to donate is fear of disfigurement and/or mutilation of a loved one's body. A survey assessing the knowledge, attitude, and behavior of university students in relation to organ donation, organ procurement, and transplantation was performed in Turkey. Although a large proportion of the 275 students expressed a willingness to donate their organs after death (49.5%), a much smaller percentage (13.8%) had already signed organ donation cards. The most common reason that students gave for not wanting to donate organs was that they did not have a clear understanding of the concept of brain death (24.0%). Possible inappropriate use of harvested organs was another common reason for the decision not to donate. Regarding the decision of whether to donate the organs of a brain-dead relative, about 41.5% of respondents said they would not approve of donation. The main reasons for opposition included suspicion about premature withdrawal of advanced life support (24.0%), worry about possible inappropriate use of the body or individual organs (22.0%), and concern about disfigurement (22.0%).[40]

It is a natural human reaction to continue to hope for a miracle that might save a loved one's life, even after brain death has occurred. It is often difficult to persuade a family that they are facing an irreversible situation, and that the dead will not return to life. Rumors circulate, and the media break sensational stories about questionable declarations of brain death, untimely declarations of death, and the stealing of organs without familial consent. Such fabrications serve only to increase reluctance on the part of families to donate. Refusal to donate is also more likely in cases in which the wishes of the deceased with regard to organ donation are unknown or are deliberately withheld.[36] Public misunderstanding of brain death criteria is among the other cited reasons for familial refusal.[41] Public opinion polls show that people are often more dedicated to donating their own organs and those of family members before they are faced with the actual situation. The initially positive attitudes of those who are somewhat aware of transplantation and use of DDs suddenly change when the time comes to making a decision.[42]

## CONCLUSION

The supply of LD organs is limited by delicate ethical and immunologic concerns. This shortage has spurred more rigorous and effective promotion of DD transplants, because they do not involve as many sensitive concerns. However, the issue is still complex. Attitudes toward removing organs from a loved one's body are driven mostly by culture, tradition, religion, and law. Although some commonalities exist in human nature and behavior across different people, many important distinctions remain between countries, ethnic groups, and even individuals within a given society. Differences in the various facets of society worldwide dictate the impossibility of universal remedies for the organ shortage. Efforts to develop and increase DD transplants in MESOT countries require time and patience, but will eventually reduce the need for LD transplants, which have their own set of risks and limitations.

Next to immunologic barriers, legal and ethical issues are the major concerns in LD transplants. The problem of the underground organ trade is already increasing and certainly represents the largest threat to the acceptance and success of LD transplants. Unfortunately, there are signs that the underground trade has spread all over the world: now there are even Web pages that offer black-market organs. LD transplants are currently limited to the kidney and more recently, the partial liver; the partial pancreas LD is used very rarely. LD grafts have advantages, including better graft survival rates. In most Middle Eastern and mid-Asian countries, LD kidney transplants outnumber DD kidney transplants. In contrast, in most Western countries, the DD organ shortage is comparably less. Further efforts and new strategies must be developed and implemented to enhance use of DDs in the Middle East and mid-Asia.

Except for "presumed consent" laws, in effect in some Western countries, legislation does not directly impact the rate of donation. The applicability of "presumed consent" laws in the Middle East would be highly questionable: there, familial or next-of-kin approval is clearly necessary for donation.

Ultimately, legislation cannot be expected to change deeply rooted traditions or religious, social, and ethical values. Instead, education in all facets of transplantation is the first and essential step. Better education of the public and of medical personnel is the key to increasing organ donation. For example,

Baskent University's recently established television and radio channels and periodicals have been mobilized for such education in Turkey. Both medical personnel and the public must be convinced that transplants (whether LD or DD) represent a priceless gift of life.

## References

1. Bilgin N. Message from the president. *MESOT Newsletter* 1998(Issue 1).
2. The World Bank Group Data and Statistics. Country Classification. www.worldbank.org
3. Ghods AJ. Should we have live unrelated donor renal transplantation in MESOT countries? *Transplant Proc* 2003;35(7):2542–2544.
4. Rizvi SAH, Naqvi SAA, Hashmi A, et al. Improving kidney and live donation rates in Asia: Living donation. *Transplant Proc* 2004;36(7):1894–1895.
5. Groth CG. Presidential address 2002: Organ transplantation as a patient service worldwide. *Transplantation* 2003;75(8):1098–1100.
6. Boobes Y, Al Daker NM. Should we have live unrelated donor transplantation in the MESOT countries? Islamic perspective. *Transplant Proc* 2003;35(7):2539–2541.
7. Chugh KS, Jha V. Commerce in transplantation in Third World countries. *Kidney Int* 1996;49(5):1181–1186.
8. al-Mousawi M, Hamed T, al-Matouk H. Views of Muslim scholars on organ donation and brain death. *Transplant Proc* 1997;29(8):327.
9. Haberal M, Moray G, Karakayali H, Bilgin N. Ethical and legal aspects, and the history of organ transplantation in Turkey. *Transplant Proc* 1996;28(1):382–383.
10. Haberal M, Demirag A, Cohen B, et al. Cadaver kidney transplantation in Turkey. *Transplant Proc* 1995;27(5):2768–2769.
11. Shaheen FAM, Souqiyyeh MZ. How to improve organ donation in the MESOT countries. *Ann Transplant* 2004;9(1):19–21.
12. Daar AS. Organ donation—world experience; the Middle East. *Transplant Proc* 1991;23(5):2505–2507.
13. Daar AS. Paid organ procurement: pragmatic and ethical viewpoints. *Transplant Proc* 2004;36(7):1876–1877.
14. Khajehdehi P. Living non-related versus related renal transplantation––Its relationship to the social status, age and gender of recipients and donors. *Nephrol Dial Transplant* 14 1999;(11):2621–2624.
15. Mahawar K, Sharma A, Angral R, et al. Altruism and living-related renal transplantation in India. *Transplant Proc* 2003;35(1):24–25.
16. Spital A. The shortage of organs for transplantation: Where do we go from here? *N Engl J Med* 1993;325(17):1243–1246.
17. Haberal M. Historical evolution of kidney and liver transplantation in Turkey. *Transplant Proc* 1995;27(5):2771–2774.
18. Masri MA, Haberal M, Shaheen FAM, et al. Middle East Society for Organ Transplantation (MESOT) Registry. *Exp Clin Transplant* 2004;2(2):217–221.
19. Haberal M, Moray G, Karakayali H, et al. Transplantation legislation and practice in Turkey: A brief history. *Transplant Proc* 1998;30(7):3644–3646.
20. Haberal M, Kaynaroğlu V, Belgin N. Ethics in organ procurement in Turkey. *Int J Artif Organs* 1992;15(5):61–263.
21. Larijani B, Zahedi F, Taheri E. Ethical and legal aspects of organ transplantation in Iran. *Transplant Proc* 36(5):1241–1244.
22. Ghods AJ. Renal transplantation in Iran. *Nephrol Dial Transplant* 2002;17(2):222–228.
23. Ghods AJ, Ossareh S, Khosravani P. Comparison of some socioeconomic characteristics of donors and recipients in a controlled living unrelated donor renal transplantation program. *Transplant Proc* 2001;33(5):2626–2627.
24. El-Meteini M, Fayez A, Fathy M, et al. Living related liver transplantation in Egypt: An emerging program. *Transplant Proc* 2003;35(7):2783–2786.
25. Haberal M, Karakayali H, Buyukpamukcu N, et al. Liver transplantation in Turkey. *Transplant Proc* 1995;27(5):2616–2617.

26. Haberal M, Gulay H, Karpuzoglu T, et al. Multiorgan harvesting from heart-beating donors in Turkey. *Transplant Proc* 23(5):2566–2567.

27. Shaheen FAM, Souqiyyeh MZ. Increasing organ donation rates from Muslim donors: Lessons from a successful model. *Transplant Proc* 2004;36(7):1878–1880.

28. Al-Sebayel M, Khalaf H. Starting the liver transplant program at King Faisal Specialist Hospital and research Center in Saudi Arabia: Early experience and future expectations. *Transplant Proc* 2003;35(7):2781–2782.

29. Sells RA. What is transplantation law and whom does it serve? *Transplant Proc* 2003;35(3):1191–11194.

30. Warren J. Commerce in organs acceptable in some cultures, guidelines needed, ethics congress recommends. *Transplant News* 2003;13:1.

31. Eric CA, Harris J. An ethical market in human organs. *J Med Ethics* 2003;29 (3):137–138.

32. Broumand B: Living donors: the Iran experience. Nephrol Dial *Transplant* 1997;12(9):1830–1831.

33. Daar AS, Gutmann TH, Land W. In: Collins GM, Dubernard JM, Persijn GG, Land W, eds. *Procurement and Preservation of Vascularized Organs.* New York: Kluwer; 1997.

34. Al-Khader AA. The Iranian transplant commune: Comment from an Islamic perspective. *Nephrol Dial Transplant* 2003;17(2):213–215.

35. Zargooshi J. Iranian kidney donors: Motivations and relations with recipients. *J Urol* 2001;165 (2):386–392.

36. Bilgin N. The dilemma of cadaver organ donation. *Transplant Proc* 1999;31(8):3265–3268.

37. Hassaballah AM. Minisymposium. Definition of death, organ donation and interruption of treatment in Islam. *Nephrol Dial Transplant* 1996;11(6):964–965.

38. Steinberg A. Minisumposium: Ethical issues in nephrology—Jewish perspectives. *Nephrol Dial Transplant* 1996;11(6):961–963.

39. Zycinski JM. Minsymposium. Bioethical issues from a Roman Catholic perspective. *Nephrol Dial Transplant* 1996;11(6):966–968.

40. Akgün S, Tokalak I, Erdal R. Attitudes and behavior related to organ donation and transplantation: a survey of university students. *Transplant Proc* 2002;34(6):2009–2011.

41. Caplan AL, Welvant P. Are required request laws working? Altruism and the procurement of organs and tissues. *Clin Transplant* 1989;3(3):170–176.

42. Tokalak I, Basaran O, Emiroglu R, et al. Health care professionals' knowledge of procedural issues in transplantation: the need for continuing education programs. *Transplant Proc* 2004;36(1):14–16.

## 3.3  THE EUROPEAN PERSPECTIVE

*Thomas Gutmann, PhD, MA, Walter G. Land, MD*

Ethical arguments do not stop at national frontiers. Therefore, no specific European perspective exists on the ethics of living donor (LD) transplantation. There are, however, different medicoethical cultures and a broad spectrum of national legal approaches to LD transplants in Europe, with intense debates concerning their appropriateness and moral justification.

### DIFFERENT DYNAMICS

LD kidney transplants have become established worldwide, given the increased use of genetically unrelated LDs. In the United States, the number of LD kidneys has exceeded the number of deceased donor (DD) kidneys since 2001,[1] but the situation in European countries differs widely. The rate of LD kidney transplants in 2003 ranged from 1 (Belgium) to 19.2 (Norway), as compared to 22.1 in the United States (Figure 3.3-1). Among the multiple reasons for the divergences in national approaches to LD transplants are distinct medical cultures and sociocultural attitudes,[2] differences in the efficiency of national procurement systems for DD organs (seen most clearly looking at Spain, the uncontested European leader in postmortem organ procurement), and, most prominently, different sets of legal restrictions.

In most European countries, the last 15 years have been characterized by a growing number of LD kidney transplants, Germany being a typical example (Figure 3.3-2), with parallel developments in the United Kingdom, the Netherlands, and Switzerland.

LD liver transplants in Europe have, with some delay, followed the U.S. pattern: a fast-growing number of right-lobe LDs among adults until 2002, followed by a decrease and stagnation since. In

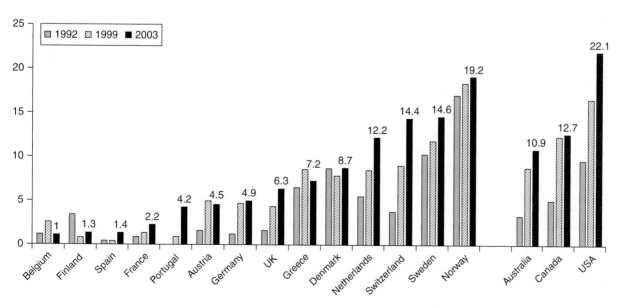

**FIGURE 3.3-1**

Living Donor Kidney Transplant Rates (pmp) 1992, 1999 and 2003 (for data cf. 3, 8)

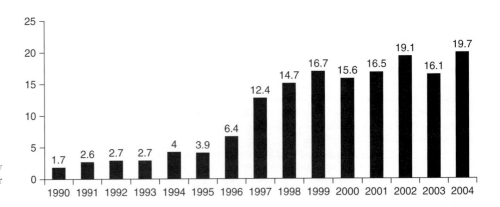

**FIGURE 3.3-2**

Share of Living Donor Kidneys in Kidney Transplantation in Germany 1990–2004 (for data cf. 40, 8)

2003, at least in some European countries, LD liver transplants were a significant proportion of overall liver transplants (in Austria, Italy, and Sweden, about 4%; France, 5%; Germany, 8.7% [vs 12.5% in 2001], Belgium, 14.3%).[3] But in other countries such as Great Britain, LD liver transplants are almost nonexistent. Again, the reasons for these divergences are manifold. Although there is no legal barrier against LD liver transplants in the United Kingdom, LD liver transplants simply are not routinely available in the UK National Health System.[4]

## LEGISLATION

Almost all (at least Western) European countries have passed acts and decrees to establish legal regulations in the field of organ transplantation. Most such provisions also addressed organ donation by living adults or even minors. The Council of Europe proposed a common regulatory framework for Europe with the 1997 Convention on Human Rights and Biomedicine[5] and its Additional Protocol concerning Transplantation of Organs and Tissues of Human Origin in 2002.[6(cf.7)] Analyses of European legislative patterns[7–10] found some common underlying principles and a common approach to most, if not all, of the ethical and social issues involved.

The main concern of European legislation on LDs is to ensure that informed consent is voluntarily given. Of course, most of the legislation explicitly requires that the physician inform the potential donor of the nature, consequences, and risks of the operation as well as of alternatives. In most of the legislation, formal requirements are spelled out for the donor's consent; in most cases, it must be given either in written form or before an official body. Some countries (eg, France, Spain, Italy, and Great Britain) require state authorities to supervise or authorize LD transplants generally or at least in specific cases. In general, the removal of organs and tissues, especially when they are nonregenerative, is only allowed for diagnostic or therapeutic purposes. Beyond that, some statutes focus on the recipient's need for the transplant. Many national enactments allow LD transplants only where no alternative treatment of comparable efficacy exists. Nearly all countries forbid organ removal if there is an increased risk for the LD. But the wording is usually vague when defining the allowed degree of risk, leaving the question of an acceptable risk–benefit ratio to physicians' discretion.

Finally, there is a broad European consensus on the ban of organ sales, as well as against other financial incentives. In Europe, market models for the procurement of transplantable organs have been debated by philosophers and economists during

the last 20 years. Nonetheless, most European countries that have passed legislation in the field of organ transplantation stipulate that the human body and its parts must not be subject to commercial transactions. Article II-3 of the Draft Treaty establishing a Constitution for Europe[11] prohibits making the human body and its parts a source of financial gain, following the almost identical Art. 21 of the Council of Europe's 1997 Convention on Human Rights and Biomedicine.[5] Most national policies against organ trade provide that persons violating these laws are liable to punishment.

Still, quite a number of Europeans seem to buy kidneys abroad, and reports of trafficking in organs are growing from Europe. In 2003, a Council of Europe investigation focused especially on Moldavia.[12] Many statutes, including the 1978 model code of the Council of Europe,[13] expressly allow refunds for any earnings lost and any expenses incurred by the organ removal or any related medical examinations. The Council of Europe's Additional Protocol makes clear that the provision that the prohibition of financial gain for LDs does not prevent compensation for loss of earnings and for any other justifiable expenses incurred by organ removal or related medical examinations; does not prevent payment of a justifiable fee for legitimate medical or related technical services rendered in connection with transplantation; and does not prevent compensation in case of undue damage resulting from the removal of organs or tissues from LDs.[6]

Yet not too many *national* policies address LDs' financial security. Moreover, throughout Europe, there is almost no satisfying approach to the problem of adequate insurance for LDs and their families against the risk of death and disability caused by donation. In many countries, for example, France and Germany, LD are protected by social insurance schemes, but Switzerland was the first country to create a legal duty of transplant centers to provide "adequate insurance" for LDs.[14]

### Genetically Unrelated LDs

The increasing use of genetically unrelated LDs is an important factor in the development of living kidney donation. The legal acceptability of certain categories of LDs is a key element. Three degrees of restrictions imposed by law can be distinguished in Europe: strong restrictions, moderate restrictions, and no restrictions at all.[8]

Strong restrictions once in place in France, where until 2003 the LD had to be genetically related. Only in emergency situations was a spouse—but no other emotionally related person—accepted as well. The 2003 reform added the possibility of living organ donation for recipients "with close ties" to the donor.

Moderate restrictions can be found in countries such as Germany, Italy, United Kingdom, and (since 2003) France. Biologically nonrelated but emotionally related organ donation is permitted in principle. Yet certain categories of potential LDs (like altruistic strangers or crossover donors) are excluded. The German Transplantation Act, like the French law, accepts living nonrelated donation of nonregenerative tissues by spouses, fiancés and fiancées, and other persons in an obvious close personal relationship with the recipient. Some countries provide, or have provided, procedural safeguards. For instance, in the United Kingdom, until 2004, a committee—the "Unrelated Live Transplant Regulatory Authority" (ULTRA)—had to evaluate and permit exceptions to the requirement for a biological relation between donor and recipient under certain conditions.

The limitation of living organ donation to related recipients has been heavily criticized[8] as being sociologically, medically, and ethically unjustifiable. The available evidence suggests that decisions about the acceptability of living unrelated donors should be made on a case-by-case basis. This is reflected by the Council of Europe's proposal that "organ removal from a living donor shall only be carried out for the benefit of a recipient with whom the donor has an appropriate relationship as defined by law, or otherwise with the approval of an appropriate independent body."[6] The possibility of case-to-case decisions is necessary because it does seem impossible "to frame a law or rule that properly defines all those who may have a good reason for wishing to donate."[15] In this sense, the International Congress on Ethics in Organ Transplantation in Munich 2002 passed resolutions that nondirected living kidney donation is ethically acceptable and should be permitted, that kidneys derived from nondirected donation should be allocated using the standard DD allocation criteria, and that the suitability of living related and unrelated organ donors should be assessed by the same criteria.[16]

As long as it is virtually impossible to provide all potential recipients with a DD organ within a reasonable period, it seems hard, if not impossible, to justify withholding a possibly lifesaving organ from a medically suitable, altruistically motivated, voluntarily consenting, yet genetically unrelated LD. The potential recipient has a moral right not to be excluded from therapeutic measures without compelling reasons. As long as we do not violate other basic moral principles, we have the duty to maximize the recipient's chances of receiving curative, palliative, or even lifesaving treatment. In this regard, the recent European history in transplant law is about breaking unjustified barriers. Nevertheless, in 2005, a German Parliamentary Commission still expressed strong disapproval of attempts to legalize kidney exchange and nondirected kidney donation in Germany.[17]

Most European countries do not have legal restrictions that require a relationship between LDs and their recipients. No such restriction is to be found, for example, in Spain, Austria, Switzerland, and the Netherlands, where unrestricted living organ donation is possible and judgments are to be made on a case-to-case basis. The 2004 Swiss legislation[14] appears to be the most advanced and most ambitious project of legislation in Europe, characterized by the renunciation of any kind of restriction on the potential pool of LDs. The Swiss act provides that a relationship of any kind between the donor and the recipient is not a condition *sine qua non* for the acceptance and permission of LD transplants. So, nondirected donation and crossover donation are not excluded. Kidneys derived from nondirected donation are to be allocated using the standard DD allocation criteria.

In sum, it can no longer be said that Europe, regarding legal regulations in the field of LD organ transplantation, suffers from a disease called HIL ("highly inappropriate legislation").[18] However, apart from the famous case of the German transplant surgeon Jochem Hoyer, who in 1996 donated one of his kidneys to a stranger in Munich,[19] no cases of nondirected donation are known in Europe. Nor are there a significant number of cases of crossover donation (kidney exchanges), except for the small, but successful, program in the Netherlands.[20,21]

## Minors and Mentally Disabled Persons

In the United States from 1993 to 2002, 35 minors, ages 11 to 17 years, were LDs.[1] But most, if not all, European countries ban organ removal from minors or from mentally disabled persons. Some countries allow it on certain conditions and attempt to provide procedural safeguards, stressing a heavy presumption against using children and mentally retarded persons as sources of nonregenerative organs, because they are usually unable to give valid consent. All European countries afford a high degree of protection to minors and incompetent adults. In most European countries, donation of nonregenerative organs by minors or incompetent adults is forbidden. On the one hand, total prohibition has the advantage of certainty and maximizes the overall legal protection of these groups of persons. On the other hand, removal of a body part from a minor can be ethically justified in exceptional cases, total prohibition can be unjust because its inflexibility fails to take into account the difference between mature and immature minors. In Norway, the country with the highest percentage of kidney LDs in Europe (Figure 3.3-1), persons under 18 years of age may give their consent, with the endorsement of their guardian and the person who has parental custody under special circumstances, if the operation is also approved by the Directorate of the Health Services. In Sweden, no distinction is made between organs that regenerate and those that do not; under extraordinary circumstances, the National Board of Health and Welfare may give permission for organ removal from a minor or a person unable to give consent, if the operation is not against the donor's own desire.

Most national policies are more restrictive and provide exceptions only in the case of regenerative tissues. Article 19, Section 2, of the Council of Europe's 1997 Convention on Human Rights and Biomedicine provides that, exceptionally and under the protective conditions prescribed by law, the removal of regenerative tissue from a person who does not have the capacity to consent may be authorized if there is no compatible donor available who has the capacity to consent and if the recipient is a brother or sister of the donor. The donation must have the potential to be lifesaving for the recipient. The authorization of his or her representative (or of an authority, person, or body provided for by law) must have been given specifically and in writing, in accordance with the law and with the approval of a competent body, and the potential donor must not object.[5]

## Bioethical Discourse

Claiming that there is no specific European perspective on the ethics of LD transplants is not to deny the different traditions of ethical discourse to be found in Europe. Nowadays, the idea that autonomy (or self-determination) is the most fundamental value to be respected in health care decisions is widely shared among bioethicists and the public in many European countries, such as

Germany, the Netherlands, and Switzerland. Yet in France, for example, stronger paternalistic tendencies seem to give more weight to the doctrine of inviolability and inalienability of the human body than to the principle of respect for the autonomy of patients.[7]

During the last 2 decades, a comprehensive discussion has taken place in the field of medical ethics, internationally, and also in Europe. "Biomedical ethics" emerged as an interdisciplinary approach of philosophical moral theory and medicine. This development reflects not only the complex ethical questions raised by rapid changes in the biological sciences and in health care but also the fact that traditional Hippocratic ethics with its maxim of *primum non nocere* (first do not harm) proved to be inadequate as the sole guideline. Traditional professional ethics, to a large extent, gave way to more complex modes of moral reasoning.[22] As a part of this process, the problems of LD transplants have been thoroughly reevaluated.

Of course, no single or unified moral theory exists today. Moral reasoning and approaches to medical ethics are as pluralistic as our societies are. Different types of ethical theory start from different, partly incompatible sets of premises and intuitions, with different strengths and weaknesses. To create a common ground for intertheoretical moral discussion, mainstream medical ethics today must work at the level of principles as a process of reasoning. The most relevant of these principles are (1) *respect for persons,* including their autonomous choices and actions; (2) *beneficence,* including both the obligation to benefit others (positive beneficence) and to maximize good consequences, that is, to do the greatest good for the greatest number (utility); (3) *justice,* the principle of fair and equitable distribution of benefits and burdens; and finally (4) *nonmaleficence (non nocere),* the obligation not to inflict harm.[23,24] In case of conflict, these principles must to be applied to specific circumstances and balanced against each other.

## Respect for Autonomy

Of course, the balancing of the donor's autonomy with the societal need not to inflict harm is one of the basic ethical problems with LD transplants. Taking autonomy seriously, we need to see that the risk–benefit ratio of any proposed LD transplant is determined not just by medical (or psychological) facts, but ultimately by personal value judgments; these judgments should generally be made by the one most affected by the outcome, that is, the prospective LD.[25,26] He or she is the one to decide what is worth the risk in order to attain a certain good—a thesis with special importance for right-lobe liver donation and other types of LD transplants with higher peri- and postoperative risks for the donor.

In the Western liberal tradition of ethical and political thought, respect for autonomy means respect for individuals' voluntary choice as the sole rightful determinant of their actions, except where the interests of others need protection from them. The ethical principle of respect for autonomy underlies the requirement of informed consent to medical treatment. Autonomous human beings do not only have "experiential" interests (including interests in health and integrity of the body), but also, and most importantly, "critical" interests that reflect their personality and the goal of giving meaning to their life through their own (maybe risky) choices.[27] Persons have an interest to decide for themselves how to live their lives. In bioethical discussions today, the widespread consensus is that it is important to start with a general presumption in favor of the principle of respect for autonomy.[28]

This principle sets limits on the justifiability of medical paternalism, that is, a physician's refusal to accept or to acquiesce to a patient's or donor's wishes, choices, and actions for that person's benefit.[23,25,26] In short, a potential LD has a moral right to take a reasonable risk in order to achieve substantial benefit for the recipient (even if the donor and the recipient are not related).[24,25]

Does this mean that LDs have a moral right to be allowed to donate regardless of the transplant center's assessment of the risk–benefit ratio? No. LD transplants involve more than the LD, but requires the participation of the transplant center as well. The physician has no moral duty to satisfy the patient's desires if he or she finds them incompatible with acceptable medical practice. Donor autonomy does not overrule medical judgment and decision making.[24,29,30] Taking patients and LDs seriously, however, means at least that the transplant center has a fundamental obligation to not deny the LD transplant without a compelling reason.[31(cf.25)]

Thus, it is often ethical to participate in acts of individual risk and sacrifice that are performed to benefit others.[31,32] However, the problem of how to deal with persons who volunteer to be bodily harmed poses a special challenge. Certainly a distinction can be drawn between allowing a person to risk harm and encouraging it.[33] It is questionable whether donation of a liver lobe or lung segment should ever be solicited by a transplant center.

This assessment also implies that the general rule, in several European countries such as Germany, is that LD organ removal is only permitted if a suitable organ from a DD is not available. But that general rule cannot be ethically justified, because the LD and the recipient may have good and sufficient reasons to an LD organ (especially kidney) transplants, even if a DD graft is available. There is no morally sound reason for pushing DD grafts against the will of LDs and their intended recipients.

To be able to give valid consent, the competent LD must, beforehand, be given appropriate information as to the purpose and nature of organ removal as well as its consequences and risks. Consent must be voluntary, that is, free from coercion and undue pressure. It is important to see that voluntariness does not presuppose "having an easy choice." Medical ethicists, in general, are very reluctant to acknowledge a genuine moral obligation to be an LD, but many individuals do feel the responsibility to restore a close person to good health. This form of "moral causation" is not taken to be coercion, unless all duties and responsibilities in life are labeled so. Still, even if the general goal is to ensure that the LD's consent is voluntarily given, family members probably are more vulnerable to undue pressure than friends or strangers. We always have to question the "myth of informed consent"— even, perhaps especially, in the case of LD transplants between genetic relatives.

## Donor Safety

LD kidney transplants may contribute to expansive, complicated organ procurement. Every case is different, and we should concentrate on further developing rational procedures to deal with this fact. All we can rely on are procedural safeguards for case-to-case decisions. A transplant physician has the moral and legal duties to make sure of the conditions of the LD's valid consent and must make reasonable efforts to establish the LD's motives and reasons. Measures taken to establish whether the LD is competent and to investigate the voluntariness of the decision to donate are generally required and justified. Confirmation of accurate donor understanding of risks, benefits, and alternatives is a fundamental obligation of the transplant center.[31] To minimize the appearance of a conflict of interest,[31] transplant centers should make efforts to assure that the medical and psychosocial assessments and the decision to donate incorporate health-care professionals not involved in the care of the recipient.[29] Especially in situations involving a high risk of donor and recipient mortality, a donor advocate is essential to protect both the donor and the recipient.

From an ethical point of view, the most important task today is to implement counseling procedures, to ensure that both the donor and the recipient make a self-responsible decision whether to proceed. In this context, we should acknowledge the transplant center's duty to be "autonomy enhancing" rather than simply show deference to patient autonomy.[32] Decision-making procedures must protect the donor and recipient's option to choose not to participate without being stigmatized by anyone. Responsibility for LDs and recipients requires transplant centers to institutionalize careful, comprehensive screening procedures and to make use of all the psychological knowledge we have for evaluating and guiding LDs and recipients.[34,35]

## CURRENT ISSUES

Despite the consensus on basic principles, a lot still must be done, and many questions remain unsolved. Among the tasks that the European and the international transplant community face today is developing an international standard of care and responsibility for LDs.[cf.29,36] We also must decide how far the transplant center's responsibility for LD reaches posttransplant.[29]

Furthermore, given the changing spectrum of risk–benefit in LD transplants, especially in LD liver transplants, we must define the minimal benefits to recipients that warrant the use of a determined LD. We must decide whether the use of LDs is justified for extended recipient indications and for marginal recipient benefit (eg, very limited life extension posttransplant).[37] Vexing questions include the following. Has the potential LD recipient been identified as acceptable for a DD transplant and been listed for such a transplant? If the risk–benefit ratio for the intended LD transplant is now very good, do we acknowledge or accept a potential LD with sound reasons to provide benefits to a recipient who, given scarce resources, is not eligible for a DD transplant? Moreover, what can be done to promote LD autonomy when the recipient has fulminant hepatic failure, where the LD can undergo only a "quick" evaluation, with only a short time to decide? Should (1) nondirected ("Good Samaritan") donation of a right liver lobe or (2) directed donation of a right liver lobe to a stranger be considered? What about LD and DD kidney exchange programs,[38] which are nonexistent in Europe? What is the normative significance of gender imbalance in LD transplants?[39] How can basic equality of access to LD transplants be achieved?

## References

1. U.S. Organ Procurement and Transplantation Network and the Scientific Registry of Transplant Recipients (OPTN/SRTR): 2003 *Annual Report.* http://www.optn.org/AR2003/default.htm.

2. EUROTOLD Project Management Group: *Questioning Attitudes to Living Donor Transplantation. European Multicentre Study: Transplantation of Organs from Living Donors—Ethical and Legal Dimensions.* Leicester; 1996.

3. Council of Europe: *Newsletter Transplant 9* (2004) *Nr. 1. International Figures on Organ Donation and Transplantation—2003.* http://www.coe.int/T/E/Social_Cohesion/Health.

4. Neuberger J, Price D: Role of Living Liver Donation in the United Kingdom. *BMJ* 2003;327:676.

5. Council of Europe: *Convention for the Protection of Human Rights and Dignity of the Human Being with Regard to the Application of Biology and Medicine (Convention on Human Rights and Biomedicine).* European Treaty Series No. 164, April 4, 1997.

6. Council of Europe: *Additional Protocol to the Convention on Human Rights and Biomedicine Concerning Transplantation of Organs and Tissues of Human Origin.* European Treaty Series No. 186, January 24, 2002.

7. Guillod O, Perrenoud J. The Regulatory Framework for Living Organ Donation. In: Gutmann T, Daar AS, Land W, Sells RA, eds. *Ethical, Legal And Social Issues in Organ Transplantation.* Lengerich and Berlin: Pabst Science Publishers; 2004:157.

8. Gutmann Th, Schroth U. *Organlebendspende in Europa. Rechtliche Regelungsmodelle, ethische Diskussion und praktische Dynamik.* Heidelberg/New York: Springer; 2002.

9. Price D. *Legal and Ethical Aspects of Organ Transplantation.* Cambridge: Cambridge University Press; 2000

10. Gutmann Th, Gerok B. International Legislation in Living Organ Donation. In: Collins GM, Dubernard JM, Persijn G, Land W, eds. *Procurement and Preservation of Vascularized Organs;* Dordrecht, Kluwer; 1997:317.

11. *Draft Treaty establishing a Constitution for Europe,* adopted by consensus by the European Convention on 13 June and 10 July 2003, submitted to the President of the European Council in Rome on 18 July 2003. http://europa.eu.int/constitution/futurum/constitution.

12. Council of Europe Parliamentary Assembly. *Trafficking in organs in Europe, Report Social, Health and Family Affairs Committee.* Rapporteur: Mrs R.-G. Vermot-Mangold, Doc. 9822, 3.6.2003. http://assembly.coe.int/Documents/WorkingDocs/doc03/EDOC9822.htm.

13. Council of Europe: *Resolution 78 (29) on Harmonisation of Legislations of Member States Relating to Removal, Grafting and Transplantation of Human Substances,* 1978.

14. Swiss Transplantation Act of 8 October 2004, http://www.bag.admin.ch/transpla/gesetz/d/TxG%20FINAL%20d.pdf.

15. Council of Europe: *Explanatory Report to the Convention for the Protection of Human Rights and Dignity of the Human Being with Regard to the Application of Biology and Medicine: Convention on Human Rights and Biomedicine* (ETS No. 164). http://conventions.coe.int/Treaty/en/Reports/Html/164.htm

16. Gutmann Th, Daar AS, Land W, Sells RA, eds. *Ethical, Legal And Social Issues in Organ Transplantation.* Lengerich and Berlin: Pabst Science Publishers; 2004.

17. Enquete-Kommission Ethik und Recht der modernen Medizin des Deutschen Bundestages. *Zwischenbericht Organlebendspende.* BT-Drs. (Parliamentary Document) 15/5050, March 17, 2005. http://www.bundestag.de /parlament/kommissionen/ethik_med/index.html.

18. Nielsen L. Living Organ Donors—Legal Perspectives from Western Europe. In: Price D, Akveld H, eds. *Living Organ Donation in the Nineties: European Medico-Legal Perspectives (EUROTOLD).* Leicester; 1996:63.

19. Hoyer J. A Nondirected Kidney Donation and its Consequences. Personal Experience of a Transplant Surgeon. *Transplantation* 2003; 76:1264.

20. Kranenburg L, Visak T, Weimar W, et al. Starting a Crossover Kidney Transplantation Program in The Netherlands: Ethical and Psychological Considerations. *Transplantation* 2004;78:194.

21. de Klerk M, Keizer SW, Weimar W. Donor Exchange for Renal Transplantation. *N Engl J Med* 2004;351:935.

22. Veatch RM. Theories of Medical Ethics: The Professional Model Compared With the Societal Model. In: Land W, Dossetor JB, eds. *Organ Replacement Therapy: Ethics, Justice and Commerce.* Berlin/Heidelberg/New York: Springer; 1992:3.

23. Beauchamp TL, Childress JF. *Principles of Biomedical Ethics.* 5th ed. Oxford: Oxford University Press; 2001.

24. United Network for Organ Sharing 1991 Ethics Committee: Ethics of Organ Transplantation from Living Donors. *Transp Proc* 1992;24:2236.

25. Veatch RM. *Transplantation Ethics*. Washington: Georgetown University Press; 2000.

26. Häyry H. *The Limits of Medical Paternalism*. London: Routledge; 1991.

27. Dworkin R. *Life's Dominion*. London: Harper Collins; 1993.

28. Childress JF. The Place of Autonomy in Bioethics. *Hastings Cent Rep* 1990;20:12.

29. The Ethics Committee of the Transplantation Society: The Consensus Statement of the Amsterdam Forum on the Care of the Live Kidney Donor. *Transplantation* 2004;78:491.

30. Delmonico FL, Surman OS. Is This Live-Organ Donor Your Patient? *Transplantation* 2003;76:1257.

31. Steiner R, Gert B. Ethical Selection of Living Kidney Donors. *Am J Kidn Dis* 2000;36: 677.

32. Price D. Transplant Clinicians as Moral Gatekeepers: Is this Role Simply one of Respecting the Autonomy of Persons? In: Gutmann T, Daar AS, Land W, Sells RA, eds. *Ethical, Legal And Social Issues in Organ Transplantation*, Lengerich/Berlin: Pabst Science Publishers; 2004:143.

33. Elliott C, Doing Harm. Living Organ Donors, Clinical Research and The Tenth Man. *J Med Ethics* 1995;21:91.

34. Schneewind KA. Psychological Aspects in Living Organ Donation. In: Collins GM, Dubernard JM, Persijn GG, Land W, eds. *Procurement and Preservation of Vascularized Organs*. Dordrecht:Kluwer; 1997:325.

35. Gutmann T, Elsaesser A, Gruendel J, Land W, Schneewind KA, Schroth U. Living Kidney Donation: Safety by Procedure. In: Terasaki PI, ed. *Clinical Transplants* 1994. UCLA: Los Angeles; 1995:356.

36. A Report of the Amsterdam Forum On the Care of the Live Kidney Donor: Data and Medical Guidelines. *Transplantation* 2004;79:S53.

37. Cronin DC, Chiappori PA, Siegler M. The Changing Spectrum of Risk/Benefit in Living Organ Donation. In Gutmann T, Daar AS, Land W, Sells RA, eds: *Ethical, Legal And Social Issues in Organ Transplantation*. Lengerich/Berlin: Pabst Science Publishers; 2004:123.

38. Gilbert JC, Brigham L, Batty DS, Veatch RM. The Nondirected Living Donor Program: A Model for Cooperative Donation, Recovery and Allocation of Living Donor Kidneys. *Am J Transpl* 2005;5:167.

39. Biller-Andorno N. Gender Imbalance in Living Organ Donation. *Med Health Care Philosophy* 2002;5:199.

40. Deutsche Stiftung Organtransplantation. *Organspende und Transplantation in Deutschland* 2004. Neu-Isenburg 2005 and http://www.dso.de/.

# DONOR COUNSELING AND CONSENT

## 4.1  TEACHING AND TESTING THE KNOWLEDGE AND THINKING OF LIVING ORGAN DONORS

*Robert W. Steiner, MD, Christine A. Frederici, LCSW, Rodolfo R. Batarse, MD, Bernard Gert, PhD*

### DEVELOPING FACTUAL INFORMATION ABOUT DONOR RISK

This chapter deals with developing and teaching comprehensive factual information about risk and benefit to enable living organ donors to make defensible decisions about donation. Other complexities of living donor selection are well reviewed elsewhere.[1-5]

It will not do just to cite "risk factors" to formulate risk for donors. For example, for kidney donors, high normal blood pressure, African race, and certainly young age are "risk factors" for eventual kidney disease, but they do not preclude donation. Centers can only teach donors in a defensible fashion if they quantify risk. For example, *always in need of formulation* is the donor's predonation baseline risk of postdonation disease in the organ to be donated. Donor risk must be formulated as a risk of a *defined entity* (eg, end-stage renal disease [ESRD]) over a defined *time period* (eg, the next 20 years). For example, the lifetime risk of ESRD for unselected individuals living to their mid-70s is almost 3% for whites and 7% for blacks,[6] and most occurs well after middle age,[7] which would serve as an upper limit of risk for the healthier donor cohort. Pancreas and kidney donors should know the long-term population risk of type II diabetes and the likelihood and pace of the major complications of diabetes for themselves. (The risk of type II diabetes is now approaching 30% in the general population[8]). Many centers accept kidney donors with borderline abnormalities such as mild hypertension or nephrolithiasis,[9] and for these donors, the long-term risks for ESRD can also be formulated from literature and from population prevalence of risk factors and disease incidence.[7] Data also exist to help quantify the expected loss of postoperative function of remaining donor kidney,[10] liver,[11,12] and lung.[13,14] Formulating long term requires study and synthesis of relevant literature.[7,15] Information that is presented in other chapters of this book will greatly assist in formulating this risk. Perioperative risk has been relatively well reported for all organ donors.[11,16-23] Risks that are so derived may only be valid to the nearest log value (less than 1 in 10, less than 1 in 1,000), and these uncertainties must be com-municated to donors. As imprecise as risk estimates may be, even the most careful donor candidate will not have more complete predictive information for most other life decisions. The alternatives to semiquantifying risk are less appealing. They are either to use the ungrounded phrases "high risk" or "low risk" without any idea (and certainly not the *same* idea) of actual numerical risk by either counselor or donor candidate or to not discuss risk at all. In these cases, of course, meaningful donor education, so central to ethical donation,[1] will not occur. Donors cannot responsibly be asked to decide to donate when they have "no idea" of what they are risking, any more than they should agree to a mortgage without knowing the amount they are borrowing. The practice of transplantation continues today because centers in fact have formed general, largely subliminal appreciations of many donor risks, but these must be articulated, defended, and tested against actual population data.[24]

### DEVELOPING FACTUAL INFORMATION ABOUT RECIPIENT BENEFIT

The nature and likelihood of recipient benefit should be quantified because it is also essential to a defensible donor decision. Prospective pancreas donors, for example, would want to know: what is the expected survival (mean, 25th and 75th percentile) of transplanted pancreata and of pancreas transplant recipients? What are the quality of life, morbidity, and longevity benefits of living versus deceased pancreas donation vs. insulin treatment? What are the limitations of successful pancreas transplantation on recipient benefit (improvement of neuropathy, etc)? Data to answer many of these questions are available at www.unos.org and change little from year to year. In some studies, donors whose recipients have done poorly have the most persistent psychological problems,[25,26] suggesting the need to emphasize pretransplant the reality of unavoidable poor outcomes in a predictable fraction of recipients. In the event of graft failure or recipient death within the first year, donors should not feel that they were misled or otherwise poorly counseled.

### STRUCTURED TESTING OF LIVING ORGAN DONORS

Many centers as yet do not employ independent donor advocates to counter their inherent conflicts of interest, and it may be hard to find informed and effective outside parties to fill this role.[2,27] In any case, the center must try to be as effective and impartial in educating its donors about the decision to donate as would be a donor advocate. The Vancouver Forum produced a valuable summary of principles for care of organ donors, but it recommended repetition of facts by the center as the primary means of educating donors about risk and benefit.[1] Repetitive exposure is less effective than requiring active feedback to verify that donors have assimilated the required information. This direct testing addresses the concerns of some ethicists that donors do not "really understand" or do not "really listen," insofar as these ethical concerns relate to testable hypotheses. Some donors who are greatly affected by the plight of the recipient are romanticizing donation or are not thinking clearly for other reasons may be immune to repetition.[28] Testing requiring explicit feedback to the center identifies these "poorly educated" donors, who are not internalizing and processing new information adequately.

**TABLE 4.1-1**
**TRUE–FALSE QUESTIONS FOR KIDNEY DONORS**

No matter how strongly we might feel about helping someone with kidney failure, each of us needs to know the facts to decide if donation is right or wrong for us. This true–false test will help determine if you have learned the essential facts about living kidney donation, so you can make a good decision for yourself.

1. Kidney transplantation is usually life saving.

   (True………False……..)

2. Donors have pain after kidney donation.

   (True………False……..)

3. Half of all living kidney donor transplants work more than 15 years.

   (True………False……..)

4. Cadaver donor kidneys only last 1–2 years and are not a good option.

   (True………False……..)

5. If I develop a kidney problem later in life after kidney donation, the Transplant Center will take care of it at no charge.

   (True………False……..)

6. The waiting time for a deceased donor kidney averages 4 to 5 years.

   (True………False……..)

7. Transplantation is usually a better treatment for kidney disease than dialysis.

   (True………False……..)

8. After transplantation, the recipient must take medicine and see the doctor regularly to keep the transplant working.

   (True………False……..)

9. Results of a donor's medical evaluation should be confidential.

   (True………False……..)

10. Donating a kidney causes kidney disease.

    (True………False……..)

11. The lifetime risk for dialysis in the general population is between 3% and 7% depending on race.

    (True………False……..)

12. The Transplant Center should never refuse a willing donor.

    (True………False……..)

(Our answers: 1:F, 2:T, 3:T, 4:F, 5:F, 6:T, 7:T, 8:T, 9:T; 10:F, 11:T, 12:F)

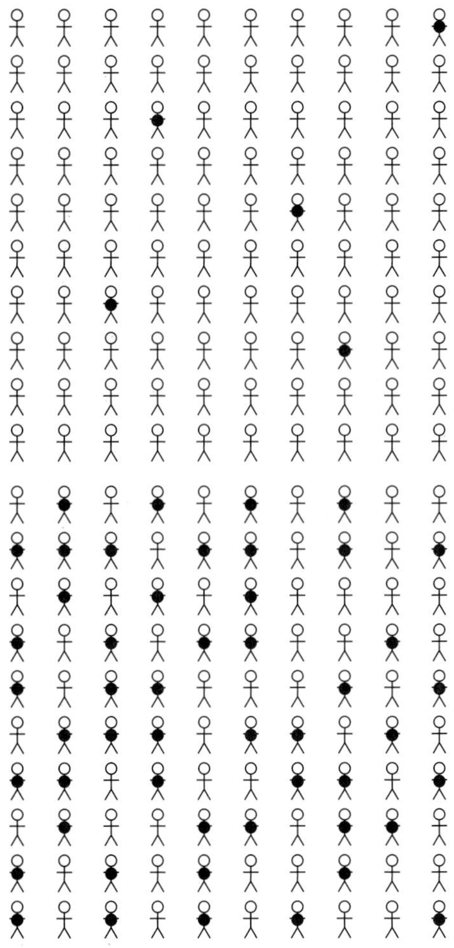

**FIGURE 4.1-1**

Conveying Essential Data Objectively to Donor Candidates by Means of Stick Figure Fields. The top panel conveys a 5% (5 per hundred) ratio and could, for example, be used to illustrate the number of living donor kidney recipients who have less than a year of graft function. The bottom panel conveys a 50% occurrence and can be used to illustrate the number of people transplanted with a deceased donor kidney at the "average" waiting time on the waiting list (about 5 years for many recipients). It also illustrates the number of recipients back on dialysis (or dead, in the case of most other transplants) at the survival half-life of the transplanted organ (about 9 years in the case of deceased donor kidneys).

## TOOLS TO TEACH DONORS ABOUT RISK AND BENEFIT

Our program requires donors to demonstrate both their mastery of basic factual knowledge and their thought processes leading to their decision to donate. We first use a true–false test containing statements about risks and benefits of deceased donor and living donor kidney transplantation (Table 4.1-1). The second donor test (Figure 4.1-1) presents quantitative data by means of a set of stick figure fields,[29] a subset of which is altered to reflect the estimated proportion of adverse outcomes (Figure 4.1-1). A field of 1,000 with two blackened reflects a 0.2% risk, for example, of liver donor perioperative mortality.[11] Risk limits and risk ranges can be presented the same way. Stick figures help emphasize the all-or-nothing nature of an event, that is, the fact that over one half of lung transplant recipients will be dead at 5 years (www.unos.org, 8/06) does not mean that all recipients will be 50%

impaired at 5 years. Presenting risk data this way, instead of by saying "low risk," avoids an implicit recommendation, that is, "low risk" means "I urge you to donate," which violates the center's neutrality.

## THE DONOR BELIEF PROFILE

There are recurring concerns among donor counselors that some donors who are acting freely seem to be informed and have an acceptable risk/benefit ratio may not have adequately thought through their decision to donate. To test the donor's ancillary beliefs and values that support the decision to donate, we ask donors' opinions on a number of statements expressing beliefs

### TABLE 4.1-2
### THE DONOR BELIEF PROFILE

#### SHOULD I DONATE A KIDNEY?

The personal decision to donate a kidney should not be made without considering all the outcomes and options. Take some time to indicate if you agree or disagree with each statement below, or if you are honestly still undecided. If you are undecided about many of these statements, or if you find you have beliefs that might make donation wrong for you, we should talk more about your wish to donate a kidney.

I can accept the pain, inconvenience, and uncertainty of a major operation.

I agree......... I disagree........I am uncertain.......

I think that kidney transplantation provides sufficient advantages over dialysis.

I agree......... I disagree........I am uncertain.......

I do not want to take any risks with my health.

I agree......... I disagree........I am uncertain.......

I feel that waiting several years for a cadaver kidney or being on long-term dialysis are reasonable and acceptable alternatives for the recipient.

I agree......... I disagree........I am uncertain.......

I can accept the fact that sooner or later my donated kidney will fail.

I agree......... I disagree........I am uncertain.......

I think that living donor kidney transplantation provides sufficient advantages over dialysis.

I agree......... I disagree........I am uncertain.......

I do not think that the recipient will take care of the kidney.

I agree......... I disagree........I am uncertain.......

I do not understand the facts surrounding kidney donation.

I agree......... I disagree........I am uncertain.......

I feel pressured to do something I really do not want to do.

I agree......... I disagree........I am uncertain.......

I can accept that if I develop kidney disease later in life, I will need dialysis at least 20% sooner if I have only one kidney.

I agree......... I disagree........I am uncertain.......

Even though I want to donate, I should think longer about such an important decision.

I agree......... I disagree........I am uncertain.......

and judgments that underlie rational decisions to donate or not to donate (Table 4.1-2). Some of these statements support and others go against donation. This nondirectional testing reminds the donor of both the ramifications of his or her decision and the intellectual processing needed to make a good decision. It helps the center see how well the donor has thought through the decision to donate. That is, to decide acceptably to donate a kidney, one should have a reasoned opinion on the preferability of kidney transplantation to chronic dialysis and the acceptability of the donor operation. Some donors seem surprised and unprepared when we ask these questions, which indicates inappropriate decision making. When taking true–false, stick figure, and belief profile tests, donors are encouraged to discuss their understanding of the questions and explain their response—particularly if it seems wrong—to display and clarify their thinking. Most take the tests in writing, but some may have the questions read to them. For the true—false and stick figure tests, a wrong answer is followed by a review of the facts that were presented to the candidate in information sessions, and the correct answer is required. Donors who perform poorly on the belief profile are not "corrected," but may withdraw or spend more time organizing their thoughts and be tested again. The tests are administered by a well-trained social worker, and the team meets periodically to rephrase or change questions and to update facts.

## REJECTING DONORS

Many centers usually just say that donors are "inappropriate" or "too risky" when they are rejected, but donor refusal is more complicated than that. Refusal of the occasional donor who wishes to take irrational risk and the complex ethical issues involved in rejecting heroic donors are discussed elsewhere.[4] For the rest, many donors are not rejected because they are known to not be deciding freely or known not to be informed or thinking rationally, but because the center is not sufficiently assured that they are informed, deciding freely, and thinking rationally.[5] Likewise, uncertainty about donor risk is a legitimate reason for donor refusal, not because that risk is known to be high, but because that risk cannot be satisfactorily estimated at all, despite the best efforts of the center. Donors with truly unknown risk cannot be counseled and, more importantly, cannot make a rational decision. The inability to formulate risk is in fact the perfectly defensible explanation for why many donors are currently rejected, not that their risk is known to be high. If their risks can be researched and comfortably estimated by centers, some of these donors may not appear to be too risky. In any case, the center should articulate its specific reasons for rejecting a given donor to try to improve its internal donor selection processes and to provide accurate feedback to the donor. Donor testing helps affirm certain donor characteristics; it removes some donors from the "uncertain" category to the "known" to be acceptable or unacceptable.

Centers should not decline to test donors because they are afraid that donors could not pass these tests. Any person who decides to give up all or part of a vital organ and cannot pass these simple tests does not have sufficient information to make a defensible decision. This may be because the donor needs more education, is incapable of understanding these basic data, or is not involved enough to be thinking clearly about the decision to donate. This may happen with donors who are receiving compensation, who need not concern themselves with outcome data, for example. In our experience, almost all legitimate donor candidates can be successfully educated and tested this way.

The true–false, stick figure, and belief profile questionnaires may be modified by individual centers according to their interpretation of the medical literature and their prioritization of important donor issues. Centers should be just as complete in addressing risks of unwanted outcomes as they are in presenting positive information about safety to donors and benefits to recipients. The goal is to develop some reasonably comprehensive but succinct standardized tools to assess donor knowledge in important areas and reinforce the donor's responsibility to learn and decide appropriately. In constructing this testing, donors should be told when centers do not agree among themselves on "factual" material. For instance, our center is fully aware of the literature on improved patient survival afforded by renal transplantation.[30] Even if we accept that these retrospective studies have adequately account for selection bias, we still feel we must explain to donors that we do not feel that kidney transplantation is a "life-saving" procedure in the same sense as transplantation of a liver, heart, or lung. Likewise, the benefits of preemptive living donor renal transplantation are difficult for us to quantify in some cases. Studies on the benefit of preemptive transplantation must use data from past eras,[31] when preemptive patients had less renal function than is the case for many preemptive transplants today. Many entirely successful preemptive kidney transplants today provide lower multiples of the level of pretransplant renal function, but require the risks of full dose immunosuppression just the same. Moreover, one retrospective database study supports young patients waiting for an optimal kidney for several years on dialysis, which supplies about 10% of normal renal function, which is counter to the supposed benefits of dialysis avoidance and renal functional improvement with early preemptive transplantation.[31]

Risk quantification in itself only provides a number; it does not tell a center whether a risk is "high" or "low," but many centers feel a risk of 1 in 100 is "small."[7] How semiquantitative estimation of risk and benefit might influence the overall donor acceptance policies of centers is outside the scope of this chapter but needs to be addressed by the transplant profession, as does moving toward a consensus on estimates of the basic risks themselves. For now, each center must make its own best decisions. In the long run, more mature, standardized living donor selection protocols, which include risk estimation and direct donor testing, seem inevitable and will evolve and improve as they gain more widespread acceptance.

## References

1. Pruett T, Tibell A, Alabdulkareem A, et al. The ethics statement of the Vancouver forum on the live lung, liver, pancreas, and intestine donor. *Transplantation* 2006;81(10):1386.
2. Wright L, Faith K, Richardson R, et al. Ethical guidelines for the evaluation of living organ donors. *Can J Surg* 2004;47(6):408–413.
3. Barr ML, Belghiti J, Villamil FG, et al. A report of the Vancouver forum on the care of the live organ donor: lung, liver, pancreas and intestine data and medical guidelines. *Transplantation* 2006;8 (10):1373–1385.
4. Steiner RW, Gert B. Ethical selection of living kidney donors. *AJKD* 2000;36(4):677–686.
5. The Authors for the Live Organ Donor Consensus Group. Consensus statement on the live organ donor. *JAMA* 2000;284:2919–2926.
6. Kiberd BA, Clase CM. Cumulative risk for developing end-stage renal disease in US population. *J Am Soc Nephrol* 2002;13:1635–1644.
7. Steiner RW, Danovitch G. The Medical Evaluation and Risk Estimation of End Stage Renal Disease for Living Kidney Donors. In: Steiner R. ed. *Educating, Evaluating, and Selecting Living Kidney Donors.* Dordrecht: Kluwer Acdemic; 2004:51–70.
8. Narayan KMV, Boyle JP, Thompson TJ, et al. Lifetime risk for diabetes mellitus in the United States. *JAMA* 2003; 290 (14):1884–1890.
9. Bia MJ, Ramos EL, Danovitch GM, et al. Evaluation of living renal donors. *Transplantation* 1995; 26: 376–398.
10. Kasiske BL, Ma JZ, Louis TA, et al. Long-term effects of reduced renal mass in humans. *Kidney Int* 1995;48(3):814–819.
11. Middleton PF, Duffield M, Lyncy SV, et al. Living donor liver transplantation—adult donor outcomes: a systematic review. *Liver Transpl* 2005;12:24–30.
12. Pomfret EA, Pomposelli JJ, Lewis WD, et al. Live donor adult transplantation using right lobe grafts. *Arch Surg* 2001;136:425–433.
13. Barr ML, Baker CJ, Schenkel FA, et al. Living donor lung transplantation: Selection, technique, and outcome. *Transplant Proc* 2001;33:3527–3532.
14. Yoon HE, Huddleston CB, Miyoshi S, et al. Pulmonary function after living donor lung transplantation. *Transplant Proc* 2001;33:1626–1627.
15. Steiner RW. Risk appreciation for living kidney donors: Another new subspecialty? *AJT* 2004;4:694–697.
16. Trotter JF, Talamantes M, McClure M, et al. Right hepatic lobe donation for living donor liver transplantation: impact on donor quality of life. *Liver Transplant* 2001;7(6):485–493.
17. Karliova M, Malago M, Valentin-Gamazo C, et al. Living-related liver transplantation from the view of the donor: a 1-year follow-up survey. *Transplantation* 2002;73(11):1799–1804.
18. Fujita S, Kim ID, Uryuhara K, et al. Hepatic grafts from live donors: Donor morbidity for 470 cases of live donation. *Transpl Int* 2000;13:333–339.
19. Broering DC, Wilms C, Bok P, et al. Evolution of donor morbidity in living related liver transplantation. *Annals Surg* 2004;240(6):1013.
20. Sharara AI, Dandan IS, Khalifeh M. Living related donor transplantation other than kidney. *Transplant Proc* 2001;33: 2745–2746.
21. Gruessner RW, Kendall DM, Drangstveit MB, et al. Simultaneous pancreas–kidney transplantation from live donors. *Annals Surg* 1997; 226(4):471–482.
22. Gruessner RWG, Sutherland DER. Living donor pancreas transplantation. *Transplant Rev* 2002;16(2):108–119.
23. Tesi R, Beck R, Lambiase L, et al. Living-related small bowel transplantation: Donor evaluation and outcome. *Transplant Proc* 1997;29:686–687.
24. Steiner RW, Mullaney SR. Estimating risk for "high risk" kidney donors. *Clin Transplant* 2006;20(16):22–23.
25. Johnson EM, Anderson JK, Jacobs C, et al. Long-term follow-up of living kidney donors: Quality of life after donation. *Transplantation* 1999;67 (5):717–721.
26. Kim-Schluger L, Florman SS, Schiano T, et al. Quality of life after lobectomy for adult liver transplantation. *Transplantation* 2002;73(10):1593–1597.
27. K, Neitzke G. Structure, methodology and ethics of German commissions on living organ donation. *Dtsch Med Wochenschr* 2006;131(22):1283–1287.
28. Biller-Andorno N, Schauenburg H. Is it only love? Some pitfalls in emotionally related organ donation. *Med Ethics* 2001;27(3):162–164.
29. Steiner RW, Gert B. A technique for presenting risk and outcome data to potential living renal transplant donors. *Transplantation* 2001; 71(8):1056–1057.
30. Ruiz-Ramon P, Hunsicker L. Outcomes for Living Donor and Cadaver Donor Kidney Transplantation. In: Steiner R. ed. *Educating, Evaluating, and Selecting Living Kidney Donors.* Dordrecht: Kluwer Acdemic Publishers; 2004:35–49.
31. Meier-Kriesche HU, Schold JD. The impact of pretransplant dialysis on outcomes in renal transplantation. *Semin Dial* 2003(Nov–Dec);18(6);499–504.
32. Schold JD, Srinivas TR, Kaplan B, et al. Younger ESRD patients may benefit from waiting for higher organ quality for renal transplantation despite of deleterious effects of dialysis. *ASN* 2005;(Abstract).

## 4.2    INFORMED CONSENT

*Aaron Spital, MD*

Family members have been donating kidneys to loved ones in need for over half a century.[1] In the early years of transplantation the vast majority of living donors were blood relatives.[2] Today, genetically unrelated volunteers make an important contribution to the living donor pool,[3,4] which now also includes people who donate extrarenal organs.[5,6] In all these cases, there is the unlikely but real possibility that the donor will experience a major complication or even death. Thus living organ donation has always been troubled by the following question: how can one justify subjecting a healthy person to the risk of major surgery for the sole purpose of benefiting another?[7] After more than 50 years of discussion and experience with thousands of living donors, this question continues to haunt us.[8–15] Indeed, concern about harming the donor is arguably the most worrying part of living organ donation.[3,9,12] This concern is actually growing because the number of living donors is increasing and because removing segments of nonrenal organs poses more risk than does nephrectomy.

One of the main justifications for allowing volunteers to donate organs despite the risk of harm is the belief that people should be free to make their own choices and to decide for themselves whether the benefit of an action is worth the risk.[16–19] This maxim is embodied in the principle of respect for individual autonomy (the right to self-rule), which is a fundamental value of free societies.[20] This major principle of biomedical ethics requires that we answer the following questions when considering a potential living organ donor: is donation consistent with this person's values and goals, and does she really want to donate despite understanding the risks involved? Asked in another way, is this person acting autonomously?[20,21] Acceptance requires that the answer be yes.

Throughout the history of transplantation, physicians have relied on the doctrine of informed consent to help make this determination.[5,6,8,10.22–28] Indeed, informed consent is generally considered an absolute requirement for accepting people as living organ donors. This approach is concordant with the principles and guidelines for the protection of human research subjects articulated in the influential Belmont Report:[29] "Respect for persons requires that subjects . . . be given the opportunity to choose what shall or shall not happen to them. This opportunity is provided, when adequate standards of informed consent are satisfied." But sometimes there are problems obtaining informed consent from donor candidates. What are these problems? Are there other acceptable mechanisms for authorizing donation? Is an autonomous genuine offer sufficient ground for accepting a potential donor? Do people have a right to donate an organ? This section tries to answer these questions. I begin with an overview of the purpose and elements of informed consent.

### WHAT IS THE PURPOSE OF INFORMED CONSENT?

The original purpose of informed consent was to protect patients and research subjects from harm and exploitation. Although these are still important goals, over the years informed consent has come to be seen primarily as a mechanism for protecting autonomous choice.[11,20(pp77)] When a person gives informed consent to living organ donation we assume that donation is consistent with

her values and goals and that the choice expressed is truly her own. To understand how informed consent allows us to reach these conclusions we need to review its components.

### THE ELEMENTS OF INFORMED CONSENT AND THEIR APPLICATION TO LIVING ORGAN DONATION

The key elements of informed consent are:[11,20] (1) competence to process relevant information and reach a reasoned decision, (2) disclosure of all relevant material, (3) understanding of what has been disclosed, (4) freedom to choose, and (5) a decision to authorize or not to authorize the action being considered. Let us now examine these elements within the context of living organ donation.

### Competence

According to Beauchamp and Childress,[20(pp71)] people are competent to make a decision "if they have the capacity to understand the material information, to make a judgment about the information in light of their values, to intend a certain outcome, and to communicate freely their wishes . . .". To be considered competent to decide about living organ donation, a person must be able to understand the risks for herself as well as the likelihood of success and the alternative treatments available for the recipient.[30] All potential living organ donors should be evaluated for competence by a skilled mental health professional,[22,25,31] who should assume that adults are competent unless proven otherwise.[32]

### Disclosure

Good decision making requires understanding of all relevant key information. In an attempt to provide guidance in this important area, The Advisory Committee on Organ Transplantation[27] and several consensus statements[22,25,31] have constructed lists of facts that should be communicated to all potential organ donors. These include (1) a description of the donor evaluation, surgery, and recuperation, including the need for postoperative physical and social support; (2) the potential short and long-term risks for the donor (physical and psychological), including the risk of death; (3) the potential impact of donation on the donor's finances, employment, and insurability; (4) the risks and probability of success for the intended recipient, including the possibility that the graft may never function; (5) alternative treatments for the intended recipient and his prognosis if the volunteer does not donate; (6) the fact that the volunteer may withdraw her offer at any time; and (7) center specific statistics regarding living donor and recipient outcomes.

Despite these guidelines, there is much variability among centers regarding the information disclosed to donor candidates.[14,33] One of the barriers to standardization here is that the risks of living organ donation have not been defined precisely, especially in cases where the volunteer is not perfectly healthy.[12,14,15] Despite these uncertainties, it is often possible to provide some quantitative estimate of risk, at least for kidney donors.[14,15] Furthermore, Price has pointed out that an incomplete database does not eliminate the possibility of informed consent as long as the uncertainty is communicated to the volunteer.[26(p281)]

To maximize the probability that potential living donors will be well informed, transplant centers should develop and distribute easily understood written and audiovisual information that is organ specific, attempts to quantify risk, and that reviews the key facts that might influence the volunteer's final decision.[25,26(p281),33] Because of the potential for conflict of interest, at least some of the professionals who educate and counsel the potential donor should function as independent donor advocates that have no vested interest in or relationship to the intended recipient.[22,25,27,31]

## Understanding

Provision of relevant information is necessary but not sufficient when counseling a potential living organ donor. Understanding and acceptance of the material presented are also essential.[14,20 p79,26(p280)] So important is understanding that some authors believe that volunteers should be rejected whenever their understanding is in doubt.[14] But given the quantity and complexity of material that must be covered, achieving full understanding may be difficult in this setting,[34] a point to which I will soon return.

## Freedom to Choose

Freedom to choose is essential for autonomous action;[20(p58),21] without such freedom, consent is invalid.[14,26(p289)] Some authors, though not all,[9,12] see this issue as the main ethical concern regarding living organ donation.[35,36] People contemplating living organ donation may experience various pressures that may limit their ability to make a completely unencumbered choice.[5,16,26 (p295),37,38] These pressures may be internal, resulting from feelings of obligation and guilt, or they may be external, as when one person (eg, the spouse of the potential recipient or a health-care professional) tries to convince another to donate an organ.

## Reaching a Decision

Two safeguards relevant to this stage of the informed consent process have been suggested. First, that consent be obtained twice: initially for the evaluation of suitability and then for the donor operation (assuming the volunteer was found to be acceptable). Second, that a short waiting period of about 2 weeks be imposed after the second consent to allow the volunteer ample time to reconsider her decision and withdraw.[5,6,25,31,39]

## BARRIERS TO INFORMED CONSENT AMONG POTENTIAL LIVING ORGAN DONORS

Determining competence of potential organ donors is important but does not pose a major barrier to informed consent. Adequate disclosure is more of a concern because discussion of every possibly relevant fact is impractical. But as long as disclosure is sufficient (see previously for what must be disclosed), the fact that it may not be entirely complete does not render consent invalid.[34] In the context of living organ donation, the elements of informed consent that are most concerning are the level of understanding of what is disclosed and the ability to choose freely.[13,38]

## Concerns About Understanding

There has long been concern that living organ donors may not fully understand the possible consequences of donating an organ

(or a part of one). Over 35 years ago, Fellner and Marshall interviewed living related kidney donors and found that most of them decided to donate immediately upon hearing of the need:[40] "Not one of the donors weighed alternatives and rationally decided." Furthermore, "With regard to the instructions and explanations offered repeatedly by the doctors of the renal transplant team in an attempt to provide the basis for an informed consent, the donors all reported that they had not really been very curious or interested in what the doctors were telling them."[41] Similar observations were made by Simmons et al. who found that 78% of 130 donors interviewed knew right away that they would donate, and 62% were classified as having made an immediate choice; only 25% decided in a way that accorded with the informed consent model.[42] Simmons and her colleagues concluded:[42] "the majority of donors volunteer immediately upon hearing of the need without any time delay or any period of deliberation." A more recent study of living kidney donors showed that this has not changed: 75% of them decided almost immediately and disclosure of relevant information did not affect their decisions.[43] These observations strongly suggest that potential organ donors often make decisions in the face of limited understanding, an observation that led Fellner and Marshall to conclude that for many donors informed consent is a myth.[40] This issue remains a concern today.[12,43,44]

## Concerns About Freedom to Choose

Another major concern regarding the validity of consent is that some living donors may offer to donate not because they really want to but because they feel they must.[12,16,26(p294),35,37,38,45,46] Although such feelings can result from pressure exerted by other people, overt external pressure is unusual[43,47,48] and can usually be detected by a skilled mental health professional during the psychosocial evaluation. More concerning is the effect of pressure that arises from within out of a sense of duty or guilt.[37,38,46,47] Because most donors are at least emotionally related to their recipients, many of them feel obligated to donate and that they have no real choice.[37,38] If a person who could donate decides to say no, how could she face her ill relative, her family, and herself?[13,47]

## MAY CONSENT THAT IS NOT FULLY INFORMED AND FREE FROM ALL PRESSURE STILL BE VALID?

In its report on the use of human tissue, The Nuffield Council on Bioethics concluded:[34] "'Fully informed consent' is . . . an unattainable ideal." Other authors have expressed similar views.[49] This limitation has been a source of appropriate concern for transplant professionals who evaluate potential living organ donors.[12, 22,25,26(p294),28] How should we respond to this important issue?

The Nuffield Council Report concluded that:[34] "The ethically significant requirement is not that consent by complete, but that it be genuine." In other words, when assessing the validity of consent of a donor candidate, what is most important is not that there be full understanding or complete freedom to choose; what is most important is that the person really wants to donate and that donation is compatible with her values and goals—that her decision is autonomous. But can a person act autonomously when understanding or freedom to choose is incomplete? Beauchamp and Childress argue that in some cases the answer is yes:[20(p59)] "For an action to be autonomous . . . it needs only a substantial degree of understanding and freedom from constraint, not a full understanding or a complete absence of influence. To restrict adequate decision making by patients . . . to the ideal of fully or completely autonomous decision-making strips their acts of any meaningful place in the practical world, where people's actions are rarely, if ever, fully autonomous."

The thesis I am trying to develop is that, while a valid consent to living organ donation does require at least some understanding and freedom to choose, it does not require full understanding and complete freedom to choose. If this is true, how can one know when the degree of understanding and freedom is sufficient?

## Addressing Concerns About Limited Understanding

To maximize the likelihood of understanding, the following steps are suggested: (1) develop a list of essential facts (including the major risks, benefits, and alternatives for the potential donor and recipient) that must be understood by all potential donors, (2) provide this information in a simple written (and ideally audiovisual) format that can be reviewed by the candidate at her leisure, (3) communicate as clearly as possible at a level consistent with the cognitive ability of the volunteer, (4) avoid unfamiliar terms, (5) present information neutrally (by a knowledgeable professional with no vested interest in the welfare of the recipient), neither encouraging nor discouraging a particular course of action,[14] (6) avoid giving too much information at one time (information overload),[20] (7) schedule as many visits as are necessary to review all information needed to reach a well-informed decision, (8) use analogies to familiar events to help explain risks, for example comparing the risk of dying from nephrectomy to the risk of dying in an automobile accident,[20(p89)] (9) employ unbiased interpreters when evaluating volunteers who do not speak the health-care team's language,[39] (10) test for comprehension of the material disclosed,[25,26,31] and (11) explore expectations and beliefs about the impact of donation on the volunteer's health and personal relationships. If the candidate has realistic expectations and is able to demonstrate comprehension of critical information, one may conclude that understanding is sufficient. But comprehension is not enough—acceptance is also essential because false beliefs can invalidate consent even in the face of understanding.[20]

In this discussion I am assuming that the volunteer is competent. Rarely, immature minors and other incompetents have been permitted to donate organs.[50] For such donors, adequate understanding is impossible. These cases raise additional ethical questions that are not addressed in this chapter.

## Addressing Concerns About Freedom to Choose

This is arguably the major concern regarding the validity of consent among potential living organ donors.[35] Some authors worry that when the health of a loved one is at stake, feelings of guilt and/or obligation may so strongly propel people to donate that informed consent is necessarily compromised.[12,51] According to Caplan,[16] "pressures [to donate] may make it impossible for someone to choose freely." "Does anyone really think parents can say 'No' when the option is certain death for their own son or daughter?" Similarly, Adams asserts:[51] "The consent of someone to donate a kidney to a near relative never occurs without some degree of coercion." While not all authors share this extreme view, concern about coercion is a theme that pervades the living donor literature.[8,16,22,25,27,31,37,39,43,46,52,53] However, contrary

to popular belief, rarely does coercion play a role in the decision to donate, at least in the Western world.

According to Beauchamp and Childress,[20(p94)] "Coercion occurs if and only if one person intentionally uses a credible and severe threat of harm or force to control another." And Faden and Beauchamp point out that there is an important difference between coercion and coercive situations.[54] Although both conditions limit freedom, "It does not follow, however, that persons in such 'coercive situations' do not act autonomously." To exemplify the difference, they note that many patients considering life saving surgery have no real choice:[54] "But this loss of freedom cannot be equated with a loss of autonomy . . . In a true situation of coercion, what controls, and thus deprives one of autonomy, is the will of another person, substituted for one's own will or desire . . . " It is reasonable to conclude that while coercion deprives people of autonomy, coercive situations do not. How does all this apply to living organ donation?

First, having a relative in need of a transplant does not necessarily create a coercive situation—some people who could donate choose not to.[42,43] Second, many living related donors, especially parents, are not ambivalent about donating and do not find the decision a difficult one to make.[47] For such volunteers there is little reason to think that their choices were not made freely. Crouch and Elliott point this out in a discussion of mother to child organ donation:[52] "We do not believe that the parent who is offered the chance to donate part of her liver to a dying child is coerced by her love for her child, or by the exhortations of her conscience . . . Neither love nor conscience constrains the mother's autonomy; rather, they give voice to her autonomy and say something about the kind of agent she is . . ." "If we are ever to get straight about the nature of voluntariness, we must recognize that moral and emotional commitments are not exceptional, are not constraints on freedom, but rather part of ordinary human life."

Of course, there are potential donors who do find themselves in coercive situations, preferring not to donate but feeling that they have no way out. But even here it would be incorrect to conclude that these people are being coerced to donate. Remember that coercion requires that the decision be forced by another person's threat of irresistible harm[20,26,55]—a rare occurrence among potential living organ donors.

This analysis indicates that feelings of obligation and coercion are not the same, and it is only the latter that deprives one of autonomy and invalidates consent. Consistent with this view, Singer et al. point out[6] that although potential donors may experience internal pressure to donate, "The need to balance selfishness and altruism is a universal feature of family relationships. We do not think it invalidates voluntary consent."

Corollaries of this critique are that the frequent reference to and great concern about "coercion" in the living donor literature is misguided and that some degree of internal pressure is acceptable. However this does not mean that we need not look for nor worry about donor candidates who experience marked pressure to donate and step forward only because they see no way out. These people should be identified and excluded.

To detect such situations and to minimize pressure exerted on or experienced by potential living donors, several safeguards should be followed. These include (1) a private exploration of the volunteer's motivation and commitment by a skilled mental health professional who has no vested interest in the welfare of the recipient; (2) disclosure of relevant information in a neutral fashion;[14] (3) giving the volunteer as much time as possible to assimilate the disclosed material and decide; (4) reminding the candidate that she may withdraw her offer at any time up to the point of surgery;[25,27,30,31] (5) maintaining confidentiality of the candidate's evaluation; and (6) communicating to the candidate the center's willingness to provide a general statement of unsuitability[22,29] that will allow her to withdraw gracefully. However, the candidate's medical record should never be falsified.[22,25,39]

## IS INFORMED CONSENT THE ONLY ACCEPTABLE MEANS FOR AUTHORIZING LIVING ORGAN DONATION?

Most discussions of living organ donation assert that all donors must give informed consent prior to proceeding.[10,22–28,30,31,56] In general, this is appropriate. However, when potential donors and recipients are very closely related, fully informed consent may not always be possible or necessary, especially when a decision must be reached quickly.[11,13,38,40,52] To understand why, we need to reconsider the purpose of informed consent and the assumptions on which it is based.

As previously discussed, informed consent is designed to ensure autonomous choice and to protect people from harm and exploitation. The interests of many of living organ donors are served well by the informed consent requirement. But informed consent has a major limitation in this setting because it assumes that the involved parties are disinterested. As Majeske et al. point out:[38] "The traditional model of informed consent is based on an impartial understanding of the requirements of autonomy that de-emphasizes personal relationships . . . In living related donation, however, partiality and personal relationships . . . importantly influence or even constitute potential donors' personal goals." Similarly, Crouch and Elliott note:[52] "The picture of the human agent as independent and self-interested . . . is an inadequate picture of the human agent within the family . . . In families, the important factor is that family members cherish each other simply for each other's sake . . . To attempt to cram a formal relation into an intimate context does violence to the morally significant aspects of the family relationship."

These observations suggest that the nature of the donor recipient relationship influences what we should require of a valid consent. When people are very closely related, such as a parent who desperately wishes to donate an organ to save her dying child, there may be no risk of exploitation at all. And for such a parent, a detailed understanding of the donation process may be much less important to her than the welfare of the sick child she loves so dearly.[13] These points are vividly demonstrated in the recollections of a set of parents, each of whom had donated a kidney to their daughter:[57] "with our daughter's life at stake, possible future risks to the donor were not a consideration. There was no question as to 'whether.' Suzy needed, and that was all there was to it." The observation that most people would accept great risk to donate to their children indicates that many parents would respond similarly.[58,59]

It seems that when the health of a loved one is at stake, many people are willing to donate a needed organ almost regardless of the risks involved simply because the person they wish to save is so important to them. Concerned relatives often decide to donate very quickly[40–43] and seem to base their decisions primarily on care and concern rather than on a careful weighing of the medical pros and cons of donating.[13,60] Rapid decisions are not surprising here given that for some volunteers all the key facts may be immediately available.[13] These are: (1) a loved one is very ill, (2) the volunteer has the opportunity to save her by donating an organ, (3) donation and transplantation are accepted and effective practices, (4) other therapeutic approaches do not exist or are less likely to be successful, and (5) making sacrifices for loved ones is a moral norm. This list includes the key ingredients thought to be necessary for "moral decision making" by potential living organ donors.[40] Additional data required by the traditional deliberative consent model may be unimportant to people who are willing to do whatever is necessary to save a loved one.

Based on these considerations, it may not make sense to require the same stringent informed consent from devoted parents and other committed relatives as we would demand from less closely related volunteers. As Majeske et al. point out:[38] "The traditional requirements of informed consent do not appear well suited to evaluations of living related donors' decision making . . . with its frequent emphasis on feelings of relatedness, interconnectedness, and obligation—a sharp contrast to the unpressured, rational decision making typically said to underlie informed consent. [In personal relationships] our actions are not a result of fixed rules or some sort of decision-making calculus but of affection and regard for the related other." Thus, rapid consent that emanates from deep affection may sometimes be just as valid as consent that is fully informed. In agreement with this view, Ubel and Mahowald assert:[61] "The medical profession should not demand that all donors base their decisions on rational reflection, but should permit immediate decision making as an expression of autonomy." Similarly, Sauder and Parker conclude:[11] "to fail to accept a prospective donor's decision because it was made too immediately or on the basis of emotion, not rational and prudential consideration of foreseeable risks and benefits, would violate the spirit of informed consent in mistaken service of the supposed letter of the doctrine's requirements. To discount or declare invalid such a decision is to largely ignore the context in which the offer was made, the relevance of the relationships of the parties involved, and the importance of those relationships for the values of the decisionmaker."

If this view is correct, how can one know if the donor–recipient relationship is such that we may accept consent that appears to emanate primarily from care and concern rather than from a careful weighing of risks and benefits? I believe that this can be determined by a skilled mental health professional during a private exploration of the potential donor's motivation and her relationship to the intended recipient. Consent that appears to derive from care and concern rather than careful deliberation may be considered acceptable only when the interviewer concludes that the volunteer is psychologically stable, closely related to the recipient, deeply concerned about her welfare, very committed to donating, not ambivalent, and free from external pressure.[13]

None of this should be interpreted to mean that we may relax our efforts to obtain informed consent from potential donors, even those who are very closely related to their intended recipients. Unquestionably, it is our job to educate all potential donors as much as possible and we should always try to obtain fully informed consent. But sometimes understanding may remain incomplete despite our best efforts to educate. When potential donors are tightly bound to their intended recipients, they may not use the traditional deliberative approach to decision making, especially if the recipient's need is urgent. In these cases, as long as the volunteer recognizes that donation carries risk of serious harm (including death) and that there is no guarantee of success, a rapid consent that emanates from care and concern may be just a valid as one that is fully informed. For volunteers who are not related to the intended recipient, fully informed consent is essential.[3,13]

# DO PEOPLE HAVE A RIGHT TO DONATE AN ORGAN?

Consider a volunteer whose offer to donate an organ is genuine and whose consent is thought to be valid. Is this person's consent sufficient ground for proceeding and does she have a right to donate? As Carl Elliott points out,[9] "in a moral framework whose dominant principle is respect for individual autonomy" the answer to these questions would seem to be yes and some authors appear to hold this view. For example, John Harris argues:[62] "If I decide that I would like to donate one of my kidneys and run the risks of the procedure . . . then it seems that this is a matter for me [to decide]. Like all other risks that I choose to run . . . these are matters of personal choice."

Although I agree that respect for autonomy is extremely important, in contrast to Harris, I believe that a decision to proceed with organ donation requires more than donor consent and that people do not have an absolute right to donate an organ.[13]

## Beyond Donor Autonomy

Beauchamp and Childress[63] define rights as "justified claims that individuals and groups can make upon other individuals or upon society; to have a right is to be in a position to determine, by one's choices, what others should do or need not do." Rights correlate with obligations, obligations not to interfere with a person's chosen action or to provide someone with that to which she is entitled. Because a person cannot nephrectomize herself, a right to donate a kidney does not mean simple noninterference; rather it implies that some physician has an obligation to remove that person's kidney upon her request. Under what circumstances, if any, does a physician have such an obligation?

When a volunteer clearly meets all medical and psychosocial criteria for kidney donation, it could be reasonably argued that given the wide acceptance of the practice, respect for autonomy obligates the evaluating physician to accept this person's offer and that she does have a right to donate.[13,14,19,51] However, clearly acceptable volunteers do not generate disagreement among the involved parties and questions about rights arise only in situations of conflict. Therefore, to delineate the limits of a right to donate an organ we must examine cases in which the evaluating team and the potential donor disagree about her suitability.

Consider a woman who strongly wishes to donate a kidney to her child even though she has a medical condition that increases her risk of donating. If the woman has an absolute right to donate this would mean that the physician would have no choice and he would be obligated to remove one of her kidneys even though he considers donation to be dangerous and ill advised. Like Ross,[18] Delmonico,[30] and Singer and Siegler,[63] I do not believe that physicians have such obligations.[13]

Those who believe that people have a right to donate seem to lose sight of the fundamental difference between a heroic deed performed by an individual alone and one that requires the help of others.[9,13,18] Living organ donation falls into the latter category and here there is more to consider than the autonomy of the volunteer—the autonomy of the responsible physicians must also be respected.[9,13,22,30,64–66] As James Childress concludes:[21] "the physician has no moral duty to satisfy the patient's desires if he finds them incompatible with acceptable medical practice. The physician's conscience merits protection too." Similarly, Carl Elliott argues:[9] "the doctor is not a mere instrument of the patient's wishes . . . [He] is also a moral agent who should be held accountable for his

actions. If a patient undergoes a harmful procedure, the moral responsibility for that action does not belong to the patient alone; it is shared by the doctor who performs it. Thus a doctor is in the position of deciding not simply whether a subject's choice is reasonable or morally justifiable, but whether *he* is morally justified in helping the subject accomplish it." Given this responsibility and the fact that most living donors are healthy people who become patients only because of their desire to help others, serious donor complications may be especially devastating for involved physicians.

This discussion should not be misconstrued as suggesting that the candidate's autonomy is unimportant. On the contrary, the views of the potential donor are so important that it may be reasonable to accept some volunteers who strongly wish to donate despite added risk.[14,65,66] But because the autonomy of physicians must also be respected, valid consent is not enough—the evaluating physician must also agree that organ donation makes sense.[3,9,13,14,22,30,64–66]

## Setting a Threshold of Acceptable Risk

If one agrees that some volunteers at added risk are acceptable, how can the evaluating team determine when the risk is too high? In my view, the answer is to assess the relative weights of risks and benefits for the donor.[65] Remember that from the point of view of the evaluating physician, the potential donor is a patient.[30] Furthermore, in keeping with the concept of an independent donor advocate team, the donor's physician must concern himself solely with the donor's welfare. Therefore, as in all other areas of medicine, before a physician can recommend organ donation to his patient, he must believe that this procedure will do more good than harm *for that patient*.[18,19,65,67] But how can people benefit from donating organs, and how can we know if they will benefit enough to justify the risk?

Although organ donation provides no physical benefit for donors (other than the occasional discovery of a treatable medical condition), it may provide psychological ones. Several studies have shown that many donors experience lasting increases in self-esteem and perhaps an improved quality of life because of the knowledge that they have made a major sacrifice to save another person's life.[40,41,43,45,47,68–70] Although not all investigators have found these psychological rewards,[71,72] there is another important benefit for living related donors that few would question: that is, seeing a loved one resurrected and then having that cherished person available to share the joys of life.[3,47,65]

These psychological benefits can be very large. This is illustrated by the reflections of a set of parental donors:[57] "There is no doubt in our minds that we, as kidney donors, have gained much more than we lost. Of inestimable value, of course, is the restoration of our daughter's life and health." The fact that the vast majority of donors are glad they donated and would do it again if they could supports the view that many people derive benefit from donating an organ.[43,45,47,48,60,68–73]

But even if we believe that a volunteer will benefit from donating, how can we know if the magnitude of that benefit is sufficient to offset the risk? Because psychological benefits are subjective they cannot be quantified precisely; and because these benefits are not physical, physicians have no special ability to estimate their value or how likely they are to occur. Therefore, perhaps more important than asking how can we estimate how much benefit a donor will experience, and whether it will be sufficient to balance the risk, is to ask who is best suited to this task?[65,66,74]

I believe the answer is usually the potential donor herself, assuming that she is competent and that she has been presented with and understands the medical risks and benefits of organ donation and transplantation.[65,66,74,75] The probability that a donor will experience psychological benefits (or psychological harm) depends heavily on individual values and life plans, the details of which are available only to the volunteer. She alone knows and understands what is most important to her. Physicians can delineate the physical risks of donation, but the experts regarding the expected psychological value of donation, which is where the possibility of benefit lies, are usually the donors themselves. As Jerome Kassirer points out:[76] "Because the patient experiences the outcome, the patient's utilities [ie, values], not the physician's, should be the ones that are incorporated [into medical decision making]."

Although the potential donor may be best able to estimate the likelihood that she will benefit from donating and best able to balance expected benefits against known risks, this does not mean that the views of the physician are unimportant. As previously discussed, because organ donation cannot be effected without the physician's help, he shares much responsibility for the outcome and his autonomy must be respected. Therefore he may and he should refuse to participate if he believes that donation would do more harm than good, even if the potential donor disagrees.[65,66]

But although the physician is never obligated to accept a potential donor at added risk, he is obligated to treat every person with respect. This means that before rejecting a volunteer, the physician must listen carefully and try to see things from that person's point of view, incorporate that vision into his own decision making process, and recognize that no one can predict the psychological value of donation for the donor better than the donor herself. Thus the volunteer's estimate of the relative size of risks and benefits should be given great weight as the physician makes his own assessment. If despite this the physician feels unable to accept the volunteer, he should advise her that other centers may disagree and he should offer her a referral for a second opinion.[77]

## CONCLUSIONS

Living organ donation always poses risk for the donor. Therefore, before proceeding, it is essential to make a concerted effort to obtain informed consent from all potential living donors. Although some candidates may feel obligated to donate, this should not be confused with coercion and usually such internal pressure does not invalidate consent. In general, volunteers who are unable to provide informed consent should not be allowed to donate. However, when the potential donor and recipient are very closely related, consent may emanate primarily from care and concern rather than from a detailed consideration of the pros and cons of donating (as required by the informed consent doctrine). In some cases such consent may be just as valid as that which is fully informed. But valid consent is not enough. Although people have a right to be heard and treated with respect, they do not have an absolute right to donate an organ. Before giving the green light for organ donation, the volunteer's health-care team must agree that donation makes sense. This professional screening and the requirement for valid consent are two critical safeguards that protect potential organ donors from harm while fostering respect for autonomy.

## References

1. Morris PJ. Transplantation—A medical miracle of the 20th century. *N Engl J Med* 2004;351:2678–80.
2. Advisory Committee to the Renal Transplant Registry. The ninth report of the Human Renal Transplant Registry. *JAMA* 1972;220:253–260.
3. The nondirected live-kidney donor: Ethical considerations and practice guidelines. *Transplantation* 2002;74:582–589.
4. Terasaki PI, Cecka JM, Gjertson DW, Takemoto S. High survival rates of kidney transplants from spousal and living unrelated donors. *N Engl J Med* 1995;333:333–336.
5. Shaw LR, Miller JD, Slutsky AS, et al. Ethics of lung transplantation with live donors. *Lancet* 1991;338:678–681.
6. Singer PA, Siegler M, Whitington PF, et al. Ethics of liver transplantation with living donors. *N Engl J Med* 1989;321:620–622.
7. Moore FD. New problems for surgery. *Science* 1964;144:388–392.
8. Cronin DC, Millis JM, Siegler M. Transplantation of liver grafts from living donors into adults—too much, too soon. *N Engl J Med* 2001;344:1633–1637.
9. Elliott C. Doing harm: Living organ donors, clinical research and The Tenth Man. *J Med Ethics* 1995;21:91–96.
10. Gutmann T, Land W. Ethics regarding living-donor organ transplantation. *Langenbeck's Arch Surg* 1999;384:515–522.
11. Sauder R, Parker LS. Autonomy's limits: Living donation and health-related harm. *Cambridge Quart HealthCare Ethics* 2001;10:399–407.
12. Shapiro RS, Adams M. Ethical issues surrounding adult-to-adult living donor liver transplantation. *Liver Transplant* 2000;6(Suppl 2):S77–S80.
13. Spital A. Ethical issues in living organ donation: donor autonomy and beyond. *Am J Kidney Dis* 2001;38:189–195.
14. Steiner RW, Gert B. Ethical selection of living kidney donors. *Am J Kidney Dis* 2000;36:677–686.
15. Steiner RW. Risk appreciation for living kidney donors: Another new subspecialty? *Am J Transplant* 2004;4:694–697.
16. Caplan A. Must I be my brother's keeper? Ethical issues in the use of living donors as sources of liver and other solid organs. *Transplant Proc* 1993;25:1997–2000.
17. Price D. *Legal and Ethical Aspects of Organ Transplantation*. Cambridge:Cambridge University Press; 2000:227.
18. Ross LF. Solid organ donation between strangers. *J Law Med Ethics* 2002;30:440–445.
19. UNOS Ethics Committee. Ethics of organ transplantation from living donors. *Transplant Proc* 1992;24:2236–2237.
20. Beauchamp TL, Childress JF. Respect for Autonomy. In: *Principles of Biomedical Ethics,* chapter 3. New York: Oxford University Press, 2001:57–112.
21. Childress JF. Who Should Decide? Paternalism in Health Care. New York: Oxford University Press; 1982:21, 59–64.
22. The Authors for the Live Organ Donor Consensus Group. Consensus statement on the live organ donor. *JAMA* 2000;284:2919–2926.
23. Daar AS, Land W, Yahya TM, et al. Living-donor renal transplantation: evidence-based justification for an ethical option. *Transplant Rev* 1997;11:95–109.
24. Merrill JP. Statement of the Committee on Morals and Ethics of the Transplantation Society. *Ann Intern Med* 1971;75:631–633.
25. New York State Committee on Quality Improvement in Living Liver Donation. A Report to: New York State Transplant Council and New York State Department of Health. December 2002. http://www.health.state.ny.us/nysdoh/liver_donation/pdf/liver_donor_report_web.pdf
26. Price D. Informed Consent. In: *Legal and Ethical Aspects of Organ Transplantation,* chapter 7. Cambridge: Cambridge University Press; 2000:269–313.
27. U.S. Department of Health and Human Services Advisory Committee on Organ Transplantation, Recommendations 1 and 2. http://www.organdonor.gov/acotrecs.html

28. World Health Organization. Guiding principles on human organ transplantation. *Lancet* 1991;337:1470–1471.

29. Belmont Report: Ethical principles and guidelines for the protection of human subjects of research. Report of the National Commission for the Protection of Human Subjects of Biomedical and Behavioral Research, 1979. http://ohsr.od.nih.gov/guidelines/belmont.html

30. Delmonico F, Surman OS. Is this live-organ donor your patient? *Transplantation* 2003; 76:1257–1260.

31. The Ethics Committee of the Transplantation Society. The consensus statement of the Amsterdam Forum on the Care of the Live Kidney Donor. *Transplantation* 2004;78:491–492.

32. Childress JF. *Who Should Decide? Paternalism in Health Care.* New York, Oxford University Press;1982:104–105.

33. Lennerling A, Nyberg G. Written information for potential living kidney donors. *Transplant Int* 2004;17:449–452.

34. Nuffield Council on Bioethics. *Human Tissue Ethical and Legal Issues.* London; 1995:45.

35. Land W. The problem of living organ donation: Facts, thoughts, and reflections. *Transplant Int* 1989;2:168–179.

36. Eurotold Project Management Group. Ethical issues affecting living donor transplantation in Europe. In: Donnelly PK, Price D, eds. *Questioning Attitudes to Living Donor Transplantation.* Leicester: UK; 1997:50–64.

37. Caplan A. Am I my borther's keeper? *Suffolk Univ Law Rev* 1995;27:901–914.

38. Majeske RA, Parker LS, Frader JE. In search of an ethical framework for consideration of decisions regarding live donation. In: Spielman B, ed. *Organ and Tissue Donation: Ethical, Legal, and Policy Issues,* chapter 8. Carbondale: Southern Illinois University Press; 1996:89–101.

39. Wright L, Faith K, Richardson R, Grant D. Ethical guidelines for the evaluation of living organ donors. *Can J Surg* 2004;47: 408–413.

40. Fellner CH, Marshall JR. Kidney donors—The myth of informed consent. *Am J Psychiatry* 1970;126:1245–1251.

41. Fellner CH, Marshall JR. Twelve kidney donors. *JAMA* 1968;206:2703–2707.

42. Simmons RG, Marine SK, Simmons RL. Gift of Life. The Effect of Organ Transplantation on Individual, Family, and Societal Dynamics. New Brunswick, NJ: Transaction Books;1987:241–254.

43. Stothers L, Gourlay WA, Liu L. Attitudes and predictive factors for live kidney donation: a comparison of live kidney donors versus non-donors. *Kidney Intern* 2005;67:1105–1111.

44. Cotler SJ, Cotler S, Gambera M, et al. Adult living donor liver transplantation: Perspectives from 100 liver transplant surgeons. *Liver Transplant* 2003;9:637–644.

45. Eisendrath RM, Guttmann RD, Murray JE. Psychologic considerations in the selection of kidney transplant donors. *Surg Gyn Obs* 1969; 129:243–248.

46. Papachristou C, Walter M, Dietrich K, et al. Motivation for living-donor liver transplantation from the donor's perspective: An in-depth qualitative research study. *Transplantation* 2004;78:1506–1514.

47. Simmons RG, Marine SK, Simmons RL. Living related donors: costs and gains. In: *Gift of Life. The Effect of Organ Transplantation on Individual, Family, and Societal Dynamics,* chapter 6. New Brunswick, NJ: Transaction Books; 1987:153–197.

48. Smith MD, Kappell DF, Province MA, et al. Living-related kidney donors: A multicenter study of donor education, socioeconomic adjustment, and rehabilitation. *Am J Kidney Dis* 1986;8:223–233.

49. Biller-Andorno N, Agich GJ, Doepkens K, Schauenburg H. Who shall be allowed to give? Living organ donors and the concept of autonomy. *Theoretical Med* 2001;22:351–368.

50. UCLA Medical Center Ethics Committee, UCLA Renal Transplant Program. Surrogate consent for living related organ donation. *JAMA* 2004;291:728–731.

51. Adams RK. Live organ donors and informed consent: A difficult minuet. *J Legal Med* 1987;8:555–586.

52. Crouch RA, Elliott C. Moral agency and the family: The case of living related organ transplantation. *Cambridge Quarterly Healthcare Ethics* 8:275–287:1999.

53. Matas AJ. The case for living kidney sales: Rationale, objections and concerns. *Am J Transplant* 2004;4:2007–2017.

54. Faden RR, Beauchamp TL. A History and Theory of Informed Consent. New York: Oxford University Press; 1986:344–345.

55. Hawkins JS, Emanuel EJ. Clarifying confusions about coercion. *Hastings Center Report,* in press.

56. Sells RA. Voluntarism and coercion in living organ donation. In: Collins GM, Dubernard JM, Land W, Persijin GG, eds: *Procurement, Preservation and Allocation of Vascularized Organs,* chapter 36. Dordrecht, Kluwer Academic Publishers, 1997, pp 295–300.

57. Pierce EG, Pierce RA. "The agony and the ecstasy." *Transplant Proc* 1973;5:1067–1068.

58. Spital A, Spital M. Living kidney donation: attitudes outside the transplant center. *Arch Intern Med* 1988;148:1077–1080.

59. Cotler SJ, McNutt R, Patil R, et al. Adult living donor liver transplantation: Preferences about donation outside the medical community. *Liver Transplant* 2001;7:335–340.

60. Crowley-Matoka M, Siegler M, Cronin DC. Long-term quality of life issues among adult-to-pediatric living liver donors: a qualitative exploration. *Am J Transplant* 2004;4:744–750.

61. Ubel PA, Mahowald MB. Ethical and legal issues regarding living donors. In: Reich WT, ed. *Encyclopedia of Bioethics.* New York, Simon Schuster Macmillan, 1995:1865–1871.

62. Harris J. Wonderwoman and Superman. *The Ethics of Human Biotechnology.* Oxford: Oxford University Press; 1992:113.

63. Beauchamp TL, Childress JF. Moral theories. In: *Principles of Biomedical Ethics,* chapter 8. New York: Oxford University Press; 2001:357.

64. Singer PA, Siegler M. Whose kidney is it anyway? Ethical considerations in living kidney donation. *AKF Nephrol Lett* 1988;5:16–20.

65. Spital A. Donor benefit is the key to justified living organ donation. *Cambridge Quart Healthcare Ethics* 2004;13:105–109.

66. Spital A. The ethics of unconventional living organ donation. *Clin Transplant* 1991;5:322–326.

67. Landolt MA, Henderson AJZ, Barrable WM, et al. Living anonymous kidney donation: What does the public think? *Transplantation* 2001;71: 1690–1696.

68. Johnson EM, Anderson JK, Jacobs C, et al. Long-term follow-up of living kidney donors: Quality of life after donation. *Transplantation* 1999; 67:717–721.

69. Marshall JR, Fellner CH. Kidney donors revisited. *Am J Psych* 1977; 134:575–576.

70. Westlie L, Fauchald P, Talseth T, Jakobsen A, Flatmark A. Quality of life in Norwegian kidney donors. *Nephrol Dial Transplant* 1993;8: 1146–1150.

71. Gouge F, Moore J, Bremer BA, McCauly CR, Johnson JP. The quality of life of donors, potential donors, and recipients of living-related donor renal transplantation. *Transplant Proc* 1990; 22:2409-13.

72. Isotani S, Fujisawa M, Ichikawa Y, et al. Quality of life of living kidney donors: the short-form 36-item health questionnaire survey. *Urology* 2002;60:588–592.

73. Fehrman-Ekholm I, Brink B, Ericsson C, Elinder CG, Duner F, Lundgren G. Kidney donors don't regret. *Transplantation* 2000;69: 2067–2071.

74. Spital A. Living organ donation: Shifting responsibility. *Arch Intern Med* 1991;151:234–235.

75. The Ethics Committee of the Transplantation Society. A report of the Amsterdam Forum on the care of the live kidney donor: data and medical guidelines. *Transplantation* 2005; 79:S53–S66.

76. Kassirer JP. Adding insult to injury: Usurping patients' prerogatives. *N Engl J Med* 1983;308:898–901.

77. Spital A. When a stranger offers a kidney: Ethical issues in living organ donation. *Am J Kidney Dis* 1998;32:676–691.

# 4.3   DONOR ADVOCACY

*David M. Kashmer, MD, Tim Schmitt, MD,*
*Ken Brayman, MD, PhD*

The gap between donor organ availability and the demand for transplantation is large and increasing. The number of potential organ donors in the United States has been estimated at more than 10500 per year.[1] Clearly, not all potential donors progress to organ procurement. As of July 22, 2006, the number of patients awaiting transplantation was 92450. More than two thirds of this list is compromised of patients awaiting renal transplantation.

Overall, less than 50% of families approached regarding donation agree to proceed.[1] A potential-to-actual donor conversion rate of 42% for 1997 through 1999 has been documented.[1] Other factors may include a family's perception of the donor process, worries regarding the appearance of their loved-one after donation, and the difficulty regarding the health-care team's change in focus from the health of their family member to the health of an unseen patient at some other location impact heavily on this decision process. The Organ Donor Collaborative is addressing many of these issues. The magnitude of the disparity between donation and recipient need has prompted the increased use of living donors, expanded criteria donors, and non-heart-beating donors to satisfy the drive to help more patients through transplantation.

Faced with the drive to help ill patients through transplantation by shrinking that gap between organ availability and need, the importance of protecting the rights of living and deceased donors has been emphasized. It is in this climate that donor advocacy has evolved to keep the healthcare team focused on the protection and the rights of any person or family to donate for the good of another.

## WHAT IS DONOR ADVOCACY?

Intuitively, "donor advocacy" may be defined as a process or instance of supporting a potential or actual organ donor. The primacy in donor advocacy is placed on protecting donors' rights to donate and the creation of representation for the donor in the decision-making process that occurs as part of transplantation evaluation and completion. This broad definition extends to each kind of donation, whether deceased or living.

Where as this broad definition satisfies intuition, in fact, much of the field of donor advocacy has grown up around the field of living donation. Regulations passed by New York State require transplant programs to appoint an independent advocacy team to evaluate, educate, and consent to all potential living liver donors as part of the transplantation progress.[2] The background behind this legislation is well known. Although the broad term *donor advocacy* applies to advocacy with regard for all donors, it is important to realize it is most commonly associated with living donation, but need not be confined to it.

## DONOR ADVOCACY, ETHICS, AND ATTITUDES

"Protection of patients' rights' and the identification of potential areas of patient abuse will continue to be a complex problem (Starzl, 1985).

The potential for coercion, lack of respect for patient autonomy, and perception of incompleteness of informed consent throughout Medicine but specifically in the field of transplantation has been identified. The purpose of establishing donor advocacy paradigms and infrastructure is to address such abuse potential.

The donor advocate works in these situations to deal with ethical concerns. For example, consensus literature indicates that donors should be competent, willing to donate, free from coercion, medically and psychosocially suitable, fully informed of the risks and benefits as a donor, and fully informed of the risks, benefits, and alternative treatment available to the recipient."[3]

Clearly, establishing each portion of the above informed consent is no small task. Donor advocates may help to confirm that patients have the capacity to donate, are free from coercion, are medically/psychosocially suitable, and are appropriately informed. In doing so, principles of autonomy, nonmaleficence, and completeness of information play central roles. As informed consent is a process, not just a signed paper, it is clear that the donor advocate assists greatly with informing the patient, over time and multiple visits, of important issues regarding the decision to donate.

Another important issue with which advocates may assist is in managing the attitudes of the health-care team toward donation. Operating-room nurses and other members of the health-care team may experience emotional distress after or during the organ procurement process.[4] This distress may be transmitted toward others and subvert organ procurement efforts.[4] The role of donor advocates in displaying compassion, reminding the team of the importance of the gift of organ donation, and taking the time to assist in framing the situation as an altruistic act cannot be overstated.

In addition, another important frontier evolving in the transplant community, in which donor advocates may play a central role, is the increased use of non-heart-beating (NHB) donors or donation after cardiac death (DCD). DCD holds the ability to greatly increase the availability of organs for transplantation. Here exists another situation where staff has expressed resentment at the intrusion of technology; they preferred brain-dead status in organ donors; they feared legal repercussions from families; they speculated about non-heart-beating cadaver donors' ability to feel pain, and they expressed concern about withdrawing life-support measures, honoring patients' wishes, allocating nursing care as a scare resource, and witnessing family members' pain.[5]

Donor advocates are of great benefit in modifying attitudes of the health-care staff toward DCD donors. Changing the health-care climate and allaying the teams' fears may help increase the use of the valuable resource of DCD donors.

## DONOR ADVOCACY AND THE DECEASED DONOR

A Virginia driver's license can denote a driver's willingness to be an organ donor. Such designation is sufficient authority to remove, following death, the driver's organs or tissues without further authority from the donor, his family, or estate.[5]

Although the law may be clear in the instance of posthumous donation where the driver's license indicates a directive to donate, people's emotions are not necessarily as defined. A family's collective emotion is often not unified. Experience confirms that if the Organ Procurement Organization (OPO) representative speaks with a donor's family before proceeding with procurement, no matter the driver's license designation, a higher level of satisfaction and trust with the process is engendered. Here, again, the donor advocate is of great use in the process. An advocacy team may play a central role in discussing with the family the donor's willingness and capacity to donate as indicated by the driver's license. As an OPO focuses on procurement, the advocacy team may help keep the focus on the donor's rights. The team may continue to answer the family's questions as the timeline to donation proceeds. Such a focus on the family's experience of organ donation may make the difference between a family member's choosing to donate or not.

As mentioned previously, there are other situations where staff attitudes may benefit from the assistance of a donor advocacy team. It is important to keep in mind that staff may have strong feelings of distress with regard to the procurement process. A donor advocacy team may indicate important tenets of organ transplantation. The team may take the time to provide inservices, materials, and resources to indicate the true nature of a donor's choice in addition to the role played by health-care providers in fulfilling that person's desire to help another.

## DONOR ADVOCACY AND THE LIVING DONOR

Virginia has very little law, either by statute or court decision, on the transplantation of organs from live donors. Only one trial court decision has been found discussing kidney donation from a minor to her sister.[6]

In the absence of statute, the donor advocate holds a particularly important job. Without clear precedent regarding what entails informed consent in the living donor, hospitals and staff do well to counsel patients over time regarding the nature of the gift of living donation. Donor advocacy, when independent of transplant staff, more optimally avoids a potential conflict of interest.

In the absence of legal precedent, the health-care provider would be well advised to strongly counsel the donor as to the risks of the procedure. Although challenging, every effort should be made to avoid pressuring the potential donor to consent to the gift.[6]

Staff dedicated to creating strong counsel, over time, also has the advantage of ensuring more complete donor information in the difficult climate left by minimal precedent.

Another obvious challenge in many cases of living donation involves making an effort to assure that the potential donor feels little or no pressure in offering the gift. After all, critics of living donation have questioned the ability of potential donors to create true informed consent in a time of what is often family crisis.[7] Time needed to explore donor questions, feelings, and motivation regarding the decision may be expended successfully by staff designated to assist in these matters.

Other states have legislated the existence of independent donor advocacy teams. As noted, New York has mandated that transplant programs appoint an Independent Donor Advocacy Team to evaluate, educate, and consent all potential living liver donors.[7] The trend, be it by statute or an institution's judgment, is to create donor advocacy teams to assist in the charged climate surrounding living donor consent and information.

In the absence of clear precedent, consensus is evolving as to who may be used as a living donor. The Amsterdam Forum, for example, indicates some consensus that minors less than 18 years of age should not be used as living donors.[8] Donor advocacy assists in the useful role of explaining to patients who is eligible to donate and why based on current trends in transplantation. The donor advocate may serve as a useful contact for further discussion from family.

Many argue that ethical issues related to simultaneous involvement with both donors and recipients, in addition to a need to ensure confidentiality, is another supporting cause for the provision of separate care providers for donors and recipients.[9] These ideas of division and independence lend themselves strongly to the model proposed and legislated by some states. Donor advocacy teams, when held independent of the recipient process, may be seen by some patients as dedicated backers who can help alleviate mistrust.

## EXPLORING BARRIERS TO DONATION AND THE DONOR ADVOCATE

Much of public policy regarding organ donation is based on two assumptions: (1) health-care providers fail to ask families to donate, and (2) if asked, families will choose to donate.[10] However, there exists evidence that these are not, in fact, the only barriers to donation. There are other barriers to donation that the donor advocate may help explore and even remove.

For example, consider African Americans and the decision not to donate. A recent attempt to model decision making regarding organ donation in this group was significantly improved when variables such as medical mistrust, bodily integrity, and religiosity were added.[11] An independent donor advocacy team may be able to address some of the mistrust that can underlie a decision not to donate. Similarly, the issues of bodily integrity and religiosity may be more completely explored.

Most information about families' experiences of the donation request is obtained from families that agreed to donation.[12] Even from these, negative feedback regarding a lack of information imparted regarding brain death, the effect of donation on funeral arrangements, a perception of healthcare provider's insensitivity, and the cost of donation is commonplace.[12] In addition to public education and other resource allocation toward donation, a donor advocate or team may have an impact in this area by spending time with the family immediately after the decision to donate is made or, when appropriate, during the process of deciding.

## DONOR ADVOCACY AND THE FUTURE

Advocacy teams have met with success. Although the majority of organ donations come from large (greater than 500-bed) hospitals, it has been shown that a donor advocacy program has the potential to greatly increase the number of donations from a community hospital.[12] This success, coupled with the drive for increased donations, may imply that donor advocacy as a field will continue to grow.

Donor advocacy has grown as a partnership between different types of health-care providers. To continue to foster a positive climate, which can often be perceived by patients, donor advocacy would do well to continue its expansion as part of a multidisciplinary transplant team.

## CONCLUSION

The gap between organ supply and demand is large, and this fact charges the ethical discussions regarding organ donation and the decision to donate. As Dr. Starzl pointed out more than 20 years ago, great potential for abuse exists in this complex system. In this environment, the donor advocacy team stands to protect the person who wishes to give a great gift of his or herself—be that person alive or deceased.

To date, the existence of donor advocacy teams is legislated in some states and, more often, the team exists due to the institution's judgment and decision. In either case, the job of the advocate is not simple. Often there is no legal precedent that mandates what must be done so as to help keep potential and actual donors free from coercion and well informed. This may leave donor advocates in a situation where guidance comes only from their respect for autonomy and other guiding ethical principles.

Donor advocacy is a field that holds the potential to greatly benefit donors and transplantation as a whole. Plainly, the potential exists to dispel barriers that plague attempts at donation. Medical mistrust, questions regarding the integrity of the body, and efforts to answer patient questions over lengthening periods of time each may be bettered by effective advocacy in the right setting.

As states begin to more fully mandate advocacy programs, and advocacy programs succeed, it seems that the field is poised to expand. The direction in which it moves should be shaped by a partnership of different types of health-care providers, such that the relationship among the health-care team continues to be amicable and effective for its patients.

# References

1. Sheehy E, Conrad C, Brigham L, et al. Estimating the Number of Potential Organ Donors in the United States. *New Engl J Med* 2003;349.

2. Rudow DL, Brown RS. Role of the independent donor advocacy team in ethical decision making. *Prog Transplant* 2005;Sep;15(3):298–302.

3. Live Organ Donor Consensus Group. Consensus Statement on the Live Organ Donor. *JAMA* 2000;284:2919–2926.

4. Wolf ZR. Nurses' responses to organ procurement from nonheartbeating cadaver donors. *AORN J* 1994;Dec;60(6):968, 971–974, 977–981.

5. Adams. *Virginia Medical Law*. Richmond, VA: Commonwealth Medico-Legal Press; 2000;99.

6. Adams. *Virginia Medical Law*. Richmond, VA: Commonwealth Medico-Legal Press; 2000:101.

7. Rudrow DL, Brown RS. Role of the independent donor advocacy team in ethical decision making. *Prog Transplant* 2005;Sep;15(3):298–302.

8. Consensus Statement of the Amsterdam Forum on the Care of the Live Kidney Donor. *Transplantation* 2004;Aug.

9. McQuarrie B, Gordon D. Separate, dedicated care teams for living organ donors. *Prog Transplant* 2003;Jun;13(2):90–93.

10. Morgan SE. Many facets of reluctance: African Americans and the decision (not) to donate organs. *J Nat Med Assoc* 2006;May;98(5):695–703.

11. Siminoff A, Arnold R, et al. Public Policy Governing Organ and Tissue Procurement in the United States. *Anl Int Med* 1995;Jul;123(1):10–17.

12. Kittur DS, McMenamin J, Knott D. Impact of an organ donor and tissue donor advocacy program on community hospitals. *Am Surg* 1990;Jan;56(1):36–39.

# NONDIRECTED AND CONTROVERSIAL DONORS

*Arthur J. Matas, MD*

## INTRODUCTION

A living donor (LD) transplant is unique—in that one individual accepts the risks of surgery entirely for the benefit of another. The donor receives no physical benefits (although there may be psychological benefits). The donor operation is associated with possible mortality, morbidity, and the potential of long-term risks of living with one kidney (see chapter 10). Thus, before proceeding with an LD operation, the donor must be fully informed of the risks, must not be coerced, and must be capable of making an independent decision.[1]

## WHY INCREASE THE NUMBER OF DONORS?

A transplant (vs dialysis) provides significantly longer life and an improved quality of life. In addition, a preemptive transplant (vs a transplant after dialysis has been initiated) provides better outcome (ie, patient and graft survival rates. For patients already on dialysis, the success of a subsequent transplant is inversely related to the number of years of dialysis—that is, the more years, the worse the outcome. Nonetheless, every patient who has been on dialysis for a number of years still benefits from undergoing a transplant (vs remaining on dialysis).

In many parts of the world, patients with end-stage renal disease (ESRD) have a choice of treatment—dialysis or a transplant. Such patients often choose a transplant because of its better survival rates and quality of life. In other parts of the world, dialysis facilities are limited in number, and a transplant becomes the only possible option. In countries without brain-death legislation, an LD transplant is the only choice. But, even in countries where deceased donation is permitted, the waiting list is growing faster than the supply of organs. As a consequence, the waiting time is getting longer.

Currently, in the United States and Canada, about 7% of wait-listed patients die annually. Increasing the number of transplants would minimize the number of such deaths on the waiting list.

## WHY INCREASE THE NUMBER OF LIVING DONORS?

Importantly, the outcome of LD transplants is better than the outcome of deceased donor (DD) transplants. The possible reasons are numerous. LD transplants usually occur earlier in the course of ESRD and are associated with better HLA matching, a longer interval for donor evaluation before acceptance, and less delayed graft function.

## WHY INCREASE THE NUMBER OF LIVING UNRELATED DONORS?

The first long-term successful LD transplants were with identical twins. Thus, it was not surprising that the better outcome of LD (vs DD) transplants was initially attributed to the benefits of human leukocyte antigen (HLA) matching.

More recent data have shown that only donors who are perfect HLA matches with their recipient (ie, identical twins and HLA-identical siblings) confer a better outcome than other LD subgroups. In fact, the outcome with all other donor subgroups—including non-HLA-identical siblings, parents, offspring, and living unrelated donors (LURDs)—is identical. Recognition of this fact has led to widespread acceptance of living unrelated donation (in many countries). Much of the increase in LD transplants in the United States in recent years has been due to the increase in the use of LURDs.

LURDs can be further subgrouped by the pretransplant relationship between donor and recipient. A number of LURDs direct the kidney to a specific individual. Such donors might be "emotionally related," for example, a spouse or longstanding friend. Or, they might be acquainted with the recipient but not have a strong emotional bond, for example, a coworker or church member. Or, they might not have met the recipient (before hearing about the need for a transplant from a mutual acquaintance).

Some LURDs do not direct the kidney to a specific individual but are instead willing to donate to anyone on the waiting list. We have termed these donors nondirected donors (NDDs).[2] Others have used the terms *altruistic* or *Good Samaritan donors,* but we prefer the term *nondirected* because we believe that all donors are altruistic.

This chapter covers nondirected donation, in general, and then specifically addresses a subgroup of potential NDDs: prisoners. It concludes with a short discussion of a potential source of increasing donation—minors.

## NONDIRECTED LIVING DONORS

Recipients of an NDD kidney have the same outcome as with any LURD kidney. In addition, because they would otherwise remain longer on the waiting list for a DD kidney, their outcome is improved by receiving an NDD kidney (vs either staying on the list or receiving a DD kidney).

NDDs have the identical surgical and postoperative risks as directed donors. However, the major difference is that NDDs do not have the opportunity to witness the short- and long-term benefits to their recipient.

Historically, the medical community has been suspicious of individuals offering to be NDDs, fearing that ultimately they might harass the individual or hospital because of their donation or assuming that such individuals are likely to be mentally unstable.[3] Yet, when Sadler reported the first NDD cases in the 1960s, he noted that these donors were emotionally stable, self-supporting, and well-educated.[4] Those first NDDs did not feel coerced, and no psychological complications developed after donation.

However, soon after Sadler's report, donations by any type of nongenetically related volunteers ceased, because it was felt that the outcomes (the then-low patient and graft survival rates) of LURD transplants (of which NDDs are a subset) did not justify the risk to the donors. But, since then, immunosuppression, as well as patient and graft survival rates, improved. As described earlier, LURD transplants have become common.

## Public Opinion and Current Practice

Since early in the history of transplantation, public opinion surveys have suggested that 11% to 29% of the general public in North America would be willing to donate a kidney to a stranger.[5–9] For example, in two studies (in 1987 and in 1999), Spital reported on the public's opinion of allowing strangers to donate;[5–7] he noted that most respondents (70% in 1987, 80% in 1999) found donating a kidney to a stranger acceptable. Importantly, 24% stated they would donate a kidney to a stranger for free. Landolt et al., in two separate surveys of British Columbia (Canada) residents, found that 26% to 29% stated they would probably or definitely be willing to donate a kidney to a stranger.[8,9] In their second study, Landolt et al. did a follow-up questionnaire and an in-depth interview of a subset of the individuals willing to donate (9): 31% of the subset were "committed" to be NDDs. Landolt et al. concluded that a significant number of individuals (8%, ie, 31% "committed" of the 26% who stated in the initial survey that they would donate to a stranger) might come forward as NDD candidates, if they were informed about the need and given unbiased information about the procedure.[9]

Although the public seems supportive, transplant centers are only beginning to consider NDDs. Spital documented the changing attitudes to use of LURDs at U.S. transplant centers. In a survey published in 1989, 48% of responding U.S. transplant centers were willing to accept friends as kidney donors;[10] in 1994, that percentage had increased to 63%; and in 2000, to 93%.[11] In the 1989 article, Spital noted that 8% of responding centers were willing to consider altruistic strangers as donors; in 1994, 15% were willing to consider altruistic strangers (but none had done such a transplant in the previous year); and in 2000, 38% said they would now consider altruistic strangers. This increasing acceptance of NDDs in the medical community was reflected in the National Kidney Foundation's sponsorship of a national conference on nondirected donation in 2001.[12]

From June to October 2003, Crowley-Matoka and Switzer contacted the 25 transplant centers doing the highest volume of LD transplants in the United States (accounting for 36% of LD transplants) and the 25 organ procurement organizations (OPOs) facilitating the highest number of transplants in the United States.[13] Of the 25 transplant centers, 24 (96%) had received inquiries from individuals interested in being an NDD; 14 (12%) centers were currently doing, or willing to do, NDD transplants.

Interestingly, 2 centers had stopped doing NDD transplants—1 because of a bad experience with a donor demanding payment posttransplant, 1 for unspecified reasons. Of the 25 OPOs, most (22) referred all inquiries to a local transplant center, whereas 3 facilitated the donations themselves.

## The Minnesota NDD Program

As of 1998, our LD program had evolved from only accepting genetically or emotionally related donors to accepting directed donors who had little or no relationship with the intended recipient. We were then contacted, in 1998, by a woman requesting to donate to anyone on the waiting list for a DD kidney. In response to her request, we developed a protocol for evaluation and possible acceptance of NDDs. The development of the program and its evolution has been described in detail.[2,14] As of May 2005, we have done 30 NDD transplants. A recent United Network for Organ Sharing (UNOS) report listed 276 NDD transplants done in the United States (Cheryl Jacobs, personal communication).

### Initial Donor Screening

When a potential NDD donor contacts our transplant center, a transplant coordinator does an initial screening interview. Because many candidates live far from our center, the screening interview helps rule out those with obvious medical or psychosocial contraindications, which are the same as for any directed kidney donor. During the interview, the surgical risks are outlined, the process is described, an approximate timetable is provided, and a clear statement is made that no payment will be made for donation. In addition, if candidates live far from our center, we may inquire whether they have contacted a closer transplant center that might be more convenient for them. (However, many centers do not have established NDD programs.)

If, at the end of the interview, the candidate is not ruled out and remains interested, he or she is mailed a packet of donor educational information (including information on surgical risks, a list of previous donors to talk to, a discussion of the decision-making process, Internet sites, a list of references to journal articles, and a description of travel resources). If still interested after reading the information, he or she must re-contact our center and forward a written, more detailed medical history, including reasons for wanting to donate. Before a full evaluation at our center, we request that a minimum number of laboratory tests be done at the candidate's local clinic (blood typing and viral studies for hepatitis B and C and for HIV), thus preventing the expense of an unnecessary full evaluation and any unnecessary trip to our center. The tests at the candidate's local clinic are paid for by our transplant center.

### Detailed Donor Evaluation

If the candidate's written medical history and local laboratory results are acceptable, he or she must then come to our center for a full medical and psychosocial evaluation. The candidate meets with an independent (ie, not involved with recipient care) donor team (surgeon, nephrologist, coordinator, clinical social worker, and psychologist). The medical evaluation does not differ from the evaluation done for directed donors, except that we insist that the one for NDDs be done at our center.

The psychosocial evaluation of potential NDDs is more extensive than that for directed donors.[14] Both a designated clinical social worker and a psychologist routinely evaluate each

NDD candidate. In contrast, our directed donors do not see a psychologist unless we have concerns about cognitive deficits or other psychological risk factors. Both the social worker and the psychologist assess each NDD candidate's psychosocial stability, ability to comprehend information, and reasons for donating.[1] The psychologist also gives the Minnesota Multiphasic Personality Inventory (MMPI), a widely used standardized diagnostic instrument, to each NDD candidate. We feel that this more extensive evaluation is warranted because the psychosocial consequences for NDDs are not yet fully understood. The evaluation establishes whether factors exist that should exclude or postpone donation.

Contraindications for donation include severe forms of depression, active grief, low self-esteem, or other underlying or untreated mental illness. Candidates are ruled out if psychosocial issues are present that could increase their vulnerability to withstand potential donor-related stresses or that could exacerbate any psychological morbidity. Additional interventions or referrals are suggested if any such factors are detected.

Candidates who are found ineligible for any reason are sent a note thanking them for their interest, and if appropriate, recommendations or referrals for additional care. They are also informed about other transplant programs if they desire another opinion.

### Waiting Interval

If, after the evaluation, the NDD candidate is accepted, we require a waiting period of at least 3 months before surgery, to allow time for donor reflection and adequate preparation.

### Recipient Selection

To select the NDD recipient, we use the same algorithm (UNOS) as for allocating DD kidneys. One advantage of NDD transplants (vs DD transplants) is the opportunity for a recipient preoperative clinic visit and reevaluation, because many prospective recipients have been on the waiting list for years. Any identified problems can be addressed before scheduling the transplant. During the clinic visit, the prospective recipient is informed of the NDD program requirements, including the need to respect the donor's anonymity. At the same time, the prospective recipient may be encouraged to write the donor a thank-you note posttransplant (to be sent via the transplant center).

### Donor Costs

Donors assume any nonmedical expenses (including the cost of two trips to our center), but may be eligible for an institutional donor grant. Such grants—which require financial screening by a social worker—are potentially available to all candidates but may only be used to help defray costs incurred as a direct result of donation (eg, travel, lodging). The maximum limit of such grants rarely covers all donor-related costs.

### Donor and Recipient Communication

The prospective NDD and recipient are not permitted to meet before surgery. We worry that meeting the recipient could make the donor feel a greater sense of obligation or even coercion. Or, the donor might renege because of an undisclosed or underlying bias against the recipient's personal situation, religion, or ethnic group.

Posttransplant, both parties may wish to communicate in writing. If so, for the first 6 months, we insist that they communicate via the transplant center. After 6 months, if mutually desired, the donor and the recipient can communicate directly or meet. If they wish, we can help facilitate the meeting, or they are free to meet on their own. Either way, we urge them to consider the potential consequences of meeting and require each of them to sign a release form before learning each other's identity.

### Results

From October 1, 1997, through February 1, 2005, we received 465 inquiries about our NDD program.

The demographic characteristics and outcome for our first 360 callers have been described in detail.[14] Of the 360 callers, 60 (17%) were deemed ineligible after the preliminary phone interview. The remaining 300 callers were sent information about donation; of these, 249 (83%) made no further contact. The other 51 came to our center for at least partial or full evaluation. Of these 51 serious candidates, 9 either were ruled out or dropped out before completing all necessary testing. So, in all, 42 candidates underwent our full evaluation. Of these 42 final candidates, 15 (36%) were ruled out; another 4 made no further contact or follow-up after their full evaluation. All of the 23 remaining candidates have now donated. Thus, the NDD process is labor-intensive: these first 360 inquiries led to 23 transplants (of the 30 that we have done).

### Donor Motivation

Of the 51 NDD candidates who completed our full or partial evaluation, 49 had their motivation assessed. They gave a combination of reasons. Most of these 49 candidates were knowledgeable about donation when they contacted our center: 33 had learned about kidney donation from the media or the Internet; 12 had known someone who was currently on dialysis or who had either undergone a transplant or died while waiting for a transplant; 3 had learned about donation from a religious organization; 2 had known someone who had been evaluated as a potential donor. Most stated that they were responding to the severe organ shortage and the need for more donors.

We found no universally stated reason for wanting to donate; NDD candidates often gave more than 1 reason. Most ($n = 29$) described what we considered to be altruistic reasons: 27 had a history of doing kind deeds, and their reasons for donating appeared consistent with those previous behaviors. Of the 49 assessed candidates, nearly a third ($n = 16$) had a strong religious conviction and believed that donating was an act of living out their faith and their dedication to serving others (ie, an act to benefit a recipient). Another 6 candidates were motivated to donate in response to their feelings about someone important in their life that had died; some saw donating as a way to effectively grieve. In addition, 2 hoped that donating might impress others significant to them; 2 thought donating might aid in publicizing organ donation; and 2 saw donating as a way to bolster their self-esteem. (We considered wanting to impress others or bolster self-esteem as contraindications to donation.)

Some of the NDD candidates felt strongly that they shouldn't have to wait to die before someone could benefit from their kidney; they also worried that they would become too old or medically ineligible in the future to be a suitable donor. Some candidates described having fulfilling, active lifestyles and said they wanted to help others experience the same level of enjoyment in their lives (ie, attain not only physical vigor but also the opportunity to see their grandchildren grow up). Several candidates simply wished to give back because a loved one had benefited from a transplant or some other type of donation.

Of note, for two NDD candidates who were accepted and went on to donate, additional motivation became clear in the postoperative period. It seemed that they sought to gain from the donation (ie, through media attention or self-promotion).

### Recipient Outcome

Of the 30 NDD grafts, 29 continue to function; 1 was lost to recurrent disease. Actuarial 1- and 2-year graft survival rates are 95%. Mean serum creatinine level (± SD) at 1 year posttransplant was $1.4 ± .5$ mg/dL; at 2 years, $1.4 ± .4$ mg/dL.

### Donor Feedback

Many NDDs thanked us for the experience and opportunity to donate. They were glad to have donated and expressed a feeling of fulfillment, without regrets. Most volunteered to speak to other NDD candidates in our program; several are volunteering in their local area in various capacities to promote organ donation. They continue to be pleased that they donated and have not reported any personal, psychological, or emotional consequences. Some NDDs reported unexpected stress (eg, in relationships or with regard to finances when they had to be out of work longer than expected). One donor did undergo marital therapy as a result of additional stress caused by the donation.

## THE WASHINGTON, DC, NDD PROGRAM

Unlike the Minnesota program, which is a single-center program, the kidney transplant centers in Washington, DC—working with the designated OPO for the area (The Washington Regional Transplant Consortium [WRTC]),—developed a cooperative NDD program.[15] The WRTC and Minnesota programs differ in two major ways. First, in the WRTC program, NDD information was posted on its Web site, and press releases were issued. Second, given the various cooperating transplant centers in the Washington, DC, area, it is possible to have the NDD nephrectomy done at a different hospital than the transplant.

When potential NDDs contact the WRTC, they are provided information about the donation process and questioned about their medical and social history and their reason for wanting to donate. They are asked to undergo a physical examination and basic laboratory tests.[15] The results are then reviewed by the living donor evaluation committee of the WRTC. If preliminarily approved, each potential NDD then has a detailed "informed consent" discussion with a WRTC staff member, and then a psychiatric examination. After psychiatric clearance, a more detailed clinical evaluation is done. The potential NDD next chooses which center he or she would prefer to go to for the surgery.

Once a center is identified, the potential NDD meets with the transplant coordinator, surgeon, nephrologist, and social worker from that center. The center's personnel review the medical and psychosocial evaluation. If approved, at this point, the potential NDD is asked to give written informed consent.

Finally, the LD evaluation subcommittee of WRTC reviews all the clinical tests and study results from the comprehensive medical evaluation, as well as the reports and recommendations from the nephrologist, renal procurement surgeon, and psychiatrist.

### Results

From January 2000 to March 2004, the WRTC program received 62 applications from potential NDDs. Of these applications, 17 were eliminated during initial review of medical history and laboratory tests. Of the remaining 45 potential NDDs, 16 did not follow through with the psychiatric examination, and another 9 were turned down because of their psychiatric examination results. At the time of a 2005 article by Gilbert et al., 10 NDD transplants had been done.[15]

## Ongoing Issues for NDD Programs

NDD programs are new and still evolving at most transplant centers. A number of issues require ongoing discussion.

First, should the kidney be allocated to the center's list, to a regional list, or, in the case of a 6-antigen match, to a national list? Good logistical reasons exist for considering only the center's list. For example, other centers within the area may not be willing to use NDDs (as was the case when we started our Minnesota program), or such donors may prefer to come to a specific center. One of the advantages of any LD kidney transplant is the short ischemic time; this advantage would be eliminated if the kidney needed to be transported. However, a regional list allows for the potential for a better HLA match and may lead to a more equitable allocation of organs. Some regional organ procurement organizations, such as the Washington program described previously, have worked out the logistical issues and have successfully developed a system to share kidneys from NDDs within a designated geographical area.

Second, should the kidney be allocated to the number one person on the waiting list, even though the most medically sick recipient would have a greater risk for a poor outcome? It could be argued that, to maximize longevity, NDD kidneys should be allocated to "ideal" recipients. In establishing our program, we felt that the balance between efficacy and equity had already been established (after years of discussion) in the UNOS allocation system for DD transplants. We elected to use the same system.

Third, should NDDs be allowed to direct the kidney to a specific subgroup? When we established our program, we identified specific subgroups (eg, children) that we could imagine defending as socially acceptable for such directions. After all, when people donate their money or goods to charity, they can designate how that gift is used. We have had five donors who would have preferred that their kidney go to a child, two who wanted to direct their kidney to an African American (citing the increased waiting time for minorities), and two who asked about designating their kidney to a single mother raising a family. In creating the protocol for our NDD program, we could not determine how to allow such directives in what we determined to be acceptable situations, without also creating the possibility of donors making requests that we felt were socially unacceptable (eg, based on religious or racial bigotry or discrimination). So we elected to allocate the kidneys of all NDDs solely according to the established UNOS algorithm. Most donors were still willing to donate after learning of that policy.

In a national telephone survey conducted by Spital on whether NDDs should or should not be allowed to direct their kidney, most respondents thought that a donor should be permitted to insist that their gift go to a child, but not to a member of a specific religious or racial group.[16] We believe that centers permitting subgroup directives need to find a consistent system, so as to eliminate potential discrimination. Importantly, the center's policy for allocation must be described upfront to all NDD candidates.

Fourth, how can centers provide better social and emotional support for NDDs? A real advantage of the NDD process is the lack of family pressure to donate. In fact, we found that family members often initially tried to discourage donation. We always recommend that partners come to the evaluation with the potential NDD, so that we can obtain firsthand information from them and receive their input; however, that is not always feasible (given the sometimes long distance from our transplant center, or family and work obligations). In addition, we counsel NDD candidates on the importance of having spousal and/or familial support for numerous reasons: assistance required after donation, increased family responsibility during recovery, and the potentially life-threatening nature of donation. In spite of our counsel, we were uncomfortable to learn that four of our NDDs were unaccompanied on their day of surgery (after we had previously been informed that support would be available).

Fifth, should transplant centers keep NDDs informed of the outcome of the transplant? Most directed donors know the short- and long-term status of their recipient. But, because of the anonymity of the NDD process, NDDs are unaware of the status of their recipient. Our program asks recipients to write a thank-you note (transmitted by the transplant center) to the donors. However, some recipients have not written such a note, and the donors have become concerned that the graft might have failed. Some donors have contacted the transplant center to ask about their recipient (and sometimes assumed that he or she was not well when they did not hear from us on a regular basis). Programs must decide how much information will be communicated, and when, to donors.

## LONG-TERM FOLLOW-UP

All LDs, including NDDs, require long-term follow-up. Long-term studies of directed donors show quality of life equal to or better than the age-matched general population.[17] Similar studies of NDDs (who do not have the benefit of seeing the result of their act) are needed. Importantly, studies of directed donors have shown that they wish that the transplant team would show more concern for them after donation.[18,19] NDDs are likely to feel similarly and may require even more support from us, especially if they have no recipient feedback or family support. Further research is needed to help identify NDDs and family members who may be at risk for psychosocial morbidity and to determine the types of interventions needed to prevent or mitigate these problems.

## PRISONERS AS DONORS

The use of prisoners as donors raises a number of ethical issues—mainly centered on whether prisoners are truly capable of making an uncoerced autonomous choice.

### Directed Donation

Prisoners have donated kidneys to family members. The evaluation and surgery are identical to that for any other donor. Two issues are important. First, it must be made clear that donation will not reduce their sentence. Second, the prison may require that guards be present during the evaluation and the entire hospitalization; at our institution, the recipient or family would have to pay for this service.

One case that received widespread attention involved an incarcerated father who had already donated a kidney to his daughter: he offered to donate his second kidney to her.[20,21] The transplant would have been the girl's third; her second graft had been

rejected as a consequence of noncompliance. There was concern that she may have been presensitized. Finances were also a major issue. Because the father was incarcerated, the state was responsible for his medical care. Removal of his second kidney would necessitate long-term dialysis for which the state would be responsible. Ultimately, the decision was made not to proceed with the transplant.

This father's offer raised a number of ethical issues. First, should one individual be allowed to give a vital organ (eg, heart) or the last of paired organs (in this case a kidney) to save a child? Clearly, a parent running into a burning building to save a child would be considered a hero. Second, should doctors be obligated or allowed to remove a vital organ or the last of paired organs?

### Organs from Executed Prisoners

Numerous proposals have suggested that organs be removed from executed prisoners; some of the first DD kidneys in France came from executed prisoners.[22] It is widely presumed that, in China, most organs are from executed prisoners.[23,24]

Using organs from executed prisoners could be done via two frameworks: (1) mandatory consent or (2) "permission" granted by the prisoners. Both entail numerous problems, independent of one's stance on capital punishment.[23,25–30] First, it is unclear whether the organs belong to the individual or to the state. Second, use of organs from executed prisoners may lead to an increase in death sentences; it is feared that this has already happened in China.[23,24] Third, some forms of execution damage the organs; other forms of execution might involve physicians playing a role in carrying out the death sentence. Fourth, even if prisoners are given the option of donating organs after death, it is not clear that they would be able to make an uncoerced decision. Even recognizing these problems, Patton argues in favor of organ procurement of executed prisoners.[26]

### Organ Donation in Exchange for Commuted Death Sentence

An alternative to removing organs from executed prisoners would be offering prisoners on death row an opportunity to donate in exchange for commuting their death sentence to life imprisonment. Death sentence or donation: a classic description of coercion. Anderson noted that if such a possibility existed, judges and juries might be more willing to dispense death sentences, knowing there would be little chance they would be carried out.[29] In addition, if the possibility of commutation existed, how would prisoners who could not be donors (eg, those with hepatitis) be treated?[29]

### Organ Donation in Exchange for Shortened Sentence

As compared with the relatively few prisoners on death row, tens of thousands of incarcerated prisoners are now serving long-term sentences. Anderson suggested that an organ donation program for "noncapital inmates is ethically superior to one limited to capital inmates because it is less likely to be subject to abuse"; it would be "compatible with traditional penal objectives, would not exploit prisoners, and would contribute to a reduction in the organ shortage"[29] Clifford Bartz, a current federal inmate, has actively campaigned for a program in which medically cleared inmates could donate in exchange for a reduced sentence.[30,31] Bartz and Anderson agree that any such program should be limited to inmates serving time for nonviolent offenses whose early release would not cause excessive worry or negative public opinion.

Kahn offered two arguments against such a proposal.[28] First, he suggested that the offer is coercive, in that the prison environment has many coercive characteristics, and thus the opportunity for less time may not be so different from coercion. Second, inmates have very few other opportunities to reduce their sentences and, therefore, this type of offer may take "advantage of their vulnerabilities in ways that can only be termed exploitive."[32]

Bartz noted that many defendants are given a choice of a plea bargain with a lesser sentence vs going to trial and risking a harsher sentence.[30] He suggested that if this type of intimidation and coercion (on the government's part) is permitted, why not organ donation in exchange for a reduced sentence? Anderson stated that the difficult living conditions in a prison can be seen as coercive, but agreed that the benefits of an organ donation program may still outweigh the disadvantages:[29] if "decent living conditions are provided" the "only possible threat would be continued incarceration for the original term of imprisonment if the prisoner chose not to sign up."[29]

Hinkle noted that public opinion does not support reduced sentences in exchange for organ donation.[23] His conclusion was based on only one survey, yet the issue is important. Currently, much of organ donation is largely based on public goodwill. If that goodwill was shattered because of a prisoner donation program, organ donation could decrease.

## MINORS AS LIVING DONORS

Experience with the use of minors as living donors is limited. Spital, in 1996, surveyed the attitudes of transplant centers regarding the use of minors.[33] Of 117 centers, 39 (33%) would allow a monozygotic twin < 18 years old to donate a kidney to his or her twin; 21% of centers would allow a nontwin minor to donate a kidney to a sibling.

Delmonico and Harmon queried the UNOS database and identified 60 living donors < 18 years old from 1987 through 2000.[34] Of these donated kidneys, 7 went to identical twins, 5 went to fraternal twins, and 15 went to HLA-identical siblings.

Three kidneys from 16- and 17-year-old females went to infants and may have represented mother-to-child transplants. Of note, however, 27 kidneys (45%) went to non-HLA-identical adults. Given that most centers do not approve of such transplants, some of these UNOS cases may actually represent data-entry errors in this enormous database.

Spital noted four clear concerns when minors are being considered as donors:[31]

> First, children are generally thought to be unable to understand and balance the risks and benefits of complicated medical procedures; if this is true, then they cannot determine whether kidney donation is in their own best interest, nor can they provide valid consent. Second, children may not feel free to say no if they fear that refusal might jeopardize parental love and support. Third, when siblings are involved, even loving parents may not be able to make a sound decision for their healthy child considering donation, because of an obvious conflict of interest. Finally, there is appropriate concern about the risks of uninephrectomy in childhood.

The Live Donor Consensus Conference suggested the following conditions under which a minor may act as a living organ donor: when the potential donor and recipient are both highly likely to benefit (as in the case of identical twins); when the surgical risk to the donor is extremely low; when all other opportunities for a transplant have been exhausted; when no potential adult LD is available, and a timely and/or effective transplant from a DD is unlikely; and when the minor freely agrees to donate without coercion, as established by an independent donor advocate.[1]

## References

1. Abecassis M, Adams M, Adams P, et al. for Live Organ Donor Consensus Group: Consensus statement on the live organ donor. *JAMA* 2000;284(22):2919–2926.
2. Matas AJ, Garvey CA, Jacobs CL, et al. Nondirected donation of kidneys from living donors. *NEJM* 2000;343:433–436.
3. Fellner CH, Schwartz SH. Altruism in dispute. Medical versus public attitudes toward the living organ donor. *N Eng J Med* 1971;284:5825.
4. Sadler H, Davison L, Carroll C, et al. The living, genetically unrelated, kidney donor. *Semin Psychiatr* 1971;3:86–101.
5. Spital A, Spital M. Living kidney donation: attitudes outside the transplant center. *Arch Intern Med* 1988;148:1077–1980.
6. Spital A. Public attitudes toward kidney donation by friends and altruistic strangers in the United States. *Transplanation* 2001;71:1061–1064.
7. Spital A: Kidney donation by altruistic living strangers. In: Gutmann T, Daar AS, Sells RA, Land W, eds. *Ethical, Legal, and Social Issues in Organ Transplantation*. Lengerich: Pabst Science Publishers; 2004:133–139.
8. Landolt MA, Henderson AJ, Barrable WM, et al. Living anonymous kidney donation: what does the public think? *Transplantation* 2001; 71(11):1690–1696.
9. Landolt MA, Henderson AJ, Gourlay W, et al. They talk the talk: Surveying attitudes and judging behavior about living anonymous kidney donation. *Transplantation* 2003;76(10):1437–1444.
10. Spital A. Unconventional living kidney donors—Attitudes and use among transplant centers. *Transplantation* 1989;48(2):243–248.
11. Spital A. Evolution of attitudes at U.S. transplant centers toward kidney donation by friends and altruistic strangers. *Transplantation* 2000; 69(8):1728–1731.
12. Adams PL, Cohen DJ, Danovitch GM, et al. The nondirected live-kidney donor: Ethical considerations and practice guidelines: A National Conference Report. *Transplantation* 2002;74(4):582–589.
13. Crowley-Matoka M, Switzer G. Nondirected living donation: a survey of current trends and practices. *Transplantation* 2005;79(5):515–519.
14. Jacobs CL, Roman D, Garvey C, et al. Twenty-two nondirected kidney donors: An update on a single center's experience. *Am J Transplant* 2004;4(7):1110.
15. Gilbert JC, Brigham L, Batty DS Jr, et al. The nondirected living donor program: a model for cooperative donation, recovery and allocation of living donor kidneys. *Am J Transplant* 2005;5(1):167–174.
16. Spital A. Should people who donate a kidney to a stranger be permitted to choose their recipients? Views of the United States public. *Transplantation* 2003;76(8):1252–1256.
17. Johnson EM, Anderson JK, Jacobs CJ, et al. Long-term follow-up of living kidney donors: Quality of life after donation. *Transplantation* 1999;67:717–721.
18. Jacobs C, Johnson E, Anderson K, et al. Kidney transplants from living donors: How donation affects family dynamics. *Adv Ren Replace Ther* 1998;5:89–97.
19. de Graff Olson W, Bogetti-Dumlao A. Living donors' perception of their quality of health after donation. *Prog Transplant* 2001;11:108–115.
20. Curriden M: Inmate's last wish is to donate kidney. *ABA J* 1996; 82(6):26.
21. Nieves E: Girl awaits father's 2d kidney, and decision by medical ethicists. *NY Times (Print)* 1998;Dec 5:A1.

22. Kass R. Human renal transplant memories: 1952 to 1981. In: Terasaki PI, ed. *History of Transplantation: Thirty-Five Recollections.* UCLA Tissue Typing Laboratory; 1991:37–60.

23. Hinkle W. Giving until it hurts: Prisoners are not the answer to the national organ shortage. *Indiana Law Rev* 2002;35(2):593–619.

24. Owen AK. Death row inmates or organ donors: China's source of body organs for medical transplantation. Comment. *Ind Int'l & Comp L Rev* 1995;5(2):495–517.

25. Banks GJ. Legal & ethical safeguards: protection of society's most vulnerable participants in a commercialized organ transplantation system. *Am J Law Med* 1995;21(1):45–110.

26. Patton L-H M: A call for common sense: organ donation and the executed prisoner. *Va J Soc Policy Law* 1995;3(1):387–434.

27. Perales DJ. Rethinking the prohibition of death row prisoners as organ donors: A possible lifeline to those on organ donor waiting lists. *St Marys Law J* 2003;34(3):687–732.

28. Coleman P. "Brother, can you spare a liver?" Five ways to increase organ donation. *Valparaiso Univ Law Rev* 1996;31(1):1–41.

29. Anderson MF: The prisoner as organ donor. *Syracuse Law Rev* 2000;951–979.

30. Bartz CE. Operation Blue, ULTRA: DION–the donation inmate organ network. *Kennedy Inst Ethics J* 2003;13(1):37–43.

31. Bartz CE. Federal inmate promises to end organ shortage within 3-5 years. Letter to the Editor. *Bioeth Exam* 2004;8(1):4.

32. Kahn JP. Three views of organ procurement policy: moving ahead or giving up? *Kennedy Inst Ethics J* 2003;13(1):45–50.

33. Spital A. Should children ever donate kidneys? Views of U.S. transplant centers. *Transplantation* 1997;64(2):232–236.

34. Delmonico FL, Harmon WE. The use of a minor as a live kidney donor. *Am J Transplant* 2002;2(4):333–336.

# CHAPTER 6

# SOCIAL ISSUES

*Thomas R. McCune, MD*

## INTRODUCTION

Living organ donors report a quality of life around the time of donation that is greater than is found in the general population. This observation has been made in Norway,[1] (1), United States,[2–5] Sweden,[6] Japan,[7] Australia,[8] and Germany[9,10] using different psychological tests for physical and emotional wellness. These observations have been made in kidney donors[1,2,4,6–9] as well as in liver donors.[3,10] It is suggested that donors for the most part have a high sense of self-esteem.[11] This is not universally found in all donors and unfortunately suicide in living kidney donors[12] and living liver donors[13] has been reported. The donation procedure is not an isolated event in the life of an individual who exhibits an elevated sense of self-esteem. Much occurs around the time of donation and afterwards that affects the emotional well-being of the donor. When presented with information concerning living kidney donation, 78% of donors in one early study felt they knew right away they would donate.[14] When potential living liver donors were interviewed about their decision to donate, 14 out of 15 felt the decision was "automatic."[15] Living kidney donors report their decision to donate was "instantaneous and immediate."[14] This seemingly immediate decision to donate is interwoven with a great deal of psychological interplay. To understand the emotional events that the donors may report after donation is important to understand the psychological factors that go into making the decision to donate. This chapter initially reviews the factors that appear to influence the potential donor. With these aspects in consideration, the remainder of the chapter presents the problems that donors either report directly through individual interviews or on surveys.

## THE DECISION TO DONATE

There appear to be three factors that go into the decision to donate. These factors are personal, recipient/family, and physical. Each of these factors represents a spectrum of emotional and physical concerns (Figure 6-1). The personal factor deals with the motivation of the potential donor. The interaction of the potential donor and the recipient and the associated families is the second factor. The final factor is the role of the transplant center plays in the process of accepting the potential donor. These represent the three important groups involved with the transplant process.

Understanding these factors may help to identify donor problems before they become critical concerns.

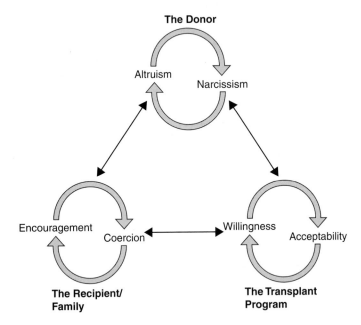

**FIGURE 6.1**

The factors that affect the decision to donate

## ALTRUISM VERSUS NARCISSISM

The personal factor of donation is the donor's question, "What's in it for me?" The spectrum of this answer ranges from the "altruism" of the anonymous donor, who wishes no contact with the recipient, to the "narcissistic" donor, who wishes to have the focus of the transplant procedure to remain solely on them. A study of potential "stranger" kidney donors and potential "relative" kidney donors conducted at Johns Hopkins compared their altruistic attitudes compared to the general population. There was essentially no difference among the general population, "stranger" and "relative" donors in their desire to help others.[16] The difference between the desires of the general population and those of the altruistic donor lays in the fact that altruistic donors are actually pursuing the opportunity to donate an organ.

The altruism of the donor may not be entirely healthy. By focusing on "a desire to help others," the potential donor may not be willing to look critically into their own personal decision for donation. One potential donor presented himself to our program in the hopes of becoming an altruistic donor and successfully competed an initial psychological screening, but requested that the donation occur before a certain date. On further questioning later in the evaluation process, it was determined that this potential donor had a court date to face the charges of vehicular hit and run. This potential altruistic donor was asked to return once the legal concerns have been resolved. The lead supporter for the donor advocate, Dr. Delmonico clearly identifies the motivation of the unacceptable narcissistic donor

1. A desire for media attention

2. A remedy for a psychological malady, such as severe depression, low self-esteem, or other underlying mental illness

3. A desire to direct the recipient selection toward a specific sex or ethnic group

4. A desire to have an involvement in the recipient's life, when the recipient does not desire it[17]

Not all donors who are motivated by personal needs can be labeled narcissistic. Dr. Papachristou has titled another type of donor whose primary reason for donating is self-centered the *egotistic*. This type of "egotistic donor"[18] approaches donation as a way to avoiding the fear of losing the recipient and not necessarily for a desire to improve the recipient's health. The egoistic donor may also be motivated to keep their position in the family. The egoistic donor looks at the relationship with the recipient solely from their point-of-view. This donor is not immediately disqualified because of the close relationship that donor and recipient have. It is important for the transplant team to differentiate between the narcissistic and egoistic donor, and within a family this may not be very obvious.

## COERCION VERSUS ENCOURAGEMENT

The second factor affecting the desire to donate is the interest of the recipient and their family. This factor asks the recipient's family's question, "What is in it for the family?" The donor can be either coerced or encouraged to proceed by the recipient or their family. The difference between coercion and encouragement is found in the promises made to the donor by the recipient or the family. If an agreement between the donor and the recipient is honored by the recipient and is felt to be adequate by the donor then the donor is encouraged. If on the other hand either the promise is not honored or the donor does not believe the promise is adequately honored, the donor can feel manipulated into donating. The best form of encouragement is that of the "black sheep of the family" who offers to donate to become reinstituted into the family.[19] Unfortunately, not all potential donors who are encouraged to donate are accepted back into the family, and in many cases the difference between coercion and encouragement may not be manifest until after the procedure occurs.

The most insidious form of donor manipulation in transplantation is financial coercion. In most countries the donation of an organ in exchange for something of financial value in against the law, but it is difficult to police. In India, selling kidneys is outlawed, but it occurs frequently enough that it can be studied. In India, selling a kidney is almost uniformly directed by the donor's desire to improve the financial status of the family.[20] Unfortunately, any financial benefit realized through selling a kidney does not result in long-term economic benefit to the family. When asked if they would donate again the majority of these donors said they would not. Financial coercion is not limited to the sale of kidneys. In the United States, donors frequently receive financial support to cover donation related expenses.[3,15,21] When the financial support exceeds the actual accrued expenses it can be argued that the donor is being coerced. Kidney donors who reported that they received financial support for more than their actual expenses from their families were 3.45 times as likely to become divorced as those donors who did not [more on this in a later section].[22] Because this form of manipulation occurs after the donation, the transplant program may not be aware it is occurring.

## WILLINGNESS VERSUS ACCEPTABILITY

The final factor affecting a potential donor's decision relates to the donor's health and well-being after the donation. This factor answers the donor's question, "Will I be healthy after donation?" The transplant center's responsibility in assessing the risks and benefits to a donor will be reviewed in other chapters. The donor who faces the prospect of major surgery may disregard the risk or be too fearful to proceed. The potential donor who is fearful about their posttransplant health may have unrealistic concerns about the potential risks. Nearly one fifth of successful donors wished that they had had more data regarding the procedure so they would have had a better understanding of the procedure as a whole.[22] Too much information could be perceived by the potential donor as pressure to donate. The potential donor who is concerned about their health, but senses that they are coerced, may experience more problems post donation. Dr. Steiner argues that the potential donor should be presented with the data related to postdonation health risks and be allowed to make the final decision.[23] This approach is acceptable when the risk of donation is low. The potential donor who approaches donation with "curiosity" and as a "personal challenge"[18] may minimize the risk of donation complications. The Johns Hopkins study of potential donors found that "stranger" donors were willing to accept a significantly greater risk of complications (average acceptable risk 64%) than related donors were willing to take (average acceptable risk 17%).[16] What seemed to separate the altruistic donor from the related donor is the increased willingness to accept the risk to his or her own health. Dr. Spital agrees that the donation process is an emotional period and that the transplant program must assume the responsibility of rejecting potential donors who have a greater risk of complications than a chance for success.[24] Just as a transplant program should not coerce a potential donor who is having exaggerated fears of complications, the donor who ignores his or her own health should not be encouraged to donate. Counselors who are acting solely as the advocate for the donor,[17] coordinators trained to present risks graphically,[25] and volunteer living-donor mentors[22] may help to alleviate these concerns. The donor advocate or mentor who has counseled and advised the potential donor of the evaluation process can also be an important ally during the period of recovery that is marked by pain, complications and the risk of depression.

There is no perfect donor. Living donation is a balance of the potential donor's motivations, the potential recipient's objectives, and the transplant program's principals. Being able to compare the compelling forces that these three groups possess can lead to a better understanding of the social concerns the donors face postprocedure.

## THE POSTDONATION PERIOD

### Stress and Depression

Most donors consider the early postdonation period stressful. Some of the first reports of the emotional concerns of kidney donors reported, "almost all donors experienced a moderately severe depression for 1 to 2 weeks following the surgery"[26]. A more recent study from the University of Heidelberg found that early posttransplant psychological strain of the kidney donor is equally attributed to their worries about their own health as to the worries of their recipient.[27] Studies from the University of Minnesota show that the psychological strain that kidney donors experience after transplantation is more related to the fact that they experienced complications.[2] The terms *depression* and *stress* are not interchangeable. Psychiatrists who are confident with the psychiatric diagnosis of depression reported the early studies of the donor's mental status and reported that donors experienced depression. Later studies by nontherapists seemed less willing to use the psychiatric diagnosis and described the donor's response to the experience as stress. It is uncertain if the level of stress reported now is equivalent with the state of depression that had been previously reported.

Depression or stress due to the anxiety of recovery is not reported in living liver donors. European studies of living liver donors show high levels of motivation and that they benefit psychologically from donation.[28] Using the SF-36, Trotter at the University of Colorado found elevated scores in mental health in living liver donors when compared to the general population.[4] It could be argued that depression can occur in living liver donors as often as it does in living kidney donors, and that these early studies of liver donors did not capture these people. Yet depression after kidney donation has been described as early as the mid-1960s[26,29] when living donation was rare, and kidney transplantation was immediately life saving, just as liver transplantation is now. In spite of the lack of definable depression or stress in liver donors, they may experience a sense of abandonment after donation. Liver donors report that they feel as though they were considered "nonpatients" when the emphasis of the transplant team shifts to the recipient.[15] The poor pain control postdonation and lack of follow-up were cited as major reasons for the perception that they were abandoned by the transplant team. Trotter attributed the lack of frustration of liver donors at the University of Colorado to the donor mentor program, which matches potential donors with previous donors of the same race, age, and life situation.[3] To relieve the abandonment experienced by the donors she interviewed, Crowley-Matoka reported that the contributing liver transplant centers for her report have now assigned a nurse coordinator/advocate to support the donor during recovery.[15]

Stress is not a uniform experience of living kidney donors. Women seem to be at risk for experiencing the greatest level of stress.[2,4,30] The University of Minnesota observed that female kidney donors between the ages of 20 and 30 experienced the highest levels of stress after transplantation. Parents who are donors are reported to have higher levels of anxiety than did other groups.[4] The concerns for a young child, as well as for your own health, can increase anxiety levels. Researchers in Germany found that donors between the ages of 31 to 40 scored the lowest on the SF-36 posttransplant. The researchers attribute the low score to poorly developed coping skills in stressful situations in these donors.[9] The researchers in Australia found that older women with lower economic levels experienced anxiety and depression postdonation. The multicenter registry of kidney donors Living Organ Donor Network (LODN) sponsored by The American Foundation for Donation and Transplantation (formerly the Southeast Organ Procurement Foundation) found that 11% of donors were prescribed antidepressants postdonation and that the majority of these patients were women.[21] Women have compared the emotional experience after kidney donation to postpartum depression.[18] In women donors, the lack of social support and fewer significant relationships have also been associated with higher rates of psychological complications.[4]

Aside from the feeling of abandonment and isolation that kidney donors feel, concerns related to disfigurement and impaired and altered sexual organ have also been reported (26). How common these fears are is unknown because these concerns are reported out of individual psychotherapy sessions. Even with the newer laparoscopic nephrectomy procedures, some kidney donors are surprised at how large their scars are.[4] In spite of the large scar, liver donors have not been found to be concerned about the extensiveness of their incision sites.[3,15] In general, living liver donors[15] and kidney donors[1,4] were grateful to have been able to donate and would do it again in spite of some negative feelings.

## FAMILY SUPPORT AFTER DONATION

The family of the donor can be the greatest source of support and the worst cause of stress to the donor. To understand the donor and how they choose to donate and deal with their recovery, the Transplant Program must understand the family. Subtle but compelling family pressures to donate have been reported by 11% of kidney donors.[14] The "urgency" of the need for a living liver donor may make the pressure to find a donor within the family greater. Pomfret suggests that when the liver recipient is a child, the stress within the family to find a donor is greater than when the recipient is an adult.[31] Fourteen percent of potential adult-to-adult liver donors she interviewed choose not to donate when they are presented to the potential risks of donation.[32]

The potential donor is also receiving pressure not to donate. In the large multicenter study of living related kidney donors sponsored by the National Kidney Foundation, it was observed that more than 14% of the donors received encouragement not to donate from the family and friends.[22] The spouse of the potential donor may be the greatest source of pressure not to donate because their family stability is at the greatest risk.[33] When the potential donor and spouse have children, the risk to the family is even greater and the marital strain is greater than when the couple have no children.[33] The donor's spouse may not only antagonize the potential donor by pressuring them not to donate, but may also alienate the "in-laws." This puts the spouse in an adversarial role, which can result in their isolation. Many potential donors are aware of this conflict and consult their spouse only after they have made the decision to donate.[34] It is interesting that pressure to donate from the family is reported by a similar percentage of donors who reports pressure not to donate. These competing pressures may allow a balance when the potential donor considers their options. Here the spouse plays an important role not only to support a potential donor's decision to donate but also to give justification not to donate.[34] Unfortunately for the potential donor, there is a risk that the decision will alienate one group of people. The donor may be forced to choose between their family of origin and their current family. This is particularly true when a married adult child donates to a member of their original family or when a parent donates to their married adult child. This situation is reported as a cause of divorce in the reviews of kidney and liver donors, which reported on divorce.[4,15,22] When the donor reestablishes a close bond with the recipient external to the marriage, loyalties may shift away from the spouse.[19] Reestablishing financial ties with the family outside the immediate family can result in marital stress. The risk for divorce and separation for the donor is also increased when they receive financial support from the family outside their marital unit.[22]

The donor is not an innocent bystander as the family dynamic is altered by transplantation. The donor frequently feels resentment to the recipient as the emphasis of the transplant team shifts from the donor to the new recipient. When this is acted out, it can be difficult for the family.[19] A parent may donate to "shield" an adult child from the need to donate.[20] A family member may donate to "protect" other family members from the need to donate, as well as from the sadness over the loss of an ill family member.[18] Siblings report the most pressure to donate[4] and they may express resentment to other family members for failing to "step up to the plate"[31]. All researches that observed these concerns encouraged an open and honest discussion of these issues in an attempt to diffuse stressful family interactions. These concerns are not the norm, and the majority of donors experience a closer relationship with the recipient in spite of family conflicts.

## FINANCIAL CONCERNS

The financial concerns of the organ donor and their family can limit the opportunities and place great stress on the recovery process. In a study from UNC Chapel Hill, the kidney transplant program found that 24% of potential donors within the family of the recipient decided not to proceed to donate due to financial concerns.[35] Pomfret at the Lahey Clinic found that 14% of potential liver donors decided not to donate due to time constraints.[32]

Donors rely heavily on support of their employers to bridge the time between the donation operation and recovery period. Employers provided sick leave, disability (both short and long terms), and leave for liver donors surveyed by the University of Colorado[3] and liver donors of the LODN.[21] The LODN survey found that 58% of kidney donors took sick leave and up to 48% took some form of disability leave.[21] Unfortunately, employers are not able to provide adequate benefits to fully support the recovery of the donor. The University of Colorado survey found that 29% of their liver donors took leave without pay (Table 6-1).[3] The LODN registry of kidney donors calculated that the average donor took 14 days of unpaid leave between the time they exhausted their employer-provided benefits and the time they were able to return to work (Table 6-2).[21] Donors also reported that the donation recovery exhausted all their accrued leave and any subsequent time from work was without pay. This period without income is not the only cause for financial concerns of the donor.

### TABLE 6.1

### FINANCIAL ASSISTANCE REQUIRED FOR LIVER DONATION

| | |
|---|---|
| Short-term disability/Sick leave | 5 |
| Long-term disability | 1 |
| Leave without pay | 7 |
| Leave with full salary | 7 |
| Financial help from friends/family | 12 |

Note: The total number sources of assistance is greater than the number of Patients (n = 24) because some patients reported more than 1 source of financial Assisstance.
Reprinted with permission: Trotter JF Liver Transplantation, Vol. 7, No 6, (June), 2001: pp. 485–493

### TABLE 6.2

### LIVING KIDNEY DONOR RECUPERTOIN

| | |
|---|---|
| Sick/Vacation days anticipated for donation | 23.8 ± 16.0 |
| Sick/Vacation days actually used | 21.3 ± 23.1 |
| Total days from donation to return to work | 46.4 ± 26.3 |
| Working days between donation and return to work | 34.0 ± 18.8 |

On average donors required 14 more days for recovery than employer benefits provided

Reprinted with permission: McCune TR. *Clin Transplant* (2004) 18(Suppl 12):33.

The NKF study of 1986 reported that medical complications of the donor subsequently contributed to the financial hardship placed on the donor and their families.[22] The range of expenses reported to the University of Minnesota was $0 to $20,000 in 1999 dollars.[2] Their donors reported paying an average $579 for expenses related to donation, but the median amount of expenses reported was $0. The average liver donor had $3,660 (in 2001 dollars) in transplant-related expenses.[3] Donors reported expenses related to travel to and from the transplant center,[3,21] lodging,[3,21] medication,[3] child care,[21] and long-distance phone bills.[15] The financial burden was so great on one liver donor family that they declared bankruptcy a year after the donation due to medical expenses.[15] The donor frequently relies on the recipient to provide support for donation-related expenses. Up to 20% of kidney donors receive financial support from their recipient for travel expenses.[21] When support was given between the donor and the recipient, it was most often parent recipients supporting their offspring who donated.[4] Parent donors were conversely least likely to support their recipient children. Donors received support from their family to cover other donation-related expenses. The LODN registry found that 24% of donors received support in paying lodging expenses from relatives.[21] Supporting the donor financially is a way for nondonor family members to contribute to the process.[4] Financial concerns of the donor seem to be a problem of U.S. kidney and liver donors. The NKF study reported that when kidney donors reported receiving support from their family and community, they also reported increased levels of financial hardship.[22] Financial stress reported by kidney donors was independent of the donor's race, sex, marital status, level of education, income, or employer benefits.

The concern about the financial burden placed on the donor is only reported from U.S. transplant centers. The financial burdens of the European and Asian donor may be less than those of the U.S. donor, or they may be underreported in the medical literature published in English.

## RECOVERY

A frequent question asked by potential donors during their decision phase is, "When will I return to my normal activities?" Many donors will also ask during recovery, "When will I feel normal again?" For the adult-to-child liver donor, they must first get out of the "crisis mode" of dealing with an acutely ill child.[15] It is only when they are confident that the worst is behind them that they report they can "return to normalcy." Adult-to-adult liver donors have a recovery phase that is independent of the recipient's recovery period as reported by the Lahey Clinic.[32]

When asked when they felt that they had achieved 100% recovery, 75% of the donors from the University of Colorado reported that they had achieved this on an average time of 3.4 months.[3]

Those donors who felt that they had not achieved full recovery on an average reported that by 4 months they had achieved approximately "82%" of recovery to normal. When Indian donors who sold their kidneys were asked to rate their health, 86% reported that nephrectomy caused a persistent decline in their health.[20] The German study of kidney donors reported by Giessing found that only 5% had not recovered completely by 1 year.[9]

Their motivation and type of job may contribute to the donors return to their previous and normal state of health. When the LODN survey asked kidney donors when they returned to work, the average was 46 +/- 26 days.[21] Ninety-six percent of liver donors at the University of Colorado returned to work on an average of 2.4 +/- 1.2 months after donation.[3] One donor in the University of Colorado survey (4%) elected to change careers postdonation. The wide statistical variants of the mean for both kidney and liver donors suggest that recovery is very variable. When counseling a potential donor on when they will return to work, it is important to stress that their return to work is totally up to them and they should not anticipate what their recovery "should be" or compare their recovery to "an average donor."

## THE DONOR IN MOURNING

The death of a recipient or the early failure of a graft is the worst outcome the organ donor can experience.[12,36–39] The reported case of a kidney donor committing suicide occurred in a woman after the death of her recipient/husband.[12] The large Norwegian study of kidney donors (n = 494) was able to identify a subgroup of 96 donors who had lost their donated kidney or the recipient.[1] The quality-of-life questionnaire observed a low reported quality of life in these unfortunate donors than was found in the remaining donors. Interestingly, the quality of life of the donors who lost their recipients was still equal to that found in the general population of Norway.

Two factors contribute to the fall in the quality of life of these unfortunate donors. The first factor is a sense of abandonment felt by the donors. In many cases the recipient was someone the donor had hoped to have a closer relationship with. Also, the abandonment by the transplant team contributes greatly to their isolation. In the Swedish study of kidney donors who lost their recipients, the donors reported that the transplant team did not initiate approach to discuss the death of the recipient.[36] Donors felt that if discussion took place, it was at their request. So complete is the abandonment of the donor, one study of kidney donors' quality of life excluded donors who had lost their recipient.[5]

The second factor that impacts the quality of life of donors is the anger and the loss of confidence in the transplant team. One living donor who offered to participate in the study from the University of Colorado was refused despite repeated phone calls to participate even 14 months after the death of the recipient.[3] Two of the 10 donors in the Swedish study expressed doubt that the best possible care was given to their recipients.[36] As uncomfortable as it may be, it is important that the transplant team maintain contact with the donor in mourning. In spite of these negative feelings, these interviewed donors were grateful for the contact with the Swedish team and were glad to donate and willing to donate again.

## CONCLUSION

The majority of donors reported in this chapter were grateful to have been given the opportunity to donate. This was even true in the studies that considered the donors who had lost their graft or recipient.[5,36] The only study, which reported regret by donors, was the study of donors in India who had sold a kidney.[20] But to improve the transplant experience of all living organ donors, the transplant community must address the concerns of the minority of donors. The part of the population that is organ donors is different than the general population from which they come. They have higher self-esteem and express a greater sense of physical and emotional wellness than is found in the general population. The tool most frequently used to evaluate the emotional and physical well-being of living donors, the RAND 36-Item Health Survey (SF-36) is an instrument for measuring health perception in a general population.[40] This survey does not include questions on the altruistic motives or narcissistic feelings of the donor, stress of coercion or sense of encouragement of the recipient and family, or the health concerns related to donation and the approach of the transplant team. To better understand how these factors affect the donors recuperation these questions need to be incorporated in future studies of donors.

Financial concerns of donors are important factors in their stress during recuperation. Donors receive financial support from employers, friends, and family. This support can be helpful or destructive depending on how it is perceived by the donor and their family. Donors should not be forced to rely on the largess of others. The U.S. government receives the greatest financial benefit from living organ donation. The U.S. government should step up and support the financial needs of donors so that no donor is faced with the possibility of bankruptcy.

Donors express a sense of abandonment after donation. Donors desire to maintain contact with the transplant team to ensure their continued good health and emotional well-being.

This sense of abandonment is greatest when the outcome after donation is not ideal. The donor advocate or volunteer mentor can play an important role keeping the donor connected with the program. This network needs to be nationwide because 36% of donors live in a different state than the one where the program is located.[21] This potential network could also provide medical follow-up on the health of the donor.

The transplant community has changed the approach to evaluate the concerns of living organ donors from individual psychotherapy with donors and their family to multicenter donor surveys. A great deal has been learned. It is time to take these concerns and criticisms and change the way the transplant community works with and supports living organ donors. We must work to create a new survey instrument to evaluate the concerns of donors, create a network to support the donor during recuperation that could include medical follow-up care, and work to remove financial disincentives that the donor must shoulder.

## References

1. Westlie L, Fauchald P, Talseth T, Jakobsen A, Flatmark A. Quality of life in Norwegian kidney donors. *Nephrol Dial Transplant* 1993;8:1146–1150.
2. Johnson EM, Anderson JK, Jacobs C. Long-term follow-up of living kidney donors: Quality of life after donation. *Transplantation* 1999;67:717–721.
3. Trotter JF, Talamantes M, McClure M, et al. Right hepatic lobe donation for living donor liver transplantation: Impact on donor quality of life. *Liver Transplant* 2001;7:485.
4. Jacobs C, Johnson E, Anderson K, et al. Kidney transplants from living donors: How donation affects family dynamics. *Advan Renal Replace Ther* 1998;5:89.

5. de Graaf Olson W, Bogetti-Dumlao A. Living donors' perception of their quality of health after donation. *Progr Transplant* 2001;11:108.

6. Fehrman-Ekholm I, Brink B, Ericson C, et al. Kidney donors don't regret. Follow-up of 370 in Stockholm since 1964. *Transplantation* 2000;69:2067.

7. Isotani S, Fujisawa M, Ishikawa Y, et al. Quality of life of living kidney donors: The short-form 36-item health questionnaire survey. *Transplantation* 2002;60:558.

8. Smith G, Trauer T, Kerr PG, et al. Prospective psychological monitoring of living kidney donors using the SF-36 health survey. *Transplantation* 2003;76:807.

9. Giessing M, Reuter S, Schonberger B, et al. Quality of life of kidney donors in Germany: A survey with the validated short form-36 and Giessen subjective complaints list-24 questionnaires. *Transplantation* 2004;78:864.

10. Pascher A, Sauer IM, Walter M, et al. Donor evaluation, donor risks, donor outcome, and donor quality of life in adult-to-adult living donor liver transplantation. *Liver Transplant* 2002;8:829.

11. Simmons RG, Klein SD, Simmons RL. *The Gift of Life: The Social and Psychological Impact of Organ Transplantation.* New York: Wiley; 1977.

12. Weizer N, Weizman A, Sharma Z, et al. Suicide by related kidney donors following the recipients' death. *Psychosom* 1989;51:216.

13. Ghobrial RM, Sammy S, Lassman C, et al. Donor and recipient outcome in right lobe adult living donor liver transplantation. *Liver Transplant* 2002;8:901.

14. Simmons RG, Marine SK, Simmons RL. *Gift of Life: The Effect of Organ Transplantation on Individual, Family, and Social Dynamics.* New Brunswick, NJ: Transaction Books;1987.

15. Crowley-Matoka M, Siegler M, Cronin DC. Long-term quality of life issues among adult-to-pediatric living liver donors: A qualitative exploration. *Am J Transplant* 2004;4:744.

16. Boulware LE, Ratner LE, Troll MV, et al. Attitudes, psychology, and risk taking of potential live kidney donors: Strangers, relatives and the general public. *Am J Transplant* 2005;5:1671.

17. Delmonico FL, Surman OS. Is this live-organ donor your patient? *Transplantation* 2003;76:1257.

18. Papachristou C, Walter M, Dietrich K, et al. Motivatio for living-donor liver transplantation from the donor's perspective: An in-depth qualitative research study. *Tranplantation* 2004;78:1506.

19. Kemph JP, Bermann EA, Coppolillo HP. Kidney transplant and shifts in family dynamics. *Amer J Psychiat* 1969;11:1485.

20. Goyal M, Mehta RL, Schneiderman LJ, et al. Economic and health consequences of selling a kidney in India. *JAMA* 2002;288:1589.

21. McCune TR, Armata T, Mendez-Picon G et al. The Living Organ Donor Network: A model registry for living kidney donors. *Clin Transplant* 2004;18(Suppl 12):33.

22. Smith MD, Kapell DF, Province MA, et al. Living-related kidney donors: A multicenter study of donor education, socioeconomic adjustment, and rehabilitation. *AJKD* 1986;8: 223.

23. Steiner RW. Risk appreciation for living kidney donors: Another new subspecialty? *Am J Transpl* (2004) 4, 694.

24. Spital A. Rejecting heroic kidney donors protects much more than the public trust. *Am J Transpl* 2004;4:1727.

25. Steiner RW, Gert B. A technique for presenting risk and outcome data to potential living renal transplant donors. *Transplantation* 2001; 71:1056.

26. Kemph JP. Psychotherapy with patients receiving kidney transplant. *Am J Psychiat* 1967;124:77.

27. Heck G, Schweitzer J, Seidel-Wiessel. Psychological effects of living related kidney transplantation-risk and chances. *Clin Transplant* 2004;18:716.

28. Danzer G, Walter M, Bonner E, et al. Leberlebendspende: Ethische reflexionen anhand erster empririscher untersuchungsergebnisse von 22 potentiellen spendern. *Med Welt* 2000;51:341.

29. Kemph JP. Renal Failure, artificial kidney and kidney transplant. *Am J Psychiatry* 1966;122:1270.

30. Morris P, St George B, Waring T, et al. Psychosocial complications in living related kidney donors: An Australian experience. *Tranplant Proc* 1987:19:2840.

31. Pomfret EA, Pomposelli JJ, Gordon FD, et al. Liver regeneration and surgical outcome of donors of right lobe liver grafts. *Transplantation* 2003;76:5.

32. Pomfret EA. What is the quality-of-life after live liver donation? *Am J Transplant* 2004;4:673.

33. Abrams HS, Buchanan DC. The gift of life: A review of the psychological aspects of kidney transplantation. *Int J Psychiatry Med* 1976–1977;7:153.

34. George CRR,Tiller DJ, Burrows SM, et al. Life with a transplanted kidney. *Med J Aust* 1970;1:461.

35. Knott RS, Levey AS, Beto JA. Psychological factors impacting patients, donors, and nondonors involved in renal transplant evaluation. *Perspectives 1996. National Kidney Foundation* 1996;15:11.

36. Haljamae U, Nyberg G, Sjostrom B. Remaining experiences of living kidney donors more than 3 yr after early recipient graft loss. *Clin Transplant* 2003;17:503.

37. Hirvas J, Enckell M, Kuhlback B, el al. Psychological and social problems encountered in active treatment of chronic uraemia. II. The living donor. *Acta Med Scand* 1976;200:17.

38. Kamstra-Hennen L, Beebe J, Stumm S, et al. Ethical evaluation of the related donation: The donor after five years. *Transplant Proc* 1981;13:60.

39. Simmons RG, Kamstra-Hennen L. The living related kidney donor: Psychological reactions when the kidney fails. *Neph Dial Transplant* 1979;208:572.

40. Brazier JE, Harper R, Jones NM, et al. Validating the SF-36 health survey questionnaire: New outcome measure for primary care. *BMJ* (1992) 305,160.

# PART II

# PAID LEGAL AND ILLEGAL
# ORGAN DONATION

# CHAPTER 7

# CURRENT
# FINANCIAL INCENTIVES

## 7.1 INCENTIVES IN WESTERN COUNTRIES: THE WISCONSIN MODEL

*Steve Wieckert, Scott Becher,*
*Hans W. Sollinger, MD, PhD*

### INTRODUCTION

The following chapter, primarily written by Wisconsin Representative Steve Wieckert and his Chief of Staff Scott Becher, demonstrates that you need a single patient who is getting the attention of an interested legislator can initiate significant changes, and even stimulate the passing of a law that will have a profound influence on organ donation. When Representative Steve Wieckert heard about Cody Monrose's situation, he was touched and became interested in potential measures to help families in similar situations. At the beginning I did not know about his efforts and found out by happenstance from a Michigan physician who visited us that a Wisconsin Legislator was trying to push a law forward that would provide some degree of compensation for live donors. I contacted Representative Steve Wieckert and expressed to him my pessimism as the justice department had indeed just a few weeks prior to our first contact indicated that any compensation for organ donors is considered to be contradictory to federal law. However, Representative Steve Wieckert, in his discussions with the justice department, could clearly determine that reimbursement for costs would not fall into this category. For this reason, he vigorously pursued work on Cody's Law and was successful in having Larry Hagman attend the first committee meeting which took place at Froedtert Hospital in Milwaukee. I had the good fortune to get to know Larry Hagman as a member of Tommy Thompson's ACOT committee, and in part I knew that Larry wanted to do me a favor by showing up at the meeting, but also he took the opportunity to attend the simultaneously occurring Harley Davidson show in Milwaukee. Needless to say, the first committee hearing was a resounding success and from there on this legislation moved forward rapidly within the Wisconsin legislature. I give all the credit to Representative Steve Wieckert; it was his idea, and while he generously gives me credit in public, I do not deserve it. I asked Representative Wieckert to write this chapter in collaboration, because he is indeed most familiar with the history of this landmark law, which is now being copied by more than a dozen other states. More important, the process that took place in Wisconsin should be a reminder to all of our patients to make sure that their voices are heard, and with a little bit of luck and persistence, they will find a legislator in their state who will take up their cause as Representative Wieckert did with Cody's Law.

Promoting organ donation and helping to save lives was the motivation for a piece of legislation introduced in the Wisconsin legislature during the 2003–2004 session, 2003 Assembly.

### BILL 477

This bill took a year to wind through the legislative process, overcoming a number of significant challenges, and became law on January 30, 2004 (2003 Wisconsin Act 119).

The bill created a state income tax deduction of up to $10,000 for expenses incurred by a living donor for the costs of travel, lodging, and lost wages associated with making a donation.

Cody Monroe, an 8-year-old boy who had received a kidney transplant from his living father, was brought to each of the committee meetings on the bill by his parents. Cody's parents provided valuable testimony. In recognition of Cody's efforts, the bill is now referred to as Cody's Law.

Since its passage, over 23 states have introduced Wisconsin's Cody's Law, and 7 states have already passed it into law.

### LEGISLATIVE PURPOSE

The authors of the legislation, including State Representative Steve Wieckert (R-Appleton) the bill's principal sponsor, believed that the act of donating an organ was sufficiently benevolent and courageous, without imposing additional costs for donating. Yet making a donation costs donors thousands of dollars in many cases, not only for the cost of travel to a transplant center, and for the hotel stays for prescreening and other medical tests, but also for the time off of work needed to recover from the donor surgery. Therefore, Cody's Law was proposed.

Fiscal analysis prepared by the Wisconsin Department of Revenue estimated that the average Wisconsin living donor had $6,000 of related expenses, of which about $4,200 was from lost wages. In 2002, Wisconsin had 213 living donors: 207 kidney donations and 6 partial liver donations. Between 30 and 40 workdays are missed by an average donor to allow for recovery time.[1]

The objective from the start was to help find solutions to the problem of the shortage of available organs for transplant. The problem defined was summed up in the statistics of 87,000 people on the waiting list for an organ transplant with over 5,200 people dying each year because of a transplant organ not being available in time.[2]

Well over a dozen potential solutions were considered, including ways to increase donations from both living and deceased individuals. All proposals had merit; but they also had limitations. There were numerous challenges: budgetary constraints, ethical and public perception considerations, and federal limitations, to name a few.

One of the advantages of Cody's Law is that it deals with living donors, who make up nearly as much of the donor pool as five deceased donors according to OPTN data as of July 8, 2005. Organs from living donors offer potentially longer useful life in the recipient as well as lower rejection rates.

## THE THREE BIGGEST CHALLENGES FOR APPROVAL

The three biggest challenges in advancing this legislation included the cost to the state treasury in terms of lost revenue, getting the legislature to give this bill priority compared to the many hundreds of bills introduced each year, and the paramount challenge of getting the federal government to acknowledge that the legislation complied with federal law.

### The Cost

In 2003, the Wisconsin state government had a very large 2-year budget deficit of over $3 billion. The chance of any legislation being approved that would either increase spending or cut revenues was, at best, unlikely. However, the authors argued the bill could help save lives, and save a lifetime of dialysis expense for Medical Assistance programs.

In addition, to help limit the loss of revenue and increase the likelihood of passage, the bill was drafted as a tax deduction instead of as a tax credit. It was originally hoped a full tax credit could be made available to a living donor for his or her expenses, so a donor would have no out-of-pocket expenses. However, prevailing budget restraints made a credit unrealistic, and a tax deduction was chosen as a less costly alternative.

The amount of the deduction was fixed at $10,000 because the amount was deemed sufficiently large to cover the highest likely expenses to be incurred by a living donor. The number is also an attention grabber. It is interesting to note that other states that have subsequently introduced Cody's Law had the option of raising or lowering the $10,000 limit based on their own needs and interests, yet all the states have used the $10,000 limit. The wheel has been invented, and it works.

### Getting Legislative Attention

Wisconsin has 132 state legislators, each with the authority to introduce legislation. During the 2003 legislative session, 1,567 bills were introduced, with the authors wanting each one to receive committee hearings and executive action, floor debate in both houses and eventually a governor's signature. To get the attention of other legislators and to get them to act on a particular piece of legislation before others is no small task. Cody's Law was rather unusual, as it was the first legislation of its kind in the country. This made advancement of the legislation even more difficult.

A number of factors contributed significantly to the legislation's visibility. First, and most important, the bill was given much needed credibility by the endorsement and active, persistent support of transplant surgeon Dr. Hans Sollinger of the University of Wisconsin Medical Center. Legislators propose a lot of ideas. Who is to say they are valuable or counter productive? Having the approval of experts in the field that the legislation affects is invaluable in gaining the support of other lawmakers.

Second, receiving positive media attention helps the bill to stand out from the others and encourages action. Miss Wisconsin 2003, Tina Sauerhammer, was the youngest medical school graduate in the history of the University of Wisconsin at age 22.[3] Her father died at the age of 45, awaiting a kidney donation, which never came. Tina dedicated her reign to the promotion of tissue and organ donation. She was an enthusiastic supporter of the bill. The media would single her out for interviews after committee meetings at which she testified.

Additionally, Larry Hagman, a famous TV celebrity who received a liver transplant and is a member of the national organ donor council through the Department of Health and Human Services actively supported passage of Cody's Law. Months were spent researching this legislation. Documentation and supporting material fill an entire file drawer in the office of the bill's author, as well as half a hard drive, he reports. During the research, the Advisory Committee on Organ Transplantation was discovered by Scott Becher, chief legislative advisor to the bill's author. Calls were made to try to locate actor Larry Hagman and get some type of indication of support for the bill. It was a long shot. The best-case scenario involved Hagman traveling to Wisconsin to testify for the bill. The likelier outcome was some show of support—a letter, or perhaps a video. But first he had to take the call.

Mr. Hagman agreed to personally testify at a committee meeting arranged in Milwaukee at the Medical College of Wisconsin. Not only did his presence give the bill much-needed attention, but also legislators and reporters at the meeting were impressed with his in-depth knowledge of the whole field of organ donation and the critical shortage our country faces.

Throughout the bill's advancement, a group of organ donors and recipients, including Cody and his parents, actively supported and testified for the legislation on more than one occasion. It was a time-consuming effort, including waiting during the committee meeting until the bill came up on the agenda for discussion. Their testimony was priceless. When they finished, there rarely was a dry eye in the room.

Because people who believed in the importance of organ donation chose to get actively involved, Cody's Law got the attention needed to advance.

### Conforming With Existing Federal and State Law

From the start, the goal of the legislation was to find ways to promote organ donation. In many of the ideas considered, federal and state laws limited what could be done. As the idea of a tax deduction started to evolve and the research calls were made, a number of different state and federal agency officials, medical experts, and legal counsels gave opinions that ranged from discouraging to "it can't be done." Usually at this point, the legislative research is put on the shelf and legislators consider other bill ideas, like highway improvements, crime prevention, and the like. However, in this case, the need for action to reduce the organ shortage was too great to let the idea fall on first review.

Awareness and acceptance did not come easily. Government officials were very sensitive to the laws against buying and selling organs. This shibboleth is considered so inviolate that some dismissed the proposal summarily. Officials from federal agencies often would refer inquires to the Department of Justice without hearing any details, and the Department would not give any opinions.

As a result, many office meetings were held at the state capitol with legal experts and agency officials. Conference calls between attorneys at the state and federal capitals were arranged. Trips to Washington to meet with Department of Health and Human Services officials were made. Former Wisconsin governor and Health and Human Services Secretary Tommy Thompson offered his support. A considerable number of changes and modifications to the original bill were drafted.

The key to success in developing the legislation was to limit the deduction for expenses to the three areas that are specifically exempt from reimbursement restrictions under federal law: travel, lodging, and lost wages. Since Wisconsin adopted Cody's Law, another state tried to pass an expanded version of the bill, covering more areas for expense deductions, but the state's Attorney General ruled against it.[4]

To be fully accurate, the law does not provide an incentive. Rather, this bill reduces a financial disincentive for organ donation. A donor will simply have less expense for donating as a result of the legislation. In many cases, a living donor will still need to spend some of his or her own money to donate, just not as much as he or she would have without this legislation, because now the expenses will be tax deductible. Someday, it would be best if the laws could evolve so that a donor would have minimal or no expense for donating, similar to a blood donor. A full tax credit would be one way to achieve that goal.

## A HELPFUL MEDIA

The fact that this was groundbreaking legislation made it difficult to develop and advance through the process, but it also made it a significant focus of media attention.

As the bill gained approval from the medical community and began to cross some legislative hurdles, the media really began to take note. Cody's Law was eventually reported in the *New York Times, The Washington Post, The Los Angeles Times, Paul Harvey News and Comment,* several cable news networks, and even in a passing comment on *The Tonight Show.* In addition, dozens of local newspapers, radio, and television stations did news reports on this law.

This media reporting was especially helpful because, as state legislators in other states across the country read about Cody's Law, they became more aware of the shortage and how they could do something about it. As a result, the bill began to spread to other states. The media deserve considerable credit for the introduction of Cody's Law in a dozen states.

## THE BENEFITS OF CODY'S LAW

The law eases the financial burden of an organ donor. Already, newspapers are reporting cases where organ donors have said the law was helpful in their own case. In addition, time after time during committee hearings, both organ donors and recipients stated how encouraging it was to them in their situation to know that the government cared about them and their plight. The law gives hope to potential recipients that the government has not forgotten about them, but is aware of the problem and is trying to help.

Also, passing the law simply creates more awareness of the need for organ donations. This can lead to more stickers on driver's licenses, more additions to living wills or Health Care Powers of Attorney, more support for awareness campaigns, as well as a host of other mutually supporting activities.

## CODY'S LAW FOR OTHER STATES

It is helpful for each state to enact this type of law. As each state does so, the disincentives for donation will be fewer, which will help lead to more organ donations, reducing the shortage and saving more lives.

Copies of the Wisconsin model can be found in the Wisconsin statutes on the State of Wisconsin Web site.[5] The author of Cody's Law has expressed his willingness to answer any questions as well.

Asking a legislator to introduce a version of Cody's Law is a good start. Most legislators are looking for good bill ideas to introduce. One of the advantages of this legislation is that it receives bipartisan support. Before introducing the bill, it may be helpful to get the support of the medical community and locate an organ donor and recipient willing to testify before a committee.

Variations of the bill are possible. However, limiting the type of tax deduction for expenses to travel, lodging, and lost wages is important to comply with federal law. Changing the deduction to an income tax credit would be of extra help for the living donor.

## References

1. Wisconsin State Legislature. Fiscal Estimate for 2003 Assembly Bill 477 [Web page]. Madison: Wisconsin Department of Revenue, 2003. http://www.legis.state.wi.us/2003/data/fe/AB-477fe.pdf . Accessed July 12, 2005.
2. 2004 Annual Report of the U.S. Organ Procurement and Transplantation Network and the Scientific Registry of Transplant Recipients: Transplant Data 1994-2003. Department of Health and Human Services, Health Resources and Services Administration, Healthcare Systems Bureau, Division of Transplantation, Rockville, MD; United Network for Organ Sharing, Richmond, VA; University Renal Research and Education Association, Ann Arbor, MI.
3. Milwaukee Journal Sentinel. A heartbeat away [Web site]. http://www.jsonline.com/news/state/sep03/171108.asp . Accessed July 12, 2005.
4. Kansas Judicial Branch. Attorney General Opinion 2000-18 [Web site]. http://www.kscourts.org/ksag/opinions/2000/2000-018.htm. Accessed July 12, 2005.
5. Wisconsin State Legislature. Wisconsin State Statute 71.05(10)(i)1. http://folio.legis.state.wi.us/cgi-bin/om_isapi.dll?clientID=33188962&hitsperheading=on&infobase=stats.nfo&record={E637}&softpage=Document. Accessed July 12, 2005.

# 7.2   INCENTIVES IN NON-WESTERN COUNTRIES: THE IRANIAN MODEL

*Ahad J. Ghods, MD*

## INTRODUCTION

In Iran, the total annual health expenditure is only 6% of its gross domestic product. Yet it has a unique, very successful (though ethically somewhat controversial), compensated, and regulated living unrelated donor (LURD) kidney transplant program. After this program was adopted in 1988, the kidney transplant waiting list was eliminated by 1999. Iran is the only country in the world without a kidney transplant waiting list.

Of the 68 million inhabitants of Iran, about 25 000 have end-stage kidney disease (ESRD), or about 368 per million, more than 50% of all ESRD patients in the country are living with a functioning kidney graft.[1]

## HISTORY OF KIDNEY TRANSPLANTATION IN IRAN

The kidney transplant program in Iran has spanned 2 distinct periods. During the first period (1967–1988) almost all kidney transplants were from living related donors (LRDs); the number of transplants performed was much lower than the national demand. In the beginning of the second period (1988–2005), attention at cultural, religious, and socioeconomic levels gave rise to a government-funded, financially compensated, and well-regulated LURD program. By providing legal financial incentives to volunteer donors, the number of transplants grew rapidly.[2]

### First Period Background

The first kidney transplant in Iran was performed in Shiraz in 1967. The number of patients undergoing dialysis steadily increased, but the kidney transplant program severely lagged behind. From 1967 to 1985, only about 100 kidney transplants were performed. In 1980, given very limited transplant activity in Iran, the Ministry of Health started allowing dialysis patients to be transplanted abroad with government funds. Any dialysis patient who had a letter of acceptance from a transplant unit abroad was approved as a transplant candidate by the Iranian government, which paid all travel and transplant expenses. As a result, a large number of patients undergoing dialysis who were

ready to be transplanted created a long kidney transplant waiting list at the Ministry of Health. From 1980 through 1985, using government funds, over 400 of these patients traveled to Europe and the United States and underwent a kidney transplant. Most of these transplants were performed in the United Kingdom with LRDs. In 1985, the high expense of kidney transplants abroad and the increasing number of patients on the kidney transplant waiting list prompted health authorities to establish transplant facilities in Iran.[3] Two kidney transplant teams were organized from 1985 to 1987; 274 kidney transplants with LRDs were performed.

### Second Period The Iranian Model

In 1988, a large number of dialysis patients needed a kidney transplant but had no LRD. A deceased donor (DD) organ transplant program had not yet been established and did not seem likely in the near future. (It was eventually launched in 2000.) So, in 1988, a government-funded, financially compensated, and carefully regulated LURD transplant program was adopted. As a result, the number of kidney transplant teams in Iran gradually increased from 2 to 25. The number of kidney transplants performed rapidly increased, so that by 1999, the waiting list was eliminated. This program was eventually named the Iranian Model. By the end of 2004, a total of 17718 kidney transplants had been performed (3196 with LRDs; 13920 LURDs; and 602, DDs). Figure 7.2-1 shows the annual number of kidney transplants in Iran from 1984 through 2004. Currently, 26 kidney transplants per million are performed in Iran each year. More than 78% of all kidney transplants in Iran have used LURDs.

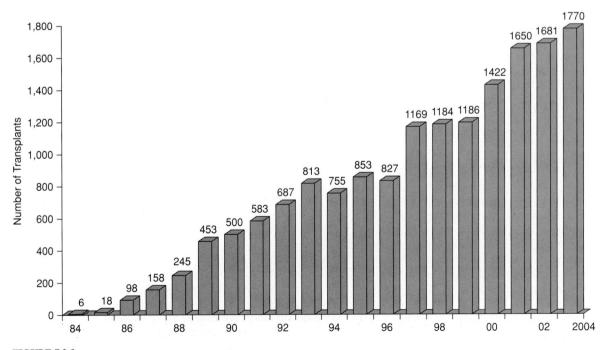

**FIGURE 7.2-1**

Annual number of kidney transplants performed in Iran, 1984–2004

## CHARACTERISTICS OF THE IRANIAN MODEL

During the initial evaluation of all kidney transplant candidates, the Iranian Model transplant physician recommends and emphasizes the advantages of undergoing an LRD (vs LURD) transplant. The physician also discusses the scarcity of DD kidneys. Candidates with no LRD are referred to the Dialysis and Transplant Patients Association (DATPA) to locate a suitable LURDs. (Those who volunteer as LURDs also contact this association.) All members of DATPA are ESRD patients; they receive no incentives for finding LURDs or for referring themselves and their LURD to a kidney transplant team. The Iranian Model has no role for a broker or an agency.

All kidney transplant teams belong to university hospitals, and the government pays all hospital expenses for kidney transplants. After the transplant, the LURD receives an award and health insurance from the government. The government also provides to the transplant recipient essential immunosuppressive drugs, such as cyclosporine (Neoral) and mycophenolate mofetil (MMF) at a greatly reduced price. Charitable organizations are also very active in providing these drugs to poor patients. Most LURDs also receive a reward or gift (arranged and defined by DATPA) from the recipient or from one of the charitable organizations. Kidney transplant teams receive no incentives in the form of gifts or government awards. The program is under the close scrutiny of the transplant teams themselves as well as of the Iranian Society of Organ Transplantation regarding all ethical issues. Foreigners are not allowed to undergo a kidney transplant with an Iranian donor, nor are they permitted to volunteer as LURDs for Iranian transplant recipients.

## ETHICAL CONSIDERATIONS

One of the arguments against models of paid kidney donation is that such donors would almost all be poor and illiterate, whereas most of their recipients would be educated and wealthy. In our study[9] of 500 LURD recipients, we found that 6% of donors were illiterate, 24.4% had attended only elementary school, 63.4% had completed high school, and 6.2% had some university training. The same education levels in their recipients were 18%, 20%, 50.8%, and 11.2%. We also grouped LURDs and their recipients according to whether they were poor, rich, or middle class. We found that 84% of LURDs were poor and 16% were middle class; 50.4% of LURD recipients were poor, 36.2% were middle class, and 13.4% were rich. Thus, more than 50% of LURD kidneys were transplanted into poor recipients. Again, the amount of financial compensation from recipients to LURDs is controlled by DATPA, and charitable organizations provide compensation on behalf of poor recipients.

The regulation in the Iranian Model prohibiting foreigners from receiving kidneys from Iranian LURDs has prevented transplant tourism. And the regulation prohibiting foreigners from volunteering as LURDs for Iranian recipients has prevented the use as LURDs of the many Afghani and Iraqi refugees residing in Iran. However, of the 2.5 million Afghani refugees in Iran, all have access to dialysis and transplant services (with Afghani donors) on an equal basis with Iranian nationals. A study conducted in 2004 showed that, of 241 Afghani refugees with ESRD, 179 were on dialysis and 62 had been transplanted in Iran. Of these 62 transplant recipients, 9 received kidneys from LRDs, (2 from spouses), 50 from Afghani LURDs, and 1 from a DD.[10]

## RATIONALE FOR THE IRANIAN MODEL

### The Use of Altruism Has Failed to Alleviate the Organ Shortage

Since the 1980s, many countries have passed legislation prohibiting monetary compensation for organ donation. All organ donations in such countries have become altruistic, meaning that donors or their families receive no financial incentive or compensation. Unfortunately, the altruistic supply of organs has been far less than adequate. Several approaches have been adopted to increase the altruistic organ supply, but the gap between supply and demand has worsened over time. The organ shortage remains the most challenging problem in transplantation today.

Only in limited circumstances are most human beings willing to show uncompensated generosity toward others; the forces of self-interest are basic for almost all of our daily activities. Providing more financial incentives to organ sources would likely increase the number of available organs for transplantation.[11]

### The Necessity of Providing Financial Incentives Is Being Accepted

Currently, in developed countries, the number of patients on kidney transplant waiting lists is steadily increasing; each year, thousands of patients die while waiting for a kidney transplant. In developing countries, more than 500000 new ESRD patients die each year because of a lack of access to dialysis and kidney transplant facilities. In addition, worldwide, several hundred thousand patients suffer on dialysis therapy while awaiting a kidney transplant. Some members of the transplant community now believe that altruism alone is not enough and that providing some financial incentives or social benefits is necessary to increase the number of donors.[1] It is increasingly accepted that, by adoption of legalized, compensated, and well-regulated LURD programs, similar to the Iranian Model, many deaths could be prevented and thousands of dialysis patients could be rehabilitated.[12] In the United States, several proposals have been submitted to the Congress to promote organ donation through incentives such as a donor medal of honor, a tax credit, or a tax refund (although several senior transplant experts have asked Congress to retain prohibition of monetary compensation for organ donation).[13] The previous severe condemnation by some ethicists against incentive-based organ donation is gradually softening; it is possible that some type of compensated LURD transplants may be legalized in the United States or other countries in the future.[14]

### The use of LURDs Is Increasing Worldwide

A gradual change in attitude has occurred since the early ethical guidelines with regard to LURDs. In 1987, a postal survey showed that only 8% of transplant centers in the United States would accept altruistic strangers as kidney donors. This percentage increased to 15% in 1993 and to 38% 1999.[15] Since 2000, in the United States, the number of living kidney donors surpassed the number of DDs. Kidney donation increased substantially in all living donor groups, but the greatest increase was in the nonspouse LURD group.[7] Interestingly, the percentage of living donors who were either a spouse or completely unrelated to the recipient increased from 5% in 1998 to 30% in 2002.[16] Reasons for this increased use of LURDs include the growing recognition by patients and their physicians that a kidney transplant, not chronic dialysis, is the treatment of choice for ESRD; that they cannot rely on the kidney transplant waiting list, because so many patients die while waiting; that LURD transplants yield better results than DD transplants; and that patients should be transplanted soon, rather than waiting for years. The shorter the period on dialysis, the better the patient and graft survival rates. Thus, many transplant centers in the United States are now accepting spouses, close friends, and altruistic strangers as kidney donors. Indeed, some patients from developed countries are traveling abroad to receive paid kidneys from strangers in developing countries.[17] If LURD transplants are increasing in the United States as a supplement to DD and LRD transplants, then their use in developing countries such as Iran with limited transplant activity is more than justified.

### Proposals of Some Ethicists Regarding the Organ Shortage Are Disappointing

Some ethicists from developed as well as developing countries are still against compensated LURD transplants. Some ethicists have proposed that the solution in developed countries is to increase DD transplants by accepting marginal donors or by passing a presumed consent law. Opponents of compensated organ donation programs need to explain why the death of thousands of patients on transplant waiting lists and why subjecting thousands of living organ donors to surgery is preferable to providing financial incentives for DDs.[11] In 2002, nearly 6 650 patients were reported to the Organ Procurement and Transplantation Network in the United States who died waiting for an organ transplant.[18] Since 2001, the number of LDs also has surpassed the number of DDs in the United States.[16] In developing countries, most transplant ethicists have proposed, first and foremost, establishing a Western model of DD kidney transplant programs, but many infrastructural deficiencies (along with cultural barriers) prevent large-scale implementation. Second, ethicists have proposed further increasing LD kidney transplants, which will surely result in coercion, particularly of female donors—a situation that is more unethical than the use of paid LURDs.[19]

The adoption of compensated LURD programs in developing countries should not be forbidden simply because all ethical issues cannot be solved. Providing financial incentives to organ sources increases the number of transplantable organs and saves or improves the lives of thousands of recipients. Condemning all forms of compensated organ transplants results in so many patient deaths and so much suffering: how can such a stance be considered ethical? Instead of condemnation, transplant experts and ethicists must organize meetings and discussions to develop ethical guidelines for the use of this type of organ donor, at least in developing countries. The Iranian Model of compensated kidney transplants has successfully eliminated the waiting list in Iran. It has prevented many patient deaths and has improved the quality of life of thousands. In this model, many (but not all) of the ethical problems related to compensated organ donation have been prevented.[20]

### Improvements Needed in the Iranian Model

In any LURD transplant program, ethical issues must frequently be revisited and possibly revised. The following revisions have been recommended in order to make the Iranian Model ethically more acceptable. (1) The entire reward and all financial incentives to LURDs should come from the government or charitable organizations, not partly from the recipient. (2) The quantity and quality of the award should have a life-changing potential. This means that, to the same extent that the donated kidney changes or improves the life of the recipient, the reward and financial incentives should also change or improve the life of the LURD. The reward also should have a long-term compensatory effect; in other words, it should not be merely cash that will only satisfy the donor short term. (3) Social benefits (in addition to financial incentives) should be provided in order to make compensated programs more attractive and meaningful. When LURDs donate a kidney to a patient with ESRD, the intent is to save or improve the life of another member of society. Therefore, the society should feel an obligation to provide compensation for this service. Just as legal and social benefits are obligatory for war-injured veterans, and for firefighters injured on duty, so should such benefits be extended to LURDs, as a token of appreciation and compensation by society.

A nondirected LURD transplant program should be implemented in such a way that LURDs and their recipient do not see or know each other, at least pretransplant. LURDs would donate their kidney directly to transplant teams or to organ procurement organizations, which would match them anonymously with transplant candidates; the organ procurement organizations would pay all financial incentives to LURDs. Given a lack of administrative expertise, this nondirected approach has not yet been tested in Iran.

### USE OF DDs

During the 1990s, several decrees allowing DD transplants were obtained from almost all senior Islamic scholars and religious leaders in Iran. After considerable effort, legislation was finally passed in April 2000 by Parliament, accepting brain death and DD transplants. But from April 2000 to April 2005, only 602 DD transplants were performed. As of yet, no financial incentives are provided for DDs or their next of kin. In 2004, DD transplants comprised 12% of all kidney transplants in Iran. The slow increase in DD transplants is also due, in part, to infrastructural deficiencies in Iran's health system.

### USE OF LRDs

Before 1988, almost all kidney transplants in Iran used LRDs. Adoption of the Iranian Model that year led to a rapid increase in LURD transplants. During the past decade 75% to 80% of all kidney transplants performed in Iran each year used LURDs. The annual number of LRD transplants has steadily decreased. In 2000, 12.2% of all kidney transplants in Iran used LRDs; 86%, LURDs; and 1.8%, DDs. In 2004, the corresponding percentages were 8%, LRDs; 80%, LURDs; and 12%, DDs (see Figure 7.2-2).

One study found that 81% of all LURD recipients in Iran had a potential LRD, who was not willing to donate, at least in part, because of the availability of LURDs.[4] With a compensated, regulated LURD program in place, it may be more ethical to perform a compensated transplant using a volunteer LURD (vs LRD or spouse who was coerced or under family pressure). Of note, some LRDs in Iran have been paid by their recipient.

### DONOR AND RECIPIENT EVALUATION

In the transplant unit of Hashemi Nejad Kidney Hospital in Tehran, the European Best Practice Guidelines for Kidney Transplantation have recently been adopted for recipient and donor selection and preparation.[5] Since 2000, this evaluation and selection

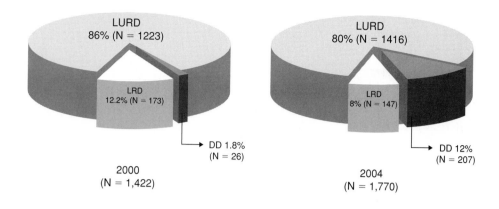

**FIGURE 7.2-2**

LURD: *living unrelated donor*     LRD: *living related donor*     DD: *deceased donor*

Sources of kidneys in Iran, 2000 and 2004

process has been carried out independently, first by transplant nephrologists and then by members of the surgical team. In selecting LRDs, priority is given to the donor who has a better *human leukocyte antigen* (HLA) match with the recipient. For LURDs, HLA matching is not practical; any donor who is ABO-compatible with the recipient is accepted.

## IMMUNOSUPPRESSIVE PROTOCOLS

Immunosuppressive therapy at Hashemi Nejad Kidney Hospital in Tehran consists of cyclosporine (Neoral) given twice daily at a dose of 4 to 6 mg/kg/day; prednisolone, initiated at a dose of 1 mg/kg/day and then tapered gradually to 15 mg/day in 4 weeks and 5 mg/day in 8 weeks; and azathioprine (AZA, at a dose of 0.5 to 1.5 mg/kg/day). Beginning in 1996, MMF was increasingly used instead of AZA; by 2004, MMF had completely replaced AZA. All recipients are also given a prophylactic dose of intravenous methylprednisolone (1 g/day) for the first 3 postoperative days. For high-risk recipients (such as those undergoing a second transplant or those with previous high panel-reactive antibody levels), induction therapy with antithymocyte globulin (ATG) and, rarely, with IL-2R antibodies is carried out. Antirejection therapy consists of methylprednisolone (1 g/day) for 3 to 5 days and, in addition, ATG for patients with steroid-resistant rejection. Tacrolimus, sirolimus, and OKT3 are nonexistent in Iran.

## RESULTS

Unfortunately, Iran has no national transplant registry to report short- and long-term kidney transplant results. Most kidney transplant teams report their own results as single-center experiences. The ESRD Office of Iran has only demographic data. The results from Hashemi Nejad Kidney Hospital (a pioneering transplant unit and one of the largest in Iran) are given below as a representative example for Iran.[6]

From April 1986 to April 2005, a total of 1881 kidney transplants were performed in this hospital: 492 (26%) with LRDs and the remaining 1389 (74%) with LURDs. Of these 1881 recipients, 695 were female; 1186, male (age range, 8–68 years). According to a recent analysis, overall patient survival rates were 93.8%, 87.8%, and 76% at 1, 5, and 10 years posttransplant; overall graft survival rates, 90.4%, 75.4%, and 52.8%. Graft survival rates did

not significantly differ for recipients of 1-HLA-haplotype-matched LRD versus LURD grafts. For LURD recipients, actuarial patient survival rates were 93.9%, 87.1%, and 72.2% at 1, 5, and 10 years posttransplant; actuarial graft survival rates were 90.5%, 74.4%, and 48.8%.

The Organ Procurement Transplant Network/United Network for Organ Sharing (OPTN/UNOS) kidney transplant registry reported higher results with LURD transplants in the United States.[7] Unfortunately, kidney transplant units in Iran are insufficiently equipped with respect to laboratory facilities, scientific consulting staff, and pharmaceuticals (including necessary immunosuppressive drugs and antibiotics).

Laparoscopic living donor (LD) nephrectomy is now being practiced by one pioneering transplant team in Iran with encouraging results.[8]

Of 17000 living donor nephrectomies that have been performed nonlaparoscopically in Iran, 3 donors have died in the perioperative period (< 0.02%).

## IMPLEMENTATION OF THE IRANIAN MODEL ELSEWHERE

In most developing countries, where an effective DD organ transplant program cannot be established because of infrastructural deficiencies, the Iranian Model can be revised according to that country's religious, cultural, and socioeconomic backgrounds.[21] It may not be necessary to adopt compensated LD programs in most developed countries, because providing financial incentives to DDs and their families will substantially increase all transplantable organs, including kidneys. In developed countries where DD transplant programs, for religious and cultural reasons, are very limited, adopting a revised form of the Iranian Model could provide superior results and successfully eliminate shortage of transplantable kidneys.

## References

1. Ghods AJ. Governed financial incentives as an alternative to altruistic organ donation. Exp *Clin Transplant* 2004;2:221.
2. Ghods AJ. Kidney transplantation in Iran. *Nephrol Dial Transplant* 2002;17:222.

3. Fazel I. Kidney transplantation in Iran: The Iranian Model In: Gutmann T, Daar AS, Sells RA, Land W, eds. *Ethical, Legal and Social Issues in Organ Transplantation*. Lengerich: Pabst Science Publishers; 2004:281.

4. Ghods AJ, Savaj S, Khosravani P. Adverse effects of a controlled living unrelated donor kidney transplant program on living related and cadaveric kidney donation. *Transplant Proc* 2000;32:541.

5. The EBPG Expert Group on Kidney Transplantation: European best practice guidelines for kidney transplantation (Part 1). *Nephrol Dial Transplant* 2000;15(Suppl 7):3, 39.

6. Ghods AJ, Ossareh S, Savaj S. Results of kidney transplantation of the Hashemi Nejad Kidney Hospital-Tehran. In: Cecka JM, Terasaki PI, eds. *Clinical Transplants* 2000. Los Angeles: UCLA Tissue Typing Laboratory; 2001:203.

7. Cecka JM. The OPTN/UNOS kidney transplant registry 2003. In: Cecka JM, Terasaki PI, eds. *Clinical Transplants* 2003. Los Angeles: UCLA Tissue Typing Laboratory; 2004:1.

8. Simforoosh N, Basiri A, Tabibi A, et al. Laparoscopic donor nephrectomy an Iranian Model for developing countries: a cost-effective no-rush approach. *Exp Clin Transplant* 2004;2:249.

9. Ghods AJ, Ossareh S, Khosravani P. Comparison of some socioeconomic characteristics of donors and recipients in a controlled living unrelated donor kidney transplantation program. *Transplant Proc* 2001;33:2626.

10. Ghods AJ, Nasrollahzadeh D, Kazemeini M. Afghan refugees in Iran Model kidney transplantation program: Ethical considerations. *Transplant Proc* 2005;37:565.

11. Mahoney JD. Should we adopt a market strategy to organ donation? In: Shelton W, Balint J, eds. *The Ethics of Organ Transplantation*. Amsterdam: Elsevier Science Ltd; 2001:65.

12. Ghods AJ. Without legalized living unrelated donor kidney transplantation many patients die or suffer—Is it ethical? In: Gutmann T, Daar AS, Sells RA, Land W, eds. *Ethical, Legal and Social Issues in Organ Transplantation*. Lengerich: Pabst Science Publishers; 2004:337.

13. Delmonico FL, Arnold R, Scheper-Hughes N, et al. Ethical incentives—not payment—for organ donation. *N Engl J Med* 2002;346:2002.

14. Harris J, Erin C. An ethically defensible market in organs. A single buyer like the NHS is an answer. *BMJ* 2002;325:114.

15. Spital A. Evolution of attitudes at US transplant centers toward kidney donation by friends and altruistic strangers. *Transplantation* 2000;69:1728.

16. Rosendale JD: Organ donation in the United States: 1988-2000. In: Cecka JM, Terasaki PI, eds. *Clinical Transplants* 2003. Los Angeles: UCLA Tissue Typing Laboratory; 2004:65.

17. The New York Times (International Edition), October 18, 2001, PA1.

18. Mc Bride MA, Harper AM, Taranto SE. The OPTN waiting list, 1988-2002. In: Cecka JM, Terasaki PI, eds. *Clinical Transplants* 2003. Los Angeles: UCLA Tissue Typing Laboratory; 2004:53.

19. Muthusethupathi MA, Rajendran S, Jayakumar M, et al. Evaluation and selection of living related kidney donors—our experience in a government hospital. *J Assoc Phys India* 1998;46:526.

20. Ghods AJ. Changing ethics in kidney transplantation: Presentation of Iran Model. *Transplant Proc* 2004;36:11.

21. Ghods AJ. Should we have live unrelated donor kidney transplantation in MESOT countries? *Transplant Proc* 2003;35:2542.

# PAID LEGAL ORGAN DONATION

## 8.1 PRO: THE CLINICIAN'S PERSPECTIVE

*Arthur J. Matas, MD*

The major arguments against sales are well defined: the vendor will suffer (short- or long-term) harm, the poor are more likely to sell than the rich, and the government and health-care system will now participate in a process where the "patient" is a vendor. We (in the transplant community and beyond) cannot deny the importance of these concerns.

However, we need to ask whether, in spite of such concerns, overriding reasons compel us to consider a policy of kidney sales—at least in some circumstances. I argue herein that if sufficient safeguards can be established to protect both the vendor and the recipient, the advantages of a *regulated system* of sales outweigh the disadvantages. In doing so, I address many of the arguments, major and minor, against sales.

In medicine, in bioethics, and in life, we often face competing principles—many of which, on their own, have merit. But, in practice, we are forced to judge the merits of each principle and then either create a balance among them or give one priority over others. A classic example in transplantation is organ allocation—should kidneys be allocated by principles of justice (equal access to everyone) or by principles of utility (the best use of each kidney)? In the United States, the United Network for Organ Sharing (UNOS) has accepted the merit of each of these two competing principles and has attempted to achieve a balance. In a similar fashion, the principles used to justify a system of sales (eg, the potential for saving lives) compete with the principles used to argue against sales.

My perspective on the issue of sales is that of a physician whose major clinical and academic focus is kidney transplantation. More detailed bioethical arguments can be found in the writings of Radcliffe-Richards,[1,2] Gill and Sade,[3] and Harris and Erin.[4]

### A REGULATED SYSTEM

By "regulated" I mean a system in which a fixed price is paid to the vendor (by the government or a government-approved agency); the kidney is allocated by a predefined algorithm similar to that used for deceased donors (DDs so everyone on the waiting list has an opportunity to receive a vendor kidney; criteria are defined for vendor evaluation, acceptance, and follow-up; and safeguards are adequate for vendor protection. In addition, as noted by Erin and Harris, the payment should not affect taxes and welfare benefits.[4] Such a system would differ from the "unregulated" markets developed elsewhere, in which the kidney may go to the highest bidder, payment is directly from the recipient, most of the payment goes to a broker, and standards for donor care are few.[5–7]

Still another, parallel approach would be to implement a system for payment for DD organs. (Because the arguments for and against this approach differ somewhat from the arguments regarding living vendors, I do not further consider this approach here.) Arguments for and against sales may be different for different geographic and socioeconomic areas of the world. I limit discussion to issues concerning a regulated system in the industrialized Western world (preferably with universal health care). Other authors have elucidated reasons to consider sales in other areas.[8,9]

It is crucial to recognize that, at least in the United States, a substantial payment (≈$100,000) could be made to a vendor and still be cost-neutral to the health-care system (because of the savings of a transplant over ongoing dialysis).[10]

### ARGUMENTS FOR SALES

The major argument for sales is that they would likely increase the number of available kidneys, shorten waiting time for a transplant, decrease the number of patients with end-stage renal disease (ESRD) who die on the waiting list, and improve patient and graft survival rates. It has long been recognized that a successful transplant provides significantly better quality of life than does maintenance dialysis.[11] Recently, considerable evidence has emerged showing that a successful transplant significantly prolongs patient survival, as compared with dialysis,[12,13] and that survival is better with a preemptive transplant (vs a transplant after initiation of dialysis).[14,15] As a consequence, more patients with ESRD are opting for a transplant rather than dialysis; waiting lists for DD transplants have grown; and the average wait for a DD kidney is now over 5 years. A major parallel development has been the recognition that outcome after living unrelated donor (LURD) kidney transplants is the same as after (non-HLA-identical) living related kidney transplants.[16]

The significant increase in waiting time for DD transplant candidates has already had dire negative consequences for them. In the United States, over 6% of waiting candidates die annually.[5,10] And, it is important to remember, these are patients who were declared to be suitable transplant recipients when they were listed. We recently studied patient deaths while on the waiting list at the University of Minnesota (unpublished data). We noted that, on average, 6.7% of patients on the list died each year. Mean age (± SD) was 54 ± 11 years. Of the deaths, 11% occurred in patients < 40 years old, 33% in those < 50, and 73% in those < 60. At the time of death, mean waiting time was 1,078 ± 847 days; 70% of the patients who died were waiting for a first transplant, and 70% had a panel-reactive antibody (PRA) level < 10%. Because the number of waiting candidates is growing steadily, and because the number of DDs has barely increased in the last decade (in North America), the waiting list and waiting times are projected to continue to increase.[12,17] Thus, even more candidates will die while waiting.

In fact, this issue alone (ie, death on the waiting list) led Radcliffe-Richards to suggest lifting the ban on sales, unless those who oppose sales can provide any reasonable arguments justifying the ban's continuation.[1] After all, currently everyone but the donor already benefits financially from the transplant (physicians, coordinators, hospitals, recipients). Moreover, ample legal precedent already exists for sales of body parts (eg, sperm, eggs) and for payments to surrogate mothers.

Gill and Sade argue a prima facie case for kidney sales based on two claims: the "good donor claim" and the "sale of tissue claim."[3] The good donor claim stems from the fact that it is already legal for a living person to donate a kidney, that is, to transfer a kidney to someone else. It then follows that kidney sales should be allowed: "If donating a kidney ought to be legal, and if the only difference between donating a kidney and selling one is the motive of monetary self-interest, and if the motive of monetary self-interest does not on its own warrant legal prohibition . . . ," then donating for money should be legal. The sale of tissue claim stems from the fact that "it is legal (and ought to be legal) for living persons to sell parts of their bodies (blood, sperm, eggs)." Thus, again, "monetary self-interest does not on its own warrant legal prohibition."

In subsequent discussions, Gill and Sade point out that if we oppose kidney sales (vs the sale of sperm or eggs) because nephrectomy is more dangerous, then we should also oppose kidney donation; if we oppose kidney sales because people should not sell body parts, then we should also oppose the sales of sperm or eggs.[3]

Another argument in favor of sales relates to current Western philosophical principles, in particular, the emphasis on autonomy.[18] The ban on sales is paternalistic and ignores the need to respect individual autonomy. In general, with "few constraints, people make personal decisions on what they wish to buy and sell based on their own values,"[3] and should be allowed to do so. In discussing the prohibition of sales, Radcliffe-Richards notes, "in a surprising contravention of our usual ideas about individual liberty, we prevent adults from entering freely into contracts from which both sides expect to benefit, and with no obvious harm to anyone else."

Finally, although most countries have laws against organ sales, a growing unregulated market for sales already exists—a market in which donors are often poorly evaluated and cared for, a market in which most of the payment goes to a broker.[5–7] Eliminating the legislative ban on sales and establishing a regulated system may well eliminate or minimize the ongoing unregulated markets,[20,21] thereby leaving people who actually do sell a kidney in a better position: better paid and better cared for. As conceded by the International Congress on Ethics in Organ Transplantation (Munich, Germany, December 2002): "The well-established position of transplantation societies against commerce in organs has not been effective in stopping the rapid growth of such transplants around the world. Individual countries will need to study alternative, locally relevant models, considered ethical in their societies, which would increase the number of transplants, protect and respect the donor, and reduce the likelihood of rampant, unregulated commerce."[22]

Of note, much of the recent discussion about sales has occurred in the bioethics and general medicine literature, with limited participation by transplant-related personnel. Two exceptions have

been the Bellagio Task Force Report on Transplantation, Body Integrity, and the International Traffic in Organs (convened under the auspices of the Center for the Study of Society and Medicine of the College of Physicians and Surgeons of Columbia University), which found no ethical principle that would justify a ban on sales under all circumstances,[23] and the report of the International Forum for Transplant Ethics, which concluded that the discussion of organ sales needs to be reopened.[2]

Clearly, if sales are to become a reality, we in the transplant community must be participants in the process—at a minimum, we must be involved in each vendor's evaluation, surgery, and care. For that reason, it is imperative that we also must more actively join in the discussion about sales (and in the formulation of any policy). We must be knowledgeable about the arguments for and against sales and about the practical concerns that would need to be addressed before any system of sales could be established.

## ARGUMENTS AGAINST SALES (AND SOME COUNTERPOINTS)

Numerous arguments—ethical, political (public policy), and practical—have been made against sales (Table 8.1-1). Yet, it is noteworthy that the debate about sales is occurring in an environment in which we accept living donation. Any effective argument against sales must be able to justify the ban on sales while simultaneously permitting donation.[1]

## AN "ARTIFICIAL" CRISIS

One argument is that "a medically invented, artificial scarcity in human organs for transplantation has generated a kind of panic and a desperate international search for them . . . "[24] No doubt, the field of transplantation is "medically invented." But it is the patients who are requesting transplants. Patients with ESRD have the choice of long-term dialysis or a transplant (at least in the industrialized world). Because a successful transplant provides longer life and better quality of life than dialysis, many patients opt for a transplant.

**TABLE 8.1-1**

**ARGUMENTS USED TO JUSTIFY THE BAN ON SALES**

1. "An artificial" crisis

2. Previous contamination of the blood supply

3. "Exploitation" of the poor

4. Society's role in protecting the marginalized

5. "Commodification" of the body (and violation of body integrity)

6. Harm to vendors

7. Lack of genuine consent

8. Difficulty in changing the law

9. Objections of organized religions

10. Desire for altruistic donation

11. Erosion of trust in the government or doctors

12. Fears of abuse of the system

## PREVIOUS CONTAMINATION OF THE BLOOD SUPPLY

Some argue that sale of blood resulted in contamination of the blood supply and in transmission of disease (specifically hepatitis C and HIV). There is no doubt that this is true. But it occurred when screening tests were not available for these viruses. Currently, LDs are screened for both hepatitis C and HIV; vendors would be similarly screened. As an extra cautionary step, vendors could be screened twice, with a 6-month interval between screening tests.

## "EXPLOITATION" OF THE POOR

The core of this argument is that risks are involved with nephrectomy, the poor are more likely to sell a kidney than the rich, and the financial offer will override their better judgment. In a broader context, the concern is that the citizens of developing countries will become vendors for citizens of industrialized countries.

The fact that uninephrectomy has risks plays an important role in this argument. For example, it was never seriously suggested that commercialization of the blood supply exploited the poor. Nevertheless, the risk of uninephrectomy, alone, cannot justify the ban on sales. As discussed earlier, if surgical risk is deemed sufficient to justify a ban on sales, then surgical risk should also be sufficient to justify a ban on donation. Moreover, our society allows the less wealthy to take many high-risk jobs that the rich are unlikely to apply for (eg, police officers, deep-sea divers, firefighters, military "volunteers," North Sea oil rig workers). And, we allow both rich and poor to engage in recreational activities that have considerably greater risk than does uninephrectomy (eg, smoking, mountain climbing, skydiving, bungee jumping).

Serious objections have never been raised about permitting financial incentives to encourage middle-class and upper-class people to be vendors.[1,25] One possible solution to the possibility of "exploitation" is to establish a minimum income for one to become a vendor. But, if it would be permissible for the middle or upper classes to sell a kidney, why should it not be permissible for the lower classes?

Thus, in a regulated system, the "exploitation" argument against kidney sales becomes, in part, the argument that the poor are more likely to be vendors than the rich. Clearly, the "exploitation" argument is not about equality. As noted by Gill and Sade, "if paying for kidneys is legalized, the ratio of poor people with only 1 kidney to rich people with only 1 kidney probably will increase."[3] This result could be seen as not being equal. But, as Gill and Sade emphasize, "the kind of equality that matters to egalitarians, however, concerns not the presence of 1 kidney vs. 2 but economic and political power. There is no reason to believe that allowing payment for kidneys will worsen the economic or political status of kidney sellers in particular or of poor people in general."[3]

In a regulated system as described previously, the "exploitation" argument is not about coercion, which is defined as "persuasion (of an unwilling person) to do something by using force or threats."[26] No potential vendor can be coerced by the opportunity to sell an organ. But when the term is (mis)used in this way, many authors argue that a payment is coercive in that it might "manipulate the victim's preferences, even if it would be rational to accept"[27] or in that "the intent of the offer is to elicit behavior that contradicts the individual's normal operative goals."[28] However, the fact of payment does not necessarily mean that the vendor's choice was not free and voluntary.[1,3,25] Moreover, Harvey

suggests that, first, if this "financial pressure" is sufficient to justify a ban on sales, then psychological or emotional pressure that may occur in related donation could justify a ban on donation and, second, a ban on sales also stops potential vendors who are not financially vulnerable.[29]

Cherry distinguishes between "coercion" and "peaceful manipulation." Coercion violates the free choice of persons, whereas peaceful manipulation "grounds the very process of negotiation through which individuals fashion consensual agreements." Cherry argues that "to be coercive, rather than peaceably manipulative, requires showing that making such an offer places potential vendors into unjustified, disadvantaged circumstances." Financial offers may be "seductive," but they "are not subtle threats."[30]

Most important, the "exploitation" argument centers on whether a regulated system of organ sales takes wrongful advantage of the calamity of others and on whether the financial offer will override the better judgment of individuals in desperate need. No doubt, a significant financial offer will provide hard choices for people in need. But there is a difference between a "hard choice" and an "involuntary choice." I do not think we are willing to say that being poor removes the ability to make rational decisions (if we believed that, we would need legal guardians to protect any decision an impoverished person makes). A regulated system is not necessarily exploitive if it pays a significant amount (an amount that has the potential to make a positive impact on the vendor's life) and if it includes procedural safeguards to ensure that vendors know what they are doing and are acting voluntarily to seek their individual best. In the case of kidney sales, the system would not be seeking the typical exploiter's "wrongful gain," but would be established to help patients in need (T. Gutmann, personal communication).

Many authors have countered the "exploitation" argument by suggesting that the ban on sales removes one potential option for the poor, and leaves them poor; whereas if they could sell a kidney, it would give them the possibility to better their lives.[1,31] There is a difference between having limited options and being able to choose rationally in one's best interests among the options available.

Clearly, the ideal solution to the problem of the poor being more likely to be vendors would be to end poverty. However, no evidence suggests that poverty will disappear in the near future, and not allowing sales does nothing to eradicate poverty. One prominent bioethicist, Veatch, once suggested that, rather than permit sales, we should prompt social change to end poverty, but he has become pessimistic about the possibility of social change and now favors sales.[25] Veatch's original concern about sales was that the (political) decision makers could, in effect, force the poor to sell their organs by withholding alternative means of addressing their problems. He has now reexamined the issue 20 years later, concluding that our society has done little to help the poor, and with "shame and bitterness" proposes that it is time to lift the ban on sales: "If we are a society that deliberately and systematically turns its back on the poor, we must confess our indifference to the poor and lift the prohibition on the one means they have to address their problems themselves."[25]

A final concern regarding "exploitation" has been that, in a government-controlled single-payer system, there would be pressure to lower the price paid for each kidney—that is, there would be institutionalized "exploitation" (as described by Veatch, previously). But a system could be defined with safeguards to prevent such institutionalized exploitation.

## SOCIETY'S ROLE IN PROTECTING THE MARGINALIZED

Many argue that a major responsibility of government in our Western industrialized society is to provide a "safety net" to protect the marginalized, and that legalization of sales would subjugate this responsibility. But governments often have competing priorities, and protecting citizens from unnecessary death (for those on the waiting list) is certainly a worthy goal. Certainly, continuing the ban on one choice for citizens (ie, to sell a kidney) does not overtly protect them; rather, it may, in fact, prevent them from financially protecting themselves.

## "COMMODIFICATION" OF THE BODY

Some argue that sales would lead to "commodification" of people, of the human body. The concern seems to be that a vendor will, in some way, lose human dignity and be seen as only worthwhile as a provider of spare parts. As Sutton phrased it, "if we allow body parts to enter the marketplace, we depersonalize and devaluate ourselves."[32]

In fact, no evidence suggests that sperm or egg donors, or surrogate mothers, have diminished self-dignity or self-worth. And, as noted in a detailed analysis by Wilkinson, "there is no necessary connection between the commodification of bodies or the commodification of persons."[33] As Gill and Sade state, "my kidney is not my humanity";[3] they continue, "humanity—what gives us dignity and intrinsic value—is our ability to make rational decisions, and a person can continue to make rational decisions with only one kidney." If, in a regulated system, vendors are treated as heroes who receive compensation for their pain (as suggested by Gutmann and Land),[34] and have their rights and interests protected, it would be quite possible to sell a kidney without loss of dignity.

Implied in the concern regarding commodification is the concept that "body integrity is highly valued."[33] The fear is that vendors would have some longstanding emotional or psychological damage because of the breaks in body integrity. Wigmore et al. argue: "violation of this integrity is not well compensated for other than by spiritual or philosophical gains such as acting in an altruistic fashion."[35] But, again, little evidence supports this concept of negative violation. Surgical procedures, a direct violation of body integrity, do not usually lead to long-term psychological harm or damage to human dignity. One could argue that surgical procedures are necessary for cure of disease and this, in some way, leads to personal justification for the violation of body integrity. But, in fact, plastic surgery done solely for cosmetic purposes requires a break in body integrity. In addition, numerous occupations and recreational activities are associated with risks to body integrity; yet, we have no compunction about limiting people's involvement in these activities. And many cultures and religions throughout the world violate body integrity as part of their beliefs (eg, piercings, male circumcision).

In reality, individuals who value their body integrity over compensation for a kidney could choose not to be vendors. Thus, the commodification argument does not justify the ban on sales.

## HARM TO VENDORS

Currently, the mortality rate associated with living kidney donation is 0.03%. If vendors are screened as thoroughly as living donors (LDs), the associated mortality rate would likely remain about 0.03%. So, on a purely rational level, the concern about vendor death does not differentiate kidney sales from donation. But, on an emotional level, death of a vendor "feels" different from death of a donor. When a donor dies because of donation, we might suggest that the death occurred while doing something "noble." Of course, a vendor might also have a "noble" use for the money. Still, the practice of transplantation requires the goodwill of the public, and it is unclear how the press or public would react to the death of a vendor.

Similarly, the surgical and long-term risks for vendors are identical to the risks for LDs. As discussed earlier, if these risks alone are sufficient to justify the ban on sales, they should also be sufficient to justify a ban on donation.

## LACK OF GENUINE CONSENT

Some argue that, because money is involved, a potential vendor cannot ever truly provide genuine informed consent. But this argument rests on a paternalistic attitude that "we" are best able to weigh the risks and benefits for others. As described earlier, this argument also ignores a fundamental tenet of current medical practice and philosophy: autonomy.

Some also argue that some potential vendors may be unable to fully understand the risks; but this worry also applies to LDs, yet we feel capable of screening and educating them. If the fact that some potential vendors may not understand the risks justifies the ban on sales, then the fact that some potential LDs may not understand the risks should justify a ban on donation.

## DIFFICULTY IN CHANGING THE LAW

Some argue that, because organ sales are currently a contentious issue, politicians (always concerned about reelection) would be reluctant to propose and fight for a change in the law. Whether or not this is true, it is not an argument either for or against sales. Certainly, it was difficult to change the law to allow emancipation of women and blacks. Presumably, if polls find that the public generally supports a regulated system of organ sales, then politicians would be willing to eliminate the ban.

## OBJECTIONS OF ORGANIZED RELIGIONS

Almost all organized religions currently support organ donation. In Judeo-Christian culture, saving lives takes precedence over other religious laws and customs. Yet, it is unclear whether organized religions would take a formal stand against sales. According to Steinberg, almost all rabbinic authorities that have expressed an opinion have stated that, from a Jewish moral point of view, there is "nothing wrong in receiving reasonable compensation for an act of self-endangerment, whereby one still adequately fulfills the most important commitment—to save life."[36]

The Catholic Church has taken a somewhat mixed stance. Capaldi argues that it is morally permissible for Catholics to participate in a market in organ sales;[37] he quotes Pope Pius XII as saying, "It would be going too far to declare immoral every acceptance on every demand of payment. The case is similar to blood transfusions. It is commendable for the donor to refuse recompense; it is not necessarily a fault to accept it."[38] In contrast, Pope John Paul II stated, "The body cannot be treated as a merely physical or biologic entity, nor can its organs and tissues even be used as items for sale or exchange. Such a reductive materialistic conception would lead to a merely instrumental use of the body, and therefore of the person."[39]

In a subsequent address to the Transplantation Society, Pope John Paul II stated, "any procedure which tends to commercialize human organs or to consider them as items of exchange or trade must be considered morally unacceptable."[40]

Clearly, individuals with religious objections can choose not to be vendors. But it will require a change in the law to eliminate the ban on sales. In theory, religious belief should not determine law and public policy,[3] yet strong opposition from organized religions could have an impact on political discussion and action.

## DESIRE FOR ALTRUISTIC DONATION

Historically, it has been felt that donation should be altruistic. But there is no reason it must be this way. With our current practice of altruistic donation, the waiting list and resultant waiting time are getting longer every year.

If there is a market in organs, some fear that altruistic living donation may decrease. But no evidence supports this concern (it is a hypothesis that can be tested). In fact, there are many reasons to believe that altruistic donation will continue. First, some recipients would continue to want to know their donor. As discussed next, there may be concerns about the "quality" of vendor kidneys. Families with these concerns might opt for donation. Second, with a regulated system of sales, waiting time is likely to be reduced but not eliminated. Outcome for kidney transplant recipients is better with a preemptive transplant,[14,15] so many recipients would still opt for preemptive transplants from altruistic donors. Third, potential vendors may be demographically different (eg, older) from potential altruistic donors, providing another reason for preferring a donor (over a vendor) kidney.

Nevertheless, in some situations, a family might rather turn to a government-regulated vendor system than to a family member or altruistic friend. If so, there could be some decrease in altruistic donation (probably related to how long the waiting list is, once a vendor system is implemented). Some of this decrease may be good. First, we do not know how much coercion is involved in living related donation; presumably a vendor system could eliminate this form of family coercion. Second, criteria for acceptance of LDs are being expanded (eg, single-drug hypertension is allowed in some centers). An expanded-criteria donor is usually accepted only if he or she is the sole available donor for an individual recipient. A large vendor system might eliminate the need to use expanded-criteria donors. Clearly, whether sales will result in a significant decrease in donation needs to be studied.

If there is a market, there is also a concern that deceased donation may decrease (again, an untested hypothesis). The great need for livers, hearts, lungs, and pancreases—all of which could never be supplied by vendors—will continue. However, it does need to be recognized that, if we eliminate the ban on organ sales, families of DDs may also lobby for a payment.

## EROSION OF TRUST IN THE GOVERNMENT OR DOCTORS

### Government

If the government (or its appointed agency) is the sole buyer of kidneys (in a regulated system), the government may be seen as preying on the poor, rather than providing a safety net.[25] And, in fact, one function of the government (providing for the needy) would be in direct conflict with the other (buying kidneys). But,

in reality, government agencies often have competing priorities (eg, consumer advocacy vs environmental protection, development of the economy vs raising the minimum wage, minimizing dependence on foreign oil vs preserving the country's wilderness). And, the goal of purchasing kidneys would be to save lives—certainly an acceptable goal for the government. It is not unreasonable to believe that a regulated system—with appropriate screening, good postoperative follow-up, and a substantial payment to the vendor—could also be managed with care and dignity so that respect (for either the government or the vendor) would not suffer.

### Doctor–Patient Relationship

Some also argue that allowing organ sales would disrupt the traditional doctor–patient relationship. But, no evidence suggests that sales would have any negative impact either on patient care or on a patient's (vendor's) expectations of the physician. No evidence suggests that medical care for surrogate mothers (analogous to vendors) has differed in any way from the current standard of practice. Presumably, in a regulated system, vendors would be given the same care as current LDs (and better care than current vendors in unregulated markets).

## FEARS OF ABUSE OF THE SYSTEM

Potential vendors might lie about their health-care status and risks. Alternatively, physicians and transplant centers (who are paid when a transplant is done) might relax acceptance criteria in order to increase the number of transplants. But, of course, such fears do not differentiate sales from living donation. The possibility of abuse is not used to justify bans on numerous other activities (eg, paying taxes, driving powerful cars). In practice, a regulated system could be established to minimize such risks (eg, rigid acceptance criteria, viral screening twice at 6-month intervals).

## SOME PRACTICAL CONSIDERATIONS

Many practical considerations are involved in establishing a regulated vendor system (Table 8.1-2). Each will require considerable discussion. Not being able to statistically address such considerations could alone justify not setting up a system.

**TABLE 8.1-2**
## SOME PRACTICAL CONSIDERATIONS

1. Determining criteria for vendors
   a. Minimum age
   b. Defined geographic area

2. Providing long-term health care for vendors

3. Following vendors long-term

4. Distributing payment

5. Verifying health status of vendors

6. Handling logistics

7. Designating price

8. Drawing the line at kidneys

1.  Determining criteria for vendors
    (a)  Should there be a minimum age?
        In North America, 18-year-olds can join the military, vote, and be LDs. However, in most states, young adults cannot legally drink until age 21 (in part because a sense of mortality is not developed until at least the mid-20s). Car rental companies, recognizing the typical poor driving record of so many young drivers, have different restrictions and rates for those under age 25. Given the many issues associated with being a young adult, it might be reasonable to set a higher minimum age for vendors than currently exists for donors.

    (b)  Should vendors be limited to a defined geographic area?
        A major concern of opponents of sales is that people from "poor" countries would come to "rich" countries to sell their kidneys. A related concern is that financial compensation would be different between countries. Harris and Erin suggest that one solution would be to confine the marketplace to a geographic area (a country or a group of countries) in which vendors or families of vendors could benefit from a policy of organ sales.[4]

        Yet, if we accept the concept of sales, is it really wrong to allow vendors to come from poor countries and provide kidneys to those in need (rich and poor) in rich countries? It could be argued that sales would allow a significant redistribution of wealth, and certainly could improve the lifestyle of each vendor. (It would be interesting to know whether opponents of sales check the labels on their clothes to determine where they were produced and whether "sweatshops" were involved.)

        Another way to limit an influx of potential vendors from poor to rich countries would be to only pay if a kidney is used. Potential vendors would likely incur some expenses in getting to a transplant center. Obviously, if they become actual vendors, the compensation could more than cover those expenses. Thus, on the one hand, it is likely that the expenses of getting to a transplant center (once for the evaluation and then for the uninephrectomy) would likely minimize the number of potential vendors crossing from one country to another. On the other hand, if a regulated system were established, it might not be surprising to see local "screening" clinics signing up vendors in poor countries; theoretically, vendors could pay the screening clinic after the uninephrectomy.

2.  Providing long-term health care for vendors
    Although the risks of uninephrectomy are small, they are not zero. In a regulated system, in a country with a universal (national) health plan, long-term care can be assured. In other countries, the payment to vendors might include payment for health insurance. However, health insurance and long-term care would be difficult to organize if vendors came from different countries.

3.  Following vendors long-term
    Clearly, if a vendor system (or a pilot trial) were initiated, it would be important to study long-term outcome. Again, this would be difficult if vendors came from different countries.

4.  Distributing payment
    Our previous study suggested that, in the United States, a payment of about $100,000 would be potentially cost-effective (some of this could be used to pay for life and health insurance and to fund long-term follow-up).[10] It might be reasonable to pay the $100,000 in a lump sum to U.S. vendors. But what if a regulated system were established that permitted vendors to come from other countries? Such vendors may have no experience in managing large sums of money; appropriate local facilities such as banks might not be available.

    In addition, regulation would have to be developed regarding whether or not payment would affect welfare benefits or taxes. Another issue is whether payment would be subject to attachment by other concerned parties (eg, creditors, ex-spouses).

5.  Verifying health status of vendors
    How to verify the health status of vendors is both an ethical and a practical issue. From a practical perspective, potential vendors could be evaluated twice (eg, viral studies), with a minimum 6-month interval between evaluations. Although two evaluations would not guarantee safety, they would minimize the risk. It could be made a federal (U.S.) offense to lie about health risks when undergoing vendor evaluation (but such a statute would have little impact on potential vendors from other countries). Potential recipients could be informed about the limitations of the evaluation process (similarly, some limitations apply to the current LD and DD pool) and sign an appropriately developed informed consent form.

6.  Handling logistics
    Numerous logistical issues would have to be resolved before a system of sales could be implemented. For example, where would potential vendors go to apply or to be evaluated? Who would do the evaluation? Would only local potential recipients be considered, or would 6-antigen matches confer priority? Would vendors have to travel to a recipient's center? Who would be responsible for long-term follow-up?

7.  Designating price
    Should there be a fixed price? If we accept sales, why not have the kidney go to the highest bidder? A government-sponsored regulated system with a fixed price paid to vendors has many advantages. The most important is that all potential recipients would have access to vendor kidneys. If some form of bartering or a "to the highest bidder" system were established, the rich would clearly benefit. Other advantages of a government-sponsored regulated system are that it could ensure adequate donor evaluation and mandatory informed consent, and could guarantee that payment goes to vendors (rather than to brokers).

    In addition, could there be a lower price for "old" (vs "young") donor kidneys, or for kidneys that have potentially worse outcome? This is a complex question that could possibly be resolved by open discussion.

8.  Drawing the line at kidneys
    If we establish a regulated system for kidney sales, should we have a system for sales of a liver lobe, a lung lobe, or a partial pancreas? Could vendors return repeatedly to sell more body parts? LD liver, lung, and pancreas transplants have been done successfully. But, for each, the potential donor morbidity is higher than after uninephrectomy. In addition, considerably more information is available on long-term follow-up after donor uninephrectomy (vs after LD liver, lung, or pancreas donation). For those reasons, it could be argued that, at this time, a vendor system should be limited to kidneys.

## WHAT DOES THE GENERAL PUBLIC THINK?

Currently, the debate about sales is taking place in the bioethics and general medicine literature, with limited involvement by transplant-related personnel. Most important, the general public has not been involved. Interestingly, two surveys have suggested that the general public is much more willing than the medical community to accept sales. In 1991, Kittur et al. found that 52% of the general public favored sales (68% of those 18 to 34 years old; 49% of those 35 to 54 years old; 31% of those ≥ 55 years old).[41] Subsequently, Guttman and Guttman found that 70% of the general public and 51% of medical students, but only 25% of surveyed physicians and nurses, favored sales.[42]

Those survey results obviously suggest that attitudes to sales may differ between the general public and the medical community. This is an important consideration. In discussing bioethics, the opinions of medical personnel are usually included—but as only one of many communities with differing perspectives. Organ sales, however, could not take place without the participation of medical and surgical personnel.

## A LIMITED CLINICAL TRIAL?

As discussed previously, careful analysis shows the shortfalls of the ethical arguments against sales. In addition, no evidence supports the argument that a regulated system of sales will have negative consequences. If additional surveys show that the public supports sales, legislators might consider repealing the prohibition.

One way to proceed would be to repeal the ban on sales and develop a national system, taking the many practical issues (Table 8.1-2) into account. Another way would be to begin a clinical trial limited to a single organ procurement area or geographic area. For the duration of the trial, potential vendors would have to come from that defined area. Standards for vendor evaluation and follow-up could be developed by a panel of physicians, ethicists, and lay personnel. Organ allocation could be by UNOS criteria; payment could include life and/or health insurance. Long-term follow-up, including psychosocial assessment, could be mandatory. Ideally, such a trial could be carried out in a culture of universal health coverage.

In addition to assessing the impact on vendors, endpoints could include the impact on the waiting list, on altruistic donation (both from LDs and families of DDs), and the impact on the use of expanded-criteria donors.

## CONCLUSION

The issue of kidney sales is not a hypothetical ethical fine point; rather, it affects the lives of people worldwide. While thinking of balancing moral principles,[34] individuals must question what their personal actions would be, should the need arise. Leon Kass writes, "I suspect that regardless of all my arguments to the contrary, I would probably make every effort and spare no expense to obtain a suitable life-saving kidney for my child–if my own were unusable. . . . I think I would readily sell one of my own kidneys, were its practice legal, if it were the only way to pay for a life-saving operation for my children or my wife."[43]

How should this topic be approached? One option would be to accept that organ sales are illegal, that the issues are complex and feelings are strong, and to end discussion. But this leaves us with the continually expanding waiting list, the probability of worse outcomes for future patients with ESRD (because of a longer wait for a transplant), and the probability of an increasing number of patients dying while waiting for a transplant.

A second option would be to open discussion about the possibility of establishing a regulated vending system. Such a discussion needs to address two (separate but intertwined) questions: (1) could a regulated vending system ever be ethically supported and (2) if so, under what circumstances? Important practical considerations must be resolved before such a system could be established.

## ACKNOWLEDGMENTS

I would like to thank Mary Knatterud for editorial assistance and Stephanie Daily for preparation of the manuscript. Much of this chapter originally was published as:

Matas AJ. The Case for Living Kidney Sales: Rationale, Objections, and Concerns. *Am J Transplant* 2004;4:2007–2017.

## References

1. Radcliffe-Richards J. Nephrarious goings on: Kidney sales and moral arguments. *J Med Philos* 1996;21:375–416.
2. Radcliffe-Richards J, Daar AS, Guttmann RD, et al. The case for allowing kidney sales. *Lancet* 1998;351:1950–1952.
3. Gill MB, Sade RM. Paying for kidneys: The case against prohibition. *Kennedy Inst Ethics J* 2002;12(1):17–45.
4. Harris J, Erin C. An ethically defensible market in organs (Editorial). *BMJ* 2002;325:114–115.
5. Scheper-Hughes N. The global traffic in human organs. *Curr Anthropol* 2000;41:191–222.
6. Goyal M, Mehta RL, Schneiderman LJ, Sehgal AR. Economic and health consequences of selling a kidney in India. *JAMA* 2002;288(13):1589–1593.
7. Daar AS. Money and organ procurement: narratives from the real world. In: Guttman TH, Daar AS, Sells R, Land W, eds. Ethical, Legal and Social Issues in Organ Transplantation. *Pabst Publishers: Lengerizh*, In Press.
8. Reddy KC. Should paid organ donation be banned in India? To buy or let die! *Natl Med J India* 1993;6(3):137–139.
9. Ghods AJ, Ossareh S, Khosravani P. Comparison of some socioeconomic characteristics of donors and recipients in a controlled living unrelated donor renal transplantation program. *Trans Proc* 2001;33:2626-7.
10. Matas AJ, Schnitzler M. Payment for living donor (vendor) kidneys: A cost-effectiveness analysis. *Am J Transplant* 2004;4(2):216–221.
11. Evans RW, Manninen DL, Garrison LP, et al. The quality of life of patients with end-stage renal disease. *N Engl J Med* 1985;312:553–559.
12. Wolfe RA, Ashby VB, Milford EL, et al. Comparison of mortality in all patients on dialysis, patients on dialysis awaiting transplantation, and recipients of a first cadaveric transplant. *N Engl J Med* 1999;341:1725–1730.
13. Schnuelle P, Lorenz D, Trede M, Van Der Woude FJ. Impact of renal cadaveric transplantation on survival in end-stage renal failure: Evidence for reduced mortality risk compared with hemodialysis during long-term follow-up. *J Am Soc Nephrol* 1998;9:2135–2141.
14. Cosio FG, Alamir A, Yim S, et al. Patient survival after renal transplantation. I. The impact of dialysis pretransplant. *Kidney Int* 1998;53:767–772.
15. Meier-Kreische HU, Port FK, Ojo AO, et al. Effect of waiting time on renal transplant outcome. *Kidney Int* 2000;58:1311–1317.
16. Gjertson DW, Cecka JM. Living unrelated donor kidney transplantation. *Kidney Int* 2000;58(2):491–499.
17. Ojo AO, Hanson JA, Meier-Kreische HU, et al. Survival in recipients of marginal cadaveric donor kidneys compared with other recipients and wait-listed transplant patients. *J Am Soc Nephrol* 2001;12:589–597.
18. Gillon R. Ethics needs principles—four can encompass the rest—and respect for autonomy should be "first among equals." *J Med Ethics* 2003; 29:307–312.
19. Xue JL, Ma JZ, Louis TA, Collins AJ. Forecast of the number of patients with end-stage renal disease in the United States to the year 2010. *J Am Soc Nephrol* 2001;12:2753–2758.

20. Friedlaender MM. The right to sell or buy a kidney: are we failing our patients? *Lancet* 2002;359:971–973.

21. Rapoport J, Kagan A, Friedlaender MM. Legalizing the sale of kidneys for transplantation: Suggested guidelines. *IMAJ* 2002;4:1131–1134.

22. Ethical, Legal, and Social Issues in Organ Transplantation. Guttman TH, Daar AS, Sells R, Land W, eds. Pabst Publishers: Lengerich (In Press).

23. Rothman DJ, Rose E, Awaya T, et al. The Bellagio Task Force report on transplantation, bodily integrity, and the international traffic in organs. *Transplant Proc* 1997;29:2739–2745.

24. Scheper-Hughes, N. *The Ends of the Body: The Global Commerce in Organs for Transplant Surgery. Organs Watch, Online Essay.* Berkeley: University of California, 1998.

25. Veatch RM. Why liberals should accept financial incentives for organ procurement. Kennedy Inst Ethics J 2003;13(1):19–36.

26. The New Oxford American Dictionary, Oxford University Press, New York, 2001.

27. Zimmerman D. Coercive wage offers. Philos Publ *Affairs* 1981;10: 121–145. Cited by Cherry NJ, reference 46.

28. Rudinow J. Manipulation. *Ethics* 1978;88:338–347. Cited by Cherry NJ, reference 46.

29. Harvey J. Paying organ donors. *J Med Ethics* 1990;16:117–119.

30. Cherry MJ. Is a market in human organs necessarily exploitative? *Public Affairs Quart* 2000;14(4):337–360.

31. Andrews LB. My body, my property. *Hastings Center Rep* 1986(October); 28–38.

32. Sutton AM. Commodification of body parts. *BMJ* 2002;235:114.

33. Wilkinson S. Commodification arguments for the legal prohibition of organ sale. *Health Care Analysis* 2000;8:189–201.

34. Gutmann T, Land W. Ethics in living donor organ transplantation. *Langenbeck's Arch* Surg 1999;384:515–22.

35. Wigmore SJ, Lumsdaine JA, Forsythe JLR. Defending the indefensible? *BMJ* 2002;325:114–115.

36. Steinberg A. Compensation for kidney donation: A price worth paying. *IMAJ* 2002;4:1139–1140.

37. Capaldi N. A Catholic perspective on organ sales. *Christian Bioethics* 2000;6(2):139–151.

38. Pius XII, Pope (1960). Papal teachings: The human body, Monks of Solemes (selected and arranged), the Daughters of Saint Paul, Boston. Cited in Capaldi *N* (ref. 56).

39. John Paul II, Pope. Blood and organ donors, August 2, 1984. *The Pope Speaks* 1985;30(1): 1–2. Cited in Capaldi N (ref. 56).

40. John Paul II, Pope. Special Address to the Transplantation Society. *Transplant Proc* 2001; 33:31–32.

41. Kittur DS, Hogan MM, Thukral VK et al. Incentives for organ donation? The United Network for Organ Sharing Ad Hoc Donations Committee. *Lancet* 1992;338:1441–1443.

42. Guttman A, Guttman RD. Attitudes of healthcare professionals and the public towards the sale of kidneys for transplantation. *J Med Ethics* 1993;19:148–153.

43. Kass LR. Organs for sale? Propriety, property, and the price of progress. *Public Interest* 1992(Spring);107:65–86.

# 8.2  PRO: THE PHILOSOPHER'S PERSPECTIVE

*Janet Radcliffe-Richards, BA, MA, Bphil*

## INTRODUCTION

When evidence of the trade in transplant organs from live vendors first filtered through to Western attention a few years ago, one of the most remarkable aspects of the immediate response was its unanimity. From widely different groups, normally hard-pressed to agree about anything, there came indignant denunciations of the whole business as a moral outrage: a gross exploitation of the poor by the rich, who were now taking the very bodies of those from whom there was nothing else left to take. Professional associations immediately pronounced it anathema, and in an extraordinarily short time most governments had rushed to make the buying and selling of organs for transplantation absolutely illegal.

This near unanimity suggests a clear-cut moral case, as did the language of exploitation in terms of which the situation was described. But in fact the issue is much more complicated than it looks. If the objectors had really been starting from their usual moral principles and applying them to a new situation, instead of going along with their immediate feelings of disgust, they could certainly not have leapt so quickly and directly to the conclusion that organ sales should be prohibited, and might not have been able to reach it at all. If the organ-selling debate is to be a serious moral inquiry, rather than a determined rationalization of prejudice, it needs to be reviewed from the foundations.

## FAMILIAR MORAL PRINCIPLES

When organ selling began it was not illegal, for the simple reason that nobody had foreseen it. But in hindsight, it should have been foreseen. Trade is just a sophisticated form of barter, and barter arises spontaneously whenever people see the possibility of mutually beneficial exchange. Anything that can be given can also be sold, and as soon as the transplant technology existed the possibility of sale necessarily arose. If one person wants money more than their spare kidney, and the other wants a kidney more than the money, exchange is bound to occur unless it is actively prevented.

Of course the fact that something will happen unless prevented does not mean that it ought to be allowed to happen. The whole point of laws and institutions is to control what would happen if people were left to their own devices. Nevertheless, the fact that two parties see some exchange as mutually beneficial is relevant to the moral question of whether it should be allowed, because it provides— by just about anyone's standards—a point in its favor. We take it for granted that buying and selling should normally be allowed for just this reason. If we start from our normal principles, there is a clear presumption in favor of allowing the exchange of money and kidneys, as of any other exchange.

This is only a presumption, of course; a presumption in favor of something may always be overridden by stronger considerations against it. The fact that a burglary may be beneficial to two conspiring burglars does not mean that burglary should be allowed. But a presumption in favor of anything is important, because it means that anyone who is against it needs to find a strong enough reason.

The general presumption in favor of allowing mutually beneficial exchange is, furthermore, only one of the ways in which our usual moral values provide a presumption in favor of allowing kidney selling. Most people, for instance—certainly all members of the medical profession—accept that there is a strong presumption in favor of saving life and preventing suffering. Because kidney transplants have the potential to save lives, or at least remove patients from the miseries of dialysis, and because organs become available through selling that otherwise would not be available, that provides an additional presumption in its favor.

The presumption is also, paradoxically, strengthened still further by a consideration usually taken to work on the other side of the debate. Many people, if not all, would agree that the worse off someone is, the stronger the presumption in favor of allowing them to improve their position. People who oppose organ selling think it is appalling that anyone should be driven by desperation to offer a kidney for sale; but you can accept that (as most of us would) and nevertheless recognize that their position might be improved by doing it. If someone sees kidney selling as their best option, they must regard their situation when that option does not exist as even worse; and the worse you think it is to have to sell a kidney, the worse you should think the position is of someone who would have chosen this option, but has had it removed.

Once again, such considerations come nowhere near settling the matter, because any *prima facie* case may be overturned by further argument. The principle of preventing suffering provides a presumption against sticking needles into people and cutting them open with knives, but doctors do these things all the time because, as most people agree, the presumptive objection is often defeated by the benefits to be achieved. So to say that most people's ordinary values support a presumption in favor of allowing organ selling is certainly not meant as a claim that they should be, all things considered, committed to allowing it.

Nevertheless, it is important to start any inquiry into the ethics of organ selling from this direction, because the strong feelings most people have against the practice usually seem to prevent their noticing that there is anything at all to be said in its favor. These likely benefits of any kidney sale were simply not mentioned in the initial outcry against the practice, and are still scarcely acknowledged by most proponents of prohibition.

This way of looking at things makes a great deal of difference to the debate, because people who are against allowing organ selling often seem to presume that their opponents must be extreme libertarians, basing their arguments on an ideology that asserts the virtues of unfettered markets and total individual freedom. The argument being developed here has no such basis. It starts with minimal values accepted by just about everyone, and claims only that these establish a *presumption* in favor of allowing organ sales. This presumption might still be defeated.

However, even though this presumption in favor of allowing kidney selling is nowhere near decisive, it is methodologically important because it puts the burden of proof on prohibitionists. In practice, because prohibition is in force in most places, and most people support it, it is opponents of prohibition who are challenged to defend their position. In moral terms, however, the case goes the other way. If you are against organ selling, but accept—as most people do—that it is on the whole a good thing to save life, alleviate suffering and poverty, and allow people to engage in mutually beneficial exchanges, the burden of proof is on you.

This makes no difference to the logic of the matter, because if opponents can raise objections strong enough to outweigh the presumption in favor, those objections will work wherever the argument starts. But it makes a great deal of difference to the conduct of an argument that usually starts from the other direction, with the conviction that organ selling must be wrong.

Schematically, the challenge for opponents is to construct an argument that starts with a presumption in favor of allowing the sale of kidneys, but reaches the conclusion that it should nevertheless be prohibited. It would have to take this form:

> There is apparently, according to our normal values, a presumption in favor of allowing the sale of kidneys,
> But . . .
>
> -----------------------------------
>
> Therefore it should be prohibited
>
> where the "but . . . " is followed either by an argument that the presumption in favor is for some reason unfulfilled or by some other claim strong enough to override it.

Setting up the argument in this way makes it clear that there is no a priori limit to the number of candidate objections that might be attempted, and in practice the refutation of one is followed quickly by the sprouting of others. However, keeping the formal structure in mind, and assessing candidate arguments one at a time, helps to prevent the kind of blur that allows a series of bad arguments to pass as cumulatively compelling. The ones that follow are some of the most commonly used.

## "BUT . . . THEY ARE INCOMPETENT TO CONSENT"

One of the first arguments to appear was that although both parties might seem to have agreed to the transaction, the consent of at least one was not valid. In populations poor enough to be tempted by kidney selling, it was claimed, would-be sellers would be too uneducated to understand the risks involved and would therefore be incompetent to consent.[1]

This line of argument is in difficulty from the start, because no one really believes the premise. Many people from well-educated populations have said they would be willing to sell if the reward were high enough, and even people from uneducated groups seem to be regarded as competent to consent to other surgical procedures—including kidney donation. The idea that anyone who wants to sell a kidney must be incompetent to do so probably depends on the question-begging assumption that wanting to sell is in itself proof of non-competence.

But even if significant numbers of potential organ sellers were incompetent to consent, this would still not support the conclusion that there should be a total prohibition. To do that you would need to add another premise, to the effect that if a significant number of people were not competent to consent to some procedure, nobody at all should be allowed to undergo it—and no opponent of organ selling seems to be willing to make such a claim. Our usual principles about autonomy and consent demand our assessing competence on a case-by-case basis, and, where noncompetence results from ignorance rather than incapacity, trying to provide enough information to bring about competence.

## "THEY ARE COERCED INTO SELLING"

A variation on the theme of invalid consent lies in the claim that the problem is not so much the sellers' competence as their situation. It is said that they are coerced into organ selling by poverty, and that coerced consent is not genuine.[2]

[1]See, for example, Sells RA. Resolving the conflict in traditional ethics which arises from our demand for organs. *Transplant Proc* 1993; 25:6(December):2983–2984; Broyer M. Living organ donation; the fight against commercialism. In: Land W, Dossetor JB, eds. *Organ Replacement Therapy: Ethics, Justice, Commerce.* Springer-Verlag; 1991:199. Some people have also argued on the same basis that the purchasers' desperation makes them incompetent to consent.

[2]See, for example, Dossetor JB, Manickavel V. Commercialization: The Buying and Selling of Kidneys. In: Land W, Dossetor JB, eds. *op cit,* p. 63: "Surely abject poverty . . . can have no equal when it comes to coercion of individuals to do things – take risks – which their affluent fellow-citizens would not want to take? Can decisions taken under the influence of this terrifying coercion be considered autonomous? Surely not . . . "; Abouna GM, Sabawi MM, Kumar MSA, Samhan M. "The negative impact of

This argument needs a metaphorical interpretation to get off the ground, because coercion typically requires a coercer, who deliberately curtails the range of options available until the best one left is the one the coercer wants the victim to choose. Poverty has no intentions. Nevertheless, it can be conceded that it does curtail options in much the same way. Nobody would choose to have a healthy kidney removed if better options were available.

However, even though most sellers' options may be severely limited by poverty, the second claim, that coerced consent is not genuine, is not —at least in any sense that supports the conclusion that the choice should be disallowed. If a kidnapper tried to coerce money out of you by threatening to kill your child, you would not have much gratitude to anyone who prevented your handing over the money on the grounds that your consent was not genuine, and left you with a dead child. The kidnapper would have reduced your range of options, but that would not make your consent to the best remaining option anything other than genuine.[3] The same applies when people are left by poverty with an unwelcome range of choices. To remove the best remaining option is actually, in the relevant sense, to coerce them still further. The only way to improve their situation is to expand their options, typically by removing by the (real or metaphorical) causes of coercion.

It should also be added that if the coercion-by-poverty argument did work it would work just as effectively against organ donation. Unpaid kidney donors are also, in this metaphorical sense, coerced into offering to donate. It is not that they like the idea of losing a kidney, but they are coerced by having to choose between that and the death of someone they care about. That threatened death suddenly makes the undesirable option of losing a kidney the best available option.

A variation of the coercion argument, which appears in other contexts as well, is that the poor can be coerced into selling by unrefusable offers:[4] more money than they could possibly get in other ways. But to this argument there is an even stronger reply. Even if coercion did generally invalidate consent, it would still be irrelevant to the issue of inducement by unrefusable offers, because this is exactly the opposite of coercion. What this does is *expand* the range of available options. The original one, of keeping the kidney, still remains; the difference is only that a better one has become available.

Perhaps the idea behind this argument is that such temptations are so great as to dazzle prospective sellers into incompetence, but if so the appropriate reply is the one given in the foregoing section. Our normal standards require us to assess competence on an individual basis and not to think of removing an option for everyone because some cannot give valid consent.

paid organ donation," *ibid* p. 166: " A truly voluntary and noncoerced consent is also unlikely . . . the desperate financial need of the donor is an obvious and clear economic coercion." It is also sometimes said that the recipient has not chosen freely either, because he is coerced by the threat of death into entering the market. This is probably enough in itself to illustrate the absurdity of the idea.

[3]This point is developed further in Radcliffe Richards, J. Nephrarious Goings On: Kidney sales and moral arguments. J Med Philos 1996: 21: 375–416.

[4]Sells RA. Voluntarism of Consent. In: Land W. and Dossetor JB (eds.) *op. cit.*; 1991:18–24.

## "THEY SHOULDN'T BE POOR"

The claim that we should not remove the best option open to the poor frequently provokes a further response. Surely, it is said, we should be abolishing poverty, not encouraging the poor to try to alleviate their situation in this particularly horrible way.

Not many people would deny that we should be trying to abolish poverty, so that premise is unlikely to be in dispute. But it does not help the argument in the least, because— even if we had any idea how to abolish poverty—there is no connection at all between the idea that we should make people less poor and that organ selling should be prohibited. For one thing, there is no reason to believe that only poverty could make people willing to sell. Most people except the fabulously rich would probably find there was some price at which they were willing to part with a kidney—especially if they could do it in secret. But, more fundamentally and more subtly, the argument fails on grounds of logic. The conclusion is supposed to be that *kidney selling should be prohibited*, so the premises need to provide a support for that conclusion. But if everyone were so well off that no one was tempted by kidney selling, no one would want to sell and prohibition would be pointless because it would have nothing to do. Conversely, as long as prohibition has anything to do, there must be people for whom selling seems a better option than any other they have, and who are therefore made worse off by prohibition.

Concern for the badly off is a very good reason for trying to make them better off, but none at all for the prohibition of organ selling.

## "THEY ARE ACTUALLY HARMED, NOT BENEFITED"

Another way to expand the "but . . . " is to argue that even though the sellers may have given genuine consent, they are simply wrong about the transaction's being to their benefit. Paternalism is now theoretically rejected in legislative and medical circles, but that does not prevent its appearance in contexts like this. Dossetor and Manickavel,[5] for instance, claim that "state paternalism grounded in social beneficence dictates that the abject poor should be protected from selling parts of their bodies to help their sad lot in life." This idea has been considerably strengthened, of late, by distressing reports from campaigning journalists and various watchdogs about the fate of people who have sold kidneys in the expectation of improving their situation, but found themselves even worse off than before.

There are questions about the accuracy of some of these reports, and also about how representative they are. The failure of some people to benefit in the way they expect, which happens in all areas of trade, is not usually regarded as sufficient to justify abolishing that kind of trade altogether. But whether or not the claims are true, there is still the question of how they could support the conclusion that kidney selling should be prohibited.

Prohibition is, after all, the situation we have now. If people are faring badly under the present system, as the reports claim, the need to protect them can hardly be used as a justification for maintaining the status quo. To make the argument work you would need to add another premise, to the effect that things would be even worse if kidney selling were legalized. But is that plausible? Live kidney donation is now so safe that many surgeons encourage it, and losing a kidney is, in itself, the same whether

[5]Dossetor JB, Manickavel V. Commercialization: The buying and selling of kidneys. In: Kjellstrand CM and Dossetor JB (eds.), *Ethical Problems in Dialysis and Transplantation*,Kluwer Dordrecht, Netherlands, 1993: 63.

it is given or sold. This means that any harm specific to selling must have to do with the surrounding circumstances. The most obvious difference in circumstances is that donation is tightly controlled and supervised, and selling, as long as it is illegal, cannot be controlled at all.

The point here is that the horror stories about exploitation, shoddy work, unfulfilled contracts, inadequate advice, lack of after care and all the rest are exactly what is to be expected when illegality forces people to resort to black markets. Properly regulated selling would be as safe for sellers as for donors. At the moment black markets provide the only option; and as long as some people are desperate for life-saving operations and others for money, the two groups will get together by some means or other. A legal market might not protect everybody, but until there is one we can protect nobody. The current abuses are among the strongest elements in the case *against* prohibition, not in its favor.

Of course there are always some risks with surgery, but the worthwhileness of any risk depends on both the nature of the risk and the value of the anticipated reward. If the rich who take up hang-gliding or mountaineering are regarded as entitled to judge their own risks, it is difficult to see why the poor, who propose to take lower risks for higher returns, should be regarded as so manifestly irrational as to need saving from themselves. *Contra* Dossetor and Mackinavel, it would seem reasonable to claim that the poorer you were, the more rational it would be to risk selling a kidney.

## "THERE IS BOUND TO BE EXPLOITATION"

Another objection is that the trade should be stopped because it involves exploitation. Even if it could in principle be rational to sell a kidney, poverty makes people vulnerable to exploitation, and the vulnerable must be protected.

Once again, there is no problem about the idea that the poor should be protected from exploitation; the problem is getting from there to the conclusion that organ selling should remain prohibited. There are innumerable problems about this one, several of which are implied in the foregoing.

One of these is implied by the arguments about coercion and inducement as ways of getting people to do what is intrinsically unattractive. Coercion works by the removal of other options until the unattractive one is the best left; and in such cases it is possible, as already argued, to protect the victim by putting a stop to the coercer's activities. But exploitation does not take this form. It works the opposite way, by adding inducements until they just tip the balance, and the intrinsically unattractive option becomes part of a package that is, all things considered, the best available. That means that if you try to abolish exploitation by abolishing the exploiting activity altogether, you may have the satisfaction of thwarting the exploiter, but you actually make things *worse* for the exploited. There are only two ways to make things better for them. One is to give them other options until this is no longer the best (in which case there is no need to prohibit it); the other is to control the trade and prevent exploitation, for which it is necessary to legalize it.

## "THE RICH SHOULD NOT GET BENEFITS DENIED TO THE POOR"

Another common claim is that allowing organ sales is wrong because it gives benefits to the rich that are not available to the poor. Like most of the arguments in the terrain, this one sounds attractive because it appeals to a benevolent-sounding principle, but it runs into the usual problems. In the first place, virtually nobody would be willing to defend, when pressed, a principle to the effect that unless everyone can have some benefit, no one should. It would rule out all the privileges enjoyed by the people in the rich world. In particular, it would certainly rule out all private medicine, which is allowed in nearly all of the countries that have banned organ selling.

But even if the principle were acceptable, it would, anyway, be irrelevant to the issue of selling as such, because it would allow the purchase of kidneys by public bodies, for distribution on the basis of need—as has been suggested by various commentators,[6] and as happens in Iran. Even if the premise were acceptable, the conclusion would still not follow.

## "SELLING BODY PARTS IS LIKE SLAVERY"

Another argument, frequently produced as decisive, is that selling parts of yourself is like selling yourself into slavery. Everyone now agrees that slavery is wrong, so they should by parity of reasoning agree that selling parts of people is also wrong.

An argument of this kind depends on the accuracy of the analogy, and the most obvious reply is that there is an enormous moral difference between allowing people to own and sell other people on the one hand, and parts of themselves on the other. But this reply is not necessary, because there is an even more obvious problem. Slavery *itself* is forbidden. We are no more allowed sell—or even give—ourselves than other people into slavery. If anything is forbidden altogether—as are, for instance, possession and use of various drugs, or murder, or living donation of vital organs such as hearts—then the outlawing of payment for such things follows a *fortiori*. Slavery cannot provide an analogy with payment for live kidney donation because live kidney donation itself is allowed, and even actively encouraged, while slavery is absolutely illegal.

This raises an important general issue in the debates about kidney selling, where objections to the procedure *as such* may be offered as objections to payment for them. For instance, it is often said that it is contrary to all the ideals of medicine to damage a healthy body. But that objection has nothing to do with selling, and would apply equally to unpaid donation. If you object to some procedure altogether, you necessarily object to payment for it. The kidney selling issue does not even arise for anyone unwilling to accept kidney donation.

This is also relevant to a version of the slippery slope argument, which regularly appears in this context. It is often argued that if you allow the sale of kidneys, there is nothing to stop you from slipping into the sale of vital organs, such as hearts. But if there were an inevitable slippery slope of this kind we would find that the permitting of kidney *donation* had led to heart donation; but we seem to have had no trouble in establishing laws that allow people to take the small risk of kidney donation, but draw the line at allowing them to do themselves serious harm. If we can stop the slippery slope in the context of giving, by saying that some procedures should not be allowed *at all*, the prevention of selling follows a *fortiori*.

[6]See, for example, Erin CA, Harris J. An ethical market in human organs. *J Med Ethics* 2003;29:137–138.

## "YOU CAN'T SELL YOUR BODY BECAUSE YOU DON'T OWN IT"

A variant on the slavery argument is the issue of ownership. It is often said that we do not own our own bodies and so cannot sell parts of them.

For anyone inclined to this line of argument, the first question is about the status of the claim. Is it intended as moral, religious, legal, or what? People with moral or religious objections to selling can always choose to refrain from doing so. The interesting question is about the law.

It is true that the legal status of bodies is often murky, but the relevant question here is what the law *should* be. Most people now think we should have the right to decide whether to *give* our kidneys, and the right to give normally implies ownership. If there is a good reason for claiming that we should have a kind of legal ownership that extends to giving but not selling, it is, to say the least, not obvious what it might be, let alone why it should be recommended.

## "THERE ARE BETTER WAYS OF GETTING KIDNEYS"

Another claim made in the kidney selling context is that there are better ways of getting kidneys. Yet again, however, this is an attractive and plausible premise that provides no support at all for the conclusion that selling should be prohibited. It might just as well be argued that because it would be better if everyone had first class health care, we should eliminate primitive clinics in the third world.

The analogy shows where the idea goes wrong. If first-class health care were available everywhere there would be no need to eliminate primitive clinics, because no one would go to them. Conversely, as long as people do want them, it shows that better ones are not available—or known to be available. Of course we should try to make enough organs available by other means (ideally obviating the need for live donation of any kind); but if that happened selling would disappear because no one would want to buy. Conversely, as long as people do want to buy, not enough are available by other means.

For this argument to work it would need an extra premise, to the effect that allowing sales would actually lessen the overall availability of transplant organs. This claim is indeed frequently made, and it raises the final kind of argument to be discussed here.

## "THERE WOULD BE CATASTROPHIC CONSEQUENCES"

It is often claimed now that if kidney selling were allowed people would stop donating organs, and even that the whole programme of transplantation would fall into disrepute.

This line of objection is quite different from the ones discussed so far. It works by claiming not that there is something inherently wrong with organ selling, but that it would lead to harm greater than any good it could achieve. There is a wide range of arguments that take this line, predicting disasters that would come about if kidney selling were legalized. It has been alleged, for instance, that if the sale of organs were allowed, "mutual respect for all persons [would] be slowly eroded,"[7] or that it would "[invite]

social and economic corruption... and even criminal dealings in the acquisition of organs for profit,"[8] or remove the incentive to overcome resistance to a cadaver programme,[9] or discourage related donors from coming forward.[10] The possibilities are endless. This kind of argument needs to be recognized as a class, because the various candidates all need the same kind of discussion.

There is obviously nothing wrong with the principle of claiming that some proposed course of action should be rejected because the resulting harms would probably outweigh the benefits, and because such arguments depend essentially on empirical claims they cannot be refuted *a priori*. Perhaps this is why, now that so many of the original arguments against organ selling have been exposed as fallacious, attempts of this second kind seem to be increasingly popular. The one about causing a decline in rates of donation and an overall lessening of the supply is particularly prevalent now.

However, although nothing can be said *a priori* about whether or not any such argument can succeed, they can be discussed in general from the point of view of methodology. Dealing with objections of this kind calls for an understanding of the difference between a genuine inquiry into the question of whether some policy would be desirable or not, and attempts rationalize—find excuses for holding on to—an existing conviction. Virtually all attempts to show that kidney selling should be prohibited come into the second category.

First, no one who started with a serious recognition that some policy had elements in its favor would think of ruling it out because of the mere *possibility* of harms that might ensue. A serious inquiry calls for a careful risk analysis, involving identifying and weighing possible goods and harms, and assessing the probability that each would come about. This must involve genuine empirical inquiry, ideally involving experiments and pilot studies. Anyone who rules out some projects on the basis of the mere possibility of harm has almost certainly decided against it on other grounds and is looking for persuasive ways to justify that decision.

Second, the appropriate response to real evidence of probable or even certain harm, in contexts where there is a presumption in favor of some policy, is not a rush to prohibition but efforts to devise ways of keeping the good elements while avoiding the bad. Nearly everything we do—including trade of all kinds—carries potential for harm, but it does not usually occur to us to abolish the whole thing rather than try to lessen or remove its dangers. When we do have such an impulse, once again, it means that we really regard the activity in question as undesirable in itself and are using the harms as an excuse to oppose it.

Third, it is most unlikely that *any* such evidence could reasonably support a conclusion that prohibition must be appropriate universally: at all times, in all places, and in all circumstances. Whether allowing payment for some kind of service would lead to harm such as a lessening of rates of donation, for instance, might well depend on the attitudes of a particular population, or the way the issue was presented.

---

[7]Dossetor JB and Manickavel V, *ibid*, 66.

[8]Abouna GM, Sabawi MM, Kumar MSA, Samhan M. The negative impact of paid organ donation. In: Land, Dossetor, eds. *Organ Replacement Therapy: Ethics, Justice, Commerce.* 1991:164–172. (171)

[9]Broyer M. Living organ donation; the fight against commercialism. In: Land W, Dossetor JB, eds. *op cit* 1991: 197–199.

[10]See, for example, Abouna *et al, ibid* p. 167; Broyer, *ibid*, p. 199.

There is far more evidence now of serious inquiry into different ways in which payment for organ donation might be implemented than there was 10 years ago, and various people have made serious attempts to think of ways to allow the good aspects of kidney selling while lessening possible harms.[11] But still, most of the arguments alleging its dangers are put forward as justifications for total prohibition. The alleged harms are, furthermore, typically backed up by no evidence at all beyond the strong feelings of their allegers; and in a context like this, where even the most flagrant logical fallacies pass unnoticed, those feelings are certainly not to be relied on.

Perhaps there are indeed good reasons for never allowing organ selling, but at the moment we have no reason to believe it. The conviction that there must be a justification for prohibition is clearly lurking in the background, systematically undermining the standards of rationality we would take for granted in a genuine inquiry.

## FEELINGS IN ETHICS

Here lies the root of the problem. The pattern of argument illustrated by these examples demonstrates a familiar phenomenon, described here by John Stuart Mill:

> For if [an opinion] were accepted as a result of argument, the refutation of the argument might shake the solidity of the conviction; but when it rests solely on feeling, the worse it fares in argumentative contest, the more persuaded its adherents are that their feeling must have some deeper ground, which the arguments do not reach; and while the feeling remains, it is always throwing up fresh entrenchments of argument to repair any breach in the old.[12]

If strong feelings come first, subsequent debate will take the form of persistent and determined attempts to justify them.

The strong feelings at the root of objections to payment showed, from the outset, in the immediacy with which those objections appeared. The outright condemnation of kidney selling came before there had been any time to consider how our usual moral principles should be applied to this new phenomenon, or any anxious weighing of pros and cons. They also show in the kinds of argument put forward. The mistakes of reasoning so far described are not obscure, of a kind that only a logician could reasonably be expected to spot. They are simple mistakes that no one would make in neutral contexts, where a genuine inquiry was being conducted.

The feelings also show themselves, more subtly, in another range of familiar justifications for prohibition: ones that invoke high-sounding ideals about altruism, human dignity, and not commodifying the human body. These ideals are introduced as though they provided independent justifications, but turn out to be nothing more than restatements of the objection.

This is most obvious in the arguments that supposedly appeal to the wrongness of commodifying the human body. Since an objection to commodification just *is* an objection to allowing payment, it cannot be used as an independent justification of it. But, less obviously, the same is true of the endlessly repeated insistence that donation must be altruistic. On the most familiar

understanding of the idea, altruism has nothing to do with the distinction between giving and selling. Many people try to sell their organs because they need the money for altruistic purposes. A Turkish man involved in the original kidney selling scandal in the UK, who was trying to buy treatment for his daughter's leukaemia, would have been regarded as a paradigm of altruism if he had wanted to give his kidney directly to his daughter; obviously he was showing exactly the same selflessness in trying to sell it for her sake. Altruism can differentiate between giving and selling only if giving is *defined* as altruistic and selling as non-altruistic. But in that case the insistence that organ giving must be altruistic is just a restatement of the claim that it must not involve selling— and therefore question begging.[13]

The same is true of arguments about human dignity. If the conclusion that payment for donation should be prohibited is to be derived from principles about human dignity, there needs to be an independent account of what human dignity is—so that we can see both whether to accept the account, and whether it really does entail that organs should not be sold. But no such account seems to be forthcoming from people who argue in this way. The wrongness of organ selling is being treated as part of the account of what human dignity is.

All this, however, raises the most fundamental question of all. If the feelings against organ selling really are so strong, and so prevalent, is that not significant in itself? Some opponents of allowing payment for body parts, when they recognize the failure of the usual lines of argument, do move into the position that Mill sees as the final retreat of his unreasoning opponents: the conviction that their feeling reflects some deeper truth, that argument cannot reach. Payment in these contexts just is wrong, and there is nothing further to be said about it.

Strong feelings do typically appear to their possessors as compelling insights into moral truth, but nobody who thinks seriously about the matter can regard mere intensity of feeling as providing the last word in matters of ethics. The fonder people are of their own moral intuitions, the more they are inclined to regard the opposing intuitions of others as prejudice and bigotry. Anyway, nobody who thinks in detail about even their own moral intuitions can fail to discover that they are full of contradictions, and cannot all be right. That is the problem here.

If the wrongness of payment for body parts is to be regarded as moral bedrock, it is indeed irrelevant that it cannot be justified in terms of other moral principles. But anyone tempted to sink with relief into this apparently comfortable position must recognize what it involves. To accept the wrongness of payment as a self-standing principle, rather than as derived from other principles, involves accepting that there are many possible circumstances in which its implications will actually *conflict* with the implications of those others, and that keeping to it will involve allowing it to override them. It must be treated as *more* important than saving life and health, respecting autonomy, increasing options, and preventing the harms done by the inevitable black market.

It is clear that most people are not willing to take this line, because if they were they would not need to engage in endless attempts to justify their opposition to organ selling *in terms* of other values. If they claim that organ selling is wrong *because* it is exploitative, or *because* people are not really choosing to do

---

[11]See, for example, Charles A Erin and John Harris, *ibid*.

[12]John Stuart Mill, *The Subjection of Women* (1869; widely reprinted), p. 1.

[13]A further objection to this line of argument is that nobody holds a general principle to the effect that if something cannot be obtained as a gift, it must not be obtained at all. If the principle is to apply to organs when it does not apply generally, a reason needs to be given.

it, or *because* it is too risky, or *because* it will dry up the supply of other organs, that implies an unwillingness to accept that it would be wrong irrespective of such considerations, let alone in spite of conflict with them. It seems that most people, at least in public and in theory, are not willing to recognize the wrongness of organ selling as a ground level moral principle, so strong that it overrides other moral considerations.

Failing to recognize the conflict is not just a matter of intellectual confusion: it has real, morally significant, practical implications. If we allow the strong feeling that organ selling must be forbidden to direct our actions, the effect will be that we try to get rid of whatever causes the feeling. If it is not reliably connected to anything that ought, morally, to be eliminated, the *only* systematic benefit of removing its cause will be the elimination of the feeling as an end in itself. This is, of course, a great advantage to all those sensitive westerners who suffer from it. Prohibition may make things worse for the Turkish father and other desperate people who advertise their kidneys, as well as for the sick who will die for lack of them; but at least these people will despair and die quietly, in ways less offensive to the affluent and healthy, and the poor will not force their misery on our attention by engaging in the strikingly repulsive business of selling parts of themselves to repair the deficiencies of the rich. But to place our own squeamish sensibilities above this real death or despair seems about as thoroughgoing an exploitation of the poor by the rich as any that has yet been discussed.

Rationality in ethics is not a matter of disregarding feelings, but of being willing to recognize conflicts between them and engaging with the question of which should be allowed to prevail. The familiar arguments against organ selling systematically dodge this confrontation by fudging connections and compatibilities between prohibition and the very moral concerns that it overrides. The result is that the feeling that organ selling must be wrong is given in practice the position it is denied in theory, and allowed to override the familiar principles in terms of which it is justified.

## CONCLUSION

The starting point of this argument makes no reference whatever to libertarian principles about individual rights and unfettered markets. It depends on nothing more than a modest *presumption* in favor of letting competent adults make exchanges they regard as mutually beneficial, strengthened, in the case of kidney selling, by the intrinsic desirability of saving life and mitigating poverty. For anyone who wants to reject these starting points the rest of the argument will be irrelevant, but these are principles that most people, including most opponents of payment in these areas, would usually accept.

This provides nothing more than a starting point, because a presumption may always be overridden by more important considerations. Nevertheless, it provides a methodological device to prevent strong feelings against payment from carrying the case unchallenged. When the arguments for prohibition are looked at in detail, it turns out that they are full of mistakes that would be glaring if they were not supporting a conclusion already believed on other grounds.

The overall conclusion is similarly modest. It is not that payment for organ donation is to be recommended as an ideal means of procurement, let alone of alleviating poverty; it is certainly not that there should be a free market; it even allows for the possibility that an outright ban might, possibly, be justified in particular times and particular places. The positive claim is only that that the strong presumption in favor of allowing some form of organ selling has not been defeated by any of the arguments offered. As long as people are dying for lack of organs, and both buyers and sellers suffer in the inevitable black market, the current total prohibition is almost certainly unjustified.

Of course we should be getting organs by other means; of course we should be doing everything we can to alleviate poverty so that no one sells through desperation. But until we achieve those things, the most obvious benefit of prohibition is to keep the desperation and exploitation of both buyers and sellers out of sight of the rich and healthy.

The issue at least needs serious debate. At the moment most of it is not serious at all, and as a result the subject is—like many other issues in biomedical ethics—in intellectual, and therefore moral, confusion.

# 8.3  CON: THE CLINICIAN'S PERSPECTIVE

*Francis L. Delmonico, MD*

The illustrative *New York Times* map that chronicled the distant travel of a kidney vendor from Brazil with a transplant recipient from Brooklyn (arranged by a broker in Israel), whose transactions were then illegally carried out in South Africa, are revealing of a highly developed system of organ trafficking that exists around the world (Figure 8.3-1).[1] The buying and selling of kidneys for transplantation has become an ethical issue for transplant clinicians everywhere.[2] Physicians who would have no part in organ trade are now responsible for the medical care of those who return to their home countries having undergone organ transplantation elsewhere from an unknown vendor. These recipients arrive at physician offices with inadequate reports of operative events and unknown risks of donor transmitted infection (such as hepatitis or tuberculosis) or a donor-transmitted malignancy.

The trafficking of body parts in the current worldwide experience is not the only kind of human trade; enterprises that traffic children and women into slavery and prostitution are known internationally.[3] This swath of human sale is all in the same mix of reprehensible activity. The ethical objection voiced against one practice of human sale is readily applied to the other. There is no ethical distinction between selling bodies and selling body parts; each violates the dignity of the human person. The opposition to organ sales is as simple and yet as profound as that fundamental principle.

Statutes have been crafted in most countries to emphasize a societal prohibition to organ sales. The European Union has condemned the practice.[4] The 1991 Resolution of the World Health Organization (WHO) on organ transplantation included a guiding principle that: "the human body and its parts cannot be the subject of commercial transactions." The recent WHO resolution has appropriately called for the international transplant community "to take measures to protect the poorest and vulnerable groups from "transplant tourism," and to bring "attention to the wider problem of international trafficking in human tissues and organs."[5]

In the United States, Section 301 of the 1984 National Organ Transplant Act (NOTA) proclaimed that: "it shall be unlawful for any person to knowingly acquire, receive or otherwise transfer any human organ for valuable consideration for use in human transplantation."[6] "Valuable consideration" is considered a monetary transfer or a transfer of valuable property among vendor, recipient, and/or organ broker in a sale transaction. Consent for organ donation as prescribed by federal law may not be induced for profit by a money payment; thus, NOTA §301 outlaws the purchase and sale of organs.

Those who would rescind this legislation in the United States have a formidable task to overcome, given the recent affirmation of Congress for NOTA by the 2004 Organ Donation and Recovery Improvement Act (P.L. 108-216). The deliberations of the transplant community with Congressional staff regarding this most recent legislation were telling in the opposition to live donor sales. However, as an initial tactic to revise NOTA, some proponents of developing a regulated market of live donor kidney sales may be considering financial incentives for deceased donation as a stepwise approach to achieving vendor sales.

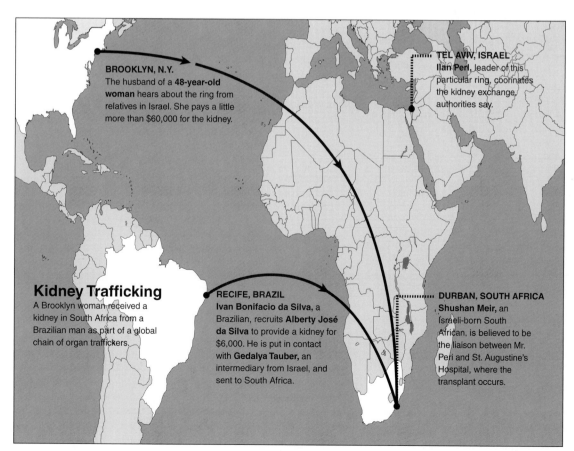

**BROOKLYN, N.Y.**
The husband of a **48-year-old woman** hears about the ring from relatives in Israel. She pays a little more than $60,000 for the kidney.

**TEL AVIV, ISRAEL**
**Ilan Peri,** leader of this particular ring, coordinates the kidney exchange, authorities say.

**Kidney Trafficking**
A Brooklyn woman received a kidney in South Africa from a Brazilian man as part of a global chain of organ traffickers.

**RECIFE, BRAZIL**
**Ivan Bonifacio da Silva,** a Brazilian, recruits **Alberty José da Silva** to provide a kidney for $6,000. He is put in contact with **Gedalya Tauber,** an intermediary from Israel, and sent to South Africa.

**DURBAN, SOUTH AFRICA**
**Shushan Meir,** an Israeli-born South African, is believed to be the liaison between Mr. Peri and St. Augustine's Hospital, where the transplant occurs.

**FIGURE 8.3-1**

## FINANCIAL INCENTIVES FOR DECEASED DONATION

At least four approaches to providing a financial incentive for a deceased's next of kin to consent to organ donation have been proposed: (1) a direct payment, (2) an income tax or estate tax credit, (3) a reimbursement for funeral expenses, and (4) a contribution to a charitable organization determined by the family or the deceased.[7]

Proponents for these approaches have argued that any of these financial incentives would be in keeping with every day transplantation practice that is market driven. Other than the live organ donor or next-of-kin who gives consent for cadaver donation, everyone in the chain of transplant care is monetarily compensated. For example, a salary is provided to the Organ Procurement Organization (OPO) coordinator who obtains family consent. The OPO charges an acquisition fee for the recovery of organs, the transplant surgeons and physicians who care for the patient are paid for their service, and finally the transplant center charges for the hospitalization.[8]

Those who are opposed to a monetary compensation for organ donation respond as follows: compensation for services rendered for the transplant recipient is ethically different from the compensation that would be provided for consent to donate or for the organs recovered. Compensation to transplant center physicians and OPO staff is accepted by our society for services in the exercise of professional responsibilities; it is for this service rendered for which physicians are compensated. Payment for organs, on the other hand, would foster an arbitrary commodification of the human body that is not referable to a professional service. Payments introduce an unacceptable commerce to the value of human life.[9] In Pennsylvania that worth of a human death could be a fixed amount, and yet in another region, for example, in Texas, that same death could have a different market value.

Polarized positions for and against financial incentives prompted the American Society of Transplant Surgeons (ASTS) to assemble a panel of ethicists in 2001 to consider whether some ethically acceptable method to increase organ donation could be conceived.[7] The panel concluded that there was a risk that such financial incentives could undermine the public trust of the transplant system. Nevertheless, the panel suggested that of the four approaches noted above, a reimbursement for funeral expenses could fulfill carefully considered ethical guidelines (Table 8.3-1). A pilot demonstration project was recommended.

However, following the presentation of a report by the ASTS Ethics Committee at the American Transplant Congress of 2002, a *Washington Post* headline read: "Surgeons Back Study of Payment for Organs Plan Aimed at Boosting Donor Rates."[10] This media headline, which mischaracterized the ASTS Ethics Committee's intent *not* to endorse payments, had a chilling effect on the transplant community's enthusiasm to recommend legislative changes. The ASTS was subsequently compelled to issue a disclaimer stating: "The American Society of Transplant Surgeons opposes payments for living and deceased donor organs ... payments would constitute the exchange of money for an organ, by the sale from a vendor not a donor. Payments would arbitrarily assign a market value to body parts, commodified and conceivably differentiated by gender, ethnicity and the social status of the vendor."

## RECENT U.S. LEGISLATION

This ASTS experience may have been influential in the final drafting of the Organ Donation and Recovery Improvement Act by Senator William Frist (R-Tennessee) a thoracic transplant surgeon trained

### TABLE 8.3-1

### RECOMMENDED CHARACTERISTICS OF A PROPOSAL TO PROVIDE FINANCIAL INCENTIVES FOR DECEASED DONATION[15]

- It should preserve the concept of the organ as a donated gift.

- It should convey gratitude for the gift.

- It should not subvert or diminish the current standard of altruism.

- It should not be an excessive inducement that would undermine personal values and alter decision making solely to receive the compensation.

- It should preserve voluntariness (eg, so that a family member is not coerced to donate by the will of another family member solely to receive the compensation).

- It should not lead to a slippery slope that fosters the sale of live human organs.

- It should honor the deceased (ie, it should not dishonor the merit of an individual's life by assigning a monetary value for the individual's organs).

- It should respect the sacred nature of the human body by not intruding or tampering without specific permission.

- It should serve the public good by maintaining the current public perception of organ donation as good.

- It should maintain public trust by the following: not altering patient care by premature life-support withdrawal from the person who might donate and not placing transplant recipients at increased health risk by jeopardizing the integrity of the organ pool.

---

at the Massachusetts General Hospital. Initially, Frist proposed that demonstration projects of financial incentives might be conducted "notwithstanding NOTA." However, the Congressional staff of Senator Edward Kennedy (D-Massachusetts), Senator Judd Gregg (R-New Hampshire), and Senator Christopher Dodd (D-Connecticut), influenced by representatives of the transplant community, objected to the language "notwithstanding NOTA" in the draft legislation. The Congressional direction was clear: there would be no overcoming of the 1984 NOTA prohibiting monetary consideration for organ donation. Further, formidable opposition prevailed from medical and religious segments of society and by prestigious organizations such as the National Kidney Foundation.[11]

Section 377 of the adopted Frist–Dodd Organ Donation and Recovery Improvement Act did call for the reimbursement of travel and subsistence expenses incurred by a living organ donor and it proposed funding of $5 million to be set aside through the Department of Health and Human Services (HHS).[10] Nevertheless, as of the 2005 Congress, there has been no funding appropriated.

## THE SLIPPERY SLOPE

Those who oppose financial incentives for deceased donation have asserted that a slippery slope would occur that sequentially takes the approval of deceased donor incentives to the sanction of a payment for live donor organs. The following practical dilemma arises in the progression from a deceased donor financial incentive to a vendor sale: how could society endorse payment for a deceased donor organ where there is no risk of donor harm (the donor is dead) and not permit payments to live donors who assume an infrequent but real risk of death? This logical transition to live donor payments has made some members of the U.S. Congress wary of demonstration projects for deceased donor financial incentives. In addition, there have been other considerations that seemed to have influenced Congressional views. Financial incentives for deceased donation could conceivably undermine the trust in the organ donor system. The donor family might withhold medical information affecting the well-being of a transplant recipient by the transmission of donor disease (malignancy or infection) to not risk loosing a donor payment. Finally, financial incentives for deceased donation could impact the decision of a family to prematurely withdraw care of a patient that does not fulfill brain death criteria.

## THE VENDOR SALE OF AN ORGAN

In the "case for allowing kidney sales," Radcliffe Richards proposed the use of direct payments to a vendor as a remedy for the poor to lift themselves out of destitution (at least temporarily).[13] Indeed, the Radcliffe Richards position has been known by the international community for nearly a decade, and yet her proposal has been repeatedly rejected.[13] In his presidential address at the 2004 Transplantation Congress, David Sutherland summarized the longstanding and consistent opposition of the Transplantation Society to organ sales.[14] Dr. Sutherland noted that the buying and selling of organs was "politically unfeasible no matter how the arguments are made."

## A REGULATED MARKET

In a statement before the Subcommittee on Health and the Environment of the Committee on Energy and Commerce, House of Representatives, 98th Congress, 1st session, on H.R. 4080 in 1984, Dr. Barry Jacobs, Medical Director, International Kidney Exchange, Ltd. proposed: "setting up a private program ... having healthy people ... to sell a kidney." At the time, Congressman Al Gore (D-Tennessee) replied: " ... just for the record Dr. Jacobs, I have heard you talk about going to South America and Africa, to Third World countries, and paying poor people overseas to take trips to the United States to undergo surgery and have a kidney removed for use in this country. That is part of your plan, isn't it?" Dr. Jacobs then responded: "Well, it is one of the proposals ... but the government would have to regulate it."

That verbal sparring of Gore with Jacobs was the eventual source of the 1984 legislation that prohibited organ sales. We are now 2 decades later and history is repeating itself. Matas and Schnitzler have recently developed proposals of organ sales with the same presumption that "the government would have to regulate it"![14] Were Congressman Gore to be questioning modern-day proponents of the regulated market of sales, one might anticipate that the same Congressional objection raised to Dr. Jacobs would be given to Matas and Schnitzler. Of course, Mr. Gore is no longer a member of Congress; however, in the drafting of the 2004 Frist legislation, the congressional staff of Senator Kennedy, Senator Gregg made clear that there would be no government program to petition the poor to sell their kidneys. Congress seemed to be well aware that a proposed government-regulated program of organ sales would not be realistically enforceable. Further, if the justification of a market in organs is to solve the organ shortage, then why should vendors be limited to a government regulated market?

If a better price is available through Internet bartering, why shouldn't vendors make their best (ie, most lucrative) deal outside of government regulation? As long as Congress is aware that the transplant community has no unanimity on a regulated market, it is highly unlikely that the proponents will see Congressional support.

## ORGAN SALES ARE NOT JUSTIFIED BY SCIENTIFIC OR ECONOMIC PRIORITIES

Attempted scientific justifications of medical benefit or economic analyses that conclude organ sales save money do not overcome the ethical objections to selling kidneys from human vendors.[15] The ethical considerations cannot be sublimated for by an economic rationale. The likely result of an increased supply of organs by purchasing kidneys does not justify using those means to do so. A consensus decision by legislators, policymakers, or the transplant community to proceed with payment for organs would have to reconcile social and professional consequences that are profound.

### The Social Consequences

Matas and Schnitzler's analysis proposes that the government be the proprietor of organ sales.[14] However, the role of the government is to provide for and protect its citizenry. Is it the proper role of government to sell body parts? Dr. Jeffrey Kahn has replied that a legislative endorsement of organ sales by the poor would represent a failure of government itself and would undermine the moral foundations of our society.[15,16] The United States would become the haven of the poor vendor with some more valuable subdivided into sold body parts (left lobe of the liver, a lobe of the lung) than kept whole. Further, it could also propel other countries to sanction an unethical and unjust standard of immense proportions, on the basis of the endorsement by the U.S. government.

The critical question for the proponents of vendor sales in the United States is whether they have the widespread support to make this case in concert to the federal government. Articles in the *American Journal of Transplantation* may be provocative academically, but proposing public policy is another matter. At the Greenwood Congressional hearings, live vendor sales were unequivocally rejected.[9]

### The Professional Consequences

A program of organ selling creates an inherent conflict for the physician's relationship with a patient. In that relationship, patients are not clients, consumers, or commodities.[16,17] The medical decision and willingness to perform a procedure may be forced on the physician not based on the best care for the "patient"; rather it is based on the dictate of the sale. The professional consequences of endorsing vendor sales are noteworthy for physicians readily compelled to accept the dictates of the organ vendor, over any "medical" judgment regarding the donation procedure. One could anticipate litigation from a potential vendor against a physician who refuses to perform a nephrectomy, thus blocking the vendor from securing $90,000 or more for the sale of their kidney!

Any attempt to assign a monetary value to the human body or its body parts, even in the hope of increasing organ supply, diminishes human dignity and devaluates the very human life physicians have nobly dedicated their careers to saving. Proponents of organ sales threaten core values of medical practice, turning physicians into "market providers" for "consumers and clients." Among the important roles of the profession that must not be lost are clear limits to engaging in or facilitating overly risky or foolhardy actions, no matter how informed and willing the vendor may be.

## REMOVING THE DISINCENTIVE TO DONATE

There is widespread sentiment in this country that live donors should not personally bear any costs associated with donation.[18] The expense reimbursement model has been proposed by Caplan and his colleagues, accompanied by live donor safeguards that are now being developed by the OPTN. Indeed, the existing NOTA legislation does not prohibit "reasonable payments associated with the removal, transportation, implantation, processing, preservation, quality control, and storage of the human organ or the expenses of travel, housing, and lost wages incurred by the human donor in connection with the donation of the organ." The Frist legislation endorses the concept of an expense reimbursement distinguished from a monetary payment that enriches a vendor.

State legislators are also addressing the need to remove financial disincentives to organ donation. Recently, the Legislature of the State of Wisconsin has enacted legislation that would provide up to a $10,000 tax deduction to cover travel expenses, lodging, and lost income.

An ad hoc live donor subcommittee of the United Network for Organ Sharing (UNOS) has proposed that employers continue the compensation for employee wages otherwise lost during the medical leave for up to 30 days following hospitalization. The difference between this approach and organ sales is that monetary profit is not the motivation for donation. However, the employee donor leave provision does not render the donor financially responsible for doing the good deed of donation. A reimbursement of expenses or a continuation of salary by an employer is an ethically acceptable approach, removing a disincentive for living donors. Finally, live donors should have some insurance against potential disability (or death) as a result of the donation procedure.

## CONCLUSION

The profession of medicine, the transplant community, and those involved in public policy have a responsibility to oppose the buying and selling of organs. It is an unethical approach to shift the tragedy from those waiting for organs to those exploited into selling them.

### References

1. *New York Times.* May 23, 2004
2. Scheper-Hughes N. Keeping an eye on the global traffic in human organs. *Lancet* 2003;361:1645–1648.
3. http://www.gtz.de/traffickinginwomen/download/svbf-organ-trafficking-e.pdf
4. By Marie-Louise Moller EU to Face Dilemma Over Buying and Selling Organs March 11, 2003.
5. Delmonico FL. The WHO Resolution on Human Organ and Tissue Transplantation. *Transplantation* 2005(Mar 27);79(6):639–640
6. Prohibition of organ purchases. The National Organ Transplant Act; 98-507 42 U.S.C. 274e. 1984. Title III §301.
7. Arnold R., Bartlett S, Bernat J, et al. Financial compensation for cadaver organ donation: an ethical reappraisal. *Transplantation* 2002;73:1361–1367.
8. Delmonico FL, Arnold R, Scheper-Hughes N, et al. Ethical incentives—not payment—for organ donation. *N Engl J Med* 2002; 346:2002–2005.
9. Okie S. Surgeons back study of payment for organs plan aimed at boosting donor rates. *Washington Post* April 30, 2002.
10. Delmonico FL. Congressional testimony on behalf of the National Kidney Foundation. Assessing Initiatives to Increase Organ Donations: The House Committee on Energy and Commerce: Subcommittee on Oversight and Investigations June 3, 2003. J. Greenwood (PA), Chair.
11. Organ Donation and Recovery Improvement Act. S 573; U.S. Senators W. Frist (TN) and C. Dodd (CT).
12. Radcliffe Richards J, Daar A, Guttmann R, et al. The case for allowing kidney sales. *Lancet* 1998;351:1950–1952.
13. Radcliffe Richards J. Nepharious goings on: Kidney sales and moral arguments. *J Med Philos* 1996;21:375–416.
14. Cosimi AB. Position of the Transplantation Society on paid organ donation. In: Cecka J, Terasaki P, eds. *Clinical Transplants*. Los Angeles, CA: UCLA Tissue Typing Laboratory; 1998:14:344–345.
15. Schnitzler M, Matas A. Paying for living donor (vendor) kidneys a cost effective analysis. *Am J Transplant* 2003.
16. *Kahn, J. Kennedy Inst Ethics J* 2003;13:1(March).
17. Kahn JP, Delmonico FL. The consequences of public policy to buy and sell organs for transplantation. *Am J Transplant* 2004;4(2):178–180.
18. Delmonico FL. Interview with Dr. Joseph Murray: A Nobel laureate and transplant pioneer reflects on the birth of clinical organ transplantation. *Am J Transplant* 2002;2:803–806.
19. Caplan A. Transplantation at any Price? *Am J Transplant* 2004;4(12): 1933.

## 8.4 CON: THE ETHICIST'S PERSPECTIVE

*Jeffrey Kahn, PhD, MPH*

### INTRODUCTION

The supply of organs for transplant remains inadequate to meet the needs of waiting patients, in spite of many programs and approaches to increase rates of donation. Over the years there have been numerous proposals to introduce schemes that would move toward outright sale of organs. Although the shortage of organs must be addressed, the social and ethical costs of a market in organs are too high, ranging from exploitation of desperate donors to the undermining of the fundamental ethic of organ donation.

After years of efforts focused on public and professional education, the existing approach of voluntary and altruistic donation still cannot provide a supply of organs sufficient to meet the needs of patients awaiting transplants, which has led to increased talk of financial incentives to give organs, including organ sales.[1–3] In this short commentary, I argue that the endorsement of policies to allow the selling of organs represents a failure itself, in that it signals a willingness to accept a policy environment that would make exploitation the rule rather than the exception. Further, an endorsement of organ sales would represent an undermining of the moral foundations of our present organ donation policies and practices.

## EXPLOITATION AS THE BASIS OF ORGAN SALES

We would expect that few would opt to sell organs if they had any other option, leaving the desperately poor with few prospects other than sale of their body parts. The problem with offers to sell one's organs is that they exploit potential donors by taking advantage of their weaknesses, regardless of whether there are other possible offers available to them. Some have argued that because many societies have foreclosed other opportunities for the desperate to address their own needs, we must at least allow them to address the desperation of their situations in the best way that they can, including selling organs if they choose.[2–4] But this approach can only lead to the prospect of increased exploitation by giving governments increased incentives to withhold social welfare alternatives, since without alternatives the motivation by the desperate to sell organs will be at their greatest. In the face of seeming indifference to the plight of the poor, is it the correct or defensible policy decision to turn our collective backs on them entirely and allow for organ selling? Using such arguments, can't we also defend prostitution, slavery, and other forms of selling one's body?

From the limited available evidence on organ selling, it seems clear that the practice takes advantage of the social and financial situations of potential sellers, playing on their unmet (and maybe unmeetable) needs. Instead of organ sales improving their situations, sellers seem to be made worse off, turning what most charitably could be termed market-driven trade into socioeconomic exploitation. Reports from India claim that selling organs makes the vast majority of donors worse off than they were before their donations—medically, socially, and even financially.[5] An unfettered system of organ sales in other parts of the world would be ripe for the same kinds of exploitation as reported from India.

Finally, such exploitation can be understood not only as unethically taking advantage of the weaknesses of potential donors, but driven by a fundamental shift in the ethics of organ procurement. A letter to the editor of JAMA in response to the report on kidney selling in India makes the point well: "The more fundamental problem . . . may simply be that the primary goal of kidney sellers is money, not benefit to recipients."[6] Such motivation runs contrary to the moral foundation of current organ donation policy and practice, threatening to undermine it. Voluntary altruistic donation and equitable access to the benefits of organ transplant are the longstanding twin principles of the organ donation system. The introduction of organ sales not only is antithetical to these principles but also may undermine the social trust on which the system depends. Without this trust, whatever increase in organ supply might be realized by organ sales could easily be offset by those unwilling to take part, even altruistically, in a suspect system. We must think very carefully before endorsing such a dubious shift in our policy priorities.

## References

1. Radcliffe Richards J. Commentary. An ethical market in human organs. *J Med Ethics* 2003(June);29(3):139–140; author reply 141.
2. Radcliffe Richards J, Daar AS, Guttmann RD, et al. The case for allowing kidney sales. *Lancet* 1998(Jun 27);351(9120):1950–1952.
3. Veatch RM. Why liberals should accept financial incentives for organ procurement. *Kennedy Inst Ethics J* 2003(Mar);13(1):19–36.
4. Hippen BE. In defense of a regulated market in kidneys from living vendors. *J Med Philos* 2005(Dec);30(6):593–626.
5. Goyal M, et al., "Economic and health consequences of selling a kidney in India," JAMA. 288(13):1589-93, 2002 Oct 2.
6. Steiner RW. Consequences of Selling a Kidney in India. (Author Reply) *JAMA* 2003;289:698–699.

# CHAPTER 9

# CHALLENGES OF PAID ORGAN DONATION FOR PUBLIC HEALTH CARE POLICY

*Mark J. Cherry, PhD*

## SOME FAILURES OF THE REGULATORY ENVIRONMENT: INTRODUCTION

Few ordeals could be more distressing than queuing for a replacement organ knowing that your life depends on receiving the transplant. Yet, the current altruism-based policies of organ procurement are not adequate to meet medical demand. In the United States alone, more than 7,000 people die every year while waiting for an organ transplant.[1] Many others endure pain and distress, at times even in hospitals on life support, while queuing for available organs. In 2005, in the United States only approximately 28,000 of the some 90,000 patients waiting for transplants received them[1]—a tragedy by any standard. Simply regarding kidney transplantation, it is predicted that by 2010 there will be some 650,000 patients in the United States who will require dialysis or transplantation, with at least 100,000 waiting for a transplant.[2,3] As demand for transplantable organs has risen, however, national growth rate of organ donation has been stagnant since 1997. Living donation has exceeded deceased donation nearly every year since 2000, with living unrelated donation accounting for some 29% of all living donation in the United States.[3]

A core policy challenge is that within bioethics the proposition that the market encourages scientific excellence and virtue in medical research and practice is usually met with considerable skepticism. Market-based research and practice, it is more typically claimed, substitutes profit-seeking behavior for truth-seeking behavior, and thus fails to protect the most fundamental interests of persons and public health. The literature does not usually regard the market as leading to the appropriate use of resources, the protection of human subjects, or the development of high quality and innovative medical products and services. To put the matter starkly, profiting from the provision of health-care services (such as transplantation) or the sale of scarce medical resources (such as human organs) is viewed as morally suspect. Calls for significant, wide-ranging, and extensive governmental regulation—including continued prohibition of the selling of human organs for transplantation—are ubiquitous. Public policy currently forbids outright any market-based solution to the scarcity of organs for transplantation.

However, realistically to assess the risks involved in market-based policy one must also consider the background risks involved in a medical enterprise bereft of the significant funds and health-care incentives of the commercial sector. To frame future public policy adequately requires critical assessment of which strategies

for procurement and allocation would most improve access to human organs, thereby saving lives, reducing human suffering, and advancing health-care outcomes, as well as increasing the efficient and effective use of scarce resources, while also avoiding significant moral harms, such as the exploitation of persons. As I argue in this chapter, each of these challenges is best met through the use of market-based systems of procurement and allocation of transplantable organs. As a result, one very promising direction for future transplantation policy is openly to craft a market in human organs for transplantation.

## IMPROVING ACCESS TO TRANSPLANTATION

The core challenge is permissibly to enhance access to transplantable organs, while also improving health-care outcomes relative to the current system of altruistic donation. The usual circumstance of transplant patients without a private donor is an evermore significant wait time. Given increased demand for human organs, and a concurrently increased queuing time, median wait times for patients with less common blood types, and highly sensitized recipients, have not been accurately calculated since 1998, because less than 50% of these patients have received a transplant since listing.[3] Yet, as queuing time for transplantable organs has increased, so too have direct and indirect health risks. Consider kidney transplantation: patients with end-stage renal failure not due to diabetes have a mortality rate of approximately 60% at 5 years, while waiting for organs; mortality rates are worse for patients whose renal failure is due to diabetes. In the Netherlands, for example, the wait time for deceased-donor kidney transplantation is in the range of four to five years.[4] Even queuing for less than 6 months has long-term negative health impacts relative to preemptive transplantation.[5,6] Over time the body becomes more fragile, creating significant risks of poor posttransplant outcomes. As median wait time continues to increase, it will eventually surpass the life span of many patients on dialysis.

Public policy that expands the number of living donors would multiply the availability of transplantable organs, such as kidneys, bone marrow, and liver segments. If such a policy also engaged families to make available organs from recently deceased relatives, this would also increase availability of nonredundant organs, such as hearts from brain-dead and cadaver donors. Expanding the pool of living and nonliving donors, including non-heart-beating donors,[7] would then save lives and reduce suffering—both worthy policy goals.

Here, market-based procurement and distribution of human organs demonstrates significant potential for improving access to transplantable organs. Policy that embraced financial incentives and other valuable benefits for donors would likely realize a considerable improvement in the number and quality of donated organs. For example, a market would allow families to sell the organs of a deceased loved one, rather than just to donate them. The knowledge that their families would benefit might persuade many more people to become organ donors. However, it would also open up other intriguing possibilities. Some individuals might be willing to consider a futures contract in which they agree to donate their usable organs upon their death to a particular buyer and have the money paid to their descendents. Others might wish to sell a redundant internal organ, such as a kidney, while still living. Some might find this a valuable way of obtaining resources to improve their life circumstances; indeed, some might view it as heroic—saving the life of another at possible risk to themselves.

Barter markets would open up related possibilities, such as organ trading, in which the families of those in need of transplant trade with each other for the necessary healthy organs; for example, a slice of healthy liver might be exchanged for a healthy kidney, or perhaps paired donor kidney exchanges.[8] At Johns Hopkins University Hospital, in July 2003, surgeons performed a "triple-swap" kidney transplant operation in which three patients, who were not tissue compatible with their own willing donors, exchanged the donor's kidney for a kidney from another of the three donors. Each donor provided a kidney to one of the three transplant patients. In a British case, a father who was not a good tissue match to donate to his son offered one of his kidneys to the British cadaveric donor pool in exchange for placing his son on the national cadaveric waiting list for a kidney. He offered a cost-neutral option for a trade in kind.[9] Other incentives, similar to those utilized to encourage blood donation, could give organ entitlements, or higher priority on the waiting list, to those families whose members donated organs. Such cases are little different from the current system of organ donation, apart from the financial compensation and other valuable consideration that donors and families would receive.

Presuming that the willingness to donate body parts is motivated by actual, rather than coerced, altruism, those who are willing to donate should still be willing to donate regardless of the existence of a market. For-profit markets in food and medicine exist side by side with food banks, charity hospitals, and other nonprofit programs. Moreover, most organ donations from living persons are to family members or close friends. The motivations underlying such donations are likely to maintain the same force regardless of the existence of a market: love, beneficence, loyalty, gratitude, guilt, or avoidance of the shame of failing to donate. For these donors, their willingness to donate stems from their relationship with the particular patient. Such donations are unlikely to change either in general character (ie, from donation to sale) or in relative number (ie, become other than driven by the need of a particular friend or relative).

Market incentives encourage persons to raise resources to further personal as well as social interests and goals. With the creation of a market, organ procurement need not be artificially limited to acts of altruism. Market incentives would very likely lead to an increase in the number of living persons willing to sell internal redundant organs to recipients, who are neither family members nor close friends. As noted, these incentives would also likely lead to the willingness of more families to have the organs of their loved ones harvested upon death. Such public policy would thereby incur significant health benefits for all those in need of a transfer.

## JUSTICE, FAIRNESS, AND EXPLOITATION

An additional challenge is that access to organ transplantation is seen as raising numerous issues of social justice, such as human exploitation and fair access to scarce health-care resources. Here market-based policy is perceived as raising particularly weighty concerns, for example, that cash payments will attract primarily poor and low-income segments of the population, including racial minorities, who will disproportionately bear the health-care complications of being donors. A common challenge to a market in human organs for transplantation is that it would exploit the poor; that it would coerce poor people into selling their organs, something that in better circumstances they would not consider.

But, why would the market necessarily be exploitative? People would be free to negotiate a bargain in which both parties would win: on the one hand, a life is saved; on the other, a family is lifted from poverty. The fear that unscrupulous entrepreneurs would coerce people to part with organs for less than the market price is likely also misplaced. Unlike illicit trading on a black market, a legally regulated market should not suffer from such behavior. For example, it should be possible as a matter of public policy to set minimum legal prices for organs to ensure that sellers are properly compensated. Countries would have to decide how best to regulate the international organ trade, but this should not be much different from the current challenges to regulate international organ donations.

Another reason why legalizing the market would discourage unscrupulous practices is that in legitimate markets, kindness and personal recognition of the other are often crucial for business, allowing partners to build up trust. Customer satisfaction and professionalism lead to long-term profits. Successful organ procurement and transplantation requires the skilled services of many professionals. Even though donor and recipient may only meet once in an organ market, reputations are built on relationships with and among surgeons, hospitals, transplant teams, and others who perform specialized services. Hospitals, as providers of highly qualified surgical teams, a suitably sterile environment, and medical follow-up, have significant professional incentives to encourage virtuous tendencies in the market. Surgeons would be unlikely to put their reputation at risk by dealing with black-market traders or con-artists. Given a good reputation, others will be much more likely to utilize their services in the future. Professional virtue and medical skill can, therefore, be seen as a profit maximizing strategy.

Perhaps the market is exploitative because there exists a moral obligation to provide assistance, such as a right to be rescued, or a duty to help others in need. If such a duty exists, then demanding compensation to fulfill one's duty may be coercive. However, it is unclear that even if the existence of such a duty could be demonstrated, that it would sustain the case against organ sales. Patients dying of organ failure would not usually be described as having special moral obligations to provide potential organ donors with financial income without asking for some good or service in return. Indeed, it may be that it is patients with end-stage organ failure who are being exploited. Contrary to the often-cited concern that a commercial organ market would exploit the poor, it may be that by offering to sell organs the poor would be exploiting the illness of the rich for personal gain. Yet, absent prior agreements or special moral obligations, it is unclear why those with healthy organs have a moral obligation to donate.

Persons have a monopoly over the use of their own bodies and its parts. Although human organs are typically characterized as a scarce medical resource, a person's monopoly ownership over his healthy organs is crucially different from monopoly ownership of natural resources. Although the second can be secured through a violation of rights, the first cannot. Most crucially, intervening in the commerce of the second can prevent exploitation. In contrast, intervening in the commerce of the first brings about exploitation by forcibly preventing others from paying the owner of the organs as much as it is worth to the owner. In short, adequately to assess claims of exploitation, and to establish policy to prevent such exploitation, one must also inquire as to who is in greater need, and thus in more threat of exploitation: the poor who need financial resources, or the patients who are dying of organ failure.

Here, critics of organ vending often claim that only the rich would be able to afford organs, and that the poor would have to suffer in extra long queues for state-funded transplants. But this consequence is unlikely for several reasons. Because the market would increase the number of organs, making transplantation more readily available, it would reduce queuing time. Consider, for example, two alternative procurement and allocation policies. On policy A, 100% of the patients spend an average of 24 months queuing for a suitable organ, with 5% mortality among patients while awaiting transplantation. On policy B, 50% of the patients spend an average of 2 months queuing, with less than 1% mortality while awaiting transplantation. The circumstance of the remaining 50% of the patients is exactly the same as that with policy A. Of the two policies, B may be worse with regard to equality, if judged solely in terms of queuing time and probability of dying while queuing. However, B is significantly better with regard to health-care outcomes: waiting time is much less for half of the patients, reducing morbidity and mortality costs. With market-based procurement, moreover, more organs would likely be available reducing queuing time for the entire wait list. Even if the organs sold predominately benefited only certain segments of the patient population, such activity would reduce the number of patients on the general waiting lists, thus reducing waiting time for others. As it is usually the poor who wait longest for scarce medical resources, it would benefit them most of all.

Second, meeting the medical needs of patients who are waiting for transplants is very costly. By reducing wait times, the market would also save financial resources, which may be particularly important for stretching the budgets of public programs that address the health-care needs of the poor. Consider: the Medicare cost of dialysis and transplantation in 2002 was $17 billion; this is expected to increase to approximately $28 billion in 2010.[2] Although these individuals only represent 0.5% of Medicare patients, they accounted for approximately 5% of the entire Medicare budget in 2002.[2,3]

Finally, even within a market system, private individuals could still donate organs for free out of charity to family members or to others in need. One might also engage other public responses to blunt the impact of the market on the impecunious: health-care policy might establish a minimum baseline of welfare or health-care benefits packages, including organ stamps, that is, federally funded organ purchase vouchers for the poor.

In general, it is difficult to count a policy as exploitative if, as in the case of legalizing organ sales, it increases the number of options open to individuals. To conclude that such circumstances are inherently exploitative, one must hold that there is something intrinsically wrong or debasing in selling one's organs, so that even if one does this freely, one has been brought to do something morally injurious to oneself. Such a conclusion is implausible, however, because the action involved in selling an organ is the same as that in donating an organ. The primary difference is that money changes hands.

## MARKETS, MEDICAL INNOVATION, AND SCIENTIFIC EXCELLENCE

An additional challenge for framing public policy is to encourage both medical innovation and scientific excellence. Here, a root concern is with potential conflicts of interest. In research, conflicts of interest arise when a researcher's judgment regarding a primary interest, such as scientific knowledge, is or may be unduly influenced by a secondary interest, such as financial gain, political viewpoints, or career advancement.[10,11] For example, physicians who are both researchers and clinicians have competing commitments. The primary goal of clinicians is generally doing what is best for one's patients within certain side-constraints, such as patient consent, institutional policy, and resource availability. Clinicians recommend treatments and interventions based on what they believe is in the best interests of their particular patients. The primary goal of researchers, on the other hand, is the discovery of answers to research questions. Researchers are constrained in how they may utilize subjects who may or may not benefit from the study design; however, the objective in a scientific inquiry is to follow a protocol to obtain data, to test a hypothesis, and to contribute to the base of scientific knowledge. The researcher's actions and decisions are not based on or directed primarily toward the interests of individual patient subjects. When clinicians/researchers enroll their own patients into clinical trials, especially if the studies include a placebo-controlled arm—in which subjects do not receive potentially beneficial medicine—a conflict of professional roles emerges since study subjects are not patients in the strict sense. Other conflicts may emerge when researchers perceive certain conclusions as supporting particular moral judgments, sociopolitical points of view, or financial gain. Here the question for transplantation policy is whether the market fares better or worse on such grounds than the current system of altruistic donation.

The central concern is that the market substitutes profit-seeking behavior for truth-seeking behavior. However, the ubiquitous calls for regulation to correct for so-called "market failures" risk enacting facile and oversimplified solutions to what is a complex problem. It is important to recognize, for example, that many of the forces that distort data are independent of the commercial market. Political, moral, and other epistemic and nonepistemic background commitments often play roles in surreptitious or unconscious distortion of scientific data so as to acquire research funding, advance one's social standing in the scientific community, or further particular sociopolitical goals. The protection of careers, as well as the furtherance of social or political goals, may at times take precedence over scientific accuracy or the protection of patients.[12–14]

Consider the example of research on human subjects. Insofar as a protocol involves research on human subjects the institutional review board (IRB) must first approve the study. IRBs are charged with ensuring that research is performed safely: with assessing the protection of human subjects and with making certain that each study meets institutional standards for scientific conduct. IRBs often also review adverse events. Importantly, this process has led to another area of concern, namely, conflicts of interest in the composition of IRBs at academic medical centers and in the use of commercial or independent IRBs.

Whereas the intent of the IRB is to harmonize the interests of clinical researchers with the protection of research subjects, the concern is that the IRB's primary function has apparently become the protection of the institution rather than the research subjects.[15] IRB membership is typically almost exclusively researchers from the particular institution, who therefore have a vested interest in the ongoing success of the institution: for example, job security, institutional prestige, or research reputation.[16,17] Grant applications may include overhead reimbursements, payments for patient care, and so forth, which for a nonprofit academic institution may be important sources of income. Similarly, members may be interested in the overall financial status of the for-profit or not-for-profit entity. The IRB is likely aware that the success of particular protocols may attract other profitable studies to the institutions. Members may be friends, mentors, or colleagues of the investigators. At times IRB members may informally coach the primary investigators on a research project regarding how best to phrase the protocol so that it will be approved. Also, members may bring a particular social, political, or moral agenda with them to the IRB; for example, members may be in favor of unfettered access to abortion or to unrestricted research on embryonic stem cells, and thus be more likely to approve even poorly designed studies that support such moral claims.

In addition to funding sources and commercial entanglements, political, moral, and other epistemic and nonepistemic background commitments often play roles in surreptitious or unconscious distortion of scientific data to acquire research funding, advance one's social standing in the scientific community, or further particular sociopolitical goals. It would be short-sighted, indeed, to overlook the pervasive and subtly nuanced conflicts that desire for renown, professional advancement, and moral worldview represent.

Here the market may fare somewhat better than governmentally controlled transplantation in that the market preserves and expands niches by providing incentives for developing high-quality or innovative products and procedures. It is in the interests of profit maximization to produce safer products and procedures as well as to support better access to transplantation. If one is in the business of selling organs, profits would generally be maximized if one provided high-quality organs with low rates of rejection. Given such circumstances, procuring organs from living persons, who usually produce better medical results, will result in higher profits than from deceased donor organs. Organs removed from living persons are more likely to be of significant use to recipients. They have greater vitality and can be screened in advance for defects, diseases, or other negative indicators. In contrast, if organs are only procured from the recently deceased, such as accident victims, one loses both vitality and screening opportunities. A central factor jeopardizing an organ's viability is the time during which it is without oxygen and other nutrients. Damage due to inadequate oxygen, or ischemia, begins immediately once the heart stops pumping. As the Institutes of Medicine Report on organ procurement from non-heart-beating donors points out, such organs have higher discard rates, which leads to increased transplant costs, as well as to the availability of fewer organs. Transplant survival data, though increasingly competitive, are not quite as good as those from heart-beating donors. An additional difficulty is rejection by the recipient. Even a well-preserved organ is more likely to be rejected after transplantation if it does not have the same genetic markers as the recipient. Such failures can be fatal. In these areas the open market will be advantaged scientifically over a system of donation: commercial sale will likely target living donors; provide adequate time to screen for organ viability, disease, and potentially deadly immunorejections; and have the flexibility to arrange for quick transference of the organ to avoid significant ischemia.

Additional legal safeguards bearing on product liability and tort gear in with market-based organ procurement and allocation of organs. The Organ Procurement and Transplantation Act of 1984, which prohibited the sale or exchange for "valuable consideration" of human organs for use in transplantation, punishing violators with a fine of not more than $50,0000 or imprisonment of not more than 5 years, or both. The law prohibits any for-profit commercial harvesting or sale of human organs for transplantation. The act defined "valuable consideration" as excluding "the reasonable payments associated with the removal, transportation, implantation, processing, preservation, quality control, and storage of a human organ or the expenses of travel, housing, and lost wages incurred by the donor."[18] As a result, any transaction with respect to organ transplantation is classified as the provision of services rather than as the sale of goods. The statute thereby directly impacts the grounds on which an individual can base a cause of action for product liability and tort with regard to organ transplantation.

Ordinarily, an individual who alleges an injury caused by a defective product can base cause of action on negligence, breach of warranty, or strict liability. Negligence can be understood in terms of a duty of the person of ordinary sense to exercise ordinary care and skill. The *Restatement (Second) of Torts* defines negligence as "conduct which falls below the standard established by law for the protection of others against unreasonable risk of harm."[19] Negligence theory requires that the injured party demonstrate that a specific defendant failed "to exercise proper care in designing, testing, manufacturing, or marketing the allegedly defective product and that, as a reasonably foreseeable and proximate result of such negligence, the plaintiff suffered injury."[20] Liability predicated on negligence theory is the standard that touches physicians. Courts have generally held that the primary purpose of the physician–patient relationship is the performance of professional medical services rather than the sale of medical products. Thus, suits against physicians for injury resulting from treatment are typically predicated on professional negligence or malpractice—that is, the failure to exercise the required degree of skill, care, or diligence required by the standard of care in treating the patient.

In contrast, an injured party predicating a cause of action on warranty need only demonstrate that the manufacturer or seller breached a promise, whether implied or expressed, that the product was both free from defects and fit for the usual purposes for which such a product is typically used. Strict liability in tort applies even stronger standards to the manufacturer or distributor of products. Liability on the part of the manufacturer or distributor follows the defective product. To establish a product liability claim under such standards, the injured party need only show that the product causing the injury was defective and unreasonably dangerous when it left the control of the manufacturer or vendor, and that as a result of this defect it caused injury.

The circumstance that any transaction with respect to human organ transplantation is classified as the provision of services, rather than as the sale of goods, creates an ongoing public policy challenge, because it effectively screens out product liability claims predicated on warranty or strict liability. Exposure to liability in this circumstance is limited to the possibility of the physician's negligence or malpractice. With the creation of an open market, product liability based on expressed or implied warranty, as well as on strict liability, becomes applicable. Individual donors as well as commercial procurement and transplantation corporations could be held strictly liability for defects that cause harm to the transplant recipient. The application of such strict product liability standards would likely motivate the development of high quality scientific procurement, screening, and transplantation techniques. Organ quality may at times be problematic precisely because of insufficient commercialization, and because of the protection from liability that donation affords those who procure and transplant organs. A central challenge of the black market, for example, is the difficulty of enforcing either appropriate medical standard of practice or quality guarantees for organs.

## CONCLUDING REFLECTIONS

Innovation, even medical innovation, is frequently driven by the profit motive. Other motives to innovate exist—scientific interest, professionalism, altruism, patriotism—however, the profit motive stimulates enhanced levels of innovation. Historically, the development of an economic sphere in which individuals and groups ventured with others, open to the possibility of success and failure, and charged whatever prices seemed likely to yield the greatest profits, offered significant incentive to innovate new products and services.[21] The open market offered both the possibility to profit from innovations as well as to raise the capital necessary for experimentation. Moreover, it diffused political and social authority, freeing innovators to compete with each other as well as to challenge the status quo. As a result, any adequate assessment of organ transplantation policies must explore whether market-based policies would, more than current altruism-based policies, successfully produce high-quality organs and develop innovative transplantation products and techniques, while encouraging virtuous behavior. David Friedman provocatively illustrates this point:

> Both barbers and physicians are licensed, both professionals have for decades used licensing to keep their numbers down and their salaries up. Governmental regulation of barbers makes haircuts more expensive; one result presumably is that we have fewer haircuts and longer hair. Governmental regulation of physicians makes medical care more expensive; one result presumably is that we have less medical care and shorter lives. Given the choice of deregulating one profession or the other, I would choose the physicians.[22]

The current regulatory environment increases costs while decreasing organ availability. Its focus on altruism, equality, and fairness leads counterproductively to less efficient organ procurement and allocation, and thereby to greater human suffering and fewer lives saved. As I have argued, market-based public policy would very likely increase both the quality and the quantity of organs available for transplant, thus leading to direct and indirect health benefits, for example, decreasing queuing times while also increasing transplant viability.

Moreover, as discussed, it is important to recognize that factors, which lead to conflicts of interest, impacting scientific excellence and medical expertise, are largely independent of the market. Political, moral, and other nonepistemic background conditions, such as career development or political goals, often play a significant role in the surreptitious or unconscious distortion of scientific data to maintain research funding and social standing in the scientific community, or to further particular social political goals. Indeed, legal safeguards from tort liability, especially product liability, become applicable with market-based organ procurement, transplantation, and scientific research. Torts predicated on warranty or strict liability are only possible if the transplanted organ is understood as a good that is being sold to the recipient. Commericalization would, therefore, introduce special legal safeguards and benefits. Finally, the market would provide significant incentives for developing high-quality and innovative transplantation products and services.

In summary, as I have argued in *Kidney for Sale by Owner: Human Organs, Transplantation, and the Market*, in more detail,[23] it is time to stop the political and social hand-wringing and honestly consider the hard facts of the public policy challenges: the current system of an altruistically based system of organ transplants is not working adequately, and a market for organ donors and recipients could save lives and considerably reduce suffering. Proper regulation might be essential to ensure that the system benefited all those in need, and that those who sold organs were adequately compensated. However, if we fail to take this opportunity, patients will continue to languish on waiting lists until they run out of time.

## References

1. UNOS. 2006 Annual Report of the U.S. Organ Procurement and Transplantation Network and the Scientific Registry of Transplant Recipients. Rockville, MD, HHS/HRS/OSP/DOT, 2006, www.optn.org/AR2006 (last accessed, 07/01/2007).
2. Xue JL, Ma JZ et al. Forecast of the number of patients with end-stage renal disease in the United States to the year 2010. *J Am Soc Nephrol* 2001;12(2):2753–2758.
3. Hippen BE. In defense of a regulated market in kidneys from living vendors. *J Med Philos* 2005;30(6):627–642.
4. de Klerk M, Keizer KM, Claas FH, et al. The Dutch national living donor kidney exchange program. *Am J Transplant* 2005;5(9):2303–2305.
5. Meier-Kriesche HU, Kaplan B. Waiting time on dialysis as the strongest modifiable risk factor for renal transplant outcomes: A paired donor kidney analysis. *Transplantation* 2002;74(10):1377–1381.
6. Abou Avache R, Bridoux F, Pessione F, et al. Preemptive renal transplantation in adults. *Transplant Proc* 2005;37(6):2817–2818.
7. Sanchez-Fructuoso A, Prats Sanchez D, Marques Vidas M, et al. Non-heart beating donors. *Nephrol Dial Transplant* 2004;(June 19; Suppl 3(iii)):26–31.
8. Delmonico FL, Morrissey PE, Lipkowitz GS, et al. Donor kidney exchanges. *Am J Transplant* 2004;4(10):1553–1554.
9. Sells RA. Paired-kidney exchange program. *New England Journal of Medicine* 1997;337:1392–1393.
10. Medical Research Council: Good research practice. In: Erickson S, ed. *Manual for Research Ethics Committees*, 6th Ed.Cambridge: Cambridge University Press, 2003:208.
11. Thompson DF. Understanding financial conflicts of interest. *New Engl J Med* 1993;329(8): 573–576.
12. Bell R. *Impure Science*. Chichester: Wiley; 1992.
13. O'Toole M. Magot O'Toole's record of events. *Nature* 1991;351, 183.
14. Cherry M. Financial conflicts of interest and the human passion to innovate. In Iltis AS, ed. *Research Ethics*. New York: Routledge, 2006: 147-164.
15. Annas G. Ethics committees: From ethical comfort to ethical cover. *Hastings Center Rep* 1991;21(3):18–21.
16. Francis L. IRBs and conflicts of interest. In Spece Jr. RG, Shimm DS, Buchanan A. *Conflicts of Interest in Clinical Practice and Research*. New York: Oxford University Press, 1996:422.
17. Slater EE. IRB reform. *N Engl J Med* 2002;346(18):1402–1404.
18. Organ Procurement and Transplantation Act of 1984, 42 U.S.C.A. §274e "Prohibition of Organ Purchases." West Supp. (1985).
19. American Law Institute. *Restatement (Second) of Torts*. Saint Paul, American Law Institute Publishers, 1965, §282.

20. Nolan RE, Schmidt WL. Products liability and artificial and human organ transplantation—A legal overview. In Cowan DH, Kantorowitz JA, Rheinstein PH, eds. *Human Organ Transplantation: Societal, Medical-Legal, Regulatory, and Reimbursement Issues.* Ann Arbor: Health Administration Press; 1987:138.

21. Rosenberg N, Birdzell Jr. LE. How the west grew rich: The economic transformation of the industrial world. In Heath E, ed. *Morality and the Market.* New York: McGraw-Hill; 2002:10-24

22. Friedman D. Should medical care be a commodity? In: Bole T, Bondenson W. *Rights to Health Care.* Dordrecht: Kluwer Academic Publishers; 1991:302.

23. Cherry M. *Kidney for Sale by Owner: Human Organs, Transplantation, and the Market.* Washington DC: Georgetown University Press; 2005.

# CHAPTER 10

# ILLEGAL ORGAN TRADE: GLOBAL JUSTICE AND THE TRAFFIC IN HUMAN ORGANS

*Nancy Scheper-Hughes, PhD*

The neoliberal readjustments of societies worldwide to meet the demands of economic globalization have been accompanied by a depletion of traditional modernist, humanist, and pastoral ideologies, values, and practices. New regulations between capital and labor, bodies and the state, inclusion and exclusion, belongs, and extraterritoriality have taken shape. Some of these realignments have resulted in surprising new outcomes (eg, the emergence and applications of democratic ideas and ideals of "medical" and "sexual" citizenship[1] in countries such as Brizil and India, which have challenged international patient laws and trade restrictions to expand the production and distribution of generic, lifesaving drugs), whereas others have reproduced all too familiar inequalities. Nowhere are these trends more stark than in the global markets in bodies, organs, and tissues to supply the needs of transplant patients who are now willing to travel great distances to procure them. But rather than lament the decline of humanistic social values and social relations, we recognize that the material grounds on which once cherished values were based have shifted today almost beyond recognition.

## ON THE TRAIL OF ORGAN STEALING RUMORS

Stephen Frears' film *Dirty Pretty Things* treats the traffic in human frailty and vulnerability in the shadowy underworld of immigrant London. In a particularly poignant scene Okwe, a politically framed, sleepless, haunted Nigerian doctor-refugee, hiding out as a hotel receptionist, delivers a freshly purloined human kidney in a Styrofoam cooler to a sleazy body-parts broker waiting in the underground parking lot of the sham hotel. "How come I've never seen you before," the tight-lipped White English broker asks Okwe before gingerly accepting the strangely animate and "priceless" parcel. Barely concealing his rage, Okwe replies between clenched teeth in finely accented Nigerian English: "Because we are the people you never see. We are the invisible people, the ones who clean your homes, who drive your taxis, who suck your cocks." And, now, he could have added, the ones who are even asked to provide you with our "spare" body parts.

Little did the London-based scriptwriter of *Dirty Pretty Things* realize how close to the mark his fictive portrayal of the global transplant underworld struck. But the film is a social thriller, not a documentary, and it toys with the theme of organ theft, blending elements of fantasy with realist scenes of human trafficking for kidneys. When Senay, a pretty Turkish waif, pledges her kidney for a passport and visa to New York City, the filmmakers unwittingly captured a real life dilemma among illegal workers from the third-world jockeying for a toehold in the North. Filipina domestic workers overseas are often lured by unsavory brokers and traffickers into selling a kidney in exchange for help with their legal status.

The Organs Watch project had its origins in another sort of popular drama, in the circulation of bizarre rumors of body snatching and organ theft in urban shantytowns, squatter camps, and refugee camps the world over in the mid-1980s. The residents of Alto do Cruzeiro, Northeast Brazil, site of my long-term anthropological research in Northeast Brazil, reported yellow vans scouring poor neighborhoods looking for street kids and other social marginals whose bodies would not be missed. The drivers were described as North American or Japanese medical agents working for large hospitals abroad. The abducted bodies, they said, would appear later on the sides of country roads or in hospital dumpsters missing vital parts, especially eyes, kidneys, hearts, and livers. "You may think this is nonsense," my ordinarily trustworthy field assistant Irene da Silva said, "but we have seen things with our own eyes in public hospitals and in police morgues, and we know better." Irene's neighbor, Beatrice, agreed: "In these days, when the rich look at us, they are eyeing us greedily as a reservoir of spare parts." Edite Cosmos added: "So many of the rich are having transplants and plastic surgeries today we hardly know anymore to whose body we are talking. Where do you think they are getting all those body parts?"

The rumors of organ theft often embellished with outlandish details, were all too easily discredited by the medical profession, who like the medical director of the police morgue in Rio de Janeiro, dismissed the charges as the ignorance of the poor who imagined that even their penises and uteruses might be taken to serve the needs of the rich. But altogether credible stories like the following, told to me by Irene Maria da Silva, a poor washerwoman from Recife, illustrate the material grounds for the profound sense of insecurity experienced by shantytown residents who are sure that almost anything can happen to themselves and to their bodies.

> When I was working in Recife, I became the lover of a man who had a large, ugly ulcer on his leg. I felt sorry for him and I would go to his house and wash his clothes for him, and he would visit me from time to time. We were lovers for several years when all of a sudden he died. The city sent for his body. I decided to follow and make sure that his body wouldn't get lost in the bureaucracy. My partner didn't own a single document, so I was going to serve as his witness and as his identification papers. But, by the time I got to the morgue it was too late; they had already sent his body to the medical school for the students to practice on.

So I followed him there and what I saw happening I could not allow. They had his body and were already cutting off little pieces of him. I demanded his body back, and after a lot of arguing they let me take it home with me.

Buried within the rumors and urban legends of kidnapping and organ stealing were real social issues and research questions that needed to be pursued on the ground and empirically. I began following the rumors in slums and shantytowns of the Third World and then following the bodies of the dead in police mortuaries and hospital morgues, and ultimately, the bodies of the living who were being recruited as kidney sellers. The dead have always had their defenders, like the Brazilian washerwoman (aforementioned) and relatives and friends have posed real obstacles to the zeal of organs and tissues harvesters. The living have to fend for themselves in a new dog-eat-dog context in which unsavory organs brokers and kidney hunters are in hot pursuit of "fresh" organs still encased in relatively healthy bodies.

## FOUNDING ORGANS WATCH

The Organs Watch project evolved from meetings of the "Bellagio Task Force on the International Traffic in Organs."[23] The Task Force, of which I was a member, was a self-appointed and freestanding study group comprised of a dozen international transplant surgeons, transplant professionals, and medical human rights workers.[2] The Task Force met in Bellagio, Italy, in 1995 and 1996 to discuss the medical, social, and bioethical consequences of the spread of organs markets and other troubling methods of organs procurement, including the use of organs from executed prisoners in China. As the sole anthropologist on the Task Force, I was "delegated" to undertake exploratory ethnographic research on the social and economic context of transplantation and organ harvesting as practiced in parts of the world where reports of organs trafficking were rift but where little on-the-ground research had been conducted. I began my work in countries and sites where I already had considerable entrée—Northeast Brazil and South Africa. Lawrence Cohen, a medical anthropological colleague, soon joined the project to explore the social and economic dynamics of debt peonage and living donor kidney sales in India.

In November 1999, with funding from the Soros Foundation's Open Society Institute in New York City, Cohen and I launched Berkeley Organs Watch as a university-based fact-finding documentation and research project designed to investigate and document the spread of commerce in tissues and body parts and of human trafficking for "fresh" organs to supply the needs of international transplant tourism. Transplant capabilities (especially kidney transplant) spread rapidly to parts of the world where new organ scarcities and demands interact with very different conceptions of medical and social ethics and in the absence of infrastructures capable of acquiring and distributing human organs by conventional means. Working together with graduate students, medical students, and local field assistants, we began documenting the social meanings and effects of buying and selling organs and tissues, investigating rumors and allegations of organ and tissue theft, and attempting to pierce the secrecy surrounding transplant waiting lists (where these exist) in response to complaints of exclusions and exceptions based on social, racial, and financial factors.

The Organs Watch project was also motivated by a more broadly theoretical concern with the body and society in late modernity, especially the particular vulnerability of the body under neoliberal globalization and the fragility of *biosociality* and *communitas* in the posthuman era. Transplant has demonstrated its awesome power to re-conceptualize and refashion the human body, the relations of (body) parts to whole, and of people and bodies to each other. Organs trafficking, within the context of transplant tourism, provides a sharp lens to view economic globalization and its effects on conceptions of "the human" and of life itself. Transplant practices, even illicit ones, provide a unique view of who we are at the present time, how we imagine our selves and our bodies in relation to others, as intimates and as strangers, and a glimpse of how we are living and under what conditions we are willing to accede to the inevitability of death.

The bioethical dilemmas and quandaries of transplant can be subsumed under the four Cs: (1) *consumption:* under what conditions is the compassionate consumption of the "body of the other" permissible; (2) *consent:* the use of vulnerable populations–the dying, prisoners, the poor, and the socially fragile—as organ donors and where fully informed consent is difficult to achieve; (3) *coercion:* the demand for sacrificial violence—bodily self-sacrifice to fulfill altruistic, kin-based, or economic survivalist needs; and, finally, (4) *commodification:* the fragmentation of the body and its parts as special objects of manipulation for sale and distribution. The exploration of these dilemmas entails a philosophical and moral quest for the elusive message in the bottle: who are we? What have we become through the globalization of new medical scarcities, desires, and needs?

## A NOTE ON UNORTHODOX METHODS

What began as a conventional exploratory research project rather quickly led to the need for new fieldwork methods and approaches that transgressed the normally discrete boundaries among anthropology, human rights work, political journalism, and detective work. My forays into the backstage scenes of organs procurement and transplantation required a different set of research skills and operating procedures, perhaps best made explicit at the outset. How does one investigate covert and criminal behavior as an anthropologist? To whom does one owe one's divided loyalties?

Under normal conditions anthropologists proceed with a kind of "hermeneutic generosity" toward the people they study. By training we tend to accept at face value, and not to second guess, much of what we are told. We try to see our anthropological subjects as friends rather than as "informants," and as collaborators in our work. The ethnographic method is qualitative and requires building trust and penetrating the "back stage" and "behind the scenes" activities and practices of everyday life. Anthropological ethnography, based on participant observation in the social settings in which we immerse ourselves—be these villages, urban slums, or hospitals and medical centers—is good at making what is generally invisible seen and heard and at revealing the secret underside of things. Anthropologists expect to win research subjects over to what is often a mutually rewarding experience. But in these ethnographic encounters in the organs trafficking underworld all the normal rules of fieldwork practice and research ethics were inadequate. These new engagements required me to enter spaces and into conversations where nothing could be taken for granted and where a "hermeneutics of suspicion" replaced earlier fieldwork modes of bracketing, cultural and moral relativism, and suspension of disbelief. In other words, this research project required a large dose of healthy skepticism, the best that a critical medical anthropology could provide.

The research sometimes required the use of semicovert methods to access information on illegal or unethical activities. In some sites I posed as a patient (or as the relative of a patient) looking to purchase or otherwise broker a kidney. I sometimes visited transplant units and hospital wards unannounced and (if anyone bothered to ask) presented myself as a confused family member of a patient looking for another part of the hospital. At other times I introduced myself to a nursing sister or orderly as Dr. Scheper-Hughes, visiting the ward or clinic, without qualifying exactly what kind of doctor I was. Posing as a kidney buyer in a flea market in Istanbul in order to understand the misery that prompts a poor person to bargain over a cup of mint tea the price and value of his kidney, I was complicit in the behavior I was studying, even though I carefully "debriefed" the person I had initially wronged and offered to help them to find an alternative solution to their desperate need. These new engagements required not only a certain militancy but also a constant self-reflexive and self-critical rethinking of professional ethics, the production of truth, and the protection of research subjects. In the end, the ethics of the "craft" of anthropology took precedence over the bureaucratic and institutional ethics of informed consent and full disclosure with one's research subjects. Our

university's Protection of Human Subjects Committee (IRB) granted an exemption to the Organs Watch project, considering it a medical human rights documentation project as well as a qualitative ethnographic research study. Because the goals of the project included preparing reports for governmental and judicial inquests and for news briefs I was given the same latitude as my colleagues in the School of Journalism at the University of California, Berkeley.

Another departure from the usual model of solitary anthropological research was the several strategic field trips I made accompanied by investigative reporters and documentary filmmakers. Anthropological fieldwork generally follows a much slower tempo, and the anthropologist is more personally intimate with, and responsible to, the people and the communities they study. But our pace is often so leisurely that, the timely moment has passed and the world has moved on to other concerns. In this instance, I felt that my findings had to be made known quickly and communicated broadly so that a public discussion of the pressing issues could begin.

The most difficult decision concerned selectively sharing with medical and other authorities—the Council of Europe, World Health Organization (WHO), parliamentary investigations, and federal police among them—some of the information on the networks of illicit human trafficking I had discovered in the

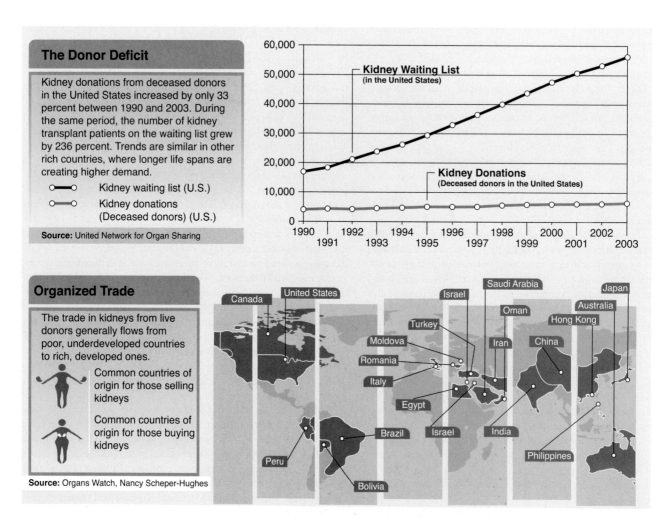

**The Donor Deficit**

Kidney donations from deceased donors in the United States increased by only 33 percent between 1990 and 2003. During the same period, the number of kidney transplant patients on the waiting list grew by 236 percent. Trends are similar in other rich countries, where longer life spans are creating higher demand.

○—○  Kidney waiting list (U.S.)

○—○  Kidney donations (Deceased donors) (U.S.)

**Source:** United Network for Organ Sharing

**Organized Trade**

The trade in kidneys from live donors generally flows from poor, underdeveloped countries to rich, developed ones.

Common countries of origin for those selling kidneys

Common countries of origin for those buying kidneys

**Source:** Organs Watch, Nancy Scheper-Hughes

**FIGURE 10-1**

course of the research. But as I came to perceive human trafficking for organs as a medical human rights abuse, I decided that being an anthropologist (and thereby committed to protecting the confidentiality of my informants) did not mean that I had to be a "bystander" to crimes committed against the bodies of vulnerable populations. Thus, I found myself in the strange situation of interviewing transplant brokers in jail who knew that my field research had contributed to their undoing. Given these research quandaries, I do not expect the Organs Watch project to become a model for engaged anthropology,[3] and I expect my refashioning of the ethnographer's craft to be greeted with lively debate and criticism.

So, take the ethnographer. She has chosen to investigate a hidden and taboo subject, as forbidden a topic as witchcraft, incest, or pedophilia. Using the traditional method of "snowballing"—one patient, one surgeon, one hospital, one mortuary, one eye bank leading to the next—she begins to uncover a string of clues that will eventually take her from Brazil to Argentina and Cuba, and from South Africa to Israel, the West Bank and Turkey, and from Moldova in Eastern Europe to the Philippines in Southeast Asia. Finally, the clues lead her back to transplant units in Baltimore, Philadelphia, and New York City. What she discovers is an extensive and illicit traffic in human organs and tissues procured from the bodies of vulnerable populations—some very dead, some in the liminal status known as brain-dead—and other, very much alive. Following new paths in the global economy, she discovers not one, but *several* organs-trade circuits and triangles circulating body parts and living bodies—buyers, sellers, brokers, and surgeons—often traveling in reverse directions. She finds that strange rumors and metaphors do at times harden into "real" ethnographic facts. She learns how effectively organ-theft jokes, science fiction novels, and urban legends conceal and distract attention from the "really real" covert traffic in humans and their body parts.

## THE DONOR DEFICIT

Millennial capitalism[4] has facilitated the spread of advanced medical procedures and biotechnologies to all corners of the world, producing strange markets and "occult economies." Together, these have incited new tastes and desires for the skin, bone, blood, organs, tissue, and reproductive and genetic material of others. Nowhere are these processes more transparent than in the field of organ transplants that now takes place in a transnational space, with both donors and recipients following new paths of capital and technology in the global economy.

The above figure shows that the demand for organ transplants in rich countries is rising exponentially producing a global donor deficit of epic proportions, a fact all too well known to the transplant world. Less well known, perhaps, are the effects of the spread of transplant technologies on creating a global scarcity of organs. This has occurred at roughly the same time that economic globalization released an exodus of displaced and "surplus" persons to do the shadow work of production and to provide bodies for sexual and medical consumption. The global market economy provided the ideal conditions for an unprecedented movement of people, including mortally sick bodies traveling in one direction and "healthy" organs (encased in their human packages) in other direction, creating bizarre new networks of international body trade.

Like any other business, the organs trade is driven by a simple market calculus of supply and demand. Its brokers organize transplant junkets that bring together affluent kidney patients from Japan, Italy, Israel, Canada, the United States, and Saudi Arabia with the stranded Moldovan and Romanian peasants, Turkish junk dealers, Palestinian refugees, away-without-leave (AWOL) soldiers from Iraq and Afghanistan, unemployed stevedores of Manila's watery slums, and Afro-Brazilians from the favelas and slums of Northeast Brazil for whom they will buy a lifesaving "spare" part.

Transplant tourism depends on four populations: desperate patients willing to travel great distances and face considerable insecurity to obtain the transplants they need, equally desperate and mobile organ sellers, outlaw surgeons willing to break the law or ignore regulations and longstanding medical norms, and organs brokers and other intermediaries with established connections to the key players in the shadowy underworld of transplant tourism. In some developing countries—China, Pakistan, the Philippines—transplant tourism is vital to the medical economies of rapidly privatizing clinical and hospital services in poorer countries that are struggling to stay afloat. The "global cities"[5] in this nether economy are not London, New York, Tokyo, and Frankfurt; but Istanbul, Lima, Lvov, Durban, Lahore, Tel Aviv, Chisenau, Bombay, Chennai, Johannesburg, and Manila. However, the United States has not been isolated from this global market that pits desperate transplant patients against equally desperate poor people, each trying to find a solution to basic problems of human survival. Transplant tourism packages, arranged in the Middle East, brought hundreds of affluent kidney patients to U.S. transplant centers for surgeries conducted with paid donors or with cadaver organs that are otherwise described as painfully scarce.[6] Until recently, the University of Maryland Medical Center advertised its kidney transplant program in Arabic, Chinese, Hebrew, and Japanese on its Web site.[7] Mt. Sinai Hospital in New York City published promotional advertisements on its transplant capabilities in the *Wall Street Journal* and in the *International Herald Tribune*. The United States is very democratic in at lease one sense—anyone with enough cash, regardless of where they come from, can become a "medical citizen" of the United States and be transplanted, even with a scarce "made-in-the-USA" transplant organ.

Americans have devised their own ways of locating and paying donors via Internet brokering. And, just as in other forms of transplant tourism, the paid donors and their recipients are willing to lie to transplant teams about the economic nature of the arrangements. North Americans (including Canadians) also travel to foreign locations for commercial transplants including China, Turkey, South Africa, and the Philippines.

On the one hand, the spread of transplant technologies, even in the murky context of illicit surgeries, has given the possibility of new, extended, or greatly improved life to a select population of mobile kidney patients from the deserts of Oman to the rain forests of Central Brazil.[8] On the other hand, the spread of "transplant tourism" has exacerbated older divisions between North and South, core and periphery, haves and have-nots, spawning, a new form of commodity fetishism in demands by medical consumers for a quality product—"fresh" and "healthy" kidneys purchased from living bodies.

In general, the circulation of kidneys follows the established routes of capital from South to North, from poorer to more affluent bodies, from black and brown bodies to white ones, and from females to males, or from poor males to more affluent males. Women are rarely the recipients of purchased or purloined organs anywhere in the world. We can even speak of organ donor versus organ recipient sites and nations. There are kidney-selling belts and entire villages and towns in which kidney selling has become central to the shadow economy.

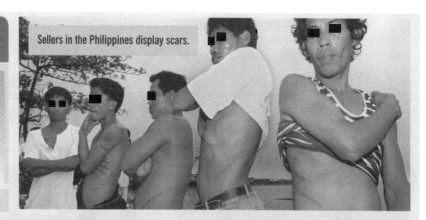

## Transplant Tourism

Kidney sellers who travel abroad for the operation—"transplant tourists"—are sometimes provided airfare, accommodation, and even sightseeing tours. Durban and Johannesburg, South Africa, emerged as common meeting points for several years, before South African authorities broke up an organ trafficking ring involving South Africans, Israelis, and Brazilians in 2003.

**Source:** Organs Watch  Nancy Scheper-Hughes

Sellers in the Philippines display scars.

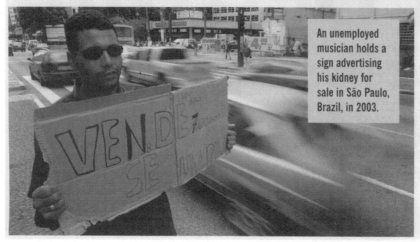

An unemployed musician holds a sign advertising his kidney for sale in São Paulo, Brazil, in 2003.

### Typical Seller (Philippines)

- Age: 28.9
- Sex: Male
- Annual Family Income: $480
- Education: 7 years

### Typical Buyer (Israel)

- Age: 48.1
- Sex: Male
- Annual Family Income: $53,000
- Education: University degree

**FIGURE 10-2**

The commodified kidney is, to date, the primary currency, in transplant tourism, the gold standard of organ sales worldwide. But markets in one cornea and part-livers from living vendors are beginning to emerge in Southeast Asia, a phenomenon I have referred to elsewhere as the "end of the body" to signal a radical historical conjuncture, a rupture in the "exceptional status" once granted by a moral philosophers to the human body as exempt from commodity candidacy, not to be reduced to an object, a mere "thing," like any other—pork butts or mechanical "weegies"—that can be bought, bartered, and sold.

In all, the strange markets, excess capital, occult medical economies, renegade surgeons,[9] and local rings of "kidney hunters" with links to an international Mafia[10] exist side by side with parallel traffic in slave workers, adoptive babies, drugs, and small arms. This confluence in the flows of immigrant workers and itinerant kidney sellers is a troubling subtext in the story of late twentieth and early-twenty-first-century economic globalization. The entry of markets (black and gray) and market incentives[11] into organs procurement has thrown into question the tired transplant rhetoric on "organs scarcity." There is obviously no shortage of desperate individuals willing to sell a kidney, a portion of their liver, a lung, an eye, or even a testicle for a pittance. But while erasing one vexing scarcity, the organs trade has produced a new one—a scarcity of transplant patients of sufficient means and independence and who are willing to break, bend, or bypass laws and longstanding codes of medical ethical conduct.

## POSTHUMAN TRANSPLANT ETHICS

From its inception, transplant medicine put severe demands on modernist conceptions of the body, the person, and the meanings of life and death. For one, transplantation demanded a radical redefinition of death, to allow the immediate harvesting of organs from bodies neither completely dead nor yet still living, which to this day still troubles many of the world's religious leaders and a surprising number of medical specialists[13]—not to mention the relatives of the nearly dead, who so often refuse to allow the term to be applied to their loved ones and prevent harvesting from taking place.

Diametrically opposed to the "softer" medical ethic of the clinic and the emergency room, based on a commitment to save the sickest, transplant ethics originally operated on the less "civil" ethic of the lifeboat and of the battlefield, based on a commitment to save the salvageable and to allow the sickest to die. But as transplant capabilities developed and the desires for transplant have "democratized," medical consumers have begun to challenge the old battlefield triage and are demanding an end to "wartime" rationing based on scarcities that could be addressed by applying neoliberal market principles to organs harvesting and thereby legally tapping into the bodies of the *living*.[12]

This move to organs markets has required a radical breach with, or a highly selective use of, classical medical ethics, based worldwide on a blend of Aristotelian theories of virtue (wisdom, courage, temperance, and justice), and the Hippocratic ethic of

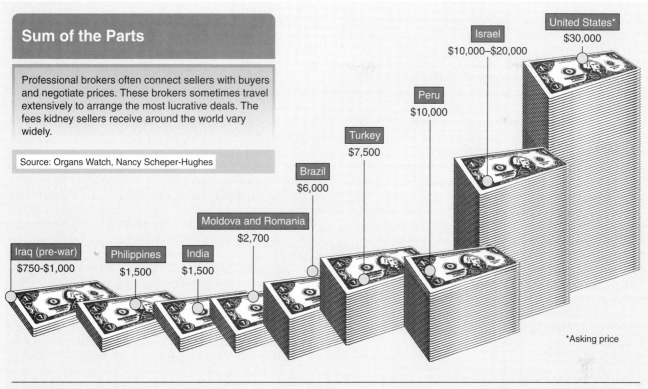

**Sum of the Parts**

Professional brokers often connect sellers with buyers and negotiate prices. These brokers sometimes travel extensively to arrange the most lucrative deals. The fees kidney sellers receive around the world vary widely.

Source: Organs Watch, Nancy Scheper-Hughes

United States*
$30,000

Israel
$10,000–$20,000

Peru
$10,000

Turkey
$7,500

Brazil
$6,000

Moldova and Romania
$2,700

Iraq (pre-war)
$750-$1,000

Philippines
$1,500

India
$1,500

*Asking price

Nancy Scheper-Hughes is professor of medical anthropology at the University of California, Berkeley, and director of Organs Watch, a center that documents the global traffic in organs.

**FIGURE 10-3**

purity, loyalty, compassion, and respect for the dignity of the individual. In the Hippocratic tradition of medical ethics, with is markedly individualist conception of physician responsibility and virtue, the physician may be seen as owing his loyalties to the patient alone, as if society—let alone the rest of the world—did not exist. In recent years, and in response to the privatization and commercialization of medicine (transplant in particular), many surgeons now espouse a frankly posthumanist utilitarian ethic based on the moral philosophy of John Stuart Mill[14] and Jeremy Bentham,[15] but stripped of their original social content and concerns.

In an essay published in *The Lancet*,[16] a few years before his untimely death, Michael Friedlaender, transplant nephrologists at Hadassah Hospital in Jerusalem, explained his about-face with respect to accepting the "greater good" that can result from adopting a utilitarian ethic with respect to the individual's right to buy (or sell) a kidney: "Recently I was told [by Nancy Scheper-Hughes] that I am a utilitarian. I had always considered myself a humanitarian, but I have since developed some doubts about my beliefs." He could not deny the growing number of kidney patients in his unit, both Jews and Arabs, who had traveled abroad for a transplant, Jews to Eastern Europe and Arabs to Iraq, returning, with a purchased kidney from a living donor. Although a few patients became seriously ill and more than one died as a result of the illicit transplant, most fared as good, and often better, than those transplanted safely at home with a cadaver kidney. "If I were ill with kidney disease I would do the same," Friedlaender said on many occasions, although he did not counsel his own patients to break the law to save themselves.

Friedlaender saw the current situation as having all the elements of a classic Skakespearean tragedy in which identifiable Ophelias, Desdemonas, King Lears, and Shylocks paraded in and out and around today's operating theatres. "The pound of flesh which I demand of him/Is dearly bought as mine, and I will have it". Friedlaender would often quote during his elegantly argued but morally tortured presentations to fellow surgeons, moral philosophers, and medical anthropologists in which he defended "the right to buy a kidney." The good doctor was all too keenly aware of the paradoxes inherent in his position. He was bold and courageous in arguing for an end to the current donor deficit impasse that had paved the way for independent brokers and black markets which have engendered antagonisms toward Israel as an unsuspecting global leader in transplant tourism. Indeed, the kidney trade evokes a timeless moral and ethical *"gray zone"*[17]—the lengths to which it is permissible to go in the interests of saving or prolonging one's own life at the expense of diminishing another person's life or sacrificing cherished cultural and political values (such as social solidarity, justice, or equity).

In the following discussion, I draw on several ethnographic sites and scenes of organ buying and selling in order to contrast the highly *variable* meanings and medical and social consequences of selling (or buying) a body part (in Israel, Moldova, the Philippines, and Brazil) with a growing consensus in the international transplant community that supports a patient-centered ethic that includes the right to purchase advanced, expensive, and experimental biomedical/surgical procedures, as well as to buy and sell body parts from the living and the dead. Both are compatible with neoliberal economics. Indeed, commercialized transplant exemplifies better than any other biomedical technology the reach of economic liberalism. Transplant technology trades comfortably in the domain of postmodern biopolitics, with its values of disposability and free and transparent circulation. The uninhibited circulation of bought and sold kidneys exemplifies a neoliberal political discourse based on juridical concepts of the autonomous individual subject, equality (at least, equality of opportunity), radical freedom, accumulation, and universalism, expressed in the expansion of medical rights and medical citizenship.

In fact, however, what makes transplant tourism possible are networks of organized crime that are responsible for putting into circulation and bringing together ambulatory organs buyers, outlaw surgeons, illicit and sometimes makeshift transplant units, and clandestine laboratories in an example of what economist Jagdish Bhagwati[18] refers to as "rotten trade." Rotten trade refers to any trade in "bads"—arms, drugs, stolen goods, and hazardous and toxic products, as well as traffic in humans, babies, bodies, and slave labor. The organs trade is fueled by a dual "waiting list," one formed by sickness, the other by misery. We have found almost everywhere a new form of globalized "apartheid medicine" that privileges one class of patients, organ recipients, over another class of invisible and unrecognized "nonpatients," about whom almost nothing is known.

## SCENES FROM THE FIELD

Avraham R., a retired lawyer of 70, stepped gingerly out of his sedan at the curb of the Beit Belgia Faculty Club at the University of Jerusalem in July 2000. The dapper gent, a grandfather of five, had been playing a game of "chicken" with me over the past 2 weeks, ducking my persistent phone calls. Each time I asked the genial grandfather for a face-to-face interview, he demurred: "It's not to protect me," he said, "but my family." Then, one afternoon, Avraham surprised me, not only agreeing to meet me but insisting that he come over to my comfortable quarters where, over a few bottles of mineral water, he explained why and how he had come to the decision to risk traveling to an undisclosed location in Eastern Europe to purchase a kidney from an anonymous "peasant," and to face transplant in a Spartan operating room ("I have more medicine in my own medicine chest than they had in that hospital," he said) rather than remain on dialysis at Hadassah Hospital, as his nephrologist had suggested.

Avraham was still eligible for a transplant, but at his age, his doctors warned, such a long operation was risky. Dialysis, they told him, was really his best option. But Avraham protested that he was not yet ready for the "medical trash-heap," which is the way he and many other Israeli kidney patients now view hemodialysis. And, like a growing number of kidney patients, he rejected the idea of a cadaver organ (the "dead man's organ") as "disgusting" and unacceptable:

> Why should I have to wait years for a kidney from somebody who was in a traffic accident, pinned under a car for many hours, then in miserable condition in the I.C.U. [intensive care unit] for days and only then, after all that trauma, have that same organ put inside me? That organ isn't going to be any good! Or worse, I could get the organ of an old person, or an alcoholic, or someone who died of a stroke. That kidney has already done its work! No, obviously, it's much better to get a kidney from a healthy person who can also benefit from the money I can afford to pay. Believe me, where I went the people were so

poor they didn't even have bread to eat. Do you have any idea of what one, let alone five thousand dollars, means to a peasant? The money I paid him was a "gift of life" equal to what I received.

Then, in December 2001, during an early snowstorm, I ducked into a small, dark, subterranean wine cave in the rustic little village of Mingir, Moldova. There, once out of earshot of his elderly father and beyond the prying eyes of disapproving neighbors, 22-year-old Vladimir, a skinny lad with a rakish metal stud in his lip, explained how he had been approached a few years earlier by Nina, a local kidney hunter, who arranged his passport, visa, and bus ticket to Istanbul, a bumpy 18-hour overnight ride. With the demise of the Soviet Union, the agricultural economy of rural Moldova collapsed in the mid-1990s. Here, in the heart of central Europe, economic globalization has meant one thing only for agricultural villagers—that 40% of the adult population has had to leave home to find work abroad. Today, Moldova is the poorest country in Europe: an indigenous "third world" within European borders. Kidney brokers stepped in and recruited, pressured, threatened and defrauded rural men (and a few women) into the kidney market. My Romanian research assistant, Calin Goiana, a graduate student in anthropology at UCLA and I together interviewed 40 kidney sellers in 11 villages of Moldova and in the capital city of Chisenau. Many other sellers refused to speak to us; some hid inside their homes and in wine cellars when we approached their home. Some 300 men traveled (with tourist visas) to Turkey, Russia, South Africa, and the United States where they sold a kidney before the Moldovan prime minister and police and other officials in several countries became involved in 2002 and 2003 in curbing the export of sad young men in thick black shoes and thin patched jackets from Moldova to supply the international transplant trade.

Once in Istanbul, Vladimir was housed in the basement of a run-down hotel facing a notorious Russian "suitcase market" in the tough immigrant neighborhood of Askary. He shared the space with several other Moldovan villagers, including a few frightened village girls barely out of high school. First, Nina (the broker) arrived to break the news to one of the girls that her "waitressing" job would be in a bar where "exotic" dancing was required. Then Vladimir was told that he was wanted for more than pressing pants. H would start by selling a few pints of his blood, and once a "match" was found, he would be taken to a private hospital where he would give up is "best" kidney for $3,000, less the cost of his travel, room and board, and the fees for his "handlers." And a few days later Vlad was told that an elderly transplant patient from Israel, who had traveled to Istanbul with his private surgeon, was matched and ready to go. When Vlad demurred, Nina arrived with her pockmarked, pistol-carrying Turkish boyfriend, who told Vladimir that he was quickly losing patience. "Actually," Vlad says ruefully, "If I had refused to go along with them, my body minus *both* kidneys, and who knows what else, could be floating somewhere in the Bosporus Strait."

Safely home again—or so they think—hapless kidney sellers such as Vladimir face ridicule and ostracism. Both kidney sellers and female sex workers are held in contempt in rural Moldova as shameless prostitutes. Months and even years later, these young men suffer from feelings of shame and regret—like Nicolae, a 26-year-old former welder from Mingir, who broke down during an interview in December 2000, calling himself "a disgrace to my family, my Church, and my country." Single male kidney sellers

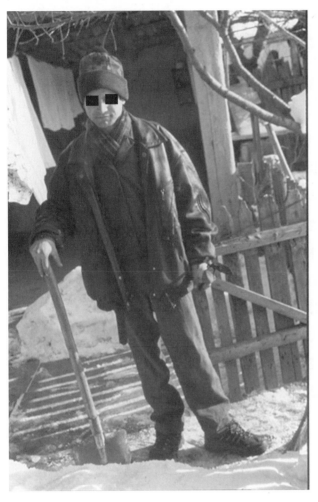

**FIGURE 10-4**

## Kidney Sellers - the Young & Naive

**Vlad was recruited from high school in rural Moldova in 2001 by a local broker promising him work in Istanbul.**

**On arrival there he learned that it was his kidney not his labor that was wanted. He was trapped.**

Source: Organs Watch, Nancy Scheper-Hughes

are excluded from marriage in rural villagers where kidney selling is viewed as male prostitution—selling one's body—and a sign of moral degeneration and criminal tendencies.

Although kidney selling is deeply stigmatized in Moldova, it is a routine event in the slums and shantytowns of Manila in the Philippines, even though the operation has put a great many young men out of work there. "No one wants a kidney seller on his work team," an unemployed kidney seller and father of three told us, while his wife fumed at him from across the room. Bagong Lupa is a garbage-strewn slum built on stilt shacks over a polluted and feces-infested stretch of the Pasig River that runs through the shantytown on its way to Manila Bay. In Bagong Lupa, "coming of age" now means that one is legally old enough to sell a kidney. But, as with other coming of age rituals, many young men lie about their age and boast of having sold a kidney when they were as young as 16 years old: "No one at the hospital asks us for any documents" they assured me. The kidney donors lied about other things as well—their names, addresses, and medical histories, including their daily exposure to the general plagues of the third world—TB, AIDS, dengue, and hepatitis, not to mention chronic skin infections and malnutrition.

In this *barangay* of largely unemployed stevedores, I encountered an unanticipated "waiting list," comprised of angry and "disrespected" kidney sellers who had been "neglected" and "overlooked" by the medical doctors at Manila's most prestigious private hospital, St. Luke's Episcopal Medical Center. When word spread that I was looking to speak to kidney sellers, several scowling and angry young men approached me to complain: "We are strong and virile men, and yet none of us has been called up to sell." Perhaps they had been rejected, the men surmised, because of their age (too young or too old), their blood (difficult to match), or their general medical condition. But whatever the reason, they had been judged as less valuable kidney vendors than some of their lucky neighbors, who now owned new VCRs, karaoke machines, and expensive pedicabs. "What's wrong with me?", a 42-year-old man asked, thinking I must be an American kidney hunter. "I registered six months ago, and no one from St. Luke's has called me—But I am healthy. I can lift heavy weights. Any my urine is clean." Moreover, he was willing, he said, to sell below the going rate of $1,300 for a fresh kidney.

When one donor is rejected, another, younger and more healthy looking, family member is often substituted. And kidney selling becomes an economic niche in some families that specialize in it. Indeed, each member of one large extended family, Bagong Lupa supplied St. Luke's Hospital with a reliable source of kidneys, borrowing strength from across the generations as first father, then son, and then daughter-in-law, stepped forward to contribute to the family income.

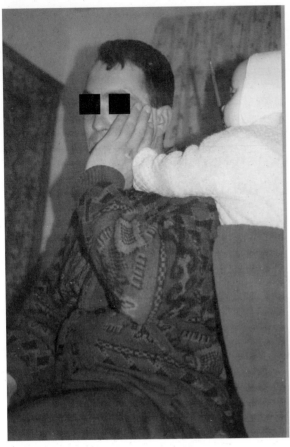

## Kidney Regret

NB, one of 17 men of Mingir, Moldova, sold his kidney to an Israeli patient in Istanbul $ 2, 700.

Two years later NB is weak, in constant pain, and excluded from his agricultural cooperative work force. He fears dying and leaving his children orphaned.

Source: Organs Watch, Nancy Scheper-Hughe

**FIGURE 10-5**

# Obligatory Sacrifice

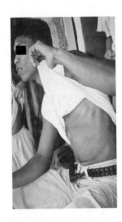

NB was 16 when his mother begged him to sell a kidney for food for his siblings and beer for her shanty-shop in a Manila slum. A good son, Osite could not refuse. Today, without a job and without a girlfriend he asks: **"What have I done to myself?"**

Source: Organs Watch, Nancy Scheper-Hughes

**FIGURE 10-6**

## THE CONSUMERS—THE EXPANSION OF MEDICAL CITIZENSHIP

Finding an available supply of organ vendors was only a partial solution to the new scarcities produced by transplant technologies. The tempting "bioavailability" of poor bodies has been a primary stimulus to the "fresh organs" trade. Today, a great many eager and willing kidney sellers wait outside transplant units; others check themselves into special wards of surgical units that resemble "kidney motels," where they lie on mats or in hospital beds for days, even weeks, watching color television, eating chips, and waiting for the "lucky number" that will turn them into the day's winner of the kidney transplant lottery. Entire neighborhoods, cities, and regions are known in transplant circles as "kidney belts" because so many people there have entered the kidney trade.

More difficult is locating patients of sufficient economic means to pay for these expensive operations, as well as sufficiently courageous to travel to the largely third-world locations where people are willing to self-mutilate in the interests of short-term survival. Here is a classic problem in microeconomics—one of supply and demand side sources separated by vast geographies, different cultures, and even by fierce religious and political hostilities.

Who, for example, would imagine that, in the midst of the longstanding religious and ethnic hostilities and an almost genocidal war in the Middle East, one of the first "sources" of living donors for Israeli kidney transplant patients would be Palestinian guest workers; or that, as recently as March 2007, Israeli patients would be willing to travel to Istanbul to be transplanted in a private clinic by a Moslem surgeon who decorates his waiting room with photos of Ataturk and a plastic glass eye to ward off evil? Or that the transplanted kidneys would be taken from impoverished Eastern Orthodox peasants from Moldova and Romania, who came to Turkey to sell smuggled cigarettes until they ran into the famous kidney brokers of Askary flea market?

New forms of social kinship and "biosociality" must be invented to link strangers, even at times political "enemies" from distant locations who are described by the operating surgeons as "a prefect match—like brothers," while they are prevented from seeing, let alone speaking to, each other. If and when these "kidney kin" meet at all, it will be by accident and like ships passing in the night, as they are wheeled, heavily sedated, on hospital gurneys into their respective operating rooms, where one surgeon *removes* the seller's kidney of the last resort and the other *inserts* the buyer's kidney of opportunity.

Transplant patient advocacy groups have sprung up in many parts of the world, from Brazil to Israel to Iran to the United States, demanding unobstructed access to transplant and to the lifesaving "spare" organs of "the other," for which they are willing to pay a negotiable, market-determined price. They justify the illicit traffic with the mantra that the purchased kidney will "save a life." That many kidney patients have refused hemodialysis, or refused to ask relatives to donate a kidney when this is an option for them, weakens the "lifesaving" argument. Today, dialysis, even as a bridge while waiting for transplant, is often viewed by sophisticated kidney activists today as unacceptable suffering. In September 2000, a 23-year-old university student from Jerusalem flew to New York City for a kidney transplant with an organ purchased from a local "donor," arranged through a broker in Brooklyn. The cost of the surgery ($200,000) was paid for by his Israeli "sick funds" (medical insurance that is guaranteed to all Israeli citizens). Noteworthy in his narrative is an almost seamless "naturalization" of living donation accompanied by a rejection of the artificiality of the dialysis machine:

> Kidney transplant from a living person is the most natural solution because you are free of the [dialysis] machine. With transplant you don't have to go to the hospital three times a week to waste your time, for three or four hours. And after each dialysis you don't feel very well, and you sleep a lot, and on weekend you feel too tired to go out with your friends. There are still a lot of poisons in the body and when you can't remove them, you feel tired. Look, it isn't a normal life. And also you are limited to certain foods. You are not allowed to eat a lot of meat, salt, fruits, vegetables. Every months you do tests to see that the calcium level is OK, and even so your skin becomes yellow. Esthetically, it isn't very nice. So, a kidney transplant from a living donor is the best, and the most *natural* solution.

Similarly, many kidney activists reject conventional "waiting lists" for organs as archaic vestiges of wartime triage and rationing, or reminiscent of hated socialist bread lines and petrol "queues." In the present climate of biotechnological optimism and biomedical triumphalism, any shortage, even of body parts, is viewed as a basic management, marketing, or policy failure. The ideology of the global economy is one of unlimited and freely circulating goods. Any of these new commodities are evaluated, like any other, in terms of their quality, durability, and market value. In today's organs market, a kidney purchased from a Filipino costs as little as $1,200; one from a Moldovan peasant, $2,700; one from a Brazilian, $6,000; and one from a Turkish worker, up to $8,000; whereas a kidney purchased from a housewife in Lima, Peru, can command up to $15,000 in a private clinic. Americans willing to donate for a fee regularly post a selling price between $20,000 and $50,000; though $30,00 seems to be the average asking price.

## BIOETHICS—HANDMAIDEN OF FREE MARKET MEDICINE?

What goes by the wayside in these new medical transactions are the modernist conceptions of bodily holism, integrity, and human dignity, not to mention traditional Islamic and Judeo-Christian beliefs in the "exceptionalism," the "sacredness" of the body. In a passage in his writings on mind–body relations, Immanuel Kant argued that the body plays a role in human cognition, linking emotion, the senses, and human thought: "Our minds reach a definite and mature status only when the fibers of our body-instrument achieve the full strength and endurance which is the completion of their development."[19] It is a strong articulation of mind–body integration.

Free market medicine requires a divisible body with detachable and demystified organs seen as ordinary and "plain things," simple material for medical consumption. But these same "plain" objects have a way of reappearing and returning like the repressed, when least expected, almost like medieval messengers and gargoyles from the past, in the form of highly spiritualized and fetishized objects of desire. As the anthropologist Veena Das once wryly observed, "An organ is *never* just an organ." Indeed, the highly fetishized kidney is invested with all the magical energy and potency that the transplant patient is looking for in the name of "new" life. As Avraham, the Israeli kidney buyer put it: "I was able to see my donor [from a village of Eastern Europe]. He was young, strong, healthy, and virile—*everything* I was hoping for."

It might be fair to ask if the life that is teased out of the body of the living donor bears any resemblance to the ethical life of the free citizen (*bios*) or whether it is closer to what Giorgio Agambern,[20] drawing on Aristotle's *Politics,* referred to as *zoe*—brute, bestial, or bare life, the unconscious, unreflective mere life of the species? Thomas Aquinas would later translate these ancient Greek concepts into medieval Christian terms that distinguished the natural life from the good life. But neither Aristotle nor Aquinas is with us. Instead, medical practitioners consult and take counsel from the new specialists in bioethics, a field finely calibrated to meet the needs of advanced biomedical biotechnologies. Even as conservative a scholar as Francis Fukuyama refers to the "community of bio-ethicists" as having "grown up in tandem with the biotech industry … and is [at times] nothing more than a "sophisticated (and sophistic) justifiers of whatever it is the scientific community wants to do."[21]

The field of bioethics has offered little resistance to the growth of markets in humans and body parts, and many now argue that the real problem lies with outdated laws, increasingly irrelevant national regulatory agencies (such as UNOS), and the archaic medical norms that are out of touch with economic realities today—and with the "quiet revolution" of those who have refused to face a premature death with equanimity and "dignity" while waiting patiently on an official waiting list for a cadaver organ. Some argue for a free trade in human organs;[22] others, like the philosopher Janet Radcliffe Richards, argue for a regulated market.[24]

In the meantime, the rupture between practice and law can be summarized as follows: although commerce in human organs is illegal according to the official legal codes of virtually all nations where transplant is practiced, nowhere are the renegade surgeons (who are well known to their professional colleagues), organs brokers, and kidney buyers (or sellers) pursued by the law, let alone prosecuted. It is easy to understand why kidney buyers and sellers would not be the focus of prosecution under the law. Compassion rather than outrage is the more appropriate response to their acts. But the failure on the part of governments, ministries of health, and law enforcement agencies to interrupt the activities of international transplant outlaws, their holding companies, money-laundering operations, and mafia connections can only be explained as an *intentional* oversight.

Indeed, some of the most notorious outlaw transplant surgeons are the medical directors of major transplant units, who serve on prestigious international medical committees and on ethics panels. None have been censured by their own profession, though a few have been investigated, and some live in self-imposed social isolation. But all practice their illicit surgeries freely, though some move their bases of international operations frequently so as to avoid medical or police surveillance. One of the transplant medicine's most notorious outlaws, Dr. Zaki Shapira, recently retired from Bellinson Medical Center near Tel Aviv, served on the prestigious international "Bellagio Task force" investigating the global traffic in organs, of which was also a member.[23] In one of his subsequent trips to Italy, he was the recipient of a prestigious human service award. Meanwhile, one of Dr. Shapira's transplant tour patients from Jerusalem provided me with copies of his medical and financial records that led to a fraudulent medical society in Bergamo, Italy, to whom the patient had sent him $180,000 that his illicit transplant (in Turkey) had cost. Shapira was arrested in Istanbul in May 2007 alongside his Turkish partner in crime, Yusef Sonmez.

The impunity of these transplant outlaws concerns more than government lassitude and obvious professional corruption. Outlaw surgeons are also protected by the charisma that accompanies their seemingly miraculous powers over life, death, and adverse circumstances. As much as his younger colleagues worry about Dr. Shapira's questionable ethics, they praise his surgical technique and his "golden hands." The head of the Turkish medical ethics committee lamented that Dr. Yusef Somnez, the "Doctor Vulture" of Istanbul fame, was one of Turkey's most celebrated transplant surgeons. "Somnez is the man who put transplant on the map in Turkey," he said.

Some transplant surgeons themselves see themselves as "above the law," a tradition they inherited from the early days of transplant, when the "founding fathers," such as Christian Bernard in South Africa and Thomas Starzl in the United States, battled against prevailing social norms and those who resisted transplant's re-definition of death to allow the removal of "fresh" organs to transplant from neomorts or quasimorts. That same sense of embattlement continues today among transplant surgeons who may publicly support international regulations against buying and selling organs, but who privately say that this is the *only solution* to organs scarcities. In the face of illicit transplants with paid donors, many surgeons simply look the other way. Others actively facilitate sales, whereas others counsel kidney patients for transplant trips overseas and care for them on their return from a trip to India, South America, South Africa, or China, where organs are purchased from the living or (as in the case of China) taken from an executed prisoner.

In the rational choice language of contemporary medical ethics, the conflict between non-malfeasance ("do no harm") and beneficence (the moral duty to perform good acts) is resolved in favor of the market and consumer-oriented principle that those able to broker or buy a human organ should be allowed to do so. Paying for a kidney "donation" is viewed as a potential "win-win" situation that can benefit both parties. Individual decision making and patient autonomy have become the final arbiters of medical and bioethical values. Social justice and notions of the "good society" hardy figure at all their discussions. In the posthumanist context, the idea of virtue in suffering and grace in dying can only appear as patently absurd. But the transformation of a person into a "life" that must be prolonged or saved at any cost has made life into the ultimate commodity fetish. A belief in the absolute value of a single human life saved or prolonged at any cost ends all ethical inquiry and erases any possibility of a global social ethic. And the traffic in kidneys reduces the human content of all the lives it touches.

## STRANGE BEDFELLOWS: TRANSPLANT MEDICINE AND THE ORGANS MAFIA

Illicit transplant transactions are obviously complex and require expert teamwork among technicians in blood and tissue laboratories, dual surgical teams working in tandem, nephrologists, and postoperative nurses. Travel, passports, and visas must be arranged. These awesome organizational requirements are arranged in many parts of the world by a new class of organs brokers, ranging from sophisticated businessmen, medical insurance agents, and travel agents to criminal networks of armed and dangerous Mafia to the local "kidney hunters" of Istanbul, Bagong Lupa, and Mingir. In Israel and the United States religious organizations, charitable trusts, and patient advocacy organizations sometimes harbor organs brokers. I have identified a large network operating between Israel and several cities in the United States on both coasts. Some have recruited organ donors locally, whereas others have recruited Russian and Moldovan immigrants, ex-prisoners, and other marginalized people who have been smuggled into the United States as tourists.

The outlaw surgeons who practice their illicit operations in rented, makeshift clinics or, just as often, in operating rooms of some of the best public or private medical centers in the city, do so under the frank gaze of local and national governments, ministries of health, regulatory agencies, and professional medical associations. In short, the illegal practice of transplant tourism, which relies on an extensive network of body brokers and human traffickers, is a public secret, one that involves some of the world's most prestigious hospitals and medical centers. Transplant crimes—even when they explode into gunfire and leave a trail of blood—(as they had in Manila several years ago)—normally go undetected and unpunished. And some of the more active and competitive surgeons can find themselves trapped and more deeply involved in "the business" than they had ever anticipated.

In addition to organized crime, military and state interests often protect organs and transplant trafficking, particularly during periods of political conflict and war. Israel became embroiled in the international kidney trade when a small market in living donors that that began in the West Bank moved to Turkey an ethics committee appointed by the Ministry of Health chastised the surgeons who were involved in the recruitment of Palestinian donors. Israelis purchase, with Iran (where kidney selling is legal), the greatest number of kidneys per capita in the world. Caught between a highly educated and medically conscious public and a very low rate of organ donation, the Israeli Ministry of Healthy has expedited the expansion of transplant tourism by allowing Israeli patients to use their national insurance to pay for transplants conducted elsewhere, even if illegally. The cost of the transplant "package" increased from $120,000 in 1998 to $200,000 in 2004. The cost includes the air travel, bribes to airport and customs officials, "double operation"

(kidney extraction and kidney transplant), the rental of operating and recovery rooms, and hotel accommodation for accompanying family members. The donor fee of between $3,000 and $10,000 (depending on the status of the donor) is also included.

Corrupt business men and their associates have formed "corporations" with ties to established medical centers and to rogue transplant units (public and private) in Turkey, Russia, Moldova, Estonia, Georgia, Romania, Brazil, South Africa, and the United States. The specific sites of the illicit surgeries are normally kept secret from transplant patients until the day of travel. And the locations are continually rotated to maintain a low profile. The surgeries are performed at night in tented operating rooms. In one plan that originated in Israel in the late 1990s, Israeli patients and doctors (a surgeon and a transplant nephrologist) were flown by a small commercial airline to a hospital in a town on the Turkish-Iraqi border for illegal transplants with kidneys procured from Iraqi soldiers and guest workers. Israeli and Turkish doctors and their patients also flew to Estonia and to Russia for commercialized transplants using unemployed workers from elsewhere in Eastern Europe. In a third and more recent scenario, in 2002-2003 kidney sellers were recruited from the slums and favelas of Recife, Northeast Brazil (by brokers including a military police officer), and sent by plane to Durban and Johannesburg in South Africa where they were met by South African brokers who "matched" these unfortunates up with Israeli patients arriving from Tel Aviv. In this instance South African surgeons operated independently, without Israeli surgeon accomplices.

The participation of South Africa's largest health maintenance organization (HMO), Netcare, and Israel's national insurance programs in the illegal multimillion dollar transplant tourism

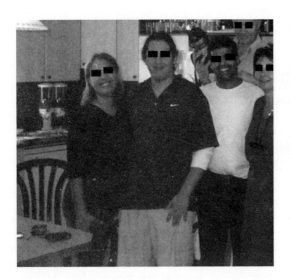

**2003: New Atlantic Body Trade Triangle linking Israel-Europe-Brazil-South Africa**

'The Above broker' entered the transplant trade following her son's 'arranged' transplant abroad. She has since organized more than 50 'budget' transplant tours to South Africa with paid and trafficked kidney donors. She fashions herself an 'equal opportunity' broker. One of her 'satisfied' kidney sellers is standing next to her son in Tel Aviv, Israel.

Source: Organs Watch, Nancy Scheper-Hughes

**FIGURE 10-7**

business, has made Israel into something of a pariah in the international transplant world and sullied South Africa's great tradition of transplant medicine. In Israel, the absence of a strong culture of organ donation, an inadequate national system of cadaver organs "capture," and the pressure exerted by angry transplant candidates have contributed to a belief (in Ministry of Health circles) that each patient transplanted abroad is one less angry and demanding client at home. The corruption of South Africa's private hospitals, surgeons, and HMOs was in part the result of the withdrawal of public support for transplant surgery, previously provided under the apartheid regime for white South Africans. The channeling of public funds for primary health care resulted in the privatization and commercialization of tertiary medical care, including transplant surgery. Indeed, if transplants are to happen at all in South Africa today, they must be paid for by private insurance. This paved the way for illicit transplant tourism. One hardly needs to explain why Northeast Brazil became the target of active recruitment of desperate and hungry kidney sellers? Despite President Lula's "Zero Hunger" program, hunger and other raw needs are still commonplace in the slums and rural villas near Recife's international airport. Most young Afro-Brazilian men were ideal candidates for kidney forfeit.

## OPERATION SCALPEL—POLICING THE TRANSATLANTIC KIDNEY SCAM

A kidney purchased from a slum dweller in Recife, from 2003 to 2004, began at $10,000 and rapidly decreased to $6,000 and then to $3,000 when police interrupted an aggressive trafficking scheme that recruited more than 100 kidney patients from Israel, Europe, and the United States; and kidney sellers from the slums of Brazil for illicit transplant transactions that took place in a private Netcare clinic of Durban's premier private medical center, St. Augustine Hospital. Among the Brazilian kidney sellers coaxed to South Africa in 2003 were dozens of undernourished and unemployed men who dreamed of finding a way out of their economic difficulties. When Gaddy Tauber, a lean and mean-looking ex-Israeli Defense Force broker, and his Brazilian side-kick, Captain Ivan, a retired military policeman, set loose rumors of $10,000 to be made in South Africa by parting with a "spare" kidney, a stampede of willing "donors" lined up to sell an "inert" part of themselves they had never thought very much about. The Brazilian sellers hoped they would be able "to see the world," even if it was no more than a "safe house" in Durban where they were kept as virtual prisoners and a shared hospital room at St. Agustine's Hospital where they tossed and turned with the agony of post operative pain. Later the hapless kidney sellers, who were actually paid between $3,000 and $6,000, grieved the loss of the "little thing" (the missing kidney) that constantly announced its absence with a tingling or itching at the site of their ugly wound. "What have I done to myself," Paulo, a house painter in a slum of Recife, asked himself aloud. Today, depressed and disgruntled, the disillusioned kidney sellers of Areas slum in Recife meet among themselves to share their anxieties about their loss of work, reputation, their strengths, and their health.

The trans-Atlantic trafficking scheme was interrupted by the Brazilian Federal Police sting called "Operation Scalpel," which put the key brokers, Gaddy Tauber and Captain Ivan, away in military brigs in Recife where they are serving long sentences (10+ years) for their crimes: fraud, organ selling, and organized crime. Taking a drag on his cigarette during Sunday visiting hours in July 2005, Gaddy was resigned and philosophical. "I broke the law," he told me in his thickly accented Israeli-English. "I deserve to be here. But in my defense I saved many Israeli lives with the kidneys the guys sold of their own free will. Did I torture them? Did I beat them up? No! Did I force them to get up on the operating table? No! They did it to themselves. So I ask: who was the victim of this victimless crime?"

Captain Ivan, housed in a small cell in another military battalion headquarters, denies his involvement in the trafficking scheme. He angrily claims that he was a fall-guy and a minor figure, duped by Gaddy Tauber and betrayed by some of the kidney sellers who, he said, became active brokers and kidney bounty hunters themselves who later turned on him to protect their own skin. As for the South African surgeons and transplant coordinators in Durban who, as Geremias, a Brazilian kidney seller puts it, "took what they wanted from us and then threw us away like garbage," are fee on bail. They are, and I hope nervously, awaiting the medical trial of the century to be held in a South African court. The surgeons and their associates have been charged with three crimes: fraud; contravening the 1983 South African Organs and Tissues Act, which prohibits the buying and selling of human body parts; and "assault to do grievous bodily harm" on the bodies of the vulnerable kidney sellers. The latter charge took the transplant world by surprise.

The trans-Atlantic organ trade triangle that brought together an unlikely group of Israeli and U.S. buyers; Brazilian and Moldovan kidney sellers; South African doctors and transnational brokers from Israel, the United States, Brazil, and South Africa may prove to be the ultimate Achilles heel that can determine the fate of commerce in living peoples' organs and whether it will be judged as something the neoliberal world can live with or as the ultimate form of human exploitation. But one fact is indisputable: it took two countries to the south—Brazil and South Africa—to challenge the power of transplant outlaws and their kidney bounty hunters. And they did so in the name of protecting and defending the vulnerable bodies of the socially disadvantaged.

## THE SOCIAL AND MEDICAL CONSEQUENCES OF SELLING A KIDNEY

Transplant surgeons have disseminated the idea of "risk-free" live donation in the absence of published, longitudinal studies of the effects of nephrectomy *among the urban poor living* anywhere in the world. The few available studies of the effects of nephrectomy on kidney sellers in India[25] and Iran[26] are unambiguous. Even under attempts (as in Iran) to regulate and control systems of "compensated gifting" by the Ministry of Health, the outcomes are devastating. Kidney sellers suffer from chronic pain, unemployment, social isolation and stigma, and severe psychological problems. The evidence of strongly negative sentiments—disappointment, anger, resentment, and even seething hatreds for the doctors and the recipients of their organs—reported by 100 paid kidney donors in Iran strongly suggests that kidney selling there represents a serious social pathology.[27]

Our research and fieldwork among kidney sellers in Moldova, Brazil, and the Philippines, which included diagnostic exams and sonograms, determined that kidney sellers face many postoperative complications and medical problems, including hypertension and kidney insufficiency, without their having access to adequate medical care or medications. Kidney sellers find themselves weakened, sick, and unemployable because they are unable to sustain the demands of heavy agricultural or construction work, the only labor available to men of their skills. Kidney sellers are often

# Israeli Broker in Jail in Brazil

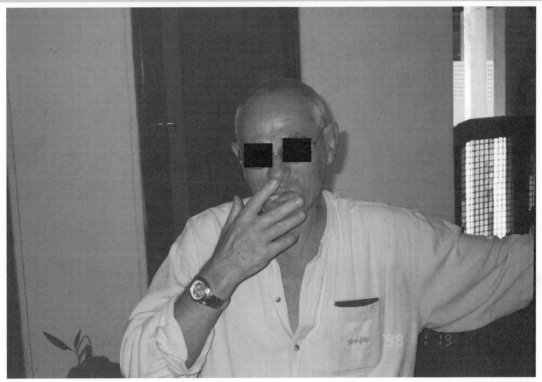

Source: Organs Watch, Nancy Scheper-Hughes

**FIGURE 10-8**

alienated from their families and coworkers, excommunicated from their churches, and excluded from marriage. The children of kidney sellers are ridiculed as "one-kidneys."

Kidney sellers in Moldova had no access to postoperative medical care following their illicit "nephrectomies" (kidney removal) in Turkey, the United States, and Russia. We had to coax young kidney sellers to accept a sonogram at the expense of Organs Watch. Some said they were ashamed to appear in a public clinic, as they had tried to keep the sale a secret. Others said they were afraid of learning negative results from the tests. If medical problems were discovered they would be unable to pay for necessary treatments or medications. Above all, they feared being labeled as "weak" or "disabled" by their employers and coworkers, or as "inadequate" by girlfriends and wives. "No young woman in the village will marry a man with the tell-tale scar of a kidney seller," a village elder in Mingir told us. Sergei said that his mother was the only person who knew the reason for the large, saber-like scar on his abdomen. His young wife believed that he had been injured in a construction accident while he was away in Turkey.

## IS A REGULATED MARKET THE SOLUTION?

*"If a living donor can do without an organ, why shouldn't the donor profit and medical science benefit?"*

Janet Ratcliffe-Richards

From the exclusively market-oriented "supply-and-demand" perspective that is gaining ground among transplant specialists and bioethicists today, the buying and selling of kidneys is viewed as a potential solution to the global scarcity in organs and as a "win-win" situation that benefits both parties.[24] In so doing, however, the human and ethical dilemmas are reduced to a simple problem in management. The problems with this rational solution are many. The arguments for "regulation" are out of touch with the social and medical realities operating in many parts of the world, but especially in second and third world nations. The medical institutions created to "monitor" organs harvesting and distribution are often dysfunctional, corrupt, or compromised by the power of organs markets and the impunity of the organs brokers, and of outlaw surgeons willing to violate the first premise of classical medical bioethics: above all, do no harm.

In 2002, then Philippine Secretary of Health, Manual Dayrit, had two proposals on his desk. The first would create a government-regulated kidney bank (to be called KIDNET) that would allow poor people to sell and deposit a kidney into a virtual "organs bank" that would then make these available to all Philippine citizens who needed them. Dayrit was reluctant to discuss how the Ministry of Health would set a "fair price" for a poor person's kidney, preferring to leave this task to the free market. The medical director of a large private hospital in Manila, where a great many commercial transplants are conducted, agreed:

"Some of our kidney 'donors' are so poor that a sack of rice is sufficient. Others want medical care for their children, and we are quite prepared to provide that for them." The second proposal was a government-sponsored program to grant death-row prisoners (most of them killers) a reprieve in exchange for donating a kidney. Their death sentence would them be replaced by life imprisonment. Those who support this proposal believe that the donor incentives program could end up convincing society that the death penalty is a terrible waste of a healthy body. "Organ donation is a medical equivalent of Catholic Lenten rites of self-flagellation," Professor Leonardo Castro, of the University of the Philippines said in defense of the prisoner organ donation incentives program.

For most bioethicists, the "slippery slope" in transplant medicine begins with the emergence of an unregulated market in organs and tissue sales. But for the critical medical anthropologist, the ethical slippery slope occurs the first time one ailing human looks at another living human and realizes that inside the other body is something capable of prolonging or enhancing his or her life. Dialysis and transplant patients are highly visible, and the media frequently reports their stories. Their pain and suffering are palpable. But although there is empathy—even a kind of surplus empathy—for transplant patients, there is little empathy for the donors. Their suffering is hidden from the general public. Few organ recipients know anything about the impact of the transplant procedure on the donor's body. If the medical and psychological risks, pressures, and constraints on organ donors and their families were more generally known, transplant patients might want to consider opting out of procedures that demand so much of the other.

In the absence of national or international registries of living donors or mandatory reporting laws concerning complications following living donation for the donor/seller, there are no reliable data on the medical/psychological risks and complications suffered by living organ donors anywhere in the world. They are an invisible clinical population, inadequately screened and without follow-up care. In the United States, kidney donors have died, and one has lapsed into a vegetative state as a result of donation. The fact that any living donors have died as a consequence of nephrectomy, no matter how few deaths have been reported, or become disabled and require a kidney transplant at a later date, sounds a cautionary note about living donation and serves as a reminder that nephrectomy (kidney removal) is not a risk-free procedure.[28]

Bioethical arguments supporting the right to sell an organ are based on Euro-American notions of contract and individual "choice." But the social and economic contexts make the "choice" to sell a kidney in an urban slum of Calcutta, or in a Brazilian *favela* or Philippine shantytown, anything but a "free" and "autonomous" one. Consent is problematic with the "the executioner"—whether on death row or at the door of the slum resident—looking over one's shoulder. Putting a market price on body parts—even a fair one—exploits the desperation of the poor, turning suffering into an opportunity. Asking the law to negotiate a fair price for a live human kidney goes against everything that contract theory stands for. When concepts such as individual agency and autonomy are invoked in defending the "right" to sell an organ, anthropologists might suggest that certain "living" things are not alienable or proper candidates for commodification. And the surgical removal of nonrenewable organs is an act in which medical practitioners, given their ethical standards, should not be asked to participate.

When the buyers and sellers are unrelated, the sellers are likely to be extremely poor and trapped in life-threatening environments

where the everyday risks to their survival are legion, including exposure to urban violence, transportation-and work-related accidents, and infectious disease that can compromise their kidney of last resort. And when that spare part fails, kidney sellers often have no access to dialysis, let alone to organ transplant. Although poor people in particular cannot "do without" their "extra" organs, even affluent people might need that "extra" organ as they age.

How can a national government set a price on a healthy human being's body part without compromising essential democratic and ethical principles that guarantee the equal value of all human lives? Any national regulatory system would have to compete with global black markets that establish the value of human organs based on consumer-oriented prejudices, such that in today's kidney market Asian kidneys are worth less than Middle Eastern kidneys and American kidneys worth more than European ones. The circulation of kidneys transcends national borders, and international markets will coexist and compete aggressively with any national, regulated systems. Putting a market price on body parts—even a fair one—exploits the desperation of the poor, turning suffering into an opportunity. And the surgical removal of nonrenewable organs is an act in which medical practitioners, given their ethical standards, should not be asked to participate. Surgeons whose primary responsibility is to provide care should not be advocates of paid self-mutilation, even in the interest of saving lives.

Market-oriented medical ethics creates the semblance of ethical choice (i.e., the right to buy a kidney) in an intrinsically unethical context. Bioethical arguments about the right to sell an organ or other body part are based on cherished notions of contract and individual "choice." But consent is problematic when a desperate seller has no other option left but to sell an organ.

The demand side of the organs scarcity problem also needs to be confronted, especially the expansions of waiting lists to include patients who would previously have been rejected. Liver and kidney failure often originate in public health problems that could be treated more aggressively preventively. Ethical solutions to the chronic scarcity of human organs are not always palatable to the public, but also need to be considered. Foremost among these are systems of educated, informed "presumed consent," in which *all* citizens are assumed to be organs donors at brain death unless they have officially stipulated their refusal beforehand. This practice, which is widespread in parts of Europe, preserves the value of organ transplant as a social good in which no one is included or excluded on the basis of their ability to pay.

## CONCLUSION—A RETURN TO THE GIFT

*"The material needs of my neighbor are my spiritual needs."*
                    Emmanuel Levinas, *Nine Talmudic Readings*
We conclude this ethnographic essay with the reminder of the radical premise entailed in organs sharing which envisioned the body as a gift, meaning also a gift to oneself. In the simplest Kantian or Wittgensteinian formulation, the body and its parts are not proper candidates for commodification and sale because they are inalienable from the body-self. The body provides the grounds of certainty for saying that one has a "self" and an existence at all. Humans both *are* and *have* a body. For those who view the body in more collectivist terms as a gift (whether following Judeo-Christian, Buddhist, or animistic religious traditions, or following a socialist ethic) the body cannot be sole, although it may be re-gifted and re-circulated in acts of generosity and care.

From its origins, transplant surgery presented itself as a complicated problem in gift relations and gift theory, a domain to which sociologists and anthropologists from Marcel Mauss to Levi-Strauss to Pierre Bourdieu have contributed mightily. The spread of new medical technologies and the artificial needs, scarcities, and the new commodities that they demand have produced new forms of social exchange that breach the conventional dichotomy between gifts and commodities and between kin and strangers. Although many individuals have benefited enormously from the ability to get the organs they need, the violence associated with many of these new transactions gives reason to pause. Are we witnessing the development of biosociality or the growth of a widespread biosociopathy?

The division of the world into organ buyers and organ sellers is a medical, social, and moral tragedy of immense and not yet fully recognized proportions.

## NOTES

1. On biological citizenship, see Adriana Petryna, *Life Exposed: Biological Citizens after Chernobyl.* Princeton University Press; 2002; on sexual citizenship, see Nancy Scheper-Hughes, "AIDS and the Social Body," *Social Science & Medicine* 1994;39(7):991–1003.

2. The members of the Bellagio Task Force are: Tsuyoshi Awaya, Professor of Medical Sociology and Law at the School of Law, Tokuyama University, Japan; Bernard Cohen, Director-Eurotransplant Foundation, Leiden, the Netherlands; Abdallah Daar, MD, Chairman, Department of Surgery, Sultan Qaboos University, Muscat, Oman; Sergei Dzemeshkevich, MD, Chief, Department of Cardiosurgery, Russian Academy of Medical Sciences, Moscow; Chun Jean Lee, MD, Professor of Surgery, National Taiwan University Medical Center, Taipei, Taiwan; Robin Monroe, Human Rights Watch/Asia, Wan Chai, Hong Kong; Hernan Reyes, MD, Medical Director, International Committee of the Red Cross, Geneva, Switzerland; Eric Rose, MD, Chairman, Department of Surgery, Columbia College of Physicians & Surgeons, New York City; David Rothman, Professor and Director, Center for the Study of Society and Medicine, Columbia College of Physicians and Surgeons, New York City; Sheila Rothman, Professor, School of Public Health, Columbia University, New York; Nancy Scheper-Hughes, Professor, Anthropology, University of California, Berkeley; Zaki Shapira, MD, Organ Transplant Department, Beilinson Medical Center, Petach Tikva, Israel; Heiner Smit, Deutsche Stiftung Organtransplantation, Neu-Isenberg, Germany; Marina Staiff, MD, Medical coordinator, Prison Detention Activities, International committee of the Red Cross, Geneva, Switzerland.

3. Nancy Scheper-Hughes, 1995. "The Primacy of the Ethical: Towards a Militant Anthropology" *Curr Anthropol* 2002;36(3):409–420; Bourdieu, Pierre. *Pour un Savoir Engage. Le Monde Diplomatique* 2002;(Feb):3.

4. Comaroff J, Comaroff, J eds. *Millennial Capitalism and the Culture of Neoliberalism.* Durham, NC: Duke University Press; 2001.

5. Sassen S. *The Global City: New York, London, Tokyo.* Princeton: Princeton University Press; 1991.

6. The United Network for Organ Sharing (UNOS) allows 5% percent of organ transplants in U.S. transplant centers to be allotted to foreign patients. However, only those centers reporting more than 15% foreign transplant surgery patients are audited.

7. See, for example, the Arabic (as well as Hebrew and Japanese) version of the university's advertisement; HYPERLINK "http://www.umn.edu/transplant/arabic.html" http://www.umn.edu/transplant/arabic.html

8. In São Paulo Hospital, Mariana Ferreira and I encountered Dombe, a Suyá Indian from the forest of Mato Grosso who, to our amazement, faced kidney transplant (including two rejection crises) with remarkable equanimity and calm. See Nancy Scheper-Hughes and Mariana Leal Ferreira, "Domba's Spirit Kidney—Transplant Medicine and Suyá Indian Cosmology," In: Ingstad B, Reynolds S, eds. *Disability in Local and Global Worlds.* Berkeley: University of California Press, 2007.

9. See Marina Jimenez and Nancy Scheper-Hughes, "Doctor Vulture—the Unholy Business of Kidney Commerce," part one of a three-part series in *The National Post* (Toronto). 2002;(March 30):B1, B4–B5.

10. Lobo F, Fangaaniello Maierovitch *W.O Mercado dos Desperados. CartaCapital* 2002;(January 16):30–34.

11. Delmononico F, Arnold R, Scheper-Hughes N, et al. Ethical Incentives—No Payment—For Organ Donation. *N Engl J Med* 2002;346(25): 2002–2005.

12. Taylor JS *Stakes and Kidneys: Why Markets in Human Body Parts are Morally Imperative.* Burlington, Vermont: Ashgate; 2005; Cherry MJ. *Kidney for Sale by Owner.* Washington, DC: Georgetown University Press; 2005.

13. For example, Alan Shewmon, a respected pediatric nephrologist at UCLA, has argued persuasively that on neurological grounds alone, although the brain-dead are incontestably and probably irreversibly dying, they are quite simply not yet dead. Margaret Lock, who has exhaustively explored the topic of breath death, refers to the brain dead as "as good as dead." Alternatively, I call them the "good enough" dead. But the point is that the brain dead are not dead in the more usual "deader than a door nail" sense of the term.

14. Stuart Mill J. Utilitarianism. In: *Ethical Theories: A Book of Readings.* Melden AI, ed. Englewood Cliffs, NJ: Prentice-Hall; 1967:391–434.

15. Bentham J. An introduction to the principles of morals and legislation. In: Melden AI, ed. *Ethical Theories: A Book of Readings.* Englewood Cliffs, NJ: Prentice-Hall; 1967:367–390.

16. Friedlaender M. The right to sell or buy a kidney: Are we failing our patients?" *Lancet* 2002(March 16):359,

17. This is a reference to Primo Levi's description, in his book *The Drowned and the Saved,* of the extent to which inmates of the concentration camps would collaborate with the enemy in order to survive.

18. Bhagwati J. Deconstructing rotten trade. *SAIS Rev* 2002;22(1):39–44.

19. Immanuel Kant. *Universal Natural History.* 1986:186; English edition, translated by Stanley Jaki Edinburgh: Scottish Academic Press Ltd. 1981(Aug).

20. Agamben B, *Homo Sacer*, 2–3, and Hannah Arendt, *The Human Condition.* Chicago: University of Chicago; 1958:12–49, treat the translation from ancient Greek to Church Latin in slightly different ways.

21. Fancis Fukuyama, *Our Postmodern Future.* New York: Farrar, Straus and Giroux; 2002:204.

22. "Offering Money for Organ Donation Ethical, HHS Committee Says," December 3, 2001.

23. Rothman D, et al. The Bellagio Task Force Report on Global Traffic in Human Organs. *Transplant Proc*1997;29:2739–2745.

24. Radcliffe-Richards J, et al. "The case for allowing kidney sales." *Lancet* 1998;352:1951.

25. Goyal M, Mehta R, Schneiderman L, Sehgal A. The economic consequences of selling a kidney in India. *JAMA* 2002;(Oct 2): 288(13):1589–1593.

26. Zangooshi J. Iranian kidney donors: Motivations and relations with recipients. *J Urol* 2001: 165:386–392; Zargooshi J. Quality of life of Iranian kidney donors. *J Urol* 2001(Nov):166(5): 1790–1799.

27. Ibid.

28. The Live Donor Consensus Conference. *JAMA* 2001;284:2919–2926.

# CHAPTER 11

# THE IMPACT OF THE INTERNET ON PAID LEGAL AND ILLEGAL ORGAN DONATION

*W. Ben Vernon, MD*

## HOW THE INTERNET FOUND A ROLE IN LIVING DONOR TRANSPLANTATION

### Forces Contributing to Recipient Demand for Living Donor Transplantation

To fully appreciate the present and future roles of the Internet in facilitating paid legal and illegal living donor organ transplants it is helpful to understand the events of the recent past that have produced the forces favoring living donation. From 1954 to 1964, successful renal transplants required isografts from an identical twin. In the first era of immunosuppression, the relatively less effective combination of prednisone and azathioprine was utilized. Favoring living donation from family members minimized alloantigen mismatch and improved graft survival. This approach was furthered for both living and deceased donor transplants by the rapid evolution of sophisticated histocompatibility techniques.

The discovery of more effective immunosuppressive agents (cyclosporine, tacrolimus, sirolimus, and a host of induction and rejection treatments) has produced a steady improvement in graft and patient survival with a concomitant reduction in the effect of histocompatibility antigen mismatch. Nevertheless, there persists a significant difference in graft survival in favor of living donor recipients. This difference can be summarized by noting that the 5-year graft survival for the least mismatched deceased donor renal transplant recipient (74.2% ± 0.8%) is not as good as for the most mismatched living donor recipient (78.6% ± 1.4%).[1] Through the 1990s laparoscopic recovery of renal allografts as well as pulmonary and hepatic grafts from living donors became safe and routine.[2,3,4]

In 1999, Wolfe et al. were able to demonstrate significant and impressive improvement in the risk of mortality for those who received a first renal transplant compared to those continued to wait for one.[5] Shortly afterwards it was observed that increasing time on dialysis prior to transplant had a negative impact on the results following transplant including acute tubular necrosis, acute cellular rejection, and graft loss.[6] The time waiting on dialysis for a kidney transplant is now the single factor with greatest impact that can be modified to positively influence the outcome of transplantation.[7]

In summary, all those with kidney transplants live longer and better than those who remain on dialysis. The less time on dialysis, the better the results following transplantation. Reduced time to transplant reduces graft loss, acute tubular necrosis,

other complications, and acute cellular rejection after transplant. All living donor kidney recipients have better graft survival than any deceased donor recipient. The only way to avoid a median wait of 38 more months on dialysis (in the US),[8] with its attendant negative impact on results posttransplant, is through living donation.

Together these forces accelerate the demand for living donor transplantation. By 2001 the number of living donors of kidneys for transplantation exceeded the number of deceased donors. Figure 11.1 details the growth in unrelated living donation for kidney transplantation. The steady increase in the number and proportion of unrelated donors demonstrates how patients with end-stage renal disease recognize the forces noted earlier. To understand the forces that drive completely unrelated individuals to use the Internet to become living donors we must explore the current legal climate and mores.

### Distribution of Living Donor Source 1991 to 2004

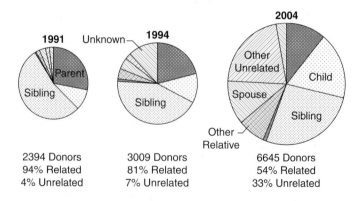

2394 Donors
94% Related
4% Unrelated

3009 Donors
81% Related
7% Unrelated

6645 Donors
54% Related
33% Unrelated

**FIGURE 11.1**

The distribution of living kidney donors has shifted from 1991 to 2004. Spouses and other unrelated donors now provide 33% of all the kidneys transplanted in 2004, compared to only 4% in 1991. The size of the circle is proportional to the total number of living donors at each time. Between "Child" and "Sibling" is a miniscule number of identical twin donors. Between "Sibling" and "Other Relative" is a small number of half-sibling donors.

## Impediments to Sufficient (Living, Traditional) Donors for Transplantation

### Biologic Impediments

The biologic impediments to living donation include blood group incompatibility between donor and recipient, recipient sensitization to donor antigens, the risk of general anesthesia required for organ recovery, pain associated with the recovery operation, immediate postoperative complications associated with organ recovery, and the long-term risk to donor health and longevity. To a great degree the introduction of laparoscopic donor nephrectomy has removed some of the pain and physical inconvenience of donating a kidney.[2] Minimally invasive recovery of the hepatic left lateral segment has similarly contributed to reducing the physical inconvenience of donating a liver graft.[9] There remains significant public concern regarding the transparency with which the transplant community has addressed these immediate physical risks and the risks to the donor's long-term health.[10]

### Psychologic and Social Impediments

The psychologic and social impediments to living donation include distance from and travel to the transplant center, inconvenience of the evaluation, recovery procedure and follow-up, expense, loss of income, and fear of injury to a living person. Recent careful investigation of the financial issues has suggested that, for most living donors, the expense involved is adequately addressed by current practices.[11] Frequently the greatest psychologic impediment to living donation can be the recipient's reluctance to receive such a gift.

### U.S. Legal Impediments

*Uniform Determination of Death Act.* This act arose from the findings of the Harvard Ad Hoc Committee on Irreversible Coma[12] and the President's Commission for the Study of Ethical Problems in Medicine.[13] It was promulgated by the National Conference of Commissioners on Uniform State Laws and passed U.S. Congress in 1982.[14] It provides for the neurologic determination of death, which is the cornerstone for deceased donor organ recovery. Although the ensuing multiple state acts produced a marvelous paradigm transition, they all (to date) require complete cessation of total brain function, including brainstem function. From today's perspective, this may be an excessively cautious requirement.[15]

In the United States, many severely brain injured individuals may not lose all brainstem function, and thus will not meet formal neurologic criteria for death. These individuals can then enter a stable, persistent vegetative state, which is an extremely undesirable outcome associated with excessive expense and family frustration. Avoidance of the persistent vegetative state is thought to be the root cause of "deceleration of treatment" through which severely brain injured individuals progress to uncontrolled cardiovascular collapse in a manner not conducive to organ recovery for transplantation.[16] Alternatively, withdrawal of support from poorly stable individuals with advanced (but not total) brain injury can occur in a process resulting in recovery of some organs ("donation after cardiac death").[17]

The present wide variation of international law surrounding neurologic criteria for death has created the opportunity for "medical tourism" through which a candidate may receive a deceased donor organ in a country with laws more conducive to rapid transplantation. The search engine Google generated 12,500 English references and three sponsored links to the query on "transplant" and "medical tourism." One of the sponsored links provides a highly competitive price for liver transplantation, and another provides information on heart and heart–lung transplantation. Examples from the Web of "medical tourism" sites include http://www.medicaltourinindia.com/medical-treatments-in-india/transplant-surgery/index.html, http://www.clalit.org.il/rabin/Content/Content.asp?CID=73&u=392, and http://en.zoukiishoku.com/.

*Uniform Anatomical Gift Act.* This act was first passed in 1968.[18] It was revised in 1987. This act provides the legal basis for the donation of organs from the deceased. Although the revised act makes clear that a living individual's documented statement to donate has legal priority over the next of kin's wishes, it took over a decade for this to become common practice among organ procurement agencies. Because this act is viewed as a cornerstone of the current organ recovery activities in the United States, it is difficult to recognize it as an impediment to obtaining adequate numbers of organs from deceased donors. For now, it remains a matter of speculation whether a system of presumed consent (in which individuals wishing to not donate organs after death are required to "opt out" in a legally binding manner) could provide more deceased donor organs than our present system.[15, 20]

*National Organ Transplant Act.* This act (NOTA) was first passed in 1984,[21] with multiple amendments since, and modified by ruling of the Secretary of Health and Human Services in 2000.[22] It stems from a concern that access to organs from deceased donors should be equitable from a geographic perspective. The concept was that deceased donors are a national resource. This act is the legal basis for the Organ Procurement and Transplant Network (OPTN), the contract for which is currently held by the United Network for Organ Sharing (UNOS).

The NOTA is the legal basis for the proscription against "valuable consideration" in exchange for organ donation. Section 42 USC 274e {OPTN Act} states, in part:

(a) Prohibition It shall be unlawful for any person to knowingly acquire, receive, or otherwise transfer any human organ for valuable consideration for use in human transplantation if the transfer affects interstate commerce.

(b) Penalties Any person who violates subsection (a) of this section shall be fined not more than $50,000 or imprisoned not more than five years, or both.

(c) Definitions

(2) The term "valuable consideration" does not include the reasonable payments associated with the removal, transportation, implantation, processing, preservation, quality control, and storage of a human organ or the expenses of travel, housing, and lost wages incurred by the donor of a human organ in connection with the donation of the organ.

(3) The term *interstate commerce* has the meaning prescribed for it by section 321(b) of title 21.[23]

As long as this statute remains in force there cannot be compensation in excess of the categories above for organ donation in the United States. It is interesting to speculate whether compensation is permitted if "interstate commerce" is not affected. It remains a matter of speculation whether compensated organ donation could increase the number of living or deceased donor organs available for transplantation.[15,24,25]

Because the initial emphasis of NOTA was on a network for organ procurement and allocation from deceased donors, an opportunity was missed for promotion of living donation transplants. The final ruling by the Secretary of Health and Human Services, the evolution of the OPTN, and the terms of contract renewal with UNOS have introduced some regulation of living donor transplants. However, a public perception remains that living donor transplants are poorly regulated, especially with respect to donor safety.[10]

### *United Nations Guidance Concerning Human Trafficking for Organ Transplantation.*

The Protocol to Prevent, Suppress and Punish Trafficking in Persons, Especially Women and Children, supplementing the United Nations Convention against Transnational Organized Crime was adopted by resolution A/RES/55/25 of 15 November 2000 at the 55th session of the General Assembly of the United Nations.[26] The United States signed the protocol December 13, 2000, and it was subsequently ratified. The protocol states:

> "Trafficking in persons" shall mean the recruitment, transportation, transfer, harbouring or receipt of persons, by means of the threat or use of force or other forms of coercion, of abduction, of fraud, of deception, of the abuse of power or of a position of vulnerability or of the giving or receiving of payments or benefits to achieve the consent of a person having control over another person, for the purpose of exploitation. Exploitation shall include, at a minimum, the exploitation of the prostitution of others or other forms of sexual exploitation, forced labour or services, slavery or practices similar to slavery, servitude or the removal of organs; . . .[27]

The most recent report from the United Nations, April 2006,[28] cites no instances of trafficking for organ transplantation. Human trafficking for sexual exploitation and forced labor remain far more common worldwide and are thought to be underreported. Trafficking for organ transplantation is probably underreported, as well. These United Nations resolutions and protocols require enforcement through national legislation and international law enforcement. The variety of national legislation and procedures surrounding organ donation and recovery provide ample opportunity for trafficking for organ transplantation.[29, 30] For example, a Web search engine generated 22,700 references in the prior year for the terms "executed," "prisoner," "China," and "organ transplant." A search of the terms "human," "trafficking," and "organ transplant" yielded 32,600 references in the past year.

The reader who imagines that Internet promotion of transplant medical tourism is limited to Web sites outside the United States should peruse www.transplantcoordinator.com and consider whether the information presented fits within our present professional framework for ethical organ transplantation. Does this site not condone or promote human trafficking? "Compensated donation" of organs for transplantation from living donors may occur in Brazil, some European states, and Asia.[31] What should be our response to those who travel to obtain a resource proscribed by law in the United States when they present for care at home?

### Current Impact of Internet on Living Donor Transplantation

To the extent that the length of time waiting for deceased donor transplantation varies from nation to nation, to the extent that this information is readily available through the Internet, and to the extent that the Internet has created a competitive, commercial, international market for transplant services, the World Wide Web has reduced the need for living organ donation. It has accomplished this with concomitant complexities. Medical tourism for deceased donor transplants reduces the transplantation of the local waiting candidates. In some transplant centers living donors for these operations may simply be paid outright for their body part. In other centers the organ may come from an executed prisoner. Although these procedures may be perfectly legal in the lands they are performed, they do not contribute to the global advance of human rights advocated by the health professions.

There exists today a single U.S. Internet site devoted to finding living donors for transplant candidates, "Matching Donors.com."[32] The idea grew from an Internet employment matching Web site and an appreciation of the mortality risk of those candidates awaiting kidney transplant on the OPTN waitlist. The organization functions under U.S. IRS code 501(c)(3) as a nonprofit corporation devoted to facilitating recognition of appropriate donor and recipient pairs. From October 2004 to May 2006, 23 kidney transplants have come to fruition throughout the United States through matchingdonors.com. Potential donors for bone marrow and liver (but not lung) transplants have registered at the site, though none of these organs have yet been transplanted through the auspices of matchingdonors.com. To date 3,000 individuals have submitted information regarding their desire to be living donors. There are presently 160 active potential recipients, for a ratio of about 20 potential donors for each potential recipient.

It is insightful to review the operation of the website, as it provides demonstration of how the impediments above are addressed in practice. Potential donors and recipients register and enter a profile (and optional photo) into the secure server. Potential donors can then review potential recipient profiles (but not vice versa). Donors may then send a private message to a secure server, and an email message is sent to the potential recipient to check their mail on the secure server. Once a relationship between potential donor and recipient has been established the further evaluation proceeds through the auspices of the potential recipient's transplant center.[33]

A monthly registration fee is charged of the recipient candidates at this site. The collected fees are used strictly for maintenance of the Web site and its operation. The fee can be waived for candidates of reduced means. Operation of this site presently is heavily subsidized by other commercial endeavors. The plan for future funding of this site is to achieve financial independence through monetary contributions with a goal that all candidates can maintain registration without fees.[34]

There is a website, www.lifesharers.com, which promotes registration of organ donors with the intent that deceased donor organs recovered from LifeSharers members are directed to recipients registered with LifeSharers. In 1996 the UNOS Board of Directors recommended that the Anatomical Gifts Act be amended so that directed donation be limited to circumstances that do not discriminate against candidates based on class membership (such as race or club membership). However, the exact forms of permitted directed donation are spelled out in the individual state anatomical gifts acts.

In some states directed donation is expressly prohibited. In others it is permitted, even to class members in some circumstances.

LifeSharers has not yet facilitated a transplant because, to date, none of its members has died in circumstances permitting organ recovery. Since its inception 4 years ago, 4,531 donors have been enrolled. LifeSharers is a 501(c)(3) nonprofit organization, staffed by volunteers. The organization relies on charitable contributions to fund its operating expenses.[35]

## LIVING ORGAN DONATION: GIFT OR ECONOMY?

### The Gift: Contributing to a Need

From the first perspective, the organ removed from a living donor is a gift. In this model the donor becomes aware of the recipient's need for an organ transplant and becomes aware that she or he has the physical and emotional capability of providing the needed organ. All that is left is finding the team to physically help with delivery of the gift. As with other true gifts, the living donor anticipates no physical return of the gift itself or repayment in any form. Those donors best at giving know how and when to give up control over the gift. For many, the gift is made before they present for evaluation as living donors. Those recipients best at receiving know there is no need to try to recompense such a gift.

Is there really no return in living donation for the donor? In those transplants involving living donation between family members, especially spouses, there may be great (intangible) rewards by improving the recipient's quality of life and recovering time from medical treatments. Living donation may be the route to increased self-esteem, self-worth, and fulfillment for the donor. Are the benefits of seeing someone you love do better really priceless?

### The Commodity: Supply Versus Demand

In the other perspective, the organ removed from a living donor is a commodity. In the Western, capitalist world the forces of the market economy press so hard on every aspect of daily life that surely living donation of an organ for transplant must be some form of economy. Maybe living donation is the cost of keeping a family intact, or what it takes to secure some advantageous real estate transaction. U.S. health-care cost accounting and the transplant literature encourage this perspective to some degree. Recent contributions have included measurements of financial break-even point, cost per quality adjusted life year gained, and cost effectiveness of paid living donors.[36] Even legislation related to deceased donation (see Uniform Anatomic Gift Act, earlier) has been written in terms of property law and property donation.

So in this market economy, why does a completely unrelated individual choose to undergo surgery to donate an organ to someone they choose not to know, as happens for the altruistic donor to a candidate on the waiting list? Are we really so mercenary as to completely miss the altruistic side of living donation?

### The Implications of Perspective on Living Donation

Is the organ removed from a living donor a gift or a commodity? This is, perhaps, the greatest remaining mystery of living donor transplant today. For one transplant more economic factors may be at play. For the next transplant, more altruistic factors may prevail. This is a complex world, and a patient-centered response must first recognize these contradictory perceptions coexist and provide for the emotional, psychological support of both donor and recipient. This is especially true when each has the other model in mind. For this reason alone, our transplant center has found routine psychological evaluation of both the living donor and the recipient to be insightful and invaluable in anticipating and managing difficulties posttransplant.

Is one perspective superior logically or ethically to the other? These discordant models of living donation are both correct. Together they provide a more robust appreciation of the living donor transplant environment. The center that is confident that none of its living donors has ever received valuable consideration for their gift is probably unaware of the myriad ways that consideration can occur. And the center that is confident that there is always something in it for everyone is probably unaware of the myriad inexplicable events occurring everyday.

## FUTURE ROLES OF THE INTERNET IN ORGAN DONATION

### Recipient Selection of Transplant Programs

Those who are facile with the biannual Internet publication of the United States' Scientific Registry of Transplant Recipients (SRTR)[37] recognize the powerful comparison-shopping guide that it represents. For those candidates able to consider alternative transplant centers why not seek the center with the best results? The Internet also provides virtually invisible limitless free counsel through innumerable chat rooms, support groups, and list servers. It appears that every transplant center and program in the United States has a presence on the Internet—frequently in a leading role for its hospital.

Now imagine the 12,500 Web pages cited previously generated by a search of "medical tourism" and "transplant." Of course, the typical site boasts of results equal to those in America or Europe achieved by the team of physicians trained abroad. To a transplant candidate interested in the reported outcomes first, and then the projected cost of the procedure, the enormously sophisticated data collection and analysis provided by the SRTR is a distant issue. That this should have been a greater concern can become evident when complications develop sometime after the recipient's return home to their principal nephrologist and a different transplant team.

The Internet has already forced a broad paradigm transition in medicine. Whereas a competent physician must stay abreast of as many topics as feasible, the patient needs to be competent in just one problem, or a few. The medical information readily available through the Internet empowers a patient, in the matter of a few hours, to become his own worst health advocate. In the United States today, the health-care system is progressing toward increased patient responsibility in benefit selection, choice of care providers, and financial coverage. As a profession, health-care providers can be hamstrung by an asymmetric ethical obligation to attend any patient who requests treatment. As providers of health care, transplant professionals must learn to politely, but intently insist on a symmetric, mutual responsibility in mapping a patient's care plan. For instance, it may be ethically appropriate, it may be ethically obligatory, to refuse to care for those who have received a transplant from an executed prisoner. What should be done for the recipient who doesn't know the source of their organ?

## Matching Living Donors to Recipients

Into the foreseeable future the demand for transplantable organs will continue to exceed the supply from deceased donors. Living donation affords the opportunity to optimize many of the variables that influence transplant outcome. Grafts from living donors continue to perform better than those from deceased donors. Not all recipients can find appropriate grafts from the limited, potential living donors available through family and traditional acquaintances. From the earliest days of deceased donor transplantation, it was recognized that the access to the largest possible donor pool is required to find appropriate grafts for some candidates.

In these circumstances living donation from Internet acquaintances will continue to flourish. The Internet affords much broader dissemination of the transplant candidate's situation and the potential donor's opportunity to meet unique needs. The Internet also provides both a forum to search for a "needle in the haystack" and timely and private opportunities—often over immense distances—to develop the personal relationship required by some for ethical living donor transplantation.

## Recognition and Reduction of Illegal Activity in Organ Transplantation

The very features that have permitted the Internet entry into living donor transplantation have a darker side. Broad access to information in a private environment provides the opportunity to enter into illegal, extralegal, and unethical arrangements that can be all but impossible for authorities to discover. The existing limited enforcement and regulation of Internet activity is presently overwhelmed by issues much greater than getting some patients off dialysis.

So, several new responsibilities fall squarely on our profession. Those centers that choose to recover organs from living donors found through the Internet are obliged to meet the highest standards in screening for potentially illegal or unethical activities. Transplant professionals must organize, develop, support, and maintain systems that search for illegal and unethical practices fostered by the Internet. Transplant professionals must work together to eliminate illegal and unethical use of the Internet in transplantation. This will require both maximal cooperation of those centers adhering to the standards and complete professional ostracism of those individuals and centers that cannot.

These responsibilities cannot wait for Internet policing to catch up with the volume of activity. Moreover, acceptance of these responsibilities will lead the transplant profession to higher moral ground. "Medical tourism"—the least of the sins noted above—is nothing but exploitation: it is exploitation of the living donor if paid, exploitation and subversion of the host nation's organ procurement and allocation system if it results in quicker transplantation from a deceased donor than at home, and exploitation of the home nation's health-care professionals who will be called upon to manage the recipient posttransplant for years to come. Yet "medical tourism" ("medical colonialism"?) exists only because the interface between medicine, law, and culture is different in different lands. The world would recognize a significant improvement in human rights everywhere were transplant professionals to advocate seriously for uniform international standards of consent, recovery, allocation, donor compensation (living and deceased), recovery from vulnerable populations (eg, children and prisoners), and mutually responsible posttransplant care.

Brighter ethical times for living donor transplantation lie ahead, and the Internet—the World Wide Web—will be one of the resources we all use to get there.

## References

1. U.S. Department of Health and Human Services. 2005 *Annual Report of the U.S. Organ Procurement and Transplantation Network and the Scientific Registry of Transplant Recipients: Transplant Data 1995-2004.* Rockville, MD: Health Resources and Services Administration, Healthcare Systems Bureau, Division of Transplantation. http://www.hrsa.gov/. Accessed April 15, 2006.
2. Ratner LE, Montgomery RA, Kavoussi LR. Laparoscopic live donor nephrectomy. A review of the first 5 years. *Urol Clinic of N Am* 2001;28:709–719.
3. Liu LU, Schiano TD. Adult live donor liver transplantation. *Clin Liver Dis* 2005;9:767–786.
4. Wells WJ, Barr ML. The ethics of living donor lung transplantation. *Thoracic Surg Clin* 2005;15:519–525.
5. Wolfe RA, Ashby VB, Milford EL, et al. Comparison of mortality in all patients on dialysis, patients on dialysis awaiting transplantation, and recipients of a first cadaveric transplant. *N Engl J Med* 1999;341:1725–1730.
6. Mange KC, Joffe MM, Feldman HI. Effect of the use or nonuse of long-term dialysis on the subsequent survival of renal transplants from living donors. *N Engl J Med* 2001;341:726–731.
7. Meier-Kreische HU, Kaplan B. Waiting time on dialysis as the strongest modifiable risk factor for renal transplant outcomes: A paired donor kidney analysis. *Transplantation* 2002;74:1377–1381.
8. Scientific Registry of Transplant Recipients. National Summaries for Select Tables by Center, Table 06: Time to Transplant for Waitlist Patients. Available at: http://www.ustransplant.org/csr/current/nats.aspx. Accessed April 26, 2006.
9. Cherqui D, Soubrane O, Husson E, et al. Laparoscopic living donor hepatectomy for liver transplantation in children. *Lancet* 2002;359:392–396.
10. CNN.com. Advocates fight for transplant rules, registry. Available at: http://www.cnn.com/2006/HEALTH/05/31/transplant.advocacy/index.html. Accessed June 6, 2006.
11. Wolters HH, Heidenreich S, Senninger N. Living donor kidney transplantation: chance for the recipient—financial risk for the donor? *Transplant Proc* 2003;35:2091–2092.
12. A definition of irreversible coma: Report of the Ad Hoc Committee of the Harvard Medical School to Examine the Definition of Brain Death. *JAMA* 1968;205:337–340.
13. President's Commission for the Study of Ethical Problems in Medicine and Biomedical and Behavioral Research. Defining death: A report on the medical, legal and ethical issues in the determination of death. Washington, DC: Government Printing Office, 1981.
14. Uniform Determination of Death Act, 12 Uniform Laws Annotated (U.L.A.) 589 (West 1993 and West Supp. 1997).
15. President's Council on Bioethics, Transcripts of April 20, 2006. Session 1: Organ Procurement and Transplantation. Available at: http://www.bioethics.gov/transcripts/april06/session1.html. Accessed June 3, 2006.
16. Hasz, RD. System changes: Successful OPO initiatives. Available at: http://www.iom.edu/Object.File/Master/27/947/RickHasz.pdf. Accessed June 3, 2006.
17. Bernat JL, D'Alessandro AM, Port FK, et al. Report of a National Conference on Donation after cardiac death. *Am J Transplant.* 2006;6:281–291.
18. Uniform Anatomical Gift Act, 8A U.L.A. 9 (1968)
19. Uniform Anatomical Gift Act, 8A U.L.A. (96 Supp.) 2 (1987)
20. Janssen A, Gevers S. Explicit or presumed consent and organ donation post-mortem: Does it matter? *Med Law* 2005;24:575–583.
21. 42 USC 273, 274 (2001).
22. 42 CFR Part 121 (1999).
23. 42 USC 274e.

24. Bryce CL, Siminoff LA, Ubel PA, et al. Do incentives matter? Providing benefits to families of organ donors. *Am J Transplant* 2005;5:2999–3008.

25. Haddow G. "Because you're worth it?" The taking and selling of transplantable organs. *J Med Ethics* 2006;32:324–328.

26. Resolution of the United Nations General Assembly, A/Res/55/25. January 8, 2001. http://daccessdds.un.org/doc/UNDOC/GEN/N00/560/89/PDF/N0056089.pdf?OpenElement. Accessed April 26, 2006.

27. Annex II, General Provisions Article 3, paragraph (a) of the Protocol to Prevent, Suppress and Punish Trafficking in Persons, especially Women and Children, which supplements the United Nations Convention against Transnational Organized Crime. Idem, 32.

28. United Nations Office on Drugs and Crime (UNODC). Trafficking in Persons, Global Patterns, April 2006. http://www.unodc.org/pdf/traffickinginpersons_report_2006-04.pdf. Accesed May 15, 2006.

29. Deutsche Gesellschaft für Technische Zusammenarbeit (GTZ) GmbH. Coerceion in the kidney trade? A background study on trafficking in human organs worldwide; Sector Project against Trafficking in Women. April, 2004. http://www.gtz.de/de/dokumente/en-svbf-organ-trafficking-e.pdf. Accessed June 3, 2006.

30. Model UN, University of Chicago. Topic Area B: Review and Regulation of Human Organ Trafficking. Available at: http://www.munuc.org/pdfs/ECOSOC_B.pdf. Accessed June 3, 2006.

31. Organs Watch. Activity related to the organ trade around the world. http://sunsite3.berkeley.edu/biotech/organswatch/pages/hot_spots.html. Accessed June 3, 2006.

32. MatchingDonors.com. Homepage. http://www.matchingdonors.com. Accessed April 26, 2006.

33. Mr Robert Volosevich, Vice President, MatchingDonors.com. May 3,2006.

34. Paul Dooley, personal communication. June 7, 2006.

35. Dave Undis, Executive Director, LifeSharers, email communication. June 7, 2006.

36. Matas AJ, Schnitzler M. Payment for living donor (vendor) kidneys: A cost-effectiveness analysis. *Am J Transplant* 2004;4:216–221.

37. Scientific Registry of Transplant Recipients. http://www.ustransplant.org/. Accessed June 3, 2006.

PART III

# ORGAN-SPECIFIC ASPECTS OF LIVING DONOR ABDOMINAL ORGAN TRANSPLANTATION

## SECTION I
## KIDNEY TRANSPLANTATION

# CHAPTER 12

# KIDNEY TRANSPLANTATION: PERSONAL REFLECTIONS

*John S. Najarian, MD*

My interest in and advocacy for living donor kidney transplants began in 1963 when I performed my first clinical kidney transplant in San Francisco. It was obvious from the first identical twin transplant (in Boston, in 1954)[1] that living donor transplants were likely to be more convenient and successful than deceased donor transplants. This continued to be true even for nonidentical twin transplants, with Imuran and prednisone as the only immunosuppressive agents.

From the outset, immediate and late results were more favorable with living related donor transplants. Moreover, the use of organs from deceased donors initially presented a difficult logistical challenge. For the most part, deceased donor transplants in the early days required that the recipient be in the university hospital awaiting the possible availability of an organ, which usually came from a separate hospital or trauma unit and had to be transported. This logistical challenge fueled our enthusiasm for attempting to persuade recipients to find living related donors whenever possible.

In 1966, after Dr. Folkert Belzer had completed his residency at the University of Oregon and was appointed a junior staff surgeon at the University of California, San Francisco (UCSF), I was asked by our chairman, Dr. Bert Dunphy, to find a suitable research project for Dr. Belzer. His primary interest was in vascular surgery; he had virtually no training in immunology. I suggested that his project in our transplantation laboratory could be to explore the possibilities of developing a technique for preserving kidneys from deceased donors. Short-term preservation would allow prospective recipients to remain at home until a deceased donor kidney became available. Furthermore, adequate time would be provided pretransplant for appropriate tissue typing of the donor kidney.

Dr. Belzer pursued this investigation in our laboratory. By serendipity, he eventually came up with a solution that would allow short-term preservation of a kidney for transplantation. One afternoon, after he had bled a series of dogs to obtain plasma for his kidney perfusion experiments, he was unable to use the plasma immediately and instead placed it in a refrigerator overnight. The next morning, he found that a layer of flocculation had formed in the plasma, which turned out to consist of lipids. He then filtered the plasma to remove the flocculent layer, so that the resultant clear plasma could be used for kidney perfusion. This "cryoprecipitated" plasma readily perfused the kidney without obstruction. In the past, perfusion of freshly drawn, unaltered plasma through the kidney had invariably resulted in vascular obstruction in the cold kidneys. Subsequently, he developed a pumping mechanism, thereby establishing perfusion preservation. This research (done in 1966) was published in the *Lancet* in 1967.[2]

Shortly thereafter, Dr. Jeffrey Collins[3] of the University of California, Los Angeles (UCLA) developed a perfusion solution now known as "Collins solution" that could be used to preserve kidneys for 12 hours at 0°C; eventually, it permitted cold storage of kidneys for up to 2 days. With kidneys that could be stored for 12 or more hours, simple transportation from one institution to another was now possible. Thanks to the Belzer technique and the Collins solution, the logistical difficulties of deceased donor kidney transplantation were primarily overcome. However, living related kidneys, when available, still remained our first choice.

On arriving at the University of Minnesota in 1967, I was pleasantly surprised to find that strong family ties in that state meant that a number of family members would frequently come forward as a possible kidney donor for a loved one in renal failure. In the Minnesota transplant program, living donation quickly increased to represent over 65% of our donors. It has remained at well over 50% ever since.

Early in the 1970s, we began transplanting younger and younger children. After attempting four kidney transplants in children under the age of 1, using deceased infant donors to obtain an appropriate size match, we unfortunately observed early rejection. All four kidney grafts were lost. It soon became apparent that such young infants possessed protective antibodies that resulted in rejection, despite our immunosuppression, which at that time included Imuran, prednisone, and Minnesota antilymphocyte globulin (MALG). Thus, we turned our attention to living related donors, whose kidney would present a lesser immunologic challenge to the recipient. Of course, only adults (such as parents or grandparents) could possibly be donors. Thus, it was important to develop surgical and metabolic techniques for transplanting these large adult kidneys into small infants. Once we did so, we began transplanting adult kidneys (typically from parents or grandparents) into infants, resulting in a very successful program in pediatric kidney transplantation.[4] We have now performed kidney transplants in about 900 children, including 50 under the age of 1 and more than 250 under the age of 2: living donors have been used in 80% of these transplants.

Currently, the United Network for Organ Sharing (UNOS) reports[5] only a slight increase in available deceased donors: from 10,000 in 1988 to 15,000 in 2002. The solid-organ transplant waiting list, however, grew from 10,000 in 1988 to almost 90,000 in 2002. Clearly, we must reexamine other sources of organs. For the same period, the use of living donors grew from 2,000 in 1988 to more than 6,000 in 2002; living donors now represent 50% of all donors. Kidney graft survival in terms of half-life (T1/2) reflects the advantage of living donors: T1/2 is now 40 years with a 3-haplotype identical sibling donor, 16 years with a 1-haplotype sibling donor, and more than 16 years with a living unrelated donor. In contrast, T1/2 is now only 10 years with a deceased donor. At Minnesota, in addition to our frequent use of living related donors, we have also increased our use of living unrelated donors (usually a spouse, distant family relative, friend, or fellow church member).

Thus, the primary increase in donor availability recently has come from the use of living unrelated donors. In addition, a novel intervention that we have used since 1997 is nondirected organ donation.[6] Nondirected organs come from individuals who want to donate a kidney to a pool (not directing it to any known individual or to any specific gender, race, or religion). We have now performed 30 nondirected living donor kidney transplants.

All of our living donors are instructed about the possible medical benefit to themselves of the donor evaluation: the screening process they undergo may yield previously unrecognized problems. In our own experience, the donor screening has uncovered cases of unsuspected diabetes, hypertension, abnormal renal function, cardiovascular disease, and six malignancies (which were all removed in curative resections). In addition, donation confers psychological benefits.

However, living donation also carries possible risks. At the present time in our own series, as well as in others, the mortality rate for living kidney donors is 0.03%; morbidity, 0.2%.[7] Most of the postoperative complications are minor and transient. In addition, we have studied the long-term results of having a nephrectomy. Studies in the 1960s, primarily in the Danish literature,[8] showed that the 25-year survival curve of individuals with one kidney was equivalent to that of age-matched controls with two kidneys. Many studies since then have also determined that there is no adverse impact, even 10 to 20 years after kidney donation. In our own studies,[9] we find no difference in renal function, in blood pressure, or in the percentage of individuals with proteinuria.

Finally, the most important aspect of living donor transplants is to make absolutely every effort to ensure that the donor is in optimal physical condition. We do not accept a donor who has an underlying adverse physical condition or who is on medications for hypertension or for any other reason. If these high standards are met, then a successful living donor program can be accomplished.

Living donors almost always experience a boost in self-esteem, a heightened quality of life, and an increased sense of well-being: in our surveys,[10] 96% felt that donation was a positive experience.

Given the operative mortality rate of 0.03%, low postoperative morbidity rate of 0.2%, and enhanced quality of life, we conclude that living donation (whether related or not) appears to be the best possible source of organs at the present time. Having said that, I just returned from Spain, whose deceased donor program is very successful, but whose living donor program unfortunately accounts for fewer than 10% of their total kidney transplants. I am pleased to add that, little by little, most of Europe is coming around to living donor transplants, as did most of the Scandinavian countries early on.

## References

1. Murray JE, Merrill JP, Harrison JH. Kidney transplantation between seven pairs of identical twins. *Annal Surg* 1958;148:343.
2. Belzer FO, Ashby BS, Dunphy JE. 24-hour and 72-hour preservation of canine kidneys. *Lancet* 1967;2:536–539.
3. Collins GM, Bravo-Sugarman M, Tersaki PI. Kidney preservation for transplantation. *Lancet* 1969;1:1219.
4. DeShazo CV, Simmons RL, Bernstein DM, et al. Results of renal transplantation in 100 children. *Surgery* 1974;75:3:461–468.
5. Cecka MJ, Terasaki PI. *Clinical Transplants 2003;* UCLA Immunogenetics Center, Los Angeles, CA.
6. Jacobs C, Roman D, Garvey C, et al. Twenty-two non-directed kidney donors: An update on a single center's experience. *Am J Transplantat* 2004;4:1110–1116.
7. Bia MJ, et al. Evaluation of living renal donors. *Transplantation* 1995;60:322–327.
8. Anderson B, et al. *Scand J Uroly Nephrol* 1968;2:91–94.
9. Kasiske BL, Ma JZ, Louis TA, Swan SK. Long-term effects of reduced renal mass in humans. *Kidney Int* 1995;48:814–819.
10. Johnson EM, Anderson JK, Jacobs C, et al. Long-term follow-up of living kidney donors: quality of life after kidney donation. *Transplantation* 1999;67(5):717–721.

# HISTORY OF LIVING DONOR KIDNEY TRANSPLANTATION

*Luis H. Toledo-Pereyra, MD, Alexander Horacio Toledo, MD*

Many medical advances occurred in 1954 in the United States, but none was more prominent than the successful living donor (LD) kidney transplant performed at the Peter Bent Brigham Hospital under the direction of Joseph Murray. The operation was performed with the strong support of the hospital administration and the leaders of the medical and surgical staff. The twin Herrick brothers accepted all known risks and consented to the pioneering surgery.

## DECEMBER 23, 1954

By 9:53 AM. the morning of that historic operation, Ronald Herrick's kidney had been removed; it waited in a basin wrapped in a cold, wet towel.[1] Hartwell Harrison, who was responsible for the donor side, knew perfectly well that the kidney without a blood supply could not tolerate being outside of the body for too long. Down the corridor, Ronald's identical twin brother, Richard, was being prepared to receive the kidney that was being maintained in the basin. Francis Moore, the chief of surgery, carried the kidney to the recipient room. Outside, nephrologist John Merrill paced the halls. In 1 hour 22 minutes, Ronald's kidney was breathing again. Murray, on the recipient side, carefully connected all the blood vessels. Blood circulated in its regular channels through the kidney by 11:15 AM.[1] The pale kidney's color turned pink and urine began to trickle from the ureter. It appeared the kidney was unmistakably functioning! A living kidney had been suspended out of the body for more than 60 minutes and returned to life, with intense blood circulation and large urinary output.

For the first time in history, a healthy monozygotic twin had successfully donated a healthy living organ to his twin brother with severely diseased and irreparable kidneys. A year before, in 1953, Michon et al.[2] had performed an LD kidney transplant, but with limited success. Two years before Michon, Kuss et al.,[3] Dubost et al.,[4] and Servelle et al.[5] had pursued kidney transplants, but with poor results. Even though some of these early groups struggled in their initial efforts, we still marvel at the bold and creative process required to conceptualize an organ transplant. Who conceived this kind of operation? How did the LD reach this pinnacle of altruism? Where did this idea come from? These were just a few questions swirling in the infancy of the modern field of organ transplantation. That 1954 milestone had been preceded by months of solid experimental work and failed attempts not only by Kuss[3] but also by other French surgeons.[2,4,5]

The results of the Herrick brothers' surgery were eagerly awaited. Surgeons and internists continuously checked the urinary output and blood work at Richard Herrick's bedside. They all took turns reaffirming that the transplanted kidney was effortlessly functioning. No evidence of infection or rejection was seen at any point. Control of uremia was at hand. Technically, this kind of surgery had been accomplished without any problems.[6–26] Now, the challenge was to repeat the same results in other transplants—not an optimistic prospect, because it was unlikely another set of identical twins were in need of a kidney transplant. What was next then?

## AFTER DECEMBER 23, 1954

Surprisingly enough, Murray et al. *did* find more identical twins with renal failure, one to two sets every year.[1,20,21,27] Success was reached every time. The critical question became how to prevent rejection and obtain some success when doing this operation between nonidentical twins.[1,22,28] To overcome the genetic dissimilarity, surgeons began using total body irradiation, learned from the experiments of John Mannick in Cooperstown, New York.[1,10,22,29] Of several non-identical-twin recipients, only one, John Riteris, received a kidney graft that worked, thanks to his fraternal twin.[1] In spite of Riteris's encouraging results, he was only one patient. New approaches needed to be intensively pursued.

In 1959, 6-mercaptopurine became an option for kidney transplants.[25,26,30,31] Murray et al., the year before, had used Thio-TEPA in rabbits receiving kidney transplants.[32] By 1960, Calne[25] and Zukowski[26] had used 6-mercaptopurine with success in dog kidney allografts. About this time, Calne, Alexandre, and Murray were testing other compounds, at Brigham Surgical Research Laboratories, obtained from Hitchings and Elion of Burroughs Wellcome Laboratories.[31] This era was one of great excitement and optimism: new pharmacologic solutions to the, thus far, overwhelming and unconquerable problem of rejection seemed ultimately attainable. Through these studies, an imidazole derivative of 6-mercaptopurine, BW-322, demonstrated the best therapeutic index. Known as azathioprine or Imuran, it would be used for decades to come in clinical organ transplants.

In March 1961, the first unrelated donor renal transplant recipient received Imuran under the surgical leadership of Murray et al. Good early results for up to 1 month were seen, until the patient died of the drug's toxic effects.[1,22,33–35] Another patient followed a similar course, but the third patient in April 1962 reached long-term success.[22]

## WELL BEYOND DECEMBER 23, 1954

Encouraged by the superb initial results of Murray and his Brigham team after their extraordinary 1954 success, other surgeons, physicians, and researchers dove into the clinical transplant arena and intensified their efforts. Among them were Küss, Hamburger, and many other French transplant leaders who had performed the surgical procedure before but with less success;[1–8] Calne, Shackman, and Woodruff from the United Kingdom;[25,31,36–38] and Hume and Goodwin from the United States.[18,39,40] All of these groups moved the emerging field of transplantation forward during the 1960s.[1,10,25,31,36–40]

On March 27, 1962, another important figure emerged: Thomas Starzl, from the University of Colorado. With painstaking detail, he began a significant series of 83 kidney transplants in humans.[41] All of these transplants used LDs except for 3 deceased donor (DD) transplants and 6 xenograft transplants. All of them were done in a short period of less than 2 years. In 1964, Starzl published his unique experience in the first extensive book on clinical and practical transplants in the United States, *Experience in Renal Transplantation*.[41] In it, he clearly outlined extraordinary findings pertaining to the surgical technique, selection of candidates, evaluation of donors, postoperative care, immunosuppressive therapy, reversal of rejection, presence of complications, immunologic studies, and pathologic responses. This unprecedented book was the fundamental basis for anyone who wanted to organize and develop a new transplant program in the United States or abroad. From 1962 to 1964, the University of Colorado transplant program was the most active in the world. It served as a Mecca where new and established transplant surgeons would learn new skills, refer patients, and seek sage and practical advice.

In the early months of 1963, few transplant programs were active in the United States. Only Boston (Brigham), Richmond (Medical College of Virginia), and Denver (University of Colorado) were consistently pursuing kidney transplantation with dedicated interest.[1,8,22,41] But in a matter of months, many other institutions began their efforts at establishing kidney transplantation. The example had been set in terms of the specialized surgical technique, the selection of candidates, the management of immunosuppression, and in some instances, the prevention or treatment of rejection. The most important sources for kidneys remained related LDs. DD transplantation was awaiting the passage of brain death legislation, beginning in the United States in 1968 and continuing until 1972. In Europe, similar laws were incorporated along the same timeline.

## MID-1960s

By the mid-1960s, related LD kidney transplantation was fairly well established. Immunosuppression consisted of Imuran and prednisone, as popularized by the pioneering efforts of Starzl in his 1962–1964 series.[41] Paul Terasaki, noted tissue-typing expert, used new and advanced histocompatibility testing to help select kidney donors for 32 recipients in Starzl's Colorado series[42] in 1964—a time when others were searching to improve the immunosuppressive methods. Franksson from Stockholm[43] introduced thoracic duct drainage for eliminating lymphocytes as a unique immunosuppressive alternative in humans. Two years later, in 1966, Starzl et al.[44] used, for the first time, antilymphocyte globulin in clinical renal transplants with good results.

In 1967, John Najarian, an inquisitive transplant surgeon with a strong immunologic background, relocated from California to revitalize the existing Minnesota transplant program. Aware of the considerable potential for antilymphocyte preparations, he developed a very effective antilymphoblast globulin, with good patient tolerance and acceptable results.[45] In many ways, the

immunosuppressive basis for the next 2 to 3 decades was established at this point in history. Other developments in patient care also included a more regimented approach to immunosuppression.

## LATE 1960s

By the late 1960s, transplanters were walking with more ease. Related LD kidney transplants were more frequent. Results were more predictable and 1-year survival rates reached 80%.[46] Surgeons had a technique they could consistently use, and the care of LDs and recipients was better defined. Immunosuppression was frequently threefold, consisting of Imuran, prednisone, and antilymphocyte preparations.[44,45,47,48]

Related LD kidneys were no longer the only source of organs. DD kidneys became more acceptable and were not a rarity. The issues and determinants of success began to change[47,49,50] As surgeons began to clear the technical hurdles of transplants, management of rejection became the paramount concern. Kidneys demonstrating a moderate to severe rejection response, particularly those that showed no rejection reversal after steroid treatment, were more likely to ultimately fail. Related LD kidneys were less prone to rejection than DD kidneys. Tissue typing was more frequently solicited, and immunologic causes began to appear as frequent problems posttransplant.

## THE 1970s AND BEYOND

The decade of the 1970s brought a more organized approach, as well as better-known immunosuppressive regimens, to transplantation. In spite of this progress, improved results were not universal.[9,10,19,24,41,47–50] Some programs reported increased mortality rates posttransplant[8–10,24,47–50] Other programs reflected on the need for better immunosuppression. Causes of the higher morbidity and mortality were related in many ways to the appearance of all sorts of infections, fueled by enhanced and increased immunosuppression.[9,10,19,24,41,47–50]

Related LD kidney transplant continued at higher numbers in the 1970s, as compared with the previous decade, even though the overall results did not consistently improve.[8–10] Dedicated transplant groups persisted in their search for new avenues of improvement in different circumstances. Starzl, in a recent review,[8] astutely labeled the 1970s as the "bleak period" of transplantation, one in which "heavy mortality and devastating morbidity" were the frequent outcomes for many transplant recipients.

As the 1970s came to a close, Calne et al.[51] published landmark work on the beneficial effect of Cyclosporin A as a single immunosuppressant in DD kidney transplants. Months later, Starzl et al.[52] further advanced the effect of Cyclosporin A by adding prednisone to the immunosuppression of DD kidney recipients, with improved results. The application of this drug to LD kidney transplants represented a natural evolution. A decade later, in 1989, Starzl et al.[53] added another promising new immunosuppressant, tacrolimus, for DD kidney, pancreas, and liver transplants.

Other drug discoveries came along, improving results. In 1992, Hans Sollinger and Fred Belzer of the Wisconsin group and Deierhoi and Diethelm of the Alabama group united forces to test the safety of mycophenolate mofetil for DD kidney recipients.[54] In a further multicenter study on refractory kidney graft rejection, a 69% rescue rate was achieved.[55] Immediately thereafter, mycophenolate mofetil was incorporated into related LD kidney transplants.

Four years later, in 1996, Barry Kahan et al. of the University of Texas Medical School in Houston introduced a new drug, rapamycin, which was evaluated in clinical trials for safety and tolerability in renal transplant patients on cyclosporine and prednisone.[56] Other controlled studies followed the Texas protocol, such as one led by Carl Groth et al. of Stockholm.[57] At the same time, Minnesota clinical researchers spearheaded by Daniel Canafax and Arthur Matas finished a similar study, with good results.[58]

These decades of progress planted the seed for the development of even better and more effective immunosuppressive drugs and regimens.[49-59] Even though these new drugs were tested initially in DD kidney recipients, it was evident that they would be very helpful when applied to related LD kidney recipients. As important as all the new synthetic immunosuppressive drugs was the landmark discovery of monoclonal antibodies: first, OKT-3 directed specifically against T-cell receptor-CD3 [59], and, next, IL-2 receptor antagonists.[59] These effective compounds were soon effectively adapted to related LD kidney transplants.

Matas et al. summarized the results of 36 years' experience from June 1963 to December 1998. That study encompassed over 2,500 LD kidney transplants at the University of Minnesota.[60] He and his group carefully reviewed their results, decade by decade, emphasizing specific changes. Of special interest in this review was that the 1970s, frequently considered by Starzl,[8] Tilney,[10] and others as the bleakest time in kidney transplantation, deserved that title well enough. Inasmuch as acute and chronic rejection were more frequently seen in the 1960s, and the immunosuppressive regimen included mostly azathioprine and prednisone, the 1970s had the highest mortality rate (42%) with graft function. Other causes of morbidity were probably associated, at least in part, with the immunosuppressive regimen used. It is also possible that many other unidentified causes were culprits. All in all, as Matas et al. rightly pointed out, since the 1960s, decade by decade, the results of LD kidney transplants have progressively improved. The incidence of graft loss from acute and chronic rejection and the number of technical complications have all decreased with time to reach 1% (acute rejection), 3% (chronic rejection), and 1% (technical complications) in the 1990s. As expected, donor source continued to be important, but the major risk factor in the 1970s was delayed graft function. Data from this Minnesota paper should be the basis for comparing other LD kidney programs in the United States.

The undeniable success of kidney transplants yielded great growth. Subsequently, the need for organ donors became more acute, and new possibilities of donor sources appeared eminently more acceptable. What was not as frequently performed in the 1950s became commonplace a decade or so afterward. For example, Starzl and his group operated on their first unrelated kidney LD on February 25, 1963.[41] The LD was the recipient's wife, who underwent the donor nephrectomy without any difficulty. The kidney graft worked initially, until rejection episodes set in at 17 and 42 days after transplant surgery. Within less than 2 years, a total of 20 unrelated kidney LDs (including 5 wives) underwent nephrectomy in Starzl's initial series of 83 kidney transplants.[41] During the same decade, the Minnesota group, both before and during Najarian's leadership, operated on 4 unrelated LDs.[60]

As time progressed, the use of unrelated LDs continued unevenly, until Terasaki issued the final verdict in his 1995 paper dealing with "high survival rates from spousal and living unrelated donors of kidney transplants."[61,62] A few years thereafter, Tony D'Alessandro and his Wisconsin group published a series on 150 unrelated kidney LDs beginning in 1981.[63] (The first report

from the Wisconsin group on 40 unrelated LDs had appeared in 1988,[64] led by John Pirsch.) The active Minnesota program reported on a similar number of unrelated LDs at about the same time.[60]

Many other dedicated transplanters, immediately before the well-known Terasaki report and definitely thereafter, actively pursued unrelated LD kidney transplantation.[65-73] In 2000, Dave Gjerston and Mike Cecka from the UCLA Immunogenetics Laboratories published data from the United Network for Organ Sharing (UNOS) Kidney Registry from 1987 to 1998.[74] In all, 2,751 unrelated LD kidney transplants had been performed by nearly 80% of all U.S. transplant centers. By 2003, 30% of all kidney LDs (2,100 donors) were in the unrelated category in the United States.[75] Overall, unrelated LD kidney transplants demonstrated excellent outcomes, practically equal to outcomes of related LD kidney transplants.[61,62,74-76]

Before anyone else, in 1986, Felix Rapaport presented a bold and imaginative proposal dealing with the continuous lack of organ donors.[77] In a clear and clever manner, he figured that two donor–recipient pairs could exchange two kidneys at different transplant centers. This new approach was ahead of its time and did not garner a great deal of initial support in the transplant community. Although this brilliant concept was simple and elegant, its application and ethics would prove more complex. However, within a few years, in 1991, Kiil Park and his group at Yonsei University in South Korea accepted Rapaport's unique challenge and moved ahead with the development of a well-structured kidney donor exchange program.[65,66]

The donor exchange idea had the goal of "relieving the pressure on the donor organ shortage."[66] In their two landmark publications in 1999, Park et al. described 110 kidney LD transplants in their exchange program, of which 86 were simple donor exchanges and 24 belonged to the LD pool exchange category.[65,66] The indications for entering the exchange were ABO incompatibility, poor human leukocyte antigen (HLA) match, and positive lymphocyte cross-match.[66] Americans and Europeans in general continued to look with jaundiced eyes on this ingenious approach; they considered it to be untested by time and fraught with potential ethical complications. But time has proven this concept to be acceptable, and others in the United States soon began to apply it in their own programs.[70-73]

In 1997, several other publications supported the concept of kidney donor exchange, as earlier espoused by Rapaport and performed by Park.[67,68] Transplant specialists and ethicists from the University of Chicago outlined an excellent supporting document on the ethics of paired-kidney exchange programs.[78-80] While presenting at the International Forum for Transplant Ethics, Bob Sells, a recognized transplant surgeon from Liverpool and a proponent of this program, concisely detailed some of the difficulties associated with the acceptance of donor exchange in the United Kingdom, where such a program would require a change in law.[67] By 2000, Matas and his group at the University of Minnesota had already performed four transplants involving nondirected donation,[69] beginning in August 1999. The Minnesota program at this stage established a strict and well-organized policy for nondirected donation.[69]

The interest in LD kidney exchange continued to gain momentum. On May 31, 2001, a group of transplant community representatives assembled in Boston to review the experience and ethical considerations concerning nondirected kidney LDs.[70] After a full day of intense discussions, the diverse conference participants wholly supported nondirected donation, assuming exact documentation on informed consent and donor safety.[70] Several years later, in 2004, a group of transplanters from UNOS Region 1 (northeast United States) described their success with 4 LD paired exchanges and 17 LD list exchange kidney transplants.[71] Nine of the 14 Region 1 transplant centers participated in the program.[71] Regional donor kidney exchange was clearly validated and could serve as the basis for similar endeavors throughout the United States.

As recently as October 5, 2005, the Johns Hopkins group led by Robert Montgomery described their admirable results with incompatible LD kidney pairs.[72] A total of 22 recipients underwent transplants through 10 paired donations, including 2 triple exchanges. All but 1 recipient had a functioning graft (median follow-up, 13 months). This study again proved the benefit of kidney paired donation and the possibility of improving the chances for kidney transplants for candidates who otherwise might not find a suitable LD.

Other significant developments have occurred in LD kidney transplantation during the last 10 years. Lloyd Ratner introduced laparoscopic kidney donor nephrectomy in 1995 at the Johns Hopkins Bayview campus.[81] The groundwork for this technique was established by the earlier innovative work of the Johns Hopkins group.[82–84] Clayman and his urological team[82,83] introduced the procedure by performing more than 10 laparoscopic nephrectomies for general urological patients. In 1994, Gill (of Clayman's group) performed laparoscopic LD nephrectomy in the pig model.[84] This novel technique offered the possibility of increased comfort and convenience with less hospitalization.[81,85] A large number of kidney transplant programs now offer this laparoscopic procedure.[85]

In summary, many advances have occurred since the extraordinary case of Murray's successful LD kidney transplant between the Herrick twins in December 1954 in Boston. Multiple hurdles were overcome throughout the years, as better immunosuppression techniques were discovered and introduced. New developments in patient selection and in donor and recipient care have also contributed to better results. The development of laparoscopic nephrectomy has helped speed donor recovery. Because of the scarcity of kidneys for transplantation, unrelated LDs have been used with a great deal of success for the last 2 decades. Recently, donor exchange programs have been accepted as another way to deal with the organ shortage.[86–89] The story of LD kidney transplants is one of positive outcomes and sustained improvements. In the future, new advances maximizing donor use and enhancing the donation process are expected.

## References

1. Murray JM. *Surgery of the Soul: Reflections of a Curious Mind*. Canton, MA: Science History Publications; 2001.
2. Michon L, Hamburger J, Economos N, et al. Une Tentative de Transplantation Renale chez L'Homme: Aspect Medicolaux et Biologiques. *La Presse Med*. 1953;61:1419.
3. Kuss R, Teinturier J, Milliez P. Quelques Essais de Greffe du Rein chez L'Homme. *Mem Acad Chir*. 1951;77:755.
4. Dubost C, Oeconomos N, Vaysse J, Hamburger J, Milliez P, Lebrigand J. Note préliminaire sur l'etude des fonctiones rénales de reins greffes chez l'homme. *Bull Soc Med Hop Paris*. 1951;67:105.
5. Servelle M, Soulié P, Rougeulle J, Delahaye G, Touche M. Greffe d'un rein de supplicié à une malade avec rein unique congénital, atteinte de nephrite chronique hypertensive azotémique. *Bull Soc Med Hop Paris*. 1951;67:99.
6. Toledo-Pereyra LH, Palma-Vargas JM. Searching for history in transplantation: Early modern attempts at surgical kidney grafting. *Transplant Proc*. 1999;31:2945-2946.
7. Groth CG. Landmarks in clinical renal transplantation. *Surg Gynecol Obstet*. 1972;134:323–328.
8. Starzl TE. The mystique of organ transplantation. *J Am Coll Surg*. 2005;201:160–170.
9. Starzl TE. *The Puzzle People: Memoirs of a Transplant Surgeon*. Pittsburgh: University of Pittsburgh Press; 1993.
10. Tilney NL. *Transplant: From Myth to Reality*. New Haven: Yale University Press; 2003.
11. Moore FD. *Transplant: The Give and Take of Tissue Transplantation*. New York: Simon and Schuster; 1972.
12. Hamilton DN, Reid WA, Yu Yu Voronoy and the first human kidney allograft. *Surg Gynecol Obstet*. 1984;159:289–294.
13. Carrel A, Guthrie CC. Anastomosis of blood vessels by the patching method and transplantation of the kidney. *JAMA*. 1906;47:1647–1651.
14. Carrel A. Transplantation in mass of the kidneys. *J Exp Med*. 1908;10:98–140.
15. Moore FD. *A Miracle and A Privilege: Recounting a Half Century of Surgical Advance*. Washington, DC: Joseph Henry Press; 1995.
16. Lawler RH, West JW, McNulty PH, Clancy EJ, Murphy RP. Homotransplantation of the kidney in the human. *JAMA*. 1950;144:844.
17. Hamburger J, Vaysse J, Crosnier J, Auvert J, Dormont J. Kidney homotransplantations in man. *Ann NY Acad Sci*. 1962;99:808–820.
18. Hume DM, Merrill JP, Miller BF, Thorn GW. Experiences with renal homotransplantations in the human: report of nine cases. *J Clin Invest*. 1955;34:327–382.
19. Gaston RS, Diethelm AG. A Brief History of Living Donor Kidney Transplantation. In: Gaston RS, Wadstrom J, eds. *Living Donor Kidney Transplantation*. London: Taylor and Francis; 2005.
20. Murray JE, Merrill JP, Harrison JH. Renal homotransplantation in identical twins. *Surg Forum*. 1955;6:432.
21. Merrill JP, Murray JE, Harrison JH, Guild WR. Successful homotransplantation of the human kidney between identical twins. *JAMA*. 1956;160:277.
22. Joseph E. Murray – Nobel Lecture. http://nobelprize.org/medicine/laureates/1990/murray-lecture.html. Accessed August 11, 2005.
23. The Nobel Prize in Physiology or Medicine 1990—Presentation Speech. http://nobelprize.org/medicine/laureates/1990/presentation-speech.html. Accessed August 11, 2005.
24. Terasaki PI. *History of Transplantation: Thirty-five recollections*. Los Angeles: UCLA Tissue Typing Laboratory; 1991.
25. Calne RY. The inhibition of renal homograft rejection in dogs by 6 mercaptopurine. *Lancet*. 1960;1:417.
26. Zukoski C, Lee HM, Hume DM. The prolongation of functional survival of canine renal homograpfts by 6 mercaptopurine. *Surgical Forum*. 1960;11:470.
27. Murray JE, Merrill JP, Harrison JH. Kidney transplantations between seven pairs of identical twins. *Ann Surg*. 1958;148:343.
28. Merrill JP, Murray JE, Harrison JH, Friedman EA, Dealy JB, Dammin GJ. Successful homotransplantation of the kidney between nonidentical twins. *New Eng J Med*. 1960;262:1251.
29. Murray JE, Merrill JP, Dammin GJ, et al. Study of transplantation immunity after total body irradiation: clinical and experimental investigation. *Surgery*. 1960;48:272.
30. Schwartz R, Dameshek W. Drug-induced immunological tolerance. *Nature*. 1959;183:1682.
31. Calne RY, Alexandre GPJ, Murray JE. A study of the effects of drugs in prolonging survival of homologous renal transplants in dogs. *Ann NY Acad Sci*. 1962;99:743.
32. Porter KA, Murray JE. Homologous marrow transplantation in rabbits after triethylenethiophosphoramide (ThioTEPA). *AMA Arch Surg*. 1958;76:906.
33. Murray JE, Merrill JP, Dammin GJ, et al. Kidney transplantation in modified recipients. *Ann Surg*. 1962;156:337.
34. Murray JE, Balankura O, Greenburg JB, Dammin GJ. Reversability of the kidney homograft reaction by retransplantation and drug therapy. *Ann NY Acad Sci*. 1962;99:768.

35. Murray JE, Merrill JP, Harrison JH, Wilson RE, Dammin GJ. Prolonged survival of human-kidney homografts by immunosuppressive drug therapy. *New Engl J Med*. 1963;268:1315.

36. Schackman R, Dempster WJ, Wrong OM. Kidney homotransplantations in the human. *Br J Urol*. 1963;35:222.

37. Woodruff MFA, Robson JS, McWhirter R, et al. Transplantation of a kidney from a brother to a sister. *Br J Urol*. 1962;34:3.

38. Woodruff MFA, Robson JS, Nolan B, et al. Homotransplantation of kidney in patients treated by preoperative local irradiation and postoperative administration of antimetabolite (Imuran); report of six cases. *Lancet*. 1963;2:675.

39. Goodwin WE, Mims MM, Kaufman JJ. Human renal transplantation—III: Technical problems encountered in six cases of kidney homotransplantations. *Trans Am Assoc Genitourin Surg*. 1962;54:116; 1962.

40. Goodwin WE, Kaufman JJ, Mims MM, et al. Human renal transplantation I: clinical experiences with six cases of renal transplantation. *J Urol*. 1963;89:13.

41. Starzl TE. *Experience in Renal Transplantation*. Philadelphia: Saunders; 1964.

42. Terasaki PI, Verdevoe DL, Mickey MR, et al. Serotyping for homotransplantations—VI: Selection of kidney donors for thirty-two recipients. *Ann NY Acad Sci*. 1966;129:500.

43. Franksson C. Letter to the eEditor. *Lancet*. 1964;1:1331.

44. Starzl TE, Marchioro TL, Porter KA, Iwasaki Y, Cerilli GJ. The use of heterologous antilymphoid agents in canine renal and liver homotransplantations and in human renal homotransplantation. *Surg Gynecol Obstet*. 1967;124:301.

45. Najarian JS, Merkel FK, Moore GE, et al. Clinical use of antilymphoblast serum. *Transpl Proc*. 1969;1:460.

46. Murray JE, Barnes BA, Atkinson JC. Fifth report of the human kidney transplant registry. *Transplantation*. 1967;5:752.

47. Najarian JS, Simmons RL, eds. *Transplantation*. Philadelphia: Lea and Febiger; 1972.

48. Salvatierra O Jr. Renal transplantation: The Starzl influence. *Transplant Proc*. 20:343.

49. Garovoy MR, Guttman RD, eds. *Renal Transplantation*. New York: Churchill Livingstone; 1986.

50. Toledo-Pereyra LH, ed. *Kidney Transplantation*. Philadelphia: F. A. Davis; 1988.

51. Calne RY, Rolles K, White DJG, et al. Cyclosporin A initially as the only immunosuppressant in 34 recipients of cadaveric organs; 32 kidneys, 2 pancreas, and 2 livers. *Lancet*. 1979;2:1033–1036.

52. Starzl TE, Weil R III, Iwatsuki S, et al. The use of cyclosporine A and prednisone in cadaver kidney transplantation. *Surg Gynecol Obstet*. 1980;151:17–26.

53. Starzl TE, Todo S, Fung J, et al. FK 506 for human liver, kidney and pancreas transplantation. *Lancet*. 1989;2:1000–1004.

54. Sollinger HW, Deierhoi MH, Belzer FO, et al. RS-61443—A phase I clinical trial and pilot study. *Transplantation*. 1992;53:428–432.

55. Sollinger HW, Belzer FO, Dierhoi MH, et al. RS-61443 (mycophenolate mofetil): A multicenter study for refractory kidney transplant rejection. *Ann Surg*. 1992;216:513–518.

56. Murgia MG, Jordan S, Kahan BD. The side effect of sirolimus: A phase I study in quiescent cyclosporine-prednisone-treated renal transplant patients. *Kidney Int*. 1996;49:209–216.

57. Brattstrom C, Tyden G, Sawe J, et al. A randomized double-blind, placebo-controlled study to determine safety, tolerance, and preliminary pharmacokinetics of ascending single doses of orally administered sirolimus (rapamycin) in stable renal transplant recipients. *Transplant Proc*. 1996;28:985–986.

58. Johnson EM, Zimmerman J, Duderstadt K, et al. A, randomized double-blind, placebo-controlled study of the safety, tolerance, and preliminary pharmacokinetics of ascending single doses of orally administered sirolimus (rapamycin) in stable renal transplant recipients. *Transpl Proc*. 1996;28:987.

59. Immunosuppressive Therapies in Organ Transplantation. http://www.medscape.com/viewarticle/437182_9. Accessed October 11, 2005.

60. Matas AJ, Payne WD, Sutherland DER, et al. 2,500 Living Donor Kidney Transplants: A Single-Center Experience. *Annal Surg*. 2001;234:149–164.

61. Terasaki PI, Cecka JM, Gjertson DW, Takemoto S. High survival rates of kidney transplants from spousal and living unrelated donors. *N Engl J Med*. 1995;333:333–336.

62. Terasaki PH, Cecka JM, Gjertson DW, Cho YW. Spousal and other living renal donor transplants. In: *Clinical Transplants 1997*, eds. Cecka JM, Terasaki PI. Los Angeles: UCLA Tissue Typing Laboratory; 1998.

63. D'Alessandro AM, Pirsch JD, Knechtle SJ, et al. Living unrelated renal donation: The University of Wisconsin experience. *Surgery*. 1998;124:604–611.

64. Pirsch JD, Sollinger HW, Kalayoglu M, et al. Living-unrelated renal transplantation: Results in 40 patients. *Am J Kidney Dis*. 1998;12:499–503.

65. Park K, Moon JI, Kim SI, Kim YS. Exchange-donor program in kidney transplantation. *Transplant Proc*. 1999;31:356–357.

66. Park K, Moon JI, Kim SI, Kim SY. Exchange donor program in kidney transplantation. *Transplantation*. 1999;67:339–348.

67. Sells RA. Paired-kidney-exchange programs. *N Engl J Med*. 1997;337:1392–1393.

68. The Authors for the Live Organ Donor Consensus Group. Consensus Statement on the Live Organ Donor. *JAMA*. 2000;284:2919–2926.

69. Matas AJ, Garvey CA, Jacobs CL, Kahn JP. Nondirected donation of kidneys from living donors. *N Engl J Med*. 2000;343:433–436.

70. Adams PL, Cohen DJ, Danovitsch GM, et al. The nondirected live-kidney donor: Ethical considerations and practice guidelines. *Transplantation*. 2002;74:582–590.

71. Delmonico FL, Morrissey PE, Lipkowitz GS, et al. Donor Kidney Exchanges. *American J Transplant*. 2004;4:1628–1634.

72. Montgomery RA, Zachary AA, Ratner LE, et al. Clinical Results From Transplanting Incompatible Live Kidney Donor/Recipient Pairs Using Kidney Paired Donation. *JAMA*. 2005;294:1655–1663.

73. Matas AJ, Sutherland DER. The Importance of Innovative Efforts to Increase Organ Donation. *JAMA*. 2005;294:1691–1693.

74. Gjertson DW, Cecka JM. Living unrelated donor kidney transplantation. *Kidney International*. 2000;58:491–499.

75. United Network for Organ Sharing: Organ Procurement and Transplantation Network Data. http://www.unos.org. Accessed October 18, 2005.

76. Matas AJ, Bartlett ST, Leichtman AB, Delmonico FL. Morbidity and Mortality After Living Kidney Donation, 1999-2001: Survey of United States Transplant Centers. *Am J Transplant*. 2003;3:830–834.

77. Rapaport FT. The Case for A living Emotionally Related International Kidney Donor Exchange Registry. *Transplant Proc*. 1986;18(suppl2):5–9.

78. Ross LF, Rubin DT, Siegler M, et al. Ethics of a Paired-Kidney-Exchange Program. *New Engl J Med*. 336:1752–1755.

79. Ross LF, Woodle ES. Ethical Issues in Increasing Living Kidney Donations by Expanding Kidney Pair Exchange Programs. *Transplantation*. 2000;69:1539–1543.

80. Ross LF, Zenios S. Practical and Ethical Challenges to Paired Exchange Programs. *Amer J Transplant*. 2004;4:1553–1554.

81. Ratner LE, Ciseck LJ, Moore RG, et al. Laparoscopic live donor nephrectomy. *Transplantation*. 1995;60:1047–1049.

82. Clayman RV, Kavoussi LR, Soper NJ, et al. Laparoscopic nephrectomy: Initial case report. *J Urol*. 1991;146:278.

83. Clayman RV, Kavoussi LR, Soper NJ, et al. Laparoscopic nephrectomy: review of the initial 10 cases. *J Endourol*. 1992;6(2):127.

84. Gill IS, Carbone JM, Clayman RV, et al. Laparoscopic live-donor nephrectomy. *J Endurol*. 1994;8(2):143.

85. Pradel FG, Limcangco R, Mullins CD, Bartlett ST. Patients' Attitudes About Living Donor Transplantation and Living Donor Nephrectomy. *Am J Kid Dis*. 2003;41:849–858.

86. Montgomery RA, Zachary AA, Racusen LC, et al. Plasmapheresis and intravenous immune globulin provides effective rescue therapy for refractory humoral rejection and allows kidneys to be successfully transplanted into cross-match positive recipients. *Transplantation*. 2000;70:887–895.

87. Jordan SC, Vo A, Bunnapradist S, et al. Intravenous immune globulin treatment inhibits crossmatch positivity and allows for successful transplantation of incompatible organs in living-donor and cadaver recipients. *Transplantation*. 2003;76:631–636.
88. Incompatible Kidney Transplant Programs. http://www.incompatiblekidneys. org. Accessed October 16, 2005.
89. Johns Hopkins Comprehensive Transplant Center. http://www. hopkinsmedicine.org/transplant. Accessed October 16, 2005.

# KIDNEY TRANSPLANTATION: GEOGRAPHICAL DIFFERENCES

*Roberto S. Kalil, MD, Lawrence G. Hunsicker, MD*

## INTRODUCTION

There has been an impressive increase in rates of living donor kidney transplant worldwide in the last two decades. In 1988, the number of living donor kidney transplants in the United States was 1,281, with only 64 (3.5%) from living unrelated donors. In 2005, 6,021 kidney transplants were from a living donor, of which, 2,040 (34%) were from unrelated living donors. This phenomenon seems to reflect a worldwide trend as described in the next sections of this chapter. But significant differences are still observed in the rates of donation within different countries and different parts of the world. In this chapter, we focus on rates of living donation (related and unrelated), in the United States, Canada, Europe, Latin America, Australia, and New Zealand. We also discuss the major differences in the public health systems with respect to reimbursement for end-stage renal disease (ESRD) treatment, incentives for organ donation, and the lack of organ allocation systems in developing nations. Finally, universal coverage for the transplant procedure and immunosuppressive therapy are available in some developing countries and completely absent in others. The complexity of these differences and their impact on living donor transplantation are only partially understood, requiring more research focused on the disparities of overall organ transplantation across the globe. Because of the availability of more reliable data, we mainly describe the rates of living donation among the nations where registry data has been available.

## UNITED STATES AND CANADA

The number of living donor kidney transplants in the United States has more than tripled between 1988 and 2005. The fraction of dialysis patients receiving transplants from deceased donors has declined due to the increased size of the waiting list with little change in the numbers of deceased kidney donors. With this, the proportion of living unrelated donors has continued to increase, with nearly 30% in 2002 and 40% in 2005, up from 5% in 1988 (Figure 14–1). The increase in living donation is observed in the minority as well as in the Caucasian non-Hispanic population. Among different racial/ethnic groups, non-Hispanic Caucasians account for 69% of living donors in 2005, with African Americans and Hispanics having similar rates of approximately 13%, consistent with their representation in the U.S. population. The total fraction of minority donors has increased from 24% in 1988 to 31% in 2005. The increase in living donation has been most prominent among donors age 20–59, with fewer donors age 60–69. Approximately 47% of all living donors are within the range of 35 to 49 years old. More women (59%) than men are living donors. Table 14.1 displays a breakdown of the demographic characteristics for U.S. living donors in 2002. The most living related donor source in the U.S. is still the blood-related

**TABLE 14.1**

**DEMOGRAPHIC CHARACTERISTICS FOR U.S. LIVING DONORS IN 2002[a]**

| | Percentage of all Living Donors |
|---|---|
| Relationship to recipient | |
| Biological, blood-related parent | 11.8 |
| Biological, blood-related child | 17.1 |
| Biological, blood-related identical twin | 0.2 |
| Biological, blood-related full sibling | 24.4 |
| Biological, related half-sibling | 1.2 |
| Biological, blood-related other relative | 7.4 |
| Nonbiological, spouse | 11.7 |
| Nonbiological, unrelated | 22.2 |
| Not reported | 4.1 |
| Age | |
| 0–17 | <0.1 |
| 18–34 | 31.5 |
| 35–49 | 47.1 |
| 50+ | 21.3 |
| Race/ethnicity | |
| White | 69.1 |
| Black | 13.4 |
| Hispanic | 12.8 |
| Asian | 3.3 |
| Other | 1.4 |
| Gender | |
| Male | 41.2 |
| Female | 58.8 |

[a]Data from UNOS-OPTN website (www.unos.org/data/).

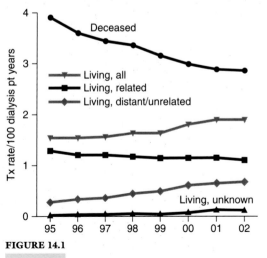

**FIGURE 14.1**

U.S. Transplant rates by year and donor type.
*Source*: USRDS 2004 ADR.[1]

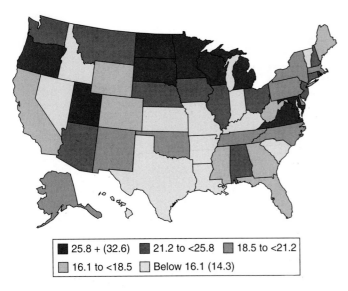

| ■ 25.8 + (32.6) | ■ 21.2 to <25.8 | ■ 18.5 to <21.2 |
| ■ 16.1 to <18.5 | □ Below 16.1 (14.3) | |

**FIGURE 14.2**

Geographical variations in living kidney donation rates (ppm), by state in 2003.
*Source*: USRDS 2004 ADR.[1]

full sibling (24%), but the total of unrelated donors (34%) now exceeds the number of full sibling donors.

There are substantial geographical differences in organ donation across the United States. The live kidney donation rate is 26.2 per million population or higher in the upper Midwest states to below 14.9 in some Southern states (Figure 14–2).[1] Because in the United States there is universal coverage for dialysis and transplantation by the federal government, it is unclear why there is such a large difference in living donation among the different regions in the United States. Differences in socioeconomic status may play a role in this difference.

In Canada, where as in the United States, all citizens have universal coverage for dialysis and transplantation, there are also large differences from province to province in the rate of live kidney donation ranging in 2004 from 24.7 per million population in Alberta to 5.8 in Quebec Province.[2]

## EUROPE

As observed in Table 14–2, there are also substantial differences across Europe in overall rates of kidney transplantation per million population (pmp), and in the fraction of living donation. High total rates of kidney transplantation are observed in Spain and Norway with rates of 49.2 and 57.6 kidney transplants pmp, respectively. The lowest rates are observed in Bulgaria, Romania, and Greece with rates of 3, 9, and 17.4 kidney transplants pmp, respectively. In general, the fraction of living donors is inverse to the rates of deceased kidney donation. The fraction of living kidney donors in Romania and Turkey was 88% and 68%, respectively, whereas the countries with the lowest fractions of living donation are Ireland, Finland, and Spain with rates of 2%, 2.5%, and 2.9%, respectively. The exceptions to this generalization were the Scandinavian countries and Netherlands with high rates of both deceased and living kidney donor transplants.[3]

These remarkable differences among the large number of nations in Europe reflect multifactorial differences including the extent of governmental financing of health-care system, presence of efficient organ procurement organizations, and cultural and religious differences. The ongoing changes in the political system in nations once belonging to the former Soviet Union will likely continue with changes in access to health care for renal replacement therapy. Due to the large number of nations in Europe, a detailed discussion of these differences is not possible in this chapter.

## LATIN AMERICA AND THE CARIBBEAN

Latin America is a conglomerate of nations with countries from North America (Mexico), Central America (Guatemala, Honduras, El Salvador, Nicaragua, Costa Rica, and Panama),

**TABLE 14.2**
## RATES OF KIDNEY TRANSPLANTATION IN EUROPE IN PER MILLION INHABITANTS (PMP) AND PERCENTAGE OF LIVING DONATION IN RELATION TO THE TOTAL NUMBER OF KIDNEY TRANSPLANTS[a]

| Country | Transplants | % (Living/Total) | Country | Transplants | %(Living/Total) |
|---|---|---|---|---|---|
| Austria | 47 | 9.8 | Latvia | 31 | 1.3 |
| Belgium | 36 | 5 | Lithuania | 17.7 | 6.6 |
| Bulgaria | 3 | 42.6 | Luxemburg | 20 | 0 |
| Croatia | 25.7 | 6 | Malta | 27.5 | |
| Cyprus | 62.8 | 65.9 | Netherlands | 41.3 | 37 |
| Czech R. | 43 | 8.6 | Norway | 57.6 | 35.8 |
| Denmark | 34.6 | 27.8 | Poland | 27.9 | 2 |
| Estonia | 28.6 | 12.5 | Portugal | 43.6 | 6.6 |
| Finland | 37.4 | 2.5 | Romania | 9 | 88.8 |
| France | 39.4 | 6.7 | Slovak R. | 18.4 | 0 |
| Georgia | 1.6 | 100 | Slovenia | 27.5 | 0 |
| Germany | 30 | 19.7 | Spain | 49.2 | 2.8 |
| Greece | 17.4 | 39.5 | Sweden | 41.3 | 38.1 |
| Hungary | 29.5 | 3.7 | Switzerland | 35.5 | 31.6 |
| Iceland | 10.2 | 100 | Turkey | 11.4 | 68.2 |
| Ireland | 37.4 | 2 | U.K. | 32.3 | 24.3 |
| Italy | 33 | 7.1 | | | |

[a]Data from Council of Europe Transplant Newsletter (5).

## TABLE 14.3

### ANNUAL NUMBER OF KIDNEY TRANSPLANTS PERFORMED IN LATIN AMERICA IN THE LAST DECADE ACCORDING TO DD DONOR TYPE

| Year | Living Donor | Deceased Donor | Total |
|------|------|------|------|
| 1990 | 1.334 | 966 | 2.300 |
| 1995 | 1.918 | 1.980 | 3.898 |
| 2000 | 3.530 | 2.890 | 6.420 |
| 2001 | 3.629 | 2.950 | 6.578 |
| 2002 | 3.299 | 3.046 | 6.345 |
| 2003 | 3.469 | 3.332 | 6.801 |

*Data from Garcia and Santiago-Delphin.[4]

three Caribbean islands (Cuba, Dominican Republic, and Puerto Rico), and South America (Argentina, Bolivia, Brazil, Chile, Colombia, Ecuador, Peru, Paraguay, Uruguay, Venezuela). The total population of these countries is 540 million, approximately 9.5% of the world population. In the 1980s, several countries developed legal support for organ donation from deceased-donor with informed consent or presumed consent, and with organ allocation systems and national registries. The growth of transplant activity in Latin America is shown in Table 14–3. As of 2002 there were over 400 transplant centers in Latin America, with at least some kidney transplants performed in each country. In the year 2000, the cumulative number of kidney transplants performed in Latin America was 63,618, approximately 13% of the total 500,545 performed worldwide. The average yearly growth in kidney transplantation between 1991 and 2001 was 10%. This growth is higher than most of the other areas of the globe. Interestingly, the rates of living donor kidney transplant have been greater than 50% for virtually this whole period, possibly related to the overall low rate of deceased donor transplants in Latin America (4.2 pmp) with a range of 0 to 16 across the continent (see Table 14–4 ).

## TABLE 14.5

### CHARACTERISTICS OF PAYMENT SYSTEM FOR TRANSPLANTATION ACCORDING TO THE PUBLIC HEALTH SYSTEM IN EACH COUNTRY*

| Universal coverage | Population With No | Coverage % |
|------|------|------|
| Argentina | Ecuador, ----------------------------------- | 85% |
| Brazil | Bolivia, ----------------------------------- | 80% |
| Chile | Paraguay, ----------------------------------- | 70% |
| Costa Rica | Peru, ----------------------------------- | 70% |
| Cuba | Colombia, ----------------------------------- | 60% |
| Panama | Venezuela, ----------------------------------- | 60% |
| Puerto Rico | Dominican Republic, ---------------------- | 60% |
| Uruguay | Guatemala, ----------------------------------- | 50% |
| | México,----------------------------------- | 40% |

*Data from Garcia VD and Santiago-Delphin E.[4]

Rates of growth in living organ transplantation have varied substantially across the continent. As observed in Table 14–5 the coverage for dialysis treatments, transplant procedure, and maintenance immunosuppressive medications vary from essentially none to universal. Also the presence of organized organ retrieval and allocation systems differs substantially, with very good governmental support in some countries and nonexistent support in others. The main obstacle to increased access to kidney transplantation in Latin American countries is lack of social support by governmental institutions. In some countries where state-supported dialysis treatment is not offered to the public, organ donation is rare because there are very few potential recipients. The other extreme is seen in countries where dialysis, transplant procedure, and medications are provided by the government (Table 14–5). The religious background across Latin American countries is similar, thus unlikely to be the cause of the highly heterogeneous rates of kidney transplantation.[4]

## TABLE 14.4

### RATES OF KIDNEY TRANSPLANTS PER MILLION PER COUNTRY DURING 2002*

| Country | Total | | Deceased-donor | | | Living donor | | | |
|------|------|------|------|------|------|------|------|------|------|
| | n | pmp | n | % | pmp | n | % | pmp | |
| Brazil | 3.126 | 18.4 | 1.342 | 42.9 | 8, 0 | 1.784 | 57.1 | 10.4 | |
| Mexico | 1.453 | 14.4 | 319 | 22, 0 | 3, 2 | 1.134 | 78, 0 | 11, 4 | |
| Argentina | 550 | 14.6 | 466 | 84, 7 | 12, 6 | 84 | 15, 3 | 2, 3 | |
| Colômbia | 387 | 9.0 | 310 | 80, 1 | 7, 2 | 77 | 19, 9 | 1, 8 | |
| Chile | 270 | 17.5 | 259 | 95, 9 | 16, 8 | 11 | 4, 1 | 0, 7 | |
| Venezuela | 209 | 8.8 | 131 | 62, 7 | 5, 6 | 78 | 37, 3 | 3, 2 | |
| Cuba | 200 | 17.9 | 186 | 93, 0 | 16, 8 | 14 | 7, 0 | 1, 1 | |
| Costa Rica | 95 | 24.4 | 39 | 41, 0 | 10, 0 | 56 | 59, 0 | 14, 4 | |
| Puerto Rico | 89 | 23.4 | 65 | 73, 0 | 17, 1 | 24 | 27, 0 | 6, 3 | |
| Uruguay | 85 | 24.8 | 79 | 92, 9 | 22, 9 | 6 | 7, 1 | 1, 9 | |
| Peru | 80 | 3, 0 | 67 | 83, 8 | 2, 5 | 13 | 16, 2 | 0, 5 | |
| Bolivia | 78 | 9, 2 | 20 | 25, 6 | 2, 4 | 58 | 74, 4 | 6, 8 | |
| Dom. Rep. | 40 | 4, 7 | 0 | — | — | 40 | 100, 0 | 4, 7 | |
| Guatemala | 44 | 3, 8 | 0 | — | — | 44 | 100, 0 | 3, 8 | |
| Panama | 28 | 9, 7 | 20 | 71, 4 | 6, 9 | 8 | 28, 6 | 2, 7 | |
| El Salvador(2000) | 25 | 3, 9 | 0 | — | — | 25 | 100, 0 | 3, 9 | |
| Ecuador | 18 | 1, 4 | 5 | 38, 8 | 0, 4 | 13 | 72, 2 | 1, 0 | |
| Paraguay (2000) | 8 | 1, 4 | 1 | 12, 5 | 0, 2 | 7 | 87, 5 | 1, 2 | |
| Honduras (1999) | 3 | 0, 5 | 0 | — | — | 3 | 100, 0 | 0, 5 | |

Data from Garcia VD and Santiago-Delphin E.[4]

In addition to differing public support for transplantation, it is important to emphasize the actual rates and causes of overall end-stage renal disease in Latin America are not well documented. Therefore, the extent of organ shortage in many Latin American countries is not clear. Another important variable when comparing Latin America to more developed nations is the life expectancy. With longer life expectancy in the United States and Western European nations, the prevalence of ESRD is increasing in the geriatric population. Conversely, in several Latin American countries there is a much shorter life expectancy due to premature death from poor access to health care, decreasing the rates of ESRD.

## AUSTRALIA AND NEW ZEALAND

Australia and New Zealand have universal coverage for ESRD and kidney transplantation. The numbers of transplants pmp in 2004 in Australia and New Zealand was 22 and 26, respectively.[5] The rates of living donor transplants are increasing, with living unrelated donation being the major component in the increase, just as in the United States (Figures 14–3 and 14–4). In the year 1995, living unrelated transplants were almost nonexistent in New Zealand and occurred at a very low rate in Australia. By 1999, the rates were up to 26% and 21% in Australia and New Zealand, respectively. In 2004, rates were 37% and 46% for living donor kidney transplants in Australia and New Zealand, respectively. The vast majority of living unrelated transplants are from spouse to spouse.

There are different native population groups among the different parts of Australia and New Zealand. Despite universal access to health care, there are significant differences in overall rates of transplantation among the different ethnic groups, just as observed in other parts of the globe. In Australia and New Zealand, the fraction of patients who were transplanted among those age 15 to 59 years receiving dialysis in 2004 was 11.9% and 7.4%, respectively. As is shown in Table 14–6, among the Australian Caucasoid patients receiving dialysis in 2004, 14.3% received a transplant, whereas among the Australian Aboriginals and Torres Strait Islanders, the corresponding transplant rate was 3.4%. This represents an increase in rate of transplantation in this minority population from 1.9% in 2003. In New Zealand

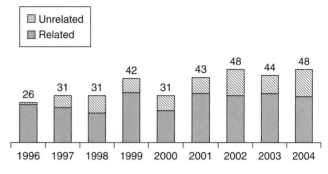

**FIGURE 14.3**

Source of Live Donor Kidney, New Zealand 1996–2004.

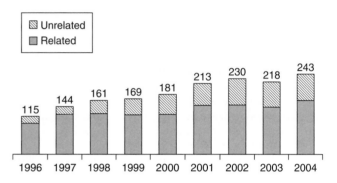

**FIGURE 14.4**

Source of Live Donor Kidney, Australia 1996–2004.

(see Table 14–7), the transplant rate for Caucasian dialysis patients was 12.9%, whereas for Maori and Pacific Islanders it was 2.1% and 4.8%, respectively. Compared to data from 1995, this was a decline in transplant rates among the Maori population (4.5% in 1995) and a stable rate for the Pacific Islanders (5.3% in 1995).

There is also a substantial variation in transplant rates among the different geographical regions of Australia, with a range in

**TABLE 14.6**
## KIDNEY TRANSPLANT RATES IN AUSTRALIA BY YEAR AND BY RACIAL/ETHNIC GROUP*

### Transplantation Rate - Age Group 15-59 years 1995–2004

| Year | Caucasoid | | | Aboriginal and Torres St. Islanders | | | All Patients | | |
|------|-----------|-----|------|----------|-----|------|----------|-----|------|
| | Dialysed | Tx | Rate | Dialysed | Tx | Rate | Dialysed | Tx | Rate |
| 1995 | 2320 | 316 | 13.6% | 345 | 13 | 3.7% | 2995 | 365 | 12.1% |
| 1996 | 2448 | 358 | 14.6% | 388 | 8 | 2.0% | 3187 | 402 | 12.6% |
| 1997 | 2527 | 359 | 14.2% | 440 | 20 | 4.5% | 3363 | 429 | 12.7% |
| 1998 | 2655 | 357 | 13.4% | 479 | 26 | 5.4% | 3555 | 436 | 12.2% |
| 1999 | 2746 | 322 | 11.7% | 513 | 19 | 3.7% | 3698 | 366 | 10.4% |
| 2000 | 2869 | 388 | 13.5% | 540 | 17 | 3.1% | 3886 | 441 | 11.3% |
| 2001 | 2947 | 391 | 13.2% | 598 | 20 | 3.3% | 4052 | 456 | 11.2% |
| 2002 | 2975 | 443 | 14.8% | 634 | 16 | 2.5% | 4151 | 511 | 12.3% |
| 2003 | 3013 | 364 | 12.1% | 678 | 13 | 1.9% | 4270 | 422 | 9.9% |
| 2004 | 3081 | 441 | 14.3% | 735 | 25 | 3.4% | 4429 | 528 | 11.9% |

*Data from the ANZDATA Registry.

TABLE 14.7

## KIDNEY TRANSPLANT RATES IN NEW ZEALAND BY YEAR AND BY RACIAL ETHNIC GROUP*

Transplantation Rate - Age Group 15-59 years 1995–2004

| Year | Caucasoid | | | Maori | | | Pacific Islander | | | All Patients | | |
|------|----------|-----|------|----------|-----|------|----------|-----|------|----------|-----|------|
| | Dialysed | Tx | Rate | Dialysed | Tx | Rate | Dialysed | Tx | Rate | Dialysed | Tx | Rate |
| 1995 | 332 | 54 | 16.2% | 240 | 11 | 4.5% | 113 | 6 | 5.3% | 725 | 78 | 10.7% |
| 1996 | 348 | 58 | 16.6% | 262 | 7 | 2.6% | 128 | 7 | 5.4% | 784 | 79 | 10.0% |
| 1997 | 372 | 73 | 19.6% | 279 | 9 | 3.2% | 134 | 3 | 2.2% | 829 | 91 | 10.9% |
| 1998 | 372 | 60 | 16.1% | 321 | 14 | 4.3% | 151 | 7 | 4.6% | 897 | 85 | 9.5% |
| 1999 | 389 | 67 | 17.2% | 318 | 16 | 5.0% | 159 | 8 | 5.0% | 928 | 98 | 10.5% |
| 2000 | 401 | 68 | 17.0% | 330 | 10 | 3.0% | 184 | 4 | 2.1% | 976 | 86 | 8.8% |
| 2001 | 414 | 64 | 15.4% | 360 | 13 | 3.6% | 213 | 5 | 2.3% | 1054 | 92 | 8.7% |
| 2002 | 435 | 60 | 13.8% | 383 | 11 | 2.8% | 225 | 14 | 6.2% | 1110 | 89 | 8.0% |
| 2003 | 433 | 57 | 13.2% | 406 | 15 | 3.7% | 227 | 12 | 5.3% | 1140 | 92 | 8.1% |
| 2004 | 440 | 57 | 12.9% | 417 | 9 | 2.1% | 227 | 11 | 4.8% | 1162 | 86 | 7.4% |

*Data from the ANZDATA Registry.[5]

2003 from 18 transplants pmp (Western Australia) to 38 (South Australia/Northern Territory) (Tables 14–6 and 14–7).[5]

In conclusion, there are large differences on living organ donation around the globe. Data are not universally available from organized registries in each region, especially in Africa and Asia. This precludes a conclusive examination of reasons for these differences. But access to health care, specific policies on organ allocation, funding for the procedure and long-term immunosuppressive therapy, and cultural and religious differences appear to account for most of the discrepancies in living (and deceased) donor organ donation.

## References

1. USRDS, Annual Data Report 2004. www.USRDS.org
2. Canadian Organ Replacement Registry (CORR), Canadian Institute for Health Information, 2005.
3. International Figures on Organ Donation and Transplantation, Council of Europe. Newsletter Transplant, Vol. 10, 1, September 2005.
4. Garcia VD, and Santiago-Delpin E: Transplantes na America Latina e Caribe.
5. ANZDATA Registry 2005 Report http://www.anzdata.org.au

# CHAPTER 15

# KIDNEY TRANSPLANTATION: THE DONOR

## 15.1 SELECTION AND WORKUP

*Mark E. Rosenberg, MD, Cathy Garvey, RN, Cheryl Jacobs, MS, LICSW*

### INTRODUCTION

The goal of this chapter is to provide guidelines for the selection and evaluation of the living kidney donor. A number of excellent reviews on this topic have been published over the years.[1–9] Important guiding principles for the care of the living kidney donor have been developed during an international forum held in Amsterdam in 2004 that included experts and leaders in transplantation from over 40 countries.[10] The goal was to develop an international standard of care regarding the responsibility of the transplant community for the living kidney donor. The recommendations of the forum are listed in Table 15.1-1 and are essential reading for anyone involved in the evaluation of the kidney donor. A similar set of guidelines was developed during a previous consensus conference of the renal and transplant communities held in Kansas City in 2000.[1] This consensus group concluded that a potential donor who consents to the donation should be "competent, willing to donate, free from coercion, medically and psychosocially suitable, fully informed of the risks and benefits as a donor, and fully informed of the risks, benefits, and alternative treatment available to the recipient."[1]

### WHO CAN BE A LIVING DONOR

When a patient is referred for a kidney transplant, the center educates and offers the recipient all options for receiving a kidney. This includes listing on the national waiting list for a deceased donor kidney, as well as the possibility of a living donor kidney transplant if there is an available donor. As the waiting times for deceased donor kidneys have continued to lengthen, transplant centers are more aggressively promoting living kidney donation. The pool of potential living donors for a given recipient has greatly expanded over the years, moving from largely first-degree relatives such as parents, siblings, and children to second-degree relatives (aunts, uncles, cousins) and emotionally related individuals such as spouses and friends. Excellent survival rates have been reported with the use of spousal and living unrelated donors.[11] More recent trends have included nondirected anonymous donors (altruistic donors) and paired organ exchanges in cases where there are willing donors but issues with ABO incompatibility or prior sensitization.[12–14] The trends in the use of donors over time are shown in Figure 15.1-1. As can be seen, the greatest increase in living donors has come from unrelated individuals.

TABLE 15.1-1

### PRINCIPLES FOR LIVING KIDNEY DONOR EVALUATION*

1. Before a living kidney donation, the donor must receive a complete medical and psychosocial evaluation to include
   - Quantification (as available) and assessment of the risk of donor nephrectomy on the individual's overall health, subsequent renal function, and any potential psychological and social consequences (including employability)
   - Assessment of the suitability of the donor's kidney for transplantation to the recipient (anatomy, function, and risk for transmissible disease)
2. Before donor nephrectomy, the potential donor must be informed of
   - The nature of the evaluation process
   - The results and consequences/morbidity of testing, including the possibility that conditions may be discovered that can impact future health care, insurability, and social status of the potential donor
   - The risks of operative donor nephrectomy. These should include, but not be limited to, the risk of death, surgical morbidities, changes in health and renal function, impact on insurability/employability, and unintended effects on family and social life
   - The responsibility of the individual and health and social system in the management of discovered conditions
   - The expected transplant outcomes (favorable and unfavorable) for the recipient and any specific recipient conditions that may affect the decision to donate the kidney
   - Disclosure of recipient specific information, which must have the assent of the recipient.
3. The potential donor should be informed of alternative renal replacement therapies available to the potential recipient.
4. The potential donor should be capable of understanding the information presented in the consent process.
5. The decision to donate should be voluntary, accompanied by
   - The freedom to withdraw from the donation process at any time
   - Assurance that medical and individual reasons for not proceeding with donation will remain confidential
6. After kidney donation, the transplant center is responsible for
   - Overseeing and monitoring the postoperative recovery process of the donor until that individual is stable, including provision of care for morbidity that is a direct consequence of donor nephrectomy
   - Facilitating the long-term follow-up and treatment of the kidney donor with preexisting or acquired conditions (related to uninephrectomy) that are thought to represent a health risk
   - Identifying and tracking complications that may be important in defining risks for informed consent disclosure
   - Working with the general health-care community to provide optimal care/surveillance of the living kidney donor

*Adopted from the consensus statement of the Amsterdam Forum on the care of the live kidney donor.[10]

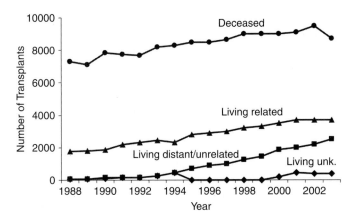

**FIGURE 15.1-1.**

Trends in the source of kidney donors.[71]

The age of the living donor remains an important issue, as increasing age is a significant determinant of poorer long-term graft survival.[15] Of the 6,647 living donors in the United Network for Organ Sharing (UNOS) database for 2004, 33% were between 18 and 34 years old; 46% were between 35 and 49 years old; and 20% were between 50 and 64 years old. Less than 1% of living donors were over age 65. Minors under age 18 should not be used as living kidney donors.[10] The upper age limit of donors remains controversial.

## INITIAL SCREENING

As planning for renal replacement therapy begins, the recipient needs to communicate the need for a kidney transplant to potential donors. Initial contact between the prospective donors and the transplant center needs to be initiated by the donor.

Ethics dictate that the evaluation of the donor and recipient needs to be as separated as possible, including different coordinators and physicians. As the evaluation proceeds, the donor should be given the opportunity to withdraw, including providing a "medical alibi." Maintaining the confidentiality of the entire evaluation process is critical. Education of the donor regarding risks of donation, the criteria used to determine eligibility, and the evaluation process is the first step before proceeding with more detailed testing. A medical history should be obtained to screen for obvious exclusions such as the presence of major medical issues or underlying kidney disease.

Confirmation of ABO compatibility between donor and recipient is critical before proceeding further, although many centers are now performing ABO-incompatible transplants. Because the kidney does not express rhesus antigens, this blood antigen system is not relevant. Blood group O is the universal donor. A preliminary crossmatch needs to be performed to test for preformed antidonor antibodies, as most centers will exclude donor–recipient pairs with a positive crossmatch. The approach to human leukocyte antigen (HLA) typing is variable. Given the expense of the test, some centers do not do HLA typing during the initial screening process because the degree of match other than HLA-identical matches is not a major consideration in selecting the donor, given the excellent outcomes of HLA-mismatched transplants.

## MEDICAL EVALUATION OF THE DONOR

The components of the medical evaluation include assessing of the current health of the kidney and determining the medical risks to the donor. Because the donation of a kidney is one of the only times in medicine that a medical procedure is carried out on a healthy individual, it is critical that the short-term and long-term risks to the donor be minimal. Therefore, a very thorough medical evaluation of the donor needs to be performed. Table 15.1-2 indicates the recommended components of the medical examination. Specific issues related to isolated medical abnormalities are discussed next. The presence of cardiac disease, particularly coronary artery disease and congestive heart failure, is usually a contraindication to donation. If there is a question whether coronary artery disease is present, then a cardiac stress test should be performed. Otherwise most centers would only obtain a resting electrocardiogram (EKG). Potential donors who smoke should be strongly encouraged to stop to increase their own general health and to reduce the incidence of postoperative respiratory complications). Donor safety remains the major consideration in the evaluation of potential donors. Absolute and relative contraindications to donation are listed in Table 15.1-3.

### Assessing the Health of the Kidney

#### *Measurement of Glomerular Filtration Rate*

Most transplant centers agree with a glomerular filtration rate (GFR) cutoff of 80 mL/min, although some centers would accept values as low as 60 mL/min.[2–4,16,17] A critical issue is what is the best method for determining GFR. Serum creatinine concentration often does not reflect the underlying GFR because it

**TABLE 15.1-2**

## DIAGNOSTIC TESTS FOR DONOR

Assessment of immunologic compatibility
- ABO blood type (done twice in some programs)
- Crossmatch

Assessment of patient health
- History and physical including careful measurement of BP and BMI, testicular or pelvic examination
- Assessment for potential nephrotoxic drugs
- Blood chemistry (electrolytes, blood urea nitrogen [BUN], creatinine, calcium, phosphorus, magnesium, liver function tests, albumin)
- Complete blood count (CBC), international normalized ratio (INR), partial thromboplastin time (PTT)
- Serologies: HIV, hepatitis C antibody, hepatitis B surface antigen, surface and core antibody, CMV antibody, EBV antibody
- Lipid profile
- Glucose tolerance test if positive family history of diabetes
- Pregnancy test
- Breast, colon, and cervical cancer screening as discussed in the text
- Chest x-ray
- EKG
- Psychosocial evaluation

Assessment of the health of the kidney
- Serum creatinine and BUN
- Urinalysis
- Urine culture
- Urinary albumin to creatinine ratio
- Estimation or measurement of GFR
- Renal imaging (CT or MR angiogram)

**TABLE 15.1-3**

## REASONS TO EXCLUDE POTENTIAL DONORS

Age < 18 and > 70*
Significant medical illness
Microalbuminuria
Proteinuria
Hematuria
Hypertension*
Recurrent nephrolithiasis
GFR < 80 mL/min/1.73 m²
BMI > 35 kg/m²
Urologic abnormalities
History of thromboembolism
Psychiatric disease
Active malignancy or previous malignancy with high metastatic potential
Untreated infectious disease
Pregnancy
Active substance abuse

*Relative contraindication.

is a function not only of creatinine clearance (which does reflect GFR) but also of creatinine production (which largely reflects muscle mass). Therefore, the same serum creatinine concentration can represent very different underlying GFRs in individuals. Many other factors can influence creatinine levels and/or creatinine secretion, including protein intake, age, sex, ethnicity, body weight, muscle mass, diet, and drugs such as cimetidine. Variation in the instrument calibration for measuring creatinine is another potential source of error.[18] Estimates of GFR based on 24-hour creatinine clearance suffer from the inaccuracies associated with these timed urine collections. Classic methods for measurement of GFR, including the gold standard inulin clearance, are cumbersome, require an intravenous infusion and timed urine collections, and are not always clinically feasible. In adults, the normal GFR based on inulin clearance and adjusted to a standard body surface area of 1.73 m² is 127 mL/min/1.73 m² for men and 118 mL/min/1.73 m² for women, with a standard deviation of approximately 20 mL/min/1.73 m². After age 30 the average decrease in GFR is 1 mL/min/1.73 m² per year.[19]

Excellent alternatives to inulin clearance include the urinary clearance of radioactive filtration markers such as $^{125}$I-iothalamate and $^{99m}$Tc-diethylenetriamine pentaacetate (DTPA). The plasma clearances of other markers such as iohexol or $^{51}$Cr-ethylene-diamine-tetraacetic acid (EDTA) have also been used to measure GFR. Availability and feasibility of these techniques limit their widespread applicability. Other methods include creatinine clearance after cimetidine to block tubular secretion and use of cystatin C (20).

Equations based on serum creatinine but factoring for sex, age, and ethnicity are the best alternative for estimation of GFR. The most commonly used formula is the Cockcroft–Gault equation. This equation was developed to predict creatinine clearance but has been used for estimating GFR. The formula is

CrCl (mL/min) = {(140-age) * weight (*0.85 if female)/72}/SCr.

The Modification of Diet in Renal Disease (MDRD) Study equation was developed using the urinary clearance of $^{125}$I-iothalamate as the gold standard.[21] The formula was derived from data in over 500 patients with a wide variety of kidney diseases and a GFR up to 90 mL/min/1.73 m². A separate group of patients was used to validate the equation. There are four different versions of this formula, all having similar accuracy. Thus, the abbreviated equation is recommended for routine use and requires only serum creatinine, age, sex, and race. This formula is

GFR (mL/min/1.73 m²) =
186 *(SCr)$^{-1.154}$ * (age)$^{-0.203}$ * (0.742 if female) * (1.210 if black).

There is some controversy regarding the validation of this formula; including the representativeness of the patient group from which it was derived and validated, its accuracy in people with normal kidney function such as kidney donors, and the lack of a component to adjust for muscle mass.

When surveyed in the early 1990s, the majority of transplant centers were using 24-hour creatinine clearance to estimate glomerular filtration rate.[17] Inaccuracies in urine collection led to alternative ways to measure GFR that were still feasible for the evaluation of potential donors.[22] In a study of 365 potential living donors referred to a single center for consideration of donation, GFR was measured using nonradiolabeled iothalamate.[23] The mean GFR in men age 20 was 129 mL/min with a fifth percentile of 100 mL/min. Women at age 20 had mean GFR of 123/min with a fifth percentile of 96 mL/min. GFR declined by 4.6 mL/min/decade in men and 7.1 mL/min/decade in women. The mean normalized GFR in this study was 101 ± 16 mL/min/1.73 m². When both the MDRD equation and the Cockcroft–Gault equation were applied to this dataset, both equations significantly underestimated GFR,[23,24] for example, in the subset of patients with a mean normalized GFR of 101 ± 16 mL/min/1.73 m² the value by the MDRD equation was 72 ± 16 mL/min/1.73 m². The Cockcroft–Gault equation performed somewhat better with a mean value of 87 ± 17 mL/min/1.73 m². This study highlights the problems with using prediction formulas based on serum creatinine. The equations were validated in populations of patients with chronic kidney disease and do not necessarily apply to the healthy population. These investigators have gone on to develop a new equation that may more accurately predict GFR.[23,24]

### Anatomic Assessment

The anatomy of the kidneys needs to be assessed to make sure there are two normal kidneys and to define the renal vasculature and ureters. The use of computed tomography (CT) or magnetic resonance angiography has replaced renal arteriography at most centers.[25] The left kidney is preferred for donation because of the longer length of the left renal vein.

### Urinalysis

The presence of proteinuria should be assessed by both urinalysis and a urinary albumin or protein to creatinine ratio. Current clinical practice guidelines recommend use of the spot urine test over a 24-hour collection because the latter is often confounded with issues of over-and undercollection.[19] Normal values are shown in Table 15.1-4. The presence of abnormal amounts of proteinuria is indicative of an underlying renal disease and is a contraindication for donation. Referral to a nephrologist for further evaluation is indicated. More controversial is the presence of microalbuminuria, defined as low levels of albumin excretion that are clearly above normal but not yet detectable by dipstick

**TABLE 15.1-4**

## DEFINITION OF PROTEINURIA AND ALBUMINURIA*

| Classification | Abnormal Values |
|---|---|
| Clinical Proteinuria | |
| 24-hour excretion | >300 mg/day |
| Protein/creatinine ratio | >200 mg/g |
| Microalbuminuria | |
| 24-hour excretion | 30–300 mg/day |
| Albumin/creatinine ratio | 17–250 mg/g (men) |
| | 25–355 mg/g (women) |
| Clinical Albuminuria | |
| 24-hour excretion | >300 mg/day |
| Albumin/creatinine ratio | >250 mg/g (men) |
| | >355 mg/g (women) |

*Data from National Kidney Foundation: K/DOQI Clinical Practice Guidelines for Chronic Kidney Disease: Evaluation, Classification, and Stratification.[19]

measurement. The presence of microalbuminuria has been most carefully studied in diabetics and is a risk factor for progression to overt nephropathy. Given the wide biological variability in albumin excretion, its presence should be confirmed by at least three measurements. If present, microalbuminuria warrants further investigation before kidney donation can be performed.

Isolated microscopic hematuria, defined as two to three red blood cells per high-power field, is not an uncommon finding and requires further investigation before approving the donor. Examining for a structural cause for the microscopic hematuria requires a CT scan of the kidney, urine cytology and culture, and cystoscopy. If the aforementioned testresults are negative, a kidney biopsy should be performed, and only if biopsy results are normal should the donor be approved.

## ISOLATED MEDICAL ABNORMALITIES

### Donor Hypertension

In the past, hypertensive individuals were excluded from being kidney donors. However, in a survey of transplant centers in 1995, a third of centers accepted donors with minor elevations in blood pressure (BP) or treated hypertensive donors if BP was controlled.[17] The reason for excluding hypertensive donors is the increased risk to these patients of developing kidney failure and the worse outcomes seen in recipients of hypertensive donor kidneys.[26,27] However, the threshold for defining hypertension was higher in these older studies. The argument has been made that low-risk individuals could be acceptable kidney donors if they have mild elevations in BP, or hypertension controlled on a single medication, along with a normal GFR and urinalysis.

The BP measurement technique can greatly influence the classification of potential donor candidates. Textor et al. evaluated 238 primarily white potential donors between 18 and 72 years of age who had normal GFR and urinary albumin excretion.[28] Different methods were used to measure blood pressure, including standard office BP measurements, overnight ambulatory blood pressure monitoring, and BP measurements performed by specialized hypertension nurses trained to follow the American Heart Association guidelines for multiple office readings. The mean

systolic and diastolic BP values increased with increasing age by all measurement techniques. Clinic BP values were higher than with the other two methods, particularly in subjects greater or equal to age 50 years old. Using cutoffs of BP values greater than 140/90 mm Hg, 36.7% of subjects would be considered hypertensive by standard clinical BP measurements, but only 11% would be hypertensive by awake ambulatory BP measurements.

These investigators went on to study blood pressure and renal function after kidney donation.[29] They demonstrated that in these white subjects with moderate essential hypertension and normal kidney function, there was no adverse affect on BP, GFR, or urinary protein excretion during the first year following living kidney donation. Treatment of hypertensive donors was done before donor nephrectomy. In another study of 18 donors who were hypertensive at the time of donation, 10 out of 18 were on antihypertensive therapy 7 years following donation.[4] There was no difference in renal function between hypertensive donors and normotensive donors when studied at the 7-year follow-up time point.

In assessing hypertensive donors, ambulatory BP monitoring should be performed in those with consistent clinic BP readings greater than 140/90 mm Hg. If average values of ambulatory BP are less than 135/85 mm Hg, then these patients could be considered for donation as long as there is no evidence for end-organ damage such as kidney disease, retinopathy, left ventricular hypertrophy, or vascular disease. Low-risk hypertensive individuals, defined as whites over age 55 with normal urinary albumin to creatinine ratio and normal GFR, could also be considered as potential donors. Antihypertensive therapy should be initiated before donation in these individuals, targeting BP less than 140/90 mm Hg. It should be appreciated that not all transplant centers would accept such donors.

### Obesity

The concern with using obese donors, defined by a body mass index (BMI) > 30 kg/m$^2$, is their potential risk for developing hypertension and renal disease over time. For example, in one study, BMI greater than 30 kg/m$^2$ was a risk factor for the development of proteinuria and renal disease when patients were followed for 10 to 20 years following unilateral nephrectomy performed for reasons other than donation.[30] The metabolic syndrome defined as the presence of three or more of the following: elevated BP, low high-density lipoprotein (HDL) cholesterol, high triglyceride level, elevated glucose level, and abdominal obesity has been associated with an increased risk of chronic kidney disease (defined as GFR < 60 mL/min/1.73 m$^2$).[31] Extending previous reports showing that dyslipidemia may be a risk factor for renal disease, Schaeffner et al. report from the Physicians' Health Study that among apparently healthy men, elevated total cholesterol levels, high non-HDL cholesterol levels, and low HDL cholesterol levels were all associated with increased risk of serum creatinine elevation.[32]

A second concern regarding the use of obese donors is their risk of developing surgical complications related to their obesity. In one study of laparoscopic donor nephrectomy, donors with BMI ≥ 35 kg/m$^2$ had longer operative times and more perioperative complications (mainly minor wound infections), yet the same low rate of major surgical complications such as conversion to open nephrectomy.[33] Also, length of stay was similar. Six to 12 months after donation, renal function and albumin excretion did not vary with preoperative BMI.

Recommendations are to measure BMI in all potential donors, evaluating for such co-morbidities as diabetes or impaired fasting glucose, vascular disease, hypertension, decreased GFR, microalbuminuria, or sleep apnea. Donation should be strongly discouraged in potential donors with a BMI $\geq$ 35 kg/m$^2$ and they should be referred to a program for weight loss reduction.

## Excluding Diabetes

Excluding diabetes is absolutely critical in the evaluation of potential donors, as progression of diabetic kidney disease will be faster in diabetics with only one kidney.[34] In patients with risk factors like obesity, gestational diabetes, and elevated fasting glucose, or those with a family history of diabetes, a fasting blood sugar and a 75-gram, 2-hour glucose tolerance test should be performed. An expert committee of the American Diabetes Association has defined normal fasting plasma glucose as less than 100 mg/dL and impaired fasting glucose as a fasting plasma glucose $\geq$ 100 to 125 mg/dL. For the diagnosis of diabetes, the fasting plasma glucose should be > 126 mg/dL, 2-hour plasma glucose > 200 mg/dL, or random plasma glucose concentration $\geq$ 200 mg/dL. Some studies have also recommended insulin levels be assessed along with the glucose measurements to detect both insulin deficiency and insulin resistance.[35,36] In women with a previous history of gestational diabetes, 35% will develop type 2 diabetes within 15 years after delivery.[37] The diagnosis of diabetes or impaired fasting glucose is a contraindication to renal transplantation, given the impact of diabetes on kidney function.

A more difficult situation is assessing the future risk of developing diabetes when the donor is from a diabetic family, given the familial clustering of diabetic kidney disease.[38,39] This is particularly true for type 2 diabetes that may develop years in the future. This form of diabetes is heterogeneous and multifactorial with both genetic and environmental factors playing an etiologic role. In rare cases, type 2 diabetes is monogenic.[40–42] It is difficult to exactly quantify the risk of developing diabetes in first-degree relatives of a diabetic recipient.[42] In a study of U.S. whites, 16% of offspring having two parents with type 2 diabetes developed diabetes when followed over an average follow-up time of 13 years.[43] The best approach is to look for risk factors that portend a greater chance of developing diabetes in the future. These include a history of gestational diabetes; impaired fasting glucose; high BMI; certain ethnic groups (there is a higher incidence such as in Pima Indians, South Asians, and Mexican Americans); poor fasting and 2-hour glucose and insulin results; and older age.

## Nephrolithiasis

A history of nephrolithiasis is not an absolute contraindication to donation.[44,45] In fact, only one third of transplant centers would exclude a potential donor with a history of nephrolithiasis.[17] In evaluating a donor with a history of kidney stones, it is critical to assess the current stone burden, the risks of recurrent stone formation, and the effects of previous stones on current renal function. A stone protocol spiral CT scan should be obtained to assess the current stone burden. Metabolic risk factors that need to be excluded and that can be screened on a 24-hour urine collection include hypercalciuria, cystinuria, hyperoxaluria, and hyperuricemia. If previous stones have been passed, records of the analysis of those stones should be obtained. Previous struvite stones suggest previous or ongoing recurrent urinary tract infections. The risk of

recurrent stone disease in patients who have undergone unilateral nephrectomy remains a concern. In one study of 50 patients followed for 5 or more years, 30% developed recurrent stones, with the greatest risk in patients with metabolic abnormalities.[46] The average time to recurrence in this study was 31 months.

The effects of loss of renal mass on the course of stone disease and renal function was examined in a cohort of 3,266 patients with nephrolithiasis, 115 of whom had only one functioning kidney.[47] The reason for the loss of renal function was variable and included infection, obstruction, agenesis, surgery, stones, and other causes. During follow-up, patients with a single functioning kidney had fewer stones than those with two functioning kidneys. The rate of loss of kidney function with age was not greater in single kidney patients vs those with two kidneys. However, subgroup analysis did reveal a greater loss of function in single-kidney males under the age of 45 years old. Measurement of GFR and the urine albumin/creatinine ratio should provide adequate information about the effects stones might have had on kidney function. The presence of a single stone in a potential donor is acceptable if the stone is < 1.5 cm in size or potentially removable during the transplant.[4,48] Contraindications for donation include bilateral stone disease or nephrocalcinosis; struvite stone formation, as these stones are associated with urinary infection; stones associated with inherited disorders such as cystinuria, primary hyperoxaluria, and distal renal tubular acidosis; stones associated with systemic disease such as sarcoidosis or inflammatory bowel disease; or patients contraindications recurrent stone disease requiring medical therapy.

## Genetic Kidney Disease

Autosomal dominant polycystic kidney disease (ADPKD) is the most common genetic renal disease affecting on average 1:1,000 individuals. ADPKD is responsible for 5% to 10% of cases of ESRD. The majority of cases involve a mutation of the polycystin gene located on chromosome 16 (PKD1 locus). Other patients have mutations at the PKD2 locus located on chromosome 4. PKD2 patients have a milder phenotype with later occurrence of cysts and renal failure. There is an as-yet-undefined third locus. The diagnosis of established ADPKD is not difficult: multiple cysts are seen in both kidneys, and most often there is a positive family history. The standard criterion for diagnosis is the presence of three to five cysts in each kidney. The number of cysts should be adjusted for the age of the patient, given that the incidence of simple renal cysts increases with age. In individuals 30, at least two unilateral or bilateral cysts should be detected; in those 30 to 59, at least two cysts in each kidney should be detected; in those > 60, four or more cysts should be detected in each kidney in order to make the diagnosis of polycystic kidney disease.[49]

In donors >30, a negative ultrasound result is very sensitive in excluding ADPKD. The more difficult situation is for younger donors. Nicolau et al. examined the sensitivity and specificity of ultrasound for the diagnosis of ADPKD by comparing ultrasound results with genetic linkage analysis in 319 at-risk individuals, 161 of whom were < 30.[50] Ultrasound had the same sensitivity as linkage analysis in individuals > 30. In those < 30, ultrasound had a sensitivity of 93% and was more sensitive in those with PKD1 than PKD2. CT with contrast and T2-weighted magnetic resonance imaging (MRI) are more sensitive in detecting renal cysts.[51] Ultrasound can detect cysts about 1 cm in size, CT 0.5 cm, and MRI 0.3 cm. Genetic testing for ADPKD by either linkage analysis or direct mutation screening is now commercially available and should be used to help select younger donors of affected family members.

Alport syndrome, also referred to as hereditary nephritis, is a disorder of the glomerular basement membrane manifesting as progressive renal failure and often hearing loss and ocular abnormalities.[52] Alport syndrome is caused by mutations in the type IV collagen gene family. Approximately 80% of cases are inherited in an X-linked fashion, 15% are autosomal recessive, and 5% autosomal dominant. The disease in males begins with asymptomatic hematuria, but progresses to end-stage renal disease (ESRD) by age 30 to 40. Female carriers have microscopic hematuria, with 12% developing ESRD by age 40 and 30% by age 60.[53,54] The reason for the lower incidence in females is related to the degree of random inactivation of the abnormal X chromosome. In evaluating potential donors, it is important to realize that if a male does not have hematuria by age 10 he is unlikely to have the disease.

Thin basement membrane disease, also known as benign familial hematuria, is a cause of asymptomatic microscopic hematuria. There is often a family history of microscopic hematuria and mutations in members of the type IV collagen gene family have been confirmed in some families. In most cases, kidney function and BP are normal, with no proteinuria or extrarenal manifestations. The diagnosis is made if renal biopsy shows diffuse thinning of the glomerular basement membrane. The differential diagnosis includes Alport syndrome, particularly in female carriers, and IgA nephropathy, which is not uncommon in certain populations. For example, in healthy Japanese donors, mesangial IgA deposition was seen in 16% of living donors on zero-hour kidney biopsy samples.[55] This finding was often associated with microscopic hematuria and, in some cases, mild mesangial proliferation. No follow-up of renal function in donors or recipients was provided in this report.[55] Most patients with thin basement membrane disease have an excellent prognosis, although some cases with progressive renal disease have been described.[56] In a potential donor with microscopic hematuria and a negative workup for structural causes of hematuria, a kidney biopsy is indicated in order to make a definitive diagnosis. In view of the uncertainty regarding the course of thin basement membrane disease or of female heterozygotes with Alport syndrome, these individuals should be excluded from being kidney donors.[57]

### Fibromuscular Dysplasia

Fibromuscular dysplasia is detected in 2% to 4% of the population.[58] In a follow-up study of 19 living donors with fibromuscular disease, of whom only one had bilateral disease, no adverse consequences were seen (donor hypertension, progressive kidney disease or proteinuria).[59] Recommendations are not to use donors with severe, diffuse, or bilateral disease.

### Malignancy

Potential donors should be free of malignancy in order to be acceptable candidates. Screening for cancer should follow standard recommendations for periodic health examinations by the United States Preventive Services Task Force (http://www.ahrq.gov/clinic/pocketgd.htm). This includes mammography every 1 to 2 years in women age 50 to 69 with some expert panels recommending beginning at age 40. Cervical cancer screening by PAP testing should be performed in all females younger than age 65 years. The exact method for colon cancer screening is debatable but should include fecal occult blood tests (two samples)

yearly after age 50 combined with flexible sigmoidoscopy every 5 years. Some expert panels recommend colonoscopy every 10 years after age 50 years especially for high-risk individuals such as those with a positive family history of colon cancer. Routine screening for prostate cancer is not recommended.

Patients with prior malignancies with a high potential for metastatic disease, even years following treatment of the tumor, should be excluded from donation. These include breast, bronchial, testicular, and renal cell cancers, as well as melanoma, cholangiocarcinoma, hematological malignancy, and monoclonal gammopathies.[60,61] In potential donors with prior malignancies, it is important to make sure prior treatment has not impaired renal function or increased the risk of donor nephrectomy. Certain low-risk malignancies that have been treated and cured do not exclude donation. These include nonmelanoma skin cancer, colon cancer (Dukes A, > 5 years ago), or carcinoma *in situ* of the cervix.

### Infectious Disease

The presence of infectious disease in the donor is a risk for both the donor and the recipient. It is important to exclude active infection with HIV, hepatitis B and C, tuberculosis, and syphilis in the donor. Other diseases common in specific geographic regions also need to be excluded. For a further discussion see the Amsterdam Forum report.[4] Most adults are cytomegalovirus (CMV) and Epstein-Barr virus (EBV) positive, and this is not a contraindication to donation. However, it is important to test for CMV and EBV antibodies to help in the care of the recipient. A prior history of a urinary tract infection does not exclude donation, unless the infections are recurrent or associated with anatomical abnormalities such as reflux. Asymptomatic bacteruria or active infection has to be treated before donation.

## PREGNANCY AFTER DONOR NEPHRECTOMY

A common question asked by potential female donors is what effects donation will have on future fertility and pregnancies. Wrenshall et al. surveyed 220 women who underwent donor nephrectomy.[62] Of the 144 who responded, 33 had a total of 45 pregnancies. The complication rate was similar to what has been noted in the general population but included a miscarriage rate of 13.3%, preeclampsia in 4.4%, hypertension during pregnancy in 4.4%, and proteinuria in 4.4%. No fetal abnormalities were noted. In another study of 23 donors who became pregnant, renal function assessed 2 to 14 years after pregnancy was not altered beyond the expected changes related to the nephrectomy.[63] The Amsterdam Forum concluded "donor nephrectomy was not detrimental to the prenatal course or outcome of future pregnancies," but did recommend waiting at least 2 months after donor nephrectomy.[4]

## THE ROLE OF THE SOCIAL WORKER IN THE EVALUATION OF THE LIVING DONOR

Clinical transplant social workers are an integral component of the recipient transplant team. Psychosocial issues associated with living donation have been increasingly recognized and necessitate similar access to social work services throughout the donor evaluation process. Fortunately, the majority of donor studies report high donor satisfaction with the experience. Most donors do not regret their decision and would donate again. They feel increased self-worth, have a better quality of life (as compared with the general population), and have a closer relationship with the recipient post transplant.[64,65] However, negative consequences have been reported as a direct result of donation, including depression, worsened relationships, and financial stress.[65] Some living donors feel forgotten. Typically, donors have little or no medical follow-up at their transplant center.

Many transplant programs are now actively attempting to enhance the experience of living donors, and to minimize any undesirable psychosocial risks, by offering comprehensive services through a designated interdisciplinary donor team. Members of the team must not be involved in the recipient's care, in order to avoid any potential conflict of interest between the commitment to the donor and the recipient.

Clinical social workers, an essential part of the donor team, provide a variety of psychosocial, educational, and supportive interventions, both before and after surgery. Discussion of all psychosocial services offered to living donors by social workers is beyond the scope of this section; instead, emphasis is on the pretransplant psychosocial evaluation—one of the most critical aspects of the entire donor process.

## Psychosocial Evaluation

The psychosocial assessment provides valuable information about a living donor's present situation and intentions about donating, and may identify potential vulnerabilities that could affect the donor's outcome. The purpose of the evaluation is not exclusively to rule out a potential donor; rather it is to maximize the donor process by tending to the individual's unique set of circumstances. The psychosocial evaluation is conducted by a trained mental health professional, often a clinical social worker experienced in transplantation. Psychosocial expertise is offered to the multidisciplinary donor team, yet the social worker frequently serves as the prospective living donor's advocate. If an individual is considered to be at greater risk (ie, has a complex psychiatric history, has a history of incarceration or substance abuse, is cognitively impaired, or is a minor), then a full evaluation may be conducted by one or more clinicians in addition to the social workers, such as a psychologist or psychiatrist. Nontraditional donor volunteers, such as coworkers, acquaintances, responders to an appeal, and complete strangers (nondirected donors), also should receive additional scrutiny because little psychosocial data are available about these populations.[12]

Most transplant programs agree that donors require a unique assessment geared towards addressing the individual's psychological, emotional, and social stability to undergo donor surgery. The social worker explores any potential personal, psychological, family, social, or financial constraints, while attempting to understand the motivations for donation. The donor's ability to develop realistic expectations and plans before and after surgery is also assessed. Key questions involve the ability to cope with potential complications, with poor recipient outcome, with changes in bodily appearance, and with changes in the relationship (if any) with the recipient.

A potential LD is usually interviewed alone to ensure that she or he is free to speak comfortably about all psychosocial, family, personal, and related issues. The prospective recipient is rarely involved in the initial interview, because some donors may respond approvingly in front of the recipient and may be less likely to express any fears and objections about donation. However, in some instances—such as when the LD has a limited or no relationship with the recipient—the spouse or partner should be permitted, and even encouraged, to participate in the interview. Cases have been reported in which spouses were displeased they were not included, leading to marital discord.[66,67] Acceptance criteria may vary by program, type of organ to be donated, and type of relationship between donor and recipient. Questions to donors must be goal-oriented with the intention of focusing on the acceptability for proceeding with donation, while also learning how the donor team might best serve the living donor over time.

## Components of a Psychosocial Assessment

### Psychosocial History

The social worker must first elicit necessary personal background information, including the individual's current situation, cognitive functioning, behavioral and emotional health, family, and significant relationships. Other important information to be obtained includes the individual's employment, living arrangements, educational level, hobbies, financial situation, legal status, family and social supports, and cultural or religious beliefs. A thorough mental health history is also essential to understand the living donor's psychological stability and whether donation would compromise it.

The presence of underlying mental illness, cognitive impairments, aberrant prosonality traits, or other factors that may interfere with the prospective donor's ability to make a reasoned decision may preclude donation. A history of anxiety, depression, marital discord, or other concerns is further discussed to determine if donation could exacerbate underlying symptoms. Present and past behaviors are explored because they may be predictors to coping with potential donor outcomes. Donors must understand how donation could affect their mental health.

### Informed Decision Making

According to Rudow et al., prospective donors "must demonstrate adequate decision making capabilities and be able to appreciate the risks and benefits of the procedure."[68] The social worker must ask questions such as these: Is the individual adequately informed about the transplant procedure and capable of understanding the potential risks and benefits of donation (both short-term and long-term)? Is consent truly, thoroughly informed? Is the individual vulnerable in any way to exploitation? Is the individual aware of alternative options for the recipient and the likelihood of the transplant's success? Does the individual recognize the possibility that future health problems related to donation may not be covered by insurance and that the ability to obtain health, disability, or life insurance may be affected? Has the individual read or heard about the potential psychosocial consequences of donation, from the existing literature and other LDs? Donors must be capable of understanding information to make a sound choice and to realistically prepare for the donation and recovery.

In the case of nondirected donation, prospective living donors must be asked their feelings about how recipients are selected and must understand the range of potential recipients who might receive their organ. They must also be aware that they might not even communicate (or meet) with the recipient if mutual consent posttransplant is not obtained.

## *Motivation*

Donation should be voluntary and reasons for donation must be thoroughly explored by the team and the donor. Donor motivation may be influenced by a variety of factors: type of relationship with the recipient, commitment to the recipient, personal beliefs and values, upbringing, religious convictions, or humanitarian reasons. Donors approach their decision from a wide range of social backgrounds, family situations, and educational levels. The social worker must assess whether the volunteer's decision is made freely without any undue pressure or coercion, and whether motivation is consistent with the donor's values and previous behaviors.

Pressure may be more likely when the recipient's death is imminent without a transplant and when no other donor options exist. This is primarily the case in liver or lung transplantation. Family relationships can influence motivation, sometimes to the point of an implied or even explicitly voiced obligation to donate. Siblings, of all relatives, reportedly feel the most pressure to donate.[64] Other family members might fear disapproval if they do not donate and may feel it is expected.[65,69] In contrast, some may be pressured to *not* donate.

Reasons for donating after a public plea on behalf of a certain recipient or for volunteering to help a complete stranger (as in the case of nondirected donation) are not yet fully understood. Motivation must be probed very carefully, but respectfully, when there is no relationship with the recipient. Until recently, the willingness to donate to a stranger was met with suspicion and thought to indicate the presence of psychopathology. Knowing how the prospective donor learned about donation and how the decision was made is important. The decision to donate can be made instantaneously or deliberatively. Some individuals (eg, parents) immediately volunteer once learning of the living donor option. Others take time to logically evaluate the situation and gather relevant information before making a decision. If the decision appears overly impulsive or self-serving, concern is appropriate.

The potential donor should be encouraged to express doubts, ambivalence, or guilt during the interview and must be assured they have the right to opt out with as little guilt as possible. If the social worker senses pressure to donate, it should be further explored. Some individuals may need permission or encouragement to decline donation.

## *Relationship with Recipient*

Donors and recipients historically had to be genetically related. Reasons for donation were more understandable when there was a close bond between the pair. As discussed previously, donors no longer need to be genetically connected for a successful outcome. Thus, psychosocial information is even more critical. Specific questions related to the donor–recipient relationship must be asked. Does the individual have a close relationship with the recipient? How does the individual know the recipient, and for how long? Did the recipient ask the individual to consider donation? If not, how did the individual learn about the option to donate? Does the individual believe the relationship will change depending on the decision to donate or not? If so, how? How does the recipient feel about the donation? Does the individual's family know the recipient? Was anything offered in return for donation?

For genetically unrelated prospective living donors, questions must be tailored to the specific situation to fully understand why the individual wishes to donate and whether expectations about the relationship are realistic.

## *Support System*

Donors must make a temporary lifestyle change and yet continue to meet personal, family, and financial obligations before and after surgery. The social worker must help the individual explore what resources and supports are required and available for donation, while assessing the ability of the individual and family to cope effectively with potential donor-related stresses. The individual must be able to identify people committed to helping throughout the donation process. If the spouse, partner, or family members disagree with the decision to donate, postoperative help may be inadequate. The employer's support is also imperative.

## *Preparedness for Donation*

Prospective donors must be able to appropriately plan to care for themselves, and any dependents, after their surgery. They must also prepare for a temporary role change within their family, social, and work environments. Moreover, they must take into account their finances, so that they are able to meet existing obligations until they have fully recovered. The recovery period may sometimes be difficult and last longer than expected.

Financial questions related to employment include whether they are eligible for any employee benefits; whether they will be able to comfortably take adequate time necessary to recover; whether they will be allowed to perform less labor-intensive interim tasks; whether they have health or life insurance benefits; and whether they are financially secure enough to donate and absorb related expenses. If finances are insufficient so donation would severely compromise a donor's financial situation, the donor team may need to highlight that concern.

The social worker must also raise the questions of necessary legal preparations: undergoing any surgery usually sensitizes people to make plans in the event of a poor outcome. Health-care directives, wills, and parental responsibilities require attention.

## *Assessment and Recommendations*

Once a comprehensive interview is completed, the social worker determines if the information satisfies the requirements of the program, or whether further intervention is necessary to optimize the donor process. Psychosocial factors such as ambivalence, guilt, major mental illness, and active substance abuse increase donor vulnerability and automatically exclude donation. Evidence for a poor support system, strong family opposition, or disregard for financial obligations are potential risk factors for donors and require further assessment.[64,65] The social worker determines if contributing risks might be modified to make donation possible. Psychosocial concerns identified during the interview are shared with the donor, thus providing an opportunity to address issues and develop a plan for resolution or understanding.

Once the social worker has fully assessed the donor's situation, she or he collaborates with the donor team members and highlights any significant findings, including any gaps in knowledge that require specific educational intervention from the team. Ultimately, the donor team must decide how the psychosocial issues will be weighed in the overall process.

## Education and Counseling

Any psychosocial issues identified during the assessment are addressed by direct social work counseling or a referral to an appropriate resource. Frequently, the social worker learns sensitive information (sometimes unrelated to donation) and must make additional recommendations (eg, for therapy for marital problems, for financial or employment assistance). Shover et al. found that the strongest correlate of donor dissatisfaction was the donor's feeling that information given preoperatively had been inadequate and that they were not psychologically prepared for surgery.[70] The social worker attempts to educate and fill any knowledge gaps and may also encourage the donor to speak with previous donors (made available by the program).

The donor social worker should remain available to donors throughout the donation process, earning their trust, helping them feel comfortable, and offering consistent support for any short- or long-term needs.

## ROLE OF THE TRANSPLANT COORDINATOR

The potential donor initiates a relationship with a transplant coordinator. Most often this is a nurse with experience with transplant patients. As the word coordinate suggests, the transplant coordinator is the person that serves as the point of contact for a potential living donor and the medical team. The coordinator is responsible for directing the donor's progress—from inquiry and evaluation to surgery and recovery. The nurse coordinator is also responsible for the education of the donor and family. As the care of the transplant patient becomes more specialized, so does the role of the transplant coordinator. It is becoming more common that transplant centers designate separate coordinators for living organ donors. This coordinator interacts with only the living donor, with the care of the potential recipient being performed by a different nurse coordinator. This allows for a designated professional to devote full attention to the needs of one patient only and avoids a possible conflict that can occur when considering the recipient's needs. A dedicated transplant coordinator often fulfills the role of a donor advocate.

When a potential kidney donor initiates contact with the center, the nurse coordinator screens each person. This is usually done by telephone and includes obtaining a general medical history. The purpose of this screening is to identify obvious contraindications to kidney donation and begin the education process for the donor. If the donor is deemed eligible to proceed, a more detailed medical history is obtained, usually in written form. This first interaction provides an opportunity to discover the motivation of a potential donor and allows the coordinator to establish a relationship between the donor and the transplant program.

The first call is also the beginning of the education process and includes a discussion of the logistics and timetable for evaluation and surgery. Written materials and additional phone and personal contact follow the initial contact. Education is provided about the time necessary to complete the evaluation, the type of medical and psychosocial evaluation that will be performed, as well as what to expect at the time of surgery and during the recovery period. The coordinator is also responsible for educating the donor and ensuring that evaluation is independent of any medical issues of the recipient. It is critical to inform the donor of the right to withdraw the offer of donation at any time.

The medical testing required of a donor is directed by the coordinator, who determines the timing and scheduling of the medical tests. The medical team and consultants that perform the donor evaluation should use the coordinator as the liaison to the patient. The coordinator oversees the completion of the evaluation and is responsible for gathering all completed testresults, arranging for final medical team review, and informing donors of the evaluation results. The coordinator is also responsible for consulting the intended recipient's coordinator or care team so that the scheduling of the transplant is done when both donor and recipient are ready to proceed.

The postoperative care of a kidney donor is often minimal, but the coordinator will continue to assist the donor during this time. Although infrequent, postoperative complications can occur in kidney donors. The coordinator needs to assist the donor and the referring medical team in addressing any postoperative problems that do arise. Finally, the coordinator is responsible for providing the required follow-up information requested by regulatory agencies such as UNOS.

## FINAL SELECTION OF THE DONOR

If there is more than one ABO-compatible, crossmatch-negative donor, then the potential donors need to work with the transplant team to identify the best individual to proceed with the detailed medical and psychosocial evaluation described earlier. The choice of this individual often involves a complex interaction of factors such as the age of the donor, the potential that the recipient will require another transplant in the future, the potential for a 6-antigen-matched donor if siblings are part of this pool, and social and logistics issues. Following the evaluation, the medical team involved with the donor should meet and make a final decision as to whether the donor is acceptable. If there are isolated medical abnormalities that present a potential future risk to the donor, then these risks need to be discussed; as Steiner advocates, quantitative risk estimation should be carried out.[7,8] A difficult issue is how much risk the donor should be allowed to take and who makes the decision (see Chapter 3). Following donor nephrectomy, the transplant center is responsible for the postoperative care related to the procedure and should be involved in the long-term monitoring of living donors.

## References

1. Abecassis M, Adams M, Adams P, et al. Consensus statement on the live organ donor. *JAMA* 2000;284(22):2919–2926.
2. Davis CL. Evaluation of the living kidney donor: Current perspectives. *Am J Kidney Dis* 2004;43(3):508–530.
3. Davis CL, Delmonico FL. Living-donor kidney transplantation: A review of the current practices for the live donor. *J Am Soc Nephrol* 2005;16(7):2098–2110.
4. Delmonico F. A report of the Amsterdam Forum on the Care of the Live Kidney Donor: Data and medical guidelines. *Transplantation* 2005;79(6 Suppl):S53–S66.
5. Kasiske BL, Bia MJ. The evaluation and selection of living kidney donors. *Am J Kidney Dis* 1995;26(2):387–398.
6. Koller H, Mayer G. Evaluation of the living kidney donor. *Nephrol Dial Transplant* 2004;19(Suppl 4):iv41-4.
7. Steiner RW. Risk appreciation for living kidney donors: Another new subspecialty? *Am J Transplant* 2004;4(5):694–697.
8. Steiner RW, Gert B. Ethical selection of living kidney donors. *Am J Kidney Dis* 2000;36(4):677–686.
9. Veitch PS. Evaluation of the potential living kidney donor. *Transplant Proc* 1996;28(6):3553–3555.
10. The consensus statement of the Amsterdam Forum on the Care of the Live Kidney Donor. *Transplantation* 2004;78(4):491–492.
11. Terasaki PI, Cecka JM, Gjertson DW, Takemoto S. High survival rates of kidney transplants from spousal and living unrelated donors. *N Engl J Med* 1995;333(6):333–336.

12. Matas AJ, Garvey CA, Jacobs CL, Kahn JP. Nondirected donation of kidneys from living donors. *N Engl J Med* 2000;343(6):433–436.

13. Ross LF, Zenios S. Practical and ethical challenges to paired exchange programs. *Am J Transplant* 2004;4(10):1553–1554.

14. Sells RA. Paired-kidney-exchange programs. *N Engl J Med* 1997;337(19):1392–1393.

15. Naumovic R, Djukanovic L, Marinkovic J, Lezaic V. Effect of donor age on the outcome of living-related kidney transplantation. *Transplant Int* 2005;18(11):1266–1274.

16. Gabolde M, Herve C, Moulin AM. Evaluation, selection, and follow-up of live kidney donors: a review of current practice in French renal transplant centres. *Nephrol Dial Transplant* 2001;16(10):2048–2052.

17. Bia MJ, Ramos EL, Danovitch GM, et al. Evaluation of living renal donors. The current practice of US transplant centers. *Transplantation* 1995;60(4):322–327.

18. Coresh J, Astor BC, McQuillan G, et al. Calibration and random variation of the serum creatinine assay as critical elements of using equations to estimate glomerular filtration rate. *Am J Kid Dis* 2002;39:920–929.

19. National Kidney Foundation. K/DOQI Clinical Practice Guidelines for Chronic Kidney Disease: Evaluation, Classification, and Stratification. *Am J Kidney Dis* 2002;39 (Suppl 1):S1–S266.

20. Dharnidharka VR, Kwon C, Stevens G. Serum cystatin C is superior to serum creatinine as a marker of kidney function: a meta-analysis. *Am J Kid Dis* 2002;40:221–226.

21. Levey AS, Bosch J, Lewis JB, Greene T, Rogers N, Roth D. A more accurate method to estimate glomerular filtration rate from serum creatinine: a new prediction equation. *Ann Int Med* 1999;130:461–470.

22. Bertolatus JA, Goddard L. Evaluation of renal function in potential living kidney donors. *Transplantation* 2001;71(2):256–260.

23. Rule AD, Gussak HM, Pond GR, et al. Measured and estimated GFR in healthy potential kidney donors. *Am J Kidney Dis* 2004;43(1):112–119.

24. Rule AD, Larson TS, Bergstralh EJ, Slezak JM, Jacobsen SJ, Cosio FG. Using serum creatinine to estimate glomerular filtration rate: accuracy in good health and in chronic kidney disease. *Ann Intern Med* 2004;141(12):929–937.

25. Kapoor A, Kapoor A, Mahajan G, Singh A, Sarin P. Multispiral computed tomographic angiography of renal arteries of live potential renal donors: A review of 118 cases. *Transplantation* 2004;77(10):1535–1539.

23. Cosio FG, Qiu W, Henry ML, et al. Factors related to the donor organ are major determinants of renal allograft function and survival. *Transplantation* 1996;62(11):1571–6.

27. Carter JT, Lee CM, Weinstein RJ, et al. Evaluation of the older cadaveric kidney donor: the impact of donor hypertension and creatinine clearance on graft performance and survival. *Transplantation* 2000;70(5):765–771.

28. Textor SC, Taler SJ, Larson TS, et al. Blood pressure evaluation among older living kidney donors. *J Am Soc Nephrol* 2003;14(8):2159–2167.

29. Textor SC, Taler SJ, Driscoll N, et al. Blood pressure and renal function after kidney donation from hypertensive living donors. *Transplantation* 2004;78(2):276–282.

30. Praga M, Hernandez E, Herrero JC, et al. Influence of obesity on the appearance of proteinuria and renal insufficiency after unilateral nephrectomy. *Kidney Int* 2000;58(5):2111–2118.

31. Chen J, Muntner P, Hamm L, et al. The metabolic syndrome and chronic kidney disease in U.S. adults. *Ann Inter Med* 2004;140:167–174.

32. Schaeffner ES, Kurth T, Curhan GC, et al. Cholesterol and the risk of renal dysfunction in apparently healthy men. *J Am Soc Nephrol* 2003;14:2084–2091.

33. Heimbach JK, Taler SJ, Prieto M, et al. Obesity in living kidney donors: clinical characteristics and outcomes in the era of laparoscopic donor nephrectomy. *Am J Transplant* 2005;5(5):1057–1064.

34. Silveiro SP, da Costa LA, Beck MO, Gross JL. Urinary albumin excretion rate and glomerular filtration rate in single-kidney type 2 diabetic patients. *Diabetes Care* 1998;21(9):1521–1524.

35. Hanley AJ, Williams K, Gonzalez C, et al. Prediction of type 2 diabetes using simple measures of insulin resistance: combined results from the San Antonio Heart Study, the Mexico City Diabetes Study, and the Insulin Resistance Atherosclerosis Study. *Diabetes* 2003;52(2):463–469.

36. Hanson RL, Pratley RE, Bogardus C, et al. Evaluation of simple indices of insulin sensitivity and insulin secretion for use in epidemiologic studies. *Am J Epidemiol* 2000;151(2):190–198.

37. Linne Y, Barkeling B, Rossner S. Natural course of gestational diabetes mellitus: Long term follow up of women in the SPAWN study. *BJOG* 2002;109(11):1227–1231.

38. Seaquist ER, Goetz FC, Rich S, Barbosa J. Familial clustering of diabetic kidney disease. Evidence for genetic susceptibility to diabetic nephropathy. *N Engl J Med* 1989;320(18):1161–1165.

39. Simmons D, Gatland BA, Leakehe L, Fleming C. Frequency of diabetes in family members of probands with non-insulin-dependent diabetes mellitus. *J Intern Med* 1995;237(3):315–321.

40. Cadaver kidney donation. *Lancet* 1973;2(7827):485–486.

41. Malecki MT. Genetics of type 2 diabetes mellitus. *Diabetes Res Clin Pract* 2005;68(Suppl 1):S10.

42. Simmons D, Searle M. Personal paper: Risk of diabetic nephropathy in potential living related kidney donors. *BMJ* 1998;316(7134):846–848.

43. Warram JH, Martin BC, Krolewski AS, Soeldner JS, Kahn CR. Slow glucose removal rate and hyperinsulinemia precede the development of type II diabetes in the offspring of diabetic parents. *Ann Intern Med* 1990;113(12):909–915.

44. Bhadauria RP, Ahlawat R, Kumar RV, Srinadh ES, Banerjee GK, Bhandari M. Donor-gifted allograft lithiasis: Extracorporeal shockwave lithotripsy with over table module using the Lithostar Plus. *Urol Int* 1995;55(1):51–55.

45. Lu HF, Shekarriz B, Stoller ML. Donor-gifted allograft urolithiasis: early percutaneous management. *Urology* 2002;59(1):25–27.

46. Lee YH, Huang WC, Chang LS, et al. The long-term stone recurrence rate and renal function change in unilateral nephrectomy urolithiasis patients. *J Urol* 1994;152(5 Pt 1):1386–1388.

47. Worcester E, Parks JH, Josephson MA, Thisted RA, Coe FL. Causes and consequences of kidney loss in patients with nephrolithiasis. *Kidney Int* 2003;64(6):2204–2213.

48. Rashid MG, Konnak JW, Wolf JS Jr, et al. Ex vivo ureteroscopic treatment of calculi in donor kidneys at renal transplantation. *J Urol* 2004;171(1):58–60.

49. Ravine D, Gibson RN, Walker RG, et al. Evaluation of ultrasonographic diagnostic criteria for autosomal dominant polycystic kidney disease 1. *Lancet* 1994;343(8901):824–827.

50. Nicolau C, Torra R, Badenas C, et al. Autosomal dominant polycystic kidney disease types 1 and 2: Assessment of US sensitivity for diagnosis. *Radiology* 1999;213(1):273–276.

51. Zand MS, Strang J, DumLao M, et al. Screening a living kidney donor for polycystic kidney disease using heavily T2-weighted MRI. *Am J Kidney Dis* 2001;37(3):612–619.

52. Kashtan CE. Familial hematuria due to type IV collagen mutations: Alport syndrome and thin basement membrane nephropathy. *Curr Opin Pediatr* 2004;16(2):177–181.

53. Jais JP, Knebelmann B, Giatras I, et al. X-linked Alport syndrome: Natural history and genotype phenotype correlations in girls and women belonging to 195 families: A "European Community Alport Syndrome Concerted Action" study. *J Am Soc Nephrol* 2003;14(10):2603–2610.

54. Jais JP, Knebelmann B, Giatras I, et al. X-linked Alport syndrome: Natural history in 195 families and genotype-phenotype correlations in males. *J Am Soc Nephrol* 2000;11(4):649–657.

55. Suzuki K, Honda K, Tanabe K, et al. Incidence of latent mesangial IgA deposition in renal allograft donors in Japan. *Kidney Int* 2003;63(6):2286–2294.

56. Nieuwhof CM, de Heer F, de Leeuw P, van Breda Vriesman PJ. Thin GBM nephropathy: Premature glomerular obsolescence is associated with hypertension and late onset renal failure. *Kidney Int* 1997;51(5):1596–1601.

57. Hudson BG, Tryggvason K, Sundaramoorthy M, Neilson EG. Alport's syndrome, Goodpasture's syndrome, and type IV collagen. *N Engl J Med* 2003;348(25):2543–2556.

58. Andreoni KA, Weeks SM, Gerber DA, et al. Incidence of donor renal fibromuscular dysplasia: does it justify routine angiography? *Transplantation* 2002;73(7):1112–1116.

59. Indudhara R, Kenney, Bueschen AJ, Burns JR. Live donor nephrectomy in patients with fibromuscular dysplasia of the renal arteries. *J Urol* 1999;162(3 Pt 1):678–681.

60. Penn I. Transmission of cancer from organ donors. *Ann Transplant* 1997;2(4):7–12.

61. Kauffman HM, McBride MA, Delmonico FL. First report of the United Network for Organ Sharing Transplant Tumor Registry: Donors with history of cancer. *Transplantation* 2000;70(12):1747–1751.

62. Wrenshall LE, McHugh L, Felton P, Dunn DL, Matas AJ. Pregnancy after donor nephrectomy. *Transplantation* 1996;62(12):1934–1936.

63. Buszta C, Steinmuller DR, Novick AC, et al. Pregnancy after donor nephrectomy. *Transplantation* 1985;40(6):651–654.

64. Jacobs C, Johnson E, Anderson K, Gillingham K, Matas A. Kidney transplants from living donors: how donation affects family dynamics. *Adv Ren Replace Ther* 1998;5(2):89–97.

65. Smith MD, Kappell DF, Province MA, et al. Living-related kidney donors: A multicenter study of donor education, socioeconomic adjustment, and rehabilitation. *Am J Kidney Dis* 1986;8(4):223–233.

66. Jacobs CL, Garvey C, Roman D, Kahn J, Matas AJ. Evolution of a nondirected kidney donor program: lessons learned. *Clin Transpl* 2003: 283–291.

67. Jacobs CL, Roman D, Garvey C, Kahn J, Matas AJ. Twenty-two nondirected kidney donors: an update on a single center's experience. *Am J Transplant* 2004;4(7):1110–1116.

68. Rudow DL, Brown RS, Jr. Evaluation of living liver donors. *Prog Transplant* 2003;13(2):110–116.

69. Pradel FG, Mullins CD, Bartlett ST. Exploring donors' and recipients' attitudes about living donor kidney transplantation. *Prog Transplant* 2003;13(3):203–210.

70. Schover LR, Streem SB, Boparai N, Duriak K, Novick AC. The psychosocial impact of donating a kidney: long-term follow-up from a urology based center. *J Urol* 1997;157(5):1596–1601.

71. USRDS 2005 Annual Data Report: Atlas of End-Stage Renal Disease in the United States, National Institutes of Health, National Institute of Diabetes and Digestive and Kidney Diseases, Bethesda, MD, 2005. 2005.

## 15.2   THE MARGINAL DONOR

*E. Steve Woodle, MD, Mahmound El Khatib, MD*

### BACKGROUND: THE ORGAN DONOR SHORTAGE

The disparity between donor kidney supply and the kidney transplant waiting list in the United States has progressively increased since the Scientific Registry of Transplant Recipients (SRTR) initiated data collection in 1988. At present, over 66,000 patients with end-stage renal disease are awaiting deceased donor kidney transplantation in the United States.[1] Recognition of this progressive disparity in donor kidney supply and demand has resulted in a remarkable increase in the application of living donor kidney transplantation in the United States. The number of living donor kidney transplants in the United States has increased from 3,088 in 1994 to 6,991 in 2004.[1]

Increasing acceptance of living donor kidney transplantation in the United States has led to an expansion of acceptance criteria for living donations. In the early 1990s, improvements in immunosupppression and in kidney allograft survival in living unrelated donors led to a progressive increase in their use as living kidney donors. More recently, altruistic living kidney donation and paired donation have enjoyed increasing acceptance in renal transplantation.[1–6]

Another approach toward increasing living donor kidney transplantation has been acceptance of "marginal" living kidney donors. This approach is analogous to the increased use of "extended criteria donors" in deceased donor transplantation. The purpose of this chapter is to describe the more common conditions encountered in living donors that connote an increased risk to either the donor or recipient in terms of renal function, kidney allograft survival, or patient survival.

### THE MARGINAL LIVING KIDNEY DONOR: UNDERLYING CONDITIONS

#### Hypertension

Hypertension is widely considered to have approached epidemic proportions in the U.S. population, with estimates exceeding 50,000,000 affected individuals. In addition, with the substantial increase in obesity in the United States, the rate of increase in hypertension incidence is also expected to rise for the foreseeable future. With the concomitant aging of the U.S. population, it is widely believed that transplant programs will be faced with a progressive increase in the proportion of willing living donors who have hypertension. Recently, a number of articles have dealt with the issue of the hypertensive living donor, however, this is a field that has yet to reach a consensus.[7–10] Although the overwhelming majority of hypertensive individuals do not develop renal failure,[11] hypertension has been shown to be a leading cause for exclusion of willing living kidney donors.[12] These observations have argued for modifications in the selection criteria for hypertensive living kidney donors.[7] Recent estimates have indicated that 17% of living donors are rejected because of hypertension or proteinuria, and that up to 40% of those rejected had mild hypertension or proteinuria and may have been acceptable for living donation.[18] This study also estimated that up to 3% of wait-listed candidates may be able to be transplanted with mildly hypertensive donors.[18]

Central to the argument for the use of hypertensive living donors are the long-term effects of living donor nephrectomy on donor blood pressure, proteinuria, and renal function. Several studies have reported long-term follow-up of living donors[13–16] (Table 15.2-1). These studies have demonstrated that there appears to be a small increase in the risk of hypertension and proteinuria in living donors; however, the risk of developing renal failure does not appear to be increased.[13–16] Two important questions must be asked if donors with hypertension are to be accepted: (1) are these donors at increased risk for exacerbation of hypertension and hypertension-related morbidity?; and (2) are the recipients of kidneys from hypertensive individuals at increased risk for allograft loss, death, or other morbidities?[17] In addition, it is recommended that programs considering using hypertensive living kidney donors maintain long-term follow-up on these donors so that meaningful data can be collected to aid in determination of long-term risks.[17]

Textor and colleagues have recently reported on experience with hypertensive living donors.[8] This experience indicated that mildly hypertensive living donors can be carefully selected using 24-hour blood pressure monitoring and careful assessment for proteinuria and microalbuminuria. Twenty-four-hour blood pressure monitoring provides a means for obtaining blood pressures

**TABLE 15.2-1**

## LONG-TERM EFFECTS OF LIVING DONOR NEPHRECTOMY

| Reference | Year | # Patients | Follow-up (yrs) | Hypertension* | Proteinuria* | ESRF (%)* |
|---|---|---|---|---|---|---|
| Najarian[13] | 1992 | 57 | >20 | ↑ | ↑ | 0 |
| Fehman-Ekhom[14] | 2001 | 402 | 12 + 8 | ↔ | ↔ | 0.3 |
| Goldfarb[15] | 2001 | 70 | >20 | ↔ | ↑ | 0 |
| Ramcharan[16] | 2002 | 464 | 20-37 | ↔ | ↔ | 0.3 |

*Compared to general population or controlled subjects.
↔ (similar), ↑ (higher), ↓ (lower).

by an automated blood pressure cuff at defined intervals (usually at 15-minute intervals while awake, and 1-hour intervals while sleeping) with recording of values. This approach provides a means for assessing blood pressure during normal daily activities. An important positive sign for potential donors is the presence of a "nocturnal dip," or reduction in blood pressure during sleep. Selected hypertensive donors are allowed to undergo transplantation after agreeing to adopt a healthy lifestyle. Textor and colleagues found that blood pressure control and microalbuminuria actually improved 1 year after living kidney donation. These data are intriguing, as they suggest that living kidney donation, when employed with the requirement for adoption of a healthy lifestyle, may actually favorably impact long-term renal function and cardiovascular risk. However, the durability of lifestyle modification in these patients remains to be demonstrated. Nevertheless, these data are encouraging and require validation by other studies.

Evaluation for hypertension in the potential living donor should include at least two blood pressure measurements by trained professionals. Elevated blood pressures should be evaluated by 24-hour blood pressure monitoring studies. At present, our recommendations for programs that wish to use donors with mild hypertension include the following:

1. Hypertension must be treated with diet, exercise, adoption of a healthy lifestyle, and at most, a single antihypertensive agent at a reasonable dose.

2. Obesity must be addressed by a weight-loss program.

3. Proteinuria and microalbuminuria must be determined.

4. Substantial microalbuminuria or proteinuria are grounds for rejection as a kidney donor.

5. Chest x-ray, electrocardiogram, echocardiogram, and fundoscopy should be performed.

6. Transplant programs and donors must agree to long-term follow-up for renal function, blood pressure, cardiovascular events, and survival.

### Advanced Age

Donors above the age of 60 are a known risk factor for delayed graft function and reduced renal allograft survival in deceased donor transplantation. Although data are not as striking in living donor kidney transplantation, renal allografts from elderly donors are clearly inferior. Comparison of 1 year results in 19 donors above the age of 60 compared to 125 donors below the age of 60

demonstrated equivalent graft survival at 1 year; however, renal function (mean serum creatinine and creatinine clearance) was lower in recipients of older donor kidneys.[19] Another study found no difference in renal allograft survival in 35 living donor renal allografts above the age of 60 compared to a control group of living donor renal allografts below the age of 60.[20] In a larger series that compared donors beyond the age of 65 ($n = 26$), a significant difference was observed in graft survival when compared to the control group (1-, 3-, 5-year Kaplan-Meier graft survival—donors 65 years of age, 88%, 79%, and 68%; donors less than 65 years of age, 90%, 82%, 74%).[21] The larger series and the use of 65 years as a cutoff rather than 60 years may explain the difference in these studies. Nevertheless, the absolute difference in 5-year graft survival was only 6%. In summary, these experiences provide evidence that living donor kidneys from donors above the age of 60 provide acceptable short- and long-term renal function.

### Obesity

Obesity is now recognized as an independent cardiovascular risk factor and has also been shown to be a significant risk factor for complications following major surgery, including living kidney donation.[22,23] Increasing experience with laparoscopic donor nephrectomy has led to a generalized recognition that nephrectomy is technically easier in obese patients than is open donor nephrectomy.[22] As a result, transplant surgeons have been less reluctant in accepting obese donors for laparoscopic donation. However, recent reports have provided evidence that obesity is a significant risk factor for end stage renal disease.[24] In addition, limited data also exist that suggest that unilateral nephrectomy is associated with increased risk of proteinuria and renal failure 10 to 20 years after nephrectomy.[25] In this study, obese patients had an average body mass index (BMI) of 31.6 kg/m$^2$ compared to 24.3 kg/m$^2$ in the nonobese group. These data are cause for a cautious approach in the use of obese living donors and also for strong advocation for adoption of a healthy lifestyle for obese donors.

### Nephrolithiasis

Opinions differ regarding the use of donors with nephrolithiasis. Clearly, any donor with nephrolithiasis and renal dysfunction should be excluded, as should donors with multiple renal stones. However, donors with one or two small stones, particularly if the stones are small (< 1.5 cm in size), and the donors of middle age or beyond may be reasonable donors. These donors should be evaluated with 24-hour urine collections for assessment of calcium, urate, and oxalate, and renal stones should be submitted, if possible, for chemical characterization. Serum calcium and parathyroid hormone levels(PTH) should also be measured. Donors with nephrolithiasis should undergo donation only after appropriate informed consent of both the donor and the recipient.

### Proteinuria

Not all proteinuria is necessarily an indication of the presence of intrinsic renal disease. Benign orthostatic proteinuria, diagnosed by split urine collection obtained while ambulatory during the day and another collection while laying down at night, is clearly not a contraindication to kidney donation. In the absence of active infection and benign orthostatic proteinuria, significant proteinuria requires a full evaluation for living donors.

### Hematuria

Persistent hematuria in living donors in the absence of urinary tract infection should first be evaluated by imaging studies, most often computed tomography (CT) or magnetic resonance imaging (MRI). An absence of lesions on imaging studies requires biopsy if the individual still wishes to donate. Previous experience in 512 living donors demonstrated that persistent, asymptomatic hematuria had a 2.7% incidence.[26] Renal biopsy in nine patients to evaluate unexplained hematuria revealed normal kidneys in two patients, thin basement membrane nephropathy in five patients, IgA nephropathy in one patient, and moderate unexplained glomerulosclerosis in one patient. Four patients (two with normal biopsies and two with thin basement membrane nephropathy) donated.[26] This experience indicates that unexplained hematuria in the absence of anatomic lesions is commonly associated with significant pathology on renal biopsy and supports the use of renal biopsy in these potential donors.

### Smoking

Smoking may be the single most significant cardiovascular risk factor in the general population. The increasing requirement for adoption of a healthy lifestyle prior to living donation has led to an increasing number of transplant programs to require potential living donors to cease smoking prior to donation. The best data on the risk of smoking and renal disease were published in a study of subjects in Okinawa, Japan.[27] The development of significant proteinuria in men was shown to be associated with the number of cigarettes smoked. Smoking was associated with proteinuria at a relative risk of 1.32, similar to the risk associated with hypertension (RR 1.56) and BMI > 25 (RR 1.45). These data argue strongly for a requirement for living donors to cease smoking prior to kidney donation.

### Drug Abuse

Drug abuse is an occasional problem encountered during evaluation of living donors. In evaluating these donors, the drug being abused and the route of administration (parenteral vs oral) are important to take into consideration. Certainly, active parenteral drug abuse by a potential donor is an absolute contraindication to living donation due to the potential risk of disease transmission, including hepatic B and C and HIV. These donors should be documented and examined and tested to prove abstinence, and many programs may require successful completion of a drug abuse rehabilitation program. Certain abused drugs, including heroin and cocaine, are associated with renal injury, and any patient with a history of abuse of these drugs should have careful evaluation of renal function.

## FAMILIAL GENETIC DISEASES

### Polycystic Kidney Disease

Autosomal dominant polycystic kidney disease (ADPKD) is a relatively common condition requiring transplantation. Living related donors for patients with ADPKD may also carry the abnormal gene; however, phenotypic expression of the gene in the form of detectable renal cysts may not occur until 30 or 40 years of age or later. The goal of screening living donors for ADPKD is to exclude the possibility that the donor will develop significant disease in the future. Living related donors for patients with ADPKD have traditionally been screened with noninvasive procedures such as ultrasound or MRI.[28] The diagnosis of ADPKD by ultrasound requires demonstration of two or more cysts on one kidney, with at least one cyst on the contralateral kidney.[29] For donors above the age of 30, ultrasound has a negative predictive value of 100%; however, in donors ages 20 to 29 years, the negative predictive value of ultrasound drops to about 96%.[28] In this age group, T2-weighted MRI has been shown to be superior.[28] Genetic testing also provides an alternative; however, these tests are not as widely available as ultrasound and MRI and take substantially longer.

### Alport Syndrome

Alport syndrome (AS) most commonly results from a heritable defect in the type IV collagen (COL4A5) gene located on the X chromosome. AS is characterized clinically by a progressive nephritis associated with hematuria, hearing loss, and ocular changes that is much less severe in women than in men. Carriers can be reliably identified by the presence of hematuria, as hematuria is present in 95% of carriers and is almost always absent in those who do not carry the defective gene.[30] In a study of 295 AS families, Jais et al. demonstrated that renal failure and deafness prior to the age of 50 is much more common in men (90% and 80%) than in women (10% and 12%). Women, however, do appear to be at increased risk of developing renal failure after the age of 60. However, prediction of risk for development of renal failure is difficult as considerable intrafamilial variation exists in phenotypic severity of disease. However, proteinuria and hearing loss do identify those at risk for developing renal failure (AS1). Our approach toward the use of donors from AS families is to assess for the presence of hematuria. If present, the patient is considered to be a carrier. All carriers should undergo evaluation for proteinuria and hearing loss. Those with proteinuria or hearing loss are excluded from living donation. Middle-aged donors without proteinuria or hearing loss may be potential candidates, and their inclusion as living donors requires appropriate informed consent from donors and recipients.

### Sickle Cell Trait

Sickle cell disease is a relatively uncommon cause of renal failure; however, patients with sickle cell disease will commonly have potential living donors that carry a single copy of the autosomal recessive sickle cell gene, a condition referred to as sickle cell trait. Sickle cell disease causes renal failure as a result of red blood cell sickling in the renal medulla, with loss of vasa recta and papillary scarring. Papillary necrosis may also be observed. The increased sickling in the medulla is due to the relatively low oxygen tension in the medulla compared to the renal cortex. These medullary lesions result in an inability to concentrate urine, which is the earliest manifestation of the disease.

Donors with sickle cell trait are at low risk of developing renal failure; however, these donors should be evaluated for early signs of sickle cell nephropathy. In addition to the standard evaluation procedures for renal function in living donors, potential donors with sickle cell trait should also undergo testing for renal concentrating ability. Evidence of significant reductions in renal concentrating ability in living donors with sickle cell trait, particularly in younger living donors, should preclude their use as living donors.

## Thin Basement Membrane Disease

Thin basement membrane disease (TBMD) is an inherited condition manifested by thinning of the glomerular basement membrane and is associated with the clinical manifestation of hematuria.[31] TBMD is relatively common, and has been estimated to affect more than 1% of the general population. In general, patients with TBMD have an excellent prognosis and are at a very low risk for renal failure; however, this risk is significantly higher than in the general population. Although less than 1% of patients with TBMD develop renal failure, development of renal failure appears to be idiosyncratic, and there are currently no means for predicting which patients are at the highest risk for developing renal failure. Patients with TBMD must be distinguished from those with Alport syndrome. The use of living related donors for patients with TBMD and renal failure is controversial, in part because the risk of donation is very difficult to define. When confronted with a patient who has developed renal failure and is demonstrated on native kidney biopsy to have TBMD, care should be taken in evaluating donors that are genetically related. The first step in evaluating related donors of patients with TBMD is microscopic examination of urinary sediment for the presence of erythrocytes and dipstick testing for hemoglobin. The most conservative course of action is to exclude donors with hematuria, even though they may be at low risk of developing renal failure even with kidney donation. When possible, use of unrelated live donors is preferable due to lack of risk of TBMD. Further advances in understanding of TBMD is needed to provide better guidance for evaluation of living donors for patients with TBMD.

## PHYSICAL ANOMALIES IN THE DONOR KIDNEY

### Cysts and Small Renal Cell Cancers

Renal cysts are not uncommonly encountered on living donor-imaging studies obtained prior to donation. Historically, small renal cysts were often missed when arteriography was used exclusively for donor imaging. However, with increasing use of MRI and CT scans, detection of isolated or a few cysts in donors is encountered not uncommonly. Once cysts are noted, they must be determined to be either simple or complex cysts by additional imaging studies if the initial study is inconclusive. The type of imaging study used to determine the presence or absence of a solid component in a renal cyst may vary among institutions. Simple cysts can be considered to be benign; however, the presence of a solid component implies a risk of malignancy, and although this risk is low, these cysts must be considered malignant until proven benign by excisional biopsy. Standard surgical approaches toward small (1- to 2-cm) complex cysts are to excise the cyst at the time of donor nephrectomy and exclude malignancy by frozen section. With a negative frozen section, preoperative informed consent,

and consultation with the recipient family following frozen section, we proceed with transplantation of these kidneys. Final pathologic diagnosis must be obtained and communicated to the donor and recipient.

Controversy exists over the malignant potential of small (< 2-cm) renal cell cancers (RCCs), as many experts do not consider these lesions to be malignant. The Israel Penn International Transplant Tumor Registry (IPITTR) has reported on a series of kidney donors with small (< 2-cm) RCCs who underwent nephrectomy *ex vivo* bench resection of the small RCCs with subsequent transplantation of the kidney.[32] No RCC recurrence has been noted to date. We currently recommend this approach for small RCCs, but only with appropriate informed consent of both donor and recipient.

### Arterial Anomalies

Almost half of the general population has single renal arteries bilaterally (REF). This implies that half of the population will have at least one kidney with more than one renal artery. For many years, the left kidney has been the preferred kidney for transplantation, as the right renal vein is substantially shorter in length than the left renal vein. However, with a significant frequency, the left kidney (or both kidneys) will have multiple vessels, requiring arterial reconstruction of accessory vessels at the time of transplantation. Many transplant programs now perform laparoscopic donor nephrectomy exclusively, thereby providing increasing technical challenges for reconstructing donor arterial vessels that have less length than those traditionally obtained by open donor nephrectomy.

In 350 consecutive laparoscopic living donors evaluated at our institution, variations in renal arterial anatomy have not precluded the use of a living donor (E. Steve Woodle and Joseph Buell, unpublished data). Three patients, however, have required use of an interposition segment of epigastric artery or vein to reconstruct an accessory artery. The primary venous anomaly that we have encountered has been a retroaortic renal vein or a periaortic renal vein collar. We have performed three left donor nephrectomies in patients with these venous anomalies.

### Fibromuscular Dysplasia

After multiple renal arteries, fibromuscular dysplasia (FMD) is the most common anatomic arterial abnormality encountered in living kidney donors. FMD has been reported to occur in 1% to 4.4 % of potential living donors.[33] A number of reports exist describing experience with kidney donation from donors with FMD.[33–36] In general, these studies indicate that carefully selected donors with FMD can provide renal allografts with reasonable graft survival rates and that the risk of progressive renal disease and renal failure is low. However, following donation, a subset of patients will require antihypertensive therapy, although the degree of hypertension was mild in most cases. The limited data on hypertension development in patients with FMD do not appear to be affected by kidney donation.

Our current recommended criteria for use of donors with FMD include evaluation by 24-hour ambulatory blood pressure monitoring and 24-hour urine collection for protein and albumin measurement. Selection of donors includes assessment of the extent of FMD in the kidney to be donated and the kidney to remain with the donor, age of the donor, menopausal status of the donor, and degree of hypertension and renal function in the donor.

# References

1. Scientific Registry of Transplant Recipients Web site. www.ustransplant.org.

2. Jacobs CL, Roman D, Garvey C, Kahn J, Matas AJ. Twenty-two non-directed kidney donors: an update on a single center's experience. *Am J Transplant* 2004;4:1110–1116.

3. Woodle ES, Boardman R, Bohnengel A, Downing K, for the Ohio Solid Organ Transplant Consortium Kidney Transplant Committee. Influence of educational programs on perceived barriers toward living donor kidney exchange programs (LDKEPs). *Transplant Proc* 2005; 37:602–604.

4. Woodle ES, Rees M, Bohnengel A, et al. A consideration of critical mass in living donor kidney exchange programs. (abstract) *Am J Transplant* 2005;5:373.

5. Delmonico FL, Morrissey PE, Lipkowitz GS, Stoff JS, Himmelfarb J, Harmon W, et al. Donor kidney exchanges. *Am J Transplant* 2004; 4:1628–1634.

6. Montgomery RA, Zachary A, Ratner LE, et al. Clinical results from transplanting incompatible live donor/recipient pairs using paired kidney donation. *JAMA* 2005;294:1655–1663.

7. Textor SC, Taler SJ, Larson TS, et al. Blood pressure evaluation among older living kidney donors. *J Am Soc Nephrol* 2003;14: 2159–2167.

8. Textor SC, Taler SJ, Prieto M, et al. Hypertensive living renal donors have lower blood pressures and urinary microalbumin one year after nephrectomy. *Am J Transplant* 2003;3:192 (abstract).

9. Torres VE, Offord KP, Anderson CF, et al. Blood pressure determinants in living-related renal allograft donors and their recipients. *Kidney Int* 1987;31:1383-1390.

10. Karpinski M, Knoll G, Cohn A, Yang R, Garg A, Storsley L. The impact of accepting living kidney donors with mild hypertension or proteinuria on transplantation rates. *Am J Kidney Dis* 2006;47:317–323.

11. Beevers D, Lip G. Does non-malignant essential hypertension cause renal damage? A clinical view. *J Hum Hypertens* 1996;10:695–699.

12. Fehrman-Ekholm I, Gab el H, Magnusson G. Reasons for not accepting living kidney donors. *Transplantation* 1996;61:1264–1265.

13. Najarian JS, Chavers BM, McHugh LE, Matas AJ. Twenty years or more of follow-up of living kidney donors. *Lancet* 1992;340:807–810.

14. Fehrman-Ekholm I, Duner F, Brink B, Tyden G, Elinder CG. No evidence of accelerated loss of kidney function in living kidney donors: results from a cross-sectional follow-up. *Transplantation* 2001;72:444–449.

15. Goldfarb DA, Matin Sf, Braun WE, et al. Renal outcome 25 years after donor nephrectomy. *J Urol* 2001;166:2043–2047.

16. Ramcharan T, Matas AJ. Long-term (20–37 years) follow-up of living kidney donors. *Am J Transplant* 2002;2:959–964.

17. Matas AJ. Transplantation using marginal living donors. *Am J Kidney Dis* 2006;47: 355–355.

18. Karpinski M, Knoll G, Cohn A, et al. The impact of accepting living kidney donors with mild hypertension or proteinuria on transplantation rates. *Am J Kidney Dis* 317–323.

19. Giessing M, Slowinski T, Deger S, et al. 20 year experience with elderly donors in living renal transplantation. *Transplant Proc* 2003;35: 2855–2857.

20. Berardinelli L, Beretta C, Raiteri M, Carini M. Early and long term results using older kidneys from cadaver or living donors. *Clin Transplant* 2001;157–166.

21. Ivanovski N, Popov Z, Kolevski P, et al. Living related renal transplantation-the use of advanced age donors. *Clin Nephrol* 2001;55: 309–312.

22. Heimbach JK, Taler SJ, Prieto M, et al. Obesity in living kidney donors: clinical characteristics and outcomes in the era of laparoscopic donor nephrectomy. *Am J Transplant* 2005;5:1057.

23. Pevavento TE, Henry ML, Falkenhain ME, Obese living kidney donors: Short term results and possible implications. *Transplantation* 1999;68: 1491–1496.

24. Hsu CY, McCulloch CE, Iribarren C, Darbinian J, Go AS. Body mass index and risk for end-stage renal disease. *Ann Int Med* 2006;144: 21–28.

25. Praga M, Hernandez E, Herrero JC, et al. Influence of obesity on the appearance of proteinuria and renal insufficiency after unilateral nephrectomy. *Kidney Int* 2000;58: 2111–2118.

26. Koushik R, Garvey C, Manivel JC, Matas JA, Kasiske BL. Persistent, asymptomatic, microscopic hematuria in prospective kidney donors. *Transplantation* 2005;80:1425–1429.

27. Tozawa M, Iseki K, Iseki C, et al. Influence of smoking and obesity on the development of proteinuria. *Kidney Int* 2002;62:956–962.

28. Zand MS, Strang J, DumLao M, et al. Screening a living kidney donor for polycystic kidney disease with heavily T2 weighted MRK. *Am j Kidney Dis* 2001;37:612–619.

29. Ravine D, Gibson RN, Walker RG, et al. Evaluation of ultrasonographic diagnostic criteria for autosomal dominant polycystic kidney disease1. *Lancet* 1994;343:824–827.

30. Jais JP, Knebelmann B, Giatras I, et al. X linked Alport syndrome: natural history and genotype-phenotype correlations in girls and women belonging to 195 families: A "European Community Alport Syndrome Concerted Action" Study. *J Am Soc Nephrol* 2003;14: 2603–2610.

31. Tonna S, Wang YY, MacGregor D, et al. The risks of thin basement membrane nephropathy. *Semin Nephrol* 2005;25:171–175.

32. Buell, JF, Hanaway MJ, Thomas MJ, et al. Donor kidneys with small renal cell cancers: Can they be transplanted? *Transplant Proc* 2005;37, 581–582.

33. Andreoni KA, Weeks SM, Gerber DA, et al. Incidence of donor renal fibromuscular dysplasia: does it justify routine angiography? *Transplantation* 2002;73:1112–1116.

34. Cragg AH, Smith TP, Thomson BH, et al. Incidental fibromuscular dysplasia in potential renal donors: Long-term clinical follow-up. *Radiology* 1989;172:145–147.

35. Kolettis PN, Bugg CE, Lockhart ME, Bynon SJ, Burns JR. Outcomes for live donor renal transplantation using kidneys with medial fibroplasias. *Urology* 2004;63:656–659.

36. Nahas WC, Lucon AM, Mazzucchi E, et al. Kidney transplantation: The use of living donors with renal artery lesions. *J Urol* 1998;160:1244–1247.

# 15.3   IMMUNOLOGIC EVALUATION

*Andrea A. Zachary, PhD*

## INTRODUCTION

The allogeneic transplant provides both a physiologic reconstitution of a patient in end-stage organ failure and an immunologic provocation. Whether one subscribes to the self/non-self-theory of immunogenicity or the "danger hypothesis,"[1] there is sufficient trauma associated with transplant surgery to account for either mechanism. It is now recognized that an injurious immunologic response to alloantigens can occur in transplants of all types of organs and most, if not all, tissues. However, the susceptibility to immunologic damage varies according to the amount of target present on the tissue (high in lung and kidney and low in liver), the tissue mass (high in liver and lung, low in pancreas), the amount of soluble antigen produced (high in liver), and the physiologic condition of the organ. This chapter focuses on immunologic aspects of the donor in kidney transplantation; however the issues discussed here can be applied to transplants of other organs as well and should always be considered in live donor transplantation.

There are several known (and almost certainly several unknown) systems of alloantigens. Both between and within these systems, antigens vary in their expression and immunogenicity. Further, the rejection risk associated with the donor's phenotype is determined not only by the nature of the donor antigens but also by the recipient's immunologic history and capability. Immunologic evaluation of the donor consists of identifying clinically relevant donor alloantigens and assessing the risk they represent, individually and collectively, for early rejection, reduced graft survival, and access to future transplantation. This chapter discusses the various known antigen systems, factors related to their roles as both sensitizing agents and targets, and methods for defining those systems in donors. It is difficult to discuss the immunologic evaluation of the donor without some discussion of the recipient. However, because immunologic issues of the recipient are the topic of another chapter in this book (see Chapter 13), discussion of recipient factors will be limited, here, to what is necessary for clarity.

## ALLOANTIGEN SYSTEMS

Three types of alloantigen systems are considered here: red blood cell antigens, human leukocyte antigens (HLA), and minor histocompatibility antigens.

### Red Blood Cell Antigens

There are several alloantigen systems that, by virtue of the way they are tested or were initially defined, are considered red blood cell antigens. Among these, the antigens of the ABO system are most relevant to renal transplantation. Antigens of the ABO system are expressed on a variety of tissues including the vascular endothelium and convoluted distal and collecting tubules of the kidney.[2] Antibodies to these antigens develop early in life, possibly as a result of exposure to microbes with cell walls bearing cross-reactive epitopes. The Lewis antigen system has also been reported to be relevant in renal transplantation.[3] Lewis blood group substances are produced in the kidney where they may serve as a target for antibodies. Early reports suggested that other red cell antigens, such as Rh, might act as minor histocompatibility antigens in transplants that are perfectly matched for HLA.[4]

### HLA: The Major Histocompatibility System

The HLA system encodes the major histocompatibility antigens, so called because a difference of a single antigen, between donor and recipient, will result in graft rejection in the absence of immunosuppression. There are nine different types of HLA antigen that are grouped into two classes based on differences in their structure, function, and phenotypic expression. There are three types of class I antigen, A, B, and Cw (the w designation has been retained to differentiate these antigens from complement components), and six types of class II antigen, those encoded by the DRB1; 3, 4, and 5 loci; DQ; and DP. Although matching for deceased donor transplants in the United States has considered only the HLA-A, -B, and -DRB1 antigens, there have been reports of hyperacute and acute rejections mediated by antibody to all but the DP antigens.[5] Individuals may vary in the number of HLA antigens they possess either by virtue of homozygosity at one or more loci or by the number of DRB loci they have on each chromosome. All chromosomes carry DRB1, and some chromosomes have another DR-encoding locus: DRB3, 4, or 5. Chromosomes carrying the DRB1-encoded antigens DR1, 8, or 10 have no other DRB locus, whereas all others have one additional DRB locus as shown in Table 15.3-1. Exceptions are the rare DR1 that also has DRB5 and the uncommon DR7 without DRB4. Thus, an

**TABLE 15.3-1**

## COMMON DR GENE COMBINATIONS

| DRB1 Antigen Present | Other DRB Loci Present | | |
| --- | --- | --- | --- |
| | DRB3 (DR52) | DRB4 (DR53) | DRB5 (DR51) |
| 1 | | | |
| 4 | | + | |
| 7 | | + | |
| 8 | | | |
| 9 | | + | |
| 10 | | | |
| 11 (5) | + | | |
| 12 (5) | + | | |
| 13 (6) | + | | |
| 14 (6) | + | | |
| 15 (2) | | | + |
| 16 (2) | | | + |
| 17 (3) | + | | |
| 18 (3) | + | | |

individual may have as few as 6 HLA antigens, if they have only one DR locus and are homozygous at all loci (an extremely rare occurrence), or as many as many as 14 HLA antigens, if they have two DR loci on each chromosome and are heterozygous for each HLA locus. The HLA system is the most polymorphic genetic system known with $1.47 \cdot 10^{17}$ different phenotypes possible at the allele level and $3.85 \cdot 10^9$ phenotypes possible at the level of serologically defined antigens (considering the HLA-A, -B, -DRB1, and -DQB loci) [calculated using data from Schreuder et al.[6]]. Corresponding antigens have not been determined for all HLA alleles; however, current, sensitive methods of antibody detection suggest that the number of serologically defined antigens is underestimated. Thus, the likelihood of an unrelated donor being well matched is very small and limited to those recipients whose phenotypes contain the most common antigens or to donors who are homozygous at several loci.

The genes encoding the HLA antigens are very closely linked and inherited from each parent as a group known as a haplotype (from haploid genotype). In transplants between a parent and a child, the donor will be haplo-identical to the recipient. Considering HLA-A, B, Cw, DR, and DQ antigens, transplants between sibs can be HLA identical, haploidentical, or completely disparate with probabilities of 0.25, 0.5, and 0.25, respectively. This is because 98% of the time, haplotypes are inherited intact without genetic recombination. The degree of antigen disparity between donor and recipient may be reduced when parents share one or more antigens. There is a high frequency of recombination between DQ and DP; therefore, sibs that are otherwise HLA identical may be disparate for DP. The immunologic relevance of DP mismatches will be discussed later.

### Other Antigen Systems

Rejection of organs from ABO-compatible, HLA-identical donors has led to investigations of other potential alloantigens. Such antigens include MICA, the series of minor histocompatibility antigens that includes HLA1-8, HB-1, and H-Y, and putative vascular endothelial cell antigens.

MICA and MICB are antigens that are encoded by genes, within the HLA gene complex, located close to the HLA-B locus. MICA antigens are found on the epithelium of the thymus and gut where they are not expressed constitutively; rather they are stress induced.

Minor histocompatibility antigens are well defined in the mouse, with different strains having 20 to 40 different minor histocompatibility antigens. It has been demonstrated in the mouse model that the effects of minor antigen mismatches are additive with multiple disparities of minor antigens being immunologically equivalent to a major histocompatibility antigen disparity. Several minor antigens have been defined in humans. As in the mouse, they are encoded by genes on different chromosomes. Interest in these antigens has been almost exclusively in the area of hematopoietic stem cell transplantation where mismatches of these antigens can result in graft-versus-host disease.

The vascular endothelium of the transplanted organ provides the first interface with the recipient. Antibody-mediated rejection that occurs in the absence of HLA disparity or the apparent absence of HLA-specific antibody has led numerous investigators to propose the existence of a series of vascular endothelial cell antigens.[5] Unfortunately, despite their potential importance in organ transplantation, these antigens remain undefined.

At present, clinical practice does not include typing of antigen systems other than ABO or HLA for several reasons. First, most transplants involve HLA mismatches which may relegate other antigen systems to a minor role in graft rejection. Second, and perhaps more importantly, typing other antigen systems represents an additional expense that is not yet justified by clinical relevance, particularly for the minor histocompatibility antigens. However, this may be different for MICA and vascular endothelial antigens which have been shown to be targets of antibody-mediated rejection.

## THE IMMUNOLOGIC IMPACT OF DIFFERENT ANTIGENS

The previous discussion provides a general overview of the different antigen systems with known relevance in transplantation. However, within each system inherent differences among the different antigens, environmental factors, recipient immunogenetics, and the recipient's immunologic history will affect the immunologic impact of a particular transplant.

### The ABO System

Considering only three blood group antigens, A1 is more immunogenic than either A2 or B. Differences in the immunogenicity of the A1 and A2 antigens are the result of both qualitative and quantitative differences with A2 expressed at lower levels than A1.[2]

### The HLA System

#### *Differences in Expression*

HLA antigens differ in their distribution and degree of expression. This, in turn, affects how readily a particular organ or tissue can sensitize a recipient and how much target it provides for immunologic destruction. HLA class I antigens are expressed on nearly all nucleated cells, whereas class II antigens are expressed constitutively only on professional antigen presenting cells. However, class II expression can be induced on a variety of tissue including, importantly, vascular endothelium. The degree of expression, or amount of antigen found on the cell surface, varies within each class, among alleles of a locus, and among individuals. Among the class I antigens, HLA-Cw is expressed at much lower levels than are A and B. Class II antigen expression is highest for the DRB1 antigens. DQ expression is lower than that of DRB1, and antigens encoded by the DRB3 and 4 genes are expressed at 15% to 20% the level of those encoded by DRB1. In addition to expression differences among the various loci, certain low-expressing alleles have been identified, and heritable reduced overall expression of HLA has been reported. Expression is also affected by zygosity, such that individuals homozygous for an antigen may have twice the amount of that antigen, as would an individual heterozygous for the antigen. HLA expression can be affected by a variety of extrinsic factors. Proinflammatory cytokines, such as the interferons and TNF, upregulate HLA expression; whereas expression is down-regulated by certain drugs such as steroids and statins[7] and in certain disease states.

### Immunogenicity

There are data suggesting HLA antigens vary in the immunogenicity,[8] but the immunologic impact of a mismatched antigen is also affected by the antigens of the recipient. The HLA molecules carry multiple antigenic epitopes, one or more of which may be unique to a single antigen, referred to as *private epitopes;* whereas others may be shared among two or more antigens and are known as *public epitopes*. Antigens that share epitopes comprise what is known as a cross-reactive group or (CREG). It has been postulated that mismatches within a CREG, where the mismatched donor antigen is cross-reactive with one of the recipient's antigens, are less immunogenic. However, such mismatches may not be equally immunogenic in both directions. For example, A2 and A28 are cross-reactive, as are B7 and B40. We have found that a CREG mismatch, in the direction of donor → recipient, is more likely to sensitize a recipient when it is A2 → A28 or B7 → B40 than when it is in the opposite direction (A28 → A2 or B40 → B7).[9] Importantly, exposure to a single HLA antigen can result in sensitization to multiple HLA antigens because of epitopes shared among those antigens.

Immunization results in the expansion of clones specific for the immunizing agent, which, in turn, permits the characteristically rapid and aggressive anamnestic response on a subsequent exposure to the antigen. A dichotomy in transplantation is that successful transplantation can often occur in the face of a crossmatch that is positive with historic sera but negative with a current serum.[5] One exception to this is when there is a repeat mismatch. There are reports of reduced survival of kidney transplants with repeat mismatches,[11,12] but there are also reports to the contrary.[13,14] It is not known whether the difference in graft survival among patients historically sensitized to an HLA antigen is due to differences in the initial response that are quantitative (ie, the extent of clonal expansion that occurred) or qualitative (eg, down-regulation or protection). A repeat mismatch of a haplotype that is identical by descent (ie, sequential transplants from two related individuals who share the mismatched haplotype) might represent a particularly troublesome scenario because additional antigens on that haplotype that are not routinely identified (such as MICA) would also be repeat mismatch.

## Other Antigen systems

As noted previously, several minor histocompatibility antigen differences, together, can be equal to the immunogenicity of a major histocompatibility antigen. In practice, however, the minor antigens are never considered in organ transplantation.

Antigens encoded by the MICA locus have been shown to be expressed on vascular endothelium.[15] In an early study, antibodies to MICA were found in sera, of some patients, collected at the time of rejection.[16] Subsequently, a larger study of renal transplant patients showed that antibodies to MICA appeared prior to clinical signs of rejection and showed a strong correlation with graft loss.[17] To date, there are no data regarding the relative immunogenicity of the various MICA antigens or of the MICA-versus-MICB antigens. However, these early studies indicate that MICA and, possibly, MICB should be considered as important transplantation antigens.

## DONOR SELECTION

### ABO Compatibility

ABO-incompatible renal transplants are performed regularly at certain transplant centers. These transplants required special treatment of the recipient to reduce isoagglutinin titers and are the subject of another chapter in this book (see Chapter 13).

### HLA Compatibility

Highly effective, modern immunosuppression and long waiting times for deceased donor transplantation have greatly diminished the interest in HLA matching for renal transplantation. However, there are several situations in which evaluating the donor HLA mismatches is extremely important. Among these are patients with several living donors from which to choose, young patients who are likely to need a second (or more) transplant, sensitized patients, and patients awaiting a regraft—particularly those who have responded aggressively to previous transplants.

Mismatches of low expressing antigens, HLA-Cw, -DR51, -DR52, and -DR53 have been ignored in deceased donor transplantation. With a few exceptions,[18] HLA-Cw has not been demonstrated to play a significant role in graft rejection. However, the DRB3-5 genes may represent a different situation because the basis for their reduced expression is different and may make them more likely to be up-regulated by extrinsic factors. Introduction of sensitive, solid-phase immunoassays has improved detection of antibodies to HLA-DR51-53, although it is usually difficult to differentiate these antibodies from antibodies to the group of associated-DRB1 antigens. We have observed several patients who have good renal function despite continued presence of antibody to DR51, DR52, or DR53; and this may be directly related to the reduced amount of target present and the failure to activate complement. However, when expression is upregulated, humoral rejection can and does occur.[19] Another factor to be considered is that patients who are mismatched for DRB1 are not necessarily mismatched for the associated additional DRB locus, but when there is a mismatch of DRB51, 52, or 53, there is also a mismatch of the associated DRB1 antigen so that mismatches of these low-expressing antigens always means a mismatch of two antigens (see Table 15.3-2).

There are conflicting data on the impact of repeat mismatches on graft survival. The detrimental effect of repeat mismatches may be dependent on other factors such as the immunogenicity of the repeated mismatch, the aggressiveness with which the patient has

**TABLE 15.3-2**

## IMMUNOLOGIC EVALUATION OF THE DONOR

| Factor | Impact on Rejection and Graft Survival | Impact on Future Access | Comments |
|---|---|---|---|
| ABO | Can cause early rejection and graft loss. | Not evaluated | Requires special recipient conditioning (see Chapter 13) |
| Low-expressing HLA | Not a significant target unless class II antigens are up-regulated by extrinsic factors. | Antibodies to DR51, -52, or -53 eliminate large portions of population for future donation. | |
| CREG match | Reduced immunologic insult compared to other mismatches. May be directional. | Sensitization is more limited because of shared epitopes. | |
| Repeat mismatch | Can result in reduced graft survival. | | Effect is variable and probably affected by recipient factors |
| Positive historic crossmatch | Majority does not have a negative impact, but exceptions include repeat mismatches and high-responder type. | | Requires good characterization of recipient's current antibodies. |
| Positive current crossmatch | Can cause early rejection and graft loss. | | Requires special recipient conditioning (see Chapter 13) |
| HLA mismatches | Vary in immunogenicity and risk for rejection and graft loss. | Common antigens and members of large CREGs can result in broad sensitization. | |
| Genetic relationship between donor and recipient | First degree relatives share one-half of all alloantigens, on average, including those those not known or tested. | | |

responded to previous transplants, and/or the historic presence of antibody to the repeat mismatch. It should be remembered that child to mother and most husband-to-wife transplants involve repeat mismatches.

Sensitization is the single largest barrier to access in transplantation. Therefore, it may be worthwhile to consider the extent of sensitization that may result from certain mismatches. The most dramatic example is the Bw4 and Bw6 epitopes present on B locus antigens. Bw4 is present on an array of HLA-B antigens as well as on HLA-A23, -24, -25, and -32. Sensitization to this epitope translates into incompatibility (ie, positive cross matches) with more than 70% of the population. As noted previously, sensitization to one antigen can result in antibodies to the entire array of antigens that share epitopes with the mismatched antigen. Therefore, sensitization to HLA-B7 may result in antibodies to any or all of the following antigens: HLA-B8, -B27, B54, -B55, -B56, -B42, -B60, -B61, and -B81. However, a CREG match (ie, the donor and recipient have different antigens within the same CREG) would reduce the number of epitopes that differ between the donor and recipient and, as such, would reduce the breadth of sensitization. A summary of the various factors to be considered when evaluating the HLA type of the donor are listed in Table 15.3-2.

## Other Antigen Systems

Until screening of antibodies to and typing for other antigen systems, such as MICA, become more feasible and their clinical importance is firmly established, these tests will be limited to research studies. However, it may be worthwhile to consider that first-degree relatives are, by default, matched for at least one half of all their genes. In turn, this means that a first degree relative is much more likely to be matched for untested alloantigens than is a relative of lesser degree or an unrelated individual and, when the ABO and HLA matches are equivalent, the first-degree relative would have fewer mismatched antigens, overall.

## TESTING DONORS

ABO typing is too well established to merit discussion here. Current methods of HLA typing include serologic testing by lymphocytotoxicity and several DNA-based methods. Commonly performed DNA-based methods are sequence-specific primer amplification (SSP), sequence-specific oligonucleotide probe hybridization (SSOP), reverse SSOP, and sequencing with SSP and reverse SSOP being the techniques most common in testing for organ transplantation. Serologic typing had been the predominant technique for HLA typing for more than 3 decades but the numerous drawbacks of the method and the diminishing supply of serologic typing reagents have made the DNA-based methods increasingly popular. Every technique in use today has shortcomings, and what is most important is that the assay be well characterized by the laboratory in which it is performed and that the necessary expertise for test performance and interpretation be available. Donors and recipients should be typed, at a minimum, for HLA-A, -B, -DR (including DR51-53), and -DQ. There are increasing anecdotal and one published reports[20] of antibodies to HLA-DP, which, if confirmed, may justify typing for the HLA-DP antigens.

At present, testing for antibodies to MICA is not standard practice. However, the reports of the involvement of MICA in antibody-mediated rejection and graft loss are likely to provoke increased of antibody-screening which, in turn, will require MICA typing of donors and recipients for clinically relevant interpretation of the antibody data.

The final assay for immunologic evaluation of the donor is the crossmatch test. These tests are almost exclusively performed using donor lymphocytes as targets and in either a lymphocytotoxicity assay or a flow cytometric assay. These tests are performed to determine the presence of antibody(ies) to donor HLA antigens. False-positive results will occur when the recipient serum contains antibodies reactive with other (non-HLA) molecules on the lymphocyte membrane, and false-negative results occur when the test sensitivity is below the threshold of detection or, in the case of the cytotoxicity assay, when the antibodies do not activate complement effectively. Therefore, crossmatch tests must be interpreted vis-a-vis data from antibody characterization assays. Solid-phase crossmatch tests using solubilized donor antigens as targets have been developed. These assays have the advantage of avoiding reactivity with non-HLA antigens. However, these tests have not been used sufficiently to know the circumstances under which the isolated molecules may be distorted and either fail to react with antibody specific for donor HLA, yielding a false-negative reaction, or acquire reactivity with other, irrelevant antibodies yielding a false-positive reaction. A positive crossmatch with current serum containing antibody-to-donor HLA has, in the past, been considered an absolute contraindication to transplantation. However, there are now protocols to eliminate donor antibody or reduce it to an acceptable level[21] (see Chapter 13) permitting successful transplantation.

## SUMMARY

The immunologic evaluation of the donor requires identifying the donor's alloantigens and determining the risk they represent, individually and collectively, for early rejection, reduced graft survival, and access to future transplants. The expanding repertoire of immunosuppressive drugs continues to be attended by increased risks of infection and malignancy, and the array of therapeutic antibodies used to rescue patients from rejection may deplete patients of cells that are necessary for autologous down-regulation of the allogeneic immune response.[22] Improving our ability to assess the immunologic of a donor's phenotype will permit a more customized approach to immunosuppression and may reduce the need for drastic rescue efforts.

## References

1. Matzinger P. Tolerance, danger, and the extended family. *Annu Rev Immunol* 1994;12:991.
2. Rydberg L. ABO-incompatibility in solid organ transplantation. *Transfusion Med* 2001;11:325.
3. Lenhard V, Hansen B, Roelcke D, et al. Influence of Lewis and other blood group systems in kidney transplantation. *Proc Eur Dial Transplant Assoc* 1983;19:432.
4. Shiramizu T, Shimbo T, Nakamura K, et al. Red blood cell types and living renal transplantation. *Tokai J Exp Clin Med* 1982;7:385.
5. Zachary AA, Hart JM. Relevance of antibody screening and crossmatching I solid organ transplantation. In: Leffell MS, Donnenberg AD, Rose NL, eds. *Handbook of Human Immunology*. Boca Raton, CRC Press; 1997:477.
6. Schreuder GM, Hurley CK, Marsh SG, et al. HLA dictionary 2004: Summary of HLA-A, B, -C, -DRB1/3/4/5, -DQB1 alleles and their association with serologically defined HLA-A, -B, -C, -DR, and -DQ antigens. *Hum Immunol* 2005;66:170.

7. Kuipers HF, Biesta PJ, Groothuis TA, et al. Statins affect cell-surface expression of major histocmpatibility complex class II molecules by distruption cholesterol-containing microdomains. *Hum Immunol* 2005;66:653.

8. Claas, FJH, Dankers MK, Oudshoorn M, et al. Differential immunogenicity of HLA mismatches in clinical transplantation. *Transplant Immunol* 2005;14:197.

9. Zachary AA, Ratner LE, Graziani JA, et al. Characterization of HLA class I specific antibodies by ELISA using solubilized antigen targets: II. Clinical relevance. *Hum Immunol* 2001;62:236.

10. Cardella CJ, Falk JA, Halloran P, et al. Successful renal transplantation in patients with T-cell reactivity to donor. *Lancet* 1982;2:1240.

11. Cecka JM, Terasaki PI. Repeating HLA antigen mismatches in renal transplants — a second class mistake. *Transplantation* 1994;57:515.

12. Opelz G. Repeated HLA mismatches increase the failure rate of second kidney transplants. Collaborative Transplant Study. *Transplant Proc* 1995;27: 658.

13. Heise ER, Thacker LR, MacQueen JM, et al. Repeated HLA mismatches and second renal graft survival in centers of the South-Eastern Organ Procurement Foundation. *Clin Transplant* 1996;10:579.

14. Farney AC, Matas AJ, Noreen HJ, et al. Does re-exposure to mismatched HLA antigens decrease renal re-transplant allograft survival. *Clin Transplant* 1996;10:147.

15. Zwirner NW, Dole K, Stastny P. Differential surface expression of MICA by endothelial cells, fibroblasts, keratinocytes, and monocytes. *Hum Immunol* 1999;60:323.

16. Zwirner NW, Marcos CY, Mirbaha F, et al. Identification of MICA as a new polymorphic alloantigen recognized by antibodies in sera of organ transplant recipients. *Hum Immunol* 2000;61:917.

17. Sumitran-Holgersson S, Wilczek HE, Holgersson J, et al. Identification of the nonclassical HLA molecules, mica, as targets for humoral immunity associated with irreversible rejection of kidney allografts. *Transplantation* 2002;74:268.

18. Chappman JR, Taylor C, Ting A, et al. Hyperacute rejection of a renal allograft in the presence of anti-HLA-Cw5 antibody. *Transplantation* 1986;42:91.

19. Schillinger K, Samaniego M, Racusen LC, et al. Relevance of DRw52-specific antibody in renal transplantation. *Human Immunol* 2000;61: S79.

20. Arnold ML, Pei R, Spriewald B, et al. Anti-HLA class II antibodies in kidney retransplant patients. *Tissue Antigens* 2005;65:370.

21. Zachary AA, Montgomery RA, Leffell MS. Desensitization protocols: improving access and outcome in transplantation. *Clin. Applied Immunol Rev* (in press).

22. Akl A, Luo S, Wood KJ. Induction of transplantation tolerance —the potential of regulatory T cells. *Transplant Immunol* 2005;14:225.

# 15.4 ANESTHESIOLOGIC CONSIDERATIONS

*David S. Beebe, MD*

## INTRODUCTION

In many ways, providing anesthesia for living related kidney donors is one of the more satisfying things anesthesiologists do. The patients who present for living donation have generally been well evaluated medically to be sure they are in proper condition to undergo donation of their organ. Patients who undergo living donation of their kidney are also almost without exception well motivated and enthusiastic about undergoing the procedure. The expectations of patients, surgeons, and nurses, as well as anesthesiologists for patients undergoing living real donation, are high, however. Patients must be safely managed in the perioperative

period so that the procedure remains one of low risk. The postoperative management of pain and nausea is important as well to minimize the discomfort and morbidity patients experience following a major surgical procedure.[1] In addition, anesthesiologists must ensure that adequate but not excessive hydration is provided to the patient during living kidney donation to try to prevent delayed graft function in the allograft. In this way the anesthetic and fluid management in the donor can also affect the outcome in the recipient. Finally with the advent of laparoscopic or laparoscopic-assisted living renal donation, anesthesiologists must understand the effects of abdominal insufflation and be prepared to treat its complications should they occur.[2]

In this section we will (1) describe the standard anesthetic and perioperative management plan for living kidney donation used at the University of Minnesota Hospital, as well as additional techniques utilized successfully at other institutions; (2) discuss the management of the renal allograft; and (3) review the effects of laparoscopy on renal function and how it affects management of the kidney donor.

## ANESTHETIC AND PERIOPERATIVE MANAGEMENT PLAN AT THE UNIVERSITY OF MINNESOTA HOSPITAL

### Preoperative Preparation

All patients undergoing elective kidney donation must have had no solids or foods by mouth for at least 6 hours prior to surgery. Patients are given medications they should continue in the perioperative period such as beta-blockers with a sip of water or juice the morning of surgery, however.

Prior to surgery the patient must undergo a thorough preoperative evaluation and review by the anesthesiologist. Although most patients who are donating their kidney are healthy, many have some conditions that require evaluation or treatment before surgery. For example, patients who have gastric reflux and/or heartburn are usually administered a nonparticulate antacid such as Bicitra® preoperatively to neutralize their stomach acid to prevent or minimize pneumonitis should aspiration occur. Another commonly occurring condition in living donors is reactive airway disease. An inhaled beta-agonist such as albuterol administered in the preoperative period can benefit these patients by preventing intraoperative bronchospasm. A patient's smoking history or past use of alcohol or drugs can affect their anesthetic management. A negative pregnancy test should be documented on female donors of appropriate age. In addition, the anesthesiologist must evaluate if there are any more recent events or conditions that may affect whether or how to proceed with the proposed procedure. For example, the presence of a fever or severe upper respiratory tract infection or dehydration from a viral gastroenteritis may mean the surgery should be delayed until these conditions resolve. The anesthesiologist should also determine whether patients have been administered a bowel preparation prior to surgery. A bowel preparation can cause significant dehydration and affect the perioperative fluid management.

In the preoperative physical the airway must be assessed to determine if tracheal intubation is likely to be difficult. The presence of limited mouth opening, obesity, or a stiff neck may mean a technique such as an awake, fiberoptic intubation is required. The patient must also be examined for conditions such as wheezing or rhonchi that could cause delay or cancellation of surgery.

Finally the laboratory values should be reviewed. Living donors usually exhibit few laboratory abnormalities. All patients should have a recent hemoglobin the day of surgery as well as a current type and screen, however, in case an intraoperative complication requiring transfusion occurs.

## Induction and Maintenance of General Anesthesia

General anesthesia with tracheal intubation is most often used for both open and laparoscopic renal donation. Intravenous propofol (2–3 mg/kg) is usually used as the induction agent because it has a rapid termination of action and antinausea effects, but intravenous agents such as thiopental (3–5 mg/kg) or etomidate (0.2 mg/kg) have been used successfully as well. In patients with no history of acid reflux, tracheal intubation is facilitated with an intermediate acting, nondepolarizing muscle relaxant such as vecuronium (0.1 mg/kg) or cis-atracurium (0.2 mg/kg). In addition, a narcotic such as fentanyl (1–3 ug/kg) is administered concurrently with propofol to blunt the hypertensive response of tracheal intubation. In patients with acid reflux disease, a formal rapid sequence induction using Sellick's maneuver to prevent regurgitation is utilized. Succinylcholine (1.5 mg/kg) is often used as a skeletal muscle relaxant in patients with acid reflux of its rapid onset. Tracheal intubation is performed in all cases regardless of whether they have reflux disease to provide for adequate ventilation of the patient in the lateral position that is used for both open and laparoscopic procedures. Tracheal intubation also protects the patient from the possibility of aspiration because of increased intraabdominal pressure from either laparoscopic insufflation or direct surgical manipulation in the abdomen with the open approach. An oral gastric tube is also placed for all living kidney donors. This empties the stomach to prevent regurgitation of gastric contents and helps with surgical visualization using either the laparoscopic or the open approach.

Following tracheal intubation anesthesia is maintained with a balanced technique using either isoflurane or desflurane with a mixture of air and oxygen with a $FiO_2$ of 50%. Fentanyl (1–2 u kg/h) is also administered in low doses throughout the procedure to reduce the inhaled anesthetic requirement and ensure the patient awakens with narcotic analgesia present. Additional skeletal muscle relaxants are administered, if required, to help with surgical visualization. Nitrous oxide was used concurrently with isoflurane or desflurane for many years during living kidney donation because of its rapid elimination, lack of renal toxicity, and minimal hemodynamic effects. It is not administered often currently because it can increase the incidence of postoperative nausea and vomiting, which is common following laparoscopy.[3] Sevoflurane is not administered to living renal donors because this agent can react with the carbon dioxide absorbant in the anesthesia machine to cause production of a potentially nephrotoxic substance called compound A.[4] Mechanical ventilation is utilized throughout either open or laparoscopic kidney donation. Ventilation is adjusted to maintain an end-tidal $CO_2$ of 35 to 40 mm Hg. Adjustments are often needed during laparoscopic donor nephrectomy, as the patient will absorb some of the carbon dioxide used for abdominal insufflation and require increased ventilation to excrete it. To prevent nausea and vomiting postoperatively, dexamethasone (0.2 mg/kg) is administered intraoperatively. Ondansetron (4 mg) is also effective to prevent nausea and vomiting.[3]

Most patients are extubated and have their oral-gastric tubes removed at the end of the operation when they are awake, strong, and maintaining normal respirations following the reversal of skeletal muscle relaxation. Analgesia is provided in the recovery room using intravenous morphine (0.1–0.2 mg/kg/h), hydromorphone (0.01–0.02 mg/kg/h), or fentanyl (100–200 ug/h). These same drugs can be used for patient controlled analgesia after discharge from the recovery.

## Other Management Techniques

Other anesthetic techniques have been successfully utilized over the years for both intraoperative and postoperative management of living kidney donors. One technique described by Sener and Torgay et al.[5] is to use combined spinal-epidural anesthesia for open living donor nephrectomy. Prior to placement of an epidural catheter through an epidural needle in a lower lumbar interspace, spinal anesthesia is administered with a small (27-gauge) spinal needle inserted through the epidural needle. An epidural catheter is placed through the same interspace. Surgery is performed with the patients awake but sedated. Additional analgesia is administered through the epidural catheter as the spinal anesthesia begins to wear off and can be used to provide postoperative analgesia. This method has been shown in a small series of patients to be as successful in maintaining graft function, but no more so, than in patients receiving general anesthesia.[5]

Other groups utilize epidural analgesia for postoperative pain management for 3 to 5 days following open donor nephrectomy. Epidural catheters are placed prior to the procedure, but general anesthesia is used for the surgery itself.[6] The epidural technique provides effective pain relief in the postoperative period, but carries the small risk of epidural hematoma in patients like renal donors who receive heparin. As a result, most institutions rely on intravenous analgesia rather than epidural techniques for postoperative pain control for both living donors and recipients.[7]

## Management of the Renal Allograft

The process of harvesting an organ and transplanting it by necessity renders it ischemic. Longer periods of ischemia increase the incidence of delayed graft function and subsequent graft loss. Although in living donation the ischemia time is much less than with cadaveric transplantation, delayed graft function and subsequent graft loss may still occur. To achieve the goals of minimal ischemic damage to the donated kidney and prompt allograft function after transplantation the anesthesiologist must (1) maintain adequate renal perfusion during dissection and harvest of the organ, (2) prepare the kidney while in the donor to tolerate the ischemic insult of harvesting without permanent damage or prolonged dysfunction, and (3) administer heparin shortly before the organ is harvested to prevent vascular thrombosis.

To maintain adequate renal perfusion during dissection and harvest adequate hydration is required. Hydration is one way the anesthesiologist helps prepare the kidney to tolerate ischemia because it ensures that blood flow and oxygen delivery to the kidney is maximized during the harvest.[7] In addition, the energy expended by the kidney is reduced if it does not have to concentrate urine because of dehydration. Initially a loading dose least 10 mL/kg of lactated Ringer's solution is administered prior to and immediately following induction of general anesthesia. Additional 10 mL/kg boluses of solution may be necessary if hypotension occurs or the urine output is inadequate. Often the surgeon can help the anesthesiologist assess the volume status of the patient by noting whether the renal vein appears collapsed indicating a low central venous pressure. Generally an infusion of at least

6 mL/kg/h of lactated Ringer's solution is required to ensure adequate hydration. If at any point the blood pressure remains 20% below the normal value in spite of adequate hydration, a vasopressor such as ephedrine (5–10 mg) or phenylepherine (100–200 $ug$) can be administered. Prolonged use of vasoconstrictors should be avoided because of their potential vasoconstrictive effects on the renal vasculature and because they are usually unnecessary in these healthy patients.[8]

Mannitol is (0.25–0.5 g/kg) also administered to the living donor. Mannitol acts as a free radical scavenger as well as a diuretic. Mannitol has been shown to lessen the incidence of acute tubular necrosis in kidney recipients, perhaps by reducing swelling in the renal tubules.[9] Furosemide may be administered as well as mannitol to further reduce absorption of fluid and minimize energy consumption. Both fluids and diuretic are utilized to try to achieve a urine output of 2 to 3 mL/kg every 15 minutes.

Finally the anesthesiologist and surgeon must communicate properly to be certain that heparin (50 U/kg) is administered prior to clamping the vessels and removing the kidney. The heparin can be reversed with a small dose of protamine (approximately 50 mg) following removal of the organ.

## EFFECTS OF LAPAROSCOPY ON RENAL FUNCTION AND MANAGEMENT OF LIVING RENAL DONORS

Patients who donate their kidneys laparoscopically have less pain, improved pulmonary function, and shorter hospitalizations than those who receive the open procedure. However, laparoscopy introduces new challenges in the anesthetic management of living renal donors. Abdominal insufflation with carbon dioxide can cause hypercarbia if the ventilation is not adjusted appropriately. Generally the ventilation must be increased at least 30% to prevent hypercarbia from absorption of carbon dioxide during laparoscopy.[10] Insufflation of the abdomen also can restrict descent of the diaphragm that can restrict ventilation in some patients, particularly the obese. Therefore the end-tidal carbon dioxide tension must be measured in all cases, and the ventilation carefully adjusted if it begins to rise.[11]

Of specific concern in living renal donation is the effect of abdominal insufflation on renal blood flow and urine output in the harvested kidney. Insufflation during laparoscopy causes a reduced urine output in most patients, including living renal donors. This probably is related to reduced renal perfusion from elevated abdominal venous pressure resulting in antidiuretic hormone release.[12] The reduced renal perfusion appears to be related to the level of insufflation pressure and may be prevented experimentally by additional fluid administration.[13] However, excessive fluid administration during surgery can impair wound healing, worsen pulmonary function, and increase the incidence of paralytic ileus.[14] Studies have not demonstrated long-term impairment in the function of living donor kidneys harvested laparoscopically in spite of generally having a lower initial urine output than those harvested with an open technique.[15] Also a recent study comparing laparoscopic donors who received greater than 10 mL/kg/h of intravenous fluid compared to those who received less showed no benefit in short- or long-term graft function in the high fluid group, although the intraoperative urine output was greater in the high-fluid group.[16] Therefore a similar fluid management regimen as the open procedure seems appropriate.

## SUMMARY

Living renal donation is becoming a common means to treat renal failure. With careful anesthetic management and the rapid advancement of surgical techniques, living kidney donation should continue to improve and help patients in renal failure with low morbidity and no mortality in the donor.

## References

1. Davis CL, Delmonico FL. Living-donor kidney transplantation: a review of the current practices for the live donor. *J Am Soc Nephrol* 2005;16:2098.
2. Biancofiore G, Amorose G, Lugi D, et al. Perioperative management for laparoscopic kidney donation. *Transplant Proc* 2004;36:464.
3. Apfel CC, Korttila K, Abdalla M et al. A factorial trial of six interventions for the prevention of postoperative nausea and vomiting. *N Engl J Med* 2004;350:2441.
4. Eger EI, Koblin DD, Bowland T et al. Nephrotoxicity of Sevoflurane versus desflurane in volunteers. *Anesth Analg* 1997;84:160.
5. Sener M, Torgay A, Akpek T, et al. Regional versus general anesthesia for donor nephrectomy: Effects on graft function. *Transplant Proc* 2004;36:2954.
6. Peters TG, Repper SM, Jones KW, et al. Living kidney donation: Recovery and return to activities of daily living. *Clin Transplant* 2000;14:433.
7. Lemmens HJM. Kidney transplantation: recent developments and recommendations for anesthetic management. *Anesthesiology Clin N Am* 2004;22:651.
8. Sprung J, KapuraL L, Bourke DL, et al. Anesthesia for kidney transplant surgery. *Anesthesiol Clin N Am* 2000;18:919.
9. Tiggeler RG, Berden JH, Hoitsma AJ, et al. Prevention of acute tubular necrosis in cadaveric kidney transplantation by the combined use of mannitol and moderate hydration. *Ann Surg* 1985;201:246.
10. Kazama T, Ikeda K, Kato T, et al. Carbon dioxide output in laparoscopic cholecystectomy. *Br J Anesth* 1996;76:530.
11. Sprung J, Whalley DG, Falcone T, et al. The impact of morbid obesity, pneumoperitoneum, and posture on respiratory system mechanics and oxygenation during laparoscopy. *Anesth Analg* 2002;94:1345.
12. Hazebroek EJ, de Vos tot Nederveen Cappel R, Gommers D, et al. Antidiuretic hormone release during laparoscopic donor nephrectomy. *Arch Surg* 2002;137:600.
13. London ET, Hung SH, Ann MC, et al. Effect of intravascular volume expansion on renal function during prolonged $CO_2$ pneumoperitoneum. *Ann Surg* 1999;231:195.
14. Holte K, Sharrock NE, Kehlet H. Pathophysiology and clinical implications of perioperative fluid excess. *Br J Anaesth* 2002;89:622.
15. Derweesh IH, Goldfarb DA, Abreu SC, et al. Laparoscopic live donor nephrectomy has equivalent early and late renal function outcomes compared with open donor nephrectomy. *Urology* 2005;65:862.
16. Bergman S, Feldman LS, Carli F, et al. Intraoperative fluid management in laparoscopic live-donor nephrectomy: Challenging the dogma. *Surg Endosc* 2004;13: [Epub ahead of print].

# 15.5   SURGICAL PROCEDURES

## 15.5.1   Open Standard Nephrectomy

*Jacques Pirenne, MD*

Nephrectomy through a flank incision has been the standard method of procuring kidney grafts from living donors (LDs) for many decades. Although laparoscopic techniques have become increasingly popular, the standard nephrectomy (SN) is the most validated method and remains extremely safe, both for the donor and for the kidney.[1]

## DONOR POSITIONING

A pivotal step in the SN is the correct positioning of the donor on the operating table, in the lateral (right or left) decubitus position. The operating table is then maximally flexed at the level of the umbilicus and the kidney rest is raised (Figure 15.5.1-1). This maneuver increases the distance between the last rib and the iliac spine. As a result, the flank becomes fully exposed. This maneuver is essential to provide as large an operating field as possible and to allow easy and safe access to the kidney.

During the positioning of the donor, extreme attention is paid to adequately support the head and the lower and upper extremities. Such support helps avoid any iatrogenic injury caused by an inappropriate movement or by compression during surgery.

The position of the donor on the operating table is then maintained by using a mattress with negative pressure and by support material.

Pulmonary embolus is a potential hazard after all types of surgery, including after living donation. Indeed, postoperative pulmonary emboli may be caused by thrombotic events during surgery. The routine use of pneumatic compression boots is strongly recommended. They are placed on the lower extremities before surgery and activated at the start of surgery.

## SURGICAL TECHNIQUE

The incision line starts in the flank at the level of the extremity of the 12th rib and from there goes downward and medially (into the direction of the umbilicus, which is used as a marker). It is easier to mark the line of incision before preparing the operative field and before draping the patient. The length of the incision is 15 cm.

The skin and subcutaneous tissue are incised. The first muscle layer is incised, starting on the top of the last rib and going downward and medially.

The tip of the 12th rib is dissected free from its periosteal membrane and is fully exposed over a distance of about 3 to 5 cm. The tip of the rib is then resected, because the kidney usually lies under the tip of the 12th rib; rib resection therefore greatly facilitates exposure and dissection of the kidney (Figure 15.5.1-2).

Once the tip of the rib has been resected, the remaining layer of the muscle is incised.

After transection of the deeper muscle, the fascia of Gerota is exposed laterally; and the peritoneum, more medially (Figure 15.5.1-2). On the medial part of the incision, care is taken to avoid disrupting the peritoneal membrane, which is thin and adherent to the posterior aspect of the rectus abdominus muscle. The fascia of Gerota and the peritoneum are separated. The fascia of Gerota is then opened, allowing access to the perirenal space (Figure 15.5.1-3).

The perirenal fat is gently removed close to the kidney capsule. This maneuver is started at the lateral aspect of the kidney and is continued downward to the lower pole and upward to the upper pole; both poles are progressively freed from their attachments. Doing so renders the kidney more mobile and facilitates further dissection of the vascular pedicle. Freeing the perirenal fat is also continued toward the kidney hilum, without entering into the fat of the kidney hilum.

At this stage, a static valve (Omnitract) is placed, lifting the upper edge of the incision upward and pulling the lower edge downward. An additional large valve is placed medially and retracts the peritoneal membrane and the abdominal contents medially, thereby exposing the kidney hilum and its vascular pedicle.

The next step is the isolation of the renal vein. *On the right side,* it is easiest to dissect the renal vein directly at its junction with the vena cava and to encircle it. It is not necessary to dissect the main trunk of the right renal vein toward the kidney hilum. That dissection can be done later on the bench if needed. It is important to free the vena cava sufficiently so that one Satinsky-type vascular clamp can be later positioned, without any additional tissue interposed in the clamp.

*On the left side,* it is easiest to directly dissect the trunk of the left renal vein, which usually clearly appears as a blue axis under a layer of peritoneum and some perirenal fat. In some donors,

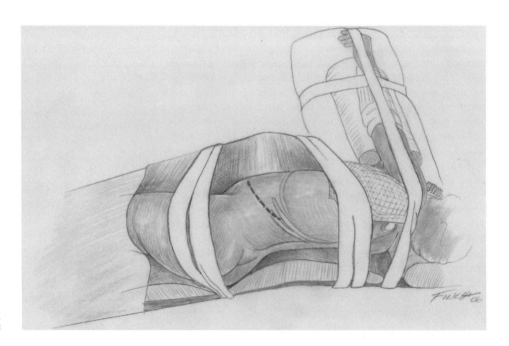

**FIGURE 15.5.1-1**

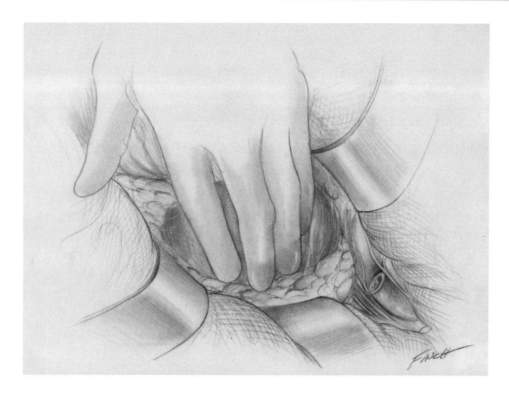

**FIGURE 15.5.1-2**

particularly if they are obese, the left renal vein is not directly visible. It is then easier to first dissect the gonadal vein (which is always easy to locate), and from there dissect upward to the junction with the inferior edge of the left renal vein.

Once the left renal vein and the gonadal vein are dissected and identified, the adrenal vein can be found at the upper edge of the left renal vein. Both the gonadal and the adrenal veins are clipped and tied; this maneuver mobilizes the trunk of the left

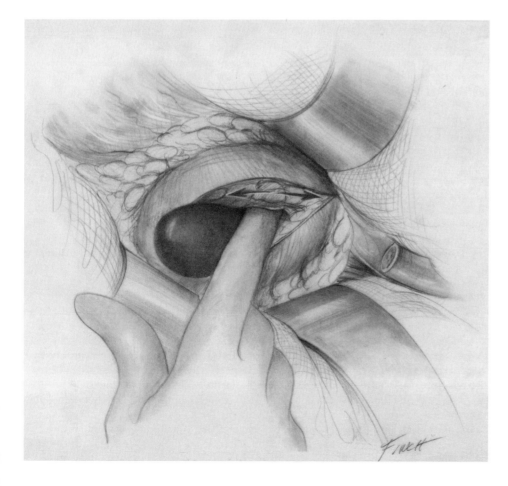

**FIGURE 15.5.1-3**

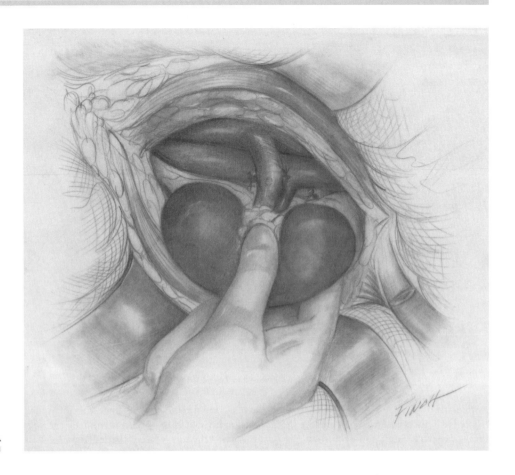

**FIGURE 15.5.1-4A**

renal vein (Figure 15.5.1-4A). The left renal vein can then be dissected more proximally to its junction with the vena cava; however, in our experience, doing so is not necessary. We usually limit the dissection of the left renal vein to the level of the adrenal and gonadal veins. Finally, and depending on the length of the renal vein to be procured and the individual donor's anatomy, lumbar veins draining onto the posterior aspect of the left renal vein may need to be clipped and tied (Figure 15.5.1-4B).

The adrenal gland is gently separated from the upper pole of the kidney using electrocoagulation. Once the renal vein is isolated and the adrenal gland has been separated, the renal artery needs to be identified. Pulsations of the renal artery are easily palpated at the posterior aspect of the renal vein. The renal artery is then gently dissected free and mobilized; extreme care must be taken to avoid causing any spasm. Any small adrenal artery taking off from the renal artery may need to be tied.

The ureter is identified and encircled, leaving the periureteral tissue in place. At the lower pole of the kidney, a triangle of perirenal fat between the kidney and the ureter is left intact, so that the ureter vascularization remains optimal.

The ureter is divided as distally as possible, usually at the place where it crosses the iliac artery (Figure 15.5.1-5). Once the ureter is divided with clips and ties, diuresis from the kidney to be procured can be controlled.

Throughout surgery, the kidney must be mobilized as little as possible, without inducing any spasm of the renal pedicle. The kidney should remain hard in consistency; diuresis should be abundant throughout the procedure. Diuresis is controlled permanently, and Lasix and mannitol are given as needed to maintain a high urine output. A high central venous pressure (~12 mm Hg) is also recommended. Before the actual procurement, it is usual to

let the kidney "recuperate" from possible manipulation for 15 to 20 minutes. If an arterial spasm is present, it can be easily handled by placing papaverine superficially on the adventitia of the renal artery (via a piece of Surgicel or a sponge). If the kidney is soft and diuresis is not optimal, it is better to wait a little more, instead of procuring an oliguric kidney that will cause delayed graft function in the recipient.

## KIDNEY RESECTION

The recipient operation is usually done simultaneously with the donor operation, so that cold ischemia time is kept as short as possible. Once the recipient is ready for implantation and the donor kidney is hard and produces abundant amounts of urine, the kidney may be procured. First, 70 U/kg of heparin is given. The renal artery and vein are clamped, and the kidney is retrieved (Figure 15.5.1-5). Certain centers use a second clamp as backup, but this can reduce the length of the renal vessels. The renal artery is cut first, the renal vein second; the kidney is then given to the recipient team. The kidney is immediately perfused with 1 L of low-potassium cold preservation solution (HTK or Euro-Collins). University of Wisconsin (UW) solution is avoided, because its high potassium content may cause heart arrhythmias after reperfusion in the recipient. Heparin is immediately neutralized by protamine. The stumps of the vessels are sewn, using a double layer of running Prolene 4/0 sutures. They are tied under the vascular clamp and clipped (Figure 15.5.1-5 inset). At the level of the right renal vein, the clamp is positioned longitudinally on the vena cava, which is partially clamped. The longitudinal venotomy is closed, using two layers of running 4/0 Prolene sutures. The vena cava should not be narrowed.

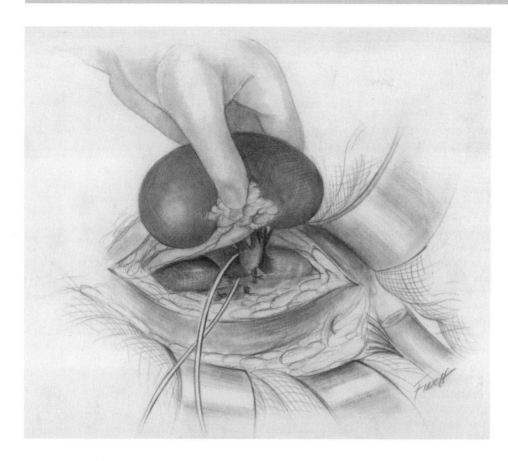

**FIGURE 15.5.1-4B**

Next, hemostasis is controlled. The operating field is filled with warm physiologic water. Positive airway insufflation is performed to exclude a pneumothorax, which can sometimes be caused by a small tear in the pleura at the posterior angle of the incision. In case of a pleural leak, the tear is identified and then simply closed under positive airway pressure. No thoracic drain is needed. Tissue-col and Surgicel are placed on the vascular stumps. An aspirating redon catheter is placed in the iliac fossa.

The muscle layers are closed in two layers, using 0-PDS. The subcutaneous tissue is closed, using interrupted Vicryl 2/0 sutures. The skin is closed, using intradermal monofilament sutures.

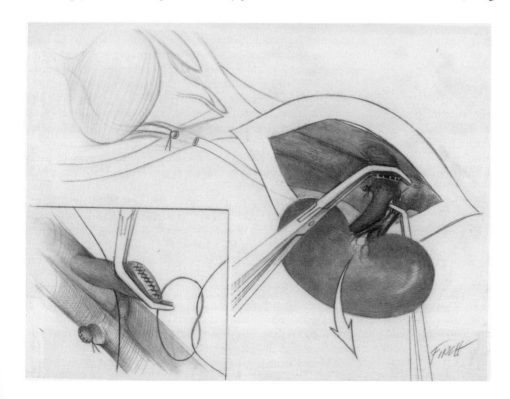

**FIGURE 15.5.1-5**

## ADVANTAGES AND DISADVANTAGES OF STANDARD NEPHRECTOMY

With the SN the length of the incision does not need to exceed 15 cm, which is no longer than the cumulative length of separate incisions required for laparoscopic procurement. And unlike with the intraperitoneal laparoscopic technique, the peritoneal cavity is not entered, so there is no risk of postoperative intraperitoneal complications (such as adhesions and intestinal obstruction, intestinal perforation, and splenic bleeding). During the SN, the absence of a pneumoperitoneum optimizes kidney perfusion and function. In addition, the absence of a pneumoperitoneum completely eliminates the risks of intraoperative pulmonary embolus caused by a small venous tear, a potential fatal hazard with laparoscopic procurement. Ureter necrosis has been described after laparoscopic kidney procurement, probably because of intraoperative manipulations and partial devascularization of the ureter—again, a complication not seen with the SN. The SN allows procurement of the right or the left kidney with the same degree of safety, whereas laparoscopic procurement of the left kidney is usually considered easier. The SN provides a longer vascular pedicle, as compared with laparoscopic procurement. With the SN, kidney extraction occurs immediately after transection of the renal artery and vein, and warm ischemia time is extremely short (less than 30 seconds). Finally, the duration of surgery is substantially shorter with the SN than with laparoscopic procurement.

One downside of the SN is the level of pain, which has repeatedly been shown to be ameliorated with laparoscopic procurement. The pain after the SN is due to the incision of the well-developed lumbar musculature. To minimize pain, the length of the incision should be kept as short as possible (a maximum of 15 cm). In addition, peridural anesthesia or patient-controlled analgesic devices are helpful and can completely control the pain. Intravenous paracetamol (at 1 g 4 times a day) is started on day 2, and the peridural is removed on day 3. Another complication that can be seen after the SN is a bulking of the incision. Again, bulking can be limited by reducing the size of the incision, by sparing the underlying muscle nerves, and by correctly closing the muscles.

## INTRAPERITONEAL OPEN APPROACH

Open intraperitoneal kidney procurement is also possible, though rarely performed. It is done via a midline or a subcostal incision. On the right side, a Kocher maneuver must first be performed to expose the right kidney and its vascular pedicle. On the left side, the kidney must be separated from the splenic flexure of the colon, the spleen, and the tail of the pancreas. Possible indications are simultaneous procurement of another abdominal organ (eg, the tail of the pancreas, a liver lobe) or the need for a rescue operation in case of failure of laparoscopic procurement.

In short, the SN remains an extremely secure technique for procuring the kidney from LDs. Because it involves an exclusively extraperitoneal approach and provides unsurpassed access to—and control of—the kidney and its vascular pedicle, it remains extremely safe for both the kidney (and thus for the recipient) and for the donor. The results of the SN should remain the gold standard to compare against the results of laparoscopic procurement.[2]

## References

1. Simmons RL, Finch ME, Ascher NL, et al. *Manual of Vascular Access, Organ Donation, and Transplantation*. New York Berlin Heidelberg Tokyo, Springer-Verlag;1984.
2. Oyen O, Andersen M, Mathisen L, et al. Laparoscopic versus Open Living-Donor Nephrectomy: Experiences from a Prospective, Randomized, Single-Center Study Focusing on Donor Safety. *Transplantation* 2005;79:1236.

## 15.5.2   A Minimally Invasive Open Donor Nephrectomy: "Mininephrectomy"

*Anil Kotru, MD, Surendra Shenoy, MD, PhD*

## INTRODUCTION

The deceased donor kidney availability has failed to keep pace with the increase in number of patients with end-stage renal disease (ESRD) eligible to receive a kidney transplant. In 2004, UNOS data showed 60,000 patients waiting on the list for the 8,000 cadaver kidneys that were available. This increasing discrepancy between the demand and supply of transplantable deceased donor organs has led to an unrealistic increase in the waiting period on the list. This organ shortage combined with the superior long-term outcome of living donor kidney transplants has resulted in a steady increase in both the percentage and the absolute numbers of living donor transplants. In the United States the number of living donors surpassed the number of deceased donors in the year 2001. In 2004, living donor kidneys accounted for 41% of all kidney transplants.

This trend of increasing living donor transplants has placed an increased responsibility of ensuring appropriateness of donor selection and safety of donor surgical procedure on the medical community.[1]

In living donation, defying the Hippocratic oath to cure only the ailing, the surgeons have to safely perform a nephrectomy on an otherwise healthy individual who has volunteered to become a donor. Following kidney donation, the health and longevity of a properly selected donor with a well-functioning single kidney is the same as that of the normal population with two kidneys. However, the procedure used for removing a kidney from the donor is associated with some short- and long-term risks. The onus of developing strategies to reduce these surgical risks rests on the surgeons.[2,3]

With growing numbers of live donations, the transplant community has revisited conventional techniques of retrieving a kidney from a living donor. This retroperitoneal donor nephrectomy technique, through a flank approach, enjoyed the best safety record. However, the pain, discomfort, and increased risk for wound-related complications with this approach were major disincentives that prompted the research for newer techniques.[4–6] The advent of minimally invasive surgical procedures using laparoscopy resulted in use of this technique to perform donor nephrectomies for the first time in 1996.[4] Since then this procedure and its variants have rapidly gained popularity.[7] Being minimally invasive, it addressed some of the complications associated with the conventional open approach. However, being a transperitoneal approach it was also associated with unique complications.[8–10] These surgical risks include injury to abdominal organs such as the spleen and intestines, hemorrhage from the renal pedicle, and incisional hernia of the abdominal wall.[11] Moreover, all transperitoneal approaches can leave the healthy donor with a lifelong risk of adhesion-related problems that could manifest at any time later. Laparoscopic procedures also need expensive instrumentation with an associated long learning curve. There is also a marginally increased risk of graft loss due to vascular or graft injury due to increased intraperitoneal pressure following $CO_2$ insufflation.[12]

The "mininephrectomy" procedure was developed with the intention of circumventing problems associated with a transperitoneal laparoscopic minimally invasive nephrectomy.[11,13] Mininephrectomy is an open minimally invasive, retroperitoneal, donor nephrectomy technique. It enjoys the safety associated with open surgical approach. While retaining the advantages of a minimally invasive approach, it eliminates the disadvantages of a transperitoneal approach. The procedure, first described in 2001, is now the preferred donor nephrectomy technique in many transplant centers.[13]

## HYPOTHESIS AND RATIONALE

"A strategically placed incision big enough to extract the donor kidney from the body should be adequate in providing exposure for successful dissection and mobilization of the organ."

Kidneys are retroperitoneal structures. The renal artery originates from the aorta, and the renal vein drains into the vena cava both of which are situated retroperitoneally. A posterior approach provides the shortest route to reach and dissect the renal vessels, the most difficult part of the surgical procedure in preparing kidneys for retrieval. The incision in a mininephrectomy procedure is placed in line with the 12th rib, that is, anatomically situated directly over the origin and insertion of the renal vessels. This provides direct exposure of the vasculature during further dissection.

## PROCEDURE

Mininephrectomy is performed under general anesthesia with the surgeon using 2.5x to 3.5x loupes and a head light with a high-intensity light source.

## Position

The donor is positioned in lateral decubitus with the kidney bridge raised between the iliac crest and the lower border of the rib cage. The lower extremity resting on the table is flexed 30 degrees at the hip and 70 degrees at the knee, thus providing stability of the field. The donor is placed in lateral position to let the abdominal panniculus fall forward. The table is flexed until the flank skin is stretched to open the space between the ribs and iliac crest (Figure 15.5.2-1). The arm resting on the table is extended, and an axillary roll is placed to relieve pressure on axillary structures. The other arm is supported with a Mayo stand or a Kraske holder.

## Incision

The length of the 12th rib and its relationship to the kidney are determined by a preoperative angiogram or similar imaging study. The 12th rib is palpated, and a 6– to 8-cm incision is marked along the course of the rib, starting 2 to 3cm (one finger's breadth) anterior to the lateral border of the sacrospinalis muscle (Figure 15.5.2-1). If the rib is absent or short, a subcostal incision is placed in the same location using the 11th rib as a guide.

A Wheatlander retractor (Aesculap, Inc., San Francisco, CA) provides exposure to deeper dissection. The latissimus dorsi and serratus posterior inferior muscles are divided to expose the 12th rib. The periosteum is dissected with electrocautery around the rib to perform an extraperiosteal rib resection (Figure 15.5.2-2).

A Thompson retractor (Thompson Surgicals) is set up with the table railpost applied to the table on the side of the operating surgeon. A cross bar is positioned parallel to the donor about 6 to 7 inches from the skin surface. The second cross bar is positioned close to the skin surface with the incision centered in between (Figure 15.5.2-3). Alternatively a Bookwalter retractor (Bookwalter Inc. Raynham, MA) may be used with the large ring positioned close to the skin surface (Figure 15.5.2-2).

The small keyhole incision does not provide exposure to the entire field of dissection in one view. This problem is overcome by modifying the use of the retractor blades to obtain adequate exposure of the area of dissection. Instead of the conventional

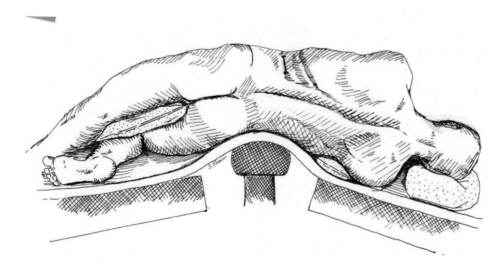

**FIGURE 15.5.2-1**

Donor positioning.

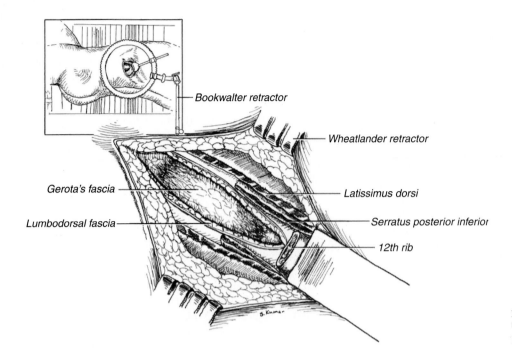

Bookwalter retractor

Wheatlander retractor

Gerota's fascia

Latissimus dorsi

Lumbodorsal fascia

Serratus posterior inferior

12th rib

**FIGURE 15.5.2-2**

Exposure of the rib and retraction.

principles of traction and countertraction using opposing blades for exposure, one or two blades on the same or adjacent sides of the incision are used to skew visualization into the area of dissection. In this fashion the upper pole, lower pole, ureter, hilum, and posterior portion of the renal pelvis are viewed and dissected sequentially.

## Dissection

On dividing the lumbodorsal fascia, extraperitoneal fat is encountered. This fat pad is excised to create working space around the kidney and to allow a longitudinal incision of Gerota's fascia. The dissection and excision of perinephric fat is commenced at the middle of the kidney posteriorly and extended superiorly to release the upper pole (Figure 15.5.2-4). Excision of the perinephric fat cre-

ates space for further dissection and maneuvering of the kidney. A self-retaining right-angle blade is used to retract the upper cut edge of the abdominal wall to facilitate dissection of the upper pole. A handheld sweetheart retractor is used to displace the kidney caudally to aid this dissection.

Next, the perinephric fat in the posterior inferior part of the kidney is excised with the retractor blade applied to the inferior edge of the abdominal wall incision. A sweetheart retractor blade is used to retract the peritoneum medially (toward the anterior abdominal wall) to aid in this process. The kidney is then gently retracted upward with a self-retaining Dever (malleable) blade. A plane is developed between the gonadal vein and ureter, preserving the periureteric plexus of vessels. The ureter is encircled with a vessel loop. With gentle traction on this loop, the ureter is dissected to a point 2 cm beyond the site where it crosses the

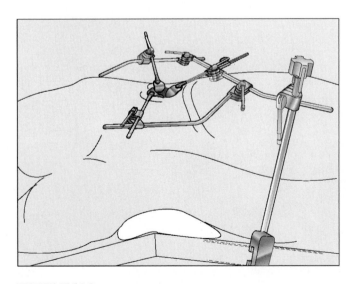

**FIGURE 15.5.2-3**

Retractor positioning for exposure.

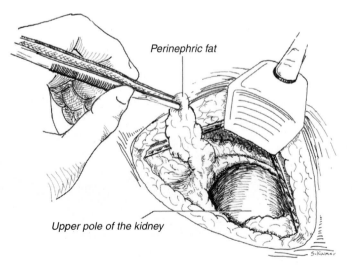

Perinephric fat

Upper pole of the kidney

**FIGURE 15.5.2-4**

Upper pole exposure.

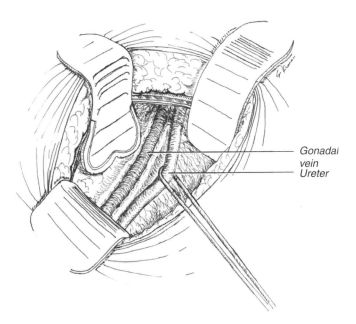

**FIGURE 15.5.2-5**

Ureteric exposure.

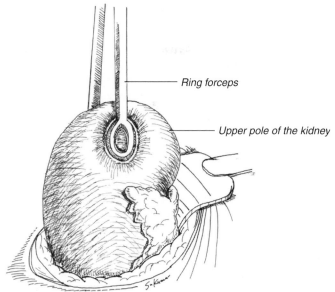

**FIGURE 15.5.2-7**

Retrieval of the kidney.

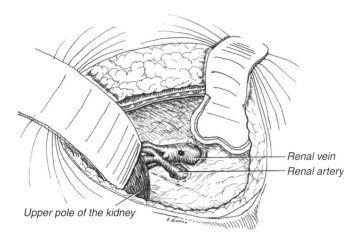

**FIGURE 15.5.2-6**

Exposure of the renal hilum.

external iliac vessels (Figure 15.5.2-5). We perform all dissection using a monopolar electrocautery with a long tip, a Debaky vascular forceps, and occasionally a right-angled forceps.

The gonadal vein is traced to its insertion into the renal vein. To aid this part of the dissection, the perinephric pad of fat anterior to the kidney is excised, and the peritoneum is retracted medially by repositioning the self-retaining sweetheart blade. Small tributaries of the gonadal vein near its entry into the renal vein are carefully divided between small Ligaclips (Ethicon Endosurgery, Inc., Cincinnati, OH). The gonadal vein is divided between medium-size Ligaclips near its insertion, leaving a generous stump on the renal vein.

The upper pole of the kidney is retracted downward (caudal) and medially (toward anterior abdominal wall) with a Dever blade. The sweetheart blade retracts the peritoneum medially. This allows complete exposure of the renal vein and it's insertion across the aorta. The dissection is then carried out to isolate, clip, and divide the adrenal vein. Next, the renal artery is dissected to its origin (Figure 15.5.2-6). This approach provides excellent exposure of the renal artery and allows dissection without any traction on this vessel. The plexus of nerves and lymphatics between the artery and the vein are divided. As the arterial dissection is completed, lumbar tributaries entering the renal vein come into view. Being a posterior approach, these veins are seen straight ahead, making it easy to clip and divide them.

The last part of the dissection requires medial retraction of the kidney with a sweetheart retractor. The variable amount of fat and areolar tissue on the posterior aspect of the hilum of the kidney is divided.

## Nephrectomy

We used 5 to 7 mg/kg of IV heparin prior to the nephrectomy. The ureter is divided first. This is done using medium Ligaclips or large Hemolock clips (Weck Closure Systems, Inc., Research Triangle Park, NC) to occlude the distal ureter.

A self-retaining sweetheart blade is used to retract the peritoneum medially. A handheld or self-retaining Dever retractor blade is used to retract the kidney downward and medially to expose the renal vein and renal artery (Figure 15.5.2-6). Vascular clamps are applied on the renal artery and vein before their division. Alternatively, the artery may be clipped between two large Hemolock clips on a right angle applicator. We do not apply vasacular clips to the renal vein to prevent the risk of vein retraction and bleeding. The kidney allograft now lies free in the retroperitoneum. The Dever blade is removed. A ring forceps is used to secure the upper pole of the kidney to deliver it vertically upward through the incision (Figure 15.5.2-7).

The renal vein stump is sutured first with a 5-0 polypropylene continuous suture followed by closure of the renal artery in a similar fashion. The arterial stump that is occluded with clips is oversewn to prevent the risk of clip dislodgement and bleeding. A laparoscopic knot pusher is used to place knots, as it is almost impossible to slide the knot down manually with the small incision.

Finally, the retroperitoneum is inspected for hemostasis and for any violation of peritoneum or pleura. If present, the peritoneal opening is closed with 4-0 absorbable suture. If a pleural opening if identified, the rent in the diaphragm is closed around a red rubber catheter. Before closure of the opening, the catheter is drained into an underwater seal to rid air in the pleural space and to expand the lung. The catheter is removed simultaneous to closure of the diaphragmatic defect.

## Closure

The lumbodorsal fascia is closed with continuous sutures as the first layer. The internal oblique, serratus posterior inferior, external oblique, and the latissimus dorsi are individually approximated with interrupted 0 Vicryl (Ethicon, Somerville, NJ) figure-of-eight sutures. Subcutaneous tissue is closed with 3-0 continuous Vicryl, and a subcuticular skin closure is performed with a 4-0 absorbable monofilament suture.

When a right nephrectomy is performed, the gonadal vein directly enters the inferior vena cava, and the renal vein is short. The retro caval arterial dissection and division of short lumbar tributaries of the inferior vena cava (if necessary) is easier with this posterior approach.

We routinely use local anesthetic pain pumps for postoperative analgesia. One infusion tube is placed in the neurovascular plain between the internal and transversalis fascia. The second tube is placed subcutaneously. This eliminates the need for narcotics and narcotic related bowel dysmotility problems in the postoperative period.

## RESULTS

Since February 2001, we have performed the mininephrectomy procedure in over 250 consecutive renal donors. The procedure enjoys the advantages of an open retroperitoneal nephrectomy. It also has the benefits of minimally invasive surgical procedures. For this report we reviewed the results of 104 consecutive procedures performed between January 2003 and December 2004 (Table 15.5.2-1). The average postoperative hospital stay for the donor was 2.5 days. No donors in this group have needed open conversion. However, we have previously converted three patients—a patient with a body mass index (BMI) >35 with extensive adhesions of perinephric fat to the kidney, and two for bleeding from the renal artery during the procedure. Even in these cases, the extended incisions were shorter (12 cm) than conventional incisions. No donor required blood transfusions. Three donors developed retroperitoneal chylocoeles (detected 3-4 weeks postoperatively) and were treated with percutaneous drains by interventional techniques. One donor had wound disruption following a fall from a horse 2 weeks following surgery and needed surgical wound repair. No other wound complications have occurred to date. There have been no complications such as abdominal wall parasthesia or muscle weakness, which are common following conventional open techniques. We feel that the transcostal approach helps us identify and preserve the intercostal neurovascular bundle thus reducing abdominal wall related complications.

In summary mininephrectomy is a minimally invasive open posterior transcostal approach, which can be used in any living renal donor. Because it is an open procedure it does not require any additional investment in special instrumentation and has a

**TABLE 15.5.2-1**
## MININEPHRECTOMY DATA 2003–2004 (*n* = 104)

| | |
|---|---|
| Follow-up (years) | 1.8 ± 0.6 |
| Age (years) (mean ± SD) | 38 ± 10 |
| Sex (m/f) | 69/35 |
| Relationship (LRD/LURD) | 80/24 |
| BMI (kg/m$^2$) < 30/ > 30 | 68/36 |
| EBL (mL) (mean ± SD ) | 150 ± 130 |
| Transfusion | 0 |
| Dissection time (min) (mean ± SD) | 150 ± 35 |
| Incision length (cm) (mean ± SD) | 6.2 ± 0.5 |
| Length of stay | 2.5 ± 1.0 |
| Postop complications | 2 |
| Readmission | 5 |
| Primary nonfunction | 0 |
| Early graft loss | 1 |

short learning curve. The retroperitoneal approach provides the safety of the conventional open technique. Unlike the transperitoneal approach, there are no foreseeable long-term risks. Thus, this procedure meets requirements for an ideal donor nephrectomy technique.

## References

1. 2004 Annual Report of he U.S. Organ Procurement and Transplantation Network and the Scientific Registry of Transplant Recipients. www.unos.org
2. Johnson EM, Remucal MJ, Gillingham KJ, et al. Complications and risks of living donor nephrectomy. *Transplantation* 1997;64:1124–1128.
3. Rohner Jr TJ, Decter RM. Upper abdominal, flank, and posterior incisions. In: Fowler Jr JE, eds. *Mastery of Surgery: Surgical Urology.* Little Brown and Co.: Boston; 1992:3–23.
4. Ratner LE, Kavoussi LR, Sroka M, et al. Laparoscopic assisted live donor nephrectomy: a comparison with the open approach. *Transplantation* 1997;63:229–232.
5. Ratner LE, Hiller J, Sroka M, et al. Laparoscopic live donor nephrectomy removes disincentives to live donation. *Transplant Proc* 1997;20: 3402–3403.
6. Schweitzer EJ, Wilson J, Jacobs S, et al. Increased rates of donation with laparoscopic donor nephrectomy. *Ann Surg* 2000;232:392–400.
7. Buel JF, Alverdy J, Newell KA, et al. Hand-assisted laparoscopic live-donor nephrectomy. *J Am Coll Surg* 2001;192:132–135.
8. Barry JM, Laparoscopic donor nephrectomy. *Transplantation* 2000;70: 1546–1548.
9. Knoepp L, Smith M, Huey J, et al. Complications after laparoscopic donor nephrectomy. *Transplantation* 1999;68.
10. Novotny MJ. Laparoscopic live donor nephrectomy. *Urol Clin North Am* 2001;28:127–135.
11. Matas AJ, Bartlett ST, Leichtman AB, Delmonico FL. Morbidity and mortality after living kidney donation, 1999-2001: Survey of United States Transplant Centers. *Am J Transplant* 2003;3:830–834.
12. Kirsch AJ, Hensle TW, Chang DT, et al. Renal effects of CO2 insufflation: Oliguria and acute renal dysfunction in a rat pneumoperitoneum model. *Urology* 1994;43:453–459.
13. Shenoy S, Lowell JA, Jendrisak M, Rmachandran V. The ideal living donor nephrectomy "Mini- Nephrectomy" Through a posterior transcostal approach. *J Am Col Surg* 2002;194(2):240–246

## 15.5.3  Transperitoneal Laparoscopic Nephrectomy

*Anand K. Khakhar, MD, Raghu Varadrajan, MD,*
*Lloyd E. Ratner, MD*

## INTRODUCTION

Transperitoneal (TP) laparoscopic live donor nephrectomy (LLDN) was the first form of purely laparoscopic donor nephrectomy reported both experimentally and clinically. To date, it remains the most commonly performed type of minimally invasive donor nephrectomy. Of note, > 70% of all the living donor nephrectomies in the United States are performed laparoscopically. In a survey conducted across 130 centers worldwide in the year 2000, 96% centers performing LLDN, preferred the TP approach, whereas approximately 4% preferred the retroperitoneal (RP) approach.[1] The centers doing TP LLDN, are split roughly equally into those that do pure LLDN and others that do hand-assisted (HA) LLDN.

Despite claims advocating open donor nephrectomy (ODN) and RP LLDN, why is TP LLDN the dominant minimally invasive donor procedure performed? Primarily, most surgeons (trained as general surgeons) are comfortable working through the peritoneal cavity; moreover, the peritoneal cavity is a naturally available potential space that can be easily inflated with pnuemoperitoneum. There is no necessity of creating a tissue dissection plane for insufflation. Also the available space for working is much more than can be availed through the retroperitoneum.[2] It allows the delivery of the kidney through a cosmetically superior and relatively less painful lower midline (vertical) or suprapubic (Pfannenstiel) incision. Because there are no tissue planes to be made for insufflation posterior or anterior to the kidney, the probability of injury to the kidney or the vasculature in the renal hilum is minimal with the TP approach. Additionally, the ability to combine concomitant abdominal surgery with LLDN is exclusively a property of the transperitoneal approach.[3] Disadvantages of LLDN include the risk of bowel injury from trocar insertion or during instrumentation, internal hernias or hernias through trocar sites, and intestinal adhesions.[4] Additionally, injuries to the lumber vein, renal artery, aorta, pneumomediastinum, splenic injury, adrenal/retroperitoneal hematomas, and so forth have been reported by larger series.[5]

In the text that follows, we discuss the necessity for LLDN, its development, and the technical aspects of TP LLDN, and we review the comparative outcome among TP LLDN, RP LLDN, and ODN. Finally we go over certain safety issues and discuss upcoming developments in LLDN.

## WHY LLDN

The primal idea of performing a minimally invasive surgery for living donor organ retrieval is geared toward removing disincentives and promoting living organ donation in an effort to bridge the precipice between the demand and the supply of organs for transplantation. Among the fears perceived by the potential employed for kidney harvesting, the possibility of future failure of the remaining kidney, size and appearance of the scar, and the postoperative analgesic requirements.[6] The Live Organ Donor Consensus Group also identified that time away from work with possible loss of income, time away from routine daily activities and family during the postoperative period, and incidental expenses[7] as possible deterrents. Anticipated outcome in transplant recipients also plays an important part in the decision-making process of certain potential donors.[8]

The standard open live donor operation is traditionally performed through a retroperitoneal approach by a flank incision, with rib resection or an anterior transperitoneal approach. This approach has witnessed considerable morbidity in terms of postoperative pain, longer convalescence, pneumothorax, and significant wound complications like hernia, diastasis of recti, and chronic pain or discomfort. There is a significant duration of absence at work and analgesic requirements associated with it. Laparoscopic donor nephrectomy (LDN) can successfully counter most of these donor disincentives. A randomized controlled trial between open donor nephrectomy (ODN) versus LLDN was undertaken at University of Michigan[9] wherein, compared to ODN, LDN was associated with greater donor satisfaction, less morbidity, and equivalent graft outcome. In this study, the resumption of light and heavy activities, driving a vehicle, and postoperative analgesic requirements were significantly better with LLDN than with ODN. Also a more direct proof of LLDN being a preferred modality among donors is available in the fact that since the advent of LLDN the rate of living donation for kidney transplantation has increased significantly.[10]

## HISTORY OF LLDN

The first LDN was performed in 1954 by Harrison for the first successful kidney transplant between identical twins.[11] The operation had not changed significantly for the next 40 years until the advent of LLDN. A revolution in laparoscopic surgery was witnessed in the late 1980s with the popularization of laparoscopic cholecystectomy. A concomitant improvement in the optical devices, cameras and laparoscopic instruments used for tissue dissection, and tissue transfixation further facilitated the development of advanced laparoscopic surgery. Clayman et al. performed the first laparoscopic nephrectomy for disease in 1990 at Washington University in St. Louis.[12] Gill et al. published the first experimental series on laparoscopic donor nephrectomy in pigs in 1994.[13] Ratner et al. reported the first successful laparoscopic donor nephrectomy (transperitoneal) in humans[14] from the Johns Hopkins Bayview Medical Center. A hand-assisted approach was first reported by Wolfe and also by Slakey for LLDN. They both argued in favor of ease and safety of the hand assisted procedure along with reduction in the learning curve.[15] Retroperitoneal laparoscopy was popularized by Rassweiler et al. in the late 1990s,[16] although Yang et al.[17] reported two cases of video-assisted extraperitoneal donor nephrectomy using special retractors and open surgery instruments in 1994. The first randomized controlled trial of ODN versus hand-assisted LLDN was published by Wolfe et al.[18] A similar trial between ODN and pure LLDN was published by Simforoosh and colleagues in Iran.[9] The retroperitoneoscopic donor nephrectomy was further reported by the Japanese authors Ishikawa, and Suzuki et al.[19] Gruessner and his team at University of Minnesota further utilized a hand-assisted laparoscopic approach for living donor distal pancreatectomy and donor nephrectomy to perform a simultaneous living donor kidney and pancreas transplantation.[20] The utility of LLDN was further enhanced by the concept of concomitant surgery with LLDN introduced by Molmenti and Ratner et al.[3]

## TECHNICAL ASPECTS OF TRANSPERITONEAL APPROACH

### Left TP LLDN

The authors place the patient in a modified lateral decubitus position with the hips rotated posteriorly to allow easy access to the lower midline for delivery of the kidney. The use of a standard kidney bridge is avoided and we break the table to hyperflex the flanks (Figure 15.5.3-1). The patient is positioned at about 45° instead of 90° and we rotate the table to compensate (Figure 15.5.3-2). The veress needle is inserted in the left subcostal region and the 1-ml saline test is done to ensure placement of the needle followed by insufflation with carbon dioxide starting low to high flow. We operate with the intraabdominal pnuemoperitoneum pressure of 15 mm Hg.

Three laparoscopic ports are employed. First we place a 12-mm port through the umbilicus; we prefer the Visiport™ (U.S. Surgical Corporation, Norwalk, CT) to incise the fascia. A second 12-mm port is similarly placed on the left lateral border of rectus slightly inferior to the level of the umbilicus. One 5-mm port is placed in the epigastrium three fingerbreadths inferior to the xiphoid in the midline. A 30° scope is used through the umbilical port. A 5-cm suprapubic Pfannenstiel incision is placed two finger-breaths above the pubic symphysis, a small hole is made into the peritoneum, and an endo-catch bag (closed) is passed into the peritoneal cavity for retraction. The peritoneal opening is sealed with a purse-string suture to prevent carbon-dioxide leakage. In the obese patients, the same configuration of port placement is moved from the midline toward the left costal margin. An additional port may be needed for retraction. We use a 5-mm port placed in the midline between the umbilical and infraxiphoid ports or alternatively in the left (or right) flank (Figure 15.5.3-3).

Dissection begins by dividing the lateral peritoneal reflection along the avascular white line of Toldt from the splenic flexure to the pelvic inlet. The colorenal attachments are divided and the left colon is mobilized medially (Figure 15.5.3-4).

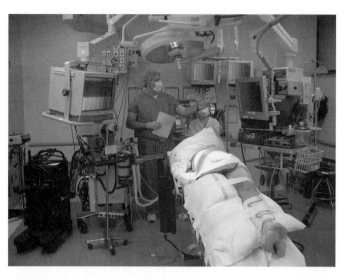

**FIGURE 15.5.3-2**

The patient is placed in a modified lateral position with the hips turned slightly posteriorly. The table is flexed, and the patient is taped securely to the table, so that the table can be rotated. Arms are crossed across the chest to allow for placement of the Aesop Robot.

At this point, a 5-cm Pfannenstiel incision is made two finger-breadths superior to the pubis. The linea alba is incised vertically, and the rectus abdominis muscles are retracted laterally. A purse-string suture of 3–0 absorbable monofilament is placed within the peritoneum. A small incision is made within the confines of the purse string, and a 15-mm Endo-catch™ bag (U.S. Surgical Corp., Norwalk, CT) is passed through the purse-string. The purse-string is tied securely to maintain pneumoperitoneum. The Endo-catch™ bag is used to retract the colon, mesentery, and duodenum

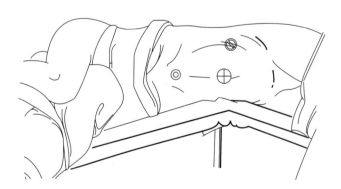

Modified Lateral Position of patient for LLDN. Flanks are hyperflexed by breaking the table.

⊕ The Umbilical 12 mm camera port

◎ Lateral rectus border 12 mm port

◎ Infra xiphoid port (5 mm)

**FIGURE 15.5.3-1**

Kidney position.

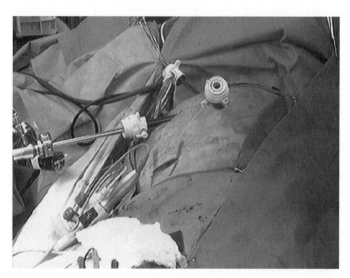

**FIGURE 15.5.3-3**

Three ports are utilized: a 12-mm port at the umbilicus, a 5-mm port 3 finger-breadths inferior to the xiphoid I the midline, and a 12-mm port along the lateral border of the rectus muscle in the lower abdomen. A 5-cm Pfannenstiel incision is made as an extraction site.

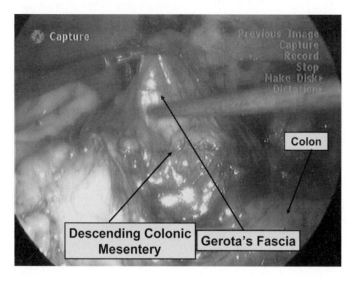

**FIGURE15.5.3-4**

The lateral peritoneal reflection is divided. The colonic mesentery is then dissected off Gerota's Fascia to expose the kidney. This can be accomplished bluntly.

medially.[21] Dissection proceeds in the plane between Gerota's fascia and the descending colonic mesentery until the left gonadal vein is identified (Figure 15.5.3-5). Just caudal to the lower pole of the kidney the soft tissues immediately medial to the gonadal vein are divided and the gonadal vein is lifted bluntly taking with it the ureter and the intervening tissues between the gonadal vein and ureter. Holding up the lower pole of the kidney on the left side, using a blunt instrument on the right side, a sweeping motion toward the pelvis is done to mobilize the ureter. This prevents devascularization of the ureter. The gonadal vein is then dissected cephalad until the left renal vein is identified. It is frequently helpful to elevate the gonadal vein, ureter, and lower pole of the kidney

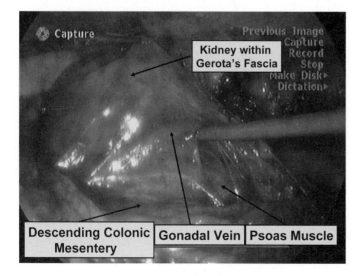

**FIGURE 15.5.3-5**

The gonadal vein and ureter are elevated off the psoas muscle posteriorly.

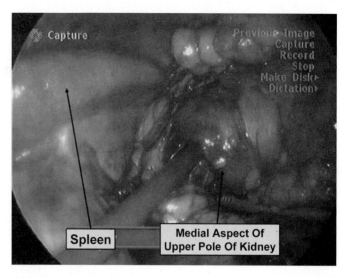

**FIGURE 15.5.3-6**

The upper pole of the kidney is dissected free from within Gerota's Fascia.

en masse anterolaterally off the psoas muscle to facilitate exposure to the renal vein and artery. Usually, a lumbar vein originating from the posterior aspect of the left renal vein at the level of the gonadal vein must be clipped and divided. This exposes the renal artery. The inferior aspect of left renal artery can be dissected down to its origin at the aorta. Next, the upper pole of the kidney is mobilized from within Gerota's fascia (Figure 15.5.3-6). Dissection proceeds along the superior border of the left renal vein until the adrenal vein is identified. The adrenal vein then is clipped and divided (Figure 15.5.3-7). The renal vein is reflected inferiorly to provide exposure to the superior border of the left renal artery. The renal artery then can be dissected from the investing lymphatic and neural tissue from the hilum to its origin at the aorta. Attachments between the renal artery and the adrenal gland are divided. Care must be taken to avoid injury to any upper pole branches. Adrenal arterial branches that emanate from the left renal artery should be clipped and divided or divided with the harmonic scalpel or ligature device. At this point, the hilar vascular dissection is complete.

The gonadal vein is dissected inferiorly to the point where it crosses the ureter and is divided. The ureter then is dissected to the level of the iliac vessels. The lateral border of the ureter is dissected inferiorly to superiorly, taking care to leave generous periureteral tissue intact, until the lower pole of the kidney is encountered. The remainder of the kidney then is freed from within Gerota's fascia. Intravenous heparin, mannitol, and furosemide are administered. The ureter is clipped distally and divided proximal to the clips. The scope is moved to the left lower quadrant port. An Endo-GIA stapler™ stapler™ (U.S. Surgical Corp., Norwalk, CT) or Endo-TA stapler™ stapler™ (U.S. Surgical Corp., Norwalk, CT) with a vascular load is passed through the umbilical port and used to divide the renal artery at its origin at the aorta (Figure 15.5.3-8). Placing the stapler through the umbilical port ensures that it is oriented posterolaterally and will not injure the superior mesenteric artery or other critical structures. The stapler is reloaded and used to divide the renal vein in a plane medial to the adrenal vein stump. The kidney is flipped over the spleen to allow room to open the Endo-catch™ bag. The kidney

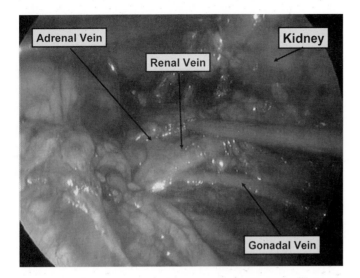

**FIGURE 15.5.3-7**

The left adrenal vein is dissected and divided. Laparoscopy affords excellent visualization and magnification of vascular structures.

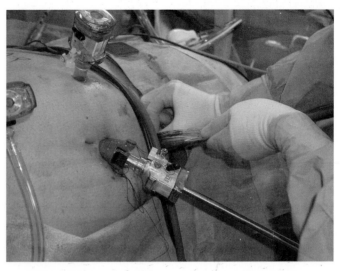

**FIGURE 15.5.3-9**

The kidney is delivered through the Pfannenstiel incision in an Endo-catch Bag.

is placed within the Endo-catch™ bag, and the purse-string is cinched securely closed. Care must be taken to ensure that the ureter is entirely within the bag before the purse-string is tightened to avoid stripping the ureter. The peritoneum is incised through the Pfannenstiel incision. The kidney is removed within the Endo-catch™ bag (Figure 15.5.3-9, Figure 15.5.3-10). The linea alba is reapproximated, and pnuemoperitoneum is reestablished. The abdomen is surveyed for hemostasis. Fascial sutures are placed at the 12-mm port sites.

## MODIFICATIONS FOR THE RIGHT KIDNEY

The right kidney may be more difficult to procure laparoscopically. An additional port may be required to retract the right lobe of the liver anteriorly for exposure. Several modifications have been employed to maximize length of the right renal vein. Division of the right renal vein with the Endo-GIA stapler™ stapler inserted through the umbilical port will result in loss of 1 to 1.5 cm of renal vein length, resulting in a vein that is short, thin, and difficult to sew. Thus the Endo-GIA stapler™ stapler is inserted through the

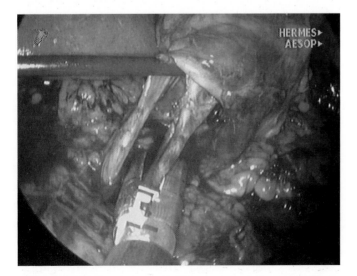

**FIGURE 15.5.3-8**

The renal artery and vein are each divided individually with a vascular stapler. It is important for safety reasons that a tissue transfixion technique is employed on the major vessels. Here the renal artery is divided at its origin at the aorta.

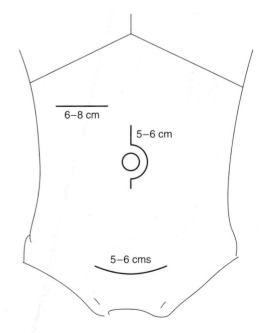

**FIGURE 15.5.3-10**

Incisions for delivery of kidney in LLDN.

port on the right lateral rectus border, and the scope is used through the umbilical port even for this part of the operation. The authors in their earlier series recommended the use of a 6-cm right upper quadrant transverse incision for an open division of the renal vasculature and delivery of the kidney,[21] but we feel that it is no longer necessary. The kidney is tented up using a blunt retractor so as to open the hilum widely. This facilitates taking a small cuff of the vena cava using the Endo-GIA™ stapler. However, if technically difficult, or if the renal vein is felt short, it may be reconstructed on the back table with a panel graft of recipient saphenous vein or an ABO-matched cadaveric vein graft if available. Inserting the stapler through the right lower quadrant port rather than through the umbilical port facilitates a more parallel line with the inferior vena cava and results in greater length of donor renal vein.[22] The length of the right renal vein can also be compensated by a more extensive mobilization of the recipient's external and common iliac veins so that it can be brought to a more superficial level. This facilitates the venous anastamosis by making it more superficial, and also prevents the kinking of a short right renal vein.

Right renal arteries that branch proximally may be problematic when approached laparoscopically. When employing the anterior transperitoneal operation, it is difficult to dissect the segment of artery that lies posterior to the inferior vena cava. If the surgeon dissects in the interaortocaval space (medial to the inferior vena cava), this maneuver can be accomplished more easily. This dissection allows division of the right renal artery at its origin at the aorta rather than at the lateral border of the inferior vena cava.[21]

## HAND-ASSISTED LAPAROSCOPY

Several surgeons have described using hand-assist devices to facilitate dissection and to extract the kidney more rapidly following devascularization.[23,24] Proponents of this technique believe that it reduces the learning curve and enables individuals with less-developed laparoscopic skills to perform the operation with a greater degree of safety.

Although different centers have placed the hand port in various locations, most have used a periumbilical, paramedian, or left/right lower quadrant transverse muscle-splitting incision (Figure 15.5.3-11a and Figure 15.5.3-11b). The one clear advantage of this technique is that it is much easier to mobilize the upper pole of the kidney manually than purely laparoscopically. Some primary surgeons place their nondominant hand into the abdomen, whereas others have an assistant place his or her hand intraperitoneally. Although hand-assist devices are relatively expensive, Wolf [25] believes that the savings achieved in operating-room time charges offsets this additional cost. Commonly employed hand-port devices include GelPort™ (Applied Medical Resources, Rancho Santa Margarita, CA), Omniport™ (Advanced surgical concepts, Wicklow, Ireland), and Lapdisc™ (Ethicon Endosurgery, Cincinnati, OH).[26]

## Tips to Ensure Safety

1.  Special attention is paid to padding the weight-bearing points on the donor. Frequent rotation of the table is used to shift the center of gravity and rotate among the weight-bearing points. We believe this protects against the potential of rhabdomyolysis during prolonged surgery, especially in obese donors.

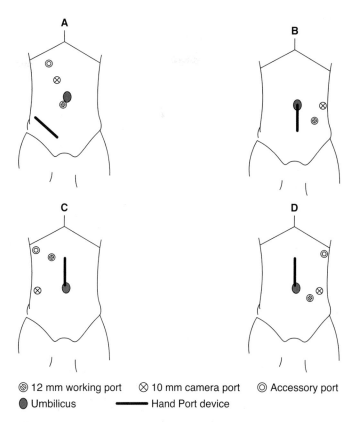

⊚ 12 mm working port    ⊗ 10 mm camera port    ◎ Accessory port
● Umbilicus              ▬ Hand Port device

Port placing strategies for HA laparoscopy: Surgeon standing contralateral to the kidney.
(**A, B**) Right and left approaches for right-handed surgeon. Using left hand through right lower-quadrant muscle-splitting incision for right nephrectomy and midline incision for left nephrectomy.
(**C, D**) Right and left approaches for right-handed surgeon. Using left hand through supraumbilical midline incision in both cases. Trocars as shown.

**FIGURE 15.5.3-11a**

Port placement for HA LLDN[50] (A,B) (C,D).

2.  The authors believe in doing blunt dissection as far as possible because this averts risk for major vascular catastrophes and also protects against inadvertent bowel injury.

3.  Also, we stress vascular transfixation using staplers or suture ligature instead of metallic clips or the plastic locking Hem-o-Lok clip™ (Weck Closure Systems, Research Triangle Park, NC) for all renal arteries and veins. Use of hemosatatic clips on the renal artery has been associated with a greater likelihood of hemorrhage resulting in severe complications and death.

4.  Dissection of the ureter should proceed from medial to the gonadal vein at the lower pole of the kidney downwards to prevent stripping of the periureteric tissues, which are vital in preventing ischemic strictures of the lower ureter.

5.  This operation should not be performed unless there is a redundancy of both disposable and nondisposable equipment available in the room for immediate access in case of equipment malfunction or failure.

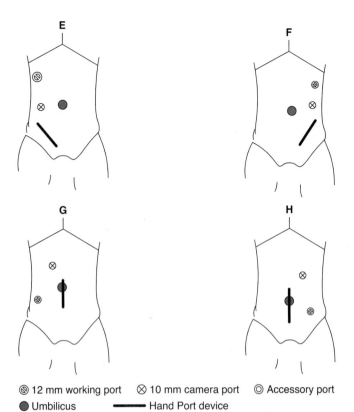

⊚ 12 mm working port   ⊗ 10 mm camera port   ◎ Accessory port

● Umbilicus                    ▬▬ Hand Port device

Port placing strategies for HA laparoscopy:
**(E, F)** Surgeon stands ipsilateral to kidney. Iliac crest incision for
hand device.
**(G, H)** Surgeon stands contralateral to kidney. University of Miami
technique with midline periumbilical hand-device incision, mirror
image with use of right hand for right nephrectomy and left hand
for left nephrectomy.

**FIGURE 15.5.3-11b**

Port placing strategies for HA laparoscopy (E,F) (G,H).

6.  The patient should be maximally relaxed for the procedure.

7.  The patient should be securely fastened to the table using
    beanbags, sticking plasters, tape, and belts as per individual
    preference. This allows rotation of the table enough to pre-
    vent rhabdomyolysis and obtain adequate exposure of the
    operating field at various stages of the operation.

8.  Finally, in case of any eventuality, the operating room
    should be fully prepared for an emergency conversion to
    open surgery including the instrument sets for open donor
    nephrectomy and emergency vascular control.

9.  During dissection of the renal artery and vein, the lateral,
    posterior and inferior (ie, ureteral) attachments to the kid-
    ney are maintained creating a 3-point fixation to the retro-
    peritoneum. These attachments are preserved until the hilar
    dissection complete to limit the mobility of the kidney and
    prevent torsion of the kidney about its vascular pedicle.

## CONTROVERSIES

Left donor nephrectomy has been accepted as the preferential
organ for LDN because of the resulting longer renal vein.[27,28]
Right donor nephrectomy is reserved for instances when the left

kidney is determined to be unacceptable for transplantation. Indications most often cited are multiple left renal arteries or veins,
early bifurcation of left renal artery/multiple left renal arteries,
smaller right kidney, a cystic mass in the right kidney, retroaortic
left renal vein, right renal artery stenosis, and ectopic right kidney.[22,29,30] Although during the early experience with LLDN,[22]
a higher incidence of thrombotic complications was noted when
right kidneys were procured. This problem was a function of the
learning curve and has been obviated by the technical modifications described previously.[21,22] A large multicenter study comparing outcomes among ODN, left LLDN, and right LLDN
demonstrated comparable outcomes in recipients at 1-year follow-up.[30] Two complications unique to the right LLDN are inadvertent injury to the liver during retraction for dissection of the
upper pole and bleeding from the vena-cava during transaction of
the right renal vein.[30]

While searching for a safer and easier approach to laparoscopic
donor nephrectomy, hand-assisted laparoscopic techniques have
been added to the surgical armamentarium by certain centers.
Slakey et al.[31] compared the outcomes among ODN, pure LLDN,
and HALLDN. There was no significant difference in the allograft
function among the three groups at 1-year posttransplant.[31] However, they found that HALLDN donors had a shorter operative
time and less warm ischemia, although there was no difference in
the short-/long-term graft outcome. Improved tactile sense and
retraction of the spleen and renal hilum contributed to the ease of
the operation and ensured access for emergency vascular control if
needed. Additionally, they found a higher incidence of ileus and
a longer incision from the hand port as compared to the kidney-
retrieval incision of pure LLDN. The analgesic requirements were
similar.

With a view to avoid the preferential use of left kidney for
LLDN, a retroperitoneal approach has been proposed to overcome the transperitoneal anatomic limitations of performing right
LLDN.[32] It is argued that the short right renal vein usually covers
the right renal artery anteriorly; thus the dissection of the right
renal artery typically entails considerable traction on both the
vein and the artery, causing technical difficulty and a potential for
vasospasm. A posterior approach obviates this at the same time
avoiding the retraction of the liver and dissection of the duodenum. A comparison between left transperitoneal LLDN and right
RP LLDN[32] revealed a longer warm ischemia time for the RP
LLDN but had a shorter operative time. There was no difference
in the hospital stay, analgesic usage, and had comparable serum
creatinine in the recipient.

## OUTCOME

Several large series from mature centers are now available to review
the outcome of donors undergoing LLDN, as well as the outcome
of those recipients receiving the laparoscopically retrieved kidneys.

Table 15.5.3-1 and Table 15.5.3-2 depict some of the largest
experiences in LLDN, whereas Table 15.5.3-3 narrates the recipient outcome for patients receiving LLDN kidneys. Table15.5.3-4
is a brief summary of the two single center studies comparing outcome of the donor and recipients undergoing ODN and LLDN
as well as HA LLDN and pure LLDN. The overall consensus is
that in experienced hands performing LLDN, the recipient outcome (S. creatinine at 6 months and incidence of DGF and allograft complications) is comparable among the ODN and LLDN
groups. Among the donors, the recuperation from surgery is faster
with LLDN, the requirements of analgesia both as inpatients and

**TABLE 15.5.3-1**

## COMPLICATIONS OF LLDN REPORTED BY CENTERS WITH SIGNIFICANT EXPERIENCE

| Investigators | Convert to open sx | Inpatient stay | Mean S.Cr. Postop mg% | Analgesia use | Mean operative time in minutes | WIT |
|---|---|---|---|---|---|---|
| Jacobs et al. Univ Maryland 738 LLDNs[33] | 12 | 64.4 ± 38.2 hr | 1.3 ± 0.3 | 74.2 ± 66.6 mg Morphine PCA | 202 ± 53 | 160–240 secs |
| Melcher et al. UCSF 530 LLDNs[49] | 1 | 3.2 ± 1.0 | | | 196 ± 43 | |
| Levanthal et al. N.W. Uni 500 LLDNs[5] | 9 | 2.0 ± 0.7 days | 1.3 ± 0.3 | | | 2.6 ± 0.6 min |
| Su et al. Johns Hopkins 381 LLDN[37] | 8 | 3.3 ± 4.5 days | | | 253 ± 56 | |

following discharge is less with LLDN, and there is no significant increase in donor morbidity with the wider application of LLDN. The complications among donors and the recipient ureteral and allograft complications have been shown to decrease as the technical details of the operation evolved and the centers mature in their experience with LLDN.[37] (Figure 15.5.3-12 and Figure 15.5.3-13).

## IMPACT

Several studies have examined the fate of the recipient of laparoscopically procured kidneys.[34,35] Studies at the Johns Hopkins University and the University of Maryland have not shown a significant incidence of delayed graft function requiring dialysis, although a recent review of the UNOS data on pediatric kidney transplant outcomes hinted at a slightly higher rate of delayed graft function in laparoscopically procured kidneys.[36] LLDN has evolved over the last decade, and a decline in the complications noted in the earlier series is apparent.[37] Advantages to the donor, as compared to ODN, are decreased postoperative pain, shorter hospital stay, a quicker convalescence, and an earlier return to work and normalcy. Fewer wages are lost for the donor and it provides a superior cosmetic outcome. It successfully removes many of the disincentives to live kidney donation and has resulted in an increased willingness of individuals to donate their kidneys including altruistic donors, living unrelated donors, church members etc.[38] A significant increase in living kidney donation has been reported by the United Network for Organ Sharing

**TABLE 15.5.3-2**

## RECIPIENT OUTCOME FROM LLDN KIDNEYS

| Investigators | S Creatinine mg% 1 week | 3 months | 1 year | Delayed Graft Function | Primary Nonfunction | Graft Loss | | Ureteral Stricture/ Necrosis |
|---|---|---|---|---|---|---|---|---|
| Jacobs et al. Univ Maryland[33] | 2 ± 1.5 | 1.6 ± 0.9 | 1.6 ± 1.4 | 19 (2.6%) | 4 (0.5%) | 3 RCC[a] Vase reconst LLDN abort | : 1 : 1 : 1 | 33 (4.4%) |
| Levanthal et al. NW Univ 500 LLDN[5] | 1.5 ± 0.2 | Not reported | Not reported | 1 (0.002%) | Nil | 4: RA thromb RA stenosis RI | : 2 : 1 : 1 | 1 (0.002%) |
| Su et al. Johns Hopkins 381 LLDN[32] | 2.6 ± 2.3 | Not reported | Not reported | 17 (4.5%) | Not reported | 9: RV thromb RA thromb Cholesterol Emb RA anast bleed | : 5 : 1 : 2 : 1 | 24 (6.3%) |

[a] Abbreviations used: RCC, renal cell carcinoma: RA renal; artery; RV renal vein; thromb: thrombosis; cholest, cholesterol; RI, renal infarct; emb, emboli; anast, anastomotic vasc: vascular; reconst reconstruction; CIA: common iliac artery. Major complications are defined as those that require repair and/or conversion to open surgery. Minor complications were manageable via laparoscopic approach and did not require conversion to open surgery nor a repeat surgery.

**TABLE 15.5.3-3**

## OUTCOME OF COMPARATIVE SERIES FROM SINGLE INSTITUTIONS

| Investigators | | Operating Time | WIT (min) | Hospital Stay (days) | L/H Work (days) | Analgesics After Discharge | Complications | | S Creat. (6 m.) mg% | Complications | |
|---|---|---|---|---|---|---|---|---|---|---|---|
| | | | | Donor Outcome | | | | | Recipient Outcome | | |
| Ruiz-Deya et al. [31] HA vs Pure LLDN | HA LLDN | 2.75 ± 0.2 hr | 1.6 ± 0.2 | 2 ± 0.1 | | | Open conversion Ileus Abd incision longer. | : 1 : 2 | 1.3 ± 0.3 | Comparable outcome in both groups. | |
| | Pure LLDN | 3.59 ± 0.2 hr | 3.9 ± 0.3 | 1.6 ± 1.3 | | | Incarcerated Hernia Deep Vein Thromb | : 1 : 1 | 1.35 ± 0.3 | Comparable outcome in both groups. | |
| Simforoosh et al. [9] ODN vs LLDN | ODN | 152.2 (80 – 260) min | 1.87 (1–5) | 2.2 (2–8) | 7.9/ 56.6 | 7.8 (0–40) | Pheumothroax Ileus Urinary Tract Infection Bleeding Re-operation for bleeding | :18 : 4 : 2 : 1 : 2 | 1.45 (0.7– 4.3) | Ureteral stricture : 2 Rvthrombosis : 1 Lymphocele : 3 Delayed graft function : 8 | |
| | LLDN | 270.8 (165–490) min | 8.7 (4–17) | 2.26 (2–5) | 5.9/34 | 33 (0–20) | Bleeding Ileus Splenic laceration Urinary Tract Infection Scotal swelling Transfusion Re-operation for bleed | : 4 : 7 : 2 : 1 : 3 : 1 : 1 | 1.41 (0.5– 9.1) | Ureteral comp :nil Vascular comp :nil Delayed graft Function :1 | |

(UNOS). In 2001, the number of living donors exceeded the number of cadaver donors.[39] By decreasing donor morbidity, the laparoscopic live donor operation has shifted the donor–recipient, risk–benefit ratio. Individuals are more willing to take greater risks on the recipient side when there is less "cost" to the donor. This effect has had a permissive role in promoting ABO blood group incompatible live donor transplants and live donor transplants across a positive crossmatch after treatment with plasmapheresis and intravenous immune globulin.[40] Several forums and opinion papers discussing methods to removing the residual donor disincentives have appeared in the literature. These incentives include a Georgia state program that discounts renewal fees for drivers' licenses for organ donors and a Pennsylvania state program that gives $300 in vouchers to living donors.[41] Various models of donor reimbursement/compensation have been proposed in this light.[42] The U.S. Congress has recommended legislative resolutions to live organ donation by accepting "Donor Leave Act." This permits federal employees, in any calendar year, to take 30 days of paid leave to serve as an organ donor. Several states, hospitals, and professional institutions have followed suit. The recently enacted Organ Donation and Recovery Improvement Act directs the Federal Health and Human Services to grant reimbursement of travel and subsistence expenses incurred by individuals in making a living organ donation to states, transplant centers, qualified organ procurement organizations, or other public or private entities for reimbursement of travel and subsistence expenses incurred by individuals in making a living organ donation.[43]

Various forms of sharing organs have been proposed among unrelated donors,[43] for instance, living donor paired exchange, living donor/deceased donor exchange, etc. The idea of minimally invasive living donor organ retrieval has subsequently been applied to liver transplantation[44] and pancreas transplantation.[20] Over and above the benefit of improved donor outcome and increased availability of organs, LLDN has invigorated a moribound academic arena of transplantation. A PubMed search on "living donor nephrectomy" yielded about 36 articles before the initial report of LLDN was published in November 1995, whereas the same search yielded about 568 articles from November 1995 to date.

## FUTURE CONSIDERATIONS

Improving precision in laparoscopic surgery using robotic technology has been done.[45] This system improves the surgeon's comfort and restores ergonomically acceptable conditions, increasing the number of degrees of freedom and recreating the three-dimensional eye–hand connection lost in video endoscopic procedures. Horgan et al[46] reported a marginally reduced hospital stay, but comparable warm ischemia time as well as operative time and blood loss using hand-assisted robotic (Da Vinci Surgical System) LLDN. The added cost (in excess of $1 million) needs justification. The author felt that motion scaling and tremor elimination enabled the performance of technically demanding procedures with extreme precision and accuracy and are potentially time saving.

**TABLE 15.5.3-4**

## COMPLICATIONS OF LLDN REPORTED BY CENTERS WITH SIGNIFICANT EXPERIENCE: DONOR COMPLICATIONS

| Investigators | Major complications | | | Minor Complications | |
|---|---|---|---|---|---|
| | Vascular injury | Visceral/other major injury | Death | | |
| Jacobs SC et al. | Renal Artery : 2 | Small Bowel :2 | Nil | Splenic injury | : 15 |
| Uni Maryland | Renal Vein : 3 | | | Liver lacerations | : 1 |
| 738 LLDNS | Common Iliac Artery : 1 | | | Pnuemothorax | : 2 |
| (33)- | Inferior Vena Cava : 1 | | | Diaphram Inj | : 2 |
| | Aorta : 4 | | | Stapler misfires | : 4 |
| | Mesenteric Vein : 2 | | | Minor vessels | : 3 |
| | 6/10 from Vascular staplers | | | Glove entrapment | : 2 |
| Melcher ML et al. | Renal Artery : 1 | | Nil | Splenic laceration | : 3 |
| UCSF | Vascular stapler | | | Bowel injury | : 2 |
| 530 LLDNs | | | | Transfusion | : 5 |
| (49) | | | | Rhabdomyolysis | : 1 |
| | | | | Wound infection | : 14 |
| | | | | DVT/PE | : 2 |
| Levanthal JR et al. | Aortic injury : 1 | | Nil | Splenic tear | : 3 |
| N.W. Uni | Renal Artery injury : 3 | | | Diaphragmatic tear | : 1 |
| 500 LLDNs | Lumbar Vein injury : 2 | | | Adrenal hematoma | : 1 |
| (5) | | | | Serosal bowel injury | : 1 |
| | | | | $CO_2$ pneumomediastium | : 2 |
| | | | | Urinary retention | : 6 |
| | | | | Wound infection | : 4 |
| Su LM et al. | Renal Artery injury : 3 | Colon injury : 1 | Nil | Splenic laceration | : 2 |
| Johns Hopkins | Renal Vein injury : 3 | Small bowel injury : 4 | | Transfusion | : 13 |
| 381 LLDN | Epigastric A. laceration : 1 | Retro Peritoneal hematoma : 8 | | Wound Infection | : 9 |
| (37) | | Testicular ischemia : 1 | | Urinary Tract Infection | : 5 |
| | | Incisional Hernia : 1 | | Retro Peritoneal Hematoma | : 3 |

Improvements in the optical instruments, particularly in telescopes, and improveresolution of cameras and development of halide light sources that afford better illumination without raising the temperature.

The author (LER) participated in a multicenter study of fatal and nonfatal hemorrhagic complications of both open and laparoscopic living kidney donation (in press). A survey of hemorrhagic complication of donor nephrectomy was sent to all members of the American Society of Transplant Surgeons (ASTS) of which 213 were returned. Over and above reporting two donor deaths and two cases of renal failure resulting from arterial control problems, the survey identified 29 conversions to open surgery for control of bleeding. A total of 66 arterial and 39 venous hemorrhage events were reported. The 33-question survey identified the methods of vascular control employed by responding surgeons, and the opinion of the surgeons was sought regarding what they thought was the safest technique for major vascular control for both open and laparoscopic donor nephrectomies. The survey concluded that locking and standard clips applied to the renal artery were associated with the greatest risks and that vascular transfixation provides the best vascular control of major vessels.

The establishment of living donor registries would contribute significantly toward the long-term health-monitoring of donors. Particularly donors that are obese and/or on single antihypertensive medications should be followed up for their blood pressure

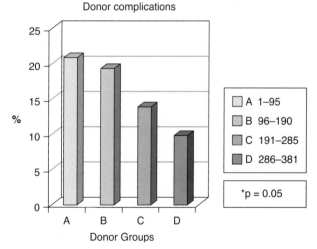

**FIGURE 15.5.3-12**

Reduction in the rate of complication among donors with improvements in LLDN.[37] An interesting observation was made by Su et al. regarding the evolution of the technique and maturity of the center in doing LLDN.[37] She documented a significant decline in the complication rate between early experience (group A) and late experience (group D); that is, p = 0.05; and a significant decline in the trend from group A to group D (p < 0.05).

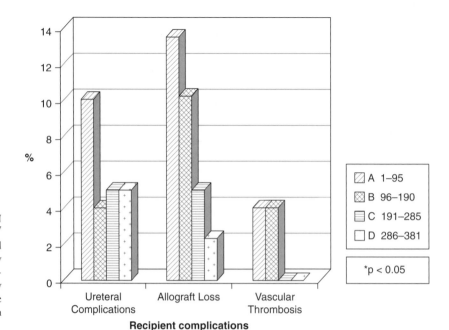

**FIGURE 15.5.3-13**

Reduction in the rate of complication among LLDN recipients with improved techniques and experience.[37] An interesting observation was made by SU LM et. al regarding the evolution of the technique and maturity of the center in doing LLDN [37]. She documented a significant decline in the complication rate between early experience (group A) vs late experience (group D) ie p = 0.05. And a significant decline in the trend from group A through D (p < 0.05).

control, proteinuria, and serum creatinine.[47,48] Over and above monitoring renal function, such registries would afford reliable long-term data on parameters like incisional pain and long-term physical/psychological sequelea (if any) among donors.

Analgesic requirements following donor nephrectomy has been improved following the adaptation of the minimally invasive approach. Further improvements have occurred from routine use of epidural catheters and patient-controlled analgesia regimes. A longer half-life of these intrathecally administered agents like ropivocaine and their ability to combine with narcotics like hydromorphone have further helped in removing donor disincentives.

## CONCLUSION

In summary, transperitoneal LLDN (either pure laparoscopic or hand-assisted) has now become the dominant mode for living donor kidney retrieval in the United States. In experienced hands the operation is safe, not deleterious for the recipient, and provides profound advantages to the donor. Early concerns about the utilization of the right kidney with LLDN are no longer valid as the operation has evolved and matured. However, there is still room to improve safety and donor comfort. Future studies should be directed toward these goals.

## References

1. Personal communication Dr Ratner LE.
2. Suzuki K, Ishikawa A, Ushiyama T, et al. Gasless laparoscopy assisted live donor nephrectomy: The initial 23 cases. *Transplant Proc* 2000; 32(4):788–789.
3. Molmenti EP, Pinto PA, Montgomery RA, et al. Concomitant surgery with laparoscopic live donor nephrectomy. *Am J Transplant* 2003; 3(2):219–223.
4. Oyen O, Andersen M, Mathisen L, et al. Laparoscopic versus open living-donor nephrectomy: experiences from a prospective, randomized, single-center study focusing on donor safety. *Transplantation* 2005; 15;79(9):1236–1240.
5. Leventhal JR, Kocak B, Salvalaggio PR, et al. Laparoscopic donor nephrectomy 1997 to 2003: lessons learned with 500 cases at a single institution. *Surgery* 2004;136(4):881–890.
6. Boulware LE, Ratner LE, Sosab JA, et al. The general public's concerns about clinical risk in live kidney donation. 2002;2:186–193.
7. Authors for the Live Organ Donor Consensus Group. Consensus statement on the live donor. *J Am Med Assoc* 2000;284:2919–2926.
8. Jones KW, Peters TG, Charlton RK, et al. Current issues in living donor nephrectomy. *Clin Transplant* 1997;11:505–510.
9. Simforoosh N, Basiri A, Tabibi A, et al. Comparison of laparoscopic and open donor nephrectomy:A randomized controlled trial. *BJU Int* 2005; 95(6):851–855.
10. Baron PW, Baldwin DD, Hadley HR, et al. Hand-assisted laparoscopic donor nephrectomy is safe and results in increased kidney donation. *Am Surg* 2004;70(10):901–915.
11. Harrison JH, Merrill JP, Murray JE. Renal homotransplantation in identical twins. *Surg Forum* 1956;6(1955):432–436.
12. Clayman RV, Kavoussi LR, Soper NJ, et al. Laparoscopic nephrectomy: Initial case report. *J Urol* 1991;146(2):278–282.
13. Gill IS, Carbone JM, Clayman RV, et al. Laparoscopic live-donor nephrectomy. *J Endourol* 1994;8(2):143–148.
14. Ratner LE, Ciseck LJ, Moore RG, et al. Laparoscopic live-donor nephrectomy. *Transplantation* 1995;60(9):1047–1049.
15. Slakey DP, Wood JC, Hender D, et al. Laparoscopic living donor nephrectomy: advantages of the handassisted method. *Transplantation* 999;68(4):581–583.
16. Rassweiler JJ, Seemann O, Frede T, et al. Retroperitoneoscopy: Experience with 200 cases. *J Urol* 1998;160(4):1265–1269.
17. Yang SC, Lee DH, Rha KH, et al. Retroperitoneoscopic living donor nephrectomy: Two cases. *Transplant Proc* 1994;26(4):2409.
18. Wolf JS Jr, Merion RM, Leichtman AB, et al. Randomized controlled trial of hand-assisted laparoscopic versus open surgical live donor nephrectomy. *Transplantation* 2001;72(2):284–290.
19. Ishikawa A, Suzuki K, Saisu K, et al. Endoscopy-assisted live donor nephrectomy: Comparison between laparoscopic and retroperitoneoscopic procedures. *Transplant Proc* 1998;30(1):165–167.
20. Tan M, Kandaswamy R, Sutherland DE, Gruessner RW. Laparoscopic donor distal pancreatectomy for living donor pancreas and pancreaskidney transplantation. *Am J Transplant* 2005;5(8):1966–1970.
21. Ratner LE, Fabrizio M, Chavin K, et al. Technical considerations in the delivery of the kidney during laparoscopic live-donor nephrectomy. *J Am Coll Surg* 1999;189:427.

22. Mandal AK, Kalligonis AN, Cohen C, et al. Should the right kidney be used in laparoscopic live donor nephrectomy [abstract]. *Transplantation* 2000;69:S403.

23. Slakey DP, Wood JC, Hender D, et al: Laparoscopic living donor nephrectomy: Advantages of the hand assisted method. *Transplantation* 1999;68:581.

24. Wolf JS, Marcovich R, Merion RM, et al. Prospective case matched comparison of hand assisted laparoscopic and open surgical live donor nephrectomy. *J Urol* 2000;163:1650.

25. Wolf JS, Tchetgen MB, Merion RM. Hand-assisted laparoscopic live donor nephrectomy. *Urology* 1998;52:885.

26. Stifelman M, Patel R. Hals Devices and Operating Room Set-Up: Pearls and Pitfalls. *J Endourol* 2004(May);18(4) 314–318.

27. Jacobs SC, Cho E, Dunkin BJ, et al. Laparoscopic live donor nephrectomy: The University of Maryland 3-year experience. *J Urol* 2000;164:1494–1499.

28. Ratner LE, Montgomery RA, Kavoussi LR. Laparoscopic live donor nephrectomy:The four-year Johns Hopkins University experience. *Nephrol Dial Transplant* 1999;14:2090–2093.

29. Arenas J, Gupta M, et al. Initial program experience with right laparoscopic donor nephrectomy. *Transplantation* 2000;69:S335.

30. Buell JF, Edye M, et al. Are Concerns over Right Laparoscopic Donor Nephrectomy Unwarranted? Annals of Surgery 233(5): 645–651, 2001.

31. Ruiz-Deya G, Cheng S, Palmer E, et al. Open donor, laparoscopic donor and hand assisted laparoscopic donor nephrectomy: A comparison of outcomes. *J Urol* 2001;166:1270–1274.

32. Ng CS, Abreu SC, Abou El-Fettouh HI, Kaouk JH, et al. Right retroperitoneal versus left transperitoneal laparoscopic live donor nephrectomy. *Urology* 2004;63(5):857–861.

33. Jacobs SC, Cho E, Foster C. Laparoscopic donor nephrectomy: The University of Maryland 6-year experience. *J Urol* 2004;171(1):47–51.

34. Nogueira JM, Cangro CB, Fink JC, et al. A comparison of recipient renal outcomes with laparoscopic versus open live donor nephrectomy. *Transplantation* 1999;67:722.

35. Ratner LE, Montgomery RA, Maley WR, et al. Laparoscopic live donor nephrectomy: The recipient. *Transplantation* 2000;69:2319.

36. Troppmann C, McBride MA, Baker TJ, et al. Laparoscopic live donor nephrectomy: A risk factor for delayed function and rejection in pediatric kidney recipients? A UNOS analysis. *Am J Transplant* 2005;5(1):175–182.

37. Su LM, Ratner LE, Montgomery RA, Jarrett TW, et al. Laparoscopic live donor nephrectomy: trends in donor and recipient morbidity following 381 consecutive cases. *Ann Surg* 2004;240(2):358–363.

38. Schweitzer EJ, Wilson J, Jacobs S, et al. Increased rates of donation with laparoscopic donor nephrectomy. *Ann Surg* 2000;232(3):392–400.

39. 2001 Annual Report of the US Organ Procurement and Transplantation Network and the Scientific Registry for Transplant Recipients: Transplant Data 1991-2000. Rockville, MD: US Dept of Health and Human Services, Health Resources and Services Administration, Office of Special Programs, Division of Transplantation; Ann Arbor, MI: United Network for Organ Sharing; Richmond, VA: University Renal Research and Education Association, 2001.

40. Ratner LE, Montgomery RA, Kavoussi LR. Laparoscopic live donor nephrectomy. A review of the first 5 years. *Urologic Clin North Am* 2001;28(4) 709–719.

41. Wiggins O. PA organ donors get $ 300 boost. *Philadelphia Inquirer.* Philadelphia 2002:A1.

42. Israni AK, Halpern SD, Zink S, et al. Incentive models to increase living kidney donation: Encouraging without coercing. *Am J Transplant* 2005;5:15–20.

43. Davis CL, Delmonico FL. Living-donor kidney transplantation: A review of the current practices for the live donor. *J Am Soc Nephrol* 2005 (Jul0;16(7):2098–2110.

44. Cherqui D, Soubrane O, Husson E, et al. Laparoscopic living donor hepatectomy for liver transplantation in children. *Lancet* 2002; 359 (9304):392–396.

45. Horgan S, Benedetti E, Moser F. Robotically assisted donor nephrectomy for kidney transplantation. *Am J Surg* 2004;188(4A Suppl):45S–451S.

46. Horgan S, Vanuno D, Sileri P et al. Robotic-assisted laparoscopic donor nephrectomy for kidney transplantation. *Transplantation* 2002;5; 73(9):1474–1479.

47. Thiel GT, Nolte C, Tsinalis D. The Swiss Organ Living Donor Health Registry (SOL-DHR). *Ther Umsch* 2005;62(7):449–457.

48. D'Cunha PT, Parasuraman R, Venkat KK. Rapid resolution of proteinuria of native kidney origin following live donor renal transplantation. *Am J Transplant* 2005;5(2):351–355.

49. Melchar ML, Carter JT, Posselt A et al. More than 500 consecutive laparoscopic donor nephrectomies without conversion or repeated surgery. *Arch Surg* 2005;140:835–840.

50. Lopez PA, Leveille RJ. Trocar Arrangement for HALS. *J Endourol* 2004;18(4) 319–325.

## 15.5.4    Retroperitoneal Laparoscopic Nephrectomy

*Jonas Wadström, MD, PhD*

### INTRODUCTION

When laparoscopic live donor nephrectomy (LDN) was introduced by L. Ratner in 1995,[1] it was at first met with some skepticism, mainly due to concerns about the safety of the procedure. The technique has, however, been demonstrated to yield equal survival rates and at the same time cause less morbidity with less pain and a shorter recuperation period than conventional open nephrectomy.[2–5] In LDN, surgery is performed on a healthy person who receives no direct therapeutic benefit. Safety issues are therefore extremely important, and the safety of the procedure is still being questioned.[6,7]

One of these safety issues concerns potential difficulties in handling major sudden bleeding, which is a life-threatening complication and the most common cause for emergency conversion.[8,9] Another severe and life-threatening intraoperative complication is intestinal injury. Intestinal injuries are often not detected intraoperatively, and the delayed diagnosis aggravates their severity and can progress into life-threatening complications.[10–12]

The most common causes for readmission are also related to gastrointestinal complications such as nausea, vomiting, dehydration, ileus, or constipation.[8–13]

Indeed, severe sudden bleeding and intestinal lesions are the two major life-threatening complications associated with the procedure and have been the cause of death in connection with laparoscopic nephrectomy.[9,14–16] A number of refinements and modifications of both the surgical instruments and the surgical technique have been introduced that increase the safety of the procedure. Two major improvements in surgical technique have been the introduction of a hand-assisted technique[17] and a retroperitoneoscopic approach.[18]

The technique described in this chapter, hand-assisted retroperitoneoscopic (HARS) LDN, combines the safety advantages of both the hand-assisted technique and the retroperitoneal approach.[19–22]

The hand-assisted technique facilitates the operation and makes it safer.[23–26] In the case of a severe sudden bleeding, a hand in the operating field allows immediate hemostasis by compression. With manual compression and manipulation of the vessels, the bleeding source can often be identified and subsequently ligated with a clip without conversion to open surgery or causing further damage to the vessels or kidney. With a pure laparoscopic technique, a massive bleeding is more difficult to handle, which puts the donor

**TABLE 15.5.4-1**

**ADVANTAGES OF COMBINED HAND-ASSISTED AND RETROPERITONEOSCOPIC NEPHRECTOMY COMPARED WITH TRADITIONAL TRANSPERITONEAL LAPAROSCOPIC NEPHRECTOMY**

- Safer trocar placement (direct vision and hand as shield)
- Reduced risk of visceral injuries (by trocars and during the operation)
- Better control of potential bleedings (immediate hemostasis with manual compression)
- Prevention of torsion of the kidney
- No risk of internal herniation
- Secure and rapid placement of vascular staplers
- Secure and rapid retrieval of the kidney
- Reduces warm ischemia time
- Reduces operating time (leads to cost reduction)
- Reduced risk of bowel obstruction
- Reduced risk of postoperative adhesions

at risk.[25,27–37] With the traditional technique, conversion to open surgery is also often necessary, which takes additional time and further prolongs the time until hemostasis can be achieved, and it can cause warm ischemia damage to the kidney.

The hand-assisted technique also facilitates the operation and the extraction of the kidney. The hand-assisted technique has thus been shown to shorten operating times as well as warm ischemia time (WIT).[25,26,30,38,39]

The retroperitoneal approach has the advantage of reducing the risk of both intra- and postoperative intestinal complications.[40–44] A detailed discussion of the advantages of the hand-assisted and retroperitoneal approach is given in reference 22. The advantages are summarized in Table 15.5.4-1.

Apart from the two major potential complications discussed previously, endoscopic nephrectomy is also associated with a number of complications that are more or less specific for endoscopic techniques. These include emphysema (including pneumomediastinum, pneumothorax, and pneumopericardium), gas embolism, trocar injuries, and malfunctioning of endoscopic instruments. It is important that the operating surgeon and anesthesiologist are well aware of these risks, as well as how they should best be avoided and treated should they occur. Some of these complications will also be addressed in the description of the procedure.

## PREOPERATIVE EVALUATION AND CHOICE OF KIDNEY

The preoperative evaluation and the grounds for accepting or rejecting a donor are essentially the same as for any other type of LDN operation.

From a surgical–technical point of view, the decision to harvest the right or left kidney may, however, influence the choice of method: endoscopic or open.

Factors influencing which kidney is harvested include: split function; arterial, venous, and ureteral anatomy; and any other renal abnormalities (eg, cysts). Extrarenal findings such as previous operations and scars or perceived difficulty in positioning on one side may also play a role. All else being equal, it is generally preferable to remove the left kidney because it has a longer renal vein, which makes the recipient operation easier. There also seems to be a lower risk for venous thrombosis with the left kidney, from both

deceased and live donors.[45] The shorter renal vein on the right side is believed to be a reason for the increased risk of graft thrombosis.[46] We have therefore only harvested right kidneys with the HARS technique when the preoperative computed tomography (CT) angiography has demonstrated a fairly long right renal vein. The number of renal arteries and veins also influences the decision of which side to harvest, but the presence of multiple vessels as such is not a contraindication for harvesting a kidney with the HARS technique. Venous abnormalities such as a retroaortic vein do not generally influence the decision of which side to harvest.[47]

## PROPHYLAXIS

Pulmonary embolus is the single most common cause of perioperative death in live donors,[48] and thromboembolism is seen in most larger series of donor follow-up.[13,49,50] Thorough assessment of risk factors for thromboembolic events must therefore be investigated thoroughly as part of the preoperative assessment.[22] From a theoretical standpoint, the increased intraabdominal pressure can be expected to compromise the venous return from the legs and thereby increase the risk or thromboembolism in connection with prolonged laparoscopic surgery such as laparoscopic LDN. Although there are only limited randomized data regarding thromboprophylaxis in laparoscopic surgery, we have adopted a policy of giving both compression stockings and low-molecular-weight heparin to all our donors. If there is any increased risk, such as heterozygote APC-resistance, we increase the dose of low-molecular-weight heparin and prolong the prophylaxis for 6 weeks postoperatively. We have not seen any bleeding complications under this policy.

All our donors are also given 24 hours of perioperative antibiotic prophylaxis.

## THE SURGICAL PROCEDURE—HARS

### Volume Loading

In increased intraabdominal pressure decreases renal blood flow, glomerular filtration rate (GFR), and can even cause oliguria.[51–53] Providing adequate intraoperative volume can, however, ameliorate the adverse effects on kidney function.[54,55] It is therefore important to ensure adequate volume loading pre- and perioperatively.

### Positioning

The patient is placed in a lateral decubitus position carefully padded and secured to the surgical table.

The table is not broken in order to maximize the retroperitoneal space and to not stretch the peritoneum.

Positioning of the patient is important because it may impact morbidity. Long operations with the patient in the decubitus position, especially with a broken table, can cause long-lasting discomfort and even lead to severe complications, such as neuromuscular injuries and rhabdomyolysis.[56–60]

### The Operation

The incision for creating the retroperitoneal space, introduction of the hand-assist device and for kidney removal is a Pfannenstiel or lower midline incision.

The skin, subcutaneous fat, and fascia are incised.

The peritoneum is left intact and a preperitoneal space is created through blunt manual dissection. Because the peritoneum is less firmly attached to the abdominal wall in this area, the dissection starts in a caudal-lateral direction toward the iliac vessels. Once the surgeon is able to feel the iliac vessels, the blunt dissection can continue in a cranial direction along the psoas muscle, and further loosening of the peritoneum from the posterior abdominal wall. A hand-assist device is then placed in the wound. The surgeon's left hand is placed between the abdominal wall and the peritoneum in order to shield the peritoneum and the viscera. A 12-mm working port is then placed immediately to the left of the hand port. Using noncutting trocars lessens the risk of injuring vessels in the abdominal wall. Gas ($CO_2$) is then insufflated into the pre-/post-peritoneal space. Gas pressure is maintained at a maximum of 12 mm Hg. Higher pressures should be avoided in order not to compromise kidney function. A 30° video laparoscope is introduced through this port. The peritoneum is further loosened by manual dissection to about 10 cm above the kidney in the cranial direction and toward the midline in the medial direction. The peritoneum gets thinner and more fragile as the dissection gets closer to the midline. Holes and tears in the peritoneum should be avoided. Should they occur, however, this is not a problem, and gas leaking into the peritoneal cavity does not reduce the retroperitoneal working space. The insufflated gas is helpful for this dissection and for finding the right plane. A second 12-mm blunt port is introduced high on the subcostal margin. The port is placed under direct vision, while the hand shields the peritoneum and viscera. The video laparoscope is moved to this second port and a third 5-mm blunt port is placed in the flank below the costal margin. The position of the patient, surgeons, and ports are depicted in Figure 15.5.4-1. The operation is performed in essentially the same manner as with the traditional laparoscopic technique.

The extraperitoneal approach, however, obviates mobilization of the colon or the spleen. The splenocolic ligament is left intact. This makes the rest of the operation easier and faster. It also brings the advantage that it prevents internal herniation through the mesocolon and into the kidney bed.[61] Throughout the operation, dissection is performed with an ultrasonic scalpel. Avoiding the use of cautery is important, especially around the ureter, because the heat and current may damage the circulation of the ureter.

Dissection of the kidney starts by opening the medioanterior portion of Gerota's fascia. The upper pole of the kidney is dissected

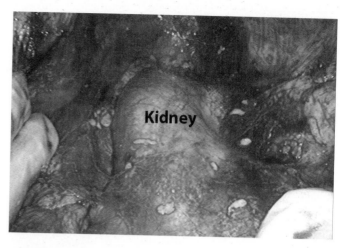

**FIGURE 15.5.4-2**

After the peritoneum has been loosened by blunt manual dissection and a retroperitoneal space is created, the kidney is found under the Gerota's fascia.

free. In most cases, this dissection is performed through the 5-mm port in the flank, which gives good access to the upper pole. The ureter is then dissected, often together with the gonadal vein, down to the iliac vessels. Once the ureter and gonadal vein have been identified, they can be lifted by an instrument introduced through the 5-mm port in the flank which facilitates this dissection. The gonadal vein is followed up to the renal vein. The vascular pedicle is then dissected starting with the vein. The dissection of the renal vein, and especially the lumbar branches, is facilitated by lifting the upper pole of the kidney by an instrument introduced through the 5-mm port in the flank. The gonadal, lumbar, and adrenal veins are divided between double clips. Smaller branches can be ligated and divided with an ultrasonic scalpel. If clips are used, if possible, they should be placed at some distance from the renal vein so that they do not come in conflict with the final stapling and division of the renal vein. The artery is then dissected and freed down to the aorta.

The lateral attachments of the kidney can be divided at any suitable time during the operation. Pictures from the intraoperative situs are shown in Figures 15.5.4-2, 15.5.4-3, 15.5.4-4.

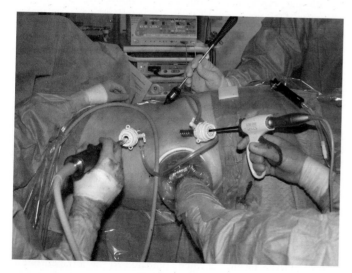

**FIGURE 15.5.4-1**

Position of the patient, surgeons, and ports.

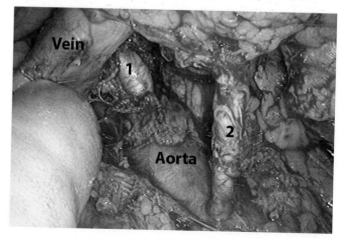

**FIGURE 15.5.4-3**

With the hand-assisted technique, the renal vein can gently be retracted allowing good access to the lumbar veins or in complex arterial dissections, here demonstrated in a case of two arteries.

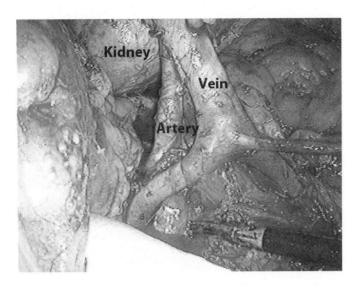

**FIGURE 15.5.4-4**

The retroperitoneal route allows good access to the renal vessels, here demonstrated by a duplicated renal vein riding over the aorta.

The ureter, the artery(ies) and the vein are then divided with an endovascular stapler. The ureter should have a lot of tissue around it to lessen the risk of ureteral necrosis. Large amounts of tissue often necessitate the use of a stapler, but the distal part of ureter can of course also be ligated with clips. The artery and vein should be ligated with a stapler; however, since a transfixational technique reduces the risk of peri- and postoperative bleeding from the divided vessels.[14]

The kidney is extracted by the hand and perfused with cold perfusion solution at a back table by a waiting surgeon. The ports are removed under direct vision in order to detect any bleeding from the port sites. The 12-mm ports are closed, but the 5-mm port in the flank is left without closure. The wound is not drained, and the abdominal wall is closed with a running suture. Skin closure is done preferably by intracutaneous sutures.

## COMMENTS

In live donor nephrectomy, the operation is performed on a healthy person who receives no direct therapeutic benefit. Every available means should be employed to reduce the risk of major complications and keep the risk of mortality to a minimum. The HARS technique, as presented here, was developed to optimize safety. It combines the advantages of hand-assisted techniques and a retroperitoneal approach. The experience so far has shown that it also is a fairly easy and quick operation, where, compared to the intraperitoneal approach, the donor experiences even less pain and with possible advantages in terms of kidney function and integrity.[19,20,21,62]

The hand-assisted technique offers a number of safety advantages. It facilitates the procedure since it provides tactile feedback that compensates for the two-dimensional picture on the video screen.[17,23,25,26,29,31,33,35,39,63] It helps to identify surgical planes and to identify structures. The tactile feedback is especially helpful in difficult cases and for surgeons in a learning phase or with limited experience, situations where complications are more likely to occur.

Sudden major bleeding is life-threatening and has led on occasion to donor mortality.[14] Bleeding can be difficult to manage

using laparoscopic instruments alone and is the most common reason for conversion to open surgery and reoperation.[8,9,13] Severe sudden bleeding can also occur with experienced surgeons, for instance, with malfunctioning of an endovascular stapler.[8,14,15] In such a situation, the hand-assisted technique is of clear advantage as it allows immediate compression to achieve hemostasis.[9,25,27,30–37]

A further advantage with the hand-assisted technique is that it has been demonstrated to shorten operative times.[25,26,30,38,39] This can be of importance because the patients are positioned in an awkward position that can cause long-lasting discomfort and even lead to severe complications such as neuromuscular injuries and rhabdomyolysis.[13,57–60] Long operative time is also generally associated with a number of postsurgical complications.

Our experience with the HARS technique indicates that the retroperitoneal approach leads to even shorter operating times because it obviates the need to mobilize the colon and spleen.[20,21] The operating time is more than 1 hour less than the presently largest single-center experience of left-sided pure laparoscopic live donor nephrectomies.[8,20,21] The hand-assisted technique also appears to shorten the operation as compared to retroperitoneal nephrectomy without hand assistance.[64]

The second set of major life-threatening complication associated with laparoscopic nephrectomy addressed with the HARS technique is gastrointestinal complications. The risk of injury to visceral organs and postoperative bowel obstruction is minimized with this technique. With the retroperitoneal approach, the risk for visceral injuries is lower.[10] Because visceral injuries can be difficult to detect during surgery, they are often discovered in the postoperative period and can progress into life-threatening complications.[10–12]

Prolonged ileus and gastrointestinal complications are indeed among the most common causes for readmission after laparoscopic live donor nephrectomy.[8,13]

It has been argued that the retroperitoneal route for endoscopic donor nephrectomy limits the working space. This is not our experience, even when gas leaks into the abdominal cavity after a tear in the peritoneum.

Gravity helps to keep the visceral organs away from the surgical site, and the peritoneum is easily moved medially with the back of surgeon's left hand.

Although HARS was introduced to optimize the safety of endoscopic LDN, we have also found that morbidity seems to be lower with the HARS technique as compared to traditional laparoscopic and open procedures.[20]

We found that the HARS procedure inflicted less pain and a shorter duration of postoperative pain than both laparoscopic and open procedures. The HARS donors also spent less time in the recovery room and did not complain of shoulder pain, which is sometimes seen after capnoperitoneum. Postoperative respiratory function was superior in the HARS group, with better peek expiratory flow measurements in the early postoperative period. These findings may be important because the ability to ventilate the lung parenchyma and early mobilization are important factors in preventing donor morbidity due to pneumonia and thromboembolic complications.

Preserving the integrity of the kidney and optimal kidney function are also important features of a donor nephrectomy. In the previously cited study, we saw less impairment to kidney function with the HARS technique when compared to the intraperitoneal technique with pneumoperitoneum.[20] The lengths of graft vessels were similar in the different techniques, but the ureters were actually a bit longer in the HARS group.

## SUMMARY

The HARS procedure optimizes the safety of endoscopic live donor nephrectomy. It combines the advantages of hand-assisted techniques and a retroperitoneal approach. The experience so far has demonstrated that it is a fairly easy operation with short operating times. Morbidity is low and kidney integrity and function is well preserved.

## References

1. Ratner LE, Ciseck LJ, Moore RG, et al. Laparoscopic live donor nephrectomy. *Transplantation* 1995;60:1047.
2. Brown SL, Biehl TR, Rawlins MC, et al. Laparoscopic live donor nephrectomy: a comparison with the conventional open approach. *J Urol* 2001; 165:766.
3. Flowers JL, Jacobs S, Cho E, et al. Comparison of open and laparoscopic live donor nephrectomy. *Ann Surg* 1997;226:483.
4. Merlin TL, Scott DF, Rao MM, et al. The safety and efficacy of laparoscopic live donor nephrectomy: a systematic review. *Transplantation* 2000;70:1659.
5. Troppmann C, Ormond DB, Perez RV. Laparoscopic (vs open) live donor nephrectomy: A UNOS database analysis of early graft function and survival. *Am J Transplant* 2003;3:1295.
6. Vastag B. Living-donor transplants reexamined: Experts cite growing concerns about safety of donors. *JAMA* 2003;290:181.
7. Barry JM. Living donor nephrectomy. *J Urol* 2004;171:61.
8. Jacobs SC, Cho E, Foster C, et al. Laparoscopic donor nephrectomy: The University of Maryland 6-year experience. *J Urol* 2004;171:47.
9. Siqueira TM Jr, Kuo RL, Gardner TA, et al. Major complications in 213 laparoscopic nephrectomy cases: The Indianapolis experience. *J Urol* 2002;168:1361.
10. Fahlenkamp D, Rassweiler J, Fornara P, et al. Complications of laparoscopic procedures in urology: Experience with 2407 procedures at 4 German centers. *J Urol* 1999;162:765.
11. El-Banna M, Abdel-Atty M, El-Meteini M, et al. Management of laparoscopic-related bowel injuries. *Surg Endosc* 2000;14:779.
12. Deziel DJ, Millikan KW, Economou SG, et al. Complications of laparoscopic cholecystectomy: A national survey of 4,292 hospitals and an analysis of 77,604 cases. *Am J Surg* 1993;165:9.
13. Matas AJ, Bartlett ST, Leichtman AB, et al. Morbidity and mortality after living kidney donation, 1999-2001: Survey of United States transplant centers. *Am J Transplant* 2003;3:830.
14. Friedman AL, Ratner LE, Peters TG. Fatal and non-fatal hemorrhagic complications of living kidney donation. *Am J Transplant* 2004; 8 (Suppl. 8):370.
15. Deng DY, Meng MV, Nguyen HT, et al. Laparoscopic linear cutting stapler failure. *Urology* 2002;60:415.
16. Parsons JK, Varkarakis I, Rha KH, et al. Complications of abdominal urologic laparoscopy: longitudinal five-year analysis. *Urology* 2004;63:27.
17. Wolf JS Jr, Tchetgen MB, Merion RM. Hand-assisted laparoscopic live donor nephrectomy. *Urology* 1998;52:885.
18. Gill IS, Rassweiler JJ. Retroperitoneoscopic renal surgery: Our approach. *Urology* 1999;54:734.
19. Wadstrom J, Lindstrom P. Hand-assisted retroperitoneoscopic living-donor nephrectomy: Initial 10 cases. *Transplantation* 2002;73:1839.
20. Sundqvist P, Feuk U, Haggman M, et al. Hand-assisted retroperitoneoscopic live donor nephrectomy in comparison to open and laparoscopic procedures: A prospective study on donor morbidity and kidney function. *Transplantation* 2004;78:147.
21. Wadström J. Hand-assisted retroperitoneoscopic live donor nephrectomy. Experience from the first 75 consecutive cases. *Transplantation* 2005;80:1060.
22. Wadström J. Living donor nephrectomy. In: Gaston RS, Wadström J, eds. *Living Donor Kidney Transplantation: Current Practices, Emerging Trends and Evolving Challenges.* London and New York, Taylor & Francis; 2005:75.
23. Velidedeoglu E, Williams N, Brayman KL, et al. Comparison of open, laparoscopic, and hand-assisted approaches to live-donor nephrectomy. *Transplantation* 2002;74:169.
24. Wolf JS Jr, Merion RM, Leichtman AB, et al. Randomized controlled trial of hand-assisted laparoscopic versus open surgical live donor nephrectomy. *Transplantation* 2001;72:284.
25. Gershbein AB, Fuchs GJ. Hand-assisted and conventional laparoscopic live donor nephrectomy: a comparison of two contemporary techniques. *J Endourol* 2002;16:509.
26. Slakey DP, Wood JC, Hender D, et al. Laparoscopic living donor nephrectomy: Advantages of the hand-assisted method. *Transplantation* 1999;68:581.
27. Lai IR, Tsai MK, Lee PH. Hand-assisted versus total laparoscopic live donor nephrectomy. *J Formos Med Assoc* 2004;103:749.
28. Tan YH, Young MD, L'Esperance JO, et al. Hand-assisted laparoscopic partial nephrectomy without hilar vascular clamping using a saline-cooled, high-density monopolar radiofrequency device. *J Endourol* 2004;18:883.
29. Stifelman MD, Sosa RE, Nakada SY, et al. Hand-assisted laparoscopic partial nephrectomy. *J Endourol* 2001;15:161.
30. Slakey DP, Hahn JC, Rogers E, et al. Single-center analysis of living donor nephrectomy: Hand-assisted laparoscopic, pure laparoscopic, and traditional open. *Prog Transplant* 2002;12:206.
31. Stifelman MD, Hull D, Sosa RE, et al. Hand assisted laparoscopic donor nephrectomy: A comparison with the open approach. *J Urol* 2001; 166:444.
32. Wolf JS Jr. Re: Editorial comment on open donor, laparoscopic donor and hand assisted laparoscopic donor nephrectomy: a comparison of outcomes. *J Urol* 2002;168:199.
33. Kercher K, Dahl D, Harland R, et al. Hand-assisted laparoscopic donor nephrectomy minimizes warm ischemia. *Urology* 2001;58:152.
34. Greenstein MA, Harkaway R, Badosa F, et al. Minimal incision living donor nephrectomy compared to the hand-assisted laparoscopic living donor nephrectomy. *World J Urol* 2003;20:356.
35. Maartense S, Idu M, Bemelman FJ, et al. Hand-assisted laparoscopic live donor nephrectomy. *Br J Surg* 2004;91:344.
36. Maartense S, Heintjes RJ, Idu M, et al. Renal artery clip dislodgement during hand-assisted laparoscopic living donor nephrectomy. *Transplant* Proc 2003;35:779.
37. Oyen O, Line PD, Pfeffer P, et al. Laparoscopic living donor nephrectomy: Introduction of simple hand-assisted technique (without hand-port). *Transplant Proc* 2003;35:779.
38. Lindstrom P, Haggman M, Wadstrom J. Hand-assisted laparoscopic surgery (HALS) for live donor nephrectomy is more time- and cost-effective than standard laparoscopic nephrectomy. *Surg Endosc* 2002;16:422.
39. Ruiz-Deya G, Cheng S, Palmer E, et al. Open donor, laparoscopic donor and hand assisted laparoscopic donor nephrectomy: A comparison of outcomes. *J Urol* 2001;166:1270.
40. Hoznek A, Olsson LE, Salomon L, et al. Retroperitoneal laparoscopic living-donor nephrectomy. Preliminary results. *Eur Urol* 2001;40:614.
41. Rassweiler JJ, Wiesel M, Carl S, et al. Laparoscopic live donor nephrectomy. Personal experiences and review of the literature. *Urologe A* 2001;40:485.
42. Buell JF, Abreu SC, Hanaway MJ, et al. Right donor nephrectomy: A comparison of hand-assisted transperitoneal and retroperitoneal laparoscopic approaches. *Transplantation* 2004;77:521.
43. Gill IS, Uzzo RG, Hobart MG, et al. Laparoscopic retroperitoneal live donor right nephrectomy for purposes of allotransplantation and autotransplantation. *J Urol* 2000;164:1500.
44. Abbou CC, Rabii R, Hoznek A, et al. Nephrectomy in a living donor by retroperitoneal laparoscopy or lomboscopy. *Ann Urol* 2000;34:312.
45. Bakir N, Sluiter WJ, Ploeg RJ, et al. Primary renal graft thrombosis. *Nephrol Dial Transplant* 1996;11:140.
46. Mandal AK, Cohen C, Montgomery RA, et al. Should the indications for laparoscopic live donor nephrectomy of the right kidney be the same as for the open procedure? Anomalous left renal vasculature is not a contraindication to laparoscopic left donor nephrectomy. *Transplantation* 2001;71:660.

47. Wadstrom J, Lindstrom P. Retroaortic renal vein not a contraindication for hand-assisted retroperitoneoscopic living donor nephrectomy. *Transplant Proc* 2003;35:784.

48. Najarian JS, Chavers BM, McHugh LE, et al. 20 years or more of follow-up of living kidney donors. *Lancet* 1992;340:807.

49. Waples MJ, Belzer FO, Uehling DT. Living donor nephrectomy: A 20-year experience. *Urology* 1995;45:207.

50. Dunn JF, Nylander WA Jr, Richie RE, et al. Living related kidney donors. A 14-year experience. *Ann Surg* 1986;203:637.

51. Lindstrom P, Kallskog O, Wadstrom J, et al. Blood flow distribution during elevated intraperitoneal pressure in the rat. *Acta Physiol Scand* 2003;177:149.

52. Razvi HA, Fields D, Vargas JC, et al. Oliguria during laparoscopic surgery: Evidence for direct renal parenchymal compression as an etiologic factor. *J Endourol* 1996;10:1.

53. Chang DT, Kirsch AJ, Sawczuk IS. Oliguria during laparoscopic surgery. *J Endourol* 1994;8:349.

54. Lindstrom P, Wadstrom J, Ollerstam A, et al. Effects of increased intra-abdominal pressure and volume expansion on renal function in the rat. *Nephrol Dial Transplant* 2003;18:2269.

55. Harman PK, Kron IL, McLachlan HD, et al. Elevated intra-abdominal pressure and renal function. *Ann Surg* 1982;196:594.

56. Wolf JS Jr, Marcovich R, Gill IS, et al. Survey of neuromuscular injuries to the patient and surgeon during urologic laparoscopic surgery. *Urology* 2000;55:831.

57. Mathes DD, Assimos DG, Donofrio PD. Rhabdomyolysis and myonecrosis in a patient in the lateral decubitus position. *Anesthesiology* 1996;84:727.

58. Kuang W, Ng CS, Matin S, et al. Rhabdomyolysis after laparoscopic donor nephrectomy. *Urology* 2002;60:911.

59. Kozak KR, Shah S, Ishihara KK, et al. Hand-assisted laparoscopic radical nephrectomy-associated rhabdomyolysis with ARF. *Am J Kidney Dis* 2003;41:E5.

60. Troppmann C, Perez RV. Rhabdomyolysis associated with laparoscopic live donor nephrectomy and concomitant surgery: a note of caution. *Am J Transplant* 2003;3:1457.

61. Knoepp L, Smith M, Huey J, et al. Complication after laparoscopic donor nephrectomy: a case report and review. *Transplantation* 1999;68:449.

62. Wadstrom J, Lindstrom P, Engstrom BM. Hand-assisted retroperitoneoscopic living donor nephrectomy superior to laparoscopic nephrectomy. *Transplant Proc* 2003;35:782.

63. Seifman BD, Wolf JS Jr. Technical advances in laparoscopy: hand assistance, retractors, and the pneumodissector. *J Endourol* 2000;14:921.

64. Tanabe K, Miyamoto N, Ishida H, et al. Retroperitoneoscopic live donor nephrectomy (RPLDN): Establishment and initial experience of RPLDN at a single center. *Am J Transplant* 2005;4:739.

## 15.5.5  Robot-Assisted Nephrectomy

*Carlos Galvani, MD, Enrico Benedetti, MD,*
*Santiago Horgan, MD*

## INTRODUCTION

Living donor (LD) kidney transplants represent an important option for patients with end-stage renal disease (ESRD) and an attractive alternative to deceased donor (DD) transplants. The introduction of laparoscopic techniques by Ratner in 1995 was an attempt to alleviate the shortage of kidneys for transplantation by replacing the conventional open approach to the donor operation.[1] The theory was that reducing the postoperative pain, hospitalization, and convalescence associated with open LD nephrectomy and offering better cosmetic results would increase the number of LDs and subsequently expand the donor pool.[2] The initial outcomes reported for the laparoscopic technique were similar to the open operation, adding all the advantages of minimally invasive

procedures.[3,4] As a consequence, the number of kidney LDs has increased considerably in the last decade, and laparoscopic donor nephrectomy now accounts for more than half of LD operations reported to the United Network for Organ Sharing (UNOS).[5]

The da Vinci® surgical system (Intuitive Surgical, Mountain View, CA) was approved by the U.S. Food and Drug Administration (FDA) in July 2000. In October 2000, at our institution, we started performing robotic hand-assisted living donor nephrectomy using the da Vinci system,[6] confident that it would offer additional benefits over conventional laparoscopic surgery. We found that the system provides all the benefits of a minimally invasive approach without giving up the dexterity, precision, and intuitive movements of open surgery. When performing robotic hand-assisted LD nephrectomy, we now follow these procedures:

## LIVING DONOR EVALUATION

The initial assessment of LD candidates is performed by a transplant nurse coordinator. Candidates could be a living relative, spouse, or close friend who is interested in donating a kidney. They must be at least 18 years of age and have a blood type compatible with the recipient's. After a compatible blood type is

**TABLE 15.5.5-1**

## PREOPERATIVE EVALUATION OF PROSPECTIVE DONORS

**Transplant Nurse Initial Assessment**
- History
- Patient education session
- HLA matching
- ABO cross-matching

**Transplant Surgeon Evaluation**
- Patient history and physical examination
- Review of transplant surgery

**Cardiac Evaluation**
- Electrocardiogram
- Dobutamine stress echocardiogram if > 50 yrs

**Pulmonary Evaluation**
- Chest x-ray
- PFT, if chest x-ray is abnormal

**Kidney Evaluation**
- 3 urinalyses and 1 urine culture
- 24-hr urine collection for creatinine and protein
- Double-spiral CT angiogram of abdomen with 3-dimensional vascular reconstruction.
- Nephrology consultation at surgeon's discretion

**Laboratory Tests**
- CBC, sickle screen (for black patients), PT/PTT, Hep B Ag and Ab, Hep B IGG core Ab; HCV, viral serology for HSV, HZV, EBV, CMV, HIV; C3, C4, IgA, IgG, IgM, ANA, RPR; glucose, uric acid, calcium; phosphorus, liver function studies, lipid profile. If family history of diabetes, glycosylated hemoglobin and glucose tolerance test

**Psychological and Social Screening**

**Final Crossmatch**
- One week before surgery

**General Surgery Consultation**
- With laparoscopic surgeon at least 1 week before surgery

**Anesthesia Evaluation**

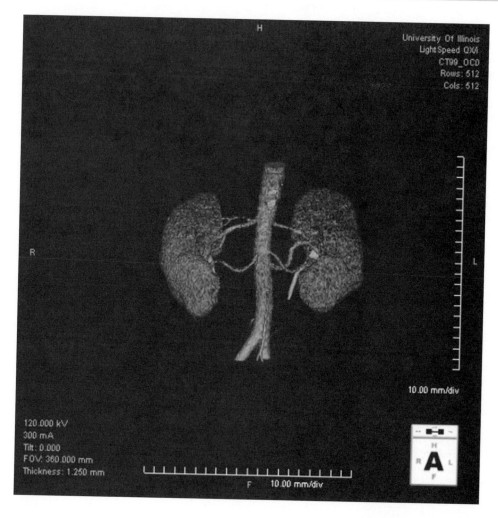

**FIGURE 15.5.5-1**

CT angiogram.

confirmed, other necessary tests include HLA tissue typing and a cross-match test for reactive HLA. If the candidate is eligible, the transplant coordinator presents the information to the transplant surgeon. Then, the candidate is screened according to a standardized protocol. A conscientious preoperative evaluation ensures that the LD is left with normal kidney function after the nephrectomy (Table 15.5.5-1). CT angiography is highly accurate for detecting vascular anomalies and for providing thorough anatomic information (Figure 15.5.5-1). The left kidney is routinely selected, regardless of the presence of vascular anomalies.

## THE ROBOTIC SYSTEM

The da Vinci(R) system has three components.

1. The surgeon operates while seated at a *console*, using four pedals, a set of console switches, and two master controls. The movements of the surgeon's fingers are transmitted by the master controls to the instrument located inside the LD. A 3-dimensional image of the surgical field is obtained using a 12-mm scope, which contains two cameras that integrate images.

2. The *control tower* is used to monitor light sources and cord attachments for the cameras.

3. The *surgical arm cart* provides four robotic arms (three instrument arms and one endoscope arm) that execute the surgeon's commands (see Figure 15.5.5-2).

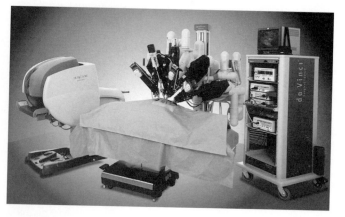

**FIGURE 15.5.5-2**

The robotic system.

## SURGICAL TECHNIQUE

### Patient Positioning

The LD is placed onto the operating room table on top of a cushioned beanbag. Pneumatic compression stockings are placed on both lower extremities. After induction of general anesthesia, a Foley catheter and an oral gastric tube are regularly placed.

Preoperative antibiotics are administered. The LD is then rolled into the right lateral decubitus position with an axillary role placed under the right axilla. The beanbag is then connected to suction. The regular use of a beanbag allows the LD to be secured to the table when it is maximally flexed, thus opening up the angle between the LD's right costal margin and the superior iliac crest. The left arm and left leg are both cushioned appropriately to protect all joints and pressure points. The abdomen is then prepared and draped in a standard sterile fashion (see Figure 15.5.5-3).

## Trocar Placement

An infraumbilical incision is made, extending from the umbilicus to 7.5-cm caudate in the midline. The midline fascia is opened, and then the peritoneum is under direct vision. A Lap Disc handport (Ethicon, Piscataway, NJ) is inserted into the abdominal cavity and secured. The handport allows the surgeon to place a hand into the abdomen to facilitate retraction and dissection and also allows for the removal of the kidney at the end of the procedure. Pneumoperitoneum is achieved with 14 mm Hg $CO_2$ insufflation. Under direct visualization, a 12-mm trocar is placed in the supraumbilical position close to the midline. A 12-mm trocar is required for the 30° robotic camera system. Two 8-mm robotic trocars are placed, one to the left of the camera trocar in the junction between the midclavicular line and the subcostal margin and the other in the midclavicular line to the right of the camera trocar. These two trocars are for the surgeon's right and left hands. An additional 12-mm trocar is placed in the left lower quadrant to assist with suction, clipping, stapling, and cutting. The da Vinci system is then brought into position, and the arms are connected to the specific trocars (Figure 15.5.5-4). Instruments specific to this system include a Maryland dissector with bipolar current for the left hand and an articulated hook cautery for the right hand.

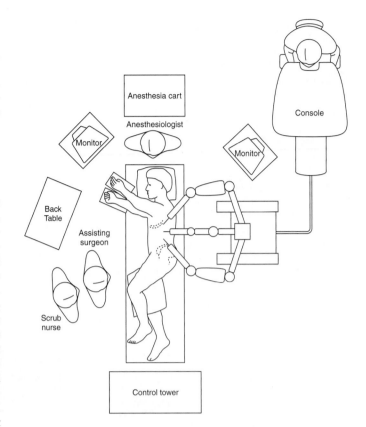

**FIGURE 15.5.5-3**

Patient positioning.

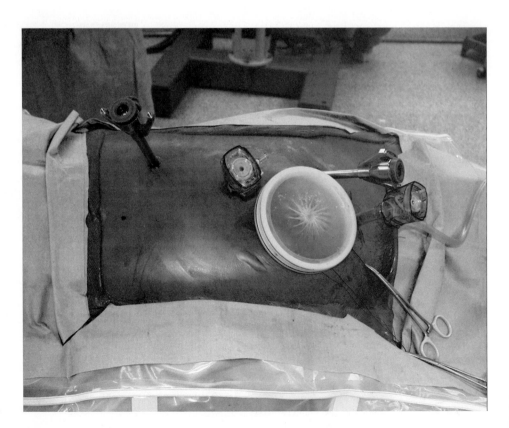

**FIGURE 15.5.5-4**

Trocar positioning.

## Mobilization of the Descending Colon and Identification of the Ureter

The surgeon's right hand is introduced into the abdominal cavity via the hand-assisted window and used to expose the left colic gutter by providing countertraction on the descending colon. The descending colon is freed from the lateral peritoneal attachments, using articulated electrocautery, and reflected medially. The splenic flexure is taken down systematically, allowing access to the kidney. After medial rotation of the colon, the psoas muscle is exposed. The three-dimensional view offered by the robotic system allows for a quick and safe identification of the left ureter. Once the left ureter is isolated, a 6-cm Penrose drain is introduced through the assistant surgeon's trocar, looped around the ureter, and then clipped to itself. The assistant surgeon uses a grasper to grab the Penrose drain and to retract the ureter laterally and anteriorly. The ureter is dissected free circumferentially in a cephalad direction, beginning at the level of the left common iliac artery. The vascular supply to the ureter must not be altered: a generous amount of fat must be preserved around it.

## Posterior Dissection of the Kidney

The posterior attachments of the kidney are taken down with the assistance of the transplant surgeon's hand, as well as the articulated robotic instruments. In this phase of the operation, the robot is particularly helpful in dissecting the upper pole of the kidney from the retroperitoneal fat and the spleen, thanks to the articulated arm that reproduces the action of the human wrist.

## Anterior Dissection of the Kidney

The gonadal vein is identified medial to the ureter and dissected off superiorly until its junction with the left renal vein. Gerota's fascia is incised superiorly, and the kidney surface is identified. Then, following a cephalad direction, a plane between the superior medial aspect of the kidney and the adrenal gland is developed. This plane of dissection is carried superiorly and laterally with the hook cautery until the kidney falls away completely from its superior pole attachments.

## Dissection of the Renal Hilum

We then turn our attention to the hilum of the kidney. The renal vein is circumferentially dissected with the hook cautery. Its tributaries (gonadal, lumbar, and left adrenal veins) are transected by the assistant using the Valleylab Ligasure® (A Division of Tyco Health Care Group, Boulder, CO). At this point, the kidney is retracted medially. The main renal artery and any accessory renal artery are identified and dissected free, up to the level of the aortic takeoff. The surgeon is then able to demonstrate that the entire kidney is free from all of its attachments (other than the vascular pedicles and the ureter). Next, the robotic system is detached from the LD, and the operation is continued laparoscopically.

## Division of the Renal Hilum and Removal of the Kidney

The ureter is clipped twice distally at the level of the iliac artery and sharply transected by the assistant surgeon. At this point, intravenous (IV) heparin at the dose of 80 U/kg is given. In our first 87 such operations, we transected the renal artery with a linear cutting vascular stapler (LCS, Ethicon, Piscataway, NJ). After experiencing three failures of the stapling device resulting in a conversion to an open procedure, we modified the technique by (1) placing a locking clip (Hem-o-Lok, Weck Closure Systems, Research Triangle Park, NC) at the takeoff of the renal artery and (2) dividing the artery with the stapling device. We continue to use the stapling device alone to transect the renal vein.

The left kidney is removed through the lower midline incision and taken to the back table, where it is flushed with cold infusion of University of Wisconsin solution (ViaSpan™ Barr Laboratories, Pamona, NY). Laparoscopic inspection of the renal bed is then performed to ensure hemostasis, while IV protamine (at an appropriate dose) is administered. After the pneumoperitoneum is evacuated, the trocars are removed, the lower midline fascia is closed with running #1 absorbable monofilament sutures. The skin incisions are closed with subcuticular 4–0 absorbable monofilament sutures and routinely infiltrated with 0.25% bupivacaine with epinephrine.

## RESULTS

For all 175 LDs who underwent this operation at our institution from October 2000 through December 2004, we evaluated intraoperative and postoperative complications, length of hospital stay, estimated blood loss, warm ischemia time, and operative time. Note that 29% of them had multiple renal arteries. We observed a significant decrease in operative time and in complications in our most recent 88 LDs ($p < 0.05$). The effect of abnormal vascular anatomy did not adversely affect our results. Conversion to open surgery was not necessary in our most recent 88 LDs because we modified several technical aspects. The estimated blood loss, warm ischemia time, and hospitalization time were not different between the first 88 LDs and the last 88 LDs of our experience.

## COMMENTS

Since the first laparoscopic donor nephrectomy was performed in 1995,[1] the open approach has all but vanished. Most transplant centers have adopted the laparoscopic technique as their preferred approach.[7] In spite of the benefits offered by laparoscopy, this technique remains challenging with a steep learning curve. Ratner et al. found that, even after 6 years of experience and 381 such operations, the mean operative time, estimated blood loss, and warm ischemia time were not significantly lower than with the open approach.[8] Furthermore, they observed a significant reduction in donor complications only after their first 285 operations (21% in the first 285 vs 10.4% after that).

On the contrary, our results show that the da Vinci robotic system clearly decreases the number of operations necessary to overcome the morbidity associated with the learning curve. Our rate of donor complications significantly decreased: from 21% in the first 105 operations to 6% in our most recent 70 operations ($p < 0.05$). Also encouragingly, our mean operative time decreased considerably after our initial experience: from 192 minutes in our first 105 operations to 114 minutes in our most recent 70 operations. According to the literature, the reported operative time for standard laparoscopic donor nephrectomy varies from 174 to 206 minutes, so our current results outperform other experienced centers.[9,10] In addition, the enhanced degree of freedom of movement of the da Vinci system's EndoWrist instruments allows surgeons with limited advanced laparoscopic skills to replicate, in the laparoscopic environment, open surgical maneuvers.

## CONCLUSION

Use of the da Vinci system for LD nephrectomy reduces the number of operations required in observing a decline in operative time and in complications, as compared with the conventional laparoscopic approach. The favorable outcome in our LDs and recipients shows that robotic hand-assisted donor nephrectomy is safe and feasible. For that reason, it has become our preferred approach.

## References

1. Ratner LE, Ciseck LJ, Moore RG, et al. Laparoscopic live donor nephrectomy. *Transplantation*1995;60:1047–1049.
2. Schweitzer EJ, et al. *Increased rates of donation with laparoscopic donor nephrectomy.* Ann Surg, 2000. 232(3): p. 392–400.
3. Lee BR, Chow GK, Ratner LE, et al. Laparoscopic live donor nephrectomy: Outcomes equivalent to open surgery. *J Endourol* 2000;14:811–819.
4. Sosa JA, Albini TA, Powe NR, et al. Laparoscopic vs. open live nephrectomy: a multivariate patient outcome analysis. *Transplantation* 1998;65(suppl):85
5. *2001 Annual Report of the U.S. Organ Procurement and Transplantation Network and the Scientific Registry for Transplant Recipients: Transplant Data 1991–2000.* Rockville, MD: Dept of Health and Human Services, Health Resources and Services Administration, Office of Special Programs, Division of Transplantation; Richmond, VA: United Network for Organ Sharing; and Ann Arbor, MI: University Renal Research and Education Association; 2001.
6. Horgan S, Vanuno D, Sileri P, Cicalese L, Benedetti E. Robotic-assisted laparoscopic donor nephrectomy for kidney transplantation. *Transplantation* 2002(May) 15;73(9):1474–1479.
7. Finelli FC, Gongora E, Sasaki TM, et al. The prevalence of laparoscopic donor nephrectomy at large US transplant centres. *Transplantation* 2001;71:1862–1864.
8. Su LM, Ratner LE, Montgomery RA, Jarrett TW, Trock BJ, Sinkov V, Bluebond-Langner R, Kavoussi LR. Laparoscopic live donor nephrectomy: trends in donor and recipient morbidity following 381 consecutive cases. *Ann Surg* 2004(Aug);240(2):358–363.
9. Philosophe B, Kuo PC, Schweitzer EJ, et al. Laparoscopic versus open donor nephrectomy: Comparing uretal complications in the recipients and improving the laparoscopic technique. *Transplantation* 1999;68:497.
10. Wolf JS, Jr, Merion RM, Leichtman AB, et al. Randomized controlled trial of hand-assisted laparoscopic versus open surgical live donor nephrectomy. *Transplantation* 2001;72(2):284–290.

### 15.5.6 Living Donor Nephrectomy Techniques: Comparative Review and Critical Appraisal

*Christoph Troppmann, MD*

Following the advent of laparoscopic nephrectomy in the mid 1990s, the field of live donor renal transplantation has undergone dramatic evolution.[1] In the United States, most transplant centers adopted laparoscopic nephrectomy rapidly, although this procedure is technically more challenging than conventional open nephrectomy. This change initially affected live donor kidneys procured for adult recipients and, shortly thereafter, also those for pediatric recipients.[2,3] The swiftness with which this shift in practice occurred in the absence of high-level evidence is nearly unrivaled in contemporary surgery. Donor and recipient expectations, the desire to decrease donor morbidity and to increase the number of available organs in order to alleviate the severe organ donor

shortage, marketing and competitive forces, and the heightened media attention were all contributing factors.

The reinvigoration of the entire field of live donor kidney transplantation over the past decade, however, has not been matched by a similar outburst of well-designed controlled studies investigating this new surgical technique and its outcomes. The level of evidence of most published studies is low.[4] To date, only four randomized controlled trials whose results qualify as Level I evidence have been conducted.[4–8] Systematic analysis of safety and efficacy of laparoscopic nephrectomy for both donor and recipient has been hampered by several factors: (1) the plethora of variations of the originally described pure laparoscopic donor nephrectomy (eg, hand-assisted laparoscopic and retroperitoneoscopic techniques) and the development of modifications of the open approach (ie, the mini-incision nephrectomy techniques) all contributed to the fragmentation of the donor population with respect to the nephrectomy technique used and thus limited comparative studies due to lack of statistical power; (2) patient selection bias, particularly in the earlier era of laparoscopic donor nephrectomy, when many transplant programs still used open nephrectomy preferentially for more complex donors (eg, those with variant renovascular anatomy), and laparoscopic nephrectomy only for lower risk, technically straightforward donors; (3) publication bias, with many significant complications not being reported in the peer-reviewed literature; (4) the prior absence of systematic, comprehensive, and mandatory reporting to national live donor registries (which even now exist mostly at nascent stages in relatively few countries and usually lack true long-term follow-up); and (5) absence of a commonly accepted, comprehensive definition and classification of live donor nephrectomy complications.[9]

In light of all above factors, meta-analyses of existing published data are also fraught with significant problems. Even the use of advanced statistical methods cannot overcome and compensate for (1) the low evidence level of the studies that would have to be used as basis for such meta-analyses and (2) the presence of the previously discussed patient selection and publication biases.[10] Statistically meaningful analysis of very significant complications, such as major intraoperative hemorrhage and patient death, is further complicated by the very low absolute incidence of these complications.[11]

Hence, in the following appraisal, only relatively few strictly evidence based recommendations can be given. Rather, this summary draws from the currently available, mostly low-level evidence, and the author's personal experience with open standard nephrectomy and with pure, hand-assisted, and robotic-assisted laparoscopic nephrectomy.

### Open Standard Nephrectomy

This procedure has the longest proven track record, with longitudinal donor follow-up for more than 40 years. Open standard nephrectomy can be done extraperitoneally via a flank approach (by far the most common open technique) or, alternatively, via a transabdominal, transperitoneal approach (nowadays only rarely used). The following comments on open nephrectomy will thus exclusively refer to the extraperitoneal flank approach.

Significant advantages of the extraperitoneal open nephrectomy technique include the significantly lower risk for intraabdominal intestinal injury, postoperative intestinal adhesion formation, postoperative internal and abdominal wall hernias and bowel obstruction, and the ability to obtain direct vascular control, if necessary, minimizing thereby the risk for potentially fatal, uncontrollable hemorrhage.[11] This technique may be advantageous for donors that have significant intraabdominal adhesions or a frozen abdomen secondary to multiple previous intraabdominal operations, as long as those operations did not involve the retroperitoneum on the side where the nephrectomy is to be performed. Open nephrectomy may also still be indicated for highly selected donors that have extreme arterial or venous variant vascular anatomy. It is undisputed that open nephrectomy is associated with the shortest warm ischemia times, and, in the hands of most surgeons, the shortest operative times of all available nephrectomy techniques.[5–7] Also, the learning curve for open nephrectomy is most favorable among all techniques; it is therefore relatively easily taught. From a recipient's perspective, the short warm ischemia time, as well as the absence of pneumoperitoneum in the donor, are advantageous in regard to postoperative graft function.[2,3]

Disadvantages of conventional open nephrectomy include the length of the incision and scar and the potential for both acute and chronic postoperative pain and neuralgia. Some patients develop a muscular bulge of the incisional area or even a frank incisional hernia (the former likely a result of denervation of the flank region). It is unequivocal that postoperative pain and donor reconvalescence are adversely affected by conventional open nephrectomy when compared with the laparoscopic approaches.[5–7,12]

In summary, for open standard nephrectomy, the main advantages include the donor's intraoperative safety; its usefulness in selected, technically complex donors; the shorter total operative time; for the recipient, the absence of adverse hemodynamic conditions during the donor operation (ie, absence of pneumoperitoneum); and the short, warm ischemia time.

## Mini-incision Open Nephrectomy

Compared with the large body of publications pertaining to both open and laparoscopic donor nephrectomy, there is relatively little published peer-reviewed evidence on outcomes of mini-incision donor nephrectomy. Analysis and comparison of previously published studies on this technique are difficult because of its numerous variations, as this operation can be done via a posterior, flank, or anterior approach.[8,13,14] The main advantages include its extraperitoneal nature; the shorter incision; the lower operating room charges than those for laparoscopic nephrectomy (because no disposable instruments are used); and, from the recipient's perspective, the absence of pneumoperitoneum with potentially better early graft function than that for laparoscopically procured kidneys.[2,3]

Mini-incision open nephrectomy has, however, several drawbacks. It is technically more challenging due to the spatially restricted operative field. Therefore, operating and warm ischemia times are longer than for open nephrectomy, and the learning curve may be steeper.[15] In the event of a significant intraoperative complication, such as massive hemorrhage, it may be more difficult to obtain vascular control; thus, donor safety may be more of an issue than with the conventional open or even with the hand-assisted laparoscopic approach. With regard to postoperative donor discomfort and quality of life, there is evidence that mini-incision nephrectomy has no advantage over conventional open nephrectomy.[14,15] Moreover, a recent randomized controlled trial and a nonrandomized retrospective study that compared mini-incision with laparoscopic nephrectomy demonstrated less donor postoperative analgesic requirements, shorter hospital stay, and better postdischarge quality of life for laparoscopic donors.[8,16] Clearly, mini-inci-

sion nephrectomy warrants further study before a more definitive assessment can be made.

## Pure Laparoscopic Nephrectomy

This was the first laparoscopic live donor nephrectomy technique to be described and has thus the longest track record of all laparoscopic techniques.[1] There is strong evidence, albeit mostly from noncontrolled, nonrandomized studies, that pure laparoscopic nephrectomy results in better cosmesis, less pain, shorter length of stay, and faster return to work for the donor, as compared with open nephrectomy.[12] This operation can be done via a true Pfannenstiel incision in a very low, suprapubic location, particularly if no hand is inserted and the kidney is extracted with a laparoscopic specimen retrieval bag. If the latter is the case, the incision for pure laparoscopic nephrectomy will always be shorter than that with the hand-assisted technique, because the incision does not need to be longer than the largest transverse diameter of the kidney (usually 4 to 5 cm), which is less than the average surgeon's transverse hand and forearm diameter.

Pure laparoscopic nephrectomy, however, is technically very challenging and associated with the steepest learning curve of all laparoscopic nephrectomy techniques. Importantly, in case of intraoperative vascular complications it does not afford any direct control. Moreover, it is a transabdominal procedure with an inherent risk for bowel, splenic, bladder injury, and postoperative hernias. It may also cause complications related to adhesions (ie, intestinal obstruction), even late postoperatively. From a survey of U.S. transplant centers, it is evident that the reoperative rate for laparoscopic donors is significantly higher than that for open donors.[11] Also, in that survey, with voluntary reporting, complications not requiring reoperation and donor readmissions were significantly more frequently reported in laparoscopic (vs open) nephrectomy donors. Operative times are also longer for pure laparoscopic nephrectomy compared with both open standard nephrectomy and hand-assisted laparoscopic nephrectomy.[17–20] As is the case for all laparoscopic techniques, operating room costs are higher than those for open standard nephrectomy due to the expenses associated with the disposable instruments and longer operating time.[21] Finally, pure laparoscopic nephrectomy may also be more difficult to carry out in obese patients, particularly in males with an unfavorable truncal body fat distribution, and in donors with significantly variant renovascular anatomy or multiple previous abdominal operations.

From a recipient's perspective, the longer operative (ie, pneumoperitoneum) time, and the longer warm ischemia time are drawbacks of this technique with regard to quality of early graft function (particularly for pediatric recipients).[2,3]

## Hand-Assisted Laparoscopic Nephrectomy

This technical modification has been applied to both transabdominal (transperitoneal) and retroperitoneoscopic approaches. A fundamental advantage of the hand-assisted techniques is the ability to control intraoperative acute hemorrhage by direct digital pressure and compression. Also, hand-assistance provides the surgeon with direct tactile feedback and allows for easier retraction and exposure, particularly in obese donors. Compared with pure laparoscopic nephrectomy, the hand-assisted procedures are easier to teach and the learning curve is not quite as steep.[20] Warm ischemia and operative times are shorter than with the pure laparoscopic technique.[17-20] The shorter pneumoperitoneum time for transabdominal hand-assisted (vs pure) laparoscopic nephrectomy may have beneficial implications for early graft function in the recipient.[2,3] The reduced operative time, when compared with pure laparoscopic and robotic-assisted nephrectomy, may also decrease the risk for neuromuscular injury and rhabdomyolysis.[22]

The disadvantages of the hand-assisted laparoscopic nephrectomy include the higher operating room cost than for open nephrectomy due to the longer operating time and use of disposable supplies and instruments. Also, hand-assisted nephrectomy requires a slightly longer incision (for hand insertion plus kidney extraction) than pure laparoscopic nephrectomy (for kidney extraction only; *vide supra*).[21]Furthermore, when choosing the surgical site for hand insertion, many surgeons favor a vertical midline fascia incision, even if the skin is incised transversally (ie, not a true Pfannenstiel incision), or place the incision off of the midline, transecting several muscular and fascial layers. Particularly in taller or more obese patients, this incision must be located further away from the pubis—and often also away from the midline—to allow the surgeon's hand and arm to reach the kidney—resulting in potentially more postoperative pain and less favorable cosmesis. As with the pure laparoscopic technique, overall surgical complication rates are higher than for open nephrectomy, and establishment of pneumoperitoneum is also required for all transabdominal cases, with the previously described potential for an adverse impact on early graft function, particularly for pediatric recipients.[2,3,6,11]

Based on the presently available evidence, there are no significant differences between the pure laparoscopic and the hand-assisted laparoscopic technique with regard to the donor's postoperative analgesic requirements, hospital length of stay and reconvalescence.[17–19]

## Retroperitoneoscopic Nephrectomy

This technical variation, which has recently become more popular, is typically performed with hand assistance and has been reported to date in larger numbers only by relatively few centers.[23,24] It offers a significant advantage in that it is extraperitoneal (as is conventional open nephrectomy) with no, or very low, risk for intraabdominal intestinal injury and postoperative intraabdominal adhesion formation.[23,24] Compared to transperitoneal laparoscopic nephrectomy, operative times are slightly shorter, and the early postoperative donor recovery (including the return of gastrointestinal function) may be faster after retroperitoneoscopic nephrectomy.[19,23–25] In addition, this technique offers all other benefits of laparoscopic nephrectomy that were described previously for the pure laparoscopic and the hand-assisted variants. Although the operative space is also insufflated with $CO_2$, there is some evidence suggesting that the renal hemodynamics may not be as adversely affected by the positive pressure created within the (retroperitoneal) operative space as by the pneumoperitoneum created during transabdominal pure laparoscopic and hand-assisted nephrectomy.[19] The absence of pneumoperitoneum may therefore at least theoretically result in better early recipient graft function, although this requires further study and confirmation. It has also been suggested that retroperitoneoscopic (vs laparoscopic) nephrectomy may potentially be associated with better postoperative pulmonary function, but this assertion remains to be corroborated by more conclusive data as well.[19]

The retroperitoneoscopic approach may not be usable in patients that have had previous operations on the side where the nephrectomy is intended to take place (eg, right kidney donation in a patient with prior suppurative perforated retrocecal appendicitis and appendectomy). Similarly, retroperitoneoscopic nephrectomy may be difficult in some female patients that have undergone previous cesarean section. For those patients, nephrectomy by a retroperitoneoscopic approach may not be feasible because of the inability to create an appropriate retroperitoneal space intraoperatively.

## Robotic-Assisted Laparoscopic Nephrectomy

This technique is currently only used by a very limited number of transplant centers.[26] Currently, there is no significant body of outcome data. The largest published experience was accumulated at a single center using a hand-assisted technique.[26] In theory, assistance by the robot allows for more precise dissection secondary to (1) the additional degrees of freedom of the laparoscopic instruments afforded by the articulating instruments available for the robotic arms, (2) the ability to scale the motion of the surgeon's hand and fingers, (3) the absence of the surgeon's tremor, and (4) the 3-dimensional view afforded by the robotic camera and the stable camera platform. For the surgeon, the operation takes place under ergonomically more favorable conditions as compared to traditional laparoscopic procedures.

Operative times tend to be longer for robotic-assisted (vs nonrobotic, hand-assisted) laparoscopic cases, in part due to the increased time required for setting up for the procedure. The purchase of the robot represents a significant investment and requires the presence of specialized personnel to help with setup and conduct of the operation. Based on published experience and anecdotal evidence, robotic-assisted laparoscopic nephrectomy requires also a larger operating room and, depending on the technique used, two qualified surgeons—one for providing hand assistance and the other for working at the controls of the robot.[26] This stands in contrast to the traditional hand-assisted laparoscopic technique, for instance, which can routinely be performed by a single surgeon with assistance by a nonsurgeon (eg, operating room technician, operating room nurse, physician assistant). Also, during pure robotic-assisted laparoscopic nephrectomy, the surgeon has no indirect or direct tactile feedback and must rely exclusively on visual cues as to the tension applied to the tissues that are being dissected, as opposed to the traditional pure laparoscopic and hand-assisted techniques. This aspect may be of particular importance during the vascular dissection. Also, the currently available robotic arm technology is not optimal for use on a patient in a lateral decubitus position (which is typically required for nephrectomy). This patient position requires a setup of the robotic equipment that can lead to crowding and interference of the robotic arms with each other. The use of the robotic technology is also somewhat limited by the extreme extent of the surgical field during laparoscopic nephrectomy, which ranges from the diaphragm and spleen to the ipsilateral crossover of the ureter with the common iliac artery, resulting in the need for major and frequent, potentially very time-consuming repositioning and readjustment maneuvers of the camera and robotic arms. Without doubt, future technological advances and innovations will ameliorate these problems.

# CONCLUSION

The ideal nephrectomy technique would (1) minimize the donor's postoperative pain and functional impairment, (2) minimize surgical and nonsurgical complication rates, (3) maximize donor safety, and (4) maximize graft quality for the recipient. The laparoscopic techniques perform distinctly better than conventional open nephrectomy in regard to the first criterion, but their equivalence with open nephrectomy in regard to all other aforementioned expectations remains to be proven. More specifically, the minimally invasive laparoscopic techniques are clearly associated with better cosmesis, less postoperative pain, shorter length of stay, and faster return to work for the donor, but at the cost of longer warm ischemia and operative times, higher operating room expenses, and higher reoperative and readmission rates.[5–7,11,12] This cost includes, at least for pediatric recipients, slower early postoperative graft function.[2,3] Also, recent evidence from a randomized controlled study suggests that among the less invasive approaches, mini-incision donor nephrectomy is associated with significantly more postoperative pain and lower quality of life when compared to the laparoscopic approaches.[8] Thus, a definitive recommendation as to an optimal donor nephrectomy technique is presently not possible.

In an ideal world, each surgeon would be proficient in performing most, if not all, nephrectomy techniques and would be able to individually tailor the operative approach to each donor's history, body habitus, and anatomy, and each recipient's specific needs. For example, a donor who has a history of previous diffuse peritonitis and multiple relaparotomies, or categorically refuses blood transfusions, might most safely undergo open nephrectomy through an extraperitoneal flank approach. Conversely, an overweight male donor with significant body fat in an unfavorable, predominantly truncal distribution might preferentially undergo hand-assisted laparoscopic or retroperitoneoscopic nephrectomy. In contrast, a thin young female patient with conventional renovascular anatomy and the strong desire to achieve an optimal cosmetic result might be best served by a pure laparoscopic approach with a very low suprapubic transverse true Pfannenstiel kidney extraction incision. Finally, if a very long renal vein is paramount for the recipient operation (eg, the transplant must be done on the left side in an obese recipient following a prior left-sided renal transplant with inability to sufficiently mobilize the left iliac vein, but the donor can only donate his or her right kidney), one might consider open donor nephrectomy which would allow to maximize right renal vein length by open application of a side-biting clamp on the inferior vena cava.

In the real world, however, individual surgeons are typically trained in open nephrectomy and at most one of the minimally invasive techniques. Hence, irrespective of the aforementioned considerations, donor nephrectomy should be performed using the technique(s) in which each individual surgeon is most proficient. Robotic-assisted nephrectomy should at this point probably only be performed at centers actively engaged in research on, and optimization of, this new technology that has yet to be fully validated for live donor nephrectomy, not the least from a resource utilization and economic perspective.

For surgeons having to choose a live donor nephrectomy technique in which to undergo (re-)training, and for transplant centers contemplating initiation of a minimally invasive live donor renal transplant program, the choice of a nonrobotic, hand-assisted laparoscopic or retroperitoneoscopic technique might, until further data is available, be most advisable for now: the hand-assisted techniques combine the advantages of a minimally invasive approach with some of the benefits of conventional open nephrectomy—resulting in an acceptable donor safety margin, at least with regard to major intraoperative complications (eg, massive hemorrhage).[11,27]

Regardless of the technique used, however, meticulous donor selection and work-up, as well as for all nephrectomies that are started laparoscopically, an appropriate and timely intraoperative decision to convert to open nephrectomy, when necessary, remain important principles for a safe, sound, and ethical surgical approach to the live kidney donor.

# References

1. Ratner LE, Ciseck LJ, Moore RG, et al. Laparoscopic live donor nephrectomy. *Transplantation* 1995;60:1047–1049.
2. Troppmann C, Ormond DB, Perez RV. Laparoscopic (vs. open) live donor nephrectomy: A UNOS database analysis of early graft function and survival. *Am J Transplant* 2003;3:1295–1301.
3. Troppmann C, McBride MA, Baker TJ, et al. Laparoscopic live donor nephrectomy: A risk factor for delayed function and rejection in pediatric kidney recipients? A UNOS analysis. *Am J Transplant* 2005;5:175–182.
4. Levels of evidence and grades of recommendation. Oxford Center for Evidence Based Medicine. www.cebm.net/levels_of_evidence.asp (accessed October 2, 2006).
5. Wolf JS Jr, Merion RM, Leichtman AB, et al. Randomized controlled trial of hand-assisted laparoscopic versus open surgical live donor nephrectomy. *Transplantation* 2001;72: 284–290.
6. Øyen O, Andersen M, Mathisen L, et al. Laparoscopic versus open living-donor nephrectomy: experiences from a prospective, randomized, single-center study focusing on donor safety. *Transplantation* 2005; 79:1236–1240.
7. Simforoosh N, Basiri A, Tabibi A. Comparison of laparoscopic and open donor nephrectomy: a randomized controlled trial. *BJU Int* 2005;95:851–855.
8. Kok NFM, Lind MY, Hansson BME, et al: Comparison of laparoscopic and mini incision open donor nephrectomy: single blind, randomised controlled clinical trial. *BMJ*, 2006; 333: 221. (Epub July 17, 2006)
9. Tan HP, Shapiro R, Montgomery RA, Ratner LE. Proposed live donor nephrectomy complication classification scheme. *Transplantation* 2006;81:1221–1223.
10. Peters JL, Sutton AJ, Jones DR, et al. Comparison of two methods to detect publication bias in meta-analysis. *JAMA* 295: 676-680.
11. Matas AJ, Bartlett ST, Leichtman AB, Delmonico FL. Morbidity and mortality after living kidney donation, 1999-2001: Survey of United States transplant centers. *Am J Transplant* 2003;3:830–834.
12. Ratner LE, Hiller J, Sroka M, et al. Laparoscopic live donor nephrectomy removes disincentives to live donation. *Transplant Proc* 1997;29: 3402–3403.
13. Shenoy S, Lowell JA, Ramachandran V, Jendrisak M. The ideal living donor nephrectomy "mini-nephrectomy" through a posterior transcostal approach. *J Am Coll Surg* 2002;194:240–246.
14. Jackobs S, Becker T, Lück R, et al. Quality of life following living donor nephrectomy comparing classical flank incision and anterior vertical mini-incision. *World J Urol* 2005;23:343–348.
15. Kok NF, Alwayn IP, Schouten O, et al. Mini-incision open donor nephrectomy as an alternative to classic lumbotomy: evolution of the open approach. *Transplant Int* 2006;19:500–505.
16. Perry KT, Freedland SJ, Hu JC, et al. Quality of life, pain and return to normal activities following laparoscopic donor nephrectomy versus open mini-incision donor nephrectomy. *J Urol* 2003;169:2018–2021.
17. Slakey D, Wood JC, Hender D, Thomas R, Cheng S. Laparoscopic living donor nephrectomy: Advantages of the hand-assisted method. *Transplantation* 1999;68:581–583.

18. Gershbein AB, Fuchs GJ. Hand-assisted and conventional laparoscopic live donor nephrectomy: a comparison of two contemporary techniques. *J Endourol* 2002;16:509–513.

19. Sundqvist P, Feuk U, Häggman M, et al. Hand-assisted retroperitoneoscopic live donor nephrectomy in comparison to open and laparoscopic procedures: A prospective study on donor morbidity and kidney function. *Transplantation* 2004;78:147–153.

20. Lindstrom P, Häggman M, Wadström J. Hand-assisted laparoscopic surgery (HALS) for live donor nephrectomy is more time- and cost-effective than standard laparoscopic nephrectomy. *Surg Endosc* 2002;16:422–425.

21. Buell JF, Hanaway MJ, Potter SR, et al. Hand-assisted laparoscopic living-donor nephrectomy as an alternative to traditional laparoscopic living-donor nephrectomy. *Am J Transplant* 2002;2:983–988.

22. Troppmann C, Perez RV. Rhabdomyolysis associated with laparoscopic live donor nephrectomy and concomitant surgery: A note of caution. *Am J Transplant* 2003;3: 1457–1458.

23. Wadström J. Hand-assisted retroperitoneoscopic live donor nephrectomy: Experience from the first 75 consecutive cases. *Transplantation* 2005;80:1060–1066.

24. Ruszat R, Sulser T, Dickenmann M, et al. Retroperitoneoscopic donor nephrectomy: Donor outcome and complication rate in comparison with three different techniques. *World J Urol* 2006;24:113–117.

25. Buell JF, Abreu SC, Hanaway MJ, et al. Right donor nephrectomy: a comparison of hand-assisted transperitoneal and retroperitoneal laparoscopic approaches. *Transplantation* 2004;77:521–525.

26. Horgan S, Vanuno D, Sileri P, Cicalese L, Benedetti E. Robotic-assisted laparoscopic donor nephrectomy for kidney transplantation. *Transplantation* 2002;73:1474–1479.

27. Friedman AL, Peters TG, Jones KW, et al. Fatal and nonfatal hemorrhagic complications of living kidney donation. *Ann Surg* 2006;243:126–130.

## 15.6  PERIOPERATIVE CARE OF THE KIDNEY DONOR

*Mark L. Sturdevant, MD,*
*Rainer W.G. Gruessner, MD*

Care of individuals volunteering for living kidney donation is a privilege and the highest priority for the surgeon who participates in the endeavor of living donor (LD) nephrectomy. Meticulous perioperative care not only allows for a smooth convalescence for most donors but also is vital in identifying complications that may threaten these previously healthy individuals. Constant vigilance coupled with specific knowledge about expected effects of uninephrectomy are paramount when serving this patient population.

### RENAL ADAPTATION

Knowledge of the expected renal adaptation to an acute loss of an entire kidney is a prerequisite in caring for LDs perioperatively. The exact biochemical processes responsible for renal adaptation are poorly understood; however, animal studies have demonstrated marked increases in ribosomal RNA, messenger RNA, and protein synthesis in the remaining kidney within 24 hours after uninephrectomy. Enhanced glomerular hemodynamics will increase the glomerular filtration rate (GFR) within 3 days; renal blood flow will increase to 70% of prenephrectomy values within 1 week. In humans, renal hypertrophy, especially of the proximal tubules, will begin within days after the operation and can be appreciated with imaging studies as early as postoperative day 4. Based on computed tomography (CT), average increases of 3% to 9% in renal length and of up to 20% in cross-sectional area can be expected.[1]

### POSTOPERATIVE RENAL FUNCTION

Renal hypertrophy with enhanced GFR precludes the 50% reduction in creatinine clearance that one might expect after removing one half of the total nephron mass. Studies of the first kidney LDs at the University of Colorado revealed early postoperative serum increases in creatinine of 33% and in BUN of 26%, along with a 30% decrease in creatinine clearance.[2] Similarly, series evaluating laparoscopic techniques showed early postoperative mean creatinine levels of 1.4 ± 0.3 and preoperative/postoperative Cr ratios equal to 1.4 even in donors older than 60 years.[3] Creatinine increases more marked than these should alert the clinician to renal dysfunction in the remaining kidney.

The most common cause of renal dysfunction in the remaining kidney is hypovolemia. A more comprehensive evaluation should ensue if there is no response to fluid resuscitation. Postoperative acute renal failure from rhabdomyolysis has been reported at several institutions and should be considered, especially in large donors. Also, one must consider the possibility of contrast nephropathy in a donor undergoing CT angiography within 3 days after the operation. At the University of Minnesota, if postoperative urine output remains acceptable (> 0.5 mL/kg/hr), serum creatinine and BUN along with electrolytes are evaluated the first postoperative day (and then not again for 6 weeks). Within several weeks, one can expect serum Cr and BUN levels to near prenephrectomy levels. But overall creatinine clearance will be permanently decreased by 17 to 21 mL/min, with no expected clinical significance.[4,5]

### FLUID MANAGEMENT

Pneumoperitoneum results in oliguria via (1) direct renal parenchymal compression (Page kidney), (2) renal vascular insufficiency from central venous compression, and (3) elevation of serum antidiuretic hormone (ADH) levels.[6] In order to optimize intravascular fluid status, donors may receive 4 to 6 L of isotonic saline intraoperatively. Renal hemodynamics will return to normal soon after desufflation; however, ADH levels are still elevated several hours postoperatively and may manifest as persistent postoperative oliguria, especially if large intraoperative diuretic doses result in hypovolemia. Such patients may require more aggressive resuscitation with isotonic saline. Most donors receive maintenance fluids in the form of D5 ½ NS with KCl 20 mEq/L at 100 to 125 mL/hr. Intravenous fluids are discontinued on the first postoperative morning if urine output is acceptable; the patient is started on a liquid diet. Several days of brisk diuresis can be expected.

### HEMODYNAMIC MONITORING

A mandatory 2-hour stay in the recovery room includes frequent (every 15 minutes) assessment of vital signs, continuous pulse oximetry, and a complete blood count (CBC), before the donor is admitted to the transplant ward. Overnight, the donor should remain on a continuous cardiac monitor and pulse oximeter. Frequent vital sign evaluation as well as a repeat CBC on postoperative day 1 allow for identification of clinically significant postoperative hemorrhage, which occurs in up to 2% of donors (50% of whom will require reexploration).[7] Retroperitoneal hematomas from dislodged clips or faulty staple lines, along with adrenal and splenic injuries, are the most likely sources of bleeding.

## PULMONARY CARE

Aggressive pulmonary toilet is paramount, with incentive spirometry, induced coughing, and early ambulation. Atelectasis and pneumothorax are relatively common complications after open donor nephrectomy. Pulmonary embolism is rare but has resulted in death after both open and laparoscopic approaches; if suspected, it should be excluded with contrast-enhanced chest CT.

## VENOUS THROMBOEMBOLISM PROPHYLAXIS

Death after LD nephrectomy has resulted predominantly from postoperative pulmonary thromboembolism (PE). Kidney LDs are typically in the moderate-risk group for thrombotic complications; their incidence of proximal deep venous thrombosis (DVT) is 2% to 4%, and their incidence of clinically evident PE is 1% to 2%.[8] Risk factors such as obesity, age > 60 years, a history of DVT, and hypercoagulable states may further place LDs into a high-risk category. During preoperative evaluation, risk factors must be identified via a thorough interview. A plan for perioperative prophylxis needs to be made. Options vary from early ambulation to the combination of intermittent pneumatic compression (IPC) plus low-molecular-weight heparin (LMWH).

Since 1984, 81% of kidney LDs at the University of Minnesota have been less than 50 years of age. Currently, about 60% are female. Women of childbearing age represent a particularly vulnerable group, given their frequent use of oral contraceptive pills (OCPs). Preoperative consultation is necessary to identify women who use OCPs, particularly estrogen-based contraception, which places surgical patients at a 2- to 11-fold increased risk of thromboembolism. Postmenopausal women using hormone replacement therapy (HRT) also incur an increased risk of thromboembolism (odds ratio, 2.1 to 3.6), as compared with age-matched controls. Estrogen-induced hepatic production of clotting factors VII and X along with fibrinogen is responsible for the hypercoagulable state; return to baseline does not occur until after 4 to 6 weeks of medication abstinence. Donors are therefore asked to discontinue their OCPs or HRT at least 1 month preoperatively. Unfortunately, many are unwilling or unable to comply, given their symptoms or fear of pregnancy. Prophylaxis in these high-risk groups includes elastic stockings, IPC, and LMWH, which is ideally administered preoperatively (< 2 hours preincision). Recommendations on the duration of LMWH prophylaxis range from the onset of normal ambulation pattern to a full 2 to 3 weeks postoperatively, but no conclusive studies are available as a guide. OCPs and HRT may be restarted safely 2 to 4 weeks after donation.

Donors without risk factors placing them in the high-risk group should undergo prophylaxis with perioperative elastic stockings and IPC until their hospital discharge. Some clinicians even suggest anticoagulation in any patient > 40 years who is undergoing an operation lasting longer than 30 minutes, but definitive evidence is lacking.

## INFECTION CONTROL

Entrance into the urinary tract places donor nephrectomy in the clean-contaminated wound class. A single dose of a second-generation cephalosporin should be given on induction. The University of Maryland reported a 2.4% wound infection rate as well as a 1.3% incidence of postoperative urinary tract infection (UTI)

in their series of almost 400 patients.[7] At the University of Minnesota, we give an additional 4-day course of trimethroprim/sulfamethoxazole, but its efficacy in UTI prophylaxis is not well studied.

## ANALGESIA

The recent evolution to minimally invasive techniques for donor nephrectomy has greatly diminished the duration and amount of parenteral analgesia. Opioid-sparing strategies are in place for LDs to receive adequate pain control and to avoid narcotic-induced nausea, vomiting, oversedation, and intestinal stasis.

### Nonsteroidal Antiinflammatory Drugs (NSAIDs)

In use since 1989, the NSAID ketorolac has been a mainstay alternative to opioid-based postoperative analgesia. Studies have consistently documented at least a 50% reduction in total opioid use in patients on ketorolac. However, potential side effects (eg, gastrointestinal and surgical site bleeding, acute renal failure) have tempered enthusiasm for using ketorolac in all surgical patients. A retrospective study by Feldman et al. documented a 1.1% incidence of acute renal failure in medical patients on ketorolac; this incidence was identical to that seen in a well-matched patient group on opioids alone. Ketorolac only became significantly nephrotoxic when used for more than 5 days.[9]

Gritsch et al. addressed the concerns of ketorolac use in kidney LDs. In a retrospective study of 83 LDs, a median cumulative dose of 210 mg was given during the first 48 hours after nephrectomy. No episodes of renal failure occurred, and only 1 surgical site hemorrhage complicated the postoperative course.[10] Creatinine clearance was slightly lower during the first 2 postoperative days, without significant long-term effects. These findings are consistent with the meta-analysis by Lee et al., who noted a statistically significant but clinically unimportant increase in early postoperative serum creatinine (0.17 mg/dL) without long-term detriment.[11]

Convinced of its safety, we prescribe ketorolac (15 to 30 mg intravenously every 6 hours) to all LDs for the first 2 postoperative days, unless they have a history of peptic ulcer disease, qualitative platelet dysfunction (eg, von Willebrand factor deficiency), or aspirin-induced asthma. Ketorolac use reduces narcotic use by almost 60%, with resultant decreases in intestinal stasis and length of hospital stay.[12]

### Acetaminophen

The analgesic effects of acetaminophen act primarily in the central nervous system (CNS), as opposed to the peripheral analgesic and antiinflammatory effects of NSAIDs.[13] Acetaminophen, given in scheduled doses (0.5 to 1.0 gm every 6 hours, orally or rectally) can decrease opioid analgesic requirements and pain scores by up to 30%. When the daily dose is limited to 4 g, side effects are very few. Acetaminophen should be used especially in those select patients unable to use NSAIDs. It should be used throughout the postoperative course to diminish the use of oral opioids and their prolonged side effects.

### Opioid-Based Analgesia

During postoperative day 1, patient-controlled analgesia (PCA) with morphine, fentanyl, or hydromorphone is provided. These three parenteral opioids, of varying potency but equivalent efficacy, may be used with only slightly different side-effect profiles. The morning after donation, most LDs are capable of tolerating oral opioids such as hydromorphone or oxycodone, so the PCA is discontinued. After 48 hours, oral opioids and acetaminophen become the sole analgesics for these patients, as ketorolac is discontinued. The duration of oral analgesia varies markedly: some LDs require none, whereas others need up to 1 to 2 weeks of treatment.

## Postoperative Nausea and Vomiting

The incidence of postoperative nausea and vomiting (PONV) is 40% to 80% in LDs. Known risk factors for PONV are female sex, nonsmoking status, and opioid use both intra- and postoperatively. All LDs receive serotonin receptor antagonists (ondansetron) intraoperatively. Postoperative symptom-triggered dosing starts within 6 hours after leaving the operating room. High-risk LDs (those with a history of PONV) should receive combination therapy, such as intraoperative dexamethasone and serotonin receptor antagonists. If such therapy is ineffective, an agent, with a different mechanism of action, such as droperidol or promethazine, should be initiated and doses titrated as needed.[14] Aggressive management of PONV is vital to facilitate introduction of a prompt oral diet and discontinuation of intravenous fluids early on postoperative day 1.

## Delayed Bowel Function

In five of six nonrandomized comparative studies, the time until first enteral intake was significantly shorter in those LDs who underwent laparoscopic donation.[15] Minimizing parenteral opioid use is the most important step toward resolving postoperative intestinal ileus. Postoperative nasogastric decompression is unnecessary. Early introduction of clear liquids followed by a regular diet is encouraged. A bowel regimen consisting of bulking agents (eg, psyllium) and stool softeners (eg, Colace) is appropriate when opioid use is ongoing. Suppositories (eg, bisacodyl) may aid in colonic decompression as well.

Delayed return of bowel function is common. But, all such delays should be evaluated with an examination of pertinent electrolytes, pancreatic enzymes, and abdominal plain film to exclude pancreatitis and frank obstruction. Mesenteric defects formed at the time of colonic mobilization and port site hernias have been reported as sources of complete small bowel obstruction. Fever and leukocytosis accompanying the intestinal ileus should raise suspicion of an occult bowel injury, a reported complication in nearly all published series, especially early in a surgeon's experience.[7]

## Discharge

When a return of gastrointestinal function and adequate oral intake are accompanied by freedom from infectious and hematologic complications, the LD is discharged, usually 2 to 4 days after laparoscopic and 3 to 5 days after open nephrectomy. At least one visit within the first 3 to 4 weeks is necessary to complete the perioperative care.

## References

1. Prassopoulos P, Cavouras D, Gourtsoyiannis N et al. CT evaluation of compensatory renal growth in relation to postnephrectomy time. *Acta Radiol* 1992;33:566–568.
2. Krohn AG, Ogden DA, Holmes JH. Renal function in 29 healthy adults before and after nephrectomy. *JAMA* 1966;196:322–324.
3. Jacobs CJ, Ramey JR, Sklar GN. Laparoscopic kidney donation from patients older than 60 years. *J Am Coll Surg* 2004;198:892–897.
4. Kasiske BL, Ma JZ, Louis TA, et al. Long-term effects of reduced renal mass in humans. *Kidney Int* 1995;48:814–819.
5. Najarian JS, Chavers BM, Matas AJ, et al. 20 years or more of follow-up of living kidney donors. *Lancet* 1992;340:807–810.
6. Nguyen NT, Perez RV, Fleming N, et al. Effect of prolonged pneumoperitoneum on intraoperative urine output during laparoscopic gastric bypass. *J Am Coll Surg* 2002;195:476–483.
7. Su LM, Ratner ER, Montgomery RA, et al. Laparoscopic live donor nephrectomy: Trends in donor and recipient morbidity following 381 consecutive cases. *Annals Surg*, 2004;240:358–363.
8. Geerts WH, Heit JA, Clagett GP, et al. Prevention of venous thromboembolism. *Chest* 2001; 119:132S–175S.
9. Feldman HI, Kinman JL, Berlin JA, et al. Parenteral ketorolac: The risk for acute renal failure. *Ann Intern Med* 1997;126:193–199.
10. Gritsch HA, Freedland MBY, Sun JC. Effect of ketorolac on renal function after donor nephrectomy. *Urology* 2002;59:826–830.
11. Lee A, Cooper MG, Craig JC, et al. The effects of renal nonsteroidal anti-inflammatory drugs (NSAIDs) on postoperative renal function: a meta-analysis. *Anaesth Intens Care* 1999;27:574–580.
12. Gritsch AH, Freedland SJ, Blanco-Yarosh, M, et al: Ketorolac-based analgesia improves outcomes for living kidney donors. *Urology* 2002;59:826–830.
13. Schug SA, Sidebotham DA, Mcguinnety. Acetaminophen as an adjunct to morphine patient-controlled analgesia in the management of acute postoperative pain. *Anaesth Analg* 1998; 87:368–372.
14. Gan JG, Meyer T, Apfel CC, et al. Consensus guidelines for managing postoperative nausea and vomiting. *Anaesth Analg* 2003;97:62–71.
15. Tooher RL, Rao MM, Scott DF, et al. A systematic review of laparoscopic live-donor nephrectomy. *Transplantation* 2004;78:404–414.

# 15.7   DONOR MORBIDITY AND MORTALITY

*Burak Kocak, MD,*
*Joseph R. Leventhal, MD, PhD*

Live kidney donation has been developed and promulgated as a means to address the growing shortage of cadaver kidneys available for transplantation. Donor nephrectomy is unique among major surgical procedures, because it exposes an otherwise healthy patient to the risks of major surgery entirely for the benefit of another person. Indeed the major risk of a living donor transplant is the risk to the donor, including perioperative morbidity and mortality, plus the long-term risk of living with a single kidney. Issues related to perioperative morbidity and mortality are especially pertinent since the recent introduction of laparoscopic donor nephrectomy, a less invasive approach to living kidney donation that has been associated with less pain and a quicker recovery time than conventional open nephrectomy. Questions have been raised as to the safety and efficacy of the laparoscopic approach, as well as to the impact of this procedure on the short-term and long-term function of the allograft.

There is a growing emphasis to inform potential donors about the inherent risks of the donor operation as part of the informed choice process. Moreover, there is no current uniformity in the reporting of complications related to living renal donation. A standardized classification for these potential complications is a necessary first step in establishing some type of regulatory process in monitoring and registering these complications. There are no mandated national or international registries except the country of Switzerland for tracking donor outcomes. A classification scheme was recently proposed to stratify negative outcomes in surgery.[1] Subsequently, this grading system has been applied to outcomes in liver transplant recipients.[2] More recently, we and others have reported on the use of serial modifications of the Clavien classification for defining the significance of complications in individuals undergoing living liver donation.[3,4]

This chapter reviews the perioperative risks of living kidney donation, drawing on published experiences with the open and laparoscopic approaches. In addition we have drawn upon our own experience with 800 living donor nephrectomies to review the incidence and type of complications encountered and to propose a standardized classification system for describing and reporting such complications.

## OPEN LIVE DONOR NEPHRECTOMY (OLDN): MORBIDITY AND MORTALITY

Najarian et al. reported over a decade ago upon the outcomes in living kidney donors with 20 years or more of follow-up at the University of Minnesota (mean 23.7) by comparing renal function, blood pressure, and proteinuria in donors with siblings.[5] In 57 donors (mean age 61 [SE 1]), mean serum creatinine was 1.1 (0.01) mg/dL, blood urea nitrogen 17 (0.5) mg/dL, creatinine clearance 82 (2) mL/min, and blood pressure 134 (2)/80 (1) mm Hg. 32% of the donors were found to be taking antihypertensive drugs and 23% had documented proteinuria. The 65 siblings (mean age 58 [1.3]) did not significantly differ from the donors in any of these aforementioned variables: 1.1 (0.03) mg/dL, 17 (1.2) mg/dL, 89 (3.3) mL/min, and 130 (3)/80 (1.5) mm Hg, respectively. Forty-four percent of the siblings were taking antihypertensives and 22% had proteinuria. To assess perioperative mortality, the authors surveyed all members of the American Society of Transplant Surgeons about donor mortality at their institutions. They documented 17 perioperative deaths in the United States and Canada after living donation, and estimated mortality to be 0.03%. In a follow-up report, Johnson et al. assessed the complications and risks of OLDN in 871 donors managed over a 10-year period.[6] The authors noted two (0.2%) "major "complications: femoral nerve compression with resultant weakness and a retained sponge requiring operative intervention. Eighty-six "minor" complications in 69 (8%) donors were described: these included 22 (2.4%) wound infections, 13 (1.5%) pneumothoraces, 11 (1.3%) febrile illness, 8 (0.9%) blood loss > 750 mL, 8 (0.9%) pneumonias, and 5 (0.6%) wound hematomas/seromas. No donor died or required ventilation or intensive care. There were no postoperative myocardial infarctions, deep wound infections, or reexplorations for bleeding. Statistical analysis identified male gender, pleural entry, and weight >100 kg as risk factors for perioperative complications. More recently, Ramcharan and Matas reported on long-term (20–37 years) follow-up of renal function in 464 living kidney donors.[7] Of the 380 donors who were alive at follow-up, 3 had abnormal kidney function, and 2 had undergone a renal transplant. The remaining donors were found to have normal renal function. The incidence of proteinuria and hypertension was similar to age-matched general population.

## LAPAROSCOPIC DONOR NEPHRECTOMY (LDN): MORBIDITY AND MORTALITY

Concerns exist as to the safety of LDN, compared with open donor nephrectomy. Tooher et al. performed a systematic review of laparoscopic LDN, including comparative studies to the open approach.[8] This metaanalysis of 44 published studies failed to demonstrate any distinct safety differences between open and laparoscopic approaches. No donor mortality was reported for either procedure, and the complication rates were similar; although the types of complications experienced differed between the two procedures. The conversion rat for LDN ranged from 0% to 13%. LDN was associated with longer operative times and longer periods of warm ischemia than the open procedure. However, this was not associated with a significantly higher incidence of delayed graft function. Donor postoperative recovery and convalescence appeared too superior for LDN, confirming earlier reports.

Matas et al. recently surveyed 234 UNOS-listed transplant programs to determine the current living donor morbidity and mortality for open nephrectomy, LDN, and hand-assisted LDN.[9] The responding 171 transplant centers performed 10,828 live donor nephrectomies between 1999 and 2001; 52.3% open, 20.7% hand-assisted LDN, and 27% LDN. Two donors (0.02%) died from surgical complications following LDN, with an additional patient undergoing LDN ending up in a persistent vegetative state. Reoperation was necessary in 22 (0.04%) open, 23 (1.0%) hand-assisted LDN, and 21 (0.9%) LDN cases (p = 0.001). Complications not requiring reoperation were reported for 19 (0.3%) open, 22 (1.0%) hand-assisted LDN, and 24 (0.8%) LDN; this did not reach statistical significance. Readmission rates were higher for LDN versus open donors (1.3 vs 0.6%), predominantly due to gastrointestinal complications.

Several large, single center-based experiences with LDN have recently been reported. Jacobs et al. described a 6-year experience with 738 consecutive LDN from the University of Maryland.[10] Conversion to the open approach occurred in 1.6% of cases, prompted primarily by occurrence of a renovascular injury. Blood transfusion was required in 1.2%. Major intraoperative complications occurred in 6.8% and major postoperative complications occurred in 17.1% of cases. Postoperative complications were most commonly associated with disturbances of bowel function. There were no donor mortalities reported.

Heimbach et al. published the Mayo clinic experience with 553 consecutive hand-assisted LDN, focusing on the impact of obesity upon donor outcomes.[11] Donors were stratified by body mass index(BMI), assessing perioperative complications and 6- to 12-month postdonation metabolic and renal function. Compared to BMI < 25, high BMI donors (> 35) had slightly longer operative times, more overall perioperative complications (wound related), yet the same low rate of major surgical complications (open conversion (1%) and reoperation) and similar length of stays. Renal function and proteinuria at 6 to 12 months did not differ with BMI. There were no donor mortalities. These authors concluded that LDN is generally safe and can be used for properly selected obese donors.

Melcher et al. have described the outcomes in 530 consecutive LDN at the University California San Francisco.[12] One open conversion, occurring within the first 10 cases performed, was described. There were no donor deaths. Five donors required perioperative blood transfusions. The overall complication rate of 6.4% included 14 wound infections, 2 bowel injuries, 1 case of prolonged ileus, 3 splenic injuries, 2 bladder infections, 1 bladder injury, 2 thromboembolic events, a case of rhabdomyolysis, a port site hernia, and 1 case of pneumonia.

## NORTHWESTERN UNIVERSITY EXPERIENCE: 1997–2005

Eight hundred LDN were performed from October 1997 through December 2005 at our center. Patient data were obtained from a combination of medical record review and doctor–patient interaction. The data collected included estimated blood loss, transfusion requirement, length of postoperative hospital stay, donor serum creatinine levels before and 1 week after the surgery, donor hemoglobin levels before, immediate after and 1 week after the surgery, intraoperative complications, postoperative recovery, and complications. Complications were defined as *untoward events* within the perioperative period that altered patient recovery, prolonged hospital stay, or represented technical deviations during the surgical procedure.

## Grading System for Complications of Live Renal Donation

A modification of the Clavien classification system describing procedure-related complications was developed and is shown in Table 15.7-1. Complications are graded in four groups as in the original classification[1]: grade 1 complications include all events, if left untreated, has a spontaneous resolution, can be cleared by the patient after instruction or needs a simple bedside procedure. This is intended to maintain grade 1 as a truly low-morbidity category. Grade 2 complications differ from grade 1 in that they are potentially life-threatening and usually require some form of intervention, which is associated with well-described complications. Grade 2 events are distinguished from grade 3 complications in that they do not produce lasting or residual disability. Grade 4 events are resulting in renal failure or deaths as a result of any complication.

## RESULTS

### Intraoperative and Postoperative Data

The estimated blood loss for the LDN procedure was $69 \pm 110$ mL. The average length of stay was $1.3 \pm 0.7$ days, which decreased to $1.1 \pm 0.5$ days in the last 100 cases. Table 15.7-2 lists intraoperative and postoperative complications. There were 11 open conversions, of which 6 were in the first hundred cases. The overall open conversion rate was 1.3%. Four conversions were elective and related to surgical technical difficulties, which included lack of exposure, donor obesity, and need for open management of multiple vessels. The remaining 7 open conversions were due to renovascular injuries, which included aortic injury, renal arterial injury, lumbar vein injury, and adrenal vein injury. There have been no open conversions in the last 200 cases at our center.

There were eight major renovascular complications (1%); all except one required open conversion. The overall rate of intraoperative complications was 2.3% (19/800 cases). There were eleven intraoperative complications other than the renovascular injuries (1.3%), of which only one was in the first hundred cases. Intraoperative complications included splenic capsular tear, a diaphragmatic injury repaired laparoscopically, adrenal hematoma, serosal bowel injury repaired laparoscopically, transient carbon dioxide pneumomediastinum and ureteral injury. The overall rate of postoperative complications was 3.3%. Postoperative complications of LDN included urinary retention, wound infection, chylous ascites, temporary lateral thigh numbness, port site granuloma with nerve entrapment, prolonged ileus, postoperative hemoglobin drop more than 2 g/dL, scrotal swelling, and postoperative intestinal obstruction secondary to internal hernia. Nine of the laparoscopic donors required readmission (prolonged ileus [4], chylous ascites [2], repair of aortic injury [1], and excision of port site granuloma [1], operation for internal hernia [1]). There was one postoperative intestinal obstruction secondary to internal hernia,

**TABLE 15.7-1**

## CLASSIFICATION OF SURGICAL COMPLICATIONS FOR LIVING DONOR NEPHRECTOMY

| Grade | Definition of Complication |
|---|---|
| Grade 1 | NON-LIFE-THREATENING COMPLICATIONS<br>An alteration from ideal postoperative course with complete recovery or which can be easily controlled and which fulfills the general characteristics, namely (1) non-life-threatening; (2) not requiring use of drugs other than analgesics, antipyretic, anti-inflammatory, and antiemetic, drugs required for urinary retention or lower urinary tract infection; (3) requiring only therapeutic procedures that can be performed at the bedside; (4) blood loss < 500 mL or Hb drop < 2 g/dL/not resulting in hemodynamic instability or Hb < 8 g/dL and (5) never associated with a prolongation of hospital stay no more than three times the expected median stay for the procedure<br>**Examples:**<br>Ileus resolving spontaneously, iatrogenic injuries not requiring any operative procedures |
| Grade 2 | NO RESIDUAL DISABILITY<br>Any complication that is potentially life-threatening but which does not result in residual disability or persistent diseases |
| Grade 2a | Complications requiring only use of drug therapy, blood loss > 500 mL or Hb drop > 2 g/dL and/or resulting in hemodynamic instability or Hb < 8 g/dL, readmission to the hospital for medical management or prolongation of hospital stay for more than three times the median length of stay |
| Grade 2b | Complications requiring additional therapeutic intervention (ie, operation for bowel obstruction, interventional radiologic procedure), readmission to the hospital for intervention<br>**Examples:**<br>Iatrogenic injuries requiring operative procedures |
| Grade 2c | Complications requiring open conversion of LDN for patient management |
| Grade 3 | RESIDUAL DISABILITY<br>Any complication with residual or lasting functional disability<br>**Examples:**<br>Organ resection caused by surgical error (eg, splenectomy secondary to splenic injury) |
| Grade 4 | RENAL FAILURE OR DEATH |
| Grade 4a | Leads to renal failure in the donor |
| Grade 4b | Leads to donor death |

treated by a laparoscopic exploration and repair. The preoperative and postoperative day #7 serum creatinine values of the donors were $1 \pm 0.2$ mg/dL and $1.3 \pm 0.2$ mg/dL, respectively.

## Grading of Complications

We observed 46 complications in our series of 800 patients (5.8%). Using the proposed classification system, 17/46 complications (37%) were defined as grade 1(adrenal hematoma [1], pneumomediastinum [2], urinary retention [8], superficial wound infection [4], transient lateral thigh numbness [1], scrotal swelling [1]). Twenty-seven of forty-six (58.7%) were classified as grade 2; these included seven prolonged ileus, four requiring rehospitalization (grade 2a), one hemoglobin drop more than 2 g/dL (grade 2a), three splenic capsular tear requiring laparoscopic intervention (grade 2b), one diaphragmatic tear requiring laparoscopic repair (grade 2b), one port site granuloma requiring operation (grade 2b), three serosal bowel injuries repaired laparoscopically, one ureteral injury, one reoperation for intestinal obstruction, one renovascular injury controlled laparoscopically, and seven renovascular injuries requiring conversion (grade 2c). One patient with post-operative chylous ascites was managed with low-fat dietary modification and interval paracentesis for symptomatic accumulation of fluid; complete resolution occurred after several weeks (grade 2b). Two additional instances of chylous ascites following living renal donation were classified as grade 3 (2.5%) due to the need for recurrent hospitalization and hospital visits for their non-operative management and poor nutritional status lasting more than six months. There were no grade 4 complications in our series. These results are summarized in Table 15.7-2.

## COMMENT

LDN has had a major impact on the field of living donor renal transplantation, and the operation has been performed in growing numbers with worldwide acceptance. As transplant centers perform more of these procedures, they will experience a higher number of complications. In recently reported large series, there has been a tendency to distinguish between "minor" and "major" complications both during and after the procedure.[10] Terms such as "major" or "minor" complications are not standardized, and therefore an informative comparison of complications is difficult. The lack of standardized definition and thus of uniform reporting of complications represents a major shortcoming in the medical literature, making interpretation of results of living kidney donation difficult. We decided to develop a classification system to assess severity of complications in order to standardize the reporting of complications of this procedure.[11] A modification of the Clavien classification system describing procedure-related complications was developed which allows us to address the specific complications of live donor nephrectomy. Clavien et al. recently proposed a modification of their original classification system which seems to be more comprehensive and universal.[12] This new classification emphasizes the risk and invasiveness of the interventions used to correct a complication, and no longer considers the length of hospital stay in the grading of complications. We would argue the particular circumstances surrounding live donor nephrectomy for inclusion of hospital stay as a metric for outcomes. Donor nephrectomy is unique among major surgical procedures, because it exposes an otherwise healthy patient to the risks entirely for the benefit of another person. Indeed, the laparoscopic approach for donor

**TABLE 15.7-2**

## INTRAOPERATIVE AND POSTOPERATIVE COMPLICATIONS AND THEIR GRADING BY SEVERITY

| Grade | | Percentage of All Complications (n = 46) | Percentage of Total series (n = 800) | Complication | No. of Points |
|---|---|---|---|---|---|
| 1 | | 37% (n = 17) | 2.1% | Urinary retention | 8 |
| | | | | Wound infection | 4 |
| | | | | Temporary Lat. Thigh numbness | 1 |
| | | | | Scrotal swelling | 1 |
| | | | | Adrenal hematoma | 1 |
| | | | | Transient $CO_2$ pneumomediastinum | 2 |
| 2 | | 58.7% (n = 27) | 3.8% | | |
| | 2a | 17.4% (n = 8) | 0.625% | Prolonged ileus | 7 |
| | | | | Blood loss > 2 g/dL | 1 |
| | 2b | 26.0% (n = 12) | 1.5% | Port site granuloma with nerve entrapment | 1 |
| | | | | Intestinal obstruction | 1 |
| | | | | Chylous ascites | 1 |
| | | | | Splenic capsular tear | 3 |
| | | | | Diaphragmatic tear | 1 |
| | | | | Serosal bowel injury | 3 |
| | | | | Ureteral injury | 1 |
| | | | | Renal vein injury | 1 |
| | 2c | 15.2% (n = 7) | 0.875% | Aortic injury | 1 |
| | | | | Renal arterial injury | 3 |
| | | | | Lumbar vein injury | 2 |
| | | | | Adrenal vein injury | 1 |
| 3 | 3 | 2.5% (n = 2) | 0.25% | Chylous ascites | 2 |
| 4 | | 0 | 0 | | 0 |

nephrectomy was introduced with the potential goal of increasing the acceptance of the donor operation by offering potential benefits such as reduced pain and a shortened hospital stay. Hospital stay thus affects the acceptability of the operation by the potential donor. Overall, we would modestly assert that our modified system for classifying outcomes is a more robust and responsive schema for specific operation.

A balance must be attained between the level detail of subclassification and the utility of the classification. The more detailed the classification is, the more it resembles a laundry list of complications and less it defines the significance of potential complications. On the other hand, if the classification is too broad, as in "major" or "minor," it assumes a subjective overtone, which minimizes the ability to objectively define the significance of the potential complications. Thus, iatrogenic injuries such as adrenal hematoma that do not require any intraoperative intervention are graded as 1. Other injuries that require further intraoperative intervention like serosal bowel injury requiring laparoscopic repair are classified as grade 2b complications. Organ resection caused by surgical error is equated with residual disability, since any organ loss due to iatrogenic injury represents a more significant complication in a donor operation (eg, splenectomy secondary to splenic injury). Conversion to open nephrectomy due to a major complication in order to manage the complication is a major departure from the initial plan for a donor operation and should be graded as a separate group (grade 2c). Conversion in the absence of a complication should not be graded here. Conversion to open donor nephrectomy is not a complication but rather a successful completion when conditions are unsuitable for laparoscopic procedure. We have observed the development of chylous ascites in three of 800 patients undergoing LDN at out institution (0.037%). Chylous ascites seems to be a potential complication of LDN owing to dissection and division of the lymphatics adjacent to the renal artery and vein. We have modified our technique to include the application of a fibrin sealant along with our previously described use of the ultrasonic scalpel to facilitate occlusion of lymphatic tissue that have been dissected during the course of vascular mobilization of the kidney after two complications. We have observed one case of chylous ascites after this refinement in our technique. In one patient this complication was successfully managed with change in diet and interval paracentesis; we elected to classify this as a grade 2b event. However, two instances of chylous ascites were classified as Grade 3 complications due to the need for recurrent hospitalization and/or hospital visits for their nonoperative management and poor nutritional status lasting more than 6 months. Although one might contend these could also have been grouped as 2b complications, we believe such complications lasting more than 6 months, requiring multiple admissions, should be graded as more severe in a healthy donor.

The recently published consensus statement on living donors underscored the need for a comprehensive discussion of potential surgical complications of the living donor operation (along with the risk of donor death), during the informed choice process by potential donors.[13] We understand that the precise reporting to assess the severity of the complication is invaluable and a grading system cannot be as revealing as reporting the precise complication. On the other hand, we believe a graded classification system for reporting complications following LDN may be useful for maintaining registry information on donor outcomes, and particularly in informing potential donors about the risks and benefits of this procedure. Clavien et al. have recently stated that an accurate assessment of the complication rate of LDN is difficult, as a standardized definition of complications is lacking.[14]

## CONCLUSION

The aggregate published experience regarding living kidney donation clearly shows this to be a procedure associated with little major morbidity and extremely rare mortalities. Clearly, the integration of laparoscopic approaches to living donation have had an impact on the acceptance of the operation for potential donors. LDN has also impacted upon the type and severity of complications seen in living donors. Regardless of the surgical approach used, the risks of nephrectomy must continue to be balanced against the better outcome for recipients of living donor transplants.

The modified classification presented here is the first of its kind for the live donor nephrectomy procedure. Although our ultimate is to propose a comprehensive and standardized classification scheme for reporting all negative outcomes of live donor nephrectomy, we acknowledge that further discussion and refinement will be required before a final classification is adopted. The development of an accepted classification constitutes an essential step in the creation of both institutional and national donor registries that would in turn be available to potential donors as part of their informed choice process.

## References

1. Clavien PA, Sanabria JR, Strasberg SM. Proposed classification of complications of surgery with examples of utility in cholecystectomy. *Surgery* 1992;111:518–526.
2. Clavien PA, Camargo CA Jr., Croxford R, et al. Definition and classification of negative outcomes in solid organ transplantation. Application in liver transplantation. *Ann Surg* 1994;220(2):109–120.
3. Salvalaggio PRO, Baker TB, Koffron AJ, et al. A comparative analysis of living liver donor risk utilizing a comprehensive grading system for severity. *Transplantation* 2004;77(11):1765–1767.
4. Ghobrial RM, Saab S, Lassman C, et al. Donor and recipient outcomes in right lobe adult living donor liver transplantation. *Liver Transplant* 2002;8(10):901–909.
5. Najarian JS, Chavers BM, McHugh LE, Matas AJ. 20 years or more of follow-up of living kidney donors. *Lancet* 1992;340:807.
6. Johnson EM, Remucal MJ, Gillingham KJ, et al. Complications and risks of living donor nephrectomy. *Transplantation* 1997;64(8):1124–1128.
7. Ramcharan T, Mata AJ. Long-term (20-37 years) follow-up of living kidney donors. *Am J Transplant* 2002;2:959–64.
8. Tooher RL, Rao MM, Scott DR, et al. A Systematic Review of Laparoscopic Live Donor Nephrectomy. *Transplantation* 2004;78(3):404–414.
9. Matas AJ, Bartlett ST, Leichtman AB, Delmonico FL: . Morbidity and Mortality After after Living Kidney Donation, 199-2001: Survey of United States Transplant Centers. *Am J Transplant* 2003;3:830–834.
10. Jacobs SC, Cho E, Foster C, et al. Laparoscopic donor nephrectomy: The University of Maryland 6-Year experience. *J Urol* 2004;171:47–51.
11. Heimbach JK, Taler SJ, Prieto M, et al. Obesity in living kidney donors: Clinical characteristics and outcomes in the era of laparoscopic nephrectomy. *Am J Transplant* 2005;5:1057–1064.
12. Melcher ML, Carter JT, Posselt A, et al. More than 500 consecutive laparoscopic donor nephrectomies without conversion or repeated surgery. *Arch Surg* 2005;140 (9):835–839.
13. Consensus Statement on the Live Organ Donor. *JAMA* 2000;284 (22):2919–2926.
14. Handschin AE, Weber M, Demartines N, et al. Laparoscopic donor nephrectomy. *Br J Surg* 2003;90:1323–1332.

# 15.8 LONG-TERM OUTCOME

*Arthur J. Matas, MD, Hassan N. Ibrahim, MD, MS*

Patients with end-stage renal disease (ESRD) have two options for renal replacement therapy: dialysis or a transplant. Those opting for a transplant must then decide whether to have a living donor (LD) transplant (if a suitable donor is available) or to go on the waiting list for a deceased donor (DD) kidney.

It has long been recognized that a successful transplant provides significantly better quality of life than does dialysis.[1] Recent data have also shown that a transplant significantly prolongs survival;[2,3] as a consequence, more patients with ESRD are opting for a transplant. In the United States, each year more patients go on the waiting list than are transplanted. Thus, the waiting list continues to grow.[4] In fact, given the current demand, it has been estimated that even if all potential DDs each year became actual donors, the need would not be met.[5]

The increasing waiting list and resultant increases in waiting time for a transplant have consequences for those going on the waiting list—a large number of transplant candidates are now dying while waiting for a kidney.[6] Thus, the organ shortage has become one of the most important issues in kidney transplantation today. A potential solution is to increase the number of LD kidney transplants. An LD kidney offers many advantages. Most important, recipients of LD kidneys have better long-term outcome (patient and graft survival) than do recipients of DD kidneys. In addition, patients can undergo a transplant earlier in the course of their disease, rather than waiting for years on dialysis. Furthermore, recipients of preemptive transplants have better outcome than those who undergo pretransplant dialysis, and outcome is inversely related to the duration of pretransplant dialysis.[7,8]

Recently, the number of LD transplants has increased, for at least three reasons. First, outcome for recipients of LD kidneys has improved steadily over the last 2 decades; thus, centers previously reluctant to recommend living donation are more willing to do so. Second, outcome for recipients of living unrelated donor (LURD) kidneys has been shown to be equivalent to that of recipients of non-human-leukocyte-antigen (HLA)-identical living related donor (LRD) kidneys.[9] The increased acceptance of LURD kidneys has appreciably expanded the potential donor pool. Third, the new option of laparoscopic donor nephrectomy is associated with less pain and a faster recovery time for the donor than is conventional open nephrectomy.[10] As a result, more potential LDs may be willing to donate, and more recipients are willing to accept an LD kidney.

An LD transplant has a significant disadvantage: the donor is required to have a major operative procedure that is associated with morbidity, mortality, and the potential for adverse long-term consequences due to living with a single kidney. Perioperative mortality after LD donation is 0.03%;[11–13] morbidity, including minor complications, is less than 10%.[14]

Only a limited number of studies have addressed the consequences of living with a single kidney. One major concern is whether unilateral nephrectomy predisposes the LD to the development of kidney disease and/or to premature death.

## LONG-TERM SURVIVAL

Anderson et al. compared the survival rates of 232 patients who underwent nephrectomy for benign disease (vs the overall Danish population). Follow-up ranged from 2 months to 26 years. If the remaining kidney was normal, survival was identical to that of the overall population.[15] In Sweden, Fehrman-Ekholm et al. found that kidney donors live longer (vs the age-matched general population).[16] Although Fehrman-Ekholm's finding may reflect the selection bias of healthy donors, both studies contradict the concept that donor longevity may be limited.

Of concern is the recent finding that mild renal dysfunction or proteinuria correlates with cardiovascular risk. All LDs lose ≥ 20% renal function; and, as discussed below, proteinuria is not uncommon after kidney donation.

## Reduced Renal Function and Cardiovascular Disease

A number of reports indicate that elevated serum creatinine may be an independent predictor of all-cause mortality and cardiovascular disease (CVD) mortality.[17–23] Those reports, however, focused on specific groups, such as hypertensive individuals,[17] older individuals,[18] patients who had a recent stroke,[19] survivors of myocardial infarction,[20] patients undergoing carotid endarterectomy,[21] patients undergoing elective cardiac valve surgery,[22] and patients with left ventricular systolic dysfunction.[23] In the Hypertension Detection and Follow-up Program (HDFP) report, for example, the 8-year mortality risk increased progressively with increasing levels of serum creatinine.[17] The risk of CVD was twofold higher in patients whose serum creatinine levels were at or above the 97th percentile (vs below it).[17]

Similarly, data from over 24,000 hypertensive participants who constituted the control groups from eight controlled trials (HDFP, MRFIT, and SHEP, among others) clearly showed that a glomerular filtration rate (GFR) was associated with an increased risk of fatal strokes, of fatal coronary events, and of cardiovascular mortality.[24] The strength of this association was similar to that of high blood pressure and of high total cholesterol.[24]

The association between chronic kidney disease and CVD in those with preexistent CVD was further analyzed using data from four publicly available community-based longitudinal studies: Atherosclerosis Risk in Communities Study, the Cardiovascular Health Study, the Framingham Heart Study, and the Framingham Offspring Study.[25] Chronic kidney disease (CKD), defined by GFR < 60 mL/min, was associated with a higher risk of cardiovascular events: 62.5% (vs 34.9% in patients without CKD).

Cross-sectional population studies also showed an association between reduced renal function and higher mortality.[26–30] Wannamethee et al. carried out a prospective study of CVD involving 7,735 men (40 to 59 years old) selected from one group's general practice in each of 24 towns in England, Wales, and Scotland.[26] After an average follow-up period of 15 years, stroke incidence was significantly increased for men whose serum creatinine levels were above the 90th percentile (vs below it, after adjustment for a wide range of cardiovascular risk factors). Major ischemic heart disease events were also significantly increased for men whose serum creatinine levels were at or above the 97.5th percentile.

More recently, serum creatinine levels were analyzed in over 6,000 adult participants in the Framingham Heart Study. Mild renal insufficiency, defined by serum creatinine levels from 1.5 to 3.0 mg/dL, was prevalent at baseline in roughly 8% of the participants (men and women combined).[27] In men (but not women), mild renal insufficiency was associated positively with all-cause mortality in age-adjusted and multivariate analysis.

Manjunath et al. reported on the relationship between renal function and CVD in 15,792 study participants from four counties in the United States.[28] After a mean follow-up of 6.2 years, participants whose GFR was 15 to 59 mL/min had a hazard ratio for atherosclerotic CDV of 1.38; those whose GFR was 60 to 89 mL/min, a hazard ratio of 1.16 (vs subjects with a GFR of 90 to 150 mL/min). Most recently, Go et al. estimated the longitudinal GFR for 1,120,295 adults in a large health-care delivery system, whose serum creatinine levels were measured from 1996 through 2000 and who had not undergone either dialysis or a kidney transplant.[29] After a median follow-up of 2.8 years, the adjusted hazard ratio for death was 1.2 for adults with a GFR of 45 to 59 mL/min (and 5.9 for those with a GFR less than 15 mL/min). The adjusted hazard ratio for cardiovascular events also increased inversely with the GFR. This large-cohort study definitely confirmed an independent, graded association between lower estimated GFR and higher risk of death. These findings were reproduced by Foley et al. in their study of a 5% sample of the U.S. Medicare population in 1998 and 1999.[30]

## IMPACT OF NEPHRECTOMY ON LONG-TERM RENAL FUNCTION

### Experimental Studies

Uninephrectomy, in humans, is followed by early compensatory changes: the GFR and renal blood flow increase to 70% of prenephrectomy values within 7 days after donation.[31–38] These compensatory hemodynamic changes, although initially beneficial, may ultimately prove deleterious;[39–45] experimental studies are therefore important.

In 1932, Chanutin and Ferris demonstrated that rats could survive after removal of one kidney as well as 50% to 70% of the contralateral kidney; however, the rats quickly developed progressive polyuria, albuminuria, nitrogenous waste retention, renal hypertrophy, hypertension, and cardiac hypertrophy.[39]

Other experimental investigators have demonstrated that the extent of glomerular sclerosis and damage are proportional to the mass of renal tissue removed.[41,44,45] Shimamura, Morrison, and others showed that, after a 5/6 nephrectomy, hyperfiltration occurs in the remaining glomeruli.[41,45,46] It was postulated that this adaptive hyperfiltration led to the subsequent deterioration. Hostetter et al. reached a similar conclusion in their study of renal structure and single nephron glomerular filtration rate (SNGFR) 1 week after an 11/12 renal ablation.[45] Remnant glomeruli show striking structural abnormalities, and a marked increase in SNGFR is caused by augmented intraglomerular pressure and renal plasma flow. Both the glomerular structural changes and the increase in SNGFR can be prevented by decreasing the "work" of the remaining nephrons with protein restriction.[47]

Thus, in the rat, extensive renal ablation leads to adaptive increase in glomerular capillary pressure and flow. Although this adaptive hyperfiltration increases the GFR, it also leads to glomerular injury. Measures that ameliorate the heightened intraglomerular pressure, namely, protein restriction and blockade of angiotensin II actions, result in preservation of glomerular structure.[48–51]

An important observation—consistently made in animal models of reduction in renal mass—is that progressive injury to remnant glomeruli is heralded by increasing proteinuria.[31,41,45] A fourfold increase in urinary protein excretion in rats was demonstrated as early as 1 week after ablation of 90% of the renal mass.[52] Because of such findings in the rat model, the reported increased incidence of proteinuria in human LDs of kidneys (discussed subsequently) has been worrisome.

The rat models used, however, required removal of 1 kidney plus significant damage to, or removal of, a large portion of the remaining kidney before progressive renal insufficiency ensued. The rat differs from many other species in that its lifespan is shorter. Also, an age-related progressive glomerulosclerosis, heralded by proteinuria, is routinely observed in laboratory rats.[53–55]

In other species, subtotal nephrectomy does not uniformly lead to the same progressive loss of renal function. One study showed that dogs undergoing three-fourths reduction in renal mass had stable renal function for over 4 years; some long-term survivors, however, did develop proteinuria.[56] Baboons undergoing a five-eighths reduction in renal mass had elevated mean blood pressure and increased protein excretion 4 months after renal mass reduction, but no additional significant damage after 4 to 12 months; biopsy results of the remnant kidney after 8 months were normal.[57]

Moreover, if more than half of the renal mass needs to be removed in the rat before compensatory changes lead to renal insufficiency, why should human LD nephrectomy be a concern? One needs to seriously consider the possibility that the "hyperfiltration damage" may be additive to the background of the "normal" loss of kidney function with age. Numerous cross-sectional studies in healthy humans have shown an age-related decrease in GFR. The GFR in men 80 to 90 years old, for example, is about half the rate in men 20 to 30 years old.[58,59] Histologic studies have also shown that after the fourth decade, the incidence of sclerotic glomeruli increases in otherwise healthy men.[60] Striker et al. noted that when unilateral nephrectomy was performed in older rats, glomerulosclerosis was more prominent in the remaining kidney.[40] Brenner et al. suggested that "age-related glomerulosclerosis poses no threat to well being.... If, however, extrinsic renal disease or surgical loss of renal tissue adds to the glomerular burden imposed by eating ad libitum, the course of glomerulosclerosis may be hastened considerably."[47]

### Proteinuria—Cause or Effect of Kidney Disease

Note that proteinuria has been incriminated as a central mediator of the progression of renal disease—rather than just being its consequence.[61] A model of reduced renal mass produced by uninephrectomy and surgical excision of both poles of the unilateral kidney (rather than infarction) is characterized by less proteinuria and subsequently less structural damage.[62] Proteinuria in humans is a significant determinant of GFR decline—in both diabetic and nondiabetic renal disease—and is also a strong predictor of both renal and all-cause mortality.[63,64] Reduction of proteinuria, either spontaneously or with pharmacotherapy, is associated with improved renal survival. Likewise, the benefit of ACE inhibitors or dietary protein restriction is somewhat directly related to the baseline level of proteinuria: the heavier the proteinuria, the greater the benefit.[63,65–66]

Numerous studies have also documented a graded association between the level of proteinuria and GFR decay in diabetic and nondiabetic renal disease alike.[65–70] Although the association of proteinuria with loss of renal function is considered causal by many, the mechanisms are not well understood. For example, it is unclear why substantial proteinuria is relatively benign in minimal-change disease, yet seems detrimental in other nephropathies. Nonetheless, numerous mechanisms have been proposed, most of which involve tubular cell injury or proliferation after increased protein trafficking in the proximal tubule.[71,72] Potentially toxic effects on the proximal tubule have been attributed to albumin, lipoproteins, oxidized LDL, transferrin-iron, protein-bound insulin growth factor-1, HDL, endothelin-1, and ammonia.[73–77] Proteins and other macromolecules such as apolipoprotein B might also cause mesangial cell injury, proliferation, and increased extracellular matrix production.[78–80] The reported increased risk of proteinuria in LDs is, therefore, worrisome and needs to be studied more carefully.

## Clinical Studies—Nondonors

In humans, evidence that a reduction in renal mass may lead to progressive renal failure comes from studies of children born with a reduced number of functioning nephrons[81–83] and from reports of focal sclerosis developing in patients with unilateral renal agenesis.[84–86] However, in those situations, it has not always been clear that the patient had one normal kidney.

Zucchelli et al. reported that 7 of 24 patients who had undergone unilateral nephrectomy, and who had a normal remaining kidney according to intravenous pyelography, developed proteinuria[87] (follow-up, 3 to 37 years). In 4 of those patients, the kidney biopsy results showed focal and segmental glomerulosclerosis. Proteinuria developed, on average, 12.2 years after nephrectomy. But after it developed, it did not increase further, and renal function, as measured by serum creatinine levels, remained stable.

Other long-term follow-up studies after nephrectomy performed for unilateral disease have not shown progressive deterioration in renal function.[88–93] In the study with the longest follow-up, Baudoin assessed patients (18 to 56 years old at the time of the study) who had undergone uninephrectomy in childhood.[92] In general, their kidney function was maintained. However, those followed ≥ 25 (vs < 25) years had a higher incidence of kidney failure, higher blood pressure, and increased urinary protein excretion.

In another study, Narkun-Burgess et al. assessed 56 World War II veterans who had lost a kidney because of trauma during the war (mean follow-up, about 45 years); results were compared with those of other World War II veterans of the same age.[93] The mortality rate was not increased in veterans who had lost a kidney; of the 28 living veterans (mean age, 64 ± 4 years; mean interval after kidney loss, 45 ± 1 years), none had serious renal insufficiency.

Similar studies, albeit with shorter follow-up, have noted small increases in blood pressure and an increased incidence of mild proteinuria after uninephrectomy. None of these shorter-term studies have suggested that proteinuria after uninephrectomy is a precursor to renal insufficiency.

Of particular interest are the case reports of patients with partial loss of a solitary kidney. Of the total of 35 such patients described in the literature, 31 reportedly had stable renal function.[94–98] However, in the largest series of case reports, Novick et al. described 14 patients (follow-up 5 to 17 years after partial nephrectomy of a solitary kidney): 12 had stable renal function, but 2 had developed renal failure and 9 had proteinuria.[97] The extent of proteinuria correlated directly with the length of follow-up and inversely with the amount of remaining renal tissue.

## Clinical Studies—Donors

Prospective LDs are screened to determine that they have two normal kidneys at the time of nephrectomy. To date, numerous studies have examined renal function, proteinuria, and hypertension.[12,14,38,99–124(reviewed in 124)] Although isolated cases of renal failure after donor nephrectomy have been reported,[114,115] no

large, single-center series has demonstrated any evidence of progressive deterioration of renal function in LDs. In recognition of this benign course, insurance companies do not increase premiums for LDs.[125] However, a limiting factor in most such studies is that mean follow-up has been < 20 years. Given that most LDs have a life expectancy of > 20 years, longer follow-up is necessary. Ellison et al. reported on 56 LDs who had subsequently been listed themselves with the United Network for Organ Sharing (UNOS) for a DD kidney transplant.[126] Some had donated before the establishment of the UNOS database, making it difficult to determine a denominator and calculate an accurate incidence. Even if such a calculation were possible, it might still underestimate the incidence of ESRD in LDs, because those who underwent an LD (vs DD) kidney transplant and those who developed ESRD but were never listed for a transplant would be missed. In the Ellison report, 86% of the LDs who were later wait-listed had donated to a sibling; the cause of ESRD was hypertensive nephrosclerosis in 36% and focal sclerosis in 16%. Clearly, careful long-term follow-up studies of LDs are imperative, in order to accurately determine their risk.

Recently, we have begun more detailed studies of renal function in LDs. To date, we have comprehensive information on > 15% of LDs who donated > 5 years ago. LDs were categorized according to the CKD staging advocated by the National Kidney Foundation.

The length of time from donation was 19.5 ± 9.6 years. The majority of LDs, 67%, were in CKD stages 2–3; in fact, overall, 32% were hypertensive, 6% were diabetic, and hyperlipidemia was present in 37%. (Note that the CKD classification system was developed for a population with two kidneys; the risks and prognosis may be different in LDs.)

Although the overwhelming majority of LDs, 87%, had an estimated GFR > 60 mL/min/1.73 m$^2$, we found that kidney donors were at least three times more likely than the general population to be categorized as CKD stage 2 or 3. Hypertension (but not diabetes and not time from donation) was an independent risk factor for having a higher CKD stage.

Using serum creatinine levels to estimate renal function has well-recognized inaccuracies and limitations. The modification of Diet in Renal Disease (MDRD) and Cockcroft-Gault (CG Cl$_{cr}$) formulas have been validated in many populations, but, to our knowledge, have not been used in LDs. We examined, in a separate analysis, the performance of these two prediction models against measured GFR in LDs. We randomly selected LDs for this study from donor lists that were stratified by time from donation. To determine GFR, we used the plasma clearance of iohexol, which has excellent correlation with inulin GFR. The mean age at the time of GFR measurement was 54.9 ± 10.2 years; mean time from donation, 13 ± 9 years (range, 3 to 33 years); 100% of these LDs were white, 29% were hypertensive, and 3% were diabetic. The mean serum creatinine level was 1.1 ± 0.19 mg/dL; mean CG Cl$_{cr}$, 70.2 ± 14.5 mL/min/1.73 m$^2$; mean MDRD GFR, 63.3 ± 15.9 mL/min/1.73 m$^2$, and mean iohexol GFR, 69.5 ± 11.1 mL/min/1.73 m$^2$. We found that the two formulas were roughly similar in their performance. Nevertheless, more information is needed regarding the ideal method of estimating GFR in kidney donors.

## Donor Follow-up ≥20 Years

We know of only three published studies reporting ≥ 20 years follow-up of LDs. In 1991, we studied our LDs ≥ 20 years after donation (range, 21 to 29 years after donation) by comparing their renal function, blood pressure, and proteinuria (vs their siblings).[12] Of 130 LDs from January 1, 1963, through December 31, 1970, we were able to locate 125; we sent them questionnaires about their current health and asked them to participate in our follow-up study. Of these 125, 78 LDs (or families) returned the questionnaire. Of the other 47 LDs, 32 were known to be alive but did not respond. For each LD, we also asked all siblings to participate. Assessments were done by local physicians.

Of the 78 LDs (or families) who returned the questionnaire, mean age at the time of donation was 43 ± 1 years (range, 16 to 70 years). Fifteen donors had died 2 to 25 years after donation; none of these 15 had had kidney disease at death. A total of 57 LDs underwent laboratory testing for our study (mean age at the time of the study, 61 ± 1 years [range, 40 to 83 years]). In addition, 65 siblings provided a history and had a physical examination; of these, 50 underwent laboratory testing. The mean age of these 65 siblings was 58 ± 1.3 years (range, 29 to 83 years).

For the 57 LDs, the mean serum creatinine level was 1.1 ± .01 mg/dL; mean BUN, 17 ± 0.5 mg/dL; mean creatinine clearance (as determined by 24-hour urine collection), 82 ± 2 mL/min.; and mean blood pressure, 134 ± 2/80 ± 1 mm Hg. We found that 32% of these LDs were taking antihypertensive drugs, and 23% had proteinuria.

The 65 siblings did not differ significantly from the 57 LDs in either demographic characteristics or outcomes of interest: mean serum creatinine level, 1.1 ± 0.03 mg/dL; BUN, 17 ± 1.2 mg/dL; measured creatinine clearance, 89 ± 3.3 mL/min.; and blood pressure, 130 ± 3/80 ± 1.5 mm Hg. Of the siblings, 44% were taking antihypertensive medications, and 22% had proteinuria.

Goldfarb et al. studied LDs 20 to 32 years (mean ± SD, 25 ± 3 years) after uninephrectomy.[120] Of 180 eligible LDs, 70 (39%) participated in the study by completing a questionnaire, having blood pressure measured, and submitting blood and urinary samples for laboratory analysis. For those 70 LDs, blood pressure and serum creatinine levels were increased at the time of the study (vs before donation), but the values were still in the normal range. The overall incidence of hypertension was comparable to the age-matched general population. Of the 70 LDs, 13 (19%) donors had a 24-hour urinary protein excretion ≥ 0.15 g per 24 hours. Donors with versus without proteinuria did not differ significantly by age, duration of follow-up, serum creatinine levels, 24-hour creatinine clearance, or prevalence of hypertension. Of note, ESRD requiring dialysis developed in two LDs.

Recently, we again studied all of our donors ≥ 20 years after donation.[122] Families of LDs who had died were asked to provide details about the health of the donor before death and about the cause of death. We were able to obtain information on 464 (60%) of 773 LDs. Of the 464 LDs, 84 have died. The cause of death was available for 27 of them; 24 had no kidney disease, but 3 were on dialysis at the time of their death. Of these 3 LDs who died with kidney failure, 1 had developed diabetes and diabetic nephropathy and started dialysis 10 years after donating a kidney and a partial pancreas, 1 had developed kidney failure secondary to hemolytic uremic syndrome at age 76 (32 years after donation), and 1 had prerenal failure secondary to cardiac disease.

In all, 380 of our LDs are known to be alive ≥ 20 years after donation. Of these LDs, 13 reported no kidney problems, but did not want to participate in our study. Another 111 stated that they were well and had no kidney problems, but did not return our questionnaire and did not provide a history or undergo a physical examination.

**TABLE 15.8-1**

**KIDNEY FUNCTION IN LDS* WHO HAD LABORATORY TESTS PERFORMED (n = 125)**

|  | Interval Postdonation | |
|  | 20–29 Years | ≥ 30 Years |
| --- | --- | --- |
| n (returned questionnaire) | 198 | 58 |
| Age (Years) | | |
| Mean (± SE) | 59.7 ± .8 | 66.7 ± 1.3 |
| Range | 38–89 | 51–89 |
| Serum creatinine level (mg/dL) | | |
| n (labs at time of study) | 74 | 29 |
| Mean (± SE) | 1.2 ± .04 | 1.3 ± .1 |
| Range | 0.7–2.5 | 0.7–2.3 |
| Proteinuria | | |
| n studied (% with proteinuria) | 92 (11%) | 21 (5%) |
| Degree proteinuria | 7 trace; 1, 1+; 1, 2+; 1, 3+ | 1, 1+ |
| Hypertension, n (%) | 72 (36%) | 22 (38%) |
| 1 Medication | 36 | 11 |
| 2 Medications | 17 | 6 |
| 3 Medications | 8 | 2 |
| Not stated | 11 | 3 |

*LDs, living donors.

† Reproduced with permission from Ramcharan T, Matas AJ. Long-term (20–37 years) follow-up of living kidney donors. *Am J Transplant* 2002;2(10):959–964.

Of the 256 LDs who returned our questionnaire, 125 also sent in records of a history and physical examination (done by their local physician), laboratory results, or both (Table 15.8-1).

In all, 198 LDs, 20 to 29 years after donation, returned our questionnaire; of these, 74 had serum creatinine levels measured (Table 15.8-1). The mean serum creatinine level was 1.2 ± .04 mg/dL(range, 0.7 to 2.5 mg/dL). Of these 198 LDs, 92 underwent urinalysis to assess for proteinuria: 82 (89%) had no proteinuria; 7 (8%), trace; 1 (1%), 1+; 1 (1%), 2+; and 1 (1%), 3+. Of these 198 LDs, 72 (36%) stated they have high blood pressure: 36 (50%) take one antihypertensive medication, 17 (24%) take two, and 8 (11%) take three (11 did not provide this information).

Another 58 LDs, 30 to 37 years after donation, returned our questionnaire; of these, 29 had serum creatinine levels measured (Table 15.8-1). The mean serum creatinine level was 1.3 ± 0.1 mg/dL (range, 0.7 to 2.3 mg/dL). Of these 58 LDs, 21 underwent urinalysis to assess for proteinuria: 20 (95%) had no proteinuria and 1 had trace proteinuria. Of these 58 LDs, 22 (38%) stated they have high blood pressure: 11 (50%) take one antihypertensive medication, 6 (27%) take two, and 2 (9%) take three (3 did not provide this information).

Of all 256 LDs who returned our questionnaire, 5 had serum creatinine levels >1.7 mg/dL. The first such LD, 69 years old at the time of the study, developed ESRD secondary to chronic glomerulonephritis and underwent a kidney transplant 24 years after donation. The second, 69, developed renal failure secondary to gout, renal stones, and repeated episodes of pyelonephritis, and underwent a kidney transplant 32 years after donation. The third, 87, had a serum creatinine level of 2.3 mg/dL (30 years after donation); he has an extensive history of cardiovascular disease, and prerenal failure has been diagnosed. The fourth, 47, had a serum creatinine level of 2.5 mg/dL (no biopsy has been done) 25 years after donation. The fifth, 66, had a serum creatinine level that vacillates from 1.7 to 2.2 mg/dL (22 years after donation); creatinine clearance (24-hour urine collection), 52 mL/mm. Kidney biopsy results reportedly showed nephromegaly with segmental and global glomerular sclerosis.

A total of 33 LDs reported 72 pregnancies after donation. Of these 33 LDs, 25 had not had pregnancies before donation. Two LDs reported having hypertension during their first pregnancy and a third had preeclampsia. Only 1 LD reported needing treatment for hypertension, during a second pregnancy.

Of interest, 250 LDs responded to our question about family history of diabetes. Of these, 87 reported a family history (20 type 1, 43 type 2, 24 not specified). After donation, 19 LDs developed diabetes; 9 of them (47%) have no other family members with diabetes. Of the 19 LDs with diabetes, 6 control it with diet alone, 5 take oral hypoglycemics, and 7 take insulin. Six have had serum creatinine level determinations (0.7, 1.1, 1.2, 1.2, 1.3, 1.8 mg/dL). Of course, this information came from respondents only, so may not reflect the true rate in the underlying population of LDs-turned-candidates. In addition, only 6 of the 19 LDs with diabetes underwent laboratory testing.

## RISK FACTORS FOR ESRD IN THE GENERAL POPULATION

Population studies have shown that smoking, obesity, elevated blood pressure, and elevated blood glucose levels are associated with increased risk for proteinuria[127–134(rev in 134)] And, as discussed above, proteinuria is an early marker for renal disease.

Whereas diabetes and hypertension are well-described causes of ESRD, the association of proteinuria with smoking and obesity is a cause for concern. Both are prevalent in the general population. In a sequential study of 5,403 men and women in Japan, Tozawa et al. noted that development of new-onset proteinuria was related to smoking and obesity.[127] In a study of Australian adults, Briganti et al. also noted an association between proteinuria and smoking.[129]

Praga et al. studied the impact of uninephrectomy (done for unilateral renal disease) on proteinuria and renal function.[133] The preoperative characteristic that determined the development of proteinuria or renal insufficiency was body mass index (BMI). The probability of proteinuria 10 years after uninephrectomy was 60% in obese patients (BMI ≥ 30) versus 7% in nonobese patients (BMI < 30); 20 years after uninephrectomy, 92% in obese patients versus 23% in nonobese patients. This finding clearly underscores the need for long-term donor follow-up with stratification for risk factors.

Presumably, in the Praga series, the patients required uninephrectomy for their disease; it is unlikely that a minimum creatinine clearance was needed before proceeding with uninephrectomy (although serum creatinine levels were reported to be normal). LDs are typically more extensively evaluated before being approved for uninephrectomy. It is important to determine whether the finding of Praga et al. also applies to long-term follow-up of LDs.

## UNINEPHRECTOMIZED HUMANS

A critical question is whether LDs who subsequently develop any form of kidney disease, even years after nephrectomy, will have an accelerated course to kidney failure. As described earlier, our long-term donor follow-up study has identified 18 LDs who developed diabetes 6 to 34 years after donation.[122]

The impact of uninephrectomy is of interest in non-LDs who develop diabetes and in non-LDs who develop polycystic kidney disease. In nine diabetic non-LDs with either unilateral agenesis or unilateral nephrectomy, none suffered accelerated kidney failure in the remaining kidney.[135,136]

Silveiro et al. studied type 2 diabetic non-LDs who underwent uninephrectomy (single-kidney diabetics, n = 20; duration of diabetes, 8.5 ± 7 years), nondiabetic non-LDs who underwent uninephrectomy (single-kidney nondiabetics, n = 17), and type 2 diabetic non-LDs with 2 kidneys (n = 184; duration of diabetes, 10 ± 7 years) (137). The single-kidney and two-kidney type 2 diabetics were matched for age, sex, and BMI. Microalbuminuria was noted in a higher proportion of single-kidney diabetics (40%) than single-kidney nondiabetics (18%) or two-kidney diabetics (20%). Macroalbuminuria was noted in a higher proportion of single-kidney diabetics (30%) than single-kidney nondiabetics (6), but no difference was found between single-kidney diabetics (30%) and two-kidney diabetics (23%). Of importance, renal function at the time of the study was not different for single-kidney patients, whether they were diabetics or nondiabetics.[137]

Zeier et al. compared 47 non-LDs with polycystic kidney disease who required uninephrectomy versus matched controls who did not undergo uninephrectomy.[138] The uninephrectomy was done for infection, stones, hemorrhage, or trauma. Both the mortality rate and the median time for serum creatinine levels to rise from 4 mg/dL to 8 mg/dL were similar in the two groups.

## FUTURE RESEARCH NEEDS

As outlined previously, numerous questions remain regarding long-term outcome for LDs.

First, and foremost, does kidney donation increase the long-term risk of developing ESRD?

Second, is the mild increase in blood pressure seen in some LDs progressive, and is it a risk for ESRD or survival?

Third, does the incidence of proteinuria increase after donation? If proteinuria develops, does it progressively worsen? Is proteinuria a marker for future renal dysfunction? Does it contribute to progressive loss of renal function?

Fourth, do LDs with a high BMI or a history of smoking have an increased risk of developing proteinuria and renal dysfunction?

Fifth, do LDs who subsequently develop type 2 diabetes or hypertension have an increased risk of developing ESRD, and does ESRD develop more rapidly?

Sixth, does the mild renal impairment, increase in blood pressure, and proteinuria associated with uninephrectomy increase cardiovascular risk?

## SUMMARY

Donor nephrectomy is a major operative procedure without physical benefit to the LD. The perioperative risks have been described in detail. Although isolated cases of renal dysfunction and ESRD have been described in LDs-turned-candidates, studies to date suggest no increase in the incidence of ESRD (vs the age-matched general population). However, long-term studies have suffered from incomplete follow-up. In addition, recent data in the non-LD population suggest that mild renal impairment increases cardiovascular risk. Long-term studies with complete follow-up are required to address these issues.

## ACKNOWLEDGMENTS

We thank Mary Knatterud for editorial assistance and Stephanie Daily for preparation of the manuscript.

## References

1. Evans RW, Manninen, DL, Garrison, LP Jr., et al. The quality of life of patients with end-stage renal disease. *N Engl J Med* 1985;312(9):553–539.

2. Wolfe RA, Ashby VB, Milford EL, et al. Comparison of mortality in all patients on dialysis, patients on dialysis awaiting transplantation, and recipients of a first cadaveric transplant. *N Engl J Med* 199;341(23):1725–1730.

3. Schnuelle P, Lorenz D, Trede M, et al. Impact of renal cadaveric transplantation on survival in end-stage renal failure: Evidence for reduced mortality risk compared with hemodialysis during long-term follow-up. *J Am Soc Nephrol* 1998;9(11):2135–2141.

4. Xue JL, Ma JZ, Louis TA, et al. Forecast of the number of patients with end-stage renal disease in the United States to the year 2010. *J Am Soc Nephrol* 2001;12(12):2753–2758.

5. Sheehy E, Conrad SL, Brigham LE, et al. Estimating the number of potential organ donors in the United States. *N Engl J Med* 2003;349(7):667–674.

6. Ojo AO, Hanson JA, Meier-Kreische H, et al. Survival in recipients of marginal cadaveric donor kidneys compared with other recipients and wait-listed transplant patients. *J Am Soc Nephrol* 2001;12(3):589–597.

7. Cosio FG, Alamir A, Yim S, et al. Patient survival after renal transplantation. I. The impact of dialysis pre-transplant. *Kidney Int* 1998;53(3):767–772.

8. Meier-Kreische HU, Port FK, Ojo AO, et al. Effect of waiting time on renal transplant outcome. *Kidney Int* 2000;58(3):1311–1317.

9. Gjertson DW, Cecka JM. Living unrelated donor kidney transplantation. *Kidney Int* 2000;58(2):491–499.

10. Wolf JS Jr, Merion RM, Leichtman AB, et al. Randomized controlled trial of hand-assisted laparoscopic versus open surgical live donor nephrectomy. *Transplantation* 2001;72(2):284–290.

11. Bay WH, Hebert LA. The living donor in kidney transplantation. *Ann Intern Med* 1987;106(5):719–727.

12. Najarian JS, Chavers BM, McHugh LE, et al. 20 years or more of follow-up of living kidney donors. *Lancet* 1992;340(8823):807–810.

13. Matas AJ, Bartlett AT, Leichtman AB, et al. Morbidity and mortality after living kidney donation in 1999-2001: A survey of United States transplant centers. *Am J Transplant* 2003;3(7):830–834.

14. Johnson EM, Remucal MJ, Gillingham KJ, et al. Complications and risks of living donor nephrectomy. *Transplantation* 1997;64(8):1124–1128.

15. Andersen B, Hansen JB, Jorgensen SJ. Survival after nephrectomy. *Scand J Urol Nephrol* 1968.2(2):91–94.

16. Fehrman-Ekholm I, Elinder CG, Stenbeck M, et al. Kidney donors live longer. *Transplantation* 1997;64(7):976–978.

17. Shulman NB, Ford CE, Hall WD, et al. Prognostic value of serum creatinine and effect of treatment of hypertension on renal function. Results from the Hypertension Detection and Follow-up Program. The Hypertension Detection and Follow-up Program Cooperative Group. *Hypertension* 1989;13(5 suppl):I80–93.

18. Damsgaard EM, Froland A, Jorgensen OD, et al. Microalbuminuria as predictor of increased mortality in elderly people. *BMJ* 1990;300(6720):297–300.

19. Friedman PJ. Serum creatinine: An independent predictor of survival after stroke. *J Intern Med* 1991;229(2):175–179.

20. Matts JP, Karnegis JN, Campos CT, et al. Serum creatinine as an independent predictor of coronary heart disease mortality in normotensive survivors of myocardial infarction. POSCH Group. *J Fam Pract* 1993;36(5):497–503.

21. Hamdan AD, Pomposelli FB Jr, Gibbons GW, et al. Renal insufficiency and altered postoperative risk in carotid endarterectomy. *J Vasc Surg* 1999;29(6):1006–1011.

22. Dries DL, Exner DV, Domanski MJ, et al. The prognostic implications of renal insufficiency in asymptomatic and symptomatic patients with left ventricular dysfunction. *J Am Coll Cardiol* 2000;35(3):681–689.

23. Anderson RJ, O'Brien M, MaWhinney S, et al. Mild renal failure is associated with adverse outcome after cardiac valve surgery. *Am J Kidney Dis* 2000;35(6):1127–1134.

24. Gueyffier F, Boissel JP, Pocock S, et al. Identification of risk factors in hypertensive patients: contribution of randomized controlled trials through an individual patient database. *Circulation* 1999;100(18): e88–e94.

25. Weiner DE, Tighiouart H, Stark PC, et al. Kidney disease as a risk factor for recurrent cardiovascular disease and mortality. *Am J Kidney Dis* 2004;44(2):198–206.

26. Wannamethee SG, Shaper AG, Perry IJ: Serum creatinine concentration and risk of cardiovascular disease: A possible marker for increased risk of stroke. *Stroke* 1997;28(3):557-563, 1997.

27. Culleton BF, Larson MG, Wilson PW, et al. Cardiovascular disease and mortality in a community-based cohort with mild renal insufficiency. *Kidney Int* 1999;56(6):2214–2219.

28. Manjunath G, Tighiouart H, Ibrahim H, et al. Level of kidney function as a risk factor for atherosclerotic cardiovascular outcomes in the community. *J Am Coll Cardiol* 2003;41(1):47–55.

29. Go AS, Cherton GM, Fan D, et al. Chronic kidney disease and the risks of death, cardiovascular events, and hospitalization. *N Engl J Med* 2004;351(13):1296–1305.

30. Foley RN, Murray AM, Li S, et al. Chronic kidney disease and the risk for cardiovascular disease, renal replacement and death in the United States Medicare population, 1998 to 1999. *J Am Soc Nephrol* 2005;16(2):489–495.

31. Ogden DA. Consequences of renal donation in man: *Am J Kidney Dis* 1983;2(5):501–511.

32. Donadio JV Jr, Farmer CD, Hunt JC, et al. Renal function in donors and recipients of renal allotransplantation. Radioisotopic measurements. *Ann Intern Med* 1967;66(1):105–115.

33. Krohn AG, Ogden DA, Holmes JH. Renal function in 29 healthy adults before and after nephrectomy. *JAMA* 1966;196(4):322–324.

34. Flanigan WJ, Burns RO, Takacs FJ, et al. Serial studies of glomerular filtration rate and renal plasma flow in kidney transplant donors, identical twins, and allograft recipients. *Am J Surg* 1968;116(5):788–794.

35. Boner G, Shelp WD, Newton M, et al. Factors influencing the increase in glomerular filtration rate in the remaining kidney of transplant donors. *Am J Med* 1973;55(2):169–174.

36. Pabico RC, McKenna BA, Freeman RB. Renal function before and after unilateral nephrectomy in renal donors. *Kidney Int* 1975;8(3):166–175.

37. ter Wee PM, Tegzess AM, Donker AJ. Renal reserve filtration capacity before and after kidney donation. *J Intern Med* 1990;228(4):393–399.

38. Anderson RG, Bueschen AJ, Lloyd LK, et al. Short-term and long-term changes in renal function after donor nephrectomy. *J Urol* 1991;145(1):11–13.

39. Chanutin A, Ferris EG. Experimental renal insufficiency produced by partial nephrectomy. *Arch Intern Med* 1932;49:767.

40. Striker GE, Nagle RB, Kohnen PW, et al. Response to unilateral nephrectomy in old rats. *Arch Pathol* 1969;87(4):439–442.

41. Shimamura T, Morrison AB. A progressive glomerulosclerosis occurring in partial five-sixths nephrectomized rats. *Am J Pathol* 1975;79(1):95–106.

42. Kaufman JM, Siegel NJ, Hayslett JP. Functional and hemodynamic adaptation to progressive renal ablation. *Circ Res* 1975;36(2):286–293.

43. Kaufman JM, DiMeola HJ, Siegel NJ, et al. Compensatory adaptation of structure and function following progressive renal ablation. *Kidney Int* 1974;6(1):10–17.

44. Purkerson ML, Hoffsten PE, Klahr S. Pathogenesis of the glomerulopathy associated with renal infarction in rats. *Kidney Int* 1976;9(5):407–417.

45. Hostetter TH, Olson JL, Rennke HG, et al. Hyperfiltration in remnant nephrons: A potentially adverse response to renal ablation. *Am J Physiol* 1981;241(1):F85–F93.

46. Morrison AB, Howard RM. The functional capacity of hypertrophied nephrons. Effect of partial nephrectomy on the clearance of inulin and PAH in the rat. *J Exp Med* 1966;123(5):829–844.

47. Brenner BM, Meyer TW, Hostetter TH. Dietary protein intake and the progressive nature of kidney disease: The role of hemodynamically mediated glomerular injury in the pathogenesis of progressive glomerular sclerosis in aging, renal ablation, and intrinsic renal disease. *N Engl J Med* 1982;307(11):652–659.

48. Meyer TW, Hostetter TH, Rennke HG, et al. Preservation of renal structure and function by long-term protein restriction in rats with reduced nephron mass. *Kidney Int* 1983;23:218 (abstr).

49. Madden MA, Zimmerman SW. Protein restriction and renal function in the uremic rat. *Kidney Int* 1983;23:217 (abstr).

50. El-Nahas AM, Paraskevakou H, Zoob S, et al. Effect of dietary protein restriction on the development of renal failure after subtotal nephrectomy in rats. *Clin Sci* (Lond) 1983:65(4):399–406.

51. Anderson S, Meyer TW, Rennke HG, et al. Control of glomerular hypertension limits glomerular injury in rats with reduced renal mass. *J Clin Invest* 1985;76(2):612–619.

52. Taal M, Brenner B. Renoprotective benefits of RAS inhibition: From ACEI to angiotensin II antagonists. *Kidney Int* 2000;57(5):1803–1817.

53. Berg BN, Simm HS. Nutrition and longevity in the rat. II. Longevity and onset of disease with different levels of food intake. *J Nutr* 1960;71:255–263.

54. Couser WG, Stilmant MM. Mesangial lesions and focal glomerular sclerosis in the aging rat. *Lab Invest* 1975;33(5):491–501.

55. Coleman GL, Barthold W, Osbaldiston GW, et al. Pathological changes during aging in barrier-reared Fischer 344 male rats. *J Gerontol* 1977;32(3):258–278.

56. Robertson JL, Goldschmidt M, Kronfeld DS, et al. Long-term renal responses to high dietary protein in dogs with 75% nephrectomy. *Kidney Int* 1986;29(2):511–519.

57. Bourgoignie JJ, Gavellas G, Hwang KH, et al. Renal function of baboons (Papio hamadryas) with a remnant kidney, and impact of different protein diets. *Kidney Int* Suppl 1989;27:S86–S90.

58. Davies DF, Shock NW. Age changes in glomerular filtration rate, effective renal plasma flow, and tubular excretory capacity in adult males. *J Clin Invest* 1950;29(5):496.

59. Rowe JW, Andres R, Tobin JD, et al. The effect of age on creatinine clearance in men: A cross-sectional and longitudinal study. *J Gerontol* 1976;31(2):155–163.

60. Kaplan C, Pasternack B, Shah H, et al. Age-related incidence of sclerotic glomeruli in human kidneys. *Am J Pathol* 1975;80(2):227–234.

61. Keane WF, Eknoyan G. Proteinuria, albuminuria, risk, assessment, detection, elimination (PARADE): A position paper of the National Kidney Foundation. *Am J Kidney Dis* 1999;33(5):1004–1110.

62. Ibrahim HN, Hostetter TH. The renin-aldosterone axis in two models of reduced renal mass in the rat. *J Am Soc Nephrol* 1998;9(1):72–76.

63. Peterson JC, Adler S, Burkart JM, et al. Blood pressure control, proteinuria, and the progression of renal disease. The Modification of Diet in Renal Disease Study. *Ann Intern Med* 1995;123(10):754–762.

64. Mogensen CE. Microalbuminuria predicts clinical proteinuria and early mortality in maturity-onset diabetes. *N Engl J Med* 1984;310(6):356–360.

65. Remuzzi G, Tognoni G for The Gisen Group. Randomised placebo-controlled trial of effect of ramipril on decline in glomerular filtration rate and risk of terminal renal failure in proteinuric, non-diabetic nephropathy. *Lancet* 1997;349(9069):1857–1863.

66. Maschio G, Alberti D, Janin G, et al. Effect of the angiotensin-converting-enzyme inhibitor benazepril on the progression of chronic renal insufficiency. The Angiotensin-Converting-Enzyme Inhibition in Progressive Renal Insufficiency Study Group. *N Engl J Med* 1996;334(15):939–945.

67. Lewis EJ, Hunsicker LG, Bain RP, et al. The effect of angiotensin-converting-enzyme inhibition on diabetic nephropathy. The Collaborative Study Group. *N Engl J Med* 1993;329(20):1456–1462.

68. Lewis EJ, Hunsicker LG, Clarke WR. Renoprotective effect of the angiotension-receptor antagonist irbesartan in patients with nephropathy due to type 2 diabetics. *N Engl J Med* 2001;345(12):851–860.

69. Brenner BM, Cooper ME, deZeeuw D: Effect of losartan on renal and cardiovascular outcomes in patients with type 2 diabetes and nephropathy. *N Engl J Med* 2001;345(12):861–869.

70. ACE Inhibitors in Diabetic Nephropathy Trialist Group: Should all patients with type 1 diabetes mellitus and microalbuminuria receive angiotensin-converting enzyme inhibitors? A meta-analysis of individual patient data. *Ann Intern Med* 2001;134(5):370–379.

71. Ledingham JG. Tubular toxicity of filtered proteins. *Am J Nephrol* 1990;10(suppl 1):52–57.

72. Burton CJ, Bevington A, Harris KP, et al. Growth of proximal tubular cells in the presence of albumin and proteinuric urine. *Exp Nephrol* 1994;2(6):345–350.

73. Kees-Folts D, Schreiner GF. A lipid chemotactic factor associated with proteinuria and interstitial nephritis induced by protein overload. *J Am Soc Nephrol* 1991;2:548 (abstract).

74. Kashyap ML, Ooi BS, Hynd RA, et al. Sequestration and excretion of high density and low density lipoproteins by the kidney in human nephrotic syndrome. *Artery* 1979;6:108121.

75. Neverov N, Ivanov A, Severgina R, et al. Cytoplasmic lipid inclusions and low density lipoprotein depositions in renal biopsies of nephrotic patients. *Nephrol Dial Transplant* 1997;10:776 (abstract).

76. Ong AC, Moorhead JF. Tubular lipidosis: Epiphenomenon or pathogenetic lesion in human renal disease? *Kidney Int* 1994;45(3):753–762.

77. Clark EC, Nath KA, Hostetter MK, et al. Role of ammonia in progressive interstitial nephritis. *Am J Kidney Dis* 1991;17(5 suppl 1):15–19.

78. Grone EF, Abboud HE, Hohne M, et al. Actions of lipoproteins in cultured human mesangial cells: modulation by mitogenic vasoconstrictors. *Am J Physiol* 263(4 pt 2):F686–F696.

79. Wheeler DC, Persaud JW, Fernando R, et al. Effects of low-density lipoproteins on mesangial cell growth and viability in vitro. *Nephrol Dial Transplant* 1990;5(3):185–191.

80. Frank J, Engler-Blum G, Rodemann HP, et al. Human renal tubular cells as a cytokine source: PDGF-B, GM-CSF and IL-6 mRNA expression in vitro. *Exp Nephrol* 1993;1(1):26–35.

81. Fetterman GH, Habib R. Congenital bilateral oligonephronic renal hypoplasia with hypertrophy of nephrons (oligoméganéphronie): Studies by microdissection. *Am J Clin Pathol* 1969;52:199.

82. Bernstein J: Renal hypoplasia and dysplasia. In: Edelmann CM Jr, ed. *Pediatric Kidney Disease*. Boston, MA, Little, Brown; 1978:541.

83. McGraw M, Poucell S, Sweet J, et al. The significance of focal segmental glomerulosclerosis in oligomeganephronia. *Int J Pediatr Nephrol* 1984;5(2):67–72.

84. Kiprov DD, Colvin RB, McCluskey RT. Focal and segmental glomerulosclerosis and proteinuria associated with unilateral renal agenesis. *Lab Invest* 1982;46(3):275–281.

85. Thorner PS, Arbus GS, Celermajer DS, et al. Focal segmental glomerulosclerosis and progressive renal failure associated with a unilateral kidney. *Pediatrics* 1984;73(6):806–810.

86. Emanuel B, Nachman R, Aronson N, et al. Congenital solitary kidney. A review of 74 cases. *Am J Dis Child* 1974;127(1):17–19.

87. Zucchelli P, Cagnoli L, Casanova S, et al. Focal glomerulosclerosis in patients with unilateral nephrectomy. *Kidney Int* 1983;24(5):649–655.

88. Goldstein AE: Longevity following nephrectomy. *J Urol* 1956;76(1):31–41.

89. Kohler B: *The Prognosis After Nephrectomy: A Clinical Study of Early and Late Results*. Stockholm, Sweden, Kungl, Boktryckeriet P.A. Norstedt & Soner, 1944.

90. Higashihara E, Horie S, Takeuchi T, et al. Long-term consequence of nephrectomy. *J Urol* 1990;143(2):239–243.

91. Robitaille P, Mongeau JG, Lortie L, et al. Long-term follow-up of patients who underwent unilateral nephrectomy in childhood. *Lancet* 1985;1(8441):1297–1299.

92. Baudoin P, Provoost AP, Molenaar JC. Renal function up to 50 years after unilateral nephrectomy in childhood. *Amer J Kid Dis* 1993;21(6):603–611.

93. Narkun-Burgess DM, Nolan CR, Norman JE, et al. Forty-five year follow-up after uninephrectomy. *Kidney Int* 1993;43(5):1110–1115.

94. Lhotta K, Eberle H, Konig P, et al. Renal function after tumor enucleation in a solitary kidney. *Am J Kidney Dis* 1991;17(3):266–270.

95. Foster MH, Sant GR, Donohoe JF, et al. Prolonged survival with a remnant kidney. *Am J Kidney Dis* 1991;17(3):261–265.

96. Rutsky EA, Dubovsky EV, Kirk KA. Long-term follow-up of a human subject with a remnant kidney. *Am J Kidney Dis* 1991.18(4):509–513.

97. Novick AC, Gephardt G, Guz B, et al. Long-term follow-up after partial removal of a solitary kidney. *N Engl J Med* 1991;325(15):1058–1062.

98. Solomon LR, Mallick NP, Lawler W. Progressive renal failure in a remnant kidney. *Br Med J (Clin Res Ed)* 1985;291(6509):1610–1611.

99. Penn I, Halgrimson CG, Ogden D, et al. Use of living donors in kidney transplantation in man. *Arch Surg* 1970;101(2):226–231.

100. Davison JM, Uldall PR, Walls J. Renal function studies after nephrectomy in renal donors. *Br Med J* 1976;1(6017):1050–1052.

101. Ringden O, Friman L, Lundgren G, et al. Living related kidney donors: Complications and long-term renal function. *Transplantation* 1978;25(4):221–223.

102. Dean S, Rudge CJ, Joyce M. Live related renal transplantation: An analysis of 141 donors. *Transplant Proc* 1982;14:657.

103. Vincenti F, Amend WJ Jr, Kaysen G, et al. Long-term renal function in kidney donors. Sustained compensatory hyperfiltration with no adverse effects. *Transplantation* 1983;36(6):626–629.

104. Weiland D, Sutherland DER, Chavers B, et al. Information on 628 living-related kidney donors at a single institution, with long-term follow-up in 472 cases. *Transplant Proc* 1984;16:5.

105. Hakim RM, Goldszer RC, Brenner BM. Hypertension and proteinuria: Long-term sequelae of uninephrectomy in humans. *Kidney Int* 1984;25(6):930–936.

106. Johnson EM, Anderson JK, Jacobs C, et al.: Long-term follow-up of living kidney donors: quality of life after donation. *Transplantation* 1999;67(5):717–721.

107. Miller IJ, Suthanthiran M, Riggio RR, et al. Impact of renal donation. Long-term clinical and biochemical follow-up of living donors in a single center. *Am J Med* 1985;79(2):201–208.

108. Tapson JS, Marshall SM, Tisdall SR, et al. Renal function and blood pressure after donor nephrectomy. *Proc Eur Dial Transplant Assoc Eur Ren Assoc* 1985;21:580–587.

109. Anderson CF, Velosa JA, Frohnert PP, et al. The risks of unilateral nephrectomy: status of kidney donors 10 to 20 years postoperatively. *Mayo Clin Proc* 1985;60(6):367–374.

110. Bohannon LL, Barry JM, Norman DJ, et al. Renal function 27 years after unilateral nephrectomy for related donor kidney transplantation. *J Urol* 1988;140(4):810–811.

111. Hoitsma AJ, Paul LC, Van Es LA, et al. Long term follow-up of living kidney donors. A two-centre study. *Neth J Med* 1985;28(6):226–230.

112. Sobh M, Nabeeh A, el-Din AS, et al. Long-term follow-up of the remaining kidney in living related kidney donors. *Int Urol Nephrol* 1989;21(5):547–553.

113. Mathillas O, Attman PO, Aurell M, et al. Proteinuria and renal function in kidney transplant donors 10-18 years after donor uninephrectomy. *Ups J Med Sci* 1985;90(1):37–42.

114. Tapson JS. End-stage renal failure after donor nephrectomy. *Nephron* 1986;42(3):262–264.

115. Ladefoged J. Renal failure 22 years after kidney donation. *Lancet* 1992;339(8785):124–125.

116. Smith S, Laprad P, Grantham J. Long-term effect of uninephrectomy on serum creatinine concentration and arterial blood pressure. *Am J Kidney Dis* 1985;6(3):143–148.

117. O'Donnell D, Seggie J, Levinson I, et al. Renal function after nephrectomy for donor organs. *S Afr Med J* 1986;69(3):177–179.

118. Talseth T, Fauchald P, Skrede S, et al. Long-term blood pressure and renal function in kidney donors. *Kidney Int* 1986;29(5):1072–1076.

119. Williams SL, Oler J, Jorkasky DK. Long-term renal function in kidney donors: A comparison of donors and their siblings. *Ann Intern Med* 1986;105(1):1–8.

120. Goldfarb DA, Matin SF, Braun WE, et al. Renal outcome 25 years after donor nephrectomy. *J Urol* 2001;166(6):2043–2047.

121. Dunn JF, Nylander WA Jr, Richie RE, et al. Living related kidney donors. A 14-year experience. *Ann Surg* 1986;203(6):637–643.

122. Ramcharan T, Matas AJ. Long-term (20-37 years) follow-up of living kidney donors. *Am J Transplant* 2002;2(10):959–964.

123. Torres VE, Offord KP, Anderson CF, et al. Blood pressure determinants in living-related renal allograft donors and their recipients. *Kidney Int* 1987;31(6):1383–1390.

124. Kasiske BL, Ma JZ, Louis TA, et al. Long-term effects of reduced renal mass in humans. *Kidney Int* 1995;48(3):814–819.

125. Spital A: Life insurance for kidney donors—An update. *Transplantation* 1988;45(4):819–820.

126. Ellison MD, McBride MA, Taranto SE, et al. Living kidney donors in need of kidney transplants: a report from the organ procurement and transplantation network. *Transplantation* 2002;74(9):1349–1351.

127. Tozawa M, Iseki K, Iseki C, et al. Influence of smoking and obesity on the development of proteinuria. *Kidney Int* 2002;62:956–962.

128. Watnick TJ, Jenkins RR, Rackoff P, et al. Microalbuminuria and hypertension in long-term renal donors. *Transplantation* 1988;45(1):59–65.

129. Briganti EM, Branley P, Chadban SJ, et al. Smoking is associated with renal impairment and proteinuria in the normal population: the AusDiab kidney study. Australian Diabetes, Obesity and Lifestyle Study. *Am J Kidney Dis* 2002;40:704–712.

130. Iseki K, Iseki C, Ilemiya Y, et al. Risk of developing end-stage renal disease in a cohort of mass screening. *Kidney Int* 1996;49:800–805.

131. Iseki K, Ikemiya Y, Iseki C, et al. Proteinuria and the risk of developing end-stage renal disease. *Kidney Int* 63:1468-1474, 2003.

132. Lhotta K, Rumpelt HJ, Konig P, et al. Cigarette smoking and vascular pathology in renal biopsies. *Kidney Int* 2002;61:648–654.

133. Praga M, Hernandez E, Herrero JC, et al. Influence of obesity on the appearance of proteinuria and renal insufficiency after unilateral nephrectomy. *Kidney Int* 2000;58:2111–2118.

134. Davis CL. Evaluation of the living kidney donor: Current perspectives. *Am J Transplant* 2004;43(3):508–530.

135. Fattor R, Silva F, Eigenbrodt E, et al. Effect of unilateral nephrectomy on three patients with histopathological evidence of diabetic glomerulosclerosis in the resected kidney. *HNO* 1987;1(3):107–113.

136. Sampson MJ, Drury PL. Development of nephropathy in diabetic patients with a single kidney. *Diabetic Med* 1990;7:258–260.

137. Silveiro SP, DaCosta LA, Beck MO, et al. Urinary albumin excretion rate and glomerular filtration rate in single-kidney type 2 diabetic patients. *Diabetes Care* 1998;21(9):1521–1524.

138. Zeier M, Geberth S, Gonzalo A, et al. The effect of uninephrectomy on progression of renal failure in autosomal dominant polycystic kidney disease. *J Am Soc Nephrol* 1992;3(5):1119–1123.

## 15.9  PSYCHOLOGICAL ASPECTS

*Annette Lennerling, RN, MSc, PhD*

### INTRODUCTION

Successful clinical kidney transplantation began with living donation. Through the years the criteria for becoming a kidney living donor (LD) have expanded: from being restricted to blood-related donors to including emotionally related donors as well as, in recent times, nondirected donors.

Nephrectomy performed in healthy individuals for the purpose of a transplant for someone else is an exceptional activity. For the recipient, a kidney transplant is not a lifesaving procedure and may therefore be questioned ethically. The use of LDs for a kidney transplant affects not only the patient with end-stage renal disease (ESRD) but also the healthy person who volunteers to donate, along with their partners, family, friends, and health-care professionals. From a clinical perspective, LD kidney transplants are very successful, but evoke a complex mix of emotions in all those involved. Thus, ethical, psychological, and social aspects must be continuously considered.

## RECRUITMENT OF LDs

The possibility of living kidney donation is rather well known to the general population. Therefore, relatives, coworkers, and friends often contact an ESRD patient's physician with a wish to begin LD assessment. However, coercion can also be involved. The role of the ESRD patient's physician in providing information and sometimes in recruiting and assessing the potential LD is problematic. For that physician, the ESRD patient's interests and well-being obviously come first and so they should. Therefore, the ESRD patient and the potential LD must be treated as two separate individuals and not as one unit.

A married couple may serve as an example. The husband has ESRD and is in need of a kidney transplant, and the wife accompanies him to his appointment with the nephrologist. While giving information about kidney transplants, his physician asks her about her health and her blood group. She feels forced to begin donor assessment, without any possibility to consider the matter.

The optimal solution is that, when the nephrologist gives initial information about transplants to the ESRD patient, another physician takes on the responsibility to inform and evaluate the potential LD (the wife in our example). In a small nephrology unit, this may not be possible; even so, the situation at the very least demands thoughtful ethical attention in order to protect the potential LD's interests.

Far too often the ESRD patient—the potential recipient—is left with the difficult task of recruiting and informing any potential LD. For the person—the potential LD—who is asked to answer.[1,2] When is the right moment to raise such a question? It is equally hard. He or she may feel extremely embarrassed and find it difficult to give an honest response. Instead, ideally, the potential recipient should give permission for family and friends to be approached by health-care professionals: perhaps a physician, a nurse, and/or a transplant specialist. Written information about living donation can be mailed and then followed by a phone call. Or, potential LDs could be invited to the hospital to hear information about the possibility of living donation, either individually or as part of a group.

After information is shared, usually one or two potential LDs step forward, and donor assessment may begin. If nobody offers to become an LD, the potential recipient should be put on the waiting list for a deceased donor (DD) kidney: doing so may be a way to reduce pressure on potential LDs.

## PREDONATION INFORMATION

In a retrospective study by Jacobs et al., about one third of LDs stated they would have appreciated more information in preparation for donation.[1] Many potential LDs look for information on the Internet and in magazines and books. They hear about donation from friends and the media. Misconceptions occur, and the procedure may be described as a small, even trivial, matter.[3]

As an introduction to the donor assessment, health-care professionals must impart both written and oral information.[4] Otherwise, the potential LD has no basis for giving informed consent. A thoroughly informed person feels secure and is less vulnerable. The concept of informed consent is perhaps an unachievable ideal;[3,5] yet great efforts at thorough communication must nonetheless be made.

The information provided must include both the benefits and the risks of living kidney donation and transplantation.[4] The psychological difficulties that may arise for LDs before, as well as after, donation are important components.

Oral information given by health-care professionals is totally dependent on their experience and commitment to living donation and is very difficult to evaluate. In contrast, the content of written information provided by a transplant center probably reflects its overall attitude to information, encapsulating the efforts made to explain the process of donation. Written information is essential to guarantee standard information; it should also be the basis for any oral information. Note that written information about donation should be given separately from written information about transplantation that is given to recipients.

When the nephrology department or transplant center is contacted by someone who offers to become a kidney LDs the written information could be sent by mail. Reading the information before the first appointment better prepares the potential LD for the in-person assessment and allows time for reflection. The potential LD should be encouraged to bring a relative or friend for the assessment. (The same holds true when written information about kidney transplantation is given to the recipient.)

## WORKUP OF LDs

A psychosocial evaluation should be included in the LD assessment in order to uncover any coercion to donate, any psychiatric disorders, and any psychological or social problems that disqualify the person.[6–9] Psychosocial difficulties may consist of the potential LD's inability to give informed consent, ambivalence, feelings of guilt, vulnerability to coercion, dependency on the recipient, substance abuse, and financial incentives.[9]

The health-care professional's discussions with the potential LD must focus on the LD's interest only. The talk could be led by a physician, a trained nurse, or a social worker—any qualified professional with a special interest and talent for this kind of work. It is an advantage if the potential LD can meet with two or more professionals, because each of them may have their own specific knowledge or competence and may thus observe the situation from a different perspective. Sufficient time must be allotted, and new meetings must be scheduled when needed. All those involved should maintain a tolerant, empathetic, and supportive attitude. The goals are to ascertain whether the potential LD has a psychosocial stability, has made the decision to donate voluntarily, and is motivated by altruism.[9] An assessment of the potential LD's ability to cope effectively with stress is also necessary: to a minor or major degree, stress always arises in connection with donation and transplantation. Older age, a lower education level, and little social support with few important relationships have all been identified as specific psychosocial risk factors for LDs.[10]

The fact that a loved one suffers from severe kidney failure and needs a kidney transplant puts a strain on the entire family. The possibility of living kidney transplantation may bring unity as well as conflicts to a family. Family roles might shift, plans for the future might have to change, social activities and contacts might diminish, and financial problems might occur. Life might appear chaotic. With all these changes, tension and conflicts in the family are not unusual.[11–14] Living kidney donation must not be regarded as a means to solve preexisting psychological problems and family conflicts. Any conflicts between the potential LD and the recipient, or among other family members, that are revealed during the assessment must be resolved before the donation proceeds.[15]

## MOTIVES AND CONCERNS

Penetrating the potential LD's motives is necessary for the purposes of assessment and for support, if needed, on an individual basis. Altruism, that is, the desire to do something significant for someone else, without expecting anything in return has been more or less taken for granted as a primary acceptable motive. But several other motives were found in a recent study involving interviews of LDs:[16]

- Identification with the recipient—*It could have been me.*

- Self-benefit from the recipient's improved health—*My husband's condition restricts our social life.*

- Logic—*You can live a normal life with one healthy kidney; it is as simple as that.*

- A feeling of moral duty, a kind of internal pressure—*I have to do it; there is nothing to discuss.*

- External pressure, that is, coercion—*I feel forced to do it.*

- Increased self-esteem or appreciation from others from doing a good deed that involves some risks—*I will be a hero.*

In addition, several retrospective studies have found two other motives for becoming a kidney LD: religious obligations and guilt from the past.[12,17,18] Guilt may be a motive for someone who has misbehaved and now sees an opportunity to be rehabilitated and regain acceptance. A parent who has left the family or a sibling with a history of social misconduct might have guilt as a motive. Of course, even if the guilt-plagued LD wants to make good, the recipient may still retain hostile feelings.

Potential LDs also have concerns that must be explored and addressed, especially their personal risks, such as having only one kidney left. They may also have fears about a poor outcome for the recipient, about the effect on other family members, about not passing the medical screening, about the lack of alternative potential LDs, about conflicting interests in the family, and about weak emotional relationship with the recipient.[2,16] On the whole, potential LDs express much more concern about the recipients than about themselves.

Factors supporting the LD's decision to donate may be previous knowledge of donation and transplantation, trust in the health-care system, satisfaction with the thorough health screening provided during the assessment, support from family and friends, and appreciation from the recipient. The long waiting time for kidneys from deceased donors (DDs) is also an important motive.

For an individual LD, all these different motives, concerns, and factors are valid in various combinations and to variable extents. A recent study in Norway and Sweden evaluated the impact of each motive in potential LDs (Figure 15.9-1).[2] The study found that the strongest motives were a wish to help, self-benefit, and identification with the recipient. In contrast, a desire for increased self-esteem, a sense of guilt from previous interactions, and religion were rare or weak motives for donation. Scandinavia is secularized; therefore, what would otherwise be seen as a religious motive was probably defined as moral duty.

For nondirected donors (NDDs), in particular, altruism must be a strong motive, coercion is probably nonexistent, and a desire for increased self-esteem might be more prevalent (as compared with blood-related or emotionally related LDs).

Given all of these motives, concerns, and factors, some LDs resort to an "optimistic fatalism" attitude;[16,19] that is, they dismiss the risks of donation by mentioning other risks in life as though they were impending.

During this phase of confused contradictory thoughts, information from the health-care professionals is key—solid basic information as well as specific responses to the individual LD's special requirements. These two difficulties are especially important to explore before the assessment ends: Coercion and unwillingness.

## Coercion

Being coerced is the only motive for donation that is not acceptable. Coercion seems to be uncommon, but should not exist at all.[16,20] Even the results of blood tests, however, might have

**FIGURE 15.9-1**

Box plots demonstrating the scores given by potential kidney donors in Sweden and Norway to various motives on a visual analogue scale (VAS) measuring 0–10 cm, where 10 is very important and naught not important. The horizontal lines indicate the 90%, 75%, 50% (median), 25% and 10% values. The circles represent individuals outside the 10% to 90% values.
With permission from Oxford University Press.

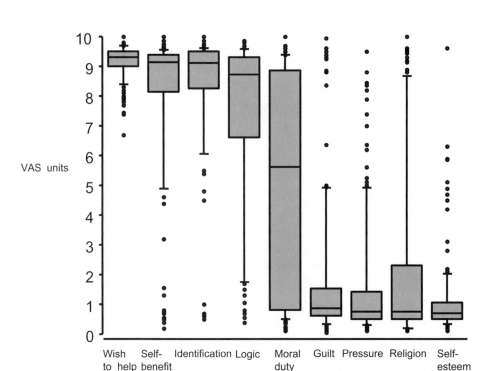

coercive effects, as in the case of a potential LD who turns out to be an human-leukocyte-antigen (HLA)-identical sibling. Therefore, no tests should be performed before the potential LD has been seen at the transplant center and has received basic information about the donation. A potential LD who indicates in any way that he or she is not proceeding voluntarily must be confidentially extricated and fully supported by the health-care professionals.

### Unwillingness

Sometimes a potential LD does not wish to donate but finds it difficult to declare this openly to the recipient and family. Some health-care professionals offer a false "alibi" for that person, for example, state that the cross-match test results turned out positive. Such "solutions" should be avoided, because false information if later exposed might disturb family relationships or might be medically harmful to the falsely excluded LD. Instead, the physician must assume responsibility and declare an unwilling potential LD unsuitable, without discussing the reason with the recipient or anyone else. In general, it is important to make recipients understand that donation must be voluntary and that loving relatives may have good reasons not to volunteer.

Likewise, when a recipient does not want a kidney from a certain relative, that relative and the health-care professionals must accept this as a fact.

## DECISION-MAKING PROCESS

The decision-making process usually starts long before the potential LD is seen by the health-care professionals.[16] At first, the process goes on under the surface, as a loved one suffers from progressive kidney failure and as the potential LD becomes increasingly aware of the role of transplants in treating ESRD. This phase may last for years.

When the time comes for the transplant, a healthy family member or friend may come forward and offer to donate a kidney, feeling this to be an instantaneous act.[6,7,16,18,20] An "instantaneous" decision is most often made emotionally, without consciously considering the pros and cons.

The decision-making process commonly ends with the view that kidney donation is the only option for this potential LD, even though other willing LDs and other forms of kidney replacement therapy may, in fact, be available.[16] For a potential LD who has come to this "only option" conclusion, upcoming problems that postpone or prevent donation are traumatic experiences. Support must be offered.

## PSYCHOLOGICAL DISADVANTAGES AFTER DONATION

The psychological effects of the transplant on the recipient mainly depend on the postoperative course and the outcome. Rejection episodes, wound complications, side effects from medications, and opportunistic infections may create very stressful situations. The recipient who encounters many obstacles can accumulate a growing anxiety and concern as to what will follow next. He or she may feel as if under constant threat. Fear of rejection is the most common long-term stressor for the recipient.[21] But eventually, most recipients adjust to life with a kidney transplant and find ways to cope with any difficulties. However, some remain deeply aware of and worried about the risks, to the point of negatively affecting their quality of life.

The LD's emotional recovery depends not only on his or her postoperative course but also on the outcome of the transplant. There is much focus on the LD before donation and much less afterward. This change occurs shortly after surgery, even though for the LD, the postoperative situation is still turbulent and full of concerns. It is a great change for the LD to go from very healthy to sick (whereas many recipients go from very sick to relatively healthy). Melancholic feelings can follow.

To show the LD appreciation and to catch psychosocial problems or prevent deep depression, a follow-up phone call or meeting with the LD must be initiated a few weeks after the hospital discharge. Any needed interventions can then begin.

Prolonged fatigue after donation is frequently reported; depression is not uncommon.[1,10,12,18,22] Such reactions may seem to be out of proportion to the donation experience, with respect to both depth and duration. The prevailing explanation is that the LD has been relieved from stress that built up during preparation for the donation. Or perhaps the LD had never before undergone such major surgery and thus had unrealistic expectations. Whatever the cause, potential LDs must be prepared for and aware of the possibility of fatigue and depression. Psychological or psychiatric help must be provided, until the LD's mental health is restored.

The LD has a double role, being both a patient and a relative to another, long-ill patient.[23] Moreover, the LD feels to some extent responsible for the recipient. In case of severe adverse events for the recipient, the LD will be distressed too.[24] Particularly in the case of graft loss, but probably also in less dramatic instances, a sense of guilt tends to afflict both parties. The recipient may feel accountable for the kidney and guilty if does not function well; the LD may feel that his or her gift was not good enough. To prevent such guilt, the health-care professionals must be prepared to intervene, providing reassuring information and helping both parties to communicate their feelings.

For both the LD and the recipient, financial problems caused by the recipient's illness and by expenses related to donation may well be causes of concern. Resolution strongly depends on how health-care and social services are organized in their particular country.[21] If health insurance and other financial support are inadequate, an extra burden is laid on both the LD and recipient.

## PSYCHOLOGICAL ADVANTAGES AFTER DONATION

Very few LDs regret their decision to donate.[7,25,26] Most remain completely content with their decision and would choose donation again if possible.[1,11,26–28] In general, LDs experience an overall better quality of life,[1,7,27,29] partly reflecting the gain made by the recipient.

An improved relationship with the recipient may be a benefit for the LD,[1,11,25] often expressed as closeness greater than before. Another psychosocial benefit for the LD is a sense of increased self-esteem.[6,14,25,30] Expressions of appreciation and gratitude from the health-care professionals are crucial in order to reinforce this effect.

## CONCLUSION

A kidney transplant is the treatment of choice for many patients with ESRD. Obtaining a kidney from an LD has a number of medical advantages for the recipient, but involves concerns for the LD. Families facing both a transplant and a donation must receive support to reduce the risk of long-term psychological morbidity, both for LD and the recipient. It is particularly important to give adequate written information to potential LDs and to appreciate how mixed their initial feelings might be concerning whether to donate. Donation is more demanding for the LD than commonly recognized.

## ACKNOWLEDGMENTS

Professor Gudrun Nyberg and Associate Professor Gunnela Nordén are acknowledged for their valuable comments.

## References

1. Jacobs C, Johnson E, Anderson K et al. Kidney transplants from living donors: How donation affects family dynamics. *Adv Ren Replace Ther* 1998;5:89.

2. Lennerling A, Forsberg A, Meyer K et al. Motives for becoming a living kidney donor. *Nephrol Dial Transplant* 2004;19:1600.

3. Dwyer J. Part of my liver. *Transplantation* 2003;76:1266.

4. Lennerling A, Nyberg G. Written information for potential living kidney donors. *Transplantation Int* 2004;17:449.

5. Spital A. Ethical issues in living organ donation: donor autonomy and beyond. *Am J Kidney Dis* 2001;38:189.

6. Fellner CH, Marshall JR. Twelve kidney donors. *JAMA* 1968;12:2703.

7. Fellner C. Renal transplantation and the living donor decision and consequences. *Psychother Psychosom* 1977;27:139.

8. Kasiske BL, Ravenscraft M, Ramos EL et al. The evaluation of living renal transplant donors: clinical practice guidelines. *J Am Soc Nephrol* 1996;7:2288.

9. Abecassis M, Adams M, Adams P, et al. Consensus Statement on the live organ donor. *JAMA* 2000;284:2919.

10. Morris P, St George B, Waring T et al. Psychosocial complications in living related kidney donors: An Australian experience. *Transplant Proc* 1987;19:2840.

11. Smith MD, Kappell DF, Province MA, et al. Living-related kidney donors: A multicenter study of donor education, socio-economic adjustment, and rehabilitation. *Am J Kidn Dis* 1986;8:223.

12. Russel S, Jacob RG: Living-related organ donation. The donor's dilemma. *Patient Educ Couns* 21:89, 1993.

13. Schover LR, Streem SB, Boparai N et al. The psychosocial impact of donating a kidney: Long-term followup from a urology-based center. *J Urology* 1997;157:1596.

14. Franklin PM, Crombie AK. Live related renal transplantation: psychological, social, and cultural issues. *Transplantation* 2003;76:1247.

15. Heck G, Schweitzer J, Seidel-Wiesel M. Psychological effects of living related kidney transplantation—risks and chances. *Clin Transplant* 2004;18:716.

16. Lennerling A, Forsberg A, Nyberg G. Becoming a living kidney donor. *Transplantation* 2003;76:1243.

17. Schumann D. The renal donor. *Am J Nurs* 1974;74:105.

18. Simmons RG, Marine SK, Simmons RL. *Gift of Life: The Effect of Organ Transplantation on Individual, Family, and Societal Dynamics.* New Brunswick, NJ: Transaction Publ; 1987.

19. Schweitzer J, Seidel-Wiesel M, Verres R, et al. Psychological consultation before living kidney donation: finding out and handling problem cases. *Transplantation* 2003;76:1464.

20. Hilton BA, Starzomski RC. Family decision making about living related kidney donation. *ANNA J* 1994;21:346.

21. Wainwright S, Fallon M, Gould D. Psychosocial recovery from adult kidney transplantation: A literature review. 22. *J Clin Nurs* 1999;8:233.

22. Lennerling A, Blohmé I, Östraat Ö, et al. Laparoscopic or open surgery for living donor nephrectomy. *Nephrol Dial Transplant* 2001;16:383.

23. Andersen MH, Mathiesen L, Oyen O et al. Living donors' experiences 1 wk after donating a kidney. *Clin Transplant* 2005;19:90.

24. Haljamäe U, Nyberg G, Sjöström B. Remaining experiences of living kidney donors more than 3 yr after early recipient graft loss. *Clin Transplant* 2003;17:503.

25. Kärrfelt HME, Berg UB, Lindblad FIE, et al. To be or not to be a living donor. *Transplantation* 1998;65:915.

26. Fehrman-Ekholm I, Brink B, Ericsson C et al. Kidney donors don't regret. *Transplantation* 2000;69:2067.

27. Johnsson EM, Anderson JK, Jacobs C, et al. Long-term follow-up of living kidney donors: quality of life after donation. Transplantation 1999;67:717.

28. Jordan J, Sann U, Janton A et al. Living kidney donors' long-term psychological status and health behavior after nephrectomy—a retrospective study. *J Nephrol* 2004;17:728.

29. Westlie L, Fauchald P, Talseth T, et al. Quality of life in Norwegian kidney donors. *Nephrol Dial Transplant* 1993;8:1146.

30. Simmons RG. Psychological reactions to giving a kidney. In: Levy N, ed. *Psychonephrology 1, Psychological Factors in Hemodialysis and Transplantation.* New York: Plenum Medical Book Company; 1981: 227–245.

# KIDNEY TRANSPLANTATION: THE RECIPIENT

## 16.1 SELECTION AND WORKUP

*Rahul Koushik, MD, Bertram L Kasiske, MD*

### INTRODUCTION

Kidney transplant recipients have reduced mortality compared to dialysis patients on the deceased donor waiting list.[1] Given the current annual increment of 20% per year, 95,000 patients are expected to be waiting for a kidney transplant by the year 2010 and 520,000 are expected be on dialysis.[2] This epidemic is largely due to an increased risk of progression to end-stage renal disease (ESRD) among patients with diabetes.[3] With the growing number of transplant candidates on the waiting list, morbidity and mortality are likely to increase, unless there is an increase in the number of living donor transplants. Although the rate of living donor transplants has been steadily increasing, the demand for organs far outstrips the supply. In any case, optimal management of Stage 4 and Stage 5 Chronic Kidney Disease (CKD) patients is necessary to improve outcomes, before and after kidney transplantation.

The goal of the pretransplant evaluation is to efficiently assess risk and to identify modifiable risk factors for adverse outcomes. The effective management of modifiable risk factors optimizes the recipient's overall chances of a successful transplant. The pretransplant evaluation also places the transplant team in a position to anticipate problems unique to a given recipient and to make a plan of action to deal with such problems, should they occur. Education is another important function of pretransplant evaluation, where the prospective recipient has a chance to meet with and directly discuss all aspects of the transplant process with the transplant team (Table 16.1-1).

### TABLE 16.1-1
### GOALS OF THE PRETRANSPLANT EVALUATION

| Goals of the Pretransplant Evaluation | Examples |
| --- | --- |
| Surgical risk assessment | Screening for CAD |
| Identification of risk factors for adverse posttransplant outcomes | High PRA |
| Setting realistic goals for modifiable risk factors | Weight loss (specify no. of kg) |
| Advance planning for patient-specific issues | Anticoagulation for metallic valve |
| Patient education | Lower risk of rejection, but increased infections in elderly recipients |

The management strategies outlined in this chapter are in accordance with published guidelines endorsed by the American Society of Transplantation,[4] the European Association of Urology,[5] and the European Renal Association-European Dialysis and Transplant Association (ERA-EDTA).[6] The goal of this chapter is to highlight the important clinical aspects of pretransplant evaluation process and provide additional insight into commonly encountered problems.

### TIMING OF THE PRETRANSPLANT EVALUATION

Outcomes after preemptive transplantation (before the need for dialysis) are better than outcomes after transplantation preceded by dialysis in adults and children.[7–11] For living donor kidney transplants, the 10-year overall adjusted graft survival was 75% for preemptive transplants versus 49% for transplants after 24 months on dialysis.[12] Perfectly timed, deceased donor transplantation is often not possible due to the long waiting times for a deceased donor kidney. Therefore, it is important to begin planning renal replacement therapy at an early stage, so that potential recipients have time to explore available options for living donors. In the United States, another benefit of timely evaluation and listing is to increase the otherwise small (15%–20%) chance that a 0-antigen-mismatched deceased donor kidney will be offered to the recipient under the Organ Procurement and Transplantation (OPTN) allocation scheme, currently managed by the United Network for Organ Sharing (UNOS).

The best time to refer potential recipients for transplant evaluation is usually 6 to 12 months before renal replacement therapy is anticipated.[13] This roughly corresponds to a glomerular filtration rate (GFR) 15 to 30 mL/min/1.73 m$^2$, or CKD Stage 4 of the National Kidney Foundation (NKF) Kidney Dialysis Outcomes Quality Initiative (K-DOQI) guidelines.[14] In the United States, it is important to counsel patients that to accrue waiting time on the UNOS waiting list they must have an estimated or measured GFR that is not more than 20 mL/min. The current NKF guidelines call for estimating GFR with a formula, which adjusts for factors other than kidney function that may influence serum creatinine.

1.  Cockcroft-Gault Formula[15]

    Estimated Creatinine Clearance (mL/min) = (140-age) × body weight in kilograms ÷ (serum creatinine in mg/dL × 72) × 0.85 if female, or

2.  Modification of Diet in Renal Disease Equation[16]

    For creatinine in mg/dL

    $GFR = 1.86 \times creatinine^{-1.154} \times age^{-0.203} \times constant$,
    where the constant is 1 for a white male, and is multiplied
    by 0.742 for white females and multiplied by 1.21 for African
    Americans.

Under special conditions, such as primary hyperoxaluria, refractory nephrotic syndrome requiring bilateral nephrectomy or, rarely, polycystic kidney disease with symptom-limiting enlargement of the kidneys requiring bilateral nephrectomy, recipients may be referred earlier to derive maximum benefit from transplantation.

## SPECIFIC CONSIDERATIONS

### Age

Children have been successfully transplanted over the age of 5 years. At the present time, there is no upper age limit for kidney transplantation. The relative survival advantage of transplantation versus dialysis is maintained for older compared to younger individuals despite the fact that the risk of death due to infections is higher for older transplant recipients as compared with wait-listed candidates.[17] Thus, from a patient's perspective, and from the perspective of a patient's physician-advocate, transplantation is generally the treatment of choice for Stage 5 CKD, regardless of age. However, it must be noted that studies of kidney transplantation in the elderly have included carefully screened and selected recipients and may not reflect the results of the entire elderly CKD population.[18] The prevalence of posttransplant cancer is fourfold higher in recipients older than 60 years of age as compared with recipients under 45 years old.[19] Thus, there may also be a role for appropriate counseling and for tailoring immunosuppression to minimize posttransplant infectious complications and cancer in elderly recipients.[20]

Long waiting times for deceased donor kidney transplantation make the use of a living donor even more attractive for an older recipient, who is more likely to die on the waiting list, than a younger recipient. The best living donor may be a healthy spouse, sibling, or biologically unrelated donor of similar age. A more difficult, ethical decision arises when the only potential donor is a much younger child of the recipient. This is because it may not always be wise to subject a healthy, young individual to the risk of donation to benefit an older recipient who has a much shorter life expectancy.

Given that there is a shortage of deceased donors, it can be argued from a societal perspective that younger patients should be given preference over older patients, because the latter have longer to live and can thereby maximize the benefit from a deceased donor kidney. In other words, society may decide to ration kidneys to younger versus older individuals, or to give older individuals only older kidneys. However, in the absence of a mandated rationing program, a physician is obligated to do what is best for his or her individual patient, and what is best is most often transplantation with a deceased donor kidney, if a living donor kidney is not available.

Given the long waiting times for a deceased donor kidney, older individuals may opt for an expanded donor kidney, to be transplanted sooner. In the United States, transplant candidates may elect to be placed on the Expanded Criteria Donor (ECD) waiting list, accepting a kidney that may function less well, in order to be transplanted sooner. Patients opting for such a program should understand that ECD kidneys may not function

as well and are statistically associated with a higher rate of graft failure and mortality after transplantation. This must be weighed against the higher risk of dying on the waiting list, compared with transplantation.[1]

### Cancer

Cancer that does not have a convincingly low chance of recurrence is generally a contraindication for LD transplantation. Transplantation most likely increases the risk of cancer recurrence, because the immunosuppression required for transplantation can be expected to reduce the recipient's immunological defense against tumor cells and/or against infectious vectors that cause cancer. The prevalence of cancer was 26% posttransplant, as compared with 1% in dialysis patients after 10 years of renal replacement therapy.[21] Reported risk factors for posttransplant cancer include older age, history of splenectomy, previous transplantation, and cigarette smoking.[19] A prospective recipient should be counseled about cancer risks at the pretransplant evaluation.

A patient with cancer may do better on dialysis than transplantation. In addition, it may not be sound ethical practice to subject a living donor to the risk of donation, if the recipient's life expectancy is significantly compromised by a high likelihood of cancer recurrence. For most cancers, an appropriate disease-free interval of 2 years after a documented cure is reasonable to reduce the risk of cancer recurrence. For some cancers, such as invasive breast cancer, invasive cervical cancer, symptomatic renal cell carcinoma, and colorectal cancer, a 5-year waiting period may be necessary. Basal cell carcinoma, cervical carcinoma *in situ,* and incidentally discovered renal cell cancers less than 5 cm size generally do not require a waiting period.

### Primary Kidney Diseases

Although many primary kidney diseases are known to have high recurrence rates in the allograft, they are not associated with graft failure in most cases. Overall, the risk of graft loss attributable to recurrent disease is about 8.4%, 10 years after kidney transplantation.[22] A notable exception is primary, idiopathic focal segmental glomerulosclerosis (FSGS), which has a 20% to 30% rate of recurrence posttransplant and a 12% to 13% risk of attributable graft loss.[22] Familial FSGS has a very low risk of recurrence.[23] In sporadic FSGS, it may be prudent to avoid living-related donors in these recipients with previous graft loss to early recurrence of FSGS.[24] Hemolytic uremic syndrome (HUS), although having a high recurrence and a 50% graft failure rate, is not considered a contraindication for transplantation. Primary hyperoxaluria is cured with combined liver–kidney transplantation if there is renal insufficiency and by isolated liver transplantation if renal function is normal. We currently recommend early referral for these patients.

### Viral Illnesses

#### Hepatitis B and C

Apart from severe cirrhotic changes in the liver biopsy, all other patients appear to be acceptable candidates for kidney transplantation. Although studies indicate that hepatitis B may not affect posttransplant survival,[25,26] hepatitis C may have a direct or indirect adverse impact on graft survival. In various studies, hepatitis C has been associated with an increase in mortality and hospitalization,[27] posttransplant diabetes,[27] cardiovascular deaths,[27] infections,[28] and liver disease.[29] Despite this, hepatitis-C-positive transplant recipients do better than their counterparts who remain on dialysis.[30] In a recent report, which included serial liver biopsies over a 10-year posttransplant period, only three cases of cirrhosis were documented in a longitudinal follow up of 51 kidney transplants with hepatitis C (antibody and HCV-RNA positive).[31] A major confounding factor in prospective kidney recipients with hepatitis is that serum transaminase elevations are not good predictors of outcome,[32] and normal serum transaminases do not exclude active liver disease.[33] Viral hepatitis may require disease-modulating therapies concurrently or prior to transplantation. This is best planned with an advance referral and can be coordinated in conjunction with a gastroenterologist. Pretransplant use of lamivudine for hepatitis B and interferon for hepatitis C appears to reduce viremia post-transplant.[34,35] Long-term efficacy of these regimens in reducing mortality due to liver disease in the kidney transplant population is not known.

### Human Immunodeficiency Virus

HIV-positive patients with a controlled viral load are not contraindicated for kidney transplantation. Highly active antiretrovirus therapy (HAART) has improved mortality in HIV-positive recipients, and HIV is the cause of 1% of all ESRD patients.[36] In one small pilot study, 10 HIV-positive kidney recipients had graft and patient survival comparable to non-HIV recipients.[37] Long-term studies on outcomes of HIV positive recipients with kidney transplant are awaited.

### Epstein Barr Virus

EBV activation posttransplant may be a risk factor for posttransplant lymphoproliferative disease (PTLD), especially in children. PTLD develops in 0.8% of adults and in 3% to 4% of children.[38] It is unclear whether pretransplant surveillance and treatment of EBV can reduce PTLD. It is important to counsel prospective recipients about the increased risk of PTLD after antibody treatment and acute rejection.

### Cytomegalovirus

CMV is the most important infection posttransplant, and prophylaxis is almost universally used in Western countries. Recipients should be counseled about CMV and its symptoms at the pretransplant evaluation.

## Coronary Artery Disease

CAD is the leading cause of death after renal transplantation.[4,39–41] In Europe, 53% of graft failures at 5 years posttransplant were attributable to CAD death with functioning allografts.[42] Risk factors for CAD after transplantation include the presence of pretransplant CAD, age, diabetes, male gender, cigarette smoking, hypertension, cholesterol, a low level of high-density lipoprotein (HDL) cholesterol, pretransplant splenectomy, and the number of acute rejection episodes.[39,40] Many of these are no different from the risk factors for CAD in the general population. However, there may also be CAD risk factors unique to the posttransplant state, including immunosuppressive agents, infections, and rejections. Indeed, graft function is likely a risk factor for CAD, and graft loss was identified as an independent risk factor for acute coronary syndromes.[43] Nevertheless,

traditional CAD risk factors appear to be risk factors for CAD after transplantation, and these are often present at the time of pretransplant evaluation. Identification and control of these risk factors will likely reduce the incidence of CAD events in the posttransplant period.

Herzog et al. found that angiographically significant lesions (> 50% stenosis) predicted CAD events posttransplant.[44] Nearly half (47%) of deaths in the immediate posttransplant period were predominantly due to CAD.[45] Kasiske et al. found that the prevalence of CAD in nondiabetic CKD recipients is also high, and it has been accepted practice among transplant centers to screen for CAD at the pretransplant evaluation.[41] Manske et al. showed that revascularization of critical coronary lesions (>75% stenosis) prior to transplantation, improved outcomes posttransplant in diabetic recipients;[46] however, only 26 patients were included in this study, and its applicability to current practice is questionable. Nevertheless, revascularization of stenotic lesions is compelling despite the lack of randomized studies to prove its efficacy.

With revascularization being an option, screening for CAD has important implications for a potential transplant recipient and adds to the risk and cost of the process. How to safely and efficiently screen for CAD is controversial. Angiography remains the gold standard. In living donor transplant candidates and especially candidates for preemptive transplants, one has to weigh the risk of radiocontrast nephrotoxicity before screening. Despite a 15% incidence of acute renal failure after radiocontrast administration,[47] the need for dialysis after coronary angiography in stable ambulatory CKD patients is low. In recent reports, with the use of adequate hydration protocols and nonionized contrast media, dialysis was needed in no more than 1% to 3% of cases.[48–50]

Noninvasive tests have gained popularity in recent years. The American Society of Transplantation (AST) guidelines recommend screening individuals at high risk with nuclear or dobutamine stress test.[4] In these guidelines, high risk is defined as

*ESRD due to diabetes,* or

*Prior history of CAD,* or

*Two or more risk factors,* where risk factors include: (1) men > 45 years, women > 55 years; (2) CAD in a first degree relative; (3) current smoker; (4) diabetes; (5) hypertension; (6) fasting cholesterol > 200 mg/dL, (g) fasting HDL cholesterol < 35 mg/dL or (h) left ventricular hypertrophy.

These guidelines further suggest that individuals with a positive noninvasive study should be considered for revascularization before elective transplant surgery.[4] However, the data from small studies using noninvasive screening are less convincing. Vandenberg et al. found that the rate of adverse peritransplant cardiac events was identical in patients with normal and abnormal pharmacologic nuclear stress tests in diabetic kidney transplant recipients.[51] Herzog et al. reported that dobutamine stress echocardiography was "less than optimal" in predicting CAD in advanced CKD.[44] There is considerable observer variation in the interpretation of these tests and nuclear and non-nuclear tests have never been compared head to head. Yet, in one study a normal dobutamine stress echocardiogram identified a very-low-risk population, with a 97% probability of being free of cardiac complications or death during a 6-month follow-up period.[52] With appropriate risk counseling, the recipients may be able to forgo an angiogram in favor of a noninvasive test performed by an experienced operator.

## Sensitization, Positive Cross Match, and ABO Blood Group Incompatibility

Acute rejection has an adverse effect on graft outcome.[53] Risk factors for acute rejection are well known (Table 16.1-2). Current immunosuppressive protocols have dramatically reduced acute rejection rates. Yet the impact of these rejections on eventual graft outcomes has remained high.[54] An important, potentially modifiable, pretransplant risk factor is sensitization. Sensitization can be thought of as the presence of preexisting immunological reactivity of the recipient to donor antigens or cells, and is usually measured by the presence of antibodies to a randomly selected panel of human lymphocytes. Sensitization increases the risk of acute rejection and consequent graft loss.[55] In a study of haploidentical living donor transplants, 5-year graft survival was 27% for recipients with a panel reactive antibody (PRA) titer 51% to 100% compared to 85% for those with 0% PRA.[56]

Preformed antibodies leading to sensitization result from pregnancies, prior transplantations, or blood transfusions. In CKD, the early use of erythropoietin and aggressive anemia management will reduce the need for transfusions. When unavoidable, leukocyte-poor transfusions may reduce the chance of sensitization. However, in a randomized study, there was no difference in the PRA levels with the use of leukocyte-poor transfusions.[57] Some studies have advocated transfusion with immunosuppression to minimize sensitization.[58]

Occasionally, a recipient will have an antibody and positive cross-match to the only potential living donor. In this situation, there are three options: (1) to forego living donor transplantation and wait for a deceased donor kidney, (2) to participate in a living donor exchange program, or (3) to undergo treatment to remove and suppress the antibody that is causing the positive cross-match. In a paired living donor exchange, recipient A (who has an antibody to a donor B) receives instead a kidney from donor D (who cannot donate to recipient C due to a positive cross match with donor D). In exchange, recipient C receives a kidney from donor B. Similar scenarios are possible with exchanges using three donor–recipient pairs. Paired living donor exchanges raise complex logistical and ethical issues, and generally require the cooperation of several transplant centers. Nevertheless, they can effectively circumvent the problem of a positive cross match. Similarly, ABO blood group incompatibilities can be overcome in a living donor exchange program.

When a living donor exchange is not an option, an attempt can be made to remove and suppress the preformed antibody that is causing the positive cross match. In the past few years, a number of centers have been using plasma exchange to remove anti-donor antibodies, and high doses of intravenous immunoglobulin to suppress antibody production.[59–63] However, the numbers of

recipients in these uncontrolled studies have been small, and long-term outcomes are uncertain. Clearly, the risk for antibody-mediated rejection is higher than that in recipients without a positive cross match. Glotz et al. also reported an increase in complications from the use of these desensitization protocols.[64] The exponential increase in the cost of transplantation, with the addition of such desensitization protocols in these high-risk recipients, also needs to be considered.

## Lifestyle Modification

Not surprisingly, cigarette smoking is associated with both cardiovascular disease and cancer after kidney transplantation.[65] Some would argue that patients who do not quit smoking endanger not only themselves but also their allograft, and therefore they should not receive a kidney transplant. However, others point out that smoking is often a way for people to cope with stress, and that smoking is more common among minorities and individuals of lower socioeconomic status. According to this argument, a policy that denies transplantation to individuals who fail to quit smoking is unjust. From a practical standpoint, it is difficult to enforce smoking cessation. Nevertheless, patients should be strongly encouraged to quit smoking, and should be offered nicotine-replacement therapy, ideally in a structured smoking-cessation program.

Alcohol abuse and chemical dependency is often associated with nonadherence to medical therapies. Therefore, it is unwise for an individual who is known to be abusing alcohol and/or drugs to undergo transplantation. Most transplant programs require individuals with active chemical dependency to be treated in a chemical dependency program, and to be documented to be drug free for at least 6 months before transplantation.

Failure to adhere to a prescribed immunosuppressive medication regimen is an all-too-frequent cause of acute rejection and graft failure. Risk factors for noncompliance can be identified and include younger age (especially adolescents), substance abuse, and a past history of nonadherence to medical therapies. However, past behaviors generally cannot predict future behaviors with enough certainty to deny someone an opportunity for a kidney transplant. For example, most would not deny transplantation to an individual who misses dialysis treatments and fails to adhere to dietary phosphorous restriction, even though such a person is at increased risk for not adhering to medications after transplantation. Even young patients who have already lost a kidney allograft due to noncompliance are often given a second chance, hoping that they have matured and "learned their lesson."

## Obesity

In parallel with trends in the general population, transplant recipients are also getting heavier.[66] Obesity has little effect on graft or patient survival, except perhaps in extremely obese recipients.[67,68] However, it is associated with increased short-term morbidity and longer hospital stays due to wound infections and incisional hernias.[69] Prospective recipients with a body mass index (BMI) greater that 35 mg/kg$^2$ are at the highest risk and should be considered for bariatric surgery before the transplantation, if other methods have not succeeded in achieving sustained weight loss. The long-term success rate of weight reduction surgery far exceeds that of diet, exercise, and medical modalities.[70] Obese recipients should be counseled about the increased risk of wound infection, dehiscence, herniation, and prolonged initial hospital stay.[71]

**TABLE 16.1-2**
### RISK FACTORS FOR ACUTE REJECTION

**Pretransplant Assessment of Factors Associated With Acute Rejection**

| | |
|---|---|
| History | Multiple pregnancies, lupus, blood product transfusions, prior transplant |
| Demographics | Black race |
| Age | < 18 years |
| Sensitization tests | Panel Reactive Antibody > 50%, positive cross match, presence of donor specific antibody |

## Peripheral Vascular Disease

Peripheral vascular disease is common in CKD, especially in prospective recipients with diabetes. Care must be taken when evaluating these recipients to screen for iliac artery disease or abdominal aortic aneurysm. Detection of these conditions may preempt steal syndrome and graft ischemia and help plan the vascular anastomosis. The potential living donor transplant recipient with signs and symptoms of peripheral vascular disease should undergo an imaging study to help the surgeon plan which vessels to use in the transplant anastomsis.

## Thrombophillic States

Thrombophillic states may be associated with deep venous thrombosis (DVT) or graft thrombosis after kidney transplant. The incidence of DVT after kidney transplantation is 6.2% to 8.3%, and approximately 25% of these patients suffer from pulmonary embolism.[72] Thrombophillic states also appear to affect long-term graft outcomes. A thrombophillic state may occur due to genetic mutations that decrease physiological inhibitors of the coagulation cascade (eg, factor V Leiden mutation) or increase activity of thrombogenic pathways (eg, prothrombin gene mutation).

Antiphospholipid antibody syndrome (APLS) is characterized by the presence of anticardiolipin antibodies (ACA) in association with thrombotic disorders of arterial and/or venous systems, spontaneous abortion(s), or thrombocytopenia. High titers of ACA are seen in 19% of transplant candidates.[73] In this study, all seven recipients with a past history of a thrombotic disorder or thrombocytopenia developed graft thrombosis within 1 week as compared with one of four who received anticoagulation with heparin.[73]

Approximately 4% of kidney transplant recipients are heterozygotes for Factor V Leiden mutation.[74] This mutation was associated with a 5-fold increased risk of deep venous thrombosis/pulmonary embolism, a 10-fold increase in slow graft function with sluggish renal vain flow, and an increased risk of graft loss due to thrombosis in a study of 202 transplants.[74] About 2% to 3% of recipients may be heterozygous for the prothrombin gene mutation (G20210A).[75] This mutation is associated with graft thrombosis[76] and decreased long-term graft survival.[75]

Given these risks, it seems reasonable to recommend preoperative screening (for thrombophillic genetic markers) and perioperative heparinization in recipients with history of previous thrombotic episodes. The recipient must understand the risks and benefits of this approach. In one study, perioperative heparinization was associated with "major bleeding" in 50% of cases.[77] It is unclear from the literature, what course should be followed for a candidate with a mutation or ACA without a past history of thrombosis.

## Psychosocial Issues

The CKD population has a high prevalence of anxiety and depression.[78] The role of the psychological counseling in the pretransplant evaluation is well established.[79] Psychological instability may lead to noncompliance, rejection, and mortality. Psychological stability and the presence of social and psychiatric support system need to be confirmed for patients with major depression and schizophrenia. A review of posttransplant economics and insurance coverage is equally important from a recipient's perspective. Whether the potential recipient will be able to pay for immunosuppressive medications should be determined prior to transplantation.

## THE PRETRANSPLANT EVALUATION PROCESS

Most transplant centers carry out a detailed evaluation of a potential living donor prior to deciding whether the patient is a candidate for transplantation. Although the details of this evaluation vary from center to center, it will most often include

1.  Consultations and interviews with

    - Kidney Transplant Surgeon

    - Transplant Nephrologist

    - Pretransplant Coordinator

    - Kidney Transplant Social Worker

    - Financial Counselor

    - Cardiologist (if symptomatic and/or high risk)

    - Other health-care professionals, as required

2.  Laboratory Testing

    - Complete blood count

    - Chemistry profile including electrolytes, blood urea nitrogen

    - Serum creatinine and estimated GFR

    - Liver enzymes, bilirubin, albumin, and international normalized ratio (INR)

    - Coagulation profile including PTT and fibrinogen levels

    - Blood grouping, tissue typing, and cross-matching

    - Serology for Hepatitis A, B, C, CMV, EBV, and HIV

    - Glycosylated hemoglobin, if diabetic

    - Fasting glucose tolerance test, if high risk for diabetes

    - Prostate specific antigen (PSA) for males age ≥ 55 or if risk factors are present

    - Serum pregnancy test for all females of child-bearing potential

    - Fasting total, low-density lipoprotein and HDL cholesterol, and triglycerides

    - Uric acid, amylase, lipase, calcium, phosphorus, and magnesium

    - Parathyroid hormone level

    - Panel reactive antibody*

    - Human leukocyte antigen (HLA) typing*

3.  X-rays, Tests, and Procedures

    - Chest x-ray

    - Pulmonary function testing for smokers or people with pulmonary symptoms

    - Electrocardiogram

    - Coronary angiogram if symptomatic or high risk (varies by transplant program)

    - Abdominal ultrasound examination (liver, gallbladder, native kidneys, etc.)

- Femoral Doppler examination if there is a history of peripheral vascular disease

- Voidind cystourethrogram if there is a history of recurrent infections, reflux, or congenital abnormalities

- Pelvic examination or Pap smear in all women, if not done within the last year

- Mammogram in all women > 40 years of age

- Colonoscopy if > 50 years of age

- Stool hemoccult (x3)

- Urinalysis

- Purified protein derivative (PPD) with controls

4.  Immunizations Updated:

- Hepatitis B vaccine, if never vaccinated or hepatitis B surface antibody negative

- Pneumocoxal vaccine, if none in the last 5 years.

- Influenza vaccine (annually)

## THE ROLE OF THE PRIMARY PHYSICIAN

The primary physician or nephrologist is critical to the pre-transplant process. He or she has an established relationship with the prospective recipient and is best suited to understand the morbidity of CKD for the individual patient. An initial information session, discussing the options of dialysis and transplantation, with their risks and benefits, is usually done once it is established the patient will someday need treatment for ESRD. At this time, important barriers to transplantation, such as ischemic heart disease, substance abuse, medication noncompliance, and behavioral issues should be identified and remedied, if possible. The patient can be referred for a pretransplant evaluation.

One of the common areas, where all the involved health personnel are encouraged to take a proactive role, is obesity and discontinuation of smoking. Both have been identified as risk factors for progressive coronary artery disease, which is the primary cause of graft loss after transplantation. The primary physician, because of his or her longitudinal relationship, can also have an important role in making a potential recipient aware of options of a donor pool for living donor transplantation. The primary physician can also conduct many aspects of donor screening and workup (Table 16.1-3).

**TABLE 16.1-3**

## ROLE OF THE COMMUNITY NEPHROLOGIST OR PRIMARY PHYSICIAN BEFORE TRANSPLANTATION

**Pretransplant Evaluation Outside the Transplant Center**

Early anticipation of renal replacement therapy
Preliminary discussion about benefits of transplant over dialysis
Identification of barriers to transplantation
Identification of potential living donors
Referral to a transplant center
Risk factor intervention for CKD patients; smoking cessation, dyslipidemia management, obesity

It is now clear that emotionally-related kidney donation by a spouse or a close friend is as good as a living related kidney in terms of long-term survival. With the advent of laparoscopic surgery, the morbidity to these donors is usually acceptable. Moreover, the waiting time on the transplant list is likely to grow as we have discussed earlier. The current time ranges between 3 and 5 years on the waiting list for a deceased donor kidney.

## PERIODIC REEVALUATION WHILE ON DIALYSIS

In some recipients, rapid progression of CKD may preclude a preemptive living donor transplant, and they may remain on dialysis for extended periods of time. These recipients frequently encounter dialysis related complications. Those on peritoneal dialysis may have peritonitis, and those on hemodialysis may have access related problems. The transplant center must be alert to notice hospitalizations, infections, or change in clinical condition that suggests CAD. All these situations could potentially call for a reevaluation of the patient's medical condition before transplantation. Good communication between the transplant center and primary physician or nephrologist can help to optimize the patient's status and avoid disappointments due to last-minute cancellations on medical grounds. For patients who remain on dialysis after initial evaluation, an annual evaluation by a cardiologist can help manage acceleration of coronary artery disease.

## SUMMARY

Preemptive living donor kidney transplantation is the best option for anyone with advanced kidney failure. The primary physician or nephrologist has a key role in the process of evaluating and preparing a potential kidney transplant recipient and exploring potential live donor options. The pretransplant evaluation is an excellent opportunity for patient education, evaluation of expectations, assessment of risks, and control of modifiable risk factors that are known to be associated with adverse outcomes after transpantation. In a careful pretransplant evaluation, an ounce of prevention is worth several pounds of cure.

## References

1. Wolfe RA, Ashby VB, Milford EL, et al. Comparison of mortality in all patients on dialysis, patients on dialysis awaiting transplantation, and recipients of a first cadaveric transplant. *N Engl J Med* 1999;341:1725–1730.
2. Xue JL, Ma JZ, Louis TA, Collins AJ. Forecast of the number of patients with end-stage renal disease in the United States to the year 2010. *J Am Soc Nephrol* 2001;12:2753–2758.
3. Jones CA, Krolewski AS, Rogus J, et al. Epidemic of end-stage renal disease in people with diabetes in the United States population: Do we know the cause? *Kidney Int* 2005;67:1684–1691.
4. Kasiske BL, Cangro CB, Hariharan S, et al. The evaluation of renal transplantation candidates: clinical practice guidelines. *Am J Transplant* 2001;1 Suppl 2:3–95
5. Kalble T, Lucan M, Nicita G, et al. EAU guidelines on renal transplantation. *Eur Urol* 2005;47:156–166.
6. European Best Practice Guidelines for Renal Transplantation (part 1). *Nephrol Dial Transplant* 2000;15 Suppl 7:1–85.
7. Awan A, Gill DG. Pre-emptive renal transplantation: the way forward. *Ir Med J* 2001;94:292–294.

8. Berthoux FC, Jones EH, Mehls O, Valderrabano F. Transplantation Report. 2: Pre-emptive renal transplantation in adults aged over 15 years. The EDTA-ERA Registry. European Dialysis and Transplant Association-European Renal Association. *Nephrol Dial Transplant* 1996;11 Suppl 1:41–43.

9. Fine RN, Tejani A, Sullivan EK. Pre-emptive renal transplantation in children: report of the North American Pediatric Renal Transplant Co-operative Study (NAPRTCS). *Clin Transplant* 1994;8:474–478.

10. Kasiske BL, Snyder JJ, Matas AJ, et al. Preemptive kidney transplantation: the advantage and the advantaged. *J Am Soc Nephrol* 2002;13:1358–1364.

11. Meier-Kriesche HU, Port FK, Ojo AO, *et al.* Effect of waiting time on renal transplant outcome. *Kidney Int* 2000;58:1311–1317.

12. Meier-Kriesche HU, Kaplan B. Waiting time on dialysis as the strongest modifiable risk factor for renal transplant outcomes: a paired donor kidney analysis. *Transplantation* 2002;74:1377–1381.

13. Steinman TI, Becker BN, Frost AE, et al. Guidelines for the referral and management of patients eligible for solid organ transplantation. *Transplantation* 2001;71:1189–1204.

14. K/DOQI clinical practice guidelines for chronic kidney disease: evaluation, classification, and stratification. *Am J Kidney Dis* 2002;39:S1–266.

15. Cockcroft DW, Gault MH. Prediction of creatinine clearance from serum creatinine. *Nephron* 1976;16:31–41.

16. Levey AS, Bosch JP, Lewis JB, et al. A more accurate method to estimate glomerular filtration rate from serum creatinine: a new prediction equation. Modification of Diet in Renal Disease Study Group. *Ann Intern Med* 1999;130:461–470.

17. Meier-Kriesche HU, Ojo AO, Hanson JA, Kaplan B. Exponentially increased risk of infectious death in older renal transplant recipients. Kidney Int 2001;59:1539–1543.

18. Doyle SE, Matas AJ, Gillingham K, Rosenberg ME. Predicting clinical outcome in the elderly renal transplant recipient. *Kidney Int* 2000;57:2144–2150.

19. Danpanich E, Kasiske BL. Risk factors for cancer in renal transplant recipients. *Transplantation* 1999;68:1859–1864.

20. Meier-Kriesche HU, Kaplan B. Immunosuppression in elderly renal transplant recipients: are current regimens too aggressive? *Drugs Aging* 2001;18:751–759.

21. Penn I. Posttransplant malignancies. *Transplant Proc* 1999;31:1260–1262.

22. Briganti EM, Russ GR, McNeil JJ, Atkins RC, Chadban SJ. Risk of renal allograft loss from recurrent glomerulonephritis. *N Engl J Med* 2002;347:103–109.

23. Conlon PJ, Lynn K, Winn MP, et al. Spectrum of disease in familial focal and segmental glomerulosclerosis. *Kidney Int* 1999;56:1863–1871.

24. Stephanian E, Matas AJ, Mauer SM, et al. Recurrence of disease in patients retransplanted for focal segmental glomerulosclerosis. *Transplantation* 1992;53:755–757.

25. Fornairon S, Pol S, Legendre C, *et al.* The long-term virologic and pathologic impact of renal transplantation on chronic hepatitis B virus infection. *Transplantation* 1996;62:297–299.

26. Rao KV, Anderson WR, Kasiske BL, Dahl DC. Value of liver biopsy in the evaluation and management of chronic liver disease in renal transplant recipients. *Am J Med* 1993;94:241–250.

27. Meier-Kriesche HU, Ojo AO, Hanson JA, Kaplan B. Hepatitis C antibody status and outcomes in renal transplant recipients. *Transplantation* 2001;72:241–244.

28. Rao KV, Ma J. Chronic viral hepatitis enhances the risk of infection but not acute rejection in renal transplant recipients. *Transplantation* 1996;62:1765–1769.

29. Batty DS, Jr., Swanson SJ, Kirk AD, *et al.* Hepatitis C virus seropositivity at the time of renal transplantation in the United States: associated factors and patient survival. *Am J Transplant* 2001;1:179–184.

30. Knoll GA, Tankersley MR, Lee JY, Julian BA, Curtis JJ. The impact of renal transplantation on survival in hepatitis C-positive end-stage renal disease patients. *Am J Kidney Dis* 1997;29:608–614.

31. Kamar N, Rostaing L, Selves J, *et al.* Natural history of hepatitis C virus-related liver fibrosis after renal transplantation. *Am J Transplant* 2005;5:1704–1712.

32. Breitenfeldt MK, Rasenack J, Berthold H, *et al.* Impact of hepatitis B and C on graft loss and mortality of patients after kidney transplantation. *Clin Transplant* 2002;16:130–136.

33. Gane E, Pilmore H. Management of chronic viral hepatitis before and after renal transplantation. *Transplantation* 2002;74:427–437.

34. Han DJ, Jung JH, Jang HJ, Kim SK, Kim SC. Impact of anti HCV (+) on renal transplantation. *Transplant Proc* 2000;32:1939.

35. Kamar N, Toupance O, Buchler M, et al. Evidence that clearance of hepatitis C virus RNA after alpha-interferon therapy in dialysis patients is sustained after renal transplantation. *J Am Soc Nephrol* 2003;14:2092–2098.

36. USRDS 2002 Annual Report; 2003.

37. Stock PG, Roland ME, Carlson L, et al. Kidney and liver transplantation in human immunodeficiency virus-infected patients: a pilot safety and efficacy study. *Transplantation* 2003;76:370–375.

38. European best practice guidelines for renal transplantation. Section IV: Long-term management of the transplant recipient. IV.11 Paediatrics (specific problems). *Nephrol Dial Transplant* 2002;17 Suppl 4:55–58

39. Kasiske BL. Risk factors for accelerated atherosclerosis in renal transplant recipients. *Am J Med* 1988;84:985–992.

40. Kasiske BL, Chakkera HA, Roel J. Explained and unexplained ischemic heart disease risk after renal transplantation. *J Am Soc Nephrol* 2000;11:1735–1743.

41. Kasiske BL, Guijarro C, Massy ZA, Wiederkehr MR, Ma JZ. Cardiovascular disease after renal transplantation. *J Am Soc Nephrol* 1996;7: 158–165.

42. Lindholm A, Albrechtsen D, Frodin L, et al. Ischemic heart disease—major cause of death and graft loss after renal transplantation in Scandinavia. *Transplantation* 1995;60:451–457.

43. Abbott KC, Bucci JR, Cruess D, Taylor AJ, Agodoa LY. Graft loss and acute coronary syndromes after renal transplantation in the United States. *J Am Soc Nephrol* 2002;13:2560–2569.

44. Herzog CA, Marwick TH, Pheley AM, et al. Dobutamine stress echocardiography for the detection of significant coronary artery disease in renal transplant candidates. *Am J Kidney Dis* 1999;33:1080–1090.

45. Ojo AO, Hanson JA, Wolfe RA, et al. Long-term survival in renal transplant recipients with graft function. *Kidney Int* 2000;57:307–313.

46. Manske CL, Wang Y, Rector T, Wilson RF, White CW. Coronary revascularisation in insulin-dependent diabetic patients with chronic renal failure. *Lancet* 1992;340:998–1002.

47. Gami AS, Garovic VD. Contrast nephropathy after coronary angiography. *Mayo Clin Proc* 2004;79:211–219.

48. Tadros GM, Malik JA, Manske CL, et al. Iso-osmolar radio contrast iodixanol in patients with chronic kidney disease. *J Invasive Cardiol* 2005;17:211–215.

49. Tadros GM, Mouhayar EN, Akinwande AO, et al. Prevention of radiocontrast-induced nephropathy with N-acetylcysteine in patients undergoing coronary angiography. *J Invasive Cardiol* 2003;15:311–314.

50. Ilkhanoff L, Carver J. Contrast-induced nephropathy and cardiac catheterization: evidence in support of using the iso-osmolar contrast agent iodixanol in patients with renal dysfunction. *J Invasive Cardiol* 2005;17:216–217.

51. Vandenberg BF, Rossen JD, Grover-McKay M, et al. Evaluation of diabetic patients for renal and pancreas transplantation: noninvasive screening for coronary artery disease using radionuclide methods. *Transplantation* 1996;62:1230–1235.

52. Reis G, Marcovitz PA, Leichtman AB, *et al.* Usefulness of dobutamine stress echocardiography in detecting coronary artery disease in end-stage renal disease. *Am J Cardiol* 1995;75:707–710.

53. Matas AJ, Gillingham KJ, Payne WD, Najarian JS. The impact of an acute rejection episode on long-term renal allograft survival (t1/2). *Transplantation* 1994;57:857–859.

54. Meier-Kriesche HU, Ojo AO, Hanson JA, et al. Increased impact of acute rejection on chronic allograft failure in recent era. *Transplantation* 2000;70:1098–1100.

55. Takemoto S. Sensitization and crossmatch. *Clin Transpl* 1995:417–432.

56. Barama A, Oza U, Panek R, *et al.* Effect of recipient sensitization (peak PRA) on graft outcome in haploidentical living related kidney transplants. *Clin Transplant* 2000;14:212–217.

57. Sanfilippo FP, Bollinger RR, MacQueen JM, Brooks BJ, Koepke JA. A randomized study comparing leukocyte-depleted versus packed red cell transfusions in prospective cadaver renal allograft recipients. *Transfusion* 1985;25:116–119.

58. Niaudet P, Dudley J, Charbit M, et al. Pretransplant blood transfusions with cyclosporine in pediatric renal transplantation. *Pediatr Nephrol* 2000;14:451–456.

59. Kupin WL, Venkat KK, Hayashi H, et al. Removal of lymphocytotoxic antibodies by pretransplant immunoadsorption therapy in highly sensitized renal transplant recipients. *Transplantation* 1991;51:324–329.

60. Schweitzer EJ, Wilson JS, Fernandez-Vina M, et al. A high panel-reactive antibody rescue protocol for cross-match-positive live donor kidney transplants. *Transplantation* 2000;70:1531–1536.

61. Jordan SC, Vo AA, Nast CC, Tyan D. Use of high-dose human intravenous immunoglobulin therapy in sensitized patients awaiting transplantation: the Cedars-Sinai experience. *Clin Transpl* 2003:193–198.

62. Jordan SC, Vo A, Bunnapradist S, et al. Intravenous immune globulin treatment inhibits crossmatch positivity and allows for successful transplantation of incompatible organs in living-donor and cadaver recipients. *Transplantation* 2003;76:631–636.

63. Jordan SC, Tyan D, Stablein D, *et al.* Evaluation of intravenous immunoglobulin as an agent to lower allosensitization and improve transplantation in highly sensitized adult patients with end-stage renal disease: report of the NIH IG02 trial. *J Am Soc Nephrol* 2004;15:3256–3262.

64. Glotz D, Antoine C, Julia P, et al. Desensitization and subsequent kidney transplantation of patients using intravenous immunoglobulins (IVIg). *Am J Transplant* 2002;2:758–760.

65. Kasiske BL, Klinger D. Cigarette smoking in renal transplant recipients. *J Am Soc Nephrol* 2000;11:753–759.

66. Weiss H, Nehoda H, Labeck B, et al. Organ transplantation and obesity: evaluation, risks and benefits of therapeutic strategies. *Obes Surg* 2000;10:465–469.

67. Meier-Kriesche HU, Arndorfer JA, Kaplan B. The impact of body mass index on renal transplant outcomes: a significant independent risk factor for graft failure and patient death. *Transplantation* 2002;73:70–74.

68. Howard RJ, Thai VB, Patton PR, et al. Obesity does not portend a bad outcome for kidney transplant recipients. *Transplantation* 2002;73:53–55.

69. Johnson DW, Isbel NM, Brown AM, et al. The effect of obesity on renal transplant outcomes. *Transplantation* 2002;74:675–681.

70. Marks WH, Florence LS, Chapman PH, Precht AF, Perkinson DT. Morbid obesity is not a contraindication to kidney transplantation. *Am J Surg* 2004;187:635–638.

71. Espejo B, Torres A, Valentin M, *et al.* Obesity favors surgical and infectious complications after renal transplantation. *Transplant Proc* 2003;35:1762–1763.

72. Andrassy J, Zeier M, Andrassy K. Do we need screening for thrombophilia prior to kidney transplantation? *Nephrol Dial Transplant* 2004;19 Suppl 4:iv64–68.

73. Vaidya S, Sellers R, Kimball P, *et al.* Frequency, potential risk and therapeutic intervention in end-stage renal disease patients with antiphospholipid antibody syndrome: a multicenter study. *Transplantation* 2000;69:1348–1352.

74. Wuthrich RP, Cicvara-Muzar S, Booy C, Maly FE. Heterozygosity for the factor V Leiden (G1691A) mutation predisposes renal transplant recipients to thrombotic complications and graft loss. *Transplantation* 2001;72:549–550.

75. Fischereder M, Schneeberger H, Lohse P, et al. Increased rate of renal transplant failure in patients with the G20210A mutation of the prothrombin gene. *Am J Kidney Dis* 2001;38:1061–1064.

76. Oh J, Schaefer F, Veldmann A, et al. Heterozygous prothrombin gene mutation: a new risk factor for early renal allograft thrombosis. *Transplantation* 1999;68:575–578.

77. Mathis AS, Dave N, Shah NK, Friedman GS. Bleeding and thrombosis in high-risk renal transplantation candidates using heparin. *Ann Pharmacother* 2004;38:537–543.

78. Kimmel PL, Peterson RA, Weihs KL, et al. Multiple measurements of depression predict mortality in a longitudinal study of chronic hemodialysis outpatients. *Kidney Int* 2000;57:2093–2098.

79. Gross CR, Kreitzer MJ, Russas V, et al. Mindfulness meditation to reduce symptoms after organ transplant: a pilot study. *Adv Mind Body Med* 2004;20:20–29.

## 16.2   ANESTHESIOLOGIC CONSIDERATIONS

*David S. Beebe, MD*

### INTRODUCTION

Renal transplantation has become the preferred method for treating renal failure due to most conditions. Renal transplantation from living donors is now performed for recipients with significant medical conditions such as those with severe diabetes that were previously considered ineligible for this operation. As a result, anesthesiologists are now required to manage patients with more complex medical conditions than in the past. On the other hand patients are coming to surgery better prepared and with more extensive evaluations of their medical conditions than ever before.[1] In this section we (1) describe the anesthetic and perioperative management of patients undergoing renal transplantation at the University of Minnesota, (2) review the monitoring required for patients undergoing this operation, (3) discuss how to manage perfusion the renal allograft provide prompt function of the transplanted kidney and prevent graft loss, and (4) describe common perioperative complications in recipients of living related renal transplants.

### ANESTHETIC MANAGEMENT OF PATIENTS RECEIVING A LIVING RENAL TRANSPLANT AT THE UNIVERSITY OF MINNESOTA

#### Preoperative Preparation

All patients receiving an elective, living related kidney must have had no solids or foods by mouth for at least 6 hours prior to surgery. Diabetics or those with other medical conditions that impair gastric emptying should have nothing to eat or drink for 8 hours prior to surgery. Patients may be given medications that they should continue in the perioperative period, such as beta-lockers with a sip of water or juice the morning of surgery.

Prior to receiving anesthesia for a living kidney transplant, the patient must undergo a thorough preoperative evaluation and review by the anesthesiologist. There are several items of concern to the anesthesiologist in renal transplant recipients. Of primary concern is the patient's reason for renal failure. Diabetes is currently the most common cause for end-stage renal disease. Diabetics have a whole list of comorbidities along with their renal failure that affect the anesthetic management including gastroparesis, autonomic neuropathy, peripheral neuropathy, cardiovascular disease, and peripheral vascular disease. Diabetics with autonomic neuropathy are at risk for severe hypotension and bradycardia with induction of general anesthesia, and of sudden death in the postoperative period.[2] Hypertension is another common cause of renal failure as well as an end result of renal insufficiency from other causes that may affect the anesthetic management. The reports of tests such as coronary angiograms or echocardiograms performed during the medical evaluation of the transplant recipient should be reviewed as well.

There also are specific items important for administration of anesthesia that must be determined. The frequency of dialysis, if it is occurring, and when the patient last dialyzed are important in determining the volume and electrolyte status of the patient prior to surgery. The last time insulin was administered in diabetic patients is important to help plan diabetes management in the perioperative period. The history of hypotension with dialysis in a diabetic patient suggests the presence of severe autonomic neuropathy that may place the patient at risk for hypotension on induction of general anesthesia. It is also important to determine if diabetic patients have symptoms of gastroparesis such as heartburn, bloating, and explosive diarrhea because they may be at risk for aspiration on induction of general anesthesia. These patients should be given a nonparticulate antacid such as Bicitra® prior to neutralize stomach acid and prevent pneumonitis should aspiration occur. Finally the type and last dose of antihypertensive medications should be noted. In general, antihypertensive medications with the possible exception of angiotensin system inhibitors should be continued until the time of surgery.[3] Angiotensin system inhibitors administered immediately before surgery have been associated with a higher incidence of hypotension on induction of general anesthesia in hypertensive patients.[4] As a result it may be beneficial to withhold these drugs in hypertensive patients undergoing kidney transplantation, particularly if they have other factors placing them at risk for hypotension on induction such as autonomic neuropathy.

The evaluation of the airway is particularly important for the anesthetic management of diabetic patients. Often patients with diabetes of long enough duration and severity develop stiff joints from glycosylation of their connective tissue from their elevated blood sugars. Inability to oppose the palms in diabetic patients is one sign that stiff connective tissue may be present. Often these patients are difficult to tracheally intubate and may require an awake, fiberoptic intubation.[5] The patient should also be examined for signs of congestive heart failure such as rales or peripheral edema. The patient should also be examined for the presence of both functioning and nonfunctioning dialysis shunts and fistulas. The presence of shunts may determine where the blood pressure can be recorded and vascular access obtained.[3]

There are several laboratory tests that should be performed at or close to the time of surgery. An electrocardiogram should be obtained in all diabetic patients and others at risk for coronary disease and compared to previous studies. A serum potassium level should be obtained in all patients as well. Since the potassium level may increase during surgery from the effects of drugs administered, blood transfusions, or from transfusion of hyperkalemic preservative solution from the new kidney, surgery may have to be delayed and dialysis or other intervention performed if the patient is hyperkalemic (> 6 mmol/L). The blood sugar level should be determined in diabetic patients because it can aid in intraoperative glucose management. Finally because patients with renal insufficiency are often anemic, all patients should have a hemoglobin level drawn and have several units of blood available for the day of surgery.[3]

## Induction and Maintenance of General Anesthesia

The choice of induction agent depends on the volume status of the patient and the presence of autonomic neuropathy and/or significant cardiovascular disease. Relatively healthy renal transplant recipients tolerate intravenous induction of anesthesia with thiopental (2.5–3 mg/kg) or propofol (2–3 mg/kg) without difficulty. Etomidate (0.2 mg/kg) is better tolerated in more hemodynamically compromised patients because it causes minimal myocardial depression and preserves autonomic tone. This is particularly important in diabetic patients with autonomic neuropathy. Often the narcotic fentanyl (50-100 μg) is administered as well to blunt the hypertensive response to tracheal intubation. Intermediate duration nondepolarizing muscle relaxants such as vecuronium (0.1 mg/kg) or cis-atracurium (0.2 mg/kg) that do not depend on renal excretion for their termination of action are administered to facilitate tracheal intubation in patients without gastroparesis or acid reflux disease. In patients with either of these disorders, a rapid sequence induction including Sellick's maneuver to prevent regurgitation of gastric contents is performed. Succinylcholine (1.5 mg/kg) has a very rapid onset depolarizing muscle relaxant that is useful for this purpose. However, the potassium level can increase 0.6 mmol/L with administration or this drug so it should be used with caution in patients with potassium levels of greater than 5.5 mmol/L.[3] Beta-blockers such as atenolol should be administered in patients with severe hypertension or suspected coronary disease if they have not received them orally prior to surgery because they help prevent perioperative myocardial infarction.[6] Caution must be exercised in administration of these agents in patients with autonomic neuropathy, however, because severe hypotension on induction of anesthesia may result.[1]

Anesthesia is maintained in most cases with the inhaled agents isoflurane or desflurane. Both agents have no nephrotoxic properties, and no deterioration of function has been noted with either agent in patients with and without renal disease.[1] Nitrous oxide also been used along with a potent inhaled agent such as desflurane or isoflurane in renal transplant procedures. It has minimal cardiovascular side effects, no renal toxicity, and rapid elimination. However, because it has been associated with increased nausea and vomiting in the postoperative period it is currently used less frequently.[7] Sevoflurane is rarely utilized for renal transplantation because it reacts with soda lime to form a substance called compound A. This substance has been shown to be nephrotoxic in animal and human studies,[8] therefore the safety in patients with renal insufficiency is unclear.[1] Additional intermediate duration, nondepolarizing skeletal muscle relaxants cis-atracurium or vecuronium are administered to provide surgical relaxation throughout the procedure. The narcotic fentanyl is administered in small amounts throughout the transplant (50–100 μg/hr) to reduce the amount of inhaled agent needed and prevent the patient from awakening in severe pain. The pharmacokinetics and pharmacodynamics of fentanyl is not altered by kidney disease significantly. A metabolite of morphine, morphine-6-$B$-glucuronide, has opioid agonist activity and is excreted by the kidneys. It can accumulate in renal failure and cause respiratory depression with long-term use. Morphine should be used cautiously in renal transplant recipients, particularly if the graft is not functioning properly. Also a metabolite of meperidine (Demerol), normeperidine, can accumulate in high amounts in patients with renal failure and cause seizures. Therefore meperidine should not be used for postoperative analgesia in renal transplant recipients.[1]

In patients with insulin dependent diabetes mellitus, blood glucose determinations are made every hour. An insulin infusion is begun if the blood glucose is greater than 90 mg/dL at 1 U/hr, and adjusted to maintain the blood sugar between 90 and 110 mg/dL. A low-dose dextrose solution ($D_5$1/2 Normal Saline at 25 mL/hr) is administered throughout the procedure, as well to provide some nutrition and help prevent hypoglycemia.[9]

At the end of surgery the antiemetic ondansetron is often administered to prevent nausea and vomiting on recovery from anesthesia. Most patients are extubated in the operating room or recovery room when they are alert, strong, and able to maintain adequate ventilation. Epidural analgesia has been used successfully in some series for postoperative analgesia in renal transplant recipients.[10] There is a small risk of an epidural hematoma when epidural analgesia is used in anticoagulated patients, however. Since most patients receive heparin intraoperatively and some in the postoperative period, intravenous analgesia is usually provided with morphine (0.1–0.2 mg/kg/hr), hydromorphone (0.01–0.02 mg/kg/hr), or fentanyl (100–200 μg/hr). These agents may be safely used for patient controlled analgesia following discharge from the recovery room as well.[1]

## MONITORING OF RENAL TRANSPLANT RECIPIENTS

Most patients undergoing renal transplantation benefit from central venous pressure measurement. Measurement of the central venous pressure helps determine if the volume status is adequate at the time of reperfusion of the allograft. It also provides a vascular access for immunosuppressive drugs that have to be administered centrally and any easy means to obtain blood samples. Rarely are pulmonary artery catheters necessary for renal transplantation except in those patients with severe cardiac disease. Similarly direct arterial catheters are rarely necessary except in compromised patients where frequent blood gases must be determined.[3]

## MANAGEMENT OF PERFUSION OF THE RENAL ALLOGRAFT

The anesthesiologist must manage the physiology of the patient to ensure the new allograft is perfused adequately and functions immediately. Immediate graft function is associated with increased allograft and patient survival. Intraoperative volume expansion prior to allograft reperfusion has been shown to increase renal blood flow and improve immediate graft function.[1] At the University of Minnesota, the central venous pressure is raised to 14 to 15 mm Hg with intravenous Normal Saline or 5% albumin prior to reperfusion of the allograft. Packed red blood cells are often used for this purpose as well if the patient begins surgery relatively anemic (Hgb < 10 g/dL).

Hypotension can cause decreased graft perfusion and delayed graft function as well. An adequate volume expansion often prevents hypotension at the time of reperfusion. Hypotension can still occur, however, from products of ischemia from the graft or lower extremity when the vascular clamps are released. The microvasculature of the graft and lower extremity also are vasodilated maximally with reperfusion following a period of ischemia and cause a low peripheral vascular resistance. Therefore it is helpful to intentionally raise the systolic blood pressure to 130 or 140 mm Hg by reducing concentration of inhaled anesthetic agents administered prior to reperfusing the allograft. Occasionally a vasopressor such as ephedrine (5–10 mg), phenylepherine (100–200 μg), or an infusion of dopamine (3–5 μg/kg/min) is required to treat hypotension following reperfusion. Dopamine has the advantage of being able to increase diuresis in the allograft. On the other hand dopamine has not been shown to increase graft survival in spite of this increased diuresis.[1]

Mannitol (0.25 to 1 g/kg) should also be administered prior to reperfusion. Mannitol administration when combined with volume expansion has been shown to decrease the incidence of acute tubular necrosis in the transplanted kidney. The mechanism by which it does this may be related to decreasing tubular swelling by its osmotic effect, its action as a free-radical scavenger, or by washing away sloughed renal tubule cells before they can cause injury by secondary obstruction.[11] Other diuretics such as furosemide can administered to cause a diuresis, but have not been shown to reduce the incidence of acute tubular necrosis in the transplanted kidney.[1]

## COMMON PERIOPERATIVE COMPLICATIONS

Reactions to agents administered for immunosuppression occasionally occur. Cyclosporine administration can result in hypomagnesemia, rhabdomyolysis, and other electrolyte disorders.[12] Some reactions to immunosuppressive agents such as to the murine monoclonal antibody $OKT_3$ can be quite severe and result in hypotension and pulmonary edema. Treatment of these reactions with antihistamines such as benadryl, vasopressors, steroids, diuresis, and postoperative ventilation may be required. Severe hypotension may also occur with reperfusion of the kidney, particularly if there is associated bleeding, and require use of a vasopressor.[3]

The most common causes of death after transplantation are cardiovascular events. Up to 6% of patients with coronary artery disease experience a cardiac complication within 30 days of transplantation.[13] Providing perioperative beta blockade, maintaining a normal hematocrit, and ensuring patients have optimum analgesia in the perioperative period are all measures that may help reduce the risk for patients with cardiac disease undergoing renal transplantation.[1]

## SUMMARY

Kidney transplantation is now the method of choice to treat patients with renal failure, even those with serious systemic disease. Careful anesthetic and perioperative management of the living organ recipient is required so that successful treatment of the patient's renal failure is achieved.

## References

1. Lemmens HJM. Kidney transplantation: recent developments and recommendations for anesthetic management. *Anesthesiology Clin N Am* 2004;22:651.
2. Usher S, Shaw A. Peri-operative asystole in a patient with diabetic autonomic neuropathy. *Anaesthesia* 1999;54:1125.
3. Sprung J, KapuraL L, Bourke DL et al. Anesthesia for kidney transplant surgery. *Anesthesiology Clin N Am* 2000;18:919.
4. Comfere T, Sprung J, Kumar MM, et al. Angiotensin system inhibitors in a general surgical population. *Anesth Analg* 2005;100:636.
5. Nadal JL, Fernandez BG, Escobar JC. The palm print as a sensitive predictor of difficult laryngoscopy in diabetes. *Acta Anaesthesiol Scand* 1998;42:199.
6. Poldermans D, Boersma E, Bax JJ. The effect of bisoprolol on perioperative mortality and myocardial infarction in high-risk patients undergoing vascular surgery. Dutch echocardiographic cardiac risk evaluation applying stress echocardiographic study group. *N Engl J Med* 1999; 341:1789.
7. Apfel CC, Korttila K, Abdalla M, et al. A factorial trial of six interventions for the prevention of postoperative nausea and vomiting. *N Engl J Med* 2004;350:2441.
8. Eger EI, Koblin DD, Bowland T, et al. Nephrotoxicity of Sevoflurane versus desflurane in volunteers. *Anesth Analg* 1997;84:160.
9. Robertshaw HJ, McAnuity GR, Hall GH: Strategies for managing the diabetic patient. *Best Pract Res Clin Anaesthesiol* 2004;18:631.
10. Akpek E, Kayhan Z, Kaya H et al: Epidural anesthesia following renal transplantation: a preliminary report. *Transplant Proc* 1999;31:3149.

11. Tiggeler RG, Berden JH, Hoitsma AJ, et al. Prevention of acute tubular necrosis in cadaveric kidney transplantation by the combined use of mannitol and moderate hydration. *Ann Surg* 1985;201:246.

12. Cavdar C, Sifil A, Sanli E, et al. Hypomagnesemia and mild rhabdomyolysis in living related donor renal transplant recipient treated with cyclosporine A. *Scand J Urol Nephrol* 1998;32:41.

13. Humar A, Kerr SR, Ramcharan, et al. Peri-operative cardiac mortality in kidney transplant recipients: incidence and risk factors. *Clin Transplant* 2001;15:154.

# 16.3   SURGICAL PROCEDURES

*Howard Sankary, MD*
*Enrico Benedetti, MD*

## HISTORY OF KIDNEY TRANSPLANTATION

Although the first successful kidney transplant was not actually performed until 50 years ago, attempts at the transplant procedures are noted as distant as 1000 BC, when tissue flaps were transferred for nasal reconstruction by Samhita, a surgeon in India.[1] Alexis Carrell was the first to receive a Nobel Prize for transplantation, for work related to anastomotic techniques.[2] In one of his experiments, a dog kidney was successfully autotransplanted in a different location.[1] The first successful experimental renal transplantation was performed in dogs by Ullmann in Vienna in 1902.[3]

Jaboulay, in France, attempted to connect the renal vessels of a sheep and pig to the brachial vessels of a human in renal failure, but neither kidney functioned. Yu Voronoy attempted to transplant cadaver kidneys into human recipients, but was not successful.[3] In 1950, Lawler, a surgeon at The Little Company of Mary Hospital in Chicago, performed an orthotopic transplant from an ABO compatible donor, but the graft failed. In 1951, Kuss transplanted for the first time an unrelated living donor kidney, and later transplanted four other cases into the iliac fossa.[4] David Hume performed a series of cadaver kidney transplants at Peter Bent Brigham Hospital without immunosuppression, but none functioned for long.[5] Later, in 1954, Murray performed the first identical-twin renal transplant.[6] It was not until the immunologic barrier was further understood that successful transfers of organs between humans could be performed. The first successful kidney transplant was performed by Murray in 1962 using the immunosuppressant azathioprine.[7]

Although the field of kidney transplantation has steadily evolved, most advances are related to modifications in immunosuppression. The initial technical design of renal transplantation is so solid that few improvements have been made in the past 30 years (Figure 16.3-1).

## Preparation

After the patient is anesthetized, prophylactic antibiotics are administered. The anesthesia team places a central venous access catheter. A urinary catheter is placed sterilely, urinary cultures are taken, and a solution of saline and methylene blue is instilled (usually 200 ml or 30 cm water pressure) into the bladder to facilitate identification of the bladder for the ureteral reconstruction. Although some suggested that intravesically applied antibiotic solution would reduce the incidence of wound complications, it has recently been determined that administration of saline alone was of similar efficacy to antibiotic solutions in minimizing the overall incidence of infectious complications.[8]

## Exposure

Kuss was the first to place kidneys into the iliac fossa (most commonly the right) with anastomosis of the kidney to the iliac vessels, after observing good function of ectopic iliac and pelvic kidneys and noting that the diameter of the internal iliac artery matched the size of the renal artery.[4] The right fossa is more desirable because of better exposure of the vessels and the bladder (Figure 16.3-2).

Although Hume initially placed the graft in the recipient's upper thigh, allowing the ureter to drain cutaneously, the successful 1954 transplant used the technique pioneered by Kuss, retroperitoneally in the iliac fossa, with anastomosis of the donor renal artery to the internal iliac artery, renal vein to the iliac vein, and ureter to the bladder.[4]

The extraperitoneal iliac approach is the most commonly used method today. This approach avoids violation of peritoneal integrity. Peritoneal dialysis can be performed without issue. Graft access for biopsy would more easily achieved. Urine leaks are more easily treated using this approach.[9,10] A curvilinear incision is made from the symphysis pubis inferiorly and medially extending 1 cm above the iliac crest going toward the costal margin. The length and exact positioning of the incision are determined by the patient's habitus. To facilitate medial exposure, we divide the ipsilateral rectus muscle, and the inferior epigastric vessels are double-ligated (Color Plates, Figure K1-6A). The oblique muscles are divided, carefully sweeping the peritoneum off the transversalis fascia to ensure a margin of fascia for closure. Some advocate a J-shaped pararectal incision that avoids division of muscle, and even a transverse incision has been shown to have an acceptable incisional hernia rate.[11] The peritoneum is then retracted medially to facilitate exposure of the appropriate vessels. For procedures where there is high risk of lymphocele formation, we routinely open the peritoneum before closure, to avoid a potential space for fluid formation.

After the fascia is divided and the peritoneum is reflected, exposure is optimized using a self-retaining retractor. We prefer the OMNI retractor (Mini-PMA200A; OMNI-Tract Surgical, St. Paul, MN). Care must be undertaken when using these devices as injuries to the femoral nerve and colon have been reported in transplant patients.[12] These injuries are most commonly a

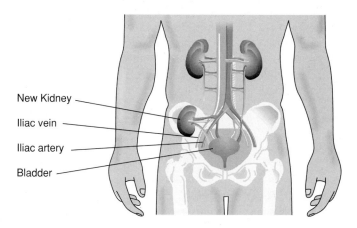

**FIGURE 16.3-1**

Schematic of transplanted kidney in reference to vessels and urologic structures.

New Kidney

Iliac vein

Iliac artery

Bladder

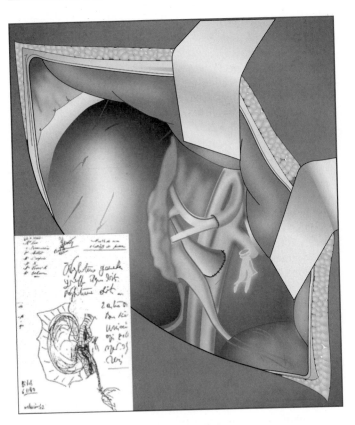

**FIGURE 16.3-2**

Original diagram by Kuss demonstrating implantation of kidney into pelvic fossa with implantation into hypogastric artery.

result of excessive tension and can be avoided with good protective packs and padded blades, and repositioning blades when the duration of the procedure is prolonged.[12]

Proper exposure would necessitate reflection of the peritoneum, recipient ureter, to the midline, division of the round ligament of the female, and mobilization of the spermatic cord in the male to allow the iliac vessels to be in the middle of the field. In some cases it may be necessary to divide the spermatic cord.[13] Adequate exposure of the external iliac artery from the crossing circumflex iliac veins to the common-internal bifurcation is usually adequate. For exposure of the iliac vein, it is not usually necessary to divide the small posterior perforating veins, although it may be necessary to divide the internal iliac vein in the event of a short renal vein[14] (Color Plates, Figure K1-6B). The lymphatics should be divided and ligated to prevent lymphocele formation with a reported incidence of .6 to 18%. A more proximal implantation of the renal graft has been advocated to decrease the incidence of lymphocele formation because the lymphatic anastomoses on the common iliac vessels are less well formed than on the external iliac.[15] Different options for arterial and venous anastomoses are depicted in the Color Plates (Figure K1-7).

### Venous Reconstruction

In performing the donor operation, we preferentially harvest the left kidney even if there are multiple renal arteries, unless removing the left kidney will compromise the donor. This is done, because failure is unlikely to be related to the arterial reconstruction, but more likely related to technical issues related to the venous reconstruction.[16,17] The right renal vein is shorter, often times

multiple, and thinner than the left renal vein, which may compromise implantation of the graft.

The anastomosis between the renal vein and the iliac vein is usually (unless the iliac artery is difficult to approach) the first vascular anastomosis to be completed (Color Plates, Figure K1-8). The first choice for this anastomosis would be to the external iliac vein.[13] If this is not feasible other strategies are possible, as described next. Choices are more limited for the right kidney because of shorter length and thinner caliber of the vein. This shorter length limits exposure, and may place the anastomosis under tension, increasing the risk of vascular complications.[18]

Although techniques for extension have been described for the cadaver right kidney, more creative approaches are necessary for a living related graft with a short renal vein, including the use of third-party extenders using cadaver iliac vessels, transposition of the iliac vein to a position lateral to the external iliac artery, and utilizing a different site for implantation.[14,19–21] Further mobilization of the iliac vein can be accomplished by ligation of the internal iliac vein more proximal.[14]

When the iliac vessels are occluded, but the inferior vena cava is open, the distal inferior vena cava is the obvious venous target, with arterial anastomosis to the common iliac artery or aorta. If the iliac vessels are open but the distal IVC is occluded, it is necessary to determine the adequacy of the collateral circulation. First a venogram should be used to define the anatomy of the collateral circulation, that is, gonadal or adrenal veins.[22] Next, the pressure should be measured in the iliac segment, and proceed with transplant if the pressure is less than 25 mm Hg.[22]

If the infrarenal IVC is occluded, the infrahepatic IVC can be used.[23] In addition, the graft can be placed in a retroperitoneal orthotopic position, attaching the transplant renal artery end to end to the splenic artery, renal artery or aorta, and renal vein to native renal vein.[24] If the entire IVC system is occluded, outflow can be directed to the portal circulation which can be accomplished using the splenic vein, IMV, or superior mesenteric vein.[22,24,25] Direct implantation into the portal vein itself is possible, but the posterior anatomic location would make for a difficult anastomosis. Since the most readily approachable vein is the superior mesenteric vein, we would preferentially use this as our first choice of "portal drainage," and prepare an arterial conduit to the iliac system or aorta, as is commonly performed when a pancreas is drained into the SMV. We have described a case where there was no access to the IVC or iliac system and where successful implantation was accomplished using the recipient splenic vessels, after performing a splenectomy.[16] Modifications to the ureteral anastomoses and arterial anastomoses may be necessary if such an approach is used, as the kidney will be in a more cephalad position.[22]

Proper position of the kidney and visualization of the kidney before closure are imperative to ensure that the vessels lie in the proper position and not kinked.[13] Failure to accomplish such may result in renal vein or arterial thrombosis. These complications usually present within the first postoperative week, and the diagnosis is established by a Doppler examination. The prognosis is poor and can rarely be remedied by immediate surgical intervention.[26]

### Arterial Reconstruction

The arterial reconstruction in the recipient receiving a living related organ might be more challenging than that of the cadaver donor, in that the artery is often shorter and does not come with a patch. Often there is more than one artery, and reconstruction may be necessary.

The first choice for reconstruction would be a direct end-to-side anastomosis between the donor renal artery and the recipient external iliac artery (Color Plates, Figures KI-9A–C and KI-12).

### Recipient Issues

Prolonged history of hypertension or diabetes that is so common in the recipients predisposes them to atherosclerotic lesions in iliac arteries, which may create technical challenges during the transplant procedure.[27] Even though there may be an adequate femoral artery pulse, the recipient may have severe disease of the iliac system. Preoperative assessment of the femoral pulses and Doppler studies are useful to delineate the degree and location of these lesions preoperatively. If there is any ambiguity, an arteriogram is necessary to determine the anatomy with specific reference to feasibility of arterial reconstruction, and need for vascular reconstruction for severe vascular disease. If disease is severe, arterial reconstruction may become problematic. If the iliac arterial system is not amenable to clamping or arteriotomy, it may be necessary to secure a segment of the external iliac artery and perform thromboendarterectomy.[28] It is imperative that no flap of plaque is raised in the distal segment, and if so, tacked. Reconstruction may necessitate patching of the arteriotomy with a segment of vein.

If the external iliac artery is not adequate for inflow, it is possible to use the hypogastric artery (Color Plates, Figures KI-9C and KI-12). This is often also involved with plaque, but if a clamp can safely be placed proximally, endarterectomy can be performed resulting in a useable vessel.[28] It has been noted in patients with an end to end internal iliac artery reconstruction that the incidence of stenosis is higher when endarterectomy is required, although other analysis have not shown such association.[29] Severe atherosclerotic changes in the external and common iliac artery may necessitate endarterectomy or bypass graft.[28,30] If a bypass is necessary, third-party donor allograft may be placed during the transplant operation. If it appears that there is need for synthetic graft, it would be safer to stage the operation, to allow incorporation of the graft, before possibly subjecting the graft to contamination during the transplant procedure. Another option is to place the graft in an intraperitoneal position if it is to be constructed at the time of the transplant operation. Intraoperative heparin is suggested for patients with severe disease necessitating extensive reconstruction.[31] Occasionally the external iliac artery becomes injured during dissection, or from clamp trauma, and continuity can be reestablished using an internal iliac artery bridge.[32]

### Donor Issues

When the anatomy of the donor renal artery is challenging, several techniques may be useful. One common challenge is the donor kidney with multiple renal arteries (Color Plates, Figure KI-10-12). According to an autopsy series the incidence of multiple renal arteries is between 18% and 30%.[33] Multiple renal arteries are theoretically associated with a higher rate of vascular complications, but in a large series with conversion to a single artery, there was not an increase in complications.[17] The renal anatomy is efficiently delineated preoperatively by computed tomography (CT) angiography, and we have rarely found conflicting anatomy at the donor operation. We preferentially use the left kidney for living donors, even with multiple arteries, but use the right kidney if the left has anatomic issues or evidence of impaired function, as it would not be appropriate to leave the donor with a compromised kidney.

Small upper polar arteries can be ligated if the distribution of the artery is less than 5% of the renal parenchyma.[17,33] Lower polar arteries are reconstructed (regardless of size) because these vessels are often the source of ureteral or pelvic blood supply.

Reconstruction of multiple arteries is influenced by the diameter, length, number, and proximity of the vessels to one another.

Multiple arteries can be joined separately to the external iliac artery, the external and internal iliac artery, or to the internal iliac artery (Color Plates, Figure KI-10-12).

Alternatively, arteries of similar diameter that are adjacent to one another can be spatulated, joined side-to-side in a "cloaca" fashion, and then anastomosed at a single arterial conduit (Color Plates, KI-12).

If the caliber of the two renal arteries is large, one third of the circumference of the two vessels can be joined to create a larger orifice (Color Plates, KI-12).

When one artery is smaller, but close in proximity to the larger vessel, the smaller vessel can be anastomosed end to side to the larger vessel (Color Plates, KI-12).

When the vessels are too distant or short for a tension free reconstruction, lengths can be extended using recipient epigastric artery, hypogastric artery, or saphenous vein.[33] The disadvantage of saphenous vein is the necessity to make a second incision. These reconstructions should be performed extracorporeally wherever possible to avoid subjecting the graft to additional warm ischemia time (Color Plates, KI-12).

For example, two arteries of large caliber can be anastomosed to the bifurcation of the internal iliac artery, which is then anastomosed to the external iliac artery (Color Plates, KI-12).

Multiple anastomoses to the iliac system can be performed in a sequential fashion, with some additional warm ischemia time, and more difficult in visibility. In this case the main renal artery is revascularized first.[16] The advantage of the sequential reconstruction is the at least two thirds of the kidney is being perfused while the accessory renal artery is addressed, avoiding global warm ischemia.[29]

### Approach to the Patient with Postrevascularization Vascular Issues

In most cases patients with vascular issues following revascularization require extracorporeal repair. The artery and vein are clamped, the kidney is flushed with preservation solution, and the repair is made. It is often necessary to extend the vascular conduit using autogenous vessel; epigastric artery, saphenous vein, and so forth.

In some cases *in situ* repair can be attempted. This can be expedited by graft cooling through a retrograde continuous perfusion using an occlusion balloon in the iliac vein, as shown next, but it is difficult to avoid warm ischemia in this situation[34] (Figure 16.3-3).

### Ureter Reconstruction (Color Plates, Figures KI-12 and 13)

Although technical issues are not usually a major issue following kidney transplantation, the ureter reimplantation can be the source of significant morbidity.[35–37]

The most common technique used at the present time involves an extravesical ureteral neocystostomy that prevents reflux into the transplanted organ. Earlier transplants were mostly performed using a Leadbetter technique, which involves a cystotomy, and creating a submucosal tunnel through the bladder, suturing the ureter to the bladder mucosa.[13] More recently extra vesicular cystostomies are preferred, using a Taguchi or Lich-Gregoir

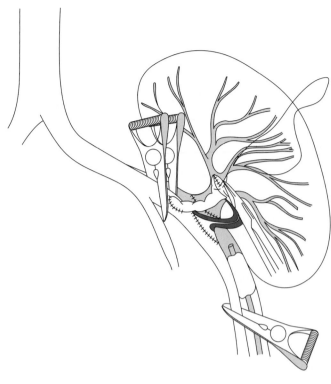

**FIGURE 16.3-3**

Illustration of retrograde *in situ* cooling for postreperfusion arterial reconstruction.

technique, as they result in a decrease of urologic complications, and are simpler to perform.[38]

The reflux associated with the Lich-Gregoir technique can be prevented by placing a full-thickness suture the toe of the ureter to the full thickness of the bladder which prevents the ureter from sliding within the submucosal tunnel[39] Figure 16.3-4).

A modification of the Lich-Gregoir anastomosis has been described in which the cystotomy is ended with an inverted y. This permitted simpler detrusor muscle approximation, avoiding strangulation of the tip of the ureter.[40]

The Taguchi procedure, as described in *The Journal of Urology* in 1968, is a stented procedure that uses a "single-stitch" technique.[38,39] This procedure has the advantage of decreased operative time (Figure 16.3-5).

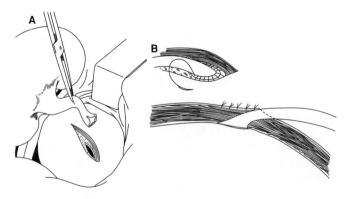

**FIGURE 16.3-4**

Schematic of Lich Gregoir ureterocystostomy.

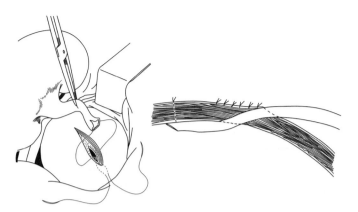

**FIGURE 16.3-5**

Schematic of Taguchi procedure with single stitch at toe of ureterocystostomy.

With both of these techniques the detrusor muscle is closed over the anastomosis creating a submucosal tunnel with an antireflux component.[38]

In complex reoperative surgery, the recipient's native ureter may be used for a conduit to the bladder, although this reconstruction is associated with a greater morbidity than extravesical ureteroneocystostomy.[13,41] A spatulated end-to-side or side-to-side anastomosis is created over a stent.

### *Stent*

Over the years there has been considerable debate whether to stent or not the ureteral anastomosis. Consensus seems to be that stents will reduce the incidence of leak and allow drainage in the event of a stricture, but has the disadvantage of necessitating a secondary procedure to remove the stent, and is associated with an increased incidence of urinary tract infections (5%–31%).[42] Stents have also been reported to migrate, cause obstruction, or cause bleeding.[42,43]

In part the difficulty of determining a role for stents relates to the fact that the complication rate from uterocystostomy is sufficiently low to yield a significant statistical power. There have been four randomized trials to help determine a role for stenting, but no consensus has been reached.[42]

In summary, there is no concrete evidence that routine stenting for the ureteral anastomosis is necessary. Nonetheless, except for the necessity of a cystoscopic procedure to remove the stent, there is little evidence that stenting causes any problem mitigating against its use.

### *Bladder Issues*

In patients with an inadequate lower urinary tract for reconstruction, a urinary diversion is an option. Early reports have described high mortality and high rates of septic complications with diversion and transplantation.[44]

Renal transplantation using an ilial conduit was first reported by Kelly[34,35] (Color Plates, Figure K1-13). Creation of the conduit before transplantation has the advantage of avoidance of contamination during the transplantation procedure. An attempt to remove all sources of infection before transplantation, often involving unilateral or bilateral nephrectomy, is made.[44] During transplantation the ileal loop is identified. The kidney is usually inverted to minimize the length of the ureter.[44] The ureterointestinal anastomosis is performed extraperitoneally through a small peritoneal window. The ureter

**TABLE 16.3-1**

| Type of Complication | Number of Complications (%) |
| --- | --- |
| Ureteral stricture, distal | 29 (2.7) |
| Urine leak | 9 (0.8) |
| UPJ obstruction | 3 (0.28) |
| Vesicoureteral reflux | 5 (0.46) |
| Clot obstruction of renal pelvis | 1 (0.1) |
| Total complications | 47 (4.3) |

is anastomosed to the conduit using nonabsorbable suture and a ureteral stent.[44,45]

The incidence of complications ranges between 1% and 10%.[46] The breakdown is demonstrated in Table 16.3-1.[47]

Early complications include obstruction ~4% and leak ~1%.[46] Ischemia is the likely cause of most urologic complications.[13] Preservation of the hilar tissue and adventitia surrounding the ureter during benching is important in preventing ischemia.[13] The LG technique has a higher incidence of permanent urinary strictures, and the T was associated with more frequent hematuria.[36]

### *Wound Closure*

Closure of the fascia is usually with a running or interrupted nonabsorbable suture, in one or two layers.[48–50]

Because of postoperative immunosuppression including steroids and or Sirolimus, the kidney transplant recipient is more prone to develop wound complications than a patient without immunosuppression. Early complications include wound dehiscence and or evisceration, and infection; whereas late complications include hernia, sinus, or incisional pain.[51]

Controversies with regard to technique involve layered versus mass closure and continuous versus interrupted closure, and suture material.

Recent published meta-analyses have confirmed a statistically significant reduction in hernia formation and dehiscence with mass closure.[51]

Although proponents of continuous closure allude to an even distribution of tension, multiple reports have shown no difference in the rate of dehiscence or hernia formation when either technique is used. One downside to the continuous closure is that suture breakage or knot disruption would be catastrophic when continuous sutures are used, and might just lead to a hernia if interrupted sutures are used.[51]

Nonabsorbable suture has the advantage of permanence but is associated with a higher incidence of sinus information. Compared to permanent sutures, the newer monofilament Polydioxanone (PDS) and polyglyconate (Maxon) are slowly absorbable and associated with no significant difference of dehiscence hernia formation or infection.[51] Sutures should be placed 2 cm from the facial edge and 2 cm for each other.[51] Factors which appear to predispose patients to would complications include obesity, lymphocele hematoma, voiding dysfunction, chronic obstructive pulmonary disease (COPD), and diabetes.[48]

### *Retransplant*

Retransplantation is most easily accomplished if nonoperated vessels can be approached. Usually the first kidney is joined to the external iliac vessels on the right side, and the left side is the

simplest approach for the second kidney. Successive retransplants can be placed more proximally on the iliac system of the recipient or more centrally if necessary. With the use of the dome cystostomy, ureteral reconstruction is not usually difficult. If there is insufficient ureter, the use of the recipient's native ureter can be attempted as described earlier.

Since retransplantation is a risk factor for lymphocele formation, some have advocated intraperitoneal approach in cases of third transplants.[58]

## CONCLUSIONS

The recipient operation in technical in living related renal transplantation is well standardized. The experience accumulated over the years helps the transplant surgeon to cope successfully with a wide range of situations related to the donor and the recipient's anatomy. With modern techniques, virtually every living donor organ in any recipient can be successfully transplanted. Attention to details and good planning are essential components to technical success.

## References

1. Doyle AM, Lechler RI, Turka LA. Organ transplantation: halfway through the first century. *J Am Soc Nephrol* 2004 ;15(12):2965.
2. Carrel A. La technique operatoire des anastomoses vasculaires et la transplantation des visceres. *Lyon Med* 1902;98:859.
3. Morris PJ: Transplantation—a medical miracle of the 20th century. *N Engl J Med* 2004;351(26):2678.
4. Cinqualbre J, Kahan BD. Rene Kuss: Fifty years of retroperitoneal placement of renal transplants. *Transplant Proc* 2002;34(8):3019.
5. Hume DM, Merrill JP, Miller BF, et al. Experiences with renal homotransplantation in the human: report of nine cases. *J Clin Invest* 1955;34:327–382.
6. Merrill JP, Murray JE, Harrison JH, et al. Successful homotransplantation of the human kidney between identical twins. *J Am Med Assoc* 1956;160:277.
7. Murray JE, Merrill JP, Harrison JH, et al.: Prolonged survival of human-kidney homografts by immunosuppressive drug therapy. *N Engl J Med* 1963;268:1315.
8. Salmela K, Eklund B, Kyllonen L, et al. The effect of intravesically applied antibiotic solution in the prophylaxis of infectious complications of renal transplantation. *Transpl Int* 1990;3:12.
9. Nahas WC, Mazzucchi E, Scafuri AG, et al. Extraperitoneal access for kidney transplantation in children weighing 20 kg. or less. *J Urol* 2000;164(2):47.
10. Adams J, Gudemann C, Tonshoff B, et al. Renal transplantation in small children—a comparison between surgical procedures. *Eur Urol* 2001;40(5):552.
11. Barone GW, Sailors DM, Ketel BL. Combined kidney and pancreas transplants through lower transverse abdominal incisions. *Clin Transplant* 1996;10:316.
12. Noldus J, Graefen M, Huland H. Major postoperative complications secondary to use of the Bookwalter self-retaining retractor. *Urology* 2002;60(6):964.
13. Odland MD. Surgical technique/post-transplant surgical complications. *Surg Clin North Am* 1998;78:55.
14. Molmenti EP, Varkarakis IM, Pinto P, et al. Renal transplantation with iliac vein transposition. *Transplant Proc* 2004;36(9):2643.
15. Sansalone CV, Aseni P, Minetti E, et al. Is lymphocele in renal transplantation an avoidable complication? *Am J Surg* 2000;179(3):182.
16. Marinov M, DiDomenico S, Mastrodomenico P, et al. Use of the splenic vessel for an ABO-incompatible renal transplant in a patient with thrombosis of the vena cava. *Am J Transplant* 2005;5:2336–2337.

17. Benedetti E, Troppmann C, Gillingham K, et al. Short- and long-term outcomes of kidney transplants with multiple renal arteries. *Ann Surg* 1995;221:406.

18. Takahashi M, Humke U, Girndt M, et al. Early posttransplantation renal allograft perfusion failure due to dissection: diagnosis and interventional treatment. *AJR Am J Roentgenol* 2003;180(3):759.

19. Dalla Valle R, Mazzoni MP, Bignardi L, et al. Renal vein extension in right kidney transplantation. *Transplant Proc* 2004;36(3):509.

20. Nakatani T, Takemoto Y, Kim T, et al. Results of cadaver kidney transplantation with right renal vein extension. *Urol Int* 2003;70(4):282.

21. Goel MC, Flechner SM, El-Jack M, et al. Salvage of compromised renal vessels in kidney transplantation using third-party cadaveric extenders: impact on posttransplant anti-HLA antibody formation. *Transplantation* 2004;77(12):1899.

22. Aguirrezabalaga J, Novas S, Veiga F, et al. Renal transplantation with venous drainage through the superior mesenteric vein in cases of thrombosis of the inferior vena cava. *Transplantation* 2002;74(3):413.

23. Pirenne J, Benedetti E, Kashtan CE, et al. Kidney transplantation in the absence of the infrarenal vena cava. *Transplantation* 1995;59:1739.

24. Gil-Vernet JM, Gil-Vernet A, Caralps A, et al. Orthotopic renal transplant and results in 139 consecutive cases. *J Urol* 1989;142:248.

25. Rosenthal JT, Loo RK. Portal venous drainage for cadaveric renal transplantation. *J Urol* 1990;144:969.

26. Mochtar H, Anis AM, Ben Moualhi S, et al. Thrombosis of the renal transplant vein. *Ann Urol* (Paris) 2001;35(1):10.

27. Galazka Z, Szmidt J, Nazarewski S, et al. Long-term results of kidney transplantation in recipients with atherosclerotic iliac arteries. *Transplant* Proc 2002;34(2):604.

28. Galazka Z, Szmidt J, Nazarewski S, et al. Kidney transplantation in recipients with atherosclerotic iliac vessels. *Ann Transplant* 1999;4:43.

29. Davari HR, Malek-Hossini SA, Salahi H, et al. Sequential anastomosis of accessory renal artery to external iliac artery in the management of renal transplantation with multiple arteries. *Transplant Proc* 2003;35(1):329.

30. Schweitzer EJ, Bartlett ST: Simultaneous PTFE reconstruction of the external iliac artery with kidney transplantation. *Clin Transplant* 1993;7:179.

31. Paduch DA, Barry JM, Arsanjani A, et al. Indication, surgical technique and outcome of orthotopic renal transplantation. *J Urol* 2001;166(5):1647.

32. Benedetti E, Baraniewski HM, Asolati M, et al. Iliac reconstruction with arterial allograft during pancreas-kidney transplantation. *Clin Transplant* 1997;11:459.

33. Makiyama K, Tanabe K, Ishida H, et al. Successful renovascular reconstruction for renal allografts with multiple renal arteries. *Transplantation* 2003;75(6):828.

34. Boggi U, Ferrari M, Vistoli F, et al. Rescue of kidney and pancreas grafts with complex vascular lesions. *Transplant Proc* 2004;36(3):505.

35. Zomorrodi A, Bahluli A. Evaluation of urologic complications in 30 cases of kidney transplantation with technique of proper exposure edge of bladder mucosa and U-stitch ureteroneocystostomy. *Transplant Proc* 2003;35(7):2662.

36. Tzimas GN, Hayati H, Tchervenkov JI, et al. Ureteral implantation technique and urologic complications in adult kidney transplantion. *Transplant Proc* 2003;35(7):2420.

37. Nane I, Kadioglu TC, Tefekli A, et al. Urologic complications of extravesical ureteroneocystostomy in renal transplantation from living related donors. *Urol Int* 2000;64(1):27.

38. Secin FP, Rovegno AR, Marrugat RE, et al. Comparing Taguchi and Lich-Gregoir ureterovesical reimplantation techniques for kidney transplants. *J Urol* 2002;168(3):926.

39. Barry JM. Re: Comparing Taguchi and Lich-Gregoir ureterovesical reimplantation techniques for kidney transplants. *J Urol* 2003; 169(5):1798.

40. Lapointe SP, Barrieras D, Leblanc B, et al. Modified Lich-Gregoir ureteral reimplantation: experience of a Canadian center. *J Urol* 1998;159:1662.

41. Benoit G. [Surgical technics of kidney transplantation]. *Prog Urol* 1996;6:594.

42. Dominguez J, Clase CM, Mahalati K, et al. Is routine ureteric stenting needed in kidney transplantation? A randomized trial. *Transplantation* 2000;70(4):597.

43. French CG, Acott PD, Crocker JF, et al. Extravesical ureteroneocystostomy with and without internalized ureteric stents in pediatric renal transplantation. *Pediatr Transplant* 2001;5(1):21.

44. Warholm C, Berglund J, Andersson J, et al. Renal transplantation in patients with urinary diversion: a case-control study. *Nephrol Dial Transplant* 1999;14:2937.

45. Surange RS, Johnson RW, Tavakoli A, et al. Kidney transplantation into an ileal conduit: a single center experience of 59 cases. *J Urol* 2003;170(5):1727.

46. Santiago-Delpin EA, Baquero A, Gonzalez Z. Low incidence of urologic complications after renal transplantation. *Am J Surg* 1986;151:374.

47. Whang M, Geffner S, Baimeedi S, et al. Urologic complications in over 1000 kidney transplants performed at the Saint Barnabas healthcare system. *Transplant Proc* 2003;35(4):1375.

48. Mazzucchi E, Nahas WC, Antonopoulos I, et al. Incisional hernia and its repair with polypropylene mesh in renal transplant recipients. *J Urol* 2001;166(3):816.

49. Humar A, Ramcharan T, Denny R, et al. Are wound complications after a kidney transplant more common with modern immunosuppression? *Transplantation* 2001;72(12):1920.

50. Kiberd B, Panek R, Clase CM, et al. The morbidity of prolonged wound drainage after kidney transplantation. *J Urol* 161:1467.

51. Ceydeli A, Rucinski J, Wise L. Finding the best abdominal closure: an evidence-based review of the literature. *Curr Surg* 2005;62(2):220.

52. Sansalone CV, Aseni P, Minetti E, et al. Is lymphocele in renal transplantation an avoidable complication? *Am J Surg* 2000;179(3):182.

# 16.4    ISCHEMIA AND REPERFUSION INJURY

*Stefan G. Tullius, MD, Nicholas L. Tilney, MD*

The primary doctrine of transplantation is that the host inevitably accepts autografts or isografts but destroys allografts via its immunological defenses. In addition to such specific antigen-dependent differences, however, antigen-independent risk factors may impact both the short and the long-term survival of the transplanted organ. This hypothesis is based on the findings that the functional survival of kidneys from living-unrelated donors is virtually identical to those of one haplotype matched living-related donor and is inevitably superior to cadaver organs, even those with comparable mismatches.[1]

The widening divergence between those seeking help and the availability of appropriate organs is forcing the initiation of new strategies to expand criteria for donor acceptance. Kidneys from living donors, both related and unrelated to the recipient, are forming a progressively larger proportion of the overall pool. At the same time and despite sustained efforts by the transplant community to keep up with the demand, the number of cadaver-donor organs has remained relatively static. As a result the demographics of the overall donor cohort, both living and deceased, are changing as organs from "high-risk" individuals, often with deleterious systemic conditions, are replacing those from more optimal sources.

## THE COMMON DENOMINATOR: ISCHEMIA/REPERFUSION INJURY

One major difference between grafts from living and grafts from cadaver donors is the time interval between removal of the organ and its placement in the recipient. While brief and generally of less consequence in the former group, it may be prolonged for many hours in the latter. The resultant non-specific-antigen-independent insult of ischemia/reperfusion (I/R) is complex, and its impact on the organ may be profound (Figure 16.4-1). Age, diabetes, hypertension, and arteriosclerosis, preexisting conditions in both donor groups, may influence its severity. The events surrounding procurement, preservation, and revascularization in the recipient are additional risk factors.

The period of ischemia entails three sequential phases. The first involves a transient period secondary to hypotension and vasoconstriction associated with donor brain death or cardiac arrest; the use of pharmacologic vasopressors to normalize blood pressure may diminish capillary tissue perfusion further. Although *in situ* cooling may improve these physiologic perturbations, surgical

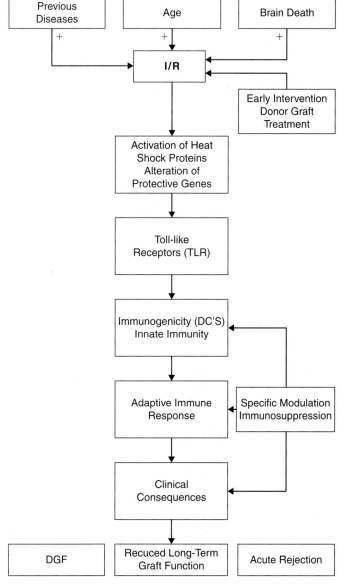

**FIGURE 16.4-1**

The consequences of I/R are orchestrated by a complex interplay of innate and adaptive immunity. Prolonged ischemia may be aggravated by additional factors as age, consequences of brain death, and previous diseases. In addition to therapeutic approaches in the recipient, clinical consequences of I/R may be prevented by treating the donor or the graft prior to transplantation.

isolation and removal of the graft may produce additional tissue assault. Laparoscopy removal of kidneys from living donors has been implicated in ischemic damage, particularly in pediatric recipients.[2] The second phase involves a prolonged interval of cold ischemia associated with storage. Third, manipulation of the organ during revascularization, while usually minor, may contribute.

The events evolving during ischemia and reperfusion are separate and distinct. The time that cells and tissues can remain undamaged or viable without blood supply is finite and varies among organs and among species. Although reperfusion restores oxygen and viability to the ischemic tissues, it is responsible for much of the overall injury is initial delayed graft function (DGF). The most obvious manifestation of this "reflow paradox" occurs in transplanted kidneys. Defined as a temporary disconnect between the functional capacity of the engrafted organ and fulfillment of the physiological needs of the recipient, DFG may increase acute rejection rates, prolong hospitalization, delay rehabilitation, and evoke higher costs.[3] Perhaps most importantly, it may increase the complexities of clinical care in assessing the coincident presence of the acute immunologic insult and its potential treatment. Nephrotoxicity of the immunosuppressive drugs used may increase ongoing renal injury. Postoperative dialysis, if necessary, may pose its own hazards and complications.

Two sequelae of I/R injury have been implicated in the context of organ transplantation: the nonspecific inflammatory response may trigger acute rejection; initial endothelial inflammation in concert with later host immunological activity may contribute to the development of chronic graft dysfunction. Although infrequent in kidneys from living donors, the incidence of DGF is generally 20% to 30% among those from cadavers and may be as high as 50%.[3] Its influence on late graft behavior is particularly difficult to ascertain accurately because of the many variables associated with transplantation.

## TISSUE AND MOLECULAR MANIFESTATIONS OF THE I/R INSULT

A series of structural, cellular, and molecular events evolve rapidly when a tissue loses its blood supply. Morphological changes of reversible acute renal failure primarily involve extensive or patchy necrosis of any or all parts of the renal tubule, although there may be little correlation between histologic damage and actual functional impairment as many nephrons may be normal microscopically.[4] With severe ischemic injury, however, tubular cells may slough, and with other debris, obstruct the lumen. The glomerular filtration rate of single nephrons may decrease, in part due to backleak of tubular fluid through denuded or disrupted basement membranes. Active transmembrane transport of ions is inhibited, energy-rich ATP stores within the ischemic cells are depleted, and calcium overload and disturbances in arachidonic acid metabolism develop. Influx of ions and water from the intravascular space causes endothelium to swell and impinge on the lumina of small vessels. Because of transmigration of water into the interstitium of the affected organ, local hemoconcentration occurs. Anoxia-driven acidosis alters the viscoelastic properties of circulating polymorphonuclear leukocytes (PMNs), T lymphocytes, and macrophages, causing them to become stiffer and obstruct the microvasculature. Passive trapping and tangling of erythrocytes accentuate the process. These factors in combination may obstruct flow on resumption of the circulation with revascularization of the organ, leading to additional ischemia and further damage to the already injured cells. Interactions between the marginating leukocytes and the endothelial cells initiate and amplify the inflammatory cascade.

## Oxygen Free Radicals

The postischemic "reflow paradoxes" may produce cell injury and death, in part at least, by the action of oxygen free radicals. These evoke inflammatory activity of the vascular endothelium during reperfusion, cell particularly sensitive to their effects.[5] The radicals may also be upregulated by hemodialysis, a treatment that becomes necessary if function of a newly transplanted kidney is delayed or inadequate to support the host.

Reoxygenation of ischemic tissue restores substrates for oxidative metabolism. One of these, hypoxanthine, becomes highly concentrated and amplifies the generation of high-energy radicals, hydrogen peroxide, superoxide radicals ($O_2^-$), and hydroxyl radicals. The postischemic endothelium is a primary producer of superoxide radicals by increasing prostaglandin H synthase and lipoxygenase in the presence of NADH or NADPH. Under physiologic conditions, these substances are generated in low enough concentrations that their normal metabolism is not deleterious to cell viability. During reperfusion, however, their rate of production overwhelms the ability of the affected cells to render them inert. Oxidative injury results. The coincident administration of nephrotoxic calcineurin inhibitors such as cyclosporine and tacrolimus may increase the insult.

Oxygen free radicals may arise from several sources and by different mechanisms. Intracellular endogenous substrate may generate radicals by auto-oxidation. Lipid peroxidation, for example, increases the presence of the molecules, particularly by oxidized low-density lipoproteins (oxLDL), a mechanism that may play a role in the later development of atherosclerosis through the binding of anti-oxLDL antibodies to the damaged vessel wall. oxLDL may also amplify tissue damage by decreasing levels of endothelial cell-produced nitric oxide, a potent vasodilatator. Hydroxy radicals may evoke cell death by interacting with iron released during ATP breakdown during ischemia. Activation and deactivation of cytoplasmatic enzymes destroy cell membranes, increase permeability, and damage DNA. Thus, rapid generation of free radicals from the I/R injury triggers a cascade of activated endothelial cells, leukocytes, and their products, all of which contribute to inflammation and remodeling of the graft vasculature.

Upregulation of MHC antigens and co-stimulatory molecules increases graft immunogenicity following I/R injury. Additional postulated mechanisms include damage to antigen presenting dendritic cells from both donor and recipient by oxygen free radicals.[6] Heat shock proteins, induced by formation of oxidized non-native proteins trigger innate host immunity. Toll-like receptors upregulated on the injured cells mediate subsequent adaptive alloimmunity via signaling pathways.

## Inflammatory Mediators

Vascular endothelial cells activated by brain death, ischemia, or other insults provoke an inflammatory cascade of remarkable complexity by expressing a range of mediators that include adhesion molecules, cytokines, and chemokines. A cytokine gradient, produced within minutes of reperfusion, promotes adhesion to circulating leukocytes by upregulating synthesis of appropriate surface receptors. Selectins are the first adhesion molecules induced after injury. E-selectin, expressed constituitively on endothelial cells, is stimulated by elevated IL-1 and TNFα levels. P-selectin, stored intracellularly in α-granules and Weibel-Palade bodies, is mobilized in response to thrombin, histamine, or hydrogen peroxide.[7] Bonding weakly with their ligands on circulating leukocytes, these acute phase proteins slow the rate of their progression and

transiently stop their progress. As the adhesive bond then breaks through shear stress, the white cell moves along the vessel wall until stopped by another selectin interaction. This intermittent sticking and release cause the marginating cells to roll along the perturbed endothelium.

Following selectin-mediated slowing, the circulating neutrophils, monocytes, and lymphocytes are immobilized on vessel walls via a series of integrins and members of the immunoglobulin superfamily. Upregulated in sequence, these create ever more secure bonds and mediate and facilitate leukocyte diapedesis and recruitment across the endothelium into the substance of the organ. ICAM-1, for instance, serves as a receptor for the integrins LFA-1 and Mac-1. Other integrins include the VLA proteins and LEUCAMs that bind to extracellular matrix molecules. In addition to ICAM-1, VCAM-1, and CD2, the immunoglobulin-like superfamily includes MHC classes I and II. As noted, these histocompatibility antigens plus various co-stimulatory molecules such as B7, activated by the nonspecific insult and putatively enhanced by Toll-like receptors on dendritic cells, increase the immunogenicity of the inflamed organ after transplantation. The subsequently enhanced host alloresponsiveness provides a continuum between initial inflammation and later immunity.

The cytokine/chemokine cascade has become well defined.[8] Ischemia increases tissue levels of a broad array of mediators that include tumor necrosis factor α (TNFα), interleukin-1 (Il-1), γ-interferon (IFNγ), platelet activating factor (PAF), leukotrienes, and complement. PAF is synthesized as rapidly as 30 minutes after ischemia and is thought to mediate early adherence of neutrophils and mononuclear cells via upregulaton of adhesion molecules. It also increases vascular permeability. The chemokine MIP-1α and RANTES, a macrophage chemoattractant, are involved in ischemia-induced reperfusion injuries. The leukotrienes and thromboxanes are chemoattractants for granulocytes. Experimentally, the accumulation of the complement protein, C1q, in ischemic myocardial segments has been associated with the dense and selective infiltration of neutrophils. Several endothelium-derived products, including the potent vasoconstrictors, the endothelins, are generated. Cyclosporine may stimulate additional endothelin production.

## Cellular Activity Involved with I/R

### Platelets

The cytoskeleton of platelets allows directional motion toward the site of a tissue insult despite the absence of a nucleus. Activated by contact with exposed collagen and peaking in number c.24 hours after injury, they are a source of various inflammatory mediators that include arachidonic acid metabolites, neutrophil-activating peptides, oxygen free radicals, serotonin, platelet factor 4, platelet-derived growth factor, and P-selectin.[9] The rapid translocation of P-selectin from intracellular storage to the cell surface is critical in interactions that attract the presence of PMNs and orchestrate deposition of fibrinogen in the site of injury.[10] Firm attachment of PMNs to the platelet membrane, at least *in vitro*, is primarily dependent on activity between the upregulated β2 integrin Mac-1 and its ligand, a process presumably important in the actual migration of these cells into platelet thrombi or areas of vascular wall injury.[11]

### Polymorphonuclear Leukocytes

The infiltration of PMNs into ischemic tissue initiates a spectrum of inflammatory changes. Entering the organ within hours after reperfusion, the majority peak around day 3 and decline around the second week. Their presence is particularly evident in necrotic tissue where they take part in phagocytosis and deposition of collagen and fibrinogen as parts of the healing process. Their obvious presence in the border zone between necrotic and intact tissue, however, may worsen local injury. Their migration through the intercellular junctions of vessel walls increases permeability, fluid extravasation, and tissue edema. Intravascular aggregation of these cells may obstruct the lumina of arterioles, capillaries, and postcapillary venules.[12]

The PMN is intimately involved with the biochemical changes of I/R injury. As metabolism shifts from aerobic to anaerobic, increased intracellular calcium activates phospholipase A and causes generation of arachidonic acid products. Besides the vasoconstrictive potential and influence of these metabolites on production of inflammatory mediators, they serve as chemotactic agents for PMN accumulation in the microvasculature.[13] Adhesion stimulated by leukotriene B4 and arachidonic acid-induced superoxide anion production can be augmented by synergistic stimulation with TNFα, escalating inflammatory reactions and tissue damage. Local release of potent mediators such as histamine, thrombin, oxygen radicals, and the complement C5b-9 complex activates vascular endothelium.[14] Selectins are expressed. P-selectin and PAF appear to act together in initiating tethering of PMNs as a first step in the adhesion cascade. Tumor necrosis factor beta (TNFβ) and oxygen radicals promote upregulation of E-selectin and Mac-1 on neutrophils and of E-selectin and ICAM-1 molecules on endothelial cells. L-selectin is believed to support flattening of migrating neutrophils under endothelial cell layers since its blockade by monoclonal antibodies (mAbs) significantly inhibits adhesion under shear flow conditions.[15] Numerous chemokines, cytokines, and chemoattractants from various sources capable of stimulating PMNs also effect integrin expression and increase avidity of the leukocytes to endothelial receptors. IL-8, for instance, promotes adhesion and transmigration of PMNs after binding to endothelial cells.

Some adherent PMNs transmigrate across endothelial cell cytoplasm or through intercellular junctions into the subendothelial matrix of the ischemic or injured organ Chemokine gradient-dependent migration of PMNs involves coordinated rearrangements in the intracellular skeleton of cells that allow them to move to and through their junctions. A cross-endothelial gradient of both CD11a/CD18 (LFA-1) and CD11b/CD18 (Mac-1) in the diapedesis of PMNs between endothelial cells also seems important, as blocking CD11b/CD18 independently of CD11a/CD18 prevents migration.[16] After repositioning in the extravascular tissue, further movement may occur after limited digestion of the basement membranes and components of the tissue matrix by elaboration in an autocrine manner a series of proteolytic enzymes that include collagenase, protease, and elastase.[8]

As noted, circulating PMNs and their products not only are responsible for tissue repair and remodeling but also may worsen the ischemic changes through inflammatory activity. Once recruited to the affected area, the phagocytic neutrophils produce oxygen free radicals that may damage structural matrix proteins irreversibly. The most potent of these, hypochlorous acid, causes cell necrosis by depleting tissue ATP.[17] Associated cytokines are also important. GM-CSF and IL-2, responsible for PMN differentiation and survival, contribute to their accumulation at the site of the injury. Their activation via CD11/CD18 also results in oxidative burst, degranulation, and increased phagocytic capabilities.[18] IL-1α and β also stimulate the respiratory burst and cause release of prostaglandins. Inducement of respiratory-burst oxydase

increases superoxide and hydrogen peroxide levels and releases more stable oxidants such as chloramines into the extracellular space, products directly involved in various cytotoxic processes. Stimulated by chemoattractants, the leukocytes release a wide range of degradative intracellular enzymes, required both for their migration through the basement membrane and for increasing their enzymatic-killing capabilities. In addition, reduction in the activity of α-1-antiprotease and α-1-antitrypsin-specific inhibition of neutrophil elastase can contribute to more extensive enzymatic damage. Stimulated PMNs secrete IL-8 as a PMN attractant and activate Th1 lymphocytes via synthesis and release of IL-12. This lymphocyte population increases alloimmunity of the injured organ by expression of MHC class II molecules.

### T Lymphocytes

The cytokines produced by T lymphocytes, including TNFα, IFNγ, GM-CSF; and IL-2, IL-4, and IL-5, make them important in stimulating and attracting neutrophils to the site of injury. In acute I/R insult of the kidney, CD4+ T cells increase in number after around 3 days; expression of their various products appears to be an integral part of the inflammatory process.[19] The concept that initial antigen-independent inflammatory events affect later lymphocyte-mediated host immune activity has been supported by the amelioration of all manifestations of I/R in a rat kidney model following blockade of the co-stimulatory molecule, B7.[20] Although the B7-CD28 interaction is an important second signal in T-cell activation by histocompatibility antigen, the striking upregulation of the signal in I/R emphasizes the interrelationship between nonspecific inflammation and the specific host immune responses

### Macrophages

Circulating monocytes, transformed into macrophages on entering the tissues, are involved in both antigen-dependent and -independent cellular host reactivity. Recruitment to an area of inflammation is the first step required for their activation. Various chemoattractants responsible for their adhesion and migration through the vascular endothelium include arachidonic acid metabolites, products of the complement cascade, extracellular matrix proteins, and chemokines such as MCP-1 and RANTES.[21] Monocytes roll on stimulated endothelial cells expressing E and L selectins; α1 and α2 integrin interactions presumably mediate subsequent tight adhesion. Their accumulation in the ischemic tissues follows neutrophil aggregation and takes place 24 to 48 hours after the initial insult. Activated cells secrete enzyme that enable their migration into the subendothelial space. IFNγ, TNFα, IL-6, GM-CSF, adhesion molecules, and arachidonic acid metabolites play a role in their inflammatory functions.[22]

Stimulated macrophages are capable of cytotoxicity, phagocytosis, and antigen presentation. Their secretory products, chemokines, cytokines, enzymes, and complement components, contribute to the development of inflammatory events as well as to the recruitment of new monocytes from the peripheral blood to the site of injury. Cytotoxic activity, increased by the production of reactive oxygen and nitrogen radicals and cytolytic proteases, may occur both nonspecifically and in the presence of antigen. Their role in modulating immunoresponsiveness is closely related to their function as antigen presenting cells interacting with the T-cell receptor (TCR)–CD4 complex. Upregulation of numerous surface accessory molecules also contributes to T-cell activation. In experimental models of I/R, macrophages are detectable up to 7 days after injury. As their fibrosis-associated products, particularly TNFα, IFNγ, and IL-6, are highly expressed within 3 days, this population may contribute to the increased inflammation at early stages after transplantation of an injured organ, influence long-term graft function by sustaining host alloimmunity, and mediate the fibrotic processes of chronic rejection.

## Innate and Adaptive Immunity

The association among nonspecific inflammatory damage, acute rejection, and the long-term consequences of I/R on graft function suggests an active role of the immune system. Indeed, the correlation between innate and adaptive immunity has been receiving increased attention. Toll-like-receptors (TLR) have been associated with linking innate and adaptive immunity by mediating pathogen recognition and immune activation of heat shock proteins (Hsp) and pathogen-associated molecular pattern structures (PAMPs).[23] PAMPs are recognized by receptors of the innate immune system so-called pattern recognition receptors (PRRs). TLRs belong to the class of PRRs expressed on the cell surface and activate signal pathways.

The expression of toll-like receptors on dendritic cells represents an additional link between innate and adaptive immunity. Triggering TLRs on DCs initiates the expression of co-stimulatory molecules on their surfaces. These, in turn, stimulate naïve T cells and initiate antigen presentation.[24] In addition to their involvement in the regulation of regulatory and memory T cells, the expression of TLR-associated cytokines is necessary for the activation of CD-4+ T cells.[25] Thus, the success of an organ transplant is already determined, at least to some extent, by the extent of the nonspecific injury of the graft at the time of transplantation. I/R is one of the major determinants of this damage, as its effects can aggravate additional risk factors such as age, brain death, and previous disease. Clinical experience with grafts from elderly donors suggests a detrimental effect of prolonged ischemia, a relationship emphasized by experimental data that show a synergistic correlation between age and severity of ischemia.[26]

The role of protective genes in antigen-independent injury and organ rejection is currently under extensive examination. The heme oxygenase system with its downstream products biliverdin, Fe, and CO may be one such system, as upregulation of HO-1 as well as its products have been associated with graft protection and prevention of rejection.[27] Of particular interest are recent findings linking hemeoxygenase-1 expression and the TLR system. An association of HO-1 upregulation and diminished TLR-4 levels is paralleled by ameliorated functional and structural changes in a liver I/R model.[28]

## Long-Term Effects of I/R Injury

The inflammatory response associated with I/R may increase host alloreactivity, providing a continuum between the antigen-independent injury and an episode of acute antigen-dependent immunological rejection that may influence the outcome of afflicted organs.[29] Although episodes of acute rejection are generally considered to predispose to chronic rejection, the presence of both early injuries may also effect later events. The influence of the initial I/R insult on long-term graft behavior has been investigated primarily in transplanted kidneys. DGF may initiate a

programmed inflammatory and fibrotic process within the organ that provokes progressive chronic changes. Both insults in combination produce a significantly less favorable graft outcome over the long-term than if either episode occurs alone or if neither develops.[30] In one clinical series, for example, the 5-year survival rate of cadaver donor kidney grafts experiencing neither insult was 85%; that of grafts experiencing both was 60%; grafts undergoing only one, regardless of whether it was antigen dependent or independent, had intermediate results.[3]

Experimentally, DFG initiates a programmed inflammatory and fibrotic process within the organ that may provoke progressive chronic changes. Prolonged (60 min) cold ischemia contributed importantly to later functional and structural abnormalities in a rat renal model of chronic rejection.[31] In another series of investigations, long-term changes in kidney isografts subjected to ischemia before engraftment were identical to those experienced by chronically rejecting allografts, although evolving at a less rapid rate.[32]

## PRESCRIPTIVE MEASURES

The importance of minimizing the insult of I/R and its influence on the ultimate fate of the graft is not only relevant to the present donor pool but also may allow utilization of currently not acceptable donor sources. Although no consistently effective measures are available to prevent the changes of I/R or to influence the development of DFG following renal transplantation, several novel approaches are intriguing. In both experimental and clinical models, cellular or molecular events in an "activated" and inflamed kidney may be diminished both at the endothelial and at the effector cell level by means of specific agents administered to the donor before organ removal, added to the perfusate, or given to the recipient immediately before and/or shortly after engraftment. Such interventions are generally less relevant to living donors, as DFG is rare and graft survival rates are excellent.

Although most treatment strategies to prolong graft survival have focused on suppressing host immunity, selective pharmacologic and biological alterations of the graft while still *in situ* may provide potential opportunities for improvement. As the immunogenicity of the inflamed organ may already be increased, immunosuppression of a donor might be initiated before its removal. Although such a strategy has produced ethical debates in the context of living donation, this treatment option may both improve the quality and increase the availability of "marginal grafts" from cadavers. Administration of steroids, for example, has resulted in significant improvements in graft function, whereas pharmacologic preconditioning with standard immunosuppressive agents has been encouraging in experimental settings.[33,34]

## Hormone Replacement Therapy

By stabilizing perturbed peripheral organs in the cadaver donor, hormone replacement therapy has been relatively effective in providing a significant increase in organs/donor useable for transplantation.[35] A major physiological change following brain death is loss of neuroendocrine function from disruption of the hypothalamic-pituitary axis. As a result, production and distribution of ACTH and the corticosteroids, thyroid hormones, vasopressin, and other substances necessary for body homeostasis cease. Donor replacement therapy with these hormones, alone and in combination, has increased substantially the use of previously unacceptable organs.

## Free Oxygen Scavengers

The activity of reactive oxygen species that occur with reperfusion of an ischemic organ has been inhibited by administering the free oxygen scavenger, superoxide dismutase (rh-SOD), to patients before revascularization of their kidney grafts. Although early effects of treatment were marginal, later (> 4 years) graft survival was superior to the untreated controls.[36]

## Blockade of Adhesion Molecules

The close interaction between adhesion molecules and cytokines in hypoxia/reoxygenation injury has been defined in experimental models. IL-1 activity, upregulated in the media of hypoxic endothelial cells and cultured *in vitro*, increases ICAM-1 expression; leukocyte adherence may be inhibited by suppressing endothelium derived IL-1.[37] Use of anti-ICAM-1 mAb is protective in ischemic kidneys in animals, although is less useful clinically.[38] The essential role that cytokines play in mediating the insult via activation of PMNs has been noted in experiments in which this leukocyte population is depleted with CD11b/CD18 (Mac 1) mAbs.[39] The results appear consistent with the sequential importance of different receptors in neutrophil/endothelial adhesion following increased periods of hypoxia. The neutrophil-based chemokine receptor, CCR1, appears particularly important in I/R injury. In contrast to severe tissue destruction in organs of wild-type animals, those of CCR1 knock-out (KO) mice were completely protected. Their inability to activate neutrophils attests to the crucial role of this population in the process.[40]

As discussed, the selectins are a group of adhesion molecules initially responsible for leukocyte endothelial cell interactions. Blockade of these acute-phase proteins by competitive inhibition prevents cell adherence to the vascular endothelium and subsequent infiltration into the injured organ. The effect of selectin blockade in renal ischemia and in brain death in rats with a recombinant P-selectin glycoprotein ligand (rPSGL-Ig), for instance, administered intravenously to the donor and/or with reperfusion after transplantation, prevented all downstream events by obviating the triggering effects of PMNs and inhibiting the subsequent infiltration of lymphocytes and macrophages.[41] There was no expression of their associated effector factors, no upregulation of MHC class II antigens, and no functional or morphologic changes secondary to the acute injury. Initial treatment with the soluble ligand also prevented all chronic changes[42] and allowed effective minimal doses of nephrotoxic calcineurin inhibitors as immunosuppression.[43]

## T-Cell Inhibitors

Several pieces of experimental evidence, including adoptive transfer of CD4+ T lymphocytes and use of an anti-CD4 mAb have suggested an antigen-independent T-cell role in I/R.[44] Additionally, a fusion protein, cytotoxic T-lymphocyte antigen-4 immunoglobulin (CLA4Ig), blocks T-cell/CD28-B7 interaction in a rat ischemia kidney model; the kidneys of treated animals never became acutely inflamed and never developed renal dysfunction or proteinuria over time.[45]

## OTHER APPROACHES

A variety of strategies have also been tested including gene therapy, cell transfer, and ischemic preconditioning. Although gene therapy has been examined primarily in extra-renal organs, there is little information, as yet, on the kidney. Direct administration of nitric oxide donor compounds and nitric oxide itself has been employed in models of I/R injury, but again, rarely in the kidney. Unlimited survival of both whole organ transplants and islet cells have been shown following HO-1 induction and CO application in donor animals prior to transplantation.[46,47] Improved methods of pulsatile perfusion of isolated organs have regained interest. Indeed, this concept may offer new avenues of organ treatment when utilized particularly for expanded donor grafts.[48] Preconditioning of the rat with low doses of cyclosporine and tacrolimus improved renal function, decreasing the tubular injury score of ischemic kidneys by inducing heat shock protein 70.[33] Pretreatment with mycophenolate mofetil protects against I/R injury.[34] This potentially cytoprotective effect may be related to decreased glycosylation of cell-adhesion molecules by its active metabolite, mycophenolic acid.

Other novel preconditioning strategies include the use of picroliv, a potent antioxidant derived from the plant *Picrorhiza kurroa*,[49] and nicaraven, a hydroxyl radical scavenger.[50] Trimetazidine has been added to University of Wisconsin or Euro-Collins perfusate solution to study the function of cold-stored and autotransplanted pig kidneys.[51] This anti-ischemic cytoprotective drug improved substantially the function and survival of the organs by impairing lipid peroxidation and reducing acidosis during cold storage and subsequent reperfusion. It also protected mitochrondrial function and reduced the intensity of interstitial and peritubular inflammation.

## SUMMARY AND FUTURE IMPLICATIONS

I/R is an important nonimmunological, antigen independent risk factor for graft outcome. In addition to its nonspecific inflammatory effects, it potentiates graft immunogenicity and increases host alloresponsiveness. Originally considered an event surrounding organ procurement, preservation, and revascularization, it has been increasingly associated with conditions unique to the cadaver donor such as brain death and asystole. However, as older and more problematic living donors are used, their kidneys are also at potential risk. Occurring early in the transplantation process, I/R initiates a cascade of molecular and cellular events that include the release of proinflammatory mediators and attraction of inflammatory cell populations into the tissues. As a consequence, the acute events may influence structural and functional changes in the organ over time that may affect eventually graft survival.

Attenuation of I/R by strategies interfering with the different processes evoked by the insult may provide means to improve overall graft outcome. The adverse contributions of prolonged ischemia, age, hypertension, and other detrimental donor-associated risk factors of chronic renal allograft dysfunction have underscored the challenges that clinicians now face in expanding the donor pool. With the use of less-than-optimal organs from "marginal" or "extended" sources, it becomes ever more imperative to bring recent advances in cytoprotection against I/R injury to the bedside. Approaches such as hormone replacement, preconditioning with immunosuppressive agents, and inhibition of adhesion or co-stimulatory molecules are being adapted clinically and tested for synergy with standard treatment. As understanding of I/R pathophysiology has improved, so are potentially promising means of targeting the underlying cellular, immunologic, and genetic events of I/R injury.

# References

1. Terasaki PI, Cecka JH, Gertson DW, et al. High survival rates of kidney transplants from spousal and living-related donors. *N Engl J Med* 1995;333:333.

2. Troppmann C, McBride MA,. Baker TJ, et al. Laparoscopic Live Donor Nephrectomy: A Risk Factor for Delayed Function and Rejection in Pediatric Kidney Recipients? A UNOS Analysis. *Transplant* 2005; 5: 175–182.

3. Troppmann C, Gillingham KJ, Benedetti E, et al. Delayed graft function, acute rejection, and outcome after cadaver renal transplantation. *Transplant* 1995;59:962.

4. Land W, Messmer K: The impact of ischemia/reperfusion injury on specific and non-specific early and late chronic events after organ transplantation. *Transplant Rev* 1996; 10:108.

5. Granger DN, Hollwarth ME, Parks DA. Ischemia-reperfusion injury: Role of oxygen-derived free radicals. *Acta Physiol Scand* 1986; 548:47(suppl).

6. Land W. Allograft injury mediated by reactive oxygen species: from conserved proteins of *Drosophila* to acute and chronic rejection of human transplants: Part III: Interaction of (oxidative) stress-induced heat shock proteins with toll-like receptor-bearing cells of innate immunity and its consequences for the development of acute and chronic allograft rejection. *Transplant Rev* 2003;17:87.

7. Springer T. Traffic signals for lymphocyte recirculation and leukocyte emigration: The multi-step paradigm. *Cell* 1994;76:301.

8. Jack RM. Function and regulation of polymorphonuclear leukocytes. In: Tilney NL, Strom TB, Paul LC, eds. *Transplantation Biology: Cellular and Molecular Aspects.* Lippincott-Raven, Phildelphia; 1996:215.

9. Leo R, Pratico D, Iuliano L, et al. Platelet activation by superoxide anion and hydroxyl radicals intrinsically generated by platelets that had undergone anoxia and then reoxygenated. *Circ* 1997;95:885.

10. Palabrica T, Lobb R, Furie BC, et al. Leukocyte accumulation promoting fibrin deposition is mediated in vivo by P-selectin on adherent platelets. *Nature* 1992;359:848.

11. Diacovo TG, Roth SJ, Buccola JM, et al. Neutrophil rolling, arrest, and transmigration across activated, surface-adherent platelets via sequential action of P-selectin and the beta 2-integrin CD11b/CD18. *Blood* 1996;88:146.

12. Friedman GB, Taylor CT, Parkos CA, Colgan SP. Epithelial permeability induced by neutrophil transmigration is potentiated by hypoxia: role of intracellular cAMP. *J Cell Physiol* 1998;176:76.

13. Abramson SB, Leszczynska-Piziak J, Weissmann G. Arachidonic acid as a second messenger. Interactions with a GTP-binding protein of human neutrophils. *J Immunol* 1991;1,147:231.

14. Lorant DE, Patel KD, McIntyre TM, et al. Coexpression of GMP-140 and PAF by endothelium stimulated by histamine or thrombin: a juxtacrine system for adhesion and activation of neutrophils. *J Cell Biol* 1991;115:223.

15. Abbassi O, Kishimoto TK, McIntire LV, et al. E-selection supports neutrophil rolling in vitro under conditions of flow. *J Clin Invest* 1993; 92:2719.

16. Arnaout MA. Structure and function of the leukocyte adhesion molecules CD11/CD18. *Blood* 1990 75:1037–1050.

17. Dallegri F, Goretti R, Ballestrero A, et al. Neutrophil-induced depletion of adenosine triphosphate in target cells: evidence for a hypochlorous acid-mediated process. *J Lab Clin Med* 1988;112:765.

18. Fantone JC, Ward PA. Polymorphonuclear leukocyte-mediated cell and tissue injury: oxygen metabolites and their relations to human disease. *Hum Pathol* 1985;16:973.

19. Takada M, Nadeau KC, Shaw GD, et al. The cytokine-adhesion molecule cascade in ischemia/reperfusion injury of the rat kidney. *J Clin Invest* 1997;99:2682

20. Takada M, Chandraker A, Nadeau KC, et al. The role of the B-7 costimulatory pathway in experimental cold ischemia/reperfusion injury. *J Clin Invest* 1997;100:1199.

21. Faruqui RM, DI Coreleto PE. Mechanisms of monocyte recruitment and accumulation. *Br Heart J* 1993;69:S19.

22. Bosco MC, Espinoza-Delgado I, Schwabe M, et al. The gamma subunit of the interleukin-2 receptor is expressed in human monocytes and modulated by interleukin-2, interferon gamma, and transforming growth factor beta 1. *Blood* 1994;83:3462.

23. Medzhitov R: Toll-like receptors and innate immunity. *Nature Rev Immunol* 2001;1: 135.

24. Pasare C, Medzhitov R. Toll-dependent control mechanisms of CD4 T cell activation. *Immunity* 2004; 21:733.

25. Medzhitov R, Janeway CA Jr. Decoding the pattern of self and non-self by the innate immune system. *Science* 2002;296:298.

26. Tullius SG, Reutzel-Selke A, Egermann F, et al. Contribution of prolonged ischemia and donor age to chronic allograft dysfunction. *JASN* 2000;11:1317–1124.

27. Buelow, R, Tullius, SG, Volk, H.-D. Protection of grafts by Heme-oxygenase-1 and its toxic product carbon monoxide. *Am J Transplant* 2001;1:313.

28. Shen, D-X, Ke, B, Zhai, Y, et al. Toll-like receptor and hemeoxygenase-1 signaling in hepatic ischemia/reperfusion injury. *Am J Transplant* 2005;5:1793–1800.

29. Shoskes DA, Parfrey NA, Halloran PF. Increased major histocompatibility complex antigen expression in unilateral ischemic acute tubular necrosis in the mouse. *Transplant* 1990;49:201.

30. Naimark DMJ, Cole E. Determinants of long-term allograft survival. *Transplant Rev* 1994:3:93.

31. Yilmaz S, Paavonen T, Hayry P. Chronic rejection of rat kidney allografts. II. The impact of prolonged ischemia on transplant histology. *Transplant* 1992;53:823.

32. Tullius SG, Heemann UW, Hancock WW, et al. Long-term kidney isografts develop functional and morphologic changes that mimic those of chronic allograft rejection. *Ann Surg* 1994;220:425.

33. Yang CW, Ahn HJ, Jung JY, et al. Preconditioning with cyclosporine A or FK506 differentially regulates mitogen-activated protein kinase expression in rat kidneys with ischemia/reperfusion injury. *Transplantation* 2003;75:20.

34. Valentin JF, Bruijn JA, Paul LC. Donor treatment with mycophenolate mofetil: protection against ischemia-reperfusion injury in the rat. *Transplant* 2000;69:344.

35. Rosendale JD, Kauffman HM, McBride MA, et al. Aggressive pharmacological donor management results in more transplanted organs. *Transplant* 2003;75:482.

36. Land W, Schneeberger H, Schleibner S, et al. The beneficial effect of human recombinant superoxide dismutase on acute and chronic rejection events in recipients of cadaveric renal transplants. *Transplant* 1994;57:211.

37. Sheeniwas R, Koga, Arakurum M. Hypoxia-mediated induction of endothelial cell interleukin-1 alpa. *J Clin Invest* 1992;90:2333.

38. Kelly KG, Williams WW, Colvin RB, Bonventre JV. Antibody to intercellular adhesion molecule-1 protects the kidney against ischemic injury. *Proc Nat Acad Sci USA* 1994;91:812.

39. Arnould T, Michiels C, Remacle J. Increased PMN adherence on endothelial cells after hypoxia:Involvement of PAF, CD18/CD 11b and ICAM-1. *Am J Physiol* 1993; 264: 1102.

40. Pratschke J, Topham PS, Paz D, et al. A new model of cold ischemia/reperfusion injury: CCR1 knockout mice are protected against renal injury. *Transplant* 1999;67:247.

41. Takada M, Nadeau KC, Shaw GD, et al. The cytokine-adhesion molecule cascade in ischemia/reperfusion injury of the rat kidney: inhibition by a soluble P-selectin ligand. *J Clin Invest* 1997;99:2682.

42. Takada M, Nadeau KC, Shaw GD, et al. Prevention of late renal changes after initial ischemia/reperfusion injury by blocking early selectin binding. *Transplant* 1997;64:1520.

43. Gasser M, Waaga-Gasser AM, Grimm MR, et al. Selectin blockade plus therapy with low-dose sirolimus and cyclosporine A prevent brain death-induced renal allograft dysfunction. *Am J Transplant* 2005; 5:662.

44. Zwacka RM, Zhang Y, Halldorson J, et al. CD4(+) T-lymphocytes mediate ischemia/reperfusion-induced inflammatory responses in mouse liver. *J Clin Invest* 1997;100:279–289.

45. Chandraker A, Takada M, Nadeau KC, et al. CD28-B7 blockade in organ dysfunction secondary to cold ischemia/reperfusion injury. *Kidney Int* 1997;52:1678.

46. Shen D-X, Ke B, Zhai Y, et al. Toll-like receptor and hemoxygenase-1 signaling in hepatic ischemia/reperfusion injury. *Am J Transplant* 2005;51:793.

47. Tullius SG, Nieminen-Kelhae M, Buelow R, et al. Inhibition of ischemia/reperfusion injury and chronic graft deterioration by a single donor treatment with Cobalt-Protoporphyrin for the induction of Heme-Oxygenase-1. *Transplant* 2005;54:1400.

48. Schold, J.D., Kaplan, B, Howard, RJ, et al. Are we frozen in time? Analysis of the utilization and efficacy of pulsatile perfusion in renal transplantation. *Am J Transplant* 2005;5:1681.

49. Singh AK, Mani H, Seth P, et al. Picroliv preconditioning protects the liver against ischemia-reperfusion injury. *Eur J Pharmacol* 2000; 395:229.

50. Yokota R, Fukai M, Shimamura T, et al. A novel hydroxyl radical scavenger, nicaraven, protects the liver from warm ischemia and reperfusion injury. *Surgery* 2000;127; 661–669.

51. Hauet T, Goujon JM, Vandewalle A, et al. Trimetazidine reduces renal dysfunction by limiting the cold ischemia/reperfusion injury in autotransplanted pig kidneys. *J Am Soc Nephrol* 2000:11:138–148.

# 16.5   PERIOPERATIVE CARE

*Mark L. Sturdevant, MD, Vincent Casingal, MD, Rainer W.G. Gruessner, MD*

## INTRODUCTION

The quality of care given to the living donor (LD) kidney recipient must match the level of selflessness exemplified by the donor and optimism felt by the patient afflicted with the ravages of end-stage renal disease (ESRD). The transplant surgeon directs a multidisciplinary team, ideally consisting of a nephrologist, transplant pharmacist, transplant-experienced nursing staff, physical and occupational therapists, social workers, and discharge and outpatient coordinators, to serve the kidney recipient during the perioperative course. Details of the preoperative evaluation and intraoperative care are discussed in accompanying chapters (Chapters 16.1 and 16.2). The following pages are devoted to the special needs of the kidney transplant recipient and the consummate care required to produce excellent outcomes.

## POSTOPERATIVE CARE

### Immediate Postoperative Monitoring

Continuous monitoring of the electrocardiogram (ECG), noninvasive blood pressure, oxygen saturation, urine output (UOP), and central venous pressure (CVP) will allow for constant reassessment of the recipient's status; in particular, intravascular volume status, cardiac function, and subsequent blood pressure must be managed appropriately to optimize early graft function. More than 95% of LD kidney recipients will have immediate graft function and brisk diuresis (often stimulated by intraoperative diuretic and mannitol), making fluctuations in volume status and electrolyte derangements commonplace. Therefore, a hemogram, electrolytes, and renal function tests are obtained every 4 hours, while troponin levels are analyzed every 8 hours during the first postoperative day; a chest x-ray (CXR) and ECG are obtained in the recovery room. The majority of recipients are cared for on a dedicated solid organ transplant unit and do not require

an intensive care unit (ICU) admission. Communication between surgeons and other team members should occur early postoperatively and address any concerns encountered during the transplant operation (eg, blood loss, kidney perfusion, anesthesia issues, and abnormal operative findings) that may affect the posttransplant course.

### Fluid and Electrolyte Management

Postreperfusion, the kidney graft often experiences a time of "dysregulation" marked by large fluid and electrolyte shifts. 40 is measured hourly after the ureteroneocystostomy is completed. During the first 24 hours, 40 is replaced milliliter-per-milliliter (mL) with D5 0.45% NS. If the UOP exceeds 500 mL per hour, the replacement fluid is changed to 0.45% NS to avoid hyperglycemia. Potassium and magnesium replacement volume can be quite high in patients who experience a large volume diuresis, especially if generous doses of loop diuretics are given. As the necessary replacement volume can be quite high (eg, 500 to 1,500 mL per hour), electrolyte replacement is separate from volume replacement. Intravascular volume management guided by constant monitoring of vital signs, 40, and CVP is paramount perioperatively; even mild, transient graft hypoperfusion can lead to profound acute tubular necrosis (ATN) with subsequent delayed graft function (DGF). During the next 48 hours, the recipient is allowed to diurese: either ½ mL-per-mL fluid replacement or standard maintenance intravenous fluids (IVFs). Daily weights are obtained to monitor cumulative changes in total body water. By the fourth postoperative day, IVFs are discontinued as the recipient prepares for discharge home.

### General Care of the Kidney Recipient

The incidence of cardiac complications posttransplant is directly proportional to the degree of underlying cardiac disease and level of postoperative graft function. Recipients with poor left ventricular function (eg, ejection fraction < 30%) may benefit from pulmonary artery catheter (PAC) placement and ICU admission to optimize their volume status. The short ischemia time and low ATN incidence noted in LD recipients lower the risk of postoperative fluid overload and cardiac dysfunction.[1] The prompt resolution of uremia leads to improved cardiac dynamics, which have been documented on an echocardiogram.[2] Unless hypotension is present, recipients on preoperative beta-blockers should restart them within 24 hours. Correction of mild to moderate hypertension (eg, systolic blood pressure < 180 mm Hg) should be judicious, to avoid any hypotension in the early postoperative course. However, markedly elevated blood pressure may be successfully managed with diuretics (eg, volume-overloaded recipient), calcium channel blockers, intravenous beta-blockers, and vasodilators; infrequently, ICU admission to initiate antihypertensive infusions (eg, sodium nitroprusside) is needed.

Pulmonary physiotherapy, as with all surgical patients, starts immediately to avoid complications related to atelectasis and pneumonia. Extended monitoring with pulse oximetry and serial CXRs may be necessary to track the course of the uncommon LD recipient who experiences DGF and resultant fluid overload. Postoperative pulmonary edema may be managed with diuretics alone; however, dialysis is usually required in those recipients who required preoperative dialytic therapy.

Appropriate management of gastrointestinal (GI) issues is crucial to avoid unnecessary morbidity and prolonged hospital stay. A major advantage to the retroperitoneal placement of the

LD kidney is the relative low incidence of postoperative ileus. Recipients are started on liquids within 24 hours of their transplant and are allowed to advance their diet if free of nausea, vomiting, and abdominal distention; most proceed to a regular diet within 2 to 3 days. Diabetics are at risk for perioperative exacerbation of gastoparesis, which may lead to a more prolonged course. The development and ubiquitous use of proton pump inhibitors (PPIs) have minimized the incidence of upper gastrointestinal (UGI) tract bleeding; historically (ie, before PPIs and H2-blockers), UGI bleeds occurred in more than 10% of kidney recipients and carried a mortality rate of up to 65%.[3,4] Kidney transplant recipients continue to be at an elevated risk for acute colonic pseudoobstruction (Ogilvie's syndrome); the 1.5% incidence is much higher than expected for an extraperitoneal operation.[5] The pathophysiologic basis for the increased risk is poorly understood, but the potentially hazardous outcome, namely, significant cecal dilation, is the usual result. Aggressive nonoperative (eg, nasogastric decompression, neostigmine) and endoscopic maneuvers are mandatory to avoid colonic perforation. A bowel regimen (eg, senna, docusate, bisacodyl) to avoid narcotic-induced constipation is started on postoperative day 1.

Infections during the first posttransplant month are essentially (> 90%) the same bacterial and fungal infections noted in the general surgical population, ie, of the surgical wound, urinary tract, lungs, and vascular-access lines.[6] An appropriately screened LD will be free of any active infection; therefore, the incidence of graft-related infection is nil. Antimicrobial prophylaxis, preoperative skin preparation with chlorhexidine, and meticulous hemostasis yield a reasonable surgical site infection incidence of 1% to 6%. Foley catheters and central venous lines are universal, but should be promptly removed when no longer needed, to decrease the incidence of urinary tract infection (UTI) and line sepsis, respectively. Aggressive pulmonary physiotherapy and early ambulation are vital in efforts to decrease the incidence of nosocomial pneumonia. If the recipient was previously immunosuppressed (eg, retransplant), a broader differential diagnosis, including the opportunistic (eg, viral, protozoan, parasite) infections, must be entertained in the evaluation of the febrile or septic posttransplant recipient. Long-term, prophylactic antimicrobials are initiated immediately posttransplant. Daily administration of sulfamethoxazole-trimethoprim (SMX-TMP) is standard prophylaxis for *Pneumocystis carinii* pneumonia, as well as for *Listeria monocytogenes* and *Nocardia* infections; starting it postoperatively also serves to minimize the incidence of UTIs. Success has been achieved in preventing cytomegalovirus (CMV) infection with prophylactic 9-(1,3-dihydroxy-2-propoxymethyl) guanine (DHPG) in parenteral (ganciclovir) or enteral (valganciclovir) forms. The efficacy of oral DHPG (valganciclovir) is equal to oral ganciclovir in preventing CMV disease in high-risk recipients but has much higher bioavailability, which allows for once-daily dosing .[7] Clotrimazole troches are used as prophylax is against oropharyngeal candidiasis.

Posttransplant hyperglycemia is prevalent due to high-dose steroids, calcineurin inhibitors, and surgical stress; also, approximately 30% to 35% of recipients are diabetic. Landmark studies in postsurgical (nontransplant) and critically ill populations now provide guidance to direct the intensity of glycemic control. Golden et al. reported significant decreases in surgical site infections without increases in hypoglycemic episodes in patients undergoing coronary bypass operations when glucose levels were kept below 150 mg/dL.[8] An actual decrease in mortality was noted by Van den Berghe et al. when critically ill patients entering the ICU had a target blood glucose level of 80 to 110 mg/dL.[9] Considering that the recipient carries the additional infectious risk factor of immunosuppression and often diabetes, tight glycemic control is prudent.

Analgesia in the early postoperative setting is accomplished with patient-controlled analgesia (PCA) until oral narcotics are tolerated. Most centers use morphine, hydromorphone, or fentanyl; meperidine should be avoided, especially in recipients with DGF, as its metabolite (normeperidine) is neurotoxic and may lead to seizure activity.

Deep venous thrombosis (DVT) prophylaxis typically consists of pneumatic stockings, sequential compression devices, and early ambulation. A recipient with additional risk factors (eg, prior DVT, hypercoagulable state) or who is noncompliant with early ambulation needs subcutaneous heparin or low-molecular-weight heparin (caregirers must follow anti-Xa levels until creatinine clearance [CrCl] is > 60 mL/min) if postoperative bleeding is not evident. The incidence of DVT is only 1% to 4% despite some evidence that high-dose steroids and the rapid resolution of uremia may place the recipient into a hypercoagulable state.[10–12] No anticoagulation regimen has proven efficacy in decreasing the incidence of graft loss to vascular thrombosis; however, many centers utilize empiric aspirin, heparin, dextran, and even long-term warfarin in an effort to diminish the incidence of this catastrophic event.

Modern immunosuppression in the early posttransplant period typically consists of a mono- or polyclonal antibody induction agent, corticosteroids, an antimetabolite (eg, mycophenolate mofetil, sirolimus), and a calcineurin inhibitor (CNI [tacrolimus, cyclosporine A]). A detailed discussion of immunosuppression is beyond the scope of this chapter (see Chapter 16.7); however, a prerequisite for optimal care of the recipient is a thorough knowledge of these medications and prompt recognition and management of their potential adverse effects. For example, hypotension secondary to Thymoglobulin can be easily corrected by decreasing the infusion rate twofold.

An 18-French Foley (3-way) catheter is placed in the operating room and serves two purposes: precise urine output monitoring and decompression of the bladder to allow for ureteroneocystostomy healing. If the bladder is healthy and no technical misadventures were experienced, the catheter is removed on postoperative day 4 when a Lich-Gregoire ureteroneocystostomy was utilized and on postoperative day 7 to 10 when the reconstruction was performed via the Leadbetter-Politano technique. Prolonged decompression may be justified when the bladder is compromised or the anastomosis technically difficult.

## THE DYSFUNCTIONAL GRAFT

### Expected Function

More than 95% of all LD kidneys will have UOP before or soon after completion of the ureteroneocystostomy. A brisk diuresis is typically noted (ie, minimum UOP 100 to 200 mL/hr) but may be an unreliable indicator of graft function due to the use of perioperative diuretics and the presence of residual function in the native kidneys or previous grafts. A downward trend in serial (every 4 hours for 24 hours) serum Cr reflects a steady improvement in overall graft function. The absolute change in Cr is less important than a consistent downward trend. As previously stated, constant monitoring of the recipient's volume status, vital signs, and electrolyte profile is mandatory in the early postoperative period and will allow the graft to function in an ideal environment.

## Evaluation

Signs of graft dysfunction in the early posttransplant period include oligoanuria or a plateau or upward trend in serum Cr despite appropriate intravascular volume and blood pressure. Risk factors for obstructive uropathy (eg, hematuria), ATN (eg, hypotension, procurement trauma, increased cold ischemia), graft thrombosis (eg, hypercoagulable state, technical difficulties), and early cellular or humoral rejection (eg, in a high immunologic risk recipient) should be reviewed to formulate a differential diagnosis for the graft dysfunction. The clinician must have a high index of suspicion for any changes in graft performance and employ a rapid, efficacious evaluation to identify the problem. Obstructive uropathy (in the form of bladder clots and resultant catheter blockage) is usually remedied with simple catheter irrigation; in refractory cases, a larger catheter (ie, 20 to 22F) is placed to facilitate manual clot evacuation. If dysfunction remains, an emergent Doppler ultrasound (US) can (1) exclude renal artery and vein thrombosis, (2) exclude hydronephrosis (eg, ureteral obstruction), (3) evaluate for a retroperitoneal fluid collection (eg, urinoma, hematoma), and (4) estimate graft size and echotexture. A thorough physical examination coupled with a high quality US should exclude graft thrombosis, obstructive uropathy, ureteral stenosis, and retroperitoneal or subcapsular hematomas with graft compression (ie, Page kidney) as diagnoses. If the US is equivocal pertaining to vascular patency, a magnetic resonance arteriogram/venogram (MRA/MRV) or reexploration is warranted to fully evaluate for thrombosis. When perigraft fluid is present, renal scintigraphy can be performed to evaluate for a urine leak; image-guided percutaneous aspiration of the fluid yielding urine confirms this diagnosis.

When these initial studies fail to produce a diagnosis in the setting of ongoing dysfunction, the two most likely culprits are ATN and acute rejection (eg, hyperacute, accelerated cellular, or humoral). If the recipient is at high immunologic risk (eg, highly sensitized, past positive crossmatch, retransplant) and low ATN risk (eg, minimal ischemia time, no hypoperfusion episodes), a percutaneous graft biopsy by postoperative day 4 or 5 would be in order. This approach avoids the possibility of ongoing, untreated rejection in the early postoperative period; the recipient should be counseled on the higher incidence of postbiopsy bleeding in this setting. If ATN is the more likely diagnosis, deferment of the graft biopsy to postoperative day 7 to 10 is a reasonable approach; the purpose of this biopsy is to exclude concomitant acute rejection. All biopsies are evaluated with standard staining (ie, hematoxylin and eosin), C4d staining (evaluates for humoral rejection), and electon micrography (EM). If ATN is present, it usually persists for 2 to 3 weeks, and graft biopsies should be performed every 7 to 10 days to exclude concomitant acute rejection. The type and severity of acute rejection dictate the treatment course.

Percutaneous graft biopsy will also be pivotal in excluding the two recurrent diseases seen in the early posttransplant period: focal segmental glomerulosclerosis (FSGS) and hemolytic uremic syndrome (HUS). Posttransplant nephrotic range proteinuria (ie, > 3.5 g/day) in a patient with known FSGS should prompt an early posttransplant biopsy, which will show diffuse foot process effacement on EM if recurrent FSGS is active.[13]

De novo HUS is poorly understood but typically presents with anemia and/or thrombocytopenia accompanied by signs of ongoing microvascular trauma (eg, depressed haptoglobin, elevated L-lactate dehydrogenase, schistocytes on blood smear). A microangiopathic process culminates in fibrin clot deposition in the afferent arterioles (confirmed on biopsy) leading to profound graft dysfunction with a high rate of graft loss.[14,15] Strong evidence implicates CNIs as causative agents in HUS; damage to the afferent arteriole endothelium has been suggested as the inciting factor.

Finally, CNIs may lead to graft dysfunction via a preglomerular vasoconstrictive mechanism.[16] Elevated CNI serum levels should prompt a temporary cessation of the drug to observe for graft function improvement.

The importance of a rapid, precise diagnosis cannot be overstated; slow recognition or a misdiagnosis may lead to the loss of a LD kidney and the immediate return of the recipient to ESRD. The definitive management of each complication is discussed in Chapter 16.6.

## Delayed Graft Function (DGF)

Regardless of etiology, the need for dialysis in the LD kidney recipient during the first posttransplant week is referred to as delayed graft function. (DGF), is suggested by a normal US coupled with a renal scintogram showing prompt perfusion and adequate parenchymal uptake of radiotracer, but poor renal excretion. Percutaneous graft biopsies every 7 to 10 days are required to exclude concomitant acute rejection during DGF; the cumulative effect of DGF and acute rejection is detrimental to both early and long-term graft survival. Communication with the nephrology team will allow for timely initiation of dialysis in order to avoid the common complications of DGF (eg, volume overload, hyperkalemia, uremia). In the deceased donor kidney recipient population, DGF is most commonly caused by ATN and 95% of such cases will resolve in time; however, due to its infrequency, less is known about the etiology and prognosis of DGF in LD kidney recipients.

## TRANSITION TO OUTPATIENT CARE

### Discharge Planning

Uncomplicated postoperative care results in the routine discharge of kidney transplant recipients by postoperative day 3 to 5. Therefore, discharge planning should begin prior to the transplant. During the latter half of the postoperative stay, plans should be made for follow-up surgical and medical care, teaching, frequent laboratory studies, and, if needed, outpatient induction immunosuppressant infusions and dialysis. A coordinated transition team consisting of both inpatient caretakers and outpatient coordinators must guide the recipient through this anxious time.

### Medication Education

Prior to discharge, the patient and family should understand and have a working knowledge of the multiple new medications that have been initiated. Compliance and its relationship to medication side effects must be emphasized; the recipient must feel confident that complaints pertaining to drug side effects will be met with an understanding, flexible attitude from the transplant coordinators and physicians.

## Monitoring

Complete blood counts, electrolytes, renal function tests, and immunosuppressant serum levels are obtained triweekly for the first several weeks (center specific). Immunosuppressant therapeutic serum levels will change depending on the incidence of rejection episodes, side effect profiles, infectious disease complications, and the time posttransplant. Stable function and therapeutic drug levels will allow for less frequent monitoring.

## Discharge

Usually by the fourth postoperative day, the recipient is ready for discharge unless complications have intervened. Typically, by this time, most recipients have adequate pain control via oral narcotics, have normal bowel function, and are tolerating a diet. Physical therapists evaluate all recipients before discharge and coordinate home therapy or rehabilitation needs if necessary.

## References

1. Hussain M, Khalique M, Askari H, et al. Surgical complications after renal transplantation in a living-related transplantation program at SIUT. *Transplant Proc* 1999;31:3211.
2. Debska-Slizien A, Dudziak M, Kubasik A, et al. Echocardiographic changes in left ventricular morphology and function after successful renal transplantation. *Transplant Proc* 2000;32:1365.
3. Troppmann C, Papalois BE, Chiou A, et al. Incidence, complications, treatment, and outcome of ulcers of the upper gastrointestinal tract after renal transplantation during the cyclosporine era. *J Am Coll Surg* 1995;180:433.
4. Sarosdy MF, Cruz AB, Saylor R, et al. Upper gastrointestinal bleeding following renal transplantation. *Urology* 1985;26:347.
5. Love R, Sterling JR, Sollinger HW, et al. Colonoscopic decompression for acute colonic pseudo-obstruction (Ogilvie's syndrome) in transplant recipients. *Gastrointest Endosc* 1988;34:426.
6. Fishman J, Rubin R. Infection in organ-transplant recipients. *NEJM* 2005; 338:24.
7. Paya C, Humar A, Dominguez E, et al. Efficacy and safety of valganciclovir vs. oral ganciclovir for prevention of cytomegalovirus disease in solid organ transplant recipients. *Am J Transplant* 2004;4: 611–620.
8. Golden SH, Peart-Vigilance C, Kao WH, et al. Perioperative glycemic control and the risk of infectious complications in a cohort of adults with diabetes. *Diabetes Care* 1999;22:1408–1414.
9. Van den Berghe G, Wouters P, Weekers F, et al. Intensive insulin therapy in critically ill patients. *NEJM* 2001;345:1359.
10. Murie JA, Allen RD, Michie CA, et al. Deep venous thrombosis after renal transplantation. *Transplant Proc* 1987;19:2219.
11. Ozsoylu S, Strauss HS, Diamond LK. Effect of corticosteroids on coagulation of the blood. *Nature* 1962;195:1214.
12. von Kaulla KN, von Kaulla E, Wasantapruck S, et al. Blood coagulation in uremic patients before and after hemodialysis and transplantation of the kidney. *Arch Surg* 1966;92:184.
13. Artero M, Biava C, Amend W, et al. Recurrent focal glomerulosclerosis: natural history and response to therapy. *Am J Med* 1992;92:375.
14. Ducloux D, Rebibou JM, Semhoun-Ducloux S etal: Recurrence of hemolyticuremic syndrome in renal transplant recipients: a meta-analysis. *Transplantation* 1998;65:1405.
15. Singh N, Gayowski T, Marino IR, et al. Hemolytic uremic syndrome in solid-organ transplant recipients. *Transpl Int* 1996;9:68.
16. Perico N, Ruggenenti P, Gaspari F, et al. Daily renal hypoperfusion induced by cyclosporine in patients with renal transplantation. *Transplantation* 1992;54:56.

## 16.6  POSTTRANSPLANT COMPLICATIONS

*Amer Rajab, MD, Anatolie Usatii, MD, Ronald M. Ferguson, MD, PhD*

### INTRODUCTION

Improvement in surgical and diagnostic techniques, cross-match testing, anesthesia, perioperative monitoring, and immunosuppressive drugs led to a significant decrease in complication rates post kidney transplantation. In fact, the current expected 1-year patient survival following kidney transplantation is near 95%. At the Ohio State University, > 90% of kidney transplant recipients undergo uncomplicated renal transplantation with immediate function and are being discharged on fourth postoperative day. Although the incidence of posttransplant complications is low, the occurrence of such complications may lead to graft loss or even patient death. The present article reviews the recipient complications following kidney transplantation. In particular, it focuses on

1. Vascular complications

2. Urologic complications

3. Infectious complications

4. Delayed graft function

### Vascular Complications

The incidence of vascular complications following renal transplantation varies between 0.8% and 15%.[1,2] During the early stages of development of the transplant procedure, vascular complication rates as high as 30% were reported.[3] Arterial complications are more frequent and more dangerous than venous misadventures. Both arterial and venous thromboses tend to occur within the first few days posttransplant, although, the adverse effects of vascular misadventures may not appear until a time well distant from the transplant operation. The early thrombosis of renal allografts can occur in approximately 2% to 8% of transplants and account for more than 25% of all early graft losses.[4–7] Improvements in immunosuppressive therapy have reduced early allograft loss due to acute rejection to very low levels. Early allograft loss, due to acute thrombotic complications, has remained constant and therefore represents a proportionally increasing percentage of early losses.

In a retrospective study of 1,200 live donor renal transplants, in 1,152 patients,[2] there were 34 vascular complications (2.8%). Stenotic or thrombotic complications were recorded in 11 cases (0.9%), including renal artery stenosis in 5 (0.4%), renal artery thrombosis in 5 (0.4%) and renal vein thrombosis in 1 (0.1%). Hemorrhagic complications were observed in 23 patients (1.9%). Although, no risk factors could be identified that were related to stenotic or thrombotic complications, grafts with multiple renal arteries were significantly associated with hemorrhagic complications (p = 0.04).

### Renal Artery Thrombosis

Arterial thrombosis occurs in approximately 1% of renal transplants, particularly when the caliber of the renal vessels is small. The usual presentation of arterial thrombosis is abrupt cessation of a previously adequate urine output. However, this sign may be masked if the native kidneys are producing urine or in cases where the patient has delayed graft function with no or low urine output.

Renal artery thrombosis can result from a variety of causes that can be classified into four categories: surgical misadventures, immunological reaction, hypercoagulability, or administration of potentially thrombogenic drugs. The vast majority of immediate postoperative thromboses are caused by surgical misadventures, such as the creation of an intimal flap in the renal artery during donor nephrectomy; occlusion due to thick plaque at the ostium of the renal artery or in the recipient iliac artery; as well as misalignment, torsion, or kinking of the anastomosis. Vascular complications were not related to the number of renal arteries.[8] In fact, only the rates of late renal artery stenosis were higher in kidneys with multiple arteries, whereas the rates of early vascular and urologic complications were not different.[9] The second-most-frequent cause of renal artery thrombosis is an immunological reaction (hyperacute rejection), a complication that is seen much less frequently in the past decade due to progress in pretransplant cross-matching. A third group of causes consists of underlying patient diseases that produce hypercoagulability, such as the production of cryoglobulins or antiphospholipid antibodies associated with active lupus erythematosus.[10] In a multicenter study, 19% of 502 renal failure patients on the kidney waiting list exhibit high titer of anticardiolipin antibodies. However, only 5% (23 of 502 patients) of the patients have antiphospholipid antibody syndrome which is characterized by the presence of anticardiolipin antibodies in association with thrombotic disorders such as lupus, frequent abortions, frequent thrombosis of arteriovenous shunts, biopsy-proven microrenal angiopathy, or thrombocytopenia.[11] Of those 23 patients, 11 received kidney transplants either with (4 patients) or without (7 patients) concomitant anticoagulation therapy. All 7 patients with the syndrome not treated with anticoagulation therapy lost their allografts within 1 week as a result of renal thrombosis. In contrast, 3 out of 4 transplant patients with the syndrome treated with anticoagulation therapy maintained their allografts for over 2 years. The fourth patient lost his graft within a week because of thrombosis. Of the remaining 70 patients with high titers of anticardiolipin antibodies but no evidence of thrombotic disorders, 37 received kidney transplants. None lost their allografts as a result of thrombosis. It was concluded that patients with antiphospholipid antibody syndrome are at high risk of posttransplant renal thrombosis, and anticoagulation therapy should be used to prevent posttransplant thrombosis.[11]

A fourth cause of renal artery thrombosis is administration of potentially thrombogenic drugs. Substantial *in vitro* data suggest cyclosporine is prothrombotic; however, an independent clinical association with allograft thrombosis is unproven. Several *in vitro* studies have shown that cyclosporine is associated with impaired fibrinolysis, increased thrombin activation, increased platelet activation, and activation of intrinsic coagulation pathways.[12–15] However, a late study showed no association between cyclosporine and vascular thrombosis.[7,16] The monoclonal antibody OKT3 has been implicated in allograft thrombosis in case reports,[17] but there were no data from clinical studies to suggest increased thrombotic risks with OKT3 or other immunosuppressive drugs.

As any patient, the posttransplant recipient with acute renal failure, post- or prerenal causes should be ruled out. Prerenal causes such as hypoperfusion due to hypovolemia or congestive heart failure should be addressed. Foley catheter and ureteral obstruction should be evaluated. The next step is to examine the vascular tree for thrombosis. One useful study is a color Doppler scan, which estimates blood flow in the renal artery and the renal

vein and allows the physician to calculate the intraparenchymal resistance index. An alternate study is a perfusion nuclear scan. Although angiogram is a valuable tool for evaluation of renal artery stenosis, it is rarely needed for vascular thrombosis. Treatment demands immediate exploration with arterial repair. Unfortunately, unless arterial thrombosis occurred during the transplant procedure, salvage is rarely achievable. The time between the occurrence of arterial thrombosis, diagnosis, and exploration is usually long, therefore, tissue infarction and necrosis have already occurred making nephrectomy necessary in the majority of cases.[3,17] If exploration reveals a patent anastomosis with cortical blood flow as evidenced by direct Doppler assessment, an intraoperative renal biopsy is indicated.

Allograft loss due to thrombosis is small but disastrous. Most transplant physicians would prefer to prevent it, but the difficult question is how to identify patients at high risk. Identifying risk factor(s) for thrombosis amenable to preventive strategies has been elusive. Epidemiological studies have attempted to define risk in terms of modifiable (drugs, dialysis modality, surgical procedure) and nonmodifiable (age, diabetes mellitus, vascular anomalies) factors. A large, case control study identified retransplantation and peritoneal dialysis as the strongest epidemiological factors associated with renal vascular thrombosis within 30 days of surgery.[6] Interventions to reduce thrombotic risk including heparin, warfarin, and aspirin have been evaluated in a retrospective case-controlled study. Studies so far used low-molecular-weight heparin (LMWH)[18–20] and unfractionated heparin[21,22] for prophylaxis of allograft thrombosis in transplant recipients. In high-risk children, enoxaparin resulted in a significant reduction in vascular thrombosis when compared with a historic control group.[18] Friedman et al. used intravenous heparin and long-term oral anticoagulation with warfarin in those with hypercoagulable state and achieved a 60% reduction in allograft thrombosis, compared with historic rates; however, they reported a very high hemorrhagic (wound) complication rate.[21] Ubhi et al.[22] randomized 70 consecutive renal transplant patients to either 5,000 U subcutaneous heparin twice daily for 7 days or no heparin. No thrombotic events occurred in the heparin group compared with six events in 5 patients in the heparin-free group, although this was not statistically significant. Alkhunaizi et al.[20] treated 120 adult kidney recipients with dalteparin 2,500 U Units daily (low-risk group) for the period of hospitalization only, or 5,000 U daily (high-risk group) for at least 1 month. High risk was defined as a hypercoagulable state (15%) or multiple vessels (31%). There were no allograft thromboses and no major hemorrhagic events. Morrissey et al.[23] reported on 235 consecutive renal allograft recipients who were screened for hypercoagulation status based on an initial clinical thrombotic risk. They identified 8 (3.4%) patients at risk. Perioperative heparinization was used in all 8 patients, and no allograft thromboses occurred in these 8 patients, or the remaining patients without clinical risk who did not receive heparin. Two patients had bleeding complications requiring intervention.[23]

Aspirin has been used for prevention of renal allograft thrombosis. Two retrospective studies from the UK have reported a significant decrease in early-graft thrombosis using aspirin as prophylaxis when compared to historical controls. The first study from Oxford[24] prescribed aspirin 75 mg/day from the day of transplant and for 1 month to all patients. The rate of allograft thrombosis prior to Aspirin prophylaxis was 5.6%; and after the introduction of Aspirin prophylaxis 1.2% (p < 0.01). The second study from Leicester[25] introduced aspirin 150 mg/day from the first postoperative day for 90 days. They reported a reduced rate of thrombosis when compared with a historic control (0% vs 5%; p = 0.03). Also no significant bleeding problem and no restriction on biopsy requirements were reported.

These trials are retrospective case control studies. Only a large, multicenoter, randomized trial can determine the safety, efficacy, and optimal duration of therapy with heparin, aspirin, or both, or other agents for the prevention of renal allograft thrombosis. In view of the low event rate, this trial would have to be very large to achieve any statistical conclusion, even if selected only for high-risk patients. In fact, even widespread screening for prothrombotic mutations is still controversial.[26,27] Patients identified in a higher clinical risk group, or with previous evidence for thrombosis, should be considered for individualized testing and prophylaxis according to these risks. For unselected patients, low-dose aspirin for routine prophylaxis appears the most pragmatic and beneficial preventive therapy at present, reserving other agents for those with a defined risk factor.

## Renal Artery Stenosis

Renal transplant artery stenosis is a relatively frequent complication after transplantation occurring in 2% to 10% of cases; however, higher incidences of up to 23% have been reported.[28] In fact, it is by far the most common vascular complication after kidney transplantation. In a report, of 154 vascular complications noted, 125 were renal artery stenosis.[29] In a series of 715 pediatric renal transplantations in the 1980s, renal artery stenosis was detected in 69 children (9.7%).[30] Fung et al.[31] retrospectively analyzed 333 pediatric renal transplantations and found renal artery stenosis in 5.7%. Bruno et al.[32] estimated the normal prevalence of arterial stenosis as 1% to 23% 3 months to 2 years after transplantation.

The gold standard for the diagnosis still remains renal arteriography. Patients may present with unexplained deterioration of renal function or an abrupt onset of refractory hypertension. On physical exam, an intense allograft bruit may be found. Most patients will undergo extensive work-up for the usual causes such as rejection or drug toxicity. Patients may remain asymptomatic. In fact, when a Doppler scan is introduced as part of routine screening, in otherwise asymptomatic renal transplant recipients, 12.4% of patients are found to have a renal artery stenosis compared with a prevalence of 2.4% when Doppler is used only to confirm the clinical suspicion in symptomatic patients.[33]

Renal artery stenosis occurs at any time posttransplantation and usually arises close to the surgical anastomosis, although pre- or postanastomotic stenoses may also occur.[29] There are three types of renal artery stenosis: anastomotic, diffuse postanastomotic narrowing of the renal artery, and a number of discrete narrowings in the distal renal arterial bed. An anastomotic stenosis is most likely related to a purse-string effect of the suture, a clamp injury, or other trauma to the donor vessels during donor organ procurement.[34] Small, subtle intimal flaps or subintimal dissections of the vascular wall precede intimal scarring and hyperplasia. Kinking or angulation of the artery produces turbulent flow with consequent anastomotic narrowing. The second type is a diffuse, postanastomotic narrowing, which may occur with any type of anastomosis. The narrowing may affect different sites along the renal artery (multiple stenoses) or the whole artery (diffuse stenoses). The third type shows a number of discrete narrowings in the distal renal arterial bed and is usually associated with chronic allograft nephropathy. Atherosclerotic diseases either of the transplant renal artery or of the adjacent proximal iliac artery usually present several years posttransplant.

The rate of late renal artery stenosis is higher in kidneys with multiple arteries.[9] Early vascular and urologic complications were not different.[9] Transplantation performed with a donor aortic patch lowered the rate of stenosis at the anastomosis (0%) compared with transplantation without a patch (7 of 140, 5.0%).[31] The use of aortic patch technique is, however, limited to cadaveric kidney transplant. Even then if shorter renal arteries are needed, a segment of the renal artery with the aortic cuff will be removed.

Renal artery stenosis leads to hypoperfusion of the transplanted kidney resulting in activation of the renin-angiotensin and sympathetic nervous systems, sodium retention, and extracellular volume expansion. Volume expansion and hypertension eventually improve renal perfusion and progressively inhibit the renin angiotensin system activity. This results in a new steady state in which hypertension is sustained mostly by extracellular volume expansion, and the plasma renin activity may be normal or even low.

Several imaging techniques are available to confirm the diagnosis (duplex-Doppler, captopril radionuclide scan, nuclear magnetic resonance, spiral computerized tomography, and angiogram), and their use depends, in part, on the center's experience.

The treatment can either be conservative (providing the stenosis is not hemodynamically significant and graft perfusion is not jeopardized) or by revascularization (surgical or percutaneous transluminal angioplasty). A 5-year follow up of 11 patients[35] who had kinks of the renal artery by Doppler ultrasound without significant pressure change and were managed conservatively has shown that the stenoses did not appear to progress and threaten renal graft function.

In pediatric transplant recipients,[31] almost 50% were treated successfully with antihypertensive drugs; the others underwent percutaneous transluminal angioplasty (PTA) with variable success. The authors concluded that PTA should be the first procedure if medication fails, and surgery should be reserved for PTA failure.[31] It was also observed that early diagnosis and treatment of renal artery stenosis does not limit survival of allografts with renal artery stenosis compared with transplants without renal artery stenosis.[31] Bruno et al.[32] showed that kidney function was restored in 60% to 90% of cases after PTA. In a retrospective study from Canada,[36] 21 interventions were performed in 18 allografts. The technical success rate of PTA/stent placement was 100%, and the clinical success rate was 94% (17 of 18 allografts). Kidney function improved significantly after treatment. One year primary and secondary patency rates were 72% and 85%, respectively. Of the 8 allografts that underwent stent placement, all 8 remained patent at last follow-up of 18.3 months. One major complication of PTA was puncture site pseudoaneurysm (5%).

The definitive approach for an anastomotic stenosis is resection with primary reconstruction, in some cases employing a patch angioplasty depending on the caliber of the vessels. For a postanastomotic stenosis, bypass grafting, using an autogenous vein graft from the external iliac to the renal artery is the preferred method. However, due to the technical difficulty of approaching vascular structures of an allograft that does not have collateral flow, the rate of graft loss after vascular reconstruction is high. When the stenoses are in the hilar or distal portion of the renal bed, PTA offers the only option.

## Renal Vein Thrombosis

Venous thrombosis early after a kidney transplant like arterial thrombosis is an infrequent but devastating complication. It occurs between 0.3% and 4.2%.[37] Of 2,003 kidney transplants performed between January 1984 and September 1998 at the University of Minnesota, 32 recipients lost their first graft early posttransplant to vascular thrombosis. Of these, 12 are due to renal vein thrombosis and 4 to renal artery thrombosis. Graft venous thrombosis usually manifests within the first 2 weeks after transplantation.[39] It presents with sudden oliguria, hematuria, and graft swelling. Renal allograft rupture[40] has been reported in four cases of renal vein thrombosis.

Multiple risk factors for renal vein thrombosis have been suggested. These included technical surgical problems, donor's right kidney, left lower quadrant allografts,[41] vessel compression by hematoma or lymphocele, or hypovolemia.[42] Also CMV infection has been associated with venous thrombosis.[43] Hypercoagulation status[44] and proximal extension of ileofemoral deep venous thrombosis have been suggested as risk factors.[45] Renal vein thrombosis tends to be more common with a right kidney graft, and in 12 recipients with renal vein thrombosis, 8 had initially received a right kidney.[39] This may be due to the short right kidney vein.

The prognosis of graft venous thrombosis is generally poor. Acute thrombosis generally results in permanent graft loss. Recently, Rerolle et al.[39] described the usefulness of catheter thromboaspiration for graft venous thrombosis. There have been reports of nonoperative salvage by streptokinase infusion,[46] although most physicians advocate intraoperative thrombectomy. However, the majority of patients suffering renal venous thrombosis experience graft infarction despite thrombectomy and require transplant nephrectomy.

## Hemorrhage

Even though end-stage renal disease patients are known to have defective coagulation due to platelet dysfunction, early post transplant bleeding is rare. Bleeding from the vascular anastomoses is extremely rare. In fact, most postoperative hemorrhage requiring exploration is due to small vascular tributaries that were not secured during back-table preparation of the allograft, and during exploration the bleeding is already stopped. Hemorrhage within the first week can occur due to transplant rupture from venous thrombosis or an uncontrolled accelerated rejection process.[40] After 1month posttransplant, the most common cause of exsanguinating hemorrhage is mycotic infection of the anastomosis. Fortunately, this is a very rare complication that results in graft and even patient loss.[47]

Hemorrahage may present as a spectrum of findings, ranging from subtle changes to shock. Pain may be an early sign of hemorrhage. Pain may be in the graft area and radiates to the back, the flank, or the rectum. Tachycardia or mild hypotension may be the only symptoms and may progress rapidly to vascular collapse. Swelling is usually difficult to recognize especially with the increasingly larger population of transplant patients. Obese patients may accumulate several units of blood without or with subtle local findings. Also the hematoma is most likely to expand into the retroperitoneal space and sometimes even communicate with the peritoneum. An ultrasound examination or CT scan can confirm the presence of a perinephric hematoma. Surgical exploration may be required to salvage the patient's life or the graft's function.

Due to improvement in surgical technique, massive intraoperative bleeding threatening the patient or the graft is rare. However, the transplant and anesthesia team should be always prepared for surgical mishap and significant blood loss. When the patient presents in extremis, and particularly when the bleeding is precipitated by ruptured mycotic psudoaneurysm of the renal artery anastomosis,

the external iliac artery may have to be ligated and blood supply to the ipsilateral lower extremity provided by an extra-anatomic bypass, such as a femoral–femoral or axillofemoral graft.

Continuous oozing into the transplant bed may be too slow to cause any early symptoms but last long enough to result in hematoma formation. The use of heparin or antiplatelet drug may contribute to this problem. Gradual drop in hemoglobin will occur; however, anemia is not an infrequent finding in the immediate posttransplant period. A mass or ecchymosis may be identified and initiate further work-up. The diagnosis will be confirmed by ultrasound, even though sometimes it is difficult to differentiate between hematoma or a lymphocele. Indications for intervention include mass effects of the hematoma including hydronephrosis or leg edema, deterioration of the renal function, or infection. A large symptomatic hematoma, in the author's opinion, is best treated by operative evacuation.

## Complications of the Transplant Bed

### Wound Complications

Wound complications are the most common surgical complication after kidney transplantations with an incidence rate of about 5%.[48] Wound complications include wound infection, wound dehiscence, and hernia. Wound complications may lead to a significant morbidity, increase hospital stay and cost, and even lower patient and graft survival.[48] In addition to the risk factors for routine surgical patients, transplant patients have an additional important factor, mainly immunosuppressive drugs. Steroid, Mycophenolate Mofetil, and recently Sirolimus all may contribute to delay healing and wound complications. Several studies have shown increased wound complications in Sirolimus-treated recipients.[49] In a prospective, randomized trial of Sirolimus-Mycophenolate Mofetil (MMF)-Prednisone versus Tacrolimus-MMF-Prednisone, the rates of perigraft fluid collections, superficial wound infections, and incisional hernias were significantly higher in the Sirolimus group.[50] In fact, Sirolimus and body mass index found to independently correlate with complications.[50] However, by decreasing or eliminating the loading dose of Sirolimus, no increase in wound complications were found.[49]

As with any general surgery, several steps before, during, and after the procedure may help to avoid wound complications. Treating any existing infection prior to transplant is important. If a remote infection is present it will provide a source of infecting organisms. Therefore, transplant procedures should be postponed until the infection is cleared. Kidney transplant incisions are clean contaminated wound since the bladder is opened during the procedure. Irrigating the bladder, especially in oliguric or anuric patients, is needed. During the procedure, adherence to common surgical principles such as good hemostasis, sharp anatomical dissection, gentle handling of the tissue, use of fine sutures and avoiding mass ligatures, pinpoint cautery coagulation to avoid thermal tissue destruction, and ligation of lymphatics surrounding the iliac vessels, may help decreasing wound complications.

Diagnosis of wound infection is based on clinical findings. Increasing local pain, erythema, swelling, drainage, and local tenderness are the whole marks. If the infection is determined to be superficial, opening the wound at bed site and antibiotics should be sufficient. Otherwise, the wound should be explored in the operating room to examine the fascia and deep tissue, and debridement should be performed to remove any necrotic tissue.

Diagnosis of wound dehiscence is easy; however, diagnosis of facial dehiscence without skin separation is difficult. The patient most likely will have a little swelling and increase drainage of serosanguinous fluid. The integrity of the facial layer is difficult to access by bed-site exam, and taking the patient to the operating room for wound exploration is safer. Although, the peritoneum remains intact and the kidney is placed in the extra-peritoneal space, bowel evisceration is not infrequent when facial dehiscence occurs. In obese patients with facial dehiscence, the only finding on exam may be mild ileus and wound drainage. Therefore, high suspicion and further investigation are needed to avoid missing the diagnosis.

## Lymphoceles

Lymphocele is a fluid collection, composed of lymph that lies between the inferior pole of the kidney and the bladder in the extra-peritoneal space. The development of a symptomatic lymphocele after kidney transplantation is a well-documented complication with a reported incidence of 0.6% to18%, making it one of the most common complications following renal transplant.[51,52] Leaks from the lymphatic channels can occur in two ways: disruption of lymphatics during iliac vessels dissection in the recipient, and lymphatics can be disrupted in the hilum of the kidney during graft procurement and preparation. Minimizing dissection around the iliac vessels and ligation of transected tissues is therefore recommended to decrease the incidence of lymphocele formation.

Peritransplant fluid collections are not infrequent finding following transplantation. The majority of recipients remain asymptomatic, and the fluid generally resorbs spontaneously and permanently. Clinically significant lymphoceles produce symptoms related to its mass effect. It may produce ureteral obstruction and allograft dysfunction with rising serum creatinine. It also may compress the bladder, iliac vein, and lower-extremity lymphatics causing significant ipsilateral leg edema.

Ultrasound imaging is a very easy and accurate test to diagnose the fluid collection. It also helps in accessing the presence of ureter compression and hydronephrosis. Lymphocele must be differentiated from other fluid collection such as urinoma, hematoma, and abscess prior to definite treatment. Fluid analysis for cell count and chemistries can easily confirm the diagnosis.

Therapeutic intervention is only required if lymphocele causes symptoms. Intervention includes percutaneous approach or surgical approach. Percutaneous therapies include simple drainage or closed drainage either with or without insertion of sclerosant. Percutaneous aspiration is simple, safe, and a bedside procedure but has a high recurrence rate of 50% to 80%.[53] Closed percutaneous drainage, which is most likely to be done in the angiographic suite, has less recurrence rate than the simple aspiration. Nevertheless it is still high[54] and carries also the possibility of infections. A number of sclerosants have been used as an adjunct to percutaneous drainage including povidone iodine,[51] tetracycline,[55] ethanol,[56] fibrin glue,[57] and bleomycin.[58] Although sclerosant therapy has a better success rate than simple aspirations, recurrence remains common. In addition, complications including acute renal failure[59] have been reported. Sclerosant induces a significant inflammatory reaction making a subsequent surgical intervention potentially hazardous. Doehn et al.[54] used a percutaneous pigtail drainage catheter for all symptomatic lymphocele patinets. In case of failure in resolving the fluid collection, the next step included sclerotherapy by instillation of tetracycline or ethanol into the lymphocele cavity. This approach failed in 61% of patients. In 19 patients with persistent lymphocele, a laparoscopic lymphocele fenestration was attempted with conversion in 2 patients and 2 recurrences.[54]

The surgical approach consists of creating a window between the extraperitoneal lymphocele and the peritoneal cavity so the fluid will flow freely into the absorptive surface of the peritoneum. The procedure can be done laparoscopically or by an open standard technique. The opening must be large enough not to collapse, yet not sufficiently large to allow herniation of the intestines. Some surgeons place omentum into the cavity, securing the edges with a few interrupted sutures. In a series of 700 renal transplant patients over 9 years, symptomatic lymphoceles occurred in 5% of patients. Laparoscopic drainage was performed in 74%, whereas open drainage was performed in 26% with one recurrence in each group.[60] In a multicenter retrospective study, laparoscopic lymphocele drainage was performed in 78 renal transplant recipients with symptomatic lymphoceles. Conversion to an open procedure was done in 8%, and during a mean follow-up of 27 months 6% had lymphocele recurrence.[52] It was concluded that laparoscopic procedure is an excellent alternative to the conventional open surgical approach.

## Urologic Complications

Urologic complications of kidney transplant recipients occur in approximately 5% to 10% of cases.[61–63] Although early reports documented high complication rates and mortality in these patients,[64,65] currently graft loss secondary to urologic complications is rare,[66,67] and long-term graft survival is not affected.[68] Out of 1,535 kidney transplant patients, 45 developed urine leak, and 54 developed ureter obstruction with an incidence rate of 6.5%.[61] Early recognition and appropriate treatment are important if major complications are to be avoided. Ureteral or pelvic necrosis, leading to urine leaks, and early and delayed ureteral strictures comprise the majority of clinically significant urologic complications, others being early ureteral obstruction by blood clots and vesicoureteral reflux.

### Techniques of Ureterovesical Anastmosis

Two techniques of ureterovesical anastomosis are known and widely used. The direct spatulated pull through Leadbetter-Politano technique and the external uretroneocystostomy. The first involves making a 3- to 4-cm cystotomy on the bladder dome and pulling the ureter directly through the bladder wall via a separate cystotomy. The ureter is spatulated and sutured to the bladder mucosa. The bladder is closed in layers. In the external uretroneocystostomy, a small incision is made in the bladder dome. The ureter is spatulated and sutured to the bladder mucosa. The bladder wall is closed to cover the anastomosis. In a prospective randomized study, the type of ureter anastomosis did not result in a significant difference in a urological complication rate.[69] Both techniques can be used interchangeably with acceptable rates of urological complications. The simplicity of the external uretroneocysrostomy technique has made it the technique of choice in our institution.

Using a ureteral stent during the transplant procedure remains controversial. Some transplant centers use stenting in every case, whereas others are more selective. Proposed benefits to stented anastomosis include avoidance of anastomotic tension due to continuous decompression of the ureter, prevention of ureter kinking, protection from narrowing, or postoperative luminal obstruction due to edema or external compression. Retrospective studies found a significant reduction in major urological complications by using prophylactic ureteral stents.[62,70,71] Several prospective randomized series have shown similar results.[72,74] On the other hand, stent can actually be a cause of obstruction through either occlusion or migration; the stent can erode through the lumen, causing hematuria, leading to increased risk of infection, thus exacerbating long-term stricturing of the anastomosis. The stents are also prone to breakage, especially if left for > 3 months, and may also migrate. The material used in the manufacturer of the stent has been suggested to affect its lithogenicity,[75] although the incidence of stent-associated calcification may be reduced by their early removal at 2 weeks after surgery.[74] In addition, the psychological trauma of subsequent cystoscopy and stent removal is also necessary to consider. We adopted the policy of select stenting in cases where there is concern about ureteric ischaemia or the anastmosis. In a prospective randomized study, patients were allocated intraoperatively to receive either routine stenting or stenting only in the event of technical difficulties with the anastomosis. There were no significant differences in major urological complications between both groups.[76] The author concluded that careful surgical technique with selective stenting of problematic anastomoses yields similar results.

## Urine Leak

Although technical failure can contribute to development of posttransplant urine leaks, in the majority of cases urine leaks and ureteral strictures are considered to be a result of ureteral ischemia, either arterial or venous. Urine leaks develop usually within the first week posttransplantation. Most of them occur in the distal ureter at, or in the immediate vicinity to, the neocystoureterostomy site. Calyceal or pelvic necrosis is a less common cause of urinary extravasation, and occurs in less than 1% of transplants.

Understanding of the anatomy of vascular supply to the collecting system of kidney plays an important role in prevention of these complications. The ureter has segmental blood supply, the minute arteries supplying the ureter branch from the renal, internal spermatic, hypogastric, and inferior vesical vessels.[77] Branches of all these arteries anastomose extensively in the ureteral adventitia.[78] All of these branches, except for branches of renal artery, are severed during organ procurement, whether it is a cadaveric or a living donor. Preservation of small branches of renal artery by avoidance of extensive dissection of renal pelvis and reimplantation of accessory renal arteries are of paramount importance if ureteral ischemia and consequently necrosis are to be prevented. Also keeping the ureter length to minimum may decrease the rate of complications.

Development of late ureteral strictures cannot be explained solely by ischemia. The role of other factors may be important. In a large retrospective review of 1,629 consecutive renal transplantations, it was demonstrated that donor age and delayed graft function are independently and significantly associated with ureteral necrosis. In this study, more CMV infections were identified in patients with ureteral necrosis than in the control population. However, a causative role of CMV in the development of ureteral necrosis was not a conclusion of the authors.[67]

Urine leak is a surgical emergency and requires immediate attention. Presence of urine in the wound predisposes to wound dehiscence and may cause serious infections and vascular anastomotic disruption. It usually becomes apparent within 1 week

of the transplantation if a technical error is the cause. Patients that present later, 1 to 3 weeks posttransplantation, are the result of ischemic necrosis and subsequent urine extravasation. Typical presenting symptoms of urine leak are elevated serum creatinine, decreased urine output, and possibly significant fluid drainage from the wound. If ureterovesical anastomosis is exposed to peritoneal cavity, patients may experience burning lower abdominal pain with urination and for some time after it. Analysis of draining fluid for BUN/creatinine usually confirms the diagnosis.[79] Disruption of ureterovesical anastomosis is best diagnosed by voiding cystogram. Urine leak can also be demonstrated by nephroscintigraphy, which will reveal extravasation of urine.[80,81]

Treatment of urine leak depends on location of leak, its severity, patient's condition, and physician's choice. Three options are available: prolonged drainage of the bladder with Foley catheter, percutaneous nephrostomy and stent placement, and reoperation. Minimal anastomotic leaks can be dealt with prolonged bladder drainage with Foley catheter. Major disruptions of the ureterovesical anastomosis require reoperation and remplantation of the ureter. Development of percutaneous minimally invasive radiological techniques was one of the major advances in management of posttransplantation patients, making graft loss secondary to urologic complications extremely rare.[82] Percutaneous interventions serve not only as a diagnostic but also as a therapeutic role. The superficial position of the transplanted kidney allows easy access for antegrade pyelography and percutaneous nephrostomy and stenting under ultrasound guidance. Nephroureteral stent is placed across ureterovesical junction and is left in place for 6 to 8 weeks after cessation of leakage to allow complete healing of the ureter and provide long-term patency. The success rate of this treatment approaches 90%.[82] In cases of pelvicaliceal leaks placement of nephrostomy alone is usually sufficient.

If percutaneous stenting fails to control the leak, definitive surgery is required. Leaks at the distal ureter can be treated with new ureterovesical anastomosis. More complex reconstructions are required if a significant ureteral necrosis or high leaks are demonstrated. Anastomosis with native ureter, Boari flap/psoas hitch, and vesicopyelostomy are a few of available options in these situations.[66]

## Ureteral Stricture and Obstruction

Ureter obstruction may be due to an external compression such as with large lymphocele, and treatment of the compressing mass alleviates the obstruction. Ureteric obstruction with no external compression is due to either ischemia or to anatomical and technical factors. Ureter obstruction secondary to ischemia becomes clinically evident late. Ureteral obstruction is usually discovered during evaluation of the recipient for elevated creatinine. Transplant ultrasound demonstrates some degree of hydronephrosis. Persistence of hydronephrosis after 24 to 48 hours of bladder drainage with indwelling catheter requires further diagnostic studies. Percutaneous pyelography will demonstrate stricture in most cases. The Whitaker test (measurement of a pressure gradient during standardized infusion of fluid in renal pelvis) is a helpful adjunct in equivocal cases to differentiate those patients with dilated but not obstructed collecting systems from those with true obstructions. Ureter obstruction due to anatomical or technical factors is likely to become evident in the early recovery period. Oligurea or anurea early after transplant must prompt work-up to rule out ureter obstruction. Hydronephrosis is not always present by ultrasound, and consequently absence of hydronephrosis does not rule out the diagnosis. Surgical intervention is most likely needed for early obstruction, whereas interventional radiology (balloon dilatation with or without temporary stent) is used for other cases. Percutaneous nephrostomy relieves obstruction and allows other uroradiologic interventions (stenting, balloon ureteroplasty). Balloon dilation of transplant ureteral strictures has been reported to be effective in up to 80% of cases.[83] When percutaneous dilatation and stenting fail or in case of recurrence, surgical correction is needed. The surgery will involve resection of the stenotic segment and creation of new uerterocystostomy. In case of long segment of ureter stenosis, the bladder can be mobilized to create new anastomosis even near the uretropelivic junction. However, if this is not feasible, the native ipsilateral or contralateral ureter should be used for a ureteroureterostomy.[84]

## Infectious Complications

Infections remain a major clinical issue in the field of renal transplantation, impacting on both graft and patient survival. Immunosuppressive medications, by virtue of its actions, entail an increased risk for infection. In the early period after transplantation and also after aggressive treatment of acute rejection patients are at the highest risk of all type of infections. Urinary tract infections with a variety of organisms and viral infections mainly with human cytomegalovirus (HCMV) are the most common.

### *Urinary*

Urinary Tract Infection. Urinary tract infection (UTI) is the most common infection in renal transplant recipients with incidence rate reported as high as 90%.[85,86] In the first 3 months posttransplant, the incidence of urinary tract infection is greater than 30%, and there is a relatively high rate of bacteremia and overt pyelonephritis of the allograft.[86] In an early study of 69 kidney transplant patients from 1980 to 1983, 26 patients developed 69 UTI episodes. Thirty-five episodes (50%) occurred within 2 months of the operation.[87] Thirteen patients presented with asymptomatic bacteriuria (55% of episodes).[87]

The widespread use of antibiotic prophylaxis with Cotrimoxazol reduces incidence of UTIs at post-renal-transplantation and delays the time of appearance of the first UTI episode. The risk of associated bacteraemia is close to 12%. UTI occurring late after renal transplantation was been considered "benign"; however, a recent analysis refuted this concept.[88] A retrospective cohort study of 28,942 Medicare primary renal transplant recipients from January 1, 1996, through July 31, 2000, showed that the cumulative incidence of UTI during the first 6 months after renal transplantation was 17% (equivalent for both men and women). The cumulative incidence of UTI at 3 years was 60% for women and 47% for men (p < 0.001). Late UTI was significantly associated with an increased risk of subsequent death.[89]

Risk factors for UTI include pretransplant UTI, a prolonged period of hemodialysis before transplantation, polycystic kidney disease, diabetes mellitus, postoperative bladder catheterization, allograft trauma, female sex, schistosomiasis, and technical complications associated with ureteral anastomosis.[89–91] Gram-negative bacteria are the most frequent causal agents (70%), although gram-positive, mainly *Enterococcus* and *Staphylococcus*, *Candida*, and some other exotic bacteria such as *Corynebacterium* are also potential etiological agents. The most commonly isolated bacteria were *Escherichia coli*, *Pseudomonas aeruginosa*, and *Proteus mirabilis*.

Clinical signs and symptoms are multiple ranging from asymptomatic bacteriuria to septic shock. Asymptomatic bacteriuria or elevated creatinines are not infrequently the only signs of UTI. Immunosuppressive medication can mask the symptoms of infection, making the diagnosis of infection based on the patient's symptoms problematic. Renal transplant recipients with UTI are at high risk of bacteremia and should receive antibiotic therapy when they exhibit asymptomatic bacteriuria. It is also imperative to rule out bladder dysfunction by measuring postvoiding residue in these patients. If patients are asymptomatic, treatment can be done at home. However, symptomatic patients especially with bacteremia need to receive intravenous antibiotics. In extreme patients and those with septic shock, minimizing their immunosuppression in addition to antibiotics may be needed.

### *CMV*

Human cytomegalovirus (CMV) is a member of the genus *Herpesvirus*. CMV is the single most frequent cause of septic complications in the early period after kidney transplantation, with overall incidences of 20% to 60%.[92–95] This wide range in the reported incidence of infection and disease results from the varying intensities of immunosuppression used and the frequency and methods used to detect CMV infection. HCMV infection is defined as isolation of CMV, or detection of CMV proteins or nucleic acid, in any body fluid or tissue specimen.[94] CMV disease is defined as detection of CMV accompanied by either CMV syndrome or organ involvement. CMV syndrome is characterized by fever, muscle pain, leucopenia, and/or thrombocytopenia. Organ involvement with CMV includes hepatitis, gastrointestinal ulceration, pneumonitis, retinitis, central nervous system disease, nephritis, myocarditis, cystitis, or pancreatitis.[94]

The incidence of CMV infection and disease during the first 100 days posttransplantation of 60% and 25%, respectively, can occur when no CMV prophylaxis or preemptive therapy is given.[92–94] Several risk factors have been reported. Concern has focused in the past mainly on avoiding CMV infection in the CMV D+/R– group because this group has been at greatest risk for severe "primary" infection during the first 3 months after transplantation.[96] A cohort study of 3,479 renal transplant recipients from July 1, 1994, to June 30, 1997, reported the highest incidence of CMV disease in D+/R– patients followed by D+/R+ compared to D–/R–.[97] Since D–/R– patients very seldom become infected by CMV with development of CMV disease, it seems inappropriate to use this group as a control group for D+/R– patients. The indirect effects of CMV infection on graft and patient survival have been increasingly recognized in recent years. Schnitzler et al. found from analyzing data from the U.S. Renal Data System and United Network of Organ Sharing (UNOS) that, by the third year, it is the D+/R+ group and not the D+/R– group that has the worst graft and patient survival.[98,99] It was suggested that there are multiple CMV virotypes and that the D+/R+ patients may have a double CMV exposure with reactivation of differing latent donor and recipient CMV.[98,99]

Acute rejection and recipient age are independent risk factors for CMV infection, whereas episodes of acute rejection and the serostatus group D+/R– are independent risk factors for CMV disease.[93,100] Antithymocyte globulin and muromonab-CD3 (OKT3) are associated with increased risks of CMV disease, especially when these agents are given as treatment of acute rejection as opposed to their use for induction therapy.[101] MMF has been suggested to increase the risk of CMV infection.[100,102] However, other studies have failed to show any association between maintenance MMF treatment and an increased frequency of CMV disease.[103,104] In fact, when MMF replaced Immuran as part of triple immunosuppressive medication, no significant increase in CMV was found.[104] In the European and tricontinental MMF studies,[105,106] the frequency of CMV tissue-invasive disease was higher in the MMF group given a high dose of 3 g/day.

CMV has been shown as a risk factor for acute rejection.[95,107] Lowance et al.[108] showed that rejections were reduced by 50% in the D+/R– serostatus group by valacyclovir prophylaxis following transplantation for 90 days. Similarly, in a retrospective register study by Opelz et al.,[109] an inhibitory effect of HCMV prophylaxis on acute rejection was suggested.

Three types of CMV management are known: prophylaxis, preemptive therapy, and CMV treatment. For prophylaxis, the antiviral agent is given to a patient population immediately after transplantation or during acute rejection treatment. Oral Gancyclovir, Valgancyclovir, and Acyclovir are used. In a multicenter study,[108] 208 CMV-negative recipients of a kidney from a seropositive donor and 408 CMV-positive recipients were randomly assigned to receive either 2 g of Valacyclovir or placebo orally four times daily for 90 days after transplantation. It was found that treatment with Valacyclovir reduced the incidence or delayed the onset of CMV disease in both the seronegative patients (p <0.001) and the seropositive patients (p = 0.03). Treatment with Valacyclovir also decreased the rates of CMV viremia and viruria. Furthermore, at 6 months, the rate of acute graft rejection in the seronegative group was 52% among placebo recipients and 26% among Valacyclovir recipients (p = 0.001). It was concluded that prophylactic treatment with Valacyclovir is a safe and effective way to prevent CMV disease after renal transplantation. Both oral Acyclovir and Gancyclovir have also been used for CMV prophylaxis. However, in a randomized study, oral Gancyclovir was found to be a more superior agent than Acyclovir.[110] Valganciclovir has now increasingly replaced oral Gancyclovir because of its higher bioavailability. Once-daily oral Valganciclovir was as clinically effective and well tolerated as oral Gancyclovir three times daily for CMV prevention in high-risk recipients.[111]

Hence, prophylaxis exposes a significant portion of patients who would never have developed disease to a prolonged course of costly antiviral therapy that may encourage viral drug resistance.[112] Furthermore, rather than prevent it, prophylaxis may only delay the onset of CMV disease in some patients. Therefore, preemptive strategies have been suggested. Preemptive treatment entails intensive surveillance for the first sign of CMV antigenemia, positive CMV PCR, or positive CMV viremia. Antiviral medications are then begun at the time of viral detection. The drawback of these strategies is that there is no perfect, easy, and fast test to confirm HCMV. Also, positive testing may not precede CMV disease. Monitoring and testing required compliant patients and are labor intensive. Steddon et al. performed weekly monitoring and found that the disease was universally preceded by positive tests for active viral replication in 62 renal transplant recipients who developed CMV disease.[113] In another study, weekly surveillance for plasma CMV PCR positivity for the first 3 months was performed in seronegative kidney recipients from seropositive donors.[114] Of patients who developed CMV disease, 40% had positive PCR before disease onset. Also, patients with CMV disease had worsened renal function and significantly more acute rejection at 1 year than those who did not. It was concluded that CMV surveillance strategies may cost slightly less but may have a deleterious effect on long-term outcome compared with prophylaxis.[114]

## Delayed Graft Function

Most transplant centers report a very low incidence of delayed graft function (DGF). Traditionally, DGF has been defined as acute renal failure after transplantation requiring dialysis. In live donor transplantation this is less than 5%, whereas 20% to 30% of cadaveric kidney transplant recipients suffer from DGF.[115] DGF induces significant distress and anxiety to the patient, increases susceptibility to infection, and increases hospital stay and cost. In addition, due to the kidney dysfunction, scheduled kidney biopsies with associated risks and costs are needed to monitor for rejection until kidney function recovered.

The pathogenesis of DGF is not fully understood. Donor factors, cold ischemia time, and recipient factors contribute to the problem. Donor factors include age, medical history, hemodynamic stability prior to donation, and the presence and length of cardiovascular arrest. The impact of cardiovascular arrest and consequently warm ischemia has become clear since kidneys from non-beating-heart donors are increasingly used.[116] Such kidneys will be subjected to a prolonged warm ischemia time resulting in significantly higher incidence of DGF.[116] Recipient factors include panel reactive antibodies, perioperative hemodynamic management, surgical complications, and use of nephrotoxic drugs such as early calcineurin inhibitors. In a retrospective study, DGF was significantly associated with greater weight and presence of an atheromatous disease in both donor and recipient, older age of donor, recipient American Society of Anesthesiology physical status category IV, cold ischemia time, and transplantation using the right kidney.[117]

Keeping preservation time (ie, cold ischemia time) to a minimum is important to decrease the incidence of DGF. Data from the U.S. Renal Data System were used to measure the relationships among cold ischemia time and delayed graft function in 37,216 primary cadaveric renal transplants (1985–1992). It was found that cold ischemia time was strongly associated with DGF, with a 23% increase in the risk of DGF for every 6-hour of cold ischemia (p < 0.001).[118] Even a relatively short increase in cold ischemic time can cause the second transplanted kidney of a pair from the same donor to have a significantly higher incidence of ATN, resulting in need for dialysis and prolongation of hospital stay.[115,119] Also the use of pulsatile perfusion preservation has been shown to decrease the incidence of DGF compared to cold storage.[120,121]

Previous retrospective or nonrandomized studies have suggested that intraoperative administration of polyclonal antithymocyte preparations may reduce the incidence of DGF, possibly by decreasing ischemia-reperfusion injury. A prospective randomized study has shown that intraoperative thymoglobulin administration was associated with significantly less DGF than postoperative administration in adult cadaveric renal transplant recipients.[122]

It is of paramount importance in approaching patients to distinguish DGF from hyperacute rejection, urological complications such as ureteral obstruction or distal ureter necrosis, and vascular complications. Radioactive renal scan or Doppler ultrasound are good tests especially to evaluate blood flow and kidney perfusion. Ureter obstruction immediately after transplant is difficult to diagnose since it is acute and no hydronephrosis will be shown. If tests showed good kidney perfusion, a kidney biopsy is needed.

The management of posttransplant DGF consists of general supportive measures, intermittent dialysis, avoidance of nephrotoxic medications, and close monitoring. Patient management can be done at home; however, it requires a good cooperative patient and his family as well as close involvement by the transplant team, the nephrologists, and the dialysis units. Weekly kidney biopsies are obtained until kidney function has recovered.

The effect of DGF on long-term outcome is somewhat controversial. Although some studies showed no impact of DGF on long-term kidney function,[123] most have shown that DGF has a negative impact on the long-term outcome of cadaveric transplants.[118,124–26] Most patients experiencing DGF will regain an adequate renal function; however, tubular dysfunction may persist. The clinical manifestations of persistent tubular dysfunction include hypercalemia, renal tubular acidosis, salt-wasting nephropathy, and hypertension.[127]

# References

1. Plainfosse MC, Calonge VM, Beyloune-Mainardi C, Glotz D, Duboust A. Vascular complications in the adult kidney transplant recipient. *J Clin Ultrasound* 1992;20:517–527.

2. Osman Y, Shokeir A, Ali-el-Dein B, et al. Vascular complications after live donor renal transplantation: study of risk factors and effects on graft and patient survival. *J Urol* 2003;169:859–862.

3. Vidne BA, Leapman SB, Butt KM, Kountz SL. Vascular complications in human transplantation. *Surgery* 1976;79:77–81.

4. Matas AJ, Humar A, Gillingham KJ. Five preventable causes of kidney graft loss in the 1990s: A single center analysis. *Kidney Int* 2002;62: 704–714.

5. Bakir N, Sluiter WJ, Ploeg RJ. Primary renal graft thrombosis. *Nephrol Dial Transplant* 1996;11:140–147.

6. Ojo OA, Hanson JA, Wolfe RA. Dialysis modality and the risk of allograft thrombosis in adult renal transplant recipients. *Kidney Int* 1999; 55:1952–1960.

7. Penny MJ, Nankivell BJ, Disney APS. Renal graft thrombosis. *Transplantation* 1994;58:565–569.

8. Mazzucchi E, Souza AA, Nahas WC, et al. Surgical complications after renal transplantation in grafts with multiple arteries. *Int Braz J Urol* 2005;31:125–130.

9. Benedetti E, Troppmann C, Gillingham K, et al. Short- and long-term outcomes of kidney transplants with multiple renal arteries. *Ann Surg* 1995;221:406–414.

10. Irish A. Hypercoagulability in renal transplant recipients. Identifying patients at risk of renal allograft thrombosis and evaluating strategies for prevention. *Am J Cardiovasc Drugs* 2004;4:139–149.

11. Vaidya S, Sellers R, Kimball P, et al. Frequency, potential risk and therapeutic intervention in end-stage renal disease patients with antiphospholipid antibody syndrome: a multicenter study. *Transplantation* 2000;69:1348–1352.

12. Baker LRI, Tucker B, Kovacs IB. Enhanced in vitro hemostasis ands reduced thrombolysis in cyclosporine-treated renal transplant recipients. *Transplantation* 1990;49:905–909.

13. Carlsen E, Prydz H. Enhancement of procoagulant activity in stimulated mononuclear blood cells and monocytes by cyclosporine. Transplantation 1987; 43: 543–548.

14. Fishman SJ, Wylonis LJ, Glickman JD, Cook JJ, Warsaw DS, Fisher CA, Jorkasky DJ, Niewiarowski S, Addonizio VP. Cyclosporin A augments human platelet sensitivity to aggregating agents by increasing fibrinogen receptor availability. *Surg Res* 1991;51:93–98.

15. Bombeli T, Muller M, Straub PW, Haeberli A. Cyclosporine-induced detachment of vascular endothelial cells initiates the intrinsic coagulation system in plasma and whole blood. *J Lab Clin Med* 1996;127:621–634.

16. Gruber SA, Chavers B, Payne WD, et al. Allograft renal vascular thrombosis—lack of increase with cyclosporine immunosuppression. *Transplantation* 1989;47 475–478.

17. Abramowicz D, Pradier O, Marchant A, Florquin S, De Pauw L, Vereerstraeten P, Kinnaert P, Vanherweghem JL, Goldman M. Induction of thromboses within renal grafts by high-dose prophylactic OKT3. *Lancet* 1992;339:777–778.

18. Louridas G, Botha JR, Meyers AM. Vascular complications of renal transplantation. The Johannesburg experience. *Clin Transplant* 1987: 240–245.

19. Broyer M, Gagnadoux MF, Sierro A, et al. Prevention of vascular thromboses after renal transplantation using low molecular weight heparin. *Ann Pediatr (Paris)* 1991;38:397–399.

20. Alkhunaizi AM, Olyaei AJ, Barry JM, et al. Efficacy and safety of low molecular weight heparin in renal transplantation. *Transplantation* 1998;66:533–534.

21. Friedman GS, Meier-Kriesche HU, Kaplan B, et al. Hypercoagulable states in renal transplant candidates: impact of anticoagulation upon incidence of renal allograft thrombosis. *Transplantation* 2001;72:1073–1078.

22. Ubhi CS, Lam FT, Mavor AI, Giles GR. Subcutaneous heparin therapy for cyclosporine-immunosuppressed renal allograft recipients. *Transplantation* 1989;48:886–887.

23. Morrissey PE, Ramirez PJ, Gohh RY, et al. Management of thrombophilia in renal transplant patients. *Am J Transplant* 2002;2:872–876.

24. Robertson AJ, Nargund V, Gray DW, Morris PJ. Low dose aspirin as prophylaxis against renal-vein thrombosis in renal-transplant recipients. *Nephrol Dial Transplant* 2000;15:1865–1868.

25. Murphy GJ, Taha R, Windmill DC, Metcalfe M, Nicholson ML. Influence of aspirin on early allograft thrombosis and chronic allograft nephropathy following renal transplantation. *Br J Surg* 2001;88:261–266.

26. Pherwani AD, Winter PC, McNamee PT, et al. Is screening for factor V Leiden and prothrombin G20210A mutations in renal transplantation worthwhile? Results of a large single-center U.K. study. *Transplantation* 2003;76:603–605.

27. Andrassy J, Zeier M, Andrassy K. Do we need screening for thrombophilia prior to kidney transplantation? *Nephrol Dial Transplant* 2004;19:64–68.

28. Buturovic-Ponikvar J. Renal transplant artery stenosis. *Nephrol Dial Transplant* 2003;18:v74–77.

29. Lacombe M. Arterial complications after renal transplantation. *Bull Acad Natl Med* 2004;188:767–778.

30. Fontaine E, Barthelemy Y, Gagnadoux MF, et al. Review of 72 renal artery stenoses in a series of 715 kidney transplantations in children. *Prog Urol* 1994;4:193–205.

31. Fung LC, McLorie GA, Khoury AE, Churchill BM. Donor aortic cuff reduces the rate of anastomotic arterial stenosis in pediatric renal transplantation. *J Urol* 1995;154: 909–913.

32. Bruno S, Remuzzi G, Ruggenenti P. Transplant renal artery stenosis. *J Am Soc Nephrol* 2004;15:134–141.

33. Wong W, Fynn SP, Higgings RM, et al. Transplant renal artery stenosis in 77 patients: does it have an immunological cause? *Transplantation* 61: 1996;215–219.

34. Fervenza FC, Lafayette RA, Alfrey EJ, Petersen J. Renal artery stenosis in kidney transplants. *Am J Kidney Dis* 1998;31:142–148.

35. Chua GC, Snowden S, Patel U. Kinks of the transplant renal artery without accompanying intraarterial pressure gradient do not require correction: five-year outcome study. *Cardiovasc Intervent Radiol* 2004; 27:643–650.

36. Beecroft JR, Rajan DK, Clark TW, Robinette M, Stavropoulos SW. Transplant renal artery stenosis: outcome after percutaneous intervention. *J Vasc Interv Radiol* 2004;15:1407–1413.

37. Englesbe MJ, Punch JD, Armstrong DR, et al. Single-center study of technical graft loss in 714 consecutive renal transplants. *Transplantation* 2004;78:623–626.

38. Humar A, Key N, Ramcharan T, et al. Kidney retransplants after initial graft loss to vascular thrombosis. *Clin Transplant* 2001;15:6–10.

39. Rerolle JP, Antoine C, Raynaud A, et al. Successful endoluminal thromboaspiration of renal graft venous thrombosis. *Transpl Int* 2000; 13: 82–86.

40. Busi N, Capocasale E, Mazzoni MP, et al. Spontaneous renal allograft rupture without acute rejection. *Acta Biomed Ateneo Parmense* 2004; 75:131–133.

41. Brown ED, Chen MY, Wolfffian NT, Ott DJ, Watson NE Jr. Complications of renal transplantation: evaluation with US and radionuclide imaging. *RadioGraphics* 2000;20: 607–622. Medline.

42. Takahashi M, Humke U, Girndt M, Kramann B, Uder M. Early posttransplantation renal allograft perfusion failure due to dissection:

diagnosis and interventional treatment. *AJR Am J Roentgenol* 2003; 180: 759–763.

43. Kazory A, Ducloux D, Coaquette A, Manzoni P, Chalopin JM. Cytomegalovirus-associated venous thromboembolism in renal transplant recipients: a report of 7 cases. *Transplantation* 2004;77:597–599.

44. Hausmann MJ, Vorobiov M, Zlotnik M, Rogachev B, Tomer A. Increased coagulation factor levels leading to allograft renal vein thrombosis. *Clin Nephrol* 2004;61:222–224.

45. Ramirez PJ, Gohh RY, Kestin A, Monaco AP, Morrissey PE. Renal allograft loss due to proximal extension of ileofemoral deep venous thrombosis. Clin Transplant. 2002; 16: 310–313.

46. Du Buf-Vereijken PW, Hilbrands LB, Wetzels JF. Partial renal vein thrombosis in a kidney transplant: management by streptokinase and heparin. *Nephrol Dial Transplant* 1998;13:499–502.

47. Garrido J, Labrador PJ, Lerma L, et al. Vascular Aspergillus infection in two recipients of kidneys from the same donor. *Nefrologia* 2004; 24:30–34.

48. Humar A, Ramcharan T, Denny R, et al. Are wound complications after a kidney transplant more common with modern immunosuppression? *Transplantation* 2001;72:1920–1923.

49. Kandaswamy R, Melancon JK, Dunn T, et al. A prospective randomized trial of steroid-free maintenance regimens in kidney transplant recipients—an interim analysis. *Am J Transplant* 2005;5:1529–1536.

50. Dean PG, Lund WJ, Larson TS, et al. Wound-healing complications after kidney transplantation: a prospective, randomized comparison of sirolimus and tacrolimus. *Transplantation* 2004;77:1555–1561.

51. Burgos FJ, Teruel JL, Mayayo T, et al. Diagnosis and management of lymphoceles after renal transplantation. *Br J Urol* 1988;61:289–293.

52. Hsu TH, Gill IS, Grune MT, et al. Laparoscopic lymphocelectomy: a multi-institutional analysis. *J Urol* 2000;163:1096–1098.

53. Teruel JL, Escobar EM, Quereda C, Mayayo T, Ortuno J. A simple and safe method for management of lymphocele after renal transplantation. *J Urol* 1983;130:1058–1059.

54. Doehn C, Fornara P, Fricke L, Jocham D. Laparoscopic fenestration of posttransplant lymphoceles. *Surg Endosc* 2002;16:690–695.

55. Pollak R, Veremis SA, Maddux MS, Mozes MF. The natural history of and therapy for perirenal fluid collections following renal transplantation. *J Urol* 1988;140:16–20.

56. Kuzuhara K, Inoue S, Dobashi Y, et al. Ethanol ablation of lymphocele after renal transplantation: a minimally invasive approach. *Transplant Proc* 1997;29:147–150.

57. Lange V, Schardey HM, Meyer G, et al. Laparoscopic deroofing of post-transplant lymphoceles. *Transplant Int* 1994;7:140–143.

58. Kerlan Jr RK, LaBerge JM, Gordon RL, Ring EJ. Bleomycin sclerosis of pelvic lymphoceles. *J Vasc Interv Radiol* 1997;8:885–887.

59. Manfro RC, Comerlato L, Berdichevski RH, et al. Nephrotoxic acute renal failure in a renal transplant patient with recurrent lymphocele treated with povidone-iodine irrigation. *Am J Kidney Dis* 2002;40:655–657.

60. Bailey SH, Mone MC, Holman JM, Nelson EW. Laparoscopic treatment of post renal transplant lymphoceles. *Surg Endosc* 2003;17:1896–1899.

61. Streeter EH, Little DM, Cranston DW, Morris PJ. The urological complications of renal transplantation: a series of 1535 patients. *BJU Int* 2002;90:627–634.

62. Mangus R, Haag B. Stented vs. nonstented extravesical ureteroneocystostomy in renal transplantation: a metaanalysis. *Am J Transplant* 2004;4:1889–1896.

63. Kocak T, Nane I, Ander H, et al. Urological and surgical complications in 362 consecutive living related donor kidney transplantations. *Urol Int* 2004;72:252–256.

64. Starzl TE, Groth CG, Putnam CW, et al. Urological complications in 216 human recipients of renal transplants. *Ann Surg* 1970;172:1–22.

65. Belzer FO, Kountz SL, Najarian JS, Tanagho EA, Hinman F. Prevention of urological complications after renal allotransplantation. *Arch Surg* 1970;101:449–452.

66. Odland MD. Surgical technique/post-transplant surgical complications. *Surg Clin North Am* 1998;78:55–60.

67. Karam G, Maillet F, Parant S, Soulillou JP, Giral Classe M. Ureteral necrosis after kidney transplantation: risk factors and impact on graft and patient survival. *Transplantation* 2004;78:725–729

68. Van Roijen JH, Kirkels WJ, Zietse R, et al. Long-term graft survival after urological complications of 695 kidney transplantations. *J Urol* 2001;165:1884–1887.

69. Pleass HCC, Clark KR, Rigg KM, et al. Urologic Complications after renal transplantation: A prospective randomized trail comparing different techniques of ureteric anastomosis and the use of prophylactic Ureteric stents. *Transplant Proc*1995;27:1091–1092.

70. Nicol DL, P'Ng K, Hardie DR, Wall DR, Hardie IR. Routine use of indwelling ureteral stents in renal transplantation. *J Urol* 1993; 150:1375–1379.

71. Lin LC, Bewick M, Koffman CG. Primary use of a double J silicone ureteric stent in renal transplantation. *Br J Urol* 1993;72:697–701.

72. Benoit G, Blanchet P, Eschwege P, et al. Insertion of a double pigtail ureteral stent for the prevention of urological complications in renal transplantation: a prospective randomized study. J Urol 1996;156: 881–884.

73. Bassiri A, Amiransari B, Yazdani M, Sesavar Y, Gol S. Renal transplantation using ureteral stents. *Transplant Proc* 1995;27:2593–2594.

74. Kumar A, Verma BS, Srivastava A, et al. Evaluation of the urological complications of living related renal transplantation at a single center during the last 10 years: impact of the Double-J stent. *J Urol* 2000;164:657–660.

75. Kohri K, Yamate T, Amasaki N, et al. Characteristics and usage of different ureteral stent catheters. *Urol Int* 1991;47:131–137.

76. Dominguez J, Clase CM, Mahalati K, et al. Is routine ureteric stenting needed in kidney transplantation? A randomized trial. *Transplantation* 2000;70:597–601.

77. Lewis WH, ed. *Gray's Anatomy of the Human Body.* Twentieth edition. XI. Splanchnology: 3b. 2. The Ureters.

78. Daniel O, Shackman R. The blood supply of the human ureter in relation to ureterocolic anastomosis. *Br J Urol* 1952;24:334–343.

79. Singh S, Aoki S, Mitra S, Berman LB. Ascites. An unusual manifestation of urinary leak in a renal allograft recipient. *JAMA* 1973;226:777–778.

80. Goodear M, Barratt L, Wycherley A. Intraperitoneal urine leak in a patient with a renal transplant on Tc–99m MAG3 imaging. *Clin Nucl Med* 1998;23:789–90.

81. Rosenberg RJ, Schweizer RT, Spencer RP. Ureteral leak after renal transplantation. *Clin Nucl Med* 1999;24:440–442.

82. Matalon TA, Thompson MJ, Patel SK, et al. Percutaneous treatment of urine leaks in renal transplantation patients. *Radiology* 1990;174:1049–1051.

83. Voegeli DR, Crummy AB, McDermott JC, Jensen SR. Percutaneous dilation of ureteral strictures in renal transplant patients. *Radiology* 1988;169:185–188.

84. Saporta F, Salomon L, Amsellem D, Patard JJ, Hozneck A, Colombel M, Chopin D, Abbou C. Results of pyeloureteral anastomoses onto the native ureter after complication of ureterovesical anastomosis in kidney transplantation. *Prog Urol* 1999;9:47–51.

85. Tolkoff–Rubin NE, Rubin RH. Urinary tract infection in the immunocompromised host. Lessons from kidney transplantation and the AIDS epidemic. *Infect Dis Clin North Am* 1997;11:707.

86. Krieger JN, Tapia L, Stubenbord WT, Stenzel KH, Rubin AL. Urinary infection in kidney transplantation. *Urology* 1977; 9:130.

87. Alexopoulos E, Memmos D, Sakellariou G, et al. Urinary tract infections after renal transplantation. *Drugs Exp Clin Res* 1985;11:101–105.

88. Abbott KC, Swanson SJ, Richter ER, et al. Late urinary tract infection after renal transplantation in the United States. *Am J Kidney Dis* 2004;44:353–362.

89. Mahmoud KM, Sobh MA, El-Agroudy AE, et al. Impact of schistosomiasis on patient and graft outcome after renal transplantation: 10 years' follow–up. *Nephrol Dial Transplant* 2001;16:2214.

90. Munoz P. Management of urinary tract infections and lymphocele in renal transplant recipients. *Clin Infect Dis* 2001;33:S53.

91. Byrd LH, Tapia L, Cheigh JS, et al. Association between Streptococcus faecalis urinary infections and graft rejection in kidney transplantation. *Lancet* 1978;2:1167.

92. Yang CW, Kim YO, Kim YS, et al. Clinical course of cytomegalovirus (CMV) viremia with and without ganciclovir treatment in CMV–seropositive kidney transplant recipients. Longitudinal follow–up of CMV pp65 antigenemia assay. *Am J Nephrol* 1998;18:373–378.

93. Sagedal S, Nordal KP, Hartmann A, Degre M, Holter E, Foss A, Osnes K, Leivestad T, Fauchald P, Rollag H. A prospective study of the natural course of cytomegalovirus infection and disease in renal allograft recipients. *Transplantation* 2000;70:1166–1174.

94. Sai IG, Patel R. New strategies for prevention and therapy of cytomegalovirus infection and disease in solid–organ transplant recipients. *Clin Microbiol Rev* 2000;13:83–121.

95. Toupance O, Bouedjoro–Camus MC, Carquin J, Novella JL, Lavaud S, Wynckel A, Jolly D, Chanard J. Cytomegalovirus–related disease and risk of acute rejection in renal transplant recipients: a cohort study with case–control analyses. *Transplant Int* 2000;13: 413–419.

96. Rubin RH, Kemmerly SA, Conti D, et al. Prevention of primary cytomegalovirus disease in organ transplant recipients with oral ganciclovir or oral acyclovir prophylaxis. *Transplant Infect Dis* 2000;2:112–117.

97. Abbott KC, Hypolite IO, Viola R, et al. Hospitalizations for cytomegalovirus disease after renal transplantation in the United States. *Ann Epidemiol* 2002;12:402–409.

98. Schnitzler MA, Woodward RS, Brennan DC, et al. The effects of cytomegalovirus serology on graft and recipient survival in cadaveric renal transplantation: Implications for organ allocation. *Am J Kidney Dis* 1997;29:428–434.

99. Schnitzler MA, Woodward RS, Brennan DC, et al. Impact of cytomegalovirus serology on graft survival in living related kidney transplantation: Implications for donor selection. *Surgery* 1997;121:563–568.

100. Sarmiento JM, Munn SR, Paya CV, Velosa JA, Nguyen JH. Is cytomegalovirus infection related to mycophenolate mofetil after kidney transplantation? A case–control study. *Clin Transplant* 1998;12: 371–374.

101. Kusne S, Shapiro R, Fung J. Prevention and treatment of cytomegalovirus infection in organ transplant recipients. *Transpl Infect Dis* 1999;1:187–203.

102. ter Meulen CG, Wetzels JF, Hilbrands LB. The influence of mycophenolate mofetil on the incidence and severity of primary cytomegalovirus infections and disease after renal transplantation. *Nephrol Dial Transplant* 2000;15:711–714.

103. Giral M, Nguyen JM, Daguin P, et al. Mycophenolate mofetil does not modify the incidence of cytomegalovirus (CMV) disease after kidney transplantation but prevents CMV–induced chronic graft dysfunction. *J Am Soc Nephrol* 2001;12:1758–1763.

104. Sarmiento JM, Dockrell DH, Schwab TR, Munn SR, Paya CV. Mycophenolate mofetil increases cytomegalovirus invasive organ disease in renal transplant patients. *Clin Transplant* 2000;14:136–138.

105. European Mycophenolate Mofetil Cooperative Study Group. Placebo–controlled study of mycophenolate mofetil combined with cyclosporin and corticosteroids for prevention of acute rejection. European Mycophenolate Mofetil Cooperative Study Group. *Lancet* 1995;345: 1321–1325.

106. The tricontinental Mycophenolate Mofetil Renal Transplant Study Group. A blinded, randomized clinical trial of mycophenolate mofetil for the prevention of acute rejection in cadaveric renal transplantation. The Tricontinental Mycophenolate Mofetil Renal Transplantation Study Group. *Transplantation* 1996;61:1029–1037.

107. Sagedal S, Hartmann A, Rollag H. The impact of early cytomegalovirus infection and disease in renal transplant recipients. *Clin Microbiol Infect* 2005;11:518–530.

108. Lowance D, Neumayer HH, Legendre CM, et al. Valacyclovir for the prevention of cytomegalovirus disease after renal transplantation. International Valacyclovir Cytomegalovirus Prophylaxis Transplantation Study Group. *N Engl J Med* 1999;340:1462–1470.

109. Opelz G, Dohler B, Ruhenstroth A. Cytomegalovirus prophylaxis and graft outcome in solid organ transplantation: a collaborative transplant study report. *Am J Transplant* 2004;4:928–936.

110. Flechner SM, Avery RK, Fisher R, et al. A randomized prospective controlled trial of oral acyclovir versus oral ganciclovir for cytomegalovirus prophylaxis in high–risk kidney transplant recipients. *Transplantation* 1998;66:1682–1688.

111. Paya C, Humar A, Dominguez E, et al. Efficacy and safety of valganciclovir vs. oral ganciclovir for prevention of cytomegalovirus disease in solid organ transplant recipients. *Am J Transplant* 2004;4:611–620.

112. Limaye AP, Corey L, Koelle DM, Davis CL, Boeckh M. Emergence of ganciclovir–resistant cytomegalovirus disease among recipients of solid–organ transplants. *Lancet* 2000;356:645–649.

113. Steddon SJ, Ball EA, Aitken C, et al. CMV prophylaxis: infection or disease as target? [abstract]. *J Am Soc Nephrol* 1999;10:766A.

114. Geddes CC, Church CC, Collidge T, et al. Management of cytomegalovirus infection by weekly surveillance after renal transplant: analysis of cost, rejection and renal function. *Nephrol Dial Transplant* 2003;18:1891–1898.

115. Giblin L, O'Kelly P, Little D, et al. A comparison of long-term graft survival rates between the first and second donor kidney transplanted the effect of a longer cold ischaemic time for the second kidney. *AJT* 2005; 5: 1071–1075.

116. Gok MA, Asher JF, Shenton BK, et al. Graft function after kidney transplantation from non–heartbeating donors according to maastricht category. *J Urol* 2004;172:2331–2334.

117. Lechevallier E, Dussol B, Luccioni A, et al. Posttransplantation acute tubular necrosis: risk factors and implications for graft survival. *Am J Kidney Dis* 1998;32:984–991.

118. Ojo AO, Wolfe RA, Held PJ, Port FK, Schmouder RL. Delayed graft function: Risk factors and implications for renal allograft survival. *Transplantation* 1997;63:968–974.

119. Tandon V, Botha JF, Banks J, et al. A tale of two kidneys—how long can a kidney transplant wait? *Clin Transplant* 2000;14:189–192.

120. Schold JD, Kaplan B, Howard RJ, et al. Are we frozen in time? Analysis of the utilization and efficacy of pulsatile perfusion in renal transplantation. *Am J Transplant* 2005;5:1681–1688.

121. Burdick JF, Rosendale JD, McBride MA, Kauffman HM, Bennett LE. National impact of pulsatile perfusion on cadaveric kidney transplantation. *Transplantation* 1997;64:1730–1733.

122. Goggins WC, Pascual MA, Powelson JA, et al. A prospective, randomized, clinical trial of intraoperative versus postoperative Thymoglobulin in adult cadaveric renal transplant recipients. *Transplantation* 2003; 76:798–802.

123. Rao KV, Anderson RC. Delayed graft function has no detrimental effect on short-term or long-term outcome of cadaveric renal transplantation. *Transplant Proc* 1995;17:2818.

124. Sanfilippo F, Vaughn WK, Spees EK, The detrimental effect of delayed graft function in cadaver donor renal transplantation. *Transplantation* 1984;38:643–648.

125. Cecka JM, Cho YW, Terasaki PI. Analysis of the UNOS scientific renal transplant registry at three years-early events affecting transplant success. *Transplantation* 1992;53:59–64.

126. Yokoyama I, Uchida K, Kobayashi T, et al. Effects of prolonoged delayed graft function on long-term out come in cadaver kidney transplantation. *Clin Transplant* 1994;8:101–106.

127. Heering P, Degenhardt S, Grabeuser B. Tubular dysfunction following renal transplantation. *Nephron* 1996;74:501–511.

## 16.7  IMMUNOSUPPRESSIVE THERAPY

*David Axelrod, MD, MBA,*
*Dixon B. Kaufman, MD, PhD*

### INTRODUCTION

Although the successful transplantation of a live donor kidney between brothers in Boston in 1954 marked the beginning of clinical transplantation, widespread use of this life-saving therapy awaited the introduction of effective immunosuppressive medications.[1] Initially

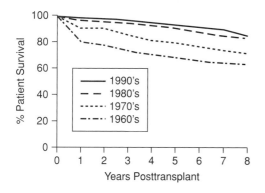

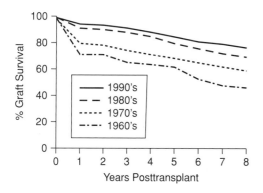

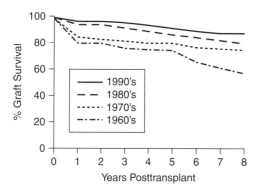

**FIGURE 16.7-1**

Improving outcome following living donation. Actuarial patient and graft survival rates by decade for primary living donor transplants: (A) patient survival, (B) graft survival, (C) death-censored graft survival. Used with permission. Matas AJ, Payne WD, Sutherland DE, et al. 2,500 living donor kidney transplants: a single-center experience. *Ann Surg* 2001;Aug; 234(2):149-64.

limited to monozygotic identical twins, over the past 5 decades, transplantation immunosuppression has advanced dramatically to the point that nonrelated, non-human-leukocyte-antigen- (HLA)- matched donor and recipient pairs can be transplanted with the expectation of 80% 5-year graft survival (Figure 16.7-1). Given the highly effective nature of currently available therapies, the goal of immunosuppressive regiments is no longer merely short-term graft survival. Although it is vital continue to prevent acute cellular rejection, physicians caring for these patients must also attempt to minimize the incidence of chronic allograft nephropathy, reduce the incidence of systemic side effects, and maximize recipient quality of life.

This chapter considers the pharmacology of immunosuppression in recipients of live donor kidney transplants. Beginning with an historical overview, currently available medications for maintenance therapy and induction treatment are reviewed in the context of standard three-drug maintenance approach. Next, results with innovative steroid or calcineurin-sparing regiments will be examined. Finally, special cases including HLA-identical transplantation and pediatric transplantation are discussed.

## HISTORY AND DEVELOPMENT OF IMMUNOSUPPRESSION

The surgical principles needed to complete a renal transplant were described as early as 1905, when Alexis Carrell[2] achieved long-term survival in a canine model of renal transplantation following bilateral nephrectomy. However, until Joseph Murray's successful transplant between identical twins in 1954, virtually all attempts at clinical transplant were doomed to acute or hyperacute rejection.[1] Aside from the success with live monozygotic twin donors, transplantation remained a limited therapy until the early experiments with whole-body irradiation. In 1958, Harvard researchers successfully transplanted a kidney from a patient's fraternal twin using irradiation and bone marrow transplant. Unfortunately, whole-body irradiation was associated with a high level of morbidity and mortality. As a result, it was not widely applied.

Discovery of the immunosuppressive effects of 6-mercaptopurine and its derivative azathioprine (AZA) revolutionized transplantation, and made successful cadaveric organ transplant possible for the first time in 1962.[3] With the addition of steroids to the armamentarium for pharmacologic immunosuppression, renal transplantation had, by the 1970s, become a practical therapy for end-stage renal disease. However, even with this steroid-based regimen, 50% 1-year graft survival remained the norm for cadaveric grafts, although better results were achieved with grafts from living donors. [4]

The success of renal transplantation was subsequently advanced by two important innovations. First was the clinical application of lymphocyte depleting antibody, initially described in kidney and liver transplantation in 1967 by Starzl et al. In 1968, researchers at the University of Minnesota catalyzed the widespread use of "induction" therapy with Minnesota antilymphocyte globulin (MALG), a polyclonal antilymphocyte preparation made from vaccinated horses.[4] With a 2-week course of MALG, 1-year graft survival rates of 79% were achieved with kidneys from live donors. A decade later, Sir Roy Calne described his success with a potent new maintenance medication, cyclosporine A (CsA).[5] Use of CsA maintenance therapy in combination with prednisone improved the 1-year survival rate of transplants from live donors from 72% to 90%.[4] After the introduction of CsA, triple-drug therapy with AZA, CsA, and prednisone was established as the standard of care with selective use of induction therapy.

The 1990s saw the rapid introduction of new compounds such as tacrolimus (Prograf®, Astellas Corporation, Chicago IL), sirolimus (Rapamune®, Wyeth Pharmaceuticals, Philadelphia, PA), and mycophenolate mofetil (MMF; CellCept®, Roche, Nutley, NJ) for maintenance therapy, as well as rabbit antithymocyte globulin (Thymoglobulin®, Genzyme, Cambridge, MA),

Muromonab-CD3 (Orthoclone OKT3®, Ortho Biotech, Raritan, NJ), and the IL-2 receptor inhibitors for induction treatment: daclizumab (Zenapax®, Roche Pharmaceuticals, Nutley, New Jersey) and basiliximab (Simulect®, Novartis, East Hanover, NJ). The immunosuppressive landscape, which was relatively uniform in the 1980s, became complex with new immunosuppressive options that could be targeted to select recipient populations. The remainder of this chapter considers the available options for immunosuppression including their established benefits and toxicities and, where available, results in the living donor transplant population.

## PHARMACOLOGY OF IMMUNOSUPPRESSION

Prolonged graft survival requires a careful balance of immunosuppressive medications to reduce or eliminate acute cellular rejection without rendering the recipient susceptible to infection or malignancy. Advances in immunosuppressive therapy have resulted in a shift from nonspecific global suppression of the immune system with corticosteroids and external beam radiation to targeted therapy that primarily affects the immune effecter cells. Available agents interfere with T-cell activation, proliferation, and cell-signaling pathways, resulting in a specific reduction in cellular immunity. Immunosuppression is generally maximal at the time of transplant, when the risk of rejection is highest, and then decreases over time as the recipient's immune system adapts to the allograft, resulting in a state of partial unresponsiveness.[6] The pharmacology of available agents for maintenance (Table 16.7-1) and induction (Table 16.7-2) agents is considered next, whereas the subsequent sections examine clinical results in living donor renal transplant recipients.

**TABLE 16.7-2**

## INDUCTION AGENTS

| Name | Target | Mechanism | Toxicity |
|------|--------|-----------|----------|
| Rabbit antithymocyte globulin | Polyclonal anti-T-cell | Complement and Fc-dependent cell lysis | Cytokine release syndrome, CMV, EBV, PTLD, serum sickness |
| Muromonab-CD3 | CD-3 protein on T cell | Opsonization of T cells with splenic/hepatic clearance | Cytokine release syndrome, CMV, EBV, PTLD |
| Daclizumab | CD-25 (IL-2 receptor) | Blocks IL-2-stimulated T-cell proliferation | None |
| Basiliximab | CD-25 (IL-2 receptor) | Blocks IL-2-stimulated T-cell proliferation | None |
| Alemtuzamab | CD-52 | Opsonization and clearance with prolonged lymphopenia | Cytokine release syndrome, rash, pulmonary edema |

## Corticosteroids

Among the first agents used in transplantation, corticosteroids have remained a cornerstone of maintenance therapy as well as the first line therapy for the treatment of acute rejection. Corticosteroids

**TABLE 16.7-1**

## MAINTENANCE IMMUNOSUPPRESSION AGENTS

| Name | Class | Therapeutic level | Toxicities |
|------|-------|-------------------|------------|
| Prednisone | Corticosteroids | N/A | Cosmetic: hirsutism, weight gain, acne, easy bruising, buffalo hump, moon facies<br><br>Metabolic: hyperlipidemia, diabetes mellitus, osteopenia, growth retardation<br><br>Cardiovascular: accelerated atherosclerosis, hypertension<br><br>Other: emotional lability, poor wound healing |
| Cyclosporine | Calcineurin inhibitor | 0–6 mos: 200–250 ng/mL > 6 mos: 150–200 ng/mL | Nephrotoxicity, hypertension, neurotoxicity, hypertrichosis, gingival hyperplasia, HUS |
| Tacrolimus | Calcineurin inhibitor | 5–15 ng/mL | Neurotoxicity, nephrotoxicity, diabetes mellitus, hemolytic uremic syndrome, Possible increased risk of PTLD |
| MMF | Antiproliferative | 1.8–4 µg/mL | Diarrhea, abdominal pain, bone marrow suppression |
| Sirolimus | TOR inhibitor | 10–14 ng/mL | Hypertriglyceridemia, mouth sores, poor wound healing, thrombocytopenia |

are lipophylic molecules that easily cross cell membranes and bind to glucocorticoid receptors (GR) within the cell cytoplasm. The GR–ligand complex moves to the cell nucleus, where it can interact with glucocorticoid response elements (GRE) in cellular DNA. Interaction with GREs appears to decrease cytokine gene expression via inhibitory effects on activator protein-1 (AP-1) and nuclear factor kB (NFkB). Following administration, corticosteroids contribute to immune nonresponsiveness due to a brief period of lymphopenia resulting from redistribution of lymphocytes into the bone marrow and other cellular compartments; changes in the expression of endothelial adhesion molecules; and lysis of immature T cells and activated T lymphocytes through apoptosis. Outside of the lymphoid system, corticosteroids have numerous effects on the function of neutrophils and macrophages. Glucorticoids inhibit neutrophil adhesion and extravasation, leading to a relative degree of neutrophilia. These drugs inhibit macrophage differentiation, decreasing class II HLA expression on activated macrophages, and also impair the release of immunomodulatory cytokines.

In general, corticosteroids (methylprednisolone) are administered intravenously at high dosages (500 to 1,000 mg) at the time of transplantation to decrease the risk of acute rejection. Subsequently, in the absence of acute rejection, the dosage is slowly tapered off using orally administered prednisone to a daily dose of 5 mg. In patients with mild to moderate rejection, pulse steroids (3–5 days of 500–1,000 mg of methylprednisolone) may be used in an attempt to reverse rejection. Furthermore, to offset the potential adrenal suppression associated with chronic steroid administration, patients undergoing operations or severe illness are often treated with "stress-dose." However, the utility of this practice in transplant patients on low-dose prednisone therapy remains controversial.[7]

The side effects of steroid therapy contribute significantly to patient morbidity after renal transplantation. Long-term steroid use has significant metabolic effects, including diabetes mellitus, hyperlipemia, salt or water retention, and osteopenia. Cosmetic changes include hirsutism, acne, easy bruising, moon facies, and the buffalo hump. Corticosteroid use contributes to weight gain and may exacerbate cardiovascular disease. Consequently, new protocols have been developed to reduce or eliminate the need for corticosteroid maintenance therapy.

## Calcineurin Inhibitors: Cyclosporine and Tacrolimus

The introduction of CsA revolutionized the field of transplantation by providing an effective means of reducing the incidence and severity of acute rejection. CsA is a cyclic peptide that enters the cell through diffusion or, at high blood concentrations, through the LDL-cholesterol receptor. In the cytoplasm, CsA binds to cyclophilin, a carrier protein; this complex subsequently binds to and inhibits calcium-activated calcineurin. When it is activated by the cellular release of calcium, calcineurin dephosphorylates multiple cytosolic targets, including the nuclear factor of the activated T-cell transcription factor (NFAT). NFAT subsequently enters the cell nucleus and binds to promoters of inflammatory cytokines (interleukin 2, interferon-g, tissue necrosis factor-a) as well as costimulatory molecules (CD40 ligand). By inhibiting calcineurin and thus limiting the production of NFAT, cyclosporine reduces IL-2 release and lymphocyte proliferation which may attenuate or abort the immune response to alloantigen.

The pharmacokinetics of cyclosporine are often patient specific and idiosyncratic, so that its use initially requires close monitoring. Although absorption of the original formulation, Sandimmune

(Novartis Pharmaceutical Corporation, East Hanover NJ), was erratic and depended on good bile flow, the newer microemulsion formulation, Neoral (Novartis Pharmaceutical Corporation, East Hanover NJ), has more predictable bioavailability.

Cyclosporine dosing is initiated at 8 to 12 mg/kg/day with the goal of attaining a 12-hour trough level of 250 to 300 ng/mL. Over time, the cyclosporine dose is reduced to achieve trough concentrations of 125 to150 ng/mL at 1 year. Recently, $C_2$ monitoring, in which the blood level is measured 2 hours after dosing, has been proposed as a more accurate method of estimating the area under the curve (AUC) for cyclosporine. Although the best dose has yet to be determined, a $C_2$ level of 800 to 1,200 appears to provide adequate protection from rejection and may diminish the incidence of hypertension and dyslipidemia after transplantation.[8] Because cyclosporine is metabolized by the P-450 system, medications that inhibit this enzyme (eg, ketoconazole) result in increases in plasma concentration, whereas compounds that increase P-450 activity (eg, phenytoin) decrease the plasma level. Clinicians must be aware of these potential interactions when managing patients on CsA.

Tacrolimus, formerly known as FK-506, is a biochemically distinct molecule that acts as a calcineurin inhibitor (CI) via an alternate pathway from that of cyclosporine. Tacrolimus, a macrolide lactone, is similar in structure to sirolimus. The molecule is lipophilic and has relatively poor bioavailability. Once absorbed, tacrolimus easily crosses the cell membrane and binds to FK-binding protein in the cytoplasm. This complex then interacts with calcineurin, inhibits its phosphatase activity, and decreases production of NFAT. Tacrolimus is metabolized by the P-450 system and, like cyclosporine, must be monitored closely with trough blood levels. Excellent results can be achieved with a blood concentration of 10 to 15 ng/mL immediately posttransplant. In the absence of rejection, levels can then be gradually lowered over the life of the graft to a goal level of 5 to 15 ng/mL.

The side effects of both CIs include neurotoxicity, nephrotoxicity, and hypertension. The nephrotoxicity of CIs is often dose related and reflects intrarenal vasoconstriction of the afferent and efferent arterioles. CIs result in increased release of endothelin-1, decreased production of nitric oxide, and increased expression of TGF-beta, that contributes to chronic allograft nephropathy (CAN).[9] CAN due to CI toxicity is histologically manifested as obliterative arteriolopathy, patchy cell necrosis, and isometric vacuolization of the proximal tubule on allograft biopsy. Cyclosporine maintenance can also have significant cosmetic side effects, including hypertrichosis and gingival hyperplasia. Tacrolimus is more likely to induce diabetes mellitus, particularly in African Americans, and may be associated with a slightly higher incidence of posttransplant lymphoproliferative disorder in children.

## Antimetabolites (Mycophenolate Mofetil, Azathioprine)

Although the introduction of AZA allowed the early performance of transplants that were not HLA identical and was recognized with a Nobel Prize, its use for maintenance immunosuppression has now been greatly reduced. Given the improved results with mycophenolate mofetil (MMF) (CellCept®, Roche Pharmaceuticals, Basel, Switzerland), most programs now use this agent as a component of a standard three-drug immunosuppressive regimen.[10]

Once absorbed, MMF is metabolized to mycophenolic acid (MPA), the active form of the drug. MPA is a potent inhibitor of the *de-novo* pathway of purine biosynthesis through its noncompetitive inhibition of the enzyme inosine monophosphate dehydrogenase (IMPDH). Lymphocytes are predominantly affected because, unlike other cell types, they lack a salvage pathway through which guanosine monophosphate (GMP) can be generated. Thus, DNA replication is limited and cell proliferation is inhibited. MMF may have additional effects on lymphocyte homing and inflammation via alterations in adhesion molecules.

MMF is orally administered twice per day at 750 to 1,500 mg per dose. These large doses are required because the drug is rapidly metabolized. MPA levels can be monitored with, as its goal level, an AUC range of 30 to 60 mg/hr/L or a $C_0$ level of 1.8 to 4 µg/mL, although the clinical utility of this approach remains to be fully established.[11] Currently, MMF is principally used as a component of a maintenance regimen that includes use of a calcineurin inhibitor with or without steroids. However, there is significant interest is using MMF as a component of a calcineurin-sparing regimen to decrease the incidence of chronic allograft nephropathy.[12]

The side effects of MMF, which are generally mild, include diarrhea and, occasionally, bone-marrow suppression. The effect of MMF on the bone marrow can be exacerbated by simultaneous treatment with antiviral agents such as valganciclovir. MMF has several important interactions with other immunosuppression agents. Co-administration of MMF and sirolimus results in MMF $C_0$ blood levels that are 2 to 4 times those in patients treated with calcineurin inhibitors.[13] This may reflect an increase in the enterohepatic recycling of MPA, which is inhibited by cyclosporine but not by sirolimus. The consequences of high MPA levels include a higher incidence of gastrointestinal toxicity, lymphocele formation, and bone-marrow suppression. Combination therapy with corticosteroids results in lower MPA levels, which increase after steroid minimization or withdrawal.[14] Corticosteroids induce hepatic glucuronyltransferase expression, thereby enhancing the activity of uridine diphosphate-GT, the enzyme responsible for MPA metabolism, and lowering systemic levels of MPA. Thus, in withdrawal protocols, MPA monitoring may assist in dose selection and monitoring.

### Sirolimus

Sirolimus is among the newest classes of immunosuppressive agents currently approved for clinical use. Like tacrolimus, sirolimus is a macrolide antibiotic that binds to the FK-binding protein. However, the sirolimus–FKBP complex does not bind to calcineurin, but instead binds to the enzyme target of sirolimus (TOR). TOR regulates the translation of mRNAs encoding for proteins crucial for regulation of the cell cycle. In experimental conditions, TOR appears to respond to the availability of nutrients and can potentiate cell division and proliferation. Clinically, sirolimus inhibition of TOR prevents cell progression from the G1 to S phase and results in potent immunosuppression.

Sirolimus is administered once per day, beginning with a loading dose of 6 mg, after which a maintenance dose of 2 mg per day is given. Drug levels should be monitored by 24-hour trough levels, with a goal of 8 to 10 ng/mL when used in combination with cyclosporine. When sirolimus is used in a calcineurin-sparing regimen, higher blood concentrations (10–12 ng/mL) are needed to achieve adequate immunosuppression. Sirolimus is metabolized through the p-450 system and, as a result, blood levels are likely to be increased by p-450 inhibitors such as ketoconazole, erythromycin, and diltiazem and reduced in the presence of anticonvulsants and rifampin. The side effects of sirolimus include hyperlipidemia, moderate thrombocytopenia, mouth ulcers, and impaired wound healing. Sirolimus may also enhance the nephrotoxic effects of cyclosporine but, by

itself, is not known to be nephrotoxic. Furthermore, because of its antifibrotic effects, sirolimus, particularly if it can be successfully used in a calcineurin-sparing regimen, may be a beneficial agent for patients at risk of chronic allograft nephropathy.

## ANTILYMPHOCYTE ANTIBODY PREPARATIONS

These preparations can be broadly divided into two general classes. One class is polyclonal preparations derived from the serum of animals immunized with human lymphocytes or thymocytes; the other is a monoclonal antibody preparation produced using a murine B cell/myeloma cell hybridoma.

The use of polyclonal antibodies in transplantation began in the 1960s. These antibodies are recognized for their broad immunosuppressive properties. The two currently available agents, rabbit antithymocyte globulin (Thymoglobulin®, Genzyme, Cambridge, MA) and horse antithymocyte globulin, act by similar mechanisms to decrease peripheral and memory lymphocytes. The polyclonal preparations bind nonspecifically to T cells, resulting in complement-dependent opsonization and lysis, Fc-dependent opsonization, or Fas-mediated apoptosis. Following the administration of these preparations, the peripheral lymphocyte count is reduced to 100 to 200/mm$^3$. Furthermore, there is preferential regeneration of the CD8+, CD57+ immunoregulatory cells, which may contribute to the lasting effects of induction therapy with these agents.

Polyclonal agents, although approved by the FDA only for treatment of rejection, have also been used as important components of induction therapy. Rabbit antithymocyte globulin (1.25–2.5 mg/kg/day) or horse antithymocyte globulin (10–30 mg/kg/day) is administered through a central intravenous catheter for 5 to 14 days, depending on the indications. Following the first several doses, patients commonly experience fever, chills, and occasionally rigors, although these symptoms can be minimized by pretreatment with acetaminophen, antihistamines, or corticosteroids. Cytokine-induced capillary leak leads to significant third spacing, so that vigorous hydration may be necessary to protect the allograft. The dosage of rabbit antithymocyte globulin or horse antithymocyte globulin should be reduced by 50% if the platelet count drops below 75,000 or if the WBC count falls to less than 3,000. The dose should be held if the platelet counts drops below 50,000 or the WBC below 2,000. Because the polyclonal agents are derived from rabbit or horse serum, up to 78% of recipients develop xenogenic antibodies. If the polyclonal agents are used for multiple courses of therapy, these xenogenic antibodies may result in serum sickness or anaphylaxis.

The monoclonal antibody treatment OKT-3 contains purified mouse antibody specific for the e-chain of the CD3 receptor on human leukocytes. Administration of OKT-3 results, preferentially, in rapid clearing of T cells as a result of opsonization and phagocytosis in the liver and spleen. On re-population, the remaining T cells have only a very low density of CD3/T-cell receptor complexes, which reduces their immunoreactivity. As with the polyclonal preparations, following the first dose of OKT-3 and other monoclonal antibody preparations, patients commonly experience a cytokine-release syndrome characterized by fever, chills, headache, and nausea. Furthermore, the resulting capillary leak can lead to pulmonary edema in patients who are severely volume loaded. Administration of corticosteroids, antihistamines, and antipyretics before the first several doses of OKT-3 treatment is recommended. The usual dose of OKT-3 is 5 mg per day for 10 to 14 days for the treatment of acute cellular rejection. Peripheral CD3 counts should be followed to achieve a goal of 10 to 25 cells/mm$^3$.

An alternative monoclonal-antilymphocyte antibody is now available as an induction agent, although this is an off-label indication. Alemtuzumab (Campath 1H®, Genzyme, Cambridge, MA) is a humanized form of the rat anti-CD52 antibody. CD52 is found on a great variety of cells, including B and T lymphocytes and mast cells. Administration of a single dose of alemtuzumab results in a reduction in peripheral lymphocytes that lasts for up to 6 months. Alemtuzumab has been used as induction therapy designed to induce near tolerance (propé tolerance) and can be combined with single- or double-agent maintenance therapy. Like all antibody preparations, alemtuzumab can cause cytokine release syndrome. Patients also develop a characteristic macular rash as a result of mast-cell lysis. This rash generally resolves without therapy.

## Monoclonal Anti-CD25 Antibody Preparations (Daclizumab, Basiliximab)

Two new agents, daclizumab (Zenapax®, Roche Laboratories, Basel, Switzerland) and basiliximab (Simulect®, Ortho Biotech, Bridgewater, NJ), have been recently incorporated into the immunosuppressive armamentarium. Both agents are monoclonal antibodies that bind to and block the IL-2 receptor, CD25, effectively limiting IL-2-driven cellular proliferation. Unlike antilymphocyte preparations, the anti-CD25 drugs do not induce either cellular lysis or cytokine release syndrome. Although they are well tolerated and efficacious as induction agents, they are not sufficiently potent to be used to treat acute rejection. The compounds differ in the timing of their administration: daclizumab is given at 1 mg/kg every 2 weeks for 5 doses beginning preoperatively; basiliximab is administered at the time of surgery and for 4 days postoperatively at a standard dose of 20 mg.

## MAINTENANCE THERAPY IN RECIPIENTS OF LIVING DONOR KIDNEY TRANSPLANTS

Immunosuppression therapy for recipients of kidneys from live donors includes a wide variety of strategies, with variable induction and maintenance strategies. (Table 16.7-3). Avoidance of acute rejection remains the most important goal of immunosuppressive therapy. Although a single episode of acute rejection is generally reversible, it can seriously impair long-term graft survival and predispose the graft to the development of chronic rejection.[15–17] Matas et al. reviewed renal allograft survival among 1,527 recipients.[18] A single episode of rejection had a profound effect on the outcome of live donor transplants, reducing 10-year graft survival from 94.6% to 52.9%. In the population of recipients of kidneys from live donors censored for death with function, a single episode of rejection was associated with a relative risk (RR) of graft failure of 9.7 P < 0.0001 compared to that in patients without rejection. However, when a single episode of rejection was accompanied by delayed graft function, the risk of graft failure increased dramatically (RR 20.2, P < 0.0001) when compared to that of patients with neither risk factor. To ensure the lowest risk of acute rejection, the standard immunosuppression regimen for recipients of kidneys from live donors has consisted of a calcineurin inhibitor, corticosteroids, and either MMF or sirolimus.

**TABLE 16.7-3**

## IMMUNOSUPPRESSIVE PROTOCOLS USED FOR RECIPIENTS OF KIDNEYS FROM LIVING DONORS

| Year | Author | N | Induction | Maintenance | Follow-Up (months) | Graft Survival (%) | Patient Survival (%) | Rejection-Free Survival (%) |
|------|--------|---|-----------|-------------|--------------------|--------------------|----------------------|------------------------------|
| 1999 | Mulloy[51] | 54 | Basiliximab | CsA/Prednisone | 12 | 94.4 | 98 | 73 (6 mo) |
| 1999 | Mulloy[51] | 51 | None | CsA/Prednisone | 12 | 98 | 98 | 53 (6 mo) |
| 1999 | Kirste[52] | 140 | ATG (selected) | CSA/MMF/Steroids | 120 | 84 | 94 | NR |
| 2003 | Bunnapradist[25] | 2,393 | NR | TAC/MMF/Steroids | 24 | 97 | 92 | NR |
| 2003 | Bunnapradist[25] | 4,686 | NR | CSA/MMF/Steroids | 24 | 97 | 94 | NR |
| 2004 | Matas[22] | 341 | RATG | CSA or TAC / MMF | 48 | 92 | 90 | 89 |
| 2004 | Wiland[35] | 136 | None | TAC/MMF/Prednisone | 12 | 95 | NR | 79 |
| 2004 | Kim[53] | 44 | None | CSA/MMF/ Steroid Withdrawal | 6 | 100 | 100 | 83 |
| 2004 | Kim[53] | 43 | None | TAC/MMF/Steroid Withdrawal | 6 | 100 | 100 | 100 |
| 2004 | Brennan[54] | 470 | Selected (anti-CD25/ anti-lymph.) | CSA or TAC/MMF/ Steroids | 31 | 92 | 97 | 80 |
| 2005 | Kaufman[31] | 97 | Basiliximab | TAC/MMF | 12 | 100 | 100 | 87.6 |
| 2005 | Kaufman[31] | 92 | Alemtuzumab | TAC/MMF | 12 | 98.9 | 96.7 | 85.7 |

Choice of the best calcineurin inhibitor to use in the setting of transplants from live donors remains largely an unanswered question. In the setting of cadaveric kidney transplants, it has been demonstrated in some multicenter randomized trials that tacrolimus provides superior results.[19–23] In the largest U.S. trial, 412 cadaveric renal transplant recipients were randomized to receive tacrolimus or cyclosporine combined with antilymphocyte antibody induction, AZA, and steroids.[20] This study demonstrated a significant reduction in the incidence of biopsy-confirmed acute rejection among patients treated with tacrolimus (30.7 vs 46.4, p = 0.001). There was also a marked reduction in steroid resistant rejection (10.7% vs 25.1%, p < 0.001). Unfortunately, the reduction in rejection did not result in a significant difference in graft or patient survival at 1 year. In addition, the improved protection from rejection afforded by tacrolimus was accompanied by a marked increase in the incidence of posttransplant diabetes mellitus (19.9% vs 4.0%, p < 0.0001). The relevance of this study's conclusions has been recently challenged because microemulsion cyclosporine and MMF were not used.

The results of large randomized trials comparing microemulsion formulations of cyclosporine with tacrolimus have demonstrated a similar reduction in the incidence of acute rejection predominantly among recipients of cadaveric renal transplants. The European Tacrolimus vs Ciclosporine Microemulsion study group reported the results of a 6-month open randomized trial involving 560 patients treated with a triple-drug regimen of calcineurin inhibitor, azathioprine, and corticosteroids.[22] Tacrolimus was again associated with a reduction in the incidence of acute rejection (19.6% vs 37.3%, p < 0.0001) and steroid-resistant rejection (9.4% vs 21%, p < 0.0001). However, as in the U.S. study, no significant difference in 1-year graft or patient survival could be demonstrated.

When compared to cyclosporine, use of tacrolimus has been shown to improve the cardiovascular risk profile.[22,23] Tacrolimus was associated with a reduction in the incidence of posttransplant hypertension 15.7% versus 23.2% in CsA-treated patients (p = 0.032) and hypercholesterolemia (4.2% vs 8.9%, p = 0.037).[22] Both posttransplant hypertension and hypercholesterolemia have been associated with an increased incidence of chronic allograft nephropathy and posttransplant cardiovascular death with function, which remains the primary cause of allograft loss among recipients of kidneys from live donors. Furthermore, cyclosporine has been associated with an increased incidence of graft fibrosis as measured by extracellular matrix density (p < 0.002).[24] Although both tacrolimus and cyclosporine have been associated with nephrotoxic effects, randomized trials suggest that patients treated with cyclosporine have a greater increase in serum creatinine at 12 months than do tacrolimus-treated patients.[19] Furthermore, for patients with declining renal function converting from treatment with cyclosporine to the use of tacrolimus can stabilize renal function.

Although multiple studies have demonstrated reduction in both the rate of acute rejection and the risk factors for chronic rejection in patients treated with tacrolimus, no prospective study of renal transplant patients has demonstrated a marked improvement in patient or graft survival in association with the choice of different calcineurin inhibitors. In fact, retrospective analysis of transplant registry data comparing results among recipients of transplants from living donors treated with either tacrolimus and MMF or microemulsion cyclosporine and MMF suggests that microemulsion cyclosporine is associated with improved long-term graft survival.[25] In a study of more than 7,000 recipients

of transplants from living donors, Bunnapradist et al. found that the mean allograft half-life of microemulsion cyclosporine-treated patients was greater (20.8 years vs 16.1 years, P < 0.001) than that in patients treated with tacrolimus.[25] Unadjusted graft survival was statistically better at 2 years (94.3% vs 92.2%, P = 0.0006). Even after adjustment for donor and recipient risk factors, most of which appeared to favor the microemulsion cyclosporine-treated group, treatment with tacrolimus was associated with an increased risk of graft loss (hazard ration [HR] = 1.28, p = 0.002). Prospective randomized trials are needed to verify or disprove the conclusions of this retrospective analysis. However, given the rapidly shifting landscape of immunosuppression, this type of study is difficult to conduct.

Until recently, corticosteroids were considered an essential component of maintenance immunosuppression, despite their well-recognized contribution to posttransplant morbidity. Although the steroid doses could be weaned to low levels, complete cessation of therapy resulted in high rates of acute rejection among patients treated with cyclosporine monotherapy or cyclosporine and MMF.[26] A randomized trial conducted in the United States was stopped by the safety monitoring committee, when there was a statistically significant increase in the rate of acute rejection in patients weaned from steroids at three months after transplant as compared to the rate in patients who remained on triple therapy (30.8% vs 9.8%).[27] However, within the context of tacrolimus-based immunosuppression, particularly with the increased use of induction therapy, corticosteroid withdrawal may now be possible.

Single-center reports have demonstrated excellent success with steroid avoidance protocols.[28–31] In 1999, Matas et al., at the University of Minnesota, began a protocol in which patients undergoing transplants from living or cadaveric donors underwent induction therapy with rabbit antithymocyte globulin followed by maintenance therapy using cyclosporine and MMF.[28] Later, the patients were randomized into groups that received either tacrolimus and sirolimus or cyclosporine and MMF. The use of corticosteroids was limited to one 500-mg dose of methylprednisolone administered at the time of transplant, followed by rapid tapering off of prednisone until postoperative day 5, at which point all steroid therapy was discontinued. Results using this protocol were compared in to 254 recipients of kidneys from live donor transplants that were treated with rapid steroid withdrawal and 180 historical live donor patients transplanted at the University of Minnesota using standard three-drug immunosuppression. In both the steroid withdrawal group and the control group, there was a 95% rate of patient survival at 36 months, whereas the respective rates of graft survival at this point were 91% and 88% (p = NS). Moreover, at 3 years after transplantation, the patients who managed without steroids had a higher acute-rejection-free graft survival rate (92% vs 77%, p < 0.001) and a trend toward a lower chronic-rejection-free graft survival rate (94% vs 90%, p = NS). Long-term results from this group, including recipients of transplants from both cadaveric and living donors, now demonstrate that they have, in comparison to historical controls, both an improved patient survival rate (92% vs 88%, p < 0.02) and an improved graft survival rate (90% vs 81%, p < 0.0001), as well as a higher acute-rejection-free graft survival rate (86% vs 77%, p = 0.0004). The benefit of steroid-free protocols for recipients of kidneys from living donors was not specifically discussed in this report.

Other approaches to steroid avoidance have included the use of IL-2 receptor antagonists or alemtuzumab. Single-center experience with the use of IL-2 receptor antagonists, rapid steroid withdrawal, tacrolimus, and MMF in 29 patients yielded a reduced incidence of acute rejection (8.3% vs 13.2%) when compared to historical controls.[30] These results have been validated in a multicenter randomized study including recipients of kidneys from both cadaveric and living donors.[32] Among patients treated with IL-2 receptor antagonist therapy, MMF, and microemulsion cyclosporine, there was little difference in the acute rejection rates of those maintained on a prednisone-free regimen and those maintained on corticosteroids (20% vs 16%, respectively). Patient and graft survival were also unaffected by the withdrawal of steroids.

Finally, using a novel approach, Calne studied the results of alemtuzumab induction followed by cyclosporine monotherapy.[33] In the absence of corticosteroids and antiproliferative agents, 29 of 31 grafts were intact and functioning at 1 year after transplantation. Furthermore, only seven episodes of rejection occurred during the year. Thus, it appears that in the context of appropriate induction therapy, long-term corticosteroid treatment may not be necessary, particularly in the lower-risk population of patients who received grafts from living donors.

The optimal final component of standard three-drug immunosuppression has evolved rapidly. Given its clear superiority over AZA, MMF appears to be the antiproliferative agent of choice. However, sirolimus may offer an attractive alternative because it provides several potential long-term benefits, including a reduction in long-term graft fibrosis. Initial studies of recipients of kidneys from cadaveric donors demonstrated a marked reduction in the rate of acute rejection in patients treated with the three-drug regimen of tacrolimus, steroids, and sirolimus as compared to control patients given only tacrolimus and steroids.[34] At present there appears to be insufficient data to choose between MMF and sirolimus. In the single randomized trial that has been reported, patient and graft survival were not statistically different between patients treated with tacrolimus, MMF, and steroids and those treated with tacrolimus, sirolimus, and steroids.[19] In both groups, the 12-month incidence of acute rejection was 4%. Although there was no difference in the incidence of infectious or wound complications, at 1 year after transplantation patients treated with sirolimus had, as expected, a greater incidence of hypercholesterolemia requiring statin treatment (54% vs 16%, P < 0.0001). Further study is needed, not only to determine if sirolimus therapy can be safely used in the absence of CIs but also to determine the subsequent impact of such therapy on the incidence of chronic allograft nephropathy.

Current immunosuppression practice appears to reflect the findings reported in the existing literature regarding the efficacy of available maintenance immunosuppressive agents. Over the last 5 years, there as been a pervasive shift from the use of cyclosporine-based immunosuppression to tacrolimus (Figure 16.7-2).

**(A)**

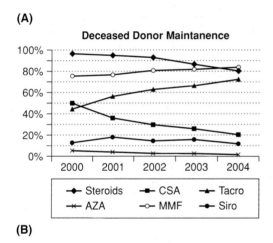

**(B)**

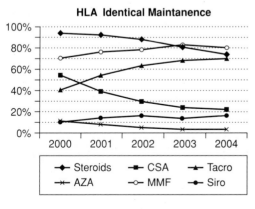

**(C)**

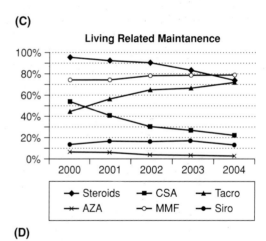

**(D)**

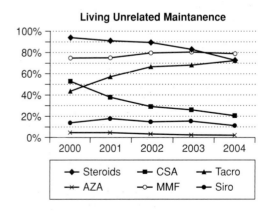

**FIGURE 16.7-2**

(**A**) Maintenance therapy in recipients of transplants from deceased donors, (**B**) HLA-identical donors, (**C**) Living related donor, and (**D**) Living unrelated donors. Data for mycophenolate sodium (Myfortic), cytoxan, and everolimus excluded due to very low use (< 1%). *Source*: Scientific Registry of Transplant Recipients; May 2005.

This shift has occurred across all populations of kidney recipients, regardless of donor source. There has also been a reduction in the use of corticosteroids, particularly for recipients of kidneys from living donors. MMF has clearly become the dominant antiproliferative agent, nearly eliminating the use of azathioprine in most regimens. The use of sirolimus appears to be steady at about 15% of the patient population.

## INDUCTION THERAPY IN RECIPIENTS OF LIVING DONOR KIDNEY TRANSPLANTS

The need for induction therapy in patients who receive kidney transplants from living donors remains controversial. After the earlier observation of dramatically better graft survival among recipients of kidneys from living related donors' kidneys compared with recipients of kidneys from deceased donors, it was believed that patients in the former group were at diminished risk of graft rejection and, therefore, the risk of cancer and CMV infection associated with induction therapy was not warranted. The introduction of new, better-tolerated induction agents, including anti-CD25 antibody therapy, has led to reevaluation of the value of induction therapy. Bartlett et al. recently reported their results comparing the outcome of cadaveric donor kidneys in patients given basiliximab induction to graft outcome from living unrelated donors who were managed without induction; all patients were given the same maintenance regimen (tacrolimus, MMF, and steroids).[35] They found that the rate of acute rejection was higher in grafts from the living unrelated donors (21.3% vs 4.0%, p < 0.0004), despite the presence of a greater number of African Americans in the group that received kidneys from cadaveric donors. The authors concluded that induction therapy is warranted for patients who receive transplants from living unrelated donors.

The effectiveness of induction with basiliximab or daclizumab has been demonstrated to be effective and well tolerated in the general renal transplant population.[36] A meta-analysis of published trials comparing IL-2R antagonists to placebo demonstrated that use of these agents resulted in a trend toward improved 1-year graft survival (RR 0.84 CI 0.64–1.10). The rates of acute rejection (RR 0.67 CI 0.60–0.75) and biopsy-proven acute rejection (RR 0.67 CI 0.59–0.76) were significantly reduced in the IL-2R antagonist group. Moreover, the reduction in acute rejection was not accompanied by an increased risk of CMV infection (RR 0.82 CI 0.65–1.03) or malignancy (RR 0.67 CI 0.33–1.36) in the induction group.

The use of induction therapy appears to have important advantages for recipients of transplants from living donors. First, it allows delayed introduction of cyclosporine without incurring the risk of acute rejection. In patients that managed without induction, failure to achieve a therapeutic cyclosporine level was associated with the risk of rejection (39% vs 15%, p = 0.16).[37] With basiliximab treatment, there was no relationship between early cyclosporine level and rejection rate (P = 0.94). Second, induction therapy appears to facilitate steroid withdrawal. As noted earlier, in the absence of induction the rate of acute rejection after steroid tapering and withdrawal exceeded 30% in patients treated with cyclosporine and AZA. Induction therapy has now been used successfully with tacrolimus and MMF maintenance. Single-center results with such induction therapy are equivalent to or better than triple drug therapy without induction.[29] Basiliximab therapy has also been used to facilitate single-drug maintenance with cyclosporine. Parrott et al.[38] reported that monotherapy was successful in 75% of patients who received basiliximab as opposed to

39% of patients treated with a placebo (p = 0.0006). However, in this study, the 1-year rate of rejection in the both the basiliximab group (29%) and the placebo group (43%) appears to be too high, given the results reported with three-drug maintenance.

The true question of which of the induction agents is preferable, if induction is going to be used for recipients of transplants from living donors, appears increasingly clear. In terms of efficacy, the recent meta-analysis of IL-2R antagonists demonstrated no significant differences in the rates of patient survival, graft survival, or acute rejection achieved with basiliximab and daclizumab.[36] Furthermore, the IL-R antagonists were equivalent to both monoclonal and polyclonal antilymphocyte treatments in the prevention of acute rejection. The IL-2R antagonists were associated with fewer side effects, reducing the incidence of fever, leucopenia, thrombocytopenia, and other adverse reactions. There was also a dramatically reduced risk of CMV infection in patients treated with IL-2R inhibitors compared with those treated with mono- or polyclonal antibody therapy (RR 0.37 CI 0.22-0.62). Although the results were not significantly different in the meta-analysis, examination of the UNOS registry demonstrated that, as compared with monoclonal or polyclonal antibody treatment, IL-R antagonists have the additional advantage of reducing the risk of post-transplant lymphoproliferative disorder (PTLD).[39] The relative risk of developing PTLD was significantly greater with monoclonal therapy than with no induction treatment (RR = 1.7, p = 0.03), and the use of polyclonal therapy was associated with a trend toward increased risk (RR = 1.3, p = 0.27). However, the IL-2R antagonists were not significantly associated with an increased risk of PTLD (RR = 1.1, P = 0.50). Thus, for the population of recipients from living donors, the IL-R antagonists appear to be the best induction agent, carrying the least risk of toxicity and late malignancy among the agents currently approved by the FDA.

Despite the potential risks associated with induction therapy, the majority of patients undergoing renal transplantation are now treated with an induction agent (Figure 16.7-3). As a result of the improved results and the potential for reduction in maintenance therapy, the use of induction has, over the past 5 years, become commonplace for recipients of renal transplants from all donor sources of renal transplantation (Figures 16.7-4A–4D). A review of these trend data suggests that the use of rabbit antithymocyte globulin has increased the most, making it now the preferred agent for the majority of recipients. The use of IL-2 receptor inhibitors

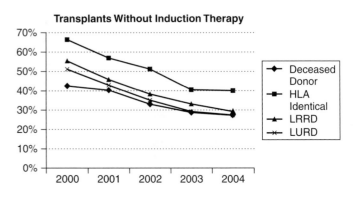

**FIGURE 16.7-3**

Incidence of no induction therapy by donor types following renal transplantation.

Source: Scientific Registry of Transplant Recipients; May 2005.

**(A)**

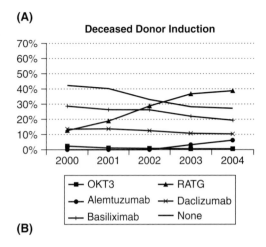

**(B)**

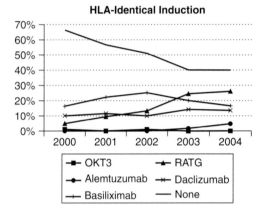

**(C)**

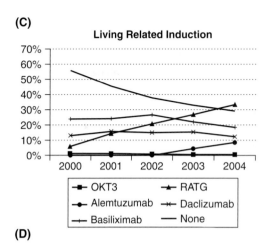

**(D)**

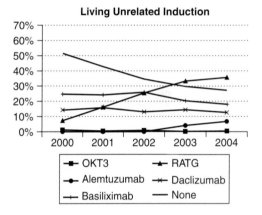

**FIGURE 16.7-4**

(**A**) Induction therapy in recipients of deceased donors, (**B**) HLA-identical donors, (**C**) Living related donors, and (**D**) Living unrelated donors. Data for horse ATG did not exceed 3.8% for any donor type in any year and were removed for clarity.
*Source:* Scientific Registry of Transplant Recipients; May 2005.

has generally remained stable, with basiliximab and daclizumab each used in about 15% of the population. It also appears that there has been a dramatic rise in the use of alemtuzumab, particularly among recipients of living donor organs.

## FUTURE DIRECTIONS IN IMMUNOSUPPRESSIVE THERAPY

The goal of reducing the acute rejection episode rate after the first year of transplant to under 15% should be almost universally achievable, given the available agents. IL2-R antagonist induction followed by triple-drug immunosuppression with tacrolimus, either MMF or sirolimus, and steroids results in rates of rejection below 5% at 1 year, with excellent patient and graft survival.[19] These results represent a remarkable improvement over graft survival rates of 50% at 1 year, which were common only 25 years ago. Unfortunately, triple-drug therapy requires the long-term use of steroids, with the attendant risks of coronary artery disease, osteopenia, cataracts, and diabetes mellitus, in addition to cosmetic changes. Similarly, lifelong calcineurin inhibitor therapy may contribute to the development of chronic allograft nephropathy and lead to premature graft loss.[40] In the next iteration of

immunosuppressive regimens, it is likely that one or both of these agents will be eliminated in favor of agents having less toxicity and producing fewer systemic effects.

### Steroid-Free Maintenance

At Northwestern University, all renal transplant recipients have been managed without the use of maintenance corticosteroids since September 1998.[30,31] During this period, two induction agents, basiliximab and alemtuzumab, have been used. The first 155 patients were given 2 doses of basiliximab and, for maintenance therapy, 3.0 g/day of MMF and tacrolimus adjusted to a 12-hour blood concentration of 7 to 8 ng/mL. Subsequent patients have been given a single dose of alemtuzumab and, for maintenance, MMF with a target of 1.5 g/day and tacrolimus adjusted to a 12-hour blood concentration of 6 to 7 ng/mL. Since the beginning of the corticosteroid-free regimen, all patients have received 3 daily doses of methylprednisolone (500 mg, 250 mg, and 125 mg) beginning at the time of transplant.

In the entire population of patients, the 1-year patient and graft survival rates have not differed with the two induction agents.[31] Specifically, the 1-year actual survival rate for patients who received alemtuzumab was 96.8%, whereas that for patients given basiliximab was 99.4% (p = ns). The 1-year actual death-censored graft survival rates for recipients given alemtuzumab and basiliximab were 99.2% and 99.4%, respectively (p = ns). Among recipients of allografts from live donors, the 1-year graft survival rates for those given alemtuzumab and basiliximab were, respectively, 98.9% and 100% (p = ns).

The 12-month actual rejection rate for recipients given alemtuzumab was 14.9%, whereas that in patients given baxiliximab was 13.5% (p = ns). However, the kinetics of rejection was very different in the two groups. The mean ± SD (median) days of rejection in the alemtuzumab group was 148 ± 82 (153 days), whereas that in the basiliximab treatment group was 51 ± 83 (10 days). For recipients of kidneys from living donors, the 12-month actual rejection rate among those given alemtuzumab was 14.3%; that among patients given basiliximab was 12.4% (p = ns). The mean ± SD days of rejection in the alemtuzumab and basiliximab treatment groups were 66 ± 53 (58 days) and 7 ± 4 (6 days), respectively.

Although all patients were managed with a prednisone-free maintenance regimen of tacrolimus and MMF, alemtuzumab induction enabled reduced use of maintenance therapy. Recipients in the alemtuzumab induction group received significantly lower doses MMF, and the mean 12-hour trough concentration of tacrolimus was 25% lower in patients treated with alemtuzumab induction.

The overall incidence and etiology of infectious disease were very similar in the two treatment groups. CMV disease occurred in 4% of recipients in the alemtuzumab group and in 5% of those in the basiliximab group. The incidence of malignancy was also similar in the induction groups. Two recipients in each group acquired PTLD.

In summary, kidney transplantation without long-term steroid maintenance can be accomplished safely with a low rejection rate and excellent short-term graft survival. In this setting, induction by the administration of a single dose of alemtuzumab appears to provide long-lasting protection against acute rejection without increasing the risk of CMV infection or PTLD. However, the efficacy of steroid avoidance in preventing or improving long-term graft survival remains untested.

### Calcineurin-Free Regimens

Kidney transplantation without the use of long-term calcineurin therapy, if successful, may allow reduction of the incidence of chronic allograft nephropathy and prolongation of allograft life. Until the introduction of sirolimus, even late withdrawal of CIs was associated with high rates of acute rejection. However, with induction therapy and sirolimus, an effective non-nephrotoxic agent, CI-free regimens now appear feasible.

Flechner et al., at Cleveland Clinic, recently reported the results of a randomized study comparing cyclosporine with sirolimus following basiliximab induction in recipients of renal transplants from cadaveric and live donors.[41,42] Patients were also given MMF and corticosteroids. Sirolimus levels were adjusted to keep the trough level between 10 to 12 ng/mL for 6 months, then reduced to 5 to 10 ng/mL. In the cyclosporine group, blood levels were maintained at 200 to 250 ng/mL throughout the study. MPA levels were monitored but were not used to adjust the dosage of the patient's MMF. At 18 months, the MPA levels in patients given sirolimus were higher than those in CI-treated patients (4.16 vs 1.93, p = 0.001) despite equivalent oral dosing.

The results, based on a mean of 36 months of follow-up, demonstrated significant advantages in the calcineurin-free group. Although there were no statistically significant differences between the sirolimus- and cyclosporine-treated groups with respect to patient (93.5% vs 100%) or graft survival (93.5% vs 93.3%), there was a trend toward a reduction in the incidence of biopsy-proven rejection (6.5% vs 16.6%) in the sirolimus treated patients. The CI-free therapy was well tolerated, with no differences in the incidence of hematologic abnormalities, hypertension, or wound healing. Patients in both groups experienced a significant increase in serum lipids, but there were no significant differences between agents.

The nephrotoxic effect of the calcineurin inhibitors appeared early and persisted throughout the study. As measured by serum creatinine levels at 6 months after transplantation, renal function was significantly better in the sirolimus-treated group than in the cyclosporine-treated group (1.29 mg% vs 1.74 mg%, p = 0.008). The same was true at 12 months (1.32 mg% vs 1.78 mg%, p = 0.004) and at 2 years (1.35 mg% vs 1.81 mg%, P = 0.008). Similar results were demonstrated when renal function was assessed using creatinine clearance, which demonstrated a 5 mL/min/year reduction in GFR in the CI-treated patients as compared with the patients given sirolimus. Interestingly, the sirolimus-treated patients appeared to have an increasing GFR, potentially reflecting graft hypertrophy. Histologic evaluation of protocol biopsy specimens at two years revealed significant differences between the two groups. As compared to cyclosporine-treated patients, transplant recipients who were treated with sirolimus were more likely to have a biopsy that was read as normal (66.6% vs 20.8%, p = 00007) and have a lower net Banff chronic allograft nephropathy (Banff CAN) score (1.48 vs 3.17, p < 0.0001). The difference in the Banff CAN scores reflects a greater degree of tubular atrophy and interstitial fibrosis in patients given CI therapy.

At the present time, no empirical data are available to guide the choice between steroid-sparing and CI-sparing regiments. Steroid-sparing regimens have the potential advantage of decreasing cardiovascular risk, which remains the major cause of post-transplant mortality. However, this may come at the expense of a higher incidence of chronic allograft nephropathy. CI-sparing regimens appear to provide better preservation of renal function at the expense of long-term steroids. Perhaps, with better induction or improved drug monitoring of MPA levels, patients can be managed with a regimen that will be free of both calcineurin and steroids. Currently, however, the only reported trial of this approach, which was used for 17 recipients, resulted in acute rejection rates of 30% in recipients of transplants from living related donors and 85% in those receiving transplants from living unrelated donors.[43]

## SPECIAL CASES

### Pediatric Recipients

Living donor renal transplantation in children offers young patients with end-stage renal disease their best opportunity for long-term growth and development. More than 50% of transplants performed on children use grafts from living donors, accounting for the majority of the growth in the pediatric transplant population. Living donation offers significant advantages including the opportunity to preemptively transplant as need for dialysis has been associated with a significant increase in the risk of graft loss (RR 1.77 P < 0.0001).[44] Acute rejection continues to present a major challenge to pediatric renal transplantation. Perhaps as a result of faster drug metabolism or a higher degree of immune responsiveness, pediatric recipients appear to have a higher incidence of acute rejection than do their adult counterparts. As in adults, a single episode of rejection can substantially increase the risk of graft failure (RR 1.31, p < 0.002) in children.[44] Thus, pediatric centers have tended to favor aggressive immunosuppressive regimens.

Although both tacrolimus and cyclosporine have been successfully used in the pediatric population, tacrolimus appears to be both more effective and better tolerated.[45] In a randomized trial of children under the age of 18 years who received transplants from living and cadaveric donors, treatment with tacrolimus, AZA, and steroids was compared with the use of CsA, AZA, and steroids.[46] Tacrolimus treatment substantially reduced the incidence of biopsy proven-acute rejection (16.5% vs 39.8%, p = 0.001) and steroid-resistant rejection (7.8% vs 25.8%, p = 0.001). Although graft loss in the two treatment groups did not differ at 1 year, graft function in the tacrolimus group was improved as determined by calculations of the GFR. Tacrolimus has the additional advantage of avoiding the cosmetic changes that occur with cyclosporine, including hairsutism and gingival hyperplasia, which can be particularly troubling to adolescents.

Registry analysis of the NAPRTCS databases confirmed that tacrolimus remains the agent of choice in combination with MMF/steroids.[47] When the use of tacrolimus was compared with similar three-drug maintenance that included CsA, it was found that tacrolimus-treated patients had improved GFRs (96.7 mL/min/1.73 m$^2$ vs 73.2 mL/min/1.73 m$^2$, p < 0.0001) at 2 years after transplantation, despite a lack of between-group differences in rates of acute rejection or graft loss.

Dosing children of all CIs can be more difficult than it is in adults due to changes in metabolism and volume of distribution with increasing age.[48] Empiric analysis of tacrolimus dosing of small children found that the AUC correlated best with the mean of the $C_0$ and $C_2$ levels, but was poorly correlated with $C_0$ levels alone, often leading to significant underdosing. In children under 5 years of age, the dose per kilogram needed in order to achieve an AUC similar to that in older children was 1.9 to 2.7 times higher. This effect was exacerbated in trials of steroid avoidance.

Pediatric transplant results may be further improved with the use of MMF, which reduces the rate of acute rejection.[49] Although MMF has been associated with a higher rate of CMV and PTLD in adults, examining the NAPRTC registry of 197 children treated with a combination of tacrolimus and MMF revealed no cases of PTLD.

Although triple therapy in children is highly effective in preventing acute rejection, prolonged exposure to corticosteroids has profound effects on growth and development. Providing adequate induction therapy with an IL-2 blocker, steroid avoidance appears to be possible without a reduction in graft survival or an increase in the rate of acute rejection. Sarwal et al.[50] have described a novel approach using 6 months of therapy with daclizumab combined with tacrolimus and MMF. After 6 months, patients were maintained on tacrolimus and either MMF or sirolimus, depending on their individual tolerance of these medications. Protocol biopsies were performed to guide therapy. The treated patients were compared with matched concurrent or historical controls on a steroid-based regimen with tacrolimus.

In this study, the advantages of steroid avoidance were clear at a mean follow-up of 20 months.[50] Both patient and graft survival were excellent (98% and 100% death-censored, respectively). Moreover, the rate of acute rejection was reduced in the steroid-avoidance

patients (8% vs 32%, P < 0.001) and the estimated creatinine clearance was improved (p = 0.004). Other advantages included an increased rate of linear growth and percentile height, a reduction in the incidence hypertension, and decreased body mass index. A finding that perhaps is more important in a childhood population was that steroid avoidance reduced the incidence of noncompliance by patients or parents from 34.8% to 10% (P < 0.001). Although these results appear promising, a true randomized controlled trial is needed for definitive establishment of the efficacy of this approach.

## HLA-Identical Donors

There is a paucity of data regarding the management of recipients of HLA-identical grafts from living donors. Although historical data clearly indicate a markedly decreased risk of rejection in these recipients, this has not been studied in the current era. Further study should be undertaken to assess the importance of induction therapy in this population and to determine if a CI free, steroid-free approach could be used. Review of data from the scientific registry of transplant recipients (SRTR) suggests that induction therapy is still commonly used in the setting of HLA identical grafts (Figures 16.7-3 and 16.7-4B). Furthermore, standard three-drug immunosuppression (tacrolimus, MMF, prednisone) appears to be the most commonly used maintenance regimen (Figure 16.7-2B). Multicenter randomized trials are needed to determine if aggressive use of CI and/or steroid-sparing regimens can be safely employed in this immunologically low-risk population.

## CONCLUSIONS

Advances in immunosuppressive therapy during the 20th century revolutionized renal transplantation. The challenge for the 21st century is to design and implement strategies to preserve allograft function, reduce CAN, and minimize the side effects of medications. As new agents are introduced, empirical evidence will become even more difficult to obtain. Given the excellent short-term outcome currently experienced by most renal transplant recipients, it is clear that only long-term studies will provide the necessary insight into the appropriate therapy for these patients.

## References

1. Morrissey PE, Madaras PN, Monaco AP. History of kidney and pancreas transplanation. In: Norman DJ, Turka LA, eds. *Primer on Transplantation*, 2nd Edition. Blackwell. 2001:411–413.
2. Carrel A. Successful transplantation of both kidneys for a dog into a bitch with removal of both nomal kidneys from the latter. *Science* 1906;23:394.
3. Merrill JP, Murray JE, Takacs F. Successful transplantation of a kidney from a human cadaver. *JAMA* 1963;185:347.
4. Matas AJ, Sutherland DER, Najarian JS. Evolution of immunosuppression at the University of Minnesota. *Transplant Proc* 2004;36:64S.
5. Calne RY. White DJG, Thiru S, et al. Cyclosporin A in patients receiving renal allografts from cadaver donors. *Lancet* 1978.
6. Halloran PF, Gourishankar S. Historical overview of pharmacology and immunosuppression. In: Norman DJ, Turka LA, eds. *Primer on Transplantation*, 2nd Edition. Blackwell. 2001:73–76.
7. Bromberg JS, Baliga P, Cofer JB, et al. Stress steroids are not required for patients receiving a renal allograft and undergoing operation. *J Am Coll Surg* 1995;180:532.
8. Stefoni S, Midtved K, Cole E, et al. Efficacy and safety outcomes among de novo renal transplant recipients managed by C2 monitoring

of cyclosporine a microemulsion: results of a 12-month, randomized, multicenter trial. *Transplanation* 2005;79:577.

9. Olyaei AJ., DeMattos AM, Bennett WM. Nephrotoxicity of immunosuppressive drugs: New insight and preventive strategies. *Curr Opin Crit Care* 2001;7:384.

10. Ojo AO, Meier-Kriesche HU, Hanson JA, et al. Mycophenolate mofetil reduces late renal allograft loss independent of acute rejection. *Transplantation* 2000;69:2405.

11. van Hest R, Mathot R, Vulto A, et al. Predicting the usefulness of therapeutic drug monitoring of mycophenolic acid: a computer simulation. *Ther Drug Monit* 2005;27:163.

12. Dudley C, Pohanka E, Riad H, et al. Mycophenolate mofetil substitution for cyclosporine a in renal transplant recipients with chronic progressive allograft dysfunction: the "creeping creatinine" study. *Transplantation* 2005;79:466.

13. Flechner SM, Feng J, Mastroianni B, et al. The effect of 2-gram versus 1 gram concentration controlled mycophenolate mofetil on renal transplant outcomes using sirolimus-based calcineurin inhibitor drug-free immunosuppression. *Transplantation* 2005;79:926.

14. Cattaneo D, Perico N, Gaspari F, et al. Glucocorticoids interfere with mycophenolate mofetil bioavailability in kidney transplantation. *Kidney Int* 2002;62:1060.

15. Almond PS, Matas A, Gillingham K, et al. Risk factors for chronic rejection in renal allograft recipients. *Transplantation* 1993;55:752.

16. Humar A, Johnson EM, Payne WD, et al. Effect of initial slow graft function on renal allograft rejection and survival. *Clin Transplant* 1997;11:623.

17. Humar A, Hassoun A, Kandaswamy R, et al. Immunologic factors: the major risk for decreased long-term allograft survival. *Transplantation* 1999;68:1242.

18. Matas AJ, Gillingham KJ, Humar A, et al. Immunologic and nonimmulologic factors: different risks for cadaver and living donor transplantion. *Transplanation* 2000;69:54.

19. Ciancio G, Burke GW, Gaynor JJ, et al. A randomized long-term trial of tacrolimus/sirolimus versus tacrolimus/mycophenolate mofetil versus cyclosporine (NEORAL)/sirolimus in renal transplantation. II. Survival, function, and protocol compliance at 1 year. *Transplantation* 2004;77:252.

20. Ciancio G, Burke GW, Gaynor JJ, et al. A randomized long-term trial of tacrolimus and sirolimus versus tacrolimus and mycophenolate mofetil versus cyclosporine (NEORAL) and sirolimus in renal transplantation. I. Drug interactions and rejection at one year. *Transplantation* 2004;77:244.

21. Pirsch JD, Miller J, Deierhoi MH, et al. A comparison of tacrolimus (FK506) and cyclosporine for immunsuppression after cadaveric renal transplantation. *Transplantation* 1997;63:977.

22. Margreiter R. Efficacy and safety of tacrolimus compared with ciclosporin microemulsion in renal transplantation: a randomised multicentre study. *Lancet* 2002;359:741.

23. Krämer BK, Zülke C, Kammerl MC, et al. Cardiovascular risk factors and estimated risk for CAD in a randomized trial comparing calcineurin inhibitors in renal transplantation. *Am J Transplant* 2003;3:982.

24. Muphy GJ, Waller JR, Sandford RS, et al. Randomized trial of the effect of microemulsion cyclosporine or tacrolimus on renal allograft fibrosis. *Br J Surg* 2003;90:680.

25. Bunnapradist S, Daswani A, Takemoto SK. Graft survival following living-donor renal transplantation: a comparions of tacrolimus and cyclosporine microemulsion with mycophenolate mofetil and steroids. *Transplantation* 2003;76:10.

26. Kasiske BL, Chakkera HA, Louis TA. A meta-analysis of immunosuppression withdrawal trials in renal transplantation. *J Am Soc Nephrol* 2000;11:1910.

27. Ahsan N, Hricik D, Matas A, et al. Prednisone withdrawal in kidney transplant recipients on cyclosporine and mycophenolate mofetil—a prospective randomized study. *Transplantation* 1999;68:1865.

28. Matas AJ, Kandaswamy R, Humar A, et al. Long-term immunosuppression, without maintenance prednisone, after kidney transplantation. *Ann Surg* 2004;240:510.

29. Khwaja K, Asolati M, Harmon J, et al. Outcome at 3 years with a prednisone—free maintenance regimen: a single-center experience with 349 kidney transplant recipients. *Am J Trans* 2004;4:980.

30. Kaufman DB, Leventhal JR, Fryer JP, et al. Kidney transplantation without prednisone. *Transplantation* 2000;69(Suppl 1):S133.

31. Kaufman DB, Leventhal JR, Axelrod DA, et al. Alemtuzumab induction and prednisone-free maintenance immunotherapy in kidney transplantation: Comparison with basiliximab induction: long term results. *Am J Trans* 2005;5:2539.

32. Vincenti F, Monaco A, Grinyo J, et al. Multicenter randomized prospective trial of steroid withdrawal in renal transplant recipients receiving basiliximab, cyclosporine microemulsion and mycophenolate mofetil. *Am J Trans* 2003;3:306.

33. Calne R, Moffatt SD, Friend PJ, et al. Campath IH allows low-dose cyclosporine monotherapy in 31 cadaveric renal allograft recipients. *Transplantation* 1999;68:1613.

34. Van Hooff J, Squifflet JP, Wlodarczyk Z, et al. A prospective randomized mulicenter study of tacrolimus in combination with sirolimus in renal transplant recipients. *Transplantation* 2003;75:1934.

35. Wiland AM, Fink JC, Weir MR, et al. Should living-unrelated renal transplant recipients receive antibody induction? Results of a clinical experience trial. *Transplantation* 77:422–425.

36. Webster AC, Playford EG, Higgins G, Chapman JR, Craig JC. Interleukin 2 receptor antagonists for renal transplant recipients: a meta-analysis of randomized trials. *Transplantation* 2004;77:166.

37. Balbontin F, Kiberd, Singh D, et al. Basiliximab widens the therapeutic window for AUC-monitored neural therapy after kidney transplantation. *Transplant Proc* 2003;35:2409.

38. Parrott NR, Hammad AQ, Watson CJ, et al. Multicenter, randomized study of the effectiveness of basiliximab in avoiding addition of steroids to cyclosporine a monotherapy in renal transplant recipients. *Transplantation* 2005;79:344.

39. Cherikh WS, Kauff HM, McBride MA, et al. Association of the type of induction immunosuppression with posttransplant lymphoproliferative disorder, graft survival, and patient survival after primary kidney transplantation. *Transplantation* 2003;76:1289.

40. de Mattos Am, Olyaei AJ, Bennett WM. Nephrotoxicity of immunosuppressive drugs: long-term consequences and challenges for the future. *Am J Kidney Dis* 2000;35:333.

41. Flechner SM, Goldfarb D, Modlin C, et al. Kidney transplantation without calcineurin inhibitor drugs: a prospective, randomized trial of sirolimus versus cyclosporine. *Transplantation* 2002;74:1070.

42. Flechner SM, Kurian SM, Solez K, et al. De novo kidney transplantation without use of calcineurin inhibitors preserves renal structure and function at two years. *Am J Trans* 2004;4:1776.

43. Oh HK, Ding P, Satmary NA. A pilot study of calcineurin inhibitor (CNI) and steroid avoidance immunosuppressive immunosuppressive protocol among living donor kidney transplant recipients. *Yonsei Med J* 2004;45:1143.

44. Ishitani M, Isaacs R, Norwood V, et al. Predictors of graft survival in pediatric living-related kidney transplant recipients. *Transplantation* 2000;70:277.

45. Kari JA, Trompeter RS. What is the calcineurin inhibitor of choice for pediatric renal transplantation. *Pediatr Transplant* 2004;8:437.

46. Trompeter R, Filler G, Webb NH, et al. Randomized trial of tacrolimus versus cyclosporine microemulsion in renal transplantation. *Pediatr Nephrol* 2002;17:141.

47. Neu AM, Ho PL, Fine RN, et al. Tacrolimus vs. cyclosporine A as primary immunosuppression in pediatric renal transplantation: a NAPRTCS study. *Pediatr Transplant* 2003;7:217.

48. Kim JS, Aviles DH, Silverstein DM, et al. Effect of age, ethnicity, and glucocorticoid use on tacrolimus pharmacokinetics in pediatric renal transplant patients. *Pediar Transplant* 2005;9:162.

49. Jungraithmayr T, Staskewtiz A, Kirste G, et al. Pediatric renal transplantation with mycophenolate-mofetil based immunosuppression without induction: results after three years. *Transplantation* 2003;75:454.

50. Sarwal MM, Vidhun JR, Alexander SR, et al. Continued superior outcomes with modification and lengthened follow-up of a steroid-avoidance pilot project with extended daclizumab induction in pediatric renal transplantation. *Transplantation* 2003;76:1331.

51. Mulloy LL, Wright F, Hall ML, et al. Simulect (basiliximab) reduces acute cellular rejection in renal allografts from cadaveric and living donors. *Transplant Proc* 1999;31:1210.

52. Kirste G. Living-donor kidney transplantation. *Langenbeck's Arch Surg* 1999;384:523.

53. Kim SJ, Lee KW, Lee DS, et al. Randomized trial of tacrolimus versus cyclosporine in steroid withdrawal in living donor renal transplant recipients. *Transplant Proc* 2004;36:2098.

54. Brennan TV, Freise CE, Fuller TF, et al. Early graft function after living donor kidney transplantation predicts rejection but not outcomes. *Am J Transplant* 2004;4:971.

# 16.8  IMMUNOBIOLOGY

*Gunilla Einecke, MD,*
*Philip F. Halloran, MD, PhD*

## INTRODUCTION

Kidney transplantation between genetically nonidentical humans leads to the activation of a large number of alloreactive lymphocytes that can exert effector functions leading to the destruction of the transplant. The two effector systems of the adaptive immune response generated during the alloimmune response are the effector T lymphocytes and alloantibodies. In most circumstances clinical rejection episodes are mediated by effector T cells, but alloantibody-mediated rejection is also common and serious.

Alloimmune responses are initiated by activation of antigen presenting cells (APCs) through innate immune recognition systems. In the graft and surrounding tissues, dendritic cells of donor and host origin become activated and move to T-cell areas of secondary lymphoid organs (SLO). Although tissue injury can trigger immune responses, injury may not be necessary: some "ticking over" of the antigen presentation system may always be occurring. In the SLO, antigen-bearing dendritic cells engage alloantigen-reactive naive T cells and central memory T cells (Figure 16.8-1). Although naive T cells are optimally triggered by dendritic cells in SLO,[1,2] previously stimulated or "antigen experienced" memory cells may be activated by other cell types, such as graft endothelium.[3] These memory cells may have been activated previously by alloantigenic stimuli or much more commonly by viral antigens that crossreact with alloantigens;[4] they recirculate between lymphoid compartments but cannot enter peripheral tissues.[5]

## THREE-SIGNAL MODEL OF THE ALLOIMMUNE T CELL RESPONSE IN THE SLO

The encounter of T cells with donor antigen occurs when host and donor APCs from the graft and the graft bed migrate to the T-cell areas of the SLO (Figure 16.8-1). An antigen on the surface of dendritic cells that triggers T cells with cognate T-cell receptors constitutes "signal 1," transduced through the CD3 complex. Dendritic cells provide costimulation, or "signal 2," delivered when CD80 and CD86 on the surface of dendritic cells engage CD28 on T cells. Signals 1 and 2 activate three signal transduction pathways: the calcium–calcineurin pathway, the RAS–mitogen-activated protein (MAP) kinase pathway, and the

nuclear factor-κB pathway.[6] These pathways activate transcription factors that trigger the expression of many new molecules, including interleukin-2, CD154, and CD25. Interleukin-2 and other cytokines (eg, interleukin-15) activate the "target of rapamycin" pathway to provide "signal 3," the trigger for cell proliferation. Proliferation and differentiation lead to a large number of effector T cells. B cells are activated when antigen engages their antigen receptors, usually in lymphoid follicles or in extrafollicular sites, such as red pulp of spleen,[7] or possibly in the transplant,[8] producing alloantibody against donor HLA antigens. Thus, within days the immune response generates the effector mechanisms that can damage the organ and mediate allograft rejection, effector T cells, and alloantibody.

## EFFECTORS AND LESIONS OF REJECTION

Rejection is a phenotype with three dimensions: clinical, immunologic, and histopathologic. *Rejection* is defined as tissue injury produced by the effector mechanisms of the adaptive alloimmune response, leading to deterioration in renal function. Increasingly new dimensions such as microarray analysis of the transcriptome are being added. There are two types of rejection: T-cell-mediated rejection (TCMR) and antibody-mediated rejection (ABMR). TCMR and ABMR can be early or late, fulminant and rapid, or relatively indolent and slow.

The cellular infiltrate observed in rejection is composed of mononuclear cells including T cells, macrophages, B cells, and plasma cells. T cells serve as the main effectors and regulators of the alloimmune response. Macrophages are possible effectors and aid in the removal of apoptotic cells. Theoretically B cells and plasma cells could contribute to the production of alloantibodies within the graft, but in fact they are seen more often in TCMR and are not per se part of the criteria for ABMR. In ABMR, the high-affinity, damaging IgG antibodies are probably made in SLO or in the marrow.

### T-Cell-Mediated Rejection

Effector T cells that emerge from SLO infiltrate the graft and orchestrate an inflammatory response including recruitment of activated macrophages. B cells and plasma cells may also be present, not as part of ABMR but because the inflamed site attracts them. The diagnostic lesions of T-cell-mediated rejection reflect mononuclear cells invading the kidney tubules (tubulitis) and the intima of small arteries (arteritis).[9] The graft displays intense interferon effects, increased chemokine expression, altered capillary permeability and extracellular matrix, and deterioration of parenchymal function.

The recruitment of the inflammatory cells into the graft is a result of expression of chemokines and adhesion molecules by the endothelium of the graft. The endothelium of postcapillary venules serves as the entry point of recipient leukocytes from the bloodstream into the allograft. Endothelial cells are activated by proinflammatory cytokines and injury to express adhesion molecules and chemokines necessary for transendothelial migration. The recruitment of leukocytes is initiated by the release of chemokines by tubular cells, interstitial cells, endothelial cells, and infiltrating recipient cells within the allograft. T cells expressing the respective chemokine receptors extravasate through the endothelium and are guided by a chemokine gradient within the graft. Binding of chemokines to their receptors induces a conformational change in integrins, which are normally present on

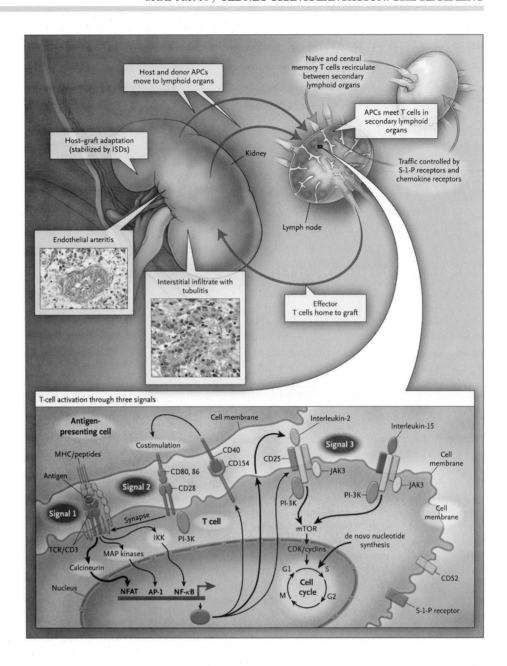

**FIGURE 16.8-1**

Steps in T-Cell–Mediated Rejection. Antigen-presenting cells (APCs) of host or donor origin migrate to secondary lymphoid organs. APCs present donor antigen to naive and central memory T cells. These T cells ordinarily circulate between lymphoid tissues, regulated by chemokine and sphingosine-1-phosphate (S-1-P) receptors.[57] T cells are activated and undergo clonal expansion and differentiation to express effector functions. Antigen triggers T-cell receptors (TCRs; signal 1) and synapse formation. CD80 (B7-1) and CD86 (B7-2) on the APC engage CD28 on the T cell to provide signal 2. These signals activate three signal-transduction pathways—the calcium–calcineurin pathway, the mitogen-activated protein (MAP) kinase pathway, and the protein kinase C–nuclear factor-κB (NF-κB) pathway— which activate transcription factors, nuclear factors of activated T cells (NFAT), activating protein 1 (AP-1), and NF- B, respectively. The result is expression of CD154 (which further activates APCs), interleukin-2 receptor  chain (CD25), and interleukin-2. Receptors for a number of cytokines (interleukin-2, 4, 7, 15, and 21) share the common  chain, which binds Janus kinase 3 (JAK3). Interleukin-2 and interleukin-15 deliver growth signals (signal 3) through the phosphoinositide-3-kinase (PI-3K) pathway and the molecular-target-of-rapamycin (mTOR) pathway, which initiates the cell cycle. Antigen-experienced T cells home to and infiltrate the graft and engage the parenchyma to create typical rejection lesions such as tubulitis and, in more advanced rejection, endothelial arteritis. However, if the rejection does not destroy the graft, adaptation occurs and is stabilized by immunosuppressive drugs. The photomicrographs of tubulitis and endothelial arteritis are taken from a mouse model in which these lesions are T-cell-dependent but independent of perforin, granzymes, and antibody. IKK denotes inhibitor of nuclear factor- B kinase, CDK cyclin-dependent kinase, and MHC major histocompatibility complex. *Source:* Halloran PF. *N Engl J Med* 2004;351:2715–2729.

circulating leukocytes in an inactive state. Tight adhesion occurs when activated integrins bind their ligands on graft cells. The most common integrins present on lymphocytes are LFA-1 that binds ICAM-1 and -2, and VLA-4 that binds VCAM-1. ICAM-1, VCAM-1 and E-cadherin are also expressed on the tubular epithelium of rejecting grafts where they may play a role in the development of tubulitis. Unfortunately, treating or preventing rejection by blocking of adhesion has not been successful, likely due to redundancy among the multiple adhesion molecules and their ligands.

An interesting but unexplained feature of rejection is that antigen-triggered effector T cells cross the donor endothelium without killing the endothelial cells. Thus TCMR can smoulder for days or weeks as an interstitial process, and the graft remains viable.

### Tissue injury in TCMR

Most rejection in clinical organ transplantation is TCMR. The main lesion for diagnosing rejection in the Banff schema is tubulitis[9] (http://tpis.upmc.edu/tpis/schema/KNCode97.html). Invasive lesions correlate with functional deterioration[10,11] and may be relevant to the tubular atrophy that often follows rejection. Tubulitis is T cell mediated: it can develop in mouse hosts lacking B cells and alloantibody[12] and is typically absent in human-alloantibody-mediated rejection.[13] Alloimmune T cells may mediate epithelial injury in kidney transplants either through direct contact or through contact-independent mechanisms. Many infiltrating cells in tubulitis lesions display cytotoxic T-lymphocyte (CTL) features.[14,15] CTL could engage epithelial cells via specialized molecules to interact with these structures and damage individual epithelial cells via cytotoxic mechanisms. Activated CTLs may kill their targets via their cytotoxic molecules perforin (Prf1) and granzymes A and B (GzmA/B). These molecules are released from stored granules, internalized, and released into the cytosol of target cells, where they initiate a cascade of events that leads to apoptosis. Alternatively, engagement of Fas on target cells by FasL on CTLs results in apoptotic death of the graft cell. However, tubulitis is not dependent on granule-associated CTL mechanisms, since it can develop in allografts rejecting in hosts lacking Prf1 or granzyme A (GzmA) and granzyme B (GzmB).[16] It has been suggested that the integrin CD103, by binding its ligand E-cadherin on epithelial cells, may permit CD8 T cells to engage the renal epithelium[17,18] and mediate invasion into tubular cells. However, mice deficient in CD103 develop tubulitis and deterioration similar to wild-type hosts, indicating that tubulitis is not dependent on this molecule.

The independence of the epithelial deterioration from CD103 and Prf1-Gzm suggests that the interstitial effector T cells and macrophages produce the epithelial changes that are the central lesion of graft rejection via contact-independent mechanisms, for example, delayed-type hypersensitivity (DTH). Activated effector T cells (CD4 or CD8) encounter antigen, possibly on host macrophages, and secrete cytokines that induce the influx of nonspecific inflammatory cells. Thus macrophages that are activated by T cells participate through DTH mechanisms,[19] but the injury remains antigen specific.[20] Mechanisms directly altering the epithelium could include the release of soluble effector T-cell or macrophage products (cytokines, Tnf superfamily members, reactive oxygen species, nitric oxide, eicosanoids, and enzymes). Additional effects may operate by changing the extracellular matrix (eg, synthesis of hyaluronic acid) or the microcirculation. Tubulitis may be a relatively late change in the epithelium, reflecting loss of epithelial integrity that permits entry of lymphocytes, which would explain the lack of requirement for cytotoxic mechanisms and the occurrence of tubulitis in atrophic tubules independent of rejection. Mechanisms of epithelial deterioration may involve parenchymal transdifferentiation into mesenchymal cells[21] and cell senescence.[22] The conditions for tubulitis may simply be inter-

stitial infiltration and compromised epithelial integrity, and the diagnostic value of tubulitis may be as an indicator of this loss of epithelial integrity.

Future research focusing on the pathogenesis of these lesions should ultimately be able to identify the molecular basis of tubulitis and endothelialitis. Our current belief is that TCMR is an interstitial inflammatory process mediated by effector T cells with cytotoxic activity but via delayed-type hypersensitivity mechanism. The epithelium deteriorates and loses its ability to exclude inflammatory cells, permitting them to enter to create tubulitis. Prf1, GzmA and GzmB, and CD103 may be supplementary but are not essential in this model.

## Antibody-Mediated Rejection

Alloantibodies against donor antigens mediate a substantial proportion of graft rejection episodes, contributing to early and late graft loss. Rejection caused by antibody is mediated by mechanisms that are different from those that mediate TCMR. Alloantibodies target capillary endothelium,[23] where they are cytotoxic through their ability to activate complement as well as recruit leukocytes to the graft. If recipients have been sensitized by previous transfusions, pregnancies, or transplants bearing donor MHC molecules, they may have preformed alloantibody against the donor. This can lead to disastrous hyperacute rejection, even on the operating table.[24] In these cases the entire endothelium of the graft is injured, and the large vessels usually fail, leading to immediate complete failure of the graft. Similar changes occur with incompatibility between donor and recipient at the ABO blood group locus. The existence of preformed alloantibodies can be detected by cross-matching prior to transplantation to prevent hyperacute rejection.

### Mechanisms of ABMR

The main antigenic targets of ABMR are MHC molecules, both class I and class II. In addition, antibodies directed against self-proteins may contribute to graft injury.[25] The B-cell response to antigens leads to the production of long-lived plasma cells, which migrate to the bone marrow where they continue to produce antibody. It is not known whether the presence of antibodies that are specific for graft antigens is maintained as a consequence of the longevity of plasma cells or as a consequence of the continuous generation of new memory B cells. Recent evidence indicates that long-term grafts might become neolymphoid organs with organized lymphoid tissue.[26] However, although examples of plasma-cell-rich rejection have been described, infiltration by B cells is not commonly seen in ABMR; the high-affinity damaging IgG antibodies are probably produced by B cells in SLO or in the bone marrow. Alloantibodies are cytotoxic through their ability to fixate and activate complement. Complement activation mediates acute graft injury by attracting inflammatory cells to the chemoattractants C3a and C5a. In addition, complement elicits spasmogenic effects by inducing the release of prostaglandin E2 from macrophages, causes edema by inducing the release of histamine from mast cells, and can induce lysis of endothelial cells. Activation of complement receptors on the surface of endothelial cells causes cytoskeletal changes and results in activation of the endothelial cells with increased expression of adhesion molecules and cytokine release. In severe cases of ABMR, thrombotic injury can dominate so that the rejection resembles thrombotic microangiopathy, with diffuse vascular injury and thrombosis.

### *Acute ABMR*

Acute alloantibody-mediated rejection is diagnosed by clinical,[27] immunologic,[28] and histologic criteria. It is classically associated with the triad of decreased renal function, the presence of alloantibody against donor antigens in recipient serum, and histological evidence of acute tissue injury (neutrophils in peritubular capillaries with endothelial damage)[13] with deposition of complement component 4d (C4d) in peritubular capillaries as an indication for the action of antibodies. However, some renal biopsies lack histological evidence of rejection and show only acute tubular injury. The demonstration of C4d deposition in peritubular capillaries has proved to be the most reliable marker of acute ABMR and is now the basis for the diagnosis of antibody-mediated rejection.[29–31]

### *Late/slow ABMR*

Recent evidence supports the hypothesis that a subset of cases of chronic allograft deterioration might be mediated by alloantibodies. Several studies have reported that *de novo* antibodies that are specific for graft HLA class I and class II molecules are a risk factor for premature graft loss as a consequence of chronic arteriopathy. Circulating HLA-specific antibodies are common in patients with long-term organ allografts and are typically present months to years before graft dysfunction, indicating that antibody-mediated graft injury might be slow to develop. The features of late/slow ABMR include duplication of the glomerular basement membrane (transplant glomerulopathy (TGP)), proliferation in the intima of arteries, and lamination of the peritubular capillary basement membrane, together with deposition of C4d in peritubular capillaries.[32–34]

## HOST–GRAFT ADAPTATION

The term *host–graft adaptation* describes the decrease in both donor-specific responsiveness and the risk of rejection in the months after a successful transplantation that is maintained with immunosuppression.[35] Changes in the organ—a loss of donor dendritic cells and a resolution of injury—contribute to the adaptation. The crucial element is a degree of anergy or clonal exhaustion: host T cells become less responsive to donor antigens when antigen persists and immunosuppression is maintained. Regulatory T cells may also contribute to stability in the control of alloimmune responses, by analogy with their ability to suppress autoimmunity,[36] although their importance in the phenomenon of host–graft adaptation remains unproven. Partial anergy (known as "adaptive tolerance" or "in vivo anergy") may be a general characteristic of T-cell responses *in vivo*, in which antigen persistence with inadequate co-stimulation triggers adaptations that limit T-cell responsiveness.[37] The resulting partial T-cell anergy is characterized by decreased tyrosine kinase activation and calcium mobilization (signal 1) and decreased response to interleukin-2 (signal 3). Adaptation in clinical transplantation resembles in vivo anergy—for example, both can occur in the presence of calcineurin inhibitors. The role of maintenance immunosuppression may be to stabilize adaptation by limiting excitation of the immune system and thus antigen presentation. In some experimental models, favorable adaptations are blocked when calcineurin is inhibited,[38] leading to suggestions that calcineurin inhibitors prevent adaptations in clinical transplantation. However, the relevance of these models to clinical adaptation, which occurs despite treatment with calcineurin inhibitors, is questionable.

## LATE SLOW DETERIORATION OF ORGAN TRANSPLANTS

Approximately 40% of late graft loss is due to nonspecific deterioration in the absence of other specific diseases and is characterized by deterioration of graft function with parenchymal atrophy and interstitial fibrosis, and in some cases with fibrous intimal thickening of arteries. The concept emerged in the early days of clinical renal transplantation that some kidneys failed late due to a type of rejection different from acute rejection, termed *chronic rejection*. Unfortunately, the term chronic rejection is ambiguous as it fails to differentiate between the presence of an active alloimmune response causing tissue damage (rejection) and the state of the transplanted tissue (eg, fibrosis and atrophy).[13] Whereas some cases of late slow graft deterioration are due to true rejection (which may be suspected in the presence of endothelialitis or tubulitis), other cases may represent the hemodynamic consequences of hypertension, accelerated senescence of the allograft, the development of an allograft glomerulopathy, or the development of chronic calcineurin toxicity or other diseases.[13,31,39–43] A new consideration is nephropathy due to BK virus.[44] Deterioration in a renal transplant thus often reflects the effects of more than one process. The degenerate term chronic rejection thus means many things to different observers and thus has little meaning on its own unless defined by the user. We have recently proposed that the term chronic rejection be replaced by accurate terms that convey whether rejection is active, the status of the parenchyma, and whether transplant glomerulopathy and other specific diseases are present.[13]

There are really two main phenomena. First, there is the widespread but nonspecific loss of nephrons and function termed *tubular atrophy/interstitial fibrosis (TA/IF)*, which occurs to a small extent in most renal transplants as a reflection of the stresses of the transplant, including T-cell-mediated rejection and CNI toxicity. It is reflected in the Banff schema by the TA/IF score. TA/IF tend to be tightly linked, suggesting a role for epithelial-mesenchymal transition (EMT). TA/IF may overlap some of the elements of aging—a type of accelerated senescence. TA/IF is not inherently progressive if the stress is terminated, for example, withdrawal of CNIs if the cause is CNI toxicity.

The second process is a specific entity, which occurs in a few kidneys but accounts for many kidneys that deteriorate late. This is what we call the "ABCD tetrad": antibody (circulating donor-specific antibody, usually anti-HLA class II or class I); basement membrane multilayering of peritubular capillaries; C4d staining of PTC; and duplication of the glomerular basement membrane (double contours),[45] indicating transplant glomerulopathy.

### *Transplant Glomerulopathy*

Transplant glomerular changes have emerged as a feature of grafts deteriorating from immunologic injury.[46–48] The term *transplant glomerulopathy (TGP)* was introduced to distinguish from glomerulonephritides characterized by deposition of immune complexes and infiltration by inflammatory cells.[49] The specific lesions of TGP are reduplication of the glomerular basement membrane owing to widening of the subendothelial space, a moderate increase in mesangial matrix, and mesangial interposition.[45] TGP occurs in many renal allografts with deteriorating renal function and has now been defined in the Banff schema. It is distinct from other entities that have been identified in renal transplants with deteriorating function, for example, rejection, allograft nephropathy, specific diseases, and accelerating factors.[9,40] TGP is often associated with peritubular capillary (PTC) basement membrane multilayering.[50,51] Both

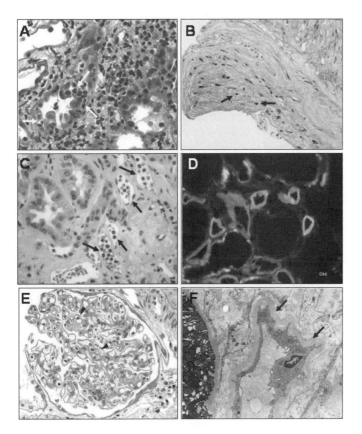

**FIGURE 16.8-2**

(**A**) Tubulitis in T-cell-mediated rejection (PAS, 40x). (**B**) Endotheli- alitis in T-cell-mediated rejection (PAS, 40x). (**C**) Infiltration of peritu- bular capillaries by polymorphonuclear cells in acute antibody-mediated rejection (PAS, 40x). (**D**) Peritubular capillaries stain positive for C4d in acute antibody-mediated rejection (**E**) Duplication of the glomerular basement membrane due to widening of the subendothelial space, indi- cating transplant glomerulopathy. (**F**) Basement membrane multilayer- ing of peritubular capillaries.

TGP and PTC basement membrane multilayering show basement membrane thickening and reduplication, suggesting common pathogenetic mechanisms, particularly endothelial cell injury.[50–53] Recent studies associate TGP with C4d deposition in PTC, sug- gesting alloantibody-mediated rejection as a pathogenesis.[33]

Many of the cases with late slow graft deterioration are thus due to late uncontrolled antibody responses and must be iden- tified and treated if possible. Better yet, they remind us of the need for lifelong immunosuppression in most renal transplant recipients, and the risks of graft loss if we excessively minimize immunosuppression. Some patients have all four elements, some have only three (eg, A,B,D), and some have only two (eg, B,D) (Figure 16.8-2). The understanding, prevention, and management of these cases are the unsolved problems and priorities in kidney transplant management.

## EFFECTS OF INJURY

Late allograft failure as a composite phenotype reflects the total burden of injury, including pretransplant factors, aging, and post- transplant-immune and -nonimmune injuries, plus limitations on organ homeostasis. Nonimmune stresses, such as brain-death- related organ injury and cold ischemia, may operate by evoking

inflammation and rejection, but also have a direct effect on paren- chyma and the circulation, acting as a challenge to homeostatic mechanisms. In renal transplant populations, the probability of late graft loss is determined by five major groups of risk factors: (1) organ characteristics (age, size, quality, and previous disease stresses, such as hypertension, cardiovascular disease, and diabe- tes, donor age); (2) brain death; (3) preservation and implanta- tion injury (cold preservation plus rewarming, reperfusion); (4) alloimmune injury (rejection): in human population data, this is rep- resented by the effect of HLA match, sensitization, immunosuppres- sive drugs, and rejection episodes; (5) and stresses in the recipient environment (infection, hypertension, proteinuria, recurrent disease, drug toxicity). In addition to understanding the mechanism of rejec- tion, the effects of age, injury, and intrinsic limitations on cell and organ survival have also emerged as important.

The basic science behind the relationships between injury and rejection is still largely incomplete. Young rats and mice a few weeks old, and even young primates 2 years of age, are not valid models of the 50-year-old human tissues we actually transplant. Nevertheless, some injury observations that are pieces of the puzzle include (1) injured kidneys are treated for rejection more frequently than those with good immediate function; (2) initial poor graft function increases the risk of late graft loss; (3) acute rejection increases the risk of late graft loss; (4) ischemic and toxic renal injury induce a stereotyped inflammatory response.

However, there are less well-appreciated complexities that make us question any easy assumptions that injury leads to im- mune responses: (1) Kidneys with DGF that recover completely have relatively little if any long term increased risk. The associa- tion between injured kidneys and increased risk of rejection may be observational: kidneys with DGF have more biopsies, and thus more opportunities for a diagnosis of rejection; (2) ABMR can induce DGF. However, rejection can occur with no new injury: the kidney on long-term immunosuppression can reject promptly when immunosuppression is stopped.

It has previously been postulated that tissue injury, by evok- ing inflammation, increases the probability of rejection.[54] Some authors propose that tissue injury causes inflammation through poorly understood pathways, probably part of the innate immu- nity mechanisms; that such inflammation activates antigen pre- sentation and thus the T-cell response; and that this could explain the poorer performance of injured organs. Thus living unrelated donor kidneys have excellent graft survival despite extensive HLA mismatching, perhaps because they lack the injury associated with brain death and prolonged cold storage that occurs in organs of deceased donors.[55] High survival rates in spousal donors support the concept that injury predisposes to immunologic recognition and rejection. The two kidneys from one deceased donor tend to show similarity in their graft survival and serum creatinine at all times posttransplant.[56] Moreover, the survival of a kidney was strongly predicted not only by its own early performance but also by the performance of the other kidney from that donor (mate effect). The probability of rejection was not paired, and rejection in the mate did not predict reduced survival of the kidney of in- terest.[56] Whereas rejection is driven mainly by nondonor factors, graft function is driven by donor factors.

These results indicate that the characteristics of the trans- planted tissue have an enduring effect on graft function and sur- vival, that early events in the mate kidney can reveal important information about the donor tissue, and that donor tissue char- acteristics are not the major factor in the probability of rejection. It is probable that donor tissue influences on the posttransplant course are heterogeneous, with immediate and long-term components. Perhaps the level of function is more influenced by long-term effects on the tissue (nephron number, senescence, capacity for repair), whereas acute injury such as cold ischemia has more influence on inflammation and rejection.

When considering effects of injury it is important to remember the direct effects of injury on the epithelium and other tissue elements, as well as the ability of injury to induce inflammation. Often direct effects of injury on the tissue are forgotten in our enthusiasm for studying the inflammatory and adaptive immune response. These direct effects are probably underestimated when rodents are used as models. The importance of peritransplant stress (brain death (in DD), surgical and temperature stress, ischemia, reperfusion, osmotic stress, etc) on the delicate renal epithelium in human renal transplantation may far outweigh its effect in eliciting inflammation and its stresses.

## Some Injury Effects May Reflect Somatic Cell Senescence Mechanisms

We are reminded of the quotation attributed to Mark Twain: to the person with only a hammer, everything looks like a nail. In transplantation, dominated by immunologists, all adverse effects tend to be attributed to immune and inflammatory mechanisms, because we know little of sciences like epitheliology. Thus effects of organ injury may be mediated through immune-inflammatory mechanisms, but this may be exaggerated and is not actually proven. The effects of tissue injury may simply be additive with rejection and not mediated through immune and inflammatory mechanisms. For example, epithelium has a finite ability to repair and sustain itself over time. Injury may simply exhaust some of this capacity. This reflects the finite limits on all somatic cells and tissue—the senescence limits that are imposed on survival of all organisms. Thus the deceased donor kidney may have exhausted part of its finite potential for repair and is more likely to manifest injury and fail when the alloimmune response occurs.

## SUMMARY

The time course of an organ transplant reflects the previous history of the organ (eg, age), its burden of injuries and stresses in the peritransplant and posttransplant period, and its intrinsic limitations on repair and homeostasis. The pathologic lesions of rejection can explain how rejection can be associated with permanent loss of the limiting elements in an organ transplant. This puts the course of an organ transplant into the same context as the general problem of repair and homeostasis of that organ in the face of normal and pathologic environmental stress. The most preventable stress is rejection, and identifying and treating all uncontrolled alloimmune injury remains the key to long-term graft stability.

## References

1. Lakkis FG, Arakelov A, Konieczny BT, Inoue Y. Immunologic 'ignorance' of vascularized organ transplants in the absence of secondary lymphoid tissue. *Nature Med* 2000;6:686–688.
2. Zhou P, Hwang KW, Palucki D, et al. Secondary lymphoid organs are important but not absolutely required for allograft responses. *Am J Transplant* 2003;3(3):259–266.
3. Biedermann BC, Pober JS. Human endothelial cells induce and regulate cytolytic T cell differentiation. *J Immunol* 1998;161(9):4679–4687.
4. Adams AB, Williams MA, Jones TR, et al. Heterologous immunity provides a potent barrier to transplantation tolerance. *J Clin Invest* 2003; 111(12):1887–1895.
5. von Andrian UH, MacKay CR. T-cell function and migration. Two sides of the same coin. *N Engl J Med* 2000;343(14):1020–1034.
6. Wang D, Matsumoto R, You Y, et al. CD3/CD28 Costimulation-Induced NF-kappaB Activation Is Mediated by Recruitment of Protein Kinase C-theta, Bcl10, and IkappaB Kinase beta to the Immunological Synapse through CARMA1. ÿÿ 2004;24(1):164–171.
7. MacLennan IC, Toellner KM, Cunningham AF, et al. Extrafollicular antibody responses. *Immunol Rev* 2003;194:8–18.
8. Sarwal M, Chua MS, Kambham N, et al. Molecular heterogeneity in acute renal allograft rejection identified by DNA microarray profiling. *N Engl J Med* 2003;349(2):125–138.
9. Racusen LC, Solez K, Colvin RB, et al. The Banff 97 working classification of renal allograft pathology. *Kidney Int* 1999;55(2):713–723.
10. Solez K, Racusen LC, Marcussen N, et al. Morphology of ischemic acute renal failure, normal function, and cyclosporine toxicity in cyclosporine-treated renal allograft recipients. *Kidney Int* 1993;43:1058–1067.
11. Solez K, Axelsen RA, Benediktsson H, et al. International standardization of criteria for the histologic diagnosis of renal allograft rejection: The Banff working classification of kidney transplant pathology. *Kidney Int* 1993;44:411–422.
12. Jabs WJ, Sedlmeyer A, Ramassar V, et al. Heterogeneity in the evolution and mechanisms of the lesions of kidney allograft rejection in mice. *Am J Transplant* 2003;3(12):1501–1509.
13. Trpkov K, Campbell P, Pazderka F, et al. Pathologic features of acute renal allograft rejection associated with donor-specific antibody. *Transplant* 1996;61:1586–1592.
14. Robertson H, Wheeler J, Kirby JA, Morley AR. Renal allograft rejection—in situ demonstration of cytotoxic intratubular cells. *Transplant* 1996;61(10):1546–1549.
15. Einecke G, Melk A, Ramassar V, et al. Expression of CTL associated transcripts precedes the development of tubulitis in T-cell mediated kidney graft rejection. *Am J Transplant* 2005;5(8):1827–1836.
16. Halloran PF, Urmson J, Ramassar V, et al. Lesions of T-cell-mediated kidney allograft rejection in mice do not require perforin or granzymes A and B. *Am J Transplant* 2004;4(5):705–712.
17. Hadley GA, Rostapshova EA, Gomolka DM, Taylor BM, Bartlett ST, Drachenberg CI et al. Regulation of the epithelial cell-specific integrin, CD103, by human CD8+ cytolytic T lymphocytes. *Transplant* 1999;67(11):1418–1425.
18. Robertson H, Wong WK, Talbot D, Burt AD, Kirby JA. Tubulitis after renal transplantation: demonstration of an association between CD103+ T cells, transforming growth factor beta1 expression and rejection grade. *Transplant* 2001;71(2):306–313.
19. Bogman MJ, Dooper IM, van de Winkel JG, et al. Diagnosis of renal allograft rejection by macrophage immunostaining with a CD14 monoclonal antibody, WT14. *Lancet* 1989;2(8657):235–238.
20. Rosenberg AS, Singer A. Cellular basis of skin allograft rejection: an *in vivo* model of immune-mediated tissue destruction. *Ann Rev Immunol* 1992;10:333–358.
21. Robertson H, Ali S, McDonnell BJ, Burt AD, Kirby JA. Chronic renal allograft dysfunction: The role of T cell-mediated tubular epithelial to mesenchymal cell transition. *J Am Soc Nephrol* 2004;15(2):390–397.
22. Halloran PF. Rethinking immunosuppression in terms of the redundant and nonredundant steps in the immune response. *Transplant Proc* 1996;28(6):11–18.
23. Racusen LC, Colvin RB, Solez K, et al. Antibody-mediated rejection criteria—an addition to the Banff 97 classification of renal allograft rejection. *Am J Transplant* 2003; 3(6):708–714.
24. Kissmeyer-Nielsen F, Olsen S, Peterson VP, Fjeldborg O. Hyperacute rejection of kidney allografts associated with pre-existing humoral antibodies against donor cells. *Lancet* 1966;2:662–665.
25. Dragun D, Muller DN, Brasen JH, et al. Angiotensin II type 1-receptor activating antibodies in renal-allograft rejection. *N Engl J Med* 2005; 352(6):558–569.

26. Colvin RB, Smith RN. Antibody-mediated organ-allograft rejection. *Nat Rev Immunol* 2005;5(10):807–817.

27. Halloran PF, Wadgymar A, Ritchie S, et al. The significance of the anti-class I antibody response. I. Clinical and pathologic features of anti-class I-mediated rejection. *Transplant* 1990;49(1):85–91.

28. Terasaki PI. Humoral theory of transplantation. *Am J Transplant* 2003; 3(6):665–673.

29. Feucht HE. Complement C4d in graft capillaries—the missing link in the recognition of humoral alloreactivity. *Am J Transplant* 2003;3(6):646–652.

30. Feucht HE, Schneeberger H, Hillebrand G, et al. Capillary deposition of C4d complement fragment and early renal graft loss. *Kidney Int* 1993;43:1333–1338.

31. Collins AB, Schneeberger EE, Pascual MA, et al. Complement activation in acute humoral renal allograft rejection: diagnostic significance of C4d deposits in peritubular capillaries. *J Am Soc Nephrol* 1999; 10:2208–2214.

32. Mauiyyedi S, Pelle PD, Saidman S, et al. Chronic humoral rejection: identification of antibody-mediated chronic renal allograft rejection by C4d deposits in peritubular capillaries. *J Am Soc Nephrol* 2001;12(3): 574–582.

33. Regele H, Bohmig GA, Habicht A, et al. Capillary deposition of complement split product C4d in renal allografts is associated with basement membrane injury in peritubular and glomerular capillaries: a contribution of humoral immunity to chronic allograft rejection. *J Am Soc Nephrol* 2002;13(9):2371–2380.

34. Vongwiwatana A, Gourishankar S, Campbell PM, Solez K, Halloran PF. Peritubular capillary changes and C4d deposits are associated with transplant glomerulopathy but not IgA nephropathy. *Am J Transplant* 2004;4(1):124–129.

35. Starzl TE, Marchioro TL, Waddell WR. The reversal of rejection in human renal homografts with subsequent development of homograft tolerance. *Surg Gyne Obs* 1963;117:385–395.

36. Sakaguchi S. Naturally arising CD4+ regulatory t cells for immunologic self-tolerance and negative control of immune responses. *Ann Rev Immunol* 2004;22:531–562.

37. Schwartz RH. T cell anergy. *Ann Rev Immunol* 2003; 21:305–334.

38. Li Y, Li XC, Zheng XX, et al. Blocking both signal 1 and signal 2 of T-cell activation prevents apoptosis of alloreactive T cells and induction of peripheral allograft tolerance. *Nat Med* 1999;5(11):1298–1302.

39. Racusen LC, Solez K, Colvin R. Fibrosis and atrophy in the renal allograft: interim report and new directions. *Am J Transplant* 2002;2(3): 203–206.

40. Halloran PF. Call for revolution: a new approach to describing allograft deterioration. *Am J Transplant* 2002;2(3):195–200.

41. Halloran PF, Melk A, Barth C. Rethinking chronic allograft nephropathy: the concept of accelerated senescence. *J Am Soc Nephrol* 1999;10(1): 167–181.

42. Bonsib SM. Acute rejection-associated tubular basement membrane defects and chronic allograft nephropathy. *Kidney Int* 2000;58(5): 2206–2214.

43. Solez K, Vincenti F, Filo RS. Histopathologic findings from 2-year protocol biopsies from a U.S. multicenter kidney transplant trial comparing tacrolimus versus cyclosporine: a report of the FK506 Kidney Transplant Study Group. *Transplant* 1998;66(12):1736–1740.

44. Nickeleit V, Klimkait T, Binet IF, Dalquen P, Del Z, V, Thiel G et al. Testing for polyomavirus type BK DNA in plasma to identify renal-allograft recipients with viral nephropathy. *N Engl J Med* 2000;342(18):1309–1315.

45. Habib R, Broyer M. Clinical significance of allograft glomerulopathy. *Kidney Int Suppl* 1993;43:S95–S98.

46. Porter KA, Dossetor JB, Marchioro TL, et al. Human renal transplants: I. Glomerular changes. *Lab Invest* 1967;16:153–181.

47. Starzl TE, Porter KA, Andres G, et al. Long-term survival after renal transplantation in humans: with special reference to histocompatibility matching, thymectomy, homograft glomerulonephritis, heterologous ALG, and recipient malignancy. *Ann Surg* 1970;172(3):437–472.

48. Merrill JP. The genesis of glomerulonephritis in renal transplants. *Adv Nephrol Necker Hosp* 1971;1:65–73.

49. Zollinger HU, Moppert J, Thiel G, Rohr HP. Morphology and pathogenesis of glomerulopathy in cadaver kidney allografts treated with antilymphocyte globulin. *Curr Top Pathol* 1973;57:1–48.

50. Monga G, Mazzucco G, Messina M, et al. Intertubular capillary changes in kidney allografts: a morphologic investigation on 61 renal specimens. *Mod Pathol* 1992;5:125–130.

51. Monga G, Mazzucco G, Novara R, Reale L. Intertubular capillary changes in kidney allografts: an ultrastructural study in patients with transplant glomerulopathy. *Ultrastruct Pathol* 1990;14(3):201–209.

52. Lajoie G. Antibody-mediated rejection of human renal allografts: an electron microscopic study of peritubular capillaries. *Ultrastruct Pathol* 1997;21(3):235–242.

53. Gough J, Yilmaz A, Miskulin D, et al. Peritubular capillary basement membrane reduplication in allografts and native kidney disease: a clinicopathologic study of 278 consecutive renal specimens. *Transplant* 2001;71(10):1390–1393.

54. Halloran PF, Homik J, Goes N, et al. The "injury response": a concept linking non-specific injury, acute rejection, and long term transplant outcomes. *Transplant Proc* 1997;29:79–81.

55. Terasaki PI, Cecka JM, Gjertson DW, Takemoto S. High survival rates of kidney transplants from spousal and living unrelated donors. *N Engl J Med* 1995;333(6):333–336.

56. Gourishankar S, Jhangri GS, Cockfield SM, Halloran PF. Donor tissue characteristics influence cadaver kidney transplant function and graft survival but not rejection. *J Am Soc Nephrol* 2003;14(2):493–499.

57. Mandala S, Hajdu R, Bergstrom J, et al. Alteration of lymphocyte trafficking by sphingosine-1-phosphate receptor agonists. *Science* 2002;296 (5566):346–349.

## 16.9   RECURRENCE OF DISEASE

*Abel E. Tello, MD,*
*Hassan N. Ibrahim, MD, MS*

### SCOPE OF THE PROBLEM

Renal transplantation is the treatment of choice for most patients with end stage renal disease. There has been significant improvement in patient and graft survival over the past 20 years. Death with a functioning graft and chronic allograft nephropathy continue to be the most common causes of graft loss. Recurrence of the native kidney disease in the renal allograft is currently estimated to account for at least 8% of allografts lost to biopsy-proven recurrent disease within 10 years of engraftment (Figure 16.9-1). This incidence depends heavily on the primary renal-disease-recipient-related factors and occasionally donor-related contributions. Studies addressing this issue have generally suffered from their small size, lack of histological confirmation of the diagnosis of the primary renal disease prior to transplantation, and the lack of histological ascertainment of the cause of graft loss posttransplantation.

In this chapter review the different studies that have addressed this issue with more emphasis on larger registry data, data that have become available in the last 3 years, and information on recurrence that has been reviewed by others elsewhere.

### RECURRENCE OF THE MAJOR GLOMERULONEPHRITIDES

#### Focal Segmental Glomerulosclerosis (FSGS)

Recurrent disease is a very important clinical problem and usually occurs within the first 6–12 months after transplantation.[1–4] Individual cases of apparent FSGS recurrence as long as 5 years after

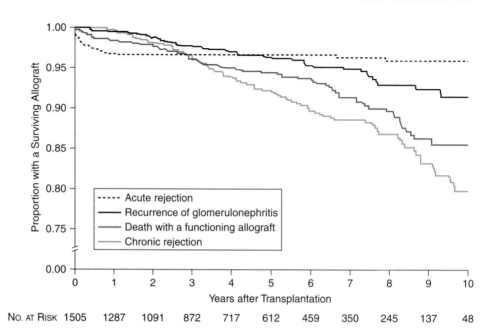

**FIGURE 16.9-1**

Kaplan–Meier Analysis of Allograft Loss Due to Recurrence of Glomerulonephritis, Acute Rejection, Chronic Rejection, and Death with a Functioning Allograft. Reprinted with permission.[8]

transplantation have also been described.[5,6] Recurrence usually manifests in the form of heavy proteinuria, hypertension, and/or loss of graft function. In patients with severe proteinuria in the course of FSGS recurrence, an increased risk of thromboembolic complications has also been noted.[7] In the largest series to date, Briganti et al. reported a 10-year incidence of graft loss in the 221 patients with biopsy-proven FSGS of 12.7% (CI 7.3-21.6%; Figure 16.9-2).[8] A slightly higher rate, 35 of 94 death-censored graft failures, were attributed to recurrent FSGS in a study by Koushik et al.[9] In this particular analysis of 228 adults and 35 children, half of the grafts lost were in repeat transplants. In addition, a report from the University of Miami indicates that 57% of the children with FSGS had confirmed recurrence.[10]

Risk factors for clinically relevant recurrence include younger age, presence of mesangial proliferation in the original biopsy, rapid progression to end-stage renal failure, and a brief duration until recurrence of proteinuria after transplantation.[1] An important issue is the question of whether a living related donor represents a higher risk for recurrence than living nonrelated or deceased donors. One study noted that in pediatric patients the benefit of a living donor is lost if the underlying disease is FSGS.[11] This was confirmed in a very large study, based on the U.S. Renal Data System (USRDS), which showed that graft failure in recipients below 20 years of age could be attributed to recurrent FSGS in 24% of living donors and in only 11% of deceased donor grafts.[12] However, in this later study, young age, but not the type of donor, was a risk factor, as in

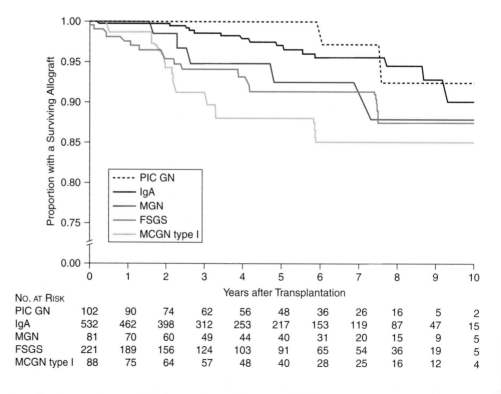

**FIGURE 16.9-2**

Kaplan–Meier Analysis of Allograft Loss Due to Recurrence of Glomerulonephritis, According to the Type of Glomerulonephritis. PIC GN, Pauci-immune glomerulonephritis; IgA, IgA nephropathy; MGN, membranous nephropathy; FSGS, focal segmental glomerulosclerosis and MCGN; MPGN, mesangiocapillary omerulonephritis. Reprinted with permission.[8]

the overall population, the benefit of a living donor over a deceased donor transplant was fully maintained. Nevertheless, even in children with underlying FSGS, living related donor transplantation has been performed in small series with reasonable results. In addition, previous literature suggests that the recurrence of FSGS may be more common in recipients who received a human-leukocyte-antigen- (HLA)-identical living related transplant. Cibrik et al. analyzed data using the USRDS and the U.S. Scientific Renal Transplant Registry between 1988 and 1997 and found 2,414 patients who had FSGS as the primary diagnosis as compared to 16,845 who had other types of glomerulonephritis.[13] FSGS patients receiving a zero mismatch living related donor kidney transplant had the lowest annually adjusted death censored graft loss per 1,000 patients. This was not significantly different than living donor zero mismatch glomerulonephritis recipients. Annual adjusted death-censored graft loss was significantly higher in FSGS recipients who received a living donor mismatch transplant. Summary of this large registry data clearly indicates that zero mismatch living related donor kidney transplants are not a risk factor for graft loss in FSGS patients, but are associated with a significantly better death-censored renal allograft survival as compared to deceased donor zero mismatch or HLA mismatch donations. In addition, data from our institution seem to indicate that, in a review over 200 patients from two centers, the risk of graft loss was around 10%, and it was unrelated to HLA mismatches.[9] Another recently recognized risk factor for recurrent FSGS appears to be white race as African Americans had significantly lower rates of graft loss attributed to recurrence.[12]

Whether antibody induction therapy is associated with heightened FSGS recurrence is controversial, but there are at least two reports that support this observation.[10,14]

Apart from supportive therapy with ACE inhibitors and/or angiotensin II receptor blockers, therapeutic options are increased immunosuppression, higher calcineurin inhibitor blood levels, and plasma exchange or immuneadsorption.[6,15–19] ACE inhibitors should be used with caution, if at all, in patients undergoing plasma exchange using AN69 filters which can lead to excess bradykinins release and hypotension. In children, prophylactic plasmapheresis prior to transplantation appears to be more effective in preventing recurrence than plasmapheresis after transplantation.[15] In children with recurrence, over half respond to plasmapheresis. However, in adults with recurrent FSGS, plasmapheresis appears less effective, but the response rate is still close to 40% to 50%.[17] The median number of treatments received is typically less, and the time from diagnosis to first treatment is greater for patients who relapse. Early institution of treatment also appears important, because the presence of sclerosis on biopsy predicts treatment failure.[6,18] Consequently, early treatment after diagnosis with a regimen of three daily plasmapheresis treatments followed by six treatments on an alternate-day basis is generally recommended but has not been vigorously tested.[17] In other cases, patients have been maintained chronically on monthly plasmapheresis treatment; as long as 6 years in one case.[6]

Alternating protein A adsorption treatment with plasma exchanges may have an additional antiproteinuric benefit.[16] The use of cyclophosphamide in conjunction with plasmapheresis has resulted in complete remission of proteinuria in 7/11 children with recurrent FSGS.[20] A different report is also consistent with the potential benefits of cyclophosphamid.[21]

Mutations in genes encoding alpha-actinin-4 and podocin (NPHS2) have been identified as causes of the hereditary forms of FSGS.[22] The presence of this mutation has also been linked to steroid resistance. Recurrence of FSGS, in one series, was noted in

35% of patients with steroid-resistant FSGS without NPHS2 mutation, whereas it occurred only in 8% of those have homozygous or compound heterozygous mutation of the NPHS2 gene.[23] This has recently been confirmed in a series of 338 patients from 272 families with steroid-resistant nephrotic syndrome.[24]

Recurrent FSGS needs to be distinguished from the pathological lesion of FSGS in the course of chronic allograft nephropathy. The latter presents late after transplantation and is seen typically in those who have had previous episodes of acute rejection, in association with arteriolar hyalinosis, and is a negative independent predictor of graft survival.

Patients who develop recurrent FSGS in the first transplant have at least a 75% change of recurrence in the second allograft with almost a 30% change of graft loss that is attributed directly to recurrent FSGS.[2–4,9,25]

## Membranoproliferative Glomerulonephritis (MPGN)

Both type 1 and the less common type 2 MPGN commonly recur after renal transplantation.[1,8,26]

### Type 1 MPGN

The rate of recurrent disease in type 1 MPGN ranges from 20% to 30%, although the incidence in children may be somewhat higher.[27–31] Perhaps the best estimate of the incidence of graft loss due to recurrent type 1 MPGN comes from a study of 1,505 renal transplant recipients with a history of end-stage renal disease due to biopsy-proven glomerulonephritis, of whom 88 had type 1 MPGN (Figure 16.9-2).[8] The incidence of allograft loss at 10 years due to recurrent type 1 MPGN was 14.4% (95% CI 7.6–26.4%).

Little data exist concerning recurrent disease in a second allograft. In one study, approximately 80% of patients in whom the first renal graft had recurrent disease experienced recurrent MPGN in the second.[32]

The presence or absence of hypocomplementemia is not helpful for either diagnosis or prognosis, as approximately 30% to 40% of these patients will lose their graft.[33]

There is no proven beneficial therapy, although the combination of aspirin and dipyridamole may stabilize renal function, similar to their anecdotal efficacy in primary MPGN. Some have suggested that the rate of recurrence has fallen from 30% to 10% after the introduction of cyclosporine.[34] There are some case reports describing successful treatment of recurrent MPGN with cyclophosphamide or plasmapheresis with modest results.[35,36]

### Type 2 MPGN

Recurrent disease is much more frequent in type 2 MPGN, ranging from 50% to 100% in different series.[26–28] Affected patients typically present within 1 year after transplantation with proteinuria that is often subnephrotic inrange. Graft loss due to recurrent disease is thought to occur in only 10% to 20% of cases, although some centers have reported rates as high as 30% to 50%.[37,38]

A retrospective comparative analysis of 75 patients with MPGN II contained in the North American Pediatric Renal Transplant Cooperative Study transplantation database has recently been published.[39] Five-year graft survival for patients with MPGN II was significantly worse (50.0 ± 7.5%) compared with the database as a whole (74.3 ± 0.6%; P < 0.001). Living related donor organs had a significantly better 5-year survival (65.9 ± 10.7%) compared with deceased donor organs ($34.1 \pm 9.8\%$; $P = 0.004$). The primary cause of graft failure in 11 (14.7%) patients was recurrent disease. Supplemental surveys were obtained on 29 (38%) of 75 patients. Analysis of these data indicate that recurrent disease occurred in 12 (67%) of the 18 patients with posttransplantation biopsies. Although there was no correlation between pretransplantation presentation, pre- or posttransplantation C3 levels, and either disease recurrence or graft failure, there was a strong association between heavy proteinuria and disease recurrence. The presence of glomerular crescents in allograft biopsies had a significant negative correlation with graft survival. At last follow-up, patients with recurrent disease had significantly higher serum creatinine and qualitatively more proteinuria than patients without biopsy-proven disease. These data indicate that recurrent MPGN II has a significant negative impact on renal allograft function and survival.

An anecdotal report in one patient found that plasmapheresis decreased the histologic changes and induced a clinical remission.[40] Institution of ACE-inhibition therapy is also generally recommended.

Little is known concerning recurrent disease among patients with type 3 MPGN who undergo renal transplantation. One case report described a patient with end-stage renal disease due to type 3 MPGN who presented with hematuria and proteinuria 16 months after undergoing renal transplantation. Renal biopsy revealed recurrent type 3 MPGN; graft loss occurred 7 years later.[41]

## IgA nephropathy (IgAN)

### Incidence of Latent mesangial IgA Deposits

Suzuki et al. assessed zero-hour biopsies in 446 living and 64 deceased donors for IgA and $C_3$ deposition.[42] IgA deposits were present in 16.1% and did not vary with donor source. Those with IgA and $C_3$ deposits were more likely to have had hematuria before donation. HLA-BW51 was more likely to be present in the donors with IgA deposits. Two separate series of a total of 12 patients noted rapid resolution of IgA deposits after transplantation in most patients.[43,44]

### Clinical Recurrence

Recurrent IgA deposition may result in a wide spectrum of manifestations, ranging from an incidentally noted histologic finding to mesangioproliferative glomerulonephritis associated with hematuria, proteinuria, and occasionally progressive renal dysfunction.

The largest reported retrospective analysis (532 allograft recipients with primary IgAN) is from Australia, where the estimated 10-year incidence of graft loss due to recurrent disease was 9.7% (95% CI 4.7–19.5%; see Figure 16.9-2). Allografts in IgA recipients exhibited a similar 10-year survival as allografts in recipients with either glomerular or nonglomerular disease.[8] In this series, recurrent IgAN was a less frequent cause of graft loss than either chronic rejection or death with a functioning graft.

Similar findings were reported in a review of 10 retrospective analyses. At a mean follow-up period of 67 months, there was a 15% incidence of significant graft dysfunction, and a 7% incidence of graft loss due to recurrent IgAN.[1] The mean time to clinical recurrence and allograft failure in most series is 31 and 63 months, respectively.

Several analyses have found no increased risk of recurrence based on living versus deceased donor status.[45–47] By comparison, other studies have reported an increased risk of recurrence in recipients of living related allografts.[48–50]

The presence of either HLA-B35 or HLA-DR4 increases the risk of recurrence in some series.[51,52] Other studies noted a higher representation of HLA-B35 and HLA-DR4 in the IgA population, but their presence had no effect on the incidence of recurrence.[46]

The likelihood of IgAN recurrence may not be affected by the type of immunosuppressive agents used. No significant difference, for example, has been observed in the incidence or severity of IgAN in studies comparing the pre- and postcyclosporine eras.[45,53] There is some evidence that the use of mycophenolate mofetil may decrease the risk of IgAN recurrence.[47] Recent data, however, challenge the notion that MMF is more beneficial than azathioprine in preventing IgAN recurrence. Chandrakantan et al. reported the Univeristy of Alabama experience with 152 kidney transplant recipients for IgAN who were at least 12 months posttransplantation.[54] Sixty-one were on aziathioprine, and 91 were on MMF. By 3 years, IgAN developed in 8.1% in MMF-treated recipients and in 10% of the azathioprine treated group (p = 0.76). Based on this information, it is difficult to make recommendations regarding the purine synthesis inhibitor of choice in subjects with IgAN. A trial of fish oil, which has been deemed safe in transplant recipients,[55] should be considered in conjunction with interruption of the renin-angiotensin system especially for IgAN recipients with heavy proteinuria.[56]

## Membranous Nephropathy

Membranous nephropathy continues to be among the most common causes of nephrotic syndrome in the nondiabetic adult. Histologically, it is characterized by basement membrane thickening with little or no cellular proliferation or infiltration. Circulating antibodies directed against endogenous antigens have been demonstrated in the Heymann experimental nephritis model of membranous nephropathy. Antibodies against megalin has received most of the attention as potential basement membrane antigen.[57]

Histological recurrence of membranous nephropathy in the transplant is not uncommon.[58–60] The mean time to recurrence, though variable, has been roughly around 1 year. Recurrence of membranous can occur in both poorly and well-matched allografts, and there is no evidence that the introduction of cyclosporine has changed the rate of recurrent disease.[61] There is some suggestion, however, that HLA-identical transplants might be more likely to have recurrent disease, though these numbers have been too small to make any meaningful conclusion regarding this issue.[59] The severity of the course of membranous nephropathy in native kidney disease seems to have no impact on the risk of recurrence. Overall, the outcome for recurrent membranous is poor. As a matter of fact, the actual risk for graft loss among patients with a recurrent membranous is 38% and 52% at 5 and 10 years, respectively.[62] Perhaps the best evidence regarding the risk of loss of the graft from recurrent disease comes, again, from Briganti et al., published in the *New England Journal of Medicine* in 2002, which estimated the incidence of graft loss due to recurrent membranous in a study of 1,505 renal transplant recipients with a history of end-stage renal disease due to biopsy proven glomerulonephritis. Among these, 81 patients with membranous disease had an incidence of allograft loss at 10 years that was at 12.5% (Figure 16.9-2).[8]

A critical issue is to be able to differentiate between recurrent and *de novo* membranous nephropathy.[59] The incidence of the latter is estimated at around 2%, but this seems to increase as the time from transplantation increases, reaching 5% at 8 years.[63] This has been shown by Schwartz et al. in their study of 1,029 renal transplants that was performed on 848 patients between 1972 and 1990.[63] *De novo* membranou nephropathy was seen in 30 biopsy specimens from 21 subjects, with 10 receiving an immunosuppressive regimen that did not include CSA. The mean time to occurrence was 62 ± 44 months. Of importance is the fact that *de novo* membranous has a very poor response to pulse steroids.

Although the pathogenesis of *de novo* membranous remains largely unknown, the presence of vascular and interstitial expansion analogous to chronic allograft nephropathy raises the possibilities that previous rejection episodes may lead to exposure of previously unrecognized glomerular antigens, possible glomerular injury due to rejection, and a possibility that the circulating antibodies directed against HLA antigens are somewhat responsible for this entity. The high likelihood of developing *de novo* membranous glomerulonephritis in second transplants has been highlighted and seems to suggest factors that are unique to the host for the development of this condition.[64] Therefore, caution and appreciation for the high risk of recurrence in repeat transplants should be taken.

Considering the observation that neither cyclosporine nor pulse steroids affect the course of recurrent membranous, there has been consideration to substituting cyclosporine with cyclophosphamide. The reports have been mixed regarding this approach and mainly anecdotal in nature, and the results do not support this approach.[65] Early surveillance for proteinuria and aggressive biopsy procedures, early initiation of ACE inhibition therapy, and protein restriction may alleviate the progression of this disease. Last, since the prevalence of viral infections, especially hepatitis C, might be higher in the transplant population than in other populations, ruling out secondary causes of membranous glomerulonephritis is always warranted.

## RECURRENCE OF DISEASES WITH A SYSTEMIC NATURE

### Systemic Lupus Erythematosus

End-stage renal disease and infection continue to contribute the most to the mortality and the morbidity associated with SLE. It is estimated that roughly 30% to 50% of all subjects afflicted with SLE will go on to develop renal manifestation. The percentage of SLE subjects with active clinical lupus decreases significantly with initiation of dialysis. A parallel reduction in serological activity also occurs.[66]

The survival of lupus patients on dialysis is similar to other patients. They do, however, seem to incur a higher mortality in the first 3 months of dialysis presumably due to sepsis and complications of high steroid therapy and cytotoxic agents.[67] Therefore, it has been a conventional approach to delay transplantation until after the first 3 months. This has three distinct advantages. First, it selects out patients who survive this critical 3-month period. Second, it may result in, as mentioned previously in reducing intensity of the serological and clinical activity of the disease. Finally, sporadic cases of complete recovery of kidney function have been described in the first 6 months of dialysis.

One of the largest series addressing the issue of recurrent SLE post transplantation comes from Mojsik et al.[6] Recurrence of lupus in the transplanted grafts was 2.7% to 3.8%, and a similar percentage resulted in graft failure. In a different series, summarizing 20 published reports, lupus patients who received living related renal transplants generally had superior graft survival rates. The 5-year graft survival rate in the cyclosporine area was 89% for living related transplants compared with 41% for deceased donor transplants. Again, the rate of recurrence was relatively rare at 2%.[67–70] Of interest, is the demonstration that pretransplant serological parameters such as complement and anti-double-stranded DNA levels appear to be unreliable predictors of the likelihood of recurrence.[71] The study that assessed histological recurrence more carefully than others comes from Stone et al.[71] In their study of 97 consecutive SLE patients who underwent a total of 106 renal transplantation and also underwent a total of 143 posttransplant biopsies. Only 9 patients had histological evidence of recurrent lupus, 6 of whom received deceased donor organs. Recurrence occurred 3.1 years after transplantation. Histological recurrence is as early as 5 days was noted. Therefore, this rate of histological recurrence of 10% is higher than what has been reported in other series. Nevertheless it again documents the excellent graft survival in lupus patients. There was one additional study that showed a higher recurrence rate and comes from Goral et al. of 54 renal transplant recipients, 31 of whom underwent biopsies because of worsening renal function and proteinuria.[72] Recurrent lupus nephritis was documented in 52% of patients who underwent biopsy and 30% of the total patients. Graft survival was worse in patients that underwent biopsy compared to those who never underwent a biopsy. Nevertheless, graft loss due to recurrent disease was rare.

### Pauci-immune Glomerulonephritis

Wegener's granulomatosis is a systemic vasculitis of the medium and small artery as well as the venules, arterioles, and very large arteries. The most classic presentation would involve the upper and lower respiratory tract infection, lower respiratory tracts, and the kidneys. Modern therapy consists of corticosteroids and cyclophosphamide induction therapy. There is a recent tendency of switching from cyclophosphamide to a less toxic immunosuppressive medication such as aziathioprine and mycophenolate mofetil once remission is achieved. Using the cyclophosphamide and prednisone, survival of 80% at 8 years with most of the deaths due to either therapy or the disease itself has been reported. Seventy-five percent achieved complete remission. More importantly, among the 98 patients followed for more than 5 years, nearly one half experienced remission that lasted at least 5 years.[72]

It has been well appreciated that both renal and extra-renal manifestations of Wegener's granulomatosis may recur after transplantation. In a series of eight patients, seven of whom did not have any evidence of systemic activity revealed that only one patient presented with a relapse episode that involved the lungs and the kidneys and was successfully treated with steroids.[74–76] In this particular series, only three patients had Wegener's granulomatosis, and none of them recurred. The patient mentioned above who recurred had microscopic polyangitis. There has been a case report of Wegener's granulomatosis also presenting as an obstructive uropathy as the disease has recurred in the ureter.[77] Data from our institution regarding eight patients with end-stage renal disease secondary to Wegener's granulomatosis revealed that seven patients were alive with a functioning graft 40–128 months posttransplantation with a mean follow-up of 91 months.[78] One patient died 126 months posttransplantation with a well-functioning graft. Posttransplant immunosuppression controlled the primary disease in all but one patient who presented with perisinusitis. Recurrent disease was not noted in any of the transplanted organs.

## Goodpastures's Syndrome

It is estimated that the incidence of recurrent linear IgG staining in renal transplant recipients with Goodpasture's syndrome may be as high as 50%.[79] The majority of these recipients are asymptomatic. The relatively low rate of recurrence is reflective of the fact that most of these patients are never transplanted until the disease is quiescent, they are usually maintained on immunosuppressant therapy, and last, the maintenance immunosuppressive therapy of kidney transplantation might be sufficient to keep the disease under control. Graft loss due to recurrent disease is extremely uncommon.[79,80]

## Scleroderma

Renal involvement in scleroderma most frequently presents as rapidly progressive renal failure with malignant hypertension.[81] It may also present as slowly progressive kidney disease characterized by proteinuria, hypertension, and renal dysfunction.[82] Although the introduction of angiotensin-converting enzyme inhibitors has alleviated the poor prognosis associated with scleroderma, a significant portion of those afflicted with renal crisis, in some series as high as 50%, may still need kidney replacement therapy.[81] The recurrence rate has been estimated to be approximately 20%.[83,84] The exact frequency of recurrent disease is difficult to ascertain, since the primary histologic changes induced by scleroderma (mucoid intimal thickening of the interlobular arteries and fibrinoid necrosis in the glomeruli) may be difficult to differentiate from acute or chronic vascular rejection. The use of cyclosporine was not a predictor of graft survival.[83–85]

In an analysis of the UNOS registry between 1995 and 2002, 258 patients with scleroderma were listed for transplantation.[86] Survival was significantly better in patients who received a transplant. Graft survival at 1 and 3 years was 68% and 60%, respectively. Early graft losses were common. Skin scores from the underlying scleroderma improved in all subjects. Although this graft survival is clearly inferior to other diseases, the improvement it offers over dialysis and the potential improvement in systemic manifestation currently warrant offering these patients a kidney transplant. In this same UNOS registry data, recurrent disease accounted for the loss of three grafts from a total of 63 losses (4%).

Renal allograft recipients with recurrent disease tend to follow a malignant course, similar to that in primary scleroderma renal crisis.[84]

## Amyloidosis

*Amyloidosis* is defined by the ability of a variety of proteins (such as immunoglobulin light chains in primary amyloidosis, amyloid A in secondary amyloidosis, ß2-microglobulin in dialysis-associated arthropathy, and amyloid beta protein in Alzheimer's disease and Down's syndrome) to form ß-pleated sheets.[87]

One- and 5-year patient survival are 68% and 30% in one study, whereas another reported a median survival of only 8.2 months in a group of patients with primary amyloid.[88,89] The outcome appears to be best in patients without cardiac involvement on two-dimensional echocardiography.[88]

Renal transplantation in renal amyloidosis is mostly limited to secondary disease, since patient survival is often relatively short in primary amyloidosis.[90–93] The largest study compared the results in 45 patients with amyloidosis (most of whom had rheumatoid arthritis) to that in a matched control group with other

disorders.[90] Three-year graft survival was similar in the two groups (53% vs 49%), although patient survival was lower in the amyloid group due predominantly to infectious and cardiovascular complications.

Recurrent amyloid deposition in the transplant occurs in 20% to 33% of cases due to continued activity of the underlying disease. However, graft loss due to recurrence is uncommon. (94). Colchicine, from the same series, can prevent the development of proteinuria.[94]

## Alport's Syndrome

Transplantation with a normal kidney into an individual with Alport's syndrome results in the presentation of a previous unrecognized antigen to the recipient leading to humoral antibody response. Therefore, recipients with Alport's may present with hematuria and graft dysfunction from this "de novo anti-GBM disease."[95–104]

The largest analysis of kidney transplantation in Alport's Syndrome comes from Byrne et al., whose analysis included 52 renal transplants in 41 patients.[104] Eighty percent of the transplant recipients were alive 10 years after transplantation and the long-term allograft survival was remarkably similar to that reported for other diseases. Of interest, men tended to have better long-term graft survival than women. Fourteen percent of allograft biopsy specimens showed linear glomerular basement membrane IgG deposits, but only 2.4% developed posttransplant anti-GBM disease. That incidence was at 3.1% in the male transplant recipients. This incidence is clearly lower than what has previously been reported. Although there is a link between HLA DR alleles and anti-GBM disease in native kidneys, this was not seen in this large series. The most common cause of graft failure in subjects with Alport's syndrome continues to be chronic allograft nephropathy and acute rejection.

Retransplantation in Alport's posttransplant anti-GBM disease has been recently studied in three cases.[105] All cases showed early antibody and complement fixation to human glomerular basement membranes. Pathological examination revealed crescentic glomerular nephritis and segmental necrosis. Netrophilic infiltrates were an early feature in all three cases. Eleven previously described cases of retransplantation in patients with Alport's Syndrome who lost their graft to anti-GBM disease followed the typical pattern of a disease that has destroyed the first allograft after months of years, the second allograft destroyed in weeks to months, and the third destroyed in days to weeks. Plasma exchange was successful in roughly 40% of all reported cases of anti-GBM disease. In conjunction with plasma exchanges, there has been the suggestion that the institution of mycophenylate mofetil and antibodies to T-lymphocytes might be of benefit.[105]

## Primary Hyperoxaluria

Combined liver–kidney transplantation is the treatment of choice for children with type 1 primary hyperoxaluria with progressive renal disease.[106] The outcome may be best if transplantation is performed when the GFR falls to 25 mL/min and prior to marked tissue oxalate deposition.

Renal transplantation has been proposed as the treatment of choice for patients who progress to end-stage renal failure, since the rate of oxalate removal with standard hemodialysis or continuous ambulatory peritoneal dialysis is insufficient to prevent systemic oxalate accumulation.[107–109]

Data from the European Dialysis and Transplant Association, for example, showed a 3-year graft survival rate of only 23% for living related donor kidneys and 17% for cadaver kidneys in a review of 98 first transplants for oxalosis.[110]

A number of manipulations have been tried to make both preventive therapy of the primary disease and renal transplantation more successful. These include: aggressive preoperative dialysis (as often as 6 days per week) to deplete the systemic oxalate pool, consideration of early transplantation (GFR $\simeq$ 20 mL/min) to minimize systemic oxalate accumulation, and the preferential use of a living related donor to reduce the risk of early acute renal failure, which will lead to oxalate retention.

## Diabetes Mellitus

Diabetic nephropathy continues to be the leading cause of end-stage renal disease in the United States and is currently the number one reason to receive a kidney transplant in isolation or in combination with pancreas transplantation.

Recurrent diabetic nephropathy develops in almost all diabetic patients undergoing renal transplantation without pancreas or islet cell transplantation.[111-113] Glomerular basement membrane thickening and mesangial expansion are seen by 2 years, followed by hyalinization of the afferent and efferent arterioles by 4 years. In contrast, the typical nodular lesions of diabetic glomerulosclerosis rarely recur in the transplant.[112]

Loss of the graft due to recurrent disease is unusual, occurring in less than 5% of cases.[113] Recurrent disease in current diabetic nephropathy was first described by Mauer et al. in 1976.[112] Trapping of proteins including immunoglobulin IgG and albumin was found in both glomerular and tubular basement membranes of renal allograft biopsy specimens of diabetic patients. These changes occurred as early as 2.5 years after renal transplantation. Another report comprising 14 diabetic renal transplant patients showed that the histologic diagnosis of diabetic glomerulosclerosis was made on average 97 months after transplantation with a range of 41 to 154 months.[114] This abnormal histologic pattern was accompanied by functional changes such as proteinuria and a decrement in GFR. In this latter study, graft survival was affected by this recurrence. Studies, however, have failed to identify the usual clinical risk factors that have been associated with the development of diabetic nephropathy in the native kidneys to that in the transplant. The notion that parameters intrinsic to the kidney must play a significant role in the development of recurrent diabetic nephropathy has also suggested by the study by Bhalla et al.[114]

Rates of recurrence of diabetic nephropathy in the renal allograft has become more difficult to study recently in view of the increasing number and availability of beta-cell-replacement therapy options for the diabetic subject. In a study of eight patients with type I diabetes without uremia had mild to advanced lesions of diabetic nephropathy kidney biopsy at the time of transplantation for 5 to 10 years.[115] The mean urinary albumin excretion rate fell from 103 mg/day before transplantation to 30 mg/day at 5 years and 20 mg/day at 10 years. Creatinine clearance declined form 108 $\pm$ 20 mL/min to 74 $\pm$ 14 mL/min at 10 years. The thickness of the glomerular basement and tubular basement membranes were similar at 5 years but decreased significantly at 10 years. In addition, the mesangial fractional volume increased from baseline to 5 years but subsequently declined. This evidence clearly suggests that pancreas transplantation can reverse the lesions of diabetic nephropathy, but reversal may require more than 5 years considering the long duration of the underlying diabetic nephropathy and some potentially adverse outcome of calcineurin inhibitor and renal histology.

## Henoch–Schonlein purpura (HSP)

Although HSP behaves somewhat similarly to IgA nephropathy, the percentage of patients progressing to end-stage renal disease seems to be distinctly lower than IgA nephropathy. In the longest follow-up of such subjects, 24 years, only 10% of children went on to develop end-stage renal disease.[116] An additional 25% had significant renal involvement as evidenced by a reduction in GFR, persistent proteinuria, or hematuria. Meulders et al. reported their own single-center data of 14 transplants that were performed in 10 patients with HSP and compared them to 64 other renal transplants that were reported in the literature prior to 1994.[117-120] Risk for renal recurrence and for graft loss due to recurrence was 35% and 11% at 5 years, respectively. Duration of the original disease of less than 36 months seems to be an independent risk factor for recurrence. Also of note is the demonstration that recurrent HSP in extra-renal sites such as the skin and abdominal pain can occur posttransplantation. There has been a suggestion that HSP may be more likely to recur in recipients of living donor kidneys.[119]

## Fabry's Disease

Fabry's disease is an X-linked glycolipid storage disease caused by deficient activity of the lysosomal enzyme alpha-galactosidase A, resulting in the accumulation and subsequent tissue deposition of globotriaosylceramide, the glycolipid substrate for alpha-galactosidase A. Although Fabry's disease has been described as an X-linked recessive disorder, affected women are increasingly recognized, suggesting X-linked dominant transmission. It commonly affects blood vessels, kidney, and heart; in the form of cardiomyopathy, skin and brain.

Fabry's disease accounts for roughly 0.017% of all causes of end-stage renal disease.[121] Although there has been initial reluctance to perform transplantation in patients with Fabry's disease considering these patients' premature cardiovascular death, an analysis from the USRDS database found 93 incident cases of end-stage renal disease due to Fabry's, who underwent renal transplantation between 1988 and 1998.[122] A case-control study of these patients, revealed that the incidence of delayed graft function and acute rejection episodes were similar to other kidney diseases. The 1-, 5-, and 10-graft survival in recipients with Fabry's were indistinguishable from the graft survival in non-Fabry recipients. The concern regarding the risk of cardiovascular disease was also alleviated by finding that the cumulative 10-year patient survival was similar to age- and gender-matched controls. Although, there are case reports of recurrence of Fabry's disease in the transplanted kidneys, it has not been shown whether disease recurrence in the allograft results in graft dysfunction or graft loss.[123-126] Of great interest is the demonstration that renal tissue well-functioning allograft from Fabry's patients examined 6 and 8 months after renal transplant has shown Fabry's inclusions in the vascular endothelium demonstrable only by electromicroscopy.[127,128] This has been proposed to represent colonization of the allograft vasculature by host endothelial cells.

In summary, the survival rates of Fabry's patients who receive an allograft are similar to age- and gender-matched controls. Whether the new introduction of alpha-galactocidase replacement therapy will be as effective in renal transplant recipients, especially in terms of extra-renal manifestations, is yet to be determined.

## Cystinosis

Cystinosis is an autosomal recessive metabolic disease that is characterized by accumulation of cystine in different organs and tissues leading to both renal and extra-renal manifestations.[129] Three forms of this disease have been described: the nephropathic form, the intermediate form, and the adult or benign form. Although the gene for the nephropathic form has been mapped to chromosome 17p13, the genes for the two other forms have not been identified. In the cases of nephropathic form, the gene, CTNS, encodes for 367 amino acid lysozomal membrane proteins named cystinosin.[130]

The earliest signs of the disease are typically manifest by 3 to 6 months of age in the form of proximal tubular defects, polyuria, polydipsia, and recurrent dehydration episodes.[129,130] Although the tubular dysfunction somewhat abates in the first few years, there is a progressive decline in GFR, and end-stage renal disease typically occurs before age 10 in the infantile form. Growth retardation, deposition of cystine in the cornea, and the conjuctiva resulting in photophobia, visual impairment, hepatomegaly, hypothyroidism, insulin-dependent diabetes, and muscular weakness. The central nervous system becomes involved with progressive loss of speech and diminution of intellectual function. The other two forms are much milder, and in the case of adult cystinosis, the patients are typically asymptomatic.

These subjects are usually treated symptomatically for their tubular defects with cysteamine, which reduces the intracellular cystine content. Unfortunately the majority will progress to end-stage renal disease. Two studies addressed renal transplantation in this population.[131,132] Thirty-six adult patients with nephropathic cystinosis underwent renal transplantation. The 1-year and 5-year graft survivals for the 30 deceased donor recipients were 90% and 75%, respectively. These subjects, however, suffered serious complications of the disease; 5 patients were legally blind, 3 had other severely impaired vision in one eye, 86% required thyroid hormone supplementation, and 20% to 30% had myopathic and neurologic complications. Eleven of these subjects only were receiving adequate cystine depleting therapy. There are no documented cases of recurrent disease in the allograft.

## Sickle Cell Disease

A recent report from the USRDS indicates that between 1992 and 1996 there were 345 new cases of ESRD caused by sickle cell renal disease.[133] A comparison of age-matched African American kidney transplant recipients with end-stage renal disease as a result of sickle cell nephropathy and all other causes reveal that incidence of delayed graft function and predischarge, acute rejection is similar in sickle cell nephropathy to other causes.[134] There was no difference in the 1-year deceased donor graft survival, and the multivariable adjusted one risk of graft loss indicated no significant effect of sickle cell nephropathy. However, the 3-year deceased donor graft survival tends to be lower in the sickle cell nephropathy group. A trend toward improved survival in sickle cell nephropathy transplant recipients compared to dialysis-treated counterparts was observed. Concerns raised regarding the widespread use of renal transplant in sickle cell nephropathy include the increased frequency of painful crisis in association with improved posttransplant hematocrit, disease recurrence in the allograft, and avascular osteonecrosis related to steroid therapy.[135–139] With regard to recurrence, there are only one or two cases that have shown histological confirmation of recurrence of sickle cell disease in the transplanted kidney at around 3 1/2 years posttransplantation. All in all, short-term graft and patient survival is comparable to other diseases. However, the long-term survival seems to be inferior to other causes. Nevertheless, sickle cell disease patients who receive a transplant tend to fare better than those who stay on dialysis.

## Hemolytic Uremic Syndrome (HUS)

Although initial reports regarding recurrence of HUS were high, more contemporary data suggest that the rate of recurrence is much lower than previously appreciated.[140–143] For example, Marika et al. reported their experience on 35 patients with end-stage renal disease caused by HUS who received 50 renal allografts.[141] Recurrence was defined, if both clinical and histological signs of thrombotic microangiopathy were present in the absence of vasculitis. After the first renal transplant, there were no cases of definite recurrence, but probable recurrence was diagnosed if there was mild evidence of vasculitis in 18 patients. In contrast, adult subjects had a 41% incidence of definite recurrence and 18% probable recurrence. The use of cyclosporine increased the risk, and the incidence of rejection was also higher in adults with HUS. The 1-year graft survival was poor at 29%; the 1-year graft survival in children with HUS was comparable to match controls. More recently, a report from the North American Pediatric Renal Transplant Cooperative Study has become available.[142] Of 68 renal allografts, HUS recurred in six allografts, occurring in five patients. Four patients had atypical HUS, and only one patient had classic HUS. HUS recurred after transplantation in 33 days or less in all but one case. In contrast to the study by Marika et al., cyclosporine had no impact on rate of recurrence. The most comprehensive evidence regarding the risk of HUS recurrence in renal transplant recipients comes from a meta-analysis that was published in *Transplantation* in 1998.[143] Encompassing the period between 1977 to June 1997, 10 studies comprising 159 grafts and 127 patients were identified. The rate of recurrence was 27.8%, and the 1-year graft survival was 76.6% in patients without recurrence and only 33.3% in patients with recurrence. Older age at onset of HUS, shorter mean interval between HUS and transplantation and shorter interval between HUS and the need for dialysis, living related donor, and the use of calcineurin were all associated with occurrence.

In summary, the rates of recurrence in children seems to be low and is not associated with adverse outcome on the graft, but that in adults is associated with very high risk of recurrence with its attendant risk of graft loss.

## Other Diseases

### *Fibrillary Glomerulonephritis*

This entity is characterized by the glomerular deposition of Congo red negative amyloid-like fibrillary material. The experience with regard to renal transplantation in this condition is quite limited. In a review of 10 patients from the literature and 4 of their own, Samaniego et al. indicate that recurrent disease was found in 43% of the patients.[144] Over follow-up of 2 to 13 years in these two cohorts, only 3 patients lost their graft due to recurrent disease.

### *Light Chain Nephropathy*

This usually presents as a nodular glomerulosclerosis with proteinuria, and in a minority of cases a crescentic glomerulonephritis might be the predominant feature. There have been at least 12 cases where the light chain nephropathy has recurred in the transplant. The underlying etiology for the light chain was monoclonal glomopathy of unknown significance in the majority of cases and multiple myeloma in the rest.[145] The majority of these patients died from infection, and none of the cases reported seem to indicate that this histological recurrence has resulted in end-stage renal failure.

### Minimal Change Disease

There has been, to our knowledge, one case of recurrence minimal change in a renal allograft.[146]

### IgM Nephropathy

This condition is defined as primary diffuse mesangial proliferative glomerulonephritis, with IgM being deposited in the mesangium as the sole or the dominant immunoglobulin. This entity was first described in 1978. There has been one case of a 9-year-old boy where proteinuria occurred 4 months after initial institution of prednisone. He was subsequently transplanted. In addition to this case, two other cases have been reported previously. These recurrences varied in time from 3 weeks to 4 years.[147]

## RISK OF RENAL ALLOGRAFT LOSS WITHOUT STEROID IMMUNOSUPPRESSION

It is not known whether steroid avoidance or rapid discontinuation of steroids posttransplantation will increase the recurrence of the different glomerulonephritides posttransplantation, which are not infrequently treated with steroids in conjunction with cytotoxic agents. Our institution has employed rapid discontinuation of steroids (5 days) over the last 5 years. We recently compared recipients of renal transplants for glomerulonephritis versus those who received their transplant for other diseases.[148] These two groups were maintained on rapid discontinuation of steroids. Graft and patient survival and the risk of recurrence were compared to a historic control group of recipients who received a transplant for glomerulonephritis between 1994 and 1999 and were maintained on long-term steroid immunosuppression. One hundred five patients comprised our GN group with no steroids, 439 concurrent controls received transplants for causes other than GN, and the third group comprised 260 transplant recipients who received an allograft for glomerulonephritis between 1994 and 1999. Follow-up ranged from 25 to 90 months. The 4-year graft and patient survival were similar in the three groups. Acute and chronic-rejection-free survivals were also similar in the groups. Two grafts were lost in the rapid discontinuation GN group from biopsy-proven recurrent GN, and 8 other subjects had evidence of histological recurrence. In contrast, the historic group of 1994 to 1999 there were 7 grafts lost from recurrence (P = 0.68). A similar experience has been reported by Alloway et al., who reported their experience with 21 recipients with FSGS who underwent early corticosteroid withdrawals.[149] Only 2 patients lost their graft from recurrent FSGS, a rate comparable to those who received long-term steroids. The data suggest that there is no penalty paid with steroid-avoidance protocols in regard to the risk of recurrent GN.

## SUMMARY

Recurrent disease has emerged as a significant cause for allograft loss in kidney transplant recipients. The recurrence rates of the different glomerulonephritides are shown in Table 16.9-1 and also in the Kaplan–Meier survival curve from Brigante et al.[8] It does not seem to depend on the source of the kidney. The type of glomerulonephritis, the gender of the recipient, and the peak

**TABLE 16.9-1**

### CAUSE-SPECIFIC INCIDENCE OF GRAFT LOSS

| Disease | n | % |
|---|---|---|
| Focal segmental glomerulosclerosis* | 221 | 12.7 |
| MPGN Type 1* | 88 | 14.4 |
| MPGN Type 2† | 75 | 14.7 |
| Membranous* | 81 | 12.5 |
| IgA Nephropathy* | 532 | 9.7 |
| Pauci-immune GN* | 102 | 7.7 |
| Others* | 481 | 3.1 |

*Incidence at 10 years.[8]
†Incidence at 5 years.[38]

level of the panel of reactive antibodies are independent predictors of the risk of recurrence.[8] Since these risk factors are not modifiable, with the exception of possibly the panel of reactive antibodies, early surveillance for recurrence by measuring urinary protein excretion rate, prompt performance of kidney biopsy, and, in the case of FSGS, the performance of pre- and peritransplant plasmapheresis should be considered. To date, there seems to be no distinct advantage for one immunosuppressive regimen over another in terms of decreasing frequency of recurrence.

## ACKNOWLEDGMENTS

We thank Andrew Johnson, Patty Johnson, and Jensina Ericksen for their expert secretarial assistance and friendship. We also thank the Catherine Watt family for their support to research in the area of immunosuppression.

## References

1. Floege J. Recurrent glomerulonephritis following renal transplantation: An update. *Nephrol Dial Transplant* 2003;18(7):1260–1265.
2. Pinto J, Lacerda G, Cameron JS, et al. Recurrence of focal and segmental glomerulosclerosis in renal allografts. *Transplantation* 1981;32(2): 83–89.
3. Tejani A, Stablein DH. Recurrence of focal segmental glomerulosclerosis post-transplantation: A special report of the North American Pediatric Renal Transplant Cooperative Study. *J Am Soc Nephrol* 1992;2(12):s258–s263.
4. Striegel JE, Sibley RK, Fryd DS, et al. Recurrence of focal segmental sclerosis in children following renal transplantation. *Kidney Int* 1986;19:S44–s50.
5. Kessler M, Champigneulles J, Heston D, et al. A renal allograft recipient with late recurrence of focal and segmental glomerulosclerosis after switching from cyclosporine to tacrolomus. *Transplantation* 1999;67:641–643.
6. Andresdottir MB, Ajubi N, Croockewit S, et al. Recurrent focal glomerulosclerosis: natural course and treatment with plasma exchange. *Nephrol Dial Transplant* 1999;14:2650–2656.
7. Biesenbach G, Janko O, Hubmann R, et al. The incidence of thrombovenous and thromboembolic complications in kidney transplant patients with recurrent glomerulonephritis is dependent on the occurrence of severe proteinuria. *Clin Nephrol* 2000;54:382–387.
8. Briganti EM, Russ GR, McNei JJ, et al. Risk of renal allograft loss from recurrent glomerulonephritis. *N Engl J Med* 2002;347(2):103–109.
9. Koushik R, Usulumarty D, Danielson B, et al. The association of focal segmental glomerulosclerosis (FSGS) with adverse outcomes after kidney transplantation (KTX). *Am J Transplant* 2005;(abst)5, suppl(11).

10. Hubsch H, Montain B, Abitbol C, et al. Recurrent focal glomerulo-sclerosis in pediatric renal allografts: the *Miami experience. Pediatr Nephrol* 2005;20(2):210–216.

11. Baum MA, Stablein DM, Panzarino VM, et al. Loss of living donor renal allograft survival advantage in children with focal segmental glomerulosclerosis. *Kidney Int* 2001;59:328–333.

12. Abbott KC, Sawyers ES, Oliver JD III, et al. Graft loss due to recurrent focal segmental glomerulosclerosis in renal transplant recipients in the United States. *Am J Kidney Dis* 2001;37:366–373.

13. Cibrik DM, Kaplan B, Campbell DA, et al. Renal allograft survival in transplant recipients with focal segmental glomerulosclerosis. *Am J Transplantation* 2003;3:64–67.

14. Raafat R, Travis LB, Kalia A, et al. Role of transplant induction therapy on recurrence rate of focal segmental glomerulosclerosis. *Pediatr Nephrol* 2000;14(3):189–94.

15. Ohta T, Kawaguchi H, Hattori M, et al. Effect of pre-and-postoperative plasmapheresis on post-transplant recurrence of focal segmental glomerulosclerosis in children. *Transplantation* 2001;71:628–633.

16. Belson A, Yorgin PD, Al-Uzri AY, et al. Long-term plasmapheresis and protein A column treatment of recurrent FSGS. *Pediatr Nephrol* 2001;16:985–989.

17. Matalon A, Markowitz GS, Joseph RE, et al. Plasmapheresis treatment of recurrent FSGS in adult renal transplant recipients. *Clin Nephrol* 2001;56:271–278.

18. Davenport RD. Apheresis treatment of recurrent focal segmental glomerulosclerosis after kidney transplantation: re-analysis of published case-reports and case-series. *J Clin Apheresis* 2001;16:175–178.

19. Belson A, Yorgin PD, Al-Uzri AY, et al. Long-term plasmapheresis and protein A column treatment of FSGS. *Pediatr Nephrol* 2001;16(12):985–989.

20. Dall'Amico R, Ghiggeri G, Carraro M, et al. Prediction and treatment of recurrent focal segmental glomerulosclerosis in renal tranplnatiaon in children. *Am J Kidney Dis* 1999;34:1048–1052.

21. Cheong HI, Han HW, Park HW, et al. Early recurrent nephritic syndrome after renal transplantation in children with focal segmental glomerulosclerosis. *Nephrol Dial Transplant* 2000;15:78–81.

22. Boute N, Gribouval O, Roselli S, et al. NPHS2, encoding the glomerular protein podocin, is mutated in autosomal recessive steroid resistant nephrotic syndrome. *Nat Genet* 2000;24(4):349–354.

23. Ruf R, Lichtenberger A, Karle S, et al. Patients with mutation in NPHS2 gene(podocin) do not respond to standard steroid treatment of nephrotic syndrome. *J Am Soc Nephrol* 2004;15(3):722–732.

24. Weber S, Bibourd O, Esquivel E, et al. NPHS2 mutation analysis shows genetic heterogeneity of steroid resistant nephrotic syndrome and low post-transplant recurrence. *Kidney Int* 2004;66(2):571–579.

25. Hosenpud J, Piering WF, Garancis JC, et al. Successful second kidney transplantation in a patient with focal glomerulosclerosis. A case report. *Am J Nephrol* 1985;5(4):299–304.

26. Denton MD, Singh AK. Recurrent and de novo glomerulonephritis in the renal allograft. *Semin Nephrol* 2000;20(2):164–175.

27. Kotanko P, Pusey CD, Levy, JB. Recurrent glomerulonephritis following renal transplantation. *Transplantation* 1997;63(8):1045–1052.

28. Mathew TH. Recurrence of disease following renal transplantation. *Am J Kidney Dis* 1988;12(2):85–96.

29. Cameron JS. Glomerulonephritis in renal transplants. *Transplantation* 1982;34(5):237–245.

30. Curtis JJ, Wyatt RJ, Bhathena D, et al. Renal transplantation for patients with type I and type II membranoproliferative glomerulonephritis. *Am J Med* 1979;66(2):216–225.

31. Glicklich D, Mata AJ, Sablay LB, et al. Recurrent membranoproliferative glomerulonephritis type I in successive renal transplants. *Am J Nephrol* 1987;7(2):143–149.

32. Andresdottir MB, Assmann KJ, Hoitsma AJ, et al. Recurrence of type I membranoproliferative glomerulonephritis after renal transplantation. *Transplantation* 1997;63(11):1628–1633.

33. Habib R, Antignac C, Hinglais N, et al. Glomerular lesions in the transplanted kidney in children. *Am J Kidney Dis* 1987;10(3):198–207.

34. Tomlanovich S, Vincenti F, Amend W, et al. Is cyclosporine effective in preventing recurrence of immune-mediated glomerular disease after renal transplantation. *Transplant Proc* 1988;20(3 Suppl 4):285–288.

35. Lien YH, Scott K. Long-term cyclophosphamide treatment for recurrent type I membranoproliferative glomerulonephritis after transplantation. *Am J Kidney Dis* 2000;35(3):539–543.

36. Muczynski KA. Plasmapheresis maintained renal function in an allograft with recurrent membranoproliferative glomerulonephritis type I. *Am J Nephrol* 1995;15(5):446–449.

37. Eddy A, Sibley R, Mauer SM, et al. Renal allograft failure due to recurrent dense intramembranous deposit disease. *Clin Nephrol* 1984;21(6):305–313.

38. Andresdottir MB, Assmann KJ, Hoitsma AJ, et al. Renal transplantation in patients with dense deposit disease: Morphological characteristics of recurrent disease and clinical outcome. *Nephrol Dial Transplant* 1999; 14(7):1723–1731.

39. Braun MC, Stablein DM, Hamiwka LA, et al. Recurrence of membranoproliferative glomerulonephritis type II in renal allografts: The North American Pediatric Renal Transplant Cooperative Study Experience. *Am Soc Neph* 2005;16:2225–2233.

40. Oberkircher OR, Enama M, West JC, et al. Regression of recurrent membranoproliferative glomerulonephritis type II in a transplanted kidney after plasmapheresis therapy. *Transplant Proc* 1988;20(1 Supp 1): 418–423.

41. Morales JM, Martinez MA, De Bustillo EM, et al. Recurrent type III membranoproliferative glomerulonephritis after kidney transplantation. *Transplantation* 1997;63(8):1186–1188.

42. Suzuki K, Honda K, Tanabe K, et al. Incidence of latent mesangial IgA deposition in renal allograft donors in Japan. *Kidney Int* 2003; 63(16):2286–2294.

43. Sanfilippo F, Croker BP, Bollinger RR. Fate of four cadaveric donor renal allografts with mesangial IgA deposits. *Transplantation* 1982;33(4): 370–376.

44. Koselj M, Rott T, Vizjak A, et al. IgA nephropathy as a donor-transmitted disease in renal transplant recipients. *Transplant Proc* 1991;23(5):2643–2646.

45. Bumgardner GL, Amend WC, Ascher NL, et al. Single-center long-term results of renal transplantation for IgA nephropathy. *Transplantation* 1998;65(8):1053–1060.

46. Frohnert PP, Donadio JV Jr, Velosa JA, et al. The fate of renal transplants in patients with IgA nephropathy. *Clin Transplant* 1997;11(2):127–133.

47. Ponticelli C, Traversi L, Feliciani A, et al. Kidney transplantation in patients with IgA mesangial glomerulonephritis. *Kidney Int* 2001;60(5):1948–1954.

48. Freese P, Svalander C, Norden G, et al. Clinical risk factors for recurrence of IgA nephropathy. *Clin Transplant* 1999;13(4):313–317.

49. Andresdottir MB, Hoitsma AJ, Assmann KJ, et al. Favorable outcome of renal transplantation in patients with IgA nephropathy. *Clin Nephrol* 2001;56(4):279–288.

50. Wang AY, Lai FM, Yu AW, et al. Recurrent IgA nephropathy in renal transplant allografts. *Am J Kidney Dis* 2001;38(3):588–596.

51. Brensilver JM, Mallat S, Scholes J, et al. Recurrent IgA nephropathy in living-related donor transplantation: Recurrence or transmission of familial disease? *Am J Kidney Dis* 1988;12(2):147–151.

52. Matsugami K, Naito T, Nitta K, et al. A clinicopathological study of recurrent IgA nephropathy following renal transplantation. *Nippon Jinzo Gakkai Shi* 1998;40(5):322–328.

53. Kessler M, Hiesse C, Hestin D, et al. Recurrence of immunoglobulin A nephropathy after renal transplantation in the cyclosporine era. *Am J Kidney Dis* 1996;28(1):99–104.

54. Chandrakantan A, Ratanapanichkich P, Said M, et al. Recurrent IgA nephropathy after renal transplantation despite immunosuppressive regimens with mycophenolate mofetil. *Nephrol Dial Transplant* 2005; 20(6):1214–1221.

55. Heide V, Bilo H, Donker J, et al. Effect of dietary fish oil and rejection in cyclosporing treated recipients of rneal transplants. *N Engl J Med* 1993;329:769–773.

56. Donadio J, Bergstrahl E, Offord K, et al. A controlled trial of fish oil in IgA nephropathy. *N Engl J Med* 1994;331:1194–1199.

57. Farquahar M, Saito A, Kerjasenki D, et al. The Heymann nephritis antigenic complex: megalin and RAP. *J Am Soc Nephrol* 1995;6(1):35–47.

58. Josephson MA, Spargo B, Hollandsworth D, et al. The recurrence of recurrent membranous glomerulopathy in a renal transplant recipient: Case report and literature review. *Am J Kidney Dis* 1994;24(5):873–878.

59. Berger BE, Vicenti F, Biava C, et al. De novo and recurrent membranous glomerulopathy following kidney transplantation. *Transplantation* 1983;35(4):315–319.

60. Cosyns JP, Couchoud C, PouteilNoble C, et al. Recurrence of membranous nephropathy after renal transplantation: Probability, outcome and risk factors. *Clin Nephrol* 1998;50(3):144–153.

61. Montagnino G, Colturi C, Banfi G. Membranous nephropathy in cyclosporine-treated renal transplant recipients. *Transplantation* 1989;47(4):725–727.

62. Truong L, Gelfand J, D'Agati V, et al. De novo membranous glomerulopathy in renal allografts: A report of ten cases and review of the literature. *Am J Kidney Dis* 1989;14(2):131–144.

63. Schwartz A, Krause PH, Offerman G, et al. Impact of de novo membranous glomerulonephritis on the clinical course after kidney transplantation. *Transplantation* 1994;58(6):650–654.

64. Heidet L, Gagnadoux MF, Beziau A, et al. Recurrence of de novo membranous glomerulonephritis on renal grafts. *Clin Nephrol* 1994;41(5): 314–318.

65. Poduval R, Josephson A, Javaid B. Treatment of de novo and recurrent membranous nephropathy in renal transplant patients. *Semin Nephrol* 2003;23(41):392–399.

66. Mojcik CF, Klippel JH. End-stage renal disease and systemic lupus erythematosus. *Am J Med* 1996;101(1):100–107.

67. Cheigh, Stenzel K. End stage renal disease is systemic lupus erythematosus. *Am J Kidney Dis* 1993;21(1):2–8.

68. Ward MM. Outcomes of renal transplantation among patients with end-stage renal disease caused by lupus nephritis. *Kidney Int* 2000; 57(5):2136–2143.

69. Bartosh SM, Fine RN, Sullivan EK. Outcome after transplantation of young patients with systemic lupus erythematosus: A report of the North American Pediatric Renal Transplant Cooperative Study. *Transplantation* 2001;72(5):973–978.

70. Stone JH, Amend WJ, Criswell LA. Outcome of renal transplantation in systemic lupus erythematosus. *Semin Arthritis Rheum* 1997;27(1): 17–26.

71. Stone JH, Millward CL, Olson JL, et al. Frequency of recurrent lupus nephritis among ninety-seven renal transplant patients during the cyclosporine era. *Arthritis Rheum* 1998;41(4):678–686.

72. Goral S, Ynares, Shappell S, et al. Recurrent lupus nephritis in renal transplant recipients. *Transplantation* 2003;75(5):651–656.

73. Hoffman GS, Kerr GS, Leavitt RY, et al. Wegener's granulomatosis: An analysis of 158 patients. *Ann Intern Med* 1992;116(6): 488–498.

74. Steinman TI, Jaffe BF, Monaco AP, et al. Recurrence of Wegener's granulomatosis after kidney transplantation. *Am J Med* 1980;68(3): 458–460.

75. Clarke AE, Bitton A, Eappen R, et al. Treatment of Wegener's granulomatosis after renal transplantation: is cyclosporine the preferred treatment? *Transplantation* 1990;50(6):1047–1051.

76. Rostaing L, Modesto A, Oksman F, et al. Outcome of patients with antineutrophil cytoplasmic autoantibody-associated vasculitis following cadaveric kidney transplantation. *Am J Kidney Dis* 1997; 29(1):96–102.

77. Rich LM, Piering WF. Ureteral stenosis due to recurrent Wegener's granulomatosis after kidney transplantation. *J Am Soc Nephrol* 1994;4(8): 1516–1521.

78. Tzardis P, Gruessner R, Matas A, et al. Long term follow-up of renal transplantation for Wegener's Disease. *Clin Transplant* 1990; 4(2):108–111.

79. Kotanko P, Pusey CD, Levy JB. Recurrent glomerulonephritis following renal transplantation. *Transplantation* 1997;63(8):1045–1050.

80. Cameron JS. Glomerulonephritis in renal transplants. *Transplantation* 1982;34(5):237–245.

81. Traub YM, Shapiro AP, Rodnan GP, et al. Hypertension and renal failure (scleroderma renal crisis) in progressive systemic sclerosis. Review of a 25-year experience with 68 cases. *Medicine (Baltimore)* 1983; 62(6):335–352.

82. Steen VD, Syzd A, Johnson JP, et al. Kidney disease other than renal crisis in patients with diffuse scleroderma. *J Rheumatol* 2005;32(4):649–655.

83. Woodhall PB, McCoy RC, Gunnells C, Seigle HF. Apparent recurrence of progressive systemic sclerosis in a renal allograft. *JAMA* 1976; 236(9):1032–1034.

84. Merino GE, Sutherland DE, Kjellstrand CM, et al. Renal transplantation for progressive systemic sclerosis with renal failure. *Am J Surg* 1977;133(6):745–749.

85. Chang YJ, Spiera H. Renal transplantation in scleroderma. *Medicine (Baltimore)* 1999;78:382.

86. Gibney EM, Parikh CR, Jani A, et al. Kidney transplantation for systemic sclerosis improves survival and may modulate disease activity. *Am J Transplant* 2004;4:2027–2031.

87. Glenner G. Amyloid deposits and amyloidosis. *N Engl J Med* 1980; 302(23):1283–1292.

88. Moroni G, Banfi G, Montoli A, et al. Chronic dialysis in patients with systemic amyloidosis: The experience in northern Italy. *Clin Nephrol* 1992;38(2):81–85.

89. Gertz MA, Kyle RA, O'Fallon WM. Dialysis support of patients with primary systemic amyloidosis. A study of 211 patients. *Arch Intern Med* 19922;152(11):2245–2250.

90. Pasternack A, Ahonen J, Kuhlback B. Renal transplantation in 45 patients with amyloidosis. *Transplantation* 1986;42(6):598–601.

91. Sobh M, Refaie A, Moustafa F, et al. Study of live donor kidney transplantation outcome in recipients with renal amyloidosis. *Nephrol Dial Transplant* 1994;9(6):704–708.

92. Sherif AM, Refaie AF, Sobh MA, et al. Long-term outcome of live donor kidney transplantation for renal amyloidosis. *Am J Kidney Dis* 2003;42(2):370–375.

93. Leung N, Lager DJ, Gertz MA, et al. Long-term outcome of renal transplantation in light-chain deposition disease. *Am J Kidney Dis* 2004;43(1):147–153.

94. Livneh A, Zemer D, Siegal B, et al. Colchicine prevents kidney transplant amyloidosis in familial Mediterranean fever. *Nephron* 1992;60(4): 418–422.

95. Kashtan CE, Michael AF. Alport syndrome. *Kidney Int* 1996;50(5): 1445–1463.

96. Tryggvason K, Zhou J, Hostikka SL, et al. Molecular genetics of Alport syndrome. *Kidney Int* 1993;43(1):38–44.

97. Hudson BG, Kalluri R, Gunwar S, et al. The pathogenesis of Alport syndrome involves type IV collagen molecules containing the a3(IV) chain: Evidence from anti-GBM nephritis after renal transplantation. *Kidney Int* 1992;42(1):179–187.

98. Querin S, Noel L, Grunfeld JP, et al. Linear glomerular IgG fixation in renal allografts: incidence and significance in Alport's syndrome. *Clin Nephrol* 1986;25(3):134–140.

99. Kashtan CE, Butkowski RJ, Kleppel MM, et al. Posttransplant antiglomerular basement membrane nephritis in related males with Alport syndrome. *J Lab Clin Med* 1990;116(4):508–515.

100. Kalluri R, Weber M, Netzer KO, et al. COL4A5 gene deletion and production of post-transplant anti-a3(IV) collagen alloantibodies in Alport syndrome. *Kidney Int* 1994;45(3):721–726.

101. Ding J, Zhou J, Tryggvason K, et al. COL4A5 deletions in three patients with Alport syndrome and posttransplant antiglomerular basement membrane nephritis. *J Am Soc Nephrol* 1994;5(2): 161–168.

102. Shah B, First MR, Mendoza NC, et al. Alport's syndrome: Risk of glomerulonephritis induced by anti-glomerular-basement-membrane antibody after renal transplantation. *Nephron* 1988;50(1):34–38.

103. Hellmark T, Johannsson C, Wieslander J. Characterization of anti-GBM antibodies involved in Goodpastures's syndrome. *Kidney Int* 1994;46(3):823–829.

104. Byrne MC, Budisavljevic MN, Fan Z, et al. Renal transplant in patients with Alport's syndrome. *Am J Kidney Dis* 2002;39(4):769–775.

105. Browne G, Brown P, Tomson C, et al. Retransplantation in Alport post-transplant anti-GBM disease. *Kidney Int* 2004;65(2):675–681.

106. Millan MT, Berquist WE, So SK, et al. One hundred percent patient and kidney allograft survival with simultaneous liver and kidney transplantation in infants with primary hyperoxaluria: a single-center experience. *Transplantation* 2003;76(10):1458–1463.

107. Watts RW, Morgan SH, Purkiss P, et al. Timing of renal transplantation in the management of pyridoxine resistant type I primary hyperoxaluria. *Transplantation* 1988;45(6):1143–1145.

108. Scheinman JI, Najarian JS, Mauer SM. Successful strategies for renal transplantation in primary oxalosis. *Kidney Int* 1984;25(5):804–811.

109. Saborio P, Scheinman JI. Transplantation for primary hyperoxaluria in the United States. *Kidney Int* 1999;56(3):1094–1100.

110. Broyer M, Brunner F, Bryuger H, et al. Kidney transplantation in primary oxalosis: data from the EDTA registry. *Nephrol Dial Transplant* 1990;5(5):L332–336.

111. Najarian JS, Sutherland DE, Simmons RL, et al. Ten year experience with renal transplantation in juvenile onset diabetics. *Ann Surg* 1979; 190(4):487–500.

112. Mauer SM, Barbosa J, Vernur RL, et al. Development of diabetic vascular lesions in normal kidney transplanted into patients with diabetes mellitus. *N Engl J Med* 1976;295(17):916–920.

113. Najarian JS, Kaufman DB, Fryd DS, et al. Long-term survival following kidney transplantation in 100 type I diabetic patients. *Transplantation* 1989;47(1):106–113.

114. Bhalla V, Nast CC, Stollenwerk N, et al. Recurrent and de novo diabetic nephropathy in renal allografts. *Transplantation* 2003;75:66–71.

115. Fioretto P, Steffes M, Sutherland D, et al. Reversal of lesions of diabetic nephrology after pancreas transplantation. *N Engl J Med* 1998; 339:69–75.

116. Ronkainen J, Nuutinen M, Koskimies O. The adult kidney 24 years after childhood Henoch-Schonlein purpura. *Lancet* 2002;360(9334):666–670.

117. Meulders Q, Pirson Y, Cosyns JP, et al. Course of Henoch-Schönlein nephritis after renal transplantation. Report of ten patients and review of the literature. *Transplantation* 1994;58(11):1179–1186.

118. Nast CC, Ward HJ, Koyle MA, et al. Recurrent Henoch-Schönlein purpura following renal transplantation. *Am J Kidney Dis* 1987;9(1):39–43.

119. Hasegawa A, Kawamura T, Ito H, et al. Fate of renal grafts with recurrent Henoch-Schönlein purpura nephritis in children. *Transplant Proc* 1989;21(1 pt 2):2130–2133.

120. Baliah T, Kim KH, Anthone S, et al. Recurrence of Henoch-Schönlein purpura glomerulonephritis in transplanted kidneys. *Transplantation* 1974;18(4):343–346.

121. Thadhani R, Wolf M, West M, et al. Patients with Fabry disease on dialysis in the United States. *Kidney Int* 2002;61:249–255.

122. Popli S, Molnar ZV, Leehey DJ, et al. Involvement of renal allograft by Fabry's disease. *Am J Nephrol* 1987;7:316–318.

123. Obrador GT, Ojo A, Thadhani R. End-stage renal disease in patients with Fabry Disease. *J Am Soc Nephrol* 2002;13:S144–S146.

124. Kramer W, Thormann J, Mueller K, et al. Progressive cardiac involvement by Fabry's disease despite successful renal allotransplantation. *Int J Cardol* 1985;7:72–75.

125. Conati D, Navario R, Gastaldi L. Natural history and treatment of uremia secondary to Fabry's disease: A European experience. *Nephron* 1987; 46:353–359.

126. Mosiner JF, Degott C, Bedrossian J, et al. Recurrence of Fabry's disease in a renal allograft eleven years after successful renal transplantation. *Transplantation* 1991;51:759–762.

127. Alroy J, Sabnis S, Kopp JB. Renal pathology in Fabry Disease. *J Am Soc Nephrol* 2002;13:S134–138.

128. Friedlaender MM, Kopolovic J, Rubinger D, et al. Renal biopsy in Fabry's disease eight years after successful renal transplantation. *Clin Nephrol* 1987;27:206–211.

129. Gahl WA, Thoene JG, Schneider JA. Cystinosis. *N Engl J Med* 2002; 347(2):111–121.

130. Bois E, Feingold J, Frenay P, et al. Infantile cystinosis in France: Genetics, incidence, geographic distribution. *J Med Genet* 1976;13(6):434–438.

131. Broyer M. Kidney transplantation in children data from the EDTA registry. The EDTA registry committee. *Transplant Proc* 1989;21(1 pt 2): 1985–1988.

132. Theodoropoulos DS, Krasnewich D, Kaiser-Kupfer MI, et al. Classic nephropathic cystinosis as an adult disease. *JAMA* 1993;270(18):2200–2204.

133. U.S. Renal Data System Annual Report, 1997. Bethesda, MD.

134. Ojo AO, Govaerts TC, Schmouder RL, et al. Renal Transplantation in end-stage sickle cell nephropathy. *Clin Transplantation* 1999; 67(2): 291–295.

135. Spector D, Zachary BJ, Sterioff S, et al. Painful crises following renal transplantation in sickle cell anemia. *Am J Med* 1978;64(5):835–839.

136. Gonzalez-Carrillo M, Rudge CJ, Parsons V, et al. Renal transplantation in sickle cell disease. *Clin Nephrol* 1982;18(4):209–210.

137. Montgomery R, Zibari G, Hills GS, et al. Renal transplantation in patients with sickle cell nephrology. *Transplantation* 1994;58(5):618–620.

138. Wong YW, Powars RD, Chan L, et al. Polysaccharide encapsulated bacterial infection in sickle cell anemia: a thirty year epidemiologic experience. *Am J Hematol* 1992;39:176.

139. Miner JD, Jorkasky KD, Perloff JL, et al. Recurrent sickle cell nephropathy in a transplanted kidney. *Am J Kidney Dis* 1987;10(4):306.

140. Artz MA, Steenbergen EJ, Hoitsma AJ, et al. Renal transplantation in patients with hemolytic uremic syndrome: high rate of recurrence and increased incidence of acute rejections. *Transplantation* 2003;76(5): 821–826.

141. Quan A, Sullivan EK, Alexander SR. Recurrence of hemolytic uremic syndrome after renal transplantation in children: A report of the North American Pediatric Renal Transplant Cooperative Study. *Transplantation* 2001;72(4):742–745.

142. Ducloux D, Rebibou JM, Semhoun-Ducloux S, et al. Recurrence of hemolytic-uremic syndrome in renal transplant recipients: A meta-analysis. *Transplantation* 1998;65(10):1405–1407.

143. Samaniego M, Nadasdy GM, Laszik Z, et al. Outcome of renal transplantation in fibrillary glomerulonephritis. *Clinical Nephrology* 2000; 55(2):159–166.

144. Short AK, O'Donoghue DJ, Riad HN, et al. Recurrence of light chain nephropathy in a renal allograft. *Am J Nephrol* 2001;21:237–240.

145. Jan CI,m Chen A, Sun GH, et al. Recurrent minimal change disease post-allograft renal transplant. *Transplant Proc* 2003;35:2888–2890.

146. Salmon AJ, Kamel D, Mathieson PW. Recurrence of IgM nephrology in a renal allograft. *Nephrol Dial Transplant* 19:2650–2652.

147. Ibrahim H, Rogers T, Casingal V, et al. Graft loss from recurrent glomerulonephritis is not increasing with a rapid steroid discontinuation protocol. *Transplantation* 2006;81(2):214–219.

148. Alloway R, Rogers C, Chaudhury R, et al. Early steroid withdrawal does not increase risk for recurrent focal segmental glomerulosclerosis [abstract]. *Am J Transplant* 2004;4(S8):595.

# 16.10 RETRANSPLANTATION

*Akinlolu O. Ojo, MD, Laura L. Christensen, MS, Fu Luan, MD*

## INTRODUCTION

Unique among all types of organ transplantation, the availability of maintenance dialysis therapy makes it possible for patients with end-stage renal disease (ESRD) and previous kidney transplantation

2. USRDS. US Renal Data System, *USRDS 2004 Annual Data Report: Atlas of End-Stage Renal Disease in the United States,* National Institutes of Health, National Institutes of Diabetes, Digestive and Kidney Disease, Bethesda, MD, 2005.

3. Hariharan S, McBride MA, Cherikh WS, et al. Post-transplant renal function in the first year predicts long-term kidney transplant survival. *Kidney Int* 2002;62(1):311–318.

4. Gjertson DW. A multi-factor analysis of kidney regraft outcomes. *Clin Transpl* 2002;335–349.

5. Ojo A, Wolfe RA, Agodoa LY, et al. Prognosis after primary renal transplant failure and the beneficial effects of repeat transplantation: multivariate analyses from the United States Renal Data System. *Transplantation* 1998;66(12):1651–1659.

# 16.11 PEDIATRIC ISSUES

## 16.11a  Medical Aspects

*Avi Katz, MD, Michael Mauer, MD*

## INTRODUCTION

Kidney transplantation is accepted as the therapy of choice for children with end-stage renal disease (ESRD). Many aspects of kidney transplantation in children parallel those of their adult counterparts. Others are unique to the pediatric recipient. Since this chapter is part of a general textbook on kidney transplantation we elected to address certain issues that are distinctive to the pediatric kidney recipient rather than provide an exhaustive review of the subject. The reader is referred to other relevant chapters in this book as well as to several recently published books, book chapters, and review articles for the aspects of pediatric kidney transplantation not considered in this chapter.[1-7]

## INFANT AND TODDLER TRANSPLANTATION

Kidney transplantation in infants and small children has the greatest potential impact on physical growth and neurologic development.[8] Preparation of an infant for kidney transplantation typically requires aggressive nutrition, frequently necessitating the use of a g-tube for night feedings, correction of acid base abnormalities, prevention or treatment of renal osteodystrophy, treatment of hypertension, prevention and treatment of urinary tract infections, and maintaining normal hemoglobin levels.[9] Beyond 6 months of age the addition of recombinant human growth hormone may further aid linear growth, as may also the intensification of dialysis support.[10,11] Age-appropriate immunizations, especially live vaccines, should be administered prior to transplantation, allowing at least 8 weeks between the final live viral immunizations and transplantation, and remembering that booster doses may be necessary in order to obtain adequate response. Canulation of the inferior vena cava (IVC) should be avoided as it risks occlusion compromising future transplantation.[12] Infants and young children at risk of IVC occlusion (eg, congenital nephrotic syndrome, bilateral Wilms' tumor, previous extensive intra-abdominal surgery) should have ultrasound/Doppler studies to document IVC patency. Exposure to blood product should be kept to a minimum. When indicated native kidneys can be removed at the time of transplantation.[8] Exceptions include children with recurrent urinary tract infections where, if urinary sterility cannot be sustained, a separate

bilateral nephrectomy is the safer approach. Children with open urinary drainage systems, such as high urinary diversions or vesicostomies, should have bilateral nephrectomies and/or bladder closure 6 weeks or more before transplantation as, otherwise, the risk of posttransplant wound infection and sepsis is too high. An alternate approach of take-down of these diversions creating a closed urinary system has been quite successful,[13] although prior nephrectomy may be required should urinary infection develop in the 6- to 8-week interval between undiversion and one-stage bilateral nephrectomy and transplantation. Done in children not yet requiring dialysis support, undiversion may occasionally precipitate a need for dialysis.[13] It is our routine to remove refluxing kidneys. This is done as two-stage procedures depending on the conditions outlined previously. Children with Vater's syndrome should have their anal repair procedures completed before undergoing renal transplantation.

Children with respiratory insufficiency secondary to massive kidneys from infantile polycystic kidney disease are often also malnourished because of associated feeding difficulties and may be best managed by initial bilateral nephrectomy followed by intensive nutritional and pulmonary rehabilitation, along with aggressive uremia support until medically prepared for subsequent transplantation. A single-stage nephrectomy/transplant procedure under these conditions confers inordinate risk.

Eagle-Barrett (prune-belly) syndrome may provide multiple challenges because of the co-existence of ineffective cough, pulmonary hypoplasia, and obstructive uropathy issues. Patency of the urethra should be verified, and abdominoplasty should be considered as it might improve pulmonary status and bladder emptying and prevent displacement of the allograft or its vascular pedicle. However, the reported outcomes[14-16] of patients with this syndrome are good. On occasion, the respiratory problems associated with severe intrauterine renal disease have led to tracheostomy placement. It is our recommendation that, if at all possible, tracheostomy removal and ostomy closure be accomplished prior to transplantation. However, in the few instances this was not possible, we have not yet encountered major problems.

Children with congenital nephrotic syndrome (CNS) or other diseases with persistent heavy proteinuria sufficient to sustain the laboratory features of nephrotic syndrome (eg, serum albumin <3 g/dL and hyperlipidemia) despite the advent of uremia, should also undergo separate bilateral nephrectomy.[6] We have long ago argued that 6 to 8 weeks are required between nephrectomy and transplantation to allow for protein repletion needed for wound healing, immunoglobulin restitution for adequate defense from infection, and reversal of the hypercoagulable state of nephrotic syndrome (NS) which could risk immediate graft thrombosis. IVIG administered after bilateral nephrectomy is retained and may be warranted, especially in patients whose NS was complicated by recurrent infections. Although antithrombin III levels could be monitored as an indicator of the complete reversal of the hypercoagulable state following nephrectomy, in practice, we have had no thrombotic complications if the aforementioned time interval between nephrectomy and transplantation is respected. Some children, despite massive proteinuria and hypoalbuminuria, may grow and gain weight and manifest no serious infectious risks. In such patients, watchful waiting is indicated since proteinuria may diminish as uremia ensues, allowing for a single-stage procedure when the NS spontaneously relents. We have set a serum albumin level of 3.0 g/dL as the cutoff for a one-stage approach. Infants or children with severe CNS may fail to thrive and have life-threatening infectious and thrombotic risks despite aggressive medical management. Bilateral nephrectomy and institution of dialysis, despite relatively intact renal filtration function, is justified in such cases. If a hemodialysis catheter is placed at this time, systemic anticoagulation is recommended to maintain its patency.

There are several situations in which respiratory problems may create renal transplant preparation issues for infants and small children. Renal conditions leading to intrauterine oligohydramnios can be associated with pulmonary hypoplasia leading to decreased pulmonary reserve and increased risks of serious consequences from pulmonary atelectasis, infection, or increased intrabdominal pressure from an adult kidney placed into a relatively small abdomen. Where children have a clear history of respiratory decompensation or distress with upper or lower respiratory infections, or following minor procedures such as line or peritoneal dialysis catheter placement, it may be wise, if at all possible, to persist with medical management, including growth hormone and vigorous dialysis (see above) in the hope that further growth will be accompanied by further pulmonary maturation and development. Should this strategy fail, transplantation may still be warranted in all but the most marginal situations, although some days or weeks of ventilatory support may then be required. The role of laparoscopic live donor nephrectomy in this age group needs to be defined.[17]

## Intraoperative Considerations

Children under 20 kg in weight almost always require intraabdominal allograft placement and end-to-side artery and vein anastomoses to the aorta and cava. If the patient is on peritoneal dialysis (PD) or the transplant is preemptive, we recommend placement of a Hickman catheter suitable for hemodialysis (HD) and removal of the peritoneal catheter at the time of surgery. The Hickman catheter would then be available should postoperative dialysis be required and could also be used for IV antibody induction treatment. If infant HD is not available, the PD catheter should be retained for possible need for dialysis support and removed as soon as good graft function is established. Abdominal infection and wound problems related to PD are the reasons for these recommendations.

Several intraoperative considerations are relevant to transplantation in these small children.[18] Hypothermia can be avoided by maintaining the room temperature at 32°C, warming all intravenous fluids and prep solutions, monitoring core temperature, and adjusting appropriate warmers. Central venous pressure (CVP) should be monitored and, prior to vascular clamp removal, raised to 15 to 18 cm $H_2O$ by colloid (usually packed red blood cell) transfusion to offset the colloid volume required to fill the kidney and cushion any anastomatic bleeding. Mannitol (250 mg/kg) and furosemide (1 mg/kg) are infused slowly (over ½ hour), with these infusions to be completed as the anastomoses are completed. Sodium bicarbonate (1 meq/kg) is also given close to clamp release to offset the lactic acid release from the aortic cross-clamping. The kidney is also warmed with saline to decrease hypothermia from the cold perfusate used to flush the kidney.

## Early Posttransplant Care

These small patients require meticulous attention to fluid and electrolyte issues, often for several days after surgery.[18] Urine output is usually replaced milliliter for milliliter, but the adult kidney can produce massive urine output relative to the small child's body mass. Thus, slight imbalance of urine versus replacement fluid volume or electrolyte composition can result in rapid development of fluid and electrolyte imbalances that are best detected and adjusted by frequent (4–6 hours) laboratory checks and constant clinical monitoring. Blood glucose should be frequently monitored and, if elevated above 180 mg/dL, the replacement solution should be switched to a 1% glucose solution. If urine output exceeds ≈15–20 mL/kg/hr and there is evidence of vascular volume overload (see below), consideration should be given to a gradual deficit in urine replacement, so that, after several hours, the urine output begins to fall. If diuretics have been ordered, these should be discontinued before the deficit urine replacement strategy is introduced. Colloid is administered to replace third space losses that can amount to 5% to 8% of the infants body weight in the first 24 to 48 hours, and bleeding losses. The goals are to maintain good peripheral perfusion and normal to slightly elevated blood pressure for age. There is no support for the idea that the adult kidney initially requires adult arterial pressure for adequate filtration function in the small child, and this misconception typically leads to serious fluid overload problems, normal to mildly elevated blood pressure (BP) for the recipient's age is the appropriate goal. A chest x-ray, which shows minimal to mild pulmonary vascular congestion without increased cardiomegaly or pulmonary edema, assures adequate vascular volume. When this state is reached, the CVP can be used as a surrogate for repeat chest x-rays. Colloid administration, until an arbitrary set CVP goal is reached, all too commonly results in pulmonary edema, prolonging intubation and ventilation requirement, or perpetrating a respiratory crises. We have seen acute renal shutdown result as often from volume overload and severe congestive heart failure as from hypovolemia and, thus, recommend avoidance of both extremes. If urine output is low despite maintaining the chest x-ray, BP, and peripheral perfusion, criteria outlined above, pushing fluids rarely helps, diuretics should be tried, and then patience should be exercised. It is our common experience that kidney function typically improves spontaneously over several hours with these hemodynamic parameters and that excess fluids are counterproductive. Again, the concept that adult kidneys require adult perfusion pressures to "function" is false and can lead to high-risk situations and even death from fluid administration aimed at achieving these blood pressure goals. Our incidence of acute tubular necrosis (ATN) is no greater in infants and young children than in older children or adults when the above fluid strategies are used.

Iatrogenic fluid overload leading to hemodilution and congestive heart failure with poor perfusion, normal to low BP, and decreased urine output can be misinterpreted as intra-abdominal bleeding. Blood transfusion in these circumstances can be lethal. This scenario is best avoided by careful review of all clinical data, including CVP changes and a chest x-ray before reflexive fluid orders are written.

A unique form of delayed oligoanuric acute renal failure associated with systemic illness (fever, thrombocytopenia, abnormal leukocyte count, and diarrhea) has been described in infants. The etiology of this entity is unclear. The picture typically develops after 1 or more days of good initial graft function. As ascites may be a component of this picture, confusion with urine leak is possible. Resolution with supportive care occurs within days to 1 to 2 weeks.[19]

# UROLOGIC ISSUES IN PEDIATRIC KIDNEY TRANSPLANTATION

## The Child with an abnormal lower urinary tract (LUT)

A urinary reservoir of adequate volume, compliance, and the ability to completely empty its content is essential for long-term optimal function of the renal allograft. These prerequisites are not met in a variety of conditions associated with ESRD in childhood. In some—extrophy/epispadias complex, urethral atresia, bladder agenesis—there are obvious anatomic abnormalities of the LUT. Others, such as neurogenic bladder, Hinman syndrome, posterior urethral valve, and prune belly syndrome—are commonly associated with abnormal bladder function.

Preparation for transplantation in children with these conditions should, therefore, include a detailed assessment of the anatomical and physiological adequacy of their LUT. This evaluation should include information regarding previous LUT surgery, the identification of abnormal voiding patterns, and imaging of the LUT by ultrasound and voiding cystourethrogram. Urodynamic testing may be added to assess urine flow, detrusor-sphincter synergy, and pressure profile during bladder filling and emptying.[3] Urodynamic evaluation may be challenging or uninterpretable in children with high-grade reflux and in those with a defunctionalized bladder. The latter condition is associated with a small-volume low-compliance bladder, at times coupled with unstable detrusor contractures, and yet, in most cases, will develop into a normally functioning reservoir following transplantation. Patients with an abnormal LUT can benefit from a variety of reconstructive procedures. Those are generally classified as continent and incontinent urinary diversion. Continent diversion may include bladder reconstruction (augmentation or rarely neobladder) or consist of an intestinal pouch functioning as a urinary reservoir (Mainz, Cock, Indiana pouch). Kidney transplantation into a reconstructed LUT has been repeatedly shown to result in short- and long-term patient and allograft survival rates that compare favorably with outcomes of kidney transplantation into a normal LUT. Importantly, reconstructive surgery, as well as transition from a incontinent to continent urinary system, can be safely performed following transplantation, optimally at a time when immunosuppression medications has been weaned.[20–31] Bladder augmentation can be safely performed in patients with ventriculoperitoneal shunts.[32] Bladder augmentation, at present, is the most common technique used for LUT reconstruction. Here, we discuss complications associated with this procedure while referring the reader to other sources for a description of alternative reconstructive techniques, their indications, and complications profiles.[33–36] Bladder augmentation is done most frequently using an intestinal segment (ileum or colon) with the transplant ureter drained in a nonrefluxing fashion into the native bladder. Continent bladder emptying is achieved via clean intermittent catheterization (CIC) either per urethra or via a supravescical intestinal conduit (eg, Mitrofanoff). UTIs are common and may cause life threatening sepsis in these immunocompromised patients. Bacterial colonization is universal in patients practicing CIC, even when maintained on daily oral antibiotics or antibiotic irrigation, and should be differentiated from acute infection. Clues for the latter include a change in urine color/odor, suprapubic tenderness, loss of continence and significant increase in mucus production, fever, increased urine WBCs and elevated creative protein (CRP). Recurrent urinary tract infections (UTIs) should prompt an assessment of the patients' compliance with CIC regimen and assure complete emptying, particularly in patients catheterizing through a continent abdominal wall stoma. The presence of stone and reflux should be ruled out. Bladder irrigation, to reduce mucus plugging, may be beneficial. Untreated colonization by urea-splitting organism may lead to stone formation.[36,37] Urolithiasis, mostly in the form of struvite stones, is not infrequent in patients with augmented bladders. Urinary stasis, ammonium generation by urea splitting bacteria, the presence of mucus, and suture lines acting as a nidus all predispose to this complication.[38] Aggressive treatment of urea-producing bacteria, adequate bladder emptying, and, possibly, bladder irrigation may decrease the incidence of this complication.

Acid resorption through the mucosa of an intestinal segment may lead to hyperchloremic metabolic acidosis, especially in cases with reduced allograft function. Chronically increased acid load, even without frank systemic acidosis, may underlie the decreased linear growth and reduced bone mineral density seen following intestinal bladder augmentation.[36,39,40] The use of a bowel segment may lead to gastrointestinal complications including intestinal obstruction, diarrhea and vitamin $B_{12}$ and bile salt malabsorption. Limiting the length of the intestinal segment used for augmentation and preservation of the terminal ileum and ileo-cecal valve greatly decrease these side effects. Diarrhea may still occur in patients with abnormal innervation. Delayed spontaneous bladder perforation is a relatively uncommon yet potentially devastating complication.[35,36,41] Perforation occurs most commonly at the intestinal–bladder anastomotic line and is thought to result from chronic ischemia aggravated by increased bladder pressure especially in patients with neurogenic bladder and in noncompliant adolescents. Symptoms of acute abdomen may be masked by immunosuppressive medications and by abnormal innervation in patients with neurogenic bladder. Diagnosis is usually made using computed tomographic (CT) cystography. Malignancy, primarily adenocarcinoma, is a well-recognized complication developing 7 to 50 years (median 20) after ureterosigmoidostomy. Patients undergoing bladder augmentation seem also at an increased risk of adenocarcinoma as well as transitional cell carcinoma of the bladder.[42–44] The influence of immunosuppressive medications on the incidence and timing of these complications is unknown. Yearly cystoscopy for tumor surveillance is currently recommended, starting 10 years postaugmentation. Finally, stomal stenosis, usually relieved by dilatation, is common when the Mitrofanoff procedure is used.[45] Given all of these potential problems, bladder augmentation should only be undertaken when the potential gains clearly outweigh the risks.

## Posterior Urethral Valves

More than 20 years ago the term *valve bladder* was coined to denote the association of a noncompliant thick-walled bladder and upper-tract dilatation in boys with posterior urethral valves (PUV).[46] Progression to ESRD following valve ablation in boys with PUV was subsequently shown to be more frequent in children with urodynamic or clinical evidence of bladder dysfunction.[47] Subsequent reports showing inferior outcome of kidney transplantation in children with PUV were therefore accepted as an extension of the concept of the deleterious effects of a "hostile" urinary reservoir on renal function. Those publications prompted some centers to routinely perform bladder augmentation prior to transplantation.[48,49] More recent series of kidney transplantation for PUV show mixed results, with some reporting inferior outcomes, whereas others report no effects of the valve bladder on allograft function.[50–56] Taken together, it seems that in only some PUV patients is the valve bladder detrimental to the long-term outcome of kidney transplantation. Development of criteria to identify the subset of patients at risk will require a more thorough understanding of the pathopysiology and natural history of the valve bladder, standardization of urodynamic studies and better-designed studies aimed at the definition of the long-term allograft outcomes in PUV.[46,57,58]

Prior to transplantation, bladder outlet obstruction due to residual valves and/or urethral stenosis should be ruled out in all PUV patients. Bilateral nephrectomy should be performed in patients with recurrent UTI and/or reflux and should be considered in markedly polyuric patients as a means to reduce the pressure in the drainage system.[59] Pretransplantation urodynamic evaluation should be reserved for patients whose history (bladder surgery, recurrent UTIs, voiding dysfunction, fast progression to ESRD) and imaging suggest severe bladder function abnormality. Following transplantation, patients should be closely monitored for evidence of valve bladder manifesting as hydronephrosis, voiding dysfunction, and/or UTI. These findings should prompt urodynamic evaluation of the bladder-storage characteristics.[60] Patients with clinical and urodynamic evidence of valve bladder are likely to benefit from the use of anticholinergic and/or alpha-receptor blocking agents, frequent and double voiding, and various regimens of bladder catheterizations or bladder augmentations.[46,59,61] All these measures can be safely instituted before or following transplantation once immunosuppressive medications are weaned to maintenance level.

## Recurrent Disease in the Renal Allograft

Involvement of the allograft with the disease originally afflicting the recipient's native kidneys accounts for almost 7% of graft loss in pediatric transplantation, far exceeding its incidence in the adult counterparts.[62,63]

## STEROID-RESISTANT NEPHROTIC SYNDROME WITH FOCAL AND SEGMENTAL GLOMERULOSCLEROSIS (SRNS/FSGS)

SRNS/FSGS, accounting for about 10% of the incidence of pediatric ESRD, is the most common glomerular disease and the third most common primary diagnosis in children requiring renal transplantation.[7] Recurrence in the allograft occurs in approximately 20% to 40% of pediatric kidney recipients with SRNS/FSGS.[64–67] Recurrence has been attributed to the action of a circulating plasma "permeability factor."[68–71] This hypothesis is supported by the rapidity with which nephrotic syndrome may recur and the purported salutary effect of both plasmapheresis and immunoglobulin adsorption therapy in these cases.[65,72,73] Furthermore, plasma fractions obtained from some patients with recurrent FSGS can induce proteinuria when injected into healthy animals.[74] Still, the exact nature of this circulating factors—whether a permeability promoting factor or, less likely, the lack of a factor essential for the maintenance of normal glomerular permselectivity—remains elusive.[68,71,75]

Recurrent SRNS/FSGS occurs more frequently in pediatric than adult patients. Age of onset over 6 years in a pediatric patient, progression from onset of nephrotic syndrome to ESRD in less than 2 years, and mesangial hypercellularity portend higher recurrence risks.[65,76]

Recurrence of SRNS/FSGN is also more frequent in nonblack patients. Given the improved outcomes with current therapies, it may no longer be appropriate to recommend against live donation to patients with high risks for recurrence of SRNS/FSGS unless the first graft is rapidly lost despite aggressive intervention.[77–80] Better understanding of the diverse mechanisms leading to the lesion of FSGS will likely result in even further improvements in outcome of kidney transplantation for this complex disease.[81]

The best predictor of recurrent FSGS is the fate of the first allograft, thus, recurrent disease is highly unlikely in second transplants when the cause for the primary allograft loss was unrelated to the underlying glomerulopathy. In contrast, recurrence in subsequent transplantation is almost universal in cases where the first allograft showed early recurrence of the nephrotic syndrome followed shortly there after by allograft loss.[65,82] Reports are conflicting regarding the ability to predict recurrence using an assay detecting changes in permeability of explanted rat glomeruli incubated with the patient's plasma.[75,83–85] More recently, mutations in the gene encoding the podocyte-specific protein, podocin (NPHS2), were identified in familial and sporadic cases of SRNS/FSGS.[86] SRNS/FSGS patients carrying homozygous and compound heterozygous podocin mutation are at a low risk for recurrent disease. The risks associated with parental-obligate carrier-donation are yet to be defined. A high rate of recurrence is reported in a small number of patients carrying heterozygous NPHS2 mutations. This observation awaits confirmation and elucidation of its pathogenesis.[71,87,88]

Recurrent SRNS/FSGS commonly manifests as nephrotic range proteinuria and hypoalbuminemia, usually within the first month after transplantation. Proteinuria, in fact, is often immediate, and early allograft biopsies are likely to show only diffuse effacement of foot processes, whereas later biopsies will show the typical FSGS lesions. Delayed allograft function has been reported to occur more frequently both in living related donor (LRD) and cadaver (CAD) transplantation for patients with recurrent SRNS/FSGS,[65,78,79] likely reflecting permselectivity barrier injury associated with the nephrotic state. Presenting as ATN without antecedent massive proteinuria, recurrence may be diagnosable only by allograft biopsy. The presence of ATN in a patient with recurrent FSGS seems to be associated with increased rate of rejection and may portend a bleak prognosis.[89] Late recurrences have been reported, including in patients with podocin mutation.[65,88]

Treatment of recurrent disease is based on the premise that a circulating permeability factor is the culprit. Removal of the inciting agent by immunoadsorption or by plasmapheresis has been associated with reduction of proteinuria or remission.[65,73,90–95] At times, maintenance of remission requires long-term plasmapheresis.[94–96] Some advocate using Cytoxan as one of the posttransplant immunosuppressive agents in addition to plasmapheresis.[97,98] An alternative approach is the use of high-dose cyclosporine.[99–102] Two recent publications report remission rates of 80% with good long-term allograft survival using high-dose oral and intravenous cyclosporine.[99,101] The authors of the latter publication propose that the intravenous administration route avoids the toxicity associated with elevated CSA peak concentrations and report a significant improvement in outcome compared to their center's historical controls.[101] Posttransplantation proteinuria provides a unique opportunity for early intervention possibly accounting for the superior remission rate compared to that of FSGS in native kidneys. There is no head-to-head comparison of the above methodologies, or their combined use, nor is there more than anecdotal support for preemptive plasmapheresis or CSA therapy instituted prior to transplantation in high-risk cases[103,104(and personal observations)].

# CONGENITAL NEPHROTIC SYNDROME OF THE FINNISH TYPE (CNF)

Congenital nephrotic syndrome of the Finnish type (CNF) is the most common form of nephrotic syndrome presenting in the first months of life. CNF is an autosomal recessive disorder due, in majority of cases, to mutation in the NPHS1 gene encoding for nephrin, a cell-adhesion protein localized to the podocyte slit diaphragm.[105–108] Two mutations, Fin-major and Fin-minor, account for more than 90% of NPHS1 mutations in Finland, whereas a myriad of other mutations prevail in infants not of Finnish descent. At present, the definitive treatment of CNF patients is bilateral nephrectomy and kidney transplantation. Nephrectomy should be performed ahead of transplantation to allow, prior to exposure to immunosuppressive medications, for correction of the hypercoagulable state induced by the severe nephrosis, as well as allow for immunoglobulin reconstitution and for correction of the protein deficiencies that could limit optimal wound healing. In some cases, proteinuria diminishes as uremia supervenes allowing the serum albumin to rise above 3 g/dL. We have then proceeded with a single-stage nephrectomy-transplant procedure. Because of the increased risk of spontaneous thrombosis, patency of the IVC should be verified prior to transplantation. Following transplantation NS recurs in approximately 40% of patients carrying a homozygote Fin major mutation. This mutation results in complete absence of nephrin in the native kidney, thus transplantation represents exposure to a "novel" antigen triggering the formation of antinephrin antibodies postulated to be responsible for alterations in the slit diaphragm of the renal allograft and proteinuria.[109] Thus, strictly speaking, this is, rather than *de novo* renal disease, akin to anti-glomular basement membrane (GBM) disease in the allograft of Alport syndrome patients. In the largest series of transplantation for CNF, time to development of NS from this cause varied from 5 days to 48 months (median 12 months). This may be preceded by an intercurrent infection.[109] Therapy, most commonly an increase in prednisone dosage combined with replacement of the antimetabolite with Cytoxan, results in remission in about 50% of cases. Failure to induce remission usually leads to loss of the allograft.[109–111] The risk for this type of *de novo* development of NS in patients carrying other NPHS1 mutations seems to be low.

# HEMOLYTIC UREMIC SYNDROME (HUS)

HUS accounts for 2% to 4% of pediatric renal transplant cases.[7] ESRD is an uncommon outcome of HUS associated with Shiga toxin (Stx)-producing strains of *Escherichia coli*.[112] In those where ESRD develop, the risk for recurrent disease is extremely low, and allograft outcome is similar to that recorded for pediatric transplantation for other primary renal diseases. Calcineurin-based immunosuppression protocols are well tolerated, and LRD transplantation should be considered.[113,114] Conversely, recurrence rate of 50% to 80%, mostly leading to allograft failure, is reported in non-Stx-HUS, with both familial and sporadic forms.[113] These contrasting outcomes underscore the importance of accurate diagnosis of the primary disease in planning for future transplantation.

Recent review of transplantation outcome in non-Stx-HUS patients evaluated for abnormalities in regulatory elements of the alternate pathway of the complement system confirms the grim outlook of transplantation for this patient subset.[115] Mutations in complement factor H (CFH) carried a 73% risk for recurrent HUS. Most recurrences were in the first year following transplantation and were resistant to therapeutic interventions. This outcome was independent of the type of factor H mutation as well as its plasma level. Simultaneous liver–kidney transplantation, aimed to correct factor H deficiency, was complicated in two cases by premature irreversible liver failure. Similar poor renal transplant outcomes were noted in few cases of HUS secondary to mutations in factor I. On the other hand, recurrent disease did not occur in four patients transplanted for HUS due to mutation of the gene-encoding membrane co-factor protein (MCP) as transplantation corrects the abnormal "local" expression of this membrane co-factor which is highly expressed in renal endothelial cells.[112] A 55% recurrence rate was seen in patients with non-Stx-HUS where no abnormalities of CFH, factor I, and MCP could be documented. Importantly, in two cases of this group, HUS developed in the living-related donor's native residual kidney within a year following donation. Thus, at present, kidney transplantation for non-Stx-HUS remains problematic, as there are no reliable strategies to prevent or treat disease recurrence. Current therapies, including plasmapheresis and fresh-frozen plasma infusions tend to provide only partial or temporary benefit. Although recurrence of HUS tends to occur in the first posttransplant year, we have seen this delayed for as long as 10 years and then appear with no discernible provocation. Importantly, recurrence needs to be differentiated from other causes of HUS in the renal allograft such as vascular rejection, calcineurin inhibitor toxicity, and malignant hypertension.

# PRIMARY HYPEROXALURIA TYPE 1 (PH 1)

PH 1 is a autosomal recessive disorder where a functional defect or absence of the liver-specific peroxisomal enzyme alanine:glyoxylate aminotransferase (AGT) results in excessive hepatic oxalate synthesis, increased urinary oxalate excretion, and calcium oxalate nephrocalcinosis and nephrolithiasis. Renal failure in PH 1 is most frequently encountered in childhood.[116–118] Organ transplantation is the only long-term solution for PH 1 patients with advanced renal disease, since, despite standard dialysis therapy, ESRD is associated with accelerated extrarenal oxalate deposition in bones, eyes, vessels, nerves, and other organs with painful debilitating and disastrous consequences.[117,119,120] The main transplant options in PH 1 are simultaneous liver–kidney (SLK), which offers correction of the metabolic lesion as well as replacement of the damaged target organ and kidney-alone transplantation (KA).[116,120] Significant improvement in transplantation outcomes have been reported in the last decade both from registries and from single-center experiences. Overall, SLK transplantation, although associated with higher short-term mortality, provides superior long-term patient and renal allograft survival compared to KA, underscoring the importance of normalized oxalate production to a favorable transplantation outcome.[121–124] SLK can be successfully performed in infants presenting with ESRD due to hyperoxaluria.[123,124] Due to size constraints, SLK in infancy may require the use of younger donors, reduced size liver transplantation, and placement of the renal allograft in the left hemiabdomen.[123,124]

A successful transplantation strategy starts with prompt diagnosis of PH 1 through familiarity with the clinical manifestations of the disease in infants and children.[125] This is followed by institution of dialysis at a GFR of 30 to 40 mL/min/1.73 m$^2$, when plasma calcium oxalate reaches supersaturation resulting in tissue oxalate precipitation. HD offers superior oxalate clearance relative to PD and should be tailored to maximize oxalate clearance (daily, nocturnal, etc).[126] Efficient oxalate removal will limit organ injury and dysfunction related to extra-renal tissue oxalate accretion and reduce posttransplantation hyperoxaluria, and is likely to result in better nutrition and growth while awaiting transplantation.[10] Plasma oxalate levels can be monitored and treatment goals of 50 µmol/L or less seem appropriate. Still, oxalate clearance provided by current dialytic modalities may only slow tissue oxalate accumulation, and prolonged dialysis is associated with inferior transplantation outcomes.[119] Prior to transplantation, the clinical and biochemical diagnosis of PH 1 should be confirmed by determination of hepatic AGT activity and its subcellular distribution or by using AGT mutation analysis. Pyridoxine responsiveness, the ability to reduce hepatic oxalate synthesis in response to pharmacologic doses of vitamin $B_6$, should be defined. In patients with significantly reduced GFR, pyridoxine responsiveness can be determined by measuring changes in blood glycolate concentration following $B_6$ challenge or deduced from results of AGT biochemical or molecular analysis.[119,127–130] One third of PH 1 patients are pyridoxine responsive, and this subset may do well with KA transplantation with pyridoxine supplementation obviating the complications associated with the combined procedure.[127,131–133]

Following transplantation the major hurdle is that of recurrent disease—calcium oxalate deposition in the renal allograft. This risk is present while hyperoxaluria continues and is increased during periods of renal allograft dysfunction. Posttransplantation hyperoxaluria due to mobilization of accrued tissue oxalate may persist for several years in spite of correction of the metabolic defect by SLK or by $B_6$ therapy in responsive cases. Prevention of recurrent disease requires reduction of urinary calcium oxalate crystal formation and avoidance of prolonged renal allograft dysfunction. The former is achieved through increased fluid intake (which may necessitate g-tube placement in infants) together with supplementation with agents that increase urine oxalate solubility (orthophosphates, magnesium, citrate) and thiazide diuretics to increase urine output without concomitant increased calciuria.[123,133,134] To avoid prolonged allograft dysfunction, organ selection and immunosuppressive protocol should aim for prompt and optimal allograft function (short ischemia time and introduction of calcineurin inhibitors [CNI] only after good graft function is established). CNI toxicity should be avoided, and investigation and treatment of allograft dysfunction should be prompt. Dialysis can be added during periods of significant reduction in allograft function. Monitoring of urinary oxalate excretion is an integral part of posttransplant management, as its normalization would permit the removal of the above measures, although $B_6$ therapy should be continued in $B_6$ responsive patients. Finally, alternative transplantation modalities, preemptive liver, and sequential liver kidney transplantation should be considered in specific situations.[120,135,136] The impact of live donation on outcome is likely to be significant in cases when organ availability is limited, since prevention of tissue oxalate accrual on long-term dialysis is a critical goal (see above).

## MALIGNANCY FOLLOWING KIDNEY TRANSPLANTATION

### Glomerulopathies Associated With Mutations in WT1 Gene

Constitutional mutations in the WT1 gene are associated with the Denys-Drash (DDS) and Frasier syndromes. Patients with these rare syndromes have abnormal gonadal differentiation, progressive glomerular disease, and, importantly for the transplantation nephrologists, a heightened risk of malignancy.[137,138] DDS is a triad composed of male pseudohermaphroditism, progressive renal disease, and Wilms' tumor. Patients may present in infancy with heavy proteinuria and often progress very rapidly to renal failure. Renal histology is eventually consistent with diffuse mesangial sclerosis.[139,140] Patients carrying an XY karyotype have either normal female or ambiguous external genitalia. Patients with a XX karyotype are mostly normal females, yet occasionally may have dysgenetic gonads (true hermaphrodites). Most DDS patients carry a dominant negative heterozygous mutation at exons 8 and 9 of the WT1 gene.[141] DDS patients are at markedly increased risk for Wilms' tumor as well as malignancy of the abnormal gonads (gonadoblastoma).[142–144] Bilateral nephrectomy and removal of all gonadal tissue should, therefore, be performed prior to or at the time of transplantation.

Frasier syndrome (FS) is defined by male pseudo-hermaphroditism and progressive glomerulopathy.[145] Patients carry an XY karyotype, have normal female external genitalia, streak gonads, and a proclivity to develop gonadoblastoma. Renal disease presents as proteinuria/nephrotic syndrome in early childhood with biopsy finding consisting with FSGS and a slow progression to ESRD. Most cases are related to mutation in an alternative splice site on intron 9 of the WT1 gene.[146] Surgical gonadectomy should be performed once the diagnosis is confirmed, and is imperative prior to exposure to immunosuppressive medications. Diagnosis of these syndromes is difficult at times due to incomplete forms of DDS and phenotypic variations associated with specific mutations.[147,148]

## Posttransplant Lymphoproliferative Disorder (PTLD)

PTLD is a spectrum of diseases of the lymphoid cell lineage most often resulting from Epstein–Barr virus (EBV)-induced B-lymphocyte proliferation in the context of a suppressed EBV specific T-cell response. The incidence of PTLD has greatly increased in recent years in parallel with the use of more aggressive immunosuppressive protocols and the concomitant decrease in acute rejection episodes. Perhaps it is worth remembering that more than one half or more of patients treated with antibody induction and Imuran and Prednisone alone for maintenance therapy never had acute rejection episodes, suggesting that at least one half of our patients are over-immunosuppressed and, consequently, exposed to increased risks without potential benefit. Clearly, there is a need to monitor immune system function other than drug levels.

PTLD is more likely to follow primary EBV infection and, thus, is most often encountered in pediatric, EBV-naïve recipients of allografts from EBV-positive donors. It most frequently occurs in the first year following kidney transplantation and may affect up to 25% of patients "at risk" receiving kidney transplantation.[149] However, there may be delays of up to 5 years before onset. Caucasian race, the use of polyclonal antibody induction, and the use of tacrolimus seem to be associated with higher incidence of PTLD in pediatric kidney transplant recipients.[150–152] The risk for PTLD seems to be further increased in patients undergoing CMV infection.[153,154]

Prevention of PTLD is limited by the lack of an effective vaccine. Induction of EBV infection in seronegative patients awaiting kidney transplantation remains anecdotal.[155] Prevention thus relies on preemptive intervention in patients thought to be at increased risk for the development of PTLD. Serial determination of EBV viral loads is currently the best tool in targeting preemptive therapy, especially in seronegative patients. Patients with persistently low or nondetectable EBV DNA are unlikely to develop EBV associated disease while increasing viral loads are frequently seen prior to the onset of PTLD.[156,157] Decreasing the intensity of immunosuppression in at-risk patients with elevated EBV viral loads resulted in decreased incidence of PTLD in pediatric liver transplant recipients.[158,159] Antiviral "prophylaxis" is widely used in at-risk patients despite the lack of sound data.[153] There are, in fact, conflicting reports regarding the effectiveness of viral chemoprophylaxis. Most recently a case control study showed decreased risk for development of PTLD in patients receiving gancyclovir, and to a lesser degree, acyclovir prophylaxis.[160] Similarly, the use of immune globulin prophylaxis for EBV related PTLD is not proven.[161,162] Beyond prevention, familiarity with the clinical manifestation and the pathologic classification (described elsewhere) of EBV-related syndromes are likely to result in improved outcome of pediatric patients inflicted by PTLD. The superior outcome of PTLD in pediatric relative to adult patients may reflect earlier diagnosis and thus a more favorable morphology that is likely to respond to reduction of immunosuppression combined with antiviral therapy without allograft rejection (personal observations).[163,164] Treatment strategies for less favorable forms of PTLD include the use of Rituximab, cancer chemotherapy, and, where indicated, surgical removal of involved organs. These aggressive malignancies are associated with inferior outcome for both patient and allograft. Retransplantation after PTLD can be performed, though optimal timing and intensity of immunosuppression are yet to be defined.[165]

## IMMUNOSUPPRESSIVE PROTOCOLS

### Therapeutic Drug Monitoring (TDM)

TDM is widely used in organ transplantation in order to address the large intraindividual and interindividual variability in pharmacokinetics (PK) of immunosuppressive medications. When coupled with outcome studies, TDM can serve as a surrogate for the elusive measurement of the level of immunosuppression. As such, data from PK studies should be applied to patients and conditions closely resembling the original study.

*Mycopholate mofetil (MMF)* MMF has been reported to be superior to azathioprine (AZA) or placebo in the prevention of acute rejection episodes both in adult and in pediatrics renal transplant recipients.[166,167] PK studies have shown significant interpatient variability and a poor correlation between MMF dose and exposure to its active metabolite mycophenolic acid (MPA), suggesting a need for TDM. Factors significantly influencing MPA levels include concomitant use of CSA and steroids, renal dysfunction, and hypoalbuminemia.[168] PK studies, in which MMF was used in combination with CSA, showed that MPA exposure correlates with risk of allograft rejection. This has led to recommendations to maintain MPA- AUC0-12 of 30 to 60 mg.h/L or MPA trough 1 to 3.5 mg/L. There does not seem to be a clear-cut association between adverse events and any single PK parameter. Ongoing trials in adults may better define the role of TDM in increasing the therapeutic potential of MMF. At present, we would recommend TDM whenever dose modification is planned, in patients with delayed graft function, rejection, opportunistic infection, or when suspecting MMF-related side effects as well as a surrogate for compliance.[168]

PK studies in pediatric transplant recipients are in accordance with the adult data suggesting a value for TDM. Pediatric-specific limited sampling algorithms that correlate well with full AUC0-12 throughout the pediatric age group are available.[169–172] Infants seem to require a higher MMF dose to obtain target MPA exposure and also seem to be more prone to its gastrointestinal (GI) side effects.[173] The use of MMF with other bone-marrow-suppressive agents (Bactrim, valganciclovir) is associated with neutropenia in a significant number of patients, especially those on steroid-free protocols. However, it makes no sense to think that WBC counts propped up by Prednisone treatment in MMF-treated patients represent improved protection from infection than lower counts in Prednisone-free protocols. A different limited sampling strategy may be needed to assess exposure to MMF when combined with other immunosuppressive medications.[172]

*Cyclosporine (CSA)* CSA microsmulsion formulation (CSA-ME; Neoral), introduced in the mid-1990s, provides increased and more consistent systemic exposure compared with the original, oil-based, CSA formulation. Neoral's maximal and most consistent immunosuppressive effect as well as the greatest variability in its absorption profile occurs in the first few hours following oral administration.[174] The 4-hour AUC (AUC0-4) was shown to highly correlate with a full 12-hour AUC and to predict early acute rejection and CSA nephrotoxicity.[175,176] The best single point surrogate for the variability of exposure during the first 4 hours after dosing in adults is the CSA concentration at 2 hours (C2). C2 monitoring was subsequently shown to be safe and efficient in the management of adult primary kidney transplants and has is replacing the traditional trough (C0) monitoring which poorly predicts AUC0-4 and rejection episodes (177-180). An additional advantage of C2 versus C0 monitoring is the reduction of variability among different CSA assays since the C2 sample has less metabolite interference. As expected, proper use of C2 monitoring in long-term management of renal transplant recipients is more difficult to institute.[181–183]

The use of Neoral in pediatric transplantation, accompanied by dose adjustment according to body surface area, largely abolished the need for age-adjusted dosing necessary while using the "classic" CSA formulation.[184,185] Similar to studies in adults, AUC0-4 seems a good indicator for the risk to develop acute rejection.[185,186] C2 monitoring has been shown by some, but not all, to reflect early-phase CSA absorption and to define risk for acute rejection in *de novo* allograft recipients[185–188]; thus, C2 monitoring may be replacing the use of trough monitoring. More data are needed to define the optimal dosing and monitoring of Neoral in infants and small children,[189] but current information supports every 8-hour dosing.

*Tacrolimus (Tac)* is monitored using trough levels. Intrapatient variability in systemic exposure is low resulting in a small number of dose changes required to maintain target blood concentration.[190] The PK accuracy of this approach has been recently questioned, suggesting that a measurement made at an additional time point during the absorption phase would be more reflective of AUC0-12 and possibly a superior predictor of clinical events.[191,192] Pediatric studies show a need for higher dosing relative to adults, mainly due to faster drug elimination. Absorption seems more consistent than that of CSA.[193–196] As suggested for adults, correlation with drug exposure may be improved by the use of sparse sampling rather than C0.[195,197]

*Sirolimus (SRL)* administration is adjusted using predose sampling, which reflects drug exposure quite well. Studies relating drug levels to clinical events are lacking.[191,198] Sirolimus drug levels are greatly increased when co-administered with CSA, yet unaffected when combined with Tac.[190,199] Adding SRL to Tac- or CSA-based immunosuppressive protocols results in reduced calcineurin inhibitor drug exposure, and, thus, a need to increase CNI dose.[190,200] The half-life of SRL is significantly shorter in children relative to that seen in adults, indicating a need for twice-daily dosing, especially in infants and young children.[194,200,201]

## STEROID-SPARING PROTOCOLS

Steroids have traditionally been a cornerstone of most immunosuppressive protocols. Nevertheless, the use of corticosteroids is associated with a myriad of side effects including a heightened risk of cardiovascular morbidity related to induction of hypertension, hyperlipidemia, and hyperglycemia; an increased propensity for infections and adverse effects on bone metabolism. Stunted growth is a feature peculiar to chronic kidney disease in infants and children. The failure of kidney transplantation to bring about catch-up growth is in substantial part related to the inhibitory effect of corticosteroids on growth velocity.[4,202] Furthermore, the cosmetic side effects related to steroid use may contribute to medication nonadherence, especially in adolescents.[203] Myriad other complications, not limited to cataracts, aseptic necroses, steroid-induced diabetes, pancreatitis, acne, and obesity, are well known. Thus, strategies aimed at reducing steroid-related side effects are of particular interest to the pediatric organ transplant recipient who is likely to be exposed to immunosuppressive medications longer than its adult counterpart. Early attempts of steroid withdrawal in adults resulted in an unacceptable increased risk for acute rejection and late graft failure. Steroid withdrawal/avoidance became feasible more recently, in conjunction with the use of more potent immunosuppressive protocols. Adults maintained on steroid-free protocols were shown to have good short- and medium-term allograft outcomes in association with an improved metabolic profile.[204–209]

The safety of administrating steroids on an alternate-day basis in pediatrics was studied by Broyer et al. Children with good allograft function and normal histology, maintained on AZA and daily prednisone, were prospectively randomized, 14 to 27 months following transplantation, to alternate-day schedule at the same cumulative dose (Prednisone at 0.25 mg/kg/day). Over the subsequent 2 years, children on the alternate-day regimen had no episodes of acute rejection, maintained normal creatinine clearance, and showed significantly improved growth velocity.[210] A similar salutary effect on growth in transplanted children maintained on alternat-day Prednisone was confirmed by single-center and registry data.[211,212] More recently, the safety of steroid withdrawal in selected pediatric recipients was shown in a case control study from Germany. During 4-year follow-up, steroid withdrawal on MMF and CSA maintenance was not associated with either acute rejection episodes or with reduced GFR, while resulting in improved growth, lower body mass index, and a decline in the use of antihypertensive medications.[213] A recent CCPT randomized controlled study showed that steroid can be safely withdrawn in rejection-free patients at 6 months following transplantation. Immunosuppression consisted of basiliximab induction and SRL and FK maintenance. Over 2 years, similar acute rejection rates were encountered in patients randomized to continue maintenance steroids and those tapered off prednisone over a 6-month

period. However, an unacceptable rate of PTLD caused early termination of the study.[149] High rates of PTLD were also encountered in other single-center reports of steroid withdrawal.[214–216] A steroid-free protocol incorporating extended induction with daclizumab for 6 months with maintenance MMF and tacrolimus was introduced by the Stanford group. A report of the initial experience with 77 patients showed lower acute rejection incidence (13%), improved height SD scores, superior BP control, and less hypercholesterolemia and lower incidence of viral infection compared with historic steroid based controls.[217,218] The protocol is currently evaluated in a multicenter prospective randomized trial. Of note, steroid-free, MMF-based protocols are associated with a high rate of neutropenia. This association reflects a higher MPA exposure under steroid-free conditions as well as reduced demargination of white blood cells, and as already noted, simply unmasks the MMF myelosuppressive effect obscured by steroid therapy. The concomitant use of myelosuppressive antiviral and antibacterial prophylaxis further accentuates this trend.[209] The above results suggest that steroid-free immunosuppression is a feasible option for the majority of pediatric recipients of kidney transplantation.

The increase incidence in recent years of PTLD, BK nephropathy, and the rate of posttransplantation hospitalization for infection and malignancy suggests that the overall intensity of present immunosuppression protocols can be reduced without a significant increase in acute rejection episodes. Whether long-term outcome of pediatric renal transplantation would benefit most from steroid avoidance, withdrawal, or a minimization of more than one agent is to be determined.

## LIVING DONATION IN PEDIATRIC KIDNEY TRANSPLANTS

Approximately 700 pediatric kidney transplantations are performed yearly representing 4% to 6% of all kidney transplantation in the United States.[219] This number has remained essentially constant over the last decade, consistent with the long-held and widespread belief among pediatric nephrologists that transplantation is the treatment of choice for children with ESRD. In fact, the rate of kidney transplantation for pediatric patients, corrected for prevalence of ESRD, is double that of adults. Overall, the best 5-year allograft survival rates, for both live (LD) and deceased donors (DD), are encountered in children ages 1to10 (similar to those of adults ages 35–49 years). The worst outcomes in the pediatric age group are in adolescents, for reasons that are not clear, but with nonadherence being a potential major contributor to increased graft loss in this age group.[220,221]

Slightly more than 50% of pediatric renal allografts come from living donors compared to 41% in adult ESRD patients. In some centers, such as the University of Minnesota (U of M) where LD transplantation is encouraged, 85% of children receive a LD primary graft. Parents comprise 81% of pediatric living donations, mothers being the parent–donor in 56% of the cases. Increasingly, at the U of M, children with unavailability of family or close relationship LD have benefited from voluntary anonymous, nondirected, renal donation,[224] sometimes in response to press coverage of the child's problems. LD transplantation offers improved allograft outcome compared to DD. The gap between the two has markedly diminished in recent years for 1-year allograft survival rates (96%–100% vs 88%–92%, respectively, for the different pediatric recipient age groups). Still, 5-year allograft outcomes are significantly superior for recipients of LD organs (79% vs 63%, respectively). Acute tubular necrosis (ATN), defined as the use of dialysis in the first transplant week, is reported in 5% of LD transplants compared with 17% for cadaver source transplantation.[221]

Living related transplantation may also result in improved posttransplantation growth, probably at least, in part, due to lower immunosuppression requirements, less acute rejection, and superior allograft function.[223] The logistics of planning for transplantation are easier when a LD is available. LD facilitates preemptive transplantation without prior exposure to dialysis, transplantation. In adults, preemptive transplantation was shown to result in improved patient and allograft outcomes.[224–226] Our own studies, which included adults and children, indicate that the detrimental effects of prior dialysis on patient and renal graft survival rates are more readily demonstrable in patients on dialysis for more than 1 year,[226] Although much easier to accomplish with LD grafts, the benefits of preemptive transplantation are also demonstrable with CAD grafts.[227] There is also a lower rate of primary nonfunction and acute rejection with this transplant strategy.[224,225] Data from NAPARTCS are also in line with these observations showing improved 3-year allograft outcome as well as lower rate of ATN in children receiving preemptive kidney transplantation compared to those undergoing dialysis prior to transplantation.[228] The patient survival advantage in this report was limited to recipients of LD allografts.[228]

Although surgical considerations of pediatric renal transplantation are covered elsewhere in this text (see Chapter 16.11b) it is worth repeating here that adult kidneys can be successfully placed in infants weighing as little as 7 to 8 kg.[229] This requires experience in surgical and postoperative management but, critically, avoids the probability of a very long waiting time for pediatric DD, since these are relatively rare. Nonetheless, current data suggest that if the increased risk of early postoperative graft thrombosis can be overcome, pediatric *en bloc* DD renal transplants can provide better long-term function than even LD transplants.[230]

Although controversial,[231,232] the use of children as LD is generally considered unethical other than in exceptional circumstances.[233] Among those may be the case of identical twins where the symbiosis of the relationship may be such that the loss of one is considered a serious threat to the other.[231]

## FUTURE PERSPECTIVES

The field of pediatric kidney transplantation has seen substantial improvements in recent years with short- and longer-term patient and allograft outcomes that are similar, or superior, to those encountered in adults. Still, for many years now, protocols employed in pediatric renal transplantation have been extensions of knowledge gained from studies in adults or based on limited, often empiric, pediatric data. One serious limitation in the evaluation of pediatric renal transplant immunosuppressive strategies is the lack of long-term follow-up into adulthood. This is particularly important because of the long life expectancy of pediatric compared to adult recipients. Thus, for example, the true impact of graft loss due to CNI toxicity may not be properly tracked by pediatric clinical investigators whose patients graduate to adult care. Similar comments may be relevant to very long-term cardiovascular malignancy, bone, and quality-of-life outcomes, among others. The formation of a body that will oversee pediatric kidney transplantation in the United States would allow us to properly address issues specific to solid organ transplantation in children. Such an organization would formulate practice guidelines and su-

pervise their implementation. It could design trials that would provide evidence-based recommendation regarding pediatric specific issues. Movement in this direction is likely to be rewarded with great improvement in the care of the pediatric kidney recipient, analogous to the gains made by our colleagues following the creation of the Pediatric Oncology Group.

## References

1. North American Pediatric Renal Transplant Cooperative Study (NAPARTCS) 2005 annual report. 2005.
2. Harmon WE. Pediatric renal transplantation. In: Pereira BJG, Sayegh MH, Blake PG, eds. *Chronic Kidney Disease, Dialysis, and Transplantation: A Companion to Brenner and Rector's the Kidney.* 2nd edition. Philadelphia, PA: Saunders; 2005:722–749.
3. Fine RN, Bajaj G. Renal transplantation in children. In: Morris PJ, ed. *Kidney Transplantation: Principles and Practice.* 5th edition. Philadelphia: Saunders; 2001: 604–657.
4. Rianthavorn p, Al-Akash SI, Ettenger RB. Kidney transplantation in children. In: Weir MR, ed. *Medical Management of Kidney Transplantation.* Philadelphia: Lippincott Williams & Wilkins; 2005:198–230.
5. Fine RN, Kelly DA, Webber SA. *Pediatric Solid Organ Transplantation.* 1st edition. Philadelphia, PA: Saunders; 2003.
6. Harmon WE, McDonald RA, Reyes JD, et al. Pediatric transplantation, 1994-2003. *Am J Transplant* 2005 Apr;5(4 Pt 2):887–903.
7. Benfield MR. Current status of kidney transplant: update 2003. *Pediatr Clin North Am* 2003 Dec;50(6):1301–1334.
8. Khwaja K, Humar A, Najarian JS. Kidney transplants for children under 1 year of age—a single-center experience. *Pediatr Transplant* 2003 Jun;7(3):163–167.
9. Parekh RS, Flynn JT, Smoyer WE, et al. Improved growth in young children with severe chronic renal insufficiency who use specified nutritional therapy. *J Am Soc Nephrol* 2001 Nov;12(11):2418–2426.
10. Katz A, Bock GH, Mauer M. Improved growth velocity with intensive dialysis. Consequence or coincidence? *Pediatr Nephrol* 2000 Aug;14 (8-9):710–712.
11. Tom A, McCauley L, Bell L, et al. Growth during maintenance hemodialysis: impact of enhanced nutrition and clearance. *J Pediatr* 1999 Apr;134(4):464–471.
12. Thomas SE, Hickman RO, Tapper D, et al. Asymptomatic inferior vena cava abnormalities in three children with end-stage renal disease: risk factors and screening guidelines for pretransplant diagnosis. *Pediatr Transplant* 2000 Feb;4(1):28–34.
13. Gonzalez R, LaPointe S, Sheldon CA, Mauer MS. Undiversion in children with renal failure. *J Pediatr Surg* 1984 Dec;19(6):632–636.
14. Fontaine E, Salomon L, Gagnadoux MF, et al. Long-term results of renal transplantation in children with the prune-belly syndrome. *J Urol* 1997 Sep;158(3 Pt 1):892–894.
15. Fusaro F, Zanon GF, Ferreli AM, et al. Renal transplantation in prune-belly syndrome. *Transpl Int* 2004 Oct;17(9):549-552.
16. Reinberg Y, Manivel JC, Fryd D, Najarian JS, Gonzalez R. The outcome of renal transplantation in children with the prune belly syndrome. *J Urol* 1989 Dec;142(6):1541–1542.
17. Troppmann C, McBride MA, Baker TJ, Perez RV. Laparoscopic live donor nephrectomy: a risk factor for delayed function and rejection in pediatric kidney recipients? A UNOS analysis. *Am J Transplant* 2005 Jan;5(1):175–182.
18. Matas AJ, Chavers BM, Nevins TE, et al. Recipient evaluation, preparation, and care in pediatric transplantation: the University of Minnesota protocols. *Kidney Int Suppl* 1996 Jan;53:S99–102.
19. Vats A, Mauer M, Burke BA, Weiss RA, Chavers BM. Delayed acute renal failure in post-transplant period in young children from unexplained etiology. *Pediatr Nephrol* 1997 Oct;11(5):531–536.
20. Mendizabal S, Estornell F, Zamora I, et al. Renal transplantation in children with severe bladder dysfunction. *J Urol* 2005 Jan;173(1):226–229.

21. Rigamonti W, Capizzi A, Zacchello G, , et al. Kidney transplantation into bladder augmentation or urinary diversion: long-term results. *Transplantation* 2005 Nov 27;80(10):1435–1440.

22. Sullivan ME, Reynard JM, Cranston DW. Renal transplantation into the abnormal lower urinary tract. *BJU Int* 2003 Sep;92(5):510–515.

23. Luke PP, Herz DB, Bellinger MF, et al. Long-term results of pediatric renal transplantation into a dysfunctional lower urinary tract. *Transplantation* 2003 Dec 15;76(11):1578–1582.

24. Surange RS, Johnson RW, Tavakoli A, et al. Kidney transplantation into an ileal conduit: a single center experience of 59 cases. *J Urol* 2003 Nov;170(5):1727–1730.

25. Nahas WC, Mazzucchi E, Arap MA, et al. Augmentation cystoplasty in renal transplantation: a good and safe option--experience with 25 cases. *Urology* 2002 Nov;60(5):770–774.

26. Hatch DA, Koyle MA, Baskin LS, et al. Kidney transplantation in children with urinary diversion or bladder augmentation. *J Urol* 2001 Jun;165(6 Pt 2):2265–2268.

27. Purohit RS, Bretan PN, Jr. Successful long-term outcome using existing native cutaneous ureterostomy for renal transplant drainage. *J Urol* 2000 Feb;163(2):446–449.

28. Warholm C, Berglund J, Andersson J, Tyden G. Renal transplantation in patients with urinary diversion: a case-control study. *Nephrol Dial Transplant* 1999 Dec;14(12):2937–2940.

29. Koo HP, Bunchman TE, Flynn JT, et al. Renal transplantation in children with severe lower urinary tract dysfunction. *J Urol* 1999 Jan;161(1): 240–245.

30. Fontaine E, Gagnadoux MF, Niaudet P, Broyer M, Beurton D. Renal transplantation in children with augmentation cystoplasty: long-term results. *J Urol* 1998 Jun;159(6):2110–2113.

31. Nguyen DH, Reinberg Y, Gonzalez R, Fryd D, Najarian JS. Outcome of renal transplantation after urinary diversion and enterocystoplasty: a retrospective, controlled study. *J Urol* 1990 Dec;144(6): 1349–1351.

32. Yerkes EB, Rink RC, Cain MP, Luerssen TG, Casale AJ. Shunt infection and malfunction after augmentation cystoplasty. *J Urol* 2001 Jun;165(6 Pt 2):2262–2264.

33. Stein R, Wiesner C, Beetz R, et al. Urinary diversion in children and adolescents with neurogenic bladder: the Mainz experience. Part II: Continent cutaneous diversion using the Mainz pouch I. *Pediatr Nephrol* 2005 Jul;20(7):926–931.

34. Stein R, Wiesner C, Beetz R, Schwarz M, Thuroff JW. Urinary diversion in children and adolescents with neurogenic bladder: the Mainz experience. Part III: Colonic conduit. *Pediatr Nephrol* 2005 Jul;20(7):932–936.

35. Stein R, Wiesner C, Beetz R, Schwarz M, Thuroff JW. Urinary diversion in children and adolescents with neurogenic bladder: the Mainz experience. Part I: Bladder augmentation and bladder substitution--therapeutic algorisms. *Pediatr Nephrol* 2005 Jul;20(7):920–925.

36. Adams MC, Joseph DB. Urinary tract reconstruction in children. In: Campbell MF, Walsh PC, Retik AB, eds. *Campbell's Urology*. 8th edition. Philadelphia, PA: Saunders; 2002:2508–2563.

37. Falagas ME, Vergidis PI. Urinary tract infections in patients with urinary diversion. *Am J Kidney Dis* 2005 Dec;46(6):1030–1037.

38. Khoury AE, Salomon M, Doche R, et al. Stone formation after augmentation cystoplasty: the role of intestinal mucus. *J Urol* 1997 Sep;158(3 Pt 2):1133–1137.

39. Wagstaff KE, Woodhouse CR, Duffy PG, Ransley PG. Delayed linear growth in children with enterocystoplasties. *Br J Urol* 1992 Mar;69(3): 314–317.

40. Mundy AR, Nurse DE. Calcium balance, growth and skeletal mineralisation in patients with cystoplasties. *Br J Urol* 1992 Mar;69(3):257–259.

41. Shekarriz B, Upadhyay J, Demirbilek S, Barthold JS, Gonzalez R. Surgical complications of bladder augmentation: comparison between various enterocystoplasties in 133 patients. *Urology* 2000 Jan;55(1): 123–128.

42. Filmer RB, Spencer JR. Malignancies in bladder augmentations and intestinal conduits. *J Urol* 1990 Apr;143(4):671–678.

43. Lane T, Shah J. Carcinoma following augmentation ileocystoplasty. Urol Int. 2000;64(1):31–2.

44. Soergel TM, Cain MP, Misseri R, et al. Transitional cell carcinoma of the bladder following augmentation cystoplasty for the neuropathic bladder. *J Urol* 2004 Oct;172(4 Pt 2):1649-1651; discussion 51–52.

45. Liard A, Seguier-Lipszyc E, Mathiot A, Mitrofanoff P. The Mitrofanoff procedure: 20 years later. *J Urol* 2001 Jun;165(6 Pt 2):2394–2398.

46. Glassberg KI. The valve bladder syndrome: 20 years later. *J Urol* 2001 Oct;166(4):1406–1414.

47. Parkhouse HF, Barratt TM, Dillon MJ, et al. Long-term outcome of boys with posterior urethral valves. *Br J Urol* 1988 Jul;62(1):59–62.

48. Churchill BM, Sheldon CA, McLorie GA, Arbus GS. Factors influencing patient and graft survival in 300 cadaveric pediatric renal transplants. *J Urol* 1988 Nov;140(5 Pt 2):1129–1133.

49. Reinberg Y, Gonzalez R, Fryd D, Mauer SM, Najarian JS. The outcome of renal transplantation in children with posterior urethral valves. *J Urol* 1988 Dec;140(6):1491–1493.

50. Salomon L, Fontaine E, Gagnadoux MF, Broyer M, Beurton D. Posterior urethral valves: long-term renal function consequences after transplantation. *J Urol* 1997 Mar;157(3):992–995.

51. Rajagopalan PR, Hanevold CD, Orak JD, et al. Valve bladder does not affect the outcome of renal transplants in children with renal failure due to posterior urethral valves. *Transplant Proc* 1994 Feb;26(1):115–116.

52. Ross JH, Kay R, Novick AC, et al. Long-term results of renal transplantation into the valve bladder. *J Urol* 1994 Jun;151(6):1500–1504.

53. Indudhara R, Joseph DB, Perez LM, Diethelm AG. Renal transplantation in children with posterior urethral valves revisited: a 10-year followup. *J Urol* 1998 Sep;160(3 Pt 2):1201–1203; discussion 16.

54. Bartsch L, Sarwal M, Orlandi P, Yorgin PD, Salvatierra O Jr. Limited surgical interventions in children with posterior urethral valves can lead to better outcomes following renal transplantation. *Pediatr Transplant* 2002 Oct;6(5):400–405.

55. Bryant JE, Joseph DB, Kohaut EC, Diethelm AG. Renal transplantation in children with posterior urethral valves. *J Urol* 1991 Dec;146(6):1585–1587.

56. Connolly JA, Miller B, Bretan PN. Renal transplantation in patients with posterior urethral valves: favorable long-term outcome. *J Urol* 1995 Sep;154(3):1153–1155.

57. Holmdahl G, Sillen U, Hanson E, Hermansson G, Hjalmas K. Bladder dysfunction in boys with posterior urethral valves before and after puberty. *J Urol* 1996 Feb;155(2):694–698.

58. De Gennaro M, Capitanucci ML, Capozza N, et al. Detrusor hypocontractility in children with posterior urethral valves arises before puberty. *Br J Urol* 1998 May;81 Suppl 3:81–85.

59. Koff SA, Gigax MR, Jayanthi VR. Nocturnal bladder emptying: a simple technique for reversing urinary tract deterioration in children with neurogenic bladder. *J Urol* 2005 Oct;174(4 Pt 2):1629–1631; discussion 32.

60. Salomon L, Fontaine E, Guest G, et al. Role of the bladder in delayed failure of kidney transplants in boys with posterior urethral valves. *J Urol* 2000 Apr;163(4):1282–1285.

61. Koff SA, Mutabagani KH, Jayanthi VR. The valve bladder syndrome: pathophysiology and treatment with nocturnal bladder emptying. J Urol. 2002 Jan;167(1):291–7.

62. Baqi N, Tejani A. Recurrence of the original disease in pediatric renal transplantation. *J Nephrol* 1997 Mar-Apr;10(2):85–92.

63. Briganti EM, Russ GR, McNeil JJ, Atkins RC, Chadban SJ. Risk of renal allograft loss from recurrent glomerulonephritis. *N Engl J Med* 2002 Jul 11;347(2):103–109.

64. Ramos EL, Tisher CC. Recurrent diseases in the kidney transplant. *Am J Kidney Dis* 1994 Jul;24(1):142–154.

65. Dantal J, Soulillou JP. Relapse of focal segmental glomerulosclerosis after kidney transplantation. *Advan Nephrol Necker Hosp* 1996;25: 91–106.

66. Tejani A, Stablein DH. Recurrence of focal segmental glomerulosclerosis posttransplantation: a special report of the North American Pediatric Renal Transplant Cooperative Study. *J Am Soc Nephrol* 1992 Jun;2(12 Suppl):S258–263.

67. Cameron JS. The enigma of focal segmental glomerulosclerosis. *Kidney Int Suppl* 1996;57(31).

68. Glassock RJ. Circulating permeability factors in the nephrotic syndrome: a fresh look at an old problem. *J Am Soc Nephrol* 2003 Feb;14(2): 541–543.

69. Ghiggeri GM, Carraro M, Vincenti F. Recurrent focal glomerulosclerosis in the era of genetics of podocyte proteins: theory and therapy. *Nephrol Dial Transplant* 2004 May;19(5):1036–1040.

70. Hoyer JR, Vernier RL, Najarian JS, et al. Recurrence of idiopathic nephrotic syndrome after renal transplantation. *Lancet* 1972;2(7773): 343–348.

71. Vincenti F, Ghiggeri GM. New insights into the pathogenesis and the therapy of recurrent focal glomerulosclerosis. *Am J Transplant* 2005 Jun;5(6):1179–1185.

72. Dantal J, Baatard R, Hourmant M, et al. Recurrent nephrotic syndrome following renal transplantation in patients with focal glomerulosclerosis. A one-center study of plasma exchange effects. *Transplantation* 1991;52(5):827–831.

73. Dantal J, Bigot E, Bogers W, et al. Effect of plasma protein adsorption on protein excretion in kidney-transplant recipients with recurrent nephrotic syndrome.[see comment]. *N Engl J Med* 1994;330(1):7–14.

74. Sharma M, Sharma R, Reddy SR, McCarthy ET, Savin VJ. Proteinuria after injection of human focal segmental glomerulosclerosis factor. *Transplantation* 2002;73(3):366–372.

75. Le Berre L, Godfrin Y, Lafond-Puyet L, et al. Effect of plasma fractions from patients with focal and segmental glomerulosclerosis on rat proteinuria. *Kidney Int* 2000;58(6):2502–2511.

76. Striegel JE, Sibley RK, Fryd DS, Mauer SM. Recurrence of focal segmental sclerosis in children following renal transplantation. *Kidney Int Suppl* 1986;19(50).

77. Abbott KC, Sawyers ES, Oliver JD, et al. Graft loss due to recurrent focal segmental glomerulosclerosis in renal transplant recipients in the United States. *Am J Kidney Dis* 2001;37(2):366–373.

78. Baum MA, Stablein DM, Panzarino VM, et al. Loss of living donor renal allograft survival advantage in children with focal segmental glomerulosclerosis. *Kidney Int* 2001;59(1):328–333.

79. Cibrik DM, Kaplan B, Campbell DA, Meier-Kriesche HU. Renal allograft survival in transplant recipients with focal segmental glomerulosclerosis. [erratum appears in *Am J Transplant* 2003 Apr;3(4):507 Note: Kriesche Herwig-Ulf Meier [corrected to Meier-Kriesche Herwig-Ulf]]. *Am J Transplant* 2003;3(1):64–67.

80. Huang K, Ferris ME, Andreoni KA, Gipson DS. The differential effect of race among pediatric kidney transplant recipients with focal segmental glomerulosclerosis. *Am J Kidney Dis* 1082;43(6):1082–1090.

81. Meyrier A. Nephrotic focal segmental glomerulosclerosis in 2004: an update. Nephrol Dialysis Transplant 2004;19(10):2437–2444.

82. Stephanian E, Matas AJ, Mauer SM, et al. Recurrence of disease in patients retransplanted for focal segmental glomerulosclerosis. *Transplantation* 1992;53(4):755–757.

83. Savin VJ, Sharma R, Sharma M, et al. Circulating factor associated with increased glomerular permeability to albumin in recurrent focal segmental glomerulosclerosis.[see comment]. New Engl J Med 1996; 334(14):878–883.

84. Cattran D, Neogi T, Sharma R, McCarthy ET, Savin VJ. Serial estimates of serum permeability activity and clinical correlates in patients with native kidney focal segmental glomerulosclerosis.[see comment]. J Am Soc Nephrol 2003;14(2):448–453.

85. Dall'Amico R, Ghiggeri G, Carraro M, et al. Prediction and treatment of recurrent focal segmental glomerulosclerosis after renal transplantation in children. *Am J Kidney Dis* 1999 Dec;34(6):1048–1055.

86. Boute N, Gribouval O, Roselli S, et al. NPHS2, encoding the glomerular protein podocin, is mutated in autosomal recessive steroid-resistant nephrotic syndrome.[erratum appears in Nat Genet 2000 May;25(1): 125]. Nature Genet 2000;24(4):349–354.

87. Weber S, Gribouval O, Esquivel EL, et al. NPHS2 mutation analysis shows genetic heterogeneity of steroid-resistant nephrotic syndrome and low post-transplant recurrence. Kidney Int 2004;66(2):571–579.

88. Bertelli R, Ginevri F, Caridi G, et al. Recurrence of focal segmental glomerulosclerosis after renal transplantation in patients with mutations of podocin. Am J Kidney Dis 1314;41(6):1314–1321.

89. Kim EM, Striegel J, Kim Y, et al. Recurrence of steroid-resistant nephrotic syndrome in kidney transplants is associated with increased acute renal failure and acute rejection. *Kidney Int* 1994 May; 45(5): 1440–1445.

90. Artero ML, Sharma R, Savin VJ, Vincenti F. Plasmapheresis reduces proteinuria and serum capacity to injure glomeruli in patients with recurrent focal glomerulosclerosis. Am J Kidney Dis 1994;23(4): 574–581.

91. Munoz J, Sanchez M, Perez-Garcia R, Anaya F, Valderrabano F. Recurrent focal glomerulosclerosis in renal transplants proteinuria relapsing following plasma exchange. *Clin Nephrol* 1985;24(4):213–214.

92. Greenstein SM, Delrio M, Ong E, et al. Plasmapheresis treatment for recurrent focal sclerosis in pediatric renal allografts. *Pediatr Nephrol* 1061;14(12):1061–1065.

93. Pradhan M, Petro J, Palmer J, Meyers K, Baluarte HJ. Early use of plasmapheresis for recurrent post-transplant FSGS. Pediatric Nephrology. 2003;18(9):934–938.

94. Belson A, Yorgin PD, Al-Uzri AY, et al. Long-term plasmapheresis and protein A column treatment of recurrent FSGS. *Pediatr Nephrol* 2001 Dec;16(12):985–989.

95. Laufer J, Ettenger RB, Ho WG, et al. Plasma exchange for recurrent nephrotic syndrome following renal transplantation. *Transplantation* 1988 Oct;46(4):540–542.

96. Haffner K, Zimmerhackl LB, von Schnakenburg C, Brandis M, Pohl M. Complete remission of post-transplant FSGS recurrence by long-term plasmapheresis. *Pediatr Nephrol* 2005 Jul;20(7):994–997.

97. Cochat P, Kassir A, Colon S, et al. Recurrent nephrotic syndrome after transplantation: early treatment with plasmaphaeresis and cyclophosphamide. Pediatr Nephrol 1993;7(1):50–54.

98. Cheong HI, Han HW, Park HW, et al. Early recurrent nephrotic syndrome after renal transplantation in children with focal segmental glomerulosclerosis. *Nephrol Dial Transplant* 2000;15(1):78–81.

99. Raafat RH, Kalia A, Travis LB, Diven SC. High-dose oral cyclosporin therapy for recurrent focal segmental glomerulosclerosis in children. *Am J Kidney Dis* 2004;44(1):50–56.

100. Srivastava RN, Kalia A, Travis LB, et al. Prompt remission of post-renal transplant nephrotic syndrome with high-dose cyclosporine. *Pediatr Nephrol* 1994;8(1):94–95.

101. Salomon R, Gagnadoux MF, Niaudet P. Intravenous cyclosporine therapy in recurrent nephrotic syndrome after renal transplantation in children. *Transplantation* 2003;75(6):810–814.

102. Ingulli E, Tejani A, Butt KM, et al. High-dose cyclosporine therapy in recurrent nephrotic syndrome following renal transplantation. *Transplantation* 1990;49(1):219–221.

103. Ohta T, Kawaguchi H, Hattori M, et al. Effect of pre-and postoperative plasmapheresis on posttransplant recurrence of focal segmental glomerulosclerosis in children. *Transplantation* 2001;71(5):628–633.

104. Gohh RY, Yango AF, Morrissey PE, et al. Preemptive plasmapheresis and recurrence of FSGS in high-risk renal transplant recipients. *Am J Transplant* 2005 Dec;5(12):2907–2912.

105. Kestila M, Lenkkeri U, Mannikko M, et al. Positionally cloned gene for a novel glomerular protein-nephrin-is mutated in congenital nephrotic syndrome. *Mol Cell* 1998 Mar;1(4):575–582.

106. Beltcheva O, Martin P, Lenkkeri U, Tryggvason K. Mutation spectrum in the nephrin gene (NPHS1) in congenital nephrotic syndrome. *Hum Mutat* 2001 May;17(5):368–373.

107. Niaudet P. Genetic forms of nephrotic syndrome. *Pediatr Nephrol* 2004 Dec;19(12):1313–1318.

108. Sako M, Nakanishi K, Obana M, et al. Analysis of NPHS1, NPHS2, ACTN4, and WT1 in Japanese patients with congenital nephrotic syndrome. *Kidney Int* 2005 Apr;67(4):1248–1255.

109. Patrakka J, Ruotsalainen V, Reponen P, et al. Recurrence of nephrotic syndrome in kidney grafts of patients with congenital nephrotic syndrome of the Finnish type: role of nephrin. *Transplantation* 2002 Feb 15;73(3):394–403.

110. Barayan SS, Al-Akash SI, Malekzadeh M, et al. Immediate posttransplant nephrosis in a patient with congenital nephrotic syndrome. *Pediatr Nephrol* 2001 Jul;16(7):547–549.

111. Lane PH, Schnaper HW, Vernier RL, Bunchman TE. Steroid-dependent nephrotic syndrome following renal transplantation for congenital nephrotic syndrome. *Pediatr Nephrol* 1991 May;5(3):300–303.

112. Noris M, Remuzzi G. Hemolytic uremic syndrome. *J Am Soc Nephrol* 2005 Apr;16(4):1035–1050.

113. Loirat C, Niaudet P. The risk of recurrence of hemolytic uremic syndrome after renal transplantation in children. *Pediatr Nephrol* 2003 Nov;18(11):1095–1101.

114. Quan A, Sullivan EK, Alexander SR. Recurrence of hemolytic uremic syndrome after renal transplantation in children: a report of the North American Pediatric Renal Transplant Cooperative Study. *Transplantation* 2001 Aug 27;72(4):742–745.

115. Bresin E DE, Castellati F, Stefanov R, et al. Outcome of renal transplantation in patients with non-shiga toxin-associated hemolytic uremic syndrome: Prognostic significance of genetic background. *Clin J Am Soc Nephrol* 2006;1:88–99.

116. Danpure C. Primary hyperoxaluria. In: Scriver C, ed. *The Metabolic & Molecular Bases of Inherited Disease*. 8th edition. New York: McGraw Hill; 2001:3323–3367.

117. Cochat P. Primary hyperoxaluria type 1. *Kidney Int* 1999 Jun;55(6):2533–2547.

118. Leumann E, Hoppe B. The primary hyperoxalurias. *J Am Soc Nephrol* 2001 Sep;12(9):1986–1993.

119. Hoppe B, Leumann E. Diagnostic and therapeutic strategies in hyperoxaluria: a plea for early intervention. *Nephrol Dial Transplant* 2004;19(1):39–42.

120. Cochat P, Basmaison O. Current approaches to the management of primary hyperoxaluria. *Arch Dis Child* 2000;82(6):470–473.

121. Cochat P, Gaulier JM, Koch Nogueira PC, et al. Combined liver-kidney transplantation in primary hyperoxaluria type 1. *Eur J Pediatr* 1999 Dec;158 Suppl 2:S75–80.

122. Cibrik DM, Kaplan B, Arndorfer JA, Meier-Kriesche HU. Renal allograft survival in patients with oxalosis. *Transplantation* 2002 Sep 15;74(5):707–710.

123. Gagnadoux MF, Lacaille F, Niaudet P, et al. Long term results of liver-kidney transplantation in children with primary hyperoxaluria. *Pediatr Nephrol* 2001 Dec;16(12):946–950.

124. Millan MT, Berquist WE, So SK, et al. One hundred percent patient and kidney allograft survival with simultaneous liver and kidney transplantation in infants with primary hyperoxaluria: a single-center experience. *Transplantation* 2003 Nov 27;76(10):1458–1463.

125. Hoppe B, Langman CB. A United States survey on diagnosis, treatment, and outcome of primary hyperoxaluria. Pediatr Nephrol. 2003 Oct;18(10):986–991.

126. Hoppe B, Leumann E. Diagnostic and therapeutic strategies in hyperoxaluria: a plea for early intervention. *Nephrol Dial Transplant* 2004 Jan;19(1):39–42.

127. Marangella M. Transplantation strategies in type 1 primary hyperoxaluria: the issue of pyridoxine responsiveness. *Nephrol Dial Transplant* 1999 Feb;14(2):301–303.

128. Monico CG, Rossetti S, Olson JB, Milliner DS. Pyridoxine effect in type I primary hyperoxaluria is associated with the most common mutant allele. *Kidney Int* 2005 May;67(5):1704–1709.

129. van Woerden CS, Groothoff JW, Wijburg FA, et al. Clinical implications of mutation analysis in primary hyperoxaluria type 1. *Kidney Int* 2004 Aug;66(2):746–752.

130. Amoroso A, Pirulli D, Florian F, et al. AGXT gene mutations and their influence on clinical heterogeneity of type 1 primary hyperoxaluria. *J Am Soc Nephrol* 2001 Oct;12(10):2072–2079.

131. Allen AR, Thompson EM, Williams G, Watts RW, Pusey CD. Selective renal transplantation in primary hyperoxaluria type 1. *Am J Kidney Dis* 1996 Jun;27(6):891–895.

132. Katz A, Freese D, Danpure CJ, Scheinman JI, Mauer SM. Success of kidney transplantation in oxalosis is unrelated to residual hepatic enzyme activity. *Kidney Int* 1992 Dec;42(6):1408–1411.

133. Monico CG, Milliner DS. Combined liver-kidney and kidney-alone transplantation in primary hyperoxaluria. *Liver Transplant* 2001 Nov;7(11): 954–963.

134. Scheinman JI, Najarian JS, Mauer SM. Successful strategies for renal transplantation in primary oxalosis. *Kidney Int* 1984 May;25(5):804–811.

135. Gruessner RW. Preemptive liver transplantation from a living related donor for primary hyperoxaluria type I. *N Engl J Med* 1998 Jun 25;338(26):1924.

136. Nakamura M, Fuchinoue S, Nakajima I, et al. Three cases of sequential liver-kidney transplantation from living-related donors. *Nephrol Dial Transplant* 2001 Jan;16(1):166–168.

137. Gubler MC. WT1, a multiform protein. Contribution of genetic models to the understanding of its various functions. *J Am Soc Nephrol* 2002 Aug;13(8):2192–2194.

138. Little M, Wells C. A clinical overview of WT1 gene mutations. *Hum Mutat* 1997;9(3):209–225.

139. Habib R, Loirat C, Gubler MC, et al. The nephropathy associated with male pseudohermaphroditism and Wilms' tumor (Drash syndrome): a distinctive glomerular lesion—report of 10 cases. *Clin Nephrol* 1985 Dec;24(6):269–278.

140. Jadresic L, Leake J, Gordon I, et al. Clinicopathologic review of twelve children with nephropathy, Wilms tumor, and genital abnormalities (Drash syndrome). *J Pediatr* 1990 Nov;117(5):717–725.

141. Jeanpierre C, Denamur E, Henry I, et al. Identification of constitutional WT1 mutations, in patients with isolated diffuse mesangial sclerosis, and analysis of genotype/phenotype correlations by use of a computerized mutation database. *Am J Hum Genet* 1998 Apr;62(4):824–833.

142. Eddy AA, Mauer SM. Pseudohermaphroditism, glomerulopathy, and Wilms tumor (Drash syndrome): frequency in end-stage renal failure. *J Pediatr* 1985 Apr;106(4):584–587.

143. Cleper R, Davidovitz M, Krause I, et al. Unexpected Wilms' tumor in a pediatric renal transplant recipient: suspected Denys-Drash syndrome. *Transplant Proc* 1999 Jun;31(4):1907–1909.

144. Bydder S, Charles A, Hewitt I, et al. Wilms tumor in a pediatric renal transplant recipient with unexpected Denys-Drash syndrome. *Transplant Proc* 2002 Dec;34(4):3203–3204.

145. Wang NJ, Song HR, Schanen NC, Litman NL, Frasier SD. Frasier syndrome comes full circle: genetic studies performed in an original patient. *J Pediatr* 2005 Jun;146(6):843–844.

146. Barbaux S, Niaudet P, Gubler MC, et al. Donor splice-site mutations in WT1 are responsible for Frasier syndrome. *Nat Genet* 1997 Dec;17(4): 467–470.

147. Heathcott RW, Morison IM, Gubler MC, Corbett R, Reeve AE. A review of the phenotypic variation due to the Denys-Drash syndrome-associated germline WT1 mutation R362X. *Hum Mutat* 2002 Apr;19(4):462.

148. McTaggart SJ, Algar E, Chow CW, Powell HR, Jones CL. Clinical spectrum of Denys-Drash and Frasier syndrome. *Pediatr Nephrol* 2001 Apr;16(4):335–339.

149. Benfield MR, Warshaw BL, Bartosh SM, et al. A randomized controlled double-blind trial of steroid withdrawal in pediatric renal transplantation: A study of the cooperative clinical trials in pediatric transplantation.; 2005: *Am J Transplant* 2005;402.

150. Dharnidharka VR, Sullivan EK, Stablein DM, Tejani AH, Harmon WE. Risk factors for posttransplant lymphoproliferative disorder (PTLD) in pediatric kidney transplantation: a report of the North American Pediatric Renal Transplant Cooperative Study (NAPRTCS). *Transplantation* 2001 Apr 27;71(8):1065–1068.

151. Dharnidharka VR, Tejani AH, Ho PL, Harmon WE. Post-transplant lymphoproliferative disorder in the United States: young Caucasian males are at highest risk. *Am J Transplant* 2002 Nov;2(10):993–998.

152. Dharnidharka VR, Stevens G. Risk for post-transplant lymphoproliferative disorder after polyclonal antibody induction in kidney transplantation. *Pediatr Transplant* 2005 Oct;9(5):622–626.

153. Green M, Webber S. Posttransplantation lymphoproliferative disorders. *Pediatr Clin North Am* 2003 Dec;50(6):1471–1491.

154. Paraskevas S, Coad JE, Gruessner A, et al. Posttransplant lymphoproliferative disorder in pancreas transplantation: a single-center experience. *Transplantation* 2005 Sep 15;80(5):613–622.

155. Babel N, Gabdrakhmanova L, Hammer M, et al. Induction of pre-transplant Epstein-Barr virus (EBV) infection by donor blood transfusion in EBV-seronegative recipients may reduce risk of post-transplant lymphoproliferative disease in adolescent renal transplant patients: report of two cases. *Transplant Infect Dis* 2005 Sep–Dec;7(3–4):133–136.

156. Green M, Bueno J, Rowe D, et al. Predictive negative value of persistent low Epstein-Barr virus viral load after intestinal transplantation in children. *Transplantation* 2000 Aug 27;70(4):593–596.

157. Stevens SJ, Verschuuren EA, Pronk I, et al. Frequent monitoring of Epstein-Barr virus DNA load in unfractionated whole blood is essential for early detection of posttransplant lymphoproliferative disease in high-risk patients. *Blood* 2001 Mar 1;97(5):1165–1171.

158. Lee TC, Savoldo B, Rooney CM, et al. Quantitative EBV viral loads and immunosuppression alterations can decrease PTLD incidence in pediatric liver transplant recipients. *Am J Transplant* 2005 Sep;5(9):2222–2228.

159. McDiarmid SV, Jordan S, Kim GS, et al. Prevention and preemptive therapy of poststransplant lymphoproliferative disease in pediatric liver recipients. *Transplantation* 1998 Dec 27;66(12):1604–1611.

160. Funch DP, Walker AM, Schneider G, Ziyadeh NJ, Pescovitz MD. Ganciclovir and acyclovir reduce the risk of post-transplant lymphoproliferative disorder in renal transplant recipients. *Am J Transplant* 2005 Dec;5(12):2894–2900.

161. Humar A, Hebert D, Davies HD, et al. A randomized trial of ganciclovir versus ganciclovir plus immune globulin for prophylaxis against Epstein-Barr virus related posttransplant lymphoproliferative disorder. *Transplantation* 2006 Mar 27;81(6):856–861.

162. Green M, Reyes J, Webber S, Rowe D. The role of antiviral and immunoglobulin therapy in the prevention of Epstein-Barr virus infection and post-transplant lymphoproliferative disease following solid organ transplantation. *Transplant Infect Dis* 2001 Jun;3(2):97–103.

163. Caillard S, Dharnidharka V, Agodoa L, Bohen E, Abbott K. Post-transplant lymphoproliferative disorders after renal transplantation in the United States in era of modern immunosuppression. *Transplantation* 2005 Nov 15;80(9):1233–1243.

164. Birkeland SA, Hamilton-Dutoit S, Bendtzen K. Long-term follow-up of kidney transplant patients with posttransplant lymphoproliferative disorder: duration of posttransplant lymphoproliferative disorder-induced operational graft tolerance, interleukin-18 course, and results of retransplantation. *Transplantation* 2003 Jul 15;76(1):153–158.

165. Karras A, Thervet E, Le Meur Y, et al. Successful renal retransplantation after post-transplant lymphoproliferative disease. *Am J Transplant* 2004 Nov;4(11):1904–1909.

166. *Ettenger R, Sarwal MM. Mycophenolate mofetil in pediatric renal transplantation. Transplantation 2005 Oct 15;80(2 Suppl):S201–210.*

167. van Gelder T, Shaw LM. The rationale for and limitations of therapeutic drug monitoring for mycophenolate mofetil in transplantation. *Transplantation* 2005 Oct 15;80(2 Suppl):S244–253.

168. van Hest RM, Mathot RA, Pescovitz MD, et al. Explaining variability in mycophenolic acid exposure to optimize mycophenolate mofetil dosing: a population pharmacokinetic meta-analysis of mycophenolic acid in renal transplant recipients. *J Am Soc Nephrol* 2006 Mar;17(3):871–880.

169. Weber LT, Shipkova M, Armstrong VW, et al. The pharmacokinetic-pharmacodynamic relationship for total and free mycophenolic Acid in pediatric renal transplant recipients: a report of the german study group on mycophenolate mofetil therapy. *J Am Soc Nephrol* 2002 Mar;13(3):759–768.

170. Payen S, Zhang D, Maisin A, et al. Population pharmacokinetics of mycophenolic acid in kidney transplant pediatric and adolescent patients. *Ther Drug Monit* 2005 Jun;27(3):378–388.

171. Filler G. Abbreviated mycophenolic acid AUC from C0, C1, C2, and C4 is preferable in children after renal transplantation on mycophenolate mofetil and tacrolimus therapy. *Transplant Int* 2004 Mar;17(3):120–125.

172. Weber LTH, Armstrong B, Oellerich VM, Toenshoff M. Validation of an abbreviated pharmacokinetic profile for the estimation of mycophenolic acid exposure in pediatric renal transplant recipients. *Ther Drug Monit* In press;2006.

173. Filler G, Foster J, Berard R, Mai I, Lepage N. Age-dependency of mycophenolate mofetil dosing in combination with tacrolimus after pediatric renal transplantation. *Transplant Proc* 2004 Jun;36(5):1327–1331.

174. Nashan B, Cole E, Levy G, Thervet E. Clinical validation studies of Neoral C(2) monitoring: a review. *Transplantation* 2002 May 15;73(9 Suppl):S3-11.

175. Mahalati K, Belitsky P, Sketris I, West K, Panek R. Neoral monitoring by simplified sparse sampling area under the concentration-time curve: its relationship to acute rejection and cyclosporine nephrotoxicity early after kidney transplantation. *Transplantation* 1999 Jul 15;68(1):55–62.

176. Mahalati K, Belitsky P, West K, et al. Approaching the therapeutic window for cyclosporine in kidney transplantation: a prospective study. *J Am Soc Nephrol* 2001 Apr;12(4):828–833.

177. Levy G, Thervet E, Lake J, Uchida K. Patient management by Neoral C(2) monitoring: an international consensus statement. *Transplantation* 2002 May 15;73(9 Suppl):S12–18.

178. Cole E, Midtvedt K, Johnston A, Pattison J, O'Grady C. Recommendations for the implementation of Neoral C(2) monitoring in clinical practice. *Transplantation* 2002 May 15;73(9 Suppl):S19–22.

179. Thervet E, Pfeffer P, Scolari MP, et al. Clinical outcomes during the first three months posttransplant in renal allograft recipients managed by C2 monitoring of cyclosporine microemulsion. *Transplantation* 2003 Sep 27;76(6):903–908.

180. Vincenti F, Mendez R, Curtis J, et al. A multicenter, prospective study of C2-monitored cyclosporine microemulsion in a U.S. population of de novo renal transplant recipients. *Transplantation* 2005 Oct 15;80(7):910–916.

181. Cole E, Maham N, Cardella C, et al. Clinical benefits of neoral C2 monitoring in the long-term management of renal transplant recipients. *Transplantation* 2003 Jun 27;75(12):2086–2090.

182. Citterio F, Scata MC, Romagnoli J, Nanni G, Castagneto M. Results of a three-year prospective study of C2 monitoring in long-term renal transplant recipients receiving cyclosporine microemulsion. *Transplantation* 2005 Apr 15;79(7):802–806.

183. Marcen R, Villafruela JJ, Pascual J, et al. Clinical outcomes and C2 cyclosporin monitoring in maintenance renal transplant recipients: 1 year follow-up study. *Nephrol Dial Transplant* 2005 Apr;20(4):803–810.

184. Hoyer PF. Cyclosporin A (Neoral) in pediatric organ transplantation. Neoral Pediatric Study Group. *Pediatr Transplant* 1998 Feb;2(1):35–39.

185. Weber LT, Armstrong VW, Shipkova M, et al. Cyclosporin A absorption profiles in pediatric renal transplant recipients predict the risk of acute rejection. *Ther Drug Monit* 2004 Aug;26(4):415–424.

186. Trompeter R, Fitzpatrick M, Hutchinson C, Johnston A. Longitudinal evaluation of the pharmacokinetics of cyclosporin microemulsion (Neoral) in pediatric renal transplant recipients and assessment of C2 level as a marker for absorption. *Pediatr Transplant* 2003 Aug; 7(4):282–288.

187. Ferraresso M, Ghio L, Zacchello G, et al. Pharmacokinetic of cyclosporine microemulsion in pediatric kidney recipients receiving A quadruple immunosuppressive regimen: the value of C2 blood levels. *Transplantation* 2005 May 15;79(9):1164–1168.

188. Vester U, Kranz B, Offner G, et al. Absorption phase cyclosporine (C(2h)) monitoring in the first weeks after pediatric renal transplantation. *Pediatr Nephrol* 2004 Nov;19(11):1273–1277.

189. Fanta S, Backman JT, Seikku P, Holmberg C, Hoppu K. Cyclosporine A monitoring—how to account for twice and three times daily dosing. *Pediatr Nephrol* 2005 May;20(5):591–596.

190. Undre NA. Pharmacokinetics of tacrolimus-based combination therapies. *Nephrol Dial Transplant* 2003 May;18 Suppl 1:i12–15.

191. Wallemacq PE. Therapeutic monitoring of immunosuppressant drugs. Where are we? *Clin Chem Lab Med* 2004;42(11):1204–1211.

192. Scholten EM, Cremers SC, Schoemaker RC, et al. AUC-guided dosing of tacrolimus prevents progressive systemic overexposure in renal transplant recipients. *Kidney Int* 2005 Jun;67(6):2440–2447.

193. Wallemacq PE, Verbeeck RK. Comparative clinical pharmacokinetics of tacrolimus in paediatric and adult patients. *Clin Pharmacokinet* 2001; 40(4):283–295.

194. Schubert M, Venkataramanan R, Holt DW, et al. Pharmacokinetics of sirolimus and tacrolimus in pediatric transplant patients. *Am J Transplant* 2004 May;4(5):767–773.

195. Kim JS, Aviles DH, Silverstein DM, Leblanc PL, Matti Vehaskari V. Effect of age, ethnicity, and glucocorticoid use on tacrolimus pharmacokinetics in pediatric renal transplant patients. *Pediatr Transplant* 2005 Apr;9(2):162–169.

196. Montini G, Ujka F, Varagnolo C, et al. The pharmacokinetics and immunosuppressive response of tacrolimus in paediatric renal transplant recipients. *Pediatr Nephrol* 2006 May;21(5):719–724.

197. Filler G, Feber J, Lepage N, Weiler G, Mai I. Universal approach to pharmacokinetic monitoring of immunosuppressive agents in children. *Pediatr Transplant* 2002 Oct;6(5):411–418.

198. Hariharan S. Recommendations for outpatient monitoring of kidney transplant recipients. *Am J Kidney Dis* 2006 Apr;47(4 Suppl 2):S22–36.

199. MacDonald A, Scarola J, Burke JT, Zimmerman JJ. Clinical pharmacokinetics and therapeutic drug monitoring of sirolimus. *Clin Ther* 2000;22 Suppl B:B101–121.

200. Filler G, Womiloju T, Feber J, Lepage N, Christians U. Adding sirolimus to tacrolimus-based immunosuppression in pediatric renal transplant recipients reduces tacrolimus exposure. *Am J Transplant* 2005 Aug;5(8):2005–2010.

201. Schachter AD, Meyers KE, Spaneas LD, et al. Short sirolimus half-life in pediatric renal transplant recipients on a calcineurin inhibitor-free protocol. *Pediatr Transplant* 2004 Apr;8(2):171–177.

202. Fine RN, Stablein D. Long-term use of recombinant human growth hormone in pediatric allograft recipients: a report of the NAPRTCS Transplant Registry. *Pediatr Nephrol* 2005 Mar;20(3):404–408.

203. Rianthavorn P, Ettenger RB. Medication non-adherence in the adolescent renal transplant recipient: a clinician's viewpoint. *Pediatr Transplant* 2005 Jun;9(3):398–407.

204. Grinyo JM. Steroid sparing strategies in renal transplantation. *Nephrol Dial Transplant* 2005 Oct;20(10):2028–2031.

205. Yang H. Maintenance immunosuppression regimens: conversion, minimization, withdrawal, and avoidance. *Am J Kidney Dis* 2006 Apr;47(4 Suppl 2):S37–51.

206. Tonshoff B, Hocker B, Weber LT. Steroid withdrawal in pediatric and adult renal transplant recipients. *Pediatr Nephrol* 2005 Mar;20(3): 409–417.

207. Matas AJ, Kandaswamy R, Humar A, et al. Long-term immunosuppression, without maintenance prednisone, after kidney transplantation. *Ann Surg* 2004 Sep;240(3):510-516; discussion 6–7.

208. Kumar MS, Heifets M, Moritz MJ, et al. Safety and efficacy of steroid withdrawal two days after kidney transplantation: analysis of results at three years. *Transplantation* 2006 Mar 27;81(6):832–839.

209. Borrows R, Chan K, Loucaidou M, et al. Five years of steroid sparing in renal transplantation with tacrolimus and mycophenolate mofetil. *Transplantation* 2006 Jan 15;81(1):125–128.

210. Broyer M, Guest G, Gagnadoux MF. Growth rate in children receiving alternate-day corticosteroid treatment after kidney transplantation. *J Pediatr* 1992 May;120(5):721–725.

211. Qvist E, Marttinen E, Ronnholm K, et al. Growth after renal transplantation in infancy or early childhood. *Pediatr Nephrol* 2002 Jun;17(6): 438–443.

212. Jabs K, Sullivan EK, Avner ED, Harmon WE. Alternate-day steroid dosing improves growth without adversely affecting graft survival or long-term graft function. A report of the North American Pediatric Renal Transplant Cooperative Study. *Transplantation* 1996 Jan 15;61(1):31–36.

213. Hocker B, John U, Plank C, et al. Successful withdrawal of steroids in pediatric renal transplant recipients receiving cyclosporine A and mycophenolate mofetil treatment: results after four years. *Transplantation* 2004 Jul 27;78(2):228–234.

214. Shapiro R, Scantlebury VP, Jordan ML, et al. Pediatric renal transplantation under tacrolimus-based immunosuppression. *Transplantation* 1999 Jan 27;67(2):299–303.

215. Chakrabarti P, Wong HY, Scantlebury VP, et al. Outcome after steroid withdrawal in pediatric renal transplant patients receiving tacrolimus-based immunosuppression. *Transplantation* 2000 Sep 15; 70(5): 760–764.

216. Silverstein DM, Aviles DH, LeBlanc PM, Jung FF, Vehaskari VM. Results of one-year follow-up of steroid-free immunosuppression in pediatric renal transplant patients. *Pediatr Transplant* 2005 Oct;9(5):589–597.

217. Sarwal MM, Vidhun JR, Alexander SR, et al. Continued superior outcomes with modification and lengthened follow-up of a steroid-avoidance pilot with extended daclizumab induction in pediatric renal transplantation. *Transplantation* 2003 Nov 15;76(9):1331–1339.

218. Chao AB SS, Salvatierra O, Sarwal MM. Expended analysis of steroid free immunosuppression supports study safety and efficacy. *Am J Transplant* 2005;5(s11):402.

219. North American Pediatric Renal Transplant Cooperative Study (NAPARTCS) 2005 annual report. 2005.

220. Rianthavorn P, Al-Akash SI, et al. *Kidney Transplantation in Children. Medical Management of Kidney Transplantation.* In: Weir MR, ed. Philadelphia: Lippincott Williams & Wilkins; 2005:198–230.

221. Harmon WE, McDonald RA, et al. Pediatric transplantation.1994-2003. *Am J Transplant* 2005;5(4 Pt 2):887–903.

222. Matas AJ, Sutherland DER. The importance of innovative efforts to increase organ donation. *J Am Med Assoc* 2005;294(13):1691–1693 (editorial).

223. Pape L, Ehrich JH, et al. Living related kidney donation as an advantage for growth of children independent of glomerular filtration rate. *Transplant Proc* 2006;38(3):685–687.

224. Meier-Kriesche HU, Schold JD. The impact of pretransplant dialysis on outcomes in renal transplantation. *Semin Dial* 2005;18(6) 499–504.

225. Goldfarb-Rumyzntzev A, Hurdle JF, Scandling J, Wang Z, Baird B, Barenbaum L, et al. Duration of end-stage renal disease and kidney transplant outcome. *Nephrol Dial Transplant* 20(1):167–175, 2005.

226. Matas AJ, Payne WD, Sutherland DER, et al. 2,500 Living donor kidney transplants: A single-center experience. *Ann Surg* 2001;234(2) 149–164.

227. Kasiske BL, Snyder JJ, Matas AJ, et al. Preemptive kidney transplantation: The advantage and the advantaged. *J Am Soc Nephrol* 2002;13:1358–1364.

228. Vats A, Donaldson NL, et al. Pretransplant dialysis status and outcome of renal transplantation in North American children: a NAPRTCS Study (North American Pediatric Renal Transplant Cooperative Study). *Transplantation* 2000;69(7):1414–1419.

229. Miller LC, Lum CT, Bock GH, et al. Transplantation of the adult kidney into the very small child. Technical considerations. *Am J Surg* 1983; (2):243–247.

230. Sureshkumar KK, Reddy CS, Nghiem DD, Sandroni SE, Carpenter BJ. Superiority of pediatric en bloc renal allografts over living donor kidneys: A long-term functional study. *Transplantation* 2006;82(3): 348–353.

231. Fost N. Children as renal donors. *N Engl J Med* 1977;296(7):363-367.

232. Webb NJ, Fortune PM. Should children ever be living kidney donors? *Pediatr Transplant* 2006;10(7):851–855.

233. Delmonico FL, Harmon WE. The use of a minor as a live kidney donor. *Am J Transplant* 2002;2(4):333–336.

## 16.11b  Surgical Technique and Complications

*Christoph Troppmann, MD*

### INTRODUCTION

Transplantation of kidneys from adult live donors into smaller pediatric recipients, on which this chapter mainly focuses, is unique in the field of live donor organ transplantation in several regards. First, these procedures can entail the most significant donor-to-recipient size and weight mismatch of all live donor transplants (with a donor-to-recipient weight ratio as high as 20:1): kidney graft size—as opposed to liver and intestinal graft size—cannot be adapted to recipient size. Transplantation of such large kidney grafts into small recipients poses unique surgical challenges, yet is very desirable from a functional perspective. Second, small pediatric recipients experience high early technical graft loss rates and the highest graft thrombosis rates of any live donor transplant recipients. In a recent United Network for Organ Sharing (UNOS) analysis, nearly 30% of grafts lost in that group were lost from thrombosis and early technical complications.[1,2] Nevertheless, long-term outcomes of live donor kidneys in small recipients are better than those of most other live donor organ transplants—provided that early technical complications can be avoided.[3–5] Third, the small recipients' hemodynamics may result in intra- and postoperative graft hypoperfusion and may compound any preexisting procurement- and implantation-related ischemic graft injury.[6] There is histologic evidence that these grafts may also suffer adverse long-term consequences due to the small recipients' inability to appropriately perfuse adult-sized kidneys (a "large-for-size" syndrome, as opposed to the "small-for-size" syndrome in live donor liver transplantation).[7,8] Thus, even relatively minor intraoperative hemodynamic alterations and suboptimal surgical technique can set the stage for poor long-term outcomes of adult-sized kidneys.

In light of all these factors it is not surprising that pediatric kidney transplants had initially lower graft survival rates, and were not universally accepted as the optimal treatment modality for most children with end-stage renal disease (ESRD) until well into the 1980s.[8–11]

This chapter focuses on the technical–surgical aspects of live donor kidney transplantation in pediatric recipients, addressing surgical considerations, strategies and techniques, postoperative complications and their risk factors, as well as preventive strategies. Pretransplant recipient selection, work-up, and medical management, as well as perioperative immunosuppression and postoperative medical care are discussed in Chapters 16.1 and 16.5–16.7.

## IMPACT OF LIVE DONOR NEPHRECTOMY TECHNIQUE ON RECIPIENT OPERATION AND OUTCOME

Kidneys from live donors have traditionally been procured by open nephrectomy, most commonly by a retroperitoneal flank approach. However, since its first description 1995, laparoscopic nephrectomy has rapidly become the technique of choice for procurement of kidneys from live donors for transplantation into adult recipients.[12–14] With a delay—that is analogous to the later introduction of renal transplantation as the treatment modality of choice for pediatric patients with ESRD—a similar trend has taken place in pediatric live donor kidney transplantation.[14–21] As a result, the vast majority of kidneys from live donors for pediatric recipients in the United States is now procured laparoscopically, too.[14]

This significant recent change in surgical practice has implications for the recipient surgeon and for postreperfusion graft function. Some of the consequences of laparoscopic procurement, particularly with regard to graft function, are only beginning to emerge and remain the subject of ongoing investigation.[14]

### Implications of Donor Procurement Technique for the Pediatric Recipient Operation

Kidney grafts from live (vs deceased) donors have shorter renal arteries and veins to begin with.[22–24] With the advent of *laparoscopic* nephrectomy, vessel length has even further decreased.

This is due to the widespread use of laparoscopic vascular staplers, which require more of the available blood vessel length to transfix the vessel as compared to the standard clamping-and-oversewing technique that can be used during open nephrectomy.[22] With respect to renal vein length, the inability to use a side-biting clamp on the inferior vena cava has also resulted in shorter right renal veins.[22,24–26] At the beginning of the laparoscopic era, these shorter right renal veins were thought to be responsible for the initially observed increased graft thrombosis rates of laparoscopically procured right kidneys.[24–26]

Kidney grafts from live (vs deceased) donors have also more frequently multiple arteries, as multiple renal arteries of live donor grafts cannot be procured and implanted on a single, common aortic Carrel patch, as is possible for many grafts from deceased donors. Moreover, because of the absence of aortic Carrel patches, arterial vascular reconstruction options for live donor kidneys with multiple renal arteries are also more limited and do not allow, for example, to create a single Carrel patch by joining two separate Carrel patches of a kidney with two renal arteries. With the advent of *laparoscopic* nephrectomy, the rate of live donor kidney grafts with multiple renal arteries has further increased for at least two reasons.[22] First, although laparoscopic procurement of right kidneys has by now become standardized and has been shown to be safe for both donor and recipient,[26] some transplant centers still prefer to laparoscopically procure the left rather than the right kidney—often irrespective of the left kidney's number of renal arteries.[25] This preference is related to the longer renal vein that is available with the left kidney and that facilitates graft implantation. Second, in cases of an early renal arterial bifurcation in close proximity to the aortic renal artery origin, a judiciously placed vascular clamp during open nephrectomy, just central to the early renal artery bifurcation, may frequently still allow to procure the renal artery as a single vessel. In contrast, laparoscopic port positioning may only allow for suboptimal vascular stapler alignment with the abdominal aorta and may therefore yield a kidney with two arteries.[22] Laparoscopic procurement of such kidneys results also more frequently in multiple renal arteries because of the extra vascular length that is used by the laparoscopic staplers.[22] Nonetheless, with increasing experience and the use of appropriate surgical techniques for reconstruction of multiple renal arteries, there is no evidence that laparoscopically procured kidneys with multiple renal arteries have worse outcome.[22,23,26]

### *Optimization of Laparoscopic Nephrectomy Technique to Maximize Graft Vessel Length and Minimize Number of Renal Arteries*

The use of TA staplers rather than GIA staplers may be advantageous. A GIA stapler places two rows of staples, cuts in between those two rows, and requires that the row of staples on the graft side of the transected and stapled vessel be cut off prior to implantation, thereby shortening usable vascular length on the graft side even further.[22] In contrast, TA staplers place only a single row of staples on the donor's vessel side, leaving the full remaining length of the graft vessel available for the recipient surgeon.[22] Nontransfixing clips to secure the renal artery and vein stumps in the donor may increase available graft vessel length, too; however, they entail a higher likelihood for serious intraoperative complications.[27]

Furthermore, optimal laparoscopic port position is paramount, because it facilitates placement of the laparoscopic vascular stapler as close and as parallel as possible to the large axial vessel(s) (eg, to the aorta during left-sided nephrectomy; to the inferior vena cava during right-sided nephrectomy). This maneuver does not only maximize vessel length but also helps to minimize the number of grafts with multiple renal arteries.[22]

Also, the hand-assisted (vs purely) laparoscopic technique may allow for more optimal positioning of the stapler relative to the renal artery and vein, because the surgeon's hand within the abdomen may facilitate manipulation and optimal positioning of these vessels between the stapler jaws.

Judicious use of all these techniques should obviate the need to have to resort to semiopen procedures that include open application of a Satinsky clamp to the inferior vena cava at the right renal vein takeoff during laparoscopic-assisted right donor nephrectomy.[25] That approach may also obviate some of the advantages of the laparoscopic technique for the donor with respect to reduction of postoperative morbidity.[28,29]

Finally, modifications of the operative technique on the back table and in the recipient (eg, lengthening of the graft renal vein; full mobilization of the recipient iliac vein, with or without lateral transposition) may facilitate the use of kidneys with short right renal veins as well.[25,30–35] These techniques are discussed in more detail later.

In summary, currently available evidence suggests that with the use of appropriate and meticulous surgical techniques in the donor and recipient, vascular complication rates for laparoscopically procured right and left kidneys are comparable to those that have been previously described for openly procured kidneys.[13,22,26]

## Implications of Procurement Technique for Pediatric Recipient Graft Function

The pneumoperitoneum that is created during laparoscopy is known to be associated with adverse hemodynamic effects on, and acutely decreased blood flow to, *native* kidneys.[36–38] Hence, it is not surprising that some studies of adult live donor kidney graft recipients suggested slower early graft function for laparoscopic (vs open) donor kidneys—without any effect, however, on delayed function, acute rejection incidence, and long-term graft survival.[13,39–42]

In contrast, for pediatric recipients of adult laparoscopic donor kidneys, a recent UNOS database analysis of 995 transplants demonstrated a higher incidence of acute rejection for laparoscopic versus open donor grafts at 6 months and at 1 year, particularly in small recipients (0 to 5 years old).[14] Delayed graft function rates were also significantly higher for laparoscopic versus open recipients (0–5 years old, 12.8% vs 2.5%; and 6–18 years old, 5.9% vs 2.8%).[14] In a multivariate analysis, significant independent risk factors for acute rejection included laparoscopic procurement and delayed graft function. Short-term graft survival was comparable for both procurement modes. These findings raised some concern, because any injury inflicted on a kidney graft during procurement may be exacerbated by the postreperfusion hemodynamic challenges encountered in pediatric recipients.[14,43] A small pediatric recipient is only able to perfuse an adult kidney graft with approximately 60% of the donor's renal blood flow prior to nephrectomy.[6] It is now well established that any early graft injury, manifested either by slow early function or delayed graft function, can be associated with increased rates of acute rejection and chronic allograft nephropathy for both adult and pediatric recipients.[44–48] Thus, even a modest degree of added initial nonspecific injury due to the adverse hemodynamic conditions created by the pneumoperitoneum may portend poorer long-term graft survival. This may be compounded further by the increased immunoreactivity of pediatric (vs adult) recipients. Any increased graft immunogenicity as a result of a nonspecific procurement injury

may, therefore, potentiate likelihood for adverse immunologic long-term outcome in pediatric recipients and lead to more graft losses from chronic rejection.[14,47,48] At present, it remains to be seen whether some of these observations are, at least in part, due to the laparoscopic learning curve and center effects. Clearly, these results warrant further study and longer follow-up.

In pediatric live donor kidney transplantation, laparoscopic nephrectomy has undoubtedly also contributed to the increase of available live donor kidney grafts.[14,29,49,50] Hence, advocating for return to more widespread use of open nephrectomy based on the aforementioned functional results would likely only decrease the overall number of available kidney grafts for pediatric recipients—a patient group that benefits most from receiving a kidney transplant in a timely fashion.[51] Rather, the potential adverse effects of laparoscopic procurement on outcome in pediatric recipients underscore the importance of aggressively implementing supportive measures that have been shown to be renoprotective in the donor and the recipient.[52–54] For donors, previous experimental and clinical studies have suggested that intraoperative volume loading and some pharmacologic agents can improve intraoperative renal blood flow during the pneumoperitoneum phase.[52,54] For recipients, hemodynamics must be optimized, including the provision of adequate preload and systemic blood pressure at the time of graft reperfusion, particularly in very small recipients.[4,6,53] Some transplant programs have advocated admitting pediatric recipients to the hospital on the day before the planned transplant in order to proceed with vigorous rehydration well ahead of the transplant operation.[20] Aggressive implementation of these principles by some centers may also explain why certain single-center studies reported no significant differences with respect to the quality of early graft function, delayed graft function incidence, and rejection rates in pediatric recipients of laparoscopically (vs openly) procured kidneys.[15–20]

## SURGICAL PRETRANSPLANT RECIPIENT EVALUATION, PREPARATION, AND MANAGEMENT

### General Considerations

Most centers that perform renal transplants in infants require a minimum age of 6 months and a minimum body weight of 6 kg. Infants less than 6 kg definitely benefit from prior management with other forms of renal replacement therapy while awaiting further growth. This requires close cooperation with the infant's pediatric nephrology team. There is, however, no universal consensus, and optimal recipient age and size remain somewhat controversial.[3]

The recipient's blood vessels that are intended for the vascular anastomoses must be of sufficient caliber and must be able to provide unimpeded in- and outflow for the graft.[55] Moreover, in infants, the abdominal cavity must be able to accommodate an adult-sized kidney. When evaluating prospective infant recipients of adult-size kidney grafts, it is important to evaluate the abdominal domain by physical examination, independent of absolute age and weight. Some prospective recipients may be very small for age or may have suffered significant loss of abdominal domain (eg, due to massive intestinal resection secondary to necrotizing enterocolitis or diffuse mesenteric thrombosis). In such patients, awaiting further growth or proceeding with at least unilateral native nephrectomy may be necessary to make sufficient space for the kidney graft and to ensure that the recipient's abdomen can be closed primarily and without undue tension after graft implantation.

Preoperative assessment of the recipient's nutritional status is paramount. If it is suboptimal and may potentially result in higher surgical posttransplant complication rates and poorer long-term graft outcome, strong consideration must be given to optimizing nutritional status prior to transplantation, for example, by high caloric nasogastric or gastrostomy feedings.

Finally, if applicable, surgical pretransplant recipient evaluation includes also assessment of the peritoneal dialysis catheter position and inspection of the catheter exit site to rule out any site infection.

## Assessment of Inferior Vena Cava

Pretransplant evaluation of the inferior vena cava should be routine for every pediatric recipient.[56,57] Particularly in infants and small children, transabdominal ultrasonography suffices in most instances to ascertain the presence of a suitable patent inferior vena cava and iliac vein system. If the ultrasonography is nondiagnostic or inconclusive, and partial or complete occlusion or absence of the inferior vena cava cannot be definitively ruled out, additional imaging studies are indicated. Magnetic resonance venography, computed abdominal tomography, or conventional inferior vena cavography (the gold standard) are options to further assess the status of the inferior vena cava and iliac veins preoperatively. The choice of the imaging technique depends in large part on the patient's residual native renal function and whether dialysis has already been instituted, and on institutional experience with, and availability of, these imaging techniques. If any significant venous abnormalities are documented, preoperative planning must be modified accordingly. The section "Absent and Occluded Inferior Vena Cava" contains a description of surgical techniques and options that may be helpful in recipients with an abnormal inferior cava and iliac venous system.

## Pretransplant Urologic Evaluation and Management of Recipients With an Abnormal Urinary Tract

According to current registry data (North American Pediatric Renal Transplant Cooperative Study [NAPRTCS] report), approximately 25% of pediatric transplant recipients have urinary tract abnormalities.[3] Therefore, in every transplant candidate, a detailed urologic system review and history of any prior interventions on the urinary tract must be obtained and correlated with the findings on physical examination (eg, previous incisions, presence of uretero- or vesicostomy).[58,59]

In prospective recipients with upper urinary tract abnormalities (eg, hydronephrosis and megaureters), a decision must be made as to the indication for, and timing of, bilateral native nephroureterectomy prior to transplantation (as discussed in detail under Native Nephrectomy).

Most prospective pediatric kidney transplant recipients should be evaluated routinely with a voiding cystourethrogram,[60] unless the nature of the kidney disease and the clinical course preclude abnormalities of the urinary outflow tract. For example, a voiding cystourethrogram would not be indicated in an adolescent with IgA nephropathy and no symptoms related to the urinary tract.

In patients in whom lower urinary tract abnormalities (including bladder extrophy, neuropathic bladder [eg, from meningomyelocele, spinal cord trauma, or neurologic diseases], posterior urethral valves, prune belly syndrome, and vesicouretal reflux) have been diagnosed in the past, or in whom these must be suspected until proven otherwise (eg, in patients with the diagnosis

of obstructive uropathy and reflux nephropathy, bladder dysfunction is common), obtaining a full history of the voiding pattern prior to the development of renal failure is important and can be helpful in determining the need for specific additional pretransplant investigations. For these patients, a basic urodynamic assessment (including measurement of urinary flow rate and estimation of the postvoid urinary residual intravesical volume by ultrasonography) should be routine. Normal average urinary flow rate is age dependent and should be at least 10 mL/sec for patients 4 to 7 years of age, 12 mL/sec for patients 8 to 13 years of age, and 18 mL/sec for patients over 13 years of age. Postvoid residual volume should be < 30 mL.[61] Besides a voiding cystourethrogram and the basic urodynamic studies, a cystometrogram and a video cystourethrogram may be indicated to further assess the degree of bladder dysfunction. Urethral obstruction (eg, from posterior ureteral valves or strictures) can be assessed by urethroscopy and cystoscopy. Bladder dysfunction is common in these patients and must be ruled out (*vide supra*). Any residual obstruction must be ruled out and corrected prior to transplantation.[58,62] In these patients with lower urinary tract abnormalities, further evaluation and possibly intervention in preparation for transplantation may be warranted.[58–60] This may require additional interdisciplinary consultation with a pediatric urologist, if not already done at the time of referral for transplantation.

For the transplant surgeon, perhaps the most important (and at times most complex) pretransplant assessment and decision that pertains to the urinary tract is whether the patient's bladder is usable. The two main criteria for a usable bladder are (1) an adequate actual or potential capacity and (2) low end-filling pressures.[58,61,63] Most prospective pediatric transplant recipients have a urinary bladder that will eventually adapt to the physiologic amounts of urine that are produced by a functioning kidney graft.[58] Even very small, long-term defunctionalized bladders can be successfully used.[58,59,61,63] Usually, these small bladders distend with usage over time. It is important, however, that any neurogenic component be ruled out pretransplant. The use of the native bladder should also be routinely considered in patients with prior urinary diversion. In a substantial proportion of these patients, including those with a continent urinary diversion using an appendiceal stoma (Mitrofanoff procedure), successful use of the bladder after appropriate pretransplant assessment is still possible.[61,63] Only the very rare small, noncompliant, fibrotic, and nondistensible bladder (eg, due to multiple previous surgical interventions or chronic infection [eg, tuberculosis]) is unlikely to distend over time and cannot be considered for use at the time of transplantation.[61,63] Overall, a pretransplant augmentation cystoplasty is only rarely necessary and should be reserved for patients with truly very low (fixed) bladder capacity or very high end-filling bladder pressures.[63–65] If indicated, the augmentation cystoplasty is preferably done using urothelial (eg, native megaureter) rather than intestinal segments (stomach, small bowel, or colon).[66]

For patients with neurogenic bladders, preparation for transplantation should include an attempt at instituting a clean intermittent self-catheterization regimen. If an intermittent self-catheterization program has already been carried out before the onset of ESRD and good compliance has been shown, the use of the native bladder can be considered.[63] In these patients, intermittent catheterization must be continued indefinitely posttransplant. For patients in whom such an approach is not feasible or unsuccessful, urinary diversion involving, for example, creation of an ileal conduit must be considered.[63,65] In the pediatric transplant setting, other, often less preferable, alternatives to an ileal conduit include continent urinary diversion procedures, and cutaneous pyelostomy, ureterostomy, and vesicostomy.[58,63–65]

Patients with significant congenital urinary tract abnormalities that are not amenable to pretransplant bladder reconstruction, bladder augmentation, substitution cystoplasty, and urethral reconstruction, must also be considered candidates for urinary diversion.[58,63–65] Total or partial reconstruction of the bladder and urethra is, however, only very rarely required to begin with in prospective transplant recipients.[58]

It is important that all patients with abnormal bladders and with a history of bladder outlet and urethral obstruction be followed and monitored throughout the life of the transplant for possible late urologic complications. This will minimize the risk for preventable graft losses if these problems were to worsen or recur.[58,61]

## THE TRANSPLANT OPERATION

### General Intraoperative Recipient Management Principles

Successful pediatric renal transplantation requires close cooperation between the anesthesia and surgical teams to ensure optimal hemodynamic and other physiologic conditions for the kidney graft. A central venous line and an arterial line are placed after induction of general anesthesia. The recipient is placed in a supine position on the operating table. A warming blanket is placed under the recipient, and the operating room temperature must be maintained at $\geq 32°C$. The recipient is prepped from the chest to the midthigh area, leaving the access to the urethra within the sterile surgical field, which is particularly important in small recipients and infants. A urinary catheter is placed, and the bladder is filled with antibiotic solution and the Foley catheter is clamped. Prior to incision, prophylactic intravenous antibiotics and immunosuppressants are given as per protocol.[55]

Throughout the operation, the recipient's temperature is monitored and any degree of hypothermia is aggressively corrected by use of the warming blanket, an appropriate operating room temperature set point, administration of warmed intravenous fluids, and, if necessary, use of warm saline abdominal lavage (in cases of intraabdominal transplants).[55]

Prior to graft reperfusion, as the vascular anastomoses are completed, mannitol (250 mg/kg) and furosemide (1 mg/kg) are infused slowly intravenously.

### Operative Technique and Principles (Color Plates, Figure K1-14 and 15)

#### General Technical Considerations

*Kidney graft implantation site* Recipient size determines the site of the graft placement, unless considerations pertaining to the establishment of venous graft drainage (see Native Nephrectomy) dictate otherwise.[55] Adult-sized kidney grafts from live donors are most frequently placed intra-abdominally (intraperitoneally) if the recipient weighs $\leq 15$ kg. Extraperitoneal graft placement in children weighing < 10 kg is relatively rare and has been reported in only few series.[67,68] Nonetheless, even these extraperitoneal grafts were still revascularized using the abdominal aorta and inferior vena cava, as is done for intraperitoneal grafts.[67,68] In most other small pediatric (>15 kg) and adolescent recipients, the kidney is placed extraperitoneally into the right or left iliac fossa.

The extraperitoneal grafts in those recipients must be placed the more cephalad the smaller the recipient. In small recipients >15 kg, this may entail a retroperitoneal, rather than an iliac fossa position. The final decision as to the graft implantation site (extra- vs intraperitoneal) rests with the surgeon and depends in large part on the preoperative recipient evaluation (see also under General Considerations). In children weighing 15 to 20 kg, physical examination and inspection of the prospective recipient's body habitus and abdominal domain are key in determining the optimal implantation site.

*Vascular anastomoses* Particularly in the laparoscopic era, live (vs deceased) donor grafts have more commonly multiple and shorter renal arteries and renal veins for the reasons discussed in detail above (see under Implications of Donor Procurement Technique for the Pediatric Recipient Operation).[22,24]

Transplant surgeons must be prepared to handle these vascular anatomical variations appropriately so as to minimize the risk for postoperative partial or complete graft thrombosis. The use of previously described sound surgical techniques can help to safely accomplish this goal.[23]

Arterial reconstruction of multiple renal arteries of live donor grafts can be more challenging due to the absence of an aortic Carrel patch. Although no prospective randomized comparison between the various surgical–technical options available for grafts with multiple renal arteries is available, anecdotal evidence suggests that end-to-side or side-to-side renal artery reconstruction techniques, which can be performed under optimal, controlled conditions on the back table, may be preferable.[23] In contrast, separate, direct anastomoses of at times very small accessory renal arteries to the recipient's vasculature (eg, to the external iliac artery or the recipient's inferior epigastric artery to provide inflow for a small lower polar renal artery) may portend higher vascular complication rates. In one recent report, where such reimplantation techniques were predominantly used, increased ureteral complication rates, potentially due to ureteral ischemia from thrombosis of smaller renal arteries, were observed.[69]

Live donor kidney grafts tend also to have shorter veins than deceased donor kidney grafts (see under Implications of Donor Procurement Technique for the Pediatric Recipient Operation).[22–26] Some additional renal vein length can be gained through careful retrograde dissection of the renal vein towards the renal hilum on the back table, ligating as many small venous side branches as possible. Further surgical options and technical maneuvers that allow to safely transplant grafts with short renal veins are described below, according to recipient size category.

*Ureteral anastomosis* The ureteroneocystostomy in infants and very small children is often created using the intravesical Leadbetter–Politano technique.[55–70] Frequently, an externalized transplant ureteral stent is used in that recipient age group. The externalized stent is typically removed at the bedside within the first week posttransplant, sometimes following a radiographic stent contrast study.

The ureteroneocystostomy in older children and adolescents is most frequently created using an extravesical technique (eg, Gregoir–Lich, "single stitch" technique).[71–73] Benefits of extravesical techniques include less ureteral length with better preserved ureteral blood supply in the ureteral remnant, minimal bladder dissection and manipulation, no separate cystostomy, and relative technical ease.[71–73]

Two recent meta-analyses (reviewing previous studies that involved mostly adult kidney recipients) suggested that stenting of extra- and intravesical ureteroneocystostomies may decrease ureteral complication rates (eg, leaks, stenoses).[74,75] In selected recipients, the transplant ureter must be drained into a native ureter, a previously created ileal conduit, or into an augmented bladder. Anecdotal evidence suggests that these recipients benefit from stenting of their ureteral anastomosis, too. For recipients with focal segmental glomerulosclerosis (FSGS), the use of an externalized ureteral stent may be advantageous, albeit for a different reason. These externalized stents, typically brought out separately through the urethra in addition to the Foley catheter, allow to selectively monitor the graft's proteinuria. In recipients with early, aggressive FSGS recurrence, as evidenced by significant graft proteinuria, early therapy may then be initiated.

An important postoperative management principle for recipients with very small bladders is prolonged bladder decompression (for 4 to 8 weeks) with a Foley catheter (or, less commonly, by creation of a suprapubic cystostomy). This provides sufficient time for appropriate healing of the ureteroneocystostomy prior to the small bladder being subjected to large volumes (and potentially high pressures) of the urine that is produced by a normally functioning transplant kidney (thus minimizing the risk for early urinary leaks).

### Operative Technique in Infants and Small Children ≤ 15 kg (Intra-abdominal, Intraperitoneal Graft Implantation)

The transplant is performed through a midline incision that extends from the xiphoid to the pubis. The cecum and the right colon are mobilized and reflected towards the patient's left upper abdomen.[55] At this stage, native uni- or bilateral nephrectomy can be performed, if necessary (see Native Nephrectomy for indications). The infrarenal abdominal aorta and inferior vena cava are circumferentially dissected free, and looped proximally and distally with soft vessel loops. These vessel loops also facilitate the subsequent retraction that is necessary to safely isolate the lumbar branches of the abdominal aorta. All lumbar branches are ligated and divided. The periaortic vascular dissection is extended to include the proximal right and left common iliac artery. The inferior mesenteric artery is dissected free at its origin and encircled with a vessel loop as well. The inferior vena cava is mobilized in a similar fashion from the left renal vein down to the left and right common iliac vein (Color Plates, Figure K1-14). These veins are encircled with vessel loops, too. The donor kidney is readied for transplantation on the back table. Next, the aorta and inferior vena cava are cross-clamped proximally. This can be done either separately or, advantageously, by placing a single Fogarty vascular clamp that extends across both vessels. The previously placed distal vessel loops around the common iliac vessels and inferior mesenteric artery are snared and maintained under tension for distal vascular control.

Next, the intended position of the kidney, as well as the alignment of the graft vessels with the abdominal aorta and inferior vena cava, are tested and optimized prior to beginning the vascular anastomoses. This operative step is of critical importance. Both renal artery and vein must lie tension- and torsion-free. Any redundant length cannot be tolerated.[59] Since the kidney is usually placed infrahepatically on the recipient's right side (in the immediate vicinity of the inferior vena cava), the renal vein of the

kidney graft may even need to be shortened in order to meet this technical requirement. The venous anastomotic site is usually located on the lower inferior vena cava. In some cases, the venous anastomosis may extend into the right common iliac vein.[55,59] For left kidneys, the optimal renal arterial anastomotic site on the abdominal aorta is often located inferior to the inferior mesenteric artery take-off. Right kidney grafts tend more often to require a renal arterial anastomotic site slightly superior to the inferior mesenteric artery take-off on the abdominal aorta. In any event, if arterial and venous anastomotic sites are adequately chosen, the artery and the vein do not cross over each other and have a straight course from the kidney hilus to their respective anastomotic site.[55,59]

For the venous anastomosis, the anterior surface of the inferior vena cava is incised and four corner sutures of 6–0 polypropylene are placed. The kidney is brought into the field and the four corner sutures are placed into the renal vein and tied. The anastomosis is done with running sutures on the right and the left side. During the anastomosis, gentle traction on the lateral holding sutures prevents inadvertent inclusion of the posterior wall (opposite to the side where the vascular suturing is taking place). An end-to-side anastomosis is performed in a similar fashion between the donor renal artery and the infrarenal abdominal aorta or right common iliac artery, depending on recipient size. For very small recipients, this may require 7–0 polypropylene sutures. When the anastomoses are complete, the proximal clamp(s) and the distal occluding vessels loops are released (Color Plates, Figure K1-15). At the time of reperfusion, it is of utmost importance in small children to maintain the central venous pressure at 15 to 18 cm $H_2O$ and an adequate aortic blood pressure at least close to, or at, the recipient's baseline arterial blood pressure prior to induction of anesthesia. Immediately after reperfusion, the kidney is irrigated with copious amounts of warm saline solution for rapid rewarming. In the reperfusion phase, aggressive volume replacement is important due to the amount of the small recipient's circulating blood that is required to fill the large kidney graft.

Attention is then brought to the ureteral anastomosis. For the ureteroneocystostomy in infants, a Leadbetter-Politano technique is preferred (Color Plates, Figure K1-12), although alternative techniques have been successfully used for these small recipients as well.[70–73,76–79] The previously filled bladder is incised anteriorly and three retractors are placed at 120° intervals. The bladder trigone is visually identified and a site for the anastomosis near the trigone on the right posterolateral aspect of the bladder is chosen. A submucosal tunnel is created by initial injection of saline solution to develop a submucosal plane. The mucosa in the area of the planned anastomosis is incised and a spacious tunnel is made. The second opening of the tunnel is made on the posterolateral outside surface of the bladder toward the right side. A clamp is passed from the distal mucosal opening intravesically through the tunnel and brought out through the right posterolateral wall of the bladder. A feeding tube is brought back through the tunnel, and the distal end is sutured to the distal ureter. The feeding tube is used to pull the ureter through the tunnel into the bladder. The ureter is shortened as appropriate, and spatulated. Next, the anastomosis to the bladder mucosa is created, with 8 to 10 interrupted 5–0 absorbable polyglyconate sutures.[55]

At this point, a ureteral stent is placed.[55] A 5 or 8 French pediatric feeding tube is secured to the urinary catheter and the catheter and stent are advanced together through the urethra into the bladder. The stent is then freed from the catheter and advanced through the ureteroneocystostomy to the pelvis of the kidney. Injecting a small amount of saline solution into the stent and aspirating it confirm the stent position. If the stent is not in the renal pelvis, the fluid cannot be aspirated. The Foley catheter must be pulled back into normal position, and stent position must be reconfirmed before the stent is secured to the Foley catheter outside the body in a definitive fashion. Alternatively, an internalized double-J stent can be placed into the pelvis of the kidney and transplant ureter and brought out into the bladder. However, this will require an invasive posttransplant reintervention for stent removal in a very small patient. Therefore, the use of externalized stents that can be removed at the bedside or in clinic is preferred in this recipient age group.

The bladder is closed in two layers of running and one layer of interrupted sutures using 4–0 or 5–0 monofilament absorbable polyglyconate suture.

### Operative Technique in Children >15 kg and Adolescents Extra-abdominal (Extraperitoneal Graft Implantation)

Operative technique for older children and adolescents is similar to that for adults as described in Chapter 16.3. The kidney graft is placed into the right or left iliac fossa. In most cases, the right iliac fossa is preferred due to the more superficial course of the common and external iliac vein on the right side.

It is important to place the kidney graft as proximally as possible. This principle is particularly relevant in small recipients >15 kg that have a shallow pelvis with a short anterior-posterior distance between the anterior abdominal wall and the bony surface of the iliac fossa. Graft placement that is too distal in a small recipient can set the stage for graft thrombosis: upon closing the abdominal fascia over the kidney graft, vascular compression and kinking, particularly of the renal vein, can ensue. In contrast, more proximal kidney graft implantation provides for a better kidney position in the iliac fossa or the retroperitoneum, with the kidney lying on its side. The renal artery and vein can align optimally and will not be prone to compression by the kidney graft itself upon wound closure. Thus, the smaller, narrower, and shallower the pelvis, the more proximal implantation must occur. A more proximal location of the venous anastomotic site (and of the kidney graft) is facilitated by graft implantation on the right side (*vide supra*).

With the extraperitoneal approach, the venous anastomosis can be done to the external iliac vein, the common iliac vein, or the inferior vena cava. Depending on the recipient's size and pelvic anatomy, the arterial anastomosis can be done to the external iliac artery, the internal iliac artery, or the distal abdominal aorta.

If the donor renal vein is too short to allow for a sufficiently proximal graft position and for a tension-, kink-, and torsion-free position and course of the renal vein, several surgical techniques can be used to facilitate implantation and to minimize the risk for postoperative graft thrombosis. These techniques may be especially helpful when transplanting right kidneys into the left iliac fossa.

First, it is possible to gain additional mobility of the recipient's common and external iliac vein by meticulously ligating and dividing all internal iliac vein branches.[30–32] This must be accomplished with great caution to avoid any bleeding that may be extremely difficult to control. Loss of control over a divided internal iliac vein is a potentially lethal complication. Complete mobilization of the external and, if necessary, of the common iliac vein

also allows transposing the iliac vein lateral to the external iliac artery.[30–32] In many cases, this maneuver significantly facilitates optimal anastomosis and positioning of the graft renal vein (Color Plates, Figure K1-6B).[32]

Second, especially on the left side, mobility of the common and external iliac vein can be further enhanced by ligating and dividing the internal iliac artery.[30,31]

Third, in very rare circumstances, if none of the aforementioned techniques alone would result in appropriate alignment and positioning of the renal vein, it is possible to lengthen the renal vein using spiral grafts and panel grafts or straight third-party vein segments.[33,34] Spiral grafts and panel grafts can be fashioned using autologous (or third-party) saphenous or gonadal veins.[33,34] Finally, in cases of unilateral or bilateral native nephrectomy done concomitantly with the renal transplant, a segment of the excised autologous renal vein may be employed for the lengthening of the graft's renal vein, too.[35] Although there are no controlled studies on this subject available in the renal transplant literature, it can be inferred from the experience with other organ transplants that venous extension grafts increase the risk for graft thrombosis.[30,31] They should therefore be avoided and only used as a last resort.

In the extremely unusual case that a short renal artery of a live donor graft must be lengthened, or additional material is necessary for vascular reconstruction, a native ipsilateral internal iliac artery segment or an undiseased native renal artery segment (in case a native nephrectomy is done at the time of transplantation) are potential options for creating arterial extension conduits.

Similar to the transplantation of adult recipients, the ureteroneocystostomy in larger children and adolescents is often created by an extravesicular technique (eg, Gregoir–Lich, single stitch technique; Color Plates, Figure K1-12).[71–73,79] If the anastomosis is stented (usually by inserting an internalized double-J stent), the stent is removed within 2 to 8 weeks posttransplant.

## SPECIAL OPERATIVE CONSIDERATIONS AND PROBLEMS

### Native Nephrectomy

An important pretransplant surgical decision pertains to the necessity for, and the timing of, native nephrectomy. In selected patients with the following diagnoses and problems (bilateral) native nephrectomy may be indicated: reflux nephropathy, particularly with recurrent infection; polycystic kidney disease (due to kidney size or cyst hemorrhage); hypoplasia with hypertension not amenable to satisfactory medical management; congenital nephrotic syndrome (see discussion below); and the need for creating additional room within the abdominal cavity to accommodate an adult-sized kidney graft (eg, in small children and infants). If nephrectomy is to be performed for the latter indication, only unilateral nephrectomy, depending on the child's and the diseased kidney's size, may be necessary (for both intra- and extraperitoneal transplants).[55]

Consideration of native nephrectomy is particularly important in children with congenital nephrotic syndrome that experience the onset of massive proteinuria at, or shortly after, birth. This may result, among other complications, in serious infections, poor nutrition, and significant arterial and venous thrombotic episodes because of hypercoagulability. For these patients, whose mortality can be excessive if left inadequately treated, rapid preparation for transplantation is essential.[58,59,80–83] Preemptive bilateral nephrectomy and initiation of dialysis (frequently via the peritoneal route) are paramount. After achieving an appropriate nutritional state, one can then proceed with renal transplantation from a live donor, usually at the earliest 6 weeks after bilateral nephrectomy.[58,59,80–83] In patients with other renal diseases that are associated with a secondary nephrotic syndrome, a decision whether bilateral nephrectomy is indicated prior to transplantation must be made on a case-by-case basis in close coordination with the patient's pediatric nephrologist.

For most patients without significant nephrotic syndrome in whom bilateral nephrectomy is indicated, operative timing is dictated by the prospective recipient's age and size, and by the intended kidney implantation site. In small recipients and infants (≤ 15 kg), bilateral nephrectomy may be advantageously performed at the time of transplantation. Since their transplant entails an intra-abdominal operation, it is easy and safe to perform nephrectomy at the time of transplantation. Moreover, performing the nephrectomy at the time of the transplant will also obviate scar and adhesion formation in the vicinity of the intended vascular anastomotic sites (ie, abdominal aorta and inferior vena cava) as would be the case if nephrectomy were to be done beforehand. In older children and adolescents (>15 kg), bilateral nephrectomy is usually performed at least 6 weeks prior to the transplant, since native nephrectomy would normally require an additional incision and additional dissection besides the right or left lower quadrant incision required for the extraperitoneal implantation of the kidney graft. The main disadvantage of staged nephrectomy and transplantation consists of the need to institute dialysis during the anephric interval (for patients with significant residual function in their diseased native kidneys).

Bilateral nephrectomy in transplant recipients follows surgical principles similar to those that apply to nephrectomy for other indications for benign diseases. The origin of the respective renal artery and renal vein need not to be identified. Rather, these vessels can be ligated in proximity to the kidney. In kidney diseases with normal ureters (eg, hypoplastic kidneys with hypertension), the native ureters should be left in place, since they may provide a useful option for draining the graft ureters, either at the time of the transplantation or at the time of a later ureter revision. Conversely, if the native ureters are diseased (eg, hydro- or megaureters in patients with reflux nephropathy, particularly with a history of recurrent infection), complete bilateral ureterectomy to the level of the bladder is indicated, unless a megaureter is needed for augmentation cystoplasty.[66]

## Absent and Occluded Inferior Vena Cava

Agenesis of the inferior vena cava is very rare and often associated with cardiac and other visceral malformations (eg, polysplenia syndrome, malrotation, and dextrocardia).[84–86] In addition to partial or complete inferior vena cava absence, several congenital inferior vena cava variants (eg, left-sided, bilateral or in association with renal vein anomalies) have been described. Although an absent inferior vena cava is generally attributed to embryological dysgenesis, it may also occasionally be the consequence of acquired perinatal renal vein and subsequent inferior vena cava thrombosis.[85] Other etiologies of acquired absence of the inferior vena cava secondary to occlusion include hypercoagulable states (eg, from nephrotic syndrome, protein C and S deficiency, antiphospholipid syndrome), trauma, previous placement of an inferior vena caval filter or clip, and insertion of an indwelling venous catheter, particularly into the lower extremity veins.[57,87] In one study, over 6%

of infants younger than 12 months of age had developed inferior vena caval thrombosis after insertion of central venous total parenteral nutrition catheters.[87] Other risk factors for inferior vena caval thrombosis include a history of multiple intraabdominal surgical procedures, dehydration, Wilms' tumor, hepatocellular carcinoma, testicular carcinoma, ulcerative colitis, chronic pancreatitis, and Budd–Chiari syndrome complicating Behçet's disease.[57]

Key to the successful management of these patients is early preoperative diagnosis, which allows devising an adequate surgical strategy for the transplant operation. Screening for absence or occlusion of the inferior vena cava should therefore be part of the pretransplant evaluation of every pediatric recipient (see under "General Considerations").[56,57]

Several surgical strategies allow proceeding with kidney transplantation in case of an absent or occluded inferior vena cava. First, iliac veins that drain through collaterals, and these collateral veins themselves (eg, the ovarian vein), have all been successfully used to provide venous drainage for kidney grafts.[85,86,88–90] For recipients with a partially or totally occluded inferior vena cava, a lower extremity and iliac venogram should be obtained preoperatively in order to assess caliber and outflow of these iliac and collateral veins (if those are contemplated as potential venous anastomotic sites). It is unclear, if any intraoperative parameters may indicate suitability of such iliac or collateral veins to provide adequate venous drainage for a kidney graft. It has been suggested that vigorous back-bleeding from the proximal iliac vein may predict adequacy of venous drainage in such circumstances.[88] But others have proposed measuring inferior vena caval pressures and postulated that "high" (eg, >25 mm Hg) pressures in the iliac or collateral vein may suggest nonsuitability for renal vein anastomosis.[86,89,98] In yet another report, normal venous pressure measurements and observation of respiratory variations on the venous pressure tracing were felt to have been important predictors for the success of subsequent renal transplants.[89]

Second, depending on extent and location of the absent segment of the inferior vena cava, it may be possible to drain the kidney into a juxtahepatic segment of the infrahepatic inferior vena cava, or into the retrohepatic inferior vena cava, with arterial inflow provided by the aorta.[84]

The third possible approach entails orthotopic graft placement, most often on the left side.[91–96] In older pediatric recipients, this can be done through an extraperitoneal approach.[93] Venous drainage of such orthotopically placed kidneys on the left side may be achieved via the native left renal vein (after ipsilateral native nephrectomy).[92,97] The venous anastomosis may be facilitated by creating a branch patch from the recipient's native left renal vein-left adrenal vein-left gonadal vein confluence, which can then be anastomosed to the graft's renal vein.[97] Alternatively, venous outflow for kidneys in a left orthotopic position may also be obtained by anastomosis to the splenic vein (with or without splenectomy).[93–96] Arterial inflow for orthotopic left kidney grafts may be either from the aorta or from the (divided) splenic artery.[86,91–94,96,97] The use of the native left renal artery for arterial inflow is discouraged, because of the smaller diameter of that vessel and the potential presence of arterial disease.

Fourth, the kidney graft may also be drained into the superior or inferior mesenteric vein.[98–100] Portal venous drainage of kidney grafts (ie, into the portal, splenic or mesenteric veins) may theoretically confer an immunologic advantage, based on experimental results obtained in small animal models.[101] The presentation of portally delivered antigen to the liver would be, if it were to result in at least partial tolerance, particularly advantageous for the more immunoreactive pediatric recipients. However, to date there is no evidence that portal kidney graft drainage confers any clinical benefit in clinical kidney transplantation.[91,93–96,98–101] This is mirrored by the observation that with current immunosuppressive drugs, even in the setting of a relatively more immunogenic pancreas transplant, portal (vs systemic) drainage exerts no measurable effect with regards to achieving a state of, or close to, operational tolerance.[101]

Fifth, in exceptional circumstances, one may consider draining the live donor kidney into a third-party conduit that bypasses the recipient's occluded distal inferior cava and iliac venous systems.[102] At least one successful transplant with this technique has been described.[102]

For older pediatric recipients and adolescents, transplantation of kidneys in a more cephalad position than usual may also require alternative techniques for draining the transplant ureter because of the greater distance between kidney graft and recipient bladder. Ureters of live donor kidney grafts may compound this problem further, because they are shorter than ureters of deceased donor kidneys. Creation of a ureteroureterostomy, a pyelopyelostomy, or drainage into an intestinal conduit are all potentially viable options to compensate for a graft ureter that does not reach the native bladder.[93,95,103–106]

Complications that are specific to implantation of kidney grafts using one of these alternative renal venous drainage sites include a higher graft thrombosis rate, although the risk for this complication is not quantifiable based on the presently available scant evidence in the literature. Exact assessment of this risk is very likely also hampered by a publication bias (ie, preferential reporting of successful outcomes). For similar reasons, it is also unknown whether those recipients benefit from routine short- and long-term anticoagulation.

In recipients with more cephalad kidney graft placement than usual, one has also to anticipate a higher rate of urologic complications as a result of increased ureteral length or the use of the graft's renal pelvis, rendering the blood supply of the urinary anastomosis more tenuous. With left-sided orthotopic implantation, particularly when the splenic artery and/or splenic vein are used for graft revascularization, pancreatitis or a pancreatic fistula may ensue from partial mobilization and manipulation of the pancreas.[93]

Overall, the key to good outcomes and avoidance of intra- and postoperative graft losses from graft thrombosis is preoperative recognition of absence or occlusion of the inferior vena cava, followed by careful preoperative delineation of the venous vascular anatomy and judicious planning of the surgical approach.

## SURGICAL COMPLICATIONS

### Graft Thrombosis

#### Incidence and Risk Factors

In pediatric recipients, thrombosis of a live or deceased donor kidney graft is the most significant and devastating surgical complication.[1–3,107] It usually results in irreversible graft failure. The overall incidence of this complication, which is more frequent in pediatric than in adult renal transplant recipients, still ranges between 3% and 8%, with significantly increased thrombosis rates for certain subgroups.[1,3,107] According to recent UNOS and NAPRTCS database analyses of pediatric renal transplants, kidney graft thrombosis is the third most common cause of graft loss, behind acute and chronic

rejection.[1,3] Thrombotic events leading to graft losses are particularly common in infants less than 2 years old, where grafts lost from thrombosis represent nearly 30% of all grafts lost in those recipients in the United States, contributing significantly to the steep 15% immediate postoperative dropoff in kidney graft survival.[1,2] Those losses are particularly disturbing, because in that age group most kidney grafts are from live donors.[1,3] Fortunately, kidney grafts from live donors have an overall lower risk for graft thrombosis than kidneys from deceased donors.[1,3,107]

Risk factors for graft thrombosis in pediatric live donor recipients include recipient, surgical, and other perioperative risk factors (Table 16.11b-1). Decreasing recipient age unequivocally increases thrombosis risk.[1,107] The recipient's primary renal disease may affect graft thrombosis rates, too. Besides the congenital nephrotic syndrome (*vide infra*), the prune-belly syndrome constitutes a risk factor for graft thrombosis as well.[80,108,109] At least one case of thrombosis of a live donor graft in a recipient with prune-belly syndrome has been reported.[108] It is assumed that the laxity of the abdominal wall can result in excessive mobility of the kidney graft and lead to torsion of the renal vascular pedicle with subsequent graft thrombosis.[108,109] Recipient risk factors for postoperative graft thrombosis in live donor pediatric recipients include also retransplant status and obesity[107,110] (Table 16.11b-1).

In patients on dialysis at the time of transplantation, dialysis mode is a significant risk factor. Peritoneal dialysis confers an increased risk for graft thrombosis.[111,112] Peritoneal dialysis

TABLE 16.11b-1

## RISK FACTORS FOR, AND CAUSES OF, EARLY POSTOPERATIVE VASCULAR KIDNEY GRAFT THROMBOSIS IN PEDIATRIC RECIPIENTS

**Recipient factors**
- Small size
- Low age
- Obesity
- (Congenital) nephrotic syndrome
- Prune belly syndrome
- Pretransplant peritoneal dialysis
- Retransplant status
- Immobilization
- Dehydration
- Inflammation/sepsis
- Endothelial damage
- Polycythemia
- Sickle cell syndrome
- Defined hypercoagulable states, including factor V Leiden (G1691A) and prothrombin (G20210A) gene mutations, antithrombin deficiency, protein C and S deficiency, antiphospholipid antibody syndrome
- Oral contraceptives

**Intra- and perioperative factors**
- Suboptimal surgical technique and graft position
- Impeded venous graft drainage (eg, chronic partial or complete inferior vena cava or iliac vein occlusion)
- Suboptimal intra- and postoperative hemodynamic management (particularly of infant recipients)

**Immunosuppression**
- Non-use of antilymphocyte antibody or IL-2 receptor antibody for induction
- Cyclosporin A, sirolimus (?)

patients have significantly higher concentrations of thrombogenic apolipoprotein(a). They also have higher procoagulant activity of factors II, VII, VIII, IX, X, XI, and XII, whereas endogenous anticoagulants, such as protein C and antithrombin, are not altered.[113,114] Peritoneal dialysis is also associated with higher hematocrit levels due to reduction of extracellular volume, so patients may be at greater risk for being hemoconcentrated.[114] In addition, peritoneal dialysis may also constitute a surrogate marker for loss of hemodialysis access options due to repetitive thrombosis of dialysis access grafts and fistulas secondary to a hypercoagulable state. Several other procoagulant states, some of which have a genetic basis, have also been identified as risk factors for graft thrombosis (Table 16.11b-1).[115,116]

Operative-surgical risk factors include the use of suboptimal technique. Important surgical–technical considerations have been described in detail in the section on the recipient implantation technique (see Operative Technique and Principles). Briefly, for intra-abdominal transplants, perfect positioning of the graft's renal artery and vein is important. No redundancy of these vessels can be tolerated, because otherwise they may kink. For extraperitoneal transplants into the iliac fossa, an as proximal as possible position of the kidney graft is paramount. Anastomosis of the donor vessels, particularly of a short donor renal vein, may be technically easier to the distal iliac vasculature, but this more distal graft position confers a higher thrombosis risk: Upon closing the fascia over the kidney, a graft position that is too distal can lead to compression, kinking, and occlusion of the graft vessels. Optimal hemodynamic and intravascular volume management of the small recipient are important to maintain appropriate postreperfusion graft blood flow. Any intra- or postoperative hypotension, irrespective of its etiology, can increase risk for graft thrombosis (Table 16.11b-1).

Peri- and postoperatively, immunosuppressive agents may impact graft thrombosis rates. A retrospective analysis of the NAPRTCS database suggested that perioperative use of interleukin-2 (IL-2) receptor antibody may decrease graft thrombosis risk.[117] The beneficial effects of IL-2 receptor blockade may be explained by mitigation of IL-2-related procoagulant effects such as (1) endothelial cell and platelet activation and (2) the microvascular thrombosis that has been observed with IL-2 administration.[117] In another registry review, non-use of antilymphocytic antibody induction therapy was noted to be associated with an increased risk for graft thrombosis.[107] Also, use of cyclosporin A was reported to be associated with higher graft thrombosis rates in some recipients.[118] Experimental evidence suggests that cyclosporin decreases prostacyclin synthesis. In addition, cyclosporin A may cause direct endothelial damage, increased thromboxane $A_2$ production, and adversely alter fibrinogen, circulating monocyte procoagulant activity, protein C, factor-VIII-related antigen, factor VIII coagulant activity, and adenosine diphosphate (ADP)-induced platelet aggregability.[30,119–122] Experimentally, the combination of preservation injury and subsequent administration of cyclosporin A increases thromboxane $A_2$ production.[123] In that regard, however, the relative contribution of preservation injury in the setting of live donor kidney transplantation is likely minimal. Finally, chronic exposure to cyclosporin A and steroids may also exhaust prostacyclin formation pathways (Table 16.11b-1).[30,123]

The potential impact of other, newer immunosuppressive agents, such as sirolimus, on graft thrombosis rates has yet to be established. For example, a recent multicenter liver transplant study reported an increased incidence of early hepatic artery thrombosis in adult recipients that were started on sirolimus early postoperatively.[124]

## Clinical Diagnosis, Treatment, and Prevention

Most early graft thromboses in pediatric recipients occur within the first 24 to 72 hours posttransplant. Over 75% of all graft thromboses are assumed to be venous. Clinical symptoms of graft thrombosis include rapidly declining or suddenly completely absent urine output, failure of the serum creatinine levels to decrease appropriately, graft tenderness (particularly for venous thromboses), unexplained hemoperitoneum (after venous thrombosis of intraperitoneal transplants), perigraft hematoma (after venous thrombosis of extraperitoneal transplants), and marked hematuria (with venous thrombosis). The first line diagnostic study to assess for graft thrombosis is transplant duplex ultrasonography. Diagnosis can also be established by a radionuclide scan, which is expected to reveal a photopenic defect with no uptake by the transplant kidney. Conventional angiography (the gold standard) is only rarely used because it is more invasive and complication-prone. In some cases, when imaging studies are inconclusive, relaparotomy, open inspection of the kidney graft, and open biopsy, as well as direct assessment of the renal vasculature will ascertain the diagnosis.

With extremely rare exceptions (eg, successful graft salvage in cases of partial renal vein thrombosis), the graft must be removed once the diagnosis of acute graft thrombosis has been made.

Unfortunately, there are only few preventive measures to minimize graft thrombosis rates. Although it was never formally studied, in recipients with congenital nephrotic syndrome bilateral pretransplant nephrectomy likely diminishes graft thrombosis risk by correcting at least partially the hypercoagulable state.[80–83] In recipients with prune-belly syndrome, it is advisable to proceed with nephropexy at the time of transplantation to minimize the risk for postoperative renal vascular pedicle torsion.[108,109] Besides avoiding or minimizing the impact of the aforementioned demographic risk factors (see section Incidence and Risk Factors and Table 16.11b-1) and optimizing surgical technique, there are no evidence-based guidelines as to the use of additional prophylactic measures to prevent graft thrombosis. Initial perioperative anticoagulation with heparin, followed by indefinite oral anticoagulation with coumadin, is recommended for all recipients in whom a hypercoagulable or thrombophilic state is suspected preoperatively (by laboratory studies or by clinical history).[115,116,125–127] It is unclear if patients that are only heterozygous for genetic abnormalities that have been associated with thrombophilic states should routinely receive specific perioperative thrombosis prophylaxis.

A typical empiric protocol for postoperative systemic heparinization includes observation of the recipient for a short time period after graft reperfusion. If no surgical bleeding is apparent, the patient is initially anticoagulated with a continuous intravenous heparin infusion at 50 to 200 U per hour. Over the following 2 to 3 days, the infusion rate is then gradually increased, targeting a prolongation of the PTT to 1.5 to 2 times of the upper limit of the normal PTT range.[31] Prior to discharge from the hospital, oral coumadin is instituted.[31]

Although suggested by one group, routine indefinite posttransplant prophylaxis with oral acetylsalicylic acid (ASA) has never been studied in a systematic fashion.[128]

## Other Surgical Complications

The exact incidence of posttransplant surgical complications in pediatric recipients is unknown. Overall incidence ranges between 10% and 20%, with the proportion of vascular complications increasing as recipient age decreases.[1,129–131]). The most common nonvascular surgical complications include ureteral complications (urine leak and ureteral obstruction), lymphoceles, and superficial and deep wound infections.[129,130,132] Complications that are specific to infants and small children with intraabdominal, intraperitoneal kidney grafts include small and large bowel injury as a consequence of the surgical mobilization and manipulation. The small bowel injury can occur as proximal as the duodenum and must be recognized early to avoid deleterious outcomes. In the rare case of orthotopic left-sided graft placement, native pancreatitis or a pancreatic fistula may occur as a result of the surgical manipulation during the dissection and should be treated conservatively.[93]

### Risk Factors

Poor nutrition is a risk factor for wound-healing complications. Therefore, the recipient's nutritional status warrants specific attention pretransplant. Particularly in children with nephrotic syndrome and significant urinary protein losses, pretransplant optimization of the nutritional status, in close coordination with the pediatric nephrology team is of utmost importance. In selected cases, pretransplant bilateral nephrectomy may be indicated to achieve that goal.[58,59]

Obesity, which is increasingly frequently encountered in pediatric kidney recipients, is—in addition to being a risk factor for graft thrombosis—also a risk factor for wound-healing complications.[110]

Sirolimus, particularly when given in combination with steroids for immunosuppression, is associated with a higher incidence of surgical complications, such as wound dehiscences, wound infections, and lymphoceles (with extraperitoneally placed kidney grafts). Avoidance of sirolimus "loading," delayed introduction of sirolimus (eg, 4–8 weeks posttransplant) and steroid-sparing or-avoiding immunosuppressive protocols may all help to minimize the adverse effects of this drug with regard to early posttransplant surgical wound complication incidence.[133]

### Lymphoceles

A recent report described a higher lymphocele incidence with the use of low-molecular-weight heparin in adult recipients.[134] Pediatric transplant recipients, who are overall at higher risk for graft thrombosis, tend to receive perioperative graft thrombosis prophylaxis with heparin more frequently than their adult counterparts. This finding would therefore be expected to be particularly relevant for pediatric recipients with an extraperitoneally placed graft that requires anticoagulation with heparin. As discussed above, sirolimus is also a significant risk factor for lymphocele formation.[133]

If symptomatic lymphoceles following extraperitoneal graft placement occur, one can first attempt nonoperative treatment (lymphocele aspiration, percutaneous drainage, with or without sclerosing therapy [eg, by injection of tetracycline or povidone iodine solution]). Symptomatic lymphoceles that fail, or are not amenable to, nonoperative treatment must be revised surgically. Laparoscopic lymphocele fenestration with or without marsupialization constitutes definitive treatment for those pediatric recipients.[135]

Preventive strategies for lymphocele formation include meticulous ligation of all perivascular lymphatic vessels prior to their division during the transplant operation and avoidance of sirolimus during the early posttransplant phase.[133] Routine peritoneal fenestration at the time of the transplant operation has been suggested for recipients of extraperitoneally placed

kidneys.[136] Potential disadvantages of this technique, however, include intraperitoneal spread of any perigraft infection, diffuse intraperitoneal urine extravasation in cases of a urinary leak, and the potential for intraabdominal adhesion formation and bowel obstruction due to the presence of intestine in the immediate vicinity of the graft site.

### Urologic Complications

Urologic complications include urinary leak, obstruction (eg, from ureteral stenosis), and stone formation. The reported overall incidence of urological complications in pediatric recipients ranges from 3% to 15%.[132] In general, these complications are managed as in adult recipients.

Briefly, small ureteral leaks may be stented (either antegrade or retrograde) in conjunction with prolonged bladder decompression by Foley catheter and percutaneous urinoma drainage. All other leaks, including those not resolving under conservative treatment, require operative reintervention.

Ureteral strictures have frequently an ischemic etiology and may be related to suboptimal live donor nephrectomy technique. Acute and chronic rejection may contribute to this process by also affecting the ureteral vasculature and blood supply. Importantly, the differential diagnosis of kidney graft ureteral obstruction must also include lymphoceles.

Isolated, short-segment ureteral strictures may be managed initially by an attempt at nonoperative balloon dilatation (balloon stricturoplasty). In selected recipients, ureteral strictures may be managed long-term by insertion of transanastomotic internal double-J ureteral stents. These stents require, however, periodic (eg, every 6 months) exchanges, which necessitate bladder instrumentation. This latter approach is therefore preferred in recipients that are not amenable to operative reintervention for anatomical reasons or because of an excessive operative risk, and for recipients whose graft has a relatively short anticipated remaining survival time and in whom a major operative reintervention would therefore not be justifiable. If transplant ureteral strictures involve multiple or (a) long(er) segment(s) (eg, in case of extensive proximal and/or distal ureteral ischemia), ureteral reimplantation (for distal strictures only), ureteroureterostomy (between the native and transplant ureter, for more proximal strictures) or pyelopyelostomy may be indicated. In patients whose native ureters are not usable and that have a very short remnant of undiseased ureter, creation of a new ureteroneocystomy may require creation of a Boari flap or the use of the psoas hitch technique.[137] Calyceal fistulas are rare and have frequently an ischemic etiology as well. They usually require surgical correction. The choice of surgical technique depends on localization and extent of the renal pelvis' ischemia and necrosis, and may involve the use of the recipient's native proximal ureter and ureteropelvic junction, or of the small bowel.[103–106]

## References

1. Ishitani M. Isaacs R, Norwood V, et al. Predictors of graft survival in pediatric living-related kidney transplant recipients. *Transplantation* 2000;70:288–292.
2. Salvatierra O Jr. A wake-up call for new strategies to improve living donor graft outcomes in pediatric kidney recipients. *Transplantation* 2000;70:262–263.
3. North American Pediatric Renal Transplant Cooperative Study (NAPRTCS). 2005 Annual Report. http://spitfile.emmes.com/study/ped/resources/annlrept2005.pdf

4. Sarwal MM, Cecka JM, Millan MT, et al. Adult-size kidneys without acute tubular necrosis provide exceedingly superior long-term graft outcomes for infants and small children. *Transplantation* 2000;70: 1728–1736.

5. Millan MT, Sarwal MM, Lemley KV, et al. A 100% 2-year graft survival can be attained in high-risk 15-kg or smaller infant recipients of kidney allografts. *Arch Surg* 2000;135:1063–1069.

6. Salvatierra O Jr, Singh T, Shifrin R, et al. Successful transplantation of adult-sized kidneys into infants requires maintenance of high aortic blood flow. *Transplantation* 1998;66:819–823.

7. Qvist E, Krogerus L, Rönnholm K, et al. Course of renal allograft histopathology after transplantation in early childnood. *Transplantation* 2000;70:480–487.

8. Salvatierra O Jr, Sarwal M: Course of renal allograft histopathology after transplantation in early childnood. *Transplantation* 2000;70:480 (editorial). *Transplantation* 2000;70:412–413.

9. Fine RN. Renal transplantation of the infant and young child and the use of pediatric cadaver kidneys for transplantation in pediatric and adult recipients. *Am J Kidney Dis* 1998;12:1–10.

10. Papalois VE, Najarian JS. Pediatric kidney transplantation: Historic hallmarks and a personal perspective. *Pediatr Transplant* 2001;5:239–245.

11. Davis ID, Bunchman TE, Grimm PC, et al. Pediatric renal transplantation: indications and special considerations. *Pediatr Transplant* 1998;2:117–129.

12. Ratner LE, Ciseck LJ, Moore RG, et al. Laparoscopic live donor nephrectomy. *Transplantation* 1995;60:1047–1049.

13. Troppmann C, Ormond DB, Perez RV. Laparoscopic (vs. open) live donor nephrectomy: A UNOS database analysis of early graft function and survival. *Am J Transplant* 2003;3:1295–1301.

14. Troppmann C, McBride MA, Baker TJ, et al. Laparoscopic live donor nephrectomy: A risk factor for delayed function and rejection in pediatric kidney recipients? A UNOS analysis. *Am J Transplant* 5: 175–182, 2005.

15. Troppmann C, Pierce JL, Wiesmann KM, et al: Early and late recipient graft function and donor outcome after laparoscopy vs open adult live donor nephrectomy for pediatric renal transplantation. *Arch Surg* 137: 908–916, 2002.

16. Kim DY, Stegall MD, Prieto M, et al: Hand-assisted laparoscopic donor nephrectomy for pediatric kidney allograft recipients. *Pediatr Transplant* 8: 460–463,2004.

17. Shafizadeh F, Ashcraft E, Baillie GM, et al: Laparoscopic donor nephrectomy for adults for pediatric living donor kidney transplantation. *Am J Transplant* 2001;1(Suppl 1):302.

18. Abrahams HM, Meng MV, Freise CE, et al. Laparoscopic donor nephrectomy for pediatric recipients: outcomes analysis. *Pediatr Urol* 2004;63:163–166.

19. Kayler LK, Merion RM, Maraschio MA, et al. Outcomes of pediatric living donor renal transplant after laparoscopic versus open donor nephrectomy. *Transplant Proc* 2002;34:3097–3098.

20. Singer JS, Ettenger RB, Gore JL, et al. Laparoscopic versus open renal procurement for pediatric recipients of living donor renal transplantation. *Am J Transplant* 2005;5:2514–2520.

21. Hsu TH, Su L-M, Trock BJ, et al. Laparoscopic adult donor nephrectomy for pediatric renal transplantation. *Urology* 2003;61:320–322.

22. Troppmann C, Wiesmann K, McVicar JP, et al. Increased transplantation of kidneys with multiple renal arteries in the laparoscopic live donor nephrectomy era. *Arch Surg* 2001;136:897–907.

23. Benedetti E, Troppmann C, Gillingham K, et al. Short- and long-term outcomes of kidney transplants with multiple renal arteries. *Ann Surg* 1995;221:406–414.

24. Ratner LE, Kavoussi LR, Chavin KD, et al. Laparoscopic live donor nephrectomy: technical considerations and allograft vascular length. *Transplantation* 1998;65:1657–1658.

25. Mandal AK, Cohen C, Montgomery RA, et al. Should the indications for laparoscopic live donor nephrectomy of the right kidney be the same as for the open procedure? Anomalous left renal vasculature is not a contraindication to laparoscopic left donor nephrectomy. *Transplantation* 2001;71:660–664.

26. Buell JF, Edye M, Johnson M, et al. Are concerns over right laparoscopic donor nephrectomy unwarranted? *Ann Surg* 2001;233:645–651.

27. Friedman AL, Peters TG, Jones KW, et al. Fatal and nonfatal hemorrhagic complications of living kidney donation. *Ann Surg* 2006;243:126–130.

28. Ratner LE, Hiller J, Sroka M, et al. Laparoscopic live donor nephrectomy removes disincentives to live donation. *Transplant* Proc 1997; 29:3402–3403.

29. Troppmann C, Johnston WK III, Pierce JL, et al. Impact of laparoscopic nephrectomy on donor preoperative decision-making and postoperative quality of life and psychosocial outcomes. *Pediatr Nephrol* 2006;21:1052–1054.

30. Troppmann C, Gruessner AC, Benedetti E, et al. Vascular graft thrombosis after pancreatic transplantation: univariate and multivariate operative and nonoperative risk factor analysis. *J Am Coll Surg* 1996;182:285–316.

31. Troppmann C. Surgical complications. In Gruessner RWG, Sutherland DER, eds. *Pancreas Transplantation*. New York: Springer-Verlag Publishers; 2005:206–237.

32. Molmenti EP, Varkarakis IM, Pinto P, et al. Renal transplantation with iliac vein transposition. *Transplant Proc* 2004;36:2643–2645.

33. Nghiem DD. Spiral gonadal vein graft extension of right renal vein in living renal transplantation. *J Urol* 1989;142:1525.

34. Reissman P, Anner H, Lias S, et al. A simple technique for the use of a variable length compilation vein graft in major venous injury. *J Am Coll Surg* 181:175–177,1995.

35. Rosenblatt GS, Conlin MJ, Soule JL, et al. Right renal vein extension with recipient left renal vein after laparoscopic donor nephrectomy. *Transplantation* 2006;81:138–139.

36. Nguyen NT, Perez RV, Fleming N, et al. Effect of prolonged pneumoperitoneum on intraoperative urine output during laparoscopic gastric bypass. *J Am Coll Surg* 2002;195:476–483.

37. Chiu AW, Chang LS, Birkett DH, et al. The impact of pneumoperitoneum, pneumoretroperitoneum, and gasless laparoscopy on the systemic and renal hemodynamics. *J Am Coll Surg* 1995;181:397–406.

38. McDougall EM, Monk TG, Wolf JS Jr, et al. The effect of prolonged pneumoperitoneum on renal function in an animal model. *J Am Coll Surg* 1996;182:317–328.

39. Ratner LE, Montgomery RA, Maley WR, et al. Laparoscopic live donor nephrectomy. the recipient. *Transplantation* 2000;69:2319–2323.

40. Nogueira JM, Cangro CB, Fink JC, et al. A comparison of recipient renal outcomes with laparoscopic versus open live donor nephrectomy. *Transplantation* 1999;67:722–728.

41. Velidedeoglu E, Williams N, Brayman KL, et al. Comparison of open, laparoscopic, and hand-assisted approaches to live-donor nephrectomy. *Transplantation* 2002;74:169–172.

42. Troppmann C, Cors C, Perez R, et al. Laparoscopic vs. open live donor nephrectomy: an OPTN database analysis of long-term kidney graft function and survival of 5532 transplants with >5 years follow-up. *Am J Transplant* and *Transplantation* (Suppl): 6: 804, abstract # 2231, World Transplant Congress, 2006.

43. Salvatierra O, Sarwal M. Vulnerability of small pediatric recipients to laparoscopic living donor kidneys. *Am J Transplant* 2005;5:201–202.

44. Troppmann C, Gillingham J, Benedetti E, et al. Delayed graft function, acute rejection, and outcome after cadaver renal transplantation. *Transplantation* 1995;59:962–968.

45. Humar A, Ramcharan T, Kandaswamy R, et al. Risk factors for slow graft function after kidney transplants: a multivariate analysis. *Clin Transplant* 2002;16:425–429.

46. Tejani A, Sullivan EK. The impact of acute rejection on chronic rejection: A report of the North American Pediatric Renal Transplant Cooperative Study. *Pediatr Transplant* 2000;4:107–111.

47. Matas AJ. Impact of acute rejection on development of chronic rejection in pediatric renal transplant recipients. *Pediatr Transplant* 2000;4:92–99.

48. Halloran PF, Melk A, Barth C. Rethinking chronic allograft nephropathy: The concept of accelerated senescence. *J Am Soc Nephrol* 1999;10: 167–181.

49. Kuo PC, Johnson LB. Laparoscopic donor nephrectomy increases the supply of living donor kidneys. *Transplantation* 2000;69:2211–2213.

50. Schweitzer EJ, Wilson J, Jacobs S, et al. Increased rates of donation with laparoscopic donor nephrectomy. *Ann Surg* 2000;232:392–400.

51. McDonald SP, Craig JC: Long-term survival of children with end-stage renal disease. *N Engl J Med* 2004;350:2654–2662.

52. London ET, Ho HS, Neuhaus AMC, et al. Effect of intravascular volume expansion on renal function during prolonged CO2 pneumoperitoneum. *Ann Surg* 2000;231:195–201.

53. Carlier M, Squifflet J-P, Pirson Y, et al. Maximal hydration during anesthesia increases pulmonary arterial pressures and improves early function of human renal transplants. *Transplantation* 1982;34:201–204.

54. Wiesmann KM, Gallay BJ, Foster S, et al. Hypertonic saline infusion during laparoscopic donor nephrectomy increases renal prostaglandin production and COX-1 transcription: implications for renoprotection. *Am J Transplant* 2002;2(Suppl 3):415 (abstract #1100).

55. Simmons RL, Najarian JS. Kidney transplantation. In: Simmons RL, Finch ME, Ascher NL, Najarian JS, eds: *Manual of Vascular Access, Organ Donation, and Transplantation.* New York: Springer-Verlag; 1984:292–328.

56. Yata N, Nakanishi K, Uemura S, et al. Evaluation of the inferior vena cava in potential pediatric renal transplant recipients. *Pediatr Nephrol* 2004;19:1062–1064.

57. Thomas SE, Hickman RO, Tapper D, et al. Asymptomatic inferior vena cava abnormalities in three children with end-stage renal disease: Risk factors and screening guidelines for pretransplant diagnosis. *Pediatr Transplant* 2000;4:28–34.

58. Salvatierra O Jr, Tanney D, Mak R, et al: Pediatric renal transplantation and its challenges. *Transplant Rev* 11:51–69,1997.

59. Salvatierra O Jr, Alexander SR, Krensky AM. Pediatric kidney transplantation at Stanford. *Pediatr Transplant* 1998;2:165–176.

60. Ramirez SPB, Lebowitz RL, Harmon WE, et al. Predictors for abnormal voiding cystourethrography in pediatric patients undergoing renal transplant evaluation. *Pediatr Transplant* 2001;5:99–104.

61. Rudge CJ. Transplantation and the abnormal bladder. In: Morris PJ ed. *Kidney Transplantation, 5th ed.* Philadelphia: Saunders;2001:173–183.

62. Lopez Pereira P, Jaureguizar E, Martinez Urrutia MJ, et al. Does treatment of bladder dysfunction prior to renal transplant improve outcome in patients with posterior urethral valves? *Pediatr Transplant* 2000;4:118–122.

63. Luke PPW, Herz DB, Bellinger MK, et al. Long-term results of pediatric renal transplantation into a dysfunctional lower urinary tract. *Transplantation* 2003;76:1578–1582.

64. Koo HP, Bunchman TE, Flynn JT, et al. Renal transplantation in children with severe lower urinary tract dysfunction. *J Urol* 1999;161:240–245.

65. Rigamonti W, Capizzi A, Zacchello G, et al. Kidney transplantation into bladder augmentation or urinary diversion: long-term results. *Transplantation* 2005;80:1435–1440.

66. Mitchell ME. Bladder augmentation in children: where have we been and where are we going? *Br J Urol* 2003; 92(Suppl 1):29–34.

67. Fangmann J, Oldhafer K, Offner G, et al. Retroperitoneal placement of living related adult renal grafts in children less than 5 years of age—a feasible technique? *Transpl Int* 1996;9(Suppl 1):S73–S75.

68. Tanabe K, Takahashi K, Kawaguchi H, et al. Surgical complications of pediatric kidney transplantation: a single center experience with the extraperitoneal technique. *J Urol* 160: 1212–1215,1998.

69. Carter JT, Freise CE, McTaggart RA, et al: Laparoscopic procurement of kidneys with multiple renal arteries is associated with increased ureteral complications in the recipient. *Am J Transplant* 2005;5:1312–1318.

70. Politano VA, Leadbetter WF. An operative technique for the correction of vesicoureteral reflux. *J Urol* 1958;79:932–941.

71. Lich R, Howerton LW, Davis LA. Recurrent urosepsis in children. *J Urol* 1961;86:554.

72. Shanfield I. New experimental methods for implantation of ureter in bladder and conduit. *Transplant Proc* 1972;4:637–638.

73. Sumrani NB, Lipkowitz GS, Hong JH, et al. Complications of "one stitch" extravesical ureteric implantation in renal transplants in the cyclosporine and precyclosporine eras. *Transplant Proc* 1989;21(1 Pt 2):1957–1959.

74. Mangus RS, Haag BW. Stented versus nonstented extravesical ureteroneocystostomy in renal transplantation: a metaanalysis. *Am J Transplant* 2004;4:1889–1896.

75. Wilson CH, Bhatti AA, Rix AA, et al. Routine intraoperative ureteric stenting for kidney transplant recipients. *Cochrane Database Syst Rev* 2005;19;(4):CD004925.

76. Salvatierra O Jr, Sarwal M, Alexander S, et al. A new, unique and simple method for ureteral implantation in kidney recipients with small, defunctionalized bladders. *Transplantation* 1999;68:731–738.

77. Mesrobian HG, Miller CG, Hatchett RL, et al. Modified extravesical ureteral reimplantation in pediatric renal transplantation: 5 years of experience. *J Urol* 1992;147:1340–1342.

78. LaPointe SP, Charbit M, Jan D, et al. Urological complications after renal transplantation using ureteroureteral anastomosis in children. *J Urol* 2001;166:1046–1048.

79. Hakim NS, Benedetti E, Pirenne J, et al. Complications of ureterovesical anastomosis in kidney transplant patients: the Minnesota experience. *Clin Transplant* 1994;8:504–507.

80. Kim MS, Stablein D, Harmon WE. Renal transplantation in children with congenital nephrotic syndrome: a report of the North American Pediatric Renal Transplant Cooperative Study (NAPRTCS). *Pediatr Transplant* 1998;2:305–308.

81. Mahan JD, Mauer SM, Sibley RK, et al. Congenital nephrotic syndrome: evolution of medical management and results of renal transplantation. *J Pediatr* 1984;105:549–557.

82. Holmberg C, Antikainen M, Ronnholm K, et al. Management of congenital nephrotic syndrome of the Finnish type. *Pediatr Nephrol* 1995;9:87–93.

83. Kim MS, Primack W, Harmon WE. Congenital nephrotic syndrome: preemptive bilateral nephrectomy and dialysis before renal transplantation. *J Am Soc Nephrol* 1992;3:260–263.

84. Pirenne J, Benedetti E, Kashtan CE, et al. Kidney transplantation in the absence of the infrarenal vena cava. *Transplantation* 1995;59:1739–1742.

85. Arrazola L, Long A, Moss A, et al. An absent inferior vena cava in a pediatric renal transplant recipient. *Clin Transplant* 2000;14:360–362.

86. Badet L, Lezrek M, Alves Saraiva W, et al. Techniques de transplantation rénale chez des enfants présentant un trouble de la perméabilité de la veine cave inférieure ou des veines iliaques. *Urologie Pédiatrique* 2005;15:285–290.

87. Mulvihill SJ, Fonkalsrud EW. Complications of superior versus inferior vena cava occlusion in infants receiving central total parenteral nutrition. *J Pediatr Surg* 1984;19:752–757.

88. Waltzer WC, Zincke H, Sterioff S. Renal transplantation. *Arch Surg* 1980;115:987–988.

89. Stippel DL, Bangard C, Schleimer K, et al. Successful renal transplantation in a child with thrombosis of the inferior vena cava and both iliac veins. *Transplant Proc* 2006;38:688–690.

90. Hajivassiliou CA, Wilkinson AG, Azmy A, et al. Renal transplantation in a child with iliac vein thrombosis and absence of superior and inferior venae cavae. *Nephrol Dial Transplant* 1997;12:1269–1270.

91. Wolf P, Boudjema K, Ellero B, et al. Transplantation rénale en cas de thrombose de la veine cave inférieure. Implantation de la veine du greffon dans la veine porte. *La Presse Médicale* 1988;17:957–959.

92. Mozes MF, Kjellstrand CM, Simmons RL, et al. Orthotopic renal homotransplantation in a patient with thrombosis of the inferior vena cava. *Am J Surg* 1976;131:633–636.

93. Gil-Vernet JM, Gil-Vernet A, Caralps A, et al. Orthotopic renal transplant and results in 139 consecutive cases. *J Urol* 1989;142:248–252.

94. Talbot-Wright R, Carretero P, Alcaraz A, et al. Complex renal transplant for vascular reasons. *Transplant Proc* 1992;24:1865–1866.

95. Marinov M, Di Domenico S, Mastrodomenico P, et al. Use of the splenic vessels for an ABO incompatible renal transplant in a patient with thrombosis of the vena cava. *Am J Transplant* 2006;5:2336–2337.

96. Shapira Z, Yussim A, Savir A, et al. The use of portal system for the transplantation of a neonate kidney graft in a child with Wilms' tumor. *J Pediatr Surg* 1985;20:549–551.

97. Hayes JM. The transplantation of difficult donor kidneys and recipients: helpful surgical techniques. *J Urol* 1993;149:250–254.

98. Aguirrezabalaga J, Novas S, Veiga F, et al. Renal transplantation with venous drainage through the superior mesenteric vein in cases of thrombosis of the inferior vena cava. *Clin Transplant* 2002;74:413–415.

99. Rosenthal JT, Loo RK. Portal venous drainage for cadaveric renal transplantation. *J Urol* 1990;144:969–971.

100. Patel P, Krishnamurthi V. Successful use of the inferior mesenteric vein for renal transplantation. *Am J Transplant* 2003;3:1040.

101. Troppmann C, Gjertson DW, Cecka JM, McVicar J, Perez RV. Impact of portal venous pancreas graft drainage on kidney graft outcome in pancreas-kidney recipients reported to UNOS. *Am J Transplant* 2004;4:544–553.

102. Gibel LJ, Chakerian M, Harford A, et al. Transplantation using inverted renal unit and donor vena cava-iliac vein conduit to bypass recipient distal vena cava and iliac venous systems. *J Urol* 1988;140:1480–1481.

103. Blaszak RT, Dunn JF, Finck CM. Use of appendix for complete transplant ureteral necrosis. *Pediatr Transplant* 2003;7:243–246.

104. Furtwangler A, el Saman A, Pisarski P, et al. Temporary small bowel interposition for urinary drainage after partial necrosis of the renal graft pelvis following living related renal donation. *Transplant Proc* 2003;35:944–945.

105. Wolters HH, Palmes D, Brockman J, et al. Therapeutical options in ureteral necrosis following kidney transplantation. *Transplant Int* 2006; 19:516–518.

106. Wolters HH, Palmes D, Krieglstein CF, et al. Reconstruction of ureteral necrosis in kidney transplantation using an ileum interposition. *Transplant Proc* 2006;38:691–692.

107. Singh A, Stablein D, Tejani A. Risk factors for vascular thrombosis in pediatric renal transplantation. A special report of the North American Renal Transplant Cooperative Study. *Transplantation* 1997;63:1263–1267.

108. Abbit PL, Chevalier RL, Rodgers BM, et al. Acute torsion of a renal transplant: cause of organ loss. *Pediatr Nephrol* 1990;4:174–175.

109. Marvin RG, Halff GA, Elshihabi I. Renal allograft torsion associated with prune-belly syndrome. *Pediatr Nephrol* 1995;9:81–82.

110. Hanevold CD, Ho P-L, Talley L, et al. Obesity and renal transplant outcome: a report of the North American Pediatric Renal Transplant Cooperative Study. *Pediatrics* 2005;115:352–356.

111. Vats AN, Donaldson L, Fine RN, et al. Pretransplant dialysis status and outcome of renal transplantation in North American children: a NAPRTCS study. *Transplantation* 2000;69:1414–1419.

112. McDonald RA, Smith JM, Stablein D, et al. Pretransplant peritoneal dialysis and graft thrombosis following pediatric kidney transplantation: a NAPRTCS report. *Pediatr Transplant* 2003;7:204–208.

113. Jones CL, Andrew M, Eddy A, et al. Coagulation abnormalities in chronic peritoneal dialysis. *Pediatr Nephrol* 1990;4:152–155.

114. Ojo AO, Hanson JA, Wolfe RA, et al. Dialysis modality and the risk of allograft thrombosis in adult renal transplant recipients. *Kidney Int* 1999;55:1952–1960.

115. Dick AA, Lerner SM, Boissy AR, et al. Excellent outcome in infants and small children with thrombophilias undergoing kidney transplantation. *Pediatr Transplant* 2005;9:39–42.

116. Wheeler MA, Taylor CM, Williams M, et al. Factor V Leiden: a risk factor for renal vein thrombosis in renal transplantation. *Pediatr Nephrol* 2000;14:525–526.

117. Smith JM, Stablein D, Singh A, Harmon W, McDonald RA. Decreased risk of renal allograft thrombosis associated with interleukin-2 receptor antagonists: A report of the NAPRTCS. *Am J Transplant* 2006;6: 585–588.

118. Vanrenterghem Y, Roels L, Lerut T, et al. Thromboembolic complications and haemostatic changes in cyclosporine-treated cadaveric kidney allograft recipients. *Lancet* 1985;1(8436):999–1002.

119. Mackie IJ, Blewitt S, Clarke P, et al. The effects of long-term cyclosporin A therapy postrenal transplantation on haemostasis. *Br J Haematol* 1986;64 812–813.

120. Neild GH, Reuben R, Hartley RB, et al. Glomerular thrombi in renal allografts associated with cyclosporine treatment. *J Clin Pathol* 1985;38: 253–258.

121. Neild GH, Rocchi G, Imberti L, et al. Effect of cyclosporin A on prostacyclin synthesis by vascular tissue. *Thromb Res* 1983;32:373–379.

122. Perico N, Remuzzi G. Thromboembolic complications during cyclosporin A therapy: Possible causes and incidence. In: Remuzzi G, Rossi EC, eds. *Haemostasis and the Kidney.* London: Butterworth & Co.; 1989:321–330.

123. Odor-Morales A, Lopez RM, Varela G, et al. Increased thromboxane production by the pancreas after 24-hour preservation in UW-1 solution. *Transplant Proc* 1991;23:1643–1644.

124. Wiesner R, Klintmalm G, McDiarmid S, et al. Sirolimus decreases acute rejection rates in de novo orthotopic liver transplant recipients. *Liver Transplant* 2002;8(Suppl): C-16

125. Morrissey PE, Ramirez PJ, Gohh RY, et al. Management of thrombophilia in renal transplant patients. *Am J Transplant* 2002;2:872–876.

126. Segel GB, Francis CW. Anticoagulant proteins in childhood venous and arterial thrombosis: a review. *Blood Cells Molecules Dis* 2000;26: 540–560.

127. Friedman GS, Meier-Kriesche H-U, Kaplan B, et al. Hypercoagulable states in renal transplant candidates: impact of anticoagulation upon incidence of renal allograft thrombosis. *Transplantation* 2001;72: 1073–1078.

128. Robertson AJ, Nargund V, Gray DWR, et al. Low dose aspirin as prophylaxis against renal-vein thrombosis in renal-transplant recipients. *Nephrol Dial Transplant* 2000;15:1865–1868.

129. Sheldon CA, Churchill BM, Khoury AE, et al. Complications of surgical significance in pediatric renal transplantation. *J Pediatr Surg* 1992;27:485–490.

130. Shokeir AA, Osman Y, Ali-El-Dein B, et al. Surgical complications in live-donor pediatric and adolescent renal transplantation: Study of risk factors. *Pediatr Transplant* 2005;9:33–38.

131. Harmon WE, Stablein D, Alexander SR, et al. Graft thrombosis in pediatric renal transplant recipients. *Transplantation* 1991;51:406–412.

132. Nuininga JE, Feitz WFJ, van Dael KCML, et al. Urological complications in pediatric renal transplantation. *Eur Urol* 2001;39:598–602.

133. Troppmann C, Pierce JL, Ghandi MM, et al. Higher surgical wound complication rates with sirolimus immunosuppression after kidney transplantation: a matched-pair pilot study. *Transplantation* 76: 426–429,2003.

134. Lundin C, Bersztel A, Wahlberg J, et al. Low molecular weight heparin prophylaxis increases the incidence of lymphocele after kidney transplantation. *Upsala J Med Sci* 2002;107:9–15.

135. Dammeier BG, Lehnhardt A, Glüer S, et al. Laparoscopic fenestration of posttransplant lymphoceles in children. *J Pediatr Surg* 2004;39: 1230–1232.

136. Zaontz MR, Firlit CF. Pelvic lymphocele after pediatric renal transplantation: a successful technique for prevention. *J Urol* 1988;139:557–559.

137. Cranston D, Little D. Urological complications after renal transplantation. In: Morris PJ, ed. *Kidney Transplantation, 5th ed.* Philadelphia: WB Saunders Co.; 2001:435–444.

# 16.12 PREEMPTIVE LIVING TRANSPLANTATION: THE IDEAL THERAPEUTIC MODALITY FOR END-STAGE RENAL DISEASE

*Herwig-Ulf Meier-Kriesche, MD, Jesse D. Schold, MStat, MEd*

Based on the premise of the large survival advantage conferred by kidney transplantation as a treatment modality for end-stage renal disease (ESRD) compared to maintenance dialysis, it is not surprising that overall prognoses improve if patients get transplanted as soon as they approach ESRD. As the demand for renal transplantation has increased, and the consequent organ shortage has prolonged waiting times for deceased donor organs, the only way to ensure a timely preemptive transplant is to rely on a living donation. The additional benefit of a living donation is the higher quality of the organ, which portends significantly longer graft life expectancy on average, and enhances the overall prognosis of the recipient over a deceased donor transplant.

In this chapter we discuss in detail the data pertinent to the survival advantage of kidney transplantation over dialysis, the variability in donor kidney quality, the damaging and long-lasting harmful effects of maintenance dialysis, potential mechanisms of damage in patients with very limited renal clearance, and finally the economic and quality-of-life considerations of living donor transplantation. These considerations together highlight that in the current situation in the United States, and likewise in many other countries, preemptive living donor kidney transplantation is the optimal treatment option for patients with approaching ESRD.

## THE SURVIVAL BENEFIT OF RENAL TRANSPLANTATION

The prevalence of ESRD in the United States has increased dramatically over the past 30 years. Although the vast majority of patients with ESRD are treated with dialysis, this time period has witnessed the growth of kidney transplantation as a viable treatment option for this population. The development of immunosuppressive therapies, increased understandings of immunology, clinical-care improvements, and enhanced surgical techniques have led to major advances in the utility of renal transplantation. The role of transplantation as the preferred therapy for ESRD patients and the timing of transplantation in the ESRD process have subsequently undergone a paradigm shift in the modern era.

Although the advantages of transplantation had been suspected for many years, concrete evidence that transplantation is superior to dialysis therapy was not formalized until the landmark publication by Wolfe et al. in 1999.[1] As this research elucidated, renal transplantation for deceased donor recipients was shown to portend a highly significant benefit for patient survival relative to a control group of patients medically cleared for transplantation and placed on the waiting list (Figure 16.12-1). In addition, the survival advantage applied to all categories of patients by age, race, and primary cause of renal disease. Furthermore, these results have been demonstrated in countries outside of the United States, which present variations in

health-care systems and patient demographics.[2–4] The protective nature of transplantation has additionally been replicated across patient body mass index groups and in transplantation of lower quality donations.[5,6] This analysis by Ojo et al. importantly demonstrated that a survival advantage persisted among transplant recipients of lower quality kidneys; however, the magnitude of this advantage was substantially reduced relative to standard kidneys.

## DELETERIOUS EFFECTS OF PRETRANSPLANT DIALYSIS

As kidney transplantation confers a survival advantage over maintenance dialysis, it is expectable that prolonged dialysis treatments will be harmful to patients. The additional question to be answered would be if maintenance dialysis confers a lasting damage imprint in patients with ESRD. In fact, the duration of dialysis has been demonstrated in a variety of contexts to be associated with outcomes following transplantation. In a single-center study, Cosio et al. were able to demonstrate that pretransplant dialysis was a significant risk factor for posttransplant death (p = 0.0003) and overall graft loss (p = 0.0003).[7] Results derived from another single-center experience from 1980 to 1995 indicated that the advantages of preemptive transplantation were particularly noteworthy among living donor transplant recipients.[8] A U.S. Renal Data System (USRDS) registry analysis extended this concept by demonstrating that not only did preemptive transplantation confer a survival advantage but also that time on dialysis was a dose-dependent risk factor for graft loss and patient death after both living and cadaveric transplantation.[9] This analysis reported that as little as 6 to 12 months of pretransplant dialysis was associated with a 37% increase in long-term graft loss as compared to preemptive transplants (Figure 16.12-2). This study also suggested that the effect of pretransplant dialysis on posttransplant survival was not attributable to disease lead time, as a proportionally equal effect was observed in patients with ESRD secondary to diabetes, glomerulonephritis, and hypertension. In addition, this analysis demonstrated that the impact of pretransplant dialysis time on graft survival was mediated by a direct effect on patient survival, and to a minor, but still clinically important degree, by its effect on death-censored graft survival. In a similar analysis, Mange

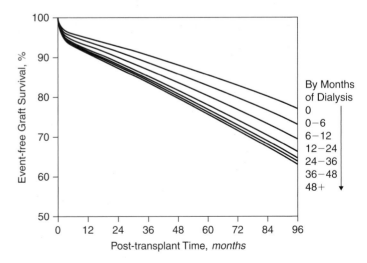

**FIGURE 16.12-2**

Increasing pretransplant dialysis time as a risk factor for graft loss. Reproduced with permission from *Kidney International* 2000;58(3):1311–1317.

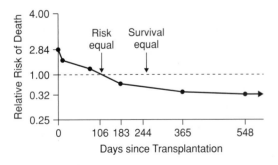

**FIGURE 16.12-1**

Survival advantage of renal transplantation over maintenance dialysis. Figure represents the relative risk of death associated with transplantation (solid line) relative to patients who have been placed on the waiting list for transplantation on dialysis (dotted line) over time. Reproduced with permission from *The New England Journal of Medicine* 1999; 341(23):1725–1730.

et al. confirmed this direct association between the duration of pretransplant dialysis and the rate of allograft loss in living transplant recipients utilizing registry data in the United States.[10] These studies emphasized the importance for patients with severe chronic renal failure to be transplanted as soon as possible, preferably before starting dialysis.

Despite of all the emerging evidence that pretransplant dialysis had a strong negative impact on prospective transplant candidates, there remained concern that part of the explanation for these results might be the willingness of prospective recipients to accept marginal kidneys when faced with extensive waiting time. This concern was addressed in a retrospective population-based paired kidney analysis.[11] In this study, only kidney pairs were analyzed, of which one kidney went into a recipient who had been on dialysis for less than 6 months, whereas the mate kidney was transplanted to a patient that had been on dialysis for more than 2 years. This study design eliminated the possibility of donor selection bias. As displayed in Figure 16.12-3, recipients with less than 6 months of pretransplant dialysis had significantly greater 10-year graft survival as compared with patients with greater than 24 months pretransplant dialysis (63% vs 29%, p < 0.0001). Patient survival was also superior in the cohort transplanted after a shorter period of dialysis. Despite the elevated risk for death and graft loss in patients who had been dialyzed for extended periods prior to transplant, even patients on dialysis for more than 4 years have improved survival expectancy compared to dialysis patients of the same vintage who remain on the waiting list. Similarly, results from a North American Pediatric Renal Transplant Cooperative Study found improved graft survival (p = 0.0003) and reduced rates of acute tubular necrosis (ATN; p < .0001) associated with preemptive transplantation in pediatric recipients as compared to patients who received either hemodialysis or peritoneal dialysis prior to transplantation.[12]

Pretransplant dialysis time has also been shown to impact patient survival following graft loss. In a retrospective study, more than 2 years of pretransplant dialysis was associated with more than a twofold relative risk for overall and for cardiovascular related death after graft loss (DAGL) based on U.S. registry data from 1988 to 1998.[13] Infections as a cause of graft loss were also

highly associated with DAGL (RR = 1.64, p < 0.0001). Of equal importance, the study did not find an association between the times that patients retained their transplant prior to graft loss and DAGL, supporting the notion of dialysis-mediated damage as the primary contributor to DAGL. These results indicate that exposure to dialysis persist in the long-term and has potentially irreversible consequences on patient mortality. As mentioned above, cardiovascular disease progression might be delayed or even reversed as long as patients have a functioning transplant, but the overall cardiovascular disease burden of a patient who has been on dialysis longer prior to transplant is higher, and that elevated risk expressed even after the patients lose their grafts. One might have expected that (assuming similar comorbidities) patients maintaining graft function longer would die sooner after graft loss than those who lose their grafts quickly because the former group is exposed to the risk of cardiovascular disease for a longer time. The fact that the risk of DAGL is unaffected by the length of time that a graft functions supports the concept that transplantation is protective. This might be explained by the intrinsic cardiovascular benefits conferred by a functioning transplant. As expected, there was a marked increase in cardiovascular death rates once the patients had lost the protective effect of the kidney transplant. Cardiovascular death rates are increased more than 10-fold in patients after allograft loss compared to patients with a functioning transplant. The late increase in cardiovascular death rates by transplant vintage is in fact due to increasing graft loss, as this phenomenon is not observed as long patients keep a functioning transplant.

These observations are consistent with the hypothesis that extended exposure to dialysis subjects patients to the adverse effects of chronic kidney disease, such that patients are in a relatively disadvantaged state by the time they undergo the transplant procedure. These effects may include altered concentrations of homocysteine, lipids, and advanced glycosylation end products as well as a generalized inflammatory state. These biochemical changes may predispose patients to cardiovascular damage and vascular damage to the allograft. Patients on dialysis also tend to suffer from poor nutrition and may be less tolerant of immunosuppressive agents after transplantation.[14]

Although the data presented indicate that maintenance dialysis is harmful to patients, this must be taken in proper context, as only a minor fraction of the dialysis population are candidates for transplantation. For those patients deemed unsuitable for transplantation, dialysis is obviously life saving.

## THE KIDNEY TRANSPLANT WAITING LIST

The perceived efficacy of kidney transplantation and the increasing incidence and prevalence of ESRD in the United States have contributed to an increased demand for the procedure. As a result, the waiting list for transplantation has expanded at a precipitous rate. In comparison, despite a significant surge in living donations, the overall rate of available donations has not been able to match the increasing demand for kidney transplantation (Figure 16.12-4). As a consequence, waiting times for a deceased donor transplant have increased significantly. Projections estimate a continued acceleration of the wait-list volume with approximately 100,000 patients listed for kidney transplantation by the year 2010.[15] Particularly for patients with poor prognoses on dialysis, such as older patients or for those patients listed at centers with extended waiting lists, the appeal of a living transplant that can be done preemptively is that much stronger. Figure 16.12-5 illustrates this point, as progressively older patients are more likely

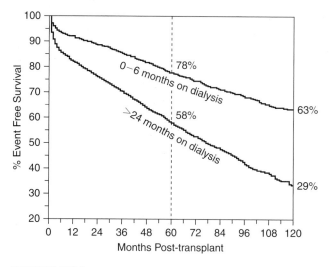

**FIGURE 16.12-3**

Paired kidney study for impact of pretransplant dialysis on long-term graft survival. Reproduced with permission from Tran*splantation* 2002;74(10): 1377–1381.

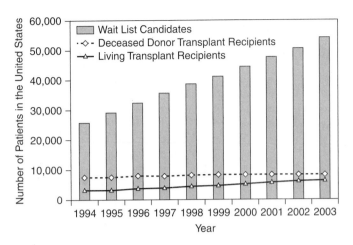

**FIGURE 16.12-4**

Number of patients transplanted and waiting for transplant 1994–2003. Data derived from 2004 SRTR Annual Report.

to die while on the waiting list, and consequently the longer expected time to transplant in older transplant candidates reflects the relative unlikelihood of older patients reaching transplantation before death. In addition, the most rapidly expanding wait-listing group consists of older candidates, who may have the greatest incentive to seek a preemptive living donation.[16]

## RELATIONSHIP BETWEEN RENAL FUNCTION AND CARDIOVASCULAR DISEASE PROGRESSION

The association between renal failure and cardiovascular disease is explained in part by predisposing factors shared by the two illnesses, such as hypertension, dyslipidemia, and diabetes (Table 16.12-1). Substantial evidence also indicates that renal insufficiency itself may predispose patients to the development and progression of cardiovascular disease. Epidemiological studies in chronic kidney disease cannot discern the common risk factors for renal disease and cardiac disease and extrapolate renal function as an independent factor driving the progression of heart disease. Perhaps a part of the explanation for the association between mild renal failure and increased cardiovascular risk is that the processes that caused renal failure also damage the cardiovascular system. On the other hand, kidney transplantation offers an ideal oppor-

**TABLE 16.12-1**

**UNADJUSTED SURVIVAL RATES BY TRANSPLANT MODALITY**

| Transplant Type | 3-Month Survival Rate | 1-Year Survival Rate | 3-Year Survival Rate | 5-Year Survival Rate |
| --- | --- | --- | --- | --- |
| Living | 97.0 | 94.6 | 87.4 | 79.2 |
| Non-ECD* Deceased Donor | 94.8 | 90.5 | 79.3 | 68.9 |
| ECD Deceased Donor | 88.9 | 80.1 | 66.5 | 51.4 |

*Source:* 2004 SRTR Annual Data Report.

*ECD, expanded criteria donors.

tunity to test the hypothesis that renal function itself is linked to cardiovascular disease progression, as the quality of the donor kidney and the resulting kidney function of the recipient are independent of the cardiovascular disease burden of the patient. This association was demonstrated in a national study of patients transplanted between 1988 and 1998, in which 1-year posttransplant renal function was strongly and inversely associated with subsequent cardiovascular death rates.[17] Although this study does not address how, and through which potential mediators, renal function impacts cardiovascular risk, it shows a direct relation of impaired renal function to cardiovascular disease progression.

If decreased renal function is a major driving force for cardiovascular disease progression, one might expect that the cardiovascular risk profile of the patients with ESRD would be favorably influenced by restoration of renal function. A retrospective study addressing this issue compared wait-listed dialysis patients to transplant patients and showed a progressive increase in the incidence of cardiovascular death by dialysis vintage even in the highly selected dialysis patients on the transplant waiting list as displayed in Figure 16.12-6.[18] However, after successful kidney transplantation, the cardiovascular death rate decreased progressively by

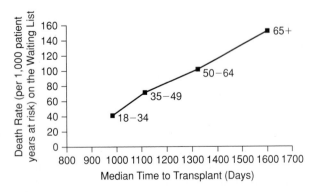

**FIGURE 16.12-5**

Death rate on the kidney waiting list versus median time to transplant by age group—1999. Source: 2004 SRTR Annual Report.

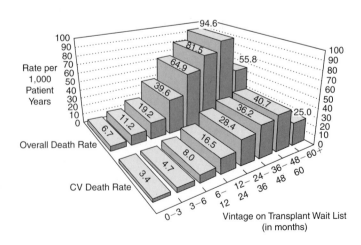

**FIGURE 16.12-6**

Overall and cardiovascular death rates by wait-list vintage 1995–2000 (censored at transplant) . Reproduced with permission from *Am J Transplant* 2004;4(10):1662–1668.

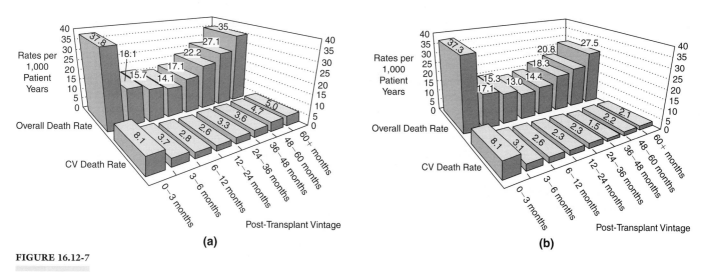

**FIGURE 16.12-7**

(a) Overall and cardiovascular death rates by posttransplant vintage for living donor transplant recipients 1995–2000. Reproduced with permission from *Am J Transplant* 2004;4(10):1662–1668. (b) Overall and cardiovascular death rates by posttransplant vintage for living donor transplant recipients 1995–2000 (censored at graft loss). Reproduced with permission from *Am J Transplant* 2004;4(10):1662–1668.

transplant vintage, and remained low in the long term, provided patients retained their grafts as displayed in Figures 16.12-7 (a) and (b).

## POTENTIAL MECHANISMS OF THE DAMAGING EFFECTS OF RENAL FAILURE AND DIALYSIS

Several risk factors associated with chronic renal failure and dialysis can be implicated in the link between decreased renal function and cardiovascular disease progression. These phenomena occur with increased frequency in patients with chronic renal failure and uremia and are either established or at least biologically plausible cardiovascular risk factors. Identification and reduction of uremia-related risk factors in patients with kidney disease is now recommended, in parallel with targeting of traditional risk factors. It is reasonable to presume that many of the uremia-mediated risk factors themselves cause damage and contribute to the elevated risk for patients undergoing kidney transplantation after extended periods of maintenance dialysis.

## DONOR KIDNEY QUALITY

Clearly there is a wide variability in the quality of the organs available for transplantation. One of the most important prognostic variables for the survival expectancy of the graft is in fact the quality of the transplanted organ. As patient survival is crucially linked to a functioning transplant, it is not surprising that also patient survival increases significantly with better quality transplant kidneys. Several studies have demonstrated a marked association between deceased donor quality and graft and patient survival.[19,20] Advanced donor age is regarded as perhaps the strongest individual risk factor for overall graft loss and patient death; however, other donor factors such as history of disease, race, cause of death, and donor creatinine level have also been shown to affect long-term outcomes. In addition donor and recipient human leukocyte antigen matching, donor and recipient cytomegalovirus status, and duration of cold ischemia time significantly contribute to the level of risk associated with the transplant. In deceased donor transplants, the cumulative

effect of these donor factors can translate to a nearly threefold risk for graft loss with the lowest 5% of donations relative to the highest donor quality. Outcomes for recipients of living donor transplants are consistently superior to recipients of deceased donor transplants (Table 16.12-2). In fact, this advantage of living transplantation is likely partially explained by the quality of the donor organ. Living donors, who have undergone extensive screening and evaluation, represent a healthier organ pool with significantly diminished risk factors for the transplant outcome. However, even within living transplants there exists significant variability in quality, and to some extent the growth of living transplants as a treatment modality in recent years has been a function of more high-risk donor characteristics.[21] In addition to the quality of the transplant organ, the

**TABLE 16-12-2**

## TRADITIONAL AND NONTRADITIONAL CARDIOVASCULAR RISK FACTORS IN CHRONIC KIDNEY DISEASE

| Traditional Risk Factors | Nontraditional Risk Factors |
| --- | --- |
| Older age | Albuminuria |
| | Hyperhomocysteinemia |
| | Anemia |
| Male gender | Abnormal calcium/ |
| | phosphate metabolism |
| Hypertension | Extracellular fluid volume |
| | overload and electrolyte |
| Higher total cholesterol | imbalance |
| Higher LDL cholesterol | Oxidative stress |
| Lower HDL cholesterol | Inflammation |
| Diabetes | Malnutrition |
| Smoking | Thrombogenic factors |
| Physical inactivity | Sleep disturbances |
| Menopause | Altered nitric oxide/endothelin balance |
| Family history of | |
| cardiovascular disease | Lp(a) lipoprotein |
| Left ventricular hypertrophy | |

Reproduced with permission from *Am J Kidney Dis* 2000; 35(4 Suppl 1):S117–S131.

ability to optimally schedule a surgical procedure, minimize ischemic time, and complete pretransplant candidate evaluations that are generally associated with a living transplant procedure provide a relatively ideal scenario for long-term success.

An additional explanation for the increased patient and graft life expectancy for the living transplant recipient, relative to the deceased donor recipient, is that living recipients have significantly less time of pretransplant dialysis. On average, patients who receive a living transplant are transplanted earlier in the ESRD process and as such are subjected to fewer of the insults associated with dialysis.

## INCIDENCE OF PREEMPTIVE KIDNEY TRANSPLANTATION

Incidence rates of living preemptive transplants by year derived from data from the Scientific Registry of Transplant Recipients (SRTR) are displayed in Figure 16.12-8. There has been mild increase in preemptive living transplant rates, with an apparent peak in 2000. Kasiske et al. reported similar rates from 1995 to 1998.[22] According to this study, characteristics of transplant recipients associated with receipt of a preemptive transplant included pediatric age, caucasian race, non-Hispanics, private insurance, high education, and type-II diabetes. The study concluded that that although preemptive transplantation appears efficacious, the procedure is not acquired uniformly to all eligible candidates.

## QUALITY OF LIFE AND ECONOMIC IMPLICATIONS OF PREEMPTIVE TRANSPLANTATION

The advantage of preemptive transplantation is not limited to better patient and graft survival. One of the commonly cited benefits of kidney transplantation is improvement in quality of life. Freedom from the burden of dialysis was a common justification for transplantation even before the survival benefits of transplantation were known.

Based on a single-center study, Laupacis et al. estimated that almost all health-related quality-of-life measures had improved in renal transplant recipients as compared to pretransplantation.[23] Similar results were seen in type-I diabetics.[24] These studies and

others helped to quantify the improved quality of life associated with transplantation and provided an additional incentive for preemptive transplantation.[25,26]

From an economic perspective, transplantation has been shown to be less expensive than maintenance dialysis.[27–30] Most studies suggest that transplantation is more cost-effective than dialysis following the first-year posttransplant and the cost savings increase progressively as long as the graft survives. Thus, preemptive transplantation offers a long-term economic benefit in addition to a survival advantage relative to receiving a transplant following initiation of dialysis. Although preemptive transplantation prior to the onset of uraemia may temporarily increase costs, it is likely that early high costs are minor compared to the long-term savings associated with transplantation; in addition, the extended graft survival and reduced likelihood of future comorbidities eventually lead to a clear economic advantage with preemptive transplantation.

## CONCLUSIONS

The cumulative evidence to date suggests that preemptive living donor kidney transplantation is the treatment modality of choice for eligible patients with ESRD. Life expectancy, quality of life, and economics are all vastly superior in living preemptive transplantation compared to all other treatment modalities for ESRD. In particular, patients with longer expected waiting times for a deceased donor transplant and those patients especially vulnerable to the adverse effects of dialysis have the strongest incentive to receive a preemptive living transplant. Overall, while transplantation is considered the preferred therapeutic option for ESRD patients, even more decidedly, preemptive living donor transplantation is the optimal teatment modality for this rapidly expanding population.

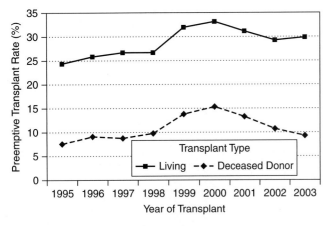

**FIGURE 16.12-8**

Incidence rates of preemptive primary transplants by donor type 1995–2003. The figure describes the percentage of all kidney transplants performed preemptively according to donor type. Figure derived from data supplied by the Scientific Registry of Transplant Recipients.

## References

1. Wolfe RA, Ashby VB, Milford EL, et al. Comparison of mortality in all patients on dialysis, patients on dialysis awaiting transplantation, and recipients of a first cadaveric transplant. *N Engl J Med* 1999;341:1725–1730.
2. McDonald SP, Russ GR. Survival of recipients of cadaveric kidney transplants compared with those receiving dialysis treatment in Australia and New Zealand, 1991-2001. *Nephrol Dial Transplant* 2002;17:2212–2219.
3. Oniscu GC, Brown H, Forsythe JL. How old is old for transplantation? *Am J Transplant* 2004;4:2067–2074.
4. Rabbat CG, Thorpe KE, Russell JD, Churchill DN. Comparison of mortality risk for dialysis patients and cadaveric first renal transplant recipients in Ontario, Canada. *J Am Soc Nephrol* 2000;11:917–922.
5. Glanton CW, Kao TC, Cruess D, Agodoa LY, Abbott KC. Impact of renal transplantation on survival in end-stage renal disease patients with elevated body mass index. *Kidney Int* 2003;63:647–653.
6. Ojo AO, Hanson JA, Meier-Kriesche HU, et al. Survival in recipients of marginal cadaveric donor kidneys compared with other recipients and wait-listed transplant candidates. J Am Soc Nephrol 2001; 12:589–597.
7. Cosio FG, Alamir A, Yim S, et al. Patient survival after renal transplantation: I. The impact of dialysis pre-transplant. *Kidney Int* 1998; 53:767–772.
8. Asderakis A, Augustine T, Dyer P, et al. Pre-emptive kidney transplantation: the attractive alternative. *Nephrol Dial Transplant* 1998;13:1799–1803.
9. Meier-Kriesche HU, Port FK, Ojo AO, et al. Effect of waiting time on renal transplant outcome. *Kidney Int* 2000;58:1311–1317.
10. Mange KC, Joffe MM, Feldman HI. Effect of the use or nonuse of long-term dialysis on the subsequent survival of renal transplants from living donors. *N Engl J Med* 2001;344:726–731.

11. Meier-Kriesche HU, Kaplan B. Waiting time on dialysis as the strongest modifiable risk factor for renal transplant outcomes - A paired donor kidney analysis. Transplantation 2002:74:1377–1381.

12. Vats AN, Donaldson L, Fine RN, Chavers BM. Pretransplant dialysis status and outcome of renal transplantation in North American children: a NAPRTCS Study. North American Pediatric Renal Transplant Cooperative Study. *Transplantation* 2000;69:1414–1419.

13. Kaplan B, Meier-Kriesche HU. Death after graft loss: an important late study endpoint in kidney transplantation. Am J Transplant 2002:2: 970–974.

14. Sarnak MJ. Cardiovascular complications in chronic kidney disease. *Am J Kidney Dis* 2003;41:S11–S17.

15. Xue JL, Ma JZ, Louis TA, Collins AJ. Forecast of the number of patients with end-stage renal disease in the United States to the year 2010. *J Am Soc Nephrol* 2001;12:2753–2758.

16. US Transplant—Scientific Registry of Transplant Recipients. 2004 OPTN/ SRTR Annual Report. 2004. Ann Arbor, MI.

17. Meier-Kriesche HU, Baliga R, Kaplan B. Decreased renal function is a strong risk factor for cardiovascular death after renal transplantation. *Transplantation* 2003;75:1291–1295.

18. Meier-Kriesche HU, Schold JD, Srinivas TR, Reed A, Kaplan B. Kidney transplantation halts cardiovascular disease progression in patients with end-stage renal disease. *Am J Transplant* 2004;4:1662–1668.

19. Schold JD, Kaplan B, Baliga RS, Meier-Kriesche HU. The broad spectrum of quality in deceased donor kidneys. *Am J Transplant* 2005;5: 757–765.

20. Metzger RA, Delmonico FL, Feng S, et al. Expanded criteria donors for kidney transplantation. *Am J Transplant* 2003;3 Suppl 4:114–125.

21. Schold JD, Fujita S, Bucci M, et al. Assessment of the Quality of Living Donor Kidneys. *Am J Transplant* 2004;4(Suppl 8), 369.

22. Kasiske BL, Snyder JJ, Matas AJ, et al. Preemptive kidney transplantation: the advantage and the advantaged. *J Am Soc Nephrol* 2002;13: 1358–1364.

23. Laupacis A, Keown P, Pus N, et al. A study of the quality of life and cost-utility of renal transplantation. *Kidney Int* 1996;50:235–242.

24. Knoll GA, Nichol G. Dialysis, kidney transplantation, or pancreas transplantation for patients with diabetes mellitus and renal failure: a decision analysis of treatment options. *J Am Soc Nephrol* 2003;14:500–515.

25. Manns B, Meltzer D, Taub K, Donaldson C. Illustrating the impact of including future costs in economic evaluations: an application to end-stage renal disease care. *Health Econ* 2003;12:949–958.

26. Whiting JF, Kiberd B, Kalo Z, Keown P, Roels L, Kjerulf M. Cost-effectiveness of organ donation: evaluating investment into donor action and other donor initiatives. *Am J Transplant* 2004;4:569–573.

27. de Wit GA, Ramsteijn PG, de Charro FT. Economic evaluation of end stage renal disease treatment. *Health Policy* 1998;44:215–232.

28. Karlberg I, Nyberg G. Cost-effectiveness studies of renal transplantation. *Int J Technol Assess Health Care* 1995;11:611–622.

29. Loubeau PR, Loubeau JM, Jantzen R. The economics of kidney transplantation versus hemodialysis. *Prog Transplant* 2001;11:291–297.

30. Whiting JF, Zavala EY, Alexander JW, First MR. The cost-effectiveness of transplantation with expanded donor kidneys. *Transplant Proc* 1999;31:1320–1321.

# 16.13 LONG-TERM OUTCOME

*J. Michael Cecka, PhD*

## HISTORICAL PERSPECTIVE

Long-term kidney graft survival has increased remarkably during the past 30 years, mainly due to substantial reductions in early rejection and graft losses within the first few months after transplantation. Still, grafts that continue to function 1 year after transplantation fail at an inexorable rate of about 5% per year such that, on average, half of all primary kidney transplants that survive the first posttransplant year will be lost within 13 years. Surprisingly, the rate of late graft failure has changed little over the years, despite the improvements in 1-year graft survival. Although few factors that affect the long-term rate of graft loss have been identified, recipients of living donor kidney grafts have consistently had lower rates of late graft failure than recipients of kidneys from deceased donors. It was apparent even among recipients of kidney transplants in the earliest period of transplantation that the long-term results of living donor transplants were superior to those of deceased donor transplants. In the United States, about 22% of living donor kidney transplants performed before 1980 survived 25 years compared with only 5% of kidneys transplanted from deceased donors.[1] That figure is in line with excellent long-term results that were recently reported from Japan,[2] where most transplants have been from living donors.

The reasons for the high, long-term graft survival rates among recipients of living donor kidneys are not well understood, but there are certainly benefits of elective surgery, when the donor and recipient are in optimal health, and of using healthy kidneys with minimal ischemia that may very well play important roles in the superior outcomes of these transplants. This chapter focuses on some of the factors that may influence long-term survival of living donor kidneys and some unexpected lessons that have been learned from the rapid expansion of living donor transplantation in the United States. There is not an exhaustive literature dedicated to the topic of long-term graft survival among recipients of living donor transplants, and so I have used data from the Organ Procurement and Transplantation Network/United Network for Organ Sharing (OPTN/UNOS) to illustrate many of the points for this chapter. The figures and tables are labeled, but most of the data are from primary kidney transplants performed at U.S. centers between 1998 and 2002. Graft survival curves are unadjusted and include patient deaths as graft losses.

Recipients of living donor kidney transplants have many distinct advantages compared with patients who do not have the option of a willing and medically suitable living donor, excellent long-term graft survival rates among them. More than 24,000 patients received their first transplant from a living donor between 1998 and 2002 according to OPTN/UNOS statistics (www.unos.org). The actuarial 5-year patient and graft survival rates were 90% and 82%, respectively. When projected to 10 years, 80% of the recipients will still be alive and nearly 70% of living donor grafts should still be functioning (Fig 16.13-1). These long-term results are clearly better than those for recipients of deceased donor kidneys during the same period. The graft half-lives, the number of years until half the grafts surviving at 1 year are lost were 18 years for recipients of living donor kidneys and 10 years for recipients of deceased donor kidneys, suggesting that the living donor transplants will function nearly twice as long.

The kidney source is the dominant determinant of long-term survival. During the past 10 years, advances in immunosuppression, patient selection and management, and long-term care have increased graft survival rates by about 13% at 10 years[3] (Fig. 16.13-2). The result has been consistently observed for grafts from living donors, grafts from deceased donors that belong to the recently designated category of expanded donors,[4] and those from younger healthier deceased donors. Living donor grafts had 35% better 10-year graft survival rates than expanded criteria deceased donor grafts and 15% higher graft survival rates than recipients of standard criteria grafts, comparing transplants done between 1988 and 1992 and those done between 1998 and 2002.

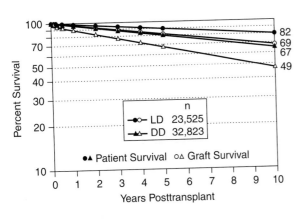

**FIGURE 16.13-1**

Long-term patient and graft survival rates for recipients of living (LD) and deceased donor (DD) primary kidney transplants between 1998 and 2002 projected to 10 years. The graft survival rates were projected to 10 years assuming a constant failure rate after the first year. The calculated graft half-lives were 17.9 years and 10.3 years for LD and DD transplant recipients, respectively. (Based on OPTN/UNOS data as of December 4, 2004.)

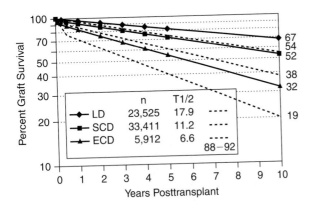

**FIGURE 16.13-2**

Actuarial and projected graft survival rates for kidney transplant recipients in 2 eras according to the donor source. The categories were: living (LD), standard criteria deceased donor (SCD), or expanded criteria deceased donor (ECD). The legend refers to transplants during the 1998–2002 period, and the dashed lines show survival results for the same donor categories transplanted during 1988–1992. There was a 13% to 14% improvement in 10-year graft survival rates for each category comparing the 2 intervals. (Modified from ref 3, with permission.)

## THE ROLE OF HISTOCOMPATIBILTY

Until the mid-1990s, better histocompatibility was generally presumed to be mainly responsible for the superior long-term results using living donor grafts as most were from human leukocyte antigen (HLA)-identical siblings or from parents or siblings who differed from the recipient for one HLA haplotype. Among first-degree relatives, other minor histocompatibility genes would likewise be shared at some level. Although many centers had performed less compatible transplants and even a few transplants from genetically unrelated living donors,[5,6] most had limited experience with these, and it was a multicenter analysis showing that

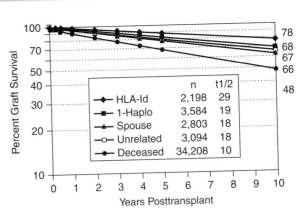

**FIGURE 16.13-3**

Long-term primary kidney graft survival rates according to the donor's relationship to the recipient (1998–2002). The figure shows survival curves for primary transplants between HLA-identical and 1-haplotype-matched siblings, from spouses and other genetically unrelated living donors and from deceased donors. (Reproduced from ref 3, with permission.)

497 transplants between spouses and from other genetically unrelated donors performed at 97 transplant centers had graft survival rates that were more similar to those for one-haplotype-related grafts than to deceased donor transplants[7] that really changed that perception. Spouse transplants performed during the more recent period (1998–2002) had similar results to those published in 1995, as did transplants from other genetically unrelated individuals (Fig. 16.13-3).

## HLA-Identical Sibling Transplants

Transplants from HLA-identical siblings have the best long-term graft survival rates. Genotypically HLA-identical kidneys are matched with the recipients for the major targets of immunological rejection, so there are fewer problems with rejection and fewer immunological graft losses. The graft half-life for HLA-identical sibling transplants during 1998 to 2002 was 29 years. The recipients of these kidneys had the lowest rate of late graft failure and a very high long-term graft survival rate projected to be 78% at 10 years. However, immunosuppression is still required for transplants between HLA-identical siblings (unlike between identical twins). These grafts are rejected despite their HLA compatibility. This suggests that when the major targets of immune rejection are eliminated, other histocompatibilty differences play an important role in long-term outcomes.[8] Patients who have been exposed to allogeneic tissues by pregnancies, previous transplants, or blood transfusions often produce anti-HLA antibodies against the foreign HLA antigens, but generally do not develop antibodies to their own HLA antigens, nor to those of a genetically HLA-identical graft, yet broadly sensitized patients reportedly have poorer graft survival rates than unsensitized patients even when the donor is an HLA-identical sibling.[9] Whether such losses are due to the action of antibodies against non-HLA antigens or are a reflection of heightened immunity in general is not clear, nor are the targets of non-HLA immune responses.

There are many candidate "minor" histocompatibility antigens, including male (Y-chromosome) antigens that appear to influence the results of HLA-matched bone marrow transplants[10] and that have been implicated in the more rapid rejection of male livers by female recipients.[11] These minor antigens may also play a role in

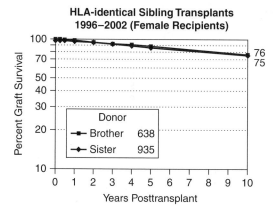

**FIGURE 16.13-4**

Long-term survival of HLA-identical sibling transplants from brother to sister or from sister to sister (1995–2002). There was no apparent difference in long-term graft survival rates when sisters received a kidney from their HLA-identical brother or sister indicating a very limited role for a male minor histocompatibility antigen. (Based on OPTN/UNOS data as of December 4, 2004.)

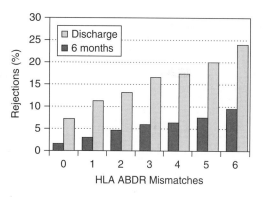

**FIGURE 16.13-5**

Incidence of early rejection episodes among living donor kidney recipients according to the number of HLA-mismatched antigens (1998–2002). The percentage of primary transplant recipients who were treated for rejections before the hospital discharge or within the first 6 months increased as the number of HLA-A,B,DR antigens mismatched between the donor and recipient increased. (Based on OPTN/UNOS data as of December 4, 2004.)

kidney rejection, but their role is not well established. The potential importance of a male antigen can be assessed by analysis of HLA-identical sibling transplants between brothers and sisters where the role of a male antigen should be more evident in the absence of stronger histocompatibility differences. Figure 16.13-4 shows there was no notable difference in graft survival rates comparing HLA-identical brother-to-sister transplants (with potential male antigen exposure) with those between sisters (no male antigen exposure). The result does not mean that male y-chromosome antigens are not important minor histocompatibility antigens in some patients, but suggests that they do not have a major impact on long-term graft survival.

## HLA Mismatches in Transplants From Other Living Donors

Some controversy still exists about the remaining role of histocompatibility in living donor transplantation. Except for HLA-matched sibling grafts, the survival rates for transplants mismatched for one, two, or three HLA antigens appear not to be different from grafts with four, five, or six antigens mismatched. Although patients with preformed antibodies to HLA antigens may be incompatible with donors that express those HLA antigens, HLA compatibility has not been widely used to select which parent would be a better donor for their child, for example. Interestingly, however, early rejection rates still correlate with the number of HLA mismatches for all living donor transplants in the U.S. experience (Fig. 16.13-5), even though these differences are apparently not reflected in poorer graft survival.[12] This seemingly paradoxical lack of a clear association between rejections and survival has been noted for recipients of deceased donor grafts as well.[13] It is not difficult to understand that although recipients who experience rejection are more likely to lose their grafts, the number with rejections is small, and not all those who experience rejection actually lose their grafts. Thus, the impact of a reduction in the incidence of rejection episodes is not manifested in notably higher overall graft survival rates. Nevertheless, a higher incidence of rejection might translate to poorer graft survival rates among poorly matched recipients in some centers or in countries where rejections are more difficult to manage. Opelz

et al.[14] reported some years ago that graft survival rates correlated with the number of mismatched HLA antigens among recipients of unrelated living donor transplants based on data reported to the Collaborative Transplant Study Registry, which includes many international transplant centers. This result has been updated subsequently at international meetings, but no subsequent report has been published. In the United States, no such correlation with graft survival has been found.[15]

## Transplants Between Parents and Offspring or Husband and Wives: Potential Immune Exposures

Transplants from offspring to their mothers and from husbands to their wives are interesting because they carry a risk that the recipient has been sensitized to the HLA antigens of the donor during pregnancy and birth. On the other hand, there is also good evidence that mothers may carry viable cells from their offspring (ie, they are microchimeric) for many years after the birth of the child,[16] and microchimerism may predispose to tolerance,[17] rendering the recipient less likely to reject a graft from the offspring donor. Is there evidence that mothers are more (or less) reactive when transplanted with a kidney from an offspring or from the father of the child? There have been anecdotal reports of accelerated rejection in these types of transplants,[18] raising the possibility that immunization has occurred. However, there have been no large-scale studies to show a correlation between microchimerism and a reduced incidence of rejection or of a lack of microchimerism when accelerated rejection occurred in these types of cases. A small Norwegian study[19] found no survival benefit for recipients who were the mother of the kidney donor. Interestingly, there were fewer rejections in very young pediatric patients who received a graft from their mother than those grafted from their father,[20] suggesting that very early in the child's development there may be diminished responsiveness to HLA antigens of the mother. Long-term graft survival results were not substantially different when comparing mothers and fathers as recipients of kidneys donated by their offspring or when comparing husbands and wives as recipients of their spouse' kidney (Figures 16.13-6 and 16.13-7). There was

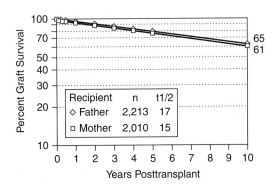

**FIGURE 16.13-6**

Long-term graft survival of offspring to parent transplants stratified by the sex of the recipient (1998–2002). Prior exposure of mothers to their childrens' paternal HLA antigens did not appear to affect long-term graft survival rates when the kidney donor was an offspring. (Based on OPTN/UNOS data as of December 4, 2004.)

a slight advantage for wives who received a kidney from their husband projected to be about 4% to 14% at 10 years, which is the reverse of what might be expected by immunological considerations alone. However, the subset of wives with more than one pregnancy who received a kidney from their husband had an intermediate survival rate and mothers had no better graft survival rates than fathers who received a kidney from an offspring donor, providing no evidence for a tolerogenic effect of potential prior exposure to donor HLA antigens among women who might have microchimerism as a result of childbirth. Immunization through pregnancies probably does occur and may partly explain the limited number of multiparous wives who have received a kidney from their husband either because they have produced antibodies against their husband's HLA antigens or because centers are reluctant to transplant in cases when donor-specific immunity is a concern.

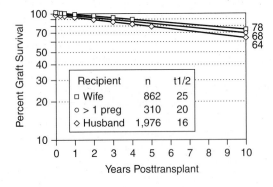

**FIGURE 16.13-7**

Long-term graft survival of spousal transplants stratified by sex and pregnancies (1998–2002). Prior exposure of mothers to their childrens' paternal HLA antigens did not appear to affect long-term survival rates when the kidney donor was the husband. The figure shows the results of transplants from the husband to the wife, a subset when the wife had more than one pregnancy with the husband and husbands who received their wife's kidney. The observation that many fewer wives were transplanted than husbands suggests that some wives produce antibodies against their children's mismatched paternal HLA antigens and are prevented form receiving the husband's kidney by a positive crossmatch. (Based on OPTN/UNOS data as of December 4, 2004.)

## TRENDS IN LIVING DONOR TRANSPLANTATION

Since 1995, the number of living donor transplants has markedly increased[21] (Figure 16.13-8) as a result of the growing confidence in superior long-term outcomes for genetically unrelated donors and a severely limited supply of deceased donor kidneys. The numbers of transplants from HLA-identical sibling donors and from parents have remained relatively constant as these transplants were generally acceptable to most transplant centers and were utilized whenever there was an opportunity. The major new growth has been in transplants between spouses, offspring to their parents, less histocompatible relatives and unrelated donors who are not spouses. Among these, all but the offspring-to-parent transplants are due to the growing acceptance of histoincompatible donors. The increase in offspring donors more likely reflects an effort to avoid the prolonged wait for a deceased donor transplant for aging parents. Kidneys transplanted from each of these donor categories resulted in superior long-term survival. Overall the results are better for recipients of completely HLA-mismatched living donor kidneys than for recipients of HLA-matched grafts from deceased donors (Fig. 16.13-9).

The confidence in long-term success rates in transplants from living unrelated donors has now reached a state of acceptance when "registries" are being established and allocation models are being offered to facilitate exchange transplants when suitable living donors are ABO or crossmatch incompatible with the intended recipient allowing them to exchange kidneys with another pair who are similarly incompatible.[22,23]

## FACTORS AFFECTING LONG-TERM SURVIVAL

If the difference in outcomes is not due to histocompatibility, why do living donor transplants have better long-term success than transplants from deceased donors? The answer is not yet clear and may be quite complicated, but there are several differences that may contribute to the superior long-term outcomes.

### Demographic Differences

There are persistent demographic differences between the recipients of living and the recipients of deceased donor transplants. A smaller percentage of blacks than whites receive living donor

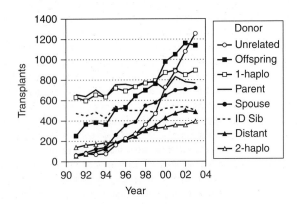

**FIGURE 16.13-8**

Increasing number of transplants from living donors according to their relationship to the recipient. The largest annual increase has been in the number of genetically unrelated nonspouse donors. (Reproduced from ref 21, with permission.)

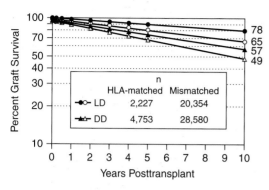

**FIGURE 16.13-9**

Long-term graft survival rates for HLA-matched and HLA-mismatched recipients of kidneys from living (LD) and deceased donors (DD) (1998–2002). HLA-mismatched living donor transplants had better long-term survival than HLA-matched transplants from deceased donors. (Based on OPTN/UNOS data as of December 4, 2004.)

kidneys (long-term survival tends to be lower among blacks), recipients are generally younger (older recipients have shorter remaining life expectancies), less often broadly sensitized (a lower immunological risk), and have spent less time on dialysis.[24] Living donors tend to be younger and can be more carefully evaluated as evidenced by the much better graft survival rates that are reported for transplants of older living donor kidneys.[25,26] Still, even when demographic differences are accounted for, recipients of living donor transplants have better long-term survival than those who get deceased donor grafts.[24]

## Preemptive Transplantation

Nearly one fourth of patients who received a living donor transplant in the United States between 1995 and 1998 were not dialyzed before transplantation.[27] Even those who were dialyzed were transplanted sooner after initiating dialysis treatment than recipients of deceased donor kidneys[3] Figure 16.13-10). The recipients of preemptive kidney transplants had better patient and graft survival rates and a lower rate of early graft dysfunction than their counterparts who had spent time on dialysis before their transplant. Patients transplanted before they begin dialysis or after only a short time on dialysis have several advantages over their counterparts who wait for years on dialysis.[27,28]

Preemptive transplant recipients had fewer acute rejection episodes during the first year, perhaps because of lower immune reactivity in patients who can avoid dialysis.[28] The survival advantage for preemptive transplants, however, may not be simply due to a reduction in acute rejection or graft dysfunction, because even when these factors were accounted for the rate of decline in estimated glomerular filtration rate was lower in preemptive transplant recipients.[29] Patients who are transplanted preemptively avoid the morbidity and mortality associated with long-term dialysis and also represent a substantial cost saving by avoiding dialysis. As the number of living donor transplants grow, the opportunities for preemptive transplantation increase. Preemptive transplantation has been rare among deceased donor kidney recipients (mostly children) and the United Network of Organ Sharing (UNOS) requirement that patients must have an estimated creatinine clearance less than 20 mL/min in order to begin accruing waiting time no doubt limits this option to patients with a suitable living donor.

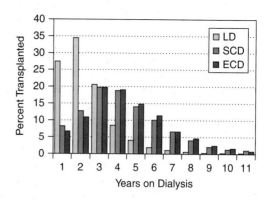

**FIGURE 16.13-10**

Recipients of living donor kidneys are transplanted earlier in their disease than recipients of deceased donor grafts. More than half of living donor transplants were performed within the first year after the patient started dialysis (27% preemptively with no dialysis) compared with fewer than 20% of deceased donor kidney recipients (only 7% preemptively). (Reproduced from ref 3, with permission.)

## Brain Death and Ischemia

There are at least two fundamental differences between kidneys from living and deceased donors: brain death in the donor and a period of cold ischemia for the kidney after removal. Although living donors are carefully screened and selected to be healthy and the surgery can be scheduled to ensure optimal conditions, there are intriguing data that suggest brain death itself may affect the deceased donor kidney,[30] increasing cytokines and proinflammatory elements and rendering kidneys from deceased donors more immunogenic and more susceptible to immunological damage in the early posttransplant period. Living donor kidneys are transplanted immediately on removal from the donor, whereas deceased donor kidneys are maintained in cold storage or on a pump until a suitable recipient is located and surgery can be scheduled. The time between removal from the deceased donor and reanastomosis of the kidney in the recipient averages about 22 hours.[31] These two factors are strongly associated with an important difference between living and deceased donor kidneys—the incidence of early graft dysfunction. Approximately 24% of deceased donor kidney recipients require dialysis during the early posttransplant period, whereas only about 4% of living donor kidney recipients have such a requirement, and many of those because of graft thrombosis from which the graft does not recover. Important factors that predispose to early dysfunction of deceased donor kidneys are prolonged ischemia, increasing donor age, and donor death due to cerebrovascular accident.[31]

Among recipients of living donor kidneys early dysfunction has been associated with laparoscopic nephrectomy,[32] particularly during the early experience with this approach,[33] but the dysfunction was not associated with poorer graft survival in these cases. Much of the early graft dysfunction in recipients of deceased donor kidneys resolves, but long-term graft survival rates are substantially reduced among patients with delayed graft function.[34]

## Other Factors

Very few factors that are generally identified in transplant registry analyses seem to affect graft survival of living donor transplants.[24,25] The transplant center may influence long-term

**TABLE 16.13-1**

## THE EXTENT OF ASSIGNABLE VARIATION IN LIVING DONOR GRAFT OUTCOMES*

| 1-year, n=21, 830 | | 5-year, n=21,003 | |
|---|---|---|---|
| Factor | Percent Variation | Factor | Percent Variation |
| Transplant center | 57.5 | Transplant center | 26.5 |
| Recipient work status | 5.8 | Donor relationship | 19.9 |
| HLA-ABDR 0mm | 5.4 | Recipient sex | 13.5 |
| Induction therapy | 5.2 | Recipient age | 12.1 |
| Recipient obese | 4.4 | Recipient black | 11.6 |
| Recipient black | 4.1 | Donor age | 6.9 |

* The transplant center was the strongest identifiable factor among 20 pretransplant variables that affected survival of living donor transplants at 1 year and between 1 and 5 years. Other long-term factors included the donor's relationship, the recipient's sex, age, and race, and the donor age. Even considering this large number of variables only 8% of the total long-term variability was predictable. (Modified from ref 35, with permission.)

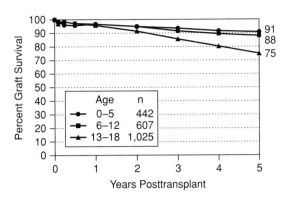

**FIGURE 16.13-11**

Five-year graft survival of pediatric recipients of living donor transplants stratified by the recipient's age (1998–2002). Pediatric recipients of living donor kidneys who survive the early posttransplant period had excellent 5-year graft survival except those who were transplanted as adolescents (ages 13–18) whose grafts began to fail at an accelerated rate after the first year. (Based on OPTN/UNOS data as of December 4, 2004.)

outcomes as shown in Table 16.13-1, although it is difficult to account for statistical variation when few transplants have been performed at many centers. Long-term graft survival rates differed among different transplant centers more than any other pretransplant variable that was analyzed. Differences in the donor relationship, recipient sex, age, and race and the donor's age accounted for 84% of the assignable variation in long-term (5-year) survival rates. Of course, the analysis could only account for a small percentage of the variation that was observed and thus, these factors probably play a relatively minor role in predicting the long-term outcome. The results suggest that the real differences are probably more subtle and reside in patient and donor characteristics that are not or cannot be collected by multicenter registries.

The elective nature of the living donor transplant ensures that the patient can be in optimal medical condition at the time of transplant. Transplantation from a deceased donor has been described as "... an urgent procedure performed in an elective population."[36] Ideally the deceased donor recipient should also be in optimum condition at the time of transplant; however, the unpredictable nature of deceased donor kidney allocation may result in a kidney offer for a patient who is not. In most cases of this type, the offer would be declined, but some may be accepted because of long waiting times. It is more likely that patients who are not ready would receive a deceased than a live donor kidney, and this may explain the slightly higher early mortality rates observed among recipients of deceased donor grafts (Fig. 16.13-1). Thorough preparation and assessment of candidates for a living donor transplant prior to transplantation provides long-term advantages when cardiovascular disease, hypertension, and other medical problems associated with long-term patient survival are treated and controlled.

## PEDIATRIC TRANSPLANTATION

Pediatric recipients represent a special group among the recipients of living donor kidneys. Pediatric recipients represent about 5% of all transplants performed in the United States each year, and 50% to 60% receive living donor kidneys, mostly from a parent (www.unos.org). They differ from adult recipients in many important ways that may affect long-term graft survival. Their underlying diseases or defects are generally associated with fewer

cormorbid conditions and systemic diseases are uncommon. Cardiovascular problems are rare, although obesity is a growing concern among children and appears to impact long-term patient survival after transplantation.[37] Obviously, their young age makes long-term graft survival an important concern. Graft loss is likely to be accompanied by broad sensitization limiting chances for retransplantation, but waiting for a well-matched kidney is not a reasonable option for most because of growth and developmental retardation associated with dialysis and uremia.

Young children and preteens have excellent long-term graft survival rates (Fig. 16.13-11).[38,39] When their grafts survive the early posttransplant period, the half-lives are comparable to those for HLA-identical siblings.[38] Teens, on the other hand, tend to lose their grafts at an accelerated rate.[38,40] In fact, the recipient's age and race are the major factors affecting long-term survival of younger recipients. These observations are independent of whether the kidney is from a living or deceased donor. The reasons for this accelerated late graft loss rate in teens has not been well established. Poor medication compliance[41,42] and a high incidence of recurring focal segmental sclerosis[43] among adolescent recipients have been reported. Although graft half-lives for very young pediatric patients are high, suggesting high long-term graft survival rates for this population, little information is available about what happens to these young patients as they pass through puberty and the teenage years. If the major reason for poor long-term survival for adolescent recipients is medication noncompliance, are younger patients more prone to accelerated graft loss when they reach adolescence as well? Clearly more long-term follow-up is needed to assess long-term graft survival in pediatric recipients.

## CONCLUDING REMARKS

Living donor transplants provide superior long-term graft function in addition to the advantages of early transplantation in an elective setting. The two main causes of late graft failure (after the first posttransplant year) are patient death and chronic deterioration of graft function.[3] Improving long-term graft survival rates requires addressing both of these causes. With an aging population of transplant recipients, some deaths are anticipated and when the graft continues to function until the patient dies, many of these late graft losses should be considered successes. However, some deaths that are due to modifiable behaviors such as smoking or conditions such as obesity, hypertension, cardiovascular disease, or infection are amenable to interventions that would prolong patient and graft survival. Long-term deterioration of graft function is a poorly understood constellation of processes that may include disease, immune responses, aging, and toxicities. Some of these conditions may also be slowed or reversed by appropriate interventions through treatment or modification of immunosuppression. Long-term survival rates for both living and deceased donor kidney grafts can still improve through reduction of late mortality and deterioration of graft function. However, while the donor surgery remains safe, with a low risk of complications, living donor transplantation is the best option for those with a willing and suitable donor.

# References

1. Cecka JM. The OPTN/UNOS Renal Transplant Registry - 2000. In: Cecka JM, Terasaki PI, eds. *Clinical Transplants 2000*. Los Angeles: UCLA Immunogenetics Center, 2001:1.

2. Yoshimura, N Akioka K, Ushigome H, et al. Twenty-five year survival of living related kidney transplants: Thirty-five year experience. *Transplant Proc* 2005;37:687.

3. Cecka JM. The OPTN/UNOS Renal Transplant Registry - 2003. In: Cecka JM, Terasaki PI, eds. *Clinical Transplants 2003*. Los Angeles: UCLA Immunogenetics Center; 2004:1.

4. Port FK, Bragg-Gresham JL, Metzger RA, et al. Donor characteristics associated with reduced graft survival: An approach to expanding the pool of kidney donors. *Transplantation* 2002;74:1281.

5. D'Allesandro AM, Sollinger HW, Knechtle SJ, et al. Living related and unrelated donors for kidney transplantation: a 28-year experience. *Ann Surg* 1986;222:353.

6. Park K, Kim SI. Kim YS, et al. Results of kidney transplantation from 1979-1997 at Yonsei University. In: Cecka JM, Terasaki PI, eds. *Clinical Transplants 1997*. Los Angeles: UCLA Tissue Typing Laboratory; 1998:149.

7. Terasaki PI, Cecka JM, Gjertson DW, Takemoto S. High graft survival rates of spousal and living-unrelated donor kidney transplants. *N Engl J Med* 1995;333.

8. Terasaki PI. Deduction of the fraction of immunologic and non-immunologic failure in cadaver donor transplants. In: Cecka JM, Terasaki PI, eds. *Clinical Transplants 2003*. Los Angeles: UCLA Immunogenetics Center; 2004:449.

9. Opelz G; Collaborative Transplant Study. Non-HLA transplantation immunity revealed by lymphocytotoxic antibodies. *Lancet* 2005; 365:1570.

10. Miklos DB, Kim HT, Miller KH, et al. Antibody responses to H-Y moinor histocompatibility antigens correlate with chronic graft-versus-host disease and disease remission. *Blood* 2005:105:2973.

11. Candinas D, Gunson BK, Nightingale P, et al. Sex mismatch as a risk ractor for chronic rejection of liver allografts. *Lancet* 1995;346:1117.

12. Fuller TF, Feng S, Brennan TV, et al. Increased rejection in living unrelated versus living related kidney transplants does not affect short-term function and survival. *Transplantation* 2004;78:1030.

13. Meier-Kriesche HU, Schold JD, Srinivas TR, Kaplan B. Lack of improvement in renal allograft survival despite a marked decrease in acute rejection rates over the most recent era. *Am J Transplant* 2004;4:378.

14. Opelz G. The impact of HLA compatibility on survival of kidney transplants from unrelated live donors. *Transplantation* 1997;64:1473.

15. Gjertson DW, Cecka JM. Living unrelated donor kidney transplantation. *Kidney Int* 2000;58:491.

16. Bianchi DW, Zickwolf GK, Weil GJ, DeMaria MA. Male fetal progenitor cells persist in maternal blood for as long as 27 years postpartum. *Proc Nat Acad Sci USA* 1996;62:705.

17. Starzl TE, Demetris AJ, Trucco M, et al. Chimerism and donor-specific non-reactivity 27-29 years after kidney allotransplantation. *Transplantation* 1993;55:1272.

18. Rosenberg JC, Jones B, Oh H. Accelerated rejection following offspring-to-mother and husband-to-wife transplants. *Clin Transplant* 2004;18:729.

19. Flesland O, Leivestad T, Solheim BG. Survival of renal allografts from living donors and the importance of being the mother of the organ donor. *Transfus Apheresis Sci* 2005;32:13.

20. Cecka JM, Gjertson DW, Terasaki PI. Pediatric Transplantation - A review of the UNOS data. *Pediatr Transplant* 1997;1:55.

21. Cecka JM. The OPTN/UNOS Renal Transplant Registry. In: Cecka JM, Terasaki PI, eds. *Clinical Transplants 2004*. Los Angeles: UCLA Immunogenetics Center; 2005:1.

22. de Klerk M, Keizer KM, Claas FHJ, et al. The Dutch National Living Donor Kidney Exchange Program. *Am J Transplant* 2005;5:2302.

23. Segev DL, Gentry SE, Warren DS, Reeb B, Montgomery RA. Kidney paired donation and optimizing the use of live donor organs. *JAMA* 2005;293:1883.

24. Gjertson DW. Explainable variation in renal transplant outcomes: A comparison of standard and expanded criteria donors. In: Cecka JM, Terasaki PI, eds. *Clinical Transplants 2004*. Los Angeles: UCLA Immunogenetics Center; 2005:303.

25. Johnson SR, Khwaja K, Pavlakis M, Monaco AP, Hanto DW. Older living donors provide excellent quality kidneys: a single center experience (older living donors). *Clin Transplant* 2005;19:600.

26. De La Vega LS, Torres A, Bohorquez HE, et al. Patient and graft outcomes from older living kidney donors are similar to those from younger donors despite lower GFR. *Kidney Int* 2004;66:1654.

27. Kaiske BL, Snyder JJ, Matas AJ, et al. Preemptive kidney transplantation: the advantage and the advantaged. *J Am Soc Nephrol* 2002;13:1358.

28. Gill JS, Tonelli M, Johnson N, Pereira BJ. Why do preemptive kidney transplant recipients have an allograft survival advantage? *Transplantation* 2004;78:873.

29. Mange KC, Joffe MM, Feldman HI. Effect of the use or nonuse of long-term dialysis on the subsequent survival of renal transplants from living donors. *N Engl J Med* 2001;344:726.

30. Nijboer WN, Schuurs TA, van der Hoeven JA, et al. Effect of brain death on gene expression and tissue activation in human donor kidneys. *Transplantation* 2004;78:978.

31. Ojo AO, Wolfe RA, Held PJ, Port FK, Schmouder RL. Delayed graft function: risk factors and implications for renal allograft survival. *Transplantation* 1997;63:968.

32. Vats HS, Rayhill SC, Thomas CP. Early postnephrectomy donor renal function: laparoscopic versus open procedure. *Transplantation* 2005; 79:609.

33. Troppmann C, Ormond DB, Perez RV. Laparoscopic (vs open) live donor nephrectomy: a UNOS database analysis of early graft function and survival. *Am J Transplant* 2003;3:1295.

34. Shoskes DA, Cecka JM. Deleterious effects of delayed graft function in cadaveric renal transplant recipients independent of acute rejection. *Transplantation* 1998;27;66:1697.

35. Gjertson DW. Center and other factor effects in recipients of living-donor kidney transplants. In: Cecka JM, Terasaki PI, eds. *Clinical Transplants 2001*. Los Angeles: UCLA Immunogenetics Center; 2002:209

36. Danovitch GM, Cecka JM. Allocation of deceased donor kidneys: Past, present and future. *Am J Kidney Dis* 2003;42:882.

37. Hanevold CD, Ho PL, Talley L, Mitsnefes MM. Obesity and transplant outcome: A report of the North American Pediatric Renal Transplant Cooperative Study. *Pediatrics* 2005;115:352.

38. Gjertson DW, Cecka JM. Determinants of long-term survival of pediatric kidney grafts reported to the United Network for Organ Sharing kidney transplant registry. *Pediatr Transplant* 2001;5:5.

39. Harmon WE, McDonald RA, Reyes JD, et al. Pediatric transplantation 1994-2003. *Am J Transplant* 5:874, 2005.

40. Smith JM, Ho PL, McDonald RA. Renal transplant outcomes in adolescents: A report of the North American Pediatric Renal Transplant Cooperative Study. *Pediatr Transplant* 2002;6:493.

41. Jarzembowski T, John E, Panaro F, et al. Impact of non-compliance on outcome after pediatric kidney transplantation: an analysis in racial subgroups. *Pediatr Transplant* 2004;8:367.

42. Furth SL, Hwang W, Neu AM, Fivush BA, Powe NR. Effects of patient compliance, parental education and race on nephrologists recommendations for kidney transplantation in children. *Am J Transplant* 2003;3:28.

43. Baum MA, Ho M, Stablein D, Alexander SR. North American Pediatric Renal Transplant Cooperative Study. Outcome of renal transplantation in adolescents with focal segmental glomerulosclerosis. *Pediatr Transplant* 2002;3:488.

# 16.14 IMMUNOLOGIC ISSUES

*Junchao Cai, MD, PhD, Paul Terasaki, PhD*

The recipient's immune response to mismatched donor antigens remained, for decades, a major obstacle to successful transplants. Highly polymorphic human leukocyte antigens (HLAs) have been recognized as major players in meditating graft rejection. However, the effect of non-HLA antigens in organ transplantation began to receive increasing attention,[1] in view of the fact that immunologic rejection still widely occurred after HLA-identical sibling transplants.[2,3] Analyzing the kidney transplant registry database of the United Network for Organ Sharing (UNOS), we investigated short (1 year) and long-term (5 years) graft survival after HLA-mismatched and after HLA-identical sibling donor kidney transplants. In addition, we investigated the occurrence of immunologic rejection (hyperacute, acute, and chronic) after HLA-mismatched and after HLA-identical sibling donor kidney transplants in recipients who lost their allografts within or after 1 year posttransplant.

Between genetically identical donors and recipients, organ transplants can be 100% successful, certainly in the first year. Our UNOS database analysis showed that the graft survival rate at 1 year posttransplant was 100% when the recipient's donor was his or her identical twin (Figure 16.14-1); at 5 years, 91%

(Figure 16.14-2). Of these recipients, 9% lost their graft because of the recurrence of their original disease or because of death with a functioning graft, with no evidence of immunologic rejection.

Interestingly, our UNOS database analysis showed that 3% of HLA-identical sibling donor kidney transplant recipients lost their graft within 1 year posttransplant; 7% of sibling donor kidney transplant recipients with all six HLA antigens mismatched lost their graft within 1 year (Figure 16.14-1). If we assume no significant difference, in other variables that may affect graft survival, between these HLA-identical and 6-antigen-mismatched recipient groups, we may conclude that within 1 year posttransplant, 4% of that 7% graft loss rate was due to mismatched HLA-mediated immune reactions, whereas the remaining 3 percentage points might be associated with mismatched non-HLA antigens.

To analyze the long-term effect of antigen mismatching on graft survival, we excluded kidney transplant recipients who lost their graft within 1 year posttransplant (Figure 16.14-2). We found that 17% of 6-antigen-mismatched recipients lost their graft within 5 years posttransplant; 7 percentage points of that 17% were due to mismatched HLA antigens. Mismatched non-HLA antigens may also play a role. We found that only 3% of HLA-identical recipients lost their graft 1 year posttransplant (Figure 16.14-1); of those who survived for more than 1 year, 10% lost their graft within 5 years. Given these survival data, we cannot conclude that non-HLA-mismatched in HLA-identical donor-recipient pairs are the major cause of all graft failures, since disease recurrence, severe infection, death with a functioning graft, and other causes account for a certain percentage of graft failures.

The most important evidence of the deteriorating effect of mismatched non-HLA antigens on graft survival is that immunologic rejection (hyperacute, acute, and chronic), according to our UNOS database analysis often occurs after HLA-identical sibling transplants (Figures 16.14-3 and 16.14-4). For primary HLA-identical transplant recipients, immune-related graft loss accounted for 19.7% (hyperacute, 1.6%; acute, 12.8%; and chronic, 5.3%) of graft failure within 1 year posttransplant; for recipients who survived more than 1 year posttransplant, immune-related

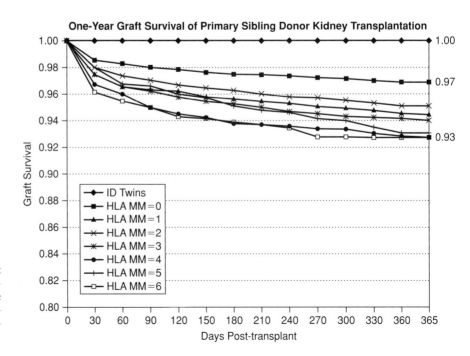

**FIGURE 16.14-1**

Effect of HLA mismatches (mm) on 1-year graft survival after sibling donor primary kidney transplants. For recipients with an ID twin donor, the graft survival rate was 100% within 1 year posttransplant; for HLA-ID recipients, 97%; for 6 antigen-mismatched recipients, 93%.

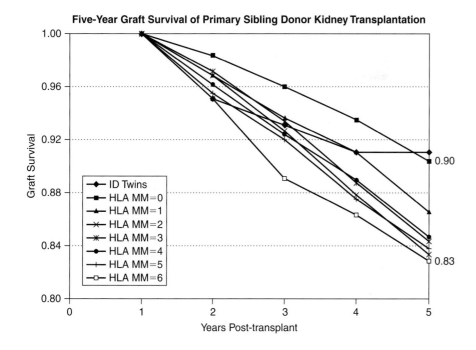

**FIGURE 16.14-2**

Effect of HLA mismatches (mm) on 5-year graft survival after sibling donor primary kidney transplants. For recipients with an ID twin donor, the graft survival rate was 100% at 5 years posttransplant; for HLA-ID recipients, 97%; for 6 antigen-mismatched recipients, 93%. Note: recipients who lost their graft within 1 year posttransplant were excluded.

graft loss accounted for 45.7% (acute, 6.1%; chronic, 39.6%) of graft failure (Figure 16.14-3). For retransplant HLA-identical transplant recipients, immune-related graft loss accounted for 25% (acute, 16.7%; chronic, 8.3%) of graft failure within 1 year posttransplant; for recipients who survived more than 1 year posttransplant, immune-related graft failure accounted for 45.3% of graft failures (acute, 9.5%; chronic, 35.8%) (Figure 16.14-4).

For HLA-identical transplant recipients, the rate of graft failure caused by acute rejection within 1 year posttransplant is about 12.8%; chronic rejection 24.2%. However, after 1 year posttransplant (with chronic rejection as the major cause of graft failure), chronic rejection associated with mismatched non-HLA antigens accounted for 39.6% of all graft failure. A very similar percentage (41.4%) of primary HLA-mismatched transplant recipients lost their graft because of chronic rejection after 1 year posttransplant. In the HLA-mismatched recipient group, not only HLAs but also some non-HLA antigens might be mismatched between the donor and the recipient. The 41.4% just cited represents an additive effect of both mismatched HLAs and non-HLA antigens. Yet surprisingly, as compared with the incidence of (39.6%) chronic rejection-related graft loss in the HLA-identical group, the 41.4% is not significantly higher. Our UNOS database analysis strongly suggests that immunologic rejection remains a major cause of graft failure after kidney transplants. Both HLA mismatches and non-HLA mismatches play a role in mediating graft rejection. Immunologic reactions to non-HLA mismatches (as compared with HLA mismatches) might be more important in long-term graft survival.

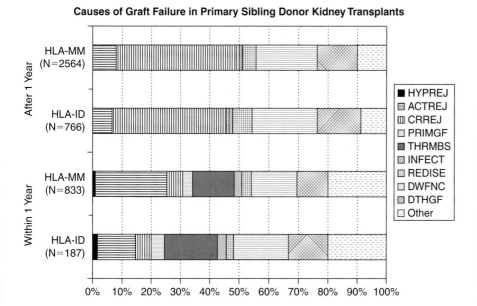

**FIGURE 16.14-3**

Causes of graft failure after sibling donor primary kidney transplants. Within 1 year posttransplant, for primary HLA-ID recipients, hyperacute rejection accounted for 1.6% of all graft failure; acute, 12.8%; and chronic, 5.3%. For primary HLA-mm recipients, the corresponding percentages were 0.7%; 24.2%; and 5.8%. For HLA-ID recipients who survived more than 1 year posttransplant, acute rejection accounted for 6.1% of all graft failure; chronic, 39.6%. For HLA-mm recipients who survived more than 1 year posttransplant, the corresponding percentages were 7.5% and 41.4%.

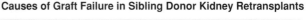

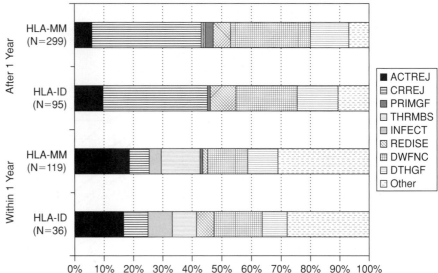

**FIGURE 16.14-4**

Causes of graft failure after sibling donor kidney retransplants. Within 1 year posttransplant, for HLA-ID retransplant recipients, acute rejection accounted for 16.7% of all graft failure; chronic, 8.3%. For HLA-mm retransplant recipients, the corresponding percentages were 18.5% and 6.7%. For HLA-ID recipients who survived more than 1 year posttransplant, acute rejection accounted for 9.5% of all graft failure; chronic, 35.8%. For HLA-mm recipients who survived more than 1 year posttransplant, the corresponding percentages were 5.7% and 37.5%.

## References

1. Opelz G. Non-HLA transplantation immunity revealed by lymphocytotoxic antibodies. *Lancet* 2005;365(9470):1570.
2. Al-Kerithy M, Salazar A, Kiberd B, et al. Impact of acute rejection on long-term graft survival in HLA-identical living-related kidney transplants. *Transplant Proc* 2001;33(6):2982.
3. Kalil J, Guilherme L, Neumann J, et al. Humoral rejection in two HLA identical living related donor kidney transplants. *Transplant Proc* 1989; 21(1 Pt 1):711.

## 16.15 LIVING DONOR KIDNEY TRANSPLANTATION AND MALIGNANCY

*E. Steve Woodle, MD, Thomas G. Gross, MD,
Rita Alloway, Pharm D, Amit D. Tevar, MD,
Joseph Buell, MD*

### KIDNEY TRANSPLANT-RELATED MALIGNANCIES

The association of transplantation and an increased risk of malignancy have been known since Penn reported the first posttransplant lymphomas in 1968.[1] Since this time, additional reports have established the increased risk of malignancy associated with immunosuppressive therapy required to prevent allograft rejection. Although it is widely believed that immunosuppressive therapy increases the risk of *de novo* transplant malignancies, the risk of malignancy recurrence, and alters the biologic behavior of malignancies in transplant recipients, the mechanisms by which this occurs are not known. In this chapter, we describe a number of transplant-related malignancies with a focus on practical guidelines for managing patients who are faced with malignancy-related issues.

Living donor transplant recipients are advantaged over deceased donor transplant recipients with respect to the threat posed by malignancy, as they generally require less immunosuppression

following transplantation, particularly highly matched living donor transplant recipients. However, antiviral prophylaxis is also very important for even highly matched transplant recipients to reduce the risk of virally driven malignancy, particularly posttransplant lymphoproliferative disorder (PTLD). Little data exist regarding the level of risk associated with living donor versus deceased donor recipients, and given that living donor recipients face the same issues posed by posttransplant immunosuppression, we cover all transplant-related malignancies and point out unique aspects of living donor transplantation where these data exist.

### LIVING DONORS WITH A HISTORY OF MALIGNANCY

#### General Considerations

Although encountered very infrequently, transplant programs on occasion have to consider potential living donor candidates who have a history of malignancy. In general, the most conservative approach is to consider as living donors only those individuals who are considered cured of their cancer. However, there remain some individuals who have high chances of cure, that are not quite 100%, who advocate strongly for an opportunity to donate their kidney to a loved one, and whose loved ones may be willing to assume this risk. In general, some experiences exist with these issues, and as such, brief consideration of these issues is provided.

#### Breast Cancer

A recent report from the IPITTR has examined a small number of cases of donors with a history of breast cancer.[2] This analysis found a 29% tumor transmission rate. Tumor transmission was limited to patients with invasive breast cancer. Breast cancer transmission was not observed in donors with a history of noninvasive breast cancers, including lobular carcinoma *in situ* and ductal carcinoma *in situ*. Based on this experience, we currently recommend not allowing breast cancer patients with a history of invasive breast cancer to become living kidney donors. Very early, small breast cancers treated with surgery and radiation that are associated with high cure rates may represent a population of potential donors; however, no evidence currently exists to support or contraindicate the use of these donors.

## Donor Kidneys With Small Renal Cell Cancers

Historically, small renal cell lesions (<2 cm diameter) were not considered malignant, primarily because they rarely exhibited malignant behavior. However, the distinction between benign and malignant renal cell lesions is now determined solely by histology. Nevertheless, the very benign behavior of these lesions raises the possibility that donor kidneys with these lesions may be transplanted with minimal risk of malignancy transmission.

Donor kidneys with small mass lesions or those with complex cystic lesions may be encountered at the time of deceased donor nephrectomy. They may also be encountered at the time of live donor nephrectomy, but with increased use of computed tomography (CT) scanning and magnetic resonance imaging (MRI) for determination of living donor anatomy, these occurrences may likely become of historical interest only. When faced with such a lesion in a living donor kidney, often the recipient will be under anesthesia, with an open abdominal incision. In these circumstances, the decision whether to use the kidney is time pressured and coercive because of the living donation. However, with deceased donor transplants, time is not an issue, and even permanent sections for pathology can often be obtained.

The lesion should first be managed by excisional biopsy with adequate margins. Frozen section should be performed to determine the presence or absence of malignancy. The absence of malignancy on frozen section is ample evidence for proceeding with transplantation. Concern does exist when the lesion appears malignant on biopsy. Recent examination of experience with small renal cell cancers (RCCs) that were noted at the time of kidney procurement, excised *ex vivo* and transplanted has noted an absence of tumor transmission in 14 recipients with median follow-up of 69 months.[3] This experience provides reassurance for those who wish to proceed with transplantation of these kidneys.

## RECIPIENTS WITH A HISTORY OF MALIGNANCY

### Preexisting Malignant Melanoma

In the United States in 1996, the incidence of melanoma was 13.8/100,000 persons. Mortality rates due to melanoma were 2.3/100,000 persons.[4] In practice the only malignant melanomas that can be considered cured are *in situ* lesions. All other lesions, regardless of depth have the potential for death. Because melanoma can recur many years following apparently successful therapy, and also because melanoma appears to be a cancer in which immune surveillance plays an important role in determining survival, recommendation to proceed with transplantation in a patient with a history of melanoma is a very serious and often difficult lesion.

The IPITTR experience with transplantation in patients with a history of melanoma includes 48 patients: 36 kidney, 10 heart, 1 lung, 1 liver transplant recipient. Of these 48 patients, 32 were male, 16 were female, and 83% were Caucasian. Median time between melanoma diagnosis and transplant was 92 months (range 0–479 months). A total of 10 recurrences (21%) were observed at a median time to recurrence of 47 months range (2–83 months). Of those patients with recurrence, 2 are alive with disease, 3 are alive without disease, and 5 died due to recurrent melanoma, giving a disease-specific death rate of 11%. These data indicate that even with long waiting times, melanoma can still recur in a relatively small, but significant fraction of patients. Current IPITTR recommendations for recipients with a history of melanoma with CIS or Clark level 1 lesions are that most are reasonable transplant candidates. Clark level 1 patients should preferably have at least a 5-year wait. Other patients should have longer waiting periods, and patients with a history of nodal disease should be strongly cautioned of the significant risk of recurrence even with long wait times.

## Preexisting Posttransplant Lymphoproliferative Disorders

Posttransplant lymphoproliferative disorders (PTLD) are a heterogeneous group of B-cell hyperplasias and malignancies that occur in a small percentage of transplant recipients. Although uncommon, clinicians are occasionally confronted with a patient who developed PTLD following renal transplantation, and subsequently lost their kidney transplant who present for retransplantation. The decision regarding candidacy for renal transplantation in these patients is a difficult one, in part because the risk of recurrent PTLD is not well known. However, there are a few reports of transplantation in patients with a prior history of PTLD.[5–8] These reports include a total of 15 patients who underwent retransplantation following PTLD. All of these patients were surviving at the time of last follow-up, and a substantial number had received antirejection therapy. The absence of recurrence in the largest group suggests that the risk of PTLD recurrence following retransplantation may be low. Presently, tools that include Epstein–Barr Virus (EBV) viral load monitoring, new immunosuppressive agents, and anti-EBV prophylaxis may provide a safety net for patients with PTLD who wish to be retransplanted. A review of these experiences with careful consideration is necessary for any program considering retransplantation of patients with a history of PTLD.

## Preexisting Genitourinary Cancers: Kidney Cancers

Renal cell cancers (RCCs) were divided by Dr. Penn into two classes: asymptomatic lesions (that were discovered incidentally) and symptomatic lesions (presented usually with pain or hematuria). Because the IPITTR lacks sufficient staging data, recurrence risk was based on these criteria. Asymptomatic RCC treated prior to transplantation were associated with a recurrence risk of < 7%. In contrast, the recurrence rate with RCC that presented with clinical signs or symptoms exceeded 25%. These observations led Dr. Penn to recommend 2-year waits for asymptomatic RCC and 5-year waits for symptomatic RCC.

Small < 2.5-cm lesions that are found incidentally and treated by radical nephrectomy may be considered at even lower risk, and patients with these lesions may be allowed to proceed with transplantation with full informed consent. These considerations may be of particular importance in patients who are in urgent need of kidney transplantation. Finally, because asymptomatic RCC in end-stage kidneys may be associated with RCC in the contralateral kidney in up to 10% of cases, many surgeons recommend bilateral nephrectomy for suspected RCC in an end-stage kidney.

## Preexisting Genitourinary Cancers: Prostate Cancers

Prostate cancer is the second leading cause of death due to cancer in men. With widespread application of prostate-specific antigen (PSA) testing, prostate cancer is being diagnosed and treated with increasing frequency. With the additional effect of aging of the U.S. population, the numbers of transplant candidates with a history of prostate cancer will likely increase for the foreseeable future. IPITTR has recently reported on its experience with prostate cancer prior to transplantation.[9] In this experience, 90 patients with a prior history of prostate cancer were identified who had undergone solid organ transplantation. In this study, tumor recurrence and disease-specific death rates increased with increasing tumor stage. Tumor recurrence rates in Stage I, II, and III disease were 14%, 16%, and 36%. Mortality due to recurrent prostate cancer was 2.9%, 6.8%, and 27.3%. These data argue strongly for avoidance of transplantation in prostate cancer patients with Stage III disease. However, with earlier diagnosis as a result of PSA testing, it is likely that increasing numbers of patients with good prognoses will be seen who will be reasonable candidates for transplantation. Additional data regarding Gleason score and PSA levels are needed in selecting patients with previous prostate cancer for transplantation.

## Preexisting Genitourinary Cancers: Bladder Cancer

Bladder cancer is common in the general population of the United States, with approximately 92% of lesions being transitional cell cancer (TCC). The IPITTR experience with transplantation in patients with a history of bladder cancer consists of 81 patients: 67 kidney, 9 heart, 2 liver, 1 lung, and 1 kidney pancreas transplant recipients. Mean age at diagnosis of bladder cancer was 47 years, and mean age at transplant was 54 years. Median waiting time from bladder cancer diagnosis to transplant was 34 months. The overall recurrence rate was 18% and the death rate due to recurrent bladder cancer was 12%. The recurrence rate did not appear to be influenced by the length of time between cancer diagnosis and transplantation: wait time < 2 years had a recurrence rate of 17%, 2- to 5-year wait time had a recurrence rate of 18%, and > 5-year wait time had a recurrence rate of 20%. These data indicate that patients with a history of bladder cancer experience significant recurrence rates following transplantation, consistent with the natural biologic behavior of bladder cancer in the general population.

## Preexisting Genitourinary Cancers: Testicular Cancer

In the IPITTR database, a total of 27 patients (16 kidney transplant recipients) were identified who were transplanted with a previous history of testicular cancer. Testicular cancer was diagnosed at a median of 153 (range 13–379) months before transplantation. Mean age at cancer diagnosis was 29.8 (range 8.3–50.7) years, and mean age at transplantation was 43.5 (range 20.4–61.3) years. Twenty-five patients (92.5%) were transplanted at more than 35 months after cancer diagnosis. Median follow-up after transplantation was 19 (range 1.7–171) months. Histologic types included seminoma (n = 8), nonseminomatous germ cell tumor (NSGCT; n = 5), and unknown in 14 patients. Cancer therapy included radical orchiectomy (n = 27), retroperitoneal lymphadenectomy (RPLND; n = 7), received external beam radiotherapy (n = 10), and chemotherapy (n = 9). At available follow-up, no patient experienced testicular cancer or treatment-related mortal-

ity. A total of 1 (4%) patient recurred. This patient, whose primary histology was seminoma, was transplanted 157 months after initial diagnosis. He recurred 13 months after transplantation, underwent radical lymph node dissection without alteration in immunosuppression, and was alive without evidence of disease at brief (4 months) follow-up. This experience suggests that patients with a history of successfully treated testicular cancer are generally reasonable candidates for transplantation.

## Preexisting Gastrointestinal Cancers: Colon Cancer

Following lung cancer, colon cancer is the second most common malignancy that results in death in the United States, affecting both men and women with relatively high frequencies. The IPITTR experience with preexisting colon cancer consists of a total of 56 patients: 34 kidney, 7 heart, and 15 liver transplant recipients. It is believed that the relatively high representation of liver transplant recipients may be a reflection of the relatively high incidence of liver transplant recipients with a history of ulcerative colitis and sclerosing cholangitis. The mean age at diagnosis of colon cancer in patients with a history of preexisting colon cancer was 47 years. Their mean age at transplant was 53 years. The median wait time from colon cancer diagnosis to transplant was relatively long at 75 months. Despite this relatively long pretransplant wait, the overall recurrence rate was high at 23%. Table 16.15-1 provides Dukes staging of preexisting colon cancers for each transplant type with wait time, recurrence rates, and 5-year survival rates. Despite the relatively high recurrence rate, the 5-year survival rate was high at 82%. The relatively high survival may be a result of assiduous monitoring for colon cancer recurrence following transplantation.

## Preexisting Hematologic Malignancies: Leukemias

Experience with solid organ transplantation in patients with a history of leukemia is relatively small. The IPITTR experience consists of 11 patients with a mean age at the time of leukemia diagnosis of 23 ± 16 years and a mean age at the time of transplant of 30 ± 15 years. Seventy-three percent were female, 91% were Caucasian, 36% were kidney transplant recipients, 36% were heart transplant recipients, 18% were liver transplant recipients, and 9% were lung transplant recipients. Sixty-four percent of patients had an interval from leukemia diagnosis to transplant of greater than 5 years, 18% waited 2 to 5 years, and 9% waited less than 2 years (9% of waiting periods were not known). These

**TABLE 16.15-1**

### PREEXISTING COLON CANCER

|  | Kidney | Liver | Heart | Total |
|---|---|---|---|---|
| Dukes Stage A | 4 | 3 | 0 | 7 |
| Dukes B1 | 19 | 3 | 2 | 24 |
| Dukes B2 | 3 | 7 | 3 | 13 |
| Dukes C | 8 | 2 | 2 | 12 |
| Median wait to transplant (months) | 74 | 54 | 50 | 75 |
| Recurrence rate (%) | 12 | 47 | 29 | 23 |
| 5-year Survival rate (%) | 94 | 60 | 71 | 82 |

data suggest that clinicians are likely to ask for long waiting times in patients with a history of leukemia. During a mean follow-up of 20 ± 25 months after transplantation, there were no recurrences of leukemia; however, one liver transplant recipient developed lymphoma after transplant, and expired from the malignancy within 5 months posttransplant. In summary, with long wait times, leukemia recurrence may be low, but it is possible that other malignancies, such as lymphoma, may arise following transplantation.

## Hematologic Malignancies: Lymphomas

Hodgkin's and non-Hodgkin's lymphomas account for approximately 9% of new cancer cases annually in the United States. Non-Hodgkin's lymphomas (NHL) are eight times more frequent than Hodgkin's lymphomas. With improving therapies and results of treatment of these lymphomas, increasing numbers of patients with a history of prior lymphomas are presenting as candidates for kidney transplantation. In deciding candidacy for these patients, one must be familiar with the risk of recurrence following transplantation so that appropriate decision making and informed consent can be achieved.

A recent review from the IPITTR analyzed experience in 91 patients with prior Hodgkin's disease (HD) and 53 patients with NHL who underwent solid organ transplantation.[10] With a median follow-up of 99 months after lymphoma diagnosis, and a medial follow-up of 25.7 months following transplantation, 9% of HD experience recurrent disease and 1% of NHL patients experienced recurrent disease. Survival following recurrence was poor (1/3 HD and 1/5 NHL) and brief (median survival 6.8 months). The only factor that appeared to correlate with risk of recurrence was the disease free interval between lymphoma diagnosis and transplantation. Of substantial interest was the observation of an overall recurrence rate of 10%, which is almost identical to that observed by the University of Pittsburgh group in their group of patients with PTLD. In summary, the relatively low incidence of recurrence of HD and NHL following transplantation indicates that a prior history of these diseases should not necessarily preclude transplantation, particularly lifesaving transplants. Patients with relatively long disease-free intervals prior to transplantation, in particular, may experience lower recurrence rates.

## Preexisting Gynecologic Cancers

IPITTR experience in transplant patients with a history of prior cervical cancer consists of a total of 48 patients. Eight patients waited less than 2 years from the time of cervical cancer diagnosis until transplant, 5 had a waiting time of 2 to 5 years, 11, had a waiting time of 5 to 10 years, and 24 had a waiting time greater than 10 years. Recurrence rates according to pretransplant waiting times were: < 2 years 13%, 2 to 5 years 0%, 5 to 10 years 27%, and > 10 years 13%. These data suggest that the risk of cervical cancer recurrence does not appear to be related to waiting time, and that cervical cancer can recur even with relatively long waiting times before transplantation.

IPITTR experience in transplant patients with a history of prior uterine cancer consists of a total of 24 patients. Five patients waited less than 2 years from the time of uterine cancer diagnosis until transplant, 5 had a waiting time of 2 to 5 years, 3 had a waiting time of 5 to 10 years, and 11 had a waiting time greater than 10 years. Recurrence rates according to pretransplant waiting

times were: < 2 years 20%, 2 to 5 years 0%, 5 to 10 years 33%, and >10 years 9%. These data suggest that the risk of uterine cancer recurrence does not appear to be related to waiting time, and that uterine cancer can recur even with relatively long waiting times before transplantation.

IPITTR experience in transplant patients with a history of prior vulvar cancer consists of a total of 19 patients. Three patients waited less than 2 years from the time of vulvar cancer diagnosis until transplant, 3 had a waiting time of 2 to 5 years, 5 had a waiting time of 5 to 10 years, and 8 had a waiting time greater than 10 years. Recurrence rates according to pretransplant waiting times were: < 2 years 33%, 2 to 5 years 33%, 5 to 10 years 40%, and >10 years 13%. These data suggest that the risk of vulvar cancer recurrence is high regardless of the length of waiting time, and that vulvar cancer can recur even with relatively long waiting times before transplantation.

## Preexisting Breast Cancer

IPITTR experience in transplant patients with a history of prior breast cancer consists of a total of 93 patients. Eleven patients waited less than 2 years from the time of breast cancer diagnosis until transplant, 31 had a waiting time of 2 to 5 years, 26 had a waiting time of 5 to 10 years, and 25 had a waiting time greater than 10 years. Recurrence rates according to pretransplant waiting times were: < 2 years 18%, 2 to 5 years 19%, 5 to 10 years 12%, and >10 years 8%. These data suggest that the risk of breast cancer recurrence is relatively high even with waiting times out to 5 years. After 5 years, the waiting time appears to decrease; however, even with waiting times up to 10 years, the recurrence rate remains as high as 8%. As in the general population, breast cancer can recur even with relatively long waiting times before transplantation. IPITTR breast cancer data indicate that the risk of recurrent breast cancer following transplantation is related to the stage at diagnosis: stage I, 6% recurrence rate; stage II, 8%; and stage III, 64% (with a 5-year survival rate of 14%). These observations argue strongly for careful evaluation of these patients with appropriate informed consent prior to proceeding with transplantation.

## Preexisting Thyroid Cancer

Most thyroid cancers, except anaplastic lesions, demonstrate relatively indolent biologic behavior. Description of their behavior and response to immunosuppressive therapy in transplant recipients has been limited to a small number of patients. A recent IPITTR study described the results in 27 patients with a history of thyroid cancer that subsequently underwent transplantation.[11] The great majority of these patients (n = 23) underwent kidney transplantation. The median time from thyroid cancer diagnosis to transplantation was 40 months (range 0.8–415 months), and median follow-up following transplantation was 26.5 months (range 0.8–207 months). Tumor histology included: papillary (56%), follicular (11%), and unspecified (33%). Two patients had positive nodes (1 papillary and 1 follicular). All patients were treated surgically. Recurrence rate was 7.8% with one patient (3.2%) dying of recurrent disease. Overall death rate was 18.5%, with four of five deaths unrelated to the preexisting thyroid cancer. This experience indicates that patients with thyroid cancer, if carefully selected, appear to be reasonable candidates for kidney transplantation, and that most deaths are due to causes other than recurrent thyroid cancer.

## *DE NOVO* TUMORS FOLLOWING RENAL TRANSPLANTATION

### Virally Driven Malignancies: Posttransplant Lymphoproliferative Disorders

PTLD was first reported by Israel Penn in 1968.[1] This first recognition of the unusual occurrence of lymphomas was noted by a temporal clustering of lymphomas in three young renal transplant recipients. The original report included these patients and also others from transplant centers in Europe. PTLD is actually a spectrum of lymphoproliferative disorders ranging from primary EBV infection-driven polyclonal B-cell proliferations, to frankly malignant lymphomas. The great majority of lymphomas that occur in transplant recipients are EBV positive and of B-cell origins. PTLD is observed with varying rates in solid organ transplant recipients with the lowest rates in kidney transplant recipients, and the highest rates in pediatric recipients of liver and small bowel transplants.[12] The increased PTLD risk in children is thought to be due to their lack of immunity/exposure to EBV and their high rate of receipt of adult organs, most of which come from EBV seropositive donors.[13] Recent data in adult transplant recipients have confirmed these observations in children, as adult EBV-seronegative recipients are at substantially higher risk of PTLD.[14] These observations have argued strongly for routine prophylaxis for EBV seronegative recipients of organs from EBV seropositive donors, and for routine monitoring of EBV viral loads in the peripheral blood. Recent studies have shown the efficacy and utility of EBV prophylaxis and viral load monitoring.[14]

PTLD most often presents with mass lesions including painless lymphadenopathy on physical exam or on imaging studies. The first step in diagnosing PTLD is to obtain biopsy specimens of suspected lesions. At the time of biopsy it is important to send the specimen for several studies, including cell-surface phenotyping for leukocyte markers, gene-rearrangement studies (to determine clonality), EBV markers, EBV viral loads, and serology studies in previously seronegative recipients. The patient should undergo staging studies including a neurologic examination. Brain imaging by CT or MRI is necessary for patients with any CNS symptoms or signs. All patients should have CT or MRI imaging of the chest, abdomen, and pelvis. In addition, because PTLD demonstrate a high degree of allograft tropism (regardless of allograft type), an allograft biopsy should be strongly considered. Finally, patients should undergo a bone marrow biopsy as a part of staging. Management of patients depends on the results of these studies. Patients with benign appearing lesions should be treated primarily with immunosupppression reduction. In general, an overall reduction in immunosupppression of 30% to 50% at a minimum is an appropriate first step. Serial staging studies should be conducted at 6-week intervals to determine the response to therapy.

Recently, anecdotal reports and two prospective trials have evaluated Rituximab, a CD20-specific monoclonal antibody approved for treatment of lymphomatous malignancies, for PTLD therapy.[15–18] In general, Rituximab has provided partial or complete remission rates approximating 50% when combined with immunosupppression reduction as first-line therapy for PTLD. These trials, however, used Rituximab in combination with immunosuppression reduction, and without a control limb consisting of immunosuppression reduction alone, the efficacy of Rituximab cannot be determined. In addition, recurrence rates after Rituximab therapy are relatively high (20%–40%), and therefore, Rituximab should be used as an adjunctive agent to immunosupppression reduction or chemotherapy.

Malignant PTLD require chemotherapy. Recent studies from the IPITTR and other reports of chemotherapy for PTLD indicate that treatment of malignant PTLD with chemotherapy is usually associated with poor survival rates, often less than 50% at 1 year. Although the proximate cause of death may be difficult to determine in these patients, IPITTR data suggest that 20% to 30% of patients with malignant PTLD may die primarily of the adverse effects of chemotherapy. It is important that when myeloablative chemotherapy is used to treat PTLD (or any other cancer) in solid organ transplant recipients, that all immunosupppression be discontinued until marrow recovery is well established.

Risk factors that determine survival in renal transplant recipients with PTLD have been recently described in an IPITTR report.[19] This study demonstrated that age and number of sites involved were statistically significant determinants of survival from PTLD in kidney transplant recipients.

CNS involvement by PTLD is a particularly ominous condition.[20] Of the various presentations of PTLD, CNS involvement is associated with the lowest survival rates, approximating 10% at 1 year following diagnosis. Immunosuppression reduction in these patients must be aggressive, and it appears that radiation therapy alone gives the best results (PTLD4).

### Virally Driven Malignancies: Kaposi Sarcoma

Kaposi sarcoma (KS) is a rare cancer that is most commonly found in patients of Middle Eastern descent that is thought to be virally driven by human herpes virus 8. KS is generally considered a low-grade malignancy and most commonly involves the skin and gastrointestinal tract (KS1). KS may present with isolated skin (60% of cases) or GI involvement, with both (mixed pattern). Whenever GI involvement is present, the prognosis is substantially worse. IPITTR data suggest that GI involvement is associated with a 41% disease specific mortality.[21] When KS is diagnosed, a careful examination of the oral cavity, and upper and lower GI endoscopy should be performed. KS is usually treated by a combination of local therapy and immunosupppression reduction. Cutaneous lesions can be treated by surgical excision and/or radiation therapy.

### Virally Driven Malignancies: *De Novo* Cervical and Vulvar Cancer

An increased incidence of cervical and vulvar cancers have been observed in solid organ transplant recipients.[22] Human papillomavirus (HPV) has been linked to cervical cancer in the general population, and two HPB serotypes (16 and 18) have been associated with cervical cancer in transplant recipients.[22]

A total of 87 patients in the IPITTR developed *de novo* cervical cancer following transplantation: 72 kidney, 7 heart, and 6 liver transplant recipients. Seventy patients received surgery, 12 received radiation therapy, and 9 received chemotherapy. Five-year survival in patients with *de novo* cervical cancer appeared to be strongly related to the stage at cancer diagnosis: Stage I, 87%; Stage II, 84%; Stage III, 50%; and Stage IV, 20%.

A total of 79 patients were identified in the IPITTR with *de novo* vulvar cancer following transplantation: 66 kidney transplants, 7 heart, 5 liver, and 1 pancreas transplant. Most patients[67] received surgical therapy, 23 received radiation therapy, and 16 received chemotherapy. Five-year survival rates according to stage included: Stage I, 96%; Stage II, 95%; Stage III, 80%; and Stage IV, 65%. These data indicate that *de novo* vulvar cancer in transplant recipients has high survival rates even in those with Stage IV disease.

## Non-Virally-Driven *De Novo* Malignancies: Nonmelanoma Skin Cancer

The development of skin cancer in transplant recipients is related to exposure to ultraviolet rays and to the duration of immuno-suppression exposure.[23,24] Basal cell carcinoma (BCC) and sqamous cell carcinoma (SCC) are by far the most common skin cancers encountered in the general population and in transplant recipients. Recent update of the IPITTR experience with BCC and SCC has recently been published.[25] In this experience, 2,018 skin cancers were identified in transplant recipients and classified as SCC, BCC, or mixed SCC/BCC. The ratio of SCC to BCC was 1.9 to 1. Recurrence rates for BCC, SCC, and SCC/BCC were 12%, 20%, and 48%. Cancer-specific mortality was lowest for BCC (11%), followed by BCC/SCC (15%), and SCC (18%). Median time to diagnosis posttransplant for each group was beyond 4 years. Although skin cancers can be readily treated in transplant recipients, their clinical behavior appears to be more aggressive than in the general population. Lymph node metastasis has been reported in approximately 6% of transplant patients.

## *De Novo* Malignant Melanoma

The frequency of malignant melanoma is almost twice as high in transplant recipients as in the general population. As in the general population, survival rates with malignant melanoma correlate with Clark and Breslow levels.[26] In the IPITTR, a total of 96 transplant recipients developed *de novo* malignant melanoma. The median time to diagnosis of malignant melanoma posttransplant was 35 months (range 1–145 months). Median of patients at the time of *de novo* melanoma diagnosis was 56 years (range 21–69 years). Seventy-six percent of patients were male and 82% were Caucasian. Clark levels were available in 28 of the 96 patients (29%): Level 1, 2 patients; Level 2, 7 patients; Level 3, 7 patients; Level 4, 11 patients; and Level 5, 1 patient. Survival according to Clark levels were: Level 1, 100%; Level 2, 57%; Level 3, 43%; Level 4, 27%, Level 5, 0%. These data indicate that *de novo* malignant melanoma tends to present with a relatively high stage and has high mortality rates.

## *De Novo* Genitourinary Cancers: Kidney Cancer

Most renal cell cancers (RCCs) in patients with end-stage kidney disease are now diagnosed incidentally on imaging studies (usually CT or MRI) performed to evaluate a wide variety of clinical problems. IPITTR experience with *de novo* RCC consists of 160 cases. In this series, the mean age at diagnosis was 51 years, and the median time to diagnosis of *de novo* RCC following renal transplantation was 61 months. In this series, 149 RCC occurred in native kidneys, and 11 occurred in the renal allograft. Twenty percent of patients developed metastatic disease, and overall mortality was 53%. In addition, 30 percent of patients presented with advanced disease, being stage III or IV at the time of diagnosis.

## *De Novo* Genitourinary Cancers: Prostate Cancer

Prostate cancer is the second leading cause of cancer related deaths in the United States. Because of increased application of PSA testing, more men are being diagnosed with prostate cancer prior to and after solid organ transplantation. Biological behavior of *de novo* prostate cancer in solid organ transplant recipients, though, has not been defined. The cancers were staged according to American Joint Committee on Cancer (AJCC) criteria. A total

of 312 patients were reported to the IPITTR with a median time to diagnosis of 43.4 months, range (0.5–305 months). These 312 transplant recipients included 221 kidney, 82 heart, 7 liver, and 1 lung transplant recipient. Median follow-up post diagnosis was 11.8 months and overall cancer specific mortality was 13.1% (41/312 patients). Stages at diagnosis included: Stage 1, 4 %; stage 2, 76%; stage 3, 16%; stage 4, 4%. Cancer-specific mortality correlated with stage: Stage 1, 6%; stage 2, 4%; stage 3, 20%; stage 4, 48%. These findings indicate that surveillance for prostate cancer in transplant recipients is very important, as prognosis is markedly influenced by the stage at diagnosis.

## *De Novo* Genitourinary Cancers: Bladder Cancer

The IPITTR series of transplant recipients with *de novo* bladder cancer following transplantation consists of 241 patients (222 kidney transplant recipients) diagnosed at a median of 77 (range 1–344) months following transplantation. Histologic types included transitional cell cancer (TCC) (n = 151), squamous cell cancer (SCC; n = 22), adenocarcinoma (n = 13), and bladder sarcoma (n = 3). Histology was unspecified in 52 recipients. All patients underwent staging transurethral resection of bladder tumor (TURBT). Cystectomy was performed in 41 patients, radiation therapy in 29 patients, and chemotherapy in 57 patients. Immunosuppression was discontinued in 5/34 (15%) recipients and reduced in 2 (6%) after cancer diagnosis. A total of 34 patients (14%) developed recurrent bladder cancer. Seventy-seven patients (32%) eventually died of bladder cancer at a mean of 13 (range 0–104) months after diagnosis of bladder cancer.

## *De Novo* Genitourinary Cancers: Testicular Cancer

*De novo* testicular cancer following renal transplantation is a very infrequent event. IPITTR experience consists of a total of 19 patients (18 of whom were renal transplant recipients) who developed *de novo* testicular cancer at a mean of 45 (range 2–30 months) following. Follow-up intervals following testicular cancer diagnosis included a mean of 41 and a median of 19 (range 1–153) months. Histologic types included: seminoma (n = 13), nonseminomatous germ cell tumor (NSGCT; n = 3), Leydig cell tumor (n = 1), and unrecorded in 2 patients. All patients underwent radical orchiectomy, 9 received external beam radiotherapy, and 7 received chemotherapy. One patient experienced a recurrence at 15 months after original testicular cancer diagnosis. This patient was alive with seminoma 66.5 months after transplantation and 53 months after original diagnosis. Four (19%) patients died of metastatic cancer (n = 2) or complications of cancer therapy (n = 2).

## *De Novo* Gastrointestinal Cancers: Colon Cancer

A recent IPITTR report examined the results of *de novo* colon cancer in solid organ transplant recipients: 93 kidney, 29 heart, 27 liver, and 1 lung transplant recipient.[27] When compared to SEER data, transplant patients were younger at diagnosis (58 vs 70 years, p < 0.001) and had a worse overall 5-year survival (44 vs 62%, p < 0.001). In addition, by Dukes staging, transplant recipients had lower survival for each stage: Dukes A and B, 74 vs 90%; Dukes C, 20 vs 66%; and Dukes D, 0 vs 9%. This experience suggests that colon cancer demonstrates a more aggressive behavior in immunosuppressed transplant patients than in the general population. Clinicians should be aware of these tendencies in caring for solid organ transplant recipients.

## *De Novo* Gynecologic Cancers: Ovarian

The IPITTR experience with *de novo* ovarian cancer following transplantation consists of 19 patients, 16 of whom received kidney transplants. Median age at diagnosis was 44.3 years, and median time to diagnosis of ovarian cancer was 29 months after transplantation. Stage at diagnosis included: Stage I (4) 21%, Stage II (3) 16%, Stage III (7) 37%, Stage IV (5) 26%. Tumor histology revealed adenocarcinoma 10 (53%), papillary 4 (21%), and other 5 (26%). Lymph node involvement occurred in 2 (10%) patients; and distal metastases, in 7 (37%). Surgical debulking was performed in 16 (84%), and chemotherapy 10 (53%). Actuarial 1-, 3-, and 5-year survivals were: 68%, 63%, and 43%. Data based on cancer staging are presented in Table 16.15-2.

## *De Novo* Gynecologic Cancers: Uterine

In the IPITTR registry, 33 patients were identified with uterine cancer at a mean of 53 months (range 1–141) following transplantation. These patients included 26 kidney transplants, 5 heart transplants, 1 liver transplant, and 1 lung transplant. Treatment included surgery (28 patients), chemotherapy (3 patients), and radiation (2 patients). Five-year patient survival strongly correlated with the stage at diagnosis: Stage I, 92%; Stage II, 82%; Stage III, 64%; and Stage IV, 0%. These data argue strongly that stage at diagnosis is a strong determinant of survival in transplant recipients with *de novo* uterine cancer.

## *De Novo* Breast Cancer

In North America, breast cancer is the most common malignancy in women, accounting for 27% of female malignancies. In addition, over 18% of female cancer deaths are secondary to breast cancer. In general, the incidence of *de novo* breast cancer in transplant recipients appears similar to the general population.[28] In the IPITTR experience, 114 U.S. renal transplant recipients with *de novo* breast cancer have been reported. Of these, 96% were female and 90% Caucasian transplant recipients. The median age

**TABLE 16.15-2**
### DE NOVO OVARIAN CANCER DATA

|  | Stage I (n = 4) | Stage II (n = 3) | Stage III (n = 7) | Stage IV (n = 5) |
|---|---|---|---|---|
| Median time to Dx | 45 months | 113 months | 22 months | 9 months |
| Adenocarcinoma | 0 | 02 (67%) | 6 (86%) | 2 (40%) |
| Papillary | 2 (50%) | 1 (33%) | 0 | 1 (20%) |
| Cystadenoma | 1 (25%) | 0 | 0 | 0 |
| Granulosa cell | 1 (25%) | 0 | 0 | 0 |
| Embryonal cell | 0 | 0 | 1 (14%) | 0 |
| Signet cell | 0 | 0 | 0 | 1 (20%) |
| Unspecified | 0 | 0 | 0 | 1 (20%) |
| Surgery | 4 (100%) | 3 (100%) | 5 (71%) | 5 (100%) |
| Chemotherapy | 1 (25%) | 0 | 5 (71%) | 4 (80%) |
| Metastasis | 0 | 0 | 3 (43%) | 4 (80%) |
| Lymph node (+) | 0 | 0 | 1 (14%) | 1 (20%) |
| Death | 0 | 1(33%) | 4 (57%) | 3 (60%) |

**TABLE 16.15-3**
### DE NOVO BREAST CANCER DATA

|  | Stage I | Stage II | Stage III | Stage IV |
|---|---|---|---|---|
| **No. Patients** | 57 | 37 | 10 | 1 |
| Histology |  |  |  |  |
| Ductal | 60% | 73% | 44% | 60% |
| Unspecified | 24% | 11% | 33% | 20% |
| Lobular | 10% | 16% | 22% | 20% |
| Treatment |  |  |  |  |
| Surgery | 100% | 100% | 78% | 0% |
| Chemo | 9% | 78% | 89% | 100% |
| XRT | 24% | 24% | 11% | 0% |
| Lymph node involvement | 0 | 38% | 100% | 100% |

at presentation was 46 years (range 16–74 years) and the median time from transplant to diagnosis was 56 months range (2–299 months). Histologic tumor types included (Table 16.15-2): infiltrating ductal carcinoma 72 patients (62%), lobular carcinoma 16 patients (14%), and unspecified in 26 patients (24%). Lymph node involvement was present at the time of diagnosis in 24 patients (21%), and distant metastases in 1 patient. Stages at the time of presentation included: stage 1, 55%; stage II, 35%; stage III, 9%; and stage IV, 1%. Survival according to stage is presented in Figure 16.15-1.

## *De Novo* Hematologic Malignancies: Leukemia

The largest series of *de novo* posttransplant leukemias comes from the IPITTR. A total of 32 patients with *de novo* leukemia had a mean age of 43 ± 15 years at time of transplant, and were predominantly male (78%) and Caucasian (75%). Leukemias were evenly divided between chronic and acute forms as well as the lymphocytic and myelogenous types. Most recipients were kidney (60%) or heart (34%) transplant recipients. The mean time from transplant to leukemia diagnosis was 66 ± 44 months. Intervention included chemotherapy alone (50%), no intervention

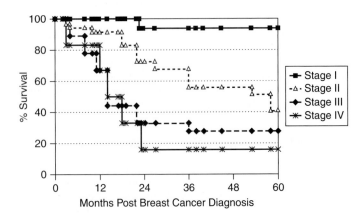

**FIGURE 16.15-1**

Survival with *de novo* breast cancer by stage in transplant recipients.

(28%), immunosuppression minimization (9.5%), combination therapy (9.5%), and immunotherapy alone (3%). Death occurred in 20/32 patients (63%), with 65% of deaths due to malignancy. Mean time to death after leukemia diagnosis was 5 ± 7 months (range 0.1–26 months).

## Thyroid Cancer

*De novo* thyroid cancers are seldomly diagnosed following transplantation. A total of 41 solid organ transplant recipients were identified in the IPITTR database with *de novo* thyroid cancer, the great majority of whom were kidney transplant recipients (n = 38). The median time from transplant to *de novo* thyroid cancer diagnosis was 29 months (range 3.5–213.5 months). Median follow-up following thyroid cancer diagnosis was 17.7 months (range 0–149 months). Tumor histology included papillary (85%), follicular (5%), and unspecified (10%). Four patients had a prior history of neck irradiation. All 41 patients underwent partial or complete thyroidectomy. Nine patients had positive nodal disease and underwent postoperative adjuvant therapy. At follow-up, 83% of patients were alive and free of disease. Disease-specific mortality was 2.4%. This experience indicates that *de novo* thyroid cancer following transplantation has a reasonable short-term prognosis and is likely effectively treated by standard therapy.

## MALTomas

Mucosa-associated lymphoid tissue lymphomas (MALTomas) are B-lymphocyte tumors that are associated with *Helicobacter pylori* infection in the gastrointestinal tract, usually the gastric mucosa.[29] MALTomas tend to be indolent tumors that are substantially less aggressive than posttransplant lymphoproliferative disorders. They usually present with benign histology, but can progress to frank lymphomas and or gastric adenocarcinoma.[31] A recent report and literature review from the Penn tumor registry indicated that most MALTomas that occur in transplant recipients are readily treated by treatment of the underlying *H. pylori* infection with or without concomitant immunosupppression reduction. Repeat gastric endoscopy with biopsy and CT scanning at regular intervals (6–8 weeks) are necessary to assure prompt eradication of the tumor and to identify development of histologically more aggressive lesions at an early point in the course of therapy.[29]

## References

1. Penn I, Hammond W, Brettschneider L, Starzl Te. Malignant lymphomas in transplantation patients. *Transplant Proc* 1968;1:106–112.
2. Friedman AL, Muthiah C, Beebe TM, Woodle ES, Buell JF. Collective experience with renal transplantation from donors with a history of breast cancer. (Abstract 537) *Am J Transplant* 2003;3:288.
3. Buell JF, Hanaway MJ, Thomas M, et al. Donor kidneys with small renal cell cancers: can they be transplanted? *Transplant Proc* 2005; 37: 581–582.
4. *Epidemiology in Cancer 2001, Eds Devita, Hellman, Rosenberg; Cancer PPO; 229*
5. Hickey D, Nalesnik M, Vivas C, et al. Renal retransplantation in patients who lost their allografts during management of a previous post-transplant lymphoproliferative disease. *Clin Transplant* 1990;4:187–190.
6. Demircin G, Rees L. Retransplantation after post-transplnat lymphoproliferative disease. *Pediatr Nephrol* 1997;11: 358–360.
7. Birkeland S, Hamilton-Dutoit S, Bendtzen. Long-term followup of kidney transplant patients with PTLD. Duration of PTLD-induced operational graft tolerance, interleukin-18 course and results of retransplantation. *Transplantation* 2003;76:153–158.
8. Karras A, Thervet E, Meur YL, et al. Successful renal retransplantation after posttransplant lymphoproliferative disease. *Am J Transplant* 2004;4: 1904–1909.
9. Woodle ES, Gupta M, Buell JF, et al. Prostate cancer prior to solid organ transplantation: the Israel Penn International Transplant Tumor Registry Experience. *Transplant Proc* 2005;37:958–959.
10. Trofe J, Buell JF, Woodle ES, et al. Recurrence risk after organ transplantation in patients with a history of Hodgkin disease or non-Hodgkin's lymphoma. *Transplantation* 2004;78:972–977.
11. Gupta M, Merchen T, Trofe J, et al. Pre-existing thyroid cancer is associated with a low risk of recurrence following solid organ transplantation. *Am J Transplant* 2003;3:344.
12. Pearlman LS. Posttransplant viral syndromes in pediatric patients: a review. *Prog Transplant* 2002;12:116-124.
13. Boubeneider S, Hiesse C, Goupy C, et al. Incidence and consequences of post-transplantation lymphoproliferative disorders. *J Nephrol* 1997;10: 136-145.
14. Lee TC, Savoldo B, Rooney CM, et al. Quantitative EBV viral loads and immunosuppression alterations can decrease PTLD incidence in pediatric liver transplant recipients. Am J Transplant. 2005 Sep;5(9):2222-8.
15. Oertel SH, Verschuuren E, Reinke P, Zeidler K, Papp-Vary M, Babel N, Trappe RU, Jonas S, Hummel M, Anagnostopoulos I, Dorken B, Riess HB. Effect of anti-CD 20 antibody rituximab in patients with post-transplant lymphoproliferative disorder (PTLD). *Am J Transplant* 2005 Dec;5(12):2901–2906.
16. Choquet S, Leblond V, Herbrecht R, et al. Efficacy and safety of rituximab in B-cell post-transplant lymphoproliferative disorders: results of a prospective multicentre phase II study. *Blood* 2005;Oct 27.
17. Blaes AH, Peterson BA, Bartlett N, Dunn DL, Morrison VA. Rituximab therapy is effective for posttransplant lymphoproliferative disorders after solid organ transplantation: results of a phase II trial. *Cancer* 2005 Oct 15;104(8):1661–1667.
18. Elstrom RL, Andreadis C, Aqui NA, et al. Treatment of PTLD with rituximab or chemotherapy. *Am J Transplant* 2006 Mar;6(3):569–576.
19. Trofe J, Buell JF, Beebe TM, et al. Analysis of factors that influence survival with post-transplant lymphoproliferative disorder in renal transplant recipients: the Israel Penn International Transplant Tumor Registry experience. *Am J Transplant* 2005 Apr;5(4 Pt 1):775–780.
20. Buell JF, Gross TG, Hanaway MJ, et al. Posttransplant lymphoproliferative disorder: significance of central nervous system involvement. *Transplant Proc* 2005 Mar;37(2):954–955.
21. Penn I. Sarcomas in organ allograft recipients. *Transplantation* 1995;60: 1485–1491.
22. Brown MR, Noffsinger A, First MR, Penn I, Husseinzadeh N. HPV subtype analysis in lower gential tract neoplasms of female renal transplant recipients. *Gynecol Oncol* 2000 Nov;70 (2):220–224.
23. Gupta AK, Cardella CJ, Haberman HF. Cutaneous malignant neoplasms in patients with renal transplants. *Arch Dermatol* 1986;122:1288-1293.
24. Penn I. Post-transplant kidney cancers and skin cancers (including Kaposi sarcoma). In: Schmahl D, Penn I eds. *Cancer in Organ Transplant Recipients*. Berlin: *Springer-Verlag*; 1991:46–53.
25. Buell JF, Hanaway MJ, Thomas M, Alloway RR, Woodle ES. Skin cancer following transplantation: the Israel Penn International Transplant Tumor Registry Experience. *Transplant Proc* 2005;37:962–963.
26. Penn I. Immunosuppression and skin cancer. *Clinics Plastic Surg* 1980; 7(3):361–368.
27. Papaconstantinou HT, Sklow B, Hanaway MJ, et al. Characteristics and survival patterns of solid organ transplant patients developing *de novo* colon and rectal cancer. *Dis Colon Rectum* 2004;47:1989–1903.
28. Penn I. Cancers in renal transplant recipients. *Adv Ren Repl Ther* 2000; 7:147–156.
29. Aull MJ, Buell JF, Peddi VR, et al. Maltoma: a helicobacter pylori-associated malignancy in transplant patients. *Transplantation* 75:225–228, 2003.

# 16.16 STRATEGIES TO MAXIMIZE THE DONOR POOL

## 16.16.1   Living Donor Exchange

*Kiil Park, MD, PhD, Jong Hoon Lee, MD, PhD*

## INTRODUCTION AND BACKGROUND

### Organ Shortage

Although a kidney transplant is now accepted as the best treatment option for patients with end-stage renal disease (ESRD), the donor organ shortage is a major barrier. Even in countries with a relatively large supply of deceased donor (DD) kidneys, the gap between the number of organ donors and the number of potential recipients continues to widen. Therefore, more than 50% of all transplanted kidneys worldwide are now obtained from living donors (LDs). The use of LDs continues to increase in the United States.[1]

In South Korea, a country with limited DD transplants, the kidney donor shortage is worsening. Despite social and legal consensus on brain death, the number of kidney transplants is limited by the number of both LDs and DDs. The total number of patients in South Korea waiting for a kidney transplant was 642.3 per million population in 2001; it increased to 700.6 per million in 2002. In 2002, the number of new transplant candidates was 129.5 per million, of whom only 15.2 per million actually underwent a kidney transplant.[2]

### Efforts to Increase Donations

Various efforts have been made in South Korea to increase the number of kidneys available for transplantation. For DD transplants, the use of non-heart-beating donors and the institution of a promotional program were proposed. For LD transplants, marginal donors and unrelated donors have been used. Several trials of kidney transplantation between ABO-incompatible donors and recipients with plasmapheresis produced reasonable results, but these trials were small; such transplants are not routinely per-

formed.[3] Crossmatch-positive donors have also been used, after conversion to negative status with plasmapheresis, intravenous immunoglobulin, and potent immunosuppression[4]; however, these methods did not succeed in all cases, and were associated with large medical costs and risks.

## DONOR EXCHANGE PROGRAMS

For many years, only first-degree relatives, that is, parents, adult children, and siblings who matched the recipient at one or more HLA haplotype, were deemed to be suitable LDs. Kidneys from genetically unrelated but emotionally motivated donors (living unrelated donors or LURD—eg, spouses, close relatives, common-law partners, close friends, well-motivated voluntary donors—were discouraged, because of relatively poor results and the fear of commercialization. Now, however, LURDs are commonly used, and excellent short- and long-term results have been achieved.[5,6]

In 1986, Rapaport et al. proposed the idea of paired-kidney exchanges in an attempt to increase the availability of organs for transplantation.[7] The proposal was to use LD kidneys that were incompatible with their designated recipient through an exchange arrangement between two donor–recipient pairs. Such an approach seemed attractive to many transplant centers, but has not been widely implemented because of social, legal, cultural, and financial issues.

### Swap and Swap-Around Programs

In South Korea, to expand the donor pool given the satisfactory results of LURD transplants, an exchange donor program was developed in 1991.[8]

A direct donor exchange (swap) was offered to patients who had a family member who was willing to donate, but was unsuitable because of positive lymphocyte crossmatching or incompatible ABO blood groups. The first swap between two families in South Korea was successfully performed in 1991; the reason for donor–recipient incompatibility was a positive crossmatch, so two patients exchanged their donor kidneys.

The second phase of our program was prompted by this initial success. The swap-around program, as it is called, entails listing many kinds of potential LDs—close friends, spouses, distant

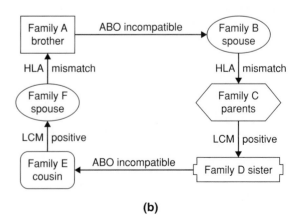

**(a)**                                                      **(b)**

**FIGURE 16.16.1-1**

Overview of exchange living donor program (swap program). (a) Direct swap program: Donor–recipient pairs exchange their donors directly. (b) Indirect swap-around program: Several donor-recipient pairs are rearranged within the donor pool. (Park K, Lee JH, Huh KH, et al. Exchange living-donor kidney transplantation: Diminution of donor organ shortage. *Transplant Proc* 2004;36:2949. Used with permission.)

relatives, emotionally motivated volunteers—in our database, after careful screening. Groups of two or more donor–recipient pairs are assembled within this pool, according to the degree of HLA match and ABO compatibility. Potential donors and recipients are then informed of availability for exchange donation (Figure 16.16.1-1).[9-11]

Since 1995, Park et al. have promoted this swap-around program and achieved excellent patient and graft survival rates at Severance Hospital, Seoul, South Korea.[9-11] Given the successful results by Park et al. for more than 10 years, many centers have recently shown interest in such a program. The United States has some experience with donor exchange. In Europe, donor exchange, at the time of this writing, has been attempted only in Romania, the Netherlands, and Israel; in Asia, only in Turkey.

## Crossover Living Donor Exchange

Successful LD swap and swap-around exchange programs require a large pool of donor–recipient pairs who are incompatible. For this purpose, several South Korean transplant centers developed a joint, *crossover* program.[9] This program provides for LD exchanges among the transplant centers.

In the Netherlands, all the kidney transplant centers participate in the crossover exchange program. This has led to a national crossover pool. To ensure an equal chance for all participating donor–recipient pairs, matching is performed by a national organ procurement and allocation organization, the Dutch Transplantation Foundation.[12]

## List-Paired Exchange

Another variation of paired-exchange programs is termed *list pairing*. Again, a potential LD, incompatible with the chosen recipient, agrees to donate a kidney to a suitable transplant candidate identified from the waiting list. In return, the original recipient is given priority on the waiting list for the next available, ABO-compatible, DD kidney. Such a list-paired program was recently instituted in the United States, within the domain of the New England Organ Bank, and resulted in 17 LD kidneys being added to the pool from 2001 through 2003.[13] List pairing, at least within the United States, requires the consent of all transplant programs within a service area, as well as authorization of a "variance" in allocation procedures from the national United Network for Organ Sharing (UNOS) policies.[14]

## SELECTION OF EXCHANGE DONORS

Selection of appropriate donors (and recipients) for a donor exchange program is of critical importance. Many criteria must be met, such as complete lack of any HLA-matched or ABO-matched living related donor or of any DD; informed consent of the donor and recipient and their families, without compulsion; minimum age of 20 years; no evidence of a commercial transaction; ethical approval; and thorough investigation of the need for the recipient's kidney transplant.[15]

As for other LURDs, potential exchange donors must undergo a preoperative clinical workup to ensure their safety and suitability. Moreover, even before the clinical workup, they must be evaluated by a team of social workers under the guidance of the ethics committee, in order to obviate any possibility of commercial organ donation. Routine psychiatric evaluation is also recommended to give potential exchange donors another opportunity to decide on their

commitment to the donation process: potential exchange donors must be able to say no, despite any earlier commitment or possible coercion. The evaluation helps to pinpoint potential donors' level of commitment and to document the absence of perceived coercion.

The only way to ensure that both recipients in a paired-exchange program actually receive their graft (ie, that neither donor withdraws from the exchange agreement) is to perform the transplants simultaneously.

To minimize the appearance of possible interfamilial conflicts, transplant centers must make efforts to assure that the medical and psychosocial evaluations of potential donors and the entire decision-making process involve health-care professionals who are not involved in the care of the recipient.

In South Korea, swaps are arranged to preferentially facilitate HLA matching, so that the donor and the recipient share at least two class I and one class II alleles if possible. In the LD pool exchange transplants that have been performed, chosen donors shared even more alleles with their recipient: at least three antigens of HLA class I (A+B) or at least one antigen of HLA class II (DR).[9-11] In addition to the degree of HLA match, many other factors should be considered (eg, socioeconomic status, gender, age, any relationship, body weight, and donor kidney function) in order to minimize any significantly different outcome between the pairs.[13]

## CURRENT RESULTS

### Donor Types

In South Korea, about 800 kidney transplants are now performed annually. Most of them use living related donors (LRDs; about 40%), followed by LURDs (about 40%) and then DDs (< 20%).[2]

The number of exchange LD kidney transplants has increased dramatically over the last 10 years: they were 1.5% of all LD transplants (4.2% of LURD) in 1995; 4.1%(10.4%) in 1997; 25.5% (46.6%) in 1999; 11.5% (40.0%) in 2000; 10.8% (44.0%) in 2002; and 13.4% (30.0%) in 2004 (Figure16.16.1-2). The main reasons for donor exchange were ABO blood-type incompatibility (76.3%), positive lymphocyte crossmatch (21.4%), and poor HLA match between spouses (2.3%).[11]

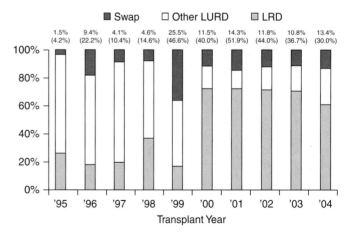

% of swap donors among living donors, ( ) % of swap donors among LURD

**FIGURE 16.16.1-2**

Exchange living donor kidney transplants, by donor type, over a 10-year period. (Park K, Lee JH: Living donor exchange program for kidney transplantations. *Transplantation and Immunology Letter* 2005;XXI(1):4. used with permission.)

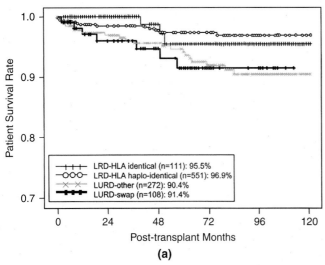
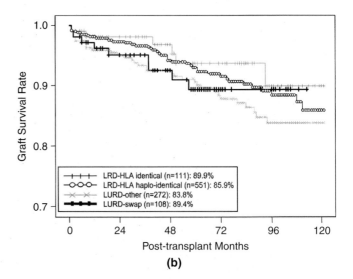

**(a)**     **(b)**

**FIGURE 16.16.1-3**

Patient and graft survival rates. There was no difference in (a) patient and (b) graft survival rates among swap, other LURD, HLA-haploidentical, or HLA-identical transplants. (Park K, Lee JH. Living donor exchange program for kidney transplantations. *Transplantation and Immunology Letter 2005*;XXI(1):4. Used with permission.)

## Patient and Graft Survival

The selection criteria (including HLA matching) used in studies of LD exchange programs were comparable to those adopted for LURD or HLA haploidentical LD transplants.[9-11] Park et al. retrospectively studied 1,051 kidney recipients, by donor type, who underwent their transplant from January 1995 through December 2004. Of the 671 LRD kidney transplants, 111 donor-recipients pairs were HLA-identical, 551 were HLA-haploidentical, and only 9 had no HLA matches. In addition, 108 LURD kidney transplants occurred in the swap program, as well as 272 other LURD kidney transplants. Park et al. found no statistically significant differences, by donor type, in 10-year patient and graft survival rates ($p > 0.05$ for patient survival, $p > 0.05$ for graft survival)[11] (Figure 16.16.1-3).

## Acute Rejection

As was expected, Park et al. found no statistically significant differences, by donor type, in acute rejection episodes in terms of frequency or severity. The incidence of acute rejection in the first year

posttransplant was 28.7% with exchange LDs, 32.4% with other LURDs, and 27.6% with HLA haploidentical LRDs ($p > 0.05$). The frequency of severe acute rejection requiring antibody treatment was 8.3% with exchange LDs, 7.7% with other LURDs, and 7.4% with HLA haploidentical LRDs ($p > 0.05$) (Table 16.16.1-1). Of the exchange LD kidney transplants, 9 grafts failed (8.3%) during the study period; the most common cause of graft failure was death with a functioning graft (55.5%). One recipient lost the graft because of irreversible acute rejection.[11]

## ADVANTAGES AND DISADVANTAGES OF DONOR EXCHANGE PROGRAMS

The principal advantage of LD exchange program is that, after arrangements are made and consent obtained, an uncomplicated ABO-compatible transplant is performed under standard immunosuppression with excellent results.[9-11] Expensive interventions such as intravenous immunoglobulin and plasmapheresis are avoided. Such transplants can be electively and preemptively

**TABLE 16.16.1-1**

### ACUTE REJECTION EPISODES, FIRST YEAR POSTTRANSPLANT, BY DONOR TYPE (FROM PARK K, LEE JH: LIVING DONOR EXCHANGE PROGRAM FOR KIDNEY TRANSPLANTATIONS. TRANSPLANTATION AND IMMUNOLOGY LETTER XXI (1): 4, 2005; USED WITH PERMISSION)

|  | Frequency | | | | Severity | |
| --- | --- | --- | --- | --- | --- | --- |
|  | 1 | 2 | 3 | Total | Antibody use | Graft Loss[‡] |
| LURD*-swap (%) | 27(25.0) | 3(2.8) | 1(0.9) | 31(28.7) | 9(8.3) | 1(0.9) |
| LURD-other (%) | 70(25.7) | 16(5.9) | 2(0.7) | 88(32.4) | 21(7.7) | 5(1.8) |
| LRD[†]-HLA haplo-identical (%) | 131(23.5) | 13(2.3) | 0(0) | 144(27.6) | 41(7.4) | 3(0.5) |
| LRD-HLA identical (%) | 9(8.2) | 1(0.9) | 1(0.9) | 11(10.0) | 2(1.8) | 1(0.9) |

*LURD = living unrelated donor; [†]LRD = living related donor; [‡]Graft Loss = graft loss due to acute rejection

**TABLE 16.16.1-2**

## ABO BLOOD TYPE, BY DONOR TYPE, OF RECIPIENTS VS. CANDIDATES

| Type | LURD*-swap (%) | LURD-other (%) | LRD[†] (%) | KONOS list[‡] (%) |
|---|---|---|---|---|
| A | 41 (37.9) | 103 (37.8) | 227 (33.8) | 492 (33.3) |
| B | 10 (9.3) | 39 (14.3) | 100 (14.9) | 397 (26.8) |
| O | 29 (26.8) | 70 (25.7) | 187 (27.9) | 423 (28.6) |
| AB | 28 (25.9) | 60 (22.1) | 157 (23.3) | 165 (11.2) |
| Total | 108 | 272 | 671 | 1477 |

*LURD=living unrelated donor; [†]LRD=living related donor; [†]KONOS list=newly registered ESRD patients for transplantation on KONOS (Korean network for organ sharing) list in 2003; *p-value=0.213* (calculated by Chisquare). From Park K, Lee JH: living donor exchange program for kidney transplantations. Transplantation and immunology letter xxi (1): 4, 2005; used with permission.

performed in a timely fashion, which may reduce or obviate the need for pretransplant dialysis.

In addition, previously unusable kidneys can be used, allowing other transplant candidates with ESRD to be removed from the waiting list. Thus, the benefit not only accrues for the original recipients, but also for candidates remaining on the list. If such transplants help alleviate the donor shortage, they may help remove incentives for or the need to consider commercial donation.

Another advantage is the emotional and psychological benefit for donors. Even if the transplant fails, donors know that they did everything possible to help a loved one. Since the donation is indirect in exchange transplants, the emotional and psychological benefits may be more diffuse. Yet, in the South Korean program, almost all the families knew each other, especially in the case of direct exchange. In fact, donor exchange must be managed carefully to avoid interfamilial conflicts; it is essential to thoroughly explain the entire procedure and the possible results pretransplant so that all expectations are realistic. Nonetheless, there is no reason to believe that the emotional and psychological benefits of exchange donation would vary substantially from those documented in more conventional programs.[16–18]

The potential disadvantages of LD exchange include psychological stress to donors and their families; possible conflicts between the donor's and the recipient's families, especially in the event of significant discrepancies in posttransplant results; and the general risks assumed by all LDs.

In addition, blood group O transplant candidates might be seen as having less opportunity to find an exchange donor Blood group O candidates require a blood group O donor. But blood group O donors are universal donors and can give to any ABO type recipient. In South Korea, blood group O is the second most common blood type in the general population as well as in ESRD patients waiting for a DD.[2] According to Park et al., LD exchange kidney recipients' ABO types were as follows: A, 37.9%; B, 9.3%; O, 26.8%; and AB, 25.9%. Of note, these percentages did not significantly differ from the other types of donor transplants (eg, with LURDs or with LRDs) or from the ESRD patients still waiting for a DD transplant ($p$ = .213; Table 16.16.1-2). Thus, blood group O recipients have the same chance of a kidney transplant—including with an exchange LD—as those with other blood types.[11]

One true disadvantage of LD exchange is the ethical and logistic complexity of the transaction. Informed consent requires greater explanation of risks and benefits for multiple parties. Documentation of thorough understanding by many different people is essential.

## SUMMARY

Exchange LD kidney transplant programs may prevent the current loss of a significant number of suitable LDs, and may thereby have a significant impact on the current acute shortage of donor organs (especially in countries without well-developed DD organ procurement systems or without established brain death statutes). All kinds of LDs—relatives, spouses, close friends, and voluntary donors—are potentially available.

With proper screening, ethics, and informed consent, the net result is a relatively uncomplicated transplant from an immunologic perspective. Posttransplant outcomes are comparable to transplants with more standard LD allografts. In fact, it is even possible to facilitate the most favorable donor–recipient combinations for long-term success.

Potential LDs should not be excluded because of a positive lymphocyte crossmatch or ABO blood type incompatibility; rather, they should be encouraged to exchange within these incompatible groups. However, they should undergo a careful predonation evaluation.

In conclusion, LD exchange programs are a viable way to help relieve the current donor organ shortage and offer good posttransplant results.

## References

1. Rosendale JD. The UNOS renal transplant registry. *Clin Transpl* 2003;65.
2. The Korean Society of Nephrology Registry. Renal replacement therapy in Korea. *Korea J Nephrol* 2003;22s:S353.
3. Tanabe K, Tokumoto T, Ishida H, et al. ABO-incompatible renal transplantation at Tokyo Women's Medical University. *Clin Transplant* 2003;175.
4. Schweitzer EJ, Wilson JS, Vina MF, et al. A high panel-reactive antibody rescue protocol for cross-match positive live donor kidney transplants. *Transplantation* 2000;70:1531.
5. Spital A. Unrelated living kidney donors. An update of attitudes and use among US transplant centers. *Transplantation* 1994;57:1722.
6. Spital A. Unconventional living kidney donors—attitudes and use among transplant centers. *Transplantation* 1989;48:243.
7. Rapaport FT. The case for a living emotionally related international kidney donor exchange registry. *Transplant Proc* 1986;18(Suppl 2):S5.
8. Kwak JY, Kwon OJ, Lee KS, et al. Exchange-donor program in renal transplantation: a single-center experience. *Transplant Proc* 1999;31:344.

9. Park K, Moon JI, Kim SI, et al. Exchange donor program in kidney transplantation. *Transplantation* 1999;67(2):336.

10. Park K, Lee JH, Huh KH, et al. Exchange living-donor kidney transplantation: Diminution of donor organ shortage. *Transplant Proc* 2004;36:2949.

11. Park K, Lee JH. Living donor exchange program for kidney transplantations. *Transplant Immunol Lett* 2005;XXI(1):4.

12. Keizer KM, de Klerk M, Haase-Kromwijk BJ, et al. The Dutch algorithm for allocation in living donor kidney exchange. *Transplant Proc* 2005;37(2):589.

13. Delmonico FL. Exchanging kidneys – advances in living donor transplantation. *N Engl J Med* 2004;350:1812.

14. Delmonico FL, Morrissey PE, Lipkowitz GS, et al. Donor kidney exchanges. *Am J Transplant* 2004;4:1628.

15. Hiraga S, Tanaka K, Watanabe J, et al. Living unrelated donor renal transplantation. *Transplant Proc* 1992;24:1320.

16. Jacobs C, Johnson E, Anderson K, et al. Kidney transplants from living donors: how donation affects family dynamics. *Adv Ren Replace Ther* 1998;5:89.

17. Johnson EM, Anderson JK, Jacobs C, et al. Long term follow-up of living kidney donors: quality of life after donation. *Transplantation* 1999;67:717.

18. Smith MD, Kappell DF, Province MA, et al. Living-related kidney donors: a multicenter study of donor education, socioeconomic adjustment, and rehabilitation. *Am J Kidney Dis* 1986;8:223.

## 16.16.2a    The History of ABO-Incompatible Living Donor Kidney Transplantation

*Jean-Paul Squifflet, MD, PhD*

### PREHISTORY

ABO-incompatible kidney transplants were first reported by Hume et al. in 1955, by Murray et al. in 1960, and by Starzl et al. in 1964.[1–3] Although long-term graft survival was observed in some initial cases, the overall experience indicated that hyperacute rejection could occur; therefore, crossing the ABO barrier was generally not done.

During the late 1970s and early 1880s, bone marrow transplants were already being performed when the donor completely matched the recipient in major antigens, that is, human leukocyte antigens (HLAs). In that setting, the risk of transplanting ABO-incompatible bone marrow was sometimes considered unavoidable: bidirectional ABO incompatibility could be present when both isoagglutinins and isoantigens were incompatible between donor and recipient (eg, A donor to B recipient; B donor to A recipient).[4] The immediate risk was hemolysis of red blood cells (RBCs) contained in the graft: therefore, bone marrow grafts were usually depleted of donor RBCs by various cell separation techniques. Delayed complications included hemolysis and RBC aplasia, the persistence of not only host isoagglutinins but also hemolysis of recipient RBCs (mediated by antibodies [Abs] produced by donor lymphocytes contained in the graft). Therefore, depletion of recipient circulating Abs was also performed.[5] The outcome after ABO-incompatible bone marrow transplants varied from series to series. But the outcome was not different from ABO-compatible bone marrow transplants, demonstrating that ABO-incompatible bone marrow transplants could be safely performed with adequate recipient preparation.[6]

The concept of depleting anti-AB Abs in kidney transplant recipients was probably first introduced by Slapak et al. in 1981,[7] when a kidney transplant patient with major donor–recipient blood group incompatibility (A1-incompatible) was successfully treated for rejection with modified plasmapheresis. Eventually, in 1990, the same group reported on pretransplant immunoadsorption and plasmapheresis for ABO-incompatible transplant recipients,[8] with a survival rate as high as 87%.

### PIONEERING ERA

In March 1981, an ABO-incompatible deceased donor (DD) kidney transplant was inadvertently performed at our institution because of an error in donor ABO typing. Despite the $A_1$ to O major ABO incompatibility and a basic immunosuppressive therapy regimen—including despite a short course of polyclonal Ab with azathioprine (AZA) and steroids without calcineurin inhibitors or additional treatments—the kidney graft functioned well and is still functioning 25 years later. Noteworthy was the good histocompatibility matching between donor and recipient with two DR-matched antigens. The graft was allocated through Eurotransplant.

Based on that successful DD kidney transplant and on the ABO-incompatible allogenic bone marrow transplant experience, a living donor (LD) ABO-incompatible kidney transplant program was initiated by Professor Guy P. J. Alexandre in June 1982. Pretransplant removal of Abs with plasmapheresis prevented Ab-mediated hyperacute rejection; the immunosuppressive regimen was started 3 days pretransplant.[9,10] The surgical procedure included a splenectomy on the day of the transplant.[11] However, despite chronic immunosuppression, antidonor- blood-group Abs returned and persisted, even after successful transplants.[12,13] In most recipients—except the three who did not undergo splenectomy—the graft continued to function well, despite the continued presence of these Abs and the persistence of the target antigen in the kidney.[14] Therefore, that situation was termed "accommodation" by Bach et al.[15] Splenectomy was proposed as a prerequisite for successful human ABO-incompatible kidney transplants by Alexandre et al.[11]

Even today, the gap continues to grow between the number of patients waiting for kidney transplants and the number of DD organs available. This gap became a major challenge throughout the world, especially in countries like Japan, where brain death criteria were not legally recognized. To help overcome this gap, LD kidney transplants across ABO blood-group barriers became more frequent.[16] Refinements in immunosuppression and patient selection increased both short- and long-term graft survival of such transplants, with success rates at 5 years posttransplant approaching those of DD and other LD transplants.[16–18] Nonetheless, the mechanism by which the kidney graft can protect itself from Abs still remains unclear.

### FIRST SERIES: 20 YEARS LATER

From June 1982 through November 1983, during Periods I and III (Table 16.16.2a-1), 39 ABO-incompatible LD kidney transplants were performed in 38 recipients who also underwent splenectomy.[14] Of those 38 recipients, 25 were male and 13 female; 1 boy received his first ABO-incompatible transplant from his mother and a second from his uncle. The recipient mean age was 23 ± 10 years. A total of 35 first transplants, 3 second, and 1 third were performed. The donor mean age was 42 ± 9 years. All kinds of ABO incompatibilities were encountered: A to O (n = 4); $A_1$ to B (n = 11); $A_2$ to O (n = 4); B to O (n = 11); B to $A_1$ (n = 1); $A_1$ to B (n = 3); $A_1$B to $A_1$ (n = 1); $A_1$B to B (n = 3); and $A_1$B to O (n = 1). Of the LDs, 31

**TABLE 16.16.2a-1**

## RECIPIENT CHARACTERISTICS, FIRST SERIES OF ABO-INCOMPATIBLE LIVING DONOR (LD) KIDNEY TRANSPLANTS

| | Period I<br>n = 6 | Period II<br>n = 3 | Period III<br>n=33 |
|---|---|---|---|
| Pre- or Peritransplant splenectomy | 6/6 | No | 33/33 |
| CsA | No | 3/3 | 33/33 |
| Donor platelet infusion | 4/6 | 3/3 | 17/33 |
| Plasmapheresis | 6/6 | 3/3 | 33/33 |
| Polycloclnal Abs from Day – 3 | 6/6 | 2/3 | 30/33 |
| AZA | 6/6 | 3/3 | 26/33 |
| Pred | 6/6 | 3/3 | 33/33 |
| Unrelated | 0/6 | 1/3 | 8/33 |

were related: mother to child (n = 20); father to child (n = 7); sister to sibling (n = 3); and uncle to nephew (n = 1); 8 were unrelated: wife to husband (n = 7) and husband to wife (n=1).

Pretransplant therapies included donor platelet infusion (21/39), 2 to 5 plasmapheresis sessions (39/39), cyclosporin A (CsA) with or without AZA (33/39) and with polyclonal Abs (36/39), including antilymphocytic (27/39) or antithymocytic (9/39) globulins and splenectomy at the time of the transplant (37/39). The 2 last recipients had already undergone splenectomy, at the time of a previous transplant and after a trauma. After the last plasmapheresis session, when the level of ¼ (ABO Abs) was reached, all recipients received 5 mL of substance A or B (depending on the incompatible blood group; blood-group-specific substances were extracted from porcine stomachs, Behasil Corporation, Miami, FL) diluted in 50 to 100 mL of saturated solution of plasma proteins, administered over 30 to 60 minutes.

Postoperatively, the immunosuppressive regimen included AZA-prednisolone (Pred) (n = 6), CsA-Pred (n = 7), and CsA-AZA-Pred (n = 26).

To these 39 recipients from Periods I and III, a small group of 3 nonsplenectomized recipients must be added: Period II (Table 16-16.2a-1). In all 3, the kidney graft was hyperacutely rejected during the first postoperative week, leading primarily to the conclusion that splenectomy could be a prerequisite for successful ABO-incompatible LD transplants (11).

The outcome of recipients from Period I (no CsA and pre- or peritransplant splenectomy, n = 6) and Period III (CsA and splenectomy, n = 33) is summarized in Table 16.16.2a-2 and in the following analysis. The 31 ABO-incompatible related LD graft recipients are alive. Graft losses occurred from acute or hyperacute rejection in 5 recipients (mean time to graft losses, 11 ± 3 days; no recipient under 15 years of age) and from chronic rejection in 8 recipients (mean time to graft losses, 9.5 ± 4.8 years).

By contrast, among the 8 ABO-incompatible unrelated LD graft recipients, 2 died early from sepsis after having been treated for rejection (2 and 3 months earlier); 2 lost their graft from hyperacute rejection, and 3 from chronic rejection. Twenty years later (Table 16.16.2a-2), only 1 recipient (husband to wife, 2 DR matches) has a functioning graft (creatinine, 1.0 mg/dL).

Noteworthy is the 9-year-old boy who received a first ABO-incompatible kidney from his mother after 20 months on dialysis. The cause of his kidney failure was a cortical necrosis after a traumatic spleen rupture (see above). He lost his first graft to chronic rejection without any acute rejection episode. After another 2 months on dialysis, he was transplanted with a second ABO-incompatible kidney grafts from his uncle. At the time of his second transplant, a laparotomy was performed, and accessory hypertrophic spleen tissue was removed, 17 years later, his kidney function remains excellent, with a creatinine level of 1.3 mg/dL.

In this small series of patients (Periods I and III), only 1 B-cell lymphoma was encountered. Of the 39 recipients, 21 underwent donor platelet infusions (Table 16.16.2a-1); the remaining 18, random blood transfusion. But no difference was seen in their

**TABLE 16.16.2a-2**

## OUTCOME OF 39 ABO-INCOMPATIBLE RELATED AND UNRELATED LIVING DONOR (LD) KIDNEY TRANSPLANTS, PERIODS I AND III

| | n | Mean Age | NO RRT*<br>Before Tx | Death | Graft Losses | | n | Functioning graft | |
|---|---|---|---|---|---|---|---|---|---|
| | | M ± SD | % | | HA<br>Rejection | Chronic<br>Rejection | | Follow-up<br>(years)<br>m + SD | Creatinine<br>(mg/dL)<br>m + SD<br>(median) |
| **Related** | | | | | | | | | |
| Time to graft loss | 31 | 20 ± 7 | 35 | 0 | 5<br>11 ± 3 days | 8<br>9.5 ± 4.8 yrs | 18 | 17 ± 3 | 1.9 ± 1.3 (1.5) |
| < 15 years<br>Time to graft loss | 9 | 11 ± 2 | 55 | 0 | 0 | 2<br>5.5 ± 4.8 yrs | 7 | 16 ± 2 | 1.8 ± 0.6 (1.7) |
| > 15 years<br>Time to graft loss | 22 | 23 ± 6 | 28 | 0 | 5<br>11 ± 3 days | 6<br>11 ± 4 yrs | 11 | 18 ± 3 | 2.0 ± 1.6 (1.4) |
| **Unrelated** | 8 | 37 ± 9 | 12 | 2 | 4 | 3 | 1 | 20 | 1.0 |

*RRT, Renal replacement therapy; Tx, transplant; HA, hyperacute.

postoperative outcome or long-term survival rates.[12] The ABO isoagglutinin titer was reduced below 1/4 with the two to five plasmapheresis sessions in all recipients and almost to 0 by the administration of substance A or B. Postoperatively, it increased more or less rapidly over the preoperative value, but it could not be correlated with the grade, incidence of rejection, or long-term outcome, given the small number of patients.[12,13]

Graft survival was also studied in two subgroups of ABO-incompatible related LD graft recipients. Graft survival rates at 2, 5, 10, and 15 years posttransplant were 100%, 89%, 78%; and 78% in the subgroup < 15 years old; 77%, 77%, 64%, and 59% in the subgroup > 15 years old (NS). Moreover, the graft survival rates of the 8 recipients < 15 years old and on CsA compared favorably with the graft survival rates of 38 ABO-compatible related LD graft recipients of the same age who underwent transplants during the same period (June 1982– November 1989) and who were also on CsA.[14]

Therefore, that series of 39 ABO-incompatible LD kidney represents the first successful attempt to overcome ABO incompatibility. In preparing the LD graft recipient by plasmapheresis (3 to 5 sessions) along with intravenous injection of substance A and/or B as part of pretransplant immunosuppression, isoagglutinins can be eliminated pretransplant. Peri- or pretransplant splenectomy could have played a role, as illustrated by the poor outcome of the three nonsplenectomized recipients during Period II. By contrast, the posttransplant recovery of isoagglutinin titers and the time to recovery could not predict posttransplant outcome, especially with regard to the incidence of early acute or hyperacute rejection.[12,13] After a critical period of 3 weeks, isoagglutinin titers could increase over the original level without jeopardizing the kidney tissue, even with the presence of antigens[13]—the phenomenon eventually termed "accommodation" by Bach et al.[15]

## MODERN ERA

Today, more than 20 years later, each part of the original protocol has been further assessed or modified by different groups, but prospective randomized studies are still lacking. Indeed, plasmapheresis was replaced by immunoadsorption columns by Tanabe et al.,[16] Tyden et al.,[19] and others.[20,21] A major drawback was the cost–benefit ratio of immunoadsorption, which had no demonstrable advantage on the hyperacute or acute rejection rate.[16]

Pretransplant immunosuppression was also extended for longer periods. Galili et al.[22] found that preventing the anti-Gal response may decrease the posttransplant immune rejection rate of ABO-incompatible allografts. That is why plasmapheresis is also used in desensitization protocols for crossmatch-positive LD candidates.

By contrast, the efficacy of substance A or B to delete the last circulating isoagglutinins can no longer be assessed. Substance A and B are no longer used for human therapeutic purposes, given their animal origin. Therefore, to eliminate Abs, intravenous immunoglobulins are currently used by Park et al.[23] and others,[16,20,21,24] along with new, more potent drugs such as tacrolimus and mycophenolate mofetil.[23] Another approach by Olausson et al.[25] is to transplant a partial heterotopic liver graft from the same donor, before kidney implantation.

The need for peri- or pretransplant splenectomy remains controversial.[19,24] During the pioneering era of ABO-incompatible LD transplants especially Period I when CsA was not yet widely used, splenectomy was also proposed by others[26] for DD kidney

transplants. The rationale for splenectomy is that the spleen is an IgM-IgG–producing B-cell reservoir. But today, splenectomy is often avoided, especially in children at risk for pneumococcal infections. Indeed, several authors have avoided splenectomy for $A_2$ to O donor-recipient pairs.[23] Others propose the use of anti-CD 20 (rituximab) monoclonal Ab infusion.[19,27]

The best clinical results seen in the first series in well-matched LD kidney transplants in recipients under 15 years have been confirmed by Tanabe et al.[16] Identical results were also reported by Yanza et al. in liver transplants[28] and also by West et al.[29] in heart–lung transplants. Preformed natural Abs (isoagglutinins) against AB antigens are present at birth as IgG, as a result of transport of maternal Abs through the placenta, but not as a result of self-production. Maternal Abs disappear from neonates after 2 weeks, but at about 8 to 12 weeks, newborn infants start producing IgM and IgG on their own. Adult levels are reached by the age of 5 to 10 years. Although the stimulus for producing Abs to A and/or B determinants remains uncertain, a common hypothesis is that it is a response to the presence of A and/or B saccharides on bacteria or other microorganisms that colorize the infant gastrointestinal tract.[30]

For the above reasons, today, crossing the ABO barrier in LD kidney transplants is feasible with the use of plasmapheresis or immunoabsorption along with potent new immunosuppressive drugs. The preparation techniques are also being successfully used in desensitization protocols for hyperimmunized recipients with positive crossmatches. Crossing the ABO barrier is also a step toward xenotransplantation.

## References

1. Hume DL, Merrill JP, Miller BF, Thorn GW. Experiences with renal homotransplantations in the human: report of nine cases. *J. Clin Invest* 1955; 34: 327–382.
2. Murray JE, Merrill JP, Dammin GJ, Dealy JB Jr, Walter CW, Brooke MS et al. Study on transplantation immunity after total body irradiation; clinical and experimental investigation. *Surgery* 1960; 48: 272–284.
3. Starzl TE, Marchioro TL, Holmes JH, Hermann G, Brittain RS, Stonington OH et al. Renal homografts in patients with major donor-recipient blood group incompatibilities. *Surgery* 1964; 55: 195–200.
4. Buckner CD, Clift RA, Sanders JE, Williams B, Gray M, Storb R et al. ABO-Incompatible marrow transplants. *Transplantation* 1978; 26: 233–238.
5. Bensinger WI, Buckner CD, Baker DA, Clift RA, Thomas ED. Removal of specific antibody in vivo by whole blood immunoadsorption: preliminary results in dogs. *J Clin Apheresis* 1982; 1: 2–5.
6. Stussi G, Seebach L, Muntwyler J, Schanz U, Gmur J, Seebach JD. Graft-versus-host disease and survival after ABO-incompatible allogenic bone marrow transplantation: a single-centre experience. *Br J Haematol* 2001; 113: 251–253.
7. Slapak M, Naik RB, Lee HA Renal transplant in a patient with major donor-recipient blood group incompatibility: reversal of acute rejection by the use of modified plasmapheresis. *Transplantation* 1981; 31: 4–7.
8. Slapak M, Digard N, Ahmed M, Shell T, Thompson F. Renal transplantation across the ABO barrier – a 9 year experience. *Transplant Proc.* 1990; 22: 1425–1428.
9. Alexandre GPJ, De Bruyere M, Squifflet JP, Moriau M, Latinne D, Pirson Y. Human ABO-incompatible living donor renal homografts. *Neth J Med* 1985; 25: 231–234.
10. Alexandre GPJ, Squifflet JP, De Bruyere M, Latinne D, Moriau M, Carlier M, Pirson Y, Lecomte Ch. ABO-incompatible related and unrelated living donor renal allografts. *Transplant Proc* 1986; 18: 452–455.

11. Alexandre GPJ, Squifflet JP, De Bruyere M, Latinne D, Moriau M, Ikabu N. Splenectomy as a prerequisite for successful human ABO-incompatible renal transplantation. *Transplant Proc* 1985; 17: 138–143.

12. Reding R, Squifflet JP, Latinne D, De Bruyere M, Pirson Y, Alexandre GPJ. Early postoperative monitoring of natural anti-A and anti-B isoantibodies in ABO-incompatible living donor renal allografts. *Transplant Proc* 1987; 19: 1989–1990.

13. Alexandre GPJ, Latinne D, Gianello P, Squifflet JP. Performed cytotoxic antibodies and ABO-incompatible grafts. *Clin Transplantation* 1991; 5: 583–594.

14. Squifflet JP, De Meyer M, Malaise J, Latinne D, Pirson Y and Alexandre GPJ. Lessons learned from ABO-Incompatible Living Donor Kidney Transplantation: 20 years later. *Experimental and Clinical Transplantation* 2004; 2: 208–213.

15. Bach FH, Ferran C, Hechenleitner P, Mark W, Koyamada N, Miyatake T et al. Accommodation of vascularized xenografts: host Th 2 cytokine environment. *Nat Med* 1997; 3: 196–204.

16. Tanabe L, Takahashi K, Sonda K, Tokumoto T, Ishikawa N, Kawai T. Long-term results of ABO-incompatible living kidney transplantation. *Transplantation* 1998; 65: 224–228.

17. Reding R, Squifflet JP, Pirson Y, Jamart J, De Bruyere M, Moriau M et al. Living related and unrelated donore kidney transplantation: comparison between ABO-compatible and incompatible grafts. *Transplant Proc* 1987; 19: 1511–1513.

18. Malaise J, Baldi A, Setola P, Mourad M, Pirson Y, Squifflet JP. Renal transplantation in children: a comparative study between parental an well-matched cadaver grafts. *Br J Surg* 1995; 82: 128.

19. Tyden G, Kumlien G, Fehman I. Successful ABO-incompatible kidney transplantations without splenectomy using antigen-specific immunoadsorption and rituximab. *Transplantation* 2003; 76: 730–731.

20. Shimmura H, Tanabe K, Ishikawa N, Tokumoto T, Takahashi K, Toma H. Role of anti A/B antibody titers in results of ABO-incompatible kidney transplantation. *Transplantation* 2000; 70: 1331–1335.

21. Katayama A, Kobayashi T, Uchida K, Goto N, Matsuoka S, Sato T et al. Beneficial effect of antibody removal and enhanced immunosuppression in few cytometry crossmatch-positive and ABO-incompatible renal transplantation. *Transplant Proc* 2002; 34: 2771–2772.

22. Galili U, Ishida H, Tanabe K, Toma H. Anti-Gal A/B, a novel antiblood group antibody identified in recipients of ABO-incompatible kidney allografts. *Transplantation* 2002; 74: 1574–1580.

23. Park W, Grande J, Ninova D, Nath K, Platt J, Gloor J et al. Accommodation in ABO-incompatible kidney allografts, a novel mechanism of self-protection against antibody-mediated injury. *Am J Transplant* 2003; 3: 952–960.

24. Ishida H, Koyama I, Sawada T, Utsumi K, Murakami T, Sannomiya A et al. Anti-AB titer changes in patients with ABO incompatibility after living related kidney transplantations. *Transplantation* 2000; 70: 681–685.

25. Olausson M, et al. Cross Match Positive Living Donor Candidates. *Am J Transplantation* 2006; 6: in press.

26. Sutherland DE, Fryd DS, So SK, Bentley FR, Ascher NL, Simmons RL, Najarian JS. Long-term effect of splenectomy versus no splenectomy in renal transplant patients. Reanalysis of a randomized prospective study. *Transplantation* 1984; 38: 619–624.

27. Sawada T, Fuchinoue S, Teraoka S. Successful A1-to-O ABO-incompatible kidney transplantation after a preconditioning regimen consisting of anti-CD20 monoclonal antibody infusions, splenectomy, and double-filtration plasmapheresis. *Transplantation* 2002; 74: 1207–1210.

28. Yandza T, Lambert T, Alvarez F, Gauthier F, Jacolot D, Huault G et al. Outcome of ABO-incompatible liver transplantation in children with no specific alloantibodies at the time of transplantation. *Transplantation* 1994; 58: 793–800.

29. West LJ, Pollock-Barziv SM, Dipchand AI, Lee KJ, Cardella CJ, Benson LN et al. ABO-incompatible heart transplantation in infants. *N Engl J Med* 2001; 344: 793–800.

30. Wu A, Buhler L, Cooper DKC. ABO-incompatible organ and bone marrow transplantation: current status. *Transplant Int* 2003; 16: 291–299.

## 16.16.2b    ABO Incompatibility

*Kazunari Tanabe, MD, PhD*

### INTRODUCTION

Recent advances in potent immunosuppressive drugs have dramatically improved the results of kidney transplants enabling the transplant community to try expanding the donor pool by overcoming immunologic barriers, such as ABO incompatibility and high recipient sensitivity.

However, ABO-incompatible kidney transplants are not a new idea: they have been tried since the early 1970s.[1,2] In 1974, Rydberg et al. introduced A2-incompatible kidney transplants using conventional immunosuppression without any pretransplant treatment, not even plasmapheresis. Of 20 A2-incompatible kidney transplant recipients, 8 lost their grafts within 1 month after surgery, whereas 12 grafts functioned long term.[1,2] Slapak et al.[3] reported 3 successful A1-to-O kidney transplants using pretransplant immunoadsorption and plasmapheresis treatment. Alexandre et al.[4] reported their first experience of 26 cases of elective ABO-incompatible living donor (LD) kidney transplants (ABO-ILKTs). Their immunosuppressive treatment included steroids, azathioprine, cyclosporine, antilymphocyte globulin, donor-specific platelet transfusion, and splenectomy at the time of the transplant. These promising clinical data stimulated Japanese transplant surgeons to perform ABO-ILKTs because of the serious shortage of deceased donor (DD) kidneys in their country. Although their short-term ABO-ILKT results were not quite as good as the results of ABO-compatible LD kidney transplants, the long-term patient and graft survival rates showed no significant difference.[5–7]

Recent ABO-ILKT results are better than during the early experience. Some transplant centers have started new ABO-ILKT programs with excellent outcomes. Newly developed potent immunosuppressive agents, such as tacrolimus (FK), mycophenolate mofetil (MMF), IL2 receptor blockers, and rituximab seem to have contributed to the marked improvement in short-term results of ABO-ILKT results.[8–13]

### PRETRANSPLANT CONDITIONING AND IMMUNOSUPPRESSION

Removal of anti-ABO antibodies (anti-ABO Abs) is mandatory to prevent hyperacute rejection, because preexisting antibodies against blood group A/B antigens cause antibody-mediated rejection. Thus, at most transplant centers, plasmapheresis or immunoadsorption is employed to remove the anti-ABO Abs pretransplant. Recipients are treated pretransplant with concomitant immunosuppression, such as FK, MMF, steroids, intravenous immunoglobulin (IVIg), and rituximab.[8–13]

Our pretransplant conditioning for ABO-ILKT recipients is quite simple. It basically consists of immunosuppression and plasmapheresis. We usually employ 7-day pretransplant immunosuppression, using FK, MMF, and methylprednisolone (MP), with two to four concomitant sessions of pretransplant plasmapheresis or double-filtration plasmapheresis (DFPP)[13] (Figure 16.16.2b-1). To remove anti-A and/or anti-B antibodies, we give recipients three or four sessions of DFPP and/or some sessions of regular plasmapheresis, starting 7 days pretransplant. All three drugs are started 7 days pretransplant. FK is initiated at a dose of 0.1 mg/kg and reduced

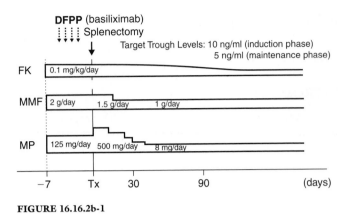

**FIGURE 16.16.2b-1**

Immunosuppressive protocol at Tokyo Women's Medical University. To remove anti-A and/or anti-B antibodies, recipients underwent 3 or 4 sessions of double-filtration plasmapheresis and/or some sessions of regular plasmapheresis, starting 7 days pretransplant. All three drugs (tacrolimus, mycophenolate mofetil, and methylprednisolone) were started 7 days pretransplant. Tacrolimus was started at 0.1 mg/kg and reduced according to the target trough levels (around 10 ng/mL before surgery). MMF was started at 1,000 to 2,000 mg/body and continued until surgery, barring adverse events. MP was started at 80 to 125 mg/day and increased to 500 mg/day on the day of the transplant.

according to the target trough levels, which are around 10 ng/ml before surgery. MMF is started at a dose of 1,000 to 2,000 mg/day; the same dose is continued until surgery, unless adverse events occur. MP is started at a dose of 20 to 125 mg/day and increased to 500 mg/day on the day of the transplant. Recipients undergo splenectomy at the time of the transplant.[13] Since January 2005, we have employed a nonsplenectomy protocol for ABO-ILKT recipients. They are treated with 1 dose of rituximab (375 mg/m²) with concomitant immunosuppression, including FK, MMF, and MP. They also undergo DPFF and/or plasmapheresis, in order to remove anti-ABO Abs. Short-term outcomes have been excellent (unpublished data).

The Johns Hopkins group and the Mayo Clinic group have both employed low-dose IVIg during pretransplant plasmapheresis and immunosuppression. The treatment protocol of the Johns Hopkins group is shown in Figure 16.16.2b-2.[12] They reported performing 4 to 5 sessions of plasmapheresis pretransplant to remove anti-ABO Abs. At the time of plasmapheresis, they employed either 5% albumin solution or fresh-frozen plasma as a replacement solution; they administered CMVIg (Cytogam) at 100 mg/kg after each plasmapheresis treatment. Pretransplant plasmaphresis or CMVIg was given until an ABO Ab titer < 16 was achieved. A single dose of rituximab was given (375 mg/mm²) after the last pretransplant plasmapheresis or CMVIg treatment. Then, FK (0.1 mg/kg/day) and MMF (2 g/day in 2 to 4 divided doses) were started at the initiation of the preoperative plasmapheresis or CMVIg treatments. Daclizumab (2 mg/kg before reperfusion, then 1 mg/kg every other week for 4 doses) and steroids (MP, 500 mg intraoperatively, then 125 mg every 6 hours for 6 doses, followed by prednisolone, 30 mg/day) were begun at the time of the transplant. When FK reached the target levels (10 to 12 ng/mL) posttransplant, the prednisolone dose was decreased to 20 mg/day. Posttransplant, protocol plasmapheresis and CMVIg treatments were given on postoperative days 1, 3, and 5.

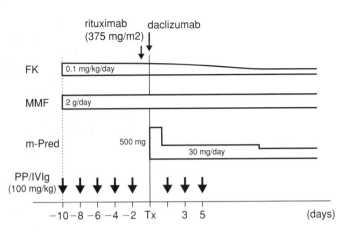

**FIGURE 16.16.2b-2**

Immunosuppressive protocol at Johns Hopkins University. The Johns Hopkins group performed 4 to 5 sessions of plasmapheresis IVIg treatment pretransplant to remove anti-ABO Abs. At the time of plasmapheresis, they employed either 5% albumin solution or fresh frozen plasma as a replacement solution. CMVIg (Cytogam) was administered at 100 mg/kg after each plasmapheresis treatment. A single dose of rituximab was given (375 mg/mm²) after the last pretransplant plasmapheresis IVIg treatment. FK (0.1 mg/kg/day) and MMF (2 g/day in 2 to 4 divided doses) were started at the initiation of the preoperative plasmapheresis IVIg treatments. Daclizmab (2 mg/kg before reperfusion, then 1 mg/kg every other week for 4 doses) and steroids (MP, 500 mg intraoperatively, then 125 mg every 6 hours for 6 doses, followed by prednisolone, 30 mg/day) were begun at the time of the transplant. Posttransplant, protocol plasmapheresis IVIg treatments were given on postoperative days 1, 3, and 5.

The Mayo Clinic group[10] employed a similar protocol. FK, MMF, and steroids were used as pretransplant immunosuppression. Thymoglobulin was added as the induction therapy. In addition, the Mayo Clinic group administered 375 mg/m² of rituximab 1 week pretransplant, instead of splenectomy.

The Stockholm group employed a blood group antigen-specific immunoadsorbent for the removal of anti-ABO Abs and also used rituximab to replace splenectomy. They used a low-molecular carbohydrate column with an A or B blood-group antigen linked to a Sepharose matrix (Glycosorb ABO, Glycorex Transplantation, Lund, Sweden) as a new antigen-specific immunoadsorbent.[8,11] The column effectively and specifically depleted anti-ABO Abs without any apparent side effects.[8,11] They performed 4 sessions of immunoadsorption pretransplant to achieve an 8x dilution of the anti-ABO Ab titer. Their preoperative desensitization protocol is shown in Figure 16.16.2b-3. They reported that adsorption of anti-ABO Abs with the Glycosorb ABO carbohydrate column was effective, lowering the antibody titers by approximately 2 to 4 steps at each session.[11] Since antigen-specific immunoadsorption depletes only anti-ABO Abs, they reported no side effects associated with conventional plasmapheresis, no coagulation disorders, and no removal of antiviral and/or antibacterial antibodies that patients had previously obtained. At least 4 sessions of pretransplant immunoadsorption were needed to achieve the target anti-ABO antibody level, which was 1:8 dilution.

Recently, Rydberg et al. examined various functions of Biosynsorb ABO, such as removal of antibody and side effects. They reported that the columns showed a high capacity to remove anti-ABO Abs and could remove more than 90% of anti-ABO Abs at 1 session. Nonspecific adsorption of proteins, such as

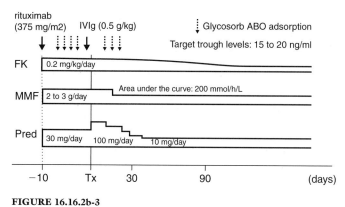

**FIGURE 16.16.2b-3**

Immunosuppressive protocol at Karolinska University. The immunosuppressive protocol consisted of 1 dose of rituximab (375 mg/m²) given 2 to 4 weeks pretransplant. Immunosuppression consisted of FK (0.2 to 0.3 mg/kg, with a target trough level of 15 to 20 ng/mL), MMF (2 to 3 g), and prednisolone (30 mg/day). All 3 drugs were started 1 week before immunoadsorption. Preoperatively, the anti-ABO Abs were removed by antigen-specific immunoadsorption. In most recipients, 4 sessions of immunoadsorption were performed pretransplant, and 0.5 g/kg of intravenous immunoglobulin was given after the last pretransplant session of immunoadsorption.

serum albumin, IgA, IgG, and IgM, was not observed. An immune complex did not form during absorption. Although the column caused activation of complements, the grade of activation was the same as that observed in patients who were undergoing hemodialysis. They concluded that the Biosynsorb ABO can successfully remove the anti-ABO Abs with minimal side effects.[14]

Tyden et al.[8,11] also employed rituximab instead of splenectomy. Their immunosuppressive protocol consisted of 1 dose of rituximab (375 mg/m₂) given 2 to 4 weeks before immunoadsorption. This was followed by FK-based immunosuppression, consisting of FK (0.2 to 0.3 mg/kg/day, with a target tough level of 15 to 20 ng/mL), MMF (2 to 3 g/day, aiming at an area under the curve [AUC] of 200 mmol/h/L), and prednisolone (30 mg/day, starting 1 week pretransplant).

## RITUXIMAB AND SPLENECTOMY

Splenectomy is one of the major controversial issues in ABO-incompatible kidney transplants. Nelson et al.[15] reported that 41 patients who underwent A2-incompatible DD kidney transplants without pretransplant plasmapheresis showed excellent graft survival without splenectomy. However, only selected patients who had low titers of anti-A2 Abs were enrolled in this study.

Alexandre et al.[4] emphasized that splenectomy is a prerequisite for successful ABO-incompatible kidney transplants. All 3 patients who did not undergo splenectomy experienced hyperacute graft rejection in the first week posttransplant, whereas 10 of 11 patients who underwent splenectomy had functioning grafts.

Toma[5] reviewed 155 ABO-incompatible kidney transplant recipients reported in the literature. Of these 155 recipients, 103 underwent splenectomy, 83 (80.5%) of whom survived more than 1 year after surgery, whereas only 17 (32.7%) of 52 grafts in patients who did not undergo splenectomy survived. However, when patients who had no pretreatment with plasmapheresis or immunoadsorption were excluded from the 52 nonsplenectomized patients, the 1-year graft survival rate was 72.7% (16 of 22), which

is no different from that of splenectomized patients. Toma speculated that splenectomy might be unnecessary in ABO-ILKTs.

Recently, a new immunosuppressive agent, the anti-CD 20 Ab rituximab, has been successfully used for ABO-incompatible kidney transplants without splenectomy. As we described before, Tyden et al.[8] used 1 dose of rituximab (375 mg/m²) instead of splenectomy, with excellent short-term graft survival. Sawada et al.[16] also employed rituximab as a preconditioning treatment for ABO-ILKT candidates and administered 3 to 4 doses of rituximab pretransplant. They also performed splenectomy and found plasma cells in the spleen on histologic examination. They concluded that splenectomy is necessary to remove any plasma cells that may still remain in the spleen after rituximab treatment and that could produce anti-ABO Abs. However, Tyden et al.[11] and other groups[10,12] employed rituximab instead of splenectomy and successfully desensitized the recipients, obtaining excellent long-term graft function after ABO-ILKTs. Since January 2005, we have employed nonsplenectomized pretransplant conditioning with rituximab administration for ABO-ILKT recipients or highly sensitized recipients. According to our limited experience, 1 dose (375 mg/m²) of rituximab completely eliminated B cells from the peripheral bloodstream and spleen. We have applied this protocol for 5 recipients since January 2005, with no rejection episodes. Clearly, rituximab can successfully desensitize recipients preoperatively and can suppress Ab production after ABO-ILKTs without splenectomy, although plasma cells still exist in the spleen.[17]

However, Vieira et al.[18] recently reported a significant reduction in anti-HLA Ab levels after a single dose (3 different dosages: 50, 150, and 375 mg/mm²) of rituximab. They reported that after elimination of B cells by rituximab, the levels should decrease over time, at a rate controlled by the half-life of Ig and of plasma cells. Yet, they also reported that B-cell depletion via rituximab therapy in end-stage renal failure patients has been shown to have minimal impact on in vitro T-cell function and cytokine release.[19]

The effectiveness of rituximab in suppressing Ab production seems to be due to the suppression of B-cell proliferation to plasma cells after second-set immunologic stimulation caused by ABO-ILKTs. Furthermore, Tokunaga et al.[20] used rituximab to treat systemic lupus erythematosus which (refractory to conventional treatment). They showed that rituximab significantly improved clinical manifestations (eg, consciousness disorder, seizures, progressive sensory disorder, hemolytic crisis), cardiac function, and laboratory test results. Rituximab not only reduced B-cell numbers and IgG levels but also down-regulated costimulatory molecules (eg, CD40 and CD80) on B cells. They suggested that rituximab may block T-cell activation through these costimulatory molecules.[20]

In theory, anti-ABO Abs should be removed before ABO-ILKTs to prevent Ab-mediated rejection. Many investigators have tried to reduce preoperative Ab titers to 8x or 16x dilutions.[10–12] However, in our experience, patients with Ab titers of 32x dilution underwent successful transplants using ABO-incompatible kidney donors, with good long-term kidney function posttransplant.[12,17,21] We do not know the acceptable upper limit of Ab titers for preventing of hyperacute rejection in ABO-ILKT recipients. We are certain that 32x dilution of anti-ABO Abs at the time of the transplant is a safe upper limit for successful ABO-ILKTs.[17]

The recent results of ABO-ILKTs under potent immunosuppression are excellent. The Johns Hopkins group reported excellent outcome in six ABO-ILKT recipients. All recipients obtained excellent graft function without any Ab-mediated rejection episodes (Table 16.16.2b-1). The Johns Hopkins group

**TABLE 16.16.2b-1**

| Case | Blood group D → R | Preoperative antibody titers | Rejection | S-Cr (mg/dl) |
|------|-------------------|------------------------------|-----------|--------------|
| 1 | B  → O | 32 | No rej. | 1.6 |
| 2 | A2 → O | 128 | No rej. | 1.3 |
| 3 | A2 → B | 8 | No rej. | 1.3 |
| 4 | AB → A | 32 | IIA | 1.5 |
| 5 | A1 → O | 128 | No rej. | 1.1 |
| 6 | B  → O | 128 | No rej. | 1.1 |

also reported the first successful transplant of patients who were both ABO-incompatible and crossmatch-positive with their only available donor. Their preconditioning regimen included splenectomy in all three such recipients at the time of the transplant. One patient received a rituximab injection at the time of the transplant. Posttransplant immunosuppression was the same as for ABO-ILKTs. No recipients experienced any hyperacute rejection. But one patient experienced Ab-mediated rejection, which was successfully reversed by plasmapheresis/IVIG and rituximab administration.[21]

Tyden et al. recently reported their updated ABO-ILKT results. Eleven recipients treated with rituximab as well as FK, MMF and steroids had good kidney function—without any rejection episodes or any serious infectious complications (Table 16.16.2b-2).[11]

Our recent ABO-ILKT results are also excellent. From January 2000 through March 2003, 45 adult patients underwent ABO-ILKTs at our institution. DFPP and/or plasmapheresis were carried out to remove anti-ABO Abs pretransplant. In 2000, 13 recipients were treated with FK, MMF, and MP without 7 days of pretransplant immunosuppression (group 1). Since January 2001, we have administered FK (0.1 mg/kg/day), MMF (1 to 2 g/day), MP (125 mg/day) concomitantly with plasmapheresis, starting 7 days pretransplant; this protocol has been applied in 32 recipients (group 2). The patient survival rate was 100% in both treatment groups. The graft survival rate was 92% in group 1 and 97% in group 2. One group 2 recipient lost the graft because of severe humoral rejection. The incidence of acute rejection was 56% in group 1 and 19% in group 2. Although the graft survival rate was good, without any significant difference between the 2 treatment groups,

the incidence of acute rejection in group 1 was significantly higher than in group 2. Pretransplant immunosuppression for 7 days using FK, MMF, and steroids in ABO-IKT recipients provided an excellent outcome, without any severe infectious complication.

Since January 2005, we have employed a new protocol for ABO-ILKTs, which includes regular immunosuppression (FK, MMF, and MP), 1 dose of rituximab (375 mg/m$^2$), and basiliximab induction without IVIg. We successfully applied this protocol for 5 ABO-ILKT recipients without any graft loss or rejection episodes. We treated these ABO-ILKT recipients with anti-donor-specific HLA Ab using the same pretransplant conditioning protocol and performed splenectomy at the time of the transplant. Our preliminary data under the new protocol, including rituximab treatment, showed that short-term results were excellent, with no graft loss and no rejection episodes (unpublished data).

No significant rejection has occurred with anti-A/B Abs and an intact complement system, although transplanted ABO-incompatible grafts expressed blood group A/B antigens in various tissues of the kidney according to several studies.[22,23] This phenomenon has been described as "accommodation" by Platt et al.[24] The titers of anti-A/B Ab sometimes increase to much higher than the pretransplant levels after surgery, but in most cases, no significant rejection occurrs. Park et al.[25] reported that accommodation in ABO-incompatible kidney transplants may be caused by alterations in signal transduction, in cell–cell adhesion, and in T-cell activation pathways and by the prevention of apoptosis. Takahashi et al. suggested that accommodation will be established within a couple weeks after ABO-ILKTs.[26] However, the exact mechanisms for "accommodation" have not been clarified.

## CONCLUSIONS

Short-term and long-term outcomes for ABO-incompatible kidney transplant recipients seem to be excellent, according to recent reports.[8–13] For such recipients, rituximab can be used safely to replace splenectomy.[11,12] The immunoadsorbent Glycosorb seems to be very promising, because it removes anti-ABO Abs effectively and specifically, but does not remove other essential proteins (and, obviously, no fresh-frozen plasma is needed as the replacement fluid). Preconditioning protocols without splenectomy that include immunoadsorption will make ABO-ILKTs simpler, safer, and easier.

**TABLE 16.16.2b-2**

| Case | Blood group (D/R) | Antibody titers before adsorption | S-Cr (mml/L) |
|------|-------------------|-----------------------------------|--------------|
| 1 | A2/O | 64 | 80 |
| 2 | B/O | 32 | 168 |
| 3 | B/A | 16 | 120 |
| 4 | A1/O | 64 | 123 |
| 5 | A2/O | 64 | 168 |
| 6 | A1/O | 128 | 98 |
| 7 | A2/O | 64 | 120 |
| 8 | B/A | 8 | 131 |
| 9 | B/O | 2 | 22 |
| 10 | A1B/B | 16 | 91 |
| 11 | A1/O | 16 | 102 |

## References

1. Rydberg L, Breimer ME, Samuelsson BE, Brynger H. Blood group ABO-incompatible (A2 to O) kidney transplantation in human subjects: a clinical, serologic, and biochemical approach. *Transplant Proc* 1987;19:4528–4537.
2. Rydberg L. ABO-incompatibility in solid organ transplantation. *Transfusion Med* 2001;11:325–342
3. Slapak M, Evans P, Trickett L, et al. Can ABO-incompatible donors be used in renal transplantation? *Transplant Proc* 1984;16:75–79.
4. Alexandre GPJ, Squifflet JP, De Bruyere M, et al. Present experiences in a series of 26 ABO-incompatible living donor renal allografts. Transplant Proc 1987; 19: 4538–4542.
5. Toma H. ABO-incompatible renal transplantation. *Urol Clin North Am* 1994;21:299–310.
6. Tanabe K, Takahashi K, Sonda K, et al. Long-term results of ABO-incompatible living kidney transplantation. *Transplantation* 1998;65:224–228.

7. Takahashi K, Saito H, Takahara S, et al. Excellent long-term outcome of ABO-incompatible living donor kidney transplantation in Japan. *Am J Transplant* 2004;4:1089–1096.

8. Tyden G, Kumlien G, Fehrman I. Successful ABO-incompatible kidney transplantations without splenectomy using antigen-specific immunoadsorption and rituximab. *Transplantation* 2003;76:730-743.

9. Fidler ME, Gloor JM, Lager DJ, et al. Histologic findings of antibody-mediated rejection in ABO blood-group-incompatible living-donor kidney transplantation. *Am J Transplant* 2004;4:101-107.

10. Gloor JM, Lager DJ, Moor SB, et al. ABo-incompatible kidney transplantation using both A2 and non-A2 living donors. *Transplantation* 2003;7:971–977.

11. Tyden G, Kumlien G, Genberg H, et al. ABO-incompatible kidney transplantation without splenectomy using antigen-specific immunoadsorption and rituximab. *Am J Tranplant* 2004.

12. Sonnenday CJ, Warren DS, Cooper M, et al. Plasmapheresis, CMV hyperimmune globulin, and anti-CD20 allow ABO-incompatible renal transplantation without splenectomy. *Am J Transplant* 2004;4:1315–1322.

13. Tanabe K, Tokumoto T, Ishida H, et al. Excellent outcome of ABO-incompatible living kidney transplantation under pretransplantation immunosuppression with tacrolimus, mycophenolate mofetil, and steroids. *Transplant Proc* 2004;36:2175-2177.

14. Rydberg L, Bengtsson A, Samuelsson O, Nilsson K, Breimer ME. In vitro assessment of a new ABO immunosorbent with synthetic carbohydrates attached to sepharose. *Transplant Int* 2005;17:666–672.

15. Shimmura H, Tanabe K, Ishikawa N, Tokumoto T, Takahashi K, Toma H. Role of anti-A/B antibody titers in results of ABO-incompatible kidney transplantation. *Transplantation* 2000;70(9):1331–1335.

16. Nelson Pw, Shield III CF, Muruve NA, et al. Increased access to transplantation for blood group B cadaveric waiting list candidates by using A2 kidneys: Time for a new nation system. *Am J Transplant* 2002;2:94–99.

17. Sawada T, Fuchinoue S, Teraoka S. Successful A1-to-O ABO-incompatible kidney transplantation after a preconditioning regimen consisting of anti-CD20 monoclonal antibody infusions, splenectomy, and double-filtration plasmapheresis. *Transplantation* 2002;74:1207-1210. Incompatible Solid Organ Transplantation (Eds Segev and Montromery) (in press)

18. Tanabe, K. ABO-incompatible transplantation. Current Opinion in Organ Transplantation (in press).

19. Vieira CA, Agarwal A, Book BK, et al. Rituximab for reduction of anti-HLA antibodies in patients awaiting renal transplantation: 1. Safety, pharmacodynamics, and pharmacokinetics. *Transplantation* 2004;77:542–548.

20. Rydberg L, Bengtsson A, Samuelsson O, Nilsson K, Breimer ME. In vitro assessment of a new ABO immunosorbent with synthetic carbohydrates attached to sepharose. *Transplant Int* 2005;17:666–672.

21. Agarwal A, Vieira CA, Book BK, et al. Rituximab, anti-CD20, induces in vivo cytokine release but does not impair ex vivo T-cell responses. *Am J Transplant* 2004;4:1357–1360.

22. Tokunaga M, Fujii K, Saito K, et al. Down-regulation of CD40 and CD80 on B cells in patients with life-threatening systemic lupus erythematosus after successful treatment with rituximab. *Rheumatology* 2005;44:176–182.

23. Warren DS, Zachary AA, Sonnenday CJ, Successful renal transplantation across simultaneous ABO incompatible and positive crossmatch barriers. *Am J Transplant* 2004;4:561–568.

24. Bannett AD, McAlack RF, Morris M, Chopek MW, Platt JL. ABO-incompatible renal transplantation: a qualitative analysis of native endothelial tissue ABO antigens after transplantation. *Transplant Proc* 1989;21:783–785.

25. Yamashita M, Aikawa A, Ohara T, et al. Local immune states in ABO-incompatible renal allografts. *Transplant Proc* 1993;25:274-276.

26. Platt JL, Bach FH. The barrier to xenotransplantation. *Transplantation* 1991;52:937–947.

27. Park WD, Grande JP, Ninova D, et al. Accommodation in ABO-incompatible kidney allografts, a novel mechanism of self-protection against antibody-mediated injury. *Am J Transplant* 2003;3:952–960.

28. Takahashi K. A new concept of accommodation in ABO-incompatible kidney transplantation. *Clin Transplant* 2005;19(Suppl. 14):76–85.

## 16.16.3a   Options Available to Recipients with Incompatible Donors

*Robert A. Montgomery, MD, PhD, J. Keith Melançon, MD, Daniel S. Warren, PhD*

### INTRODUCTION

Donor–recipient incompatibilities have become one of the most significant barriers to further expansion of live donor kidney transplantation. Based on blood group frequencies in the United States there is a 35% chance that any two individuals will be blood-type incompatible. Up to one third of potential donors may be eliminated on this basis. Thirty percent of the patients waiting on the deceased donor list are sensitized to human leukocyte antigen (HLA) molecules. HLA sensitization results from previous exposure to allogeneic tissue in the form of pregnancies, blood transfusions, and tissue or solid organ transplants. We estimate that there are currently 6,000 patients on the deceased donor waiting list who have willing but incompatible living donors.[1] As many as 3,500 patients present each year with an incompatible donor.[2] At a time of a deepening crisis in organ availability, new strategies must be designed to utilize donors who are excluded on the basis of incompatibility.

There are now several options available to patients with incompatible live donors. At our institution these options include, desensitization, kidney-paired donation (KPD), domino-paired donation (DPD), or kidney-paired donation followed by desensitization. Determining which modality provides the best option for an individual patient is dependent on a careful evaluation and assessment of the breadth and strength of the patient's human leukocyte antigen HLA or ABO reactivity, donor and recipient blood types, and risk of antibody-mediated rejection (AMR).

### THERAPEUTIC OPTIONS TO ALTER DONOR SPECIFIC REACTIVITY

There are a number of therapeutic agents and modalities that appear to reduce humoral immune responsiveness (Figure 16.16.3a-1). These agents or interventions work by depleting or modulating B-cells, plasma cells, or soluble antibody (Figure 16.16.3a-2). They can be used in desensitization protocols to overcome either ABO or HLA incompatibilities.

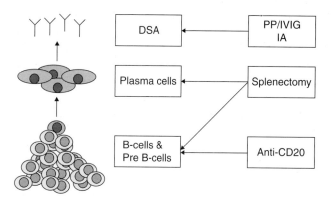

**FIGURE 16.16.3a-1**

Therapeutic Targets to Reduce Donor Specific Humoral Responses

**Pre-transplant Plasmapheresis (PP) and IVIg**
- PP reduces antibody titer to a level in which hyperacute rejection is unlikely.
- Low dose IVIg repletes lost antibody, suppresses de novo Ab production, and is immunomodulatory.
- FK 506 and MMF reduces T and B-cell responses

**B-cell Ablative Therapy**
- Splenectomy reduces plasma cell burden, precursor cells, B-cell immune surveillance capabilities
- Anti-CD20 rapidly depletes the peripheral B-cell compartment but not plasma cells

**Post-transplant Plasmapheresis (PP) and IVIg**
- PP prevents rebound, maintaining antibody titer at a safe level until tolerance or accommodation occurs.
- IVIg, FK 506, and MMF promotes engraftment (tolerance vs accommodation).

**Induction**
- Agents like ATG and anti-IL-2 receptor Ab reduce T-cell responsiveness and T-cell help

**Maintenance Immunosuppression**
- Fk 506, Rapamycin, MMF/DSG, and steroids, reduce the risk of cellular rejection and some have anti-B-cell properties

**FIGURE 16.16.3a-2**

The Goals Of Preconditioning For Incompatible Kidney Engraftment

## Splenectomy

Alexandre et al. reported that patients who did not undergo pre-transplant splenectomy lost their grafts acutely to AMR and thus established the historic basis for splenectomy of ABOi recipients.[3] This practice was adopted by the Japanese groups and in the largest series published to date of 441 ABOi kidney transplants performed at 55 Japanese centers, 98% of the patients underwent splenectomy.[4] Unfortunately, the need for splenectomy has not yet been addressed in a large series. Splenectomy is thought to reduce the risk of AMR by reducing immune surveillance capabilities and de-bulking lymphoid mass including donor-reactive plasma cells. Due to the potential infectious complications, especially among immunosuppressed patients, splenectomy has been a barrier to wider acceptance of ABOi in the West. Several groups have reported small series of patients in which the B-cell ablative monoclonal antibody, anti-CD20 has been substituted for splenectomy.[5,6] We now have a series of 14 patients successfully transplanted across and ABOi barrier without splenectomy or anti-CD20.[7]

Although our use of splenectomy for ABOi has diminished, we continue to use this intervention to allow successful transplantation of high-risk positive crossmatch patients. Splenectomy has been associated with a reduction in DSA and can be performed prior to the initiation of PP for patients with high-titer DSA or at the time of transplant for high-risk patients. We have also used splenectomy as a salvage procedure for patients who develop sudden oliguria from severe AMR during the first week after desensitization for a positive crossmatch (+XM). All ABOi and positive crossmatch patients are immunized against pneumcoccus, menigiococcus, and HFlu (pediatric dose), and receive a tetnus booster. Those that receive a splenectomy also receive a 1-year course of penicillin for bacterial prophylaxis.

## Anti-CD20

Originally approved for the treatment of non-Hodgkin's lymphoma, anti-CD20 has been quickly adopted by the transplant community for off-label use in the prevention and treatment of AMR. The theoretical advantage of anti-CD20 is that its effect is temporary and, if given prior to transplantation, coincides with the time in which the risk of AMR is greatest. The B-cell compartment eventually reconstitutes in the presence of an intact spleen, minimizing the life-long risk of infection associated with splenectomy. However, the majority of germinal center B-cells, plasmablasts, and long-lived plasma cells are resistant to anti-CD20 therapy.[8] In our experience, reduction in de novo isohemagglutinin or donor specific anti-HLA antibody production after a single dose of anti-CD20 is modest if it occurs at all. This drug may be effective in conjunction with plasmapheresis (PP) or immunoabsorption (IA) to reduce the risk of AMR. We no longer routinely use either splenectomy or anti-CD20 for preconditioning in ABOi transplantation but have expanded its use as a B-cell induction therapy for high-risk +XM patients. In this case we use it in combination with plasmapheresis and intervenous immune globulin (PP/IVIg) to either lower high-titer DSA or reduce the risk of AMR among moderate-to-high risk +XM patients. For patients who are felt to be at very high risk we will often use both anti-CD20 and splenectomy. The optimal timing for anti-CD20 administration is not known. There are experimental data that suggest that some B cells may only be susceptible to killing when they are recirculating which can take as long as 1 month.[8] In some cases we have given a dose of anti-CD20 the night before transplant; and in others, 1 month before beginning desensitization.

## PP and IA

Without antibody reduction, high-titer DSA or isohemagglutinins can result in the very rapid destruction of an incompatible graft. Thus, the need to reduce titers to safe levels becomes paramount. There are several effective methods of reducing DSA and isohemagglutinins. PP lowers antibody titers in a predictable manner. IA with protein A or synthetic blood group A or B columns also provides efficient removal of donor-directed antibodies.[5,9] PP depletes coagulation factors, and this limits the number of blood volumes that can be cleared with each treatment. Patients undergoing desensitization regimens that include PP are at increased risk of bleeding from invasive procedures and renal biopsies. This risk can be reduced by using fresh frozen plasma rather than albumin as the replacement fluid for PP treatments that take place within 24 hours of a procedure. PP removes antibody in a nonselective manner and this may have the effect of increasing the individual's susceptibility to infectious complications. With IA several blood volumes can be absorbed and a higher percentage of DSA or isohemagglutinin cleared without removal of coagulation factors. However, the efficiency of antibody removal drops significantly after 1 blood volume is surpassed. At our institution, PP is performed on an every-other-day basis. This provides optimal redistribution of IgG between the interstitial and vascular compartments.

## IVIg

The utility of IVIg in ABOi preconditioning protocols has not been established. Most successful protocols in the West do include either multiple low doses of IVIg or a single high dose.[10,11] There is not evidence that IVIg alone is sufficient to protect the ABOi graft and efficacy has only been demonstrated when IVIg is combined with PP or IA. IVIg either in low or high doses has been shown to be efficacious for reducing panel reactive antibodies (PRA) and lowering DSA.[12–14] There are many putative mechanisms for IVIg including the activation of anti-idiotypic networks and the suppression of endogenous antibody production.[reviewed in 15] In our protocol we use CMVIg as our source of IVIg, with 100 mg/kg administered immediately following each PP. Low-dose CMVIg is well tolerated and free of thrombotic and fluid overload complications associated with higher doses (1–2 g/kg). The putative advantages of CMVIg are that there is a professional donor pool which reduces batch-to-batch variability and that it is enriched with antimicrobial antibodies, affording more protection from infectious complications. Low-dose CMVIg does not interfere with cell-based or solid-phase assays that employ anti-human globulin.

## Immunosuppression

There are currently multiple maintenance immunosuppressive agents with varying mechanisms of action that have been used by groups performing ABOi and positive crossmatch transplants. Agents like MMF and deoxyspergualin have anti-B-cell properties and may be very important components of prophylactic therapy. It has been suggested that improved results for ABOi transplants by groups in Japan, Europe, and the United States may be related to the inclusion of MMF in preconditioning and maintenance regimens. The Japanese groups have had extensive experience with deoxyspergualin in the ABOi setting, but most have switched to MMF in recent years.[16]

Agents like calcineurin inhibitors, steroids, and rapamycin that are associated with T-cell modulation may also be important to successful engraftment of ABO- and HLA-incompatible kidneys. Additionally, suppression of T-cell function may be important for the prevention of B-cell activation. Our standard preconditioning and maintenance therapy includes FK506, MMF, and steroids. For induction we use anti-IL-2 receptor antibodies but we are currently comparing clinical efficacy to ATG.

## ABO INCOMPATIBILITY

### The Initial Evaluation: Compatibility Testing and Interpretation

The blood type of the donor and recipient are determined using standard serologic testing.[17] Eighty percent of the blood group A

**TABLE 16.16.3a-1**

## # OF PLASMAPHERESIS TREATMENTS VS ISOAGGLUTININ TITER

| Isoagglutinin titer by AHG | # of PreTx Treatments | # of PostTx Treatments |
|---|---|---|
| 16 | 0 | 2 |
| 32 | 3 | 4 |
| 64 | 4 | 4 |
| 128 | 5-6 | 5 |
| 256 | 7-8 | 5 |
| 512 | 9-10 | 6 |
| >512 | >10 | 6 |

population in the United States is subtype A1 and the donor blood type may be important in terms of the risk of AMR. ABO blood group antigens are expressed on tissues throughout the body. The density of endothelial cell ABO antigen expression varies between blood types (A1 > B > A2). It is thought that a higher density of targets for recipient antibody binding increases the likelihood of AMR. Although this seems theoretically plausible it has not been well substantiated by recent data from centers performing ABOi kidney transplants in the United States.[6,18,19]

Recipient ABO antibody titers are measured using serial dilutions of the patient's plasma with group A or group B indicator cells and are converted to the anti-human globulin (AHG) test phase. The titer end points are the reciprocal of the highest dilution demonstrating agglutination at the AHG phase. The importance of IgM is unclear, but most centers perform ABOi guide therapy based on IgG antibody monitoring (AHG isohemagglutinin titers). Moreover, IgM is primarily intravascular and is efficiently removed with a single plasmapheresis treatment.

Higher anti-blood group antibody titers increase the degree of difficulty of antibody removal. The kinetics of plasmapheresis are predictable and the number of treatments necessary to bring the titer to a safe level (dilution 1:16) to proceed with transplantation can be estimated from the initial isohemagglutinin titer (Table 16.16.3a-1). It is also thought that patients who start with higher anti-blood group titers are at greater risk for AMR due to reexpansion of antibody during the first weeks following ABOi transplants. In our experience the initial titer clearly determines the number of pretransplant plasmapheresis treatments and as a rough estimate, each treatment reduces the titer by about 1 dilution. However, we have not observed a higher rate of AMR in high titer patients. We believe posttransplant plasmapheresis is important for preventing the rebound among high titer patients.

### Establishing a Risk Profile

The data collected from the initial isohemagglutinin testing are integrated and a risk profile is generated (Figure 16.16.3a-3). Additional considerations including a history of sensitization, co-morbid conditions, vascular access problems, and hypercoagulable states are factored in to the assessment. Patients with A1 donors or high titer isohemagglutinins are currently considered to be at higher risk for AMR. Patients with high initial titers will require more treatments and desensitization will be more costly among these patients. Co-morbid conditions, previous transplants, and a history of sensitization further increase the complexity, cost, and risk of rejection. It is not unusual for highly sensitized patients to

**Factors Associated With Increased Risk Of AMR: ABOi**
Donor blood type (A1 > B > A2)
Isoagglutinin titer
History of sensitization, previous transplant,
high risk donor/recipient pair

**Factors Associated With Increased Risk Of AMR: (+) XM**
# of previous transplants
Breadth of anti-HLA Ab--estimated by (PRA)
Initial DSA titer
Previous early graft losses
# of repeat mismatches
Multiple sensitizing events--Ab response to each
Rising titer or rebound between treatments

**FIGURE 16.16.3a-3**

present with an ABOi donor after several failed live donor transplants from blood-type-compatible donors. It is feasible to cross both barriers in select patients, but this does represent a higher immunologic risk. [20]

## Treatment Plan

Where possible, consideration should be given to enrolling higher-risk patients into kidney paired donation (KPD) programs in order to bypass rather than cross the more challenging incompatible barriers. Donor and recipient pairs with blood types A and B are best suited for KPD. ABOi pairs in which the recipient is blood type O are less likely to find a match in KPD pools as they can only exchange with a positive crossmatch pair in which the donor is blood type O. The other option is List Donation (LD) but there have been ethical challenges to entering O recipients into list donation because this causes an exodus of O deceased donors kidneys from the list and further disadvantages O patients on the list.[21,22] Until there is widespread pooling of potential live donor KPD patients, ABOi pairs with O recipients should be considered for desensitization.

Once the decision to proceed with ABOi transplantation has been made, a treatment plan can be developed based on the risk profile of the transplant. Reduction of anti-A or anti-B antibody below an AHG titer of 16 prior to transplantation is considered to be essential for successful engraftment of an ABOi kidney, and this goal can be accomplished by either PP or IA. We believe that protocol posttransplant PP or IA, with the objective of maintaining anti-blood group antibodies at or below 16 until accommodation has occurred significantly improves outcomes. Once thought to be essential to successful engraftment of an ABOi kidney, splenectomy is rarely performed at our institution when the blood group barrier is crossed. Anti-CD20 has been used in lieu of splenectomy in a limited number of high-risk patients but is no longer routinely administered.[6]

Our algorithm for preconditioning is shown in Table 16.16.3a-2. Recipients of A2 kidneys with titers < 16 do not require preconditioning. Close posttransplant monitoring is critical and PP/IVIg is performed only in the circumstances where there is a rise in titers of two or more dilutions above baseline. Patients with A2 donors and anti-A titers $\geq$ 32 receive PP/IVIg to lower their anti-A titer to 16 or less. For non-A2 donor organs up to a titer of 128 we use every other day PP/IVIg treatments to lower the

**TABLE 16.16.3a-2**

## THERAPEUTIC ALGORITHM FOR ABOi TRANSPLANTATION

| A2 donor | Initial isoagglutinin titer $\leq$ 16 | No preconditioning. Quadruple immunosuppression* |
| | Initial isoagglutinin titer $\geq$ 32 | No splenectomy or anti-CD 20 Precontitioning** Quadruple Immunosuppression* |
| Non-A2 donor | Initial isoagglutinin titer $\leq$ 128 | No splenectomy or anti-CD 20 Precontitioning** Quadruple Immunosuppression* |
| | Initial isoagglutinin titer 256 or 512 | No splenectomy Anti-CD 20 Precontitioning** Quadruple Immunosuppression* |
| | Initial isoagglutinin titer $\geq$ 1024 or high titer AB donor into O recipient | Splenectomy Anti-CD 20 Precontitioning** Quadruple Immunosuppression* |

*IL-2R Ab, FK 506, MMF, Prednisone
**PP/CMVIg # based on titer

titer to 16 prior to transplant. For non-A2 transplants in which the recipient anti-A or anti-B titer is $\geq$ 256, we recommend including anti-CD20 in the preconditioning regimen in addition to PP/IVIg. When isoagglutinin titers are $\geq$ 1,024 or when the donor is AB and the recipient is O with titers $\geq$ 512 we recommend splenectomy prior to commencing preconditioning or on the day of transplant.

## Preconditioning for ABOi Transplantation

After establishing the treatment plan, the date of the transplant is set. The preconditioning regimen must then be accomplished prior to that date. The number of treatments necessary to reach the target titer of 16 can be estimated from the starting titer (Table 16.16.3a-1). Optimal antibody clearance is achieved using every other day single volume exchanges. Once the number of treatments is determined we work backwards from the date of surgery. For example, if we estimate five treatments will be required, we begin PP/IVIg 10 days before the planned transplant (Figure 16.16.3a-4). MMF and FK506 are initiated on the first day of PP with the goal of rapidly reaching therapeutic drug levels. For FK506, the target is 8 to 10 ng/dL. Some patients on dialysis will not be able to tolerate full-dose MMF (2 g/day) due to GI toxicity. In this case an attempt should be made to raise the dose to 2 g/day after transplantation. Splenectomy and/or anti-CD20 are part of the preconditioning regimen for high-risk patients only. The optimal timing for these interventions has not been established. We generally give anti-CD20 on the day prior to surgery. When indicated, splenectomy is performed laparoscopically just prior to transplantation during the same period of anesthesia. Patients receive induction with daclizumab (2 mg/kg initial dose and 1 mg/kg every 2 weeks for 5 total doses). A single 100-mg dose of dexamethasone is given prior to reperfusion.

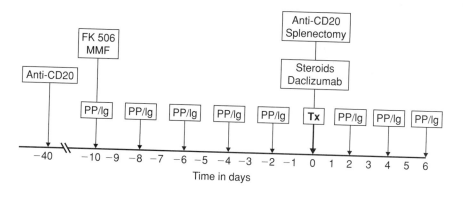

**FIGURE 16.16.3a-4**

This is a fusion representation which includes all of the possible interventions. Splenectomy and anti-CD20 are only given to high-risk patients. The majority of (+) XM patients receive PP/IVIg and standard immunosuppression only.

## Posttransplant Immunosuppression and Monitoring

Dexamethasone, 25 mg, is administered every 6 hours for 6 doses postoperatively, followed by prednisone 30 mg/day. Tacrolimus is continued and titrated to target levels of 10 to 12 ng/mL. Prednisone is reduced to 20 mg/day when therapeutic tacrolimus levels are achieved, and slowly tapered thereafter. We believe that MMF is a critical component of the post-transplant immunosuppression and every attempt should be made to achieve a daily dose of 2 g.

We perform at least 2 posttransplant PP/IVIg treatments by protocol with additional sessions added for high risk or high titer patients. The goal of posttransplant PP/IVIg treatments is to maintain the blood group antibody titers < 16 for 2 weeks in order to allow accommodation to occur. Titers are determined before and after each treatment. Once PP/IVIg is discontinued, weekly titers are checked for the first 4 weeks, monthly for the first 6 months, and then bimonthly. We perform protocol biopsies at 1, 3, 6, and 12 months posttransplant. Subclinical cellular or antibody-mediated rejection is treated.

## Acute Rejection

A rise in titer by 2 dilutions, with or without deterioration in renal function, triggers a biopsy. PP/IVIG is reinitiated when evidence of AMR is present in histologic sections (margination of neutrophils in the pericapillary tubules, fibrin thrombi, or necrotizing vasculitis). Most AMR has a cellular component, and patients are treated with a pulse of steroids followed by a taper. It should be noted that approximately 75% of our protocol biopsies of patients who have received an ABOi graft are positive for C4d but lack histologic features of AMR and clinical dysfunction.[23] If severe AMR develops consideration should be given to either splenectomy or anti-CD20 rescue. Cellular rejection is treated with either steroids or antilymphocytic antibody preparations. Most clinical rejections occur in the first 2 weeks after ABOi transplantation.

## TRANSPLANTATION OF HIGHLY SENSITIZED PATIENTS

### The Initial Evaluation: HLA Testing and Interpretation

There is no single antibody detection assay, which will provide all the information necessary to manage sensitized patients. When a patient is being assessed for HLA compatibility with a specific donor, we believe that the only important antibody is antibody directed against that donor. Third-party antibody may be impor-

tant for the determination of risk of AMR or graft loss but desensitization is only necessary if DSA is present. Currently, the risk of AMR can only be assessed by the presence of current or historic DSA, although the absence of DSA does not eliminate the risk of AMR from an anemnestic response. There are promising new approaches to measuring precursor B-cell frequency using tetramers but they remain experimental at this point.

There are three important questions that must be answered when evaluating a patient for desensitization: (1) Is there DSA? (2) What is the antibody specificity? (3) What is the strength of the antibody? The cytotoxic crossmatch (CXM) using recipient serum and donor lymphocytes with or without anti-human globulin (AHG) is a good starting point. If positive, the CXM can be titered and the strength of the antibody estimated. If the CXM is negative, a flow cytometric crossmatch (FCXM) is performed to detect lower level DSA. We use mean channel shifts relative to a standard to quantify DSA in a FCXM. Since the presence of autoantibody can result in a (+) XM, an autologous recipient XM should be performed. Non-HLA antibodies can produce (+) XMs and further testing is often necessary to determine the relevance of the XM.

Solid-phase assays that use purified HLA molecules as targets can be used to further define and characterize the DSA. These assays are considerably more sensitive and specific when compared to lymphocyte-based assays. We generally use combinations of cell-based and solid-phase assays to obtain a complete picture of the patient's immunologic risk and formulate a treatment plan.

### Establishing a Risk Profile

The results of the HLA testing and the patients history are synthesized to establish the patient's immunologic risk (Figure 16.16.3a-3b). The mode of sensitization seems to be important. In our series, patients with previous transplants are at increased risk for AMR. This risk seems to increase incrementally with each additional previous transplant. Patients who have been sensitized by homografts, bone transplants, or other composite-tissue transplants appear to be at higher risk for AMR. Sensitization from pregnancy and blood transfusions is more easily managed with the exception of spousal and child-to-mother transplants in which there is a repeat haplotype mismatch.

We will only desensitize patients who have documented DSA. Third-party antibodies do not cause AMR and removing them with PP does not appear to be of value. Furthermore, the presence of a +XM is not sufficient to warrant treatment unless it can be demonstrated that DSA is present. Positive crossmatches (especially B-cell) that are not due to the presence of DSA are common, and further characterization of the patient's anti-HLA antibody is essential to establish risk and the need for pretransplant antibody removal therapy. Once it has been established that DSA is present, the abundance of antibody needs to be determined. We precondition with PP/IVIg prior to transplant if any DSA is detected even reactivity strengths that would only be detectable by the most sensitive assays.

Other factors that contribute to immunologic risk are the presence of multiple donor reactive HLA-specific antibodies, repeat mismatches from previous transplants, or pregnancies, DSA that is rising at the time of desensitization or rebounding between PP/IVIg treatments (Figure 16.16.3a-3b). If there are multiple DSA specificities, each must be monitored during the desensitization process. All must be at a safe level prior to transplantation. An attempt is made to obtain records of the HLA typing of all previous allografts as well as the paternal HLA information for pregnancy-induced sensitization. Even in the absence of detectable antibody, repeat mismatches do appear to increase risk for AMR. We have observed the phenomenon of expanding specificities during AMR episodes in which antibody not detected at baseline suddenly appears to repeat mismatched antigens.

## Nonimmunologic Risk

Much of the increased incidence of co-morbid conditions in the highly sensitized population results from prolonged dialysis. These conditions can complicate pre- and posttransplant patient care and increase the risk of a poor outcome. Insufficient vascular access is a common challenge and, when present, adds a great deal of complexity to desensitization and subsequent management. Many of the patients in our cohort have either groin or lumbar catheters. Line sepsis and the inability to gain vascular access for dialysis, antibiotics, and other medications is the most common cause of morbidity and mortality in our experience. Among the patients who have poor vascular access, superior vena cava syndrome is common and can cause significant arm and head swelling posttransplantation. We have found that a magnetic resonance venography at the time of initial evaluation can be helpful in planning vascular access strategies.

Many patients that we see have been on dialysis in excess of 10 years. Resting hypotension, presumably due to autonomic dysfunction, is a common finding among these patients. This condition is frequently recalcitrant to pharmacologic intervention and is associated with a greater incidence of delayed graft function (DGF) or slow graft function after transplantation. Since clinical function is a key indicator of the onset of AMR, DGF eliminates an important early warning signal. Resting hypotension may resolve after successful transplantation.

Nephrogenic fibrosing dermopathy (NFD) is a condition that we have found in varying degrees of severity in up to 10% of sensitized patients. The most common phenotype is tight skin in the hands and forearm, but we have also seen pulmonary fibrosis and pancreatitis associated with FND. Although it is not clearly associated with prolonged dialysis, in our experience it is clustered in the subgroup of patients that have experienced long cumulative dialysis exposure. FND may improve after successful transplantation.

In our experience, hematologic hypercoagulability is also a common feature among highly sensitized patients, although the reasons for this are unclear. The cohort may be biased toward patients who have been sensitized by previously thrombosed allografts or perhaps hypercoagulability is associated with a hyperresponsive humoral immune system in a subset of patients. Whatever the cause, anticoagulation must be maintained throughout the preconditioning and posttransplant periods, and this offers further challenges to the clinical team especially with respect to PP and the coagulopathy that it induces. Our index of suspicion is very high during the evaluation process and hematologic work ups are triggered by: previous allograft thrombosis, repeated vascular access thrombosis, multiple miscarriages, deep venous thrombosis, or pulmonary emboli. In over 100 positive crossmatch transplants we have not had a vascular thrombosis, although many patients with confirmed hypercoagulable conditions have been transplanted while on therapeutic heparin.

Not surprisingly, co-morbid conditions associated with dialysis are exaggerated in this group. Cardiovascular, bone, infectious, hematalogic, hepatic, and metabolic disorders are increased. Patients must be carefully screened for co-morbid conditions that might reduce their ability to tolerate desensitization or transplantation.

## Treatment Plan

After establishing the patient's risk profile the therapeutic desensitization plan is formulated. All patients will receive PP/IVIg and quadruple sequential immunosuppression (FK506, MMF, daclizumab, steroids). The FK506 and MMF are started on the first day of pretransplant PP/IVIg and daclizumab and steroids are added on the day of transplant. The number of pretransplant PP/IVIg treatments can be estimated from the starting titer (Table 16.16.3a-3). The goal is to reduce DSA to a level that is safe and will not result in hyperacute rejection. Most patients will have a (-) CXM at the time of surgery. However, some patients, especially those with very high starting titers, will be resistant to complete elimination of DSA. In this case, a decision must be made whether or not to proceed to transplant with a low titer (+) CXM. If PP/IVIg is discontinued, DSA will usually rebound, often to levels higher than the starting titer. Thus, it may be harmful to initiate desensitization unless there is a reasonable expectation that the patient can be transplanted. We have transplanted patients with CXM titers as high as 16 on the day of surgery after prolonged PP/IVIg. Hyperacute rejection has not occurred, but most of these patients have developed early AMR requiring an extended course of posttransplant PP/IVIg treatment. Based on our experience, we no longer consider a starting titer of > 256 (AHG-CDC) to be amenable to desensitization.

**TABLE 16.16.3a-3**

## # OF PLASMAPHERESIS TREATMENTS FOR POSITIVE CROSSMATCH TRANSPLANTATION

| DSA Titer by AHG CDC XM | # of PreTx Treatments | # of PostTx Treatments |
|---|---|---|
| (+) Flow, (-) AHG | 2 | 2 |
| 1-4 | 3 | 3 |
| 8-16 | 4 | 3 |
| 32-64 | 5 | 4 |
| 128 | 6-7 | 4 |
| 256 | 8-10 | 5 |
| 512 | 11-15 | 6 |
| >512 | >20 | 6 |

**TABLE 16.16.3a-4**

## THERAPEUTIC ALGORITHM FOR (+) XM TRANSPLANTATION

| Risk Level | Example | Therapeutic Plan |
|---|---|---|
| Low-to-Moderate | Primary Tx: pregnancy induced | Preconditioning**<br>No splenectomy or anti-CD<br>20 Quardruple immunosuppression* |
| Moderate | 2nd or 3rd Tx: low titer, no repeat mismatches | Anti-CD 20<br>No splenectomy<br>Preconditioning**<br>Quardruple immunosuppression* |
| Moderate-to-High | Multiple txs: broad sensitization, multiple repeat mismatches | Splenectomy<br>No Anti-CD20<br>Preconditioning**<br>Quardruple immunosuppression* |
| High | Multiple txs: broad sensitization, multiple repeat mismatches, high titer DSA | Splenectomy<br>Anti-CD20<br>Preconditioning**<br>Quardruple immunosuppression* |

*IL-2R Ab, FK 506, MMF, Prednisone        **PP/CMVIg # based on titer

Patients who are deemed to be at low-to-moderate risk will receive PP/IVIg and quadruple sequential immunosuppression (Table 16.16.3a-4). Patients with moderate immunologic risk will have anti-CD20 added to their induction therapy. High-risk patients undergo pre-transplant splenectomy and may also receive anti-CD20. The optimal timing of the administration of anti-CD20 remains unclear. There are experimental murine data suggesting a benefit to initiating therapy 1 month prior to PP.[8] We have given the drug both 1 month and 1 day prior to transplantation and not observed a difference in outcome.

The last PP/IVIg treatment is usually performed on the day before transplant. The first posttransplant treatment is performed on postoperative day 2. FFP is used for replacement in both cases. On the day of transplant, patients receive 2mg/kg of daclizumab and solumedrol 500 mg prior to reperfusion. The mean number of pretransplant PP/IVIg treatments for our cohort is 4. DSA is monitored throughout the treatment period.

### Follow-up

PP/IVIg is discontinued when DSA is either eliminated or has stabilized at a low level and the patient is clinically well. AMR is treated with reinitiation of PP/IVIg and a steroid pulse. AMR is often accompanied by histologic evidence of cellular rejection. When AMR does occur, the rise in Cr may be preceded by a rise in DSA. A biopsy may be helpful for investigating a rise in DSA that does not produce an increase in Cr. If the biopsy demonstrates C4d and neutrophil margination in the preitubular capillaries, PP/IVIg is instituted. A change in the patient's clinical condition is investigated with a biopsy and a measurement of DSA. Resolution of AMR is tracked by frequent biopsies and DSA determinations. Cellular rejection is usually treated with pulse steroids but ATG may be necessary for more severe rejections.

Among patients with stable Cr, we perform protocol biopsies at 1, 3, 6, and 12 months. Assays for DSA are performed before and after each PP treatment, at weekly intervals for the first

month posttransplant, every 2 weeks for the first 3 months, and monthly during the remainder of the first year. When DSA or serum creatinine is discordant, the biopsy is used to resolve the disparity.

### KIDNEY-PAIRED DONATION

First described by Rapaport in the mid-1980s, Kidney-Paired Donation (KPD) involves two patients with incompatible donors agreeing to exchange donors so that each recipient receives a compatible organ.[24] In conventional KPD, a donor/recipient pair with blood types A and B are matched with the opposite blood type incompatibility (B and A) so that each recipient receives a blood type compatible kidney (Figure 16.16.3a-5). Unfortunately, these are the rarest combinations of blood types and conventional KPD will only benefit 3% to 5% of patients on the list. The possibility of including blood type O patients in exchanges would be predicted to greatly expand the impact of KPD. By matching ABOi patients with HLA-incompatible pairs, it becomes feasible for a patient with a positive crossmatch, blood type O donor to enter into a KPD (Figure 16.16.3a-6). These so-called unconventional KPDs allow virtually every patient with an incompatible donor to potentially benefit from KPD.

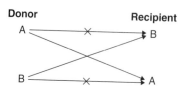

**FIGURE 16.16.3a-5**

Conventional KPD
Only ABOi pairs A/B or B/A (3% of donor/recipient pairs eligible)

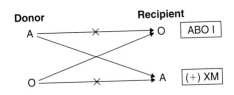

**FIGURE 16.16.3a-6**

Unconventional KPD
(all ABOI and + XM donor/recipient pairs eligible)

We recently reported the successful transplantion of 22 patients using KPD.[25] Twelve patients were transplanted in conventional KPDs, whereas 10 patients received kidneys through unconventional KPD. As expected the results have been comparable to those achieved nationally through standard live donor transplants. The unconventional KPDs included patients with PRAs > 80, but negative donor-specific crossmatches, and there were no cases of AMR. Most of the sensitized patients who participated in unconventional exchanges were offered this modality because their DSA titers with their intended donor exceeded levels that could be safely and effectively treated with desensitization. Thus, KPD can be offered as an alternative modality for patients who are not good candidates for desensitization.

At various times our KPD pool has consisted of between 50 and 75 incompatible pairs. After transplanting the patients who matched easily in either conventional or unconventional KPDs, our pool became enriched with patients who were broadly sensitized to HLA antigens or had difficult-to-match blood types. We have recently relaxed the requirement for completely compatible pairings and matched patients to donors for whom they had low titer DSA or were ABOi. These patients were then desensitized to their KPD donor and transplanted. In these cases, patients who were not candidates for desensitization with their intended donors were matched to KPD donors with whom desensitization was a viable option.

By adding living nondirected donors (LNDD) to our KPD pool, we have been able to generate what we have referred to as domino-paired donations (DPD). In a DPD the LNDD is matched to a recipient who has an incompatible donor who is in turn matched to a patient at the top of the UNOS list (2-way DPD; Figure 16.16.3a-7) or another recipient with an incompatible donor who gives their kidney to a patient on the deceased donor list (3-way DPD). We have performed both 2- and 3-way DPD, some of which have also involved desensitization, with successful outcomes.[26] Instead of the LNDD being matched with one recipient in a traditional allocation paradigm, DPD allows the LNDD's gift to be multiplied because several transplants that would not have been possible occur. The likelihood of finding a match in a DPD is enhanced because the pairing of a LNDD to a recipient in the KPD pool is not limited by the need to find a reciprocally matched donor. LNDDs are able to match with recipients who would not normally find a partner, freeing up their donor to give to another patient. In this way, allocating LNDD kidneys to DPD produces both quantitative and qualitative benefits.

KPD and DPD provide additional solutions for patients with incompatible donors. They can be used in concert with desensitization or as an alternative. We have estimated that applying an optimized algorithm applied to a national KPD list would match about 47% of the pairs.[1] The remaining unmatched pairs will consist primarily of difficult-to-match patients, and desensitization with either their intended donor or incompatible KPD donor will be their best alternative.[27]

## References

1. Segev DL, Gentry SE, Warren DS, Reeb B, MontgomeryRA. Kidney paired donation and optimizing the use of live donor organs. *JAMA* 2005;293:1883–1890.
2. Gentry SE, Segev DL, Montgomery RA. A comparison of populations served by kidney paired donation and list paired donation. *Am J Transplant* 2005;5:1914–1921.
3. Alexandre GP, Squifflet JP, De Bruyere M. Present experiences in a series of 26 ABO-incompatible living donor renal allografts. *Transplant Proc* 1987;19:4538–4542.
4. Takahashi K, Saito K, Takahara S, et al. Excellent long-term outcome of ABO-incompatible living donor kidney transplantation in Japan. *Am J Transplant* 2004;4:1089–1096.
5. Tyden G, Kumlien G, Fehrman I. Successful ABO-incompatible kidney transplantations without splenectomy using antigen-specific immunoadsorption and rituximab. *Transplantation* 2003;76:730–731.
6. Sonnenday CJ, Warren DS, Cooper M, et al. Plasmapheresis, CMV hyperimmune globulin, and anti-CD20 allow ABO-incompatible renal transplantation without splenectomy. *Am J Transplant* 2004;4:1315–1322.
7. Segev DL, Simpkins CE, Warren DS, et al. ABO incompatible high-titer renal transplantation without splenectomy or anti-CD20 treatment. *Am J Transplant* 2005;5: 2570–2575.
8. Gong Q, Ou Q, Ye S, et al. Importance of cellular microenvironment and circulatory dynamics in B cell immunotherapy. *J Immunol* 2005;174:817–826.
9. Higgins RM, Bevan DJ, Carey BS, et al. Prevention of hyperacute rejection by removal of antibodies to HLA immediately before renal transplantation. *Lancet* 1996;348:1208–1211.
10. Tyden, G, Kumlien, G, Genberg, H, et al. ABO incompatible kidney transplantations without splenectomy, using antigen-specific immunoadsorption and rituximab. *Am J Transplant* 2005;5:145–148.
11. Sonnenday CJ, Ratner LE, Zachary AA. Preemptive therapy with plasmapheresis/intravenous immunoglobulin allows successful live donor renal transplantation in patients with a positive cross-match. *Transplant Proc* 2002;34:1614–1616.
12. Glotz D, Haymann JP, Sansonetti N, et al. Suppression of HLA-specific alloantibodies by high-dose intravenous immunoglobulins (IVIg). A potential tool for transplantation of immunized patients. *Transplantation* 1993;56:335–337.
13. Jordan SC, Vo A, Bunnapradist S, et al. Intravenous immune globulin treatment inhibits crossmatch positivity and allows for successful transplantation of incompatible organs in living-donor and cadaver recipients. *Transplantation* 2003;76:631–636.

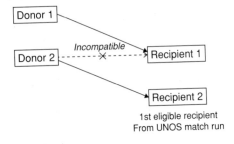

**FIGURE 16.16.3a-7**

2-Way Domino Paired Donation

1st eligible recipient
From UNOS match run

14. Montgomery RA, Zachary AA, Racusen LC, et al. Plasmapheresis and intravenous immune globulin provides effective rescue therapy for refractory humoral rejection and allows kidneys to be successfully transplanted into cross-match-positive recipients. *Transplantation* 2000;70:887–895.

15. Kazatchkine MD, Kaveri SV. Immunomodulation of autoimmune and inflammatory diseases with intravenous immune globulin. *N Engl J Med* 2001;345:747–755.

16. Shimmura, H, Tanabe, K, Ishida, H, Tokumoto, T, Ishikawa, N, Miyamoto, N, Shirakawa, H, Setoguchi, K, Nakajima, I, Fuchinoue, S, Teraoka, S, Toma, H. Lack of correlation between results of ABO-incompatible living kidney transplantation and anti-ABO blood type antibody titers under our current immunosuppression. Transplantation 2005; 80: 985–988

17. Technical Manual. 2002; 792

18. Gloor, JM, Lager, DJ, Moore, SB, Pineda, AA, Fidler, ME, Larson, TS, Grande, JP, Schwab, TR, Griffin, MD, Prieto, M, Nyberg, SL, Velosa, JA, Textor, SC, Platt, JL, Stegall, MD. ABO-incompatible kidney transplantation using both A2 and non-A2 living donors. *Transplantation* 2003; 75: 971–977

19. Haas M, Rahman MH, Racusen LC, Kraus Es, Bagnasco SM, Segev DL, Simpkins CE, Warren DS, King KE, Zachary AA, Montgomery RA. C4d and C3d staining in biopsies of ABO-and HLA-incompatible renal allografts: Correlation with histologic findings. *Am J Transplant.* 2006; 6(8): 1829–1840.

20. Warren, DS, Zachary, AA, Sonnenday, CJ, King, KE, Cooper, M, Ratner, LE, Shirey, RS, Haas, M, Leffell, MS, Montgomery, RA. Successful renal transplantation across simultaneous ABO incompatible and positive crossmatch barriers. *Am J Transplant* 2004; 4: 561–568.

21. Ross, LF, Woodle, ES. Ethical issues in increasing living kidney donations by expanding kidney paired exchange programs. *Transplantation* 2000; 69: 1539–1543

22. Delmonico, FL, Morrissey, PE, Lipkowitz, GS, Stoff, JS, Himmelfarb, J, Harmon, W, Pavlakis, M, Mah, H, Goguen, J, Luskin, R, Milford, E, Basadonna, G, Chobanian, M, Bouthot, B, Lorber, M, Rohrer, RJ. Donor kidney exchanges. *Am J Transplant* 2004; 4: 1628–1634

23. Haas, M, Rahman, H, Racusen, LC, Kraus, E, Bagnasco, SM, Segev, DL, Simpkins, CE, Warren, DS, King, KE, A., ZA, Montgomery, RA. C4d and C3d Staining in Biopsies of ABO- and HLA-Incompatible Renal Allografts: Correlation with Histologic Findings. *American Journal of Transplantation* 2006; in press:

24. Rapaport, FT. The case for a living emotionally related international kidney donor exchange registry. *Transplant Proc* 1986; 18: 5–9

25. Montgomery, RA, Zachary, AA, Ratner, LE, Segev, DL, Hiller, Houp, J, Cooper, M, Kavoussi, L, Jarrett, T, Burdick, J, Maley, WR, Melancon, JK, Kozlowski, T, Simpkins, CE, Phillips, M, Desai, A, Collins, V, Reeb, B, Kraus, E, Rabb, H, Leffell, MS, Warren, DS. Clinical results from transplanting incompatible live kidney donor/recipient pairs using kidney paired donation. *Jama* 2005; 294: 1655–1663

26. Montgomery, RA, Gentry, SE, Marks, WH, Warren, DS, Hiller, J, Houp, J, A., ZA, Melancon, JK, Maley, WR, Rabb, H, Simpkins, CE, Segev, DL. Domino paired kidney donation: A strategy to make best use of live non-directed donation. *Lancet* 2006; 368(9533):419–421.

27. Montgomery, RA, Simpkins, CE, Segev, DL. New options for patients with donor incompatibilities. *Transplantation* 2006; 82(2): 164–165.

## 16.16.3b Desensitization Protocols for High-PRA Recipients

*James M. Gloor, MD, Mark D. Stegall, MD*

## AN APPROACH TO TRANSPLANTATION OF THE SENSITIZED PATIENT

People who have developed anti-HLA antibodies, generally following blood transfusion, pregnancy, or prior transplant, are said to be sensitized.[1] Anti-HLA antibodies with donor specificity (DSA) have been recognized as an important risk factor for allograft loss since the early days of transplantation. In 1969 Patel and Terasaki demonstrated in a retrospective analysis of 225 kidney transplants that detectable DSA at the time of transplantation ("positive crossmatch") was associated with allograft loss within hours in the majority of cases, a phenomenon they termed "hyperacute rejection."[2] Since that report, the identification of DSA has been an important component of pretransplant patient preparation. One of the primary goals in transplantation of sensitized patients is to avoid allograft injury due to humoral rejection. This goal can be achieved by avoiding donor–recipient combinations in which the recipient has donor specific antibodies (DSA). Nevertheless, some recipients with DSA can be successfully transplanted, although interventions to avoid antibody mediated allograft injury are needed.[3-7] The unique needs of sensitized kidney transplant candidates can be categorized in four areas: (1) DSA detection and characterization, (2) pretransplant preconditioning, (3) posttransplant DSA monitoring and treatment, (4) treatment of humoral rejection.

### DSA Detection and Characterization

Kidney transplant candidates with anti-HLA antibodies need to be identified prior to transplantation.[8] Historically, this has been done by exposing a "panel" of T lymphocytes collected from blood donors whose HLA tissue antigens have been determined to sera from the transplant candidate. Using either cytotoxicity or flow cytometry-based techniques, patients with positive panel reactions are determined to have HLA antibodies. Calculation of the percentage of positive reactions/panel assigns a "percent panel reactivity" or PRA. Candidates with high PRA percentages are considered to have a wide array of anti-HLA antibodies. By comparing the pattern of HLA antigens present in positive and negative reactions, an assessment of anti-HLA antibody specificity can often be calculated. Nevertheless, individuals with a wide array of antibodies may react with nearly all the panel ("high PRA"), resulting in inability to assign anti-HLA specificity. This method of detection and characterization of HLA antibodies suffers from several shortcomings. By confining the assay to T lymphocytes, antibodies with HLA class II specificity are not identified. As newer techniques of antibody detection have become available, it has become increasingly clear that these HLA class II antibodies are capable of producing severe, even hyperacute humoral rejection.[9] Analyses based on cell panels are dependent on the sensitivity of the assay used, and may be too insensitive to detect low levels of HLA antibodies. Finally, the specificity of the assay may be questionable, with some positive reactions potentially caused by the interaction of antibodies with antigens irrelevant to transplantation.[10] In current practice, the characterization of anti-HLA antibody status can be thought to consist of three determinations. (1) Are there anti-HLA class I or II antibodies present? (2) If present, for which HLA antigens do they have specificity? (3) If present, how high is the level of antibody activity? Since no one technique or assay satisfactorily answers all three questions, comprehensive antibody characterization requires a combination of techniques.

### Are Anti-HLA Class I or II Antibodies Present?

Given the fact that detection of antibodies is an essential first step in characterization of antibody status, it is important that the assay used to detect these antibodies be as sensitive as possible, and not affected by non-HLA interactions. Currently, solid-phase assays in which multiple purified HLA class I or II antigens are bound to synthetic flow beads or wells are available, economical, and lend themselves to high throughput screening.[11,12] Fluorochrome-labeled synthetic beads coated with a wide array of HLA antigens can be incubated with recipient sera and analyzed with flow cytometry, whereas antigens bound to wells in testing trays can be assayed with enzyme-linked immunosorbent assay (ELISA)-based techniques. Positive reactions in these tests indicate that antibodies with HLA specificity are present, but do not allow determination of which HLA antigens are targeted. Conversely, patients with negative reactions can confidently be considered to be nonsensitized to HLA antigens.

## What Is the HLA Specificity of the Antibodies?

Patients testing positive for anti-HLA antibodies (class I or II) using solid-phase multiantigen testing methods undergo further testing to determine the specificity of these antibodies. Using similar assays as those described above, beads or wells coated with single specific HLA antigens bound to solid phase substrates can be analyzed by flow cytometry or ELISA, and donor specificity identified if present.[13]

## What Is the Level of DSA Activity?

If antidonor antibodies are identified using sensitive and specific solid-phase assays, it is important to determine the level of DSA activity in order to formulate the best approach to pretransplant conditioning. This can be achieved through a combination of complement dependent cytotoxicity (CDC) and flow cytometric crossmatches using both T and B lymphocytes. Individuals with CDC positive crossmatches are considered to have high levels of DSA activity, whereas those with negative CDC but positive flow cytometric crossmatches are considered to have low levels.

### Pretransplant Conditioning

The goal of pretransplant conditioning is to prevent immediate allograft injury produced by high levels of DSA activity. On completion of the pretransplant antibody evaluation, candidates can be characterized as having high or low levels of HLA class I, class II, or both DSA. The approach to pretransplant conditioning is dependent on whether an individual transplant candidate has a potential living kidney donor or awaits deceased kidney donation.

### Deceased Donor Candidates

Currently, in the United States there are over 7,000 individuals awaiting kidney transplantation with PRA antibodies exceeding 80% (2004 OPTN/SRTR Annual Report 1994–2003. HHS/HRSA/HSB/DOT; UNOS; URREA). Annually, approximately 300 of these individuals are transplanted, typically with a zero HLA mismatched kidney.[14] The estimated waiting time for these patients is significantly prolonged compared to nonsensitized candidates despite efforts to prioritize organ allocation based on PRA, and patients with a wide array of anti-HLA antibodies may be essentially nontransplantable using traditional methods. Given this situation, different approaches have been developed with the goal of lowering the level of anti-HLA antibodies and improving the likelihood of obtaining an acceptably matched kidney. In a randomized, double-blind, placebo controlled study of 101 sensitized deceased donor kidney transplant candidates,

periodic administration of 2 g/kg intravenous immunoglobulin was effective in lowering PRA and increased the rate of transplantation compared to placebo.[15] In another investigation of 9 highly sensitized patients awaiting transplantation, administration of the genetically engineered chimeric murine/human anti-CD20 monoclonal antibody Rituximab resulted in a modest decrease in alloreactivity measured by flow cytometry.[16] Nevertheless, the interventions that are currently available for reducing allosensitization in deceased donor kidney transplant candidates have not been predictably effective in many patients.

### Living Donor Transplant Candidates

*High DSA.* Transplant candidates with high DSA (positive CDC and FXM crossmatch) require therapy prior to transplant to lower the level of antidonor antibody activity to a level below that which causes allograft injury. Currently there are two approaches to achieving this goal. Administration of high-dose intravenous immunoglobulin (typically in the range of 2 g/kg body weight) has been shown to be successful in ameliorating a positive complement dependent cytotoxicity crossmatch, and permitting successful transplantation.[4,6] Patients who fail to respond to one dose of IVIG may subsequently respond to repeated doses. The likelihood of an individual responding to high dose IVIG therapy may be predicted by performing a crossmatch between the donor–recipient pair in question after adding IVIG to the sera to be studied. Conversion of the positive crossmatch to negative in this *in vitro* system is reported to be predictive of a similar response when performed *in vivo* after administration of IVIG. Although the mechanism of intravenous immunoglobulin in producing a negative crossmatch is not completely delineated, it is proposed that the presence of exogenous immunoglobulin with antiidiotypic action inactivate DSA. Other mechanisms include the stimulation of synthesis of blocking antibodies, complement inhibitory activity, interaction with helper T cells, and interactions with antibody presenting cells.[17] Using this method, Jordan et al. have reported that 75% of patients with DSA detected using a complement dependent cytotoxicity crossmatch are found to be "*in vitro* responders," and in that group 90% are successfully converted to a negative crossmatch. In a series of 47 patients transplanted, the 1-year allograft survival was 80%, with a humoral rejection rate of 40%. Similarly, Glotz et al. report successful desensitization and transplantation of 4 patients with cytotoxic DSA levels.[6]

Another approach to transplantation of patients with high levels of DSA incorporates a series of plasmapheresis treatments, followed by administration of a lower dose of IVIG (typically 5–10 g based on body weight).[3,5,7] In this approach the goal of plasmapheresis is to physically remove DSA prior to transplantation and thus obtain a negative crossmatch at the time of transplantation. The IVIG in this approach prevents hypogammaglobulinemia and its associated profound immunosuppression, although it is possible that it provides some of the immunomodulatory effect described above as well.

Individuals with high levels of DSA have been successfully transplanted using both high dose IVIG as well as plasmapheresis based regimens. Both approaches have advantages and disadvantages. Preconditioning with intravenous immunoglobulin has the advantage of ease of administration and relative low cost compared to other methods. Nevertheless, some adverse effects have been recognized, typically associated with the administration of large volumes of colloid solution to anuric renal failure patients, as well as rare thrombotic complications. Plasmapheresis followed by low-dose IVIG is expensive, and requires considerable time during the period preceding transplantation. If not already present, intravenous access is required. Although the optimum approach to positive crossmatch transplantation is not yet defined, some information is available permitting comparison of high dose IVIG and plasmapheresis-based protocols. Stegall et al. report a comparison of high dose IVIG and two plasmapheresis-based protocols in a series of 37 positive crossmatch kidney transplants as defined using an anti-human globulin enhanced CDC crossmatch.[18] In that experience, both high-dose IVIG and plasmapheresis protocols were effective in producing a negative crossmatch in patients with lower levels of DSA (AHG-CDC T cell crossmatch titer ≤ 1:4). Neither high-dose IVIG nor plasmapheresis was effective in producing a negative crossmatch in patients with crossmatch titers exceeding 1:16. In patients with titers of 1:8–1:16, however, high-dose IVIG rarely produced a negative crossmatch, whereas plasmapheresis-based protocols predictably did so.

*Low DSA.*   Individuals with low levels of DSA (CDC crossmatch negative/FXM positive) are at low risk for hyperacute rejection since the levels of DSA required to produce severe allograft injury typically result in a positive cytotoxicity crossmatch. Therefore these individuals do not require the intensive preconditioning used in the preparation of high DSA patients for transplantation. Nevertheless, low DSA patients are at high risk for humoral rejection during the first days to weeks after transplant.[19] This rejection occurs as a result of the anamnestic memory response produced by exposure of the recipient memory B lymphocytes to circulating donor antigen shed from the allograft. An important objective in transplantation of patients with low levels of DSA is to prevent this memory response. Although the optimum method of achieving this objective is currently not well defined, different approaches have been utilized. High-dose IVIG has been shown to be effective in individuals with high DSA levels. This approach has also been utilized in patients with low levels of DSA.[20.] Akalin et al. report a series of 8 patients with positive FXM treated with pretransplant high-dose IVIG as well as antithymocyte antibody induction.[21] In that group no humoral rejection occurred. Similarly, Gloor et al. report a series of 18 patients in whom FXM was positive and CDC XM was negative who received high-dose IVIG and antithymocyte induction. Humoral rejection was diagnosed in 11% of patients.[20]

Another potential approach to prevention of posttransplant increase in DSA may be the use of the anti-CD20 antibody, rituximab. Although this agent has been used in high-DSA patients as part of a protocol incorporating the use of plasmapheresis, its major role may be in preventing the recruitment of naïve and memory B lymphocytes (CD20+) into the DSA-secreting plasma cell population.[3]

Activation of B lymphocytes with the subsequent evolution into plasma cells typically is thought to require an interaction with T lymphocytes. Thus, measures to deplete T lymphocytes such as antithymocyte antibody induction may represent effective therapy in prevention of B-cell activation and plasma cell development. Although the approach appears rational, further investigation is needed.

## POSTTRANSPLANT MONITORING AND THERAPY

A major goal in transplantation of sensitized patients is to achieve a level of circulating DSA sufficiently low to avoid allograft injury. Patients with high DSA at baseline have undergone preconditioning to achieve this level, whereas low DSA patients

may not require preconditioning. Nevertheless, identification of an increase in circulating DSA level and implementation of therapy prior to allograft injury is a key component of protocols for positive crossmatch kidney transplantation. In protocols that do not incorporate antithymocyte induction, crossmatch testing can detect increases in DSA, and routine posttransplant testing is standard. [7] In protocols in which antithymocyte induction is utilized, measures must be taken to remove these antibodies prior to crossmatching to prevent interference with the test interpretation.[22] Once detected, therapy to lower DSA levels can be implemented. Similar to the pretransplant conditioning regimens, both high-dose IVIG and plasmapheresis/low-dose IVIG have been used to achieve this. Importantly, low levels of DSA are commonly identifiable following transplantation using sensitive crossmatch techniques such as flow cytometry. [13,23] Nevertheless, a positive CDC crossmatch occurring in the first weeks after transplant is typically followed by a humoral rejection episode unless measures are taken to intervene. Although therapy with plasmapheresis is generally effective in lowering the level of DSA to below that resulting in a positive CDC crossmatch, these antibodies are still typically detectable by flow cytometry.

Acute humoral rejection most commonly occurs during the first weeks following transplantation. Typically, patients who have not developed humoral rejection during the first 2 weeks after transplantation do not do so later, despite the presence of low levels of DSA detectable in peripheral blood. The phenomenon of detectable DSA without demonstrable allograft injury has been termed *accommodation* in the setting of ABO blood group incompatible transplants.[24] Although the exact mechanism is not known, changes in gene expression at the level of the allograft have been demonstrated.[25] Additionally, upregulation of protective genes such as BCL-XL and BCL 2 have been reported in some transplant recipients with circulating DSA.[26]

## TREATMENT OF HUMORAL REJECTION

Significant advances have been made in the diagnosis of humoral rejection, primarily due to the recognition that the histologic appearance of humoral rejection differs significantly from that of acute cellular rejection.[27,28] The identification of the complement degradation product C4d as a marker for the interaction of antibody, antigen, and complement system has permitted more timely and accurate diagnosis of humoral rejection[29–31]. The Banff 97 classification for allograft histology has been modified to take these factors into account.[32] Currently, the approach to the treatment of humoral rejection is based on removal or inactivation of circulating DSA, as well as efforts to decrease antibody production.

## INACTIVATION/REMOVAL OF DSA

Similar to the preconditioning regimens used to prepare for transplantation, both plasmapheresis and high-dose IVIG have been used to treat humoral rejection.[33,34] Early reports on the efficacy of plasmapheresis in treating humoral rejection gave contradictory results.[35,36] Nevertheless, in these older reports, the criteria used to define humoral rejection were not standardized. Additionally, in many reports therapy was delayed after the diagnosis of rejection, and plasmapheresis was implemented after the rejection episode had been unsuccessfully treated using other modalities. More recent studies report successful reversal of humoral rejection in most patients treated with plasmapheresis-based protocols, although chronic allograft nephropathy may follow.[3,7] Pascual et al. report successful reversal of humoral rejection using a combination of plasmapheresis and increased maintenance immunosuppression.[34] Similarly, high-dose IVIG has been shown to be effective in reversing humoral rejection in small numbers of patients.[37] Doses used are similar to those utilized in pretransplant conditioning regimens.

## INHIBITION OF FURTHER DSA PRODUCTION

In addition to removal or inactivation of DSA, further efforts to decrease production appear rational, since the persistence of high levels of DSA are associated with poor outcome.[13] DSA are thought to be produced by long-lived plasma cells located predominantly in the bone marrow and spleen.[38] Depletion of these cells using currently available immunosuppressive medications is ineffective. Nevertheless, recruitment of new antibody secreting cells from the memory B-cell population likely.[39] Given that these cells express CD20 to a greater or lesser degree, the use of anti-CD20 antibody appears to be a rational approach to decreasing DSA production.[40] In addition, the development of new antibody-secreting cells likely requires T-cell support, thus measures to deplete T cells likely give some benefit.[39] Individuals who have not received antithymocyte induction who develop humoral rejection frequently have an associated component of acute cellular rejection, which may also be effectively treated using antithymocyte antibody therapy. Finally, some individuals with humoral rejection recalcitrant to other therapeutic interventions appear to respond to splenectomy.

## CONCLUSION

Transplantation of sensitized individuals is a challenging procedure which is justified by the fact that these patients are often otherwise unlikely to receive a transplant. In addition, years of prior hemodialysis while awaiting transplant often leaves these patients with precarious dialysis access. Although the long-term outcome of transplants performed in the presence of DSA is not well characterized currently, short- to intermediate-term outcomes appear favorable and lend further support to efforts to overcome the barrier.

## References

1. Moore SB, Sterioff S, Pierides AM, Watts SK, Ruud CM. Transfusion-induced alloimmunization in patients awaiting renal allografts. *Vox Sanguinis* 1984;47:354–361.
2. Patel R, Terasaki PI. Significance of the positive crossmatch test in kidney transplantation. *New Engl J Med* 1969;280(14):735–739.
3. Gloor JM, DeGoey SR, Pineda AA, et al. Overcoming a positive crossmatch in living donor kidney transplantation. *Am J Transplant* 2003;3(8):1017.
4. Jordan SC, Vo AA, Tyan D, Nast CC. Desensitization therapy with high-dose intravenous gammaglobulin: applications to treatment of antibody-mediated rejection. *Pediatric Transplantation* 2004.
5. Schweitzer E, Wilson JS, Fernandez-Vina M, et al. A high panel-reactive antibody rescue protocol for cross-match-positive live donor kidney transplants. *Transplantation* 2000;70(10):1531–1536.
6. Glotz D, Antoine C, Julia P, et al. Desensitization and subsequent kidney transplantation of patients using intravenous immunoglobulin. *Am J Transplant* 2002;2:758–760.
7. Montgomery RA, Zachary AA, Racusen LC, et al. Plasmapheresis and intravenous immune globulin provides effective rescue therapy for refractory humoral rejection and allows kidneys to be successfully transplanted into cross-match-positive recipients. *Transplantation* 2000;70(6):887–895.
8. Gebel HM, Bray RA. Sensitization and sensitivity: defining the unsensitized patient. *Transplantation* 2000;69(7):1370–1374
9. Scornik JC, LeFor WM, Cicciarelli JC, et al. Hyperacute and acute kidney graft rejection due to antibodies against B cells. *Transplantation* 1992;54(1):61–64.
10. Lobashevsky A, Senkbeil R, Shoaf J, et al. Specificity of preformed alloantibodies causing B cell positive flow crossmatch in renal transplantation. *Clinical Transplantation* 2000;14:533–542.
11. Gebel HM, Bray RA, Nickerson P. Pre-transplant assessment of donor-reactive HLA-specific antibodies in renal transplantation: Contraindication vs. risk. *Am J Transplant* 2003;3:1488–1500.
12. Zachary AA, Delaney NL, Lucas DP, Lefell MS. Characterization of HLA class I specific antibodies by ELISA using solubilized antigen targets: 1. Evaluation of GTI QuikID assay and analysis of antibody patterns. *Human Immunology.* 2001;62:228–235.
13. Gloor JM, DeGoey S, Ploeger N, et al. Persistence of low levels of alloantibody after desensitization in crossmatch positive living donor kidney transplantation. *Transplantation* 2003;78(2):221–227.
14. Stegall MD, Dean PG, McBride MA, Wynn JJ, Organ Procurement and Transplantation Network/ UnitedNetwork for Organ Sharing Kidney/Pancreas Transplantation Committee. Survival of mandatorily shared cadaveric kidneys and their paybacks in the zero mismatch era. *Transplantation* 2002;74(5):670–675.
15. Jordan SC, Tyan D, Stablein DM, et al. Evaluation of intravenous immunoglobulin as an agent to lower allosensitization and improve transplantation in highly sensitized adult patients with end-stage renal disease: report of the NIH IG02 trial. *J Am Soc Nephrol* 2004;15(12):3256–3262.
16. Vieira CA, Agarwal A, Book BK, et al. Rituximab for reduction of anti-HLA antibodies in patients awaiting renal transplantation: Safety, Pharmacodynamics, and Pharmacokinetics. *Transplantation* 2004;77(4):542–548.
17. Jordan S, Tyan D, Czer L, Toyoda M. Immunomodulatory actions of intravenous immunoglobulin (IVIG): potential applications in solid organ transplant recipients. *Pediatric Transplantation* 1998;2:92–105.
18. Stegall MD, Gloor JM, Winters J, Moore SB. A Comparison of Plasmapheresis vs High-Dose IVIG Desensitization in Renal Allograft Recipients with High Levels of Donor Specific Alloantibody. *Am J Transplant* 2006; 6(2): 346–351.
19. Karpinski M, Rush D, Jeffery J, et al. Flow cytometric crossmatching in primary renal transplant recipients with a negative anti-human globulin enhanced cytotoxicity crossmatch. *J Am Soc Nephrol* 2001;12:2807–2814.
20. Gloor JM, Mai ML, DeGoey S, et al. Kidney transplantation following administration of high dose intravenous immunoglobulin in patients with positive flow cytometric / negative enhanced cytotoxicity crossmatch. *Am J Transplant* 2004;4(suppl 8):256.
21. Akalin E, Ames S, Sehgal V, et al. Intravenous immunoglobulin and thymoglobulin facilitate kidney transplantation in complement-dependent cytotoxicity B-cell and flow cytometry T- or B- cell crossmatch positive patients. *Transplantation* 2003;76(10):1444–1447.
22. Bearden CM, Book BK, Sidner RA, Pescovitz MD. Removal of therapeutic anti-lymphocyte antibodies from human sera prior to anti-human leukocyte antibody testing. *J Immunologic Methods* 2005;300:192–199.
23. Zachary AA, Montgomery RA, Ratner LE, et al. Specific and durable elimination of antibody to donor HLA antigens in renal transplant patients. *Transplantation* 2003;76(10):1519–1525.
24. Saadi S, Platt JL. Immunology of xenotransplantation. *Life Sciences* 1998;62(5):365–387.
25. Park WD, Grande JP, Ninova D, et al. Accommodation in ABO-incompatible kidney allografts. *Am J Transplant* 2003;3(8):952.
26. Salama AD, Delikouras A, Pusey CD, et al. Transplant accomodation in highly sensitized patients: a potential role for Bcl-xL and alloantibody. *Am J Transplant* 2001;1(3):260–269.

27. Mauiyyedi S, Crespo M, Collins AB, et al. Acute humoral rejection in kidney transplantation: II. Morphology, immunopathology, and pathologic classification. *J Am Soc Nephrol* 2002;13:779–787.

28. Trpkov K, Campbell P, Pazderka F, et al. Pathologic features of acute renal allograft rejection associated with donor-specific antibody. Analysis using the Banff Grading Schema. *Transplantation* 1996;61(11): 1586–1592.

29. Feucht HE, Schneeberger H, Hillebrand G, et al. Capillary deposition of C4d complement fragment and early renal graft loss. *Kid International* 1993;43:1333–1338.

30. Nickeleit V, Zeiler M, Gudat F, Thiel G, Mihatsch MJ. Detection of the complement degradation product C4d in renal allografts: Diagnostic and therapeutic implications. *J Am Soc Nephrol* 2002;13:242–251.

31. Herzenberg AM, Gill JS, Djurdev O, Magil A. C4d deposition in acute rejection: an independent long-term prognostic factor. *J Am Soc Nephrol* 2002;13:234–241.

32. Racusen LC, Colvin RB, Solez K, et al. Antibody-mediated rejection criteria- an addition to the Banff '97 classification of renal allograft rejection. *Am J Transplant* 2003;3:708–714.

33. Jordan SC, Quartel AW, Czer LSC, et al. Posttransplant therapy using high dose human immunoglobulin (intravenous gammaglobulin) to control acute humoral rejection in renal and cardiac allograft recipients and potential mechanism of action. *Transplantation* 1998;66(6): 800–805.

34. Pascual M, Daidman S, Tolkoff-Rubin N, et al. Plasma exchange and tacrolimus-mycophenolate rescue for acute humoral rejection in kidney transplantation. *Transplantation* 1998;66(11):1460–1464.

35. Allen NH, Dyer P, Geoghegan T, et al. Plasma exchange in acute renal allograft rejection: a controlled trial. *Transplantation* 1983;35(5): 425–428.

36. Cardella CJ. Renal allograft and intensive plasma exchange: A critical assessment. In: Liss AR, ed. *Therapeutic Apheresis and Plasma Perfusion.* New York: Alan R. Liss; 1982:283–290.

37. Jordan SC, Vo A, Toyoda M, Tyan D, Nast CC. Post-transplant therapy with high-dose intravenous gammaglobulin: applications to treatment of antibody-mediated rejection. *Pediatr Transplantation* 2005;9: 155–161.

38. Slifka MK, Ahmed R. Long-lived plasma cells: a mechanism for maintaining persistent antibody production. *Current Opinion in Immunology* 1998;10:252–258.

39. Bernasconi NL, Traggiai E, Lanzavecchia A. Maintenance of serological memory be polyclonal activation of human memory B cells. *Science* 2002;298(5601):2199–2202.

40. Pescovitz MD. B cells: a rational target in alloantibody-mediated solid organ transplantation rejection. *Clin Transplantation* 2005;DOI: 10.1111/j.1399-012.2005.00439x.

## Chapter 16.16.3c   Auxiliary Liver Transplants for Highly Sensitized Kidney Recipients

*Michael Olausson, MD, PhD*

## SENSITIZED PATIENTS

After rejection of a deceased donor (DD) or living donor (LD) kidney graft, patients sometimes acquire HLA or non-HLA antibodies and become sensitized to a portion of the population. Their sensitization makes it more difficult to find another suitable DD or LD kidney, so the candidate often remains on the DD waiting list for a long time.[1] Once a new kidney does become available, the candidate's serum is tested against the prospective DD's or LD's lymphocytes pretransplant. A positive crossmatch test result indicates the presence of alloreactive HLA antibodies in the candidate's serum and is usually considered a contraindication

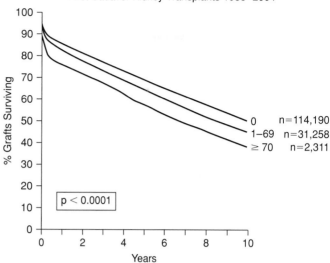

**FIGURE 16.16.3c-1**

Graft survival rates and PRA levels in highly sensitized primary DD kidney transplant recipients, 1985-2004. DD, deceased donor; PRA, panel-reactive antibody.

to that kidney transplant, given the high risk of hyperacute or severe acute rejection episodes leading to poor graft survival.[2] Data from the Collaborate Transplant Study group (CTS) demonstrated inferior graft survival rates in first and retransplant recipients with a high panel-reactive antibody (PRA) level (Figure 16.16.3c-1, Figure 16.16.3c-2).

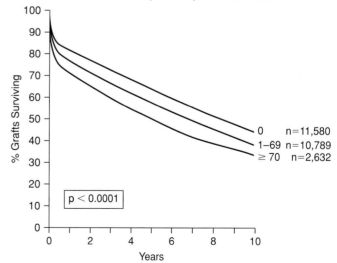

**FIGURE 16.16.3c-2**

Graft survival rates and PRA levels in highly sensitized retransplant DD kidney recipients, 1985-2004. DD, deceased donor; PRA, panel-reactive antibody.

Other organs such as the heart and lungs carry similar risks for rejection in such candidates. However, the liver seems to tolerate a positive crossmatch much better.[3-6] A combined DD whole liver and kidney transplant can be performed without the same risk for rejection as a kidney transplant alone.[6-13]

## KIDNEY TRANSPLANTS ALONE

To overcome the harmful effects of the antibodies, various schemes for removing them–plasmapheresis, protein A adsorption, and high doses of immunoglobulins[14-16] have been tried, so far with limited success. In most protocols, a living related kidney transplant is performed, preceded by extensive treatment of the recipient to achieve a negative crossmatch (see Chapter 16.16).

Usually, a negative crossmatch using both the cytotoxic technique (CDC) and the more specific flow cytometric technique (Flow) is required. Often, the procedure must be postponed or canceled because of failure to achieve a negative crossmatch. Frequently, prospective living related donors cannot donate because of problems with the crossmatch.

Recipients with a 70% or higher PRA level and a negative crossmatch have a significantly lower graft survival rate at 1 year posttransplant and later, as compared with recipients with a lower PRA level and a negative crossmatch (Figure 16.16.3c-3). This difference is even more pronounced in retransplanted recipients (Figure 16.16.3c-4). Results for heart and lung transplant recipients are even more discouraging, short- and long-term (Figure 16.16.3c-5 and Figure 16.16.3c-6).

### Crossmatch of First Cadaver Kidney Transplants 1995–2004

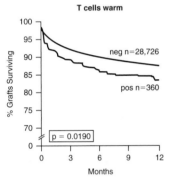 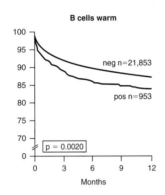 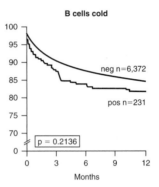 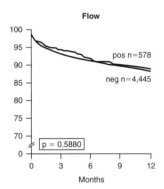

**FIGURE 16.16.3c-3**

Impact of a positive crossmatch on graft survival rates in highly sensitized primary DD kidney transplant recipients, 1995–2004. DD, deceased donor; Flow, flow cytometric technique.

### Crossmatch of First Cadaver Kidney Retransplants 1995–2004

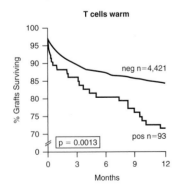 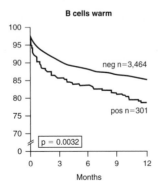 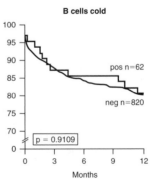 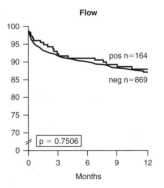

**FIGURE 16.16.3c-4**

Impact of a positive crossmatch on graft survival in highly sensitized retransplant recipients, 1995–2004. DD, deceased donor; Flow, flow cytometric technique.

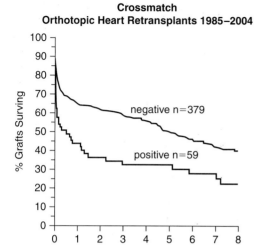

**Crossmatch**
**Orthotopic Heart Retransplants 1985–2004**

negative n=379

positive n=59

**FIG 16.16.3c-5**

Impact of a positive crossmatch on graft survival rates in heart retransplant recipients, 1985–2004.

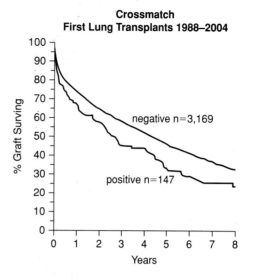

**Crossmatch**
**First Lung Transplants 1988–2004**

negative n=3,169

positive n=147

**FIG 16.16.3c-6**

Impact of a positive crossmatch on graft survival rates in primary lung transplant recipients, 1988–2004.

## COMBINED PARTIAL AUXILIARY LIVER AND KIDNEY TRANSPLANTS

In a recent publication, we showed that transplanting a partial liver as an auxiliary graft and a kidney from the same donor protected the kidney from rejection in 70% of the recipients, despite a positive pretransplant CDC crossmatch.[17] (This combined procedure can be performed from both LDs and DDs.) Our first combined LD transplant used a brother as the LD for his sister. She received segments 2 and 3 of his liver together with his right kidney, despite a positive crossmatch. No rejection was seen. Both organs are still functioning 3 years posttransplant. The brother had been previously turned down as a donor because of the positive crossmatch.

## Donor Operation

The surgical technique that we used for the donor operation is as follows: the lateral 2 segments of the donor liver are removed, using an *in situ* split technique in both a DD and LD. Dissection is carried out with a Cavitron Ultrasonic Surgical Aspirator (CUSA). The segment 4 artery is saved. In a DD, the remaining right lobe can be used for a liver transplant for an adult recipient.

Next, the right or the left kidney from the same DD or LD is removed, flushed, and stored in cold University of Wisconsin (UW) solution (Figure 16.16.3c-7).

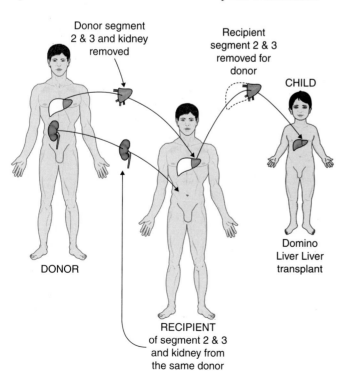

Donor segment 2 & 3 and kidney removed

Recipient segment 2 & 3 removed for donor

CHILD

DONOR

RECIPIENT of segment 2 & 3 and kidney from the same donor

Domino Liver Liver transplant

**FIG 16.16.3c-7**

Illustration of an auxiliary liver and combined kidney transplant followed by a domino segmental liver transplant.

## Recipient Operation

The lateral two segments of the recipient are removed, leaving a clamp on the left hepatic vein, left portal trunk, and left hepatic artery.

The donor liver is then connected to these vessels in an end-to-end fashion, using 5-0 (for the left hepatic vein), 6-0 (for the left portal trunk), and 7-0 (for the left hepatic artery) Prolene sutures. A Roux-en-Y loop is connected to the bile ducts of segment 2 and 3 bile ducts.

After the liver transplant is done, the kidney is transplanted into the left or right lower abdominal quadrant, using a retroperitoneal approach (Figure 16.16.3c-7).

## DOMINO LIVER TRANSPLANTS

We have also used the native liver segments 2 and 3 from recipients of combined partial auxiliary liver and kidney transplants for domino liver transplants. These domino transplants were performed in a "piggy back" fashion, as in regular LD liver transplants.

Our first such domino liver transplant used segments 2 and 3 of the liver from the first recipient for a 3-year-old child with liver failure (Figure 16.16.3c-7). That case was, to our knowledge, the world's first domino liver transplant using a liver from a patient with kidney disease. In effect, the recipient thus became a LD for a nonrelated recipient.

## ETHICAL CONSIDERATIONS

We described the ethical considerations involved with combined partial auxiliary liver and kidney transplants in recipients with kidney failure and multispecific antibodies in the *American Journal of Transplantation*.[17] As emphasized in that article, our donor and recipient operations were uneventful, without complications or major blood loss. Even though we removed several liver grafts from LDs, their kidney function was unaffected.[17]

As we stated in that article, this combined procedure carries an obviously increased risk of surgical morbidity. But this increased risk must be compared to the risks and benefits of long-term dialysis and other desensitizing treatments. No controlled studies have been done in this area, however. Still, we believe that the surgical risk can be reduced by carefully selecting patients and by limiting this procedure to centers with great experience in liver surgery. In our series, we used a previously well-described technique for auxiliary partial orthotopic liver transplants.[18] This technique has predominantly been applied for small grafts from LDs,[18] but it has also been used to treat patients with acute liver failure and metabolic disorders.[19,20]

An ethical concern with DDs is the need for a split-liver graft, which complicates organ procurement and may increase the morbidity of recipients of the right liver lobe. However, because of the organ shortage, especially for pediatric transplant candidates, *in situ* split procedures with DDs are already widely accepted; they are performed at many centers with good results for both recipients.[21] *In situ* split procedures with LDs should not be a problem; on the contrary, they potentially add organs to the pediatric liver donor pool. Furthermore, the removed left lateral liver lobe in kidney recipients with healthy livers have now been used as grafts in domino procedures in Japan as well.[22] In our series in Sweden, we have so far used 9 (out of our total of 19 livers from combined transplants) for domino liver transplants. Because we do not have a centralized organ allocation system in Sweden,

combined transplants can never impair any child's chances on the DD liver waiting list, since pediatric recipients are always our highest priority.

Using LDs in combined transplants also raises this question: is combined kidney and partial liver donation far too risky to be justified for a recipient without an immediate life-threatening disease? Given our vast experience with left lateral liver resections for cancer patients and donors, and assuming that donors undergo a thorough workup and receive complete information, we believe that their morbidity and mortality risk can be kept acceptably low. Moreover, considering the low quality of life and obvious morbidity and mortality of patients on long-term dialysis, we also believe that the high probability of doing good for recipients, their families, and society outbalances the low probability of doing harm for the LDs.

## References

1. Doxiadis IIN, Smits JMA, Th Schreuder GM, et al. Association between specific HLA combinations and probability of kidney allograft loss: the taboo concept. *Lancet* 1996;348:850–853.
2. Terasaki PI. Humoral theory of transplantation. Am J Transplant. 2003 Jun;3(6):665–673.
3. Gordon RD, Fung JJ, Markus B, et al. The antibody cross-match in liver transplantation. *Surgery* 1986 Oct;100(4): 705–715.
4. Manez R, Kelly RH, Kobayashi M, et al. Immunoglobulin G lymphocytotoxic antibodies in clinical liver transplantation: Studies toward further defining their significance. *Hepatology* 1996 May;21(5):1345–1352.
5. Hathaway M, Gunson BK, Keogh AC, Briggs D, McMaster P, Neuberger JM. A positive cross-match in liver transplantation -no effect or inappropriate analysis? A prospective study. *Transplantation* 1997;Jul;15;64(1):54–59.
6. Neuman UP, Lang M, Moldenhauer A, et al. Significance of a T-lymphocytotoxic cross-match in liver and combined liver-kidney transplantation. *Transplantation* 2001;71(8) 1163–1168.
7. Flye MW, Duffy BF, Phelean DL, Ratner LE, Mohanakumar T. Protective effects of liver transplantation on a simultaneously transplanted kidney in a highly sensitised patient. *Transplantation* 1990 Dec;50(6):1051–1054.
8. Eid A, Moore SB, Wiesner RH, et al. Evidence that the liver does not always protect the kidney from hyperacute rejection in combined liver-kidney transplantation across positive lymphocyte cross-match. *Transplantation* 1990;Aug;50(2):331
9. Saidman SL, Duquesnoy RJ, Demetris AJ, et al. Combined liver-kidney transplantation and the effect of preformed lymphocytotoxic antibodies. *Transplant Immunol* 1994;(2):61-67.
10. Mjörnstedt L, Friman S, Bäckman L, Rydberg L, Olausson M. Combined liver and kidney transplantation against a positive cross match in a patient with multispecific HLA-antibodies. *Transplantation Proc* 1997;29:3164–3165.
11. Morrissey PE, Gordon F, Shaffer D, et al. Combined liver-kidney transplantation in patients with cirrhosis and renal failure: effect of a positive cross-match and benefits of combined transplantation. *Liver Transpl Surg* 1998 Sep;4(5):363–369.
12. Pollack MS. The very rapid loss of donor specific antibodies from the circulation after liver transplantation allows successful kidney transplantation from the same donor for even the most highly sensitized patients. *Hum Immunol* 2003 Oct;64(10 Suppl):S62.
13. Gutierrez A, Crespo M, Mila J, Torregrosa JV, Martorell J, Oppenheimer F. Outcome of simultaneous liver-kidney transplantation in highly sensitized, cross-match-positive patients. *Transplant Proc* 2003 Aug;35(5):1861–1862.
14. Higgins RM, Bevan DJ, Carey BS, et al. Prevention of hyperacute rejection by removal of antibodies to HLA immediately before renal transplantation. *Lancet* 1996;348: 1208–1211.

15. Glotz D, Antoine C, Julia P, et al. Intravenous immunoglobulins and transplantation for patients with anti-HLA antibodies. *Transpl Int* 2004 Jan;17(1):1–8.
16. Vieira CA, Agarwal A, Book BK, et al. Rituximab for reduction of anti-HLA antibodies in patients awaiting renal transplantation: 1. Safety, pharmacodynamics, and pharmacokinetics. *Transplantation* 2004 Feb 27;77(4):542–548.
17. Olausson M, Mjörnstedt L, Nordén G, et al. Successful combined partial liver and kidney transplantation in highly sensitized cross-match positive recipients. *Am J Transplant* 2006 Jan; 7(1): 130–136.
18. Gubernatis G, Pichlmayr R, Kemnitz J, Gratz K. Auxiliary partial orthotopic liver transplantation (APOLT) for fulminant hepatic failure: first successful case report. *World J Surg* 1991;Sep-Oct;15(5): 660–666.
19. Ikegami T, Shiotani S, Ninomiya M, et al. Auxiliary partial orthotopic liver transplantation from living donors. *Surgery* 2002 Jan;131(1 Suppl):S205–S210.
20. Burdelski M, Rogiers X. Liver transplantation in metabolic disorders. *Acta Gastroenterol Belg* 1999 Jul-Sep;62(3):300–305.
21. Rogiers X, Malago M, Gawad K, et al. In situ splitting of cadaveric livers. The ultimate expansion of a limited donor pool. *Ann Surg* 1996 Sep;224(3):331–341.
22. Hashikura Y, Ikegami T, Nakazawa Y, et al. Delayed domino liver transplantation: use of the remnant liver of a recipient of a temporary auxiliary orthotopic liver transplant as a liver graft for another patient. *Transplantation* 2004 Jan 27;77(2):324.

# CHAPTER 17

# KIDNEY TRANSPLANTATION: COST ANALYSIS

*Mark A. Schnitzler, PhD, Thomas Burroughs, PhD, Steven K. Takemoto, PhD*

Kidney transplantation enjoys some of the most comprehensive health economic analyses available in medicine today. This is due in no small part to the existence of the United States Renal Data System (USRDS). In this chapter we describe recent contributions to our understanding of the economics of living donor kidney transplantation using the USRDS database. We also consider the existing holes in our knowledge and suggest future studies that may fill in these gaps leading to more informed practice decisions and policy.

## HEALTH CLAIMS ANALYSIS OF TRANSPLANT COSTS

Comprehensive health economic studies without health claims data are among the most difficult of clinical studies to perform well. Although traditional clinical endpoints, such as treatment success or survival, are generally measurable, cost is an extensive and nebulous composite outcome. Patients see many providers with diverse financial arrangements. Although patients have consented to participate in studies, their providers usually have not consented to provide financial information to the study and often refuse to submit data. Although it is possible to collect complete financial records for a limited set of providers in studies of major treatments such as transplant, such studies are nearly impossible when long-term follow-up is required. The numbers of discrete providers involved tends to grow rapidly with time following the initial intervention. The solution to these problems, which we and others have employed with great success in transplantation, is the use of clinical data linked to health claims data.

The scientific value of linked health insurance claims to transplant registry data for economic analysis can be seen clearly in our article that demonstrated recipients of zero HLA-antigen-mismatched kidney grafts had 3-year total medical costs that were 25% less than those who received six HLA-antigen-mismatched kidney grafts.[1] With subsequent studies we have demonstrated the cost-effectiveness of kidney transplantation over dialysis by examining costs for nonoptimal kidney transplants,[2,3] demonstrated the economic benefit for alternative methods of HLA matching,[4,5] assessed the cost associated with donor and recipient cytomegalovirus sero-pairing after renal transplantation,[6] assessed costs associated with development of new onset diabetes after renal transplantation,[7] demonstrated the cost-effectiveness of extending Medicare coverage past the current 3-year cut-off for transplant recipients,[8] and assessed the economic value of living donors.[9] Here we will provide examples demonstrating the richness of health-care claims data and explain details used for economic analyses.

Health insurance claims provide a wealth of information not collected in the survey forms that comprise the transplant registry database maintained by the Organ Procurement Transplant Network (OPTN). For instance, posttransplant diabetic complications were first studied in medical claims.[10] When hospitals, clinics, physicians, or other health-care providers file for reimbursement for services performed, they justify the cost by providing the patient diagnosis using International Classification of Disease ninth revision (ICD-9) codes, and often itemize specific procedures performed using Current Procedural Terminology fourth edition (CPT-4) codes. In addition to our studies of the economics of transplantation, we have used health claims data to examine the epidemiology and outcomes associated with a number of complications and comorbidities associated with transplantation. We have shown how health-care claims data could be used to obtain more detailed information about diabetes,[11] posttransplant hepatitis-C[12] gastrointestinal complications,[13] avascular necrosis,[14] and cardiovascular[15] complications than data collected by the transplant registry. Some of the ICD-9 and CPT-4 codes that we have used to derive endpoints in transplantation are shown in Table 17-1.

One advantage of using claims over transplant surveys is the flexibility of the data. It is not necessary for survey designers to anticipate future complications that may be important for a condition. Every condition that occurs in a patient is captured. OPTN forms collect information regarding complications and medications on yearly follow-up forms. Medical claims contain detailed information describing interventions and therapies. Prescription claims indicate brand names of dispensed drugs and their doses making it possible to compare the efficacy of alternative treatments and to examine temporal implications of dose changes. Procedures such as insertion of stents, dialysis, and infusions are coded, making it possible to define dates of complication endpoints. Thus, with medical claims, it is possible to define the date of the office visit when complications are first observed. Knowing endpoint dates makes it possible to perform time to event and time-varying analyses.

Many types of medical claim data are available for study. Most analyses in transplantation have used data from Medicare since this information was linked to the USRDS database. Patients older than age 65 and those with chronic debilitating conditions including dialysis are eligible for Medicare. Individuals with levels of income below the poverty levels receive health-care benefits through Medicaid. Private payers are a third major provider of health-care coverage in the United States. Individuals receiving health-care coverage from their employer or purchasing health coverage are included in this group. Major providers of private payer coverage in the United States include Wellpoint, United Healthcare, and Kaiser.

**TABLE 17.1**

| Complication | ICD-9 diagnosis code | CPT-4 procedure code |
|---|---|---|
| Chronic kidney disease | 016.0, 095.4, 189.0, 189.9, 223.0, 236.91, 250.4, 271.4, 274.1, 283.11, 403.x1, 404.x2, 404.x3, 440.1, 442.1, 447.3, 572.4, 580–588, 591, 642.1, 646.2, 753.12–753.17, 753.19, 753.2, 794.4 | |
| Dialysis | | 36145, 36488, 36489, 36490, 36491, 36800, 36810, 36815, 49420, 49421, 75790, 90747, 90935, 90937, 90945, 90947, 90989, 90993, 90999, 93990 |
| Cardiovascular disease | 276.6, 394–398.99, 401–405, 410–420, 423–438, 440–459 | |
| Congestive heart failure | 398.91, 425, 428, 402.x1, 404.x1, 404.x3 | |
| Diabetes | 250, 357.2, 362.0x, 366.41 | |
| Hypertension | 362.11, 401.x–405.x, 437 | |
| Anemia | 280.x, 281.x | |
| Proteinuria | 791.0 | |

## COST-EFFECTIVENESS OF LIVING DONOR KIDNEY TRANSPLANTATION

We examined the economic value of living donation using data provided by the USRDS. A total of 2,757 recipients of living unrelated donor (LURD) kidneys and 24,333 wait-listed dialysis patients with linked and complete clinical and Medicare health claims data.[9] This allowed us to estimate both cost and outcome simultaneously and, of most importance, determine average total cost of medical care for patients experiencing certain events or treatments. Specific costs of interest included, for example, transplant hospitalization or transplant failure events, and costs across specific intervals, for example, the states of first and second years posttransplant or a year of maintenance dialysis. These estimates have the advantage of being actual costs of medical care for these patients from the perspective of Medicare, the payer, instead of literature derived estimates or ad hoc constructs. Specific cost averages from the cohorts of patients used in this study are provided in Table 17-2.

We used a Markov model with the cost and survival estimates for LURD kidney transplant as representative costs of transplant from a potential donor shown in Table 17-2. A tree diagram representation of this model is presented in Figure 17-1 showing the possible outcomes considered for patients on the waiting list versus receiving a vendor kidney. In each period following transplantation, a patient and his or her allograft will survive to the next period, the allograft will fail with the patient returning to dialysis, or the patient will die with allograft function. An additional organ transplant from any source shortens the waiting times for a string of patients limited by the death rate while waiting. This averages to one expected lifetime on dialysis for a wait-listed patient. Therefore, outcomes for the reference patient are calculated for a lifetime on dialysis. Each period for this patient will end with continued dialysis or death.

The model is partitioned into a period of 1 year in length. Patient and graft survival rates provide all calculation of the fractions of patients experiencing an event or in any given state for each period. Costs are simply multiplied across these proportions,

**TABLE 17.2**
## LURD RECIPIENT COSTS

| | |
|---|---|
| Initial cost (transplant hospitalization) | $29,201 |
| Organ Procurement cost | $15,000 |
| Initial cost (first 12 months excluding transplant hospitalization) | $28,492 |
| Total first year cost transplantation | $72,693 |
| Maintenance cost-transplantation(month 12–24) | $12,814 |
| Cost first year post graft loss | $136,338 |
| Excess cost of graft loss over dialysis | 94,508 |
| Maintenance cost-dialysis: year prior to transplant | $41,830 |
| Annual increase in dialysis maintenance costs | $268 |
| Cost Year Prior to Death on Dialysis | $93,985 |
| Excess cost of Death on Dialysis | $52,155 |
| Cost Year Prior to death with graft function | $83,471 |
| Excess cost of death with function | $70,657 |
| **Transplant Graft Survival** | |
| LURD graft survival at year 1 (not ECD) | 94.3% |
| LURD graft survival at year 2 (not ECD) | 91.8% |
| LURD graft survival at year 3 (not ECD) | 89.1% |
| LURD graft survival at year 5 (not ECD) | 82.0% |
| Long Term Graft Loss Rate (Calculated from year 3 *to* year 5) | 4.1% |
| **Other Transplant Survival Parameters** | |
| Rate of graft failure due to death with function | 42.5% |
| Death risk after graft loss (within 1 year) | 16.8% |
| Death risk after graft loss (through year 2) | 24.6% |
| Death risk after graft loss (after 1 year) | 7.8% |
| **Wait-List Survival** | |
| Four year patient survival on the wait list given 2-year survival | 87.1% |
| Long term death rate on the wait list (Calculated as rate from year 2 to year 4) | 6.7% |
| **Utility Scores** | |
| Dialysis | 0.68 |
| Transplantation | 0.84 |
| **Discounting and Willingness to Pay** | |
| discount factor for QALYs | 5.0% |
| discount factor for costs | 5.0% |

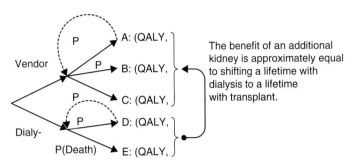

**FIGURE 17-1**

Markov model tree diagram for a living donor transplant.

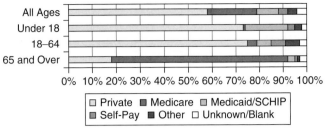

**FIGURE 17-2**

Type of medical insurance coverage by age of insured.[16]

discounted to present value, and summed to determine the current economic value of the cost of care. Quality-adjusted life years (QALYs) are calculated similarly using the utility estimates for states presented in Table 17-2. The utility estimates are based on time trade offs and are referenced against a period of time in perfect health. An individual with a health utility score of 0.84 would be willing to trade the duration of their remaining expected life in that state for 84% of that duration in perfect health. By performing a similar calculation for dialysis, we can compare transplant to dialysis.

Our model was set to a time horizon of 20 years and we estimated that transplantation from an LURD saved $94,579 (U.S. 2002 dollars) and provided 3.5 quality-adjusted life years (QALYs) gained relative to dialysis. Further, adding the value of QALYs, a LURD transplant saves $269,319, assuming society values additional QALYs from transplantation at the rate paid per QALY while on dialysis. We concluded that at the minimum, a vender program saves society >$90,000 per transplant and increases the number of QALYs for the ESRD population. Thus, society could break even while paying $90,000/kidney vendor.

It is important to note that we were unable to directly estimate changes in the long-term cost of medical care in this study. We assumed there was no long-term economic effect beyond the costs associated with graft failure, resumed maintenance dialysis, and death. However, this has not been proven, but could be assessed with the data generated by more extensive claims based research. Although Medicare coverage ends at 36 months posttransplant due to legal enrollment restrictions without meeting a non-ESRD eligibility criterion, private payers do have these enrollment restrictions.

Further, while it is consistent with the existing literature to assume the long-term impact of donation on donors' health costs is zero, this has not been measured directly. The next section discusses potential study designs that could address this critical element in the living donation cost-effectiveness equation.

## POTENTIAL STUDIES OF LONG-TERM LIVING DONOR HEALTH COSTS

The distribution of type of insurance coverage by age of individuals is shown in Figure 17-2. Seventy-five percent of working-age individuals are enrolled in private payer health plans. Since more than 80% of living donors were age 18 to 49 and 99% were younger than age 65 at the time of donation,[17] private payer health-care claims will likely be the most informative for economic studies of living donors.

Private payer claims from many health plans include laboratory results that make it is possible to stage renal impairment using standards advocated by the National Kidney Foundation (NKF).[18] These data will be important for future studies since most examinations into the safety of kidney donation have compared rates of end-stage renal disease or transplantation as their benchmark demonstrating the safety of organ donation. The NKF defines impaired kidney function as kidney damage or glomerular filtration rates lower than 90 (Table 17-3). GFR can be calculated from serum creatinine values found in laboratory results.[19] Results from the Third National Health and Nutrition Examination Survey (NHANES III) conducted during 1988 to 1994 by the Centers for Disease Control and Prevention established the prevalence of impaired kidney function in the United States.[20] According to these statistics, patients with kidney failure represent only 1.5% (300,000/19.5 million) of individuals with impaired kidney function (Table 17-3). Thus, a kidney failure endpoint may not accurately reflect risks associated with donation since impaired kidney function is associated with significant morbidity.

A recent report examined GFR 5 or more years after donation for 389 of 2643 kidney donors from a single center.[21] Two thirds had GFR consistent with stage 2–3 chronic kidney disease, 26% were hypertensive, 2% were diabetic, and 40% were taking lipid-lowering agents. In another large study of over 400 donors, no accelerated loss of kidney function was observed.[22] Five donors had impaired renal function as defined by NKF guidelines.[18] Renal function deteriorated with increasing age, but rates of impaired kidney function for donors were similar to what is seen among normal healthy subjects. A study of living donors with more than 20 years of follow-up from the University of Minnesota also seems to indicate that donation does not have an impact on long-term kidney function.[23] Of 773 who donated a kidney between 1963 and 1979, they could find current information for 464 (60%). Of these, 84 died, 3 with kidney failure. Of the 380 who were alive,

**TABLE 17.3**

| Stage | Description | GFR* | Prevalence N(1000s) | % |
|-------|-------------|------|---------------------|---|
| 1 | Kidney damage with normal or GFR | 90 | 5,900 | 3.3 |
| 2 | Kidney damage with mild GFR | 60-89 | 5,300 | 3 |
| 3 | Moderate GFR | 30-59 | 7,600 | 4.3 |
| 4 | Severe GFR | 15-29 | 400 | 0.2 |
| 5 | Kidney Failure | <15 or dialysis | 300 | 0.1 |

*GFR-Glomerular filtration rate in mL/min/1.73 m2.

67% returned questionnaires and 33% provided laboratory results to assess kidney function. Although this study indicated impaired renal function was not increased in living donors, it illustrated a potential problem with current studies of living donors: high dropout rates due to loss of contact and nonresponse.

Although one would expect the contact information to be accurate for the donors at the time of their surgical procedure, we expect a large proportion of donors moved and are difficult to contact. In the 5-year period between 1995 and 2000, 45% of the U.S. population moved at least once.[24] These patterns of migration vary with age, marital status, and education,[25] all of which are related to health status. Failure to locate individuals who have moved can contribute to substantial bias. In a prospective study of 20,051 childhood cancer survivors, treatment clinics had current addresses for 65%.[26] A commercial tracing firm was employed to contacting the remaining 35%. Compared to individuals who were contacted without tracing, who did not have a current address, were associated with a number of health-status-associated risk factors, including

- Lower health-care utilization during the previous 2 years (odds ratio [OR] 0.7 95% confidence interval (CI)I: 0.6–0.8)

- Higher smoking incidence (OR 1.4, CI: 1.3–1.4)

- Higher rates of obesity (OR 1.3, CI: 1.1–1.4)

- Increased reports of seizures or blackouts (OR 1.4, CI: 1.3–1.7)

  - poor general health (OR 1.3, CI: 1.0–1.4)

  - moderate to severe pain from their disease (OR 1.3, CI: 1.1–1.4)

  - moderate to severe functional status limitations (OR 1.3, CI: 1.1–1.4)

  - moderate to severe activity limitation (OR 1.3, CI: 1.1–1.4)

Investigators concluded that if the extra effort was not exerted to find subjects in this study, results would have indicated better average health status. Interestingly, the 65% of childhood cancer survivors that did not require tracing was a similar fraction to the 60% contact rate reported in the long-term follow-up study of living donors by the Minnesota group.[23] With cancer survivors, one might expect patients with complications to have more regular chart entries. With living donors, one might expect it is easier to find donors when the recipient is alive with a functioning graft. Recipient contact has been used to find donors in a previous study.[23] However, donors whose recipients have lost grafts and/or died may be at risk of impaired psychosocial and health status.

Issues that should be addressed in well designed economic analysis in transplantation have been clearly laid out.[27] One of the most important aspects of an economic analysis is the perspective or point of view from which the analysis is undertaken. Typical perspectives are those of society, insurers, hospitals, physicians, and patients. We have typically adopted the societal point of view, but studies from the donor's point of view are necessary to clearly describe the risks involved in donation.

## CONCLUSIONS

Our understanding of the costs associated with treatment options for end-stage renal disease has been greatly enhanced by the existence of linked clinical and claims data managed by the USRDS.

The Medicare claims linked to OPTN registry data have given us insights unavailable in most other areas of medicine. That renal transplantation, either deceased or living donor, reduces average recipient health expenditures is accepted as fact. This is a somewhat unique situation in medicine, where a complex and advanced intervention is not merely cost-effective, providing improved benefits at some additional cost, but cost saving. This leaves open the possibility of a number of important policy initiatives that may be "funded" through the savings from additional or more successful transplants including lifetime Medicare immunosuppression coverage,[8] reimbursement for living donor expenses, and paid living donation.[9]

However, significant challenges remain. We have extensive and increasing knowledge of the costs associated with dialysis, transplantation, graft failure, and early posttransplant maintenance. Yet, the costs of long-term maintenance of the transplant recipient and factors that lead to differences in these costs have not been well described. Further, we know very little about the long-term costs associated with living donation. Further understanding of these and other aspects of the economics and finances of living donor kidney transplantation will facilitate more informed practice and policy formation.

## References

1. Schnitzler MA, Hollenbeak CS, Cohen DS, et al. The economic implications of HLA matching in cadaveric renal transplantation. *N Engl J Med* 1999;341:1440–1446.
2. Whiting JF, Woodward RS, Zavala EY, et al. Economic cost of expanded criteria donors in cadaveric renal transplantation: analysis of Medicare payments. *Transplantation* 2000;70:755–760.
3. Schnitzler MA, Whiting JF, Brennan DC, et al. The expanded criteria donor dilemma in cadaveric renal transplantation. *Transplantation* 2003;75:1940–1945.
4. Hollenbeak CS, Woodward RS, Cohen DS, et al. The economic benefit of allocation of kidneys based on cross-reactive group matching. *Transplantation* 2000;70:537–540.
5. Mutinga N, Brennan DC, Schnitzler MA. Consequences of eliminating HLA-B in deceased donor kidney allocation to increase minority transplantation. *Am J Transplant* 2005;5:1090–1098.
6. Schnitzler MA, Lowell JA, Hardinger KL, et al. The association of cytomegalovirus sero-pairing with outcomes and costs following cadaveric renal transplantation prior to the introduction of oral ganciclovir CMV prophylaxis. *Am J Transplant* 2003;3:445–451.
7. Woodward RS, Desai NM, Baty JS, Gage BF, Brennan DC. Cost-effectiveness of new onset diabetes mellitus among U.S. wait-listed and transplanted renal allograft recipients. *Am J Transplant* 2004;4:590–598.
8. Yen EF, Hardinger K, Brennan DC, Woodward RS, Desai NM, Crippin JS, et al. Cost-effectiveness of extending Medicare coverage of immunosuppressive medications to the life of a kidney transplant. *Am J Transplant* 2004;4:1703–1708.
9. Matas AJ, Schnitzler M. Payment for living donor (vendor) kidneys: a cost-effectiveness analysis. *Am J Transplant* 2004;4:216–221.
10. Kasiske BL, Snyder JJ, Gilbertson D, Matas AJ. Diabetes mellitus after kidney transplantation in the United States. *Am J Transplant* 2003;3:178–185.
11. Woodward RS, Schnitzler MA, Baty J, et al. Incidence and cost of new onset diabetes mellitus among U.S. wait-listed and transplanted renal allograft recipients. *Am J Transplant* 2003;3:590–598.
12. Abbott KC, Lentine KL, Bucci JR, et al. Impact of diabetes and hepatitis after kidney transplantation on patients who are affected by hepatitis C virus. *J Am Soc Nephrol* 2004;15:3166–174.

13. Hardinger KL, Brennan DC, Lowell J, Schnitzler MA. Long-term outcome of gastrointestinal complications in renal transplant patients treated with mycophenolate mofetil. *Transpl Int* 2004;17:609–16.

14. Abbott KC, Koff J, Bohen EM, et al. Maintenance immunosuppression use and the associated risk of avascular necrosis after kidney transplantation in the United States. *Transplantation* 2005;79:330–6.

15. Lentine KL, Brennan DC, Schnitzler MA. Incidence and predictors of myocardial infarction after kidney transplantation. *J Am Soc Nephrol* 2005;16:496–506.

16. Woodwell D. National Ambulatory Medical Care Survey: 2002 Summary. National Center for Health Statistics, 2004.

17. Living Donors Recovered in the U.S. by Donor Age. January 1, 1988 - March 31, 2005. United Network for Organ Sharing, 2005.

18. K/DOQI clinical practice guidelines for chronic kidney disease: evaluation, classification, and stratification. *Am J Kidney Dis* 2002; 39:S1–266.

19. Manjunath G, Sarnak MJ, Levey AS. Prediction equations to estimate glomerular filtration rate: an update. *Curr Opin Nephrol Hypertens* 2001;10:785–792.

20. Jones CA, McQuillan GM, Kusek JW, et al. Serum creatinine levels in the US population: third National Health and Nutrition Examination Survey. *Am J Kidney Dis* 1998;32:992–999.

21. Ibrahim H, Rogers T, Humar A, Matas A. [566] Prevalence of chronic kidney disease years after donor nephrectory using measured GFR. American Transplant Congress. Seattle, 2005.

22. Fehrman-Ekholm I, Duner F, Brink B, Tyden G, Elinder CG. No evidence of accelerated loss of kidney function in living kidney donors: results from a cross-sectional follow-up. *Transplantation* 2001;72:444–449.

23. Ramcharan T, Matas AJ. Long-term (20-37 years) follow-up of living kidney donors. *Am J Transplant* 2002;2:959–964.

24. Schachter J, Franklin R, Perry M. Migration and geographic mobility in metropolitan and nonmetropolitan America: 1995 to 2000. In: U.S. Department of Commerce EaSA, ed: U.S. Census Bureau, 2003.

25. Franklin R. Migration of the Young, Single, and College Educated: 1995 to 2000. Census 2000 Special Reports. In: U.S. Department of Commerce EaSA, ed: U.S. Census Bureau, 2003.

26. Mertens AC, Walls RS, Taylor L, et al. Characteristics of childhood cancer survivors predicted their successful tracing. *J Clin Epidemiol* 2004; 57:933–944.

27. Whiting JF. Standards for economic and quality of life studies in transplantation. *Transplantation* 2000;70:1115–1121.

# PANCREAS TRANSPLANTATION

# CHAPTER 18

# HISTORY OF AND RATIONALE FOR PANCREAS TRANSPLANTATION

## 18.1 HISTORY OF LIVING DONOR PANCREAS TRANSPLANTATION

*David E. R. Sutherland, MD, PhD,*
*John S. Najarian, MD, Rainer W.G. Gruessner, MD*

The pancreas was the first extrarenal organ that was transplanted successfully from a living donor (LD),[1] done as a segmental graft (distal pancreas—body and tail) from a mother to her diabetic daughter at the University of Minnesota Hospital on June 20, 1979, restoring insulin independence,[2] the objective of the procedure. An earlier attempt at an extrarenal LD transplant—of a small bowel segment—by Ralph Deterling in Boston in 1964 was not successful because the recipient died within 12 hours (Chapter 32).[3]

The first LD segmental pancreas transplant was done 11½ years after the world's first deceased donor (DD) pancreas transplant (also segmental), also done at the University of Minnesota by Kelly and Lillehei et al.[4] in December 1966 (Table 18.1-1). In the interval between the first deceased and first LD pancreas transplants, (1) a series of 13 more DD pancreas transplants (all whole organ; only one functioned >1 year, the others failed from either technical problems seemingly related to the duodenum or from rejection) were done by Lillehei et al.[5] at the University of Minnesota, with the last in 1973[6]; (2) pancreas transplant programs began at a few other centers[7] in the United States[8,9] and Europe,[10,11] predominantly using DD segmental grafts[9-11]; (3) a clinical islet transplant program began in 1974 at the University of Minnesota,[12,13] initially and mainly from deceased but with two from LDs,[1,14] in the hope that a minimally invasive

**TABLE 18.1-1**

**LANDMARKS IN LIVING DONOR SEGMENTAL PANCREAS TRANSPLANTATION**

| Date | Landmarks–1 | References |
|---|---|---|
| Dec 16, 1966 | World's **first clinical pancreas transplant,** done at the University of Minnesota (U MN) by William Kelly and Richard Lillehei as a segmental graft (body and tail) from a **deceased donor** (DD) on a vascular pedicle of spleen artery and vein, a technique adaptable for the living donor (LD) segmental pancreas transplants initiated 12½ years later, also at the U MN. *[The subsequent 13 DD pancreas transplants done by Lillehei (1966–73) were whole organ (pancreaticoduodenal), but in this interval and up to the first LD case in 1979 at the U MN, the few centers (Montefiore Hospital in New York, Huddinge Hospital in Stockholm, Herriot Hospital in Lyon) doing pancreas transplants, including the U MN when pancreas transplants were resumed at this institution with 5 cases in 1978, did predominantly segmental grafts from deceased donors. Whole organ or pancreaticoduodenal transplants were resurrected in the early 1980s and by the mid-1980s had become dominant, but segmental grafts have never disappeared and are, of course, the only option for LD transplants.]* | (4) (5,6) (1,2) (9-11) (16) |

| Date | Landmarks–2 | References |
|---|---|---|
| Sept 27, 1977 | World's **first LD distal pancreatectomy for transplantation** purposes, done at the U MN, with islets isolated from the excised segment infused intraportally from an HLA-identical sister to her diabetic brother, a recipient of a previous renal allograft from a different sibling. The recipient became C-peptide positive for six weeks but was never insulin-independent. *[A second LD islet after kidney [IAK] transplant was done at the U MN on July 12, 1978; same donor(SD) as the kidney; recipient was insulin-independent only during the third week posttransplant, following which she had a rejection episode of the renal allograft (she had one prior to the IAK as well), with concomitant loss of islet function.]* *[Both of these cases were part of a series of 18 IAK allografts in 14 recipients done at the U MN during 1974–78, the others from DDs. Islet autografts, akin to an LD transplant, at the time of total pancreatectomy for benign disease, had also been successfully initiated at the U MN on Feb 14, 1977, 7 months prior to the first LD islet allograft (see chapter 22).]* *[On July 25, 1978, 2 weeks after the 2nd LD islet allograft, and after a 5-year hiatus, the U MN resumed doing pancreas transplants with 5 segmental grafts from DDs that year as a prelude to the first LD case the following year.]* | (1) (14) (16) |

| Date | Landmarks–3 | References |
|------|-------------|-----------|
| June 20, 1979 | World's **first LD immediately vascularized segmental pancreas transplant,** open duct (OD), done at the U MN after previous kidney (PAK) from the same donor (mother) to diabetic daughter. Functioned 4 years before failing from recurrence of disease (selective beta cell loss on biopsy, no isletitis). *[First of 124 MN LD cases through 2006, and **first** of 5 **OD** in the first 8 MN LD cases.] [Also **first LD PAK** and **first** from the **same donor (SD)** as the kidney. Of the 33 LD PAK transplants in 32 patients in the MN series to date, each had the prior kidney from an LD, 25 from the SD and 8 from a different donor, including one with a primary PAK from the SD (sister) and a PAK retransplant from a different donor (mother).] [In the U MN series of 1912 pancreas transplants from 1978 to 2006, 6.5% are from LDs. Of ~26,000 pancreas transplants reported to the International Pancreas Transplant Registry as of 2006, only 152 (including the MN cases) were from LDs, or ~0.6%.]* | (1,2) (17) (See Chapter 20.5) |
| Mar 18, 1980 | World's **first LD pancreas transplant alone** (PTA), enteric-drained **(ED),** done at Huddinge Hospital, Stockholm, Sweden. Early rejection, graft removed day 24. *[Fourth LD pancreas transplant in the world, preceded by 3 LD PAK transplants at the U MN]. [The Stockholm program did two more LD PTAs (ED) in 1985.]* | (46) (1) (53) |

| Date | Landmarks–4 | References |
|------|-------------|-----------|
| Oct 14, 1980 | World's **first identical (ID) twin pancreas transplant,** first duct injection **(DI)** in LD graft. Second LD **PTA** done at the U MN, third in world. Recipient nonimmunosuppressed and insulin-independent for 6 wks; graft failed from recurrence of disease (isletitis) but not recognized initially on biopsy because DI induced changes assumed to be the cause (5th MN LD case). *[Ten ID twin pancreas transplants have been done in the MN series to date, of which 3 thrombosed. Of the 7 technically successful, 3 non immunosuppressed grafts initially functioned 1 ½, 1, and 7 months before recurrence of disease (RD); of the 4 prophylactically immunosuppressed grafts, 2 functioned 5 and 8 years before RD while 2 are currently functioning at >19 and >16 years.] [Of the 124 MN LD pancreas transplant cases to date, 53 have been PTA. Ten PTA outside of MN have been reported to the Registry.]* | (41) (41, 62-67, 78, 79) (17, 42, 92) (66-67, 76, 78-80) (17) (See Chapter 20.5) |
| Nov 17, 1980 | World's **first LD simultaneous pancreas and kidney** (SPK) transplant with both organs from SD, OD, done at the University of Miami. Technical failure. *[Seventh LD pancreas transplant in the world (preceded by 3 PAKs and 2 PTAs at U MN and 1 PTA at Stockholm).]* | (52) (See Chapter 20.5) |
| Dec 3, 1980 | **First LD pancreas transplant with decades of function** (recipient insulin-independent 24 years), PAK with DI from HLA-identical sibling, SD as kidney done 2 years earlier at U MN, kidney still functioning at 28 years. Pancreas probably ultimately failed from DI-induced fibrosis or RD (no biopsy). (6th MN LD case) | (41, 17) |

| Date | Landmarks–5 | References |
|------|-------------|-----------|
| Mar 19, 1981 | First LD (brother) PTA (DI) with subsequent (1 year later) kidney transplant (1st **KAP**) from different LD (mother). Pancreas functioned 2 months, kidney 2 years, before rejecting (7th MN LD case). *[11 of 53 LD PTA recipients at U MN from 1979 to 2005 went on to have a KAP, 3 from different LDs, 4 from the same LDs, and 4 from DDs with a pancreas retransplant (SPK); one of the latter had a subsequent LD kidney retransplant, making 12 LD KAPs in the series to date.]* | (49, 61) (17) |
| Aug 20, 1981 | First **ED** LD pancreas transplant at U **MN,** PTA from sister, functioned for 4 years (9th MN LD case). *[Of the 124 MN LD cases, 57 have been done with ED, including the 122nd.]* | (49, 63) (17) |
| Oct 8, 1981 | **First recognized case of RD** (selective beta cell destruction) in pancreas graft, LD PTA from HLA-identical sibling, resumed insulin at 2 months, biopsy at 6 months showed normal islets except for nearly complete loss of beta cells (11th MN LD case, third with ED). | (63, 67, 74-80) |
| Jan 6, 1982 | First LD (brother) PTA (ED) with subsequent (7 ½ years later) DD kidney (**KAP**) as an SPK transplant (both graft functioned 11 years; LD (wife) kidney retransplant done a year after the first kidney graft failed, currently functioning >5 years). LD pancreas functioned 6 years, failed from atherosclerotic occlusion of iliac artery (15th MN LD case). | (44, 64, 92) |
| Nov 4, 1982 | **First PTA LD** (sister) pancreas transplant (ED) **with decades of function** (recipient still insulin-independent at >24 years) (24th MN LD case). | (17, 63, 92) |

| Date | Landmarks–6 | References |
|---|---|---|
| Mar 16, 1983 | First **ID** twin *PAK* (SD) transplant, ED, again non immunosuppressed, and **first** LD transplant where RD **with isletitis and selective beta cell destruction recognized** at 6-week biopsy. Beta cell loss complete at 1 year in spite of transient addition of immunosuppression. Kidney graft still functioning at > 24 years (28th MN LD case). | (62, 66, 67, 78, 79) |
| July 26, 1983 | First **ID** twin (PTA) recipient **propylactically immunosuppressed** (azathioprine). Insulin-independent > 5 years before graft failed from RD (32nd MN LD case). | (44, 78, 79) |
| June 21, 1984 | First LD (father) pancreas transplant (PTA) to a **pediatric** recipient (17 years old), ED, at U MN functioned > 5 years (37th MN LD case). *[Of 6 pediatric (<18 years old) pancreas transplant recipients (4 PTA, 2 SPK) in the MN series, 2 are from LDs, this one and an SPK in 1995.]* | (42) (86, 92) |
| Feb 19, 1985 | First **LD PAK** in which the pancreas came from a **different donor** than the kidney, both from HLA-identical sisters (akin to the first IAK); currently functioning > 21 years (16th LD PAK and 42nd MN LD case overall). *[There are 8 different donor LD PAKs in the MN series to date, in contrast to 25 from the SD.]* | (44) (17) |
| Feb 26, 1985 | First **LD** (father) pancreas **retransplant,** ED PTA done 17 months after the primary LD (brother) pancreas transplant and 8 months after rejection of the first; the second also failed, of thrombosis. The patient had a subsequent LD (sister) KAP, so 3 family members were LDs to the same recipient (43rd MN LD case). *[This is 1 of 3 LD retransplants in the MN series; the others, a PAK (sister first, then mother) and a PTA (sequential siblings).]* | (44) (93) |

| Date | Landmarks–7 | References |
|---|---|---|
| Oct 15, 1985 | First LD PTA (ED) in **USA outside of U MN** reported to the registry *(and second USA LD pancreas transplant that had been reported at all outside of U MN),* at St. Luke's Medical Center in Phoenix *(done same day as third LD PTA in the Stockholm series).* The Phoenix graft functioned 9 ½ years. | (See Chapter 20.5) |
| Mar 20, 1986 | First LD PTA followed by a **KAP** from the **same LD** after the **pancreas failed** for immunological reasons; the kidney is currently functioning > 15 years. LD pancreas failed from rejection or RD at 3 years; a DD pancreas retransplant placed 3 years before the KAP functioned 5 years and another DD pancreas retransplant is currently functioning > 7 years (48th MN LD case). | (44) (17) |
| June 5, 1986 | First LD (sister) PTA followed (1 year later) by a **KAP** from the **same LD** with the **pancreas** still **functioning.** Both grafts still functioning at 20 and 19 years (50th MN LD case). *[Of the two subsequent LD SD KAP recipients, the first had both grafts function for 13 and 11 years before dying; the other has both grafts currently functioning at 6 ½ and 4 ½ years.]* | (44) (17) |
| Dec 23, 1986 | First LD (brother) pancreas transplant done with **bladder drainage (BD),** PAK from SD done 5 months after the kidney. Both organs currently functioning > 20 years (55th MN LD case). *[Of the 124 MN LD cases, 45 have been done with BD, including the 121st; since introduction of BD for LD pancreas transplants, only 14 of 69 have been ED.]* | (72) (17) |
| May 12, 1987 | First LD pancreas transplant (PTA with ED) reported to the Registry from **Asia** *(65th case in the Registry),* at Hallym University Medical Center in Seoul, Korea; the series continued with 8 more cases (5 SPK, 3 PTA) at Asan Medical Center Ulsan University from 1992 to 2006. *[The next Asian center to report a series of LD pancreas transplants was Tokyo Women's Medical College beginning in 2004 with at least 3 SPKs as of 2006.]* | (See Chapter 20.5) |

| Date | Landmarks–8 | References |
|---|---|---|
| May 13, 1987 | First **ID twin** (sister) pancreas transplant with **long function,** PTA (ED), currently > 19 years on immunosuppression since transplant (cyclosporine/azathioprine) (60th MN LD case). *[Next longest function of ID twin pancreas transplant is currently > 16 years (73rd MN LD case).]* | (44,79,93) (17,93) |
| Oct 15, 1989 | First LD pancreas transplant (PAK from SD, DI) reported to the Registry from the **Middle East,** at University of Kuwait *(78th case in the Registry).* The pancreas was done 6 months after the kidney. Both organs functioned until 1991 and were then rejected when immunosuppression became unavailable during the Gulf War. | (55) (See Chapter 20.5) |
| Jan 22, 1991 | First LD (brother) pancreas transplant with **portal drainage** via inferior mesenteric vein, PTA (ED), a technique used at the U MN for 5 DD segmental grafts in the mid-1980s. Currently functioning 15 years (75th MN LD case). | (42,93) (17) |
| July 7, 1992 | First genetically **unrelated LD** (wife) pancreas transplant, PAK 1 ½ years after LD kidney from SD. Also, **first LD** pancreas with exocrine drainage via **ureter** *(3 subsequent cases to date).* Pancreas currently functioning > 14 years, kidney failed at 12 years with immediate LD kidney retransplant, currently functioning (76th MN LD case). | (42,93) (17) |

| | | |
|---|---|---|
| March 10, 1994 | First LD (mother) **SPK** transplant (DI) at U MN *(second in world after the one at U Miami in 1980)*. Pancreas and kidney functioned >10 years, with LD kidney retransplant now functioning >2 years (81st MN LD case). *[As of 2006, 38 LD SPK transplants had been done at U MN and 17 outside of MN reported to the Registry.]* | (48)<br><br>(17,94) |

| Date | Landmarks–9 | References |
|---|---|---|
| Aug 15, 1995 | First LD (mother) **SPK** transplant (BD) to a **pediatric** recipient (14 years old) with diabetes and renal failure secondary to hemolytic uremic syndrome. The pancreas is currently functioning >11 years; the kidney failed from calcineurin-inhibitor toxicity at 9 years followed by a kidney retransplant, currently functioning (86th MN LD case). *[Second pediatric LD pancreas transplant in the MN series, the other a PTA in 1986.]* | (86)<br><br><br>(42) |
| May 1, 1996 | First **offspring** (daughter)-**to-parent** (mother) LD pancreas (SPK) transplant (BD). Both grafts currently functioning >10 years (91st MN LD case). | (17,93) |
| June 13, 1997 | First LD pancreas transplant (SPK, BD) initiating a series at a USA institution other than the U MN, at the **University of Illinois in Chicago** *(113th case in the Registry)*, with >8 cases to date including identical twin transplants. | (56-58)<br>(See Chapter 20.5) |
| Oct 16, 1998 | First **non-spouse genetically unrelated** (friend) LD pancreas (SPK) transplant. Also **first ABO-incompatible** LD pancreas transplant (AB to B). Both grafts functioning >8 years. *[Second ABO-incompatible LD SPK transplant was done in 2000 (A to O), with pancreas functioning at 6 ½ years.]* | (93)<br><br>(17) |
| Feb 3, 1999 | First LD pancreas (SPK) recipient (BD) with successful **pregnancy** 4 years posttransplant, but with acute rejection episode in third trimester. Kidney functioned but pancreas failed at 5 years; kidney currently functioning >7 years (108th MN LD case). | (17) |
| May 23, 2000 | First LD pancreas transplant (SPK, ED) at a second center in Europe (after Stockholm), at University of Oslo. | (See Chapter 20.5) |

| Date | Landmarks–10 | References |
|---|---|---|
| Nov 22, 2000 | First laparoscopic (hand-assisted) distal pancreatectomy for LD pancreas (SPK) transplant (BD), both grafts functioning >6 years (118th MN LD case). *[All six LD pancreas transplants done at U MN since this one have been done with laparoscopic distal pancreatectomy (and in SPK donors the kidney as well)—3 SPK (1 BD, 1 ED, 1 DI), all currently with pancreas function at >1 ½, 3, and 5 years; 2 PTA, with 1 functioning >4 years; and 1 SD PAK (DI) functioning >1 year. All 7 donors are euglycemic. The University of Illinois also began doing LD distal pancreatectomies laparoscopically in 2005.]* | (51)<br><br><br><br>(94) |
| Jan 19, 2005 | Third LD islet allograft, done at Kyoto University Hospital in Japan *(an interval of 28 years since the first and 26 ½ years since the second LD islet transplant at the U MN)*. The Kyoto case was mother to daughter (diabetes secondary to chronic pancreatitis); the recipient was insulin-independent for at least 7 months. | (See Chapter 20.5) |
| Sept 15-16, 2005 | The Vancouver Forum on The Care of Live Organ Donors for Lung, Liver, **Pancreas**, and Intestine Transplants was held. This international conference of transplant surgeons and physicians and allied health professional was convened by the Transplantation Society Ethics Committee, with subsequent publication of data and medical guidelines for living organ donation, including the pancreas. | (103) |

approach could replace solid organ pancreas transplantation for beta cell replacement therapy in diabetes (it has not yet, but the islet program continues to this day[15]); and (4) deceased donor pancreas transplants (initially with segmental grafts) were resumed at the University of Minnesota in 1978,[16] a program that also continues to this day.[17]

Thus, even though the first LD solid organ pancreas (segmental) transplant was done in 1979, this seminal event was preceded by two LD islet allografts done 21 and 11 months earlier in a pair of diabetic recipients, the islets being isolated from the distal (body and tail) pancreas excised in a manner identical to that done in the first LD segmental pancreas transplant case.[1] The rationale to do LD islet allografts was based on the unsatisfactory results with our initial DD islet allografts—only transient reduction in insulin requirements or a temporary period of C-peptide positivity,[13,14] while at the same time our first islet

autograft in early 1977 (preceding the first LD islet allograft by 6 months) preserved insulin independence after a total pancreastectomy for chronic pancreatitis, an outcome duplicated in another patient 5 months before our second LD islet allograft.[14] At that time (late 1970s) it was not clear whether the failure to ameliorate diabetes in recipients of DD islets was for technical reasons (inadequate organ preservation prior to or injury during isolation) or for immunological reasons. However, the successful islet autografts led us to believe that the technical problems could be overcome if rejection could be prevented.[14] Autologous islets were isolated immediately after pancreastectomy, eliminating prolonged preisolation preservation as a factor in outcome, and the use of an LD hemipancreas for islet allotransplantation did the same. Islet autografts could not be rejected, a situation that could only be duplicated with an isograft. However, even though the possibility of rejection of allogenic islets was not eliminated by using LDs, we knew from our experience with renal allografts that the incidence of rejection episodes or losses was lower in organs that came from living rather than from deceased donors.[18] Thus we thought that LD islet allografts had a reasonable probability of succeeding and that we would gain an understanding or the causes of failure of islet allografts from DDs.[1]

The first LD islet transplant was done on September 27, 1977; the second on July 12, 1978,[1] just short of 2 weeks before pancreas transplants were resumed at the University of Minnesota on July 25, 1978.[16] The latter ended a 5-year hiatus in pancreas transplantation at our institution since the last case in the Lillehei series.[5,6]

The courses of the two recipients of LD islets were described in detail in 1980 in a paper in *Diabetes* on a series of islet allografts and autografts at the University of Minnesota presented at a Kroc Foundation Conference in 1979.[14] The paper in *Diabetes*[14] focused on our initial islet autografts (three cases) and our second series of islet allografts, 8 transplants in 7 patients, since the initial series of 10 DD islet transplants in another 7 recipients had been described in detail previously.[13] In the *Diabetes* article,[14] the two islet allografts from LDs were identified as Patient Nos. 3 and 6 in the second series of cases.

In regard to the living islet donors, the operation and their courses were first described (along with a summation of the recipients' courses) in a separate paper (Figure 18.1-1), the first paper ever on living pancreas donors, published as part of the proceedings of the First International Symposium on Transplantation of the Pancreas held in Lyon, France, in March 1980.[1] In the same paper the courses of the first three LDs of segmental pancreas grafts were described,[1] with the courses of the first three recipients of LD

pancreas recipients described in this[1] and a companion paper on the first 12 recipients (9 DD grafts) of pancreas transplants in the new Minnesota series.[2] But the living islet donor story comes first.

## LIVING DONOR ISLET TRANSPLANTS

Both LD islet allograft recipients done at the University of Minnesota had had previous LD kidney transplants, in the first case from a different and in the second from the same sibling.[1] In the first case, we had a technical problem with the islet isolation when our mechanical tissue chopper malfunctioned during the tissue preparation and had to be repaired, resulting in prolonged ischemia. Nevertheless, the recipient became C-peptide-positive after the transplant and his insulin needs decreased, but he could not be withdrawn from insulin. He was already on azathioprine and prednisone at the time of the islet transplant because of the renal allograft placed more than 3 years previously and had been rejection-free, but nevertheless, since it was a different donor, he was given a course of Thymoglobulin. Predictably, in this pre-antiviral drug era, at 4 weeks, he developed a cytomegalovirus infection. Immunosuppression was reduced, but during the next month his C-peptide levels declined to the pretransplant baseline, indicating the islets had failed. He subsequently (2 years later) received a DD pancreas graft that functioned for 5 years and ultimately (24 years later) required a kidney retransplant that is currently functioning, and he remains diabetic.

The second recipient of an LD islet allograft was severely vasculopathic and thus a better candidate for an islet than a pancreas transplant, prompting us to try again.[1] She had received a kidney

---

## Living-Related Donor Segmental Pancreatectomy for Transplantation

### D. E. R. Sutherland, F. C. Goetz, and J. S. Najarian

CLINICAL application of pancreas transplantation has been difficult for a variety of reasons, but rejection is a major cause of graft failure. The pioneers in the field transplanted whole pancreaticoduodenal grafts, mandating the use of cadaver donors.[1-3] In recent years, almost all grafts have been segmental, in which the tail and body of the pancreas to the left of the portal vein is transplanted based on a vascular pedicle of the splenic artery and vein.[4-6] Various techniques have been applied, more or less successfully, for handling the pancreatic duct and its secretion, including anastomoses to the bowel[5,7] or ureter,[4,7] injection of synthetic polymers,[6,8] or free drainage into the peritoneal cavity.[9]

Since, in normal individuals, most of the pancreas can be excised without the induction of diabetes,[10] we have used the technique of segmental pancreatectomy for transplantation from living donors. This step is an extension of the use of related donors for kidney transplantation and was approved by our University Committee on the Use of Human Subjects in Research.

beta cells can compensate for the loss, just as a normal kidney can compensate for the loss of a contralateral kidney. Use of related donors for pancreas transplantation should substantially reduce the chance of rejection, and with HLA-identical siblings, less immunosuppression would be needed than with transplantation of mismatched grafts.

#### HISTORICAL EVOLUTION AND OUTCOME IN RECIPIENTS OF ISLET OR PANCREAS ALLOGRAFTS FROM RELATED DONORS

The tail and part of the body of the pancreas (approximately 50%) was removed from 5 related donors for islet or pancreas transplantation between September 27, 1977 and January 17, 1980 (Table 1). In the first 2 instances, the pancreas were processed for islet transplantation to the portal vein of the recipient. In 3 instances, the excised segment was transplanted as an intact graft to the peritoneal cavity, with anastomoses of the splenic vessels of the donor to the iliac vessels of the recipient.

*Islet Recipients*

**FIGURE 18.1-1**

Title page of first report on living donor (LD) segmental pancreatectomies for islet and pancreas allografts, from the University of Minnesota, in proceedings of the International Conference on Pancreas Transplantation held in Lyon, France, 1980 (from reference 1).

allograft 3 years earlier from her sister and had had a severe rejection episode during the first year, so the islet allograft was done in the face of presensitization to her donor even though the crossmatch was negative with the techniques used at the time. Nevertheless, the patient became C-peptide-positive and was insulin-independent during the third week posttransplant, before abruptly becoming hyperglycemic with loss of C-peptide and need to resume exogenous insulin at her pretransplant dose.[1,14] She died a few years later of a myocardial infarct.

Both of the LD islet allografts were considered early failures.[1] The first may have been partly for technical reasons, something we were trying to avoid so we could interpret our previous DD islet allograft results, though most likely rejection occurred after reduction in immunosuppression to allow recovery from the CMV infection.[2] Because of our experience in the second patient, we decided that related donors who had previously given a kidney should not be a donor for a pancreas or islet transplant if the prospective recipient had had a previous rejection episode of the kidney.[1]

Although the success with two of our first three islet autografts[14] had been one factor that prompted us to do the LD islet allografts, the next six islet autografts prevented insulin dependence in only one patient.[19] We were concerned that the technical aspects of islet preparation were not satisfactorily solved, and in 1978, transplantation of immediately vascularized pancreatic deceased grafts was resumed at the University of Minnesota,[16] followed a year later by initiation of LD pancreas transplants,[1] as described later in this chapter (Table 18.1-1).

The fact that the first two LDs of a pancreas segment for islet isolation did not have surgical complications, retained their spleens, and did not develop diabetes or even glucose intolerance encouraged us to go ahead with LD segmental pancreas transplants.[1] The literature on major pancreatic resections at that time indicated that most of the pancreas could be removed from a normal individual without the occurrence of diabetes,[20–22] so the outcome in our two islet donors was not surprising, but the presumption did need to be confirmed and thus both LD islet donors and the subsequent living pancreas donors were serially studied, a task ably carried out by our endocrinologist colleagues over the years,[23–26] allowing us to refine the criteria for living pancreas donation as we uncovered risk factors for glucose intolerance or diabetes (see Chapter 19.3).

Our first publication (Figure 18.1-1) on living related donor segmental pancreatectomy for transplantation included a table outlining the technical details of the surgery (Figure 18.1-2); an

**Table 2.   Technique for Living-Related Donor Segmental Pancreatectomy for Transplantation**

( 1 ) Distal pancreas (body and tail) removed (50%)
( 2 ) Splenic artery and vein ligated at hilum of spleen
( 3 ) Spleen not removed (survives on short gastric vessels)
( 4 ) Pancreas transected at neck (over portal vein)
( 5 ) Proximal pancreas stapled
( 6 ) Splenic artery divided at origin from celiac axis and splenic vein at junction with portal vein
( 7 ) No drain

**FIGURE 18.1-2**

Table from the first paper (1980) gives the technical details of living donor segmental pancreatectomy for islet or pancreas transplantation. (from reference 1).

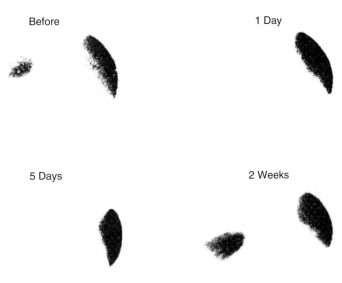

Before       1 Day

5 Days       2 Weeks

**FIGURE 18.1-3**

Figure from the first paper (1980) on living pancreas and islet donors showing serial spleen scans in the world's second living islet donor before and after distal pancreastectomy and ligation of the splenic artery and vein in the hilum. After initial loss of ability to take up radioactive technetium, the uptake became normal by 2 weeks (from reference 1).

illustration of serial spleen scans postdonation showing an initial loss and then a regain of full function by two weeks (Figure 18.1-3); and the results of predonation and 1 to 3 years postdonation metabolic studies, including the first living islet (Figure 18.1-4) and first living pancreas (Figure 18.1-5) donors.[1]

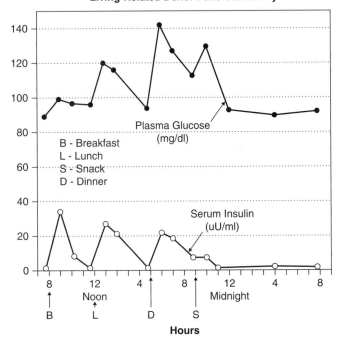

**Living-Related Donor Pancreatectomy**

B - Breakfast
L - Lunch
S - Snack
D - Dinner

Plasma Glucose (mg/dl)

Serum Insulin (uU/ml)

8    12 Noon   4    8   12 Midnight   4    8
B        L          D       S

**Hours**

**FIGURE 18.1-4**

Figure from the first paper (1980) on living pancreas and islet donors showing normal 24-hour metabolic profile of glucose and insulin values >2 years after distal pancreastectomy in the first living islet donor (still alive and nondiabetic 29 years later) (from reference 1).

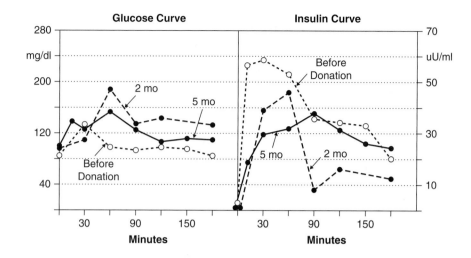

**FIGURE 18.1-5**

Figure from the first paper (1980) on living pancreas and islet donors showing oral glucose tolerance tests before and after distal pancreatectomy in the first living donor for segmental pancreas transplant (called the third donor because of the two previous living islet donors). The glucose levels were slightly higher and the insulin levels slightly lower after donation, but were near or within the normal range. The donor is still alive and nondiabetic 27 years later (from reference 1).

However, to continue the discussion on islet transplants, as expected, technical advances over time improved the results of islet autografts (see Chapter 22), so by the 1990s, with adequate yields, insulin independence could be achieved in 70% of pancreatectomized patients if more than 300,000 islets were transplanted.[27] Although not achieving yet the efficiency of pancreas transplants,[29,29] the results of islet allografts also improved over time,[30] and, at least at our center, in some cases islets from a single donor could induce insulin independence in a recipient,[31,32] raising the possibility that LD islet allografts could be done again.

Indeed, a third LD islet allograft (mother to daughter, diabetic due to chronic pancreatitis) has been recently reported.[33] It was done by Shinichi Matsumoto (a former islet research fellow at the University of Minnesota) and colleagues at the University of Kyoto on January 19, 2005, more than a quarter-century after the second case,[1] but the one in Kyoto was successful in that the recipient was insulin-independent for at least 7 months.[34,35]

In the interim, between the years of the first (1977) and most recent (2005) LD islet allograft (total of 3 cases), more than 150 LD segmental pancreas transplants were done, including 124 at the University of Minnesota (see Chapter 20.5; 1 Minnesota case and 7 other cases were reported after the Registry analysis in the chapter). The story of the early application of LD segmental pancreas transplants, the circumstances prompting their application, and their evolution over time is told in the remainder of this chapter with the sequence of events summarized in Table 18.1-1.

## LIVING DONOR SEGMENTAL PANCREAS TRANSPLANTS

The first LD pancreas transplant was done as a segmental graft (body and tail) from a mother to her diabetic daughter at the University of Minnesota on June 20, 1979, with the duct left open.[1,2] The mother had donated a kidney to her daughter 2 ½ years previously, so the second donation and operation was in the pancreas after kidney (PAK) transplant category. It was the sixth pancreas transplant in a new Minnesota series[2] that had begun 11 months previously, on July 25, 1978,[16] a half-decade after the last case of Lillehei in his series at the same institution.[6] The LD case was reported at the March 1980 Lyon meeting as part of 12 segmental pancreas transplants that had been done in the new Minnesota series up to that time (Figure 18.1-6), including 2 more (both PAKs) from LDs.[2]

At the time of the Lyon meeting nearly all DD pancreas transplants were being done by the segmental technique, with various methods of duct management, as can be seen by perusal of the published proceedings.[36] Duct management was controversial, but most centers just getting into pancreas transplantation were either using enteric drainage, as promoted by the Stockholm group,[10] or the duct-injection technique introduced by the Lyon group.[11] While at Minnesota we were leaving the pancreatic duct open to drain into the peritoneal cavity.[37] We had done segmental pancreas transplants in canines, leaving the duct open as a control against duct injection and other techniques; we found that as long as the pancreatic enzymes remained inactive (not exposed to enterokinase), the secretions were absorbed with a remarkably low peritonitis or technical failure rate,[38] and thus applied the technique clinically.[12,37] The bladder drainage technique, developed by Hans Sollinger et al. at the University of Wisconsin,[39] as a variation of the urinary drainage technique pioneered by the Montefiore group,[9] was to come later.[42]

The open-duct technique was technically successful in half of our clinical cases,[2,37] and indeed our very first recipient of an open-duct DD graft done in July 1978[16] went on to enjoy insulin independence for 17 years until she died with a functioning graft after being thrown off a horse.[17] But after 13 cases, including 4 LD open-duct grafts,[40] it was apparent that this method of exocrine drainage was tolerated better in canines than in humans, and we gave it up.[41] We went on to use all duct management techniques for DD and LD cases alike, as summarized in a 1993 article, written after > 500 total and >75 LD pancreas transplants had been done, describing the evolution of transplantation for diabetes up to that time at the University of Minnesota.[42] Following the lead of Starzl et al.,[43] we resumed using whole pancreaticoduodenal grafts from most DDs in 1985,[44] as did nearly every center,[45] but of course LD pancreas transplants continued to be segmental.[42] (Of our 124 LD pancreas transplants through 2006,[17] exocrine secretion management was by open duct in 5, duct injection in 13, enteric drainage in 57, bladder drainage in 45, and ureteral drainage in 4.)

At the time of the Lyon meeting, only 105 pancreas transplants in 98 patients were known to have been done in the world,[7] and the first LD case was approximately the world's 80th pancreas transplant since the very first.[4] At the Lyon meeting, 4 LD pancreas transplants were reported, the 3 from Minnesota[1,2] and 1 from Stockholm—the first LD pancreas transplant alone (PTA)—done by Carl Groth and associates on March 18, 1980,[46]

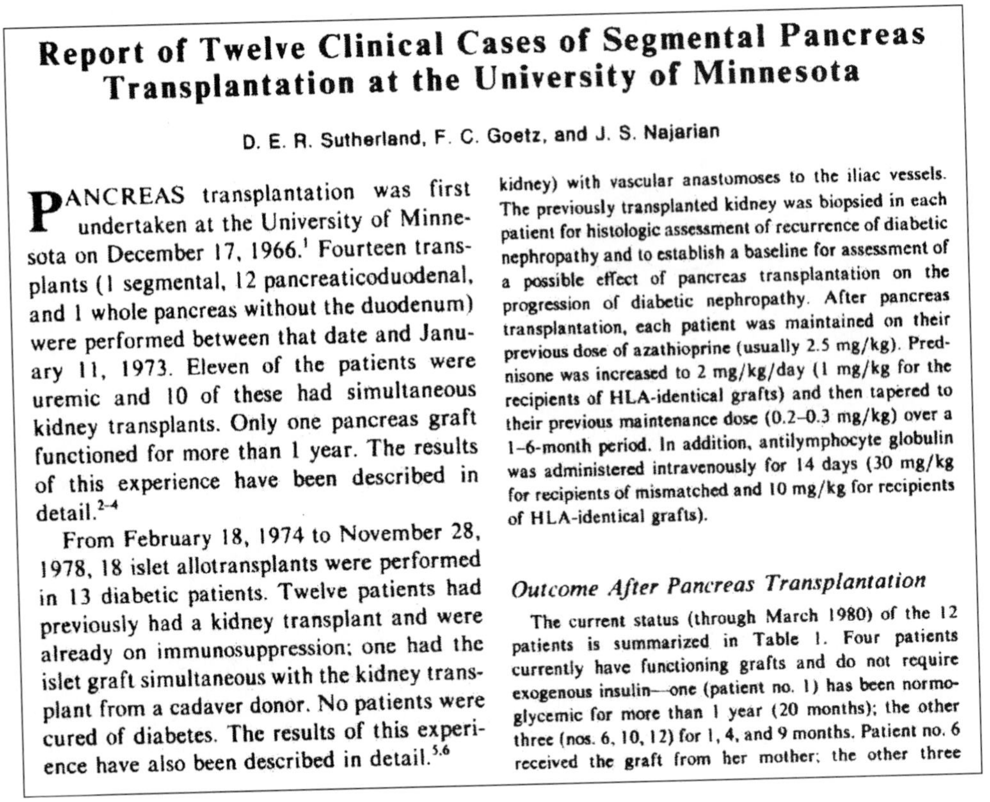

## Report of Twelve Clinical Cases of Segmental Pancreas Transplantation at the University of Minnesota

D. E. R. Sutherland, F. C. Goetz, and J. S. Najarian

**P**ANCREAS transplantation was first undertaken at the University of Minnesota on December 17, 1966.[1] Fourteen transplants (1 segmental, 12 pancreaticoduodenal, and 1 whole pancreas without the duodenum) were performed between that date and January 11, 1973. Eleven of the patients were uremic and 10 of these had simultaneous kidney transplants. Only one pancreas graft functioned for more than 1 year. The results of this experience have been described in detail.[2-4]

From February 18, 1974 to November 28, 1978, 18 islet allotransplants were performed in 13 diabetic patients. Twelve patients had previously had a kidney transplant and were already on immunosuppression; one had the islet graft simultaneous with the kidney transplant from a cadaver donor. No patients were cured of diabetes. The results of this experience have also been described in detail.[5,6]

kidney) with vascular anastomoses to the iliac vessels. The previously transplanted kidney was biopsied in each patient for histologic assessment of recurrence of diabetic nephropathy and to establish a baseline for assessment of a possible effect of pancreas transplantation on the progression of diabetic nephropathy. After pancreas transplantation, each patient was maintained on their previous dose of azathioprine (usually 2.5 mg/kg). Prednisone was increased to 2 mg/kg/day (1 mg/kg for the recipients of HLA-identical grafts) and then tapered to their previous maintenance dose (0.2–0.3 mg/kg) over a 1–6-month period. In addition, antilymphocyte globulin was administered intravenously for 14 days (30 mg/kg for recipients of mismatched and 10 mg/kg for recipients of HLA-identical grafts).

### Outcome After Pancreas Transplantation

The current status (through March 1980) of the 12 patients is summarized in Table 1. Four patients currently have functioning grafts and do not require exogenous insulin—one (patient no. 1) has been normoglycemic for more than 1 year (20 months); the other three (nos. 6, 10, 12) for 1, 4, and 9 months. Patient no. 6 received the graft from her mother; the other three

**FIGURE 18.1-6**

Title page of first report[2] on recipients of living donor (LD) segmental pancreas transplants, from the University of Minnesota, in proceedings of the International Conference on Pancreas Transplantation held in Lyon, France, 1980. (from reference 2).

< 2 weeks before the meeting. The Stockholm recipient rejected the LD pancreas graft within a month, which was unfortunate since one of the original rationales for LD pancreas transplants was to decrease the probability of rejection, given the high rate of early rejection in the technically successful DD pancreas transplants done to date.[7,8–12] Our initial approach of doing an LD PAK from the same donor as the kidney for a recipient with no prior rejection episodes of the kidney (and thus a confirmed nonresponder to the donor) was designed to thwart the high pancreas allograft rejection rate the other groups, as well as our own,[16] were experiencing.

At the time of the Lyon meeting, the first Minnesota LD pancreas transplant had been functioning 9 months, and metabolic studies in the recipient showed excellent graft endocrine function (Figure 18.1-7). The residual pancreas of the donor also showed excellent function on metabolic testing (Figure 18.1-5). Our first LD pancreas transplant recipient differed from the first Stockholm case not only by being a PAK, but a PAK from the same donor (SD) as for her renal allograft, which had not undergone any rejection episodes, a favorable situation since the recipient was demonstrably immunologically unreactive to the donor under the immunosuppressive regimen in use (in her case azathioprine and prednisone). The risk of rejection was much higher for the Stockholm LD PTA case, at least as high as that of an HLA-mismatched LD kidney transplant at the time, and the risk of graft loss was probably higher given that hyperglycemia was known as a late sign of rejection in animal models, making efforts at reversal less likely to succeed.[47] Nevertheless, at Minnesota we went on to do LD PTAs within 2 months of the Lyon meeting,[40] while continuing to do LD PAK transplants[41] and ultimately LD (1994) SPK transplants.[17,48]

The technique of LD distal pancreastectomy was outlined at the Lyon meeting (Figure 18.1-2), but the first illustration of the

surgical (open laparotomy) technique (Figure 18.1-8) was published 2 years later,[49] after our 8th LD case (out of 35 total from July 1978 to October 1981). This publication[49] also contained data on metabolic studies in the LD pancreas donors and their recipients (Figures 18.1-9 and 18.1-10).

Indeed, the pancreas recipient (our 6th LD case, PAK from SD, duct-injected, done December 3, 1980) whose metabolic studies at 6 months are illustrated in Figure 18.1-9 had the longest duration of insulin independence (23 ½ years) in our series until recently eclipsed by a PTA recipient, (our 24th LD case, ED, done November 4, 1982), now insulin-independent >24 years[17] (see Table 18.1-1).

The surgical technique for LD pancreatectomy we described at the beginning of our series[1,49] remained standard[50] until the year 2000 (Table 18.1-1) when we began to do the operation laparoscopically.[51] There have been no technical failures to date (eight cases) with the laparoscopic approach, with or without concomitant donor nephrectomy (see Chapter 19.3).

Except for the LD PTA at Stockholm in 1980,[46] and an unpublished but Registry reported,[52] single LD SPK transplant (open-duct) at the University of Miami in November 1980 that failed for technical reasons (Table 18.1-1), no LD pancreas transplants outside of Minnesota were published or reported to the Registry until the Stockholm group did two more PTA cases in October and November 1985.[53] Neither the second nor third Stockholm LD pancreas transplants achieved long-term function, but it is not clear from their publication as to the causes of loss.[53] They did publish detailed metabolic studies on the LDs that showed a decline in insulin secretory capacity at 3 months with some recovery at 1 year, and all three Stockholm donors were insulin-independent at the time of the report.[54] After the Stockholm cases in 1985 (only the third and fourth outside of Minnesota), seven centers (1 European, 1 Middle East, 2 U.S.,

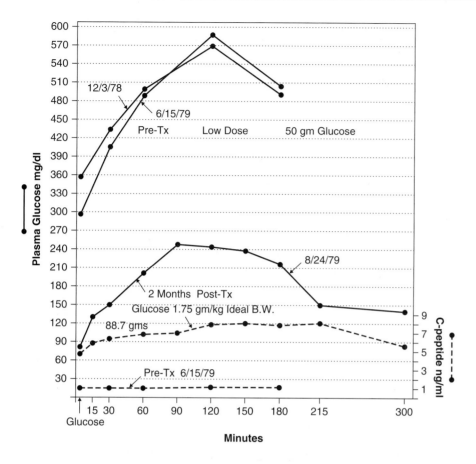

**FIGURE 18.1-7**

Figure from the first report[1] (1980) from the University of Minnesota on recipients of living donor (LD) segmental pancreas allografts, showing results of oral glucose tolerance tests (GTTs) before and 2 months after transplantation in the first recipient ever of an LD (mother) pancreas transplant. Prior to transplantation the recipient had a very abnormal GTT with absence of C-peptide, while posttransplant the GTT glucose values were normal or only slightly above normal and C-peptide was present. The recipient was insulin-independent for 5 years before the pancreas graft failed from recurrent disease (selective loss of beta cells on biopsy). She survived > 24 years from the pancreas transplant before dying with a renal allograft (from the same LD) that functioned for >26 years (from reference 2).

and 3 Asian) either published[55,56] or reported 24 more cases as of 2006, for a total of 28 outside of Minnesota (see Chapter 20.5 for a tabulation of 21 of the non-Minnesota cases).

The most significant series of LD pancreas transplants outside of the University of Minnesota is that of Enrico Bendedetti and colleagues at the University of Illinois in Chicago (Table 18.1-1), with more than 10 LD pancreas transplants to date (only 7—all SPK—reported to the Registry as tabulated in Chapter 20.5).

They have published the results of their series,[56–58] including successful transplants from identical twin donors with recurrence of disease (autoimmune destruction of beta cells) prevented by immunosuppression,[57] and successful transplantation of ABO-incompatible LD pancreas–kidney transplants by antibody reduction protocols,[58] advancing the steps taken in these areas earlier at the University of Minnesota.[17,42]

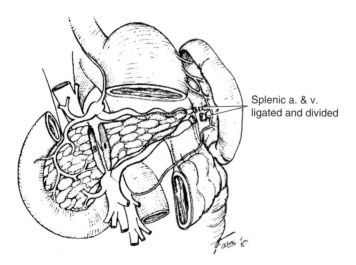

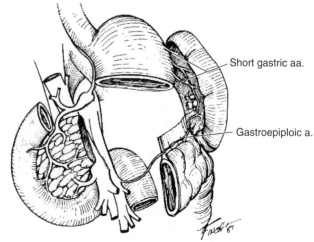

**FIGURE 18.1-8**

Figure from the first publication[1] (1982) illustrating of the surgical technique for spleen-sparing, distal pancreatectomy from a living donor (LD) for segmental transplantation. Of the 35 Minnesota pancreas transplants described from July 1978 to October 1981, 12 were from LDs (from reference 49).

**FIGURE 18.1-9**

Figure on metabolic studies in a recipient of a living donor (LD) segmental pancreas transplant from the same publication (1982) first illustrating the surgical technique (see Figure 18.1-8). The patient was the recipient of the 6th LD pancreas transplant (December 1980) in the Minnesota series, duct-injected, and was insulin-independent > 23 years; a kidney transplanted from the same LD (HLA-identical sister) 2 years prior to the pancreas transplant is currently functioning > 28 years (from reference 49).

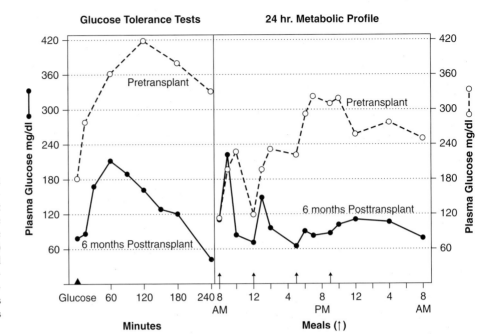

It is apparent that LD pancreas transplants have been done predominantly at the University of Minnesota (Table 18.1-1), 124 cases through 2006, nearly 7% of our pancreas transplants since 1978 (see Chapter 20.5). The outcomes of and protocols for LD pancreas transplants at the University of Minnesota have been sequentially published as the series expanded,[2,16,17,22–26,37,40–42,44,48,51,59–94] now over more than a quarter-century since the first case.[1]

The proportion of LD pancreas transplants at Minnesota has decreased with time as the results with DDs got better.[17] The number of DDs available for solitary pancreas transplants can still meet the demand—though this scenario could change if more candidates are listed—but an LD pancreas transplant is definitely a bonus for the sensitized candidate who finds a volunteer to whom he or she has a negative crossmatch. In addition, an LD SPK from the same donor still allows a fixed date for the transplant and a single operation to place both organs and preempt dialysis in the nephropathic diabetic. Although an SPK from a deceased pancreas and living kidney donor achieves the one-operation goal,[42] it does not allow a fixed date with a guarantee that a deceased pancreas donor will be available.[95,96] An open date means the donor has to also be on call, and the probability of attaining a DD pancreas on a fixed date for an LD kidney transplant is relatively low. Thus, we offer a menu (one that has historically evolved, see Table 18.1-1) to the uremic diabetic: an LD SPK with both organs from the same donor; an LD kidney on a fixed date with hope that a DD pancreas will be available if not, subsequent to the LD kidney the recipient can be placed on the list for a DD PAK); an LD kidney done urgently when a DD pancreas is allocated to the recipient; and the waiting list for a DD SPK for both organs for those who do not have an LD for either.[17]

A few unique aspects of our LD pancreas transplant experience warrant comments or notation, including the original rationale for the procedure[1,41,42]: our observations on recurrence of autoimmune disease (selective beta cell destruction, isletitis) in LD pancreas grafts,[61,62,66,74,76,79,80] that were later followed by rare, but similar, observations of DD grafts[97–101]; the use of paren-

tal donors for the rare pediatric recipient[42,86]; the introduction and development of laparoscopy for LD segmental pancreatectomy[51,94]; the importance of metabolic studies before and after surgery in living pancreas donors for refining the criteria to be a donor[23,93]; the shift in LD pancreas transplant categories from predominantly PTA and PAK to SPK cases as the results of solitary pancreas transplant improved,[17,85,92] with another shift occurring as the option of doing an SPK from a deceased pancreas and a living kidney donor[42] expands in application[17,95,96]; the need for kidney after pancreas (KAP) transplants in some PTA recipients with LDs done for some[17,42]; the role of the Registry in tracking LD pancreas transplants around the world[102]; and the ethical issues surrounding LDs, including of the pancreas,[82,103] and the need for guidelines on donor selection and follow-up care.[103] The sequence of events relevant to these topics is outlined in Table 18.1-1.

## PERSPECTIVES

The *rationale* to use LDs for transplantation of any organ is twofold, either to get better outcomes than those with DDs or to alleviate a shortage of DD organs, or both. Initially for pancreas transplants the main rationale was for better outcomes (see Chapter 18.2 for a full discussion).

The early rationale for LD pancreas transplants was to lower the rejection rates,[1,41,42] and that objective was achieved,[63] but more so for PAK than PTA recipients in the precyclosporine (1978–1984) era.[91] In the cyclosporine era (1984–1994), PTA as well as PAK immunological failures were less with LDs than DDs,[84] but after tacrolimus was introduced in 1994,[85] the results of LD versus DD solitary pancreas transplants were not much different.[92] Indeed we did find that technically successful graft survival rates were higher with LDs even in the early part of the new series of pancreas transplants at the University of Minnesota,[41,63] but much more so for PAK than PTA transplants, primary because the rejection rates were so much lower for same-donor LD PAK than LD PTA transplants.[92] Not until the cyclosporine era

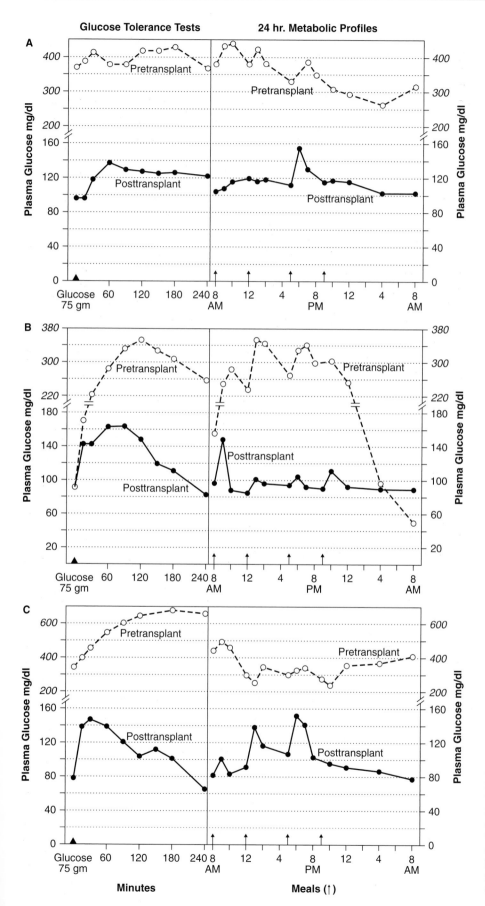

**FIGURE 18.1-10**

Figure on metabolic studies in recipients of the 9th, 11th, and 12th living donor (LD) segmental pancreas transplants in the Minnesota series, all done with enteric drainage in 1981; from the same publication (1982) first illustrating the surgical technique (see Figure 8). One pancreas transplant alone (PTA) recipient (a) was insulin-independent > 2 years before rejecting; the other (b) was until recurrence of disease (selective beta cell loss) at 2 months, while the pancreas after kidney (PAK) recipient was insulin-independent > 8 years; the latter has a kidney transplanted a year prior to the pancreas from the same LD still functioning > 26 years (from reference 49).

were the LD PTA pancreas transplant survival rates significantly higher than those with DDs.[77,84] Once we began using tacrolimus the difference in outcomes between LD and DD outcomes became less.[84,92] Thus, we began doing SPK transplants from the same LD for recipients who wanted a fixed date and one operation for both organs,[87–94] as opposed to a fixed-date LD kidney followed by a DD PAK, or an unfixed date with a kidney LD on call for when a DD pancreas became available for a simultaneous transplant.[17,42] We have also succeeded with ABO-incompatible LD SPK transplants (Table 18.1-1), the incentive being to preempt dialysis and correct diabetes with one operation.[17]

Initially, we had preferred sequential kidney and pancreas (PAK) transplants for the uremic diabetic, keeping the magnitude of the operation low relative to combined placement of both organs.[2,41,42] Because we had done renal allografts routinely in diabetic patients during the 1970s,[18] a large recipient pool was available for both DD and LD PAK transplants when the current Minnesota series began in 1978.[2,16,42] In 1986 we resumed SPK transplants at the University of Minnesota,[44] either with both from the same DD or with a DD for the pancreas and an LD for the kidney,[42] and began doing LD SPK transplants with both organs from the SD beginning in March 1994.[48] The LD SPK program rapidly expanded in the next few years.[87–94] As of 2006 we had done 38 LD SPK transplants,[17] and 9 have functioned >10 years. During this period (1994–2006) we did only 4 PTAs and 2 PAKs from LDs, a shift in our approach compared to 1979–1994 when we did 49 PTAs and 31 PAKs from LDs.[17] The shift occurred because the results of DD PTA and PAK transplants improved[92] so there was less incentive to use LDs purely for outcome, and the waiting times for solitary pancreas transplants from DDs remain relatively short for unsensitized candidates.

Currently at our center, LD PTA and PAK transplants are done mainly in patients who have HLA antibodies, making finding a DD difficult, but who have a negative crossmatch to a suitable LD volunteer. In the case of LD PAK transplants, they can be from the same or different donor. The SD does give an immunological advantage, but we have recipients in both categories with long-term function (Table 18.1-1).

The *recurrence of disease* in pancreas transplants was a surprise to us, as noted in the early citations,[61,62,66,67,74,76,78,79] but perhaps should not have been since an autoimmune cause of type 1 diabetes was proposed, though still controversial. Our observations of rapid recurrence of autoimmune beta cell destruction in nonimmunosuppressed identical twin transplants was the trigger of realization,[66,67] but indeed we had already had at least two cases in immunosuppressed LD recipients[61]; we were just uncertain of the cause in the face of immunosuppression. It is now obvious that in some recipients of pancreas grafts, the autoimmune response to beta cells is greater than that to the histocompatibilty antigens, given that recurrence of disease occurs in a percentage of recipients of DD[97–101] as well as LD pancreas transplants (see Chapter 20.4).

Pancreas transplantation in children is rare, but diabetic children may develop renal disease independent of diabetes and thus be candidates for an SPK or PAK, and with severe lability for a PTA. We have done children in the SPK and PTA categories, with one each from LD,[42,86] both with parental donors (Table 18.1-1). Although the LD PTA graft from the father functioned only 5 years, the recipient (type 1 diabetes) thereafter was no longer labile, so the transplant served its purpose to get him through adolescence and beyond. The pancreas graft in the LD SPK case (dia-

betes and renal failure secondary to hemolytic uremic syndrome) is still functioning >11 years, though a kidney retransplant was required at 9 years. We remain open to doing more pediatric pancreas transplants with LDs.

In regard to LDs of pancreas segments, our first concern is having the least surgical complications possible, and our second and equal concern is selecting volunteers who have sufficient beta cell mass to stay nondiabetic postdonation. The surgery complication rate has been low (see Chapter 19.3), and the laparoscopic approach allows rapid recovery.[94] However, the metabolic effect of hemipancreatectomy is less predictable[23–26] than we originally thought,[1] and 3% to 5% of donors may eventually become diabetic even with the current criteria outlined in Chapter 19.3. We continue to work with our endocrinologists to find the screening tests that will lower the risk. Currently we use the criteria as outlined at the Vancouver forum on living donors.[103]

The future of LD pancreas or islet transplants remains uncertain. The short waiting time for DD solitary pancreas transplants currently limits the incentive to use LDs, a thought that may change since there is little reason for PAK candidates not to be listed, and PTA transplants are probably also underutilized. A DD shortage could trigger a resurgence of LD solitary pancreas transplants. There are alternatives to LD SPK transplants with the use of an LD kidney and DD pancreas, simultaneously or sequentially, but again, a shortage of DDs could increase the incentive for same-donor LD SPK transplants.

The history of pancreas transplantation is in its fourth decade, with living pancreas donors used nearly two-thirds of that time.[104] We think the application will continue.

## References

1. Sutherland DERS, Goetz FC, Najarian JS. Living-related donor segmental pancreatectomy for transplantation. *Transplant Proc* 1980;12(Suppl. 2):19–25.
2. Sutherland DER, Goetz FC, Najarian JS. Report of 12 clinical cases of segmental pancreas transplantation at the University of Minnesota. *Transplant Proc* 1980;12 (No. 4, Suppl. 2): 33–39.
3. Deterling R. Comment on living donor intestinal transplantations. In: Alican F, Hardy JD, Cayirli M, et al, eds. Intestinal transplantation: laboratory experience and report of a clinical case. *Am J Surg* 1971;121:150–159.
4. Kelly WD, Lillehei RC, Markel FK, Idezuki Y, Goetz FC. Allotransplantation of the pancreas and duodenum along with the kidney in diabetic nephropathy. *Surgery* 1967;61:827–835.
5. Lillehei RC, Simmons RL, Najarian JS, et al. Pancreatico-duodenal allotransplantation: experimental and clinical experience. *Ann Surg* 1970;172:405–436.
6. Lillehei RC, Ruiz JO, Aquino C, Goetz FC. Transplantation of the pancreas. *Acta Endocrinol* 1976;83(suppl 205):303–320
7. Sutherland DER. International human pancreas and islet transplant registry. *Transplant Proc* 1980;12 (No. 4 Suppl. 2):229–236.
8. Connolly JE, Martin RC, Steinberg J, et al. Clinical experience with pancreaticoduodenal transplantation. *Arch Surg* 1973;106:489–493
9. Gliedman ML, Gold M, Whittaker J, Rifkin H, Sobreman R, Freed S, Tellis V, Veith FJ. Clinical segmental pancreatic transplantation with ureter-pancreatic duct anastomosis for exocrine drainage. *Surgery* 1973; 74:171–180
10. Groth CG, Lundgren G, Arner P, et al. Rejection of isolated pancreatic allografts in patients with diabetes. *Surg Gynecol Obstet* 1976;143: 933–937
11. Dubernard JM, Traeger J, Neyra P, et al. A new method of preparation of segmental pancreatic grafts for transplantation: trials in dogs and in man. *Surgery* 1978;84:633–640

12. Najarian JS, Sutherland DER, Matas AJ, et al. Human islet transplantation: A preliminary experience. *Transplant Proc* 1977;9:233–236

13. Sutherland DERS, Matas AJ, Najarian JS. Pancreatic islet cell transplantation. *Surg Clin No Am* 1978;58:365–382

14. Sutherland DER, Matas AJ, Goetz, FC, Najarian JS. Transplantation of dispersed pancreatic islet tissue in humans: autografts and allografts. *Diabetes* 1980;29:31–34

15. Hering BJ, Kandaswamy R, Ansite JD, et al. Single-donor, marginal-dose islet transplantation in patients with type 1 diabetes. *JAMA* 2005;293:830–835

16. Sutherland DER, Goetz FC, Najarian JS. Intraperitoneal transplantation of immediately vascularized segmental pancreatic grafts without duct ligation: A clinical trial. *Transplantation* 1979;28:485–491

17. Sutherland DER, Gruessner RW, Dunn DL, Matas AJ, Humar A, Kandaswamy R, Mauer SM, Kennedy WR, Goetz FC, Robertson RP, Gruessner AC, and Najarian JS. Pancreas Transplantation at the University of Minnesota: 1966–2005. In: Corry RJ, Shapiro R, eds. *Pancreatic Transplantation*. New York 2007: Informa Healthcare, pages 279–332

18. Najarian JS, Sutherland DER, Simmons RL, et al. Ten-year experience with renal transplantation in juvenile onset diabetics. *Ann Surg* 1979;l90:487–500.

19. Najarian JS, Sutherland DER, Baumgartner D. Total or near total pancreatectomy and islet autotransplantation for treatment of chronic pancreatitis. *Ann Surg* 1980;192:526–542

20. Yellin AE, Vecchione TR, Donovan AJ. Distal pancreatectomy for pancreatic trauma. *Am J Surg* 1972;124:135–141

21. Stephanini P, Carboni M, Patrassi N, Basoli A. Beta-islet tumors of the pancreas: results of a study on 1,077 cases. *Surgery* 1974;75:597–609

22. Griffin W. In: Buchwald H, Varco RC, eds. *Metabolic Surgery*. New York: Grune & Stratton; 1978:111

23. Kendall DM, Sutherland DER, Goetz FC, Najarian JS. Metabolic effect of hemipancreatectomy in living related pancreas transplant donors: Preoperative prediction of postoperative oral glucose tolerance. *Diabetes* 1989;38 (Suppl. 1):101–103

24. Kendall DM, Sutherland DER, Najarian JS, Goetz FC, Robertson RP. Effects of hemipancreatectomy on insulin secretion and glucose tolerance in healthy humans. *N Engl J Med* 1990;322:898–903

25. Seaquist ER, Robertson RP: Effects of hemipancreatectomy on pancreatic alpha and beta cell function in healthy human donors. *J Clin Invest* 1992;89:1761–1766

26. Robertson RP, Sutherland DE, Seaquist ER, Lanz KJ. Glucagon, catecholamine, and symptom responses to hypoglycemia in living donors of pancreas segments. *Diabetes* 2003;52:1689–1694

27. Wahoff DC, Papalois B, Najarian JS, et al. Autologous islet transplantation to prevent diabetes after pancreatic resections. *Ann Surg* 1995;222 (No. 4):562–579

28. Frank AM, Barker CF, Markmann JF. Comparison of whole pancreas and isolated islet transplantation for type 1 diabetes mellitus. Chapter 7. *Advan Surg* 2005;39:137–162

29. Sutherland DER. Beta-cell replacement by transplantation in diabetes mellitus: which patients at what risk, which way (when pancreas, when islets), and how to allocate deceased donor pancreases. *Curr Opinions in Organ Transpl* 2005;10:147–149

30. Merani S, Shapiro AMJ. Current status of pancreatic islet transplantation. *Clin Scie* 2006;110:611–625

31. Gores PF, Najarian JS, Stephanian, E, et al. Insulin independence in type I diabetes after transplantation of unpurified islets from a single donor with 15-deoxyspergulain. *Lancet* 1993;34:19–21

32. Hering BJ, Kandaswamy R, Harmon JV, et al. Transplantation of cultured islets from two-layer preserved pancreases in type 1 diabetes with anti-CD3 antibody. *Am J Transplant* 2004;4:390–401

33. Matsumoto S, Okitsu T, Iwanaga Y, et al. Insulin independence after living-donor distal pancreatectomy and islet allotransplantation. *Lancet* 2005;365(9471):1642–1644

34. Matsumoto S, Okitsu T, Iwanaga Y, et al. Insulin independence of unstable diabetic patient after single living donor islet transplantation. *Transplant Proc* 2005;37(8):3427–3429

35. Matsumoto S, Okitsu T, Iwanaga Y, et al. Follow up study of the first successful living donor islet transplantation. Supplement to *American Journal of Transplantation* and *Transplantation* 2006; World Transplant Congress Abstract No. 808, page 339

36. Dubernard JM, Traeger J, eds. *Transplantation of the Pancreas*. New York, Grune and Stratton; 1981. Hardcover edition of the December 1980 issue (Volume XII, No. 4, Suppl. 2) of *Transplantation Proceedings*

37. Sutherland DER, Baumgartner D, Najarian JS. Free intraperitoneal drainage of segmental pancreas grafts: Clinical and experimental observations on technical aspects. *Transplant Proc* 1980;12(No. 4, Suppl. 2):26–32

38. Baumgartner,D, Sutherland DER, Najarian JS. Studies on segmental pancreas autotransplants in dogs. Technique and preservation. *Transplant Proc* 1980;12(No. 4, Suppl. 2):163–171

39. Sollinger HW, Cook K, Kamps D. Clinical and experimental experience with pancreaticocystostomy for exocrine drainage in pancreas transplantation. *Transplant Proc* 1984;16:749–751

40. Sutherland DER, Goetz FC, Najarian JS. Review of the world's experience with pancreas and islet transplantation and results of intraperitoneal segmental pancreas transplantation from related and cadaver donors at Minnesota. *Transplant Proc* 1981;13: 291–297

41. Sutherland DER, Goetz FC, Rynasiewicz JJ, et al. Segmental pancreas transplantation from living related and cadaver donors: A clinical experience. *Surgery* 1981;90:159–169

42. Sutherland DER, Gores PF, Farney C, et al. Evolution of kidney, pancreas and islet transplantation for patients with diabetes at the University of Minnesota. *Am J Surg* 1993;166:456–491

43. Starzl TE, Iwatsuki S, Shaw BW Jr., et al. Pancreaticoduodenal transplantation in humans. *Surg Gynecol Obstet* 1984;159:265–272

44. Sutherland DER, Dunn DL, Goetz FC, et al. A 10-Year experience with 290 pancreas transplants at a single institution. *Ann Surg* 1989;210: 274–285

45. Sutherland DER, Chow SY, Moudry-Munns, KC. International Pancreas Transplant Registry Report—1988. *Clin Transplant* 1989;3: 129–149

46. Groth CG, Lundgren G, Gunnarsson R, Hardstedt C, Ostman J. Experience with nine segmental pancreatic transplantations in preuremic diabetic patients in Stockholm. *Transplant Proc* 1980;12 (Suppl. 2):68–71

47. Sutherland DER. Pancreas and islet transplantation. 1. Experimental Studies. *Diabetelogia* 1981;20:161–185

48. Gruessner RWG, Sutherland DER. Simultaneous kidney and segmental pancreas transplants from living related donors - the first two successful cases. *Transplantation* 1996;61:1265–1268

49. Sutherland DER, Goetz FC, Elick BA, Najarian JS. Pancreas and islet transplantation in diabetic patients with long-term follow-up in selected cases. In: Friedman EA, L'Esperance FA, eds. *Proc. Diabetic Renal-Retinal Syndrome, Prevention and Management*. New York: Grune and Stratton; 1982:463–494

50. Sutherland DER, Ascher NL. Distal pancreas donation from a living relative. In: Simmons RL, Finch ME, Ascher NL, Najarian JS, eds. *Manual of Vascular Access, Organ Donation, and Transplantation*. New York: Springer-Verlag; 1984:153–164

51. Gruessner RW, Kandaswamy R, Denny R. Laparoscopic simultaneous nephrectomy and distal pancreatectomy from a live donor. *J Am Coll Surg* 2001;193:333–337

52. Sutherland DER. Pancreas and islet transplantation. II. Clinical trials. *Diabetologia* 1981;20:435–450

53. Groth CG, Tyden G. Segmental pancreatic transplantation with enteric drainage. In: Groth CG, ed. *Pancreatic Transplantation*. London: Grune & Stratton Ltd; 1988:99–112

54. Bolinder J, Gunnarson R, Tyden G, Brattstrom C, Groth CG. Metabolic effects of living related pancreatic graft donation. *Transplant Proc* 1988;20(3):4475–478

55. Abouna GM. Current status of pancreas transplantation for the treatment of diabetes mellitus. *J Kuwait Med Assoc* 1997 (Dec);29 (4): 394–395

56. Zielinski A, Nazarewski S, Bogetti D, et al. Simultaneous pancreas-kidney transplant from living related donor: a single-center experience. *Transplantation* 2003;76:547–552.

57. Benedetti E, Dunn T, Massad MG, et al. Successful living related simultaneous pancreas-kidney transplant between identical twins. *Transplantation* 1999;67:915–918.

58. Sammartino C, Pham T, Panaro F, et al. Successful simultaneous pancreas kidney transplantation from living-related donor against positive cross-match. *Am J Transplant* 2004;4:140–143.

59. Sutherland DER, Najarian JS, Greenberg BZ, et al. Hormonal and metabolic effects of a pancreatic endocrine graft: Vascularized segmental transplantation in insulin-dependent diabetic patients. *Ann Intern Med* 1981;95:537–541

60. Rynasiewicz JJ, Sutherland DER, Ferguson RM, et.al. Cyclosporin A for immunosuppression: Observations in rat heart, pancreas and islet allograft models and in human renal and pancreas transplantation. *Diabetes* 1982;31(Suppl. 4):92–108

61. Sutherland DER, Goetz FC, Elick BA, Najarian JS. Experience with 49 segmental pancreas transplants in 45 diabetic patients. *Transplantation* 1982;34:330–338

62. Sutherland DER, Sibley RK, Chinn P, et al. Identical twin pancreas transplants: reversal and recurrence of pathogenisis in type 1 diabetes. *Clin Res* 1984;32(2):561A

63. Sutherland DER, Goetz FC, Najarian JS. Pancreas transplants from living related donors. *Transplantation* 1984;38:625–633

64. Sutherland DER, Goetz FC, Najarian JS. One hundred pancreas transplants at a single institution. *Ann Surg* 1984;200:414–440

65. Sutherland DER, Goetz FC, Najarian JS. Recent experience with 89 pancreas transplants at a single institution. *Diabetologia* 1984;27:149–153

66. Sutherland DER, Sibley RK, Xu XZ, et al. Twin-to-twin pancreas transplantation: Reversal and reenactment of the pathogenesis of Type I diabetes. *Trans Assoc Am Phys* 1984;97: 80–87

67. Sibley RK, Sutherland DER, Goetz FC, Michael AF. Recurrent diabetes mellitus in the pancreas iso- and allograft: A light and electron microscopic and immunohistochemical analysis of four cases. *Lab Invest* 1985;53:132–144

68. Sutherland DER, Goetz FC, Kendall DM, Najarian JS. Effect of donor source, technique, immunosuppression, and presence or absence of end-stage diabetic nephropathy on outcome in pancreas transplant recipients. *Transplant Proc* 1985;17:325–330

69. Sutherland DER, Goetz FC, Najarian JS. Surgery and possible complications in the living donor for the pancreas transplant, short and long term. In: Touraine JL, ed. *Transplantation and Clinical Immunology XVI.* Amsterdam: Elsevier Science Publishers B.V; 1985:7–15

70. Sutherland DER, Casanova D, Sibley RK. Role of pancreas graft biopsies in the diagnosis and treatment of rejection after pancreas transplantation. *Transplant Proc* 1987;19: 2329–2331

71. Prieto M, Sutherland DER, Fernandez-Cruz L, Heil JE, Najarian JS. Experimental and clinical experience with urine amylase monitoring for early diagnosis of rejection in pancreas transplantation. *Transplantation* 1987;43:71–79

72. Prieto M, Sutherland DER, Goetz FC, Rosenberg ME, Najarian JS. Pancreas transplant results according to the technique of duct management: Bladder versus enteric drainage. *Surgery* 1987;102:680–691

73. Prieto M, Sutherland DER, Fernandez-Cruz L, Heil JE, Najarian JS. Experimental and clinical experience with urine amylase monitoring for early diagnosis of rejection in pancreas transplantation. *Transplantation* 1987;43:71–79

74. Sibley RK, Sutherland DER. Pancreas transplantation: An immunohistologic and histopathologic examination of 100 grafts. *Am J Pathol* 1987;128:151–170

75. Sutherland DER, Goetz FC, Najarian JS. Experience with single pancreas transplantation compared with pancreas transplantation after a kidney transplantation; and with transplantation with pancreas grafts from living related compared with cadaveric donors. In: Groth CG, ed. *Pancreatic Transplantation.* London: Grune & Stratton Ltd; 1988:175–189

76. Sibley R, Sutherland DER. Recurrence of diabetes mellitus in the pancreas graft. In: Groth CG, ed. *Pancreatic Transplantation.* London: Grune & Stratton Ltd; 1988:339–355

77. Sutherland DER, Kendall DM, Moudry KC, et al. Pancreas transplantation in nonuremic, Type I diabetic recipients. *Surgery* 1988;104:453–464

78. Sutherland DER, Sibley RK. Recurrence of disease in pancreas transplants. Chapter 2. In: Van Schilfgaarde R, Hardy MA, eds. *Transplantation of the Endocrine Pancreas in Diabetes Mellitus.* Amsterdam: Elsevier Science Publishers B.V; 1988:60–66

79. Sutherland DER, Goetz FC, Sibley RK. Recurrence of disease in pancreas transplants. *Diabetes* 1989;38 (Suppl. 1):85–87

80. Nakhleh RE, Gruessner RWG, Swanson PE, et al. Pancreas transplant pathology. A morphologic, immunohistochemical and electron microscopic comparison of allogeneic grafts with rejection syngeneic grafts, and chronic pancreatitis. *Am J Surg Pathol* 1991;15:246–256

81. Sutherland DER, Goetz FC, Kendall DM, et al. Experience with pancreas transplants from living related donors. In: Abouna GM, Kumar MSA, White AG, eds. *Organ Transplantation 1990.* Dordrecht, The Netherlands: Kluwer Academic Publishers; 1991:383–388

82. Sutherland DER, Goetz FC, Gillingham KJ, Moudry-Munns KC, Najarian JS. Medical risks and benefit of pancreas transplants from living related donors. In: Land W, Dossetor JB, eds. *Organ Replacement Therapy: Ethics, Justice and Commerce.* Berlin, Heidelberg: Springer-Verlag; 1991:93–101

83. Santamaria P, Nakhleh RE, Sutherland DER, Barbosa JJ. Characterization of T lymphocytes infiltrating human pancreas allograft affected by isletitis and recurrent diabetes. *Diabetes* 1992;41:53–61

84. Sutherland DER, Gruessner RWG, Moudry-Munns KC, Gruessner A, Najarian JS. Pancreas transplants from living related donors. *Transplant Proc* 1994;26(2):443–445

85. Gruessner RWG, Sutherland DER, Najarian JS, Dunn DL, Gruessner A. Solitary pancreas transplantation for nonuremic patients with labile insulin-dependent diabetes mellitus. *Transplantation* 1997;64:1572–1577

86. Bendel-Stenzel MR, Kashtan CE, Sutherland DER, Chavers BM. Simultaneous pancreas-kidney transplant in two children with hemolytic-uremic symptom. *Pediatr Nephrol* 1997;11: 485–487

87. Gruessner RWG, Kendall DM, Drangstveit MB, Gruessner A, Sutherland DER. Simultaneous pancreas-kidney transplantation from live donors. *Ann Surg* 1997;226:471–482

88. Humar A, Gruessner RWG, Sutherland DER. Living related donor pancreas and pancreas-kidney transplantation. *Brit Med Bull* 1997;53:879–891

89. Gruessner RWG, Leone JP, Sutherland DER. Combined kidney and pancreas transplants from living donors. *Transplant Proc* 1998;30:282

90. Sutherland DER, Najarian JS, Gruessner RWG. Living versus cadaver donor pancreas transplants. *Transplant Proc* 1998;30:2264–2266

91. Kandaswamy R, Stillman AE, Granger DK, Sutherland DER, Gruessner RWG. MRI is superior to angiography for evaluation of living-related simultaneous pancreas and kidney donors. *Transplant Proc* 1999;31:604–605

92. Sutherland DE, Gruessner RW, Dunn DL, et al. Lessons learned from more than 1,000 pancreas transplants at a single institution. *Ann Surg* 2001;233:463–501

93. Gruessner RW, Sutherland DE, Drangstveit MB, Bland BJ, Gruessner AC. Pancreas transplants from living donors: short- and long-term outcome. *Transplant Proc* 2001;33:819–820

94. Tan M, Kandaswamy R, Sutherland D E, and Gruessner R W. Laparoscopic donor distal pancreatectomy for living donor pancreas and pancreas-kidney transplantation. *Am J Transplant* 2005;5:1966–1970.

95. Farney AC, Cho E, Schweitzer EJ, et al. Simultaneous cadaver pancreas living-donor kidney transplantation: a new approach for the type 1 diabetic uremic patient. *Ann Surg* 2000;232:696

96. Boggi U, Vistoli F, Del Chiaro M, et al. Simultaneous cadaver pancreas-living donor kidney transplantation. *Transplant Proc* 2004;36:577

97. Tyden G, Reinholt FP, Sundkvist G, Bolinder J. Recurrence of autoimmune diabetes mellitus in recipients of cadaveric pancreatic grafts [see comments] [published erratum appears in *N Engl J Med* 1996 Dec 5;335(23):1778]. *N Engl J Med* 1996;335:860–863

98. Burke GW, Ciancio G, Miller J, Allende G, Pugliese A. Hyperglycemia occurring 5–8 years after simultaneous pancreas-kidney (SPK) transplantation associated with the prior development of islet cell antibodies. *Am J Transplantat* 2003;380(3):A889.

99. Pugliese A, Allende, G, Laughlin R, et al. Reurrence of autoantibodies and autorreactive T cells in patients with type 1 diabetes following pancreas transplantation. *Diabetes* 2004;53(Suppl 2):A69

100. Sisino G, Dogra R, Allende G, et al. Evidence for ductal cell to ß-cell trans-differentiation and proliferation in the transplanted pancreas of patients with type 1 diabetes and recurrence of islet autoimmunity. *Diabetes* 2006;55 (Suppl 1):A32.

101. Reijonen H, Geubtner K, Allende G, et al. Identification of islet-autoantigen specific CD4+ T-cells in the pancreatic lymph nodes and pancreas of a pancreas-kidney transplant patient with recurrence of Autoimmunity. *Diabetes* 2006;55(Suppl 1):A88.

102. Gruessner AC, Sutherland DE. Pancreas transplant outcomes for United States (US) and non-US cases as reported to the United Network for Organ Sharing (UNOS) and the International Pancreas Transplant Registry (IPTR) as of June 2004. *Clin Transplant* 2005;19:433–455

103. Pruett TL, Tibell A, Albdulkareem A, et al. The ethics statement of the Vancouver forum on live lung, liver, pancreas, and intestine donor. *Transplantation* 2006;81:1386

104. Sutherland DER, Gruessner RWG. History of Pancreas Transplantation. In: Gruessner RWG, Sutherland DER, eds. *Transplantation of the Pancreas.* New York: Springer-Verlag; 2004:39–68

## 18.2   RATIONALE FOR LIVING DONOR PANCREAS TRANSPLANTS

*Rainer W.G. Gruessner, MD*

The rationale for pancreas transplants using living donors (LDs) has shifted over time. Initially, in the azathioprine (AZA) and cyclosporine A (CSA) eras, LDs were used because of better graft survival, as compared with deceased donors (DDs). In the University of Minnesota series, the 1-year graft survival rate for technically successful pancreas after kidney (PAK) transplants from January 1, 1979, to March 21, 1994 (AZA and CSA eras) was 78% with LDs versus 57% with DDs; for technically successful pancreas transplants alone (PTAs), 61% with LDs versus 56% with DDs. Better graft outcome with LDs was mainly due to the significantly lower rate of graft loss from rejection: at 5 years, 49% of PAK and PTA recipients with LDs lost their grafts from rejection vs. 67% with DDs.[1,2]

The immunologic advantage was partly offset by a higher thrombosis rate, given the overall small size of the splenic artery and vein. But, because the technical failure rate in the AZA and CSA eras was lower for LD transplants than the immunologic failure rate for DD transplants, the probability of long-term function was significantly higher with LD (vs DD) transplants.[1,2]

With the introduction of tacrolimus (TAC) and mycophenolate mofetil (MMF) and their combined use in the mid-1990s, the graft survival rate improved markedly for DD pancreas recipients because of the reduced graft loss rate from rejection.[3] Thus, the immunologic advantage of LD pancreas transplants in the

TAC era was no longer as distinct as it had been in the AZA and CSA eras. The incentive for using LDs subsequently also waned, because a DD pancreas shortage did not exist. As a result, at the University of Minnesota, LDs of solitary pancreas grafts (PAK and PTA) in the TAC era have been used only if the recipient (1) is highly sensitized (panel-reactive antibody level [PRA] > 80%) and has a low probability of receiving a DD graft, (2) must avoid high-dose immunosuppression, or (3) has a nondiabetic identical twin or a 6-antigen-matched sibling.

As the number of LD pancreas transplants in the solitary categories (PAK, PTA) decreased, interest in simultaneous pancreas and kidney (SPK) transplants using LDs increased. In the AZA and CSA eras, SPK transplants using LDs had not been performed because of concern about the magnitude of the procedure: thus, PAK recipients and their LDs had to undergo surgery and anesthesia twice. With improved surgical techniques, use of aggressive anticoagulation, and refined immunosuppressive regimens, SPK transplants using LDs have been performed successfully since 1994.[4,5] Such transplants are now promoted for three reasons: (1) about 41% of SPK candidates die within 4 years of being listed on the waiting list[6], not because of the lack of DD pancreas grafts, but because of the high demand for DD kidney grafts; (2) the number of candidates on the pancreas waiting list is more than twice the actual number of pancreas transplants done each year, and the waiting list continues to grow by more than 15% annually[7]; and (3) morbidity and mortality are higher, and quality of life is lower, for diabetic (vs nondiabetic) patients on dialysis, but priority for a kidney transplant is usually not given to diabetic patients.[8,9]

SPK transplants using LDs have also been promoted for yet another reason: given the high, unmet demand for DD SPK transplants, pancreas transplant professionals frequently recommend use of an LD for the kidney transplant, followed later by a DD pancreas transplant (thus, shifting emphasis from the SPK to the PAK category).[10–12] That way, however, the recipient must undergo two operations, including receiving anesthesia twice. And, even though long-term kidney graft outcome is better with an LD (vs DD), long-term pancreas graft outcome with a DD in the PAK category is less favorable than in the SPK category.[13] For these reasons (ie, the shortage of DD kidney donors and the less favorable long-term pancreas outcome in the PAK category), the use of LDs for SPK recipients can be recommended, especially if the donor and the recipient are HLA-identical.[4,5,14] Furthermore, according to the International Pancreas Transplant Registry (IPTR), from 1996 through 2005, 46% of all SPK transplants using LDs were done preemptively versus only 20% of SPK transplants using DDs.[15] A preemptive kidney transplant costs only about a third of the cost of dialysis.[8]

Pancreas transplants using LDs (like any other transplant using an LD) are performed electively when both the recipient and the donor are in optimal condition. If a living related donor is used, other advantages include good HLA matching, lower immunologic risk, less immunosuppression, lower risk of infection and posttransplant malignancies, and shorter preservation time.

Unlike with a DD pancreas, the donated distal pancreas from an LD does not undergo the stress and trauma inherent with DD pancreas procurement and preservation.[16] Granted, a DD has to be sustained on ventilated support, and pancreas donation after cardiac death is only recommended under optimal conditions. Still, an LD distal pancreas provides healthy tissue without the need for extended preservation and can be quickly transplanted into the diabetic recipient. Also, an LD can typically be cleared of any tendency toward developing type 1 or 2 diabetes, thanks to antibody testing and intravenous glucose-induced insulin secretion testing. Such testing cannot be done in a timely fashion with a DD. Although only half of the LD pancreatic mass is used, the segment itself is much more likely to contain a sufficient number of viable islets to render the recipient normoglycemic.[17]

In summary, pancreas (and kidney) transplants using LDs decrease the number of deaths of diabetic patients on dialysis and of candidates on the waiting lists; help overcome the organ shortage; reduce morbidity; improve quality of life for patients formerly on dialysis or with debilitating side effects of diabetes mellitus; reduce the risk of graft loss from rejection; and may provide superior long-term outcome.

## References

1. Sutherland DER, Gruessner R, Dunn D, et al. Pancreas transplants from living-related donors. *Transplant Proc* 1994;26:443–445.

2. Gruessner RWG, Najarian JS, Gruessner AC, Sutherland DER. Pancreas transplants from living related donors. In: Touraine JL, Traeger J, Bétuel H, et al, eds. *Organ Shortage – The Solutions.* Dordrecht, The Netherlands: Kluwer Academic; 1995:77–83.

3. Gruessner RW, Burke GW, Stratta R, et al. A multicenter analysis of the first experience with FK506 for induction and rescue therapy after pancreas transplantation. *Transplantation* 1996;61:261–273.

4. Gruessner RWG, Sutherland DER. Simultaneous kidney and segmental pancreas transplants from living related donors – the first two successful cases. *Transplantation* 1996;61:1265–1268.

5. Benedetti E, Dunn T, Massad MG, et al. Successful living related simultaneous pancreas-kidney transplant between identical twins. *Transplantation* 1999;67:915–918.

6. Gruessner RWG, Sutherland DER, Gruessner AC. Mortality assessment for pancreas transplants. *J Transplant* 2004;4:2018–2026 www.unos.org, accessed July 2006. www.usrds.org, accessed July 2006.

7. Gruessner RWG. Should priority on the waiting list be given to patients with diabetes: pro. *Transpl Proc* 2002;34:1575–1576.

8. Larson TS, Bohorquez H, Rea DJ, et al. Pancreas-after-kidney transplantation: an increasingly attractive alternative to simultaneous pancreas-kidney transplantation.[Miscellaneous Article] *Transplantation* 2004;77:838–843.

9. Hariharan S, Pirsch JD, Lu CY, et al. Pancreas after kidney transplantation. *J Am Soc Nephrol* 2002;13:1109–1118.

10. Gruessner AC, Sutherland DER, Dunn DL, et al. Pancreas after kidney transplants in posturemic patients with type I diabetes mellitus. *J Am Soc Nephrol* 2001;12:2490–2499.

11. Gruessner AC, Sutherland DER. Pancreas transplant outcomes for United States (US) and non-US cases as reported to the United Network for Organ Sharing (UNOS) and the International Pancreas Transplant Registry (IPTR) as of June 2004. *Clinical Transplantation* 2005;19(4):433–455.

12. Gruessner RWG, Kendall DM, Drangstveit MB, et al. Simultaneous pancreas-kidney transplantation from live donors. *Ann Surg* 1977; 226:471–482.

13. Gruessner A. Personal communication. International Pancreas Transplant Registry (IPTR). September 2006.

14. Contrearas JL, Eckstein CA, Smyth MT, et al. Brain death significantly reduces isolated pancreatic islet yields and functionality in vitro and in vivo after transplantation in rats. *Diabetes* 2003;52:2935–2942.

15. Robertson RP. Chapter 15: Endocrine function and metabolic outcomes in pancreas and islet transplantation In: Gruessner RWG, Sutherland DER, eds. *Transplantation of the Pancreas.* New York: Springer-Verlag; 2004: 441–454.

# CHAPTER 19

# PANCREAS TRANSPLANTATION: THE DONOR

## 19.1 SELECTION AND WORKUP

*Elizabeth R. Seaquist, MD,*
*Rainer W.G. Gruessner, MD*

## INTRODUCTION

*Type 1 diabetes* is a chronic medical condition associated with significant morbidity, increased mortality, and a substantial impact on overall quality of life. The use of intensive insulin regimens to achieve near-normal levels of glycemia has been clearly shown to reduce the overall risk for the development of the microvascular complications of the disease, but such regimens are difficult for some patients to master and are associated with an increased risk of hypoglycemia. Indeed, hypoglycemia has become the limiting factor preventing the widespread implementation of intensive insulin regimens to normalize hypoglycemia in patients with type 1 diabetes. This is particularly true because patients with repeated episodes of hypoglycemia lose their ability to detect hypoglycemia before they develop frank neuroglycopenia. This hypoglycemia unawareness creates a situation where patients become reliant on others to recognize and treat episodes of hypoglycemia. Not only does this have a substantial impact on a patient's autonomy, but also it may increase the risk of injury during hypoglycemia and have a deleterious effect on long-term cognitive function.

Successful pancreas and islet transplants have allowed some patients with type 1 diabetes to achieve normoglycemia and insulin independence. Because they do not need to control their diabetes with insulin, they are no longer at risk for recurrent hypoglycemia and the development of hypoglycemia unawareness. Therefore, some have advocated that patients with hypoglycemia unawareness and/or early diabetes complications are ideal candidates for pancreas or islet transplants because, if successful, they will achieve the normoglycemia necessary to slow the rate of progression or reverse their microvascular complications while preventing the occurrence of life-threatening hypoglycemia.

The use of living related donors for organ transplantation is advocated by many transplantation experts because of the generally improved long-term survival of grafts from living related donors. In kidney transplantation, graft survival continues to be about 10% greater if a living donor is used than if the kidney comes from a deceased donor.[1] However, the benefits of living related donation in pancreas transplantation do not appear to be as significant. Indeed, because of the technical failure rate associated with living related donation, the 3-year survival rate is approximately the same for deceased and living related pancreas transplants.[2,3] Nonetheless, living related donation is still offered at a few institutions because of the logistic benefits it offers some recipients. Pancreas-kidney transplant recipients who opt for a living related kidney donation because of the improved graft survival associated with this kind of donation may decide to accept a pancreas from the same living kidney donor in order to receive both organs at the same time. Potential pancreas recipients with rare tissue types or related problems with immunological matching may also opt for a living donor in order to avoid a very long wait on the transplant list for a suitable deceased donor.

The potential risk of hemipancreas donation may be substantial and donors must be carefully evaluated before a decision can be made to permit the donation of a hemipancreas to a family member or friend. In the subsequent paragraphs, the risks of hemipancreas donation and the preoperative evaluation that should be done to determine the suitability of a candidate to donate a hemipancreas will be reviewed. From the outset, it must be emphasized that based on long-term survival rates, living related pancreas donation does not appear to have an advantage over deceased donation and that even with sophisticated metabolic testing it is impossible to determine if a potential donor will retain normal glucose tolerance after surgery. Consequently, living related pancreas donation should only be considered in very unusual and uncommon situations.

## EXPERIENCE WITH HEMIPANCREAS DONATION AT THE UNIVERSITY OF MINNESOTA

The University of Minnesota has the greatest experience with living hemipancreas donors in the world, although other centers have also reported their experience with this technique.[4,5] More than 115 such operations have been performed at the University of Minnesota to date, although long-term follow-up of these individuals has been extremely limited, given an inability to contact donors after they have left the institution because of lack of a forwarding address.[3] The most comprehensive evaluation of the impact of hemipancreas donation on metabolic function was reported by Kendall et al. in 1990.[6] In this investigation, 28 donors were examined before and 1 year after the organ donation. All had normal fasting glucose concentrations, normal results on oral glucose tolerance tests, and normal 24-hour serum glucose profiles prior to donation. Three of the 28 experienced surgical complications, including 1 who required a splenectomy for splenic vascular compromise and another who developed a collection of sterile intraabdominal fluid at the resection site that required drainage. One year after surgery, all demonstrated an increase in glucose concentration and a reduction in insulin levels (see Table 19.1-1).

**TABLE 19.1-1**

## METABOLIC EFFECTS OF HEMIPANCREAS DONATION*

|  | Fasting Glucose (mg/dL) | Fasting Insulin (µU/mL) | Blood Glucose 2 Hours After Oral Glucose Load | Percentage With Abnormal Response on Oral Glucose Tolerance Test |
|---|---|---|---|---|
| Before donation | 88 ± 7 | 6.4 ± 4 | 117 ± 18 | 0 |
| One year after donation | 97 ± 16[a] | 5.5 ± 4[b] | 156 ± 53[c] | 25% |

*Data from reference 6.

[a]$p < 0.003$; [b]$p < 0.05$; [c]$p < 0.001$

In addition, 25% displayed abnormal glucose tolerance on an oral glucose tolerance test. Subsequent evaluation of normoglycemic donors 1 or more years after donation demonstrated that all had a significant reduction in stimulated insulin and glucagon secretion with a reduction in functional beta cell reserve.[7] Normoglycemic donors were also found to have hyperproinsulinemia[8] even though insulin sensitivity was not altered.[9] The presence of hyperproinsulinemia generally suggests that pancreatic islet cells are under increased demand to provide sufficient insulin to maintain normal glucose homeostasis and may be seen in individuals with type 2 diabetes. The observation that normoglycemic donors have hyperproinsulinemia is very concerning because it suggests they may be at higher risk for developing diabetes than was previously thought.

In 2001, University of Minnesota donors who underwent surgery between January 1978 and August 2000 were contacted to learn the impact of hemipancreas donation on health. Ten of the 46 who responded (22%) reported that their hemoglobin $A_{1c}$ was elevated,[3] implying that they had developed diabetes. In a more recent examination of metabolic function, 5 of 6 donors with presumed normal glucose tolerance who returned to the University of Minnesota for evaluation were found to have impaired glucose tolerance or frank diabetes (Seaquist, unpublished data). These observations suggest that between 25% and 80% of donors with normal glucose tolerance before hemipancreas donation will develop abnormal glucose tolerance or diabetes after undergoing the procedure.

## SELECTION CRITERIA FOR DONORS

In 1996, in an effort to reduce the rate at which hemipancreas donors developed diabetes after the procedure, strict endocrinological criteria were developed to use in the selection of living donors for pancreas transplantation at the University of Minnesota (see Table 19.1-2). These criteria recognized the importance of both personal and family history of endocrine disease in establishing risk and the role of obesity and other conditions associated with insulin resistance in unmasking beta cell dysfunction after donation. We now recommend that potential donors with any of the exclusion criteria listed in Table 19.1-2 be excluded from donating because their own risk of developing diabetes after donation

**TABLE 19.1-2**

## EXCLUSION CRITERIA FOR LIVING HEMIPANCREAS DONORS AT THE UNIVERSITY OF MINNESOTA

### Historical and clinical criteria

1. History of type 2 diabetes in any first-degree relative (parent, sibling, child)
2. Personal history of gestational diabetes
3. Additional first-degree relative with type 1 diabetes (other than proposed recipient)
4. Body mass index greater than 27 kg/m²
5. Age greater than 50 years
6. Age of the donor within 10 years of the age at which type 1 diabetes was diagnosed in the proposed recipient
7. Clinical evidence of diseases associated with insulin resistance (eg, polycystic ovarian syndrome, hypertension)
8. Personal history of an autoimmune endocrine disorder involving the thyroid, adrenal, pituitary, gonads
9. History of or active diseases of the exocrine pancreas (eg, active or chronic pancreatitis)
10. Active or uncontrolled psychiatric disorders
11. Heavy smoking, alcoholism, or excessive alcohol use
12. Hypertension, cardiac disease
13. Active infections or malignant disorders

### Metabolic criteria

1. Any glucose value above 150 mg/dL during standard oral glucose tolerance tests
2. Hemoglobin $A_{1c}$ greater than 6%
3. Glucose disposal rate calculated from data collected during intravenous glucose tolerance tests less than 1.0%
4. Presence of elevated titer of islet cell autoantibodies or anti-GAD antibodies
5. Acute insulin response to intravenous glucose or intravenous arginine of less than 300% of basal
6. Glucose potentiation of arginine-induced insulin secretion of less than 300% of basal

is deemed to be unacceptably high. In addition, potential donors with metabolic abnormalities uncovered during preoperative testing are excluded because of uncertainty over whether their hemipancreas would provide adequate function for the recipient. Although we believe that these exclusion criteria have been helpful in eliminating high-risk donors from consideration of hemipancreas donation, we do not have any evidence to suggest that we have reduced the risk of developing diabetes following hemipancreatectomy. Future investigation will be necessary to determine if these criteria are successful in reducing diabetes following hemipancreas donation.

The metabolic testing (Table 19.1-3) performed in the evaluation of potential pancreas donors includes a standard oral glucose tolerance test, hemoglobin $A_{1c}$, and measurement of antibodies associated with type 1 diabetes. In addition, a comprehensive insulin secretory test is done in the fasting state. In this test, both arginine- and glucose-induced insulin secretion are measured under basal conditions. Functional beta cell reserve is then measured by the glucose potentiation of arginine induced insulin secretion test (GPAIS) in which the arginine stimulation test is repeated after glucose has been administered intravenously at a rate of 900 mg/min for 60 minutes.

**TABLE 19.1-3**

## METABOLIC TESTING FOR LIVING DONOR PANCREAS CANDIDATES*

1. **Fasting glucose level (post 10- to 16-hour fast)**

2. **Hemoglobin $A_{1c}$ level**

3. **Oral glucose tolerance test (OGTT):**
   A > 150 g carbohydrate diet is given for 3 days prior to the test and usual physical activity. After a 10- to 16-hour fast (water is permitted, smoking is not), a 75-g oral glucose load in 250–300 ml of water is given over 10 minutes. The end of the drink time is time 0. Measurement of glucose and insulin is performed at the following intervals: -10, -5, 0, 15, 30, 60, 90, 120, 150, 180, 240, and 300 minutes.

4. **Arginine stimulation test (AST):**
   A >150 g carbohydrate diet is given for 3 days prior to the test and usual physical activity. After a 10- to 16-hour fasting period (water is permitted, smoking is not), the test is commenced between 0730 and 1000 hrs., 5 g of arginine (arginine HC1 10%) via IV push is given over 30 seconds. Time 0 is at the end of the bolus. Measurement of glucose, insulin, glucagon, and C-peptide is performed at the following intervals: -10, -5, 0, 2, 3, 4, 5, 7, 10, 25, and 30 minutes. AIR to arginine is defined as the mean of the peak 3 insulin values between 2 and 5 min following the arginine injection with the basal value subtracted.

5. **Intravenous glucose tolerance test (IVGTT):**
   35 min after the arginine injection, 209m glucose is given IV over 30 seconds. The end of the infusion is time 0. Glucose, insulin, glucagon, and C-peptide are measured at the following intervals: -5, 0, 1, 3, 4, 5, 10, 15, 20, 25, and 30 minutes.
   Acute insulin response (AIR) to glucose is defined as the mean of the 3-, 4-, and 5-minute insulin values following the glucose injection with the basal value subtracted. Glucose disposal rate (kg) is defined as the slope of the natural log of glucose values between 10 and 30 min after injection. First-phase insulin release (FPIR) is defined as the sum of insulin levels at 1 and 3 min.

6. **Glucose potentiation of arginine-induced insulin secretion (GPAIS):**
   145 minutes after the last blood draw in the above test, a glucose infusion (D20W) at 900 mg/min is started through an IV pump. The infusion is maintained for 70 minutes. At minute 60, 5 g of arginine (10% arginine HCL) IV is given over 30 seconds. The end of the bolus is time 0. Measurement of glucose, insulin, glucagon, and C-peptide is performed at the following intervals: -10, 0, 2, 3, 4, 5, 7, and 10 minutes. Acute insulin response at 900 mg/min glucose potentiation (AIR-900) is defined as the mean of the 3 peak insulin values between 2 and 5 min with the basal value subtracted.

7. **Insulin autoantibodies (IAAS):**
   Measured by fluid-phase radioassay incorporating competition with cold insulin and precipitation with polyethylene glycol.

8. **GAD 65 autoantibodies (GAAS):**
   Measured in triplicate by radio-assay, using in vitro transcribed and translated recombinant human GAD (65-kDa isoform) and precipitation with protein A-sepharose.

9. **Islet cell antigen 512 autoantibodies (IC512):**
   ICA512 is measured by radio immunoassay in duplicate using a 96-well plate format with a recombinant ICA512 protein.

Figure 19.1-1 provides an example of the flow sheet used for such a secretory test. The secretory responses on this test are determined by calculating the mean of the 3 highest consecutive insulin values obtained in the first 5 minutes after the acute injections of glucose or arginine and then subtracting the basal values obtained before the acute injection from the mean value. A normal response should be greater than 300% of the basal. Those with a secretory response less than 300% of basal is informed that their risk of developing diabetes after hemipancreatectomy is high.

The principles for accepting a potential pancreas donor are not different from those for other solid-organ transplants. The potential donor must understand the nature of the procedure and the risk to his or her health, must not be coerced, must provide voluntary consent, must be mentally competent, and must be of legal age. All potential donors undergo a thorough medical, social, and, frequently, psychological evaluation. Initial screening usually rules out volunteers with major health problems, for example, current or previous disorders of the pancreas, active infections or malignancies, major personality disorders, and drug or alcohol dependence. Single parents of minor children are also excluded. The social and psychological evaluations assess the donor's voluntarism and altruism as well as the dynamics of the donor–recipient relationship.

The medical evaluation of potential pancreas donors includes both the pancreas-nonspecific and -specific tests. The former are the same as for kidney donation. They include the following: electrocardiogram (ECG) and chest radiograph; ABO blood typing and tissue typing; leukocyte crossmatch and panel-reactive antibody (PRA) tests; biochemistry profile (eg, electrolytes, serum creatinine and clearance, blood urea nitrogen, uric acid, serum protein, and albumin); liver function, tests; lipid profile; complete blood count; coagulation profile; hepatitis A, B, and C tests; cytomegalovirus (CMV), Epstein-Barr virus (EBV), human immunodeficiency virus (HIV) and rapid plasma reagin (RPR) testing; urine analysis and urine culture; in women ≤ 55 years old, serum pregnancy tests; in women ≥ 40 years old, mammogram and Pap smear; in all women, pelvic and breast examination; and, in men > 50 years, prostate-specific antigen (PSA) test. In addition, all potential donors must undergo a history and physical examination; SPK donors must also undergo serial blood pressure measurements.

In kidney transplantation, because of the extreme shortage of donor organs (in particular for blood group O recipients), transplants have been done using blood group $A_2$ (20% of all blood group A) donors and blood group O recipients. The results have been successful, explained by the low expression of A determinants in $A_2$ (vs $A_1$) kidneys (see Chapter 16.16.3c). If ABO isoagglutinins are eliminated by plasmapheresis (or immunoadsorption) and splenectomy of the recipient, kidney transplants using $A_1$ donor organs and blood group O recipients have also been successful. In the University of Minnesota series, two blood-"incompatible" pancreas transplants from living donors have been performed. In one case, the donor blood group was AB, and the recipient, B; in the other, the donor was $A_2$, and the recipient, O. Splenectomy was not performed in either case; baseline titers were < 1:128 and reduced with plasmapheresis to < 1:8 at the time of the transplant. In both SPK recipients, all grafts are functioning, although one kidney graft was recently diagnosed with chronic rejection. Pancreas transplants with a positive B-cell crossmatch have also been successfully performed after peritransplant administration of intravenous immunoglobulin (IVIG) and plasmapheresis.[10,11]

Once the potential donor has cleared all of the above tests, he or she still needs to undergo a radiographic study to determine the anatomic suitability of the pancreas. In contrast to living kidney donors in whom arterial variations are common, the blood supply to the distal pancreas via the splenic artery shows

| UNIVERSITY OF MINNESOTA Pancreas donor insulin secretion study AST/IVGTT/GPAIS |
|---|

**Place IV Lines before −45 min. Place heating pad on blood drawing arm. Total blood volume: 93ml**

| | Time | Sample # | Glucose (1 mL) | Insulin (2 mL) | Comments |
|---|---|---|---|---|---|
| | −10 | 1 | | | |
| | −5 | 2 | | | |
| | 0 | 3 | | | |

**At 0 minutes (after blood draw), give a Arginine 5 grams IV push over 30 seconds.**
**Time 0 is midpoint of bolus.**

| | Time | Sample # | Glucose | Insulin | |
|---|---|---|---|---|---|
| | +2 | 4 | | | |
| | +3 | 5 | | | |
| A | +4 | 6 | | | |
| S | +5 | 7 | | | |
| T | +7 | 8 | | | |
| | +10 | 9 | | | |
| | +25 | 10 | | | |
| | +30 | 11 | | | |

**At +35 minutes, give D50W (dextrose) 20 grams (40 cc) IV push over 30 seconds.**
**Re-zero stopwatch at mid-bolus.**

| | Time | Sample # | Glucose | Insulin | |
|---|---|---|---|---|---|
| I | +3 | 12 | | | |
| V | +4 | 13 | | | |
| | +5 | 14 | | | |
| G | +7 | 15 | | | |
| T | +10 | 16 | | | |
| T | +15 | 17 | | | |
| | +20 | 18 | | | |
| | +25 | 19 | | | |
| | +30 | 20 | | | |

**Patient may remove heating pad for the next hour (+30 to +90 mins).**

| | Time | Sample # | Glucose | Insulin | |
|---|---|---|---|---|---|
| | +120 | 21 | | | |
| | +125 | 22 | | | |

**At minute +125 begin dextrose (D10W) infusion @ 540 cc/hr (which will be 900 mg/min).**

| | Time | Sample # | Glucose | Insulin | |
|---|---|---|---|---|---|
| 9 | +175 | 23 | | | |
| 0 | +180 | 24 | | | |
| 0 | +185 | 25 | | | |

**At minute +185, give arginine 5 grams IV push over 30 seconds.**
**Re-zero stopwatch at mid-bolus.**

| | Time | Sample # | Glucose | Insulin | |
|---|---|---|---|---|---|
| G | +2 | 26 | | | |
| P | +3 | 27 | | | |
| A | +4 | 28 | | | |
| I | +5 | 29 | | | |
| S | +7 | 30 | | | |
| | +10 | 31 | | | |

**FIGURE 19.1-1**

Flowsheet used at the University of Minnesota during comprehensive insulin secretory study.

little variation. But, even in the presence of an anatomic variation (eg, splenic artery off the suprarenal aorta), a distal pancreatectomy is usually technically feasible. Until the mid-1990s, aortography was the gold standard for assessing the vascular anatomy of the donor's pancreas (and kidney, if both organs were to be donated at the same time). Since the mid-1990s, magnetic resonance imaging (MRI) and angiography (MRA) have become increasingly popular because of their less invasive nature. In addition, MRI/MRA studies provide details of parenchymal structure and allow 3D reconstruction of not only arterial but also venous anatomy. An alternative to MRI/MRA is computed tomography (CT) angiography (CTA), which also allows 3D vascular reconstruction. Thus, aortography is no longer used routinely, eliminating complications associated with this procedure, including pseudoaneurysms or hematomas at the arterial puncture site or, albeit rarely, artery thrombosis around the puncture site.

If several medically suitable pancreas donors are available, the final selection is based on the histocompatibility result: an HLA-identical sibling is the ideal choice (providing all other criteria for pancreas donation are met). If serologic and endocrinologic evaluation identifies several equally suitable donors, the volunteer with the least reactive mixed lymphocyte reaction (MLR) result is usually chosen. But, selection must also be determined by other factors, such as age and the donor-recipient relation.

Only a few pancreas transplants have been performed using living unrelated donors, primarily spouses. Altruistic donors have not yet been used in pancreas transplantation.[10]

The same inclusion and exclusion criteria as for pancreas donors apply for islet donors (see Chapters 20 to 23).

## FUTURE DIRECTIONS

Pancreas transplantation has become a standard from of therapy for patients with type 1 diabetes and advanced diabetic nephropathy who are considering or have received a kidney transplant. In addition, pancreas transplants alone or islet cell transplants have become therapies that successfully reverse hypoglycemia unawareness in patients with type 1 diabetes while making them insulin-independent. The availability of donor organs is and will continue to be a major factor limiting the number of pancreas and islet transplants that can be performed. Because of the shortage of donor organs, many have begun to advocate for expanding the use of living related donors in pancreas and islet transplantation.[12,13] However, whether preoperative testing can accurately eliminate those potential donors who are at risk to develop diabetes after hemipancreatectomy is still not clear. The interesting observations of Butler et al. (in which the apoptotic rates of beta cells were increased in humans with type 2 diabetes while the rates of beta cell replication were normal[14]) predict that insulin secretory rates at one point in time may be inadequate to determine if an individual can maintain normal glucose tolerance following a surgical reduction in beta cell mass. In the future, consideration may be given to postoperative administration of drugs like the GLP-1 analog exenatide that are known to regulate beta cell proliferation in animals,[15] but the effect of such agents on beta cell mass in humans is unknown. At the present time, potential donors and their families are best served by undergoing an intensive metabolic evaluation to ensure they have normal beta cell function before donation and by thorough counseling about the risks associated with hemipancreatectomy.

## References

1. U.S. Renal Data System USRDS. *Atlas of End-Stage Renal Disease in the United States*. Bethesda, MD, National Institutes of Health, National Institute of Diabetes and Digestive and Kidney Diseases; 2004.
2. Gruessner AC, Sutherland DE. Pancreas transplants for United States (US) and non-US cases as reported to the International Pancreas Transplant Registry (IPTR) and to the United Network for Organ Sharing (UNOS). *Clin Transpl* 1997;45,.
3. Gruessner RW, Sutherland DE, Drangstveit MB, Bland BJ, Gruessner AC. Pancreas transplants from living donors: short- and long-term outcome. *Transplant Proc* 2001;33:819.
4. Bolinder J, Gunnarsson R, Tyden G, et al. Metabolic effects of living related pancreatic graft donation. *Transplant Proc* 1988;20:475.
5. Zielinski A, Nazarewski S, Bogetti D, et al. Simultaneous pancreas-kidney transplant from living related donor: a single-center experience. *Transplantation* 2003;76:547.
6. Kendall DM, Sutherland DE, Najarian JS, Goetz FC, Robertson RP. Effects of hemipancreatectomy on insulin secretion and glucose tolerance in healthy humans. *N Engl J Med* 1990;322:898.
7. Seaquist ER, Robertson RP. Effects of hemipancreatectomy on pancreatic alpha and beta cell function in healthy human donors. *J Clin Invest* 1992;89:1761.
8. Seaquist ER, Kahn SE, Clark PM, Hales CN, Porte D, Jr., Robertson RP: Hyperproinsulinemia is associated with increased beta cell demand after hemipancreatectomy in humans. *J Clin Invest* 1996;97:455.
9. Seaquist ER, Pyzdrowski K, Moran A, Teuscher AU, Robertson RP. Insulin-mediated and glucose-mediated glucose uptake following hemipancreatectomy in healthy human donors. *Diabetologia* 1994;37:1036.
10. Gruessner RWG. Living donor pancreas transplantation. In: Gruessner RWG, Sutherland DER, eds. *Transplantation of the Pancreas*. New York: Springer-Verlag; 2004:423–440.
11. Barr ML, Belghiti J, Villamil FG, et al. A report of the Vancouver Forum on the care of the live organ donor: lung, liver, pancreas and intestine: data and medical guidelines. *Transplantation* 2006;81 (10):1373–1385.
12. Matsumoto S, Okitsu T, Iwanaga Y, et al. Insulin independence after living-donor distal pancreatectomy and islet allotransplantation. *Lancet* 2005;365:1642.
13. Shapiro AM, Lakey JR, Paty BW, et al. Strategic opportunities in clinical islet transplantation. *Transplantation* 2005;79:1304.
14. Butler AE, Janson J, Bonner-Weir S, et al. Beta-cell deficit and increased beta-cell apoptosis in humans with type 2 diabetes. *Diabetes* 2003;52:102.
15. Brubaker PL, Drucker DJ. Minireview: Glucagon-like peptides regulate cell proliferation and apoptosis in the pancreas, gut, and central nervous system. *Endocrinology* 2004;145:2653.

## 19.2   SURGICAL PROCEDURES AND PERIOPERATIVE CARE

### 19.2.1   Standard Open Distal Pancreatectomy

*José Oberholzer, MD, José G. Avila, MD,*
*Enrico Benedetti, MD*

Living organ donation has experienced a steady increase since the first successful living related kidney transplant was performed between identical twins by Joseph Murray in 1954 in Boston.[1] Based on information reported in December 2002 to the United Network for Organ Sharing (UNOS) there were 6,535 living donors recovered in 2001, representing a 258% increase over those recovered in 1988 in the United States.[2] This increased activity in living organ transplantation is mainly due to the increasing gap between patients on the waiting list and available cadaveric donors with desperately increasing waiting times. The increase in living organ donation may also be the consequence of improved and less invasive donor operations, and optimized perioperative care for donors and recipients.[3] The improvement in short-term patient and graft survival is largely due to the decrease in surgical complications; the advent of new immunosuppression therapies has not yet had the expected impact on long-term graft survival.[4]

Organs procured from living donors are in general of better quality than those procured from a cadaver donor. Other benefits of living donation are the possibility of prospective cross match with the option of using desensitization protocols, potentially better HLA matching and reduced period of organ preservation and ischemia time. All these factors may allow for using less immunosuppression with consequently lower rates of posttransplant infections and malignancies. Of course living donation also alleviates the current organ shortage and reduces waiting time for recipients. On the other hand, these advantages for the recipients are facing obvious disadvantages for the donor undergoing a substantial operation for altruistic reasons with possible long-term consequences and complications.

Diabetic patients with end-stage renal disease (ESRD) manifest the highest mortality of any group of patients on dialysis[5] and early transplantation is possibly of greatest benefit for this patient population.[6] According to the Diabetes Control and Complications Trial (DCCT),[7] having an intense regimen of external insulin therapy can decrease the incidence of secondary complications of diabetes, but considerably increases the risk of hypoglycemia. In addition, other groups have shown that despite an aggressive exogenous insulin therapy, long-term life-threatening complications including nephropathy can still develop in diabetic patients.[8] The most accurate glycemic control and insulin independence can be achieved by endocrine replacement in the form of either whole pancreas[6,9] or islet transplantation.[10,11]

The first pancreas transplant using a living donor was performed in June 20, 1979, at the University of Minnesota.[12] Since then, according to the International Pancreas Transplant Registry (IPTR), as of October 2001, 142 pancreas transplants had been performed worldwide, of which 135 were performed in the United States with 0% mortality.[13] The three main surgical strategies to utilize living donors in diabetic patients are (1) pancreas after living donor kidney transplant (PAK), (2) simultaneous cadaver pancreas and living donor kidney (SCPLDK), and (3) living donor simultaneous pancreas and kidney transplant (LDSPK). In the future, pancreata procured from living donor may also represent a source for islet transplantation, although islet isolation techniques have to become more reliable before this can be considered on a larger scale.[14]

Simultaneous pancreas and kidney transplants using a cadaver donors has become the standard method of treatment of uremic diabetic patients,[3] performed more commonly than PAK,[15] which has driven a highly, unmet demand for cadaver SPK donors. Because of the shortage of cadaver kidney donors and the less favorable long-term pancreas transplant outcomes in PAK compared to SPK, the use of LDSPK transplants has been advocated.[16–19] Current techniques have shown a high degree of safety for the donor and low morbidity in the recipient.[18]

Current immunosuppression, plasmapheresis with or without splenectomy allows for further expanding the indications for living organ donation by reducing immunological barriers such as positive crossmatch or ABO incompatibility between recipient and donor.[20–22] Although kidney transplantation in the presence of positive crossmatch or ABO incompatibility has been performed by several centers, ABO-incompatible pancreas transplantation from a living donor has only been recently performed successfully.[23]

The main indication for the use of living donors for pancreas transplantation may present the highly presensitized recipient who would otherwise have a very long waiting time and significant risk of dying while on the waiting list.

## DONOR SURGICAL PROCEDURE

### Standard (Open) Procurement of the Distal Pancreas from a Living Donor

Distal pancreatic resection for transplantation is distinct from distal resection for other causes in that the manipulation of the pancreas should be as gentle as possible in order to avoid the development of pancreatitis in the donor and the recipient; the splenic artery and vein must be well preserved, and the spleen should not be removed.

After the induction of general anesthesia, the placement and management of the patient on the table follow the same routine guidelines as for any type of major procedures (nasogastric suction, Foley catheter bladder drainage, and prophylactic antibiotics). Either a bilateral subcostal or a supraumbilical midline incision is performed. The peritoneal cavity is opened, and from the surgical field the nasogastric tube can be adjusted along the greater curvature of the stomach facilitating decompression. Following, the stomach can be reflected upward and the transverse colon downward; the gastrocolic ligament is divided close to the transverse colon from the pylorus toward the splenic flexure of the colon (Figure 19.2.1-1). Most of the short gastric vessels should be preserved and also the right gastroepiploic artery to assure appropriate blood flow to the spleen. Once access is obtained to the retroperitoneal plain through the division of the gastrocolic ligament, the body and tail of the pancreas and the superior pole of the spleen can be reached.

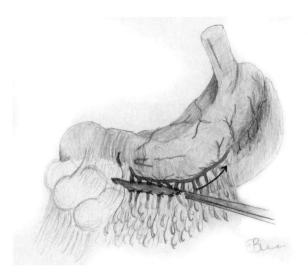

**FIGURE 19.2.1-1**

Division of the gastrocolic ligament with preservation of the gastroepiploic artery, the short gastric vessels, and the splenocolic ligament.

The inferior margin of the distal pancreas can be mobilized by dissecting the retroperitoneal attachments, ligating, dividing small arteries and veins that pass from the pancreas to the mesocolon and retroperitoneum, although the retropancreatic plane is mostly avascular. At the level of the transition between the pancreatic body and tail, the superior border of the pancreas is avascular. A peritoneal incision can be made at this level approaching from a small tunnel created along the posterior surface of the pancreas. A large vessel loop can be passed through to allow for the retraction of the tail to protect it during dissection of the splenic hilum (Figure 19.2.1-2). At this point, a peritoneal incision is made over the splenic hilum and the pancreas is dissected off from it. The main trunks of the distal splenic artery and vein are ligated and divided (Figure 19.2.1-2 and Color Plates, Figure PA-1) followed by ligation and division of the smaller branches of splenic artery and vein as close to the tail of the pancreas as possible in order to help preserve the collateral blood flow to the spleen from gastroepiploic, short gastric, and left gastric arteries. The splenic artery should always be divided first to avoid venous congestion of the spleen.

After dissection of the tail of the pancreas from the splenic hilum, the superior margin can be mobilized. The splenic artery and vein must be retained intact throughout the body and the tail of the pancreas (Figure 19.2.1-3). Care must be taken to ligate and divide all of the lymphatic and small blood vessels that course between the pancreas and the retroperitoneal tissues. Once this is performed, the pancreas can be elevated from its bed. The inferior mesenteric vein is ligated and divided at its junction with the splenic vein (Figure 19.2.1-3). If the inferior mesenteric vein does not drain directly into the splenic vein, it should be preserved. The junction of the superior mesenteric and splenic veins, and the most proximal portion of the portal vein are located directly behind the neck of the pancreas, which is the site of surgical division of the gland. The superior mesenteric vein is isolated inferiorly to the pancreas, and the portal vein is isolated at the superior margin of the pancreas, taking care of not damaging the hepatic and gastroduodenal arteries or the common bile duct. At this point, a finger should be able to encircle the neck of the pancreas by passing along the avascular plane behind the pancreas and anterior to the portal vein (Figure 19.2.1-4). After this, the splenic artery should

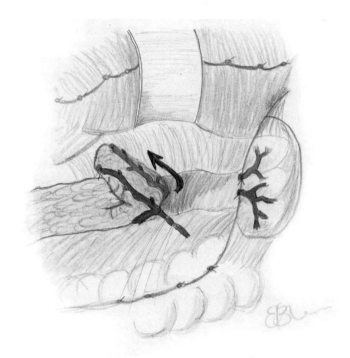

**FIGURE 19.2.1-3**

Medial mobilization of the posterior surface of the tail of the pancreas; the inferior mesenteric vein is ligated and divided.

be dissected all the way up to the celiac artery. Alternatively, the common hepatic artery can be identified distally in order to prevent a proximal spasm, but neither the common hepatic nor the left gastric artery dissection is required if the splenic artery can be identified unequivocally.

Once the vascular structures are securely identified and freed, the pancreas is divided at the level of the neck (anterior to the portal vein) (Figure 19.2.1-5 and Color Plates, Figure PA-2). It is suggested that the pancreatic parenchyma is divided between ligatures of 4–0 or 3–0 absorbable sutures placed at the upper and

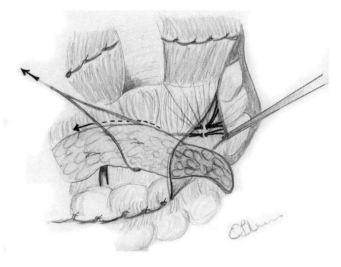

**FIGURE 19.2.1-2**

Ligation and division of the distal splenic artery and vein. A loop is placed around the tail of the pancreas for anteriomedial traction.

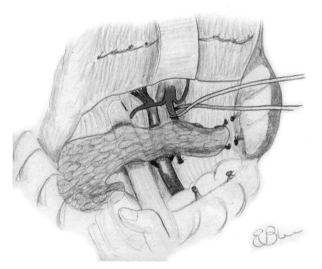

**FIGURE 19.2.1-4**

Isolation of the pancreatic neck and the proximal splenic artery (looped).

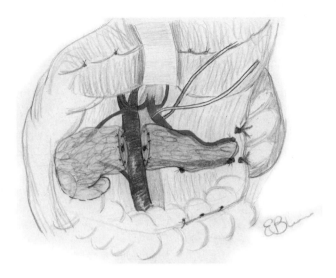

**FIGURE 19.2.1-5**

Division of the pancreatic head.

lower margin of the pancreas, followed by identification of the pancreatic main duct, which is divided with a scalpel and its proximal end sewn with 5–0 or 6–0 nonabsorbable suture.

Heparin, 70 U/kg, is given intravenously after complete dissection of the pancreas. Then, a vascular clamp is placed on the splenic artery approximately 0.5 to 1 cm distal to its origin from the celiac artery and then divided (Figure 19.2.1-6). Another vascular clamp should be placed occluding partly the superior mesenteric and portal veins, then the splenic vein should be divided where it enters the superior mesenteric vein (Color Plates, Figure PA-3). Once this is done, the distal pancreas can be removed. At this point, protamine sulfate should be given to the patient in order to reverse the effect of heparin.

The donor splenic artery and vein are sewn with 5–0 nonabsorbable sutures, making sure not to cause narrowing of the celiac artery or the superior mesenteric vein (Figure 19.2.1-6). The

cut surface of the proximal pancreas is oversewn with interrupted 4–0 nonabsorbable sutures in a U-type fashion to avoid leakage of pancreatic fluids coming from smaller ducts.

Once the distal pancreas is removed, it should be stored and flushed (low pressure) through the splenic artery with approximately 200 mL of UW solution at 4ºC on the back-table.

Assessment of the spleen should be performed after the donor procedure is completed, and only in the case of major bleeding form the splenic hilum or from the spleen itself, it should be removed. After homeostasis is ensured, closure of the abdomen is performed by standard techniques, and usually the placement of drains is not necessary. Once in the recovery room, the donor is extubated and returned to the general surgery ward.

### Standard (Open), Simultaneous Procurement of the Left Kidney and Distal Pancreas from a Living Donor

If the living donor procurement includes the left kidney, a xifoumbilical midline laparotomy incision is performed. After opening the abdominal cavity, the nasogastric tube is adjusted along the greater curvature of the stomach as described above. It is suggested that whenever possible, the left kidney should be procured because of simultaneous mobilization of the distal pancreas, greater length of the renal vein, and avoidance of liver mobilization.[23] In order to expose the kidney, the attachments of the descending colon to the lateral peritoneum are divided from the splenocolic ligament down to the sigmoid colon and the mobilization continues to the level of the aorta and vena cava. The ureter is identified at the level of the common iliac artery and dissection is continued toward the lower pole of the kidney. The gonadal vein can be identified at the same level as the ureter and should be ligated and divided at its junction with the left renal vein. Also, the left adrenal vein is ligated at its junction with the left renal vein. The anterior and posterior aspects of the left renal vein are dissected. Lumbar veins tributaries to the left renal vein should also be ligated and divided at their junction. Posterior, and most commonly superior from the left renal vein, the renal artery is dissected up to its origin in the aorta. After a lateral incision of Gerota's fascia, the kidney is mobilized from its superior pole down. First, the lateral and anterior aspects of the kidney should be completely dissected free, then, the retroperitoneal attachments to the posterior aspects of the kidney are dissected. Finally, the left adrenal gland is dissected off from the upper pole of the kidney. At this point, mannitol and furosemide are given intravenously, keeping in mind that central venous pressure and urine output should be constantly monitored. Only the distal part of the ureter is ligated at the level where it crosses the iliac vessels in order to see directly the urine output from the kidney; heparin is given intravenously at a dose of 70 U/kg. First the renal artery is clamped with vascular clamps; then the renal vein and the kidney is excised. Protamine is given intravenously to counteract the heparin. The renal artery and vein are sewn with 5–0 nonabsorbable sutures. Following, the dissection of the pancreas should be initiated and the distal pancreatectomy performed as previously described.

### Postoperative Care

Postoperative care of living pancreas donors is similar to that of any patient undergoing a major abdominal procedure. Once the donor is placed back in the general surgery ward where vital signs, urine output, and blood glucose levels are closely monitored

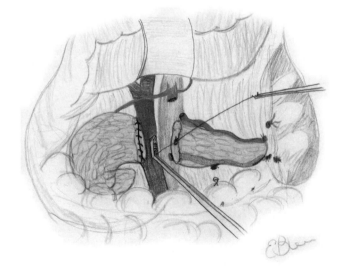

**FIGURE 19.2.1-6**

Removal of the distal pancreas; suture ligation of the proximal splenic artery and splenic vein.

throughout the night or over the first 12 hours, serial hemoglobin levels are determined to monitor for possible postoperative bleeding. In order to assess integrity and the function of the remaining pancreas, serum amylase, lipase, and blood sugar levels are measured. The nasogastric tube remains connected to a low suction, but can be removed once bowel function returns. Oral intake usually resumes within the first 3 days. Donors with postoperative shoulder or left flank pain should undergo splenic radionuclide or CT scans to ensure viability of the spleen or formation of an abscess. The prophylactic use of octreotide at a dose of 100 μg subcutaneously every 8 hours for 5 days starting during the surgery has been shown to reduce the incidence of pancreatic leaks.[24–26] The discharge of the donor from the hospital takes place usually 7 ± 4 days after the operation.

## References

1. Harrison JH, Merrill JP, Murray JE. Renal homotransplantation in identical twins. *Surg Forum* 1956;6(1955):432–436.
2. Rosendale JD, Dean JR. Organ donation in the United States: 1988-2001. *Clin Transpl* 2002;93–104.
3. Sutherland DE, Gruessner RW, Dunn DL, et al. Lessons learned from more than 1,000 pancreas transplants at a single institution. *Ann Surg* 2001;233(4):463–501.
4. Meier-Kriesche HU, Schold JD, Srinivas TR, et al. Lack of improvement in renal allograft survival despite a marked decrease in acute rejection rates over the most recent era. *Am J Transplant* 2004;4(3):378–383.
5. Jukema JW, Smets YF, van der Pijl JW, et al. Impact of simultaneous pancreas and kidney transplantation on progression of coronary atherosclerosis in patients with end-stage renal failure due to type 1 diabetes. *Diabetes Care* 2002;25(5):906–911.
6. Cicalese L, Giacomoni A, Rastellini C, et al. Pancreatic transplantation: a review. *Int Surg* 1999;84(4):305–312.
7. Diabetes Control and Complications Trial (DCCT). Update. DCCT Research Group. *Diabetes Care* 1999;13(4):427–433.
8. Rayhill SC, D'Alessandro AM, Odorico JS, et al. Simultaneous pancreas-kidney transplantation and living related donor renal transplantation in patients with diabetes: is there a difference in survival? *Ann Surg* 2000;231(3):417–423.
9. Fioretto P, Steffes MW, Sutherland DE, et al. Reversal of lesions of diabetic nephropathy after pancreas transplantation. *N Engl J Med* 1998;339(2):69–75.
10. Shapiro AM, Lakey JR, Ryan EA, et al. Islet transplantation in seven patients with type 1 diabetes mellitus using a glucocorticoid-free immunosuppressive regimen. *N Engl J Med* 2000;343(4):230–238.
11. Kessler L, Passemard R, Oberholzer J, et al. Reduction of blood glucose variability in type 1 diabetic patients treated by pancreatic islet transplantation: interest of continuous glucose monitoring. *Diabetes Care* 2000;25(12):2256–2262.
12. Sutherland DE, Goetz FC, Najarian JS. Living-related donor segmental pancreatectomy for transplantation. *Transplant Proc* 1980;12(4Suppl2):19–25.
13. Gruessner AC, Sutherland DE. Report for the international pancreas transplant registry-2000. *Transplant Proc* 2001;33(1-2):1643–1646.
14. Matsumoto S, Okitsu T, Iwanaga Y, et al. Insulin independence after living-donor distal pancreatectomy and islet allotransplantation. *Lancet* 2005;365(9471):1642–1644.
15. Gruessner AC, Sutherland DE. Analysis of United States (US) and non-US pancreas transplants reported to the United network for organ sharing (UNOS) and the international pancreas transplant registry (IPTR) as of October 2001. *Clin Transpl* 2001;41–72.
16. Benedetti E, Dunn T, Massad MG, et al.: Successful living related simultaneous pancreas-kidney transplant between identical twins. *Transplantation* 1999;67(6):915–918.
17. Benedetti E, Rastellini C, Sileri P, et al.: Successful simultaneous pancreas-kidney transplantation from well-matched living-related donors. *Transplant Proc* 2001;33(1-2):1689.
18. Zielinski A, Nazarewski S, Bogetti D, et al. Simultaneous pancreas-kidney transplant from living related donor: a single-center experience. *Transplantation* 2003;76(3):547–552.
19. Sammartino C, Pham T, Panaro F, et al. Successful simultaneous pancreas kidney transplantation from living-related donor against positive cross-match. *Am J Transplant* 2004;4(1):140–143.
20. Thielke J, DeChristopher PJ, Sankary H, et al. Highly successful living donor kidney transplantation after conversion to negative of a previously positive flow-cytometry cross-match by pretransplant plasmapheresis. *Transplant Proc* 2005;37(2):643–644.
21. Montgomery RA, Zachary AA, Racusen LC, et al. Plasmapheresis and intravenous immune globulin provides effective rescue therapy for refractory humoral rejection and allows kidneys to be successfully transplanted into cross-match-positive recipients. *Transplantation* 2000;70(6):887–895.
22. Segev DL, Simpkins CE, Warren DS, et al. ABO Incompatible High-Titer Renal Transplantation without Splenectomy or Anti-CD20 Treatment. *Am J Transplant* 2005;5(10):2570–2575.
23. Gruessner R. Living Donor Pancreas Transplantation. In: Guessner R, Sutherland D, eds. *Transplantation of the Pancreas.* New York: Springer-Verlag; 2004:423.
24. Benedetti E, Coady NT, Asolati M, et al. A prospective randomized clinical trial of perioperative treatment with octreotide in pancreas transplantation. *Am J Surg* 1998;175(1):14–17.
25. Benedetti E, Coady NT, Asolati M, et al. Value of perioperative treatment with sandostatin after pancreas transplantation: a prospective randomized trial. *Transplant Proc* 1998;30(2):432–433.
26. Berberat PO, Friess H, Uhl W, et al. The role of octreotide in the prevention of complications following pancreatic resection. *Digestion* 1999;60(Suppl2):15–22.

### 19.2.2 Laparoscopic Donor Distal Pancreatectomy

*Rainer W.G. Gruessner, MD*

## INTRODUCTION

The advent of laparoscopic technology has offered an alternative to open surgical procedures. In the field of transplant surgery, the viability of this new technology was first demonstrated by laparoscopic donor nephrectomy,[1] which rapidly became the procedure of choice for kidney donation (see Chapter 15.5). Laparoscopic donor nephrectomy is associated with reduced hospital stay, decreased need for pain medications, and more rapid convalescence. Cosmetically, it is more appealing to potential donors, as compared with the traditional flank incision used for open nephrectomy. Equally important, it is equivalent to the open procedure regarding donor safety and allograft quality.[2–6] The laparoscopic approach has even become an option for selected liver donors (see Chapter 29.3.3), specifically for pediatric recipients.[7]

Laparoscopic procedures are increasingly used to treat a variety of pancreatic pathologies.[8–11] Laparoscopic distal pancreatectomy for benign or malignant lesions appears to be safe, with the additional benefits of reduced hospital costs, accelerated postoperative recovery, early resumption of oral nutritional intake, and decreased need for pain medications.

As with other laparoscopic procedures, distal pancreatectomy can be done using either the hand-assisted or full laparoscopic approach. I prefer the hand-assisted (vs full) laparoscopic approach for distal pancreatectomy from a living donor (LD), because having tactile feedback greatly facilitates safe dissection of the key vascular structures (ie, the celiac axis and the splenic/superior mesenteric vein confluence).[12] In contrast to laparoscopic distal pancreatectomy for pancreatic pathologies or even for LD islet transplants, safe retrieval of the vascular structures is paramount for the success of LD segmental pancreas transplants. An additional, albeit minor, advantage of the hand-assisted (vs full) approach is the shorter extraction time of the distal pancreas. The hand-assisted procedure can be accomplished with a single 6-cm periumbilical incision and only two 12-mm ports, whereas the full laparoscopic approach usually requires placement of ≥ 3 ports and a 6-cm (preferably Pfannenstiel) incision for safe extraction of the distal pancreas.

The first laparoscopic distal pancreatectomy from an LD (in combination with a simultaneous left nephrectomy) was performed at the University of Minnesota on November 22, 2000.[12] As of September 15, 2006, a total of seven such operations have now been performed at the University of Minnesota; our initial experience with the first five laparoscopic LDs was published in 2005.[13]

In the "open technique" era, we had already shown that a distal pancreatectomy in an LD could be done without a concurrent splenectomy. A spleen-preserving distal pancreatectomy was first described by Sutherland et al. in 1980 for a pancreas LD[14]: they showed that spleen preservation is possible if the blood supply via the right gastroepiploic vessels, the short gastric vessels, and the splenic ligaments (eg, splenocolic, gastrocolic) is left intact. Nuclear medicine studies by other researchers showed that, despite markedly decreased or absent uptake in the immediate postoperative period, splenic blood flow can return to normal or near-normal by 2 weeks.[15] Later, in 1988, Warshaw described spleen-preserving pancreatectomies in 22 of 25 patients with benign or malignant pancreatic disorders[16]; in that series, spleen scans proved splenic viability and function. The first laparoscopic distal pancreatectomy from an LD was also accomplished with spleen preservation[12]; only one of the seven subsequent operations in the University of Minnesota experience required a laparoscopic splenectomy at the time of the distal pancreatectomy.[13] Increasingly, laparoscopic distal pancreatectomies for benign or malignant pancreatic disorders are also performed with spleen preservation.[17–20]

## OPERATIVE PROCEDURE

After induction of general anesthesia, the donor is placed on the operating table in a supine position, in order to allow occasional rotation to a slightly right lateral decubitus position. Central venous access, nasogastric suction, Foley catheter bladder drainage, and sequential compression devices are all used. Prophylactic antibiotics are administered intravenously before the incision is made and repeated every 4 hours during the procedure.

The operating surgeon and the scrub nurse stand on the donor's right; the assistant and camera operator, on the left. Standard laparoscopic instrumentation and at least two television monitors are used. A periumbilical incision (about 7 cm long) is made, providing a better cosmetic result and more maneuvering space for the inserted left hand, as compared with a supraumbilical incision. A Gel-port (Applied Medical, Rancho Santa Margarita, CA) is placed to allow for hand assistance. The first 12-mm trocar is placed about 3 cm lateral and caudad to the umbilicus, along the lateral edge of the left rectus muscle, for insertion of a 30-degree laparoscope and camera. After a pneumoperitoneum (12 to 14 mm Hg) is created, the second trocar is placed in the left upper midabdomen in the plane of the anterior axillary line. This second "working" port allows insertion of the Ultracision Harmonic Scalpel (Ethicon Endo-Surgery, Inc., Cincinnati, OH) or ultrasonic shears, laparoscopic scissors, and other instruments (Color Plates, Figure PA-4).

The dissection begins by mobilizing the left curvature of the colon and the descending colon from the abdominal wall, using the harmonic scalpel. The colon is retracted medially, exposing the left lateral edge of the abdominal aorta. The inferior margin of the pancreas is separated from the left Gerota's fascia and the adrenal gland with the harmonic scalpel. This inferior approach, which involves dissecting first along the inferior margin of the pancreas, avoids dividing the gastrocolic ligament and increases the chances of leaving the right gastroepiploic vessels intact.

The inferior mesenteric vein is then identified, ligated with clips, and divided near its insertion into the splenic vein. However, dissection and mobilization of the inferior mesenteric vein are not required if it drains directly into the superior mesenteric vein.

A retropancreatic tunnel is created between the inferior and superior margin of the pancreas. Care is taken to include the splenic artery (which runs posteriorly and cranially to the upper border of the pancreas) in this plane of dissection. The newly created tunnel allows passage of the left index finger along the underside of the pancreas (Figure PA-5). It also allows placement of a vessel loop around the tail of the pancreas (including the splenic vessels), in order to facilitate atraumatic anteromedial retraction of the pancreas (Color Plates, Figure PA-5).

The avascular plane of the superior margin of the pancreas is taken down laterally toward the spleen, using the harmonic scalpel. Retracting the distal pancreas anteriorly and medially separates the tail of the pancreas from the spleen, thereby exposing the most medial short gastric veins and the splenic hilum. The splenic artery and vein are individually dissected free in the hilum, then clipped twice on both sides and divided. The remaining tissue (including the medial short gastric veins) is divided using a 35-mm vascular stapler (ETS Flex Endoscopic Articulating Linear Cutter, Ethicon Endo-Surgery, Inc.; Figure 19.2.2-1C). In the process of dissecting the superior margin of the pancreas and taking down the splenic hilum, care is taken not to disturb the (lateral) short gastric veins and right gastroepiploic vessels, because they constitute the major remaining blood supply to and from the spleen. Likewise, the lateral and inferior attachments of the spleen are preserved.

The posterior surface of the distal pancreas is freed from its retroperitoneal attachments to the level of the portal vein, using electrocautery. The splenic vein is dissected free circumferentially at its confluence with the superior mesenteric vein, taking care to preserve all small tributaries from the distal pancreas. Finally, the splenic artery is traced back to its takeoff from the celiac axis and also circumferentially dissected free (Figure 19.2.2-1D). The neck is now completely mobilized above the anterior surfaces of the superior mesenteric and portal veins.

The pancreas is then stapled across, using a 45-mm ETS Flex Linear Articulating Stapler (Color Plates, Figure PA-6; Ethicon Endo-Surgery, Inc.). Depending on the size of the neck of the pancreas, 1 reload may be necessary (Figure 19.2.2-1E). The donor is now given 70 U/kg of heparin intravenously. The splenic artery is clipped twice and divided about 0.5 to 1 cm distal from its origin in the celiac artery in order to avoid any stenosis of the common hepatic artery (Figure 19.2.2-1F). The splenic vein is also clipped twice (Figure 19.2.2-1G), about 0.5 cm distal to the portal confluence, and divided with laparoscopic scissors. After

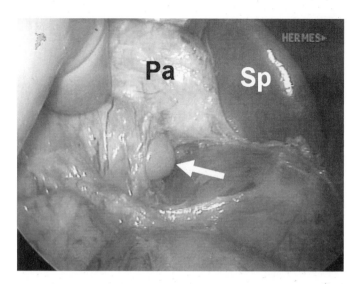

**FIGURE 19.2.2-1A**

Retroperitoneal attachments between the pancreas (Pa) and the spleen (Sp) have been taken; the tip of the surgeon's index finger (arrow) is passed around the superior margin of the distal pancreas.

the vessels are divided, protamine (10 mg/1,000 U heparin) is administered intravenously.

The distal pancreas is extracted by hand through the periumbilical midline incision and passed off to the recipient team. After the pneumoperitoneum is restored, hemostasis is achieved. The staple line of the proximal pancreas is oversewn in a running fashion with a 4–O nonabsorbable suture, not only to achieve hemostasis but also to prevent leakage from the pancreatic duct or the cut surface (Figure 19.2.2-H). If the pancreatic duct can be identified in the staple line, it is individually oversewn with a 5–O nonabsorbable suture or clipped (Color Plates, Figure PA-7).

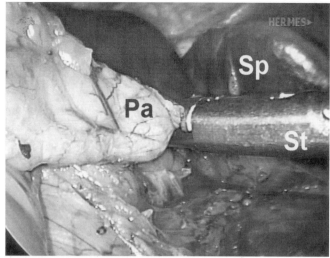

**FIGURE 19.2.2-1C**

The splenic hilum is stapled across with a 35-mm endovascular stapler (St), thereby separating the distal pancreas (Pa) from the spleen (Sp).

Hemostasis is ensured and the viability of the spleen is assessed. After the distal splenic artery and vein are divided, the consistency of the spleen is soft, and the color frequently turns from pink to purple because of the significantly diminished blood flow. The spleen rarely has to be removed for bleeding. A drain is left in the abdomen, right next to the spleen, only in the event of major capsular tear(s) or ongoing bleeding from the splenic surface.

The abdomen is irrigated and the port sites are closed under direct vision using O-polyglactin sutures on a suture passer (Endoclose system, Autosuture, Tyco Healthcare Group LP, Norwalk, CT). The midline fascia is closed using 0-looped polypropylene sutures.

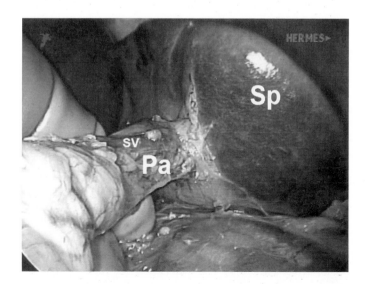

**FIGURE 19.2.2-1B**

Medial retraction of the distal pancreas (Pa) exposing the space between the Pa and the spleen (Sp). The main trunks of the splenic artery and splenic vein (SV) have been clipped and divided. A bridge containing soft tissue and smaller branches still connect the distal Pa and Sp.

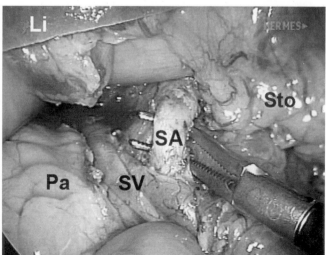

**FIGURE 19.2.2-1D**

A laparoscopic right angle is passed around the splenic artery (SA) at its takeoff from the celiac axis. In this case, the splenic vein (SV) was located on the anterior surface of the pancreas (Pa). The liver (Li) and stomach (Sto) are in close proximity.

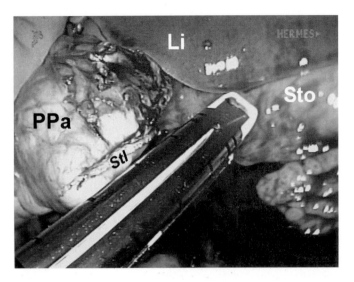

**FIGURE 19.2.2-1E**

The pancreatic neck has been stapled across with a 45-mm stapler (Stl = staple line). The proximal pancreas (PPa), the liver (Li), and the stomach (Sto) are also shown. The splenic artery (SA) and vein (SV) are not yet divided.

The median operative time for LDs undergoing both a distal pancreatectomy and a nephrectomy with the open technique was 6 hours and 50 minutes; with the laparoscopic technique, 7 hours and 15 minutes. The actual operative time, however, was probably shorter than reported, because the donor surgeons usually have to wait about 1.5 to 2 hours intraoperatively for the recipient team to prepare to receive the organs. When a distal pancreatectomy is performed, the pneumoperitoneum is aborted during the waiting time.

## OPERATIVE VARIATIONS

If the distal pancreas is procured along with a kidney, the left kidney (assuming normal anatomy) is preferred. Advantages for the

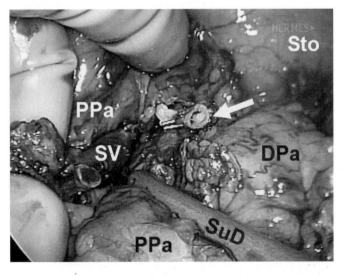

**FIGURE 19.2.2-1F**

The splenic artery is clipped twice at its takeoff from the celiac axis (white arrow). A suction device (SuD) removes the blood between the divided splenic artery and the splenic vein. The splenic vein and the distal pancreas (DPa) are pulled in a caudad direction.

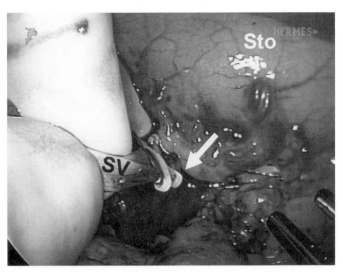

**FIGURE 19.2.2-1G**

The splenic vein (SV) is clipped twice at its confluence with the superior mesenteric vein. The SV is divided with endoscopic scissors.

donor operation of using the left (vs the right) kidney include the following (1) concurrent mobilization of the inferior margin of the pancreas, as part of the dissection of the upper pole of the kidney; (2) only minor donor rotation from the standard right to a slightly right lateral decubitus position, which facilitates mobilization of the pancreas; (3) avoidance of at least two additional port sites; and (4) avoidance of mobilization of the ascending colon and right colonic flexure. For the recipient operation, the left kidney is also preferable because of the longer renal vein.

### Left Kidney

If the left kidney is procured laparoscopically along with the distal pancreas, the operating table is flexed at a point midway between the donor's iliac crest and rib cage and rotated 45 degrees (right

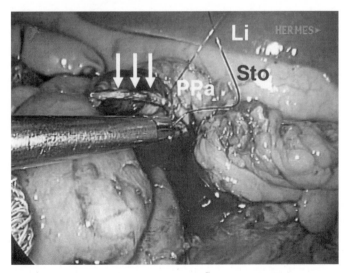

**FIGURE 19.2.2-1H**

The proximal pancreatic stump (PPa) (arrows showing the staple line) is oversewn with a 4–0 absorbable suture in a running fashion. The liver (Li) and the stomach (Sto) are shown in close proximity.

decubitus position) to open up the left subcostal space and to facilitate access to the left kidney (Color Plates, Figure PA-4).

The kidney is dissected and removed first. The technique is described in detail in Chapter 12.5.3. In brief, the left colonic flexure and the descending colon are first mobilized medially, to the level of the aorta. Then, the left ureter and the left gonadal vein are identified and dissected circumferentially at the level of the left common iliac artery. The ureter and the left gonadal vein are then mobilized up to the lower pole of the kidney.

Next, the left gonadal vein is ligated with clips and divided close to its entrance in the left renal vein. Likewise, the left adrenal vein is identified, clipped, and divided on the opposite side of the left renal vein. The left renal vein is circumferentially dissected free, down to and partly across the aorta. Any lumbar veins draining posteriorly into the renal vein are also clipped on both sides and divided. Complete mobilization of the left renal vein usually provides some exposure of the renal artery. The proximal renal artery is dissected free circumferentially down to its origin in the aorta. (Overlying lymphatic and ganglionic tissues are divided with the harmonic scalpel.) After the main vascular structures of the left kidney are completely dissected free, Gerota's fascia is incised anterolaterally, and all perinephric adhesions are taken down from the lower to the superior pole of the kidney. The adrenal gland is dissected off the upper pole with the harmonic scalpel. To maintain good urine output intraoperatively, mannitol and furosemide are given.

Once the kidney is completely mobilized, the ureter is clipped distally twice. Then, heparin (70 U/kg) is administered intravenously. The renal artery is clipped 2 or 3 times at its origin in the aorta and divided. The renal vein is divided proximal to the clipped stump of the left adrenal vein with a 35-mm vascular stapler (see above). The heparin effect is reversed with protamine sulfate (see above). The kidney is removed through the periumbilical midline incision and passed off to the recipient team. After the pneumoperitoneum is reestablished, hemostasis is achieved.

As attention is turned to the pancreas, it becomes evident that, during the dissection of the left kidney, most of the inferior margin of the pancreas has already been mobilized. The laparoscopic distal pancreatectomy continues as described above.

### Right Kidney

If the right kidney is to be removed, the donor is initially placed in the left lateral decubitus position. A peri- or infraumbilical midline incision (about 7 cm long) is made. The laparoscope/camera port site (using a 12-mm trocar) is about 3 cm below the umbilicus at the level of the lateral edge of the right rectus muscle. A second (working) port (for a 12-mm trocar) is usually placed between the umbilicus and the rib cage, about 3 cm to the right of the midline incision; this site is used to introduce the laparoscopic instruments. A third port (for a 5-mm trocar) is inserted laterally in the posterior axillary line, midway between the iliac crest and rib cage; this site allows insertion of a liver retractor. As on the left side, the colon is mobilized first by taking down all attachments to the lateral abdominal wall and mobilizing it medially to the level of the vena cava and the duodenum. The technique is described in detail in Chapter 12.5.3; note that the dissection of the renal vein is easier on the right (vs left) side because of the absence of tributaries (the right adrenal and gonadal veins drain separately into the vena cava). Other than that one note, the dissection, mobilization, and procurement are no different for the right (vs left) kidney. After extracting the right kidney and assuring hemostasis, the port sites are closed with the Endoclose system (Autosuture,

Tyco Healthcare Group LP, Norwalk, CT). The location of the port sites on the left sides are described above.

## POSTOPERATIVE CARE

Postoperative care of LDs undergoing laparoscopic distal pancreatectomy is similar to that of any patient undergoing a major laparoscopic procedure. The donor is usually extubated either in the operating room or in the recovery room. After an appropriate observation time, the donor is transferred to the general surgery or transplant ward. Vital signs are monitored closely over the first 12 hours. Serial hemoglobin levels are obtained to monitor for possible postoperative bleeding. Serial serum amylase levels are obtained to assess exocrine function; serial plasma glucose levels, to assess endocrine function. Only donors with postoperative shoulder or left flank pain (a rare development) should undergo splenic radionuclide or CT scans, in order to ensure viability of the spleen and to rule out formation of an abscess. Sequential $^{99mn}$Tc-sulfur colloid scans of the spleen have shown markedly decreased uptake initially, with normalization within 2 weeks postoperatively.[15]

In our series of laparoscopic distal pancreatectomies, all LDs were out of bed and ambulating within the first postoperative day. Most tolerated normal oral intake by postoperative day 3. Furthermore, all were back to their preoperative state of health and back to work within several weeks. Donor satisfaction was high from a cosmetic perspective. In our series, none of the LDs experienced pancreatitis, leak, or pseudocyst formation. The only perioperative complication was in one donor who required a splenectomy at the time of the initial distal pancreatectomy secondary to a completely infarcted spleen. Hemoglobin $A_{1c}$ levels have remained normal in all of our LDs, but the longest follow-up has only been 4 years.

## FUTURE DEVELOPMENTS

We prefer the hand-assisted laparoscopic approach, although the full laparoscopic approach may be similarly effective and safe. Nonetheless, as of September 15, 2006, the full approach has not been used in any LD, at our institution or elsewhere. Since the pancreas needs to be removed through an incision, the only advantage of the full laparoscopic procedure appears to be retraction of the distal pancreas through a Pfannenstiel (vs midline) incision, resulting in a better cosmetic outcome. But a potential disadvantage of the full laparoscopic approach is the lack of tactile feedback (particularly at the celiac axis and the splenic/superior mesenteric vein confluence)—a lack that would increase the difficulty of the vascular dissection. The lack of 3-dimensional visualization, inherent in laparoscopy, can be overcome with robot devices, such as the da Vinci surgical system (Intuitive Surgical, Sunnyvale, CA) (see Chapter 15.5.5).[21] As of September 15, 2006, one living donor pancreas and kidney procurement using the da Vinci surgical system has been done at the University of Illinois Medical Center (S. Horgan, personal communication, August 2006).

## References

1. Ratner LE, Ciseck LJ, Moore RG, et al. Laparoscopic live donor nephrectomy. *Transplantation* 1995;60:1047–1049.
2. Schweitzer EJ, Wilson J, Jacobs S, et al. Increased rates of donation with laparoscopic donor nephrectomy. *Ann Surg* 2000;232:392–400.

3. Leventhal JR, Kocak B, Salvaggio PR, et al. Laparoscopic donor nephrectomy 1997 to 2003: lessons learned with 500 cases at a single institution. *Surgery* 2004;136 (4):881–890.

4. Jacobs SC, Cho E, Foster C, Liao P, Bartlett ST. Laparoscopic donor nephrectomy: the University of Maryland 6-year experience. *J Urol* 2004;171:47–51.

5. Buell JF, Lee L, Martin JE, et al. Laparoscopic donor nephrectomy vs. open live donor nephrectomy: a quality of life and functional study. *Clin Transplant* 2005;19(1):102–109.

6. Melcher ML, Carter JT, Posselt A, et al. More than 500 consecutive laparoscopic donor nephrectomies without conversion or repeated surgery. *Arch Surg* 2005;140(9) 835–839; discussion 839–840.

7. Cherqui D, Soubrane O, Husson E, et al. Laparoscopic living donor hepatectomy for liver transplantation in children. *Lancet* 2002;359 (9304):392–396.

8. Cushieri A. Laparoscopic surgery of the pancreas. *JR Coll Surg Edinb* 1994;39:178–184.

9. Gagner M, Pomp A. Laparoscopic pylorus-preserving pancreatoduodenectomy. *Surg Endosc* 1994;8:408–410.

10. Dulucq JL, Wintringer P, Stabilini C, et al. Are major laparoscopic pancreatic resections worthwhile? A prospective study of 32 patients in a single institution. *Surg Endosc* 2005;19(8):1028–1034.

11. Mabrut JY, Fernandez-Cruz L, Azagra JS, et al. Hepatobiliary and Pancreatic Section (HBPS) of the Royal Belgian Society of Surgery; Belgian Group for Endoscopic Surgery (BGES); Club Coelio. Laparoscopic pancreatic resection: results of a multicenter European study of 127 patients. *Surgery* 2005;137(6):597–605.

12. Gruessner RWG, Kandaswamy R, Denny R. Laparoscopic simultaneous nephrectomy and distal pancreatectomy from a live donor. *J Am Coll Surg* 2001;193(3):333–337.

13. Tan M, Kandaswamy R, Sutherland DER, Gruessner RWG. Laparoscopic donor distal pancreatectomy for living donor pancreas and pancreas-kidney transplantation. *Am J Trans* 2005;5:1966–1970.

14. Sutherland DER, Goetz FC, Najarian JS. Living-related donor segmental pancreatectomy for transplantation. *Transplant Proc* 1980;12:19–25.

15. Crass JR, Frick MP, Loken MK. The scintigraphic appearance of the spleen following splenic artery resection. *Radiology* 1980;136:737–739.

16. Warshaw AL. Conservation of the spleen with distal pancreatectomy. *Arch Surg* 1988;123:550–553.

17. Ueno T, Masaaki O, Nishihara K, et al. Laparoscopic distal pancreatectomy with preservation of the spleen. Brief clinical report. *Surg Laprosc Percutan Tech* 1999;9:290–293.

18. Vezakis A, Davides D, Larvin M, McMahon MJ. Laparoscopic surgery combined with preservation of the spleen for distal pancreatic tumors. *Surg Endosc* 1999;13:26–29.

19. de Wilt JH, van Eijck CH, Hussain SM, Bonjer HJ. Laparoscopic spleen-preserving distal pancreatectomy after blunt abdominal trauma. *Injury* 2003;34(3):233–234.

20. Fernandez-Cruz L, Martinez I, Gilabert R, et al. Laparoscopic distal pancreatectomy combined with preservation of the spleen for cystic neoplasms of the pancreas. *J Gastrointest Surg* 2004;8(4):493–501.

21. Horgan S, Benedetti E, Moser F. Robotically assisted donor nephrectomy for kidney transplantation. *Am J Surg* 2004;188(4A):45S–51S.

# 19.3  MORBIDITY, MORTALITY, AND LONG-TERM OUTCOME

*Rainer W.G. Gruessner, MD*

## INTRODUCTION

According to the International Pancreas Transplant Registry (IPTR), pancreas transplants using living donors (LDs) are performed at only a few centers in the United States and Asia.[1] The reluctance to use LDs is based on the anatomy of the pancreas (an unpaired organ) and on the risk of serious organ-specific complications (eg, pancreatitis, leak, pseudocyst). Furthermore, possible deterioration of glucose metabolism in the LD, as a result of hemipancreatectomy, remains a lifelong concern. Nonetheless, it is important to emphasize that, according to IPTR and United Network for Organ Sharing (UNOS) data, no LD has died as a result of the surgical procedure.

## SURGICAL COMPLICATIONS

Overall, surgical complications are rare; < 5% of all LDs require a relaparotomy.[2–4] Surgical complications are most commonly related to the spleen: bleeding usually occurs intraoperatively (although capsular tears are mostly controllable after the splenic vessels have been ligated and divided); ischemia can occur intra- and postoperatively (although splenectomy due to ischemia is more commonly performed postoperatively). The incidence of intra- and postoperative splenectomy ranges from 5% to 15%. That is a low rate, yet LDs should still receive, 2 weeks preoperatively, polyvalent pneumococcus, meningococcus, streptococcus, and hemophilus B vaccine, in order to protect against the occurrence of overwhelming postsplenectomy infection (OPSI). A postoperative perisplenic or subdiaphragmatic abscess is frequently associated with clinical symptoms (eg, pain, fever, hiccups) and can initially be treated with percutaneous drainage, but may eventually require splenectomy, washout, and/or drainage.

Complications related to the pancreas are also uncommon, observed in ≤ 5% of LDs. Such complications include pancreatitis, pancreatic leak or fistula, pancreatic abscess, and pancreatic pseudocyst. Selective ligation of the main pancreatic duct and oversewing of the cut surface of the pancreas reduce the risk of leak, fistula, and abscess. Percutaneous peripancreatic drainage frequently helps to resolve such complications; < 3% of LDs require a relaparatomy.[2–4] LDs who develop a pancreatic leak, fistula, or pancreatitis should be placed on octreotide to speed recovery. Sterile pancreatic fluid collections or sterile pancreatic pseudocysts are usually spontaneously absorbed or can be successfully treated by percutaneous aspiration or drainage. Serum amylase levels usually return to normal range within 3 to 5 days (Figure 19.3-1), but for LDs with pancreatic complications, hyperamylasemia usually persists.

If the splenic artery and vein are double-ligated (open technique) or double-clipped (laparoscopic procedure), postoperative bleeding is uncommon, because of the diminished arterial flow; if it occurs, it usually stops on its own. Of greater concern are bleeding complications that originate from the short gastric veins; the risk of such bleeding is diminished if meticulous hemostasis in the left upper quadrant is achieved before closure of the abdomen.

Because any reported blood loss is only about 300 mL,[4,5] < 5% of LDs require blood transfusions. Despite the low incidence, I recommend autologous blood transfusion: 1 or 2 U of the LD's blood is usually stored up to 6 weeks before the scheduled surgery.

A late, rare complication is the development of upper gastrointestinal bleeding secondary to esophageal or gastric varices (in the absence of portal hypertension) from venous collateralization in donors in whom the spleen was left inside. A splenectomy is required and is curative.

Despite the advent of laparoscopic distal pancreatectomy, the spectrum of complications in LDs has not changed. A recent report on a series of laparoscopic donor distal pancreatectomies

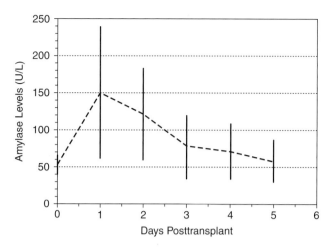

**FIGURE 19.3-1**

Serum amylase levels before and after (5 days) distal pancreatectomy.

noted one splenectomy at the time of the initial donor surgery for a nonviable spleen, but no postoperative pancreatic leaks or pancreatitis. Of note, conversion to an open pancreatectomy was not required for any of the 7 LDs.[5]

Simultaneous removal of a kidney increases the spectrum of complications, but only slightly increases the overall risk of surgical complications.

Complications that are not unique to (open or laparoscopic) distal pancreatectomy include, but are not limited to, wound infection (< 3%), incisional hernia (< 2%), and small bowel obstruction (cumulative risk of about 1% per year).

## MEDICAL COMPLICATIONS

As with any other type of abdominal surgery, pancreas LDs can develop a variety of medical complications postoperatively, such as atelectasis, urinary tract infection, and prolonged bowel dysfunction (in particular, if the kidney was removed simultaneously and the left colonic flexure and ascending colon had to be mobilized). These conditions are usually reversible by the time the LD is discharged from the hospital (usually in 5 to 9 days). Serious medical complications such as pneumonia, deep vein thrombosis, or pulmonary embolism have not been reported.[2–5]

## METABOLIC COMPLICATIONS

The effects of donor distal pancreatectomy on insulin secretion, glucose metabolism, and pancreatic α- and ß-cell function have been studied at various time points postdonation.[6–11]

The first study by Kendall et al[6] in 28 LDs demonstrated deterioration of insulin secretion and of glucose tolerance at 1 year postdonation. Specifically, the LDs' mean fasting serum glucose level was significantly higher 1 year after distal pancreatectomy (97 ± 16 mg/dL), as compared with baseline (88 ± 7 mg/dL). Fasting serum insulin levels and the area under the insulin curves during oral glucose tolerance tests (OGTTs) were significantly lower at 1 year; their mean 24-hour serum glucose-profile value was significantly higher at 1 year. Correspondingly, the 24-hour urinary C-peptide excretion was lower at 1 year.[6] Of the 28 LDs studied, 25% had abnormal glucose tolerance, with modest impairment of early insulin secretion during the OGTT at 1 year.

Interestingly, although most of their serum glucose levels were higher postoperatively than preoperatively, their mean postoperative 24-hour glucose-profile value did not exceed the range established in nondiabetic individuals.[7]

Given that LDs generally maintain normoglycemia after distal pancreatectomy, despite diminished insulin secretion, Seaquist and Robertson suggested that healthy humans may compensate for distal pancreatectomy by increasing glucose disposal.[8] Their study demonstrated that first-phase insulin secretion in response to glucose, insulin secretory response to arginine, and first-phase glucagon secretion in response to intravenous (IV) arginine were significantly decreased in LDs, as compared with controls matched for age, sex, and body mass index. Moreover, donors of a distal pancreas had significantly less insulin secretory reserve than the matched controls.[7,8]

The observation of diminished ß-cell function in donors of a distal pancreas who were still able to maintain normal plasma glucose levels (fasting state) and normal hemoglobin $A_{1c}$ ($HbA_{1c}$) levels led to this hypothesis: such donors might have compensated for decreased ß-cell mass by increasing insulin sensitivity in the liver and/or soft tissues (muscle or fat tissue). However, neither insulin- nor glucose-mediated glucose uptake was increased after distal pancreatectomy.[7,9] But a follow-up study by Seaquist et al.[10] showed that fasting serum concentrations of proinsulin and its metabolites were higher in LDs than in matched controls. The ratio of total proinsulin to immunoreactive insulin was directly correlated with fasting plasma glucose and demonstrated a significantly inverse relationship to insulin secretory reserve in LDs. The findings of Seaquist et al. support the hypothesis that disproportionate hyperproinsulinemia may result from increased ß-cell demand in LDs.[10]

The relationship between diabetes and obesity 9 to 18 years after distal pancreatectomy in LDs was studied by Robertson et al. in eight donor–recipient pairs.[11] No differences between the two groups (LDs and recipients) were noted in any of these values: fasting plasma glucose, $HbA_{1c}$, fasting insulin or C-peptide, acute insulin or C-peptide responses to arginine and to glucose, or ß-cell secretory reserve. However, eight patients were obese; this subgroup included all patients who developed mild diabetes (4 LDs and 2 recipients). The study's conclusion was that obesity should be a contraindication to donation of a distal pancreas and that LDs should assiduously avoid becoming obese.

Robertson et al., in another study,[12] also assessed glucagon, catecholamines, and symptom responses to hypoglycemia in LDs. As shown before, some LDs acquired diminished insulin and glucagon responses to intravenous agonists. Few developed diabetes or required treatment for hyperglycemia. However, these LDs became at risk for hypoglycemia, when treated with sulfonylureas and insulin. Stepped hypoglycemic clamps were applied in 7 LDs who had varying degrees of glycemic control (as compared with 16 controls), in order to assess the impact of distal pancreatectomy on islet α-cell responses to hypoglycemia. Although glucagon responses to arginine and insulin responses to glucose and arginine were diminished in distal pancreas LDs, no deficiencies in glucagon responses were detected during hypoglycemia. The LDs also had significantly higher peak epinephrine responses (vs controls) during the clamp, but there were no significant differences in epinephrine levels or symptom responses. Of note, these results contrast with previous findings that LDs have diminished ß-cell responses to glucose and to arginine and diminished α-cell responses to arginine. These somewhat contradictory results could, however, be due to the small number of LDs (n = 7) tested.

A larger study in 46 LDs assessed $HbA_{1c}$ levels at various points postdonation. In 10 LDs who underwent distal pancreatectomy through August 31, 1996, elevated $HbA_{1c}$ levels were noted; 3 of those 10 required insulin > 6 years postdonation. All 3 had causes of elevated $HbA_{1c}$ levels that are now considered contraindications for pancreas donation (gestational diabetes, increased body mass index, undisclosed history of alcohol abuse). In that study, all LDs who underwent distal pancreatectomy after September 1, 1996, have shown normal $HbA_{1c}$ levels.[13]

These results demonstrate the importance of a meticulous metabolic evaluation of LD candidates. Modifications have frequently been necessary over the last 2 decades. Over time, acceptance criteria have become more stringent (see Chapter 19.1), in order to avert any negative impact on the LD's metabolic outcome. Ultimately, only 15% to 20% of all potential LDs now qualify. But for those who do qualify, pancreas donation can now be performed with a relatively low risk. According to some of the most current data, avoidance of obesity postdonation diminishes the risk of long-term metabolic complications.

## QUALITY OF LIFE STUDIES

As with all other types of organ LDs, the vast majority of pancreas LDs stand by their decision to donate. In a retrospective study, 43 of 46 pancreas LDs stated that they had made the correct decision. But about 20% of LDs have also experienced social, marital, financial, and/or employment problems. A more detailed analysis of psychosocial outcome after pancreas donation is warranted.[2,13]

## References

1. Gruessner AC, Sutherland DE. Pancreas transplant outcomes for United States (US) and non-US cases as reported to the United Network for Organ Sharing (UNOS) and the International Pancreas Registry (IPTR) as of June 2004. *Clin Transplant* 2005;19:433–455.

2. Gruessner RWG, Kendall DM, Drangstveit MB, et al. Simultaneous pancreas-kidney transplantation from live donors. *Ann Surg* 1997;226: 471–482.

3. Zielinski A, Nazarewski S, Bogetti D, et al. Simultaneous pancreas-kidney transplant from living related donor: a single-center experience. *Transplant* 2003;76:547–552.

4. Gruessner RWG. Living Donor Pancreas Transplantation. In: Gruessner RWG, Sutherland DER, eds. *Transplantation of the Pancreas*. New York: Springer-Verlag; 2004, Ch14:423–440.

5. Tan M, Kandaswamy R, Sutherland DER, et al. Laparoscopic donor distal pancreatectomy for living donor pancreas and pancreas-kidney transplantation. *Am J Trans* 2005;5:1966–1970.

6. Kendall DM, Sutherland DER, Najarian JS, et al. Effects of hemipancreatectomy on insulin secretion and glucose tolerance in healthy humans. *N Engl J Med* 1990;322:898–903.

7. Robertson RP. Endocrine Function and Metabolic Outcomes in Pancreas and Islet Transplantation. In: Gruessner RWG, Sutherland DER, eds. *Transplantation of the Pancreas*. New York: Springer-Verlag; 2004, Ch 15:441–454.

8. Seaquist ER, Robertson RP. Effects of hemipancreatectomy on pancreatic alpha and beta cell function in healthy human donors. *J Clin Invest* 1992;89:1761–1766.

9. Seaquist ER, Pyzdrowski K, Moran A, et al. Insulin-mediated and glucose-mediated glucose uptake following hemipancreatectomy in healthy human donors. *Diabetologia* 1994;37: 1036–1043.

10. Seaquist ER, Kahn SE, Clark PM, et al. Hyperproinsulinemia is associated with increased ß cell demand after hemipancreatectomy in humans. *J Clin Invest* 1996;97:455–460.

11. Robertson RP, Lanz KJ, Sutherland DER, et al. Relationship between diabetes and obesity 9 to 18 years after hemipancreatomy and transplantation in donors and recipients. *Transplantation* 2002;73:736–741.

12. Robertson RP, Sutherland DER, Seaquist ER, et al. Glucagon, catecholamine, and symptom responses to hypoglycemia in living donors of pancreas segments. *Diabetes* 2003;52:1689–1694.

13. Gruessner RWG, Sutherland DER, Drangstveit MB, et al. Pancreas transplants from living donors: Short- and long-term outcome. *Transplant Proc* 2001;33:819–820.

# PANCREAS TRANSPLANTATION: THE RECIPIENT

## 20.1 SELECTION AND WORKUP

*Raja Kandaswamy, MD*

### INTRODUCTION

Options for treatment of type 1 diabetes mellitus include (1) exogenous insulin administration and (2) beta cell replacement by pancreas or islet transplantation.

Exogenous insulin administration, with intensive monitoring, showed decreased glycosylated hemoglobin levels and secondary complications in the diabetes control and complications trial.[1,2] However, with intensive insulin therapy there was an increased risk of hypoglycemia and its attendant risks.

Pancreas transplantation offers the advantage of insulin independence and protection from secondary complications of diabetes without the risk of hypoglycemia. However, the risks of surgery and immunosuppressive therapy have to be taken. The success rates of pancreas transplantation have steadily improved over the last 20 years.[3] Today pancreas transplantation is accepted as the standard of care for treatment of insulin-dependent diabetic uremic recipients who need a kidney transplant. The pancreas transplant may be performed simultaneously or sequentially after a kidney transplant from a living or deceased donor. Pancreas transplants are also performed in nonuremic diabetics with hypoglycemia unawareness or other secondary complications of diabetes.

Islet transplantation, first performed in 1977,[4] has been less successful.[5] In the last 10 years, there have been tremendous advances in the field with early insulin independence achieved consistently, both with multiple donors at the University of Alberta[6] and with single donors at the University of Minnesota.[7,8] However, long-term insulin independence rates, even with modern protocols, appear to be low.[9] Therefore, currently, pancreas transplants offer the best chance of long-term insulin independence in type 1 diabetic recipients.

Pancreas transplantation from a living donor (LD) was first performed in 1979 at the University of Minnesota.[10] Since then, LD pancreas transplants have been performed regularly over the last 25 years. Because the waiting time for a deceased donor (DD) pancreas transplant is not long (usually a few months for a nonsensitized recipient), there has been less of a need to perform large numbers of LD transplants as in kidney transplantation. However, this might change with time as islet transplants become more successful, creating greater demand for DD pancreases.

### RECIPIENT SELECTION

LD pancreas transplantation is suitable for virtually all pancreas transplant recipients. The rate-limiting step, as in kidney transplantation, is the availability of a suitable donor. Because the donor surgery carries significant risks (more so than kidney donation), and the waiting time for a deceased pancreas is not long, there are fewer pancreas LDs.

Most pancreas donors today are simultaneous kidney donors,[11–14] and with the advent of laparoscopy in pancreas donation,[15] a minimally invasive option is now available for potential donors.

There are some situations where a LD pancreas transplant may be strongly considered:

1. Recipient with a rare tissue type who has a well-matched LD
2. High panel-reactive antibody level 1 with a negative crossmatch to an LD
3. Recipient in whom an elective transplant is strongly preferred due to medical or personal considerations
4. Recipient who desires tissue or organs from people he or she is related to or familiar with
5. HLA-identical siblings (although recurrent disease is a consideration)

### RECIPIENT CATEGORIES

There are three main recipient categories in pancreas transplantation:

1. Simultaneous pancreas-kidney transplants (SPK). Most pancreas transplants including LD transplants fall under this category. The DD waiting time for this category is quite long because of the kidney. Thus, to avoid a long wait, an LD can be used; this option is only available at selected centers.[2,16]
2. Pancreas after kidney transplant (PAK). In a uremic diabetic who has undergone a kidney transplant, usually from an LD, a sequential PAK transplant can be done. This is usually from a DD, although it can be performed with an LD as well. The disadvantage of PAK transplants is that the recipient undergoes two operations. However, in some high-risk recipients this may be preferred since the two procedures separately are smaller than a combined transplant. The interval between the kidney and the pancreas transplant varies depending on recipient recovery and donor availability. PAK is the most frequently performed category at the University of Minnesota.[17–19]
3. Pancreas transplant alone (PTA). This is performed in nonuremic diabetics with either an LD or DD. Most candidates

have severe glycemic control problems, hypoglycemia unawareness, and frequent insulin reactions. APTA not only makes the recipient insulin-independent but also obviates glycemic control problems and may ameliorate secondary complications, thus increasing its applicability.[17,20]

## INDICATIONS FOR PANCREAS TRANSPLANTS

Most pancreas transplants are performed in recipients with diabetic nephropathy who also need a kidney transplant. The risks of immunosuppression are taken by having a kidney transplant; therefore, the addition of a pancreas poses no additional immunosuppressive risks.[21] Renal transplant recipients who are insulin-dependent even if they have type 2 diabetes have successfully received a pancreas transplant.[22]

The indications for pancreas transplants have expanded as the results have improved. The ADA position statement[13] on pancreas transplants (Table 20-1) is, at best, conservative. A pancreas transplant is indicated for patients who have developed secondary complications of diabetes. Neuropathy has been shown to improve[11,23–25] posttransplant. Nephropathic changes of the glomeruli show improvement, interstitial expansion is reversible, and atrophic tubules can be reabsorbed.[26] Advanced retinopathy and vascular disease are unchanged.[27] However, atherosclerosis and endothelial function improve.[28]

A pancreas transplant can be offered early to patients prior to the onset of secondary complications if they understand the risks of immunosuppression and prefer it over the risk of diabetic complications.

Contraindications to transplants include malignancy, active infections, noncompliance, serious psychosocial problems, and prohibitive cardiac risk. Although it was clear that uremic diabetics with a kidney and pancreas transplant enjoyed a survival benefit, it was questioned for solitary pancreas transplants (PTA) by one study.[29] However, a more comprehensive reanalysis showed that solitary pancreas transplant recipients also had a survival benefit over wait-listed patients.

## PRETRANSPLANT EVALUATION

The pretransplant evaluation should comprise a medical, psychological, and social evaluation. Prior to the evaluation, the recipient must be well informed about the risks and benefits of the procedure and understand the basic aspects of the evaluation. At the University of

Minnesota, this is done by mailing an information booklet to the potential recipient well before the evaluation.

As part of the medical evaluation, a cardiac risk assessment is performed because diabetes is a major risk factor for coronary artery disease (CAD). Coronary angiograms are done in most candidates, although cardiologists are increasingly using noninvasive methods. In long standing diabetics, noninvasive methods are not sensitive for CAD and poorly predictive of postoperative outcome.[30,31] In young patients with short duration of diabetes, dobutamine stress echocardiograms are used for cardiac evaluation.[32] If significant CAD is detected, aggressive revascularization, be it by stenting, angioplasty, or bypass surgery, is promptly done. With the use of iso-osmolar contrast, the risk of contrast-induced nephropathy is minimized in patients with kidney dysfunction.[33] Revascularized transplant candidates do better than those treated by medical therapy alone.[34]

Another key component of the medical evaluation is the vascular exam. If significant lower extremity vascular insufficiency is found, it may need to be corrected pretransplant, because the transplant may further diminish lower extremity arterial flow. Vascular disease of the iliac arteries, if suspected, should be looked for using a Doppler ultrasound. A follow-up magnetic resonance angiogram (MRA) or a contrast angiogram may be indicated.

Pulmonary function tests are indicated in chronic smokers and patients with chronic airway disease. Perioperative bronchodilator therapy and ICU monitoring may be indicated in some patients.

Liver function tests should be performed to rule out cirrhosis or active hepatitis. The diagnosis of viral hepatitis (B or C) is associated with poor outcome after extra hepatic transplantation.[35] A liver biopsy may be needed if cirrhosis is a contraindication to a pancreas transplant.

A gastrointestinal evaluation to look for significant autonomic dysfunction should be performed. Some immunosuppressive agents have significant GI side effects. A prokinetic agent may be indicated. In some cases, a gastric pacemaker device has been used.

A urologic evaluation is important for patients in whom bladder drainage is planned. Bladder dysfunction can pose a risk to the anastomosis and increase the risk of graft pancreatitis.

## CONCLUSION

Every person on the pancreas waiting list should be considered a potential candidate for an LD transplant. Advantages include elimination of waiting time, elective surgery, decreased rejection rates, and minimal ischemic time. Disadvantages include increased technical complications and need for anticoagulation (for 6 months). Recently, an LD islet transplant was reported from Japan.[17] As the applicability of islet transplantation increases, unless alternative sources of islets are available, LD pancreas and islet transplants may be performed more frequently.

**TABLE 20-1**

## SUMMARY OF AMERICAN DIABETES ASSOCIATION (ADA) RECOMMENDATIONS FOR INDICATIONS FOR PANCREAS TRANSPLANTS

1. Established ESRD in patients who have had, or plan to have, a kidney transplant

2. History of frequent, acute, and severe metabolic complications (eg, hypoglycemia, hyperglycemia, ketoacidosis)

3. Incapacitating clinical and emotional problems with exogenous insulin prescription

    Consistent failure of insulin-based management to prevent acute complications

## References

1. DCCT Research Group. Diabetes control and complications trial (DCCT): The effect of intensive diabetes treatment in long-term complications in IDDM. *N Engl J Med* 1993;329:977–986.
2. DCCT Research Group. Lifetime benefits and costs of intensive therapy as practiced in the diabetes control and complications trial. The Diabetes Control and Complications Trial Research Group. *JAMA* 1997; 277:372.

3. Gruessner AC, Sutherland DER. Pancreas transplant outcomes for United States (US) cases reported to the United Network for Organ Sharing (UNOS) and non-US cases reported to the International Pancreas Transplant Registry (IPTR) as of June 2004. *Clin Transplant* 2005; 19(4):433–455.

4. Najarian JS, Sutherland DER, Matas AJ, et al. Human islet transplantation: a preliminary report. *Transplant Proc.* 9(1):337-9, 1977.

5. Hering BJ and Ricordi C. Islet transplantation for patients with type I diabetes. *Graft* 2(1):12–27, 1999.

6. Shapiro AM, Lakey JR, Ryan EA, et al. Islet transplantation in seven patients with type 1 diabetes mellitus using a glucocorticoid-free immunosuppressive regimen. *N Engl J Med* 2000;343(4):230–238.

7. Hering BJ, Kandaswamy R, Harmon JV, et al. Insulin independence after single-donor islet transplantation in type 1 diabetes with hOKT3-1 (ala-ala), sirolimus, and tacrolimus therapy. *Am J Transplant* 2001; 1(1):180–180.

8. Hering BJ, Kandaswamy R, Ansite JD, et al. Single-donor, marginal-dose islet transplantation in patients with type 1 diabetes. *JAMA* 293(7): 1594.

9. Shapiro AM, Ricordi C, Hering BJ, et al. International trial of the Edmonton protocol for islet transplantation. *N Engl J Med* 2006;355(13): 1318–1330.

10. Sutherland DE, Goetz FC, Najarian JS. Living-related donor segmental pancreatectomy for transplantation. *Transplant Proc* 1980;12(4 Suppl 2): 19–25.

11. Gruessner KR, Kendall DM, Drangstveit MB, et al. Simultaneous pancreas- kidney transplantation from live donors. *Ann Surg* 1997;226(4): 471–480.

12. Gruessner RW, Sutherland DE. Simultaneous kidney and segmental pancreas transplants from living related donors - the first two successful cases. *Transplantation* 1996;61(8):1265–1268.

13. Sutherland DE, Najarian JS, Gruessner R. Living versus cadaver donor pancreas transplants. *Transplant Proc* 1998;30(5):2264–2266.

14. Gruessner RWG, Sutherland DE, Drangstveit MB, et al. Pancreas transplants from living donors: Short-and long-term outcome. *Transplant Proc* 2001;33:819–820.

15. Gruessner RWG, Kandaswamy R, Denny R. Laparoscopic simultaneous nephrectomy and distal pancreatectomy from a live donor. *J Am Coll Surgeons* 2001;193(3):333.

16. Farney AC, Cho E, Schweitzer EJ, et al. Simultaneous cadaver pancreas living-donor kidney transplantation: a new approach for the type 1 diabetic uremic patient. *Ann Surg* 2000;232(5):696–703.

17. Sutherland DE, Gruessner RW, Dunn DL, et al. Lessons learned from more than 1,000 pancreas transplants at a single institution. *Ann Surg* 2001;233(4):463–501.

18. Gruessner AC, Sutherland DE, Dunn DL, et al. Pancreas after kidney transplants in posturemic patients with type I diabetes mellitus. *J Am Soc Nephrol* 2001;12(11):2490–2499.

19. Humar A, Ramcharan T, Kandaswamy R, et al. Pancreas after kidney transplants. *Am J Surg* 182(2):155–161, 2001.

20. Sutherland DER, Gruessner RWG, Humar A, et al. Pretransplant immunosuppression for pancreas transplants alone in nonuremic diabetic recipients. *Transplant Proc* 22001;33:1656–1658.

21. Sutherland DER, Stratta R, Gruessner A. Pancreas transplant outcome by recipient category: single pancreas versus combined kidney-pancreas. *Curr Opin Organ Transplant* 1998;3:231–241.

22. Light JA, Sasaki TM, Currier CB, et al. Successful long-term kidney-pancreas transplants regardless of C- peptide status or race. *Transplantation* 2001;71(1):152–154.

23. Sutherland DER, Groth CG. *History of Pancreas Transplantation.* 2002; In Press.

24. Kennedy WR, Navarro X, Goetz FC, et al. Effects of pancreatic transplantation on diabetic neuropathy. *N Engl J Med* 1190;322:1031–1037.

25. Solders G, Tyden G, Persson A, et al. Improvement of nerve conduction in diabetic neuropathy. A follow-up study 4 yr after combined pancreatic and renal transplantation. *Diabetes* 1992;41(8):946–951.

26. Fioretto P, Sutherland DER, Najarfian B, et al. Remodeling of renal interstitial and tubular lesions in pancreas transplant recipients. *Kidney Int* 2006;69(5):907–912.

27. Stratta RJ. Impact of pancreas transplantation on complications of diabetes. *Curr Opin Organ Transplant* 1998;3:258–273.

28. Fiorina P, La Rocca E, Venturini M, et al. Effects of kidney-pancreas transplantation on atherosclerotic risk factors and endothelial function in patients with uremia and type 1 diabetes. *Diabetes* 2001; 50(3):496–501.

29. Venstrom JM, McBride MA, Rother KI, et al. Survival after pancreas transplantation in patients with diabetes and preserved kidney function. *JAMA* 2003;290(21):2817–2823.

30. Vandenberg BF, Rossen JD, Grover-McKay M, et al. Evaluation of diabetic patients for renal and pancreas transplantation: noninvasive screening for coronary artery disease using radionuclide methods. *Transplantation* 62(9):1230–1235.

31. Herzog CA, Marwick TH, Pheley AM, et al. Dobutamine stress echocardiography for the detection of significant coronary artery disease in renal transplant candidates. *Am J Kidney Dis* 1999;33(6): 1080–1090.

32. Bates JR, Sawada SG, Segar DS, et al. Evaluation using dobutamine stress echocardiography in patients with insulin-dependent diabetes mellitus before kidney and/or pancreas transplantation. *Am J Cardiol* 1996; 77(2):175–179.

33. Tadros GM, Malik JA, Manske CL, et al. Iso-osmolar radio contrast iodixanol in patients with chronic kidney disease. *J Invasive Cardiol* 2005; 17(4):211–215.

34. Manske CL, Wang Y, Rector T, et al. Coronary revascularisation in insulin-dependent diabetic patients with chronic renal failure. *Lancet* 1992; 340(8826):998–1002.

35. Robertson RP, Sutherland DER., Lanz KJ. Normoglycemia and preserved insulin secretory reserve in diabetic patients 10-18 years after pancreas transplantation. *Diabetes* 1999;48:1737–1740.

# 20.2  SURGICAL PROCEDURES

*Rainer W.G. Gruessner, MD*

## GENERAL ASPECTS

Pancreas transplants can be performed either as solitary transplants in nonuremic or posturemic (ie, after a previous kidney transplant) patients or as simultaneous pancreas and kidney transplants in uremic patients with insulin-dependent diabetes mellitus. Before 1994, living donor (LD) pancreas transplants were done only as a pancreas transplant alone (PTA) or as a pancreas after kidney (PAK) transplants because of the concern that multiorgan retrieval (ie, pancreas and kidney) from LDs might entail too much morbidity[1]; with that approach, dual-organ LDs had to endure two separate procedures, which many were loath to do. Since 1994—after it was shown that multiorgan donation could be done safely[1-3]—most LD pancreas transplants have been done simultaneously with the kidney from the same LD (SPK), with no or only very little added morbidity.

In contrast to whole-organ transplants from deceased donors (DDs), only about 50% of the pancreas is procured from LDs. Nonetheless, the technical aspects and considerations with regard to management of exocrine pancreatic secretions are similar. The two most common techniques are bladder drainage and enteric drainage. Other techniques for management of exocrine pancreatic secretions, such as ureteral drainage, duct injection, or duct ligation, are rarely used.[3,4]

The two main advantages of bladder drainage are (1) the ability to monitor urinary amylase levels as a marker for rejection[4-6] and (2) containment of surgical complications to the right (or left) lower abdominal quadrant.[7-9] Monitoring exocrine pancreatic function has proven to be effective: it has been shown that exocrine rejection (hypoamylasuria) precedes endocrine rejection (hyperglycemia) by several days, with most rejection episodes being reversible after initiation of treatment for exocrine rejection.[5,6,10] Monitoring urinary amylase levels is particularly crucial for PTA and PAK recipients; in SPK recipients, serum creatinine levels can be used for rejection monitoring.[10] In SPK recipients, it has been shown that hypercreatinemia precedes hyperamylasuria by several days and that > 90% of all rejection episodes affect either the kidney alone or the kidney and the pancreas simultaneously; isolated pancreas rejection episodes are rare.[10,11]

Despite its monitoring advantages, bladder drainage is also associated with unique metabolic and urologic complications. In contrast to whole-organ pancreaticoduodenal transplants, complications of bladder drainage are usually less serious in recipients of segmental pancreas grafts from LDs, because of the absence of the donor duodenum. Still, even in bladder-drained LD recipients, the loss of exocrine pancreatic secretions in the urine can lead to bicarbonate deficiency and electrolyte derangements, causing chronic (hyperchloremic) metabolic acidosis and dehydration; such recipients can be saddled with permanent bicarbonate supplementation and the need for increased fluid intake. However, recipients rarely require fludrocortisone for water and sodium retention, or acetazolamide or octreotide for bicarbonate reduction and pancreatic juice production. Transplantation of only the distal pancreas and the absence of the donor duodenum typically diminish the posttransplant risks of severe fluid and electrolyte imbalances.

Urologic complications, also not uncommon with bladder drainage, include (recurrent) bacterial urinary tract infections, hematuria, chemical cystitis, urethritis, bladder stones, and graft pancreatitis (secondary to reflux of urine into the pancreatic ducts).[12] These complications, thought to be the consequences of altered urothelial integrity and a change to an alkaline pH of the urine, can usually be managed nonoperatively (eg, with placement of Foley catheter, antibiotics, urinary tract analgesics). But serious, albeit rare, complications have been described, such as perineal excoriation; ureteral disruption and strictures; and autodigestion of the glans penis, major labia, and urethra.[13,14] Of note, malignancies caused by exposure of pancreatic enzymes to the urothelium have not been described after LD transplants.

The operative therapy of choice for persistent or refractory bladder drainage-related complications is conversion to enteric drainage. Because a segmental pancreas graft has a smaller immunologic reserve than a whole-organ graft, we recommend conversion from bladder to enteric drainage if the LD and recipient are not HLA-identical and the recipient has been rejection-free for at least 6 months posttransplant.[15,16]

The most physiologic technique for draining pancreatic exocrine secretions is enteric drainage, which is associated with no technique-related metabolic or urologic complications. Only if the pancreaticoenterostomy was made in the distal ileum do recipients occasionally complain about diarrhea. Thus, the preferred location for a pancreaticoenterostomy is the jejunum. The major disadvantage of enteric drainage, however, is the inability to monitor exocrine pancreatic secretions other than in the serum. The sensitivity of pancreatic serum parameters for diagnosing rejection is generally lower and enteric drainage remains associated with a higher immunologic graft loss rate than bladder drainage in solitary pancreas transplant recipients.[10,17] Another concern with enteric drainage is the possible development of (diffuse) peritonitis in case of an anastomotic leak. This particular complication appears to be less grave if a Roux-en-Y loop, rather than a side-to-side pancreaticoenterostomy, was created.[10]

With LD transplants (unlike with whole-organ pancreas transplants), the use of portal (vs systemic) vein drainage is not a true alternative. Portal vein drainage would require the use of vascular extension graft(s); this modification and drainage into the low-flow portal circulation might increase the risk of graft thrombosis. Thus, systemic drainage is the technique of choice for segmental grafts. No convincing evidence exists today that systemic vein drainage places pancreas recipients at a higher risk for developing arteriosclerosis due to peripheral hyperinsulinemia.[18,19] Furthermore, comparable metabolic control is achieved with portal and systemic vein drainage.[20–22]

Segmental pancreas grafts have been placed both intraperitoneally and extraperitoneally. The increasing consensus among pancreas transplant surgeons seems to be that the preferred placement for both whole-organ and segmental grafts is intraabdominal.[23,24]

## OPERATIVE PROCEDURES

The dissection of the recipient iliac vessels is as extensive for LD transplants as for whole-organ transplants, because of the importance of creating tension-free anastomoses. In contrast to whole-organ transplants, the external iliac vein is positioned medially to the external iliac artery (Color Plates, Figure PA-8): doing so reflects the natural position of the donor splenic artery and vein. In general, in order to decrease the risk of thrombosis, extension grafts should not be used. The following is a detailed description of the operative procedure and the surgical variants.

The recipient is placed on the operating table in the supine position. After general endotrachial anesthesia is induced, Foley catheter bladder drainage begins, an arterial line is placed for constant blood pressure monitoring, nasal gastric suction is instituted, prophylactic antibiotics are given (repeated every 4 hours during the course of the procedure), and sequential compression devices are used. The recipient is prepped and draped in standard fashion for a lower midline incision. As mentioned above, the pancreas is placed intraabdominally, preferably on the right side of the pelvis, because the iliac vessels are more superficial there than on the left side. The recipient is then placed in a slight Trendelenburg position.

The abdomen is entered through the midline incision extending from a point slightly above the umbilicus down to the pubic bone. The abdomen is first explored for any pathologic findings. If the abdominal contents appear normal, the dissection is started by mobilizing the cecum and distal portion of the ascending colon medially. Doing so creates a comfortable retroperitoneal bed for the graft and also allows exposure to the proximal common iliac artery and vein. As part of this initial dissection, the right native ureter is identified, isolated, and fully mobilized to a point midway between the iliac vessels and the bladder.

The right common, external, and internal iliac arteries are dissected free, all the way from the aortic bifurcation until just proximal to the inguinal ligament (Color Plates, Figure PA-8). Care is taken not to injure any nerve structures at the aortic bifurcation. Next, the right common, external, and internal iliac veins are mobilized. Major lymphatic vessels and lymph nodes overlying the iliac vessels are ligated; the gonadal or ovarian vein may also be ligated, in order to prevent possible impingement on the venous graft anastomosis. To create tension-free anastomoses, all internal iliac (hypogastric) veins (sometimes including the first right lumbar vein) are ligated, stick-tied, and divided; for optimal alignment, it may also be necessary to ligate and divide the internal iliac artery. This extensive dissection facilitates the venous graft anastomosis technically, makes unnecessary the use of extension grafts, and, as mentioned, decreases the risk of creating a venous anastomosis under tension.

The lower abdominal dissection is completed by mobilizing the bladder. Its lateral attachments are divided. In women, the round ligament is divided; in men, care is taken to preserve the spermatic cord. Dissection of the bladder can be limited to its right anterolateral portion: the bladder's close proximity to the right iliac vessels allows creation of a pancreaticocystostomy with little mobilization.

Once the dissection in the recipient is completed, along with the benchwork preparation (ie, flushing of the LD's splenic artery, identification of the pancreatic duct, ligation of vessels and ducts on the cut surface), heparin is given intravenously (40 U/kg for nonuremic, 30 U/kg for posturemic, and 20 U/kg for uremic recipients). In our experience, intraoperative heparinization—even in uremic recipients—helps decrease the rate of thrombosis.

The proximal common iliac artery and vein and the distal external iliac artery and vein are clamped with atraumatic vascular clamps. The internal iliac artery (if not ligated and divided earlier; see above) is separately clamped with a short atraumatic vessel clamp (eg, bulldog clamp) (Color Plates, Figure PA-8). Because of the varying degree of atherosclerotic disease in recipients, clamps on the proximal and distal arteries should be placed at plaque-free locations. When clamping the iliac vessels, it is important to position the external iliac vein medially to the artery (in contrast to whole-organ transplants, where the iliac vein is positioned laterally to the iliac artery). The venotomy is usually made first and irrigated with heparin-containing solution. Four double-armed 6–0 nonabsorbable sutures are placed at the corners and sides of the venotomy. The segmental pancreas from the recipient is brought into the operative field. The 6–0 nonabsorbable venotomy stitches are taken to their respective points on the LD's splenic vein. They are tied as the pancreas is lowered into the operative field. The end-to-side venous anastomosis is completed by running the 6–0 nonabsorbable corner sutures continuously from one end to the other and tying them at the corners. Likewise, the arteriotomy is made in the external iliac artery lateral and proximal to the venotomy (Color Plates, Figure PA-9). The arteriotomy is irrigated with heparin-containing solution. Four double-armed 6–0 or 7–0 nonabsorbable sutures are placed at the corners and sides of the arteriotomy. Any intimal dissections or plaques are tagged at this time, usually with interrupted 7–0 nonabsorbable sutures. The end-to-side arterial anastomosis is completed by running the 6–0 or 7–0 nonabsorbable corner sutures continuously from one end to the other and tying them at the corners.

If the diameter of the splenic artery is small, the anastomosis should be accomplished with interrupted 6-0 or 7-0 nonabsorbable sutures. If the external iliac artery cannot be used because of severe atherosclerotic disease, the LD's splenic artery can also be anastomosed end-to-end to the internal iliac artery.

At the beginning of the arterial anastomosis, mannitol (0.5 to 1.0 g/kg body weight) and octreotide are given to the recipient to diminish the inflammatory response which usually manifests itself as graft edema. After the vascular anastomosis is completed, all vascular clamps on the iliac artery and vein are removed. Any bleeding sites, particularly on the cut surface of the pancreas, are identified and carefully controlled with fine suture-ligation techniques.

Given the proximity of the external iliac vessels to the bladder, a tension-free bladder anastomosis can easily be constructed. Two techniques for *bladder drainage* are used: pancreaticocystostomy and ductocystostomy.

If a *pancreaticocystostomy* (Color Plates, Figure PA-9) is created, the cut surface of the pancreas is anastomosed to the bladder by using the invagination ("telescope") technique, as described for the Whipple procedure. First, an outer layer is begun with interrupted nonabsorbable 4–0 sutures between the posterior surface of the pancreas and the bladder wall. The stitches are anchored in the pancreas about 1 to 2 cm distal to the cut surface. The bladder is then transversely incised, over a length of 2 to 4 cm, and opened. An inner layer of running 4–0 absorbable sutures is run around the entire circumference of the pancreas and the cystotomy, anchored in the cut surface line on the pancreas side, thus invaginating the cut surface of the pancreas into the bladder. Before the inner running suture line is completed, a stent is passed into the pancreatic duct and tagged with interrupted 7–0 absorbable sutures to the tip of the pancreatic duct. The anterior outer layer is finished with interrupted 4–0 nonabsorbable sutures, anchored 1 to 2 cm distal to the cut surface on the pancreatic side.

If a *ductocystostomy* (Color Plates, Figure PA-9) is created, a direct anastomosis is constructed between the pancreatic duct and the bladder urothelium. The seromuscular layer of the bladder is transversely incised down to the urothelium (2 to 4 cm in length). An outer layer is begun with running or interrupted nonabsorbable sutures between the posterior surface of the pancreas and the bladder wall. A small incision, about the size of the lumen of the pancreatic duct, is made in the bladder urothelium (0.5 cm), and the bladder is opened (Color Plates, Figure PA-9). The posterior row of the inner anastomosis is done between the pancreatic duct and the bladder urothelium with interrupted 7–0 absorbable sutures. Before the posterior inner layer is completed, a stent is passed through the duct-to-urothelium anastomosis. The stent is tagged at the tip of the pancreatic duct with interrupted 7–0 absorbable sutures. The inner anterior layer of the anastomosis is completed with interrupted 7–0 absorbable sutures over the stent. The outer anterior layer between the seromuscular bladder wall and the anterior surface of the pancreas is done with 4–0 nonabsorbable sutures in running or interrupted fashion. A variant of the outer layer is the creation of an anterior and posterior muscular flap (each 2 cm wide) after the bladder is incised (and while the urothelium is intact). This dissection results in a collar of bladder muscular tissue surrounding a broader area of the proximal and middle portion of the segmental graft.[25]

Irrespective of whether a pancreatico- or ductocystostomy is created, the stent is either spontaneously excreted through the urether or cystoscopally removed 4 weeks posttransplant.

For *enteric drainage* (Color Plates, Figure PA-10) of segmental grafts, a Roux-en-Y loop is usually used. In preparation for the pancreaticoenterostomy, the recipient's proximal small bowel is drawn to the level of the cut surface of the pancreas, to ensure that the mesentery of the jejunum is long enough to reach the graft. The pancreatico- or ductojejunostomy should be made as proximally as possible (ideally, 40 to 80 cm distal to the ligament of Treitz) to establish near-normal physiology and to prevent the development of diarrhea (which has been noted if the anastomosis is created more distally in the small bowel). Once the appropriate loop of jejunum is identified, the jejunum is divided with the gastrointestinal anastomosis (GIA) stapler. The stapled distal end of the divided jejunum is oversewn with 4–0 absorbable sutures. The proximal end is anastomosed end-to-side or side-to-side about 40 cm distal to the distal end of the divided jejunum. The jejunojejunostomy is a two-layer anastomosis, either handsewn or stapled.

If a *pancreaticojejunostomy* is created, the Roux-en-Y loop is anastomosed to the whole cut surface of the pancreas by using the invagination ("telescope") technique. The anastomosis can be created end-to-side (by using the antimesenteric side just distal to the jejunal stump end) or end-to-end (by using the jejunal stump itself after resection of the staple line). The two-layer anastomosis is begun with an outer posterior layer with interrupted 4–0 nonabsorbable sutures. If the side, and not the distal stump itself, is used, the jejunum is incised transversely on the antimesenteric side over the length of 3 to 4 cm. An inner layer between the cut surface of the pancreas and the jejunal wall (full-thickness bites) is constructed circumferentially with running 4–0 absorbable sutures. Doing so allows the whole cut surface of the distal pancreas to invaginate into the Roux-en-Y limb. An outer posterior layer of interrupted 4–0 nonabsorbable sutures completes the anastomosis.

If a *ductojejunostomy* is created, interrupted 4–0 nonabsorbable sutures are placed on the posterior surface of the pancreas (1 to 2 cm distal to the cut surface) and the jejunum, to construct the posterior outer layer of the anastomosis. A stab wound (0.5 mm) is made through all layers of the antimesenteric wall of the jejunum, approximately equaling the diameter of the pancreatic duct. The pancreatic duct is then anastomosed to the full thickness of the jejunal wall with interrupted 6–0 or 7–0 nonabsorbable sutures. The anterior outer layer is completed between the anterior surface of the pancreas (1 to 2 cm distal to the cut surface) and the jejunum with 4–0 nonabsorbable sutures.

Irrespective of whether a pancreatico- or ductojejunostomy is created, a stent is placed in the pancreatic duct and tagged with absorbable 6–0 sutures. The stent extends into the jejunal lumen and usually passes with the enteric contents within a few weeks.

## VARIATIONS IN OPERATIVE PROCEDURES

### Diversion of Exocrine Pancreatic Secretions

Aside from bladder drainage and enteric drainage, two other techniques have been used in LD segmental pancreas transplants: ureteral drainage and duct injection.

*Ureteral drainage* was originally described in 1973 by Gliedman et al,[26] who anastomosed the pancreatic duct of a DD, systemic-drained, segmental graft to the ipsilateral ureter of the recipient. The native ureter can be used if the recipient is uremic, is on dialysis, and produces no or only very little urine. The ductoureterostomy is a one-layer anastomosis, with 6–0 or 7–0 absorbable sutures over a stent that extends into the bladder. The stent is tagged with a 6–0 absorbable suture so that it can be removed cystoscopically if it does not pass spontaneously. Ureteral drainage is not widely used, because of its relatively high anastomotic complication rate (leaks, strictures). Of note, leaks can occur not only at the anastomotic site itself but also at the cut surface of the pancreas. Nonetheless, ureteral drainage is an option if the pancreatic duct and the ipsilateral native ureter are a good size match and if bladder or enteric drainage cannot be used (because of a short pancreatic neck and because of concern about injuring the LD's splenic vessels when constructing an outer, second anastomotic layer).

*Duct injection* was first described by Dubernard et al in 1978 for DD segmental grafts.[27] After revascularization, 3 to 5 mL of a synthetic polymer (neoprene, prolamine, polyisoprene, silicon) is injected into the main pancreatic duct.[28–30]

Duct injection can also be performed on the bench. The pancreatic duct is cannulated with a small blunt-tipped catheter (Color Plates, Figure PA-11). Spillage of the polymer should be avoided. After injection of the polymer, the pancreatic duct is oversewn with a single 5–0 absorbable suture. The cut surface can also be oversewn, again with a single 4–0 absorbable suture. Duct injection is now rarely used, because of its higher complication rate (as compared with bladder or enteric drainage). In particular, duct-injected recipients develop graft pancreatitis obligatorily; pancreatic fistulas with infections are not uncommon. However, duct injection can be used as a rescue conversion technique for recipients with surgical complications after bladder- or enteric-drained pancreas transplants.[23]

### Positional Variations

If a previous kidney graft was placed on the right side, the pancreas can be engrafted to the left iliac vessels. Again, intraperitoneal placement via a midline incision is preferred. The dissection of the common, external, and internal iliac vessels is done laterally to the sigmoid colon. As on the right side, the external iliac vessels are used for anastomosis, because their relatively distal position allows creation of a tension-free bladder anastomosis. Because the external iliac vessels are deeper on the left side than on the right side, it is advisable to ligate and divide the internal iliac artery as well as all hypogastric veins, in order to maximize mobilization and to create a tension-free venous anastomosis. The technique for vascular engraftment of the segmental pancreas on the left side does not differ from the technique on the right side. The arterial anastomosis is lateral and proximal to the venous anastomosis. Likewise, the technique of the pancreaticocystostomy or ductocystostomy is identical to the technique on the right side.

If bladder drainage is not used, the segmental pancreas does not have to be placed in a caudad position as described above, but can also be placed in a cephalad position, thus making the enteric anastomosis technically easier. In this case, the proximal common iliac vessels are used for revascularization. The splenic vein is anastomosed end-to-side to the common iliac vein or to the distal inferior vena cava, using 6–0 or 7–0 nonabsorbable sutures in running fashion. Likewise, the arterial anastomosis is between the splenic artery and the proximal common iliac artery. On the right side, the arterial anastomosis is medial and caudad to the venous anastomosis. In the cephalad position, the segmental pancreas graft is easily anastomosed to the proximal jejunum about 40 to 80 cm distal to the ligament of Treitz, either side-to-side or with a Roux-en-Y loop. The enteric anastomotic technique is the same as described above for the caudad position.

If the pancreas graft is placed on the left side in the cephalad position, the common iliac artery and vein are used for anastomosis. The dissection of the common iliac vessels can be done either laterally or medially to the sigmoid colon. The lateral dissection is as described for the caudad position. If the pancreas graft is placed in the medial position, the dissection has to be carried out through an avascular window between the vessel-bearing arcades of the mesocolon. According to the natural position of the common iliac artery and vein on the left side, the venous anastomosis is made medially and proximally to the arterial anastomosis.

### Portal Vein Drainage

Portal vein drainage has been described for DD segmental pancreas transplants, but not for LD segmental pancreas transplants. For DD segmental transplants, both the superior and the inferior mesenteric vessels have been used for arterial anastomosis.[31,32] Another technical variant is venous drainage of a segmental graft via the portal vein by constructing an end-to-side anastomosis between the donor's splenic vein and the recipient's superior mesenteric vein; for the arterial anastomosis, an extension graft needs to be anastomosed to the recipient's common iliac artery and anastomosed to the donor's proximal or distal splenic artery. Portal vein anastomosis of segmental pancreas transplants cannot be done with bladder drainage.

## Posttransplant Care

Immediately posttransplant, recipients are brought to the postanesthesia care unit (PACU) or intensive care unit (ICU). As with any surgical procedure, hemodynamic and ventilatory assessment is essential during recovery. The endotracheal tube is usually removed in the operating room. On transfer from the operating room, blood tests, a chest x-ray, and an electrocardiogram (ECG) are routinely obtained. Blood pressure, pulse rate, and urine output are monitored. Initially, a complete blood count, a complete chemistry panel, and coagulation profiles are also obtained in the PACU or ICU.

The first 24 to 48 hours posttransplant are most crucial[33]: the recipient undergoes the physiologic response to surgical trauma; the transplanted pancreas is in a varying degree of ischemic or reperfusion injury; and immunosuppression begins. Initially, vital signs and laboratory parameters (in particular, plasma glucose, serum amylase and lipase, urinary amylase, hemoglobin, and PTT) are monitored every 4 hours. For fluid and electrolyte management, recipients are usually placed on ½ normal saline with 10 meq/$HCO_3^-$. Bicarbonate replacement is especially important for bladder-drained recipients, but even enteric-drained SPK recipients can initially develop acidosis that requires bicarbonate replacement. Intravenous fluids are usually infused at an In = Out ratio once hemodynamic stability is obtained; after the first 24 hours, recipients are usually placed on a straight rate (75 to 150 mL/hour) that should also take the central venous pressure into account (target, 8 to 14 mm Hg). In general, SPK recipients have larger fluid requirements than do PTA or PAK recipients. In the immediate posttransplant stage, dextrose (D5W) infusion is usually avoided, so as not to interfere with pancreas graft function. An insulin drip is started if blood sugar levels exceed 150 mg/dL, so as not to further stress the insulin-producing cells on top of the preservation and ischemic injury.

One of the most crucial elements in the immediate posttransplant care of LD segmental pancreas recipients is anticoagulation.[2,4] During the transplant procedure, they receive 20 to 40 U/kg of heparin (see above). While still in the operating room, before closure of the abdominal incision, recipients are started on a heparin drip (usually 200 U/hour). The target PTT within the first 24 hours is 40 to 50; thereafter, 40 to 60. In addition, recipients are started on Coumadin on posttransplant day 3 (and continue for up to 6 months). The heparin drip is usually discontinued on posttransplant day 5. Close monitoring of hemoglobin levels is imperative: postoperative hemorrhage is not infrequent after a pancreas transplant. Fluid and blood product substitution has to be adjusted accordingly. Obviously, it is better to surgically explore the recipient for bleeding (in case of over-anticoagulation) than for thrombosis, which is equivalent to graft loss. I do not recommend early use of low-molecular-weight heparin, because its effect is more difficult to correct.

Antimicrobial prophylaxis, usually initiated perioperatively, consists of antibacterial, antifungal, and antiviral medications. Broad-spectrum antibiotics are given intraoperatively, every 4 hours, and up to 48 hours posttransplant. Antifungal medications (eg, fluconazole) are administered for 5 to 7 days. Antiviral medications,

in particular cytomegalovirus (CMV) prophylaxis, are first given intravenously in the immediate postoperative period, then orally when the recipient tolerates a regular diet. Depending on the recipient's and LD's CMV status, CMV prophylaxis is continued for up to 6 months posttransplant. In addition, sulfamethoxazole/trimethoprim is given as long-term prophylaxis against *Pneumocystis carinii* and *Nocardia* infections.

Immunosuppression is initiated in the operating room; the first dose of antibody therapy is usually given before graft reperfusion. Standard immunosuppressive protocols consist of quadruple immunosuppression for induction and triple immunosuppression for maintenance therapy. For induction, anti-T-cell agents are given in combination with a calcineurin inhibitor, an antimetabolite, and steroids. Administration of the calcineurin inhibitor may be delayed if a kidney was transplanted simultaneously with the pancreas and if early kidney graft dysfunction (ie, acute tubular necrosis) is diagnosed. The most common calcineurin inhibitor used for pancreas recipients is tacrolimus; early target levels (within the first 3 months posttransplant) are 10 to 13 ng/mL; thereafter, 5 and 10 ng/mL. The most commonly used antimetabolite is mycophenolate mofetil (MMF), usually given at a dose of 2 to 3 g per day; more recently, MPA level monitoring has been used (target, 1.0 to 1.5 ng/dL). Steroids are no longer used routinely, because of their numerous side effects and their negative impact on glucose metabolism.

Posttransplant graft function is usually assessed by closely monitoring plasma glucose levels; insulin must be administered if plasma glucose levels exceed 150 mg/dL. For bladder-drained grafts, urinary amylase levels are followed (beginning on posttransplant day 1). The extent of ischemic or reperfusion damage is assessed with serum amylase and lipase levels. Because serum amylase and serum lipase levels can be elevated despite good glucose control and good endocrine function, octreotide can be used to minimize the pancreatic inflammatory response to the underlying ischemic or reperfusion and injury.

In bladder-drained recipients, the Foley catheter remains in place for about 2 to 3 weeks. Initial episodes of hematuria may require initiation of continuous bladder irrigation through a three-way system, in order to prevent formation of obstructive clots. Once recipients report bowel movement, oral intake is initiated. Most recipients, in the absence of complications, are discharged from the hospital within 7 to 10 days posttransplant.

## References

1. Gruessner RWG, Sutherland DER. Simultaneous kidney and segmental pancreas transplants from living related donors – the first two successful cases. *Transplantation* 1996;61:1265–1268.
2. Gruessner RWG, Kendall DM, Drangstveit MB, et al. Simultaneous pancreas-kidney transplantation from live donors. *Ann Surg* 1997; 226: 471–482.
3. Gruessner AC. International Pancreas Transplant Registry (IPTR) data, personal communication, November 2005.
4. Gruessner RWG. Living Donor Pancreas Transplantation. In: Gruessner RWG, Sutherland DER, eds. *Transplantation of the Pancreas*. New York: Springer-Verlag; 2004, Ch 14:423–440.
5. Gruessner RWG, Nakhleh R, Tzardis P, et al. Differences in rejection grading after simultaneous pancreas and kidney transplantation in pigs. *Transplantation* 1994;57:1021–1028.
6. Benedetti E, Najarian JS, Sutherland DER, et al. Correlation between cystoscopic biopsy results and hypoamylasuria in bladder-drained pancreas transplants. *Surgery* 1995;118: 864–872.

7. Sollinger HW, Cook K, Kamps D, et al. Clinical and experimental experience with pancreaticocystostomy for exocrine pancreatic drainage in pancreas transplantation. *Transplant Proc* 1984;16:749–751.

8. Prieto M, Sutherland DE, Goetz FC, et al. Pancreas transplant results according to the technique of duct management: Bladder versus enteric drainage. *Surgery* 1987;102:680–691.

9. Gruessner RW, Sutherland DE, Troppmann C, et al. The surgical risk of pancreas transplantation in the cyclosporine era: An overview. *J Am Coll Surg* 1997;185:128–144.

10. Gruessner RWG. Immunobiology, Diagnosis, and Treatment of Pancreas Graft Rejection. In: Gruessner RWG, Sutherland DER, eds. *Transplantation of the Pancreas.* Neew York: Springer-Verlag; 2004:Ch11;349–380.

11. Gruessner RWG, Dunn DL, Tzardis PJ, et al. Simultaneous pancreas and kidney transplants versus single kidney transplants and previous kidney transplants in uremic patients and single pancreas transplants in nonuremic diabetic patients: Comparison of rejection, morbidity, and long-term outcome. *Transplant Proc* 1990;22:622–623.

12. Troppmann C. Surgical Complications. In: Gruessner RWG, Sutherland DER, eds. *Transplantation of the Pancreas.* New York: Springer-Verlag; 2004:Ch9.2.2;206–237.

13. Tom WW, Munda R, First MR, et al. Autodigestion of the glans penis and urethra by activated transplant pancreatic exocrine enzymes. *Surgery* 1987;102:99–101.

14. Mullaney JM, DeMeo JH, Ham JM. Enzymatic digestion of the urethra after pancreas transplantation: a case report. *Abdom Imag* 1995;20:563–565.

15. West M, Gruessner AC, Sutherland DE, et al. Surgical complications after conversion from bladder to enteric drainage in pancreaticoduodenal transplantation. *Transplant Proc* 1998;30:438–439.

16. Gruessner RWG, Stephanian E, Dunn DL, et al. Cystoenteric conversion after whole pancreaticoduodenal transplantation. *Transplant Proc* 1993;25:1179–1181.

17. Gruessner AC, Sutherland DE. Pancreas outcomes for United States (US) and non-US cases as reported to the United Network for Organ Sharing (UNOS) and the International Pancreas Transplant Registry (IPTR) as of June 2004. *Clin Transplant* 2005;19:433–455.

18. Diem P, Abid M, Redmon JB, et al. Systemic venous drainage of pancreas allografts as independent cause of hyperinsulinemia in type I diabetic recipients. *Diabetes* 1990;39:534–540.

19. Hughes TA, Gaber AO, Amiri HS, et al. Kidney-pancreas transplantation. The effect of portal versus systemic venous drainage of the pancreas on the lipoprotein composition. *Transplantation* 1995;60:1406–1412.

20. Cattral MS, Bigam DL, Hemming AW, et al. Portal venous and enteric exocrine drainage versus systemic venous and bladder exocrine drainage of pancreas grafts: Clinical outcome of 40 consecutive transplant recipients. *Ann Surg* 2000;232:688–695.

21. Stratta RJ, Shokouh-Amiri MH, Egidi MF, et al. A prospective comparison of simultaneous kidney-pancreas transplantation with systemic-enteric versus portal-enteric drainage. *Ann Surg* 2001; 233:740–751.

22. Petruzzo P, Laville M, Badet L, et al. Effect of venous drainage site on insulin action after simultaneous pancreas-kidney transplantation. *Transplantation* 2004;77:1875–1879.

23. Gruessner RWG. Recipient Procedures. In: Gruessner RWG, Sutherland DER, eds. *Transplantation of the Pancreas.* New York: Springer-Verlag; 2004:Ch 8.2.2;150–178.

24. Zielinski A, Nazarewski S, Bogetti D, et al. Simultaneous pancreas-kidney transplant from living related donor: a single-center experience. *Transplantation* 2003;76:547–552.

25. Frisk B, Hedman L, Brynger H. Pancreaticocystostomy with a two-layer anastomosis technique in human segmental pancreas transplantation. *Transplantation* 1987;44:836–838.

26. Gliedman ML, Gold M, Whittaker J, et al. Pancreatic duct to ureter anastomosis for exocrine drainage in pancreatic transplantation. *Am J Surg* 1973;125:245–252.

27. Dubernard JM, Traeger J, Neyra P, et al. A new method of preparation of segmental pancreatic grafts for transplantation: Trials in dogs and in man. *Surgery* 1978;84:633–639.

28. Land W, Gebhardt C, Gall FP, et al. Pancreatic duct obstruction with prolamine solution. *Transplant Proc* 1980;12:72–75.

29. McMaster P, Gibby OM, Evans DM, et al. Human pancreatic transplantation with polyisoprene and cyclosporine A immunosuppression. Proc. 1980 EASD satellite symposium on islet-pancreas transplantation and artificial pancreas. *Horm Metab Res* 1981;22:151–156.

30. Sutherland DE, Goetz FC, Elick BA, et al. Experience with 49 segmental pancreas transplants in 45 diabetic patients. *Transplantation* 1982; 34:330–338.

31. Tyden G, Lundgren G, Ostman J, et al. Grafted pancreas with portal venous drainage. *Lancet* 1984; 1: 964–965.

32. Sutherland DE, Goetz FC, Moudry KC, et al. Use of recipient mesenteric vessels for revascularization of segmental pancreas grafts: Technical and metabolic considerations. *Transplant Proc* 1987; 19: 2300–2304.

33. Leone JP, Christensen K. Postoperative Management: Uncomplicated Course. In: Gruessner RWG, Sutherland DER, eds. *Transplantation of the Pancreas.* New York: Springer-Verlag; 200:Ch 9.1;179–190.

## 20.3 PERIOPERATIVE CARE, IMMUNOSUPPRESSIVE THERAPY, AND POSTTRANS-PLANT COMPLICATIONS

*Raja Kandaswamy, MD*

### PREOPERATIVE EVALUATION

This has been discussed previously in Chapter 20.1

### Pancreas Preservation

In living donor (LD) pancreas transplants, since the organ is transplanted soon after retrieval, back-table flush is usually done using Ringer's Lactate (LR) solution. If the cold ischemic time is expected to be an hour or longer flushing with University of Wisconsin (UW) solution or HTK solution may be considered. Advantages of the HTK solution include lower viscosity, lower potassium, and decreased cost.[1]

### Anesthetic Considerations

Concomitant systemic complications of long-standing diabetes mellitus can be a challenge for the anesthesiologist.[2] Dysautonomic response to hypoxia and drugs can lead to morbidity[3] and mortality.[4] Awareness of these risks and familiarity with immunosuppressive side effects are important. Anti-T-cell agents are often started in the operating room. They have significant systemic side effects from the cytokine response. In addition, steroids are given which may affect blood pressure and glucose.

Significant blood loss may be encountered in a procedure such as LD pancreas or kidney–pancreas transplant. Prompt replacement with blood or colloids should be instituted to avoid hypovolemia and hypoperfusion of vital organs. Careful monitoring of blood glucose levels with continuous intravenous (IV) insulin therapy is required to maintain tight control. Perioperative beta-blockade should be used or long-standing diabetics with significant cardiac history. Perioperative anticoagulation may be started in the operating room especially in hypercoagulable patients.

### Operative Procedure

This has been discussed previously in Chapter 20.2.

## Postoperative Case

After an uncomplicated pancreas transplant, the recipient is transferred to the postanesthesia care unit (PACU) or the surgical intensive care unit (SICU). Centers that have a specialized monitored transplant unit (with central venous and arterial monitoring capabilities) transition the postoperative recipients through the PACU to the transplant unit. Others transfer directly to the SICU for the first 24 to 48 hours. Care during the first few hours posttransplant is similar to care after any major operative procedure. Careful monitoring of vital signs, central venous pressure, oxygen saturation, and hematologic and laboratory parameters is crucial. The following factors are unique to pancreas recipients and should be attended to.

1. Blood glucose levels. Any sudden, unexplained increase in glucose levels should raise the suspicion of graft thrombosis. An immediate ultrasound examination must be done to assess blood flow to the graft. Maintenance of tight glucose control (< 150 mg/dL) using an intravenous insulin drip is important to "rest" the pancreas in the early postoperative period.

2. Intravascular volume. Because the pancreas is a "low flow" organ, intravascular volume must be maintained to provide adequate perfusion to the graft. CVP monitoring is used to monitor intravascular volume status. In some cases, such as patients with depressed cardiac function, pulmonary artery catheter monitoring may be required during the first 24 to 48 hours. If the hypovolemia is associated with low hemoglobin levels, then washed packed red blood cell transfusions should be given. Otherwise, colloid or crystalloid replacement can be used.

3. Maintenance intravenous (IV) fluid therapy. The choice of IV fluid is usually $D_5\frac{1}{2}$ NS. The use of dextrose is not contraindicated and may be of benefit, as long as IV insulin is used to maintain good blood glucose control. In SPK recipients, whose IV rate is based on urine output, dextrose should be eliminated if the urine output is high (>500 mL/hr). Maintenance solution for BD recipients should include 10 mEq of $HCO_3$ added to each liter to account for the excess $HCO_3$ loss.[95] Sodium lactate can be used as an alternative.[7]

4. Antibiotic therapy. Broad-spectrum antibiotic therapy (with strong gram-negative coverage) and antifungal therapy are instituted before the incision is made in the OR, then continued for 3 days (for antibiotics) and 7 days (for antifungal). At the University of Minnesota, since the introduction of this protocol, we have noted a decrease in postoperative abdominal infections.[8] Cytomegalovirus (CMV) and antiviral prophylaxis is similar to that for other solid organs.

5. Octreotide. The use of octreotide in pancreas recipients helps reduce the incidence of technical complications.[9] This benefit should be weighed against evidence, in rat studies, that shows decreased pancreatic islet blood flow with octreotide use,[10] although clinically no detrimental effects of octreotide use have been documented. A dose of 100 to 150 μg IV/SQ tid is administered for 5 days posttransplant. Dose adjustments may be made for nausea, which is the predominant side effect.

6. Anticoagulation. Although perioperative anticoagulation is generally used in all pancreas transplants, it is especially important in LD pancreas transplants due to the higher thrombotic risk. This is due to the smaller blood vessels in segmental pancreas profits.[11,12] Heparin (70 U/kg) is

administered intraoperatively prior to vascular clamping. Postoperative heparinization is titrated to a PTT of 40 to 70 for days. Aspirin 81 mg once a day (for life) and Coumadin therapy (target INR of 2 to 2.5) for 6 months is started on postoperative day 1 and 3, respectively.

Immunosuppression is essential to thwart rejection in all allotransplant recipients.[13] Before the advent of cyclosporine in the early 1980s,[14] azathioprine and prednisone were the mainstays of immunosuppression. From the early 1980s to the mid-1990s cyclosporine was added to the mix and resulted in significant improvement in immunologic outcomes.[15] Since the mid-1990s, tacrolimus and mycophenolate mofetil have replaced cyclosporine and azathioprine as the main drugs, resulting in even better pancreas graft survival rates.[15–17] In addition, steroids have been successfully withdrawn from some pancreas recipients[18] and, in some cases, avoided.[19] Using rapamycin in combination with tacrolimus, steroids have been successfully avoided in some pancreas recipients.[20,21] At the University of Minnesota, MMF used in combination with tacrolimus has also been successful in eliminating steroids.

Anti-T-cell therapy has always remained a part of the induction protocol for pancreas recipients.[22] With the recent emphasis on steroid withdrawal or avoidance, anti-T-cell-therapy has taken on added importance to avoid rejection. Anti-CD-25 antibodies are also used frequently as induction therapy.[23] Avoidance of calcineurin inhibitors has been attempted in pancreas transplantation. When combined with steroid avoidance, this required prolonged anti-T-cell therapy, which increases the risk of infection without adequately controlling rejection.[24]

For PTA recipients, whose rejection rates are the highest of all categories, pretransplant immunosuppression has decreased rejection rates and graft loss from rejection.[25] Heavy use of immunosuppression may increase the infection rate, but effective antimicrobial prophylaxis has helped ameliorate this problem.[26,27]

## INTRAVENOUS IMMUNOGLOBULIN (IVIG) AND PLASMAPHERESIS

IVIG has many applications in transplantation. It has been used successfully to decrease anti-HLA antibodies in transplant recipients on the waiting list and to shorten their waiting times.[28,29] It can also be used to control acute humoral rejection in kidney and heart allograft recipients.[30] Plasmapheresis has been used to decrease humoral antibody titers in ABO-incompatible liver and kidney recipients.[31,32] It has also been used to control hyperacute or accelerated acute rejection in positive-crossmatch kidney recipients[33,34] and lung[35] recipients. At the University of Minnesota, for ABO-incompatible ($A_2$ to O, B or AB) and positive-crossmatch (T-cell) pancreas recipients, the treatment protocol consists of intraoperative IVIG (0.5 mg/kg) followed by a course of 5 to 7 days in combination with daily plasmapheresis. For B-cell-positive crossmatch recipients, IVIG may be used without plasmapheresis.

## Surgical Complications

1. Bleeding. The risk of bleeding in LD pancreas transplants is higher than that in deceased donor pancreas transplants due to more aggressive anticoagulation. The incidence of bleeding is already high in deceased donor transplants ranging from 6% to 8%.[8,36] Frequent physical examinations and monitoring of hemoglobin help detect bleeding early.

Heparin should not be suspended preferentially. Early relaparotomy in uncontrolled bleeding may prevent morbidity of excessive blood loss.

2. Thrombosis. The incidence of thrombosis posttransplant ranges from 5% to 13%.[36,37] This risk is higher in LD pancreas transplants due to the small caliber of the blood vessels.[38] Most thromboses are due to technical reasons. An ultrashort splenic vein in the segmental graft or atherosclerotic arteries (either in patient or graft) increases the risk of thrombosis. In the recipient, a deeply placed iliac vein, technically difficult vascular anastomosis, kinking of the vein by torsion of the graft, significant postoperative bleeding with compressing hematoma, and a hypercoagulable state (HCS) are some factors that increase the risk of thrombosis. The most common form of HCS in Factor V Leiden mutation in the Western world. Incidence ranges from 2% to 5% but may be as high as 50% to 60% in patients with a family history of thrombosis.[39] Other causes of HCS include antithrombin (ATIII) deficiency, protein C+S deficiency, resistance to activated protein C, and anticardiolipin antibodies.[40]

    Thrombosis usually occurs in the first 2 weeks after transplant and is manifested by a sudden increase in insulin requirement or a sharp drop in urine amylase levels. Venous thrombosis may be associated with a swollen, tender graft, hematuria, and lower-extremity edema ipsilaterally. Diagnosis is usually confirmed by Doppler ultrasound. Early exploration and graft pancreatectomy is indicated.

3. Pancreatic leaks. In LD pancreas, the absence of donor duodenum increased the incidence leaks. The cut surface of the pancreatic hemigraft is anastomosed to either bladder or bowel. While doing enteric drainage, a Roux-En-Y loop is preferred to minimize the adverse consequences of a leak and to increase the chances of salvage with primary repair leak rates with whole organ pancreas ranging from 4% to 6%.[8,36] The incidence in LD pancreas transplants is higher.

    A leak from an enteric anastomosis almost always leads to a laparotomy. Graft pancreatectomy is indicated if there is significant peritoneal contamination. Diagnosis is made by elevated pancreatic enzymes associated with a tender abdomen. Differential diagnosis includes pancreatitis, acute rejection, and intraabdominal abscess.

    Leaks in bladder-drained grafts can be managed conservatively with bladder decompression (Foley catheter). Large leaks may require operative intervention for repair or enteric conversion.[41]

4. Intra-abdominal infections. The incidence of intraabdominal infections requiring reoperation ranges from 4% to 10%.[8,36] Opening the duodenal segment intraoperatively, with associated contamination, predisposes to this high rate. Fungal and gram-negative infections predominate. With the advent of advanced interventional radiologic procedures to drain intraabdominal abscesses, the incidence of reoperations is fast decreasing. If the infection is uncontrolled or widespread, then graft pancreatectomy followed by frequent washouts may be necessary.

5. Others. Other surgical complications that may require laparotomy include wound dehiscence, severe pancreatitis (sometimes hemorrhagic or neurotic), pseudoaneurysms, and arteria-venous AV fistula in the graft, and severe painful rejection. The overall incidence of laparotomy decreased

from the 1980s (about 32%) to the 1990s (about 19%). The mortality rate in recipients requiring relaparotomy also decreased from 9% to 1%. Improved anti-infective prophylaxis, surgical techniques, immunosuppression, and advances in interventional radiology have all contributed to this decrease.[8]

## Nonsurgical Complications

1. Pancreatitis. The incidence of posttransplant pancreatitis varies based on the type of exocrine drainage. BD recipients with abnormal bladder function are at increased risk secondary to incomplete bladder emptying or urine retention causing resistance to the flow of pancreatic exocrine secretions. Other causes of pancreatitis include drugs (corticosteroids, azathioprine, cyclosporine), hypercalcemia, viral infections (CMV or HCV), and reperfusion injury after prolonged ischemia. Pancreatitis is usually manifested by an increase in serum amylase and lipase with or without local signs of inflammation. The treatment usually consists of catheter decompression of the bladder for a period of 2 to 6 weeks depending on the severity. In addition, octreotide therapy may be used to decrease pancreatic secretions. The underlying urological problem, if any, should be treated. If repeated episodes of pancreatitis occur, an enteric conversion of exocrine drainage may be indicated.[42–44]

2. Rejection. The incidence of rejection is discussed in the Results section earlier in this chapter. The diagnosis is usually based on an increase in serum amylase and lipase and a decrease in urine amylase in BD recipients. A sustained significant drop in urinary amylase from baseline should prompt a pancreas biopsy to rule out rejection.[45] In ED recipients one has to rely on serum amylase and lipase only. A rise in serum lipase has recently shown to correlate well with acute pancreas rejection.[46] Other signs and symptoms include tenderness over the graft, unexplained fever, and hyperglycemia (usually a late finding). Diagnosis can be confirmed by a percutaneous pancreas biopsy.[47,48] In cases, where percutaneous biopsy is not possible due to technical reasons, empiric therapy may be started. Rarely, open biopsy is indicated. Transcystoscopic biopsy, which was frequently used in the past, has been largely abandoned.

3. Others. These include infections complications such as CMV, HCV, extra-abdominal bacterial or fungal infections, posttransplant malignancy such as posttransplant lymphoproliferative disorder, and other rare complications such as graft-versus-host disease that occur in pancreas transplantation. The diagnosis and management of these complications is similar to those of other solid organ transplants.

## Radiologic Studies

1. Ultrasonography. This is the most frequent study used in pancreas recipients. Noninvasive, portable, and relatively inexpensive, it provides prompt information regarding blood flow to the pancreas; the presence of arterial or venous occlusion, thrombi, pseudoaneurysms, or AV fistulas; resistance to blood flow within the pancreas (suggestive of either rejection or pancreatitis); and peripancreatic fluid collections.

2.  CT scan. A computed tomography (CT) scan provides more detail of pancreatic and surrounding anatomy. Use of PO, IV, and bladder contrast (in BD recipients) is recommended. Thus, a CT cystogram can be combined with an abdominal CT scan. A CT scan is frequently used as a guide in pancreas biopsies or in placement of directed intra-abdominal drains.

3.  Fluoroscopy. A contrast cystogram can be performed under fluoroscopy and can be used instead of, or in addition to, a CT cystogram to look for bladder leak. The combination of the tests increases the sensitivity for detecting leaks.

4.  Magnetic resonance angiogram (MRA). An MRA is done if vascular abnormalities are suspected on the ultrasound and if the patient's kidney function is inadequate to perform standard angiography with contrast. MRA provides resolution comparable to a CT angiogram, without the risk of contrast nephropathy, but it is inferior to standard angiography in providing fine vascular detail.

5.  Angiography. This is the gold standard test for evaluating details of arterial anatomy in and around the pancreas. However, it is rarely employed, except in cases where angiographic intervention (such as angioplasty, stenting of a stenotic segment, or coiling of an AV fistula or pseudoaneurysm) is planned. Contrast nephropathy is feared in a diabetic kidney, and reasonable alternatives (such as ultrasound and MRA) are available.

## Minimizing Surgical Complications

Although complications can never be totally avoided, they can be minimized by

1.  Proper donor and recipient selection

2.  Meticulous surgical techniques

3.  Careful postoperative care

These factors are applicable to any transplant, but more so to LD pancreas transplants in view of their increased complexity and risk of complications. As the organ-shortage problem expands into pancreas transplants, LD pancreas transplants will increase, and careful adherence to the above principles will help increase their applicability.

## References

1. Agarwal A, Murdock P, Pescovitz MD, et al. Follow-up experience using histidine-tryptophan ketoglutarate solution in clinical pancreas transplantation. *Transplant Proc* 2005;37(8):3523–3526.

2. Hogan K, Rusy D, Springman, SR. Difficult laryngoscopy and diabetes mellitus. *Anesth Analg* 1988;67(12):1162–1165.

3. Burgos LG, Ebert TJ, Asiddao C, et al. Increased intraoperative cardiovascular morbidity in diabetics with autonomic neuropathy. *Anesthesiology* 1989;70(4):591–597.

4. Page MM, Watkins PJ. Cardiorespiratory arrest and diabetic autonomic neuropathy. *Lancet* 1978;1(8054):14–16.

5. Elkhammas EA, Henry ML, Tesi RJ, et al. Control of metabolic acidosis after pancreas transplantation using acetazolamide. *Transplant Proc* 1991;23(1 Pt 2):1623–1624.

6. Schang T, Timmermann W, Thiede A, et al. Detrimental effects of fluid and electrolyte loss from duodenum in bladder-drained pancreas transplants. *Transplant Proc* 1991;23(1 Pt 2):1617–1618.

7. Peltenburg HG, Mutsaerts KJ, Hardy EL, et al. Sodium lactate as an alternative to sodium bicarbonate in the management of metabolic acidosis after pancreas transplantation. *Transplantation* 1992;53(1):225–226.

8. Humar A, Kandaswamy R, Granger DK, et al. Decreased surgical risks of pancreas transplantation in the modern era. *Ann Surg* 2000;231:269–275.

9. Benedetti E, Coady NT, Asolati M, et al. A prospective randomized clinical trial of perioperative treatment with octreotide in pancreas transplantation. *Am J Surg* 1998;175(1):14–17.

10. Carlsson P O, Jansson L. The long-acting somatostatin analogue octreotide decreases pancreatic islet blood flow in rats. *Pancreas* 1994; 9(3):361–364.

11. Humar A, Gruessner RWG, Sutherland DER. Living related donor pancreas and pancreas-kidney transplantation. *Brit Med Bull* 1997;53(4): 879–891.

12. Benedetti E, Rastellini C, Sileri P, et al. Successful simultaneous pancreas-kidney transplantation from well- matched living-related donors. *Transplant Proc* 2001;33(1-2):1689–2001.

13. First MR. Current clinical immunosuppressive agents and their actions. Transplant Proc 2002;In Press.

14. Calne RY, Rolles K, White DJ, et al. Cyclosporin A initially as the only immunosuppressant in 34 recipients of cadaveric organs: 32 kidneys, 2 pancreases, and 2 livers. *Lancet* 1979;2(8151):1033–1036.

15. Stratta RJ. Simultaneous use of tacrolimus and mycophenolate mofetil in combined pancreas-kidney transplant recipients: a multi-center report. The FK/MMF Multi-Center Study Group. *Transplant Proc* 1997; 29 (1-2):654–655.

16. Gruessner AC, and Sutherland DER. Analysis of the United States (US) and Non-US pancreas transplants as reported to the International Pancreas Transplant Registry (IPTR) and the United Network for Organ Sharing (UNOS). *Clin Transplant* 1998;53–71.

17. Gruessner RW, Sutherland DE, Drangstveit MB, et al. Mycophenolate mofetil and tacrolimus for induction and maintenance therapy after pancreas transplantation. *Transplant Proc* 1998;30(2):518–520.

18. Gruessner RWG, Sutherland DER, Parr E, et al. A prospective, randomized, open-label study of steroid withdrawal in pancreas transplantation - A preliminary report with 6-month follow-up. *Transplant Proc* 2001;33:1663–1663.

19. Kaufman DB. Steroid-free immunosuppression for pancreas transplantation. In Press 2001.

20. Salazar A, McAlister VC, Kiberd BA, et al. Sirolimus-tacrolimus combination for combined kidney-pancreas transplantation: effect on renal function. *Transplant Proc* 2001;33(1-2):1038–1039.

21. Kaufman DB, Leventhal JR, Koffron AJ, et al. A prospective study of rapid corticosteroid elimination in simultaneous pancreas-kidney transplantation: comparison of two maintenance immunosuppression protocols: tacrolimus/mycophenolate mofetil versus tacrolimus/sirolimus. *Transplantation* 2002;73(2):169–177.

22. Gruessner AC, Sutherland DER. Pancreas transplant outcomes for United States (US) cases reported to the United Network for Organ Sharing (UNOS) and non-US cases reported to the *International Pancreas Transplant Registry (IPTR)* as of October 2000. 2001;(4):45–72.

23. Stratta RJ, Alloway RR, Lo A, et al. A multicenter trial of two daclizumab dosing strategies versus no antibody induction in simultaneous kidney-pancreas transplantation: interim analysis. *Transplant Proc* 2001;33 (1-2):1692–1693.

24. Gruessner RW, Kandaswamy R, Humar A, et al. Calcineurin inhibitor- and steroid-free immunosuppression in pancreas-kidney and solitary pancreas transplantation. *Transplantation* 2005;79(9):1184–1189.

25. Sutherland DER, Gruessner RWG, Humar A, et al. Pretransplant immunosuppression for pancreas transplants alone in nonuremic diabetic recipients. *Transplant Proc* 2001;33:1656–1658.

26. Rubin RH. A new beginning. *Transpl Infect Dis* 1999;1:1–2.

27. Villacian JS, Paya CV. Prevention of infections in solid organ transplant recipients. *Transpl Infect Dis* 1999;1(1):50–64.

28. Tyan DB, Li VA, Czer L, et al. Intravenous immunoglobulin suppression of HLA alloantibody in highly sensitized transplant candidates and transplantation with a histoincompatible organ. *Transplantation* 1994;57(4):553–562.

29. Glotz D, Haymann JP, Niaudet P, et al. Successful kidney transplantation of immunized patients after desensitization with normal human polyclonal immunoglobulins. *Transplant Proc* 1995;27(1):1038–1039.

30. Jordan SC, Quartel AW, Czer LS, et al. Posttransplant therapy using high-dose human immunoglobulin (intravenous gammaglobulin) to control acute humoral rejection in renal and cardiac allograft recipients and potential mechanism of action. *Transplantation* 1998;66(6): 800–805.

31. Watanabe H, Misu K, Kobayashi T, et al. ABO-incompatible auxiliary partial orthotopic liver transplant for late- onset familial amyloid polyneuropathy. *J Neurol Sci* 2002;195(1):63–66.

32. Shishido S, Asanuma H, Tajima E, et al. ABO-incompatible living-donor kidney transplantation in children. *Transplantation* 2001; 72(6): 1037–1042.

33. Montgomery RA, Zachary AA, Racusen LC, et al. Plasmapheresis and intravenous immune globulin provides effective rescue therapy for refractory humoral rejection and allows kidneys to be successfully transplanted into cross-match-positive recipients. *Transplantation* 2000; 70(6):887–895.

34. Takeda A, Uchida K, Haba T, et al. Acute humoral rejection of kidney allografts in patients with a positive flow cytometry crossmatch (FCXM). *Clin Transplant* 2000;14 Suppl 3:15–20.

35. Bittner HB, Dunitz J, Hertz M, et al. Hyperacute rejection in single lung transplantation—case report of successful management by means of plasmapheresis and antithymocyte globulin treatment. *Transplantation* 2001;71(5):649–651.

36. Reddy, K. S., Stratta, R. J., Shokouh-Amiri, M. H. et al. Surgical complications after pancreas transplantation with portal- enteric drainage. *J.Am.Coll.Surg.* 189(3):305–313, 1999.

37. Kandaswamy R, Humar A, Gruessner A, et al. Vascular graft thrombosis after pancreas transplantation: Comparison of the FK 506 and cyclosporine eras. *Transplant Proc* 1999;31:602–603.

38. Gruessner RWG, Sutherland DER. Simultaneous kidney and segmental pancreas transplants from living related donors - the first two successful cases. *Transplantation* 1996;61:1265–1268.

39. Wuthrich RP, Factor V Leiden mutation: potential thrombogenic role in renal vein, dialysis graft and transplant vascular thrombosis. *Curr Opin Nephrol Hypertens* 2001;10(3):409–414.

40. Friedman GS, Meier-Kriesche HU, Kaplan B, et al. Hypercoagulable states in renal transplant candidates: impact of anticoagulation upon incidence of renal allograft thrombosis. *Transplantation* 2001;72(6): 1073–1078.

41. Eckhoff DE, Ploeg RJ, Wilson MA, et al. Efficacy of 99mTc voiding cystourethrogram for detection of duodenal leaks after pancreas transplantation. *Transplant Proc* 1994;26(2):462–463.

42. Del Pizzo JJ, Jacobs SC, Bartlett ST, et al. Urological complications of bladder-drained pancreatic allografts. *Br J Urol* 1998;81(4): 543–547.

43. Kaplan AJ, Valente JF, First MR, et al. Early operative intervention for urologic complications of kidney- pancreas transplantation. *World J Surg* 1998;22(8):890–894.

44. Troppmann C, Gruessner AC, Dunn DL, et al. Surgical complications requiring early relaparotomy after pancreas transplantation: a multivariate risk factor and economic impact analysis of the cyclosporine era. *Ann Surg* 1998;227(2):255–268.

45. Kuo PC, Johnson LB, Schweitzer EJ, et al. Solitary pancreas allografts. The role of percutaneous biopsy and standardized histologic grading of rejection. *Arch Surg* 1997;132(1):52–57.

46. Papadimitriou JC, Drachenberg CB, Wiland A, et al. Histologic grading of acute allograft rejection in pancreas needle biopsy: correlation to serum enzymes, glycemia, and response to immunosuppressive treatment. *Transplantation* 1998;66(12):1741–1745.

47. Klassen DK, Weir MR, Cangro CB, et al. Pancreas allograft biopsy: safety of percutaneous biopsy-results of a large experience. *Transplantation* 2002;73(4):553–555.

48. Malek SK, Potdar S, Martin JA, et al. Percutaneous ultrasound-guided pancreas allograft biopsy: a single-center experience.

## 20.4  THE IDENTICAL TWIN TRANSPLANT EXPERIENCE: RECURRENCE OF DISEASE

*Rainer W.G. Gruessner, MD*

The autoimmune cause of diabetes mellitus is based on several independent observations, including (1) the presence of a lymphocytic infiltrate in the islets ("isletitis"), (2) the appearance of a series of autoantibodies coupled with a progressive loss of insulin secretion, (3) the specificity of pancreatic ß-cell destruction, and (4) recurrence of type 1 diabetes mellitus in patients transplanted with identical twin pancreas grafts in the absence of immunosuppressive therapy.[1]

In the University of Minnesota experience, nine pancreas transplants were performed between monozygous twins. Of those, seven were technically successful. The first four such transplants were performed in the precyclosporine (CSA) era, between October 1, 1980, and July 31, 1983.[2]

The first three recipients were not given any induction or maintenance immunosuppression. Each of the three recipients demonstrated normal glucose metabolism early posttransplant, but remained insulin-independent for only 5 to 12 weeks. Once progressive hyperglycemia was diagnosed in the first recipient, no attempt was made at graft salvage, and antirejection treatment was not initiated. In the second recipient, azathioprine (AZA) was started 6 weeks posttransplant, but in the absence of clinical improvement, the drug was stopped 6 weeks later. In the third recipient, antirejection treatment was started with Minnesota antilymphocyte globulin (ALG), and azathioprine (AZA) was given, but efforts were discontinued in the absence of clinical improvement.[2,3]

Pancreas graft biopsies at the time of decline in graft function in those three recipients revealed mononuclear cell infiltrates in the islets consisting of T11 (pan T), OKT8 (suppressor/killer), OKT9 (transferrin receptor), OKT10 (activated), and HLA-DR-reactive mononuclear cells, as well as 63D3 and OKM1 reactive monocytes.[4] Further immunohistopathologic analysis showed that the isletitis was mostly constituted by $CD8^+$/T-lymphocyte receptor α, ß ($TCR_{\alpha,\beta}{}^+$) T lymphocytes surrounding and infiltrating the affected islets. $CD4^-$/$CD8^-$/$TCR_{\gamma,\delta}{}^+$ T lymphocytes were observed within the islets.[5]

Pancreas graft biopsies obtained after loss of graft function in two of these three recipients revealed resolution of the inflammatory process and selective destruction of all ß cells; in the third recipient, a mononuclear cell infiltrate was noted in islets containing demonstrable ß cells, but no infiltrate was noted in islets without ß cells. Because no immunohistologic evidence of humoral-mediated immune reaction was seen in any of the biopsies, it was postulated that selected ß-cell destruction was a consequence of ß-cell-mediated immunity leading to recurrent diabetes mellitus.[3,4,6]

The fourth identical twin pancreas recipient was prophylactically given AZA posttransplant. A biopsy at 6 weeks posttransplant, however, showed mild isletitis without ß-cell destruction. At 36 months posttransplant, mild hyperglycemia developed. A biopsy showed resolution of isletitis, but destruction of ß cells in 70% of the islets. At the time, cyclosporine had become available in clinical practice and was added to the immunosuppressive regimen. The recipient temporarily required only a relatively low amount of exogenous insulin, but 5 years posttransplant, became fully insulin-dependent.[2,3]

Of the last three identical twin pancreas transplants done between May 1, 1987, and September 30, 1990, 2 recipients were given induction therapy with Minnesota ALG, and all three were maintained on CSA-based maintenance therapy. All three recipients were alive as of September 2006. Of those, two have remained normoglycemic for over 15 years. The third recipient, on lower-dose immunosuppressive therapy, developed biopsy-proven isletitis at 1 year posttransplant and became fully insulin-dependent 8 years posttransplant, despite intermittent anti-T-cell therapy.

This unique clinical experience, in itself, lends strong surgical evidence to diabetes mellitus being an autoimmune disease. It also demonstrates that the disease recurrence in the absence of immunosuppressive therapy can occur as early as several weeks posttransplant and that low-dose immunosuppressive therapy cannot prevent disease recurrence. Furthermore, immunosuppression given late (ie, months or years after the clinical onset of diabetes mellitus) does not allow ß-cell regeneration—there are new reports in diabetic kidney transplant alone recipients that would indicate reversal of diabetes mellitus even if recipients were immunosuppressed for up to decades. The fact that immunosuppression prevents recurrence of disease in pancreas transplant recipients means that it should also prevent progression of disease in *de novo* autoimmune diabetes mellitus if applied early enough. Such a study, preferably done in children who carry a genetically high risk to develop diabetes mellitus, has not been done because of the concern of immunosuppressive side effects.

Except for the cases presented herein, all other cases of recurrent diabetes mellitus after pancreas transplantation have been noted in pancreas grafts obtained from deceased donors. It remains a relatively rare occurrence overall (< 1%), and the overall relatively small number of living donor pancreas transplants might be the reason that it has not been observed in nontwin living related transplants.

# References

1. Gruessner RWG. Immunology in pancreas transplantation—Autoimmune reactivation. In: Gruessner RWG, Sutherland DER, eds. *Transplantation of the Pancreas*. New York: Springer-Verlag; 2004:393–397.
2. Sutherland DER, Sibley RK, Xu XZ, et al. Twin-to-twin pancreas transplantation: Reversal and reenactment of the pathogenesis of Type I diabetes. *Trans Assoc Am Phys* 1984;97: 80–87.
3. Sutherland DER, Goetz FC, Sibley RK. Recurrence of disease in pancreas transplants. *Diabetes* 1989;38:85–87.
4. Sibley RK, Sutherland DER, Goetz F, et al. Recurrent diabetes mellitus in the pancreas iso- and allograft. A light and electron microscopic and immunohistochemical analysis of four cases. *Lab Invest* 1985; 53:132–144.
5. Santamaria P, Nakhleh RE, Sutherland DER, et al. Characterization of T lymphocytes infiltrating human pancreas allograft affected by isletitis and recurrent diabetes. *Diabetes* 1992;41:53–61.
6. Nakhleh RE, Gruessner RWG, Swanson PE, et al. Pancreas transplant pathology. A morphologic, immunohistochemical, and electron microscopic comparison of allogeneic grafts with rejection, syngeneic grafts, and chronic pancreatitis. *Am J Surg Pathol* 1991;15:246–256.

# REGISTRY REPORT AND
# LONG-TERM OUTCOME

*Angelika C. Gruessner, PhD*

## INTRODUCTION

From the first pancreas transplant using a deceased donor (DD) on December 17, 1966, through December 31, 2005, almost 25,000 pancreas transplants were reported to the International Pancreas Transplant Registry (IPTR).[1] The IPTR has been maintained since its inception at the University of Minnesota. The record on pancreas transplants in the United States and in European countries associated with Eurotransplant is complete because reporting is mandatory to the United Network for Organ Sharing (UNOS) and to Eurotransplant. For all other countries, reporting is voluntary and, therefore, may not be complete.

Figure 21-1 shows the overall development of pancreas transplantation over time (1966–2005). More than 75% of all pancreas transplants through June 30, 2006, were performed in the United States, where, because of improving outcome, the number of pancreas transplants continuously increased from 1979 to 2000. Since 2001, the number of pancreas transplants in the United States has remained stable. Outside the United States, the rate of pancreas transplants is lower. Next to the United States, most reports to the IPTR have come from Europe.[2]

Outside the United States, the majority of pancreas transplants are done in combination with a simultaneous kidney transplant (SPK); in the United States, the SPK total has remained stable, but solitary pancreas transplants are performed with increasing frequency. This trend is noted for both pancreas trans-

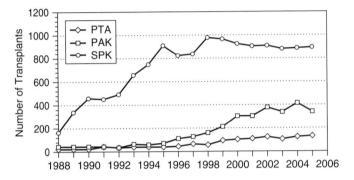

**FIGURE 21-2**

Annual number of U.S. pancreas transplants, by recipient category.

plants alone (PTA) as well as for pancreas after kidney transplants (PAK) (Figure 21-2).

Of the 24,655 pancreas transplants reported worldwide through 2005, a total of 495 (2%) were multiorgan transplants, that is, with the addition of a liver and/or intestinal graft (for nondiabetic reasons). Of the remaining 24,160 pancreas transplants in diabetic patients, 18,893 (78%) were SPK; 3,579 (15%), PAK; and 1,688 (7%), PTA.

## LD PANCREAS TRANSPLANTS

The first pancreas transplant using a living donor (LD) was a PAK transplant performed at the University of Minnesota, Minneapolis, on June 20, 1979. The first LD PTA was done at Huddinge Hospital, Stockholm, Sweden, on March 18, 1980; the first LD SPK, at Jackson Memorial Hospital, Miami, Florida, on November 12, 1980.

Through 2005, a total of 144 segmental pancreas transplants using LDs (0.6%) were reported to the IPTR, from six countries (Table 21-1). Most reports came from the United States (93%), where 85% (n = 123) of the LD transplants were performed at the University of Minnesota.

Table 21-2 shows the different categories of LD pancreas transplants performed from 1976 to 2005. The time period from the very first pancreas transplant (in 1966) on was arbitrarily divided into 4 decades for comparison with DD transplants. In the first decade (1966–1975), LD pancreas transplants were not performed.

The 3 following decades differed in immunosuppressive protocols and surgical techniques. In the second decade (1976–1985) the most common immunosuppressive protocol for maintenance

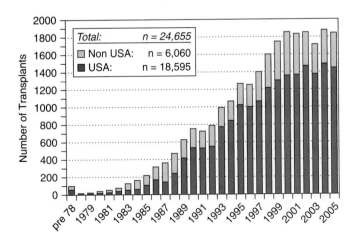

**FIGURE 21-1**

Annual number of U.S. and non-U.S. pancreas transplants reported to the IPTR (1966–2005). Reporting for 2005 is not complete for non-U.S. transplants.

### TABLE 21-1

## COUNTRIES THAT REPORTED LD PANCREAS TRANSPLANTS TO THE IPTR, BY RECIPIENT CATEGORY

|  | PAK | PTA | SPK | Total |
|---|---|---|---|---|
| United States | 33 | 54 | 47 | 134 |
| Sweden |  | 3 |  | 3 |
| South Korea |  | 2 |  | 2 |
| Kuwait | 1 |  |  | 1 |
| Norway |  |  | 1 | 1 |
| Japan |  |  | 3 | 3 |

LD, living donor; IPTR, International Pancreas Transplant Registry; PAK, pancreas after kidney; PTA, pancreas transplant alone; SPK, simultaneous pancreas–kidney.

therapy consisted of azathioprine (AZA) and prednisone. In the third decade (1986–1995), cyclosporine (CSA) was added to the standard immunosuppressive protocol. In the fourth decade (1996–2005), the most common immunosuppressants were tacrolimus (TAC, as a replacement for CSA) and mycophenolate mofetil (MMF, as a replacement for AZA).

The absolute number of LD pancreas transplants per decade did not change over time; however, relative to the total number of pancreas transplants, the rate decreased from 7% in the second decade to 0.3% in the fourth decade. During the second and third decades, the emphasis was on solitary pancreas transplants; during the fourth decade, most LD pancreas transplants were in the SPK category, a clear shift from solitary to combined pancreas–kidney transplants.

Of note, of the 31 LD PAK transplants at the University of Minnesota, 24 used a kidney and segmental pancreas from the same LD.

Over the decades, recipient and donor characteristics in LD pancreas transplants worldwide remained relatively stable (Table 21-3). The mean age of solitary LD pancreas (PTA, PAK) recipients was 33 ± 7 years, as compared with 37 ± 9 years for LD SPK recipients. Solitary LD pancreas recipients tended to be younger than their DD transplant counterparts, but the difference was not statistically significant.

### TABLE 21-2

## LD PANCREAS RECIPIENT CATEGORIES, BY TIME PERIOD

|  | PAK | PTA | SPK | Total |
|---|---|---|---|---|
| 1966–1975 (1st decade) | 0 | 0 | 0 | 0 |
| 1976–1985 (2nd decade) | 18 | 32 | 1 | 51 |
| 1986–1995 (3rd decade) | 14 | 24 | 7 | 45 |
| 1996–2005 (4th decade) | 2 | 3 | 43 | 48 |
| Total | 34 | 59 | 51 | 144 |

LD, living donor; PAK, pancreas after kidney; PTA, pancreas transplant alone; SPK, simultaneous pancreas–kidney.

### TABLE 21-3

## PATIENT CHARACTERISTICS

|  | PAK | PTA | SPK | Overall |
|---|---|---|---|---|
| Recipient age (years) | 33 ± 7 | 32 ± 7 | 37 ± 9 | 34 ± 8 |
| LD age (years) | 39±13 | 36±10 | 42±10 | 39±11 |
| LD gender (%) |  |  |  |  |
| Female | 74% | 67% | 63% | 67% |
| Male | 26% | 33% | 37% | 33% |
| LD relationship to recipient (%) |  |  |  |  |
| Parent | 27% | 18% | 22% | 22% |
| Sibling | 69% | 82% | 53% | 65% |
| Child |  |  | 4% | 2% |
| Other |  |  | 4% | 2% |
| Unrelated | 4% |  | 17% | 9% |

LD, living donor; PAK, pancreas after kidney; PTA, pancreas transplant alone; SPK, simultaneous pancreas–kidney.

The overall mean age at donation of LDs was 39 ± 11 years, as compared with 28 ± 11 years for DDs. Thus, LDs were significantly older than DDs. Although 66% of DDs were male, the majority of LDs (66%) were female. Most frequently, LDs were sisters, followed by mothers. Of unrelated LDs, spouses donated most frequently.

Along with the immunosuppressive protocol, the duct management technique is one of the most influential factors in posttransplant outcome. Table 21-4 shows the diverse spectrum of techniques used in LD pancreas transplants. Enteric drainage was the most frequent technique in the second and third decades, followed by duct injection. But in the fourth decade, bladder drainage was used in 83% of all LD pancreas transplants, followed by enteric drainage (8%) and duct injection (8%).

## PATIENT AND GRAFT SURVIVAL

Short- and long-time patient survival rates for LD (vs DD) pancreas recipients were high, irrespective of the analyzed decade. Overall patient survival rates for PAK recipients were 92% at 5 years, 76% at 10 years, and 60% at 20 years. As of June 30, 2006, one PAK recipient was alive 25 years posttransplant. For PTA recipients, overall patient survival rates were 91% at 5 years, 82% at 10 years, and 52% at 20 years. As of June 30, 2006, one PTA recipient was alive 25 years posttransplant. Because LD SPK

### TABLE 21-4

## DUCT MANAGEMENT TECHNIQUE IN LD PANCREAS TRANSPLANT RECIPIENTS, BY TIME PERIOD

|  | 1976–1985 | 1986–1995 | 1996–2005 | Total (%) |
|---|---|---|---|---|
| Bladder drainage | 0 | 17 | 40 | 57 (40) |
| Duct injection | 6 | 3 | 4 | 13 ( 9) |
| Enteric drainage | 39 | 3 | 4 | 13 ( 9) |
| Open duct | 6 | 21 | 4 | 64 (44) |
| Ureterostomy | 0 | 0 | 0 | 6 ( 4) |
|  | 0 | 4 | 0 | 4 ( 3) |

LD, living donor.

transplants were mainly performed in the fourth decade, the possible follow-up time is shorter than for LD PAK and LD PTA recipients. The overall SPK recipient survival rate was 98% at 5 years.

Table 21-5a shows LD and DD patient survival rates by recipient category and decade. Statistical comparison is difficult: the number of LD transplants was very small, as compared with DD transplants. Still, the patient survival rate for solitary (PTA, PAK) pancreas recipients was significantly higher for LD (vs DD) recipients, particularly in the second decade. The patient survival rate was also higher for LD (vs DD) SPK recipients in the fourth decade.

In all, only 30 LD pancreas recipients were reported to have died. Of those 30 recipients, 7 died with a fully functioning pancreas graft. The most common causes of early and late death were cardiovascular ailments, followed by infections.

Table 21-5b shows the LD and DD graft survival rates by recipient category and decade. Pancreas graft survival rates, in general, improved over time, because of a decrease in technical failures and in immunologic graft loss.[2] In the second decade, the graft survival rates for solitary (PAK, PTA) LD pancreas recipients were clearly superior, as compared with DD recipients. In the third decade, for PAK recipients, the graft survival rates after LD versus DD transplants were comparable; for PTA recipients, the graft survival rate was higher after LD (vs DD) transplants. In the fourth decade, for SPK recipients, graft survival rates after LD versus DD transplants were comparable. Note that overall long-term graft function was significantly better for solitary LD (vs DD) pancreas recipients.

The technical failure rate in the second decade was 31%. In the third and fourth decades, it decreased to 6%, comparable to the technical failure rate for DD transplants.[2] This reduction in technical failures was the result of (1) aggressive anticoagulation (using systemic heparinization perioperatively and Coumadin for up to 6 months posttransplant), (2) better antimicrobial prophylaxis and therapy to avoid postoperative intraabdominal infections, and (3) improved surgical techniques.

The immunologic graft loss rate at 1 year posttransplant for solitary (PTA, PAK) LD pancreas recipients decreased from 40% in the second decade to 17% in the fourth decade. For technically successful LD SPK transplants, the immunologic graft loss rate at 1 year was 5%, resulting in a 5-year graft function rate of 88%. This reduction in immunologic graft loss was due to (1) the advent of more potent, less toxic immunosuppressive agents in the mid-1990s (TAC, MMF, sirolimus) and superior immunosuppressive protocols; (2) improved diagnosis of rejection (via computed tomography [CT] or ultrasound-guided pancreas graft biopsies); and (3) superior antirejection protocols.

Table 21-5c shows the kidney graft survival rates for LD SPK versus DD SPK recipients. In the last 2 decades (1986–2005), kidney graft function in LD SPK recipients was excellent; in the fourth decade, the difference between LD versus DD kidney graft survival in SPK recipients almost reached significance.

**TABLE 21-5a**

## PATIENT SURVIVAL RATES (AT 1, 5, AND 10 YEARS POSTTRANSPLANT) FOR LD VERSUS DD PANCREAS GRAFTS, BY TIME PERIOD AND RECIPIENT CATEGORY

|  | Tx Year | Donor Type | N | 1 Year | 5 Years | 10 Years | p |
|---|---|---|---|---|---|---|---|
| PAK | 1976–1985 | LD | 17 | 100% | 87% | 61% | 0.01 |
|  |  | DD | 110 | 79% | 57% | 40% |  |
|  | 1986–1995 | LD | 14 | 100% | 100% | 100% | 0.01 |
|  |  | DD | 379 | 93% | 77% | 50% |  |
|  | 1996–2005 | LD | 2 | 100% | — | — | — |
|  |  | DD | 2408 | 95% | 84% | — |  |
| PTA | 1976–1985 | LD | 30 | 90% | 90% | 85% | 0.05 |
|  |  | DD | 103 | 79% | 66% | 61% |  |
|  | 1986–1995 | LD | 23 | 90% | 90% | 78% | 0.22 |
|  |  | DD | 332 | 92% | 80% | 61% |  |
|  | 1996–2005 | LD | 3 | 100% | — | — | — |
|  |  | DD | 1020 | 97% | 86% | — |  |
| SPK | 1976–1985 | LD | 1 | — | — | 42% | — |
|  |  | DD | 407 | 71% | 56% |  |  |
|  | 1986–1995 | LD | 7 | 100% | 100% | 100% | 0.01 |
|  |  | DD | 6124 | 91% | 80% | 68% |  |
|  | 1996–2005 | LD | 43 | 100% | — | — | — |
|  |  | DD | 12042 | 95% | 86% | — |  |

Tx, transplant; LD, living donor; PAK, pancreas after kidney; PTA, pancreas transplant alone; SPK, simultaneous pancreas–kidney.

**TABLE 21-5b**

**PANCREAS GRAFT SURVIVAL RATES (AT 1, 5, AND 10 YEARS POSTTRANSPLANT) FOR LD VERSUS DD GRAFTS, BY TIME PERIOD AND RECIPIENT CATEGORY**

|  | Tx Year | Donor Type | N | 1 Year | 5 Years | 10 Years | p |
|---|---|---|---|---|---|---|---|
| PAK | 1976–1985 | LD | 17 | 53% | 41% | 18% | 0.004 |
|  |  | DD | 110 | 20% | 3% | 3% |  |
|  | 1986–1995 | LD | 14 | 43% | 34% | 34% | 0.33 |
|  |  | DD | 379 | 46% | 31% | 16% |  |
|  | 1996–2005 | LD | 2 | 100% | — | — | — |
|  |  | DD | 2,408 | 77% | 55% | — |  |
| PTA | 1976–1985 | LD | 30 | 33% | 20% | 13% | 0.001 |
|  |  | DD | 103 | 17% | 4% | 3% |  |
|  | 1986–1995 | LD | 23 | 57% | 39% | 39% | 0.04 |
|  |  | DD | 332 | 43% | 21% | 12% |  |
|  | 1996–2005 | LD | 3 | 100% | — | — | — |
|  |  | DD | 1,020 | 75% | 49% | — |  |
| SPK | 1976–1985 | LD | 1 | — | — | — | — |
|  |  | DD | 407 | 41% | 23% | 13% |  |
|  | 1986–1995 | LD | 7 | 71% | 43% | 43% | 0.65 |
|  |  | DD | 6,124 | 74% | 61% | 46% |  |
|  | 1996–2005 | LD | 43 | 88% | 77% | — | — |
|  |  | DD | 12,042 | 84% | 70% | — |  |

Tx, transplant; LD, living donor; PAK, pancreas after kidney; PTA, pancreas transplant alone; SPK, simultaneous pancreas-kidney.

## LONG-TERM GRAFT SURVIVAL

According to the IPTR, 4 LD pancreas recipients have had a functioning graft for ≥ 20 years; 13, for ≥ 15 years; 23, for ≥ 10 years; and 54, for ≥ 5 years. Table 21-6 shows long-term graft function by recipient category. Of the 4 LDs whose recipients have had a functioning graft for ≥ 20 years, 3 were HLA-identical and 1 was HLA-nonidentical; of the 13 LDs whose recipients have had a functioning graft for ≥ 15 years, 9 were HLA-identical and 4

HLA-nonidentical; and of the 23 LDs whose recipients have had a functioning graft for ≥ 10 years, 15 were HLA-identical and 8 were HLA-nonidentical. Particularly in the second decade, the results of HLA-identical (vs HLA-nonidentical) transplants were significantly better. Thus, the best long-term outcome was clearly achieved with HLA-identical grafts. With the advent of new immunosuppressive drugs, the advantage of HLA-identical donors became, at least for short-term outcome, no longer statistically significant.

**TABLE 21-5c**

**SPK KIDNEY GRAFT SURVIVAL RATES (AT 1, 5, AND 10 YEARS POSTTRANSPLANT) FOR LD VERSUS DD GRAFTS, BY TIME PERIOD**

|  | Tx Year | Donor Type | N | 1 Year | 5 Years | 10 Years | p |
|---|---|---|---|---|---|---|---|
| SPK | 1976–1985 | LD | 1 | — | — | — | — |
|  |  | DD | 407 | 55% | 35% | 22% |  |
|  | 1986–1995 | LD | 7 | 100% | 86% | 57% | 0.66 |
|  |  | DD | 6 124 | 83% | 67% | 46% |  |
|  | 1996–2005 | LD | 43 | 100% | 84% | — | 0.06 |
|  |  | DD | 12,042 | 91% | 75% | — |  |

Tx, transplant; LD, living donor; PAK, pancreas after kidney; PTA, pancreas transplant alone; SPK, simultaneous pancreas-kidney.

**TABLE 21-6**

## LONG-TERM LD PANCREAS GRAFT FUNCTION, BY RECIPIENT CATEGORY

|        | ≥ 5 Years | ≥ 10 Years | ≥ 15 Years | ≥ 20 Years |
|--------|-----------|------------|------------|------------|
| PAK    | 11        | 7          | 4          | 2          |
| PTA    | 16        | 12         | 9          | 2          |
| SPK    | 27        | 4          | —          | —          |
| Total  | 54        | 23         | 13         | 4          |

Tx, transplant; LD, living donor; PAK, pancreas after kidney; PTA, pancreas transplant alone; SPK, simultaneous pancreas-kidney.

## References

1. Gruessner AC, Sutherland DER, Gruessner RWG. International Pancreas Transplant Registry In: Gruessner RWG, Sutherland DER, eds. *Transplantation of the Pancreas.* New York: Springer-Verlag; 2004:539–582.
2. Gruessner AC, Sutherland DER. Pancreas transplant outcomes for United States (US) and non-US cases as reported to the United Network for Organ Sharing (UNOS) and the International Pancreas Transplant Registry (IPTR) as of June 2004. *Clin Transplant* 2005;19(4):433–455.

# COLOR PLATES

*Illustrations by Martin Finch*

# KIDNEY

Figures KI-2 to 8, 9B to 11, 13 to 15, and 16B reproduced from: *Manual of Vascular Access, Organ Donation, and Transplantation*. Eds.: Simmons RL, Finch ME, Ascher NL, Najarian JS. Springer-Verlag, New York (1984). With kind permission of Springer Science and Business Media.

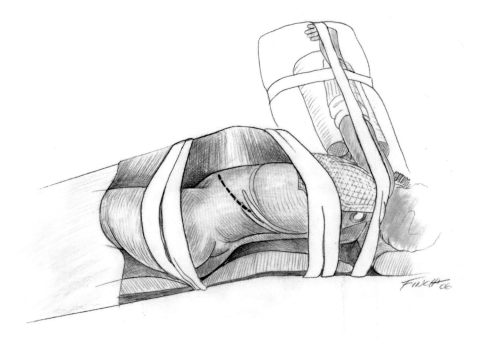

**COLOR PLATES, FIGURE KI-1**

The donor is placed on the right or left side on the operating table. A "beanbag" (Vac-Pac®, Olympic Medical, Seattle, WA, USA) is placed underneath the body to secure its position while tilting the table for optimal exposure; in addition, the body is secured with tapes as shown. The table is flexed and the kidney rest is raised to achieve maximal distance between the lowest rib and the iliac crest. The incision is made from slightly posterior to the tip of the 12th rib to the lateral rectus muscle border.

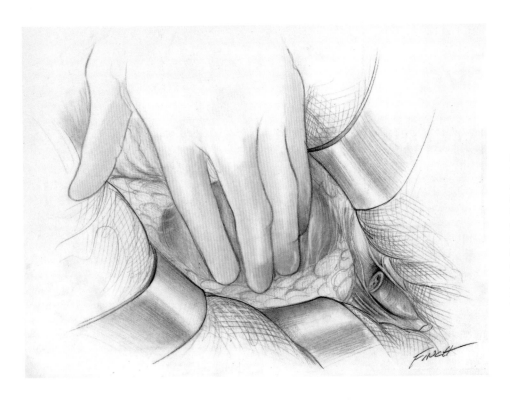

**COLOR PLATES, FIGURE KI-2**

After dividing the oblique and transverse muscles as well as the transversalis fascia, the peritoneum is peeled off anteromedially to expose Gerota's fascia in the retroperitoneal space. The tip of the 12th rib is resected without entering the pleural space. If the pleural space has been entered, it should be oversewn after the lungs have been maximally insufflated by the anesthesiologist; a chest x-ray needs to be obtained immediately postoperatively to assess the need for chest tube placement. In donors with a high ribcage, resection of the tip of the 12th rib may not be necessary.

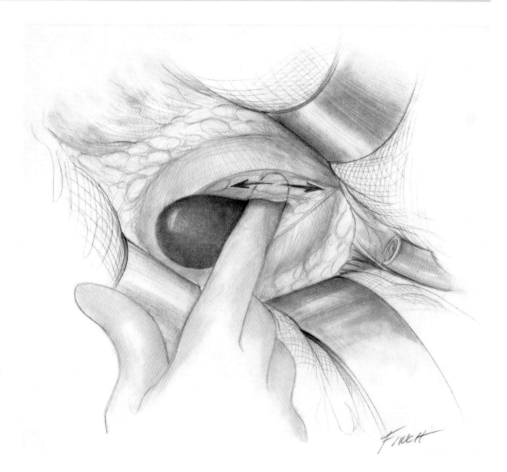

**COLOR PLATES, FIGURE KI-3**

Gerota's fascia is incised and the kidney is exposed anteriorly in its entire length from its greater curvature to the hilum. Blunt or sharp dissection can be used. The ureter is exposed, taking care to leave periureteral tissue with the accompanying blood vessels intact.

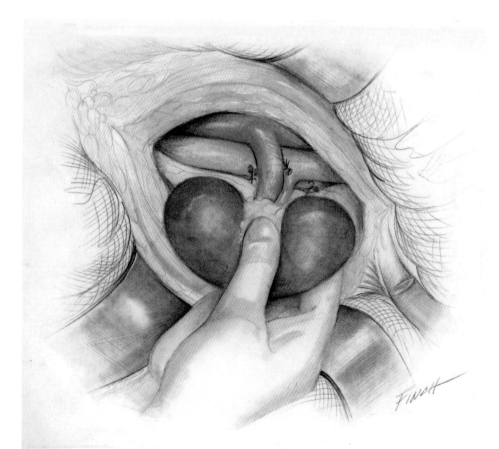

**COLOR PLATES, FIGURE KI-4A**

Anterior dissection of the renal vessels: The renal vein is dissected in its entire length toward the vena cava. On the left side, the left gonadal and adrenal veins are ligated and divided. On the right side, those veins do not need to be ligated, because they usually enter the vena cava directly. After the renal vein is completely mobilized circumferentially, the renal artery is dissected free, its origin off the aorta is identified, and the perilymphatic and nerve tissue is divided.

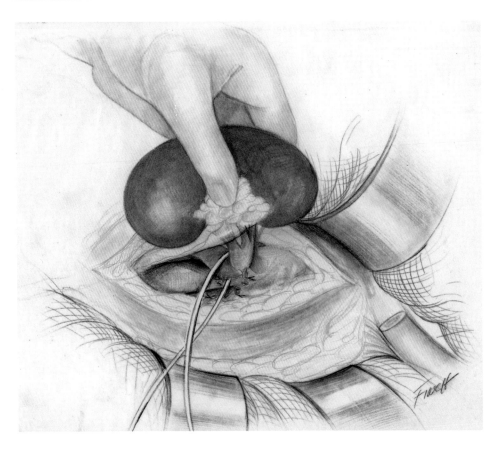

**COLOR PLATES, FIGURE KI-4B**

Posterior dissection of the renal vessels on the left side; ligation and division of the lumbar vein(s): The kidney is now completely mobilized and remains attached only by the renal artery, renal vein, and ureter. Excessive traction on the renal artery needs to be avoided, to prevent arterial spasm and intimal disruption.

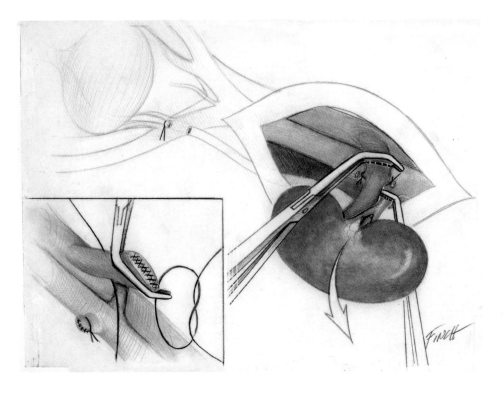

**COLOR PLATES, FIGURE KI-5**

The kidney is removed by distal ligation and by division of the ureter as it crosses the common iliac artery. The renal artery is clamped about 5 to 10 mm distal from its takeoff from the aorta; a rim of vena cava is clamped around the orifice of the renal vein. Both renal vessels are divided, leaving a stump of about 5 to 10 mm behind. The kidney is removed and handed to the recipient team. The vessels are then oversewn, clipped, and/or doubly ligated. After hemostasis is obtained, the wound is closed in layers.

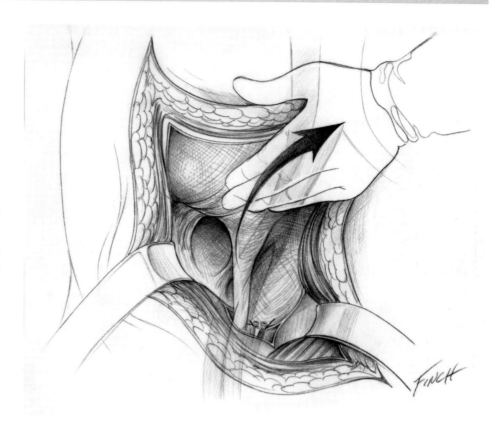

**COLOR PLATES, FIGURE KI-6A**

A curved ("hockey-stick") incision is made (starting at the level of the umbilicus along the lateral margin of the rectus muscle toward the pubic bone) to expose the recipient's iliac vessels. The insertion of the oblique and transverse muscles into the rectus sheath is divided, as is the transversalis fascia. The peritoneum is gently moved medially. A plane is developed parallel to the lateral abdominal wall and above the psoas muscle to expose the iliac vessels. In the process, the inferior epigastric vessels and, in women, the round ligament are divided and ligated; in men, the spermatic cord is identified and a loop is placed around it.

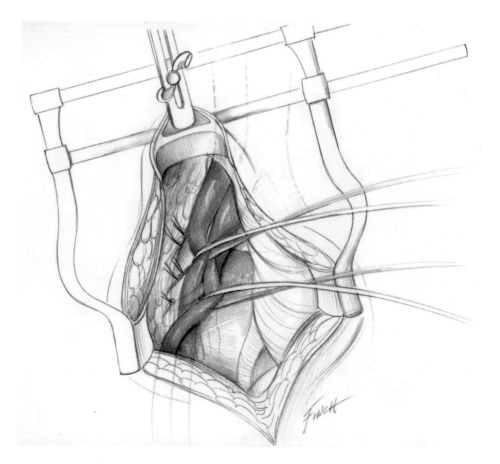

**COLOR PLATES, FIGURE KI-6B**

The iliac artery and vein are dissected out, so that all lymphatic vessels located anteriorly are ligated and divided, to prevent development of a lymphocele. Lateral lymphatic vessels which do not cross the iliac vessels are left intact; also, the lymph nodes that underlie the inguinal ligament are preserved. Rarely, the internal iliac veins need to be ligated and divided (as shown); this maneuver may be indicated in an obese recipient with a deep pelvis or if a short right renal vein has to be anastomosed to a deep and tethered external iliac vein. Dissection of the iliac vessels is usually not necessary proximal to the bifurcation of the common iliac artery.

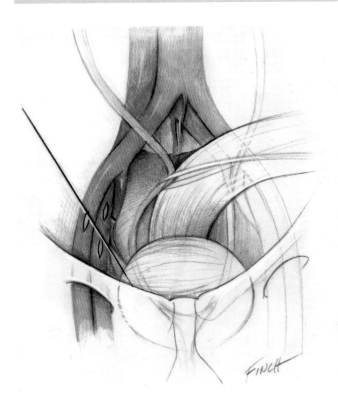

**COLOR PLATES, FIGURE KI-7**

Two options for vascular anastomoses are shown.
Option 1: <u>End-to-side</u> anastomosis between the donor's renal vessels and the recipient's external iliac vessels; the venous anastomosis is slightly distal to the arterial anastomosis.
Option 2: <u>End-to-end</u> anastomosis between the donor's renal artery and the recipient's internal iliac artery; the venous anastomosis is constructed slightly more proximal than in Option 1. If the internal iliac (hypogastric) artery is used, the internal iliac vein(s) may need to be ligated and divided, to bring the external and common iliac veins to a more superficial position.

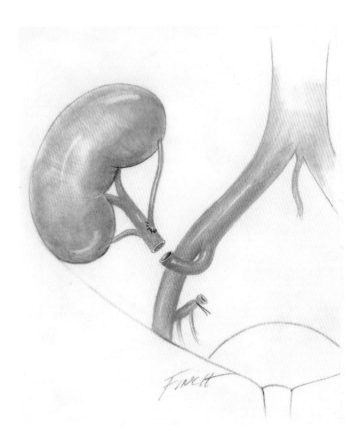

**COLOR PLATES, FIGURE KI-8**

The venous anastomosis is usually constructed first. Two corner and 2 side stitches (nonabsorbable 5-0 or 6-0 sutures) are placed at equal intervals around the circumference of the venotomy. The corner stitches are tied and run from one corner to the other on both the anterior and posterior wall of the renal vein.

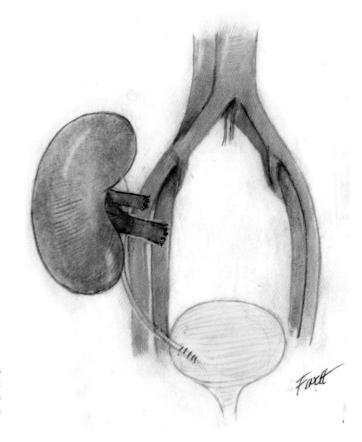

## COLOR PLATES, FIGURE KI-9A

The donor's renal artery is anastomosed <u>end-to-side</u> to the recipient's external iliac artery. The construction of the anastomosis is identical to that described for the renal vein, using 2 corner and 2 side stitches (nonabsorbable 6-0 sutures). If the renal artery is very small, the sutures may be placed in interrupted (rather than running) fashion.

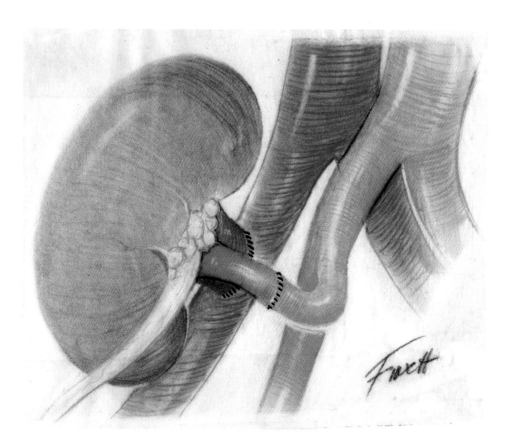

## COLOR PLATES, FIGURE KI-9B

If the donor's renal artery is anastomosed <u>end-to-end</u> to the recipient's internal iliac artery, the anastomosis is constructed between 3 sutures that are placed at equal intervals around the circumferences. Or, if the vessels are small, the anastomosis may be constructed in interrupted fashion. The use of the hypogastric artery was initially preferred over the external iliac artery, because of concern of compromised blood flow to the leg. Over time, as the incidence of technical complications greatly diminished, the end-to-side technique became the preferred anastomotic technique. After completion of the arterial and venous anastomoses, the clamps are removed and blood flow is restored.

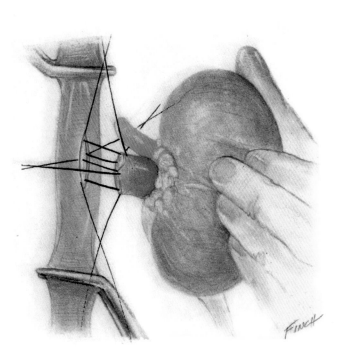 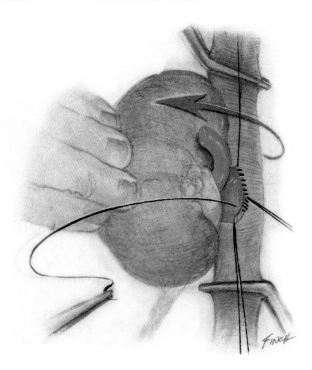

**COLOR PLATES, FIGURE KI-10**

If the donor has multiple renal veins, they can usually be dealt with by ligating the smaller vein(s), because of the venous collaterals in the kidney. If the donor has multiple renal arteries, multiple in situ or ex situ anastomoses are required.

Figure KI-10 shows the different options for ex situ reconstruction of the donor's multiple arteries that require only 1 anastomosis to the recipient's artery.

**FIGURE KI-10A**

The end of a small renal artery (supplying the upper pole) is anastomosed to the side of a larger renal artery, either directly or via an interposition graft (of epigastric artery, internal iliac artery [or a branch], or saphenous vein).

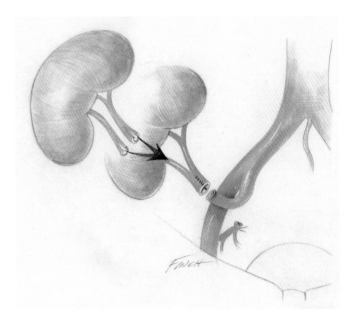

**FIGURE KI-10B**

Two equal-sized renal arteries are sutured together to create 1 opening.

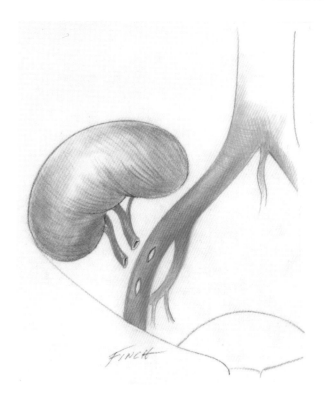

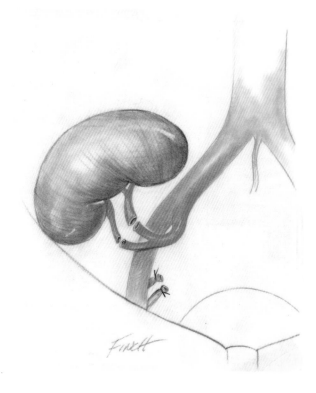

**COLOR PLATES, FIGURE KI-11**

Different anastomotic options for multiple arteries are shown.

**FIGURE KI-11A**

Both of the donor's renal arteries are separately anastomosed end-to-side to the recipient's external iliac artery.

**FIGURE KI-11B**

Both of the donor's renal arteries are separately anastomosed end-to-end to the recipient's 2 internal iliac arteries.

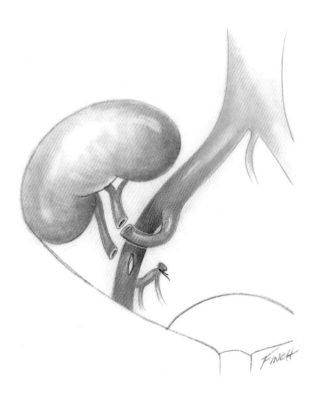

**FIGURE KI-11C**

One of the donor's renal arteries is anastomosed end-to-side to the recipient's external iliac artery, the other, end-to-end to the recipient's internal iliac artery.

| Arterial Anastomoses | | | Ureteral Anastomoses |
|---|---|---|---|
| Single Artery/Single Anastomoses | Multiple Arteries/Single Anastomoses | Multiple Arteries/Mutiple Anastomoses | |
| **End-to-Side** 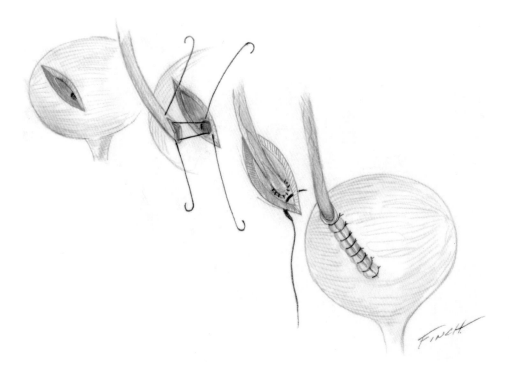 | | | **Lich-Technique** |
| **End to End** | | | **1-Stitch-Technique** |
| | | | **Politano-Leadbetter Technique** |
| | | | |

**COLOR PLATES, FIGURE KI-12**

Different options for arterial and ureteral anastomoses.

**COLOR PLATES, FIGURE KI-13A**

Extravesical ureteroneocystostomy (Lich technique): The spatulated ureter is anastomosed to the urothelium with running 6-0 or 7-0 absorbable sutures (stents are infrequently used). The divided muscle layer is then repaired using interrupted or running 5-0 absorbable sutures over the distal ureter, thereby creating a submucosal ureteral tunnel.

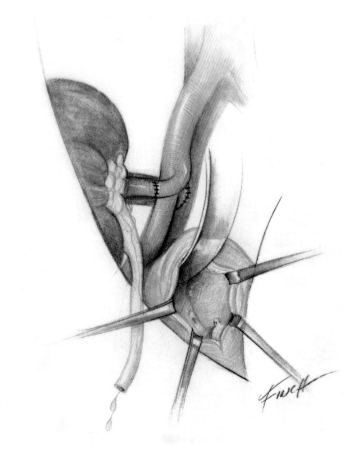

**COLOR PLATES, FIGURE KI-13B**

Intravesical ureteroneocystostomy (Leadbetter-Politano technique): After opening the bladder anterolaterally, a transverse incision is made on the posterior lateral bladder wall. The ureter is pulled inside the bladder through a submucosal tunnel (2 to 4 cm) without tension. The tip of the ureter is anastomosed to the urothelium circumferentially, in interrupted fashion, using 5-0 or 6-0 absorbable sutures (stents are infrequently used). The bladder is closed in 3 layers.

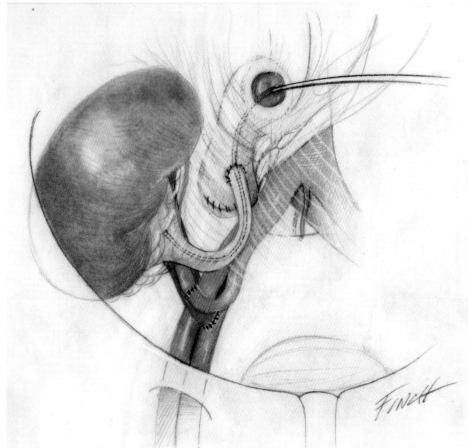

**COLOR PLATES, FIGURE KI-14**

Anastomosis between ureter and ileal loop: In recipients without a bladder or with severe neurogenic bladder abnormalities, an anastomosis between the ureter and the ilial loop may be required. A 10-cm loop, on a mesenteric pedicle with an external Brooke ileostomy, is constructed, either several weeks before or at the time of the transplant. In adult recipients, the kidney graft is placed via the standard retroperitoneal approach in the iliac fossa; the tip of the ureter is anastomosed toward the bottom of the ilial loop. The anastomosis is constructed by taking full-thickness bites, in running or interrupted fashion. Tension needs to be avoided; placement of a stent is rarely indicated.

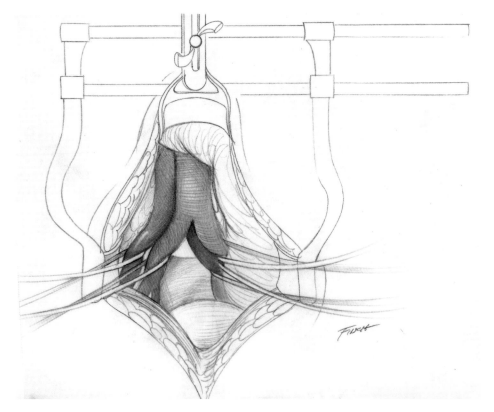

Exposure for a pediatric kidney transplant: The native kidneys are usually removed first, to create more space. In the process, the right colon and the mesenteric attachments at the level of the iliac vessels are mobilized, to expose the distal abdominal aorta and the vena cava. The colon and the small bowel are reflected cranially and laterally. The distal aorta and vena cava are dissected free, from the takeoff of the renal vessels to the level of the common iliac bifurcations. The inferior mesenteric artery, lumbar arteries and veins, and the midsacral vessels are doubly looped for temporary occlusion. Clamps or elastic vessel loops are placed around the abdominal aorta and cava and the common iliac vessels, for in- and outflow obstruction in preparation for graft implantation.

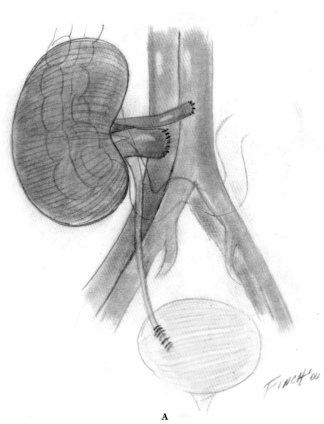

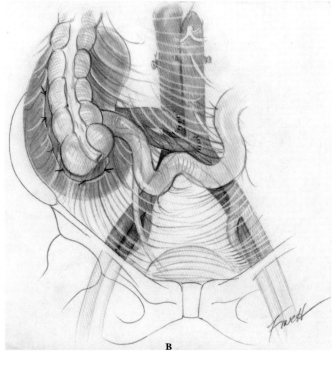

A

B

**COLOR PLATES, FIGURE KI-16**

Pediatric kidney transplant: The donor's renal artery and vein are anastomosed to the recipient's distal aorta and vena cava in end-to-side fashion. The kidney can be placed intraabdominally (Figure 16A) or retroperitoneally (Figure 16B) with the colon on top of it. Intraabdominal placement allows for better biopsy access.

# PANCREAS

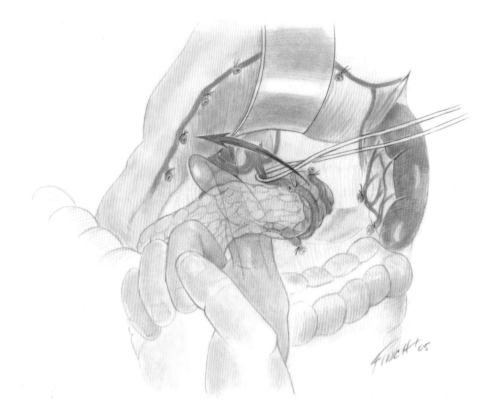

**COLOR PLATES, FIGURE PA-1**

Division of the distal splenic vessels, posterior mobilization of the tail of the pancreas off the retroperitoneum, and mobilization off the pancreatic neck (index finger): The proximal splenic artery is looped. The spleen is preserved along with the gastroepiploic vessels, the short gastric vessels, and the ligament attachments of the spleen.

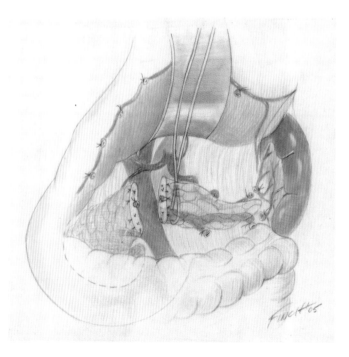

**COLOR PLATES, FIGURE PA-2**

Division of the pancreatic neck as it overlies the superior mesenteric and portal veins: The parenchyma is divided, using multiple small ligatures to avoid leakage from the cut surface. The pancreatic duct is ligated on the recipient side and tagged with a suture on the graft side. The splenic vein is circumferentially dissected free and looped close to its confluence with the superior mesenteric vein.

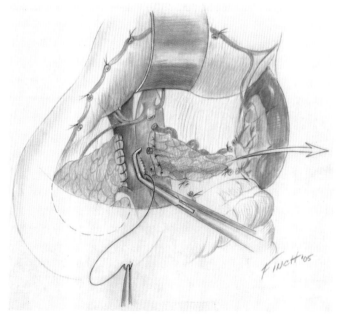

**COLOR PLATES, FIGURE PA-3**

Removal of the distal pancreas: The proximal splenic artery is clamped and divided. The remaining stump in the recipient is oversewn, using nonabsorbable 5-0 or 6-0 sutures in running fashion, taking care not to narrow the lumen of the celiac artery. A rim of portal/superior mesenteric vein, right at the orifice of the splenic vein, is clamped; the splenic vein is divided. The transection line is oversewn with nonabsorbable 5-0 or 6-0 sutures in running fashion.

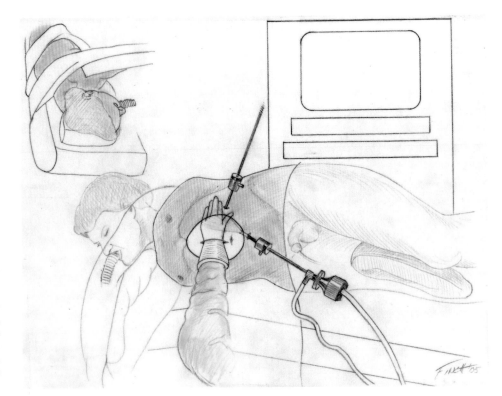

**COLOR PLATES, FIGURE PA-4**

Hand-assisted laparoscopic distal pancreatectomy: The donor is placed in the right lateral decubitus position. The surgeon's hand is inside the abdomen via a supraumbilical midline incision (6 to 8 cm). Two ports are placed: the first, perirectally, 2 cm below and slightly left of the donor's umbilicus (for the laparoscope and camera); the second, in the mid left abdomen (anterior axillary line). The monitors are shown behind the operating table.

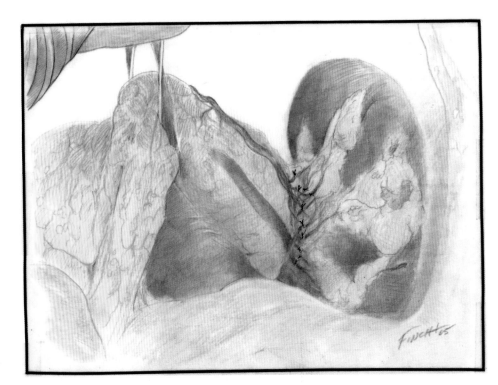

**COLOR PLATES, FIGURE PA-5**

Hand-assisted laparoscopic distal pancreatectomy: A vessel loop is passed around the distal pancreas, to allow for retraction of the tail of the pancreas and for separation between the pancreas and spleen. Several smaller vessels have already been individually clipped in the splenic hilum.

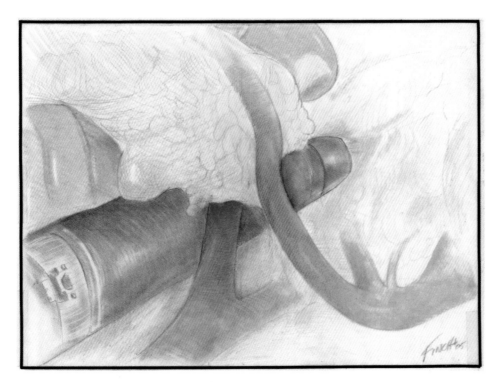

**COLOR PLATES, FIGURE PA-6**

Hand-assisted laparoscopic distal pancreatectomy: A 45-mm stapler has been placed across the neck of the pancreas. The splenic artery (SA) and splenic vein (SV) are dissected free and isolated; they are shown at the level of the celiac axis (CA) (HA = hepatic artery, LGA = left gastric artery) and the portal vein confluence (SMV = superior mesenteric vein, PV = portal vein).

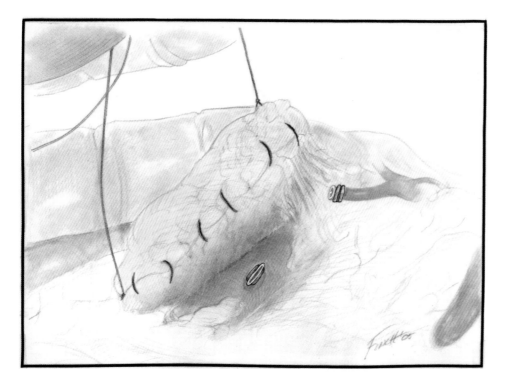

**COLOR PLATES, FIGURE PA-7**

Hand-assisted laparoscopic distal pancreatectomy: The proximal pancreatic stump is oversewn with 4-0 absorbable sutures in running fashion. The clip is shown on the pancreatic duct. The stumps of the splenic artery and splenic vein are shown in proximity to the celiac axis and the superior mesenteric vein.

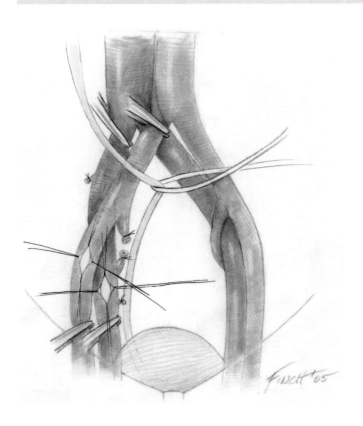

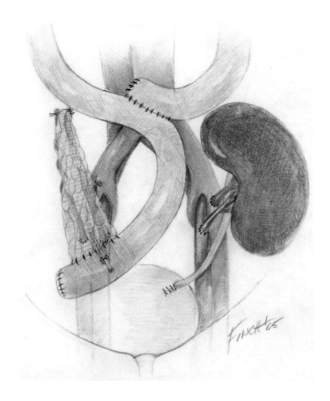

**COLOR PLATES, FIGURE PA-8**

Dissection of the recipient's right iliac vessels: The internal iliac veins are ligated and divided. The internal iliac artery is also ligated and divided. The external iliac artery is placed lateral to the external iliac vein. The arteriotomy is made proximal to the venotomy. The ureter is looped and retracted medially and cranially to the common iliac artery.

**COLOR PLATES, FIGURE PA-10**

Living donor (LD) segmental pancreas transplant with systemic vein and bowel exocrine drainage via a Roux-en-Y loop: The donor's splenic artery and vein are anastomosed end-to-side to the recipient's external iliac artery and vein. The splenic artery anastomosis is lateral and proximal to the splenic vein anastomosis. A 2-layer ductojejunostomy or pancreaticojejunostomy (telescope or invagination technique) is constructed end-to-side; about 40 cm distal to that anastomosis, a jejunojejunostomy is created in standard fashion. The ureter of the simultaneously transplanted kidney is implanted into the bladder, using the extravesical ureteroneocystostomy (Lich) technique.

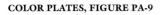

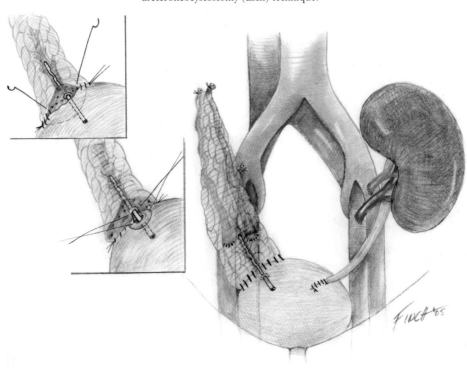

**COLOR PLATES, FIGURE PA-9**

Living donor (LD) segmental pancreas transplant with systemic vein and bladder exocrine drainage: The donor's splenic artery and vein are anastomosed end-to-side to the recipient's external iliac artery and vein. The splenic artery anastomosis is lateral and proximal to the splenic vein anastomosis. A 2-layer ductocystostomy (inset A) is constructed. The pancreatic duct is sutured to the urothelial layer (inner layer) using interrupted 7-0 sutures over a stent. Alternatively, a 2-layer pancreaticocystostomy can be constructed (inset B): the cut surface of the pancreas is invaginated into the bladder (telescope anastomosis). The ureter of the simultaneously transplanted kidney is implanted into the bladder, using the extravesical ureteroneocystostomy (Lich) technique.

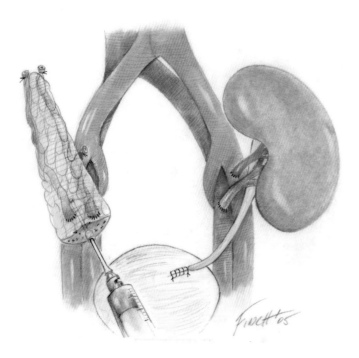

**COLOR PLATES, FIGURE PA-11**

Living donor (LD) segmental pancreas transplant with systemic vein drainage and duct injection: The donor's duct is injected with a synthetic polymer that causes fibrosis of the exocrine tissue. Note the meticulous ligation of the vascular and exocrine structures on the cut surface of the pancreas. The ureter of the simultaneously transplanted kidney is implanted into the bladder, using the extravesical ureteroneocystostomy (Lich) technique.

# LIVER

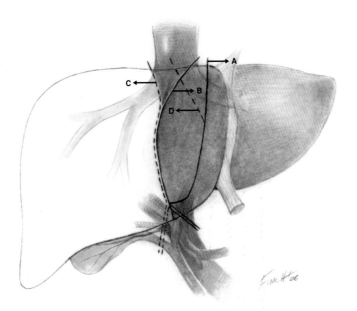

**COLOR PLATES, FIGURE LI-1**

Types of donor grafts: (A) left lateral segments (2 and 3), including the left hepatic vein, the left portal vein, the left hepatic artery, and the left bile duct; (B) left lobe segments (1 through 4 or 2 through 4), including the left and middle hepatic veins, the left portal vein, the left hepatic artery, and the left bile duct; (C) right lobe segments (5 through 8), including the right hepatic vein, the right portal vein, the right hepatic artery, and the right bile duct; (D) extended right lobe segments (4 through 8), including the right and middle hepatic veins, the right portal vein, the right hepatic artery, and the right bile duct.

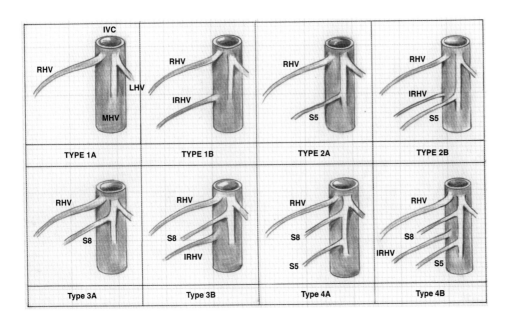

**COLOR PLATES, FIGURE LI-2**

Classification of the right hepatic vein anatomy adapted from: Varotti G, Gondolesi GE, Goldman J, et al.: Anatomic variations in right liver living donors. J Am Coll Surg 2004; 198(4): 577-582. IVC, inferior vena cava; RHV, right hepatic vein; LHV, left hepatic vein; MHV, middle hepatic vein; IRHV, inferior right hepatic vein; S5, segment 5 vein; S8, segment 8 vein.

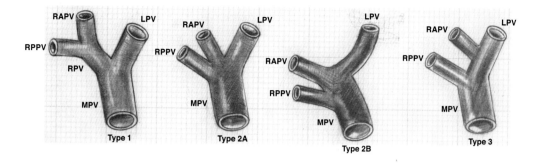

**COLOR PLATES, FIGURE LI-3**

Classification of the portal vein anatomy adapted from: Varotti et al., J Am Coll Surg 2004; 198: 577-582, and Macdonald DB, Haider MA, Khalili K, et al.: Relationship between vascular and biliary anatomy in living liver donors. Am J Roentgenol 2005; 185(1): 247-252.

RPV, right portal vein; LPV, left portal vein; MPV, main portal vein; RAPV, right anterior portal vein; RPPV, right posterior portal vein.

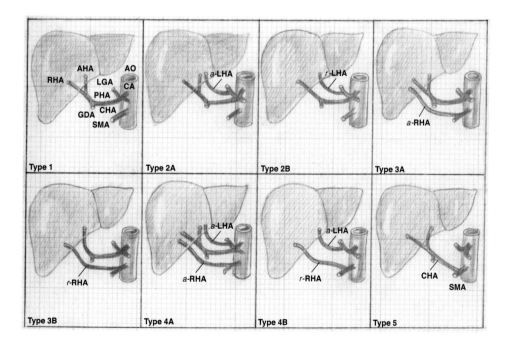

**COLOR PLATES, FIGURE LI-4A**

Classification of hepatic artery anatomy adapted from: Varotti et al.: J Am Coll Surg 2004; 198: 577-582.
AO, aorta; CA, celiac axis; CHA, common hepatic artery; SMA, superior mesenteric artery; LGA, left gastric artery; PHA, proper hepatic artery; GDA, gastroduodenal artery; RHA, right hepatic artery; LHA, left hepatic artery; a, accessory; r, replaced.

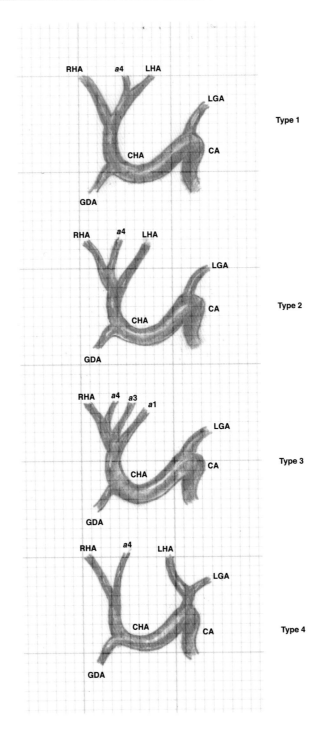

**COLOR PLATES, FIGURE LI-4B**

Classification of left hepatic artery anatomy adapted from: Shinohara H, Tanaka A, Hatano E, et al.: Anatomic and physiological problems of Segment IV: liver transplants using left lobes from living related donors. Clin Transplant 1996; 10: 341-347.

CA, celiac axis; CHA, common hepatic artery; LGA, left gastric artery; GDA, gastroduodenal artery; RHA, right hepatic artery; LHA, left hepatic artery; a2, a3, a4, arterial supply to segments 2, 3, and 4.

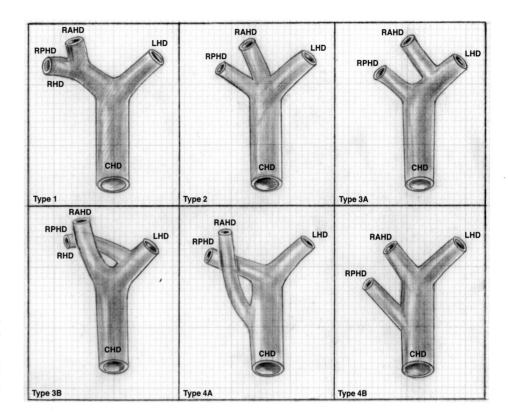

**COLOR PLATES, FIGURE LI-5**

Classification of bile duct anatomy adapted from: Varotti et al., J Am Coll Surg 2004; 198: 577-582.
CHD, common hepatic duct; RHD, right hepatic duct; LHD, left hepatic duct; RAHD, right anterior hepatic duct; RPHD, right posterior hepatic duct.

**COLOR PLATES, FIGURE LI-6**

Parenchymal transection of the liver for (right or left) lobe removal using the CUSA [Cavitron ultrasonic surgical aspirator] (Tyco Healthcare, Mansfield, MN) or the Hydrojet (Erbe, Tübingen, Germany). An umbilical tape (orange) is placed behind the liver for determining the ideal resection line.
IVC, inferior vena cava; RHV, right hepatic vein; LHV, left hepatic vein; MHV, middle hepatic vein; MPV, main portal vein; PHA, proper hepatic artery; CBD, common bile duct; CA, cystic artery; CD, cystic duct; FL, falsiform ligament.

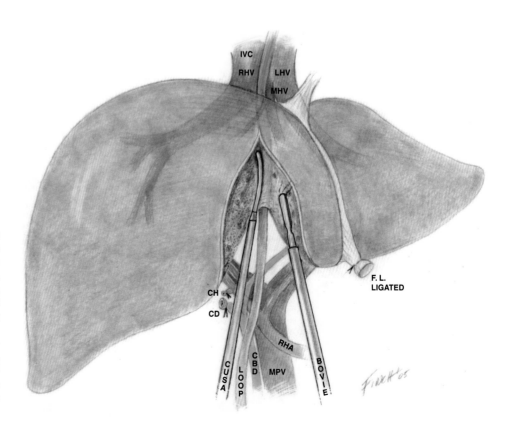

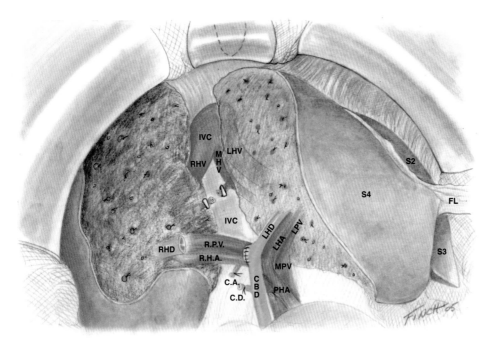

**COLOR PLATES, FIGURE LI-7**

Hepatic transection completed for right lobe removal.

IVC, inferior vena cava; RHV, right hepatic vein; MHV, middle hepatic vein; LHV, left hepatic vein; RPV, right portal vein; RHA, right hepatic artery; RHD, right hepatic duct; LPV, left portal vein; LHA, left hepatic artery; LHD, left hepatic duct; MPV, main portal vein; PHA, proper hepatic artery; CBD, common bile duct; CA, cystic artery; CD, cystic duct; S2, S3, S4, segments 2,3, and 4; FL, falsiform ligament.

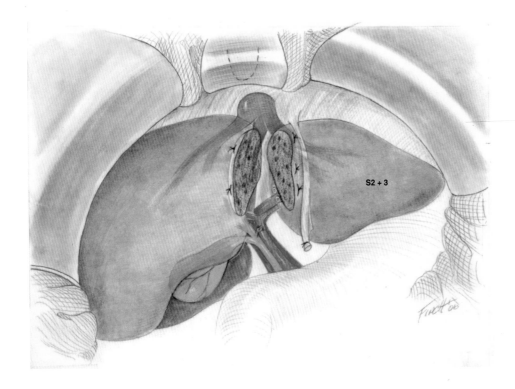

**COLOR PLATES, FIGURE LI-8**

Hepatic transection completed for removal of left lateral segments (2 and 3). The bile ducts to segments 2 and 3 are divided; the vascular structures are still intact.

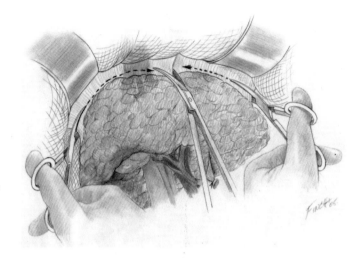

**COLOR PLATES, FIGURE LI-9**

The ligamentous attachments (falsiform ligament, triangular ligament) of the liver are taken down, and the liver is dissected off the diaphragm; prominent diaphragmatic veins may be ligated and divided at this time. The suprahepatic IVC and the hepatic veins are identified by taking down overlying attachments.

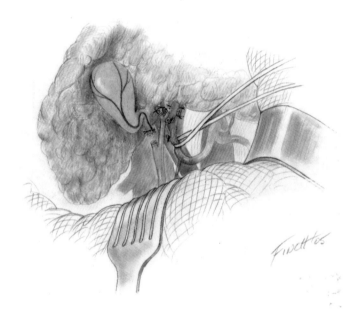

**COLOR PLATES, FIGURE LI-10A**

Hilar dissection: The cystic duct and artery are transected distal to the common bile duct and the proper hepatic artery (in case their respective stumps are used for anastomoses in the recipient). The hepatic artery and the hepatic duct are divided in the hilum as high as possible, usually beyond their respective bifurcations. For the high hilar dissection (HHD), the hepatic ducts and arteries are cut intrahepatically at the 3rd level of their pedicles or beyond; HHD increases the number of options for arterial and ductal reconstruction.

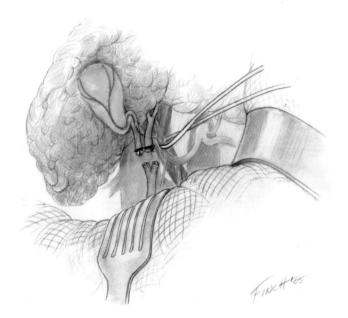

**COLOR PLATES, FIGURE LI-10B**

Hilar dissection: If the right and left bile ducts cannot be individually transected in the hilar plate, the hepatic duct and the cystic duct are transected individually; both stumps may be used for anastomoses in the recipient.

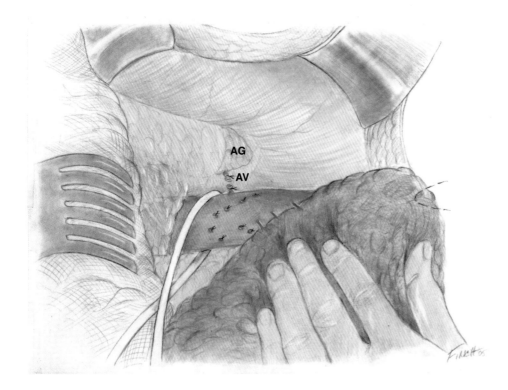

**COLOR PLATES, FIGURE LI-11**

Recipient hepatectomy: The right lobe is moved medially and cranially; the retrohepatic veins are individually ligated and divided; the right adrenal vein (AV) is ligated and divided (the adrenal gland [AG] is shown; the infrahepatic vena cava is encircled with a vessel loop proximal to the renal veins).

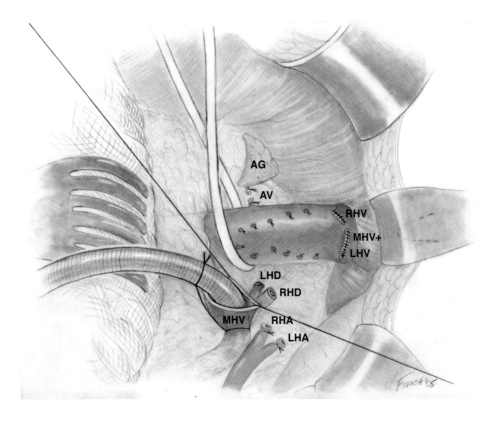

**COLOR PLATES, FIGURE LI-12**

Recipient operation: The native liver is removed. All retrohepatic veins are ligated and divided, as is the right adrenal vein. The stumps of the right hepatic vein and the middle and/or left hepatic veins are oversewn or stapled. The piggyback technique leaves the inferior vena cava intact. A cannula is shown in the main portal vein (secured with a tie); the recipient is placed on portal bypass. The hepatic artery and bile duct are transected beyond their respective bifurcations.

AG, adrenal gland; AV, adrenal vein; RHV, right hepatic vein; MHV, middle hepatic vein; LHV, left hepatic vein; MPV, main portal vein; RHA, right hepatic artery; LHA, left hepatic artery; RHD, right hepatic duct; LHD, left hepatic duct.

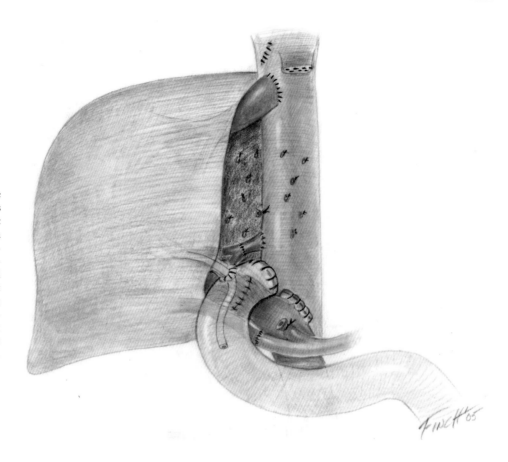

**COLOR PLATES, FIGURE LI-13**

Implantation of the donor's right lobe *without* the middle hepatic vein (segments 5 through 8): The donor's right hepatic vein is anastomosed to the recipient's vena cava, just distal to the stump of the recipient's right hepatic vein; the donor's retrohepatic segment 5 vein is anastomosed to the recipient's vena cava, using a short segment of the recipient's saphenous vein; the donor's right hepatic artery is anastomosed end-to-end to the recipient's right hepatic artery (the recipient's left hepatic artery is ligated); the donor's right portal vein is anastomosed end-to-end to the recipient's right portal vein (the recipient's left portal vein is oversewn); the donor's right hepatic duct is anastomosed to the recipient's Roux-en-Y loop and internally stented.

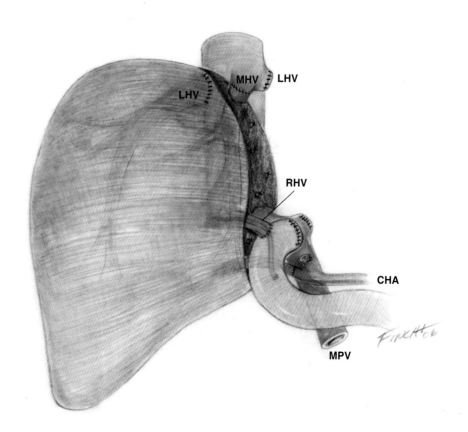

**COLOR PLATES, FIGURE LI-14**

Implantation of the donor's right lobe *with* the middle hepatic vein (segments 4 through 8): The donor's right hepatic vein is anastomosed as shown in Figure LI-13; the donor's middle hepatic vein is anastomosed end-to-end in triangular fashion to the recipient's middle hepatic vein stump (alternatively, to the recipient's middle and left hepatic vein trunk); the donor's right portal vein and the donor's right hepatic artery are anastomosed end-to-end to the recipient's right portal vein and right hepatic artery. The donor's right bile duct is anastomosed to the recipient's Roux-en-Y loop and internally stented.

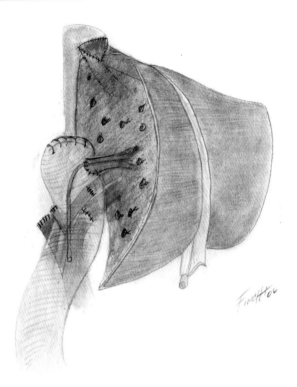

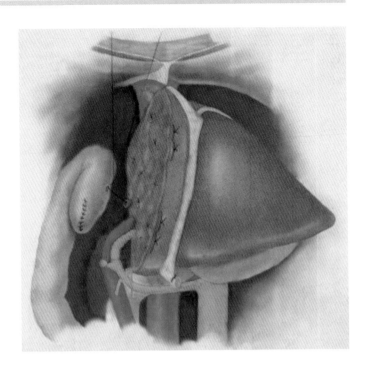

**COLOR PLATES, FIGURE LI-16**

Implantation of the donor's left lateral segments (2 and 3): The donor's left hepatic vein is anastomosed to the recipient's middle and left hepatic vein trunk (in triangular fashion); the donor's left portal vein and left hepatic artery are anastomosed end-to-end to the recipient's left portal vein and left hepatic artery. The donor's left bile duct(s) is anastomosed to the recipient's Roux-en-Y loop and internally stented.

**COLOR PLATES, FIGURE LI-15**

Implantation of the donor's left lobe (segments 2 through 4 or 1 through 4): The donor's left and middle hepatic veins are anastomosed to the recipient's middle and left hepatic vein trunk (in triangular fashion); the donor's left portal vein and the donor's left hepatic artery are anastomosed end-to-end to the recipient's left portal vein and left hepatic artery. The donor's left bile duct is anastomosed to the recipient's Roux-en-Y loop and internally stented.

| Hepatic Vein | Portal Vein | Hepatic Artery | Bile Duct |
|---|---|---|---|
| | | | |
| | | | |
| | | | |
| | | | |

**COLOR PLATES, FIGURE LI-17**

Anastomotic variations for hepatic veins, portal veins, hepatic arteries, and bile ducts. Adapted from: Tanaka K, Inomata Y, Kaihara S: *Living-donor liver transplantation*. Prous Science, Barcelona, Spain. (2003).

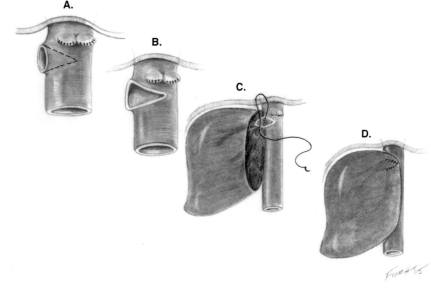

## COLOR PLATES, FIGURE LI-18

Variants to avoid venous outflow obstruction.

### FIGURE LI-18-A

Extended right lobe engraftment (segments 4 through 8): A common orifice of the donor's right and middle hepatic veins is created and anastomosed to the cava in triangular fashion. Adapted from: Liu CL, Zhao Y, Lo CM, Fan ST: Hepatic venoplasty in right lobe live donor liver transplantation. Liver Transplantation 2003; 9(12): 1265-1272.

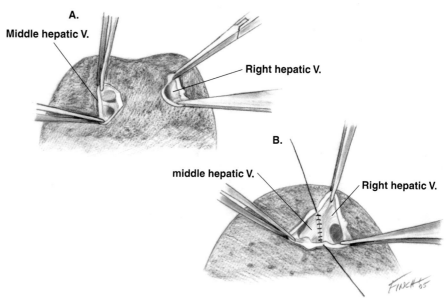

### FIGURE LI-18B

Approximation of the right and middle hepatic vein orifices, with creation of a triangular venoplasty. Adapted from: Liu et al., Liver Transplantation 2003; 9(12): 1265-1272.

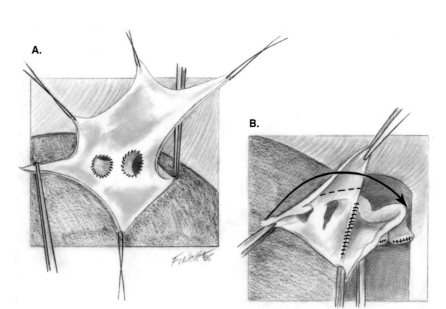

### FIGURE LI-18C

Use of cryopreserved or stored deceased donor vascular allografts to enlarge the venous outflow tract: The graft is anastomosed to a large triangular cava orifice with horizontal and caudal extension. Adapted from: Malago M, Testa G, Frilling A, et al.: Right living donor liver transplantation: an option for adult patients: single institution experience with 74 patients. Ann Surg 2003; 238(6): 853-863.

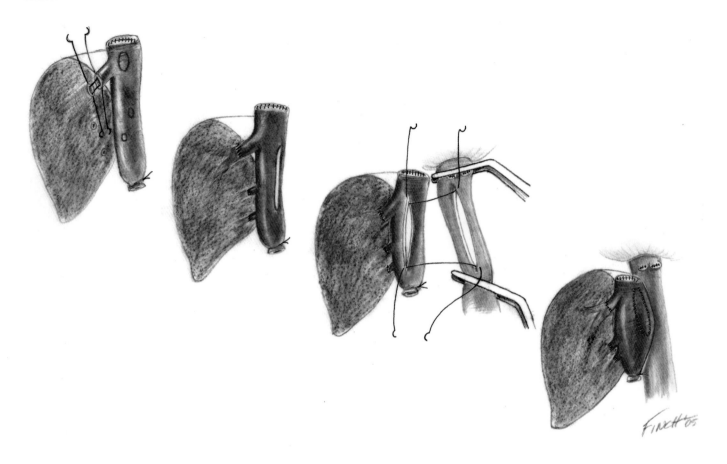

**FIGURE LI-18D**

Double vena cava technique: A cryopreserved or deceased donor vena cava allograft is used for anastomosis with the donor's right hepatic vein and segments 5 and 8 veins; the caval allograft is then anastomosed side-to-side to the recipient's vena cava, after the stumps of the right, middle, and left hepatic veins are oversewn. Adapted from: Sugawara Y, Makuuchi M, Akamatsu N et al., Liver Transplantation, 2004; 10(4): 541-547.

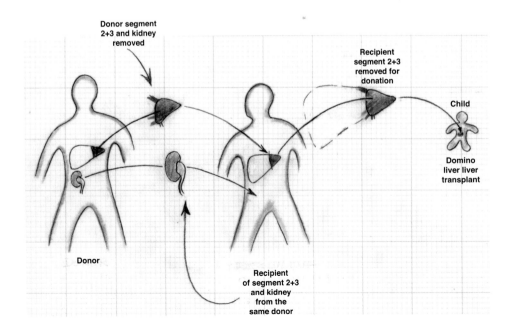

**COLOR PLATES, FIGURE LI-19**

Auxiliary liver transplants for highly sensitized kidney transplant recipient: Illustration of an auxiliary liver and combined kidney transplant (adult-to-adult), followed by a domino segmental liver transplant (adult-to-child).

# INTESTINE

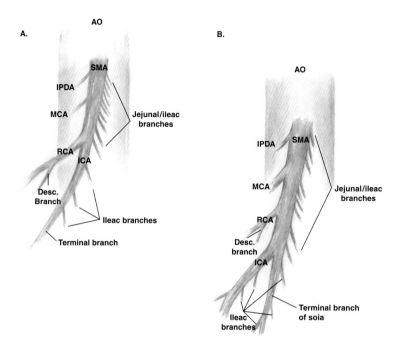

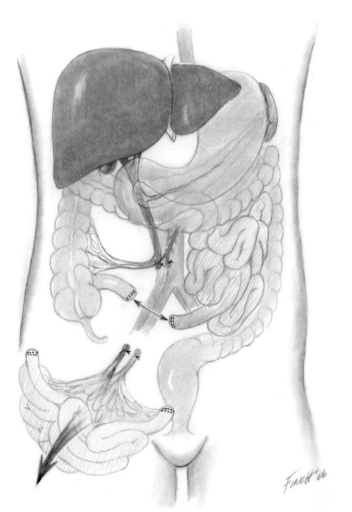

## COLOR PLATES, FIGURE IN-1

Two anatomic variants of arterial supply for living donor (LD) intestinal grafts are shown.

### FIGURE IN-1A

The ileocolic artery (ICA) is the distal extension of the superior mesenteric artery (SMA), consisting of the terminal branch and several distal ileal arteries. The ICA is transected just distal to the takeoff of the right colic artery (RCA) from the SMA. Note that the descending branch of the RCA is always preserved and stays with the donor.

### FIGURE IN-1B

The ileocolic artery (ICA) and the terminal branch of the superior mesenteric artery (SMA) are separate, independent blood vessels. If the terminal branch of the SMA stays with the intestinal graft, the ICA and right colic artery (RCA) are preserved and remain in the donor. The terminal branch is transected just distal to the ICA's takeoff from the SMA.
AO, aorta; IPDA, inferior pancreaticoduodenal artery; MCA, middle colic artery; desc., descending

## COLOR PLATES, FIGURE IN-2

Donor operation: About 180 to 200 cm of distal donor ileum on a vascular pedicle comprising the ileocolic artery and vein are removed. The donor's ileocolic artery and vein stems are ligated and divided. Note that the right colic artery and vein with their descending branches are preserved, to provide blood supply to the cecum and terminal ileum (which remain in the donor). An ileoileostomy between the proximal ileum and the terminal ileum (20 to 40 cm of which remain in the donor) is created to restore small bowel continuity in the donor.

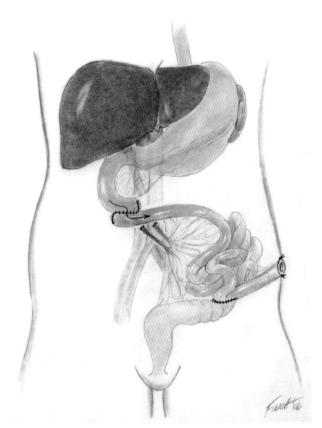

**COLOR PLATES, FIGURE IN-3**

Recipient operation: The donor's ileocolic artery and vein (or the terminal branches of the donor's superior mesenteric artery and vein) are anastomosed end-to-side to the recipient's infrarenal aorta end cava. The position of the arterial anastomosis is distal to the venous anastomosis. The arterial anastomosis is usually constructed in interrupted fashion; the venous anastomosis, in running fashion. Note that different marking sutures are placed during the donor operation to distinguish the proximal and distal bowel ends.

**COLOR PLATES, FIGURE IN-4**

Recipient operation: The donor's ileocolic artery and vein (or the terminal branches of the donor's superior mesenteric artery and vein) are anastomosed end-to-side to the recipient's infrarenal aorta and vena cava. A 2-layer, side-to-side (functional end-to-end) donor duodenum-to-recipient ileum anastomosis is constructed. A Bishop-Coop ileostomy is created. A side-to-end anastomosis from the donor's distal ileum to the recipient's sigmoid colon is constructed.

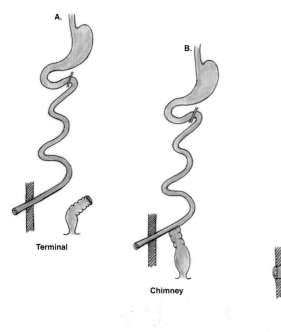

**A.**

Terminal

**B.**

Chimney

**C.**

Loop

**D.**

End to end
anastohosis

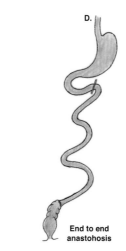

**COLOR PLATES, FIGURE IN-5**

Recipient operation: Different types of ileostomies used in intestinal transplant recipients include (1) terminal or end-ileostomy without construction of a distal anastomosis; (2) Bishop-Coop ("chimney" spout) ileostomy and anastomosis of the donor's distal ileum to the recipient's proximal colon; (3) loop-ileostomy and anastomosis of the donor's distal ileum to the recipient's proximal colon; and (4) primary distal anastomosis (ileocolostomy), usually only used for HLA-identical transplants.

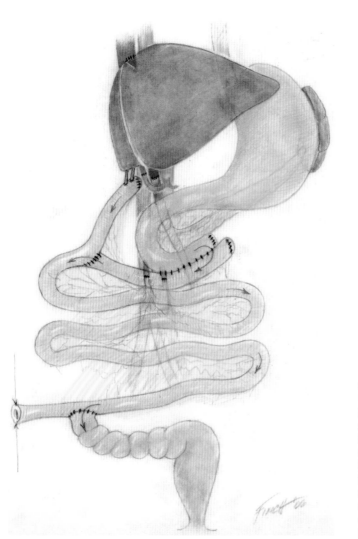

**COLOR PLATES, FIGURE IN-6**

Recipient operation: For a combined living donor (LD) liver and intestinal transplant in a pediatric recipient, liver segments 2 and 3 are implanted in standard fashion (the donor's left hepatic vein to the recipient's vena cava, the donor's left hepatic artery to the recipient's proper or common hepatic artery, the donor's left portal vein branch to the recipient's portal vein trunk). The donor's ileocolic artery and vein are anastomosed to the recipient's infrarenal aorta and cava. In the recipient, a duodenum-to-donor ileum anastomosis and a distal Bishop-Coop ileostomy are constructed to reestablish bowel continuity. A very short Roux-en-Y loop (10 to 20 cm) is anastomosed to the donor's bile duct(s).

# ISLET AUTOTRANSPLANTATION AFTER PANCREATECTOMY: HISTORY AND OUTCOMES

*David E.R. Sutherland, MD, PhD, Takashi Kobayashi, MD, Bernhard J. Hering, MD, Tun Jie, MD, Annelisa M. Carlson, MD*

## INTRODUCTION

Autografts of any kind are essentially living donor transplants, even though the recipient is the source of the tissue. Islet autografts, to maintain beta cell mass in patients undergoing pancreatic resection so as to prevent or minimize postpancreatectomy diabetes, are of special interest in this context. They have their allograft counterparts as beta cell replacement therapy in patients with *de novo* diabetes, including living donor segmental pancreas transplants, as covered in previous chapters. Islet allografts, the minimally invasive alternative to a pancreas transplant, have also been done from living donors, with three cases reported, two in the late 1970s from the University of Minnesota[1,2] and one in 2005 from Japan.[3,4]

Islet autotransplants (autografts, IATs) concomitant with total (TP) or partial pancreatectomy have been performed for nearly 30 years[5] to preserve beta cell mass and prevent or minimize surgical diabetes.[6] The concept is shown schematically in Figure 22-1. As experience with the technique has grown, metabolic outcomes have improved.

The main criterion for success of the islet autograft per se is whether insulin independence is maintained or whether postsurgical diabetes is made milder by preserving beta cell mass. The overall outcome, however, depends on the response to pancreatic resection, particularly in those with chronic pancreatitis, in whom the degree by which pain is reduced or eliminated, narcotic analgesics withdrawn, and quality of life improved is as important as the metabolic measurements.

The major application of IATs has been in patients with chronic pancreatitis who undergo resection to alleviate pain refractory to medical or prior surgical interventions, and who would otherwise become dependent on exogenous insulin. The largest series of IATs is at the University of Minnesota, but several centers worldwide, all cited in this chapter, have reported on their experience with islet autografts. Ultimately, understanding the factors that lead to the success of islet autografts may improve the metabolic outcomes of islet allografts for patients with type 1 diabetes mellitus.

## HISTORICAL CONTEXT

The first IAT was done at the University of Minnesota in 1977 and clearly demonstrated that free islets could engraft and function in humans and establish an insulin-independent state.[5] An allogenic islet transplant program had already been initiated at Minnesota (1974) for patients with type 1 diabetes, but at the time the first IAT was done, none of the islet allografts had induced insulin independence in the recipients.[1,5,7] Thus, the initial attempts were aimed at increasing the understanding of factors that might affect the success of allogenic islet transplants.

The first recipient in the Minnesota series underwent an intraportal IAT after near-total pancreatectomy and remained insulin-independent and pain-free until she died of an unrelated cause 6 years later.[6,8,9] This case proved that a viable islet preparation could be made from a freshly excised human pancreas. It

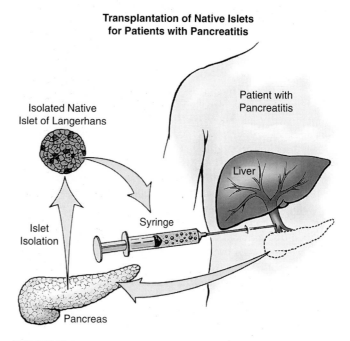

**Transplantation of Native Islets for Patients with Pancreatitis**

Isolated Native Islet of Langerhans

Patient with Pancreatitis

Liver

Islet Isolation

Syringe

Pancreas

**FIGURE 22-1**

Sequence of events to preserve beta cell mass in patients undergoing total pancreatectomy for benign disease. The resected pancreas is dispersed by collagenase digestion followed by islet isolation. Autologous islets are then embolized to the patient's liver via the portal vein.

also showed that the previous failures with islet allografts were either due to low viability related to preservation of the deceased donor pancreas or to rejection. Since the initial reports,[5,6,9] the Minnesota IAT experience has been published in a series of papers.[8,10–17]

Shortly after the initial reports on IATs from Minnesota, several centers worldwide began performing them. The world literature as of 2006 reflects a collective experience of about 300 IATs, including the Minnesota cases cited above and those done elsewhere.[18–28] Since the first case nearly 30 years ago, IATs have been performed by more than 20 centers worldwide.

Segmental pancreatic autotransplantation is another method for preserving beta cell mass after pancreatic resection.[29–33] The first segmental pancreatic autotransplant was performed around the time of the first IAT.[29] This approach appears to be used less frequently than IATs to preserve beta cell mass after total pancreatectomy, and indeed there are no reports in the literature on segmental pancreas autotransplants for the past decade.

## PATIENT SELECTION AND PAIN SYNDROME

At the University of Minnesota, pancreatic resection rather than surgical drainage procedures is the main approach to treatment of chronic pancreatitis with intractable pain.[14,34] If endoscopic procedures, including pancreatic duct sphincterotomies and stent placement, do not permanently relieve the pain, as is often the case,[35] we go right to resection. A Whipple procedure can be tried first, and if pain persists, a completion pancreatectomy with an IAT is done later. A distal pancreatectomy is done only if there is one mid-duct stricture, and it is likely that only the body and tail are involved with chronic pancreatitis. The majority of patients with chronic pancreatitis referred for surgical treatment have longstanding intractable pain requiring narcotic analgesics, and most want the most definitive procedure that can be done, total pancreatectomy and, if nondiabetic, an IAT in order to preserve insulin independence or minimize the severity of postpancreatectomy diabetes.

The severity of the gross morphologic changes associated with pancreatitis, as detected by imaging studies, including computerized tomography (CT) scans, endoscopic retrograde cholangiopancreatography (ERCP), or endoscopic ultrasound (EUS), does not necessarily correlate with the degree of pain the patient is experiencing.[36,37] Minimal-change chronic pancreatitis was first described by Walsh et al.[38] in patients who had severe abdominal pain with minimal gross morphologic changes but clear histopathologic changes in the gland, with resolution of pain in most patients following pancreatectomy. Layer et al[39] have also described two forms of chronic pancreatitis, relatively early-onset where pain precedes by years the gradual development of gross pathology, and late-onset where gross changes are detectable when the patient presents with pain. In our own series, we have 15 cases of minimal gross changes in the pancreas on EUS where chronic pancreatitis was confirmed histopathologically on the resected specimen (Gupta, K, unpublished observations, submitted in 2006 to the *American Society Gastroenterology*, for the 2007 *Digestive Disease Week*).

There are several articles on the pain of pancreatitis, which indicate that the cause is multifactorial.[40–43] Even when there is increased ductal pressure, it is not necessarily the cause of the pain,[44] and pain in patients with chronic pancreatitis exists in the absence of increased ductal pressure. Indeed, microscopic pathology with intrinsic neuritis had the best correlation in at least one study.[41] Some patients have increased sensitivity to pain of central origin, perhaps explaining the symptoms in minimal-change chronic pancreatitis.[45]

Thus, at Minnesota we are very liberal at applying total pancreatectomy and IATs in patients with chronic pancreatitis and intractable pain, no matter how minimal or severe the morphologic findings. Many patients have a history of acute relapsing pancreatitis evolving to chronic pancreatitis, where elevations in serum amylase and lipase cease to exist. Past history associated with even minimal criteria for chronic pancreatitis on EUS leads us to recommend the operation in patients requiring narcotics to manage their pain.[14] Some patients with chronic pancreatitis have diabetes when referred for surgical consultation, and in these, the decision for resection is easy, especially when exocrine deficiency also exists as is often the case. However, most patients are seen when diabetes does not exist; thus the total pancreatectomy must be undertaken with the acceptance of diabetes as a tradeoff for relief of pain and the chance to wean off narcotics. If the IAT prevents diabetes, it is a bonus. However, when a total pancreatectomy is done for chronic pancreatitis in a nondiabetic patient, an IAT to preserve beta cell mass should be done whenever possible.

## SURGICAL CONSIDERATIONS

During resection, the blood supply to the pancreas should be preserved as long as possible to minimize the detrimental effects of warm ischemia on the islets.[10,46,47] The pylorus and spleen are usually spared whenever possible, though the benefits can be questioned, particularly of retaining the pylorus. Recent information from the bariatric surgery literature suggests that activity of the intestinal hormone glucagon-like peptide (GLP-1) may be affected by the type of intestinal reconstruction selected.

At the University of Minnesota, the early series included cases in which the entire duodenum was preserved (95% pancreatectomy; Figure 22-2A), but the complication rate was actually lower

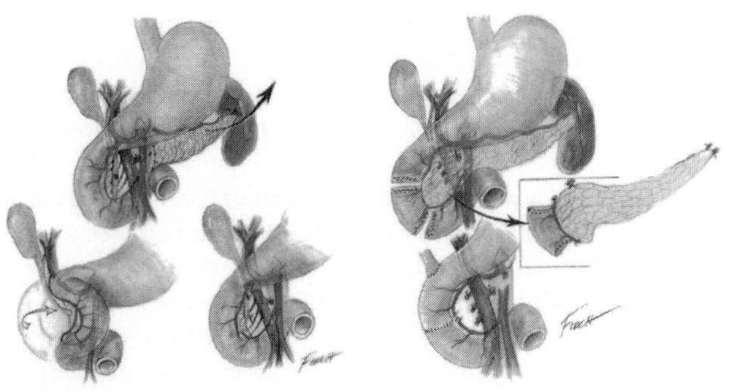

Near-total pancreatectomy          Total pancreatectomy

**FIGURE 22-2 A, B**

Two surgical techniques for pancreatectomy followed by islet autotransplantation, as described by Farney et al, *Surgery* 1991;110:427. (A) Duodenal-sparing 95% pancreatectomy attempting to preserve blood supply to entire duodenum. (B) Total pancreatectomy and pylorus- and distal-sparing duodenectomy with orthotopic reconstruction via duodenoduodenostomy and choledochoduodenostomy. We prefer this approach and believe it has fewer complications.

in those who had part or all of the duodenum resected *en bloc* with the pancreas.[8] Thus, for the past 15 years, we have routinely done a pancreaticoduodenectomy, pylorus- and fourth portion-sparing, whenever possible with orthotopic reconstruction via a duodeno-duodenostomy and choledochoduodenostomy (Figure 22-2B).

Since the splenic artery and vein are usually included with the pancreas specimen to preserve islet blood supply during the procedure, the spleen must survive on the often-marginal collateral circulation if it is to be spared. There are cases in our series of late gastric or esophageal varices requiring subsequent splenectomy (unpublished observations), so we leave the spleen only if its appearance is unchanged by the pancreatectomy.

## METABOLIC CONSIDERATIONS

In patients with painful chronic pancreatitis referred for resection, baseline metabolic studies should be routine, including fasting and postprandial glucose levels, baseline and stimulated C-peptide levels, and glycosylated hemoglobin levels, to evaluate existing beta cell function. Patients with long standing disease often have symptoms of exocrine insufficiency (steatorrhea); though formal evaluation of exocrine insufficiency is usually not done, all candidates for islet autografts at our center are counseled that exocrine deficiency will persist, be made worse, or be induced by the operation.

GLP-1 is produced by L cells in the distal intestinal tract and acts as a powerful incretin. Studies of patients with Roux-en-Y gastric bypass have shown increased levels of GLP-1 with concomitant improvement in diabetes, results not seen in patients with restrictive bariatric procedures.[48,49] Therefore, increased levels of GLP-1 might occur by resecting the pylorus at the time of total pancreatectomy and mirror the positive impact on insulin independence seen in the bariatric surgery literature. A decreased islet mass may thus be sufficient to sustain insulin independence. Although not yet applied clinically, current evidence suggests that GLP-1 agonists may help maintain or improve beta cell function after islet transplants. In one animal model, GLP-1 agonists improved glucose tolerance by increasing beta cell mass.[50,51] Expanded and regenerated beta cell mass was also seen with GLP-1 after 90% pancreatectomy in animals.[52] The beneficial effects of GLP-1 agonists may even extend to islet neogenesis[51,53–55]; however, this hypothesis remains to be tested.

## ISLET ISOLATION AND INFUSION CONSIDERATIONS

Islet isolation must be done in a laboratory that meets all of the FDA criteria for processed tissue, something that exists at only a few medical centers currently, though more and more are acquiring the technology. The islet isolation laboratory at the University of Minnesota is located in a building dedicated to molecular and cellular therapeutics.

After resection, the pancreatic duct is cannulated and the organ is taken to the islet isolation facility. There it is dispersed by collagenase digestion using the modified Ricordi technique as previously described.[16,56]

We do not routinely purify the preparation because of concerns about reducing the islet yield.[57] If the final crude tissue volume exceeds 15 mL, we reduce the volume by purifying all or part of the islet preparation, so that infusion via the portal vein can occur without undue rise in portal pressure.[58,59] If portal pressure reaches 30 cm water, or if the recipient previously had prior portal vein occlusion or preexisting portal hypertension, excessive islets or the whole preparation can be freely dispersed in the peritoneal cavity or transplanted beneath the kidney capsule or submucosal layer of the stomach in the hope that they engraft, even though no studies have been done to ensure that this occurs.[10,60]

Clinical observations and animal studies indicate that the liver (via the portal vein) is the most efficient site for islet engraftment.[61,62] It is the only site in humans associated with achieving insulin independence.[10] Other sites have been used, such as the renal capsule,[63–66] spleen,[62,67] omentum,[68] and peritoneal cavity,[69,70] but have rarely been associated with function of islet autografts in humans.[71,72] At any site, including the portal vein, the islets initially survive by nutrient diffusion and during this period have reduced functional capacity, a function that presumably improves once neovascularization occurs.[73,74]

Before islet infusion, we administer heparin (70 U/kg) to prevent intraportal clotting from tissue thromboplastin (which is assumed to be in the preparation).[75] We have administered heparin since our very first cases in the 1970s.[6,10] Nearly all of the reports of complications related to portal infusion of islets[75–79] were published before the development of standardized semiautomated pancreas dispersion techniques and before the routine use of heparinization before islet infusion.

In a series of 50 consecutive allogenic islet infusions into the portal vein reported by the Edmonton group, Doppler ultrasound evaluation revealed a 4% rate of radiologically detected but clinically insignificant portal vein thrombosis.[58] In our series, we have not seen portal vein thrombosis as a clinical entity, but we have always administered heparin before islet infusion and have continued it after infusion if portal pressures were high. Liver function tests typically show a transient rise in serum enzyme levels during the early postoperative period,[56] with no implication for future hepatic dysfunction.

## INTRA- AND POSTOPERATIVE CONSIDERATIONS

Intraoperative management must focus on maintaining euglycemia, normothermia, and hemodynamic stability. We handle glucose monitoring of islet autotransplant recipients in a manner similar to that of diabetic pancreas transplant recipients.[80] Animal studies have shown a decrease in islet engraftment with hyperglycemia; furthermore, glucose toxicity may cause structural lesions in the transplanted islets.[81–83] Severe hyperglycemia at the time of allogeneic islet transplants in one animal model impaired graft function.[84] We continue to promote islet engraftment posttransplant by an exogenous insulin drip to maintain euglycemia, minimizing the need for insulin secretion from the freshly infused islet autograft and theoretically decreasing islet stress.

## EXPANDING APPLICATION

A few centers have recently reported on islet autografts after resection for benign pancreatic processes, including pancreatic pseudocyst with compressive symptoms,[26] cystic neoplasms of the pancreas,[85,86] insulinomas,[86,87] and, in one case, a neuroendocrine tumor of the pancreas.[86] Pathologic evaluation was completed prior to autologous islet infusion in all recipients to confirm that the lesions were benign.

In the Minnesota series, IATs have been done at the time of distal pancreatectomy for benign cystic tumors in four cases (unpublished observations). In these cases it is uncertain as to how well the intrahepatic islets are functioning because those in the native pancreatic remnant are also functioning, but presumably the future risk of diabetes is reduced, particularly from weight gain, or if a completion pancreatectomy should be required. There are also 10 cases of chronic pancreatitis in our series where an IAT was done after only a distal pancreatectomy, with the head remaining; a few recipients required a completion pancreatectomy at a later date, none of whom became diabetic, indicating good engraftment at the initial IAT (unpublished observations).

An islet autograft has also been reported in a patient with pancreatic adenocarcinoma[88]; that patient underwent a pylorus-preserving pancreaticoduodenectomy, complicated by an anastomotic leak at the pancreaticojejunostomy. The leak was treated by an urgent completion pancreatectomy with an IAT. The patient died 2.5 years later of recurrent disease.[89]

Transplants of islets isolated from pancreas allografts excised for technical problems or allograft pancreatitis ("islet autoallografts") have also been performed, at least at our institution, with one case published.[90] In this case the islet yield was > 8000 islet equivalents (IEQs)/kg body weight. The patient remained insulin-independent for > 1 year while on immunosuppression and up to the time of the report, indicating successful engraftment and maintenance of islet "autoallo" function, but ultimately had to take exogenous insulin, indicating decline or loss of islet function for immunologic or nonimmunologic reasons (unpublished observation).

## ISLET AUTOTRANSPLANTS IN CHILDREN

Chronic pancreatitis is less common in children than in adults, but should be treated the same way. The aim must be to relieve pain, eliminate the need for narcotics, and preserve beta cell mass. As of December 2006, we have performed 25 IATs in children; the youngest was 5 years of age. We reported our first pediatric case in detail.[91] In a subsequent report of our initial cases, we had a 50% rate of insulin independence and all of the children became pain-free.[14] Our most recent follow-up demonstrates a 54% rate of insulin independence in the 13 pediatric patients with long-term information available (Bellin M et al. abstract submitted to the 2007 Pediatric Academic Society annual meeting).

## LITERATURE REVIEW

The largest series published to date on patients undergoing pancreatectomy and IATs have come from the University of Minnesota,[1,6,8–10,14,16,17,56] the University of Cincinnati,[19,20,92] and the University Hospitals of Leicester in the United Kingdom.[26–28] Reports have focused on metabolic outcomes, quality of life, and pain reduction.

## INSULIN INDEPENDENCE

The ability to achieve insulin independence after IATs appears to correlate directly with the number of IEQs infused. IEQs serve as an indirect measurement of beta cell mass, but there is much overlap in that a small percentage of patients receiving < 2000 IEQs/kg will become insulin-independent, whereas some receiving > 5000 IEQs/kg will not.[17,19] We have shown that islet yields are poorest in patients with prior pancreatic resections (distal pancreatectomies or surgical drainage procedures such as the Puestow

procedure).[16,93] In addition, fewer islets are recovered as pathologic fibrosis increases.[10,16] The timing of the procedure may have a direct impact on islet yield. Maximal islet yield and insulin independence may be more easily attained if the IAT is performed earlier in the disease course, as recently reported by the Cincinnati group.[20,94]

## Minnesota Series

In the 1995 report on the Minnesota series,[10] the lowest islet yields were in patients with a prior Puestow procedure, with only an 18% insulin independence rate in this group, in contrast to a 71% insulin independence rate in patients without a prior resection or drainage procedure. In a later update of the Minnesota series, at a time when we were much more likely to treat even mild hyperglycemia, and nearly all cases were total pancreatectomies, insulin independence was achieved in only 16% of patients with prior resections versus 40% in those without prior resections.[16] A prior Whipple operation has less effect on the islet yield than a prior distal pancreatectomy.[14]

As of mid-December 2006, 195 IATs had been done at the University of Minnesota; more than half of them, since 2000 (Figure 22-3). Our latest published outcome analysis encompassed 134 patients from 1977 through 2004, of whom 120 had sufficient follow-up for analysis.[17] The age range was 5 to 70 years old (Figure 22-4), and the duration of disease from 1 to 30 years (Figure 22-5). The etiology of the pancreatitis was idiopathic in nearly half of the patients (Figure 22-6). Most had had previous operations, a third directly on the pancreas (Figure 22-7). More than three-fourths underwent a total or completion pancreatectomy at the time of the IAT (Figure 22-8). This analysis[17] confirmed the correlation between the degree of pancreatic fibrosis and a history of a prior Puestow procedure with attainment of low islet yields (Figure 22-9). Again, we found a strong correlation between islet yield and insulin independence. Of patients receiving > 2 000 IEQs/kg, 47% were completely insulin-independent, whereas 25% required intermittent insulin.

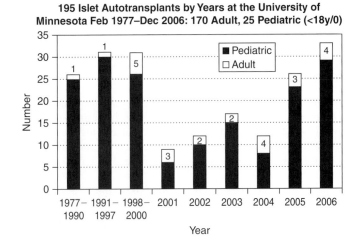

**195 Islet Autotransplants by Years at the University of Minnesota Feb 1977–Dec 2006: 170 Adult, 25 Pediatric (<18y/0)**

**FIGURE 22-3**

Islet autograft experience at the University of Minnesota by era/year includes 195 cases (170 adults, 25 children <19 years old) from February 1977 to December 2006.

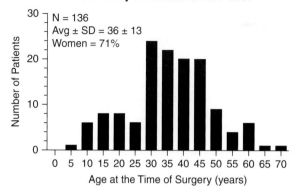

**FIGURE 22-4**

Age and gender (71% female) distribution of 136 patients undergoing islet autotransplantation at the University of Minnesota from 1977 to 2004. From presentation by Jie et al. *J Am Col Surg* 2005;201(3 Suppl):S14.

From 2000 to 2004, there were 43 complete pancreatectomy patients in the Minnesota series in whom the metabolic status could be assessed relative to islet yield (Figure 22-10). About a third had little, or no, islet function and were fully insulin-dependent. Another third had mild diabetes and needed insulin only intermittently or long-acting insulin once daily to maintain euglycemia. The other third were insulin-independent. The mean islet yield was lowest in the completely insulin-dependent group and highest in the completely insulin-independent group, with the mean in the intermittent insulin group in between, but there was much overlap between the groups—showing that factors other than pure islet yield affect function and outcomes.[17]

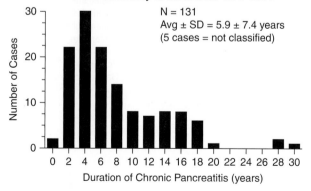

**FIGURE 22-5**

Best estimated duration of chronic pancreatitis in 136 patients undergoing total pancreatectomy and islet autotransplantation at the University of Minnesota from 1977 to 2004. From presentation by Jie et al. *J Am Col Surg* 2005;201(3);(Suppl):S14.

### Etiology of chronic pancreatitis in 136 patients undergoing total pancreatectomy and islet autotransplantation at the University of Minnesota 1977–2004*

- Idiopathic            59 (43%)
- Alcohol               21 (15%)
- Divisum               17 (13%)
- Familial              15 (11%)
- Biliary               14 (10%)
- Iatrogenic            4 (3%)
- Cystic Fibrosis       3 (1%)
- Trauma                2
- Congenital cyst       1

**FIGURE 22-6**

Presumed etiology of chronic pancreatitis in 136 patients undergoing total pancreatectomy and islet autotransplantation at the University of Minnesota from 1977 to 2004. From presentation by Jie et al. *J Am Col Surg* 2005;201(3);(Suppl):S14.

### Previous operations in 136 patients undergoing total pancreatectomy and islet autotransplantation at the University of Minnesota 1977–2004*

- Hx of abdominal operations  – 126 (93%)
- Hx of cholecystectomy       – 57 (42%)
- Hx of pancreatic operations – 45 (33%)
  - Puestow:    17
  - Duval:      1
  - Whipple:    9
  - Distal:     12
  - Combined:   6 (partial resection + Peustow)

**FIGURE 22-7**

Previous operations in in 136 patients undergoing total pancreatectomy and islet autotransplantation at the University of Minnesota from 1977 to 2004. From presentation by Jie et al. *J Am Col Surg* 2005;201(3); (Suppl):S14.

### Operation performed in 136 patients undergoing total pancreatectomy and islet autotransplantation at the University of Minnesota 1977-2004*

- Complete pancreatectomy    – 105 (77%)
- Near-total pancreatectomy  – 21 (15%)
- Distal pancreatectomy      – 10 (7%)
- OR time: 10 ± 1.7 hours
  – (2 – 4 hours waiting time for islet isolation)
- Estimated blood loss – 1500 cc (50 cc – 30 L)
- Length of stay – 22 days (1 day – 89 days)*

**FIGURE 22-8**

Type of procedure performed in 136 patients undergoing pancreatectomy and islet autotransplantation at the University of Minnesota from 1977 to 2004. From presentation by Jie et al. *J Am Col Surg* 2005;201(3);(Suppl):S14.

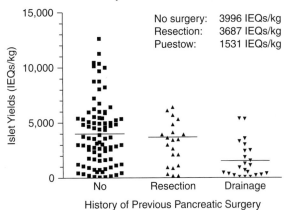

**FIGURE 22-9**

Islet isolation yield by previous surgery in 136 patients undergoing total pancreatectomy and islet autotransplantation at the University of Minnesota from 1977 to 2004. From presentation by Jie et al. *J Am Col Surg* 2005;201(3);(Suppl):S14.

## Leicester Series

The latest report from the Leicester series did not show any correlation between islet yield and insulin independence.[26] But these results may be due to the underlying cause of pancreatitis and possibly to patient compliance issues with follow-up care: the largest proportion of patients had chronic pancreatitis from alcoholism.[26]

## Cincinnati Series

Recent data from Cincinnati showed a 40% rate of insulin independence overall, regardless of whether patients had undergone prior resections or drainage procedures (mean follow-up, 18 months).[19] Factors that the Cincinnati group correlated with postoperative insulin independence included the recipient's weight, body mass index, and gender.[20] Patients with a body mass index > 28 had a higher chance of insulin dependence.[20] It may be advisable for patients to reach their ideal body weight before undergoing the procedure, to minimize preexisting insulin resistance and to maximize the chance for insulin independence. Last, the Cincinnati group reported that insulin-independent recipients had lower mean insulin requirements during the first 24 hours posttransplant, possibly relating to the detrimental effect of hyperglycemia on islet function.[94]

## General

Insulin independence is only partially the goal of an IAT, since preserving any beta cell mass at all is beneficial. Indeed, islet allograft recipients who remain insulin-dependent but have beta cell function and are C-peptide-positive are metabolically more stable and less prone to hypoglycemic unawareness than those who have no beta cell function.[95–97] Administration of C-peptide in addition to insulin in type 1 diabetics results in reduction in secondary complications of diabetes.[98–100] We extrapolate these findings to autograft recipients to assume that those who are C-peptide-positive even with an insulin requirement will have an improved metabolic outcome. In our series, about a third of autograft recipients are insulin independent, but another third have sufficient islet yield and engraftment so near-normoglycemia is maintained with exogenous insulin, often just one injection of the long-acting variety (Lantus).[17]

Although a third of our islet autograft recipients become fully diabetic because of inadequate islet yield,[14,17] as long as pain is relieved or improved, we consider the operation a success. We only offer islet autografts to patients who are fully informed about the risk of becoming diabetic, and who accept this risk in exchange for reasonable chances at both pain reduction and narcotic withdrawal.

**FIGURE 22-10**

Short-term metabolic outcome according to islet yield in 43 patients undergoing complete pancreatectomy and islet autotransplantation at the University of Minnesota from 2000 to 2004. The mean islet yield is higher in insulin-independent than insulin-dependent recipients but there is considerable overlap. From presentation by Jie et al. *J Am Col Surg* 2005;201(3); (Suppl):S14.

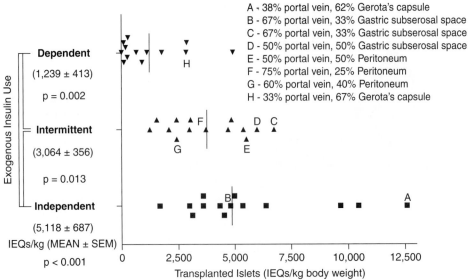

## LONG-TERM METABOLIC OUTCOMES

One long-term study of metabolic outcomes in six recipients from our center reported that islet autografts prevented diabetes mellitus for up to 13 years (mean follow-up, 6.2 ± 1.7 years).[15] Islet function was assessed by measuring fasting plasma glucose, intravenous glucose disappearance rate ($\kappa G$), hemoglobin $A_{1c}$, insulin responses to intravenous (IV) glucose and arginine, and insulin secretory reserve. Stable insulin secretory reserve was maintained, but insulin responses to glucose tended to decrease over time; the IV glucose disappearance rate significantly correlated with the number of islets transplanted.[15] However, despite normoglycemia and insulin independence, another Minnesota study showed reduced functional beta cell secretory reserve in autograft recipients, as compared with normal individuals.[21] A third Minnesota study showed that intrahepatic islet grafts (despite secreting glucagon in response to arginine) failed to secrete glucagon in response to sustained hypoglycemia, a peculiarity that may be site-dependent.[101] Nonetheless, intraportal autografts of as few as 265,000 islets can result in release of insulin and glucagon, at appropriate times, and result in prolonged insulin independence.[102]

## QUALITY OF LIFE AND PAIN

Health-related quality of life is significantly worse in patients with chronic pancreatitis, as compared with a gender- and age-adjusted general population.[103] Our primary goal in performing pancreatectomy and IATs is to improve quality of life by alleviating pain and giving the patients a chance to withdraw from narcotics, while preventing or minimizing surgical diabetes as much as possible. Studies evaluating health-related quality of life outcomes in this population are limited. In the 2003 series from Cincinnati, quality of life was measured using a standardized assessment tool (SF-36); at an average follow-up of 19 months postoperatively, quality of life had significantly improved.[20] Prospective studies are needed.

In the Cincinnati series, unremitting abdominal pain refractory to high-dose narcotics was the indication for surgery in all patients who underwent total pancreatectomy and IATs.[19,20,92] Narcotic independence was achieved in 58% of the most recent 26 patients, with a marked reduction in postoperative narcotic use as measured by morphine equivalent determinations done pre- and postoperatively.[19]

These findings are similar to those reported in the 1995 Minnesota series of 46 patients; in 83%, pain resolved or improved, and 81% were able to withdraw from narcotics.[10] In our recent review of 120 patients through 2004, 63% showed pain resolution or improvement.[17] In a recent small series from a group in Tennessee, 100% of patients who underwent total pancreatectomy for chronic pancreatitis without IATs became narcotic-independent (median follow-up, 46 months).[104]

Narcotic independence may not be obtainable in patients with opioid-induced hyperalgesia (OIH). Such patients, after receiving narcotics for chronic pain, paradoxically become more sensitive to pain, via mechanisms originating in afferent neurons and in the spinal cord.[105–111] Future studies are needed to identify patients at risk of OIH and to develop effective strategies for narcotic weaning. OIH in patients referred for pancreatectomy and IATs may be highly prevalent; accordingly, an endpoint such as narcotic independence may not be ideal for assessing postoperative success.

## FUTURE DIRECTIONS

A basic but important limitation to a more widespread clinical application of islet autografts after pancreas resection is the limited number of centers with the facilities and technology to isolate and prepare pancreatic islets for human recipients. A few centers, including our own, have successfully used distance processing for both allogenic and autologous islets.[112–114] The feasibility of this approach is enhanced by improvements in preservation methods that have extended ischemic pancreas preservation time and increased islet yield and viability from suboptimal pancreases.[115–119]

The long-term success of islet autografts in patients with chronic pancreatitis[15] contrasts with the apparently less favorable long-term results for islet allotransplants in patients with type 1 diabetes mellitus.[96] In the Edmonton islet allograft series, only 20% of recipients who achieved insulin independence remained so at 5 years, but nearly all remained C-peptide-positive,[96] indicating survival of beta cells. The difference in outcomes may be due to the rejection rate of islet allografts, or if not rejected, to the necessity of immunosuppressive therapy (calcineurin inhibitors). However, a controlled study comparing long-term function of islet auto- and allografts of comparable beta cell mass remains to be done.

Autologous islets are as fresh as possible. They are procured from a pancreas that, though diseased, is not under the stress of brain death and is not subjected to prolonged ischemia or to hours of cold preservation before isolation (as is the case for allogenic islets). In animals, islet yields and islet functionality are negatively affected by brain death, presumably because of activation of proinflammatory cytokines that occurs during brain death.[120] Additional research is needed to develop strategies to minimize the biochemical effects of brain death on allogenic islet function.[120]

Single-donor islet allografts have resulted in insulin independence in diabetic recipients at Minnesota,[121] yet in most cases, multiple donors are required.[122] Even when a single-donor islet allograft results in insulin independence, the insulin reserve may be marginal. Increasing islet viability for transplants is important; one possibility is to use a living donor.[1–4] This approach is almost certain to be effective, given the good outcomes in autograft recipients with an islet mass well below that required for a successful outcome with deceased donor islet allografts.

## CONCLUSION

Currently, an IAT is a safe, effective procedure to prevent or minimize surgical diabetes after pancreatectomy for benign disease. Pancreatic resection (even partial) with an islet autograft should always be considered the primary surgical option for patients with chronic pancreatitis and intractable pain refractory to medical therapy. Relief of pain to allow withdrawal from narcotics is the primary objective and the prevention of diabetes a secondary goal. Long-term follow-up studies are needed to evaluate and compare differences in islet durability between islet auto- and allografts of the same beta cell mass. Such a comparison may allow us to make a distinction between immunologic and nonimmunologic factors that affect declines in or sustenance of islet graft function over time.

# References

1. Sutherland DE, Matas AJ, Goetz FC, Najarian JS. Transplantation of dispersed pancreatic islet tissue in humans: autografts and allografts. *Diabetes* 1980;29(Suppl 1):31–44.

2. Gores PF, Najarian JS, Sutherland DER. Clinical Islet Allotransplantation: The University of Minnesota Experience. In: Ricordi C, ed. *Pancreatic Islet Cell Transplantation*. Austin: Landers Company; 1992:423–433.

3. Matsumoto S, Okitsu T, Iwanaga Y, Noguchi H, Nagata H, Yonekawa Y, et al. Insulin independence after living-donor distal pancreatectomy and islet allotransplantation. *Lancet* 2005;May 7-13;365(9471):1642–1644.

4. Matsumoto S, Okitsu T, Iwanaga Y, et al. Insulin independence of unstable diabetic patient after single living donor islet transplantation. *Transplant Proc.* 2005;Oct;37(8):3427–3429.

5. Sutherland DE, Matas AJ, Najarian JS. Pancreatic islet cell transplantation. *Surg Clin North Am* 1978;Apr;58(2):365–382.

6. Najarian JS, Sutherland DE, Matas AJ, Goetz FC. Human islet autotransplantation following pancreatectomy. *Transplant Proc* 1979; Mar; 11(1):336–340.

7. Najarian JS, Sutherland DE, Matas AJ, et al. Human islet transplantation: a preliminary report. *Transplant Proc* 1977;Mar;9(1):233–236.

8. Farney AC, Najarian JS, Nakhleh RE, et al. Autotransplantation of dispersed pancreatic islet tissue combined with total or near-total pancreatectomy for treatment of chronic pancreatitis. *Surgery* 1991;Aug;110(2):427–437; discussion 437–439.

9. Najarian JS, Sutherland DE, Baumgartner D, et al. Total or near total pancreatectomy and islet autotransplantation for treatment of chronic pancreatitis. *Ann Surg* 1980;192(4):526–542.

10. Wahoff DC, Papalois BE, Najarian JS, et al. Autologous islet transplantation to prevent diabetes after pancreatic resection. *Ann Surg*1995;Oct;222(4):562-75; discussion 575–9.

11. Wahoff DC, Papalois BE, Najarian JS, et al. Clinical islet autotransplantation after pancreatectomy: determinants of success and implications for allotransplantation? *Transplant Proc* 1995;Dec;27(6):3161.

12. Farney AC, Hering BJ, Nelson L, et al. No late failures of intraportal human islet autografts beyond 2 years. *Transplant Proc* 1998;Mar; 30(2):420.

13. Hering BJ, Wijkstrom M, Eckman PM. Islet transplantation In: Gruessner RWG, Sutherland DER, eds. *Transplantation of the Pancreas*. New York: Splinger-Verlag; 2004.

14. Sutherland DER, Gruessner RWG, Tun J, et al. Pancreatic islet autotransplantation for chronic pancreatitis. *Clin Transplant* 2004;18 (Suppl 13):17.

15. Robertson RP, Lanz KJ, Sutherland DE, Kendall DM. Prevention of diabetes for up to 13 years by autoislet transplantation after pancreatectomy for chronic pancreatitis. *Diabetes* 2001 Jan;50(1):47–50.

16. Gruessner RW, Sutherland DE, Dunn DL, et al. Transplant options for patients undergoing total pancreatectomy for chronic pancreatitis. *J Am Coll Surg* 2004 Apr;198(4):559-567; discussion 568–569.

17. Jie T, Hering BJ, Ansite JD, et al. Pancreatectomy and auto-islet transplant in patients with chronic pancreatitis. *ACS* 2005;201(3(Supp)):S14.

18. Watkins JG, Krebs A, Rossi RL. Pancreatic autotransplantation in chronic pancreatitis. *World J Surg* 2003;Nov;27(11):1235–1240.

19. Ahmad SA, Lowy AM, Wray CJ, et al. Factors associated with insulin and narcotic independence after islet autotransplantation in patients with severe chronic pancreatitis. *J Am Coll Surg* 2005;Nov;201(5):680–687.

20. Rodriguez Rilo HL, Ahmad SA, D'Alessio D, et al. Total pancreatectomy and autologous islet cell transplantation as a means to treat severe chronic pancreatitis. *J Gastrointest Surg* 2003;Dec;7(8):978–989.

21. Teuscher AU, Kendall DM, Smets YF, Leone JP, Sutherland DE, Robertson RP. Successful islet autotransplantation in humans: functional insulin secretory reserve as an estimate of surviving islet cell mass. *Diabetes* 1998;Mar;47(3):324–330.

22. Jindal RM, Fineberg SE, Sherman S, et al. Clinical experience with autologous and allogeneic pancreatic islet transplantation. *Transplantation* 1998;Dec 27;66(12):1836–1841.

23. Oberholzer J, Triponez F, Mage R, et al. Human islet transplantation: lessons from 13 autologous and 13 allogeneic transplantations. Transplantation 2000;Mar 27;69(6):1115–1123.

24. Farkas G, Pap A. Management of diabetes induced by nearly total (95%) pancreatectomy with autologous transplantation of Langerhans cells. *Orv Hetil* 1997;Jul 20;138(29):1863–1867.

25. Sarbu V, Dima S, Aschie M, et al. Preliminary data on post-pancreatectomy diabetes mellitus treated by islet-cell autotransplantation. *Chirurgia (Bucur)* 2005;Nov-Dec;100(6):587–593.

26. Clayton HA, Davies JE, Pollard CA. Pancreatectomy with islet autotransplantation for the treatment of severe chronic pancreatitis: the first 40 patients at the Leicester General Hospital. *Transplantation* 2003;Jul 15;76(1):92–98.

27. White SA, Davies JE, Pollard C, et al. Pancreas resection and islet autotransplantation for end-stage chronic pancreatitis. *Ann Surg* 2001;Mar; 233(3):423–431.

28. White SA, Dennison AR, Swift SM, et al. Intraportal and splenic human islet autotransplantation combined with total pancreatectomy. *Transplant Proc* 1998;Mar;30(2):312–313.

29. Hogle HH, Reemtsma K. Pancreatic autotransplantation following resection. *Surgery* 1978;Mar;83(3):359–360.

30. Rossi RL, Soeldner JS, Braasch JW, et al. Segmental pancreatic autotransplantation with pancreatic ductal occlusion after near total or total pancreatic resection for chronic pancreatitis. Results at 5-to 54-month follow-up evaluation. *Ann Surg* 1986;Jun;203(6):626–636.

31. Tamura K. Segmental autotransplantation of the pancreas for pancreatic cancer or chronic pancreatitis. *Nippon Geka Hokan* 1993;Nov 1;62(6): 285–286.

32. Dafoe DC, Naji A, Perloff LJ, Barker CF. Pancreatic and islet autotransplantation. *Hepatogastroenterology* 1990;Jun;37(3):307–315.

33. Fukushima W, Shimizu K, Izumi R, et al. Heterotopic segmental pancreatic autotransplantation in patients undergoing total pancreatectomy. *Transplant Proc* 1994; Aug;26(4):2285–2287.

34. Carlson AM, Kobayashi T, Sutherland DER. Islet autotransplantation to prevent or minimize diabetes after pancreatectomy. pending publication.

35. Dite P, Ruzicka M, Zboril V, Novotny I. A prospective, randomized trial comparing endoscopic and surgical therapy for chronic pancreatitis. *Endoscopy* 2003;Jul;35(7):553–558.

36. Noh KW, Wallace MB. EUS in the diagnosis of chronic pancreatitis. *VHJOE* 2006 2006;5(1):6.

37. Sahai AV, Zimmerman M, Aabakken L, et al. Prospective assessment of the ability of endoscopic ultrasound to diagnose, exclude, or establish the severity of chronic pancreatitis found by endoscopic retrograde cholangiopancreatography. *Gastrointest Endosc* 1998;Jul;48(1):18–25.

38. Walsh TN, Rode J, Theis BA, Russell RC. Minimal change chronic pancreatitis. *Gut* 1992 Nov;33(11):1566–1571.

39. Layer P, Yamamoto H, Kalthoff L, et al. The different courses of early- and late-onset idiopathic and alcoholic chronic pancreatitis. *Gastroenterology* 1994;Nov;107(5):1481–1487.

40. Malfertheiner P, Buchler M, Stanescu A, Ditschuneit H. Pancreatic morphology and function in relationship to pain in chronic pancreatitis. *Int J Pancreatol* 1987;Feb;2(1):59–66.

41. Keith RG, Keshavjee SH, Kerenyi NR. Neuropathology of chronic pancreatitis in humans. *Can J Surg*1985;May;28(3):207-211.

42. Di Sebastiano P, Fink T, Weihe E, et al. Immune cell infiltration and growth-associated protein 43 expression correlate with pain in chronic pancreatitis. *Gastroenterology* 1997;May;112(5):1648–1655.

43. Di Sebastiano P, di Mola FF, Buchler MW, Friess H. Pathogenesis of pain in chronic pancreatitis. *Dig Dis* 2004;22(3):267–272.

44. Manes G, Buchler M, Pieramico O, Di Sebastiano P, Malfertheiner P. Is increased pancreatic pressure related to pain in chronic pancreatitis? *Int J Pancreatol* 1994;Apr;15(2):113–117.

45. Buscher HC, Wilder-Smith OH, van Goor H. Chronic pancreatitis patients show hyperalgesia of central origin: a pilot study. *Eur J Pain* 2006;May;10(4):363–370.

46. Corlett MP, Scharp DW. The effect of pancreatic warm ischemia on islet isolation in rats and dogs. *J Surg Res* 1988;Dec;45(6):531–536.

47. White SA, Robertson GS, London NJ, Dennison AR. Human islet autotransplantation to prevent diabetes after pancreas resection. *Dig Surg* 2000;17(5):439–450.

48. le Roux CW, Aylwin SJ, Batterham RL, et al. Gut hormone profiles following bariatric surgery favor an anorectic state, facilitate weight loss, and improve metabolic parameters. *Ann Surg* 2006;Jan;243(1):108–114.

49. Greenway SE, Greenway FL 3rd, Klein S. Effects of obesity surgery on non-insulin-dependent diabetes mellitus. *Arch Surg* 2002;Oct;137(10):1109–1117.

50. Xu G, Kaneto H, Lopez-Avalos MD, Weir GC, Bonner-Weir S. GLP-1/exendin-4 facilitates beta-cell neogenesis in rat and human pancreatic ducts. *Diabetes Res Clin Pract* 2006;Jul;73(1):107–110.

51. King A, Lock J, Xu G, Bonner-Weir S, Weir GC. Islet transplantation outcomes in mice are better with fresh islets and exendin-4 treatment. *Diabetologia* 2005;Oct;48(10):2074–2079.

52. Xu G, Stoffers DA, Habener JF, Bonner-Weir S. Exendin-4 stimulates both beta-cell replication and neogenesis, resulting in increased beta-cell mass and improved glucose tolerance in diabetic rats. *Diabetes* 1999;Dec;48(12):2270–2276.

53. Stoffers DA, Kieffer TJ, Hussain MA, et al. Insulinotropic glucagon-like peptide 1 agonists stimulate expression of homeodomain protein IDX-1 and increase islet size in mouse pancreas. *Diabetes* 2000;May;49(5):741–748.

54. Bonner-Weir S, Sharma A. Are there pancreatic progenitor cells from which new islets form after birth? *Nat Clin Pract Endocrinol Metab* 2006;May;2(5):240–241.

55. Bonner-Weir S, Weir GC. New sources of pancreatic beta-cells. *Nat Biotechnol* 2005;Jul;23(7):857–861.

56. Farney AC, Sutherland DER. Islet autotransplantation. In: Ricordi C, ed. Pancreatic Islet Cell Transplantation. Austin: R.G. Landes Publishing Co., 1992:291-312.

57. Gores PF, Sutherland DE. Pancreatic islet transplantation: is purification necessary? *Am J Surg* 1993;Nov;166(5):538–542.

58. Casey JJ, Lakey JR, Ryan EA, et al. Portal venous pressure changes after sequential clinical islet transplantation. *Transplantation* 2002;Oct 15;74(7):913–915.

59. Robertson RP. Pancreatic islet cell transplantation: likely impact on current therapeutics for type 1 diabetes mellitus. *Drugs* 2001;61(14):2017–2020.

60. Cameron JL, Mehigan DG, Broe PJ, Zuidema GD. Distal pancreatectomy and islet autotransplantation for chronic pancreatitis. *Ann Surg* 1981;Mar;193(3):312–317.

61. Warnock GL, Rajotte RV, Procyshyn AW. Normoglycemia after reflux of islet-containing pancreatic fragments into the splenic vascular bed in dogs. *Diabetes* 1983;May;32(5):452–459.

62. Gray DW. Islet isolation and transplantation techniques in the primate. *Surg Gynecol Obstet*. 1990 Mar;170(3):225–232.

63. Gray DW, Cranston D, McShane P, Sutton R, Morris PJ. The effect of hyperglycaemia on pancreatic islets transplanted into rats beneath the kidney capsule. *Diabetologia* 1989 Sep;32(9):663–667.

64. Gray DW, Sutton R, McShane P, Peters M, Morris PJ. Exocrine contamination impairs implantation of pancreatic islets transplanted beneath the kidney capsule. *J Surg Res* 1988;Nov;45(5):432–442.

65. Matarazzo M, Giardina MG, Guardasole V, et al. Islet transplantation under the kidney capsule corrects the defects in glycogen metabolism in both liver and muscle of streptozocin-diabetic rats. *Cell Transplant* 2002;11(2):103–112.

66. Vargas F, Julian JF, Llamazares JF, et al. Engraftment of islets obtained by collagenase and Liberase in diabetic rats: a comparative study. *Pancreas* 2001;Nov;23(4):406–413.

67. Sutton R, Gray DW, Burnett M, et al. Metabolic function of intra-portal and intrasplenic islet autografts in cynomolgus monkeys. *Diabetes* 1989;Jan;38 Suppl 1:182–184.

68. Ao Z, Matayoshi K, Lakey JR, Rajotte RV, Warnock GL. Survival and function of purified islets in the omental pouch site of outbred dogs. *Transplantation* 1993;Sep;56(3):524–529.

69. Wahoff DC, Sutherland DE, Hower CD, Lloveras JK, Gores PF. Free intraperitoneal islet autografts in pancreatectomized dogs—impact of islet purity and posttransplantation exogenous insulin. *Surgery* 1994;Oct;116(4):742–748; discussion 748–750.

70. Wahoff DC, Hower CD, Sutherland DE, Leone JP, Gores PF. The peritoneal cavity: an alternative site for clinical islet transplantation? *Transplant Proc* 1994;Dec;26(6):3297–3298.

71. Fontana I, Arcuri V, Tommasi GV, et al. Long-term follow-up of human islet autotransplantation. *Transplant Proc* 1994;Apr;26(2):581.

72. White SA, London NJ, Johnson PR, et al. The risks of total pancreatectomy and splenic islet autotransplantation. *Cell Transplant* 2000;Jan-Feb;9(1):19–24.

73. Andersson A, Korsgren O, Jansson L. Intraportally transplanted pancreatic islets revascularized from hepatic arterial system. Diabetes 1989;Jan;38(Suppl 1):192–195.

74. Korsgren O, Christofferson R, Jansson L. Angiogenesis and angioarchitecture of transplanted fetal porcine islet-like cell clusters. *Transplantation* 1999;Dec 15;68(11):1761–1766.

75. Mehigan DG, Bell WR, Zuidema GD, Eggleston JC, Cameron JL. Disseminated intravascular coagulation and portal hypertension following pancreatic islet autotransplantation. *Ann Surg* 1980;Mar;191(3):287–293.

76. Memsic L, Busuttil RW, Traverso LW. Bleeding esophageal varices and portal vein thrombosis after pancreatic mixed-cell autotransplantation. *Surgery* 1984;Feb;95(2):238–242.

77. Mittal VK, Toledo-Pereyra LH, Sharma M, et al. Acute portal hypertension and disseminated intravascular coagulation following pancreatic islet autotransplantation after subtotal pancreatectomy. *Transplantation* 1981;Apr;31(4):302–304.

78. Toledo-Pereyra LH, Rowlett AL, Cain W, et al. Hepatic infarction following intraportal islet cell autotransplantation after near-total pancreatectomy. *Transplantation* 1984 Jul;38(1):88–89.

79. Walsh TJ, Eggleston JC, Cameron JL. Portal hypertension, hepatic infarction, and liver failure complicating pancreatic islet autotransplantation. *Surgery* 1982;Apr;91(4):485–487.

80. Manciu N, Beebe DS, Tran P, et al. Total pancreatectomy with islet cell autotransplantation: anesthetic implications. *J Clin Anesth* 1999;Nov; 11(7):576–582.

81. Korsgren O, Jansson L, Andersson A. Effects of hyperglycemia on function of isolated mouse pancreatic islets transplanted under kidney capsule. *Diabetes* 1989;Apr;38(4):510–515.

82. Clark A, Bown E, King T, Vanhegan RI, Turner RC. Islet changes induced by hyperglycemia in rats. Effect of insulin or chlorpropamide therapy. *Diabetes* 1982 Apr;31(4 Pt 1):319–325.

83. Dohan FC, Lukens FDW. Lesions of the pancreatic islets produced in cats by the administration of glucose. *Science* 1947;105:183–183.

84. Makhlouf L, Duvivier-Kali VF, Bonner-Weir S, et al. Importance of hyperglycemia on the primary function of allogeneic islet transplants. *Transplantation* 2003;Aug 27;76(4):657–664.

85. Lee BW, Jee JH, Heo JS, Choi SH, Jang KT, Noh JH, et al. The favorable outcome of human islet transplantation in Korea: experiences of 10 autologous transplantations. *Transplantation* 2005;Jun 15;79(11):1568–1574.

86. Berney T, Mathe Z, Bucher P, et al. Islet autotransplantation for the prevention of surgical diabetes after extended pancreatectomy for the resection of benign tumors of the pancreas. *Transplant Proc* 2004;May;36(4):1123–1124.

87. Oberholzer J, Mathe Z, Bucher P, et al. Islet autotransplantation after left pancreatectomy for non-enucleable insulinoma. *Am J Transplant* 2003;Oct;3(10):1302–1307.

88. Liu X, Forster S, Adam U, et al. Islet autotransplantation combined with total pancreatectomy for treatment of pancreatic adenocarcinoma. *Transplant Proc* 2001;Feb-Mar;33(1-2):662–663.

89. Forster S, Liu X, Adam U, Schareck WD, Hopt UT. Islet autotransplantation combined with pancreatectomy for treatment of pancreatic adenocarcinoma: a case report. *Transplant Proc* 2004;May;36(4):1125–1126.

90. Leone JP, Kendall DM, Reinsmoen N, Hering BJ, Sutherland DE. Immediate insulin-independence after retransplantation of islets prepared from an allograft pancreatectomy in a type 1 diabetic patient. *Transplant Proc* 1998;Mar;30(2):319.

91. Wahoff DC, Paplois BE, Najarian JS, et al. Islet autotransplantation after total pancreatectomy in a child. *J Pediatr Surg* 1996;Jan;31(1): 132–135; discussion 135–136.

92. Islet auto transplants at the University of Cincinnati. A 5 Year Experience. *Clinical and Exp Islet Transplant I*; July 26, 2006.

93. Wahoff DC, Leone JP, Farney AC, Teuscher AU, Sutherland DE. Pregnancy after total pancreatectomy and autologous islet transplantation. *Surgery* 1995;Mar;117(3):353–354.

94. Ahmed SA, Wray C, Rilo HL, et al. Chronic pancreatitis: recent advances and ongoing challenges. *Curr Probl Surg* 2006;Mar;43(3): 127–238.

95. Paty BW, Senior PA, Lakey JR, Shapiro AM, Ryan EA. Assessment of glycemic control after islet transplantation using the continuous glucose monitor in insulin-independent versus insulin-requiring type 1 diabetes subjects. *Diabetes Technol Ther* 2006;Apr;8(2):165–173.

96. Ryan EA, Paty BW, Senior PA, et al. Five-year follow-up after clinical islet transplantation. *Diabetes* 2005;Jul;54(7):2060–2069.

97. Ryan EA, Lakey JR, Paty BW, et al. Successful islet transplantation: continued insulin reserve provides long-term glycemic control. *Diabetes* 2002;Jul;51(7):2148–2157.

98. Johansson BL, Borg K, Fernqvist-Forbes E, et al. Beneficial effects of C-peptide on incipient nephropathy and neuropathy in patients with Type 1 diabetes mellitus. *Diabet Med* 2000;Mar;17(3):181–189.

99. Kamiya H, Zhang W, Sima AA. C-peptide prevents nociceptive sensory neuropathy in type 1 diabetes. *Ann Neurol* 2004;Dec;56(6): 827–835.

100. Ekberg K, Brismar T, Johansson BL, et al. Amelioration of sensory nerve dysfunction by C-Peptide in patients with type 1 diabetes. *Diabetes* 2003;Feb;52(2):536–541.

101. Kendall DM, Teuscher AU, Robertson RP. Defective glucagon secretion during sustained hypoglycemia following successful islet allo- and autotransplantation in humans. *Diabetes* 1997;Jan;46(1):23–27.

102. Pyzdrowski KL, Kendall DM, Halter JB, et al. Preserved insulin secretion and insulin independence in recipients of islet autografts. *N Engl J Med* 1992;Jul 23;327(4):220–226.

103. Berney T, Rudisuhli T, Oberholzer J, Caulfield A, Morel P. Long-term metabolic results after pancreatic resection for severe chronic pancreatitis. *Arch Surg* 2000;Sep;135(9):1106–1111.

104. Behrman SW, Mulloy M. Total pancreatectomy for the treatment of chronic pancreatitis: indications, outcomes, and recommendations. *Am Surg* 2006;Apr;72(4):297–302.

105. Angst MS, Clark JD. Opioid-induced hyperalgesia: a qualitative systematic review. *Anesthesiology* 2006;Mar;104(3):570–587.

106. Chu LF, Clark DJ, Angst MS. Opioid tolerance and hyperalgesia in chronic pain patients after one month of oral morphine therapy: a preliminary prospective study. *J Pain* 2006;Jan;7(1):43–48.

107. Gardell LR, King T, Ossipov MH, et al. Opioid receptor-mediated hyperalgesia and antinociceptive tolerance induced by sustained opiate delivery. *Neurosci Lett* 2006;Mar 20;396(1):44–49.

108. Liang DY, Liao G, Wang J, Usuka J, Guo Y, Peltz G, et al. A genetic analysis of opioid-induced hyperalgesia in mice. *Anesthesiology* 2006;May; 104(5):1054–1062.

109. Mao J. Opioid-induced abnormal pain sensitivity. *Curr Pain Headache* Rep 2006;Feb;10(1):67–70.

110. Dogrul A, Bilsky EJ, Ossipov MH, Lai J, Porreca F. Spinal L-type calcium channel blockade abolishes opioid-induced sensory hypersensitivity and antinociceptive tolerance. *Anesth Analg* 2005;Dec;101(6): 1730–1735.

111. Mercadante S, Arcuri E. Hyperalgesia and opioid switching. *Am Hosp Palliat Care* 2005; Jul–Aug;22(4):291–294.

112. Langer RM, Mathe Z, Doros A, et al. Successful islet after kidney transplantations in a distance over 1000 kilometres: Preliminary results of the Budapest-Geneva collaboration. *Transplant Proc* 2004;Dec; 36(10):3113–3115.

113. Rabkin JM, Olyaei AJ, Orloff SL, et al. Distant processing of pancreas islets for autotransplantation following total pancreatectomy. *Am J Surg* 1999;May;177(5):423–427.

114. Rabkin JM, Leone JP, Sutherland DE, et al. Transcontinental shipping of pancreatic islets for autotransplantation after total pancreatectomy. *Pancreas* 1997;Nov;15(4):416–419.

115. Matsuda T, Suzuki Y, Tanioka Y, et al. Pancreas preservation by the 2-layer cold storage method before islet isolation protects isolated islets against apoptosis through the mitochondrial pathway. *Surgery* 2003;Sep;134(3):437–445.

116. Fujino Y, Kuroda Y, Suzuki Y, et al. Preservation of canine pancreas for 96 hours by a modified two-layer (UW solution/perfluorochemical) cold storage method. *Transplantation* 1991;May;51(5):1133–1135.

117. Fraker CA, Alejandro R, Ricordi C. Use of oxygenated perfluorocarbon toward making every pancreas count. *Transplantation* 2002;Dec 27; 74(12):1811–1812.

118. Tsujimura T, Kuroda Y, Avila JG, et al. Influence of pancreas preservation on human islet isolation outcomes: impact of the two-layer method. *Transplantation* 2004 ;Jul 15;78(1):96–100.

119. Tsujimura T, Kuroda Y, Churchill TA, et al. Short-term storage of the ischemically damaged human pancreas by the two-layer method prior to islet isolation. *Cell Transplant* 2004;13(1):67–73.

120. Contreras JL, Eckstein C, Smyth CA, et al. Brain death significantly reduces isolated pancreatic islet yields and functionality in vitro and in vivo after transplantation in rats. *Diabetes* 2003 Dec;52(12):2935–2942.

121. Hering BJ, Kandaswamy R, Ansite JD, et al. Single-donor, marginal-dose islet transplantation in patients with type 1 diabetes. *JAMA* 2005;Feb 16;293(7):830–835.

122. Sutherland DE, Gruessner A, Hering BJ. Beta-cell replacement therapy (pancreas and islet transplantation) for treatment of diabetes mellitus: an integrated approach. *Endocrinol Metab Clin North Am* 2004;Mar; 33(1):135–48.

# CHAPTER 23

# ISLET TRANSPLANTATION USING LIVING DONORS

*Juliet Emamaullee, PhD, James Shapiro, MD, PhD*

## INTRODUCTION

### Therapeutic Options for Patients With Type 1 Diabetes

Diabetes is a disease that results from impaired glucose metabolism, either due to a complete loss of the insulin producing β-cells within the islets of Langerhans of the pancreas (type 1 diabetes mellitus; "T1DM"), or due to a defect in insulin production and/or utilization (type 2 diabetes mellitus; "T2DM"). Currently, there are more than 200 million patients with diabetes worldwide, and it is projected that more than 5% of the world's adult population will be afflicted with diabetes by the year 2025.[1] T1DM is often referred to as juvenile-onset diabetes, as approximately 13000 children are diagnosed with T1DM each year in the United States, making T1DM the most prevalent chronic childhood disease.[2] Although careful blood glucose monitoring and insulin administration can provide patients with T1DM with a relatively good quality of life, the long-term impact of this disease remains significant. For patients that are diagnosed with T1DM as children, it has been estimated that approximately 15% will die before their 40th birthday, a mortality rate that exceeds 20 times that of the general population.[2] Causes of death related to T1DM include acute complications, such as hypoglycemic coma, and chronic secondary conditions, such as nephropathy or cardiovascular disease.[2] Patients with T1DM also face many chronic complications, including nephropathy, retinopathy, peripheral neuropathy, coronary ischemia, stroke, amputation, erectile dysfunction, and gastroparesis.[2] It has been determined that patients with diabetes represent 8% of those who are legally blind, 30% of all patients on dialysis due to end-stage renal disease, and 20% of all patients receiving kidney transplants in the United States.[2] In an effort to prevent these long-term complications in patients with diabetes, the Diabetes Control and Complications Trial (DCCT) was conducted to examine the benefit of intensive blood glucose regulation by frequent insulin injection or pump.[3–5] Results from the DCCT clearly demonstrated that this approach improved glycosylated hemoglobin levels and significantly protected against nephropathy, neuropathy, and retinopathy.[4,5] However, the penalty for improved glycemic control was a threefold increased risk of serious hypoglycemic events, including recurrent seizures and coma.[4,6]

It has thus become clear that the restoration of an adequate islet mass would provide the best glucose regulation and long-term health outcome for patients with T1DM. The first efforts directed at addressing this issue have involved whole pancreas transplantation. Currently more than 25000 pancreas transplants have been performed worldwide for end-stage renal disease (simultaneous kidney pancreas or pancreas after kidney transplantation) or occasionally for severe hypoglycemic unawareness (pancreas transplant alone). Recent improvements in surgical technique (portal venous and enteric endocrine drainage) maintenance immunosuppression have substantially improved the risk profile and enhanced long-term outcomes with this approach.[7,8] However, only 50% of patients who have undergone pancreas-alone transplantation still maintain evidence of graft function (insulin independence) at 5 years, according to the International Pancreas Transplant Registry.[9] Also, recent data from the United Network for Organ Sharing (UNOS) has shown that only 28% of the approximately 6000 cadaveric pancreata donated each year are transplanted, since the organ must conform to strict donor criteria and requirements for short cold ischemic time to be considered suitable for transplantation.[9,10] Despite strong evidence that the procedure can prolong life, reverse established nephropathy, and improve quality of life, pancreas transplantation is not felt to be suitable for diabetic patients that are early in the evolution of their disease. Compared to vascularized pancreas transplantation, β-cell replacement via transplantation of isolated pancreatic islets offers a simpler procedure that avoids risks associated with major surgery.[9]

## BACKGROUND

Experimental islet transplantation first made its mark when Paul Lacy successfully reversed chemical diabetes in rodents in 1972.[11] Attempts to translate these findings to the clinic initially met with failure and occasionally with serious complications including portal vein thrombosis, portal hypertension, and disseminated intravascular coagulation when impure islets were infused into the portal vein.[12] The first subject to achieve insulin independence for 1 month was reported by Lacy's group in 1989.[13] Camillo Ricordi developed a method for high-yield isolation of human islets using the so-called Ricordi Chamber, and subsequently reported 50% insulin independence rates at 1 year in subjects who underwent cluster islet-liver transplants for abdominal malignancies in the setting of surgical-induced (nonautoimmune) diabetes.[14] Groups in Giessen, Germany, and in Milan, Italy, achieved insulin independence in approximately half of their treated subjects in the late 1990s. However, of the total world experience of over 450 attempts at clinical islet transplantation at this time, fewer than 8% of subjects achieved insulin independence. After 3 decades of research, the 1-year insulin independence rates in clinical islet transplantation were still too low to justify the risks associated with portal infusion and lifelong immunosuppression in most patients with T1DM.[15–19]

## The Edmonton Protocol

A new protocol developed by Shapiro et al. in 1999 was designed for patients with "brittle diabetes" who experienced extreme difficulty in managing their blood glucose levels ("glucose lability") and/or severe hypoglycemic unawareness.[20] Compared to previous clinical islet transplantation studies, the Edmonton Protocol emphasized avoidance of corticosteroids; use of potent immunosuppression with combined sirolimus, tacrolimus, and anti-CD25 antibody to protect against rejection and recurrent autoimmunity; and use of two (or occasionally more) fresh islet preparations to provide a mean islet implant mass of approximately 13000 islet equivalents (IE)/kg recipient body weight.[20] For the first time, dramatic improvements in islet allograft survival were observed, and all of the first seven patients achieved sustained independence from insulin.[20] Since 2000, more than 85 consecutive patients have received islet transplants at the University of Alberta, and the 1-year insulin independence rate remains steady at approximately 80% after completed transplants. An international multicenter trial (Immune Tolerance Network) has replicated the results obtained at the University of Alberta, but has shown a broad spectrum of success based on the center's previous experience and skill in islet isolation and immunosuppressive management.[21] The Miami group has demonstrated that islets can be cultured for up to 3 days prior to being transplanted, with similar success when transplanted using Edmonton-like immunosuppression.[22] The Miami group also showed that islets could be successfully shipped and transplanted at a remote facility (Houston).[22,23] A Swiss–French consortium (the GRAGIL Network) also demonstrated the benefits of centralized islet processing facilities servicing a broader network of centers throughout Europe.[19,24]

Islet transplantation has been funded in Alberta, Canada, as accepted clinical standard of care since 2001. In the U.S. large registration trials are currently moving forward to secure a Biological License and therefore reimbursement, which will make a significant difference to the availability of islets for transplantation in that country. The breakthrough data obtained in Edmonton have encouraged many centers around the world to implement clinical islet transplantation, and since 2000 more than 550 patients have been transplanted using recent variants of the Edmonton Protocol in almost 50 centers worldwide.[25]

Despite this success, islet-alone transplantation remains restricted to patients with severe hypoglycemia or glycemic lability, and is presently unsuitable for the majority of patients with T1DM. It has also not been explored yet in patients with T2DM. Most patients require two or occasionally three islet implant procedures in order to achieve insulin independence, although insulin independence following single donor infusion has been reported in a cohort of patients at the University of Minnesota.[26,27] Although C-peptide secretion (> 0.5 ng/mL) has been maintained in 88% of islet graft recipients beyond 3 years in Edmonton, emerging data on the long-term insulin independence rates have shown that after 3 years, only 50% of recipients remain off insulin, and at 5 years posttransplant this number falls to approximately 10%.[28] Although the exact cause of the disconnect between loss of insulin independence and maintenance of C-peptide status has not been fully elucidated to date, it is likely that multifactorial events are contributing to this observation. Although rejection (acute or chronic) and recurrent autoimmunity may be responsible for graft loss, it is also likely that other nonimmune events contribute, including chronic toxicity from sirolimus/tacrolimus, failure of islet regeneration, or transdifferentiation (again due to antiproliferative effects of sirolimus). Perhaps even more importantly, islet "burn-out" from constant metabolic stimulation could result in decayed function, because only a marginal mass of islets actually engraft in most subjects. Although the risk of malignancy, posttransplant lymphoma, and life-threatening sepsis has been very low in patients treated to date, fears of these complications limit a broader application in patients with less severe forms of diabetes including children. Moreover, a number of immunosuppression-related side-effects have been encountered, which can be dose or drug limiting in some patients.[29] It is clear therefore that although outcomes have improved substantially after islet transplantation, extensive refinements in clinical protocols are needed both to improve safety and to enhance success with single donor islet infusions.

## Living Donor Islet Transplantation: The Next Step

Living donor islet transplantation, which is currently an experimental procedure, provides a unique opportunity to treat many more patients with unstable forms of T1DM (outlined in Figure 23-1). In an attempt to meet the demand for donor organs and to improve clinical outcomes, living donor programs have moved forward successfully in kidney, liver, and lung transplantation at most leading transplant centers worldwide. Given the rapid, global implementation of cadaveric islet transplantation over the past 5 years, it seems inevitable that living donor islet transplantation will become routine eventually. Despite remarkable success in clinical islet transplantation since 1999, islet supply and functional viability remain to be significant challenges when islets are derived from cadaveric organ donors.[30] Living donor islet transplantation represents a unique opportunity to overcome donor organ shortage and procure the islet tissue under perfect conditions, with closer HLA matching between donor and recipient. Furthermore, opportunities for pretransplant recipient conditioning for specific donor tolerance induction protocols could be developed in the living donor islet transplant setting.

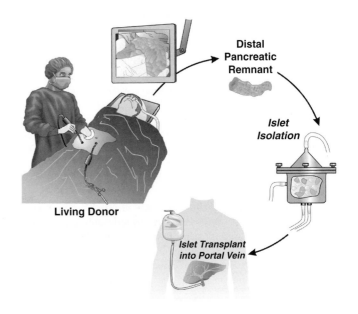

**FIGURE 23-1**

Future potential for living donor islet transplantation.

There has been precious little previous clinical experience with living donor islet allotransplantation, with only three reported cases in the literature (Figure 23-2).[31,32] Two clinical attempts at living donor islet allotransplantation were carried out more than 25 years ago by Sutherland et al. at the University of Minnesota in 1978.[31] Although neither recipient achieved sustained islet function, these pioneering efforts were truly remarkable given the early stage of clinical islet transplant development at the time. The immunosuppression available was primitive by current standards (azathioprine and high-dose steroids), and the islets were isolated using suboptimal conditions. The first successful living donor islet transplantation case was carried out at the University of Kyoto in early 2005, in a collaboration between the Japanese and Edmonton programs.[32] The recipient, a 27-year-old female, developed C-peptide-negative, unstable diabetes following chronic pancreatitis as a child. The donor, her 56-year-old mother, underwent open surgical resection of the distal half pancreas (47% as measured preoperatively by CT volumetry). There were no surgical complications in either donor or recipient. The islet mass was 408 114 IE (8 200 IE/kg) in a volume of 9.5 mL after tissue digestion, and was transplanted unpurified into the portal vein using the percutaneous approach under full systemic heparin. Immunosuppression was started pretransplant with the Edmonton Protocol style using sirolimus and low-dose tacrolimus (started 7 days pretransplant), combined with anti-IL2R antibody (given 4 days pretransplant and on the day of transplant) and anti-TNF blockade induction (infliximab; given 1 day pretransplant). The recipient was successfully weaned off insulin at 22 days posttransplant and continues to be insulin independent with excellent glycemic control and a normal HbA1C as of late 2005. The donor has continued to have normal HbA1c values and no evidence of glucose intolerance since the procedure.

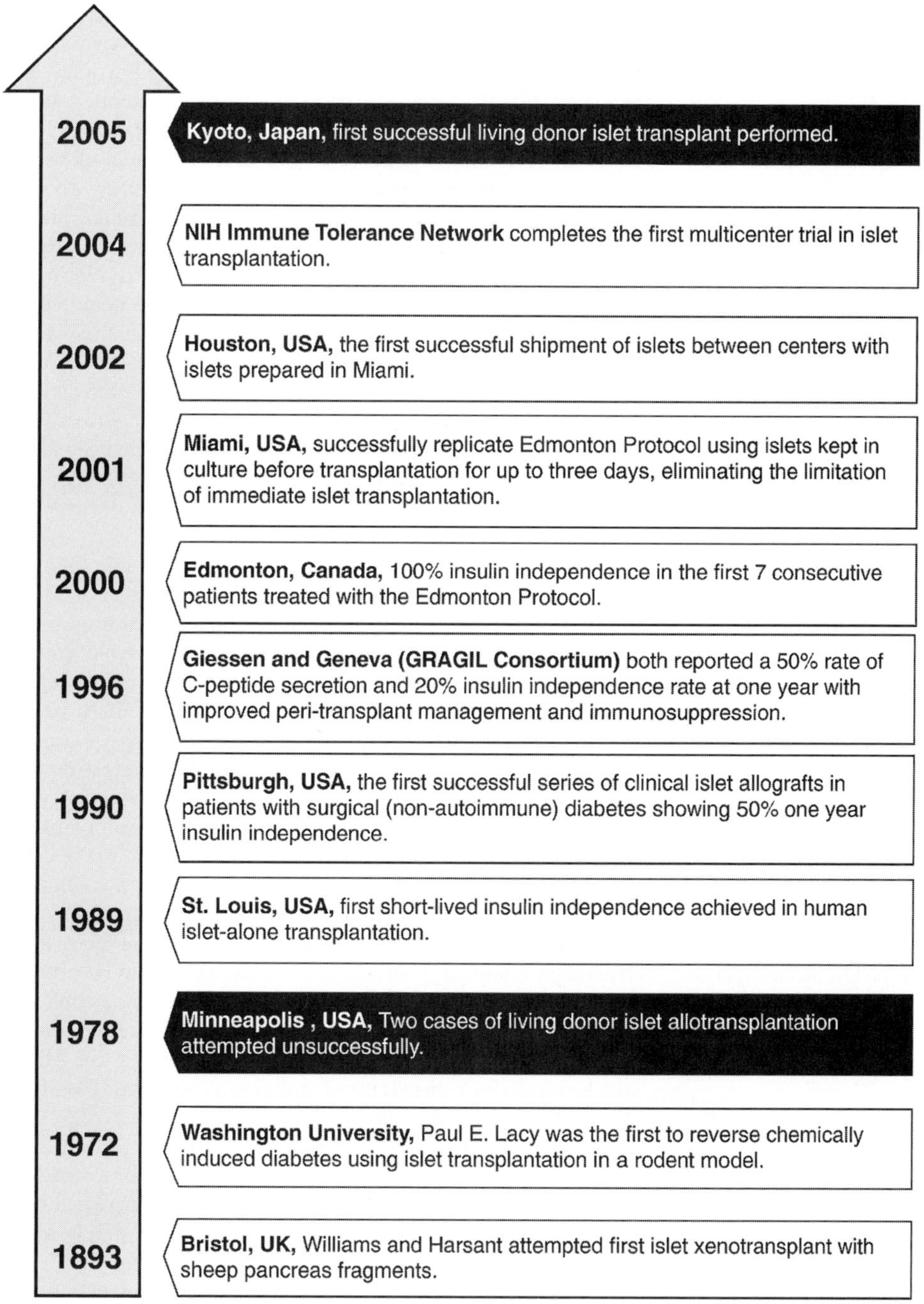

**2005** Kyoto, Japan, first successful living donor islet transplant performed.

**2004** NIH Immune Tolerance Network completes the first multicenter trial in islet transplantation.

**2002** Houston, USA, the first successful shipment of islets between centers with islets prepared in Miami.

**2001** Miami, USA, successfully replicate Edmonton Protocol using islets kept in culture before transplantation for up to three days, eliminating the limitation of immediate islet transplantation.

**2000** Edmonton, Canada, 100% insulin independence in the first 7 consecutive patients treated with the Edmonton Protocol.

**1996** Giessen and Geneva (GRAGIL Consortium) both reported a 50% rate of C-peptide secretion and 20% insulin independence rate at one year with improved peri-transplant management and immunosuppression.

**1990** Pittsburgh, USA, the first successful series of clinical islet allografts in patients with surgical (non-autoimmune) diabetes showing 50% one year insulin independence.

**1989** St. Louis, USA, first short-lived insulin independence achieved in human islet-alone transplantation.

**1978** Minneapolis , USA, Two cases of living donor islet allotransplantation attempted unsuccessfully.

**1972** Washington University, Paul E. Lacy was the first to reverse chemically induced diabetes using islet transplantation in a rodent model.

**1893** Bristol, UK, Williams and Harsant attempted first islet xenotransplant with sheep pancreas fragments.

**FIGURE 23-2**

Historical context of clinical attempts at living donor islet transplantation (highlighted in white), compared to cadaveric islet transplantation. The poor clinical results observed in cadaveric islet transplantation prior to the introduction of the Edmonton Protocol in 2000 discouraged extensive investigation into living donor islet transplantation, which was attempted (unsuccessfully) twice in the late 1970s. However, the first living donor islet transplant attempted in early 2005 has proven to be successful.

Although it is difficult to make any substantial conclusions from this single successful case of living donor alloislet transplantation, results from living donor islet autotransplantation suggest that the insulin independence may be achieved routinely with a far lower islet transplant mass that has been required for cadaveric allografts to date. Typically in an islet autotransplant, over 70% of patients will remain insulin free if an islet mass exceeding 300000 IE ($\geq$ 2500 IE/kg) is returned.[33] A major caveat of the islet autograft data is that robust long-term follow-up is lacking.

Living donor islet autotransplantation is an established and accepted surgical procedure for selected patients with severe pain from chronic pancreatitis, and active living donor islet autotransplant programs exist at several institutions. The islet yield obtained from the autografted pancreas is inversely related to the degree of preexisting fibrosis from chronic pancreatitis. The success of islet autotransplantation may be due in part to the use of nonpurified islet preparations, resulting in less islet loss, as well as the absence of diabetogenic antirejection medications and lack of underlying autoimmunity.

The controlled nature of the living donor setting would be of particular benefit in islet transplantation, especially in opening up the limited donor supply. Waiting times for clinical islet transplantation have increased substantially in the Edmonton program since 1999, and this will become more acute as other islet programs move forward and as whole pancreas transplant programs seek access to the more stable donors. Presently, clinical islet programs rely entirely on a scarce supply of pancreas organs derived from heart-beating, brain-dead cadavers. Organs obtained for islet transplantation tend to be more "marginal" and come from older, less stable donors. Furthermore, the pancreas is particularly susceptible to toxicity from the circulating products of severe brain injury, hemodynamic instability, and inotropic support in a brain-dead organ donor, and is compounded by cold ischemic injury during transportation, which inevitably results in islet damage and loss. Contreras et al. demonstrated a marked reduction in islet recovery and in islet viability in experimental islet transplantation using tissue derived following brain death compared to healthy rodent donors, highlighting this issue, and recently his group has confirmed these findings using human islets.[30] Similarly, Lakey et al. demonstrated a strong relationship between islet recovery and donor stability.[34] The extensive processing and purification steps during isolation cause further islet destruction and loss, often resulting in at best 60% recovery of the estimated $10^7$ IE/pancreas.[35] For this reason, nearly all islet recipients require islets prepared from two cadaveric donors, who, combined with reduced tissue viability, may result in alloantigenic priming of the recipient's immune system. In the living donor setting, the distal half-pancreas is procured in "ideal" circumstances, without exposure of the pancreas to hemodynamic instability or inotropic drugs, and the pancreas is processed immediately without prolonged cold ischemia. Thus, the potency of islets derived from a living donor source is assumed to be far superior to cadaveric tissue.

## DONOR CONSIDERATIONS

### Assessment and Selection

Based on the Minnesota experience in living donor pancreas transplantation, an extensive set of donor selection criteria has been established that should apply equally to living donor islet transplantation.[36] Donor safety must be paramount throughout the selection process and subsequent surgical intervention. As with all living

donor organ transplantation, the potential donor should understand the procedure and its associated risks, must not be coerced, and must be of legal age and competence to provide voluntary consent. A thorough complete history and physical examination should be taken by the surgical team, screening in particular for comorbidities that would exclude a potential donor from surgery (eg, history of pancreatic disorders or insulin resistance, active infections, or drug or alcohol dependence). The physical exam should include standard biochemical and coagulation profiles, cardiac profiling with electrocardiogram, and virology screening (HBV, HCV, CMV, EBV, HIV). Immunological compatibility between a potential donor and a recipient should be assessed with ABO blood grouping, crossmatching, and PRA testing.

In the case of living pancreas donation for islet transplantation, potential ABO-compatible donors should be selected based on standard criteria used to minimize the risk of postsurgical metabolic dysfunction (summarized in Table 23-1). Donor safety and avoidance of diabetes induction in a healthy donor as a result of distal pancreatectomy is paramount. Overweight or obese donors (body mass index < 27 kg/m$^2$) should be avoided, as they have increased risk of developing type 2 diabetes. Potential donors should be evaluated with oral glucose tolerance tests (OGTTs) to assess the maximum insulin secretion and functional insulin secretory reserve of the pancreas, to be sure that distal pancreatectomy does not disrupt metabolic function. Acceptable values include fasting blood glucose <110 mg/dL, 2-hour postingestion values < 140 mg/dL, and no other glucose value > 200 mg/dL during the 2-hour testing period.[36] Further assessment of the potential donor's $\beta$-cell reserve function should be evaluated using either the acute response to insulin (AIR) or the Insulinogenic Index. AIR is calculated as the mean of the serum insulin concentrations at times 1, 3, 4, 6, 8, and 10 minutes during an intravenous glucose tolerance test (IVGTT). For prospective donors, AIR values should be > 300% of the basal insulin secretion in the fasting state. An alternative to AIR is the Insulinogenic Index, an index of first-phase insulin secretion which is calculated as the ratio between changes in plasma insulin concentrations during the first 30 min following an oral glucose load and changes in plasma glucose concentrations over the same period.[37] Plasma HbA1C should be measured in all potential donors as a measure of chronic hyperglycemia, and values < 6% are considered to be compatible with donation. Finally, autoantibody titers should be determined for GAD, ICA512, and mIAA antibodies, which are associated with increased susceptibility to T1DM.[38] In the case where the potential pancreas donor is a sibling of the recipient with T1DM, the Minnesota group has implemented the requirement that the potential donor must be >10 years older than the recipient was at diabetes onset and that no other first-degree relatives have T1DM, in order to reduce the possibility of late onset T1DM in the donor postdonation.[36] After a potential donor has been evaluated by the surgical team, an independent complete assessment of the donor should be obtained using a staff internal medicine consultant that is not connected with the islet program (ie, following the same procedure used in most liver transplant programs). Using these criteria, the Minnesota living donor pancreas program has reported that 15%–20% of the candidates qualify to donate.[36]

Once a suitable potential donor has been identified, imaging with ultrasound followed by CT volumetry may be carried out to determine the anatomical suitability of the pancreas for donation. Although anatomical variation in vascular supply to the recipient is not a concern for islet transplantation, this is still necessary to further reduce the risk of surgical diabetes by ensuring

**TABLE 23-1**
## SUMMARY: DONOR AND RECIPIENT EVALUATION CRITERIA SPECIFIC TO LD ISLET TRANSPLANTATION

**Donor Selection**

| Test | Acceptable Range | Purpose |
|---|---|---|
| 1. Body Mass Index | < 27 kg/m$^2$ | Avoidance of donors with a propensity for type 2 diabetes |
| 2. Oral Glucose Tolerance Test | Fasting blood glucose < 110 mg/dL, 2-hour postingestion values < 140 mg/dL, and no other glucose value > 200 mg/dL during the 2-hour testing period. | Confirmation of a completely normal baseline insulin secretory reserve, ruling out undiagnosed type 2 diabetes or underlying glucose intolerance |
| 3. AIR or Insulogenic Index | AIR: >300% of basal insulin values Insulin ogenic Index: > 0.5 | Further assessment of beta-cell reserve function |
| 4. HbA1C | <6% | Indicator of chronic hyperglycemia |
| 5. Autoantibody screen for GAD, ICA512 and mIAA antibodies | No evidence of elevated serum titers | Rule out donors with a potential to develop T1DM |

**Recipient Selection**

| Test | Acceptable Range | Purpose |
|---|---|---|
| 1. Body Mass Index | BMI <30 kg/m$^2$ or weight < 90 kg | Donor: recipient metabolic imbalance |
| 2. HYPO Score and Lability Index (LI) | Hypo score: > 1047 (90th percentile) LI: >433 mmol/L$^2$/hr week$^{-1}$ (90th percentile) Composite: HYPO score >423 (75th percentile) and LI >329 (75th percentile) | Selection of recipients whose risk for adverse hypoglycemic events outweighs the risks of islet transplantation and life long immunosuppression |
| 3. HbA1C | <10% | Elimination of recipients with either poor compliance or inadequate insulin therapeutic regimen |
| 4. Cardiac Function Assessment | BP <160/100 mm Hg; No myocardial infarction 6 months prior to assessment; no angiographic evidence of noncorrectable coronary artery disease; LVEF >30% as measured by echocardiogram | Avoidance of cardiac death in the recipient within 5–10 years of transplant |
| 5. Kidney Function Assessment | No proteinuria (< 1 g/24 hr); GFR >80 (male), >70 (female) mL/min/1.73 m$^2$; Serum creatinine <115 μM (male), <125 μM (female) | Eliminate recipients who are better candidates for simultaneous kidney–pancreas transplantation and/or those who may experience adverse renal function as a result of calcineurin inhibitor or sirolimus therapy |
| 6. Panel Reactive Antibody (PRA) | <20% by flow cytometry | Reduce incidence of antibody-mediated graft rejection |

that the pancreas remnant volume will be at least 50% and to evaluate the pancreas for evidence of any underlying disease. Because the possibility exists that vascular supply to the donor spleen may be compromised, resulting in splenectomy, the living donor should receive standard presplenectomy immunizations at least 2 weeks prior to surgery to protect against encapsulated organisms and to reduce the risk of postsplenectomy sepsis.

## Living Pancreas Donation Procedure

Two options exist for procurement of the distal pancreas: an open laparotomy with a bilateral subcostal incision, or a hand-assisted laparoscopic approach. The open approach is more established, but surgical experience with laparoscopic distal pancreatectomy is now considerable and may be more appealing from a donor's standpoint. Once the pancreas has been dissected from the retroperitoneal bed and the splenic hilum, the distal splenic artery and vein are divided and ligated at the level of their respective origins. The distal pancreatic parenchyma should be divided to resect < 50% of the pancreatic volume, which generally can be achieved by dividing the pancreas to the left side of the superior mesenteric vein. Because preservation of the pancreatic duct for anastomoses is not an issue in islet transplantation, the pancreas can be divided using a vascular stapler, and the staple line in the proximal pancreas should be oversewn (and also possibly infiltrated with tissue fibrin glue) to prevent the development of fistula or leakage postoperatively in the donor. Furthermore, prophylactic octreotide may be given preoperatively in an attempt to further diminish this risk. It is possible to preserve the spleen on its smaller vascular supply via the short gastric vessels, but on occasion the spleen may become markedly congested, infarct, or tort when preserved in this way. Therefore, if a splenic-preserving approach is chosen, careful further visualization of the spleen should occur once the distal pancreas has been removed to be sure it is still viable.

To prepare the distal pancreas specimen for islet isolation, the splenic arterial and venous stumps are reopened (if stapled during retrieval), and the splenic artery is cannulated and flushed with chilled UW solution. The pancreatic duct is then cannulated and flushed with approximately 60 mL of ductal preservative solution (in the Kyoto case, University of Kyoto solution was infused).[32] The pancreas is then transported on two-layer oxygenated perfluorochemical-UW (preferably) to a cGMP islet isolation facility where processing is initiated as soon as possible. The pancreas should be digested using an optimal blend of Liberase collagenase enzyme that has been validated in previously successful clinical islet isolations.[39] The tissue digest should be washed extensively. At this juncture, a decision is made regarding purification—generally if the islet digest sediment is less than 10 cc in packed tissue volume, then no purification is required. Infusion of unpurified pancreatic digest exceeding 10 cc may increase the risk of portal thrombosis, and therefore appropriate judgment is needed together with full systemic anticoagulation and continuous monitoring of portal pressure.

The recipient should be concurrently prepared for islet transplantation to minimize cold ischemic time, and the islets either may be infused using the percutaneous approach to the portal vein in interventional radiology or transplanted using surgical access via a minilaparotomy if indicated. If a large volume of pancreatic digest is to be infused in an unpurified state, it may be safer to administer therapeutic anticoagulation in the more controlled open operating room environment rather than use a percutaneous approach. The donor should be monitored postoperatively for evidence of bleeding (decreased serum hemoglobin values) and serum lipase and amylase should be monitored to rule out pancreatitis or pancreatic fistula. A Doppler ultrasound examination of the donor should be performed before discharge home (or at 7–14 days postsurgery if discharged earlier) to rule out a possible pancreatic fistula and to confirm patency of the portal vein.

## Risks to the Donor

### Surgical Complications

The surgical procedure for distal pancreatectomy is relatively straightforward, is considered a substantially less risky procedure than living donor right lobe liver transplantation, and is perhaps comparable in risk to a living donor kidney procedure in terms of risk. Surgical resection of the distal half of the pancreas is a standard procedure in patients with a variety of conditions including a variety of benign or malignant pancreatic neoplasms and chronic pancreatitis. The potential risks associated with the surgery have been clearly defined previously. Complications include the general risks of anesthesia and surgery (chest infection, wound infection, deep vein thrombosis, pulmonary embolism), as well as the specific risks of the pancreatic resection, including pancreatic fistula, impaired glucose tolerance or rarely diabetes, splenic, and/or portal vein thrombosis, and the potential risks associated with the asplenic state if the spleen is removed concurrently. A review of more than 200 patients undergoing distal pancreatectomy at Johns Hopkins, which represents the largest single-center experience with this procedure, suggests that the outcome and complication rates clearly vary with the nature of the underlying pancreatic disease.[40] In this series, the perioperative mortality rate was 0.9%, and 69% of the patients had no postoperative complications. The overall complication rate was 31%, which included new-onset diabetes (8%), pancreatic fistula (5%), intraabdominal

abscess (4%), small bowel obstruction (4%), and postoperative hemorrhage (4%).[40] These incidence of surgical complications are consistent with those observed in the Minnesota living pancreas donor program, which has had a 0% mortality rate to date.[36]

### Metabolic Complications

The incidence of new-onset diabetes after distal pancreatectomy reflects the loss of islet cell mass associated with the resection. Indeed, an extensive review of the literature on the effects of pancreatic resection on glucose metabolism suggests that little change in metabolic status of the surgical patient occurred postoperatively unless more than 80% of the pancreas parenchyma was excised, or if more than 50% was excised in patients with underlying diffuse pancreatic disease.[41] The series of living donor segmental pancreas transplants at the University of Minnesota suggest that living pancreas donation for islet transplantation may pose a minimal risk to the donor.[36,42] Initial experience suggested a modestly increased donor risk of procedural complications, impaired glucose tolerance, or, more seriously, new diabetes induction in healthy donors followed up long-term (up to 5%).[43] More recently, careful avoidance of obese donors, those with a preresectional impairment of glucose tolerance or those at increased risk of diabetes as a result of positive serological autoimmune antibody markers, has largely eliminated this risk, with no new cases of postsurgical diabetes since 1996.[36]

## RECIPIENT CONSIDERATIONS

### Assessment and Selection

Clinical islet transplantation is associated with a number of risks, including bleeding or portal vein thrombosis in the short term or lifelong immunosuppression in the longer term. Consequently, much effort is made in assessing potential islet transplant recipients. In particular, individuals at high short-term risk from their diabetes, often because of frequent, severe, and recurrent hypoglycemia, are considered to be suitable candidates for islet transplantation. Unstable blood glucose control, despite an optimized insulin regimen, or progressive secondary complications of diabetes have also been identified as potential indications for islet transplantation.

When potential recipients are considered for islet transplantation, their metabolic status and diabetes-related secondary complications should be carefully evaluated to select for those patients who would receive the greatest benefit despite the requirement for lifelong immunosuppression (Table 23-1). Currently, islet transplantation is reserved for patients with C-peptide negative (< 0.3 ng/mL) T1DM. Recipients with elevated BMI (> 30 kg/m$^2$) or those > 90 kg are generally avoided, as their metabolic demand may not be met by the transplanted islet mass. The current indications for islet-alone transplantation include severe hypoglycemic unawareness and/or glycemic lability. To assess these symptoms, Ryan et al developed an objective scoring system to measure the severity of both hypoglycemia (the HYPO score) and the Lability Index (LI), which is based on the changes in blood glucose over time.[44] Current selection criteria for islet-alone transplantation include a HYPO score > 1047 (90th percentile), LI > 433 mmol/L$^2$/hr week$^{-1}$ (90th percentile), or a composite with the HYPO score > 423 (75th percentile) and LI >329 (75th percentile).[28] Plasma HbA1C should be < 10% in all potential recipients to exclude those with poor diabetes compliance or an inadequate baseline insulin regimen. Clearly if diabetes control can be improved by a more optimized insulin and monitoring regimen then this negates a need for islet transplantation. In terms of secondary diabetes complications, the patient's cardiac and renal function should be assessed. Selected recipients should have adequate cardiac function including blood pressure < 160/100 mm Hg, no evidence of myocardial infarction in the 6 months prior to assessment, no angiographic evidence of noncorrectable coronary artery disease, and left ventricular ejection fraction (LVEF) > 30% as measured by echocardiogram. To eliminate patients who are better candidates for simultaneous kidney–pancreas transplantation or those who may experience adverse renal function as a result of tacrolimus or sirolimus therapy, selected recipients should have no evidence of macroscopic proteinuria (< 300 mg/24 hr), calculated glomerular filtration rate (GFR) > 80 (> 70 in females) mL/min/1.73 m$^2$. It is important to ensure that subjects do not have unstable proliferative retinopathy at the time of transplant, as acute correction of glycemic control may lead to accelerated retinopathy. Potential recipients should be screened for panel reactive antibody assays (PRA) and determined to be <20% to reduce the incidence of antibody-mediated graft rejection.

## Islet Transplantation Procedure

Purified islets can be implanted into the liver by way of the portal vein using two accepted approaches. In cadaveric islet transplantation, the percutaneous transhepatic approach is most often utilized to implant donor islets.[28] This procedure is performed using local anesthesia, combined with opiate analgesia and hypnotics given as premedication. Although intravenous heparin administration is not routinely used for cadaveric islet transplantation, therapeutic heparinisation may be required for living donor islet transplants, since large volumes of unpurified islet tissue will be infused, increasing the risk for portal vein thrombosis. Access to the portal vein is achieved by percutaneous transhepatic approach using a combination of ultrasound and fluoroscopy to guide the radiologist. A branch of the right portal vein is cannulated, and a catheter is positioned proximal to the confluence of the portal vein. A portal venogram is performed routinely to confirm the position of the catheter.[45] Unfractionated heparin (70 U/kg) is mixed with the islet preparation immediately prior to infusion to reduce the risk of portal vein thrombosis. Islets are then infused, aseptically, into the main portal vein under gravity, with regular monitoring of portal venous pressure (by an indirect pressure transducer) before, during, and after the infusion. Islet infusion should not proceed if initial pressure is > 20 mm Hg.[45] Higher peak postinfusion portal pressures may be more acceptable in the living donor islet transplant setting, where there is much greater concern for the nonuse of retrieved tissue. This may only be accomplished safely when full therapeutic heparinization is initiated and continued throughout the early postoperative period. The following day, an ultrasound examination is performed to rule out intraperitoneal hemorrhage and to confirm that the portal vein is patent and has normal flow. The ultrasound should be repeated at 1 week to exclude any late portal vein thrombosis.

An alternative approach involves surgical laparotomy and cannulation of a mesenteric venous tributary of the portal system. This approach should be considered if a patient is anticoagulated prior to transplantation or if a hemangioma is present on the right side of the liver that may be at risk for puncture and bleeding if the percutaneous approach were to be used. A main advantage of this approach is that it can be carried out with complete surgical control in order to prevent uncontrolled bleeding. Another

advantage includes the potential for use of a dual-lumen catheter for cannulation of a mesenteric vein (ie, dual-lumen 9Fr Broviac line), which allows for continuous monitoring of portal pressure during islet infusion. This surgical approach does present several disadvantages, such as the requirement for a surgical incision, adhesion formation, and the risk of wound infection and wound herniation, which may be exacerbated when the drug sirolimus is used posttransplant, as this drug interferes with wound healing.

## Risks to the Recipient

### Surgical Complications

There are two potentially serious surgical complications in islet transplantation: bleeding from the catheter tract created by the percutaneous transhepatic approach and portal vein thrombosis, particularly when large volumes of tissue are infused. In the Edmonton program, adverse bleeding events occurred early in the development of the program, but have been completely avoided in the past 40 consecutive procedures with the routine use of effective methods to seal and ablated the transhepatic portal catheter tract on egress when the catheter is withdrawn. The combination of coils and tissue fibrin glue (Tisseel®) was used previously, but more recently we have preferred Avitene® paste (1 g Avitene powder mixed with 3 cc of radiological contrast media and 3 cc of saline—approximately 0.5 cc to 1.0 cc of this paste is injected into the liver tract).[46] Main portal vein thrombosis has not been encountered in Edmonton with the use of purified islet allograft preparations, but thrombosis of a right or left branch, or peripheral segmental vein, has been encountered in approximately 5% of patients. Other rarely observed procedural side effects include fine-needle gallbladder puncture, arteriovenous fistulae (which may require selective embolisation), or steatosis in the hepatic parenchyma, which generally does not present any clinical complications or require intervention.

### Immunosuppressive Therapy and Complications

Successful islet transplantation for T1DM requires immunosuppression which can effectively control both alloimmunity and the autoimmunity which lead to diabetes in the first place. A further challenge is the avoidance of agents known to be toxic to islets, particularly corticosteroids, which have been the mainstay of immunosuppression since successful allotransplantation was first developed. In the current version of the Edmonton Protocol, the induction agent daclizumab (anti-CD25 (IL-2 receptor) antibody) is administered intravenously immediately prior to transplantation (1 mg/kg), with a second dose given at 2 weeks posttransplant. Maintenance immunosuppression is achieved using sirolimus and a low-dose of tacrolimus. Sirolimus appears to be associated with less nephrotoxicity and diabetogenicity than calcineurin inhibitors (ie, cyclosporine and tacrolimus). A loading dose of sirolimus (0.2 mg/kg) is given prior to transplant, followed by 0.15 mg/kg and then adjusted subsequently to achieve trough levels between 10–12 ng/mL for the first 3 months and 7–10 ng/mL subsequently. A low dose of tacrolimus can be used and adjusted to maintain trough levels between 3 and 6 ng/mL. The success of this regimen described initially at the University of Alberta has been replicated at other centers as part of a multicenter ITN trial.[21,47]

Other successful regimens have been reported by Hering et al. from the Minnesota Group, including antithymocyte globulin and etanercept (antitumor necrosis factor alpha antibody) induction with a combination of sirolimus and mycophenolate mofetil ± low dose tacrolimus for maintenance, or hOKT3 γ 1(Ala–Ala) (humanized anti-CD3 antibody) and sirolimus induction with sirolimus and reduced-dose tacrolimus for maintenance.[26,27] Other immunosuppressive agents have been used in some cases because of drug intolerance or other side effects. The risk of renal dysfunction resulting from calcineurin inhibitor therapy has been reduced using low-dose tacrolimus-based regimens, but renal function in islet recipients receiving any tacrolimus should be carefully monitored, as these patients often possess mild preexisting renal impairment. It has also recently become apparent that the drug sirolimus may also have nephrotoxic side effects, and that this may be compounded when used in combination with a calcineurin inhibitor drug.[48,49] The gastrointestinal side-effects of tacrolimus are not infrequent and may lead to episodic diarrhea. Neurotoxicity may be seen with tacrolimus but is less frequent with low-dose regimens.[50] Neutropenia from sirolimus and the risk of mouth ulceration may be reduced by using a lower target trough level and a tablet rather than a liquid formulation. Sirolimus has also been associated with a number of side effects in islet recipients including peripheral edema, development of ovarian cysts in female recipients, menstrual cycle irregularities, small bowel ulceration, and dyslipidemia.[28,51]

The risk of all types of malignancy are increased in chronically immunosuppressed individuals, but squamous epithelial cancers are the most common and most readily treatable. The lifetime risk of lymphoma is estimated to be 1% to 2% in transplant recipients, but this risk may be an overestimate for islet recipients, in whom glucocorticoids and OKT[3] are avoided.

## CONCLUSIONS

In summary, living donor islet transplantation offers the potential for a far less limited donor pool to serve patients with T1DM. There are potential and real risks for a living donor in terms of surgically induced diabetes and potential for surgical complications, but with stringent selection criteria and careful surgical technique and postoperative monitoring, these risks may be minimized. Islet transplantation is still in its relative infancy compared to solid organ transplantation, and concerns relating to the long-term durability of an islet graft still need to be addressed. It is likely that an islet transplant derived from a living donor source will be far more potent (and less injured) than islets isolated from cadaveric pancreata. If tolerance induction is to be applied in clinical islet transplantation, avoidance of islet injury and enhanced donor antigen exposure may be particularly important.

## References

1. King H, Aubert RE, Herman WH. Global burden of diabetes, 1995–2025: prevalence, numerical estimates, and projections. *Diabetes Care.* Sep 1998;21(9):1414–1431.
2. National Diabetes Data Group (U.S.). National Institute of Diabetes and Digestive and Kidney Diseases (U.S.), National Institutes of Health (U.S.). *Diabetes in America.* 2nd ed. [Bethesda, Md.]: National Institutes of Health, National Institute of Diabetes and Digestive and Kidney Diseases; 1995.
3. The effect of intensive treatment of diabetes on the development and progression of long-term complications in insulin-dependent diabetes mellitus. The Diabetes Control and Complications Trial Research Group. *N Engl J Med* Sep 30 1993;329(14):977–986.
4. Keen H. The Diabetes Control and Complications Trial (DCCT). *Health Trends* 1994;26(2):41–43.
5. Diabetes Control and Complications Trial (DCCT). Update. DCCT Research Group. *Diabetes Care.* Apr 1990;13(4):427–433.
6. Adverse events and their association with treatment regimens in the diabetes control and complications trial. *Diabetes Care* 1995;18(11):1415.
7. Kendall DM, Rooney DP, Smets YF, Salazar Bolding L, Robertson RP. Pancreas transplantation restores epinephrine response and symptom recognition during hypoglycemia in patients with long-standing type I diabetes and autonomic neuropathy. *Diabetes* Feb 1997;46(2):249–257.
8. Newell KA, Bruce DS, Cronin DC, et al. Comparison of pancreas transplantation with portal venous and enteric exocrine drainage to the standard technique utilizing bladder drainage of exocrine secretions. *Transplantation* Nov 15 1996;62(9):1353–1356.
9. Larsen JL. Pancreas transplantation: indications and consequences. *Endocr Rev* Dec 2004;25(6):919–946.
10. Statistical Data Reported by the U.S. Scientific Registry of Transplant Recipients and the Organ Procurement and Transplantation Network. Available at: www.unos.org. Accessed April 2005.
11. Ballinger WF, Lacy PE. Transplantation of intact pancreatic islets in rats. *Surgery* Aug 1972;72(2):175–186.
12. Walsh TJ, Eggleston JC, Cameron JL. Portal hypertension, hepatic infarction, and liver failure complicating pancreatic islet autotransplantation. *Surgery* Apr 1982;91(4):485–487.
13. Scharp DW, Lacy PE, Santiago JV, et al. Insulin independence after islet transplantation into type I diabetic patient. *Diabetes* Apr 1990;39(4):515–518.
14. Ricordi C, Tzakis AG, Carroll PB, et al. Human islet isolation and allotransplantation in 22 consecutive cases. *Transplantation* Feb 1992;53(2):407–414.
15. Brendel M HB, Schulz A, Bretzel R. International Islet Transplant Registry Report. *University of Giessen, Germany.* 2001:1.
16. Hering B RC. Islet transplantation for patients with Type 1 diabetes: results, research priorities, and reasons for optimism. *Graft* 1999;2(1):12.
17. Gross CR, Limwattananon C, Matthees BJ. Quality of life after pancreas transplantation: a review. *Clin Transplant* Aug 1998;12(4):351–361.
18. Secchi A, Di Carlo V, Martinenghi S, et al. Effect of pancreas transplantation on life expectancy, kidney function and quality of life in uraemic type 1 (insulin-dependent) diabetic patients. *Diabetologia* Aug 1991;34 Suppl 1:S141–144.
19. Benhamou PY, Oberholzer J, Toso C, et al. Human islet transplantation network for the treatment of Type I diabetes: first data from the Swiss-French GRAGIL consortium (1999-2000). Groupe de Recherche Rhin Rhjne Alpes Geneve pour la transplantation d'Ilots de Langerhans. *Diabetologia* Jul 2001;44(7):859–864.
20. Shapiro AM, Lakey JR, Ryan EA, et al. Islet transplantation in seven patients with type 1 diabetes mellitus using a glucocorticoid-free immunosuppressive regimen. *N Engl J Med* Jul 27 2000;343(4):230–238.
21. Shapiro AM, Ricordi C, Hering B. Edmonton's islet success has indeed been replicated elsewhere. *Lancet* Oct 11 2003;362(9391):1242.
22. Goss JA, Schock AP, Brunicardi FC, et al. Achievement of insulin independence in three consecutive type-1 diabetic patients via pancreatic islet transplantation using islets isolated at a remote islet isolation center. *Transplantation* Dec 27 2002;74(12):1761–1766.
23. Goss JA, Goodpastor SE, Brunicardi FC, et al. Development of a human pancreatic islet-transplant program through a collaborative relationship with a remote islet-isolation center. *Transplantation* 2004;77(3):462–466.
24. Kempf MC, Andres A, Morel P, et al. Logistics and transplant coordination activity in the GRAGIL Swiss-French multicenter network of islet transplantation. *Transplantation* 2005;79(9):1200–1205.
25. International Islet Transplant Registry. Available at: http://www.med.uni-giessen.de/itr/ITN/itn.html.
26. Hering BJ, Kandaswamy R, Ansite JD, et al. Single-donor, marginal-dose islet transplantation in patients with type 1 diabetes. *JAMA* 2005;293(7):830–835.

27. Hering BJ, Kandaswamy R, Harmon JV, et al. Transplantation of cultured islets from two-layer preserved pancreases in type 1 diabetes with anti-CD3 antibody. *Am J Transplant.* Mar 2004;4(3):390–401.

28. Ryan EA, Paty BW, Senior PA, et al. Five-year follow-up after clinical islet transplantation. *Diabetes* Jul 2005;54(7):2060–2069.

29. Ryan EA, Lakey JR, Paty BW, et al. Successful islet transplantation: continued insulin reserve provides long-term glycemic control. *Diabetes* Jul 2002;51(7):2148–2157.

30. Contreras JL, Eckstein C, Smyth CA, et al. Brain death significantly reduces isolated pancreatic islet yields and functionality in vitro and in vivo after transplantation in rats. *Diabetes.* Dec 2003;52(12):2935–2942.

31. Sutherland DE, Matas AJ, Goetz FC, Najarian JS. Transplantation of dispersed pancreatic islet tissue in humans: autografts and allografts. *Diabetes* 1980;29 Suppl 1:31–44.

32. Matsumoto S, Okitsu T, Iwanaga Y, et al. Insulin independence after living-donor distal pancreatectomy and islet allotransplantation. *Lancet* May 2005;365(9471):1642–1644.

33. Gruessner RW, Sutherland DE, Dunn DL, et al. Transplant options for patients undergoing total pancreatectomy for chronic pancreatitis. *J Am Coll Surg* Apr 2004;198(4):559–567; discussion 568–559.

34. Lakey JR, Warnock GL, Rajotte RV, et al. Variables in organ donors that affect the recovery of human islets of Langerhans. *Transplantation* Apr 15 1996;61(7):1047–1053.

35. Tsujimura T, Kuroda Y, Avila JG, et al. Influence of pancreas preservation on human islet isolation outcomes: impact of the two-layer method. *Transplantation.* Jul 15 2004;78(1):96–100.

36. Gruessner RW, Sutherland DE. Living Donor Pancreas Transplantation. *Transplant Reviews.* April 2002;16(2):108–119.

37. Kosaka K, Kuzuya T, Hagura R, Yoshinaga H. Insulin response to oral glucose load is consistently decreased in established non-insulin-dependent diabetes mellitus: the usefulness of decreased early insulin response as a predictor of non-insulin-dependent diabetes mellitus. *Diabet Med* Sep 1996;13(9 Suppl 6):S109–119.

38. Franke B, Galloway TS, Wilkin TJ. Developments in the prediction of type 1 diabetes mellitus, with special reference to insulin autoantibodies. *Diabetes Metab Res Rev.* Sep-Oct 2005;21(5):395–415.

39. Barnett MJ, Zhai X, LeGatt DF, Cheng SB, Shapiro AM, Lakey JR. Quantitative assessment of collagenase blends for human islet isolation. Transplantation. Sep 27 2005;80(6):723–728.

40. Lillemoe KD, Kaushal S, Cameron JL, Sohn TA, Pitt HA, Yeo CJ. Distal pancreatectomy: indications and outcomes in 235 patients. *Ann Surg May* 1999;229(5):693–698; discussion 698–700.

41. Slezak LA, Andersen DK. Pancreatic resection: effects on glucose metabolism. *World J Surg.* Apr 2001;25(4):452–460.

42. Kendall DM, Sutherland DE, Najarian JS, Goetz FC, Robertson RP. Effects of hemipancreatectomy on insulin secretion and glucose tolerance in healthy humans. *N Engl J Med* Mar 29 1990;322(13):898–903.

43. Robertson RP, Lanz KJ, Sutherland DE, Seaquist ER. Relationship between diabetes and obesity 9 to 18 years after hemipancreatectomy and transplantation in donors and recipients. *Transplantation* Mar 15 2002;73(5):736–741.

44. Ryan EA, Shandro T, Green K, et al. Assessment of the severity of hypoglycemia and glycemic lability in type 1 diabetic subjects undergoing islet transplantation. *Diabetes* Apr 2004;53(4):955–962.

45. Owen RJ, Ryan EA, O'Kelly K, et al. Percutaneous transhepatic pancreatic islet cell transplantation in type 1 diabetes mellitus: radiologic aspects. *Radiology* Oct 2003;229(1):165–170.

46. Villiger P, Ryan EA, Owen R, et al. Prevention of bleeding after islet transplantation: lessons learned from a multivariate analysis of 132 cases at a single institution. *Am J Transplant.* Dec 2005;5(12):2992–2998.

47. Shapiro AM, Lakey JR, Paty BW, Senior PA, Bigam DL, Ryan EA. Strategic opportunities in clinical islet transplantation. *Transplantation* May 27 2005;79(10):1304–1307.

48. Kaplan B, Schold J, Srinivas T, et al. Effect of sirolimus withdrawal in patients with deteriorating renal function. *Am J Transplant* Oct 2004;4(10):1709–1712.

49. Senior PA, Paty BW, Cockfield SM, Ryan EA, Shapiro AM. Proteinuria developing after clinical islet transplantation resolves with sirolimus withdrawal and increased tacrolimus dosing. *Am J Transplant* Sep 2005;5(9):2318–2323.

50. Gruessner RW, Burke GW, Stratta R, et al. A multicenter analysis of the first experience with FK506 for induction and rescue therapy after pancreas transplantation. *Transplantation* Jan 27 1996;61(2):261–273.

51. Molinari M, Al-Saif F, Ryan EA, et al. Sirolimus-induced ulceration of the small bowel in islet transplant recipients: report of two cases. *Am J Transplant* Nov 2005;5(11):2799–2804.

CHAPTER 24

# PERSONAL REFLECTIONS AND HISTORY OF LIVING DONOR LIVER TRANSPLANTATION

*Christoph E. Broelsch, MD, Silvio Nadalin, MD, Massimo Malagó, MD*

In 1983 the National Institute of Health in the United States held the Consensus Conference on Liver Transplantation (LT) to determine the fate of a procedure that has been considered to be "experimental" because of its hitherto unfavorable results. Within 20 years after the first LT performed in 1963 by the great pioneer in the field, Dr. Thomas Starzl,[1] many centers, mostly in Europe, tried the procedure but failed and aborted their attempts. There are reports, that up to 43 centers around the world did one or more procedures between 1963 and 1975, but none released accumulated data to demonstrate survival.[2] Individual surgeons, much under criticism of their fellow hepatologists or surgeons, wanted to demonstrate their skills, by mastering this most difficult surgical procedure. Virtually, it was clinically abandoned in the seventies and many of us—then younger surgeons—went back to the laboratory to explore pathomechanisms of rejection, preservation, and auxiliary transplants.

In three European centers, in Cambridge, UK, Sir Roy Calne; in Hannover, Germany, Professor Rudolf Pichlmayr; and in Groningen, Netherlands, Dr. Ruud Krom, LT became an organized clinical/experimental project based on vast experience in kidney transplantation and immunology, extended into cooperation with hepatologists, pathologists, and pediatricians. Based on approximately 300 reported cases, the conference determined LT to be a clinical procedure to be performed in selected centers.

Much of this success was driven by the results in pediatric LT, where the need for the procedure was most apparent and the results helped to overcome the dismal survival statistics in adults with end-stage liver diseases (Figure 24-1).[3] Although the first pediatric liver transplantation on Bennie Solis baby in Denver in 1963 by Dr. Starzl failed,[4] the forthcoming series of pediatric transplants was impressing successful, facilitated by new immunosuppression protocols, particularly by introduction of Cyclosporine. In 1981, as Dr. Starzl's group (Dr. Byers Shaw and Dr. Shun Iwatzuki) moved to the University of Pittsburgh, emphasis was placed on pediatric LT with the unanimous support of the Department of Pediatrics (Dr. Basil Zitelli, Dr. Malatak). This cooperation was exemplary for pediatricians to create the new subspecialty of hepatology.

Within the shadow of the two major transplant programs in Pittsburgh and Cambridge, in Hannover a most effective transplant program evolved under the leadership of Professor Pichlmayr, which I have had the privilege to supervise since 1979 in cooperation with Professor Martin Burdelski, the pediatric hepatologist. Until 1984, 12 pediatric transplants have been performed resulting in 75% survival (Table 24-1).[3]

With the growing need for transplants in children documented by mortality on the waiting list greater than 40%, the concept of

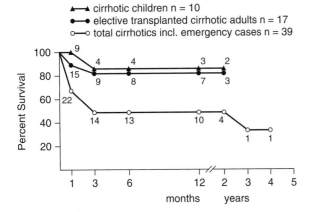

**FIGURE 24-1**

Early results of pediatric liver transplants from living donors.

**TABLE 24-1**

**COURSE OF PEDIATRIC PATIENTS FOLLOWING TIME OF INDICATION FOR LIVER GRAFTING AT THE MEDIZINISCHE HOCHSCHULE DURING THE PERIOD 1981–1983[3]**

| | |
|---|---|
| Admitted and selected for LT | n = 35 |
| Transplanted | n = 12 (alive n = 9) |
| Died on waiting list | n = 17 |
| Still waiting | n = 6 |

reduced size LT (RSLT) was introduced by the French surgeons, Prof. Henry Bismuth and Didier Houssin in 1983, using a whole left lobe (segments 1–4) as a substitute for the diseased liver.[5] Together with Peter Neuhaus and Burkhard Ringe, we reported the first two cases of RSLT of a left lateral lobe (segments 2 and 3) in two babies, 1.5 and 2 years old, respectively. Although one baby died 2 months later from a CMV infection, it could be demonstrated that a partial liver transplant was technically feasible and sufficient to expect long-term survival.[6] This technique was transferred to the University of Chicago where the first series of RSLT was reported in 1987 together with Dres. Emond and Thistlethwaite.[7] Especially, the pediatric hepatologist Dr. Peter Whitington carried the responsibility to select and treat the children from all over the United States. He collected a number of special cases and established a referral pathway from all over the world.

The application of RSLT immediately released the pretransplant mortality on the waiting list but it was heavily criticized for inferior results and the traumatization of scarce donor organs exploiting those for the preferential use in children while the need in the adult population was steadily growing. The clinical ethicist of the University of Chicago and his group, Dr. Mark Siegler, met the criticism of the procedure's initially unfavorable results by introducing "the principle of equipoise."[8] The principle justifies the application of an innovative procedure (ie, RSLT), because more children could be treated even yielding inferior results, while maintaining only a standard procedure, which would yield somewhat better results, would leave a considerable number of children untreated! Several centers were assisted by the Chicago team to enter the pediatric transplant program by using partial liver transplants and the procedure soon became popular.[9] With growing experience, the initial disadvantage of the reduced-size procedure could be overcome, and as demonstrated by a report by Professor Jean-Bernard Otte from Brussels in 1990 there was no more disadvantage in receiving a reduced-size liver versus a whole liver transplant in babies.[10]

In the meantime, it became apparent that the application of RSLT would not overcome the shortage of cadaveric organs even in children, but more significantly would only shift the shortage away from the pediatric group into the adult waiting list. Thus, in 1988 Professor Pichlmayr was the first to transplant both liver lobes from a cadaveric donor into two recipients of appropriate size, introducing the concept of split liver transplantation (SLT) for the first time.[11] Our group in Chicago, first in the United States, modeled the application of SLT into a system of need, and prepared a protocol of 20 consecutive transplants: while one recipient would receive a "standard" lobe, that is, left lateral segment (as being used in children), a second recipient would receive the residual "experimental" liver lobe in the absence of any alternative, that is, no full size cadaveric graft available. A special patient consent form was developed, and insurance coverage was also obtained together with the approval of the Institutional Ethics Board. The Chicago series was the only consecutive and prospective series performed on 18 patients according to the protocol, calling for one recipient with highest urgency and one elective one. The results turned out not to be as expected, but revealed the "Achilles heel" of the procedure: the cut edge of segment 4 and the biliary system. Hence, in the presence of a poor functioning graft, both recipients were in jeopardy and the retransplantation rate increased (Table 24-2).[12] The bottom line was no real increase in donor organ availability for both pediatric and adult recipients. For the adults, in addition, a new phenomenon was discovered: the small graft syndrome that prevented the

**TABLE 24-2**

**GRAFT AND PATIENT OUTCOME FOR 18 SPLIT LIVER TRANSPLANTATIONS AT THE UNIVERSITY OF CHICAGO FROM JULY 1988 TO JULY 1989[12]**

| Status | Incidence | Type of SLT | Follow-up (months) |
|---|---|---|---|
| Alive with primary graft | 9/18 (50%) | 5 R-SLT ; 4 L-SLT | 2–12 |
| Alive with retransplant | 3/18 (17%) | 3 L-SLT | 6–8 |
| Died | 6/18 (33%) | 4 R-SLT, 2 L-SLT | |
| Total patient survival | 67% | | |
| Total graft survival | 50% | | |

SLT, split liver transplantation; L-SLT, left SLT; R-SLT, right SLT.

expansion of the procedure of hemiliver transplants between two adults.[13] The big hope for the SLT temporarily vanished until the increasing pressure on transplant surgeons prompted them to change the extracorporeal split procedures of preserved organs into harvesting the donor organs in situ or by sophisticated *ex situ* procedures, definitely avoiding the likelihood of a nonviable transplant. The hazards and risks of a split harvest induced a drastic reduction of the split procedure to less than 20% of all donors. In addition, the logistic of sharing was another hampering factor in its broader application. Theoretically, out of 5,000 deceased donors in the United States, or 700 donors in Germany, only 10% would find a split recipient match which would serve the pediatric as well as the adult recipients. Just by numbers, for the pediatric population a sufficient number of donor organs are available by efficiently exhausting the cadaveric pool and considering this theoretical entity: arguments rise against the use of live donors for children, because of the lack of need. The criticism would call for a network of transplant centers with mutual trust into the quality of the organs harvested. Currently, most centers perform SLT under their own responsibility and within their own region to avoid long-distance shipping and extended cold ischemia time. The procedure of splitting presents a major effort on personal and institutional resources. With the same preferences or organ allocation for pediatric recipients according to all national allocation systems including Eurotransplant rules, PELD or MELD scores in the United States, only centers with a large pediatric waiting list would profit from splitting of donor organs. In fact, the majority of transplant centers have no incentive or interest in splitting the organs allocated to their adult recipients, and they refer to at least an increased postoperative morbidity of SLT recipient.

Facing the downsides of the SLT series, in 1988 at the University of Chicago, a new protocol for living donor liver transplantation (LDLT) was developed, resulting in 1989 in the first successful procedure in the United States.[13] Three other procedures preceded this series in Chicago: first in Sao Paolo, Brazil, by Silvano Reia; the second in Brisbane, Australia, by Russel Strong (the first successful); and the third in Shimane, Japan, by N. Nagasue. Prospectively, 20 procedures were anticipated according to the University of Chicago Protocol, whereby the entire left liver lobe was removed, and following preservation, segment 4 was dispatched to achieve sufficient length on the vascular pedicles. Since the segment 4 gave rise to circulation and ischemia problems resulting in several fatal outcomes in the split procedures, it seemed logical to eliminate this segment for avoiding the same complication for the live procedures. Unfortunately, after the first three left hemihepatectomies, in all live donors, a bleeding, an infection, or a biliary problem occurred. Although none of them required re-operation, the procedure shifted to the exclusive harvesting of the left lateral segment (Figure 24-2).

Four grafts out of the first 20 cases were lost: 2 children died and 2 could be rescued: one with a cadaveric graft; and the other, with a LDLT from another relative.[13] During this productive and successful time, several pediatric surgeons visited the University of Chicago, among them Professor Koichi Tanaka from Kyoto, who later started the world's largest pediatric and, somewhat later, an adult LDLT program. Recently he published a personal series of 1,000 live donor liver transplants before his mandatory retirement.14 He was followed by a number of Japanese surgeons in Tokyo (Professor Masatoshi Makuuchi) in Shinshu University (Professor J.S. Kawasaki). In Japan, The LDLT procedure is driven by the absence of cadaveric liver grafting, which is diametric opposed to the Western ethical concept: that the availability of alternatives could only provide an informed consent for an individual.

Although this is a highly esteemed criterion, even in the Western world, while the shortage of donor organs persists, decision making for live organ donation is significantly influenced by the fear to die before transplantation or to advance into a critical stage of cirrhosis. Thus, a psychological coercion cannot be completely excluded. It is still under ethical discussion, how much coercion in terms of taking a certain risk to save the life of a loved one is appropriate. The main practical argument against the rapid development and broad application of LDLT procedures, however, did not come from ethicists, but from physicians and surgeons themselves because of the hitherto inadequate exploitation of the cadaveric donor pool and in particular of the inadequate application of the split transplant procedure. Therefore, emphasis was renewed to optimize the split procedure, which, between 1990 and 1993, was virtually vanished because of its obvious difficulties. The first reports of successful split grafting appeared in 1995 by Jean de Ville de Goyet from the Brussels group,[15] and later, in 2001, by Didier Azoulay from the group of Professor Henry Bismuth in Paris.[16] Apparently, the pressures on the waiting lists became so dramatic, that means had to be found to make the split procedure adequately safe, at least in terms of survival comparable to the full size procedure. Since 1991 at the University Hospital Eppendorf in Hamburg, Germany, our group, directed by my colleagues Professors Xavier Rogiers and Massimo Malagó, undertook the task to harvest the partial organs in site from circulatory stable deceased donors—just like in the live donor procedure. The development of a clinical hepatobiliary surgical specialty within a German surgical department became the basis to familiarize our own surgeons as well as many others who came for a training period with this demanding procedure. There were clear advantages by performing the split procedures in site: first, the quality of the graft, by nature of the quality of the donor and the donor management; second, the shortening of the ischemia time at least of one part of the donor liver, and easier logistic issues. Most importantly, the dissection procedure within the donor already revealed any circulatory disturbances, anatomical abnormalities, and the homogenous perfusion of the critical segment 4 (Table 24-3).[17]

Contemporarily, reports accumulated that similar results could be obtained by a modified ex site splitting, which in turn was logistically easier, because there was little need for the use of donor hospital resources and operating room (OR) times, for which organ procurement agencies had to pay. In fact, disturbances on regular OR schedules prompted donor hospitals not to favor long procedures, and other procurement teams for heart and lungs did not always accept the extra waiting time. Clearly, the *in situ* harvesting procedures take up to 2 hours or more even by experienced teams, but as a result better and more viable organs can be obtained, simply by selection of an optimal donor. Therefore, whenever possible, our teams try to perform *in situ* procedures, obtaining the pediatric organ first while the remnant liver (lobes 4–8) remains in situ to await the flush once the heart and heart/lungs have been taken out.

At this point, it has to be clarified that the liver division into a left lateral segment and an "extended right lobe" (segments 4–8) does not represent the true split approach, because it again favors the pediatric group of recipients only while the adult side only

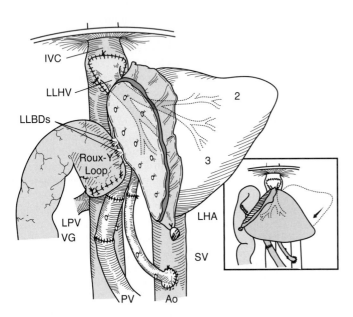

**FIGURE 24-2**

Living donor liver transplant in a pediatric recipient. (In this case, arterial and venous jump grafts were used.) Abbreviations used: AO, aorta; IVC, inferior vena cava; LLBDs, left hepatic bile ducts of segments 2 and 3; LHA, left hepatic artery;  LLHV, left hepatic vein; LPV, left portal vein;  PV, portal vein; SV, saphenous vein jump graft;  VG, venous graft.

**TABLE 24-3**

**COMPARATIVE RESULTS OF *EX SITU* VERSUS *IN SITU* SPLITTING AT THE EPPENDORF UNIVERSITY IN HAMBURG, GERMANY, BETWEEN 1994 AND 1995**[17]

|  | Ex Situ | In Situ |
| --- | --- | --- |
| Graft survival | 58% (11/19) | 86% (12/14) |
| Patient survival | 63% (12/19) | 93% (13/14) |
| Cold ischemia time (min) | 715 (505–1 005) | 580 (285–875) |
| AST max (U/dL) | 690 (168–5 588) | 516 (122–1,742) |
| PRBC (mL/Kg) | 64.8 (0–666) | 47.9 (0–125) |
| Biliary complications | 3 | 0 |
| PPF/PNF | 2/0 | 0/0 |

Abbreviations used: AS, aspartate aminotransferase; PRBC, packed red blood cells; PPF,poor primary function; PNF, primary nonfunction.

received half of the benefit. The need is clearly on the adult side more strikingly in terms of sheer numbers and variability of the diseases. Thus, the true split between adults has not yet become clinical practice, although selected cases have been reported by my colleagues Rogiers, Gundlach, and Broering in Hamburg.[18]

With both innovations, the split and the living related procedures, the pediatric cohort became sufficiently being served, and as a result, pediatric mortality on the waiting list became virtually zero. Mortality on the waiting list for adults, in contrast, is still dramatically increasing. Therefore, within a few years, the procedures of right or left hemihepatectomy for live organ donation have been performed to serve the adult population despite a significant higher morbidity and mortality risk as compared to the small left lateral hepatectomy procedure performed for children.[19] Single centers (Richmond, VA, Dr. Amadeo Marcos; Mount Sinai, New York, Dr. Charles Miller) performed more than 100 procedures within 2 years,[20,21] until the first dramatic death of a donor was reported in New York.[22] The incidence served as a milestone for the future application of the procedure: ethical consideration and surgical and institutional requirements were reconsidered with the result in order to proceed more carefully with the expansion of the procedure. However, there was no halt because the procedure turned out to be most effective and life saving. The individual rights of families are mandating this alternative for treatment, the procedure can be cost saving, and it has been shown that the risk can be minimized by appropriate evaluation. Through the live donor procedure, quality standards have been upgraded, training programs have been adapted, and medical and ethical considerations have been considered more seriously. The basis of our Western society, the respect for human life, has been more vigorously incorporated into the transplant profession. In the future, cadaveric organs will remain scarce because societies will not give up their individual rights for decisions pro or con regarding postmortem donations. On the same basis, society will have to accept the increasing demand for live organ donation. There will be no "monsters hiding" anymore[23] as long as responsible surgeons prevent coercion and commerce.

## References

1. Starzl, TE, Groth CG, Brettschneider L, et al. Orthotopic homotransplantation of the human;over/ *Ann Surg* 1968;168(3):392–415.
2. Starzl TE, Keop LJ, Halgrimson CG, et al. Fifteen years of clinical liver transplantation. *Gastroenterology* 1979;77(2):375–388.
3. Pichlmayr R, Broelsch C, Wonigeit K, et al. Experiences with liver transplantation in Hannovre. *Hepatology* 1984;1(1 Suppl):56S–60S.
4. Starzl TE. Memoirs of a transplant surgeon. *The Puzzle People*. University of Pittsburgh Press; 1992.
5. Bismuth H, Houssin D. Ruduced-size orthotopic liver graft in hepatic transplantation in children. *Surgery* 1984;95(3):367–370.
6. Broelsch C, Neuhaus P, Burdelski M, et al. Orthotopic liver transplantation of hepatic segments in infants with biliary atresia. In: Langenbechs Arch Chir 1984, Supplement,
7. Surgical Forum '84 for Experimental and Clinical Research, pp. 105–109, from the 101st Congress of the German Society for Surgery, Munich, April 25–28, 1984.
8. Broelsch CE, Then, Thistlethwaite JR, et al: [Heterotopic or orthotopic liver replacement with liver segments?] Z Gastroenterol Verh 1987, 22:66–72.
9. Singer PA, Lantos JD, Whitington PF, et al: Equipoise and the ethics of segmental liver transplantation. Clin Res 1988, 36(6):539–545.
10. Singer PA, Siegler M, Whitington PF, et al: Ethics of liver transplantation with living donors. N Engl J Med 1989, 321(9):620–622.
11. Otte JB, de Ville de Goyet J, Alberti D, et al. The concept and technique of the split liver in clinical transplantation. *Surgery* 1990;107(6):605–612.
12. Pichlmayr R, Ringe B, Gubernatis G, et al. [Transplantation of a donor liver to 2 recipients (splitting transplantation)—a new method in the further development of segmental liver transplantation]. *Langenbecks Arch Chir* 1988;373(2):127–130.
13. Emond JC, Whitington PF, Thistlethwaite JR, et al. Transplantation of two patients with one liver. Analysis of a preliminary experience with 'split-liver' grafting. *Ann Surg* 1990;212(1):14–22.
14. Broelsch CE, Whitington PF, Emond JC, et al. Liver transplantation in children from living related donors. Surgical techniques and results. *Ann Surg* ; 214(4):428–437; discussion 437–439.
15. Tanaka K, Yamada T. Living donor liver transplantation in Japan and Kyoto University: what can we learn? *J Hepatol* 2005;42(1):25–28.
16. de Ville de Goyet J. Split liver transplantation in Europe—1988 to 1993. *Transplantation* 1995;59(10):1371–1376.
17. Azoulay D, Marin-Hargreaves G, Dastaing D, et al. Ex situ splitting of the liver: the versatile Paul Brousse technique. Arch Surg 2001, 136(8):956–961.
18. Rogiers X, Malago M, Gawad K, et al: In situ splitting of cadaveric livers. The ultimate expansion of a limited donor pool. *Ann Surg* 1996;224(3):331–339.
19. Broering DC, Kim JS, Mueller T, et al. One hundred thirty-two consecutive pediatric liver transplants without hospital mortality: lessons learned and outlook for the future. *Ann Surg* 2004, 240(6):1002–1012; discussion 1012.
20. Boillot O, Dawahra M, Mechet I, et al. [Orthotopic liver transplantation from a living adult donor to an adult using the right hepatic lobe]. *Chirurgie* 1999;124(2):122–129; discussion 130–131.
21. Marcos A, Ham JM, Fisher RA, et al. Single-center analysis of the first 40 adult-to-adult living donor liver transplants using the right lobe. *Liver Transplant* 2000;6(3):296–301.
22. Miller CM, Gondolesi GE, Florman S, et al. One hundred nine living donor liver transplants in adults and children: a single-center experience. *Ann Surg* 2001;234(3):301–311; discussion 311–312.
23. Josefson D: Transplants from live patients scrutinized after donor's death. *BMJ* 2002;324(7340):754.
24. Shaw BW Jr. Where monsters hide. *Liver Transplant* 2001;7(10):928–932.

# REGIONAL VARIATIONS IN THE U.S. LIVING DONOR EXPERIENCE

*Mark Wang, MD, Irma Dixler, BSN, RN, Jonathan P. Fryer, MD*

The data and analyses reported in the 2005 Annual Report of the U.S. Organ Procurement and Transplantation Network and Scientific Registry of Transplant Recipients have been supplied by United Network of Organ Sharing (UNOS) and University Renal Research and Education Association (URREA) under contract with U.S Department of Health and Human Services (HHS). The authors alone are responsible for reporting and interpreting these data.

## INTRODUCTION

The use of live donors for solid organ transplantation has been a controversial issue ever since Joseph Murray and Hartwell Harrison successfully performed the first-ever live kidney transplant between identical twins at Boston's Peter Bent Brigham Hospital on December 23, 1954. Due to the unavailability of effective immunosuppression at that time, the decision to use a live donor was primarily based on the immunological advantage provided by using this unique donor–recipient combination. Since very few patients needing kidney transplants are fortunate enough to have an identical twin, transplants were rare events in these early days.[22]

With the development of immunosuppressive strategies, transplant could be extended to more histologically disparate donor–recipient combinations, and by the late 1960s, live related kidney transplants were performed more frequently.[22] Additionally, refinement and clarification of brain death laws enabled the use of cadaveric donors as a second source of organs, with the first success achieved by Starzl in 1967.[21] Subsequently, as organ procurement techniques improved, the majority of organ transplants were performed using deceased, brain-dead donors. However, due to complications associated with the early immunosuppressive protocols,[2] this decade was labeled by Starzl as the "bleak period" of transplantation, marked by "heavy mortality and devastating morbidity."[22]

The advent of cyclosporine as an effective immunosuppressive drug in the early 1980s revolutionized transplantation by replacing azathioprine and prednisone.[2,7] By the late 1980s, the successes achieved with cyclosporine permitted the expansion of transplantation to other abdominal organs including the liver, the pancreas, and the intestine resulting in "phenomenal increases" in the numbers of transplants and transplant centers.[4]

Unfortunately, this explosion in transplant activity eventually led to a progressive disparity between the numbers of candidates on the transplant waiting lists and the availability of deceased organ donors. Therefore, the relative shortage of deceased donor organs renewed interest in the use of living donors. This was ultimately enhanced further by the introduction of laparoscopic nephrectomy in 1995.[16,19] Laparoscopic nephrectomy is currently available in over 60% of transplant programs in the United States and has led to a dramatic increase in the number of living donor kidney transplants being performed per year. Since 2001, the number of live donors has surpassed the number of deceased donors for kidney transplants.[5] The subsequent use of living donors with other organ transplants has increased the controversy associated with the use of living donors but has led to the development of guidelines and standards for their use.[18]

Worldwide, the use of live donors for transplantation has been variable and is influenced by many individual societal standards. In Japan, the public has historically been averse to the concept of using organs from deceased donors. Although religious and spiritual beliefs are often implicated, in fact, the reasons for this societal bias appear to be largely secular and pertain to dissatisfaction with poorly defined brain death laws as well as public distrust of medical professionals. As one example, the failed heart transplant performed by Dr. Juro Wada in 1968 led him to be accused of murder after concerns arose regarding brain death of the donor and readiness of the recipient for transplantation.[10] Although organ transplantation from a brain-dead donor was officially made legal in March 1999, public opinion remains mixed and the vast majority of organ transplants continue to be performed using live donors.[10]

In Canada, as in many other countries, there is a heavy imbalance between supply and demand for organs.[6] This impasse has encouraged Canadians to take steps to increase both deceased and live donation, including considering a financial reimbursement policy for living donors, citing financial barriers as a major current obstacle in organ donation.[11] Due to such pressures and incentives,[6] the number of living donors in Canada has doubled within the past decade.[1] Deceased donor rates, however, have remained stagnant.[13,14]

The examples of Japan and Canada illustrate how the use of live donors for organ transplantation may be influenced by public opinion, cultural tradition, and supply and demand pressures. The following study will evaluate regional variability in the use of live donors for transplantation in the United States.

## OBJECTIVES

The purpose of this study is to identify and define regional variability in the use of live donors for abdominal solid organ transplantation in the United States. Numbers of living donor transplants, donors, and recipients are used as markers of living donor activity. Data are categorized by both classical U.S. regions and regions defined by the UNOS.

## METHODS

Unless otherwise specified, all data were provided by request from the Organ Procurement and Transplantation Network (OPTN) and included the number of living donor transplants performed per state, for each year spanning from 1995 to 2005, for the following organs: kidney, liver, intestine, and pancreas (based on OPTN data as of April 28, 2006). To establish if donors and recipients were traveling to other states for their transplants, analogous data were also obtained for the number of living donors and recipients per state, based on their state of residence at the time of transplant (based on OPTN data as of April 28, 2006).

Data from individual states were grouped into the four classical U.S. regions: the Northeast, Midwest, South, and West, as defined by the U.S. Census Bureau.[23] Classical regions and their included states are as follows:

**Northeast.** Connecticut, Maine, Massachusetts, New Hampshire, Rhode Island, Vermont, New Jersey, New York, Pennsylvania.

**Midwest.** Indiana, Illinois, Michigan, Ohio, Wisconsin, Iowa, Kansas, Minnesota, Missouri, Nebraska, North Dakota, South Dakota.

**South.** Delaware, District of Columbia, Florida, Georgia, Maryland, North Carolina, South Carolina, Virginia, West Virginia, Alabama, Kentucky, Mississippi, Tennessee, Arkansas, Louisiana, Oklahoma, Texas.

**West.** Arizona, Colorado, Idaho, New Mexico, Montana, Utah, Nevada, Wyoming, Alaska, California, Hawaii, Oregon, Washington.

**Puerto Rico.** Puerto Rico was included as a fifth region, owing to its unique cultural differences, for the sake of completeness.

The data from individual states were analogously grouped into regions defined by UNOS (based on OPTN data as of April 28, 2006). UNOS-defined regions and their included states are as follows:

**Region 1.** Connecticut, Massachusetts, Maine, New Hampshire, Rhode Island.

**Region 2.** District of Columbia, Delaware, Maryland, New Jersey, Pennsylvania, West Virginia.

**Region 3.** Alabama, Arkansas, Florida, Georgia, Louisiana, Mississippi, Puerto Rico.

**Region 4.** Oklahoma, Texas.

**Region 5.** Arizona, California, New Mexico, Nevada, Utah.

**Region 6.** Hawaii, Oregon, Washington.

**Region 7.** Illinois, Minnesota, North Dakota, South Dakota, Wisconsin.

**Region 8.** Colorado, Iowa, Kansas, Missouri, Nebraska.

**Region 9.** New York, Vermont.

**Region 10.** Indiana, Michigan, Ohio.

**Region 11.** Kentucky, North Carolina, South Carolina, Tennessee, Virginia.

To standardize the data obtained for individual regions, all data were presented as the rate per million population. Population data for all 50 U.S. states, the District of Columbia, and

Puerto Rico for the year 2004 were provided by the U.S. Census Bureau.[24] The fraction of transplants performed using live donors was also determined by dividing the number of live donor transplants by the total number of transplants performed per region for each of the four organs.

Finally, to assess the extent to which living donation is driven by need, data for the numbers of living donor liver transplants, total numbers of liver transplants, and average MELD/PELD scores at time of transplant were collected for the interval from 2001 to 2005 for each UNOS region (OPTN data as of July 21, 2006). The number of living donor liver transplants was divided by the total number of liver transplants to yield a percentage for each region of living donor activity. These percentages were then plotted against the average MELD/PELD scores, with each of the UNOS regions representing a data point on the graph. A line of best fit with positive slope and sufficiently high correlation coefficient would suggest that higher MELD/PELD scores had placed more pressure on centers to perform living donor liver transplants, presumably after the supply of livers from cadaveric donors was exhausted.

## RESULTS

### Classical U.S. Regions

The Midwest appears to be the most active of the classical U.S. regions in the living donor experience. Figure 25-1 indicates that overall, the number of living donor transplants performed per million population is highest in the Midwest, followed by the Northeast, the West, and finally the South. For all regions, the overwhelming majority of living donor operations are kidney transplants. The Midwest leads in the number of living donor

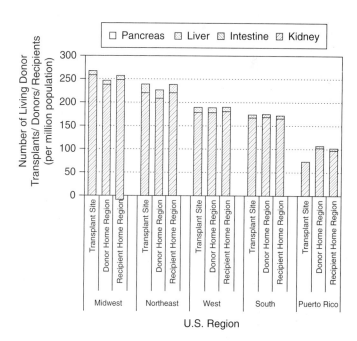

**FIGURE 25-1**

Number of living donor transplants performed, living donors, and living donor organ recipients, per million population, by classical U.S. region of transplant, by organ. The number of living donor transplants from 1995 to 2005, for each region, for each organ, was divided by the corresponding region's population in millions.

kidney transplants at 258 transplants per million population, followed by the Northeast at 220, the West at 179, and finally the South at 169. Puerto Rico, at only 75 living donor kidney transplants per million population, has performed fewer living donor transplants than any of the classical U.S. regions. Liver transplants are the second most common type of living donor transplant performed. At 19 transplants per million population, the Northeast is the dominant region in performing live donor liver transplants followed by the West, the Midwest, and the South with 10.5, 9, and 5 transplants per million population, respectively. Puerto Rico has performed no living donor liver, intestine, or pancreas transplants.

Intestine and pancreas transplants are performed much less commonly in the classical U.S. regions. Of the few that have been performed, living donor intestine transplants are predominately performed in the Midwest, although the number of such operations is minimal (0.4 per million population in the Midwest). Meanwhile, living donor pancreas transplants seem to take place exclusively in the Midwest; however, this figure is even less impressive (less than 0.1 operations per million population).

The data for the home regions of living donors and living donor organ recipients are extremely similar to the data for the transplant sites. The Midwest boasts the greatest living donor activity by providing the most living donors as well as recipients per million population, followed by the Northeast, West, and South. This is readily apparent in Figure 25-1, where the numbers of transplants, living donors, and recipients for living donors (per million population) are approximately equal within each region. This observation suggests that the number of living donor transplants performed estimates the number of living donors and recipients, and that all three factors contribute to overall living donor activity.

Puerto Rico serves as the sole exception to this observation. According to Figure 25-1, although Puerto Rico has performed only 75 living donor kidney transplants per million population, the number of living kidney donors per million population is 103, suggesting that this territory is an exporter of such organs. Additionally, there are 4 living liver donors per million population in Puerto Rico, even though no living donor liver transplants have been performed in that region. Puerto Rico supplies a comparatively high number of recipients per million population as well, with 99 patients for kidneys from living donors and 4 for livers. Such findings indicate that Puerto Rico supplies a considerably large number of not only living donors but also recipients of organs from living donors.

As another measure of living donor activity, Figure 25-2 depicts the ratio of living donor transplants to total (living plus deceased donor) transplants. With regards to kidney transplants for all regions, including Puerto Rico, this ratio lies within the narrow range of 0.34 to 0.44. For liver transplants, there is greater variability between regions regarding this ratio. At 0.08, the ratio of living donor liver transplants to total liver transplants is highest in the Northeast. The West and Midwest follow with ratios of 0.06 and 0.04, respectively, and the South trails at 0.02. Although the absolute difference between these figures for the Northeast and the South is only 0.06, the relative difference is fourfold. Last, as is evident from the same figure, living donor intestine and pancreas transplants are rare, but appear to occur most frequently in the Midwest where nearly one tenth of intestinal transplants involve a live donor. With regards to living donor pancreas transplants, the Midwest is the only region to perform such operations. No liver, intestine, or pancreas transplants take place in Puerto Rico.

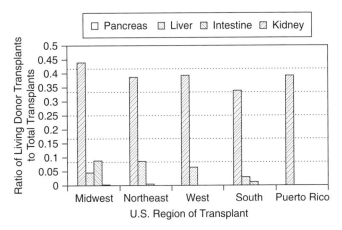

**FIGURE 25-2**

Ratio of living donor transplants to total transplants, by classical U.S. region of transplant, by organ. The number of living donor transplants was divided by the number of total (living plus deceased organ) transplants for each region, for each organ, for the period spanning from 1995 to 2005.

## UNOS-Defined Regions

In addition to classical U.S. regions, analogous data were compiled for the 11 regions defined by UNOS. Figure 25-3 depicts the number of living donor transplants per million population, by UNOS region, by organ. Again, kidney transplants comprise the overwhelming majority of living donor transplants, followed by liver, intestine, and finally pancreas transplants. The greatest number of living donor kidney transplants takes place in Region 7 at 331 per million population. Region 2 is next at 254, and Region 1 follows close behind at 247. The fewest living donor kidney transplants take place in Regions 3 and 4 at 133 and 136, respectively. With regards to living donor liver transplants, Region 9 leads at 31 transplants per million population. Regions 1, 2, 5, 7, and 8 follow, all within the narrow range of 12 to 15 transplants per million population. No living donor liver transplants were performed in Region 6. Last, as expected, living donor intestine and pancreas transplants are both undetectable in the graph due to the rarity of their occurrence.

When organized by UNOS regions, the data for the home regions of living donors and living donor organ recipients are extremely similar to the data for the transplant sites. Region 7 clearly leads in overall living donor activity by providing the most living donors and recipients per million population, followed by the Northeast, West, and South. This is readily apparent in Figure 25-3, where the numbers of transplants, living donors, and recipients for living donor organs (per million population) are approximately equal within each UNOS region. Again, this phenomenon suggests that if a region is highly active in performing living donor transplants, it will also supply a correspondingly high number of living donors and recipients for living donor organs.

As another measure of living donor activity, Figure 25-4 depicts the ratio of living donor transplants to total (living plus deceased donor) transplants. With a ratio of 0.79, Region 7 still appears to be the most active region in performing living donor kidney transplants. Regions 1, 2, 5, 6, 8, 9, 10, 11 all follow, with ratios within the surprisingly narrow range of 0.36 to 0.47. At 0.30 and 0.29, the lowest ratios belong to Regions

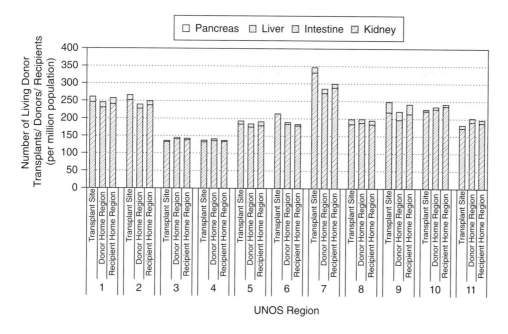

**FIGURE 25-3**

Number of living donor transplants performed, living donors, and living donor organ recipients, per million population, by UNOS region of transplant, by organ. The number of living donor transplants from 1995 to 2005, for each region, for each organ, was divided by the corresponding region's population in millions.

3 and 4, respectively. Finally, the ratio of living donor kidney transplants to total kidney transplants is relatively constant throughout nearly all UNOS regions, with Region 7 being the sole exception.

For liver operations, Region 9 boasts the highest ratio of living donor transplants to total transplants at 0.13, followed by Region 7 at 0.12 and Region 1 at 0.1. Region 6 performed the least living donor liver transplants compared to cadaveric donor liver transplants.

Although living donor intestine transplants are rare compared to living donor kidney and liver transplants, they constitute an entire third of total intestine transplants in Region 1 and four fifths of all intestine transplants in Region 7. Living donor pancreas transplants are extremely rare. The ratio of living donor pancreas transplants to total pancreas transplants is 0.005 in Region 7 and zero in every other region.

## Average MELD/PELD Scores Versus Percentage of Living Donor Liver Transplants

The number of living donor liver transplants was divided by the total number of liver transplants for each UNOS region; this percentage served as a marker of living donor activity. Based on OPTN data from July 21, 2006, the UNOS regions most active in the living donor experience were Regions 9, 1, 5, 7, and 9, at 12.34%, 13.10%, 9.39%, and 9.09%, living donor liver transplants, respectively. The highest average MELD/PELD scores (at time of transplant) for each region correspond to the same regions at 25.6, 25.4, 26.8, and 23.9, respectively. Meanwhile, the UNOS regions least active in the living donor experience were Regions 3, 4, 6, and 10 at 1.51%, 0.56%, 0.47%, and 0.00%, respectively. These regions displayed lower average MELD scores at 20.0, 21.6, 22.8, 21.7, respectively.

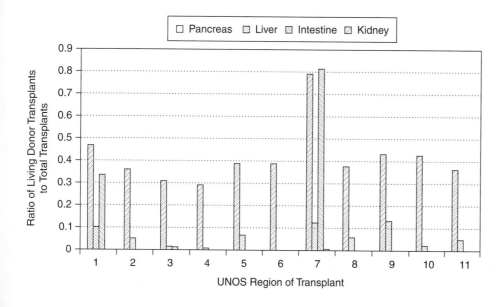

**FIGURE 25-4**

Ratio of living donor transplants to total transplants, by UNOS region of transplant, by organ. The number of living donor transplants was divided by the number of total (living plus deceased organ) transplants for each region, for each organ, for the period spanning from 1995 to 2005.

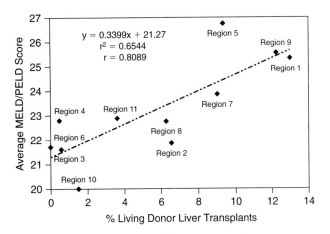

**FIGURE 25-5**

Average MELD score versus percentage of living donor liver transplants. The number of living donor liver transplants was divided by the number of total (living plus deceased organ) liver transplants, for each UNOS region, for the period spanning from 2001 to 2005, to obtain a percentage. This percentage was plotted against the average MELD score at time of transplant. Each data point represents one UNOS region for a total of 11 data points. A line of best fit was added and found to have a positive slope and a reasonably high correlation coefficient (r = 0.8089).

Average MELD/PELD scores at time of transplant were plotted against the percentage of total liver transplants that included live donors to yield Figure 25-5. Each of the data points represents one UNOS region for a total of 11 data points. A line of best fit was added and shown to have a positive slope and a reasonably high correlation coefficient (r) of 0.0809. This suggests that regions with higher average MELD/PELD scores tend to be more active in the living donor experience, whereas regions with lower average MELD/PELD scores tend to be less active. Because higher average MELD/PELD scores would put more pressure on a particular center to resort to organs from live donors, particularly after exhausting the supply of available cadaveric organs, Figure 25-5 implies that our observed trends for living donation may be driven (at least in part) by need.

## DISCUSSION

Based on the data, a number of interesting trends have been observed. Most importantly, living donor transplants are a more common phenomenon in certain regions of the country. Based on analysis of the number of living donor transplants per million population, we have found that the Midwest is more active overall than any other region in the living donor experience. The Northeast follows close behind as a second major player, followed by the West, and finally the South.

Additionally, it seems intuitive that if a particular region performs the most living donor transplants per million population, then that same region would supply the highest number of living donors as well as recipients for those organs. Our data confirm this quite convincingly; as depicted in Figures 25-1 and 25-3, the bars for region of transplant, donor home regions, and recipient home regions are of similar heights within each region (with Puerto Rico in Figure 25-1 and UNOS Region 7 in Figure 25-3 being the only notable exceptions).

Last, certain organ transplants are more common than others. Based on the number of operations per million population, living donor kidney transplants are much more common than living donor liver transplants in every region. Living donor intestine and pancreas transplants are much less common than living donor liver transplants. When the data are presented as a ratio of living donor transplants to total transplants, in the Midwest a greater fraction of organs come from living donors for intestine transplants (0.09) than liver transplants (0.04). This indicates that for the Midwest, although intestine transplants are rare compared to kidney and liver transplants, nearly a tenth of all intestine transplants are living donor operations. Nearly half of all kidney transplants in all regions are living donor operations. Pancreases, on the other hand, come almost exclusively from deceased donors; in fact, the Midwest is the only region that has performed any living donor pancreas transplants from 1995 to 2005.

Several possible explanations are offered for the regional trends observed. First, the observed trends may be center-driven. The Midwest, particularly Region 7, is home to medical centers that have pioneered living donor transplants.[9] Living kidney donation has been a common phenomenon at centers in Minnesota, Wisconsin, Illinois, and North Dakota (based on OPTN data as of April 28, 2006). New York and Boston contain several medical centers that perform living donor liver transplants frequently, conferring leadership in this field to the Northeast, particularly UNOS Region 9 (based on OPTN data as of April 28, 2006). Additionally, as one center becomes active in performing living donor transplants, other regional centers tend to follow suit in order to remain competitive. Hence, center-driven efforts and resultant local–regional competition may contribute to the observed trends seen in this study.

Second, these trends may be culturally driven. The umbrella of culture includes components such as ethnicity, tradition, and factors related to lifestyle such as mindset, religious beliefs, philosophy, diet, and exercise, among others. We have already discussed how the cultural mindset and historical traditions of Japan, for example, have led the country to reject deceased donors as an acceptable alternative. Analogously, regional variations in culture within the United States may drive regional variations in living donor transplant activity.

Thirdly, such trends may be need-driven. It is possible that centers in the South, for example, may have better access to organs from deceased donors and therefore perceive less need to utilize live donors. Meanwhile, centers in the Midwest and Northeast may lack sufficient cadaveric donors and must therefore resort to living donation. Similar reasoning can be applied for UNOS regions. Such an explanation may help to illuminate why, for Figures 25-1 and 25-3, the numbers for transplant region, donor home region, and recipient home region tend to be so similar within each region.

Additionally, Figure 25-5 suggests that regions with higher average MELD/PELD scores tend to have greater percentages of living donor liver transplants. The opposite is true for regions with lower average MELD/PELD scores. Because higher MELD/PELD scores would put more pressure on a particular center to resort to organs from living donors, particularly after exhausting the supply of available cadaveric organs, Figure 25-5 certainly supports the hypothesis that our study's observed trends for living donation may be need-driven.

Other patient-related factors may also contribute to the decision to use a live donor. In some candidates the prospect of a better outcome is an important influence. Although the effectiveness of currently available immunosuppressive agents has eliminated most advantages of HLA matching for most organ transplant candidates, live donation from a HLA-identical donor is clearly advantageous by reducing waiting time and providing the best possible post-transplant outcomes. In fact, overall kidney transplant outcomes are better when live donors are used, regardless of HLA matching. Furthermore the highly controversial concept of extending the search for optimal live donor–recipient combinations, beyond friends and family, may ultimately influence live donor activity.

In conclusion, although the use of living donors for transplantation continues to be controversial, it is becoming increasingly common. Although multiple factors may influence the use of living donors, the shortage of deceased donor organs has been a primary stimulus. Therefore, as disparities between the numbers of transplants performed and the numbers of candidates on the waiting list decrease, live donor use may plateau or decrease, as has been seen with liver transplants.[20]

# References

1. Buske L. Number of living organ donors doubled in 7 years. *Canad Med Assoc J* 2004;171(1): 24.

2. Curtis JJ. Experience with cyclosporine. *Transplant Proc* 2004;36: S54–S58.

3. Fabrizio MD. Johns Hopkins-Brady Urological Institute-Innovative Surgical Techniques. Department of Urology, Johns Hopkins Medical Institutions. Laparoscopic Live Donor Nephrectomy. 3 Jul 2006. <http://urology.jhu.edu/surgical_techniques/nephrectomy/index.html>.

4. Furukawa H, Todo, S. Evolution of immunosuppression in liver transplantation: contribution of cyclosporine. *Transplant Proc* 2004;36: S274–S284.

5. Giessing M, et al. Laparoscopy for living donor nephrectomy – particularities of the currently applied techniques. *Transplant Int* 2005;18:1019.

6. Giles S. An antidote to the emerging two tier organ donation policy in Canada: the Public Cadaveric Organ Donation Program. *J Med Ethics* 2005;31:188–191.

7. Graeb C, et al. Cyclosporine: 20 years of experience at the University of Munich. *Transplant Proc* 2004;36:S125–S129.

8. Groth CG. Landmarks in clinical renal transplantation. *Surg Gynecological Obstetr* 1972; 134:323–328.

9. Hoff M. Trailblazers. *Medical Bulletin, University of Minnesota.* 2005. Last accessed July 13, 2006. <http://www.mmf.umn.edu/bulletin/spring2005/features/trailblazers/ trailblazers1.cfm>.

10. Kita Yoshiaki, et al. "Japanese organ transplant law: a historical perspective." *Progr Transplant* 2000;10:106–108.

11. Klarenbach S, Garg AX, Vlaicu S. Living organ donors face financial barriers: a national reimbursement policy is needed. *Canad Med Assoc J* 2006.;174(6):797–798.

12. Manninen DL, Evans RW. Public attitudes and behavior regarding organ donation. *JAMA* 1985;253:3111–3115.

13. McAlister VC, Badovinac K. Transplantation in Canada: report of the Canadian Organ Replacement Register. *Transplant Proc* 2003;35(7):2428–2430.

14. McAlister VC, et al. "Transplantation in Canada: review of the last decade from the Canadian Organ Replacement Register." *Clin Transplant* 2003;101–108.

15. Middleton Philippa F, et al. Living Donor Liver Transplantation––Adult Donor Outcomes: A Systematic Review." *Liver Transplant* 2006;12:24–30.

16. Montgomery RA, et al. Renal transplantation at the Johns Hopkins Comprehensive Transplant Center. *Clin Transplant* 2003;199–213.

17. Moon, L. Japan and organ transplants. *Japan vs. U.S. in Organ Transplantation.* 2002. MiraCosta College. Last accessed July 4, 2006. <http://www.miracosta.edu/home/lmoon/Japanorgans.html>.

18. Rudow Dianne LaPointe, Brown Jr, RS. "Evaluation of living liver donors." Progr *Transplant* 2003;13:110–116.

19. Shaw Gina. The Tiniest Revolution: Minimally Invasive Methods Changing World of Surgery. *Washington Diplomat* Feb 2001. Last accessed 12 July 2006. <http://www.washdiplomat.com/02-02/c2_02_02.html>.

20. Shiffman ML, et al. Liver and intestine transplantation in the United States, 1995-2004. *Am J Transplantat* 2006;6(5pt2):1170–1187.

21. Tanaka K. Progress and future in living donor liver transplantation. Keio Medical Science Prize Symposium. Shinanomachi Campus, Keio University School of Medicine. Tokyo. Nov 29,2002.

22. Toledo-Pereyra LH, Toledo AH. 1954. *J Invest Surg* 2005;18:285–290.

23. U.S. Census Bureau. Census Bureau Region and Division Codes, State and County Federal Information Processing System (FIPS) Codes, and Minor Civil Divisions (MCD) and Places with Census and FIPS Codes. Dec 22, 2004. Last accessed June 2006. <http://www.census.gov/popest/geographic/codes02.html>.

24. U.S. Census Bureau. American Fact Finder. Oct 18, 2004. Last accessed May 2006. <http://factfinder.census.gov/jsp/saff/SAFFInfo.jsp?_pageId=gn10_select_state>.

# INSTITUTIONAL NEEDS FOR LIVING DONOR: LIVER TRANSPLANTATION

*Alan J. Koffron, MD, Michael Abecassis, MD*

## INTRODUCTION

Live donor liver transplant (LDLT), although proving itself a valuable option in the transplant armamentarium, requires vast institutional dedication, resources, and interdepartmental collaboration. In efforts to optimize donor safety and recipient outcome, all facets of the transplant process require attention, periodic evaluation, and oftentimes improvement to achieve the aforementioned goals. This chapter addresses the basic institutional and divisional needs to embark on a highly demanding arm of liver transplantation, highlighting those essential institutional components of the peritransplant process.

## BACKGROUND

In November 2002, the New York State Transplant Council's Committee on Quality Improvement in Living Liver Donation's submitted a landmark report to the New York State department of Health.[1] Over many months this committee, composed of a 17-member panel extensively analyzed and reviewed donor and recipient selection criteria; informed choice processes, preoperative, intraoperative, and postoperative care plans; as well as discharge planning procedures, in order to improve the care of live liver donors and recipients. The resulting report contains guidelines to help reduce morbidity and mortality associated with live adult liver donation (hemihepatectomy) in New York State and has subsequently been regarded by some as standard guidelines for transplant centers in the rest of the country.

These guidelines not only provide a rationale and prescribed conduct for centers performing LDLT, but also, based on past experiences, delineate the essential institutional components necessary for the successful application of this therapeutic option. These include

1. An Independent Donor Advocate Team (IDAT). A central component of optimal donor safety is the establishment of an IDAT. This team is focused on avoiding any type of conflict of interest and is designed to protect the well-being of the donor. The objectives of the IDAT include education of the potential donor through the process of informed consent, while avoiding external pressures to donate, such as coercion, and culminates in the individual's ability to make an informed choice based purely on the principles of altruism.

2. Informed choice is centered on an informed decision having received full disclosure of the risks, alternatives, and outcomes. This constitutes the desired product of both the IDAT and the transplant team working together with the potential donor and the recipient.

3. Evaluation of both the donor and recipient include medical and psychosocial assessments necessary to identify potential absolute or relative contraindications to the live donor transplant. This evaluation requires a multidisciplinary effort including surgeons, hepatologists, radiologists, and other specialties. Contraindications can exist for either the donor or the recipient in isolation and also for the pair as a unit.

4. The perioperative care required for both the donor and recipient is dependent on adequate facility support. The combined efforts of the surgical and anesthesia teams, nursing and ancillary support staff presume a coordinated approach to the care of these patients and the necessary infrastructure to ensure safety and quality outcomes.

5. Discharge planning intimates a deliberate, focused preparation of the patient, by trained individuals to ensure the readiness of the patient for discharge, in order to optimize the safety and recovery of the patient once released.

Although each of these requirements is intuitive, the integrity of the process and the requisite conduct deserve detailed review to ensure the successful application of the therapy. The New York State Guidelines provide a comprehensive description of the various components and provide a framework on which the transplant center can build a LDLT practice that falls within acceptable standards.

In order to describe the institutional needs of a LDLT center, it is important to first outline the particular needs of the donor–recipient pair.

Potential donors must be made aware that in contrast to the consent process for deceased donors, the living donor is exposed to both immediate risk and unknown future medical problems related to his or her organ system. In addition, the potential donor faces possible and unforeseen financial and emotional consequences of the donation as well as potential chronic illness. Moreover, there may be financial and emotional risks to family members and others as a result of complications suffered by the donor. Therefore, it is essential that a dedicated and committed team, particularly the IDAT make the potential donor aware of all possible outcomes.

Although many recipients are initially in favor of LDLT for obvious reasons, including decreased waiting-list mortality, most patients are unaware of the imperfections of LDLT. Recipients are largely unaware of the need to protect the confidentiality of the donor evaluation process, the inherent risks to the donor (including death), the incremental risks of a partial graft to the recipient, and of alternatives to LDLT. Also, it is incumbent on the transplant team to make the recipient aware that despite their best efforts, LDLT can result in recipient death. It is only through exhaustive education of the recipient by a committed and knowledgeable transplant team with appropriate resources that the recipient can be truly informed.

Despite the best intentions of all parties involved, the need for liver transplantation can result in coercive decision making. There can be both external and internal pressures that result in coercion. A well-trained team of psychologists/psychiatrists and social workers are essential to root out coercion.

Finally, the decision to proceed to LDLT must be made for the right reasons. There must be a high level of moral and ethical consideration that influences the team's decision to recommend LDLT. The philosophic approach to LDLT must include measures of (1) the clinical need for LDLT as compared to other clinical alternatives, including transplantation of a graft from a deceased donor; this is typically dictated by an evaluation of waiting list mortality; (2) an assessment of the team's ability to successfully perform the procedure; this is based on transplant center experience, not only in LDLT but also in associated procedures as well as a recognition of the necessary resources and infrastructure; (3) the transplant center's commitment to the development of a robust LDLT program, highlighting the fact that there is no role for token LDLT in a center where patients have no fundamental need for the procedure (short waiting times, low MELD scores at transplantation, etc). Transplant centers must resist the temptation to perform LDLT in the absence of dire need for their patients.

## INDEPENDENT DONOR ADVOCATE TEAM (IDAT)

An IDAT is a necessary component of any LDLT program. The team's primary concerns are the well-being of the live donor, the provision of an informed decision-making process, and the detection of external pressures (coercion) to donate. The IDAT should conduct their evaluation in an unobstructed and protected manner and be able to communicate their decision about a donor's candidacy without hesitation or reservation. The IDAT should have no financial or personal conflict of interest as a result of the donor's decision. In addition, members of the IDAT should have no caregiver responsibilities to the recipient. The team should consist of a physician, coordinator, psychiatrist or psychologist, and a social worker, all possessing a depth of knowledge in liver disease and transplantation, and pursue continuing education in this regard. More specifically, the psychiatrist, psychologist, or social worker (who should have a master's degree or higher) should be skilled in individual and family counseling, understand the donation process, and have knowledge of and be able to provide information on community programs for social support including temporary housing and transportation to the surgical center.

The IDATs role should exist throughout the entire transplant process including evaluation, donation, postoperative, and post-discharge periods. This role includes the assessment of pain control, facilitating optimal postoperative contact with hospital staff and ensuring that the needs of the donor are fulfilled in accordance with best medical practice.

The team should ensure the process of informed choice (and therefore emphasize that the decision to donate is not a foregone conclusion) and the well-being of the donor, provide information regarding the risks (medical, psychosocial, and financial) of live donation, explain the evaluation process and perioperative donor experience, discuss the donor's medical and psychosocial suitability, and assure continuity of care.

The IDAT must play a major role in donor candidate education, providing and discussing facts about the donation process, and help the patient reference his or her personal values to the particulars of donation.

The team should evaluate the ability of prospective donors to exercise informed choice, inform the potential donor about the risks of the medical interventions, and balance the donor's expectations (recipients' gratitude, sense of well-being from donation) against the real medical risks. It is essential that the team determine that the potential donor's decision is completely voluntary.

The transplant center must provide potential donors with access to an IDAT. The team could be within the institution, or some members of the team may be employed by other institutions. In an ideal world, no member of the IDAT should be employed by the transplant center, but this is not practical because the type of knowledge required by the IDAT is not typical of community practice physicians and social workers in the community. However, it is clearly possible to engage health-care workers in the community in the formation of an IDAT.

## INFORMED CHOICE

The forces that influence a donor are numerous and complex. The donor must be free to make an informed independent choice. The informed choice requires a thorough understanding of the technical elements of the evaluation process, surgery, recovery, and an appreciation of the unknown and unforeseeable consequences that might in the short or long run change the patient's life, health, employment, insurability, or emotional situation. The person who gives consent to be a live organ donor should be competent, willing to donate, free from coercion, medically and psychosocially suitable, and fully informed of the risks and lack of benefit of donation as well as of the alternative therapies available to the recipient. In addition, the donor must not benefit monetarily from donation. Several important principles govern informed choice: informed understanding and disclosure, a complete understanding of the risks associated with the procedure, the ability to make a free and independent choice, documentation of the process, and finally, the ability to evaluate the final decision by the donor to donate (or not).

1. Informed understanding. The donor must demonstrate informed understanding. This is best achieved with written and verbal presentation of the necessary information in lay language and in accordance with the person's educational level. The potential donor must demonstrate their understanding of the essential elements of the donation process, particularly the risks of the procedure. Adequate time should be allowed for the potential donor to absorb the information provided, ask questions, and have questions answered. This may require several consultations for the donor to absorb the information and formulate questions. Written material provided to the potential donor should serve as a basis for not only consent but also as future reference for the donor. The donor's family/loved ones should be given the opportunity to discuss their concerns.

2. Disclosure. The transplant team and the donor advocacy team should disclose their institutional affiliations to the potential donors. The relationship of the donor and the recipient should not alter the level of acceptable risk. There should be a cooling-off period between consent and the actual donation procedure. Non-English-speaking candidates and hearing-impaired candidates should be provided with a nonfamily interpreter. A member of the donor advocate team should witness the potential donor's signing of a consent document.

3. Risks. All known risks should be fully explained to the potential donor, including the physical (death, liver failure, disfigurement, or functional malady), psychological (body image; recipient death; or need for retransplantation, possibility of recurrent disease in recipient, adjustment disorder postsurgery, and impact on donor and/or recipient's family). In addition, social (change in lifestyle, ability to obtain future employment), and financial (out-of-pocket expenses for insurance, child-care costs, loss of employment costs, potential for disability benefit needs, impact on ability to obtain health and life insurance) consequences should be considered.

4. Free choice. The team must establish that there is no donor monetary compensation, no coercion to donate by family or others, and must stand ready to assist the potential donor with a "medical excuse" or general statement of unsuitability for donation if requested. However, medical information on donor should not be falsified to provide the donor with an excuse, declining donation. The process of choice should allow the donor to balance risk and benefit and to understand that he or she may decline to donate at any time. The recipient must be aware of and accept the risks to the donor.

5. Documentation. The potential donor's disclosure and consent process should be completely documented, and the donor should have a medical record separate from the recipient's to protect donor confidentiality.

6. Decision to donate. Once the IDAT determines the suitability of the donor, then, further evaluative processes such as medical and psychological assessment, assessment of the level of social support and of family dynamics. If the potential donor wishes to donate, but the independent advocate team does not agree, the donation should not occur. If the independent advocate team and the potential donor agree to donate, final review rests with the transplant team.

## EVALUATION

The details of the donor and medical evaluation are discussed in detail elsewhere in this publication. These include a gamut of specific diagnostics tailored to LDLT. In a broader sense, this pivotal portion of the process requires a coordinated institutional effort, performed by educated staff members in order to ensure the donor fulfills the following (1) absence of systemic disease or its likely occurrence, (2) absence of current or past impairment to any vital organ, (3) steps to exclude of nonseropositive hepatitis and steatohepatitis (eg, liver biopsy), (4) absence of special vulnerability to complications (eg, infection, blood loss, delayed wound healing, or peptic ulcer disease). These determinations can be made by a combination of physicians, nurses, and coordinators that include both the IDAT and the transplant team caring for the recipient.

In addition, a psychiatrist or psychologist fully versed in the donation process should evaluate the potential donor to (1) exclude the presence of coercion by those close to the donor or recipient; (2) ensure the donor is free of psychiatric disorders; (3) ensure that there is no evident profit motive in the donor's participation; (4) fully evaluate the potential impact of prior physical, sexual, or substance abuse; (5) make sure that the donor acknowledges and understands the attendant risks of LDLT; (6) restate the ability to withdraw from the donation process. Although "Good Samaritan" donation is currently not encouraged in the case of such a donor, this evaluation is necessary to assess the candidate's understanding and motivation. In addition, these specialists should be available to the transplant team throughout the perioperative course, take part in LDLT conferences, and provide the potential donor with the option of future outpatient assistance and support should an adverse event occur.

Although much of the focus of the transplant team is centered on medical evaluation and care of the donor–recipient pair, attention should be paid to the financial burden accompanying LDLT. The transplant team should include both a social worker and a financial officer versed in transplant finances, insurance policy, and the nuances of posttransplant care. These individuals must (1) ensure that the recipient insurance will provide evaluation and medical expense coverage for the donor, (2) the donor is prepared for the potential "hidden costs" of donation (lost work, travel, day care, etc), (3) the recipient has the financial wherewithal to support the posttransplant medical regime, and (4) the pair is aware of potential resources for support should difficulties arise. This important component of the team should be involved in the evaluation, decision process, and long-term follow-up of both patients. The details of the costs of LDLT are discussed elsewhere in this publication.

Not infrequently, the transplant team is faced with potential donors and recipients with circumstances of a psychosocial concern. Although these patients may be found medically appropriate for the procedure, a separate ethics committee is of considerable value in the evaluation process. This committee, comprised of a medical ethicist, psychiatrist/psychologist, physicians, and nurse coordinators, each fully educated in LDLT, should discuss these unusual circumstances to determine if potential, subtle psychosocial risks are present. This evaluation provides multidisciplinary, objective advice to the transplant team in the interest of safety for the patient.

## LIVER TRANSPLANT RECIPIENTS

The recipient indications, evaluation, and care are discussed in detail elsewhere in this communication, but there needs to be an institution-wide consensus regarding indications and contraindications for LDLT. Although the standard transplant selection committee oftentimes identifies potential LDLT recipients, these patients require the combined efforts of the LDLT team to ensure optimal outcomes given the additional potential risks of nondeceased liver transplantation. Potential LDLT recipients should meet standard eligibility criteria to be listed on the deceased transplant waiting list using United Network for Organ Sharing (UNOS) recipient criteria for transplantation.[2] These criteria should be supplemented by the following as possible exclusions for LDLT, due to the current uncertain outcomes in these circumstances, these additional criteria include: a model for end-stage liver disease (MELD) score of greater than 25, adult fulminate failure, cholangiocarcinoma, advanced hepatocellular carcinoma, complex co-morbities (eg, cardiopulmonary disease), retransplantation for hepatitis C, concommitant renal failure, and acute alcoholic hepatitis. It should be noted that this is an inclusive list, and that most transplant centers do not adhere strictly to the list. For instance, some centers consider some of these "relative contraindications" as indications for LDLT. Examples of this include cholangiocarcinoma (early stages under specific adjuvant therapy protocols) as well as hepatocellular carcinoma that exceeds the UNOS criteria but have a reasonable potential outcome.

The recipient should be informed of specific risks and benefits, alternative treatments, and expected outcome of LDLT.

## PERIOPERATIVE CARE AND FACILITY SUPPORT

An attending surgeon should accept responsibility for the donor throughout the perioperative course. Preoperatively, donors should be given the option of autologous blood donation, or have appropriate blood banked, and LDLT surgery should be scheduled only when sufficient staffing will be available for the postoperative period, including attending physician and nursing coverage during weekends/holidays.

### Operative Teams

It is widely recommended that two liver transplant attending surgeons participate in the donor hepatectomy: one present for the entire procedure, and both present for the critical portions of the procedure (eg, parenchymal transection). A third liver transplant attending surgeon should be present in the recipient operating room. This surgeon should have experience in deceased liver transplantation but does not necessarily need expertise in LDLT.

It is also recommended that three surgeons should be board certified in general surgery or an equivalent acceptable foreign certification, and be able to demonstrate experience in liver transplant surgery. Additional recommendations are experience in living donor hepatectomy (15 procedures) or major hepatobiliary resectional surgery (20 procedures) or surgical fellowship at an American Society of Transplant Surgeons (ASTS)-approved liver transplant fellowship program with demonstrated experience (15 procedures) with the live donor hepatectomy procedure. For a new program with no experience in LDLT, surgeons should have demonstrated experience in major hepatobilary resectional surgery (20 procedures) and have visited an established program, having observed a minimum of 5 cases.

As with the surgical team, there should be two separate anesthesia teams, directed by a separate anesthesia attending for the live donor and the recipient procedure. The anesthesia attendings should be present for the critical anesthetic and surgical portions of the procedures, immediately available at all other times when dual procedures exist. These anesthesiologists should have experience in liver transplant anesthesia and/or major hepatic resection surgery and/or cardiac surgery anesthesia. Fellows and or chief residents (postgraduate year 4 or 5) and qualified certified registered nurse anesthetists (CRNAs) may also fulfill these roles.

### Postoperative Care

Initially, living adult liver donors should receive intensive care (ICU or PACU), and if cleared for transfer by the transplant team, donors should recover in a surgical unit that is dedicated to the care of transplant recipients or hepatobiliary patients. The donor should be evaluated at least daily by a liver transplant attending physician, with documentation in the medical record, including pain management,

unless a pain management team is able to dispatch this responsibility. This team, including an anesthesiologist must be experienced in the care of liver donors and communicate with the transplant team regarding the pain control of the donor.

The patient-care team should be familiar with the common complications associated with the donor and recipient operations (eg, hemorrhage, gastric dilatation, wound infection, electrolyte disorders), have appropriate monitoring in place to detect these problems and clinical notification systems in place should they arise.

An attending transplant surgeon should be available, at all times, as a resource for the medial team providing continuous coverage of the transplant service. This team may consist of general surgery residents (postgraduate year 2 level or higher), transplant fellows, or physician extenders (nurse practitioners or physician assistants), dedicated to the liver transplant service and not covering other surgical and non-surgical patients. Patients with abnormalities require immediate evaluation and notification to the appropriate senior medical staff (fellow, chief resident, attending) within 30 minutes, and institutional policies should exist to assure this process occurs in all instances.

Nursing staff should have ongoing education and training in living liver transplantation nursing care (donor and recipient), including donor pain management issues. The registered nursing ratio should be 1:2 in the ICU/PACU level setting, 1:4 in the floor transplant unit on all shifts, adjusted as appropriate for the acuity level of the patients. In addition, the same registered nurse should not take care of both the donor and the recipient to avoid confusion (if identical surnames) and allow the nurse to focus solely on the needs of either the donor or the recipient.

The department of radiology should have faculty possessing experience in liver transplantation and evaluating preoperative imaging studies of potential liver donors (computerized tomography and/or magnetic resonance imaging), specifically with respect to liver volume estimates (right and left lobe) and detailed vascular anatomy.

## DISCHARGE PLANNING

Discharge planning should be viewed as a comprehensive process, beginning with the decision to donate, supported by the independent donor advocacy team, and potentially enhanced by referral to previous donors.

The discharge plan should be a written protocol, reviewed with the patient by a health-care professional (primary care nurse, social worker, or transplant coordinator), and should include restrictions on activities, activities permitted, diet, medications, wound care, 24-hour contact number (for addressing patient questions, concerns, problems) to a contact person knowledgeable about live adult liver donation, surgeon contact information, follow-up visits, instructions for family members or caregivers.

Appropriate outpatient follow-up should include visits with the transplant surgeon(s) to assess wound healing, monitor for signs/symptoms of infections, and monitor liver function; standardized assessment of liver function and morphology over time; and written summary of the patient's condition which should be provided to the patient and his or her primary care physician on the patient's discharge from the hospital, ensuring continued appropriate medical care of the patient. When appropriate, some patients may require follow-up social/psychological supports which may include measures such as social worker; a psychologist or psychiatrist; participation in a professionally run support group; participation in a center-sponsored computer donor list-serve or bulletin board to share patient concerns; and invitation to a donor recognition event, such as an annual recognition ceremony or presentation of a donor medal. Last, there may be need to provide assistance on financial/insurance concerns, possibly by the transplant center's financial coordinator.

## SUMMARY

It is clear that LDLT for adult recipients is currently in a stage of maturation as a therapy, and that there is no standardization currently implemented across transplant centers performing the procedure. The NYS Health Commission in conjunction with the transplant community has set forth some guidelines, which have been discussed in detail regarding institutional needs for LDLT.[1] UNOS has also established a committee on living donation that has made similar observations and recommendations.[2] Finally, a national study by the National Institutes of Health will examine standardized processes as part of its objectives.[3] The recommendations and guidelines discussed above should be viewed purely as that, and not as absolute rules. Each institution has certain subtleties in its structure that make it unique, and therefore these recommendations should be made to fit those peculiarities. However, it is also clear that there are certain core requirements that must be present, especially with regards to institutional resources, such as personnel, infrastructure, and processes that are necessary for the safe implementation of a successful LDLT program. This objective requires the close collaboration of physicians, surgeons, and other health-care workers, as well as of hospital administrators. Finally, two guiding principles that are essential are making sure that the procedure is necessary for the recipient population (ie, that waiting-list mortality is affected by the performance of LDLT) and, more importantly, that donor safety and well-being are considered top priorities by all parties.

## References

1. NYT guidelines (New York State Register, 10 NYCRR § 405.22(l).
2. Abecassis M, Adams M, Adams P, et al. The Live Organ Donor Consensus Group. Consensus statement on the live organ donor. *JAMA* 2000;284:2919–2926.
3. Adult to Adult Living Donor Liver transplantation Cohort Study, http://www.nih-a2all.org/

# CHAPTER 27

# ROLE OF SPLIT LIVER TRANSPLANTATION FROM DECEASED DONORS: LESSONS LEARNED

*Andrew M. Cameron, MD, PhD, Hasan Yersiz, MD,*
*Ronald W. Busuttil, MD, PhD*

## INTRODUCTION

Over 75,000 Americans develop end-stage organ failure each year. Ten percent of those who are placed on the list for transplantation die while waiting. Furthermore, United Network of Organ Sharing (UNOS) data from the year 2000 show that 10% of those awaiting liver transplantation were pediatric recipients (0–17 years old). The disparity between need and organ availability is large, growing, and acutely felt among pediatric patients.[1]

Several possible mechanisms to expand the organ pool are being pursued. These include the aggressive use of extended criteria donors, the use of non-heart-beating donors, the use of living donors, and also the use of split deceased donor transplants, which is the subject of this chapter.

The basis of splitting a cadaveric organ to transplant two recipients results from the understanding of the surgical anatomy of the liver derived from the work of Couinaud.[2] With the rapid growth of clinical liver transplantation in the 1980s following the introduction of cyclosporine, there followed an increasing demand for pediatric cadaveric organs with resultant increases in waiting times and wait-list mortality. Early efforts focused on the surgical reduction of adult cadaveric grafts, termed *reduced-liver transplantation* (RLT), were reported by both Bismuth and Broelsch in the mid-1980s.[3,4] Initially RLT was plagued by technical difficulties but later showed results equal or superior to pediatric whole grafts. Though outcomes were improving for pediatric recipients, the discard of the remnant graft after reduction and the drain this practice placed on the adult pool made RLT untenable.

These techniques were soon modified to create both a left lateral segment graft appropriate for a pediatric recipient and a right trisegment graft for an appropriately sized adult. Techniques of split liver transplantation (SLT) could also be modified for living volunteers to create living donor liver transplantation. Pichlmayr and Bismuth both reported successful SLT in 1989,[5,6] and Emond reported a larger series of nine split procedures from the University of Chicago in 1990[7] (see Table 27-1).

In these early series, overall patient and graft survival were inferior to that seen with pediatric whole grafts with higher rates of complication and need for retransplantation. However, interest was raised in the possibility of using these techniques for maximization of a stagnant donor pool. Larger series out of Europe subsequently showed improved results with elective transplants giving pediatric patient and graft survivals at 6 months of 89% and 80% respectively.[9] These data represented significant improvement over previous SLT reports and were equivalent to those for cadaveric whole organs.

TABLE 27-1

## THE FIRST ATTEMPTS AT SPLIT LIVER TRANSPLANTATION

| Center/Author | Date of Split | Recipients | Outcome |
|---|---|---|---|
| Hannover-<br>*Pichlmayr*[5] | February 1988 | L: 2yo-BA<br>R: 63yo-PBC | reOLT @ 4 months<br>Alive @ 12 years |
| Paul-Brousse-<br>*Bismuth*[6] | May 1988 | L: 45yo-FHF<br>R: 55yo-FHF | Died POD 20<br>Died POD 45 |
| Chicago-<br>*Broelsch*[4] | July 1988 | L: 3mo-FHF<br>R: 7mo-A1AT | Died POD 2<br>Alive @ 12 years |
| Brussels-<br>*Otte*[8] | Nov 1988 | L: 5yo-Tyrosinemia<br>R: 55yo-ESLD | Alive @12 years<br>Died POD 3 |

European efforts led by Pichlmayr and Bismuth advocated an *ex situ* split at the recipient institution following a conventional whole organ harvest.[5,6] This reduced time and effort spent at the donor hospital and focused efforts and expertise at the recipient institution. Potential disadvantages included long, cold ischemia times and the risk of graft rewarming during manipulation. Broelsch and Busuttil described a technical modification in which the split was performed *in situ* at the donor institution with surgical division completed in the heart-beating cadaveric donor prior to aortic cross-clamp and organ cold perfusion.[10] *In situ* splitting reduces cold ischemia, simplifies identification of biliary and vascular structures, and reduces reperfusion hemorrhage. However, *in situ* splits require specialized skills, prolonged operating room time, and increased logistical coordination at the donor institution.

Preliminary reports of *in situ* SLT data from the University of Hamburg, Germany, and the University of California, Los Angeles, showed results in both their pediatric and adult recipients equal to or exceeding whole cadaveric grafts.[10,11] Since these initial reports both universities have published expanded results confirming their earlier observations. At UCLA over 150 *in situ* splits have been performed, and this technique is the default when an optimal donor is available. This series is described in detail below. SLT now accounts for 10% of adult transplants at UCLA and 40% of pediatric transplants. It represents a complementary rather than competitive technique with living donation, with the advantage that it incurs no additional risk to a living donor.

## EVALUATION OF THE DONOR

Careful donor and recipient selection are essential to the success of SLT.[12] Potential donors are usually restricted to optimal candidates based on age (< 50), ABO compatibility, liver function, brevity of hospitalization, absence of down time, serum sodium, and size match. Prospective analysis of the relative importance of these factors has not yet been done, but conservatism seems warranted at this time to minimize the possibility of graft primary nonfunction (PNF). Evaluation by the recovering team is of high importance, not only in terms of assessing parenchymal quality but also in ascertaining vascular and biliary anatomy.

Insights into the surgical anatomy of the liver and its eight distinct segments allow for the creation of partial allografts of varying size. Division of parenchyma at the falciform ligament yields a left lateral segment graft [2,3] of approximately 250 cc, appropriate for a pediatric recipient and a right trisegment graft[1,4–8] of approximately 1,100 cc, which is appropriate for a well-selected adult recipient. Division of the parenchyma along the middle hepatic vein creates two equal-size grafts. A left lobe graft[1–4] of approximately 400 cc volume can be used for smaller adults (< 60 kg), whereas the right lobe graft will typically have a volume of around 800–1,000 cc and can be used for an adult weighing < 80 kg (see Table 27-2).

## EVALUATION OF THE RECIPIENT

Key in the process of recipient selection in SLT is estimation of how much parenchyma the patient will require to meet their immediate postoperative metabolic needs. Also to be considered is the cause of recipient liver failure, the severity of illness, and the degree of portal hypertension. In healthy humans the liver constitutes 5% of body weight in infancy and decreases to a plateau of approximately 2.5% in adults. Liver weight in males is generally greater than that in females. Normal liver regenerates successfully after right trisegmentectomy (20% remnant). Liver injured by chronic hepatitis, cirrhosis, or steatosis shows delayed or incomplete regeneration.

There are two commonly used measures to quantify graft size to recipient size. The first is to express graft weight as a percentage of the expected size of the recipient's liver, designated "standard volume." Alternatively graft weight may be quantified simply as a percentage of recipient body weight, that is, the "Graft to Recipient Weight Ratio" or GRWR. In general it is thought that recipients require grafts of 40% standard volume or approximately 1% of their body weight. Grafts that provide less than this volume more frequently manifest the "small-for-size syndrome" showing prolonged synthetic dysfunction with a cholestatic pattern. Pretransplant acuity status or original disease may negatively impact in small-for-size grafts as well.

## TECHNIQUES

### Anatomic Principles

As per Couinaud, the liver is divided into eight functional units, termed *segments* that receive separate hilar pedicles. Each pedicle contains a portal venous branch, hepatic arterial branch, and a bile duct radicle. Hepatic parenchymal dissection takes place through connective tissue "scissurae" that separate individual segments. Each segment has drainage through venous branches which are tributaries of the hepatic veins.

Prior to any split procedure standard techniques of abdominal organ procurement are used. These include a long midline incision with mobilization of the right colon and duodenum medially to expose the retroperitoneal structures. The inferior mesenteric vein (IMV) is cannulated to allow for "precool" and eventual portal flush, and control of the infrarenal and supraceliac aorta are obtained.[13] This allows for rapid progression to aortic cannulation and cross-clamping in the event of donor instability.

### Creation of a Left Lateral Segment Graft[2,3] and Right Trisegment Graft[1,4–8]

SLT is initiated with division of the falciform ligament to the caval–hepatic vein junction. The left hepatic vein is identified, isolated, and encircled with a vessel loop. A common middle and left hepatic

**TABLE 27-2**
## SLIT LIVER VOLUME CONSIDERATIONS

| Division of Graft | Products | Volumes | Recipients |
|---|---|---|---|
| | LLS[2,3] | 250 cc | Pedi (<25 kg) |
| Along Falciform Ligament: | R Triseg[1,4–8] | 1,150 cc | Adult (Average) |
| | L Lobe[1–4] | 400 cc | Adult (<60 kg) |
| Along Middle Hepatic Vein: | R Lobe[5–8] | 1,000 cc | Adult (<80 kg) |

vein will require separation after parenchymal division. Identification of independent segment 2 and 3 veins is critical and requires that both orifices are preserved on a common caval patch.

Next, hilar dissection begins at the base of the round ligament with isolation of the left hepatic artery, left portal vein, and left hepatic duct. The left hepatic artery is traced along its length with particular attention given to preservation of the origin of the segment 4 branch. If the segment 4 branch arises high off the left hepatic artery and is significant in size, it must be reanastomosed to the right trisegment's gastroduodenal artery remnant. Portal venous branches to segment 4 are ligated and divided lateral to the umbilical fissure, which results in isolation of the entire left portal vein.

With vascular control of the left lateral segment obtained parenchymal transection is initiated. The liver is scored with the electrocautery approximately 1 cm to the right of the falciform ligament. The parenchyma is divided between the left lateral segment and segment 4 and carried to 1 cm above the left bile duct in the umbilical fissure. The left hilar plate containing the bile duct is sharply transected. The left lateral segment is now separate from the rest of the parenchyma with its own vascular pedicle and venous drainage (Figure 27-1). Following organ cold perfusion the left hepatic artery, left portal vein, and left hepatic vein are sharply divided. The left bile duct is flushed with cold University of Wisconsin (UW) and stored in the standard fashion (Figure 27-2). The right trisegment graft is removed in the standard fashion and stored in cold UW solution (Figure 27-3).

Transplantation of the left lateral segment requires preservation of the recipient vena cava ("the piggyback technique"). Biliary anastomosis may be duct-to-duct but more commonly is accomplished with Roux-en-Y reconstruction. Preparation of the right trisegment graft requires closure of the left hepatic vein, left portal vein, and left hepatic artery origins. Oversewing of the left hepatic duct remnant is likewise required. The cut parenchymal edge is carefully inspected for vascular or biliary leaks, which are oversewn.

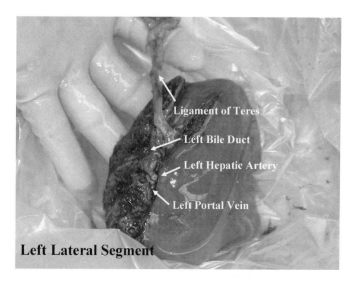

**FIGURE 27-2**

The left lateral segment[2,3] split graft.

## Creation of a Left Segment Graft[2–4] and a Right Segment Graft [1,5–8]

A larger left lobe segment[2–4] can be obtained, which is then appropriate for transplantation into larger children or adults less than 60 kg.[14] Dissection begins as above with identification of the hepatic vein origins, but now the left and middle hepatic veins are encircled with a vessel loop to guide parenchymal transection. The left bile duct, left hepatic artery, and left portal vein are identified and dissected along their extrahepatic length the level of the round ligament. Segment 4 artery branches are preserved, and the left portal vein is freed along its length via division of caudate branches

Temporary occlusion of the left hepatic artery and left portal vein will show a plane of demarcation for parenchymal transection. The plane is marked with electrocautery and proceeds to the hilar plate, ligating parenchymal vessels as encountered. At the

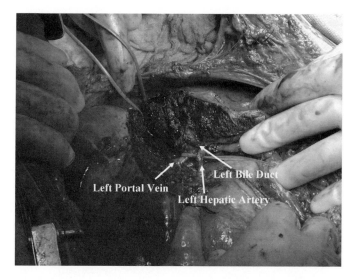

**FIGURE 27-1**

Vascular control and parenchymal division to create a left lateral segment[2,3] graft.

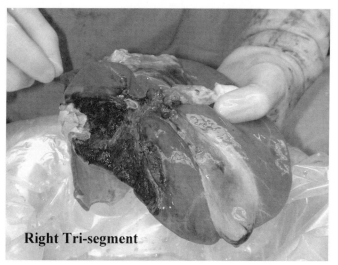

**FIGURE 27-3**

The right trisegment[1,4–8] graft.

hilar plate the left hepatic duct is transected. After organ cold perfusion the left portal vein is sharply divided just distal to the bifurcation. Next the right hepatic artery is divided just distal to its takeoff from the proper hepatic artery. The common portal vein and the common hepatic duct are thus maintained with the right graft, while the celiac axis stays with the left graft, thus maximizing arterial flow to segment 4, which may be derived from both the left and the right hepatic arteries. The left and middle hepatic veins are taken from the suprahepatic vena cava as a common cuff. The left hepatic duct is flushed with cold UW preservation solution prior to storage. The remnant right graft is procured by standard techniques. Back-table preparation may require vascular reconstruction with donor-derived conduit vessels.

## Creation of a Left Segment Graft[1–4] and a Right Segment Graft[5–8]

True left–right splits create a left lobe graft[1–4] that may be used for adults weighing up to 60 kg or more.[15] The right lobe permits transplantation into size-for-size donor-to-recipient weight ratios. The procedure begins as above with isolation of the hepatic veins and in this case looping of the right hepatic artery. The diaphragmatic attachments to the liver are released, and dissection continues along the right lobe to the inferior vena cava. Following retrograde cholecystectomy attention is turned to the hepatic hilum. The right hepatic artery is identified and exposed lateral to the common hepatic duct, avoiding skeletonization of the arterial bifurcation with subsequent compromise of segment 4 branches. The right portal vein is approached laterally and dissected to the bifurcation where it is encircled with a vessel loop. A Pringle maneuver will demonstrate the line of demarcation (Figure 27-4).

The left bile duct is sharply divided at the hilar plate, and parenchymal division is performed along the main portal fissure (Figure 27-5). On completion the right hepatic vein, right portal vein, and right hepatic artery are maintained for cold perfusion. After this, the right portal vein is divided just distal to the bifurcation and the right hepatic artery is taken distal to its takeoff from the proper hepatic artery. The right hepatic vein is divided from the suprahepatic vena cava as a patch, and the right graft is removed

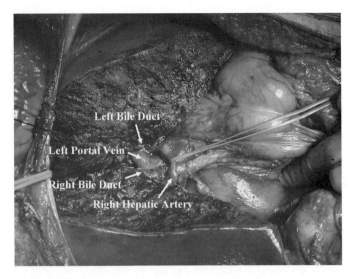

**FIGURE 27-5**

Parenchymal division in the left-right split.

(Figure 27-6). The bile duct is flushed and the graft stored. The left graft is now removed using standard recovery techniques and stored (Figure 27-7). Preparation will include closure of the right portal vein orifice, right hepatic vein orifice, and right hepatic artery orifice. Right lobe grafts 4–8 require the recipient's vena cava ("piggybacking").

## RESULTS OF SLT

### Published Results

The initial series on adult-child SLT published by Broelsch in 1990 showed recipient survival inferior to that of cadaveric whole graft recipients.[7] When a later expanded series failed to show improved results there was early skepticism about the practice. However, a subsequent report by de Ville collected from the European Split

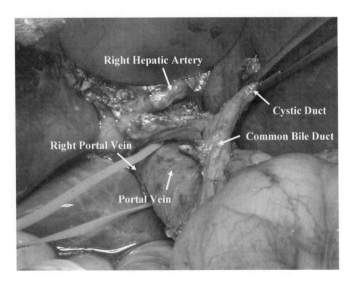

**FIGURE 27-4**

The Hilar dissection in the left–right split.

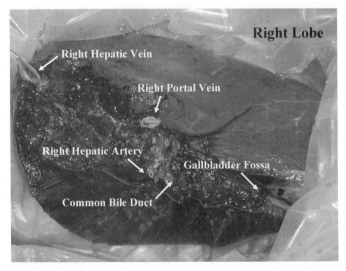

**FIGURE 27-6**

The right lobe[5–8] split graft.

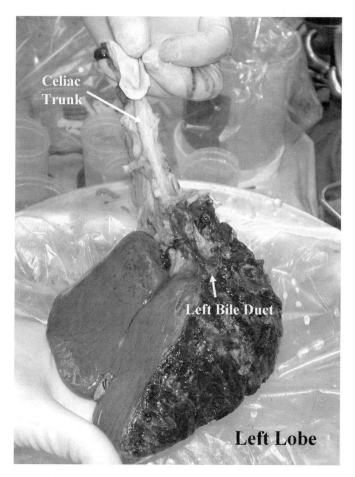

**FIGURE 27-7**

The left lobe[1-4] split graft.

Liver Registry showed success with 100 SLTs that was equivalent to whole grafts.[9] Elective SLT pediatric and adult survival at 6 months was 89% and 80%, respectively. Still complications were high with 20% of grafts lost to HAT, or portal vein thrombosis and biliary complications were present at 19%

Adult–child SLT expanded during the late 1990s with several centers reporting individual experiences of up to 78 splits. Complication rates remained high (30%) with biliary problems being the most common. Graft sharing is reported but remained infrequent, accounting for 5% of total grafts (see Table 27-3).

More recently, Renz et al. reported on ASTS survey data collected on SLT.[20] Data were obtained on 215 SLTs performed in the United States from 1994 to 2001. Forty-two of these were *in situ* procedures; 140, *ex vivo;* and 33, partial procedures. Graft failure was seen in 32% of recipients; with death, in 26%. When compared with historic control recipient results were generally comparable to "extended criteria" whole organ recipients and inferior to recipients who received organs from "optimal" donors age 18 to 40. UNOS status 1 recipients fared the worst when receiving a split right lobe graft. The SRTR data were significantly worse than those reported by UCLA (see below) and other selected single-center series.

Less has been published on adult–adult SLT. The early experience from Chicago yielded patient and graft survivals of 67% and 50%, respectively, lower than those of whole graft recipients. Paul Brousse reports on the largest series of splitting for two adult recipients with 27 SLTs that gave an approximately 80% 1-year graft survival rate.[21] These procedures were done *ex vivo*, and a 22% biliary complication rate was reported with one incidence of PNF. Biliary complications were more likely to occur in the left lobe graft; and arterial complications, in the right. Smaller North American series from Humar et al and others have given similar results (see Table 27-4).

## THE UCLA SLT EXPERIENCE

In 2003, UCLA reported on their series of SLT, which had reached 100. This series is rapidly approaching 200 and shows outcome results comparable to those seen with whole organ transplantation. Specifically, a retrospective analysis of SLTs occurring from 1991 to 2003 documented 100 SLTs, which generated transplants for 105 pediatric recipients and 60 adult recipients with sharing of 25 allografts with other centers across the United States.[16]

The incidence of biliary and vascular complications in recipients of left lateral segment grafts created by splitting was statistically no different than that seen with a historic control group of living donor left lateral segment grafts or pediatric whole graft recipients. Graft and recipient survival were also no different between these groups.

Adult right trisegment graft recipients in this series showed a 10% rate of biliary complications and 7% incidence of vascular complications. Long-term graft function was excellent with patient and graft survival equal to a control group that received cadaveric whole grafts from "optimal donors" ages 10 to 40. Predictors of graft and recipient survival were analyzed and showed an effect determined by UNOS status 1, indication for transplant, as well as donor creatinine and length of hospitalization.

**TABLE 27-3**

## RESULTS IN LEFT LATERAL SEGMENT/RIGHT TRISEG SPLIT LIVER TRANSPLANTATION

| Center/Author | Year | n | Recipient Survival | Graft Survival | Complication Rate |
|---|---|---|---|---|---|
| Los Angeles -*Yersiz*[16] | 2003 | 92 | 78% | 68% | 24% |
| Hamburg -*Broering*[17] | 2001 | 49 | 82% | 76% | 28% |
| Birmingham -*Noujaim*[18] | 2001 | 49 | N/A | N/A | 8% |
| London -*Rela*[19] | 1998 | 22 | 86% | 82% | 45% |

TABLE 27-4
## RESULTS IN LEFT LOBE/RIGHT LOBE SPLIT LIVER TRANSPLANTATION

| Center/Author | Year | n | Recipient Survival | Graft Survival | Complication Rate |
|---|---|---|---|---|---|
| Minneapolis -*Humar*[22] | 2001 | 18 | 89% | 89% | 43% |
| Villejuif -*Azoulay*[21] | 2001 | 34 | 81% | 75% | 24% |
| Hamburg -*Broering*[23] | 2001 | 12 | 93% | 85% | N/A |

## CONCLUSIONS

SLT developed in the 1980s and 1990s out of an acute need to expand availability of pediatric organs without depletion of the adult cadaveric pool, as had been the case with earlier RLT efforts. The optimism generated by the possibility of transplanting two recipients from a single donor was tempered by early series, which showed results inferior to whole graft transplantation. Improvements in technique along with experience in donor and recipient selection have resulted in large single-center series with results for both pediatric and adult recipients similar to whole grafts from "optimal donors," though a recent analysis of SRTR data still shows an overall nationwide lag in SLT graft performance and outcomes. Future directions include more widespread applicability of adult–child SLT as criteria for inclusion become more rigorously defined and more centers gain comfort with the technique. Further expansion of the use of true left–right splits to generate grafts for two adult recipients is also anticipated.

SLT from deceased donors represents a complementary, not competitive, addition to the armamentarium of the transplant surgeon, which also includes cadaveric whole organ grafting and living donor liver transplantation. Specific advantages include the fact that no extra risk is imparted to a living donor. For those recipients, both pediatric and adult, without an appropriate living donor, SLT represents a potentially life-saving option.

## References

1. Sheehy E, Conrad SL, Brigham LE, et al. Estimating the number of potential organ donors in the United States. *NEJM* 2003;349:667–674.
2. Couinaud C. *Le Foie: Etudes Anatomiques et Chirurgicales.* Paris: Masson; 1957.
3. Bismuth H, Houssin D. Reduced size orthotopic liver graft in hepatic transplantation in children. *Surgery* 1984;95:367–370.
4. Broelsch CE, Emond JC, Thistlethwaite JR, et al. Liver Transplantation with reduced size donor organs. *Transplantation* 1988;45:519–524.
5. Pichlmayr R, Ringe B, Gubernatis G. Transplantation of a donor liver to 2 recipients (splitting transplantation)—a new method in the further development of segmental liver transplantation. *Langenbecks Archiv Chir* 1989;373:127–130.
6. Bismuth H, Morino M, Castaing D, et al. Emergency orthotopic liver transplantation in two patients using one donor liver. *Br J Surg* 1989;76:722–724.
7. Emond JC, Whitington PF, Thistlethwaite JR, et al. Transplantation of two patients with one liver. Analysis of a preliminary experience with "split-liver" grafting. *Ann Surg* 1990;212:14–22.
8. Otte JB, de Ville de Goyet J, Alberti D, et al. The concept and technique of the split liver in clinical transplantation. *Surgery* 1990;107:605–612.
9. De Ville de Goyet J. Split liver transplantation in Europe, 1988-1993. *Transplantation* 1995;59:1371–1376.
10. Goss JA, Yersiz H, Shackleton CR, et al. In situ splitting of the cadaveric liver for transplantation. *Transplantation* 1997;64:871–877.
11. Rogiers X, Malago M, Gawad KA, et al. One year of experience with extended application and modified techniques of split liver transplantation. Transplantation 1996;61:1059–1061.
12. Rogiers X, Bismuth H, Busuttil RW, et al, eds. *Split Liver Transplantation: Theoretical and Practical Aspects.* New York: Springer; 2002.
13. Emre S, Schwartz M, Miller CM. Chapter 39 "The Donor Operation." In: Busuttil, Klintmalm, eds. *Transplantation of the Liver.* Chicago, IL: Sanders.
14. Yersiz H, Renz JF, Hisitake G, et al. Technical and logistical considerations of in situ split liver transplantation for two adults: Part I. Creation of a left segment II, III, IV and right segment V-VIII grafts. *Liver Transplant* 2001;7:1077–1080.
15. Yersiz H, Renz JF, Hisitake G, et al. Technical and logistical considerations of in situ split liver transplantation for two adults: Part II. Creation of a left segment I-IV and right segment V-VIII grafts. *Liver Transplant* 2002;8:78–81.
16. Yersiz H, Renz J, Farmer D, et al. One hundred in situ split liver transplantations: A single center experience. *Ann Surg* 2003;238:496–507.
17. Broering D, Mueller L, Ganschow R, et al. Is there still a need for living-related liver transplantation in children. *Ann Surg* 2001; 234: 713–722.
18. Noujaim HM, Mayer DA, Buckels JAC et al. Division of vascular pedicle and vascular complications after ex vivo split liver transplantation. European Liver Transplantation Association. 2001. Berlin, Germany.
19. Rela M, Vougas V, Muiesan P, et al. Split Liver Transplantation: King's College Hospital Experience. *Ann Surg* 1998;227:282–288.
20. Renz JF, Emond JC, Yersiz H, Ascher NL, Busuttil RW. Split Liver transplantation in the United States: Outcomes of a national survey. *Ann Surg* 2004;239:172–181.
21. Azoulay D, Castaing D, Adam R, et al. Split liver transplantation for two adult recipients: feasibility and long term outcomes. *Ann Surg* 2001;233:565–574.
22. Humar A, Kandaswamy R, Sielaff T, et al. Split Liver Transplants for 2 adult recipients: an initial experience. ATC, *Transplant 2001;* Chicago IL. May 12–16.
23. Broering D, Gundlach M, Topp S, et al. In-situ full right-left splitting: the ultimate expansion of the adult donor pool. ATC, *Transplant 2001;* Chicago, IL. May 12–16.

CHAPTER 28

# LIVER REGENERATION

*Jeroen de Jonge, MD, PhD, Kim M. Olthoff, MD*

## INTRODUCTION TO LIVER REGENERATION

The liver is the only solid organ that has the ability to proliferate in response to loss of cell mass and restore cellular architecture and function after resection, substantial toxic injury, or infection. This unique ability was recognized in the ancient Greek myth, described in Hesiod's *Theogony* (750 to 700 BC). Prometheus, a Titan, was punished by Zeus for stealing the secret of fire from the gods of Olympus and giving it to the humans. He was condemned to having a portion of his liver devoured daily by an eagle. His liver regenerated each night, thus providing the eagle with eternal food and Prometheus with eternal torture. The first successful liver resection for trauma was described by Hildanus in the 17th century; however, the first medical documentation of the ability of the human liver to regenerate was not made until 1890 by Ponfick.[1] Shortly after, the first successful planned resection was performed by Langenbuch in 1888 and the first hemihepatectomy by Wendle in 1911.[2]

In normal circumstances, cell division is rarely seen within the liver with less than 0.1‰ of hepatocytes in mitosis at any given time,[3] with the remainder staying in the G0 phase of the cell cycle. Following surgical resection, infection or toxic injury, however, this low cell turnover transforms into a sudden massive hepatocyte proliferation, in which approximately 95% of the hepatic cells reenter the cell cycle and produce recovery of functional liver mass within 2 weeks in rats and mice,[4] even after 90% hepatectomy.[5] Once a species- and age-specific ratio of liver weight to total body weight is reached (about 4.5% in rodents, 2.5% in humans), liver cell proliferation ceases.[6,7] Perhaps more remarkable than the capacity of hepatocytes to proliferate is that they do so while simultaneously performing all essential functions needed for homeostasis. Even after a 2/3 resection of the liver, the essential functions of the liver, including metabolism, synthesis, storage and redistribution of nutrients, carbohydrates, fats and vitamins, glucose regulation, synthesis of many blood proteins, secretion of bile, and biodegradation of toxic compounds are little disturbed.

## REGENERATION IN LIVER TRANSPLANTATION

Why is regeneration so important in liver transplantation? In a healthy adult liver, the background requirement for tissue repair is minimal and the majority of liver energy is expended in normal metabolism. However, posttransplantation, the balance is dramatically shifted to the critical tasks of injury recovery at the expense of normal hepatic metabolism. The success of restoring lost liver mass, repairing tissue injury, and resolving inflammation determines the ability of the liver to support normal metabolic function and thus, determines the success or failure of the graft.

In deceased donor (DD) whole organ transplantation, hepatocyte loss occurs in the form of ischemia/reperfusion (I/R) injury because of the necessary preservation period from procurement to implantation, as well as damage that may have occurred in the donor from trauma and brain death. Regenerative mechanisms are actively engaged after transplantation depending on the length and degree of preservation injury. Similarly, hepatocytes lost to the alloimmune response require replacement. Laboratory studies demonstrate that these conditions together contribute to increased injury, resulting in a complex molecular process in which cell stress, proinflammatory stimuli, and the activation of the innate immune response are acting independently and in concert.[8,9] In pediatric recipients, in a less acute process, liver growth and regeneration is necessary as the liver grows with the child.

Regeneration is, however, most required in the setting of transplanting a small-for-size graft into a larger recipient. This is clearly the case in the setting of adult-to-adult living donor liver transplantation (AALDLT). Ischemic injury is minimized in AALDLT in that the preservation period is very short. However, this technique provides a graft that is by definition too small, requiring vigorous immediate hepatocyte proliferation. By transplanting only 50% to 60% of what is the expected standard liver volume in adults, we introduce a conflict of interest: recipients (and donors) must rely on the rapid repair and regeneration of a partial liver, and at the same time this liver graft has to maintain the basic metabolic functions required of the liver. In the situation of a severely ill recipient—which requires the expenditure of an unusual amount of metabolic energy by the liver—this balance may be disrupted and lead to blunted regeneration. Similarly, when factors in the donor graft demand increased efforts for repair or regeneration of the graft, the balance tips in the opposite direction, not leaving enough energy to maintain metabolic function.[10] In either scenario, the graft functions poorly and the recipient may not recover (Figure 28-1).

## MOLECULAR AND CELLULAR CHARACTERISTICS OF LIVER REGENERATION

Recently several excellent comprehensive reviews have been published on liver regeneration.[11–13] Here we provide a brief summary of the molecular and cellular pathways elucidated in recent years.

### Models of Liver Regeneration

Liver regeneration is most clearly shown in the experimental model that was pioneered in 1931 by Higgins and Anderson.[14] In this model, a simple two-thirds partial hepatectomy (PHx) is

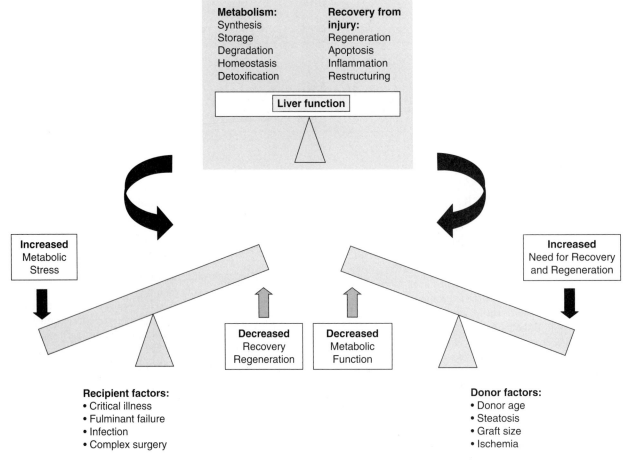

**FIGURE 28-1**

Hypothesis of the balance between liver regeneration and metabolic function. Increased metabolic requirement (recipient factors) will lead to decreased recovery/regeneration of the graft. Increased need for recovery/regeneration (donor factors) will lead to decreased metabolic support of the recipient

performed, without damage to the lobes left behind. This leads to enlargement of the residual lobes to make up for the mass of the removed lobes in 5 to 7 days. Other well-known models of liver regeneration are associated with extensive tissue injury and inflammation and include the use of hepatic toxins, such as ethanol (EtOH),[15] carbon tetrachloride ($CCl_4$)[16] and galactosamine (GalN),[17] bile duct ligation,[18] or portal vein ligation[19] and ischemia and reperfusion (I/R) injury.[20] In each model, the different toxic agents injure specific liver cell subpopulations, therefore, PHx is the preferred *in vivo* model to study the pure regenerative response. It has been demonstrated that regenerative signaling observed in a rat liver transplant model of I/R injury is similar to that observed after PHx.[21]

## General Features of Liver Regeneration

Liver regeneration after surgical resection is carried out by proliferation of existing mature cellular populations. These include hepatocytes, biliary and fenestrated endothelial cells, Kupffer cells, and cells of Ito (stellate cells).[22] The kinetics of cell proliferation and the growth factors produced by proliferating hepatocytes suggest that hepatocytes may provide the mitogenic stimuli leading to proliferation of the other cells. The degree of hepatocyte proliferation is directly proportional to the degree

of injury.[23] Immediately after liver resection, the rate of DNA synthesis in hepatocytes begins to increase as they exit the resting state of the cell cycle (G0), enter G1, traverse to DNA synthesis (S phase), and ultimately undergo mitosis (M phase). The induction of DNA synthesis in rodents occurs later in the nonparenchymal cells (at about 48 hours for Kupffer and biliary epithelial cells, and at about 96 hours for endothelial cells).[24,25] The first peak of DNA synthesis occurs at 40 hours after resection in rodents, at about 72 to 96 hours in dogs, and at 7 to 10 days in primates. In small animals, the regenerative response returns the liver to the preresection mass in 1 week to 10 days. Hepatocyte proliferation starts in the periportal areas of the lobules[26] and then proceeds to the pericentral areas by 36 to 48 hours. Liver histology at day 3 to 4 after PHx is characterized by clumps of small hepatocytes surrounding capillaries, which change into true hepatic sinusoids. The hepatic matrix composition also changes from high laminin content to primarily containing fibronectin and collagen types IV and I. After a 70% hepatectomy, restoration of the original number of hepatocytes theoretically requires 1.66 proliferative cycles per residual hepatocyte. In fact, most of the hepatocytes (95% in young and 75% in very old rats) in the residual lobes participate in one or two proliferative events.[27] However, the liver has an almost unlimited capacity to regenerate.

## Liver Stem Cells

In response to liver damage inflicted by agents such as galactosamine, hepatocytes are unable to replicate. In this situation a population of cells known as oval cells proliferates to replace the hepatic parenchyma.[28] In the human situation, oval cells participate in repopulation of the liver after acute massive necrosis and have also been identified in chronic liver disease.[29] The oval cells are thought to be derived from biliary epithelial cells.[30] These human progenitor cells seem to originate from the canals of Hering[31] and play an important role in acetaminophen-induced injury.[32]

## INDUCTION OF PROLIFERATION: PRIMING AND CELL-CYCLE PROGRESSION

Within minutes after PHx specific transcription factors, such as nuclear factor (NF)-κB, signal transducer and activator of transcription 3 (STAT3) and AP1 are activated in remnant hepatocytes.[33] The Taub group initially identified 70 immediate early genes, which are rapidly activated by normally latent transcription factors, before the onset of *de novo* protein synthesis. This list has been expanded with the help of new microarray analysis techniques to over 180 genes.[34–36] Historically, the onset of liver regeneration has been attributed to a flow-dependent response by which increased relative flow after PHx resulted in hepatocyte proliferation and hyperplasia.[37] Not until the experiments of Moolten and Buche,[38] who demonstrated the existence of humoral factors in the induction of liver growth after PHx, the realization that secreted factors are critical for liver regeneration began to emerge. Cytokines, such as IL-6 and TNF-α, have been proposed as the earliest growth factors triggering activation of several transcription factors during regeneration.[39,40] However, these cytokines alone are not sufficient for the induction of this process, as restitution of liver mass is only delayed, but not abolished, in the absence of IL-6 or TNF-α.[40,41] Therefore, other blood-derived mitogens, such as hepatocyte growth factor (HGF), were first identified as important growth factor during liver regeneration.[42] Hepatocytes in normal liver are not ready to respond to mitogenic signals without a set of "priming" events that switch them into a responsive state. This has been described by Fausto[43] who identified *priming factors*, involved in initiating and triggering of the hepatic response to injury and concomitant *growth factors* and their receptors, allowing competent hepatocytes to progress through the cell cycle (Figure 28-2). Priming is accomplished by the release of preformed cytokines that subsequently activate transcription factor complexes and allow the cell to exit $G_0$ into $G_1$ of the cell cycle.[44] This group includes TNF-α and IL-6. Growth factors would include the potent hepatocyte mitogens HGF, transforming growth factor (TGF)-α, and heparin-binding epidermal growth factor (HB-EGF). This process is further controlled by *co-mitogens* such as insulin, glucagon, steroid and thyroid hormone, and epinephrine, which facilitate activity of the mitogens and by down-regulation of growth factor inhibitors such as activin A and transforming growth factor (TGF)-β.

So far, few factors have been identified to be possibly responsible for the release of these priming cytokines and growth factors in the onset of liver regeneration. The first is endotoxin lipopoly-saccharide (LPS), produced in the gut by Gram-negative bacteria. Circulating LPS is an extremely strong signal for Kupffer cells to start the cascade resulting in hepatocyte replication (Figure 28-3).[33,35] Rats treated with antibiotics and germ-free rodents

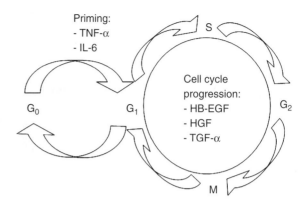

**FIGURE 28-2**

Multistep model of liver regeneration. Priming is a reversible process initiated by cytokines as well as by nutritional and hormonal signals. Priming sensitizes the cells to growth factors but is ineffective in their absence. Growth factors are required for cells to move beyond a restriction point in Gl. HGF, hepatocyte growth factor; TGF, transforming growth factor; TNF, tumor necrosis factor; IL-6, interleukin-6.

have a delayed peak of DNA replication after partial hepatectomy, confirming the importance of LPS.[46] Another major finding is the demonstration that cytokine activation and DNA replication are severely impaired in mice lacking the complement components C3a and C5a.[47] In particular, mice lacking both C3a and C5a have impaired production of TNF and IL-6 after partial hepatectomy and poor activation of NFkB and STAT3. In the initiation of growth factors, urokinase-type plasminogen activator (uPA) appears to play an important role. uPA and its downstream effector, plasminogen, increase within 1 to 5 minutes after partial hepatectomy and rapidly cleaves the HGF precursor, pro-HGF. Blocking uPA delays the appearance of HGF, thereby delaying liver regeneration, whereas blocking plasminogen-activator inhibitor (PAI) induces the release of HGF, thereby accelerating liver regeneration.[48]

## Maintaining Liver Function During Regeneration

For the patient, it is vital that the graft continues to function during regeneration. Several of the expressed early genes encode enzymes and proteins that are involved in regulating gluconeogenesis, a very important process after partial hepatectomy to compensate for the lost glycogen content and to produce sufficient glucose for the whole organism.[49,50] Liver-specific transcription factors (hepatocyte nuclear factors; HNF) have an important role in determining the level of glucose production, fatty acid metabolism, and liver-specific-secreted proteins. CAAT/enhancer binding protein (C/EBP)-α regulates expression of genes involved in hepatic glucose and lipid homeostasis, has antiproliferative proprieties and is down-regulated during liver regeneration after hepatectomy.[51,52] The C/EBP-β isoform is reported to be up-regulated and protects against hypoglycaemia.[53] In a microarray analysis of gene expression profiles after living donor liver transplantation, we recently demonstrated that C/EBP-α was down-regulated, as well as HNF-4α and the peroxisome proliferator receptor (PPAR)-α. Expression of many other liver-specific genes, such as IGFBP1, glucose 6-phosphatase, and α-fibrinogen, is regulated in the basal state by hepatic nuclear factor-1 (HNF1). The transcriptional activity of HNF1 is up-regulated during liver regeneration by

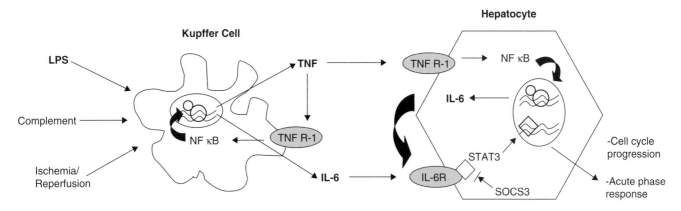

**FIGURE 28-3**

Activation of liver regeneration. After activation by LPS, complement, and I/R injury, Kupffer cells in the liver release TNF, leading to NFκB activation. NFκB regulates the transcription of many genes, including IL-6. IL-6 is secreted, binds to its receptor on hepatocytes, and activates STAT3, which activates genes involved in proliferation, the acute-phase response and its own inhibition (via SOCS3).

binding of HNF1 to the growth-induced transcription factors STAT3 and AP-1.[54] Together growth-induced and tissue-specific transcription factors enable the liver to maintain metabolic function, despite the loss of two thirds of its functional mass.

## Termination of Proliferation

The size of the liver is highly regulated and is controlled by the functional needs of the organism. The most well-known antiproliferative factors within the liver are TGF-β and related family members such as activin.[55] TGF-β is produced mainly by hepatic stellate cells and during liver regeneration hepatocytes initially become resistant to TGF-β.[13] This might be caused by the formation of inhibitory complexes of SNON and SKI with TGF-β.[56] These inhibitory complexes decrease after liver-mass restitution, increasing sensitivity to TGF-β again and returning the liver to a quiescent state. Similarly, activin A blocks hepatocyte mitogenesis and shows diminished signaling during liver regeneration when its cellular-receptor level is reduced. Its receptor level is restored once liver regeneration is terminated.[57] Suppressors of cytokine signaling (SOCS) are important negative regulators of cytokine signaling that prevent the tyrosine phosphorylation of STAT proteins. It has been shown that IL-6 signaling in the liver causes the rapid up-regulation of SOCS3, which correlates with the subsequent down-regulation of phosphorylated STAT3, thereby terminating the IL-6 signal.[58]

## THE ROLE OF THE IMMUNE SYSTEM IN LIVER REGENERATION

The (living donor) partial liver transplantation environment is unique in that the liver graft is simultaneously subjected to ischemia and reperfusion injury, metabolic stress, the need for regeneration of cell mass and the host immune response. Events early in the life of an allograft, such as significant I/R injury, may affect later graft function, allogenicity, and ultimately survival. In an experimental rat model of ischemic injury, prolonged preservation times were associated with significant up-regulation of the major histocompatibility complex (MHC) class II antigen expression and the co-stimulatory molecule B7.[1,59] Blocking of this co-stimulatory molecule with CTLA4Ig resulted in

decreased reperfusion injury.[60] Local injury and inflammation seem to act as a triggering signal and invoke a more active immune response,[61] findings confirmed in clinical studies in both kidney and liver transplantation, where a correlation between significant preservation injury and the amount of severe rejection over time was shown.[62] An increasing number of chemokines known to be involved in the alloimmune response, such as interferon-inducible protein 10 (IP-10), monokine induced by gamma interferon (MIG), and macrophage inflammatory protein 1 alpha (MIP-1α) are being recognized in liver injury and regeneration.[63] Our studies in mice indicate that compared to whole grafts, 50% partial liver grafts expressed highly induced levels of IP-10 and TCA-3 (chemokine (C–C motif) ligand 1, CCL1), with increased T-cell and neutrophil infiltration. Blocking TCA-3 expression reduced tissue injury, transaminase release, and decreased cell infiltration, demonstrating increased inflammatory response in partial grafts compared to whole liver grafts. Simultaneously, the regenerative response may be triggered by the same immune system: after reperfusion of the partial graft, increased concentrations of bacterial LPS in the portal system caused activation of the innate immune system via CD 14 (LPS receptor), and recently the importance of the Toll-like receptor (TLR)/myeloid differentiation factor (MyD88) pathway was shown.[64] This triggers activation of NFκB in the hepatic Kupffer cells, which results in production of IL-6. Thus, in this complex situation, the same cell signals that play an important role in the allograft response may also be pivotal to liver regeneration and inflammation. This implies that immunosuppression may have deleterious effects on cellular proliferation or recovery of the hepatocyte from injury. In fact, glucocorticoids, routinely used in immunosuppression protocols, have been shown to markedly inhibit cell-cycle progression in both partial hepatectomy models and in transplant models with ischemic injury.[65] Tacrolimus, a calcineurin inhibitor, is the mainstay of most immunosuppressive regimens. It is metabolized by the liver and the doses should be adjusted as various studies documented changes in pharmacokinetics and up to 25% higher trough levels.[66,67] Indeed, recipients of a partial liver graft were shown to need lower doses in the first 3 months after transplantation.[68] The effect of Cyclosporine on regeneration remains unclear, as it was shown not only to enhance proliferation in quiescent hepatocytes,[69] but also to inhibit liver regeneration after hepatectomy.[70] In an experimental transplantation model, no effect of Cyclosporine in the early postoperative phase was seen in whole or partial grafts.[71] Rapamycin (Sirolimus) is being used increasingly in liver transplant patients and may have significant effects on hepatocyte replication. It inhibits the activation of cyclin D1, thereby preventing progression through G1 and entry into the DNA-synthesis phase of the cell cycle.[72] It functions through the inhibition of target of rapamycin (TOR)—an important regulator of protein translation, ribosome synthesis, and the cell-growth machinery—which might have a significant role in cell-cycle transition.[73]

## DONOR AND RECIPIENT FACTORS INFLUENCING LIVER REGENERATION

After partial liver transplantation there is a delicate balance between regeneration and sustaining adequate metabolic needs. Numerous outside influences may interfere with this balance and may result in significant graft dysfunction, failure, or patient death. Donor age, steatosis, and ischemic injury have been shown to have a significant effect on liver regeneration in both experimental and clinical settings. The effect of the graft size and viral status of the donor on regeneration remain unclear.

### Donor Age

Older livers do not regenerate as quickly as younger livers, and show delayed regeneration after acute injury. Rodent models have shown reduced and delayed DNA-synthesizing capacity,[74] and a clinical study showed a greater graft/standard liver volume in the young donor livers compared with middle-age and older donor grafts.[75] In the transplantation setting, older grafts have poorer long-term survival when combined with longer cold ischemic times. Some early statistics from the United Network for Organ Sharing (UNOS) database show that the graft survival using older adult living donor grafts (more than 44 years) have inferior outcome compared to younger living donor grafts.[76] It is unclear if this is because of a decreased ability of older livers to regenerate while maintaining metabolic support and repair ischemic injury. It must be emphasized that age may affect the regeneration and recovery of the living donor as well as the recipient. Many liver programs limit the upper age limit of the donor, and although no definite age has been specified, 55 to 60 years old is a generally accepted upper age limit.

### Steatosis

In the prereplicative phase of rodent liver regeneration after partial hepatectomy, fatty infiltration of the remnant lobes occurs. Although this phenomenon has been observed for decades,[77] it has received renewed interest lately, as hepatic steatosis is becoming a more prevalent human disease[78] and potential donors with a body mass index of > 28 have a 78% chance of more than 10% steatosis.[79] Numerous animal studies have shown marked impairment of regeneration in steatotic livers, as well as the inability to tolerate warm ischemic injury,[80] findings that correlate with the decreased survival of patients with steatotic livers following resection[81] and in clinical transplantation setting.[82] Selzner examined the effects of steatosis on liver regeneration in a rat model of obese and normal Zucker rats.[80] They reported delayed and impaired onset of mitosis and increased mortality rate in obese rats with steatosis. IL-6 partially rescued this defect by normalizing hepatocyte entry into G1

but failed to improve subsequent S- and M-phase progression. This study suggests that steatosis impairs normal liver regeneration at multiple steps in the regenerative cycle. Although deceased donor grafts with severe macrovesicular steatosis should therefore not be used, those with less than 30% macro or microvesicular steatosis can be transplanted with immediate and long-term results similar to that of organs without fat.[83,84] Marcos showed that the function of right-lobe-living donor grafts with up to 30% steatosis did not differ from fat-free grafts, and regeneration seemed not to be impaired,[85] but many living donor programs will not use grafts with greater than 10% to 20% steatosis, and some centers will not accept any amount of steatosis in living donor grafts. Experimental data have shown that normal fat metabolism plays an important role in the regenerative phase after liver resection and help rather than hinder regeneration. Peroxisome proliferator-activated receptor α (PPAR-α), which regulates hepatic lipid turnover in rodents, appears to be necessary for normal liver regeneration.[86] Mice in which the normal accumulation of fat was prevented had a profound deficit in hepatocyte proliferation, suggesting that fat accumulation may serve as a fuelling source for the energy needed by the regeneration process.[87,88] Steatohepatitis (inflammation of the liver in the setting of fatty infiltration) carries an even greater risk and should be considered as a contraindication for donation. In those livers, lipid accumulation is associated with hepatocyte mitochondrial damage and abnormalities in cytochrome p450 induction. This is caused by free radical injury from abnormal fatty acid oxidation and accumulation of dicarboxylic fatty acids during intermediary metabolism. Both donors and recipients would be at risk in this setting, from liver failure and hepatocyte apoptosis.

### Ischemic Injury

Animal studies have shown impaired regeneration when massive hepatectomy is combined with warm ischemic injury.[89] Ischemic injury, both warm and cold, is an unavoidable component of transplantation, although ischemic injury in AALDLT is minimized by careful planning of the donor and recipient procedures. After prolonged cold ischemia of whole liver grafts, there is initiation of the cell-cycle pathways with upregulation of markers of liver regeneration. The more extensive the ischemic injury, the greater the expression and activation of cytokines, transcription factors and immediate early genes and the greater the magnitude of hepatocellular replication.[21] However, the liver can only tolerate ischemic injury up to a certain point, after which the damage is too extensive, and the graft is unable to maintain functional homeostasis and regenerative capabilities.[9] Using animal models of partial liver graft transplantation, investigators have studied the interplay between the regenerative response and the ischemic injury in the setting of 50% and 30% size partial liver grafts. The partial grafts showed a robust regenerative response if the ischemic injury was minimal, where 30% grafts showed an optimal regeneration after a 1-hour cold ischemic period.[90] Therefore, theoretically, there could be an advantage in ischemic preconditioning of the graft, as it was shown to improve liver function after liver resection.[91] However, it is apparent that when rodent partial grafts are subjected to ischemic injury of more than 10 hours, there is a significant effect on survival, with extensive hepatic necrosis, the inability to initiate or maintain the regenerative response, and decreased survival.[92] Recently Debonera demonstrated in the same model that in this situation the IL-6 / STAT3 pathway is activated, but progression of the cell cycle fails.[93] The clinical impact of CI has been demonstrated in a multicenter report of AALDLT, where every hour of additional CI added a significant risk of graft loss.[94]

## Graft Size

The amount of liver mass transplanted has been shown to be an important variable after transplantation. Early experimental studies addressing regeneration after transplantation show that a small-for-size graft will adapt to its environment and achieve a size equal to the original native liver. It must be emphasized that the state of the recipient is an important component in determining appropriate liver volume. As seen in experimental models, the accumulation of additional stressful stimuli, such as sepsis or renal failure, may push a relatively small graft into failure. Patients with fulminant hepatic failure and those with significant metabolic stress may require more liver volume than stable patients undergoing transplantation under elective conditions.[95] Although it has been performed successfully, many centers are not performing LDLT in acutely ill patients with fulminant failure because of the uncertainty of knowing whether a partial graft is enough volume to support the recovery of such a recipient. In rodents and humans there is a relationship between liver growth and body mass. In rodents, removal of up to 30% is not sufficient to cause a synchronized wave of hepatocyte proliferation, although the liver eventually regains its mass. In resections involving the removal of 40% to 70% of the liver, there is a linear relationship between the amount of tissue resected and the extent of hepatocyte proliferation,[4] but resections >70% result in increased mortality. It has been demonstrated that in mice a 30% hepatectomy elicits the priming reaction, but fails to induce cell-cycle progression.[96] In liver transplantation in animals and humans, there are also limits to the growth capacity of small transplants, so that transplanted livers that represent less than 0.8% of body mass may fail to grow or function properly, resulting in "small-for-size syndrome" and severe morbidity and high mortality. Data obtained from experiments in rodents may be relevant to this problem. We refer to chapter 30.6 for more detailed reading about the small-for-size problem.

## Hepatitis C

The processes of viral replication, alloimmune response, metabolic function, and cancer recurrence have all been correlated with cellular replication. Because the majority of liver transplant patients have hepatitis C, it is important to know if this vigorous regenerative response in the partial graft has a significant effect on the kinetics of viral replication in hepatitis C virus (HCV) positive individuals. Early results suggested that recipients of living-donor liver transplants may have an earlier and more severe recurrence of HCV when compared with recipients of whole cadaveric liver grafts [97,98]; however, this has not been confirmed in other studies.[99–101] Investigators have noted that HCV RNA replication is enhanced in proliferating cells, suggesting that viral replication is regulated by cell-cycle-dependent factors. Because the primary target cell for HCV replication *in vivo* is the hepatocyte, events that lead to hepatocyte proliferation may enhance HCV replication. Alternatively, HCV core proteins have been shown to have significant interaction with cellular promoters and regulators of cell growth, which may affect liver regeneration.

## Other Factors

There is a small array of clinical and experimental evidence that several other factors may influence the regenerative response after transplantation. In addition to the reduced cell mass of the graft itself, portal blood flow dynamics are altered and the graft is subjected to increased portal flow and pressure. The significance of this situation is unclear: increased portal flow is associated with increased recovery,[102] but increased portal pressure is associated with the so-called small-for-size syndrome, which is discussed in detail in chapter 26.6.[103,104] Poor hepatic venous drainage has been shown to inhibit regeneration and segments with poor venous drainage become atrophied with time. Female gender may have a positive effect on regeneration of partial grafts in murine models, but no human study has confirmed this finding.

## CLINICAL PRACTICE AND FUTURE PERSPECTIVES

### Clinical Practice

After living donor liver transplantation, the regenerative process remains difficult to follow in a systemic fashion. In living donor transplantation from adult to children, the graft is usually the appropriate size and grows gradually with the child. In AALDLT, most liver regeneration occurs in the first few weeks after resection or transplantation, and the time course does not appear to differ significantly in donors or recipients, according to MRI volumetry. Interestingly, Humar showed in the human partial liver transplantation setting that liver mass was restored to 120%, 114%, and 104% in recipients of a left lobe split liver, right lobe split liver, and right lobe living donor graft, respectively. In contrast, the right lobe living donors had attained only 79% of their ideal liver weight at 3 months postoperatively.[105] The hepatic function tests of the donors usually recover within the first postoperative week.[85] However, in our experience we see a slightly prolonged time to normalization of hyperbilirubinemia and hypoalbuminemia in the recipients of a partial graft, compared to recipients of a whole graft, which is in accordance with the decreased metabolic function in partial grafts during the first period of regeneration. Conventional clinical blood tests and liver biopsy are inadequate measures to really monitor hepatic regeneration, and bilirubin, albumin, prothrombin time, and platelet count only become abnormal in advanced failure. In the search for new minimally invasive liver function tests to identify failing regeneration at an earlier time point, indocyanine green monitoring, methionine breath tests, cholate clearance, and liver single-photon remission computed tomography scans are now correlated with liver volume and other donor and recipient variables. Also, serum TGF—levels have been used for evaluating regeneration after hepatectomy,[106] although not routinely used. The elucidation of serum biomarkers for liver regeneration is a goal of clinical researchers in this area.

### Future Perspectives

As we continue to expand the criteria and use more marginal donor grafts, as well as increase the use of living donor grafts, the ability of the liver to activate cell-cycle pathways and initiate regeneration becomes exceedingly important. In addition, it is becoming increasingly apparent that there is a close relation among the inflammatory response induced by I/R injury, the immune response, and regeneration. If liver regeneration could be enhanced, and inflammation controlled, still smaller grafts could be used. Recently, Fausto showed that cell proliferation can be induced by a single injection of HB-EGF.[96] Other data demonstrated that the high mortality occurring in mice after 85% hepatectomy could be greatly improved by blockage of the receptor for advanced glycation end products (RAGE). Blockage of RAGE in these animals increased TNF and IL-6 production, enhanced the expression of the anti-inflammatory cytokine IL-10, increased NFkB activation, and increased hepatocyte DNA replication.[107] In experimental models of acute liver failure[108] and the use of severely steatotic donors,[109] administration of IL-6 showed marked improvement in regeneration and survival, but so far no reports of the use of rIL-6 in the human situation were published. In the future, administration of rIL-6 may prove to be beneficial in promoting regeneration of small or steatotic grafts. Increased interest in nutrition and biochemical interventions may support the metabolic demands during regeneration, as addition of essential purines, pyrimidines, glucose, and adenosine to (intravenous) nutrition may relieve the graft from energy-costing processes and enable faster growth ("regenutrition"), especially in critically ill patients. Combinations of HB-EGF, TGF , and HGF may provide the stimuli necessary for hepatocyte survival and proliferation. Although some of these applications may still be far in the future, we should start to translate our experimental knowledge on liver regeneration into new treatment strategies. Recently, the NIH-sponsored Adult to Adult Living Donor Liver Transplant (A2ALL) multicenter study started in nine transplant centers of excellence to investigate outcomes in donors and recipients after AALDLT.[94] An important aim of this long-term study is to characterize the process of liver regeneration and function in donors and recipients of LD grafts and compare to processes within DD grafts. Hopefully clinical insights can be gained into factors that may enhance or inhibit human liver regeneration.

# References

1. Ponfick VA. Ueber Leberresection und Leberreaction. *Verhandl Deutsch Gessellsch Chir* 1890;19:28.
2. Hardy KJ. Liver surgery: the past 2000 years. *Aust N Z J Surg* 1990; 60(10):811–817.
3. Fausto N, Webber EM. Liver regeneration. The Liver: *Biol Pathobiol* 1994:1059–1084.
4. Bucher NLR. Regeneration of mammalian liver. *Int Rev Cytol* 1963; 15:245–300.
5. Gaub J, Iversen J. Rat liver regeneration after 90% partial hepatectomy. *Hepatology* 1984;4(5):902–904.
6. Van Thiel DH, Gavaler JS, Kam I, et al. Rapid growth of an intact human liver transplanted into a recipient larger than the donor. *Gastroenterology* 1987;93(6):1414–1419.
7. Fausto N. Liver regeneration: From laboratory to clinic. *Liver Transplant* 2001;7(10):835–844.
8. Diehl AM. Cytokine regulation of liver injury and repair. *Immunol Rev* 2000;174:160–171.
9. Olthoff KM. Molecular pathways of regeneration and repair after liver transplantation. *World J Surg* 2002;26(7):831–837.
10. Mann DV, Lam WW, Hjelm NM, et al. Metabolic control patterns in acute phase and regenerating human liver determined in vivo by 31-phosphorus magnetic resonance spectroscopy. *Ann Surg* 2002;235(3): 408–416.
11. Fausto N, Riehle KJ. Mechanisms of liver regeneration and their clinical implications. *J Hepato-Biliary-Pancreatic Surg* 2005;12(3):181–189.
12. Taub R. Liver regeneration: from myth to mechanism. *Nat Rev Mol Cell Biol* 2004; 5(10):836–847.
13. Koniaris LG, McKillop IH, Schwartz SI, Zimmers TA. Liver regeneration. *J Am Coll Surg* 2003;197(4):634–659.
14. Higgins GM, Anderson RM. Experimental pathology of the liver. I. Restoration of the liver of the white rat following partial surgical removal. *Arch Pathol* 1931;12:186–202.
15. Kaplowitz N. Biochemical and cellular mechanisms of toxic liver injury. Seminars in *Liver Dis* 2002;22(2):137–144.
16. Reynolds ES. Liver parenchymal cell injury. I. Initial alterations of the cell following poisoning with carbon tetrachloride. *J Cell Biol* 1963; 19:139–157.
17. Dabeva MD, Shafritz DA. Activation, proliferation, and differentiation of progenitor cells into hepatocytes in the D-galactosamine model of liver regeneration. *Am J Pathol* 1993;143(6):1606–1620.
18. Kountouras J, Billing BH, Scheuer PJ. Prolonged bile duct obstruction: A new experimental model for cirrhosis in the rat. *Brit J Exp Pathol* 1984;65(3):305–311.
19. Bilodeau M, Aubry MC, Houle R, et al. Evaluation of hepatocyte injury following partial ligation of the left portal vein. *J Hepatol* 1999;30(1):29–37.
20. Jaeschke H. Mechanisms of reperfusion injury after warm ischemia of the liver. *J Hepato-Biliary-Pancr Surg* 1998;5(4):402–408.
21. Debonera F, Aldeguer X, Shen X, et al. Activation of interleukin-6/STAT3 and liver regeneration following transplantation. *J Surg Res* 2001;96(2):289–295.
22. Gressner AM. Cytokines and cellular crosstalk involved in the activation of fat-storing cells. *J Hepatol* 1995;22(2 Suppl):28–36.
23. Bucher NLR, Swaffield MN. The rate of incorporation of labeled thymidine into the deoxyribonucleic acid of regenerating rat liver in relation to the amount of liver excised. *Cancer Res* 1964;24:1611–1625.
24. Grisham JW. Cellular proliferation in the liver. *Rec Results Cancer Res* 1969;17:28–43.
25. Widmann JJ, Fahimi HD. Proliferation of mononuclear phagocytes (Kupffer cells) and endothelial cells in regenerating rat liver. A light and electron microscopic cytochemical study. *Am J Pathol* 1975; 80(3):349–366.
26. Rabes HM, Wirsching R, Tuczek HV, Iseler G. Analysis of cell cycle compartments of hepatocytes after partial hepatecomy. *Cell Tissue Kinet* 1976;9(6):517–532.
27. Stocker E, Heine WD. Regeneration of liver parenchyma under normal and pathological conditions. *Beitr Pathol* 1971;144(4):400–408.
28. Fausto N, Campbell JS. The role of hepatocytes and oval cells in liver regeneration and repopulation. *Mech Devel* 2003;120(1):117–130.
29. Roskams T, De Vos R, Van Eyken P, et al. Hepatic OV-6 expression in human liver disease and rat experiments: Evidence for hepatic progenitor cells in man. *J Hepatol* 1998;29(3):455–463.
30. Lemire JM, Shiojiri N, Fausto N. Oval cell proliferation and the origin of small hepatocytes in liver injury induced by D-galactosamine. *Am J Pathol* 1991;139(3):535–552.
31. Theise ND, Saxena R, Portmann BC, et al. The canals of Hering and hepatic stem cells in humans. *Hepatology* 1999;30(6):1425–1433.
32. Kofman AV, Morgan G, Kirschenbaum A, et al. Dose- and time-dependent oval cell reaction in acetaminophen-induced murine liver injury. *Hepatology* 2005;41(6):1252–1261.
33. Taub R, Greenbaum LE, Peng Y. Transcriptional regulatory signals define cytokine-dependent and - independent pathways in liver regeneration. *Seminars Liver Dis* 1999;19(2):117–128.
34. Haber BA, Mohn KL, Diamond RH, Taub R. Induction patterns of 70 genes during nine days after hepatectomy define the temporal course of liver regeneration. *J Clin Invest* 1993;91(4):1319–1326.
35. Su AI, Guidotti LG, Pezacki JP, et al. Gene expression during the priming phase of liver regeneration after partial hepatectomy in mice. *Proc Natl Acad Sci USA* 2002;99(17):11181–11186.
36. Arai M, Yokosuka O, Chiba T, et al. Gene expression profiling reveals the mechanism and pathophysiology of mouse liver regeneration. *J Biol Chem* 2003;278(32):29813–29818.
37. Starzl TE, Porter KA, Francavilla JA, et al. A hundred years of the hepatotrophic controversy. *Ciba Found Symp* 1977;(55):111–129.
38. Moolten FL, Bucher NL. Regeneration of rat liver: transfer of humoral agent by cross circulation. *Science* 1967;158(798):272–274.
39. Yamada Y, Kirillova I, Fausto N, Peschon JJ. Initiation of liver growth by tumor necrosis factor: Deficient liver regeneration in mice lacking type I tumor necrosis factor receptor. *Proc Nat Acad Sci USA* 1997; 94(4):1441–1446.

40. Cressman DE, Greenbaum LE, DeAngelis RA, et al. Liver failure and defective hepatocyte regeneration in interleukin-6- deficient mice. *Science* 1996;274(5291):1379–1383.

41. Fujita J, Marino MW, Wada H, et al. Effect of TNF gene depletion on liver regeneration after partial hepatectomy in mice. *Surgery* 2001; 129(1):48–54.

42. Michalopoulos G, Houck KA, Dolan ML, Leutteke NC. Control of hepatocyte replication by two serum factors. *Cancer Res* 1984;44(10): 4414–4419.

43. Fausto N. Liver regeneration. *J Hepatol* 2000;32(SUPPL.1):19–31.

44. Webber EM, Fausto N, Godowski PJ. In vivo response of hepatocytes to growth factors requires an initial priming stimulus. *Hepatology* 1994; 19(2):489–497.

45. Aldeguer X, Debonera F, Shaked A, et al. Interleukin-6 from intrahepatic cells of bone marrow origin is required for normal murine liver regeneration. *Hepatology* 2002; 35(1):40–48.

46. Cornell RP, Liljequist BL, Bartizal KF. Depressed liver regeneration after partial hepatectomy of germ-free, athymic and lipopolysaccharide-resistant mice. *Hepatology* 1990;11(6):916–922.

47. Strey CW, Markiewski M, Mastellos D, et al. The proinflammatory mediators C3a and C5a are essential for liver regeneration. *J Exp Med* 2003;198(6):913–923.

48. Currier AR, Sabla G, Locaputo S, et al. Plasminogen directs the pleiotropic effects of uPA in liver injury and repair. *Am J Physiol Gastrointest Liver Physiol* 2003;284(3):G508–G515.

49. Haber BA, Chin S, Chuang E, et al. High levels of glucose-6-phosphatase gene and protein expression reflect an adaptive response in proliferating liver and diabetes. *J Clin Invest* 1995;95(2):832–841.

50. Rosa JL, Bartrons R, Tauler A. Gene expression of regulatory enzymes of glycolysis/gluconeogenesis in regenerating rat liver. *Biochem J* 1992; 287(Pt 1):113–116.

51. Mischoulon D, Rana B, Bucher NL, Farmer SR. Growth-dependent inhibition of CCAAT enhancer-binding protein (C/EBP alpha) gene expression during hepatocyte proliferation in the regenerating liver and in culture. *Mol Cell Biol* 1992;12(6):2553–2560.

52. Costa RH, Kalinichenko VV, Holterman AX, Wang X. Transcription factors in liver development, differentiation, and regeneration. *Hepatology* 2003;38(6):1331–1347.

53. Greenbaum LE, Cressman DE, Haber BA, Taub R. Coexistence of C/EBP alpha, beta, growth-induced proteins and DNA synthesis in hepatocytes during liver regeneration. Implications for maintenance of the differentiated state during liver growth. *J Clin Invest* 1995;96(3):1351–1365.

54. Leu JI, Crissey MA, Leu JP, et al. Interleukin-6-induced STAT3 and AP-1 amplify hepatocyte nuclear factor 1-mediated transactivation of hepatic genes, an adaptive response to liver injury. *Mol Cell Biol* 2001;21(2):414–424.

55. Derynck R, Zhang YE. Smad-dependent and Smad-independent pathways in TGF-beta family signalling. *Nature* 2003;425(6958): 577–584.

56. Macías-Silva M, Li W, Leu JI, et al. Up-regulated transcriptional repressors SnoN and Ski bind smad proteins to antagonize transforming growth factor-? signals during liver regeneration. *J Biolog Chem* 2002;277(32):28483–28490.

57. Date M, Matsuzaki K, Matsushita M, et al. Differential regulation of activin A for hepatocyte growth and fibronectin synthesis in rat liver injury. *J Hepatol* 2000;32(2):251–60.

58. Campbell JS, Prichard L, Schaper F, et al. Expression of suppressors of cytokine signaling during liver regeneration. *J Clin Invest* 2001;107(10):1285–1292.

59. Takada M, Chandraker A, Nadeau KC, et al. The role of the B7 costimulatory pathway in experimental cold ischemia/reperfusion injury. *J Clin Invest* 1997;100(5):1199–1203.

60. Olthoff KM, Da Chen X, Gelman A, et al. Adenovirus-mediated gene transfer of CTLA4Ig to liver allografts results in prolonged survival and local T-cell anergy. *Transplant Proc* 1997;29(1-2):1030–1031.

61. Matzinger P. Tolerance, danger, and the extended family. *Annu Rev Immunol* 1994;12:991–1045.

62. Howard TK, Klintmalm GB, Cofer JB, et al. The influence of preservation injury on rejection in the hepatic transplant recipient. *Transplantation* 1990;49(1):103–107.

63. Koniaris LG, Zimmers-Koniaris T, Hsiao EC, et al. Cytokine-responsive gene-2/IFN-inducible protein-10 expression in multiple models of liver and bile duct injury suggests a role in tissue regeneration. *J Immunol* 2001;167(1):399–406.

64. Seki E, Tsutsui H, Iimuro Y, et al. Contribution of Toll-like receptor/myeloid differentiation factor 88 signaling to murine liver regeneration. *Hepatology* 2005;41(3):443–450.

65. Debonera F, Krasinkas AM, Gelman AE, et al. Dexamethasone inhibits early regenerative response of rat liver after cold preservation and transplantation. *Hepatology* 2003;38(6):1563–1572.

66. Troisi R, Militerno G, Hoste E, et al. Are reduced tacrolimus dosages needed in the early postoperative period following living donor liver transplantation in adults? *Transplant Proc* 2002;34(5):1531–1532.

67. Trotter JF, Stolpman N, Wachs M, et al. Living donor liver transplant recipients achieve relatively higher immunosuppressant blood levels than cadaveric recipients. *Liver Transplant* 2002;8(3): 212–218.

68. Taber DJ, Dupuis RE, Fann AL, et al. Tacrolimus dosing requirements and concentrations in adult living donor liver transplant recipients. *Liver Transplant* 2002; 8(3):219–223.

69. Dos Reis GA, Shevach EM. Effect of cyclosporin A on T cell function in vitro: The mechanism of suppression of T cell proliferation depends on the nature of the T cell stimulus as well as the differentiation state of the responding T cell. *J Immunol* 1982;129(6): 2360–2367.

70. Yokomuro K, Miyahara S, Takahashi H, Kimura Y. Regeneration and the immune system. II. Suppressor activities of lymphocytes activated in vivo by liver regeneration and their genetic control. *Eur J Immunol* 1983;13(11):883–889.

71. Alvira LG, Herrera N, Salas C, et al. Influence of cyclosporine on graft regeneration and function after liver transplantation: trial in pigs. *Transplant Proc* 2002;34(1):315–316.

72. Nelsen CJ, Rickheim DG, Tucker MM, et al. Evidence that cyclin D1 mediates both growth and proliferation downstream of TOR in hepatocytes. *J Biol Chem* 2003;278(6):3656–3663.

73. Francavilla A, Carr BI, Starzl TE, et al. Effects of rapamycin on cultured hepatocyte proliferation and gene expression. *Hepatology* 1992; 15(5):871–877.

74. Taguchi T, Fukuda M, Ohashi M. Differences in DNA synthesis in vitro using isolated nuclei from regenerating livers of young and aged rats. *Mech Ageing Dev* 2001;122(2):141–155.

75. Ikegami T, Nishizaki T, Yanaga K, et al. The impact of donor age on living donor liver transplantation. *Transplantation* 2000;70(12): 1703–1707.

76. Abt PL, Mange KC, Olthoff KM, et al. Allograft Survival Following Adult-to-Adult Living Donor Liver Transplantation. *Am J Transplant* 2004;4(8):1302–1307.

77. Murray AB, Strecker W, Silz S. Ultrastructural changes in rat hepatocytes after partial hepatectomy, and comparison with biochemical results. *J Cell Sci* 1981;50:433–448.

78. Lonardo A. Fatty liver and nonalcoholic steatohepatitis. Where do we stand and where are we going? *Dig Dis* 1999;17(2):80–89.

79. Rinella ME, Alonso E, Rao S, et al. Body mass index as as a predictor of hepatic steatosis in living liver donors. *Liver Transplant* 2001;7(5): 409–414.

80. Selzner M, Clavien P-A. Failure of regeneration of the steatotic rat liver: Disruption at two different levels in the regeneration pathway. *Hepatology* 2000;31(1):35–42.

81. Behrns KE, Tsiotos GG, Nagorney DM, et al. Hepatic Steatosis as a Potential Risk Factor for Major Hepatic Resection. *J Gastroint Surg* 1998;2(3):292–298.

82. Todo S, Demetris AJ, Makowka L, et al. Primary nonfunction of hepatic allografts with preexisting fatty infiltration. *Transplantation* 1989; 47(5):903–905.

83. Fishbein TM, Fiel MI, Emre S, et al. Use of livers with microvesicular fat safely expands the donor pool. *Transplantation* 1997;64(2): 248–251.

84. Urena MA, Moreno Gonzalez E, Romero CJ, et al. An approach to the rational use of steatotic donor livers in liver transplantation. *Hepatogastroenterology* 1999;46(26):1164–1173.

85. Marcos A, Fisher RA, Ham JM, et al. Liver regeneration and function in donor and recipient after right lobe adult to adult living donor liver transplantation. *Transplantation* 2000;69(7):1375–1379.

86. Anderson SP, Yoon L, Richard EB, et al. Delayed liver regeneration in peroxisome proliferator-activated receptor-alpha-null mice. *Hepatology* 2002;36(3):544–554.

87. Shteyer E, Liao Y, Muglia LJ, et al. Disruption of hepatic adipogenesis is associated with impaired liver regeneration in mice. *Hepatology* 2004; 40(6):1322–1332.

88. Farrell GC. Probing Prometheus: fat fueling the fire? *Hepatology* 2004; 40(6):1252–1255.

89. Selzner M, Camargo CA, Clavien P-A. Ischemia impairs liver regeneration after major tissue loss in rodents: Protective effects of interleukin-6. *Hepatology* 1999;30(2):469–475.

90. Selzner N, Selzner M, Tian Y, et al. Cold ischemia decreases liver regeneration after partial liver transplantation in the rat: A TNF-?/IL-6-dependent mechanism. *Hepatology* 2002;36(4 I):812–818.

91. Clavien PA, Selzner M, Rudiger HA, et al. A prospective randomized study in 100 consecutive patients undergoing major liver resection with versus without ischemic preconditioning. *Ann Surg* 2003;238(6): 843–850; discussion 851–852.

92. Debonera F, Que X, Aldeguer X, et al. Partial liver grafts with prolonged cold preservation initiate blunted regenerative responses. *Am J Transplant* 2002;2(Supp l3):156.

93. Debonera F, Wang G, Xie J, et al. Severe Preservation Injury Induces Il-6/STAT3 Activation with Lack of Cell Cycle Progression After Partial Liver Graft Transplantation. *Am J Transplant* 2004;4(12): 1964–1971.

94. Olthoff KM, Merion RM, Ghobrial RM, et al. Outcomes of 385 adult-to-adult living donor liver transplant recipients: a report from the A2ALL Consortium. *Ann Surg* 2005;242(3):314–323, discussion 323–325.

95. Lo C-M, Fan S-T, Liu C-L, et al. Minimum graft size for successful living donor liver transplantation. *Transplantation* 1999;68(8):1112–1116.

96. Mitchell C, Nivison M, Jackson LF, et al. Heparin-binding epidermal growth factor-like growth factor links hepatocyte priming with cell cycle progression during liver regeneration. *J Biol Chem* 2005; 280(4): 2562–2568.

97. Gaglio PJ, Malireddy S, Levitt BS, et al. Increased risk of cholestatic hepatitis C in recipients of grafts from living versus cadaveric liver donors. *Liver Transplant* 2003;9(10):1028–1035.

98. Garcia-Retortillo M, Forns X, Llovet JM, et al. Hepatitis C recurrence is more severe after living donor compared to cadaveric liver transplantation. *Hepatology* 2004;40(3):699–707.

99. Russo MW, Galanko J, Beavers K, et al. Patient and graft survival in hepatitis C recipients after adult living donor liver transplantation in the United States. *Liver Transplant* 2004;10(3):340–346.

100. Shiffman ML, Stravitz RT, Contos MJ, et al. Histologic recurrence of chronic hepatitis C virus in patients after living donor and deceased donor liver transplantation. *Liver Transplant* 2004;10(10):1248–1255.

101. Humar A, Horn K, Kalis A, et al. Living Donor and Split-Liver Transplants in Hepatitis C Recipients: Does Liver Regeneration Increase the Risk for Recurrence? *Am J Transplant* 2005;5(2): 399–405.

102. Eguchi S, Yanaga K, Sugiyama N, et al. Relationship between portal venous flow and liver regeneration in patients after living donor right-lobe liver transplantation. *Liver Transplant* 2003;9(6): 547–551.

103. Yagi S, Iida T, Taniguchi K, et al. Impact of portal venous pressure on regeneration and graft damage after living-donor liver transplantation. *Liver Transpl* 2005;11(1):68–75.

104. Troisi R, Cammu G, Militerno G, et al. Modulation of portal graft inflow: a necessity in adult living-donor liver transplantation? *Ann Surg* 2003;237(3):429–436.

105. Humar A, Kosari K, Sielaff TD, et al. Liver regeneration after adult living donor and deceased donor split-liver transplants. *Liver Transplant* 2004;10(3):374–378.

106. Tomiya T, Hayashi S, Yanase M, et al. Serum transforming growth factor-alpha level can be a parameter for evaluating liver regeneration after partial hepatectomy in patients with liver cancer. *Semin Oncol* 1997;24(2 Suppl 6):S6-14–S6-17.

107. Cataldegirmen G, Zeng S, Feirt N, et al. RAGE limits regeneration after massive liver injury by coordinated suppression of TNF-alpha and NF-kappaB. *J Exp Med* 2005;201(3):473–484.

108. Hecht N, Pappo O, Shouval D, et al. Hyper-IL-6 gene therapy reverses fulminant hepatic failure. Mol Ther 2001; 3(5 Pt 1):683–7.

109. Gao B. Therapeutic potential of interleukin-6 in preventing obesity- and alcohol-associated fatty liver transplant failure. Alcohol 2004; 34(1):59–65.

# CHAPTER 29

# LIVING DONOR LIVER TRANSPLANTATION: THE DONOR

## 29.1 SELECTION AND WORKUP

*Abhinav Humar, MD, Cheryl Jacobs, MS, LICSW, Ann Kalis, RN*

### INTRODUCTION

The evaluation of individuals who present as possible liver donors is a crucial part of the living donor liver transplant (LDLT) process. A complete and thorough evaluation is important in minimizing the risks of the procedure for the potential donor and optimizing donor safety—the underlying principal of any living donor procedure.[1] The predonation evaluation of the potential donor, and characterization of the subsequent liver graft that they may yield, is also critical in ensuring a successful outcome for the recipient. The evaluation process may vary between donors, depending on whether the recipient is an adult or pediatric patient, the size of the planned liver resection, and the individual center's preference. But, the major steps of the process basically remain the same and essentially can be divided into three major parts: (1) medical evaluation, (2) surgical or radiologic evaluation, and (3) psychosocial evaluation. The potential donor should satisfy each of the three parts of this evaluation process before being considered an acceptable donor. The evaluation process should, at the same time as being complete, not be overly cumbersome for the donor: it should be streamlined and efficient, invasive tests should be minimized, and the process should be cost-effective.

Members of multiple teams need to be involved in the evaluation process. This should include hepatologist, surgeon, psychologist, social worker, and transplant coordinator. This chapter also includes sections from the latter two team members, who offer their unique perspective on their role in the evaluation process.

### MEDICAL EVALUATION

The medical evaluation of the potential donor has several goals and attempts to answer several important questions. One important goal is to ensure that the donor does not have underlying medical problems that would significantly increase the risk associated with a general anesthetic and a major intra-abdominal procedure. This part of the evaluation is not too dissimilar from the evaluation for any individual undergoing a major general surgical procedure. The other important part of the medical evaluation serves to identify and exclude any possibility of chronic liver disease or liver dysfunction in the potential donor. This includes the screening for viral pathogens that may impact on the donor's liver function or could potentially be significantly harmful when transmitted to the recipient.

The exact nature of the tests performed and their order will vary from center to center.[2] In principle, one should try to limit the number of invasive investigations and reserve them for the later part of the evaluation. In an effort to limit the cost associated with an evaluation, more expensive tests should generally be performed later in the evaluation process, after donors have passed through the initial screening process.

Perhaps the most useful part of the evaluation is the initial screening history—this may be performed by an experienced transplant coordinator (a phone interview is adequate), or the donor is asked to fill out a one- to two-page information sheet. Questions regarding age; height; weight; blood type (if known); past and current medical, surgical, or psychosocial problems (including a history of alcohol use); and current medication use are very useful. Donors with a significant past medical history, obese donors, and those with significant co-morbidities can be excluded with the screening history, thus avoiding a detailed and expensive evaluation process. Age is an important variable to determine at the initial screening, and potential donors falling outside the centers accepted age criteria could be excluded early. There is insufficient live donor liver data at present to define an upper age limit for donation. Many centers have chosen 55 years of age as the upper limit of acceptability, but potential donors have been considered by some centers up to the age of 60. Based on data from the general surgical literature and experimental regeneration data, the limit of 60 has been considered appropriate. The lower limit of age for donation is determined by the ability to give legal consent.

After the initial screening history, basic screening labs should be performed—all of these can be performed at a laboratory that is physically closest to the potential donor. Tests to be included are complete blood count, serum electrolyte levels, liver function tests, lipid profile, and blood type.[3] Based then on the results of the screening history and screening labs, the potential donor can be brought into the transplant center for a more thorough evaluation.

The next part of the evaluation begins with a careful history and physical examination by a physician. Some feel that a physician who is not directly involved with the transplant team, and can, therefore, provide an unbiased opinion, without knowledge of the potential recipient, should perform the examination. Individuals identified with significant underlying disorders of the cardiac, respiratory, or renal systems should be excluded from donation. Individuals with underlying risk factors for specific organ systems (eg, age > 40 and positive family history for cardiac disease) may require specialist consultation and more specific tests (eg, echocardiogram or stress test). More detailed laboratory tests should also be performed during this part of the evaluation. This should include detailed viral serologic evaluation (Hep C, Hep B, cytomegalovirus [CMV], Epstein–Barr virus [EBV], and human immunodeficiency virus [HIV]), screening for thrombophilia disorders (protein C, protein S, antithrombin III, factor V Leiden mutation, prothrombin mutation, and cardiolipid/antiphospholipids antibodies) and tests to exclude underlying chronic liver diseases (serum transferrin saturation, ferratin, α-1-antitrypsin antinuclear antibody, smooth muscle antibody, and antimitochondrial antibody). Other tests that should be performed at this initial visit include electrocardiography, chest radiography, and pulmonary function tests (if history of smoking or asthma). Additional laboratory tests and imaging studies may be needed based on abnormalities identified in the history and physical.

## Special Issues in the Medical Evaluation

### Donor Obesity

Body mass index (BMI) is a useful parameter to measure in the donor, as a number of studies have shown a good correlation between obesity (BMI > 28 kg/m$^2$) and hepatic steatosis. One recent study suggested that 78% of potential donors with a BMI > 28 kg/m$^2$ had >10% steatosis on liver biopsy. However, not all studies have shown this degree of correlation, and mild degrees of obesity may not be associated with significant steatosis in many cases. In these cases a more direct evaluation of the liver parenchyma, usually with a liver biopsy, may be necessary to rule out the possibility of hepatic steatosis.

An additional problem with the use of obese donors is the potential for increased surgical risk in the donor. Studies from the general surgery literature, suggest an increased incidence of surgical complications such as bleeding and wound problems in obese individuals. Obesity is also a risk factor for underlying cardiovascular problems, which could lead to an increased chance for medical complications posttransplant.

Because of these risk factors, most obese donors will not be suitable donors. The exact upper limit of BMI is at the discretion of the individual center. Certainly a BMI of greater than 35 would be a contraindication for virtually all centers. Many centers will exclude donors with BMI > 30, but others will selectively evaluate these donors and routinely perform a liver biopsy on these individuals to rule out the possibility of liver steatosis.[4,5]

## Hepatitis B Core Antibody-Positive Donors

The use of donors who are hepatitis B virus (HBV) core antibody positive involves consideration of two factors: risk to the donor and potential risk of transmission to the recipient.[6] Donors who are HBV core positive but surface antigen negative have had previous exposure to HBV, but do not have active infection. The proportion of potential donors that are core positive will vary depending on the geographic area. For example, in parts of Asia, more than 50% of potential donors may fall into this category. The majority of these donors will have completely normal lives, and studies from centers in Asia have shown that the risk to these donors is no higher versus non-HBV-core-antibody-positive donors. However, because these donors have had previous HBV infection, a liver biopsy should likely be performed during the evaluation process to rule out the possibility of hepatic inflammation or fibrosis.

With regard to the recipient, the issues are no different from those for a deceased donor who is core positive. A recipient, who has not been exposed to HBV in the past, can potentially acquire primary HBV infection after transplantation from these donors. However, this risk can be minimized or virtually eliminated by the use of appropriate HBV prophylaxis.

## Evaluation for Thrombophilia

Deep venous thrombosis with subsequent pulmonary embolism represents a serious postoperative complication that can be potentially life threatening. Several cases of pulmonary embolism have been reported with at least one or two cases of mortality due to this complication. Known risk factors for thromboembolic complications include obesity, use of oral hormone therapy, older age, smoking, positive family history, and an identified underlying procoagulation disorder. These risk factors should be addressed during the evaluation process, including screening tests to identify a procoagulation disorder. Tests should include testing for protein C and S and α-1-antitrypsin deficiency, checking for factor VIII elevation, evaluating for the presence of antiphospholipid or anticardiolipin antibodies, and screening for the factor V Leiden and prothrombin gene mutations.

## SURGICAL EVALUATION

This part of the evaluation is concerned with determining whether the anatomy of the liver is suitable for donation. A number of tests can be performed for this part of the evaluation, but essentially one wants to obtain information about the vascular anatomy, the liver volume (both the volume to be removed and the volume to be left behind), and the presence of any abnormalities of the hepatic parenchyma.

### Vascular Anatomy

Evaluation of the vascular anatomy predonation includes imaging of the hepatic artery, portal vein, and hepatic veins. Most centers have abandoned the use of invasive tests such as angiogram, and routinely use CT or MRI with 3-D reconstructions as a single test.[7,8] Although some vascular variations may preclude donation, most can be handled with vascular reconstruction techniques. However, preoperative knowledge of these variations is important for planning the operative procedure and performing the operative dissection. Possible vascular variations include a replaced or accessory left (or right) hepatic artery, trifurcation of the main portal vein, and accessory hepatic veins (Figures 29.1-1 and 29.1-2). Depending on which portion of the liver is to be removed, these anatomical variations either may have no impact or may significantly complicate surgery.

The billiary anatomy may be difficult to evaluate accurately preoperatively. Some centers routinely preform MRCP or ERCP as part of the evaluation process. The latter is an invasive test, whereas the former may not provide the degree of accuracy and clarity required to be of value. As a result many centers choose to perform an intraoperative cholangiogram, rather than preoperative billiary imaging. However, ongoing improvements in imaging modalities may soon allow for preoperative noninvasive imaging that is equivalent to the intraoperative cholangiogram with regards to its detail and clarity.

### Liver Volume

Two important questions need to be answered with regard to liver volume during the evaluation process (1) is the volume of the graft to be transplanted of adequate size for the recipient,

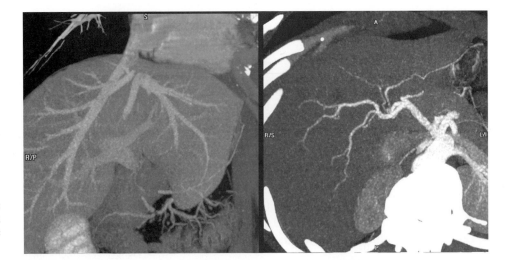

**FIGURE 29.1-1**

Vascular anatomy, including the hepatic veins, portal vein, and hepatic artery can be determined with a single noninvasive test such as a CT scan with contrast.

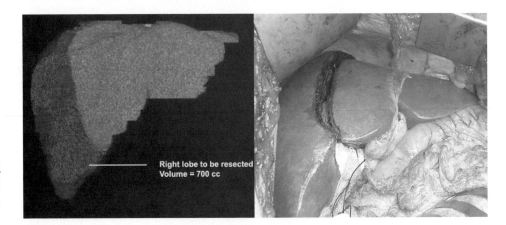

Right lobe to be resected
Volume = 700 cc

**FIGURE 29.1-2**

Determination of the volume of liver to be resected is an important component of the preoperative surgical evaluation and usually correlates well with intraoperative findings.

and (2) is the volume of liver to be left behind in the donor of sufficient size to prevent acute liver failure. Although the donor's height and weight may provide a crude estimate of liver volume, it is not very accurate. This is especially true for the left lateral segment, which can be quite variable in size. Again a computed tomography (CT) or magnetic resonance imaging (MRI) scan can provide a good estimate of the liver volume. It is often helpful for the surgeon to work closely with the radiologist in making the planned line of liver transection, to provide the most accurate assessment of graft volume (see Table 29.1-1).

For a pediatric recipient, the main issue is not usually whether the liver volume may be too small; rather the issue is whether it may be too large; this may lead to problems with closure of the abdomen in the recipient. Usually the graft-weight to recipient-weight (GW/RW) ratio should not exceed 5%. The left lateral segment is used most commonly for these recipients, and removal of this small portion of the liver should not be a concern with regard to adequate residual volume in the donor. For an adult recipient, however, volume of the graft and residual volume are more critical issues. Most centers currently use the right lobe for adult recipients. Preoperative evaluation should include measurement of the graft liver volume to ensure that it is not too small for the recipient. Most centers attempt to keep the GW/RW ratio greater than 0.8, or an estimate of graft weight as a percentage of standard liver mass to exceed 40%. Grafts that are smaller than that may lead to small-for-size syndrome in the recipient.

With regard to residual volume in the donor, an important part of the evaluation process is to make sure that the donor is not left with too small a liver volume. Liver failure has been reported postdonation, with at least one donor requiring an urgent liver transplant because of liver failure after donation. The planned

**TABLE 29.1-1**

## COMPONENTS OF LIVING DONOR EVALUATION

1) Medical Evaluation

   – Complete history and physical

   – Laboratory tests:

       a) General: Blood Type, Blood Counts, Metabolic Panel
       b) Liver: Liver function tests
       c) Infectious: CMV, GBV, HIV, Hep B, Hep C
       d) Thrombophilia: Protein C & S, AT III, Factor V Leiden, Prothrombin mutations

   – Others: Chest x-ray, EKG, PFT's (if indicated)

2) Surgical Evaluation

   – CT or MRI imaging
   – Liver Biopsy (routine or selective)
   – Other invasive tests as indicated (eg, angiogram, ERCP)

3) Psychosocial Evaluation

resection should not exceed 70% of the total liver volume; that is, the donor should be left with at least 30% of the measured total liver volume.

## Liver Parenchyma

Evaluation of the liver parenchyma predonation is best done with a liver biopsy. The role and utilization of liver biopsy, however, varies from center to center and remains controversial. Some centers routinely biopsy all potential donors, whereas others biopsy only on a selective basis.[9,10] The main purpose of the liver biopsy is to assess for the presence and degree of steatosis and rule out any possibility of underlying chronic liver disease. Steatosis may be more common in donors with a history of alcohol use, elevated triglyceride levels, higher BMI, or abnormal appearance on CT imaging. Some centers use these criteria to selectively biopsy the donors. Unfortunately, even with the use of the above selection criteria, some cases of steatosis may not be identified predonation. Additionally, other parenchymal abnormalities that are occult may be difficult to identify using the above criteria, hence the reason why some centers recommend routine biopsy for all potential donors. Liver biopsy represents an invasive test, with a potential risk for complications such as bleeding. However, the risk of complications is generally very low and may be outweighed by the benefit of identifying a potential donor with significant occult liver disease that would preclude donation. Additional studies are needed to better define the role for liver biopsy.

Liver biopsy results that would preclude donation include fibrosis, nonalcoholic steatohepatitis (NASH), steatosis > 20% (for right lobe liver donors), and histologic abnormalities such as inflammatory changes. There are some data to suggest that steatosis identified on a predonation biopsy can be reversed with a program of dieting and exercise, and rebiopsy in this situation may show the potential donor to be suitable.

## PSYCHOSOCIAL EVALUATION

This part of the evaluation assesses the donor's mental fitness and willingness to donate, ensuring that consent is obtained in a voluntary manner with the absence of coercion. The formal part of this evaluation should be conducted by a health-care professional such as a psychiatrist, psychologist, social worker, or other mental health professional. There are several components to this part of the evaluation, but basically the following issues should be addressed:[11–13]

1. Motivation for donation. The potential donor's reasons for donating need to be determined, including a careful assessment to ensure that there is no coercion or inducement involved. Some sense of the relationship with the potential recipient should also be obtained.

2. Knowledge of the process. The potential donor must fully understand the donation process, the surgery involved, the potential complications, and the recovery involved. This is important so that an informed consent can be obtained.

3. An evaluation should be made of the donor's overall mental-health status, and his or her support structures and coping strategies. This include evaluation in the following 3 categories:

i) Mental health. The mental health history of the potential donor should be obtained including underlying psychiatric disorders, history of substance abuse, and overall competence.

ii) Psychosocial history. The current psychosocial status of the potential donor should be evaluated including concurrent stressors, coping strategies, support structures, and stability of living arrangements.

iii) Work or school issues. The potential donor's work and financial status and how the surgery combined with recovery time may impact on how this should be evaluated.

## THE ROLE OF THE TRANSPLANT COORDINATOR

The liver transplant coordinator plays a central role in the evaluation of the living liver donor. This role encompasses the entirety of the donor process from initial inquiry, throughout the evaluation, and on through convalescence and follow-up. Usually he or she is a registered nurse who has specialized knowledge and or experience in the area of organ transplantation. Certification by a central governing body such as the American Board of Transplant Coordinators is optional.

Variations among different centers may determine whether a transplant coordinator is assigned solely to the care of the donor or have dual responsibility of caring for the donor and recipient. Strict adherence to confidentiality policies and concern regarding bias may become issues when the transplant coordinator is responsible to both donor and recipient. Checks and balances within the donor team act as a preventative measure. The combination of responsibilities can be advantageous in that it offers a more comprehensive view of donor–recipient dynamics. It also provides insight into appropriate timing of transplant as the coordinator has a heightened awareness of the recipient condition. A combined role can enhance communication within the donor team.

At all periods of the donation process the transplant coordinator is a crucial link among liver transplant team member, patients, families, significant others, and other health-care providers. Overall responsibilities include education of donor and significant others, gathering relevant information, facilitating the scheduling of the evaluation, reviewing of medical information, providing ongoing support and reassurance throughout the process, and assisting in monitoring recovery and postdonation follow-up.

The transplant surgeon likely first addresses the option of live donation at the time of the transplant evaluation for the recipient. Family members and significant others are often present. The transplant surgeon offers live liver donation as an alternative to deceased donor transplant. He/she explains that the use of a live donor allows for a more predictable course in that a time for transplant can be chosen and the procedure scheduled, thus alleviating much of the anxiety inherent in waiting for a deceased organ. Use of a live donor allows a recipient to be transplanted in a timely manner. It eliminates the risk of a recipient becoming too ill for transplant while awaiting a deceased donor organ.

Initial inquiry by a perspective donor candidate can begin at any time. This may be a random phone call, an impromptu meeting in the hallway, or at a scheduled appointment with the recipient. Donor exclusion criteria should be discussed. A brief health assessment can be done at this time. This will help to identify absolute contraindications to donation. It may be obvious at this point that a particular donor would not be acceptable, thus eliminating the cost of unnecessary medical testing and time commitment on behalf of the potential donor and the coordinator. Establishing good rapport at this time is essential. Material should be presented in an unhurried and understandable manner. This conversation will lay the foundation for a professional relationship that may continue through actual donation and follow-up. Every inquiry should be treated graciously. Prospective donors should be praised for this altruistic offer.

If no obvious contraindications are identified, a very brief description of the evaluation process, the surgery recovery period, and expected follow-up should be described. This information will be repeated again on a face-to-face visit with the surgeon and donor coordinator at the time of the evaluation. Potential donors need to know that the evaluation may entail several appointments to meet with all the members of the donor team. Potential donors should be informed that any member of the donor team at any point during the evaluation might turn them down for a medical or psychological reason. The impact of donation in terms of employment and family should be discussed. It is imperative that a potential donor understand that their safety and best interest are of paramount importance to all team members.

At this point, if the potential donor is still interested, a formal health history form and information packet containing educational materials should be sent. Written material should include an overview of the evaluation process, overview of the surgery, possible risks and complications of the donor operation, a description of the postoperative course, expectations regarding the postdonation follow-up, answers to frequently asked questions, and a list of all the donor team members and their contact numbers. A list of Web sites pertaining to live donation may also be helpful.

Discussion should also include the possibility that a potential recipient may deteriorate to the point of being too ill to undergo live donor liver transplant. A decision such as this should be made by the entire donor team. The potential donor should be asked to review written information, complete the health history and return it along with verification of compatible blood type and contact the donor coordinator if they wish to proceed. It is important to stress the seriousness of the decision to donate. Allow ample time for the potential donor to process the information and encourage phone calls to address questions or concerns. Potential donors should be reassured that they can "opt-out" at any point during or after the evaluation, even at the point of being deemed suitable candidates to donate if it does not feel right for them. Most donors are hearing information regarding donation for the first time and will require repetition of the information.

Enlisting the help of a primary care doctor, attending support groups, and talking with others who have previously donated help to assure thoughtful consideration that may be helpful for the potential donor in making a final decision. Caution should be taken to be sure the decision is not coerced.

On receiving completed documentation (health assessment and verification of blood type) the coordinator should review the medical information. If the potential donor meets criteria, the evaluation can begin. In cases where multiple donors have come forward it is helpful to review candidates with the donor team to select the one donor that seems most suitable. Only one candidate should be evaluated at a time.

Potential donors should be encouraged to include family members or significant others who would be impacted by their decision in the evaluation and decision making process. Strict confidentiality should be assured. The donor coordinator should be available to offer information and provide support to the po-

tential donors and significant others throughout the remainder of the donation process. Education is offered during several conversations as the patients' ability to retain information may vary throughout the evaluation. Levels of education and the degree of support available will be different for each potential donor. Competence should be assessed to ensure informed consent.

Findings during the medical and social evaluation may identify health concerns or risks. This may result in the need for lifestyle adaptations or the donor being denied. Referral to primary care may be necessary for management of abnormalities such as hyperlipidemia, hypertension, or other health concerns. Finally, patients and family need to be encouraged to talk about their hopes and fears throughout the evaluation process. Realistic outcomes should be discussed.

When the evaluation is complete the donor team reviews all medical and psychosocial information and determines candidacy. The donor coordinator communicates this decision to the donor. The decision may elicit anger, disappointment, or frustration if the potential donor is denied. Acknowledgment of these feelings is important. Appropriate referrals to social work or an appointment with a physician may be necessary to help to aid in the understanding of this decision. Acceptance of the candidate for donation allows for the scheduling of the live donor transplant. Donors will experience multiple emotions including fear, anxiety, and excitement.

Frequent and ongoing contact between the donor coordinator and the potential donor during the evaluation and pretransplant waiting period offers the donor coordinator firsthand knowledge of the home environment and social support which may help to predict and anticipate needs postdonation. This can be helpful in planning for care by the inpatient nursing staff. Information should be shared with inpatient staff to optimize care during recovery.

The coordinator should be available to family and significant other to provide updates, provide support, and answer questions on the day of surgery as well as during the postoperative period. After the surgery itself and discharge from hospital, the coordinator continues to provide ongoing support for the donor. Donors should be encouraged to talk about concerns and health-related issues as they arise during this time. Outpatient follow-up appointments allow for discussion among the donor, the donor coordinator, and the physician. Once the follow-up of the donor is finished with the transplant center, they should be encouraged to have an annual physical with their primary care physician and to contact the transplant center any time a concern arises that may relate to the liver donation.

## THE ROLE OF THE TRANSPLANT SOCIAL WORKER

Clinical transplant social workers are an integral component of the transplant team. Psychosocial issues associated with living donation have been increasingly recognized and necessitate similar access to social work services throughout the donor evaluation process. Fortunately, the majority of donor studies report high donor satisfaction with their experience. Most donors do not regret their decision and would donate again. They feel increased self-worth, a better quality of life (as compared to the general population), and have a closer relationship with the recipient posttransplant. However, negative consequences have been reported as a direct result of donation including depression, worsened relationships, and financial stress. Some living donors feel forgotten.

Many transplant programs are now actively attempting to enhance the experience of living donors and to minimize any undesirable psychosocial risks by offering comprehensive services through a designated interdisciplinary donor team. Members of the team must not be involved in the recipient's care, in order to avoid any potential conflict of interest between the commitment to the donor and the commitment to the recipient.

Clinical social workers, an essential part of the donor team, provide a variety of psychosocial, educational, and supportive interventions, both before and after surgery. Discussion of all psychosocial services offered to living donors by social workers is beyond the scope of this section; instead, emphasis is on the pretransplant psychosocial evaluation—one of the most critical aspects of the entire donor process.

The psychosocial assessment provides valuable information about a living donor's present situation and intentions about donating and may identify potential vulnerabilities that could impact on the donor's outcome. The purpose of the evaluation is not exclusively to rule out a potential donor; rather *it is* to maximize the donor process by tending to the individual's unique set of circumstances. The psychosocial evaluation is conducted by a trained mental health professional, often a clinical social worker experienced in transplantation. Psychosocial expertise is offered to the multidisciplinary donor team, yet the social worker frequently serves as the prospective living donor's advocate. If an individual is considered to be at greater risk (ie, has a complex psychiatric history, has a history of incarceration or substance abuse, is cognitively impaired, or is a minor), then a full evaluation may be conducted by one or more clinicians in addition to the social workers, such as a psychologist or psychiatrist. Nontraditional donor volunteers, such as coworkers, acquaintances, responders to an appeal, and complete strangers (nondirected donors) also should receive additional scrutiny because little psychosocial data are available about these populations.

Most transplant programs agree that donors require a unique assessment geared toward addressing the individual's psychological, emotional, and social stability to undergo donor surgery. The social worker explores any potential personal, psychological, family, social, or financial constraints, while attempting to understand the motivations for donation. The donor's ability to develop realistic expectations and plans before and after surgery is also assessed. Key questions involve the ability to cope with potential complications, with poor recipient outcome, with changes in bodily appearance, and with changes in the relationship (if any) with the recipient.

A potential living donor is usually interviewed alone to ensure that she or he is free to speak comfortably about all psychosocial, family, personal, and related issues. The prospective recipient is rarely involved in the initial interview, because some donors may respond approvingly in front of the recipient and may be less likely to express any fears and objections about donation. However, in some instances—such as when the potential donor has a limited, or no relationship with the recipient—the spouse or partner should be permitted, and even encouraged, to participate in the interview. Cases have been reported in which spouses were displeased they were not included, leading to marital discord. Acceptance criteria may vary by program, type of organ to be donated, and the type of relationship between donor and recipient. Questions to donors must be goal oriented with the intention of focusing on the acceptability for proceeding with donation, while also learning how the donor team might best serve the living donor over time.

## Psychosocial History

The social worker must first elicit necessary personal background information including the individual's current situation, cognitive functioning, behavioral and emotional health, and family and significant relationships. Other important information to be obtained includes the individual's employment, living arrangements, educational level, hobbies, financial situation, legal status, family and social supports, and cultural or religious beliefs. A thorough mental health history is also essential to understand the living donor's psychological stability and whether donation would compromise their situation.

The presence of underlying mental illness, cognitive impairments, aberrant personality traits, or other factors that may interfere with the potential donor's ability to make a reasoned decision may preclude donation. A history of anxiety, depression, marital discord, or other concerns are further discussed to determine whether donation could exacerbate underlying symptoms. Present and past behaviors are explored because they may be predictors to coping with potential donor outcomes. Donors must understand how donation could impact on their mental health.

## Informed Decision Making

The potential donor must demonstrate adequate decision-making capabilities and be able to appreciate the risks of the surgical procedure. The social worker must ask questions such as the following. Is the individual adequately informed about the transplant procedure and capable of understanding the potential risks associated with donation (both short term and long term)? Is consent truly, thoroughly informed? Is the individual vulnerable in any way to exploitation? Is the individual aware of alternative options for the recipient and the likelihood of the transplant's success? Does the individual recognize the possibility that future health problems related to donation may not be covered by insurance and that the ability to obtain health, disability, or life insurance may be affected? Has the individual read or heard about the potential psychosocial consequences of donation, from the existing literature and other living donors? Donors must be capable of understanding information to make a sound choice, in addition to realistically preparing for the donation and recovery.

## Motivation

Donation should be voluntary, and reasons for donation must be thoroughly explored by the team and the donor. Donor motivation may be influenced by a variety of factors: type of relationship to the recipient, commitment to the recipient, personal beliefs and values, upbringing, religious convictions, or humanitarian reasons. Donors approach their decision from a wide range of social backgrounds, family situations, and educational levels. The social worker must assess whether the volunteer's decision is made freely without any undo pressure or coercion, and whether motivation is consistent with the donor's values and previous behaviors.

Pressure may be more likely when the recipient's death is imminent without a transplant and when no other donor options exist. Family relationships can influence motivation, sometimes to the point of implied or even explicitly voiced obligation to donate. Siblings, of all relatives, reportedly feel the most pressure to donate. Other family members might fear disapproval if they do not donate and may feel it is expected. In contrast, some may be pressured to *not* donate.

Reasons for donating after a public plea on behalf of a certain recipient or for volunteering to help a complete stranger (as in the case of nondirected donation) are not yet fully understood. Motivation must be probed very carefully, but respectfully, when there is no relationship to the recipient. Until recently, the willingness to donate to a stranger was met with suspicion and thought to indicate the presence of psychopathology. Knowing how the prospective donor learned about donation and how the decision was made is important. The decision to donate can be made instantaneously or deliberatively. Some individuals (eg, parents) immediately volunteer once learning of the living donor option. Others take time to logically evaluate the situation and gather relevant information before making a decision. If the decision appears overly impulsive or self-serving, concern is appropriate.

The potential donor should be encouraged to express doubts, ambivalence, or guilt during the interview and must be assured they have the right to opt out with as little guilt as possible. If the social worker senses pressure to donate, it should be further explored. Some individuals may need permission, or encouragement to decline donation.

### Relationship to the Recipient

Donors and recipients historically had to be genetically related. Reasons for donation were more understandable when there was a close bond between the pair. As discussed above, donors no longer need to be genetically connected for a successful outcome. Thus, psychosocial information is even more critical. Specific questions related to the donor–recipient relationship must be asked. Does the individual have a close relationship with the recipient? How does the individual know the recipient, and for how long? Did the recipient ask the individual to consider donation? If not, how did the individual learn about the option to donate? Does the individual believe the relationship will change depending on the decision to donate or not? If so, how? How does the recipient feel about the donation? Does the individual's family know the recipient? Was anything offered in return for donation?

For genetically unrelated prospective living donors, questions must be tailored to the specific situation to fully understand why the individual wishes to donate and whether expectations about the relationship are realistic.

### Support System and Preparedness for Donation

Donors must make a temporary lifestyle change and yet continue to meet personal, family, and financial obligations before and after surgery. The social worker must help the individual explore what resources and supports are required and available for donation, while assessing the ability of the individual and family to cope effectively with potential donor-related stresses. The individual must be able to identify people committed to helping throughout the donation process. If the spouse, partner, or family members disagree with the decision to donate, postoperative help may be inadequate. The employer's support is also imperative.

### Preparedness for Donation

Prospective donors must be able to appropriately plan to care for themselves, and any dependents, after their surgery. They must also prepare for a temporary role change within their family, social, and work environments. Moreover, they must take into account their finances, so that they are able to meet existing obligations until they have fully recovered. The recovery period may sometimes be difficult and last longer than expected.

Financial questions related to employment include whether they are eligible for any employee benefits, whether they will be able to comfortably take adequate time necessary to recover, whether they will be allowed to perform less labor-intensive interim tasks, whether they have health or life insurance benefits, and whether they are financially secure enough to donate and absorb related expenses. If finances are insufficient so donation would severely compromise a donor's financial situation, the donor team may need to highlight that concern

The social worker must also raise the questions of necessary legal preparations: undergoing any surgery usually sensitizes people to make plans in the event of a poor outcome. Health-care directives, wills, and parental responsibilities require attention.

### Assessment and Recommendations

Once a comprehensive interview is completed, the social worker determines whether the information satisfies the requirements of the program, or whether further intervention is necessary to optimize the donor process. Psychosocial factors such as ambivalence, guilt, major mental illness, and active substance abuse increase donor vulnerability and automatically exclude donation. Evidence for a poor support system, strong family opposition, or disregard for financial obligations are potential risk factors for donors and require further assessment. The social worker determines whether contributing risks might be modified to make donation possible. Psychosocial concerns identified during the interview are shared with the donor, thus providing an opportunity to address issues and develop a plan for resolution or understanding.

Once the social worker has fully assessed the donor's situation, she or he collaborates with the donor team members and highlights any significant findings, including any gaps in knowledge that require specific educational intervention from the team. Ultimately, the donor team must decide how the psychosocial issues will be weighed in the overall process.

### Education and Counseling

Any psychosocial issue identified during the assessment receives direct social work counseling or a referral to an appropriate resource. Frequently, the social worker learns sensitive information (sometimes unrelated to donation) and must make additional recommendations (eg, for therapy for marital problems, for financial or employment assistance). The social worker attempts to educate and fill any knowledge gaps and may also encourage the donor to speak with previous donors (made available by the program).

The donor social worker should remain available to a donor throughout the donation process earning their trust, helping them feel comfortable, and offering consistent support for any short- or long-term needs.

### References

1. Surman OS. The ethics of partial liver donation. *New Engl J Med* 346(14): 1038.
2. Brown R Jr, Russo M, Lai M, et al. A Survey of Liver Transplantation from Living Adult Donors in the United States. *N Engl J Med* 348(9): 818–825.

3. Rudow DL, Brown RS, Jr. Evaluation of living liver donors. *Prog Transplant* 2003;13(2):110–116.

4. Evaluation of 100 patients for living donor liver transplantation. *Liver Transpl.* 2000 May;6(3):290–295

5. Trotter JF. Selection of donors and recipients for living donor liver transplantation. *Liver Transpl.* 2000 Nov;6(6 Suppl 2):S52–S58.

6. Chen YS, Cheng YF, De Villa VH, et al. Evaluation of living liver donors. *Transplantation* 2003;Feb 15;75(3 Suppl):S16–S19.

7. Alonso-Torres A, Fernandez-Cuadrado J, Pinilla I, et al. Multidetector CT in the evaluation of potential living donors for liver transplantation. *Radiographics* 2005;Jul-Aug;25(4):1017–1030.

8. Valentin-Gamazo C, Malago M, Karliova M, et al. Experience after the evaluation of 700 potential donors for living donor liver transplantation in a single center. *Liver Transplant* 2004 Sep;10(9):1087–1096.

9. Nadalin S, Malago M, Valentin-Gamazo C, et al. Preoperative donor liver biopsy for adult living donor liver transplantation: risks and benefits. *Liver Transpl.* 2005 Aug 11;(8):980–986.

10. Iwasaki M, Takada Y, Hayashi M, et al. Noninvasive evaluation of graft steatosis in living donor liver transplantation. *Transplantation* 2004; Nov 27;78(10):1501–1505.

11. Jacobs C, Johnson E, Anderson K, Gillingham K, Matas A. Kidney transplants from living donors: how donation affects family dynamics. *Adv Ren Replace Ther* 1998;5(2):89–97.

12. Pradel FG, Mullins CD, Bartlett ST. Exploring donors' and recipients' attitudes about living donor kidney transplantation. *Prog Transplant* 2003;13(3):203–210.

13. Schover LR, Streem SB, Boparai N, Duriak K, Novick AC. The psychosocial impact of donating a kidney: long-term follow-up from a urology based center. *J Urol* 1997;157(5):1596–1601.

14. Pascher A, Sauer IM, Walter M, et al. Donor evaluation, donor risks, donor outcome, and donor quality of life in adult-to-adult living donor liver transplantation. *Liver Transplant* 2002 Sep 8; (9):829–837.

15. Pomfret EA, Pomposelli JJ, Lewis WD, et al. Live donor adult liver transplantation using right lobe grafts: donor evaluation and surgical outcome. *Arch Surg* 2001 Apr;136(4):425–433.

16. Marcos A, Fisher RA, Ham JM, et al. Selection and outcome of living donors for adult to adult right lobe transplantation. *Transplantation* 2000 Jun 15;69(11):2410.

17. Brandhagen D, Fidler J, Rosen C. Evaluation of the donor liver for living donor liver transplantation. *Liver Transpl.* 2003 Oct;9(10 Suppl 2): S16–S28.

# 29.2  ANESTHESIOLOGIC CONSIDERATIONS

*Susanne Shamsolkottabi, MD,*
*Kumar G. Belani, MBBS, MS*

## INTRODUCTION

The need to accept living adults to donate a part of their liver to surgically replace the liver of a patient with end-stage liver disease (ESLD) is based on the lack of availability of a sufficient number of cadaveric organs.[1] Despite this, living donors provide portions of their livers for approximately 30% of pediatric and 5% adult liver transplants. Fortunately, approximately 50% of eligible liver recipients have an identifiable volunteer donor.[2] However, many of these prospective donors do not qualify, and therefore a significant number are unacceptable. There are numerous benefits to performing living donor liver transplantation. These include the probability of selecting the best graft (anatomically, immunologically, and functionally) and being able to plan and perform the operation electively. This allows more optimal preparation of the

recipient and significantly decreases waiting time. Graft ischemia time is also significantly reduced, thereby decreasing the likelihood of graft dysfunction due to ischemia. Living donor livers demonstrate much reduced levels of markers of inflammation following reperfusion.[3] Donor liver surgery may involve left lobectomy, segmental resection, or even right hepatic lobectomy. Dissection of the liver requires prior identification of adequate vascular inflow and outflow with satisfactory billiary drainage. The middle hepatic vein is avoided.[4] The donor operation precedes the recipient operation. Open laparotomy is the common approach. However, successful left hepatic lobe segmental resection using a laparoscopic-assisted approach has been described.[5] In this chapter, we discuss the perioperative anesthesia care and concerns of the living hepatic donor.

## SELECTION CRITERIA

The ideal candidate is a healthy individual with no organ dysfunction with a normal body mass index (BMI) or mild obesity who is able to understand the procedure (see Table 29.2-1). The donor should have stable cardiopulmonary function, no renal disease, no coagulopathy, and normal liver function. If the donor has had prior surgery, there should be no history of prior problems with general anesthesia. This includes the presence of a feasible, maskable, and easily intubatable upper airway (ie, absence of obstructive sleep apnea and airway abnormalities). They should have a normal hemogram, chest x-ray, electrocardiogram (EKG; if age > 45 years for males; > 50 years for females). A preoperative echocardiogram to rule out the presence of a patent foramen ovale (PFO) is helpful. Absence of a PFO decreases the risk of a paradoxical air-embolism that may occur during donor hepatic resection.[6]

## PREOPERATIVE ASSESSMENT

This may be done in the surgical clinic once the donor is identified. Traditionally, this is done at the time of surgical work-up of the donor. The surgical evaluation includes a detailed study of liver anatomy and its vascular supply and biliary drainage. The preoperative assessment includes a thorough review of systems to confirm candidacy as listed in Table 29.2-1 and to rule out the presence of bronchial asthma, diabetes mellitus, cardiac disease including hypertension, mitral valve prolapse, arrhythmias, neuromuscular disorders, hiatal hernia with significant reflux, and airway abnormalities. If a history of sleep apnea is present, this must be investigated to assess severity and relationship to presence or absence of a difficult upper airway. Patients using continuous positive airway pressure (CPAP) to treat obstructive sleep apnea may

**TABLE 29.2-1**

## REQUIREMENTS FOR CANDIDACY FOR LIVING DONOR LIVER RESECTION

- Healthy and willing ASA 1 or 2 adult
- Absence of active systemic disease
- Feasible upper airway for mask ventilation and endotracheal intubation
- No prior problems with anesthesia
- No patent foramen ovale
- Normal organ function including absence of coagulopathy or deep vein thrombosis

require CPAP in the immediate postoperative period. Furthermore, these patients need close vigilance including monitoring for sleep apnea. The donor is assessed for adequacy of vascular access including central venous line placement. The details of anesthesia care are discussed with the prospective donor. This should include a discussion about the possible need for blood product usage. Preoperative phlebotomy for intraoperative autologous use of the collected whole blood is not practiced at our institution. Instead, blood lost during surgery is salvaged and washed, and the separated red blood cells are made available for transfusion intraoperatively. Finally, before completing the anesthesia consent process, the list of allergies and medications used are recorded. The prospective donor is notified that intraoperatively phlebotomy may be done immediately prior to liver resection for surgical reasons. The collected blood is stored in CPDA bags for transfusion following hepatectomy. The donor is informed to be *nulla per os* (NPO) for solids for at least 6 hours prior to the procedure and instructed to take clear liquids, if necessary, until 2 hours before anesthesia induction.

## PAIN CONTROL

Living liver donors may suffer significant postoperative discomfort because of the large subcostal incision required for hepatic lobe or segment isolation. Significant pain relief can be afforded by central neuraxial blockade provided via a low thoracic epidural catheter with a combination of an infusion of local anesthetics and opioids. At many institutions including ours, this is not routine practice because of the small risk of epidural bleeding due to intraoperative low-dose heparin given immediately prior to removal of the liver lobe or segment. Instead, our patients are informed and educated about the availability of intravenous patient-controlled analgesia using opioids (morphine or dilaudid). Using this approach, and also providing nonsteroidal anti-inflammatory drugs (NSAIDs; ibuprofen, ketorolac) to decrease opioid dose, has been quite successful in providing patient comfort and encouraging early ambulation at our institution.

## ANESTHESIA CARE

The donor operation takes several hours. After confirming NPO status and placement of a large bore peripheral IV (usually 16 or 14 G), a routine general anesthesia induction is performed. Midazolam is commonly used for preoperative anxiolysis (and amnesia) during transfer from the preoperative receiving area and the operating room. The choice induction agent at our institution is propofol (the large IV with good crystalloid flow decreases the likelihood of pain on injection) followed by a nondepolarizing skeletal muscle relaxant (either cisatracurium or rocuronium). An infusion of the nondepolarizer titrated to the presence of a single twitch during train-of-four monitoring ensures the required and uninterrupted upper abdominal muscle relaxation. Anesthesia is continued with an inhalational agent, either isoflurane or desflurane. Both ensure adequate hepatic blood flow. Isoflurane has minimal hepatotoxicity, and if this is a concern, desflurane may be used. To enhance analgesia and decrease stress response, an opioid infusion is also started following a loading bolus dose (usually fentanyl).

The goals of anesthesia are listed in Table 29.2-2). To successfully achieve these goals, the living donor is prepared with a large-bore peripheral IV as indicated above. In addition, a large IV (14 g) is also placed in an antecubital vein in an

**TABLE 29.2.-2**

## GOALS OF ANESTHESIA FOR LIVING LIVER DONOR SURGERY

| | |
|---|---|
| Decrease stress response | • Ensure adequate analgesia with opioid infusion |
| Preserve hepatic blood flow and oxygenation | • Use isoflurane or desflurane<br>• Use higher $F_IO_2$ (> 50%) |
| Uninterrupted skeletal muscle relaxation | • Nondepolarizer infusion titrated with the use TOF monitoring (1 out of 4 twitches) |
| Avoid hepatic congestion/ encourage a shrunken liver | • Careful titration of maintenance crystalloid with a negative fluid balance but without promoting pre-renal azotemia. Keep CVP at 3–5 mm Hg.<br>• Rapid phlebotomy of 300–500 ml during active dissection and isolation (for lobectomy) |
| Prevent lower extremity deep vein thrombosis | • Use compressible stockings<br>• Mild hemodilution preferred<br>• Normothermia of lower extremities |
| Ensure normothermia | • Provide surface warming with upper and lower body forced-air warmers |

outstretched arm on an armboard with an upper-arm blood pressure cuff. The IV is kept open with intermittent saline flushing and used for phlebotomy when required (for donors scheduled for hepatic lobectomy). This is aided by inflating the arm cuff to above venous pressure. The blood is allowed to drain directly into a CPDA-containing bag sitting on a weighing scale to provide an estimate of volume collected. A central venous catheter via the internal jugular vein is inserted for central venous pressure (CVP) and hemoglobin monitoring when hepatic lobectomy is planned. We suggest the use of intraoperative ultrasound during central line placement. Invasive blood pressure monitoring is not standard practice at our institution. Instead, we prefer continual noninvasive monitoring of blood pressure with waveform using the Vasotrac System (Medwave Inc., Arden Hills, MN).

Blood loss during donor hepatectomy is customarily not a major issue. The surgeons trained in hepatobiliary surgery usually perform a meticulous dissection of the liver using the cavitational ultrasonic surgical aspirator (CUSA). Blood loss during left donor hepatectomy averages 562 ± 244 mL (range 300–1,100 mL) and 902 ± 564 mL (range 150–2,600 mL) for right donor hepatectomy.[7,8] The blood lost during surgery is salvaged and washed in a Cell-Saver™ (Hemonetics Laboratories, Boston, MS), and the separated red blood cells are transfused once the partial donor hepatectomy is completed.

After the donor liver dissection is completed, the lobe or segment is isolated and ready for excision. This is only accomplished when the recipient is ready to allow prompt revascularization and reperfusion. This minimizes cold ischemia time. Immediately prior to excision of the donor segment or lobe, heparin (low dose—70 U/kg IV) is administered to prevent intrahepatic thrombosis of the removed liver segment or lobe. Once the segment or lobe of the liver is removed, heparin may be reversed with protamine (usually 1 mg protamine for every 100 U heparin) after administering a test dose.

Following successful resection of a liver lobe or segment, the salvaged and/or phlebotomized blood is returned to the donor. This will improve the intravascular volume status of the donor. Urine output that may have been low (approximately 0.5 mL/kg/hr) during dissection of the liver will now improve. Additional crystalloid may be administered to increase urine flow. The muscle relaxant and opioid infusion are stopped once abdominal closure begins. As closure is completed, the patient is weaned from inhalational anesthetics, and neuromuscular blockade is reversed when train-of-four monitoring suggests that there is a ratio of 0.7 or greater. Most patients can be successfully extubated in the operating suite and are transported to the postoperative care unit breathing spontaneously. To decrease the likelihood of postoperative nausea and vomiting, we provide prophylaxis with either ondansetron alone or a combination of ondansetron and dexamethasone. These agents are given at least 30 minutes prior to emergence. Meperidine (25 to 50 mg IV) may be used to prevent/treat postoperative shivering.

## MORBIDITY AND MORTALITY

Because of the extent, location, organ involved, and duration of surgery, one can expect that there will be considerable morbidity and even mortality following living liver donor surgery. Indeed, in one report summarizing morbidity and mortality following living liver donor surgery,[9] the time to complete recovery averaged approximately 12 to 13 weeks. Morbidity reported ranged from 0% to 67%. The same authors indicated that two deaths were reported in the 1151 liver donors that made up the study population. Some of the common problems noted were abdominal discomfort, bile leak, and prolonged ileus. Postoperative duration of hospital stay ranges between 10 to 14 days.[10,11] In another review by Merritt,[12] the mortality risk is estimated to be 0.2% to 0.3%, and the risk of a catastrophic complication including mortality is estimated to be between 0.4% and 1%. There have been no anesthesia-related deaths reported, but intraoperative and nonsurgical early postoperative morbidity is summarized in Table 29.2-3.

## SUMMARY AND CONCLUSIONS

Anesthesia care for living liver donors requires a thorough assessment of adults who are willing to donate a portion of their liver. Donors need to be healthy and be free of conditions that may predispose them to increased anesthesia risk. Proper preparation

**TABLE 29.2-3.**

## INTRAOPERATIVE AND EARLY POSTOPERATIVE NONSURGICAL MORBIDITY FOLLOWING LIVING LIVER DONOR SURGERY

* Brachial plexus injury
* Postoperative respiratory depression
* Intraoperative hypertension with ST-T- wave changes (procedure cancelled)
* Severe bradycardia following induction
* Occipital alopecia (prolonged surgery with pressure on occiput)
* Over dose of muscle relaxant
* Early extubation requiring reintubation

and meticulous surgical technique including dedicated postoperative care will minimize intraoperative and postoperative morbidity. The risk for exposure to homologous blood products is small. Most donors are satisfied with their decision to donate and will return to their usual activities within 3 to 4 months.

## References

1. Testa G, Malago M, Broelsch CE. Living-donor liver transplantation in adults. *Langenbecks Arch Surg* 1999;384(6):536–543.
2. Trotter JF, et al. Adult-to-adult transplantation of the right hepatic lobe from a living donor. *N Engl J Med* 2002;346(14):1074–1082.
3. Jassem W, et al. Cadaveric versus living-donor livers: differences in inflammatory markers after transplantation. *Transplantation* 2003;76(11): 1599–1603.
4. Abdalla EK, Noun R, Belghiti J. Hepatic vascular occlusion: which technique? *Surg Clin North Am* 2004;84(2): 563–585.
5. Cherqui D, et al. Laparoscopic living donor hepatectomy for liver transplantation in children. *Lancet* 2002;359(9304):392–396.
6. Hatano Y, et al. Venous air embolism during hepatic resection. *Anesthesiology* 1990;73(6):1282–1285.
7. Lutz JT, et al. Blood-transfusion requirements and blood salvage in donors undergoing right hepatectomy for living related liver transplantation. *Anesth Analg* 2003;96(2):351–355, table of contents.
8. Beebe DS, et al. Living liver donor surgery: report of initial anesthesia experience. *J Clin Anesth* 2000;12(2):157–161.
9. Beavers KL, Sandler RS, Shrestha R. Donor morbidity associated with right lobectomy for living donor liver transplantation to adult recipients: a systematic review. *Liver Transplant* 2002;8(2):110–117.
10. Beavers KL, et al. The living donor experience: donor health assessment and outcomes after living donor liver transplantation. *Liver Transplant* 2001;7(11): 943–947.
11. Miyagi S, et al. Risks of donation and quality of donors' life after living donor liver transplantation. *Transplant Int* 2005;18(1):47–51.
12. Merritt WT, Living donor surgery: overview of surgical and anesthesia issues. *Anesthesiol Clin N Am* 2004;**22**(4): 633–650.
13. Pomposelli JJ, et al. Life-threatening hypophosphatemia after right hepatic lobectomy for live donor adult liver transplantation. *Liver Transplant* 2001;7(7):637–642.
14. Soejima Y, et al. Perioperative management and complications in donors related to living-donor liver transplantation. *Surgery* 2002;131 (1 Suppl): S195–S199.
15. Ayanoglu HO, et al. Anesthetic management and complications in living donor hepatectomy. *Transplant Proc* 2003;35(8):2970–2973.
16. Humar A. Donor and recipient outcomes after adult living donor liver transplantation. *Liver Transplant* 2003;9(10 Suppl 2): S42–S44.
17. Pomfret EA. Early and late complications in the right-lobe adult living donor. *Liver Transplant* 2003;9(10 Suppl 2):S45–S49.

# 29.3   SURGICAL PROCEDURES

## 29.3.1a   Adult Donor to Adult Recipient, Right Lobe

*Giuliano Testa, MD, Massimo Malagó, MD, Enrico Benedetti, MD*

## INTRODUCTION

In the conclusion of the paper reporting the first description of a formal right hepatectomy, Lortat-Jacob writes that this operation might in the future be applied to various pathologies of the liver.[1]

It is most possibly true that he never thought that one day the right hepatectomy would have been used not to save the person undergoing it but to save a patient in need of a liver transplant.

Reading the first description of the right hepatectomy, it is evident that through the decades not much has been changed, at least in the general design of its execution. When the operation started to be used for living donor liver transplantation, it became clear especially to very experienced hepatobiliary and transplant surgeons that major changes in its conceptual and technical approach were necessary.

The facts that the right liver must be harvested with all vessels intact, that posterior hepatic veins of greater caliber must be preserved, that a precise line or parenchymal section must be drawn, that ischemia to the hepatic ducts must be avoided, and that parenchymal transection must be performed in full perfusion of the liver make the right hepatectomy for donation definitely more challenging than the same operation performed to remove a tumor.

The description that follows attempts to describe all the important steps of the donor right hepatectomy, not as the authors preferred technique but as a summary of the techniques that have been reported in the literature.

## INCISION AND CHOLECYSTECTOMY

The operation is performed with the donor in the supine position. To facilitate the exposure the donor can be placed in slight reverse Trendelemburgh.

The incisions used are either a standard Mercedes or a right subcostal extended on the upper midline of the abdomen toward the Xiphoid process. The Falciform ligament is taken down toward the suprahepatic vena cava.

The right liver is then mobilized by dissection of the triangular ligament. None of the ligaments to the left of the Falciform are dissected.

A cholecystectomy is performed. None of the papers published describe the cholecystectomy. We like to perform the cholecystectomy in a retrograde fashion taking the cystic artery and duct last. The rationale is to limit to the minimum the dissection around the common bile duct and safely recognize any possible anatomical anomaly.

The cystic duct is not tied because it will be used for the intraoperative cholangiogram.

### Hilar Time

The hilar time starts with the dissection of the right hepatic artery. Some surgeons make a point in their report of limiting the dissection of the hepatic artery to the lateral aspect of the proper hepatic duct with the aim of leaving intact the tissue between artery and the bile duct thus preserving its vascularization.[2,3]

There is actually no hard evidence in any reports that this practice has an influence in early or delayed complications of the biliary system of the donor. The authors of this chapter have dissected the right hepatic artery to the medial aspect of the hepatic duct, completely separating the plane between the posterior face of the hepatic duct and the anterior face of the artery, in more than 150 donors, and have had no complication attributable to the extent of the dissection. The small arterial branch to segment 4 should be preserved (Figure 29.3.1a-1 and Figure 29.3.1a-2).

In practical terms it appears that the only difference in the amount of dissection is the length of the artery obtained in the graft.

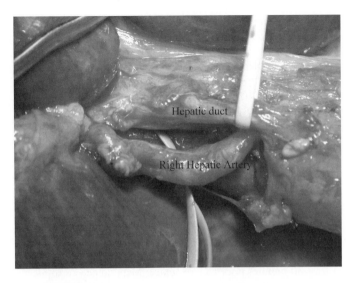

**FIGURE 29.3.1a-1**

The right portal vein is dissected next. Small branches draining the caudate lobe must be taken between locking stitches to permit full mobilization of the right branch of the portal vein. It is sufficient to dissect about 1 cm of right portal vein to obtain the necessary length for safely placing the vascular clamp at the time of removal of the right liver. The dissection of the portal vein allows the visualization of the anterior face of the hilar plate and of the caudate process of the caudate lobe. It is through this plane that the line of parenchymal resection will pass.

In the technique described by Malago the left portal vein is also dissected for a few millimeters from the confluence with the right portal vein. This maneuver is necessary in order to obtain full exposure of the anterior face of the hilar plate, allowing the early division of the right hepatic duct as described next.[4]

### Right Liver Mobilization

After dissection of the triangular ligament the liver is rotated medially and the vena cava is visualized. The posterior hepatic veins are taken between locking stitches. There is general consensus that

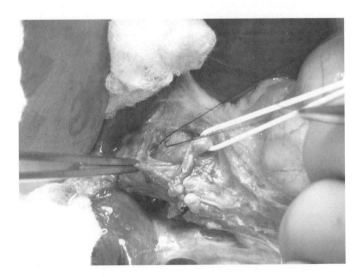

**FIGURE 29.3.1a-2**

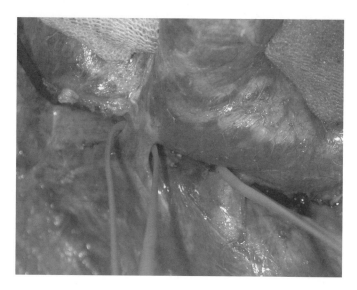

**FIGURE 29.3.1a-3**

posterior hepatic veins with a diameter larger than 0.5 cm should be eventually reanastomosed to the cava of the recipient. These veins can be primarily dissected, ligated and cut for then being reopened in the back table, or left intact and clamped at the time of the removal of the right liver. When not too cumbersome for the rest of the cava dissection it is probably better to choose the second option: It avoids unnecessary congestion of the liver and provides a longer stump for the anastomosis (Figure 29.3.1a-3).

The extent of the dissection of the retrohepatic-cava plane is not clearly described in any paper. In general it can be pictured as a longitudinal line drawn from the space between right and middle hepatic vein to the midportion of the process of the caudate lobe. It usually corresponds to half to two thirds of the anterior surface of the vena cava (Figure 29.3.1a-4).

The right hepatic vein must be circumferentially dissected. Most of the surgeons at this point will pass an umbilical tape or a mersilene band around the right hepatic vein. It will be used for the hanging maneuver during the last part of the liver parenchyma resection.

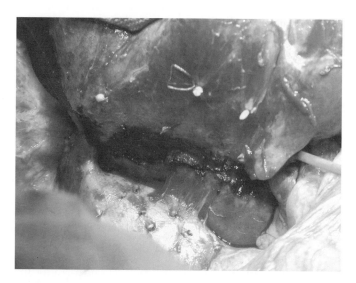

**FIGURE 29.3.1a-4**

## Cholangiogram and Intraoperative Doppler/US

The timing of these two tests is different in various publications, but there is no description of this operation without these tests.

The intraoperative cholangiogram is routinely performed through the stump of the cystic duct. When the cystic duct does not allow an easy introduction of the cholangiogram catheter, a longitudinal choledocothomy can be performed.

The rotation of the C-arm is used by many authors in order to visualize hepatic ducts that are not visible on the standard posteroanterior plane and to obtain a better comprehensive view of the anatomy of the hepatic duct confluence.

Fan has described the placement of a clip on the liver capsule to help correctly identify the confluence of the right and left hepatic ducts and the branches of the right hepatic duct.[5]

The intraoperative Doppler ultrasound is mainly performed to map the position and direction of the middle hepatic vein. It also helps localizing the hepatic veins draining segment 5 and segment 8. In some centers the Doppler is used to obtain more precise information regarding the contribution of the middle hepatic vein and its tributaries to the venous outflow of the paramedian sector of the liver and help decide whether the middle hepatic vein should be taken with the graft or not (see Chapter 30.4).

The route of the middle hepatic vein can be drawn on the anterior surface of the liver with the bovie. This line and the line of Cantlie obtained by temporarily occluding the right inflow to the liver will help the decision on where the line of parenchymal resection should lie.

## Parenchymal Resection

The line of parenchymal resection can be drawn on the anterior surface of the liver from the dome, between the right and the middle hepatic vein, to the gallbladder fossa up to the hilar plate. The line can be continued on the posterior surface of the liver by splitting with the bovie the caudate process and continuing to incise the glissonian capsule from the apex of the split to the medial side of the right hepatic vein. The groove created on the glissonian capsule will accommodate the umbilical tape at the time of the hanging maneuver (Color Plates, Figure 19.3.1a- LI-6).

Some surgeons perform the division of the right hepatic duct prior to the resection of the liver parenchyma.[2,4]

In this case the caudate process of the caudate lobe is divided in the direction of the portal vein confluence. A biliary probe is inserted in the hepatic duct to define the exact location of the hepatic duct confluence. The right portal vein and artery are pulled caudally with a vein retractor and a long Anderson clamp is passed behind the hilar plate, and its tips are directed toward the apex of the split in the caudate process. The hepatic duct is then sharply divided with an 11-blade knife (Figure 29.3.1a-5).

To facilitate the resection of the parenchyma the liver can be displaced downward and anteriorly placing laparotomy pads in the right upper quadrant. Once the parenchyma is split the two halves of the liver can be held steady and separated either by the hand of the assistant or by placing holding stitches on the parenchyma itself.

The resection of the parenchyma has been performed with multiple devices. No matter whether CUSA, Water Jet Dissector, Monopolar and Bipolar Coagulator, Tissue Link or Staple Devices are used, the ultimate goal is to resect the parenchyma with the minimal blood loss possible and respecting the anatomical structures vital to the graft and to the donor. Individual preferences

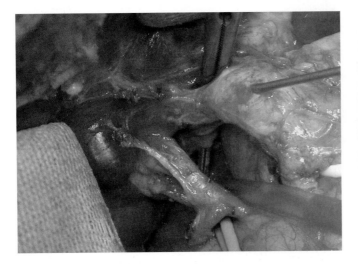

**FIGURE 29.3.1a-5**

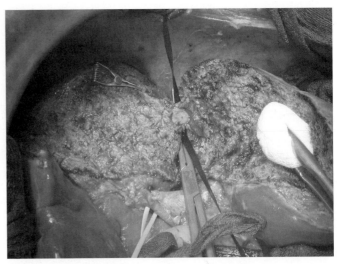

**FIGURE 29.3.1a-6**

dictate the level of comfort in relying on the aforementioned devices for hemostasis of larger vessels and prevention of bile leaks. Silk or vycril ligatures and prolene stitches are often used in support of the mechanical devices.

The plane of resection is dictated by the position of the middle hepatic vein (see Chapter 30.4). After determining the position of the middle hepatic vein with the intraoperative Doppler, some surgeons deliberately incise the parenchyma 1 cm lateral to it or simply over it.

It is normally fairly easy to resect the parenchyma starting from the anterior margin of the liver, over the gall bladder fossa, and find the branch of the middle hepatic vein veering toward segment 5 or segment 8 branches. At this point, the middle hepatic vein will dictate the plane of transection, as determined by the planned procedure: hepatectomy with or without harvesting of the middle hepatic vein.

The middle hepatic vein can be "carved out" of the liver parenchyma by gentle dissection. All affluent branches are ligated or oversewn. When the middle hepatic vein is not harvested with the graft, segments 5 and 8 vein branches can be either preserved or oversewn (see Chapter 30.4). The point of transaction of the middle hepatic vein is determined by surgeon preference and liver anatomy.

It is our preference not to pursue the middle hepatic vein to the confluence with the cava but transect it in the plane between right hepatic vein and middle hepatic vein/cava confluence. This technique requires almost universally a backbench reconstruction with an interposition graft (see Chapter 26.4) but eliminates any potential risk of injury to the left liver venous outflow.

When the middle hepatic vein is left to the donor, the veins draining segments 5 and 8 directly into the middle hepatic vein can be preserved for implantation in the recipient. In this case, control of these veins can be achieved as described by Lee: by clamping them with a bulldog clamp.[6] A careful dissection with the CUSA or the Water Jet allows a sufficient length of these veins for an accurate nonstenosing closure on the middle hepatic vein and the anastomosis in the recipient.

Most of the literature reports the division of the right hepatic duct after a various amount of the peranchymal resection has been completed.[5,7–10] The division is always performed in a sharp fashion avoiding the use of any device that may cause thermal injury to the hepatic duct (Color Plates, Figure 29.3.1a-LI-7).

The last third of the parenchymal resection can be helped by passing the umbilical tape between the transected parenchyma and the hilar structures and pulling it by both ends. In this way the liver is lifted upward and the resection is greatly facilitated. Alternatively the left hand can be placed under the liver while the dissection is continued with the right as described by Marcos[7] (Figure 29.3.1a-6).

### Removal of the Graft and Closure of the Stumps

Some surgeons leave the liver, divided and perfused, to rest for a variable length of time, up to 1 hour. There is no scientific evidence this resting time may contribute to the establishment of the intrahepatic venous connections that allow rerouting of the venous outflow after the interruption especially with the middle hepatic vein. Nevertheless like many unproven things, in medicine it makes sense, at least to some of the surgeons.

Vascular clamps are used in sequence to control the right branch of hepatic artery, portal vein, and hepatic veins.

Great care must be paid in the positioning of the clamps especially on the inflow vessels. Damage or stenosis of the main or left portal vein and of the arterial inflow may have catastrophic consequences for the donor.

Due to the limited length of the right portal vein, it is particularly important to place the clamp at the edge of the right portal vein and not on the wall of the main portal vein. Moreover the closure should be performed with fine nonabsorbable sutures placed in a transverse direction with the long axis of the portal vein.

The closure of the hepatic duct stumps is also usually done in a transverse fashion with absorbable sutures. A cholangiogram prior to the closure of the cystic duct is performed in some centers to evaluate for the presence of bile leaks and the absence of strictures of the proper and left hepatic duct[11,12] (Figure 29.3.1a-7).

The placement of a drain and the use of fibrin sealant on the resection surface is a matter of surgeon preference.

Although the left side of the liver is not mobilized, many surgeons secure the liver to the abdominal cavity with few stitches with the purpose of avoiding rotation and venous congestion.

The graft is perfused on the back table and prepared for the implantation. The preparation of the venous outflow and of the hepatic ducts is described elsewhere in this book.

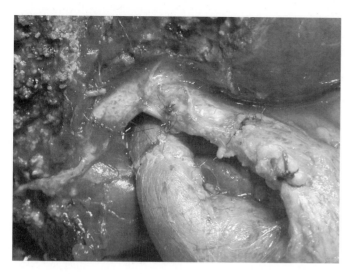

**FIGURE 29.3.1a-7**

The right hepatectomy for living donation is a challenging operation in which margin for error is minimal because the consequences can be catastrophic for the donor and the recipient.

When prepared and planned meticulously, it is currently one of the most fascinating operations that a transplant surgeon can perform.

## References

1. Lortat-Jacob JL, Robert HG. Hepatectomie Droite Reglee. *La Presse Medicale* 1952;60(26):549–551.
2. Miller CM, Gondolesi GE, Florman S, et al. One hundred nine living donor liver transplants in adults and children: A single-center experience. *Ann Surg* 2001;234(3):301–312.
3. Lo CM, Fan ST, Liu CL, et al. Adult-to-adult living donor liver transplantation using extended right lobe grafts. *Ann Surg* 1997;226(3):261–270.
4. Malago M, Testa G, Frilling A, et al. Right living donor liver transplantation: An option for adult patients. *Ann Surg y* 2003;238(6):853–863.
5. Fan ST, Lo CM, Liu CL, et al. Biliary reconstruction and complications of right lobe live donor liver transplantation. *Ann Surg* 2002;236(5):676–683.
6. Lee SG, Park K< Hwang S, et al. Modified right liver graft from a living donor to prevent congestion. *Transplantation* 2002;74(1):54–59.
7. Marcos A, Fisher RA, Ham JM, et al. Right lobe living donor liver transplantation. *Transplantation* 1999;68:798–803.
8. Bak T, Wachs M, Trotter J, et al. Adult-to-adult donor liver transplantation using right-lobe grafts: Results and lessons learned from a single-center experience. *Liver Transplant* 2001;7(8):680–686.
9. Settmacher U, Steinmuller TH, Schmidt SC, et al. Technique of bile duct reconstruction and management of biliary complications in right lobe living donor liver transplantation. *Clin Transplant* 2003;17(1):37–42.
10. Nakamura T, Tanaka K, Kiuchi T, et al. Anatomical variations and surgical strategies in right lobe living donor liver transplantation: Lessons from 120 cases. *Transplantation* 2002;73:1896–1903.
11. Dulundu E, Sugawara Y, Sano K, et al. Duct-to-duct biliary reconstruction in adult living-donor liver transplantation. *Transplantation* 2004;78(4):574–579.
12. Ishiko T, Egawa H, Kasahara M, et al. Duct-to-duct biliary reconstruction in living donor liver transplantation utilizing right lobe graft. *Ann Surg* 2002;236(2):235–240.

## 29.3.1b  Adult Donor to Adult Recipient, Extended Right Lobe

*See Ching Chan, MD, MS, Chung Mau Lo, MD, MS*

### INTRODUCTION

Although the importance of venous drainage of segments 5 and 8 is well recognized,[1] inclusion of the middle hepatic vein (MHV) in the right lobe graft remains a controversial issue for fear of donor developing liver failure. Therefore, ways to reconstruct segment 5 and 8 venous drainage for right liver grafts devoid of the MHV have been deviced.[2–4] In our center, the MHV is regularly included in the right lobe graft to provide uniform venous drainage of segments 5 and 8. The safety and necessity of including the MHV are validated.[5–6] In one center, which procured the MHV in the later part of their series, no difference in blood loss, transfusion requirements, peak serum liver enzymes, time interval from surgery to complete normalization of liver enzymes, complications, and length of hospitalization was demonstrable when comparison was made with donors in the earlier part of the series.[7] It is arguable that this conclusion could be confounded by the factor of maturation of the technique.

Outcomes of donor right hepatectomy including the MHV improved with accumulation of experience. In our series of 200 donor right hepatectomies all including the MHV, the operation time was shortened with maturity of techniques (Figure 29.3.1b-1). Similarly, blood loss improved in each era of 50 cases (500 mL, 410 mL, 286 mL, 251 mL).[8] Other centers have gradually adopted the policy of including the MHV into the right lobe graft.[6,9,10] In a study on volumetric analysis of the remnant left liver of the right liver donor, it was shown that there was less regeneration of segment 4 without the MHV. Nevertheless, the entire left liver volume is unaffected. In our own series, to assure donor safety, preservation of segment 4b hepatic vein (V4b) has become mandatory.[12]

### DONOR WORKUP

Donor workup in a stepwise fashion is to ensure that the volunteer remains psychologically and physically healthy in the long term after the organ donation. Only healthy individuals ages 18 to 60 are eligible.

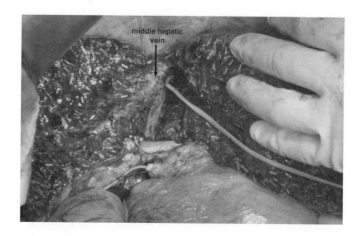

**FIGURE 29.3.1b-1**

Donor right hepatectomy with the middle hepatic vein exposed.

## Step 1

A detailed medical history is taken to identify any co-morbidities as there is a consensus in the transplant community that donors are healthy subjects.[13] Body mass index over 30 kg/m² cautions to fatty-liver- and obesity-related comorbidites. Blood group compatibility is verified. Hepatitis B and C carrier status preclude donation. Hepatitis B core antibody positivity mandates recipient lifelong prophylaxis with lamivudine.[14]

## Step 2a

A psychological assessment is performed to verify the potential donor's knowledge and coping ability of live donor liver transplantation (LDLT). This includes knowledge in donor and recipient morbidity and mortality, and the urgency of the recipient requiring the transplant.

## Step 2b

Chest radiograph and electrocardiogram are performed. Computed tomography (CT) of the liver under sodium bicarbonate cover[15] is performed. Maximum intensity projections of portal veins and hepatic veins and three-dimensional reconstruction of the hepatic artery are produced. Volumetry of the donor liver by the Heymsfield's method[16] measures the right liver and left liver volumes using the middle hepatic vein as a demarcation line for the plane between the two lobes.[12] Attenuation of the liver parenchyma on the plain film is assessed for detection of fatty change. For adult live donor liver transplant (ALDLT), the right lobe is often used unless the donor is substantially heavier than the recipient. The right lobe of the donor to the estimated standard liver volume 35% or less is associated with increased recipient mortality[17] and precludes ALDLT. Hepatic vein anatomy is determined by the axial cuts in venous phase and the easier perception by maximum intensity projections. Presence of substantial inferior hepatic vein(s) allows anticipation during operation. Attention to the presence of segment 4b hepatic vein or segment 3 hepatic vein draining into the MHV calls for a more caudal division of the MHV to preserve adequate drainage of segment 4 of the remnant left lobe.[12] The right, left, and segment 4 hepatic arteries are also illustrated by the three-dimensional reconstructions.

## Step 3

Invasive investigations such as liver biopsy and visceral angiogram are performed selectively when indicated, and only after genuineness and suitability otherwise of the potential donor are ascertained. A fatty change of up to 20% by histopathology is acceptable. In practice, the visceral angiogram is seldom necessary.

## Step 4

Informed consent including the donor and recipient morbidity and mortality as spelled out will be obtained from the potential donor.

## DONOR RIGHT HEPATECTOMY

### Exposure

Access for donor right hepatectomy is gained through a bilateral subcostal incision with upper midline extension. The incision on the right side is extended to the anterior axillary line, whereas the incision on the left side is extended only to the lateral border of the rectus muscle. The left subcostal incision could be avoided for donors with smaller anteroposterior dimensions and lower body mass index. The two curved blades of the Bookwalter retractor pull the rib cage laterally and anteriorly to open up the aperture made by the costal margins. Laparotomy pads are placed over the tissues to protect them from damage by the mechanical retractors blades. Excising the xiphoid process facilitates access to the suprahepatic IVC and the root of hepatic veins. The ligamentum teres is ligated and divided, and the falciform ligament severed. Following a careful laparotomy, intraoperative ultrasonography (IOUS) is performed to study the junction of the MHV and left hepatic vein with the IVC. The relation of the V4b to the MHV already known from CT is ascertained by IOUS. This also registers the flow characteristics of the hepatic arteries, portal veins, and hepatic veins for reference throughout the operation.

### OPERATIVE CHOLANGIOGRAM

The Calot's triangle is dissected to isolate the cystic duct and cystic artery. After cannulation of the cystic duct with a 3.5 Fr Argyle tube, the gallbladder is excised. Minimal dissection of the right liver hilum just enough to identify the right hepatic duct is done. A large-size titanium clip marks the planned line of bile duct division. The biliary tract is then outlined by real-time operative cholangiogram under fluoroscopic control using undiluted contrast. Image quality is improved by temporary occlusion of the distal common bile duct by a bulldog clamp. This supraduodenal portion of the common bile duct is isolated just enough for the clamp without disruption of the blood supply.[18] The clamp must be removed once the cholangiogram is finished to avoid ischemic damage to the duct. With the donor in supine position, the right posterior sectoral duct is revealed first, followed by the right anterior, and then by the left ductal systems. The parallax technique clarifies the anteroposterior location of the right anterior and posterior sectoral ducts. This is done by swinging the C-arm to obtain a right lateral view of the trunk, the true anteroposterior view for the liver.

### ISOLATION OF MAJOR VESSELS AND PARENCHYMAL TRANSECTION

Hilar dissection is then continued to identify and isolate the right hepatic artery and the right portal vein. The space between the right hepatic artery and the right hepatic duct should not be disrupted in order to preserve the blood supply of the latter. To gain the entire length of the right portal vein, all branches to the caudate lobe are ligated and then divided. A sizeable branch from the right portal vein may represent vessels supplying segment 6 and should not be sacrificed.

The right triangular ligament is taken down while leaving the Gerota fascia not damaged. In the normal liver, the right adrenal gland could often be freed from the liver with careful dissection using the electrocautery operated with precision. Minor bleeding from the right adrenal gland is controlled by the Argon Beam Coagulator; and more severe bleeding, by plication with sutures. Short hepatic veins on the right side of the midline of the IVC are divided between ligatures. Inferior right hepatic vein(s) larger than 5 mm are preserved. Temporary right lobe inflow control is performed to mark the line of transection, the Cantlie's line with electrocautery. The line on the inferior surface is just to the left of the gallbladder fossa and joining with the planned line of division of the right hepatic duct marked earlier.

In contrast to hepatectomy for neoplasm, continuous inflow control during liver transection is not applicable. Pringle maneuver with intermittent reperfusion of the liver is practiced by some centers. It was demonstrated that blood loss was lower for donors with Pringle maneuver. However, the difference did not reach statistical significance.[19] Possible explanations to this are that the bleeding from the hepatic vein tributaries is not controlled by inflow control and there is bleeding during the 5-minute reperfusion time. Another potential advantage of the Pringle maneuver is the down-regulation of apoptosis pathway by ischemic preconditioning for grafts with long cold ischemic time.[20] This, however, was associated with poorer initial graft functioning by a prospective trial in deceased donor liver procurement.[21] For ALDLT, prolonged cold ischemia should not be an issue because graft delivery matches the explantation of the native liver. A low central venous pressure could only be attained with good rapport with the anesthetist. This is effective in lowering blood loss.[22]

After mobilization of the right lobe from its posterior attachments, a full thickness suture at the liver edge on both sides of this line aids opening up of the transection plane by the weight of hemostats. The placement of the laparotomy pad behind the right lobe brings the transection plane to more vertical. Liver parenchymal transection is started with electrocautery for the first 1 to 2 cm of parenchyma between segments 5 and 4a. The rest of the liver transection employs the Cavitron ultrasonic surgical aspirator (CUSA) which exposes the left side of the MHV that lies two thirds of the depth from the superior surface of the liver (Figure 29.3.1b-1).[23] The CUSA at a frequency of 23 kHz is set at amplitude of 60% for the normal donor liver and irrigation with normal saline at 4 to 5 mL per minute. The liver parenchyma is disrupted by cavitation of the aerosol. When the dissector is set at lower amplitudes, there is a tendency for the operator to bring the instrument into direct contact with the liver parenchyma which will damage small and friable vessels. Suction is set to a moderately high level just enough to provide a clear operative field. Electrocautery incorporated into the CUSA allows diathermy of vessels less than 1 mm in diameter. Should the V4b insert into the MHV, transection stops to preserve this vein for draining segment.[12] We find it unnecessary to use other devices like waterjet approaching the root of the MHV as the vein becomes less and less friable. At the liver hilum, the right portal pedicle containing the right hepatic duct is also dissected out with CUSA. Line of division already marked and verified by operative cholangiogram is followed. The right hepatic duct(s) is severed with scissors, tangential to the transection plane which is often quite horizontal already developed. No attempt is made to denude the duct in order to maintain adequate blood supply. The right duct stump is repaired by 6/0 polydioxanone (PDS) suture, continuous, back-and-forth. Liver parenchyma dorsal to the MHV is cleaved mainly by sharp dissection, and the caudate lobe is transected until the inferior vena cava (IVC) is exposed. Lifting up of the caudate lobe with a cotton-tape or a right angled forceps much facilitates the transection. Care is taken to dissect in a definable plane between the liver capsule and the IVC.

### Graft Delivery

Graft delivery starts with applying a clamp onto the proximal right hepatic artery and division of the latter distal to the clamp. The right portal vein is then divided between vascular clamps applied at right angle to the course of the main portal vein. The MHV, right hepatic vein, and if present the inferior right hepatic vein are controlled with vascular stapler (TA 30, Tyco Healthcare, Norwalk, Connecticut) prior to its division by scissors. To avoid stricture of the portal vein, the right portal vein stump is sutured in

a transverse manner with 6/0 Prolene sutures continuous, back-and-forth. Biliary leakage and patency of the remnant left hepatic duct is checked with intraoperative cholangiogram and methylene blue instillation. The methylene blue of the bile ducts is flushed out with normal saline. The cystic duct is ligated twice with 2/0 Vicryl. The remnant left liver is maintained in the anatomical position by reconstitution of the falciform ligament with nonabsorbable sutures. Patency of the vessels is verified with intraoperative ultrasonography. The hepatic flexure of the colon and the corresponding portion of greater omentum are allowed to ascend into the right subphrenic space and prevent adherence of the small bowel to the transection surface of the remnant left lobe. The abdominal is closed without drainage.[24]

### BACKTABLE PROCEDURE

To shorten the cold ischemic time, the right liver graft is not delivered until the recipient is almost ready for graft implantation. Precise communication between the two teams is vital in this regard. The graft once delivered is flushed with 3 times the graft volume cold histidine–tryptophan–ketoglutarate (HTK; Dr. Franz Köhler, Chemie GmbH, Alsbach-Hähnlein, Germany) solution while immersed in an ice-sludge basin on the backtable. The right portal vein is cannulated and wall adapted to the vein wall with fingers.[25] The right hepatic artery is flushed with 50 mL cold HTK solution through a Fr 21 angiocatheter under gravity. Utmost care is taken not to damage the intimate of the artery by the angiocatheter. The right anterior and posterior sectoral ducts are also flushed with cold HTK solution. The graft is weighed and transferred to another basin with cold HTK solution. Venoplasty of the middle hepatic vein with the right hepatic vein of the graft is then performed.[26] Even though the MHV and the RHV are often at a distance of up to 2 cm, they can be drawn together for fashioning of a single venous cuff (Figure 29.3.1b-2).[26] Often misled by planar schematic drawings, there is a false perception of the inadequate length of the MHV wall portion of the venoplasty for the anastomosis to the IVC. In practice, the IVC which is tubular, with a venotomy made over the RHV stump, faces the venoplasty of the MHV and RHV. The portion of the recipient IVC in between the RHV and MHV also makes up for the deficit in length on the MHV not included in the graft to preserve the segment 4b hepatic vein for venous drainage of the remnant left lobe of the donor.

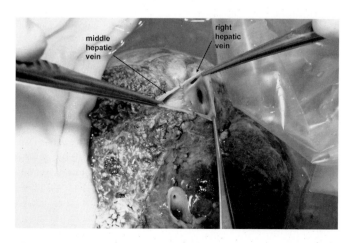

**FIGURE 29.3.1b-2**

Venoplasty of the middle and right hepatic veins to form a single cuff.

# References

1. Lee S, Park K, Hwang S, et al. Congestion of right liver graft in living donor liver transplantation. *Transplantation* 2001;71:812.

2. Sugawara Y, Makuuchi M, Sano K, et al. Vein reconstruction in modified right liver graft for living donor liver transplantation. *Ann Surg* 2003; 237:180.

3. Sugawara Y, Makuuchi M, Akamatsu N, et al. Refinement of venous reconstruction using cryopreserved veins in right liver grafts. *Liver Transplant* 2004;10:541.

4. Malago M, Molmenti EP, Paul A, et al. Hepatic venous outflow reconstruction in right live donor liver transplantation. *Liver Transplant* 2005;11:364.

5. Fan ST, Lo CM, Liu CL, et al. Safety and necessity of including the middle hepatic vein in the right lobe graft in adult-to-adult live donor liver transplantation. *Ann Surg* 2003;238:137.

6. Scatton O, Belghiti J, Dondero F, et al. Harvesting the middle hepatic vein with a right hepatectomy does not increase the risk for the donor. *Liver Transplant* 2004;10:71.

7. Shah SA, Grant DR, Greig PD, et al. Analysis and outcomes of right lobe hepatectomy in 101 consecutive living donors. *Am J Transplant* 2005;5:2764.

8. Chan SC, Fan ST, Lo CM, et al. Toward current standards of donor right hepatectomy for adult-to-adult live donor liver transplantation through the experience of 200 cases. *Ann Surg* (in press).

9. Malago M, Testa G, Frilling A, et al: Right living donor liver transplantation: an option for adult patients: single institution experience with 74 patients. *Ann Surg* 2003;238:853.

10. Kasahara M, Takada Y, Fujimoto Y, et al: Impact of right lobe with middle hepatic vein graft in living-donor liver transplantation. *Am J Transplant* 2005;5:1339.

11. Kido M, Ku Y, Fukumoto T, et al: Significant role of middle hepatic vein in remnant liver regeneration of right-lobe living donors. *Transplantation* 2003;75:1598.

12. Chan SC, Lo CM, Liu CL, et al. Tailoring donor hepatectomy per segment 4 venous drainage in right lobe live donor liver transplantation. *Liver Transplant* 2004;10:755.

13. Abecassis M, Adams M, Adams P, et al: Consensus statement on the live organ donor. *JAMA* 2000;284:2919.

14. Lo CM, Fan ST, Liu CL, et al. Safety and outcome of hepatitis B core antibody-positive donors in right-lobe living donor liver transplantation. *Liver Transplant* 2003;9:827.

15. Merten GJ, Burgess WP, Gray LV, et al. Prevention of contrast-induced nephropathy with sodium bicarbonate: a randomized controlled trial. *JAMA* 2004;291:2328.

16. Heymsfield SB, Fulenwider T, Nordlinger B, et al. Accurate measurement of liver, kidney, and spleen volume and mass by computerized axial tomography. *Ann Intern Med* 1979;90:185.

17. Fan ST, Lo CM, Liu CL, et al. Determinants of hospital mortality of adult recipients of right lobe live donor liver transplantation. *Ann Surg* 2003;238:864.

18. Fan ST, Lo CM, Liu CL. Technical refinement in adult-to-adult living donor liver transplantation using right lobe graft. *Ann Surg* 2000;231:126.

19. Imamura H, Takayama T, Sugawara Y, et al. Pringle's manoeuvre in living donors. *Lancet* 2002;360:2049.

20. Clavien PA, Yadav S, Sindram D, et al. Protective effects of ischemic preconditioning for liver resection performed under inflow occlusion in humans. *Ann Surg* 2000;232:155.

21. Azoulay D, Del GM, Andreani P, et al: Effects of 10 minutes of ischemic preconditioning of the cadaveric liver on the graft's preservation and function: the ying and the yang. *Ann Surg* 2005;242:133.

22. Jones RM, Moulton CE, Hardy KJ. Central venous pressure and its effect on blood loss during liver resection. *Br J Surg* 1998;85:1058.

23. Fan ST, Lo CM, Liu CL, et al: Safety of donors in live donor liver transplantation using right lobe grafts. *Arch Surg* 2000;135:336.

24. Liu CL, Fan ST, Lo CM, et al: Safety of donor right hepatectomy without abdominal drainage: A prospective evaluation in 100 consecutive liver donors. *Liver Transpl* 2005;11:314.

25. Chan SC, Liu CL, Lo CM, et al. Applicability of histidine-tryptophan-ketoglutarate solution in right lobe adult-to-adult live donor liver transplantation. *Liver Transpl* 2004;10:1415.

26. Lo CM, Fan ST, Liu CL, et al. Hepatic venoplasty in living-donor liver transplantation using right lobe graft with middle hepatic vein. *Transplantation* 2003;75:358.

## 29.3.1c  Adult Donor to Adult Recipient, Left Lobe

*Sander Florman, MD, Charles M. Miller, MD*

## INTRODUCTION

The disparity between the supply of deceased donor organs and the ever-growing demand for transplants has long been the impetus for pursuing living donation.[1,2] Patients, families and physicians have generally accepted that the potential risks involved with donation from a healthy, living donor are justified so that another person can have the potentially life-saving transplant opportunity. The physicians who perform these donor surgeries are also accepting a tremendous responsibility, however. Although good recipient outcome is the motivation, donor safety and the donor's long-term outcome must remain paramount.

The initial experiences worldwide with live donor liver transplantation were with the left lateral segment for pediatric recipients, for whom the likelihood of death on the deceased donor waiting list was exceptionally high.[1] Surgical techniques were refined during the early 1990s, and ultimately, the success of these procedures led to their more widespread application. Eventually, the opportunity for living donor liver transplantation was offered to larger recipients who required more functional liver mass than the left lateral segment could provide. In Australia in 1989, Strong et al reported the first left lobe live donor liver transplant in a pediatric recipient.[3] The first adult-to-adult live donor liver transplant using a left lobe graft was reported by Hashikura in 1994 in Japan. With little or no cultural provisions for deceased donation in Japan,[4] most of these early efforts were pioneered in Asia.[5,6]

For adult recipients, the left lobe was initially chosen mostly because the resection was associated with a lower risk of complications for the donors compared with a right lobe resection.[7–10] These early efforts were associated with generally poor results, however.[11] The small-for-size syndrome was described when recipients of relatively small partial grafts, at least functionally, had prolonged cholestasis, ascites, and/or encephalopathy posttransplant.[12] Some even died as a result of small-for-size syndrome. Many of these recipients were later recognized to have had excessive portal inflow that produced overperfusion of these partial grafts, resulting in poor graft function.

Consequently, surgeons attempted more formidable resections (ie, right lobectomy) to provide greater graft volumes. Even with the significantly larger right lobe partial graft, however, small-for-size syndrome may still occur.[13–15] Partial grafts have been shown to receive three or more times the normal amount of portal flow.[10] In addition, graft outflow issues can be equally critical for success. Early experiences with living donor right lobe transplants highlighted the need to understand the hemodynamics of partial liver grafts.[10,16]

It is important for the versatile live donor liver surgeon to have experience with all potential resections so that recipient outcomes can be maximized and donor morbidity minimized. When the involved principles are appropriately understood and applied, excellent outcomes are possible with relatively small graft volumes. Herein we discuss our approach to and describe techniques for live donor left lobectomy for adult recipients.

## GRAFT SELECTION

Graft selection is arguably second in importance only to surgical technique for ensuring good recipient outcomes. Consideration of a variety of factors is imperative, including but certainly not limited to the donor and recipient body weights and the degree of recipient illness (ie, portal hypertension). Calculating the standard liver volume (SLV) is an important component of estimating the necessary volume requirement for a given recipient.[13,16]

A variety of anatomic resections from live donors for transplantation have been performed, the most common being the left lateral segment (ie, segments II and III) for pediatric recipients and the left lobe (ie, segments I, II, III, and IV) or right lobe (ie, segments V, VI, VII and VIII) for larger recipients (Color Plates, Figure LI-1). In the donors, the morbidity associated with these procedures increases incrementally with larger resections.

With careful donor and recipient evaluation and an expert understanding of portal hemodynamics, the left lobe may have far greater utility for adult recipients than has previously been appreciated. Using the left lobe for a large child or even an adolescent is well accepted and appropriate when a left lateral segment would be too small. In addition, when the donor is significantly bigger than the recipient, or when the left lobe is larger than the minimum volume requirement for the recipient (generally accepted as 40% of the recipient's SLV), then a larger donor resection is likely unnecessary.[7]

Utilizing the left lobe for an adult recipient with significant portal hypertension, on the other hand, is potentially more hazardous. Furthermore, when the potential donor graft is estimated to be less than 40% of the intended recipient's SLV, more complex decision making is required to determine if the left lobe will be an adequate graft. The presence of cirrhosis and the degree of portal hypertension are critical determinants of what minimum graft volume is required for any given recipient.[15,17] In the absence of cirrhosis and with lesser degrees of portal hypertension, a graft that is 30% or more of the recipient's SLV is likely adequate, whereas in the presence of cirrhosis with greater degrees of portal hypertension at least 45% is generally required.[17] Planned recipient portal inflow modification (eg, splenectomy, shunting) may also affect the decision regarding the minimum graft size necessary for success.

Whether to include the caudate lobe as part of the left lobe resection remains controversial. In certain cases, inclusion of the caudate lobe may increase the volume by approximately 3% to 4% of the whole liver volume, corresponding to an 8% to 12% increase in the volume of the left lobe graft.[18–21] The techniques to reconstruct the main draining vein of the caudate lobe to preserve function and to prevent venous congestion of the caudate have been described.[19,22]

## DONOR EVALUATION

Donors should undergo complete evaluations including an assessment to rule out any elements of coercion. Routine use of donor biopsy has been debated, but should probably be done to ensure that no occult conditions exist.[23] Routine hematology and

chemistries as well as virologic screening should be performed. We now advocate routine computed tomography (CT) imaging with three-dimensional reconstruction for volumetry, angiography, venography, and a magnetic resonance cholangiopancreatography (MRCP) for cholangiography. The accuracy of these procedures obviates the need for more invasive, potentially hazardous testing (eg, arteriogram, endoscopic retrograde cholangiopancreatography [ERCP]).

Care must always be taken to minimize donor exposure to risk. Accurate noninvasive testing is an essential component of the donor evaluation. Initially, donors underwent invasive testing with formal angiograms and even endoscopic retrograde cholangiography. These procedures, considered gold standards for imaging of the vascular and biliary anatomy, respectively, also carry certain morbidity. We also advocate a time-out period after the donor has given informed consent and before the actual surgery, to ensure that the donor wants to proceed and is not caught up in the emotional aspects of donation. Exceptions to this time-out period are made in the case of pediatric recipients with acute hepatic failure and possibly in emergent adult cases.

## SURGICAL TECHNIQUES

### Perioperative Prophylaxis

It is imperative that all appropriate measures of prophylaxis be taken when performing elective live donor liver resections. Donors should receive intravenous perioperative antibiosis, with the first dose administered just before skin incision. Donors should have sequential compression devices in place prior to the induction of anesthesia for deep venous thrombosis protection, as well as subcutaneous low-molecular-weight heparin injections. Warming blankets should be used intraoperatively to prevent hypothermia.

It is particularly important to have expert anesthesiologists present during live donor hepatectomies, and especially during the parenchymal transection. Good communication can help to ensure limited blood loss and good donor outcomes. During the parenchymal transection, the donor should be placed in a slight Trendelenberg position, and the central venous pressure should be lowered.[24] The blood-cell saver is routinely used. These maneuvers will help to limit blood loss.

All donors have a nasogastric tube placed at the time of the procedure, to be kept in place postoperatively until normal intestinal function resumes. Standard stress ulcer prophylaxis is also strongly recommended.

### Incision and Exposure

A low right subcostal with a long vertical extension to the xyphoid is performed for optimal exposure, followed by a brief evaluation of the abdominal viscera. Hepatic ultrasonography should be performed to confirm preoperative anatomic assessments, with special attention paid to the hepatic venous anatomy.

The round ligament is divided, and the falciform ligament is taken back to the level of the suprahepatic vena cava. The falciform ligament should be left long enough on the left lobe so that it can be attached to the recipient's anterior abdominal wall to prevent graft torsion. The left triangular ligament is divided medially to the suprahepatic vena cava, exposing the lateral border of the left hepatic vein at the junction with the vena cava. The gastrohepatic ligament is examined and divided, with care taken to

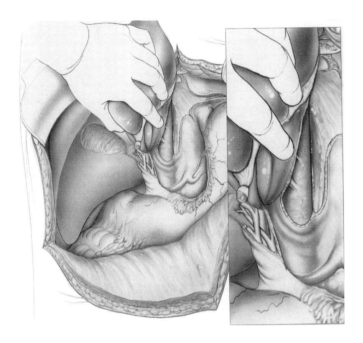

**FIGURE 29.3.1c-1**

Reflection of the left lateral segment; exposure of the caudate lobe and the left side of the retrohepatic inferior vena cava.

identify and preserve any accessory or replaced left hepatic artery coursing through this ligament. The caudate lobe is then exposed and can be gently retracted up and to the right, exposing the inferior vena cava (Figure 29.3.1c-1).

## Cholecystectomy and Cholangiography

A cholecystectomy and a cholangiogram via the cystic duct are performed. Delineating the biliary anatomy is critical and one of the more challenging parts of the live donor resection. Divide the left hepatic duct too far to the left and there are likely to be multiple ducts that may all require reconstruction in the recipient. Divide the duct too close to the bifurcation and there is the possibility of compromising or injuring the donor's remaining duct. Special attention must be paid to ensure that the right posterior hepatic duct does not drain into the left hepatic duct. In case of such an anatomical variant, the left hepatic duct must be divided to the left of the junction of the right posterior hepatic duct with the left hepatic duct. Preoperative imaging and intraoperative cholangiography should be evaluated specifically to determine if this anatomic variant is present.

## Hilar Dissection

The hilar dissection is performed with care to avoid unnecessary dissection of the right-sided structures. The left hepatic artery, left portal vein, and left hepatic duct must all be carefully isolated in such a manner that they will be transplantable in the recipient without injury to the donor. While maximizing the length of these structures to optimize the recipient procedure, care must be taken not to narrow or impinge on the remaining donor structures. There is no substitute for surgical experience and knowledge of common hepatic anatomic variations.

## Hepatic Artery Dissection

The left hepatic artery is carefully dissected proximally to the level of the bifurcation of the proper hepatic artery into right and left branches. In the case of an accessory or replaced left hepatic artery, the dissection is carried proximally to the left gastric artery and even down as far as the celiac axis. This often results in considerable extra length for the arterial reconstruction. In performing this tedious dissection, small side branches to the stomach must be individually ligated and divided. Care must be taken to evaluate the arterial supply of segment IV, which may arise from the right hepatic artery in up to 20% of donors, and is often referred to as the middle hepatic artery.[25,26] In these cases, it is important to evaluate the caliber of this segmental artery and to determine whether a separate reconstruction is necessary.

Although there is often redundant arterial supply to segment IV via the main left hepatic artery, there may be some risk of arterial insufficiency for the segmental bile duct if a separate segment IV artery is not reconstructed.[26,27] One useful method is to reassess the backflow of a separate segment IV artery after main left hepatic artery reperfusion in the recipient. If there is good backflow then there is less concern over performing an additional, often technically difficult, reconstruction that might increase the risk for hepatic artery thrombosis.[27] There are, however, some who advocate multiple arterial reconstructions regardless of the presence or absence of backflow.[25]

There are several common variations that occur with the left hepatic artery and are importantly recognized by the live donor surgeon when procuring the left lobe for transplant[27] (Color Plates, Figure LI-4B). Most commonly, the left hepatic artery is single and arises from the common hepatic artery. Less commonly, there may be a separate segment IV branch that arises from the right hepatic artery. The left hepatic artery arises aberrantly from the left gastric artery in approximately 13% of patients.[28] Least commonly, there may be three separate arteries that supply each segment (ie, segments II, III, and IV) separately. These anatomic configurations have significant implications for the hepatic arterial reconstruction that will be required in the recipient.

## Portal Vein Dissection

The left portal vein is identified medial and posterior to the left hepatic artery and dissected circumferentially. When the caudate lobe is to be included with the left lobe graft, care must be taken to preserve the small portal caudate branches that drain directly into the left portal vein. When the graft to be procured does not include the caudate lobe, these small braches can be sacrificed, thereby allowing for greater mobilization and length of the left portal vein. The left portal vein dissection may be somewhat challenging technically as a result of overlying left and middle hepatic arteries. The left portal vein has a relatively long extrahepatic course, however, thus making this dissection somewhat easier than the dissection required to expose the right portal vein.

## Hepatic Vein Dissection

The area between the middle and right hepatic veins as they enter the suprahepatic vena cava is often easily developed by dividing the loose peritoneal reflection over the vena cava and bluntly spreading in this area. When possible, it is preferable to completely dissect and encircle the common trunk of the left and middle hepatic veins just as they enter the vena cava. In some cases this is technically hazardous and should not be done until the parenchymal transection is performed. In most patients the left and middle hepatic veins will have a common trunk that enters the vena cava. It is very important to mobilize the left and middle hepatic veins to their base at the vena cava. This often necessitates mobilization of the diaphragm and ligation and transection of the left phrenic vein.

## Parenchymal Transection

The line of transection for the left lobectomy is the same as that for a right lobectomy that does not include the middle hepatic vein, namely, just to the right of the middle hepatic vein along the main portal fissure. This line should be confirmed with ultrasonography intraoperatively, just prior to and during the parenchymal transection. It is useful to line up the right border of the middle hepatic vein with the lateral border of the vena cava posteriorly to ensure that the transection is performed in the correct plane. The transection should proceed approximately 0.5 cm lateral to the right border of the middle hepatic vein, thereby keeping a protective, small rim of hepatic parenchyma on the middle hepatic vein.

When the caudate lobe is not included with the left lobe graft, the transection should proceed from the anterior surface of the liver to the hilum and the ductus venosum. When the caudate is to be included, the transection should proceed from the anterior surface of the liver to the hilum and then posteriorly to the vena cava. Care should be taken in the area of the hilum, where the parenchymal transection should proceed to the left of the common and right hepatic ducts. Periodically throughout the transection it may be useful to repeat the ultrasonography to confirm the correct plane and to reconfigure the lateral border of the middle hepatic vein with the vena cava.

For obtaining a graft with the caudate lobe, the small short hepatic veins to the caudate lobe are ligated and divided. Care is taken to identify the caudate lobe vein, the largest of the short hepatic veins draining the caudate lobe. Couinaud reported that nearly 70% of caudate lobes have a single, dominant vein that drains the caudate lobe.[29] Reconstruction of this vein in the recipient can lead to a fully functional caudate lobe,[19] and prevent venous congestion of the caudate lobe.

## Graft Removal and Preservation

At the appropriate time, once the parenchymal transection has been completed, consideration must be given to the order in which the vascular structures will be clamped and divided. The backtable should be set up and the preservation solution should be chilled and cannulated. We have generally ligated the proximal hepatic artery(ies) and divided the artery first, then the left portal vein. Application of the vascular clamp on the left portal vein must be done with care to ensure that there is no encroachment on the portal bifurcation that may subsequently lead to narrowing of the remnant donor portal vein. Following division of the left portal vein, a large vascular clamp is placed across the vena cava around the orifices of the left and middle hepatic veins and the hepatic veins are then divided.

It may be useful on the backtable to perform a left and middle hepatic vein venoplasty (Figure 29.3.1c-2) to optimize venous outflow in the recipient.

The graft is removed from the donor and passed off to the backtable where it is preserved with cold preservation solution and

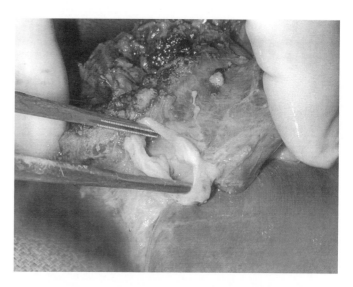

**FIGURE 29.3.1c-2**

A venoplasty between the left and middle hepatic veins to optimize graft outflow.

kept on ice (Figures 29.3.1c-3 and 29.3.1c-4). The flush continues via the stump of the left portal vein until the effluent from the hepatic veins is clear. Generally, 750 to 1000 mL of solution is required. Some have described the technique of beginning flushing with the preservation solution while *in situ* in the donor.[8] The left hepatic artery may also be flushed but care must be taken when doing so, to avoid injuring the endothelium of this small vessel.

In the donor, the stump of the left portal vein is run closed with fine suture and the defect in the vena cava is similarly closed. Care is taken to ensure good hemostasis and good flow in the

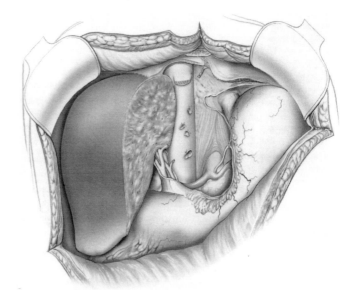

**FIGURE 29.3.1c-3**

The remnant right lobe after the left lobe graft was removed from the donor.

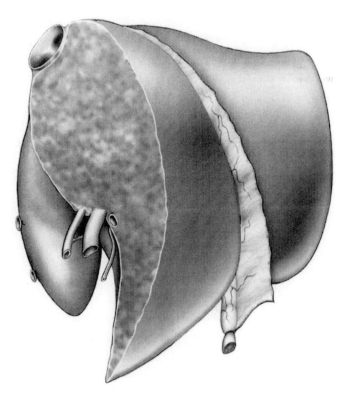

**FIGURE 29.3.1c-4**

The left lobe graft with the caudate lobe.

remnant right portal vein and hepatic artery. The stump of the left hepatic bile duct is oversewn, and a careful evaluation of the cut surface of the liver is performed, specifically looking for any small open bile ducts. Some surgeons advocate performing a final cholangiogram via the cystic duct stump prior to closure to assess and document the donor's remnant ductal anatomy and to rule out any potential leaks. Use of methylene blue or indocyanine green to assist in ruling out any small leaks from the cut surface of the remnant parenchyma has also been described.[8,30] A useful and simple technique to identify a bile leak is to gently blot the cut surface of the liver with a clean laparotomy pad looking for yellow bile staining. This is only effective after perfect hemostasis has been achieved. In addition, this technique is particularly valuable when an occult caudate duct leak is present because it may be separated from the main ductal system, making it virtually impossible to detect via cholangiography.

Once leaks have been ruled out and hemostasis is complete, a single closed-suction drain (ie, Blake, Jackson-Pratt) is placed alongside the cut surface of the liver and brought out through a separate stab incision below the main incision. The position of the nasogastric tube is confirmed. The omentum is then placed alongside the cut surface, and the fascia is then closed.

## CONCLUSIONS

The left lobe graft is anatomically far better suited for partial liver transplantation than is the larger right lobe graft, and there is considerably less morbidity for the donor. The venous drainage of the left lobe graft is superior to that of the right lobe, yet it generally has substantially less mass. The technically most challenging aspect of left lobe donor surgery is arguably the arterial dissection, as a result of highly variable arterial anatomy, especially for segment IV.

With an expert understanding of an individual recipient's portal inflow, modifications can be made to optimize graft perfusion and thereby make left lobe transplantation as, if not more successful, than right lobe transplantation. The simple calculations of graft and recipient weights are not adequate to accurately predict which graft a recipient will require. With optimal outflow and attention to the intricacies of inflow considerations, many recipients can have good outcomes with the left lobe graft while exposing their donors to potentially less morbidity with a lesser hepatic resection.

There is no substitute for surgical experience and knowledge of common hepatic anatomic variants. There is also no substitute for careful donor evaluation and operative planning to determine which graft will be best for an individual recipient, while minimizing donor risk.

## References

1. Otte JB. History of pediatric liver transplantation. Where are we coming from? Where do we stand? *Pediatr Transplant* 2002;6:378–387

2. United Network for Organ Sharing (UNOS). http://www.unos.org (accessed July 2005)

3. Strong RW, Lynch SV, Ong TH, et al. Successful liver transplantation from a living donor to her son. *N Engl J Med* 1990;322:1505–1507.

4. Hashikura Y, Makuuchi M, Kawasaki S, et al. Successful living related partial liver transplantation to an adult patient. *Lancet* 1994;343:1233–1234

5. Otte JB. The availability of all technical modalities for pediatric liver transplant programs. *Pediatr Transplant* 2001;5:1–4

6. Kawasaki S, Hashikura Y, Ikegami T, et al. First case of cadaveric liver transplantation in Japan. *J Hepatobiliary Pancreat Surg* 1999;6:387–390

7. Kokudo N, Sugawara Y, Imamura H, Sano K, Makuuchi M. Tailoring the type of donor hepatectomy for adult living donor liver transplantation. *Am J Transpl* 2005.

8. Fan ST, Lo CM, Liu CL. Donor hepatectomy for living-donor liver transplantation. *Hepato-Gastroenterology* 1998;45: 34–39

9. Kanoh K, Nomoto K, Shimura T, et al. A comparison of right-lobe and left-lobe grafts for living-donor liver transplantation. *Hepato-Gastroenterology* 2002;49:222–224

10. Shimada M, Shiotani S, Ninomiya M, et al. Characteristics of liver grafts in living-donor adult liver transplantation. *Arch Surg* 2002;137:1174–1179

11. Miller CM, Gondolesi GE, Florman S, et al. One hundred nine living donor liver transplants in adults and children: a single-center experience. *Ann Surg* 2001;234:301–311

12. Emond JC, Renz JF, Ferrell LD, et al. Functional analysis of grafts from living donors. Implications for the treatment of older recipients. *Ann Surg* 1996;224:544–552

13. Urata K, Kawasaki S, Matsunami H, et al. Calculation of child and adult standard liver volume for liver transplantation. *Hepatology* 1995;21:1317–1321.

14. Kiuchi T, Kasahara M, Uryuhara K, et al. Impact of graft size mismatching on graft prognosis in liver transplantation from living donors. *Transplantation* 1999;67:321–327.

15. Ben-Haim M, Emre S, Fishbein TM, et al. Critical graft size in adult-to-adult living donor liver transplantation: impact of the recipient's disease. *Liver Transplant* 2001;7:948–953.

16. Gondolesi GE, Florman S, Matsumoto C, et al. Venous hemodynamics in living donor right lobe liver transplantation. *Liver Transplant* 2002;8:809–813.

17. Soejima Y, Shimada M, Seuhiro T, et al. Outcome analysis in adult-to-adult living donor liver transplantation using the left lobe. *Liver Transplant* 2003;9: 581–558.

18. Hwang S, Lee S-G, Ha T-Y, et al. Simplified standardized technique for living donor liver transplantation using left liver graft plus caudate lobe. *Liver Transplant* 2004;10:1398–1405.

19. Takayama T, Makuuchi M, Kubota K, et al. Living related transplantation of left liver plus caudate lobe. *J Am Coll Surg* 2000;190:635.

20. Miyagawa S, Hashikura Y, Miwa S, et al. Concomitant caudate lobe resection as an option for donor hepatectomy in adult living related liver transplantation. *Transplantation* 1998;66:661–663.

21. Makuuchi M, Sugawara Y. Living-donor liver transplantation using the left liver, with special reference to vein reconstruction. *Transplantation* 2003;75:S23–S24.

22. Sugawara Y, Makuuchi M, Takayama T. Left liver plus caudate lobe graft with complete re-vascularization. *Surgery* 2002;132:348.

23. Nadalin S, Malago M, Valentin-Gamazo C, et al. Preoperative donor liver biopsy for adult living donor liver transplantation: risks and benefits. *Liver Transplantat* 2005;11:980–986.

24. Cunningham JD, Fong Y, Shriver C, et al. One hundred consecutive hepatic resections. Blood loss, transfusion and operative technique. *Arch Surg* 1994;129:1050–1056.

25. Suehiro T, Ninomiya M, Shiotani S, et al. Hepatic artery reconstruction and biliary stricture formation after living donor adult liver transplantation using the left lobe. *Liver Tx* 2002;8:495–499.

26. Ikegami T, Kawasaki S, Matsunami H, et al. Should all hepatic arterial branches be reconstructed in living-related liver transplantation? *Surgery* 1996;119:431–436

27. Shinohara H, Tanaka A, Hatano E, et al. Anatomical and physiological problems of Segment IV: liver transplants using left lobes from living related donors. *Clin Transplant* 1996;10:341–347.

28. Todo S, Makowka L, Tzakis AG, et al. Hepatic artery in liver transplantation. *Transplant Proc* 1987;19:2406–2411.

29. Couinaud C. The paracaval segments of the liver. *J Hepatobiliary Pancreat Surg* 1994;2:145–151.

30. Soejima Y, Shimada M, Suehiro T, et al. Feasibility of duct-to-duct biliary reconstruction in left-lobe adult-living-donor liver transplantation. *Transplantation* 2003;75(4):557–559.

## 29.3.2  Adult Donor to Pediatric Recipient

*Thomas Heffron, MD, Todd Pillen, PA, Carlos Fasola, MD*

### INTRODUCTION AND HISTORY

Living donation liver transplantation (LDLT) originated as a series of stepwise surgical solutions to satisfy a need for children dying of end-stage liver disease due to lack of donor organs. Reduced-size cadaver donor liver transplantation (RCDLT) was developed in different institutions and countries by Broelsch et al in 1984.[1] This operation was used to overcome size disparity between small recipients and large donors, and it allowed the use of a donor more than 10 times larger than the weight of the recipient. RCDLT shifts the use of donor organs from adults to children while doing nothing to increase the total number of available organs.

The four cases of split liver transplantation were performed in 1988 originally reported by Pichylmayer, Broelsch, and Emond,[2–5] and Bismuth enabled two recipients to receive a transplant from one donor liver. The inherent desirability of living related liver transplantation (LRLT) pertains from its complete independence from cadaver donors availability. The first attempted LRLT in the world was performed by Raia[6] in 1988, but resulted in recipient death. Strong et al[7] reported the first successful LRLT in 1990, but the recipient required retransplantation, from a cadaver

donor, in the first year after transplantation. Led by Christoph Broelsch, the University of Chicago team performed the first successful series in the world with over 20 patients in 1989.[8] Tanaka and Ozawa[9] started LRLT programs in Japan and quickly became world leaders in both pediatric and adult LRLT.

The major perceived obstacle prior to performing LRLT was the ethical dilemma of subjecting any adult to any risk to donate a segment of liver to save the life of a related child. In our own experience with 40 left-side hepatectomies performed by three surgeons (Broelsch, Emond, and Heffron) in noncirrhotic patients, we observed no mortality or long-term morbidity. The risk of major complications was estimated at less than 1%, and the risk of minor complications at less than 7% over a 4-year period there were no deaths or long-term complications in 85 patients undergoing liver resection by three surgeons for benign disease, including benign hepatic lesions and living related donors.[12]

Although the first three donors at the University of Chicago consisted in a full left hepatectomy—with removal of the left medial segment on the back table—the ensuing 39 involved only a left lateral resection, leaving segment four with the donor. All recipients were small children. A left hepatectomy is reserved for larger pediatric recipients who need a larger amount of liver tissue (ie, adolescents). The risk of living donor hepatectomy is directly related to the percentage of donor liver removed. Therefore, a left lateral hepatectomy should have minimal risk to the donor. This criterion necessarily limits recipients, as somewhere between 0.8% and 1% of the recipients' weight must be encompassed as viable liver parenchyma for the best chance of success. This should not usually pose a problem in pediatric liver transplantation, as the majority of patients are less than 10 kg in size. The problem pertains in finding a left lateral segment small enough (especially in the area of the thickest point) to fit in the infants' abdomen to allow the small child to perfuse the graft and fit in the abdomen while avoiding respiratory compromise. Our experience has enabled us to be very successful at Children's Hospital of Atlanta to place very large grafts in very small children. Utilizing this method in partial cadaveric segmental grafts as well as in living donors, no child has died of chronic liver disease in the last 7 years after being listed for tranplantation. Our 1-year patient actuarial survival since 1999 is 94% in 164 consecutive patients (Figure 29.3.2-1).

All prospective donors undergo a complete medical and psychiatric evaluation. Hepatic and cardiopulmonary diseases, in patients age 55 or greater, are definite contraindications to the procedure. A medical physician not immediately associated with the surgical team acts as a donor advocate. ABO blood compatibility

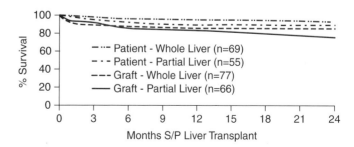

**FIGURE 29.3.2-1**

Whole versus partial liver actuarial patient and graft survival (January 1999 to September 2005).

was originally required, but our recent results with crossing blood groups now allow us to cross with impunity.[8]

A volumetric computed tomographic (CT) scan of the liver is necessary to ensure the appropriate size of the segment to be used. Probably of more importance is the width at the widest point of the hepatic segment to be resected. The preoperative estimated volume has been very accurate in our series, differing less than 50 mL from the actual weight after resection.[11] The hepatic vasculature is evaluated by CT scan in all cases, while utilizing celiac and mesenteric angiographies only selectively. Two arteries to the donor segments is not an absolute contraindication, but may increase the risk of hepatic artery thrombosis if the diameter is less than 2 mm.

Donor hepatectomy consists of either full left, or left lateral hepatectomy depending on the relative donor–recipient size ratio (Color Plates, Figure LI-1). Larger, adult-size, children may be effectively treated utilizing a right hepatectomy (as discussed elsewhere in this chapter). The majority of pediatric recipients may be treated through a left lateral hepatectomy. We restrict our discussion to left lateral hepatectomy, as other resections are covered elsewhere in this book.

## DONOR SEGMENT SIZE

The relative size of the liver graft consists of graft volume compared to the recipient body size. Graft weight (grams)/recipient body weight (grams) x 100(%). Adequate graft size, for optimum function in the recipient, has been reported to be between 1% and 3%. For example if the recipient is 10 kg, an optimal graft size should be between 100 and 300 g. A ratio of graft weight to recipient weight of over 5% has been thought to be related to poor graft perfusion and thus to poor graft survival.[12] Although some centers do not routinely use artificial meshes to close the abdominal wall, due to its perceived increased risk of infection,[13] we do, by routinely closing the abdominal wall with Goretex mesh to avoid respiratory compromise or graft necrosis in large-graft-to-recipient ratios without increased incidence of infection or graft loss. This large graft/recipient size ability is a key factor, enabling us to have no waitlist mortality in pediatric recipients at our institution for children with chronic liver disease. We feel that graft maximal thickness/recipient anteroposterior peritoneal cavity diameter as well as inflow hepatic arterial flow and volume are also important predictors of graft ischemia.

## LEFT LATERAL HEPATECTOMY (Color Plates, Figure LI-8)

The liver segment is harvested through a bilateral subcostal incision with midline extension to the xiphoid process, if necessary. The left triangular and gastrohepatic ligaments are divided with electrocautery. If a left hepatic artery arising from the left gastric artery is encountered, it is preserved. The hepatic artery is also isolated, branching off either the common hepatic or the left gastric. The left portal vein is then dissected free, ligating and dividing all posterior branches, including all branches to segment 4 and the caudate lobe. They must be handled gently to avoid traction injury. The portal vein and the hepatic artery must be dissected as long as possible. The point of the left hepatic duct division is between 2 and 3 mm to the left of the bifurcation of the right and left ducts (Figures 29.3.2-2, 29.3.2-3, and 29.3.2-4). A cholecystectomy is performed. If there is doubt about the biliary anatomy, a cystic duct cholangiogram is performed. In our experience, this

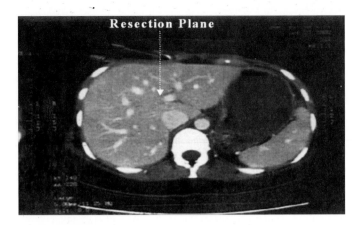

**FIGURE 29.3.2-2**

Resection plane.

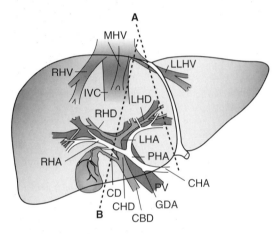

**FIGURE 29.3.2-3**

Resection planes for (A) left lateral segmentectomy and (B) left lobe resection. Abbreviations used: CBD, common bile duct; CD, common duct; CHA, common hepatic artery; CHD, common hepatic duct; GDA, gastroduodenal artery; IVC, inferior vena cava; LHA, left hepatic artery; LHD, left hepatic duct; LLHV, = left lateral hepatic vein; MHV, middle hepatic vein; PHA, proper hepatic artery; PV, portal vein; RHA, right hepatic artery; RHD, right hepatic duct; RHV, right hepatic vein.

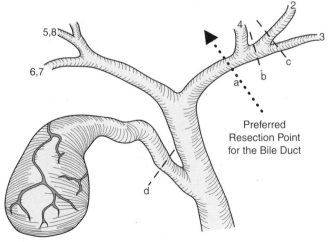

**FIGURE 29.3.2-4**

Preferred resection point for the bile duct.

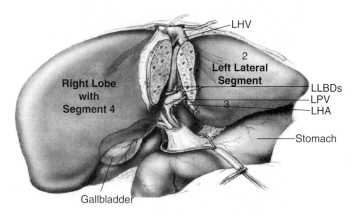

**FIGURE 29.3.2-5**

Right lobe with segment 4 and left lateral segment. Abbreviations used: LHA, left hepatic artery; LHV, left hepatic vein; LPV, left portal vein; LLBDs, left lateral bile ducts.

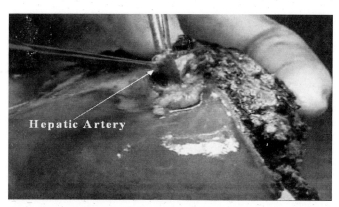

**FIGURE 29.3.2-7**

Hepatic artery.

is necessary less than 5% of the time. After the anterior segment of the left hepatic duct has been divided, the posterior duct is probed under direct vision to look for a posterior duct to the right lobe of the liver. If a duct is found, the posterior division of the left hepatic duct is directed toward the left lobe of the liver until the left hepatic duct is completely divided.

The division of the liver parenchyma includes a combination of electrocautery, a hydrojet water dissector and/or a cavitron ultrasonic surgical aspirator (CUSA) dissector. Parenchymal division proceeds from the point of bile duct division, and then 5 mm to 1 cm to the right of the falciform ligament. As the upward division of liver parenchyma (line A) is encountered, a veer to the left is undertaken before encountering the left hepatic vein, just prior to its entrance into the inferior vena cava. An important fact is that the parenchymal division involves the line of resection as it sweeps under the left portal vein and then up in the groove between the caudate and segments 2 and 3, as this line continues up toward the left hepatic vein. The dissections in these two lines are deepened, until all that is connecting the left lateral segment are the blood vessels (Figure 29.3.2-5 and 29.3.2-6). In the first series, the left hepatic vein was dis-

sected free and umbilical tape was placed around it, as one of the first steps. Recently, in over the last 100 cases, the hepatic vein is not actually seen and a pediatric curved vascular clamp is used to clamp the left hepatic veins or vein with a small rim of hepatic tissue around it. If there are two veins, the inner lip may be anastomosed together to yield one anastamosis at the time of recipient implantation (Figure 29.3.2-7). The portal vein, hepatic artery, and hepatic vein are then separately clamped, and the liver segment is immediately removed, flushing immediately the portal vein of the graft with Viospan solution, with 1:100 mixture of heparin until clear. The hepatic artery is not usually flushed due to its small size and risk of intimal flap disruption (Figures 29.3.2-8 and 29.3.2-9). One obvious advantage of this technique is to minimize warm ischemic time. Cadaveric iliac artery and vein are used as necessary for extension grafts. Using the above technique,[15] vascular complications have been minimized with optimal patient and graft survival. Extension of these concepts developed in living donor liver transplant to cadaver donor partial and split grafting have enabled optimal patient and graft survivals.

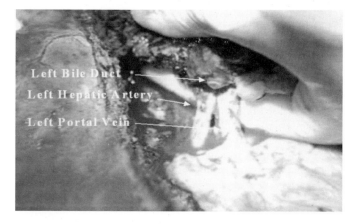

**FIGURE 29.3.2-6**

Left bile duct; left hepatic artery; left portal vein.

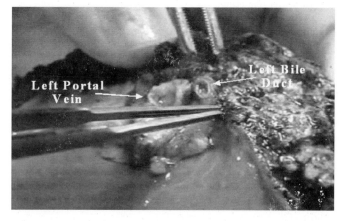

**FIGURE 29.3.2-8**

Left portal vein.

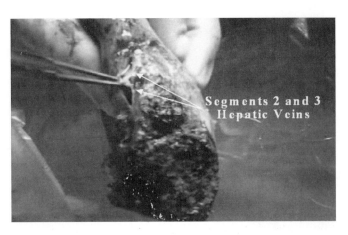

**FIGURE 29.3.2-9**

Segments 2 and 3, hepatic veins.

## References

1. Broelsch CE, Neuhaus P, Burdelski M, et al. Orthotopic transplantation of hepatic segments in infants with biliary atresia (in German).

2. Pichlmayr R, Ringe B, Gubernatis G, et al. Transplantation of one donor liver to two recipients(splitting transplantation). A new method for further development of segmental liver transplantation. Langenbec-7ks. *Arch Chir* 373:127–130. 212.

3. Emond JC, Whitington PF, Thistlethwaite JR, et al. Transplantation of two patients with one liver. Analysis of a preliminary experience with "split-liver" grafting. *Ann Surg* 1990;14–22.

4. Bismuth H, Morino M, Castaing D, et al. Emergency orthotopic liver transplantation in two patients using one donor liver. *Br J Surg* 1989; 76:722–724.

5. Otte JB, de Ville de Goyet J, Alberti D, et al. The concept and technique of the split liver in clinical transplantation. *Surgery* 1990;107:605–612.

6. Rai S, Nery JR, Mies S. Liver transplantation from live donors. *Lancet* 1989;497.

7. Strong RW, Lynch SV, Ong TH, et al. Successful liver transplantation from a living donor to her son. *N Engl J Med* 1990;322:1505–1507.

8. Broelsch CE, Emond JC, Whitington PF, et al. Application of reduced sized liver transplants as split grafts, auxiliary orthotopic grafts and living related segmental transplants. *Ann Surg* 1990;212:368–375.

9. Ozawa K, Uemoto S, Tanaka K, et al. An appraisal of pediatric liver transplantation from living relatives. Initial clinical experience in 20 pediatric liver transplantations from living relatives as donors. *Ann Surg* 1992;216:547–553.

10. Heffron T, Langnas A, Fox I, et al. Preoperative evaluation of the living related donor in pediatric living related liver transplantation. How accurate is it? *Transplant Proc.* 1994;Feb;26(1):135.

11. Heffron TG, Emond JC, Bendendo F, et al. Hepatic resection for benign and living related donors. *Gastroenterology* 1993;104:4(2) A59, #235. Presented at Digestive Disease Week in Boston, MA, May 1993.

12. Urata K, Kawasaki S, Matsunami H, et al. Calculation of child and adult standard liver volume for liver transplantation. *Hepatology* 1995;21: 1317–1321.

13. Kiuchi T, Kasahara M, Uryuhara K, et al: Impact of graft size mismatching on graft prognosis in liver transplantation from living donors. Transplantation 67:321-327,1999.

14. Tanaka K, Inomata Y. Living Related liver transplantation in pediatric recipients. PP629-646. In: Bussetil and Klintmalm, eds. *Transplantation of the Liver*. second edition. Elsevier; 2005.

15. Heffron TG, Welch D, Pillen T, et al. Low Incidence of Hepatic Artery Thrombosis After Liver Transplantation Without Systemic Anticoagulation or Microsurgery. *Pediatric Transplant* 2005;9:486–490.

### 29.3.3  Laparoscopic Donor Procedures for the Pediatric Recipient

*Kohei Ogawa, MD, Mikiko Ueda, MD, Koichi Tanaka, MD*

## INTRODUCTION

Living donor (LD) liver transplants since the first successful one in 1989 have become widely accepted as a useful treatment[1] for end-stage liver disease and genetic metabolic disorders. The use of LD livers avoids the problem of the deceased donor (DD) shortage and provides excellent-quality grafts. However, major concerns with such an invasive donor operation include postoperative complications, including a morbidity rate of 20% to 40% and an estimated mortality rate of up to 1%.[2-6] A large skin incision in LDs is needed even to obtain a left lateral segment of the liver for a small child. Large skin incisions are accompanied by severe abdominal pain and sometimes delay the return of donors to normal life.

Since the first laparoscopic cholecystectomy in France in 1987,[7,8] laparoscopic abdominal surgery has improved rapidly, thanks to technical advances, the accumulation of experience, and the development and improvement of instruments minimizing surgical invasiveness. The advantages of a laparoscopic approach include reductions in the incision size, in pain, in the risk of wound infection, in the duration of hospital stay, and in the time required for recovery. In the field of kidney transplantation, laparoscopic nephrectomy,[9-11] has contributed to a better postoperative course for LDs.

For patients with benign and malignant disorders, laparoscopic liver resections without significant morbidity or mortality have been reported by various centers.[12-18] The first laparoscopic LD hepatectomy was reported by Cherqui et al., with excellent results, in 2002.[19] Laparoscopic donor hepatectomies will inevitably lead to improvements in donor quality of life. A left lateral segmentectomy seems feasible for conversion to a laparoscopic approach, given its anatomic simplicity as compared with a right or left lobectomy. Herein we describe our experience with laparoscopic lateral segmentectomy for LDs.

## PATIENTS AND METHODS

All study protocols were approved by the Ethics Committee of Kyoto University Hospital. The laparoscopic procedure was proposed to prospective LDs who did not meet these exclusion criteria, designed to ensure their safety: body mass index > 25; fatty liver; complicated anatomy of vessels and bile duct; age > 40 years old; or past history of abdominal surgery. Obese donors were excluded because of the increased risk of pulmonary embolism. Our exclusion criteria are likely to change with accumulated experience. We described the innovative aspects and other details of laparoscopic donation to eligible LDs; those who provided written consent were enrolled in our study.

### Preoperative Anatomic Evaluation

To evaluate the LDs portal and hepatic venous systems, all laparoscopic donor candidates underwent preoperative abdominal enhanced three-dimensional computed tomography (CT). With an open left lateral segmentectomy, we usually preserve the gallbladder; therefore, we perform intraoperative cholangiography by direct puncture of the common bile duct, using a 24-G catheter-over-needle device. Because this procedure is difficult to perform safely under laparoscopy, all laparoscopic donor candidates also underwent preoperative drip-infusion cholangiography with CT (DIC-CT) or magnetic resonance cholangiopancreatography (MRCP). We preferred MRCP, because with DIC-CT, the risk of anaphylaxis against the contrast material is not particularly low.

## Donor Operation

After the induction of general anesthesia, a 16-G central venous catheter was inserted from the right internal jugular vein for sucking carbon dioxide from the right atrium in case of carbon dioxide embolism. Transesophageal echocardiography was selected for monitoring carbon dioxide embolism.

The donor was placed in a supine position with legs apart. The operator stood between the legs, and assistants stood on both sides (Figure 29.3.3-1). A 1-cm-long supraumbilical incision was made, and a 12-mm trocar was inserted. Pneumoperitoneum was created with carbon dioxide and maintained at 8 mm Hg. A laparoscope with a flexible tip was placed, and another 4 trocars were inserted (Figure 29.3.3-2). The donor was then placed in a head-up position to drop the intestine off the liver. The round and falciform ligaments were dissected to the anterior surface of the left hepatic vein with a harmonic scalpel (AutoSonix UltraShears, Tyco, USA). The left triangular and coronary ligaments were then dissected.

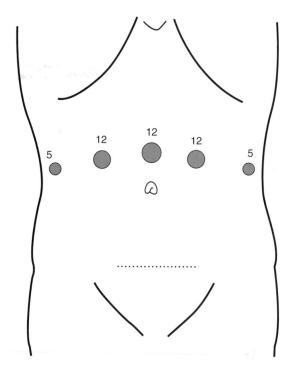

**FIGURE 29.3.3-2**

Trocar positions. Numbers represent trocar diameter (mm).

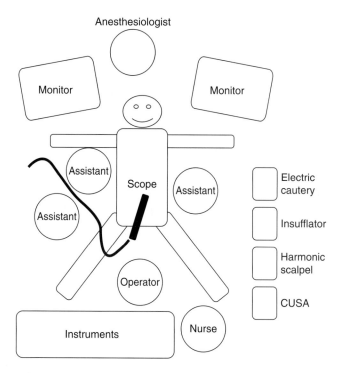

**FIGURE 29.3.3-1**

Operating-room setup for laparoscopic lateral segmentectomy.

After mobilization of the lateral segment, the dissection was moved to the hepatic hilum. The left hepatic artery was first dissected and encircled. The left branch of the portal vein was then dissected and encircled. These two encircled vessels were isolated with vessel loops for easy reidentification. Small portal branches to the caudate lobe were clipped and divided.

The hepatic parenchymal resection was started from the edge, with the harmonic scalpel. The medial segment was transected 5 mm to the right of the falciform ligament, with an ultrasonic surgical aspirator (CUSA Excel, Tyco, USA) or with the harmonic scalpel, without blood inflow occlusion or graft manipulation. The left hepatic duct was dissected and sharply divided. The remnant side of the duct was closed with a 6-0 absorbable running suture (PDS-II, Ehicon, USA). Parenchymal bleeding was controlled with bipolar electrocoagulation with dropping water (our own technique). Small vessels were sealed and divided with the harmonic scalpel; large vessels were clipped and divided. A straight suction tube was inserted between the lateral segment and the caudate lobe, as a directional guide for the cutting end of the hepatic parenchyma. After the completion of the hepatic parenchymal resection, the left hepatic vein was isolated with vessel tape. A 10-cm suprapubic skin incision was then made, and a 15-mm trocar was inserted. After systemic administration of 1000 U of heparin, the donor side of the left hepatic artery was clipped and divided, with the graft side open. The donor side of the left portal vein was divided with a linear stapler (EndoTA, Tyco, USA) and divided; the graft side was clamped with a small vascular clamp. Finally, the left hepatic vein was divided with a linear stapler (EndoTA, Tyco), with the graft side open.

A large specimen bag (Endocatch, Tyco) was then inserted through the suprapubic trocar. The graft was placed in the specimen bag. The suprapubic incision was completed; the specimen bag (with the graft) was removed through this wound. The graft was perfused on the backtable. The suprapubic wound was closed, and pneumoperitoneum was again created. The abdominal cavity was lavaged with normal saline; hemostasis was assessed. A 5-mm suction drain (J-VAC, Ethicon) was inserted from the wound farthest to the left and placed around the cut surface of the liver. The other wounds for the trocar ports were closed.

## RESULTS

From November 2002 to January 2003, we performed five laparoscopic left lateral segmentectomies in LDs. In three donors, a small laparotomy was needed because of intraoperative bleeding from the hepatic vein. The two donors who completed the full laparoscopic procedure were discharged from the hospital after 6 days without any complications; there were no wounds infections (Fig. 29.3.3-3). But two of the three donors who were converted to a small laparotomy experienced some postoperative complications. One had an adhesive ileus, which recurred and eventually required surgical treatment; the other developed bile leakage from the stump of the left hepatic duct, which was treated with endoscopic nasobiliary drainage (Table 29.3.3-1). Of the five recipients, two experienced hepatic arterial thrombosis, one of whom required surgical reconstruction. Another recipient died of sepsis caused by biliary leakage from the hepaticojejunostomy. During long-term follow-up, all four surviving recipients experienced biliary stenosis requiring percutaneous transhepatic biliary drainage (PTCD; Table 29.3.3-2).

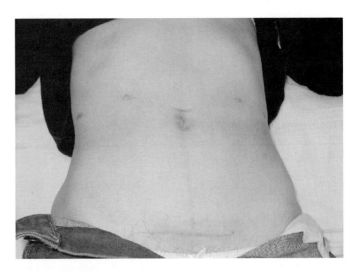

**FIGURE 29.3.3-3**

Donor abdomen after surgery.

## COMPLICATIONS

### Intraoperative Bleeding

A profound preoperative understanding of the LD's hepatic vein and portal branch anatomy is crucial to prevent intraoperative bleeding. With pneumoperitoneum, suctioning blood decreases pneumoperitoneum pressure and sometimes results in a poor visual field. With uncontrollable bleeding, conversion to laparotomy must be done without hesitation, and the bleeding must be stopped under direct visualization.

**TABLE 29.3.3-1**
**DONOR RESULTS**

| Case | Conversion to laparotomy | Hospital stay (days) | Returned to work (days) | Complications |
| --- | --- | --- | --- | --- |
| 1 | No | 6 | 16 | None |
| 2 | No | 6 | 6 | None |
| 3 | Yes | 21 | 45 | Ileus |
| 4 | Yes | 12 | 120 | Bile leakage |
| 5 | Yes | 17 | 20 | None |

**TABLE 29.3.3-2**
**RECIPIENT RESULTS**

| Case | Age (months) | Surgical complications | Outcome |
| --- | --- | --- | --- |
| 1 | 7 | Biliary stenosis | Alive |
| 2 | 9 | HAT (day 5), biliary stenosis | Alive |
| 3 | 11 | HAT (day 4), biliary stenosis | Alive |
| 4 | 9 | Bile leadage | Died (day 35) |
| 5 | 30 | Biliary stenosis | Alive |

## Gas Embolism

Some authors recommend gasless suspension laparoscopy during parenchymal dissection, given the possibility that gas might enter the bloodstream through the small vessels in the cut surface of the liver.[13,18,20,21] However, carbon dioxide is soluble in water, so small amounts entering the bloodstream represent a minimal risk.[22,23] Ricciardi et al reported that the risk of significant gas embolus under pneumoperitoneum was minimal during laparoscopic hepatic resection.[24] According to their report, hepatic venous and portal venous pressures increase with the elevation in intraabdominal pressure, and hepatic tissue blood flow decreases. These changes in intrahepatic pressure and blood flow secondary to increased intraabdominal pressure protect against carbon dioxide embolus during the hepatic resection.

Because pneumoperitoneum provides a much better visual field than gasless suspension laparoscopy, we used pneumoperitoneum throughout our five cases; we encountered no instances of gas embolism. However, we follow all needed precautions such as monitoring abdominal pressure, arterial carbon dioxide levels, performing transesophageal echocardiography, and inserting a central venous catheter for removing gas in the atrium. Gas embolism can be detected by a sudden marked fall in blood pressure and by arrhythmia (such as bradycardia). In those situations, pneumoperitoneum should be stopped immediately; pooling gas in the atrium must be evacuated with the central venous catheter.

## CONCLUSION

Laparoscopic lateral segmentectomy offers LDs the possible benefits of decreased postoperative pain and shorter recovery period, as compared with the open procedure. However, in our early series, the laparoscopic procedure could not be completed in three of five donors because of intraoperative bleeding. The frequency of hepatic artery thrombosis and biliary complications in our five recipients was not low. Intraoperative manipulation might affect vascular and biliary complications. Further development of instruments and of technical skills is necessary before this procedure can become standard.

## References

1. Strong RW, Lynch SV, Ong TH, et al. Successful liver transplantation from a living donor to her son. *N Engl J Med* 1990;322:1505.
2. Sauer P, Schemmer P, Uhl W, et al. Living-donor liver transplantation: evaluation of donor and recipient. *Nephrol Dial Transplant* 2004;19 (Suppl 4):iv11.
3. Grewal HP, Thistlewaite JR Jr, Loss GE, et al. Complications in 100 living-liver donors. *Ann Surg* 1998;228:214.
4. Yamaoka Y, Morimoto T, Inamoto T, et al. Safety of the donor in living-related liver transplantation—an analysis of 100 parental donors. *Transplantation* 1995;59:224.
5. Renz JF, Roberts JP. Long-term complications of living donor liver transplantation. *Liver Transplant* 2000;6:S73.
6. Fujita S, Kim ID, Uryuhara K, et al. Hepatic grafts from live donors: donor morbidity for 470 cases of live donation. *Transplant Int* 2000; 13:333.
7. Mouret P. How I developed laparoscopic cholecystectomy. *Ann Acad Med Singapore* 1996;25:744.
8. Dubois F, Berthelot G, Levard H. Laparoscopic cholecystectomy: historic perspective and personal experience. *Surg Laparosc Endosc* 1991;1:52.
9. Ratner LE, Ciseck LJ, Moore RG, et al. Laparoscopic live donor nephrectomy. *Transplantation* 1995;60:1047.
10. Merlin TL, Scott DF, Rao MM, et al. The safety and efficacy of laparoscopic live donor nephrectomy: a systematic review. *Transplantation* 2000;70:1659.
11. Sasaki TM , Finelli F, Bugarin E, et al. Is laparoscopic donor nephrectomy the new criterion standard? *Arch Surg* 2000;135:943.
12. Gugenheim J, Mazza D, Katkhouda N, et al. Laparoscopic resection of solid liver tumours. *Br J Surg* 1996;83:334.
13. Watanabe Y, Sato M, Ueda S, et al. Laparoscopic hepatic resection: a new and safe procedure by abdominal wall lifting method. *Hepatogastroenterology* 1997;44:143.
14. Samama G, Chiche L, Brefort JL, et al. Laparoscopic anatomical hepatic resection. Report of four left lobectomies for solid tumors. *Surg Endosc* 1998;12:76.
15. Cuesta MA, Meijer S, Paul MA, et al. Limited laparoscopic liver resection of benign tumors guided by laparoscopic ultrasonography: report of two cases. *Surg Laparosc Endosc* 1995;5:396.
16. Cunningham JD, Katz LB, Brower ST, et al. Laparoscopic resection of two liver hemangiomata. *Surg Laparosc Endosc* 1995;5: 277.
17. Ferzli G, David A, Kiel T. Laparoscopic resection of a large hepatic tumor. *Surg Endosc* 1995;9:733.
18. Kaneko H, Takagi S, Shiba T. Laparoscopic partial hepatectomy and left lateral segmentectomy: technique and results of a clinical series. *Surgery* 1996;120:468.
19. Cherqui D, Soubrane O, Husson E, et al. Laparoscopic living donor hepatectomy for liver transplantation in children. *Lancet* 2002;359:392.
20. Huscher CG, Lirici MM, Chiodini S. Laparoscopic liver resections. *Semin Laparosc Surg* 1998;5:204.
21. Hashizume M, Takenaka K, Yanaga K, et al. Laparoscopic hepatic resection for hepatocellular carcinoma. *Surg Endosc* 1995;9:1289.
22. Yacoub OF, Cardona Jr. I, Coveler LA, et al. Carbon dioxide embolism during laparoscopy. *Anesthesiology* 1982;57:533.
23. Moskop Jr. RJ, Lubarsky DA. Carbon dioxide embolism during laparoscopic cholecystectomy. *South Med J* 1994;87:414.
24. Ricciardi R, Anwaruddin S, Schaffer BK, et al. Elevated intrahepatic pressures and decreased hepatic tissue blood flow prevent gas embolus during limited laparoscopic liver resections. *Surg Endosc* 2001;15:729.

### 29.3.4   Laparoscopic Right Living Donor Hepatectomy

*Andreas J. Karachristos, MD, Amit D. Tevar, MD,*
*Dong-Sik Kim, MD, Joseph Buell, MD,*
*E. Steve Woodle, MD, Steven M. Rudich, MD*

## LAPAROSCOPIC HEPATECTOMY

Minimally invasive surgery has revolutionized many areas of general, thoracic, and gynecologic surgery during the last 20 years, allowing earlier recovery, less postoperative pain, reduced complications, and improved cosmesis. Although laparoscopic wedge liver resections and biopsies were described from the early 1990s and the first left lateral segmentectomy was performed in 1996,[1] hepatobiliary surgeons have been cautious to adopt minimally invasive approaches in hepatic surgery. Indeed, widespread application of laparoscopic techniques to liver surgery has been an area of resistance, due to the complexity of liver surgery, the rich and complex blood supply of the liver and concerns related to potential tumor cell dissemination and gas embolization. However, refinements in laparoscopic equipment, intraoperative imaging technology, better means of achieving and maintaining hemostasis, and increased familiarity of hepatobiliary surgeons with (advanced) minimally invasive techniques, have led a few groups to explore the feasibility of

**TABLE 29.3.4-1**

## LAPAROSCOPIC LIVER RESECTIONS

| Center | Number of major Resections (≥3 Couinaud Segments) | Number of Minor Resections | Conversion Rate (%) | Mortality (%) | Morbidity (%) |
|---|---|---|---|---|---|
| Montsouris Institute, Paris, France | 38 | 51 | 13 | 1 | 19 |
| Rikshospitalet, Oslo, Norway | 14 | 46 | 6 | 0 | 16 |
| Royal Brisbane Hospital, Australia | 12 | 0 | 8 | 0 | 2 |
| University of Cincinnati and Northwestern University | 31 | 69 | 0 | 1 | 23 |

laparoscopic liver surgery, not only for (smaller) wedge resections but also for larger and more complex hepatic surgeries.

Patient selection is a key component for successful outcome in laparoscopic liver surgery. Peripheral lesions are technically less demanding as limited resection is usually adequate.[2–4] However, several groups have provided evidence that major resections (≥3 Couinaud segments) are also safe.[5,6] Our group, in conjunction with a group from Northwestern University, has reported results from 100 laparoscopic liver resections, including 31 formal hepatectomies (20 right and 11 left) using a hand-assisted approach.[6] There were no conversions to open surgery; there was one mortality and significant morbidities occurred in 23% of patients. The most common complications were bile leaks and perihepatic abscesses. These results are very comparable to those achieved with open hepatic resection. Importantly, patients experienced less pain, and the mean hospital stay was 3 days, which is a marked improvement compared with traditional open hepatectomy[5] (Table 29.3.4-1).

Another group, from Australia, has reported their experience with 12 laparoscopic right hemihepatectomies.[7] In five patients,

the operation was completed entirely laparoscopically (ie, without the use of a hand-assist port), in five the operation was performed with the use of hand port, and two patients were converted to open. There were no mortalities, one patient developed a bile leak, which resolved spontaneously, and one patient developed a wound dehiscence. The average hospital stay was 8 days; for those in which the operation was completed without hand port, 4 days.[7]

As expected with any new and evolving technology, most centers reported on their experience with resection of benign lesions. However, the presence of malignancy is not a contraindication to laparoscopic liver resection. A multicenter study from Europe of 37 laparoscopic resection procedures included 2 major hepatectomies, 12 wedge resections, 9 segmentectomies, and 14 bisegmentectomies.[3] Ten patients had hepatocellular carcinoma (HCC) whereas 27 had liver metastasis. There were no deaths and morbidity was 22%, with bleeding being the most common perioperative complication. Of importance, pathologic margins were positive or inadequate in up to one third of the patients. The rate of positive margins was higher in patients where laparoscopic

**TABLE 29.3.4-2**

## TECHNIQUES OF LAPAROSCOPIC LIVER RESECTION

| Center | Reference | Patient Position | Hand-Assisted | Parenchymal Division Technique |
|---|---|---|---|---|
| University Hospital of Paris, France | 2 | Supine | No | Harmonic scalpel Ultrasonic dissector |
| Multicenter European Study | 3 | Supine | No | Crushing forceps Hook Coagulator Harmonic scalpel Stapling device |
| Royal Brisbane Hospital, Australia | 5 | Supine | Yes and No | Harmonic scalpel Stapling device |
| Rikshospitalet, Oslo, Norway | 4 | Supine | No | Ultrasonic scalpel Surgical aspirator LigaSure® Stapling device |
| University of Turin, Italy | 9 | Semidecubitus or supine | No | Ultrasonic scalpel Crushing forceps |
| Montsouris Institute, Paris, France | 7 | Supine | No | Not described in text |
| University of Cincinnati and Northwestern University | 6 | Semidecubitus or supine | Yes | Harmonic scalpel Hook coagulator Stapling device |

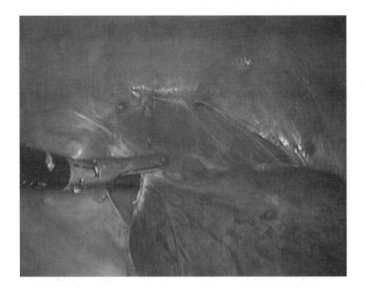

**FIGURE 29.3.4-1**

Right lobe mobilization using harmonic ultrasound dissection.

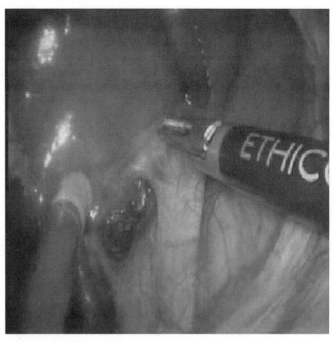

**FIGURE 29.3.4-2**

Laparoscopic dissection and mobilization of the vena cava.

ultrasound was omitted. Reported disease-free survival and overall survival for patients with HCC and colorectal metastasis resected laparoscopically is similar to those treated by open laparotomy.[7]

In summary, minimally invasive hepatic resections can be performed for both benign and malignant liver lesions and can be employed safely in peripheral small lesions as well as in larger lesions needing formal right or left hemihepatectomies. However, at this point in its current evolution, it should be avoided for large central tumors, tumors close to the porta hepatis, for repeat hepatectomies, or when there is doubt regarding the tumor margin.

The technique of laparoscopic resection varies among authors (Table 29.3.4-2). Specifically, for the right hemi-

hepatectomy, the patient is placed either in supine or in left lateral position. We prefer a left semidecubitus position with a beanbag or a left lateral position. Use of laparoscopic ultrasound is of paramount importance. Our group always uses a hand-assist device to help with vascular control and manipulation/mobilization of the liver. The falciform ligament can be divided between staples, and the ligamentum teres, coronary, and triangular ligaments can be divided using either harmonic

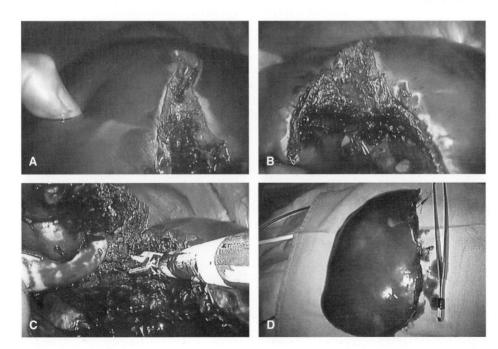

**FIGURE 29.3.4-3**

Parenchymal dissection. (**A**) Beginning the resection with harmonic scalpel. (**B, C**) Continued parenchymal division with linear staplers. (**D**) Final resection specimen.

scissors or LigaSure® (Valley Lab, Boulder, CO). Our preference is to perform most of the mobilization with the harmonic scalpel (Figure 29.3.4-1). Hand retraction is key to many aspects of this operation and allows visualization of the underlining vena cava (Figure 29.3.4-2). The inferior vena cava ligament is divided, and the right lobe is completely mobilized. Short hepatic veins are divided between clips or with the use of LigaSure®. The right hepatic vein is dissected with harmonic scissors. Dissection of the porta hepatis is performed with harmonic shears or diathermy, with hand assistance. A tape can be placed around the portal triad for intermittent application of Pringle maneuver or proximal control, in case of bleeding. The right hepatic artery and duct can be individually divided between clips, and the right portal vein is divided with a linear stapler. Alternatively, the blood supply to the right lobe can be controlled intraparenchymally using staplers.[5] Intraparenchymal dissection is performed along Cantlie's line after Glisson's capsule is scored with cautery and while maintaining a central venous pressure at or below 5 mm Hg. The method of parenchymal transection varies substantially. Laparoscopic ultrasonic dissector, TissueLink® (TissueLink Medical, Dover, NH), crushing clamps, and laparoscopic linear staplers have all been successfully employed.[2–7] We prefer a selective approach by reducing the liver parenchyma with harmonic scissors or TissueLink® and applying several staplers for intraparenchymal vascular control (Figure 29.3.4-3). Hemostasis at the transected parenchymal margin is ensured with argon beam coagulator and application of fibrin glues.

There are limited published data comparing the laparoscopic with the open approach for major hepatic resections. No prospective studies have been reported. In a case control study from France comparing open to laparoscopic 2–3 bisegmentectomy, the laparoscopic approach was associated with longer operative times, decreased blood loss and similar morbidity.[8] In a comparative study from Italy of minor resections by minimally invasive means or laparotomy, laparoscopy reduced blood loss and length of hospital stay.[9]

## LAPAROSCOPIC RIGHT LIVING DONOR HEMIHEPATECTOMY

The introduction of laparoscopic donor nephrectomy has been shown to increase available kidney donors up to 25%, to substantially the need for parenteral analgesics and to shorten length of hospital stay, and bring about quicker return to functional recovery.[12] In a relatively brief period of time from its initial introduction, this procedure has become the "standard" for live donor kidney transplantation and has stood the test of time, insofar as complications and patient morbidity.

After several groups demonstrated the safety and efficacy of laparoscopic right hemihepatectomy, the obvious next hurdle was to address the use of laparoscopy for right living donor hepatectomy. The donor, by definition, is a healthy individual, and his or her safety should and must be the primary consideration. Mortality for open right living donor hepatectomy is estimated to be 0.23% to 0.5%, although this may likely be an underestimate.[10] Morbidity ranges between 0% and 100% with a median of 16%, in which biliary and infectious complications occur most commonly. Another very important aspect of elective right donor hepatectomy are the long-term complications, such as incisional hernias, as well as the impact of the donor operation on quality of life. In one study, the mean time to complete recovery after open right donor hepatectomy was 3.4 months and the mean time to return to work 2.4 months. Importantly, up to 71% of donors reported ongoing symptoms, most commonly abdominal discomfort and scar numbness.[11] Approximately one third to one half of donors experienced more pain than expected, and nearly one third reported that their scar was larger than expected.[10] The thought of a long period of convalescence, fear of postoperative discomfort and pain, as well as fear of future insurability may all discourage potential donors.

Several groups have evaluated techniques for laparoscopic right and left living donor hepatectomies in animal models such as pig, sheep, as well as human cadavers.[13–15] These reports demonstrate that current technology facilitates safe (nondestructive) laparoscopic procurement of hepatic lobes, allowing the recovery of intact specimens with adequate length and quality of vascular and biliary structures in a timely manner, while preserving donor physiology. However, in one of these models, concerns have been raised regarding graft injury due to prolonged maintenance of pneumoperitoneum.[16]

Laparoscopic liver donation was first performed for left lateral segmentectomy, as the risk for the donor is much less than that for a right lobe donation. Recently, a group from France reported their experience with 16 laparoscopic left lateral segmentectomies for transplantation in children.[17] There was one conversion, and all grafts were adequate in size and were successfully transplanted, although one recipient needed to be retransplanted due to graft necrosis secondary to portal vein thrombosis.[17]

Two groups have recently reported transplantation of right hemilivers from living donors (Table 29.3.4-3). Koffron et al reported their experience of four laparoscopically assisted right donor hemihepatectomies.[18] All grafts were transplanted successfully, and the donors were discharged without complications after a mean length of stay of 3 days. Although the postoperative hospitalization did not differ among laparoscopic and open donors, this feasibility study demonstrated that living donor right hepatectomy could be performed with minimally invasive techniques.

**TABLE 29.3.4-3**

## LAPAROSCOPIC LIVING RIGHT DONOR HEPATECTOMY

| Center | Year | Reference | Lobectomies Right | Left | Operative Time (min) | Conversion | EBL | Mortality |
|--------|------|-----------|-------|------|----------------------|------------|-----|-----------|
| Northwestern University | 2006 | 18 | 4 | 0 | 235 | 0 | 150 | 0 |
| Nigata University | 2006 | 19 | 3 | 10 | 363 ± 32.7 | 0 | 302 ± 191 | 0 |

There are several points that merit attention in their technique that differentiates this procedure from non-donor laparoscopic right lobectomy. In the donor hepatectomy, the Pringle maneuver is avoided to ensure uninterrupted inflow to the graft. Similarly, the right hepatic artery and right portal vein are not transected until the time of graft removal from the donor. The hand port was placed through a 5 cm subxiphoid midline incision for right lobe manipulation, assistance in portal triad dissection, and graft extraction. Mobilization of the right lobe, dissection of the right hepatic vein, isolation of the right hepatic artery and right portal vein were performed in a manner identical to laparoscopic right hepatectomy. Once the right lobe was mobilized, then the hand port incision was used for cholangiography, transection of the right hepatic duct, and parenchymal transection, using standard open techniques. After transection of the vessels, the graft was retrieved from the midline incision. The principle of this technique is to ensure the integrity of the graft and vessels via standard open techniques and avoid the morbid subcostal incision through laparoscopic mobilization of the liver and vessel isolation. The authors report subjective reduction in postoperative pain using this method.

Another group from Nigata University in Japan reported their experience with 13 laparoscopically assisted living liver donor hemihepatectomies, including three right hepatectomies.[19] These authors used gasless, abdominal wall lifting laparoscopy in most of the cases, in an attempt to decrease the potential deleterious effects of pneumoperitoneum on hepatic function, as well as to minimize any potential for gas embolism, especially during parenchymal dissection. As with the Northwestern group, mobilization of the liver and vessel dissection was performed by laparoscopy, whereas the parenchyma transection, as well as the transection of the vessels, was performed in a more routine open standard fashion, through a midline 12-cm incision. Three of the recipients died in the postoperative period: two from bleeding and one from sepsis for reasons unrelated to laparoscopic graft retrieval. The laparoscopically assisted donors experienced less pain, used fewer analgesics, and had reduced long-term symptoms in comparison with a matched group of non-laparoscopic hepatic donors.

## SURGICAL PROCEDURE FOR LAPAROSCOPIC LIVING RIGHT HEMI-HEPATECTOMY

The patient is placed in a supine position, with arms adducted and standard monitoring devices placed for a major hepatic resection. Both pneumoperitoneum and gasless, abdominal-wall lifting methods have been used to gain working space. The operation can be divided into four distinct phases.

1. Laparoscopic mobilization of the right lobe and exposure of IVC and its branches into the right hemi-liver.

2. Portal dissection, with isolation of the right hepatic artery and portal vein, using either the midline hand port incision (minilaparotomy incision) or hand-assisted laparoscopy. Following cholangiography, the right hepatic duct is transected.

3. Liver parenchymal dissection, using a variety of devices. An umbilical tape, placed in the space between the IVC and overlying liver, has been found useful for rotating and making the transection plane more superficial. The transection is done without inflow occlusion with all major vascular structures being left intact during parenchymal division. Ultra-

sound is extensively used to locate the middle hepatic vein in order to direct the transection line.

4. Vessel transection and hemiliver extraction. Once the two hemilivers are separated and attached just by the major vessels, the right hepatic artery is ligated and cut lateral to the common bile duct, as is the underlying right portal vein. After lateral retraction of the graft, the right hepatic vein is stapled and divided at the IVC. The graft is allowed to decompress through the portal vein and is then slowly and carefully extracted through the midline hand-assist port. Immediately on the back table, the staple line at the hepatic vein is excised, and the right lobe graft is flushed with preservation solution. A completion cholangiogram can be performed on the donor to rule out any bile leaks as well as to document the integrity of the left-side biliary system.

Donor selection of the appropriate patient for laparoscopic living right hepatectomy is of paramount importance. Experience with laparoscopic liver surgery has shown the difficulty in managing the many variations in anatomy at the hepatic hilum, particularly the biliary, and somewhat less for the hepatic artery anatomy. As a result, only candidates with straightforward and uncomplicated anatomy at the hilum should be considered for laparoscopic live right donor hepatectomy. The donor also has to have appropriate body habitus. As much of the laparoscopic right donor hepatectomy is performed through a relatively small upper midline incision (used as the hand port during the laparoscopic portion of the operation), body habitus must play a key role in successfully performing this operation. Too large of an anterior–posterior diameter would make the "open" hilar dissection and parenchymal division extremely challenging, at best, and downright dangerous in a worst-case scenario. As in open surgery, the greatest risk of profound blood loss during laparoscopic live right hepatectomy will be during the parenchymal dissection. As currently described, this is performed through the laparoscopic hand port, using an umbilical tape to bring up the intersection between the two hemilivers to aid in the division.

Complete familiarity with parenchymal dissection is absolutely required, whether that being through the use of LigaSure®, TissueLink®, the Helix Hydrojet, or the laparoscopic cavitational ultrasonic surgical aspirator (CUSA). Caution and great care needs to be demonstrated during dissection toward the hepatic hilum, so that inadvertent bile duct or hepatic artery injury does not occur. One must also keep in mind that adequate length of these structures must be preserved for implantation. More destructive parenchymal dissection modalities, such as the TissueLink® and LigaSure®, should be minimized in dissecting biliary structures in the pedicle.

One important theoretical issue to consider in regards to laparoscopic live right donor hepatectomy is the issue of pneumoperitoneum. Is it harmful to the hepatic allograft? Ischemic hepatic graft injury secondary to long pneumoperitoneum has not been observed clinically. In the reports of laparoscopic major hepatic resections, hepatic dysfunction based upon long operative times has not been noticed. In addition, as much of the live right hepatic donor hepatectomy is performed open, through the upper midline incision, the actual time of laparoscopy is modest. As such, it is highly doubtful that pneumoperitoneum will be found very harmful for immediate or long-term allograft function.

In summary, the technical groundwork to perform a laparoscopically assisted live right donor hepatectomy has been established and living right liver donor hepatectomy has been successfully accomplished. This requires a potential donor with the proper body habitus and uncomplicated biliary and hepatic artery anatomy. Surgical confidence in advanced laparoscopic techniques, including facility with several means of transecting liver parenchyma is an absolute must. However, fewer than 10 living right liver donor hepatectomies have been performed worldwide and the procedure is in its infancy, in terms of clinical development. Substantial experience will be necessary to define its role in clinical liver transplantation. Finally this procedure should be performed only by hepatobiliary transplant surgeons familiar with both minimally invasive liver surgery and living liver donor operation.

## References

1. Azagra JS, Goergen M, et al. Laparoscopic anatomical (hepatic) left lateral segmentectomy-technical aspects. *Surg Endosc* 1996;10(7): 758-761.

2. Cherqui D , Husson E, et al. Laparoscopic liver resections: a feasibility study in 30 patients. *Ann Surg* 2000;232(6):753–762.

3. Gigot JF, Glineur D, et al. Laparoscopic liver resection for malignant liver tumors: preliminary results of a multicenter European study. *Ann Surg* 2002;236(1):90–97.

4. Mala T, Edwin B, et al. Laparoscopic liver resection: experience of 53 procedures at a single center. *J Hepatobiliary Pancreat Surg* 2005;12(4): 298–303.

5. O'Rourke N, Fielding G Laparoscopic right hepatectomy: surgical technique. *J Gastrointest Surg* 2004;8(2):213–216.

6. Buell JF, Koffron AJ, et al. Laparoscopic liver resection. *J Am Coll Surg* 2005;200(3):472–480.

7. Vibert E, Perniceni T, et al. Laparoscopic liver resection. *Br J Surg* 2006; 93(1):67–72

8. Lesurtel M, Cherqui D, et al. Laparoscopic versus open left lateral hepatic lobectomy: a case-control study. *J Am Coll Surg* 2003;196(2): 236–242.

9. Morino M, Morra I, et al. Laparoscopic vs open hepatic resection: a comparative study. *Surg Endosc* 2003;17(12):1914–1918.

10. Middleton PF, Duffield M, et al. Living donor liver transplantation––adult donor outcomes: a systematic review. *Liver Transplant* 2006; 12(1):24–30.

11. Trotter JF, Talamantes M, et al. Right hepatic lobe donation for living donor liver transplantation: impact on donor quality of life. *Liver Transplant* 2001;7(6):485–493.

12. Ratner LE, Hiller J, et al. Laparoscopic live donor nephrectomy removes disincentives to live donation. *Transplant Proc* 1997;29(8): 3402–3403.

13. Kurian MS, Gagner M, et al. Hand-assisted laparoscopic donor hepatectomy for living related transplantation in the porcine model. *Surg Laparosc Endosc Percutan Tech* 2002;12(4): 232–237.

14. Lin E, Gonzalez R, et al. Can current technology be integrated to facilitate laparoscopic living donor hepatectomy? *Surg Endosc* 2003;17(5): 750–753.

15. Pinto PA, Montgomery RA, et al. Laparoscopic procurement model for living donor liver transplantation. *Clin Transplant* 2003; 17(Suppl 9): 39–43.

16. Schemmer P, Barro-Bejarano M, et al. Laparoscopic organ retrieval for living donor liver transplantation does not prevent graft injury. *Transplant Proc* 2005;37(3):1625–1627.

17. Soubrane O, Cherqui D, et al. Laparoscopic left lateral sectionectomy in living donors: Safety and reproducibility of the technique in a single center. *Ann Surg* 2006;244(5): 815–820.

18. Koffron AJ, Kung R, et al. Laparoscopic-assisted right lobe donor hepatectomy. *Am J Transplant* 2006;6(10):2522–2525.

19. Kurosaki I, Yamamoto S, et al. Video-assisted living donor hemihepatectomy through a 12-cm incision for adult-to-adult liver transplantation. *Surgery* 2006;139(5):695–703.

## 29.4   PERIOPERATIVE CARE

*Giuliano Testa, MD,*
*Rose Luther-Campise, MD,*
*Enrico Benedetti, MD*

### INTRODUCTION

Living donor liver transplantation (LDLT) offers several advantages over cadaveric donation. It can reduce the waiting time and permits semielective scheduling of the transplant, which allows the recipient to be better prepared for surgery. The graft is harvested under optimal conditions from a healthy donor, and the cold ischemic time is reduced from the usual 8 to 12 hours to 1 hour or less,[6] which has been shown to decrease the associated markers of inflammation seen after reperfusion and may improve graft survival.[8]

These advantages, though, need to be weighed carefully against the fact that a healthy person is being exposed to a major surgical procedure with significant morbidity and even mortality.

Additionally the donor has to face financial and emotional consequences. The donation will limit the functionality of the donor for weeks or months after the surgery and may cause stress in the family.[9] This has been the topic of extensive ethical discussions, especially because the only benefit to the donor is the ability to help another person. Therefore, the safety of the donor must always take priority in LDLT.[10]

Approximately half of the patients with end-stage liver disease that are judged appropriate for a living donation will have a potential donor, though a significant percentage (potentially 40%–70%) of these will be found unsuitable.[6] Donor safety is the main focus in this process, which leads to very strict selection criteria and this high percentage of exclusions. The process of donor selection is covered elsewhere (Chapter 29.1).

### DONOR SURGERY AND ANESTHETIC MANAGEMENT

The technical details of the surgery are covered elsewhere. Currently almost all patients undergoing adult-to-adult LDLT in the United States receive a right hepatic lobe.[6]

The intraoperative management of the donor during LDLT raises legitimate concerns about perioperative complications among anesthesia providers as well as the surgical team, especially because the patient is a healthy individual who is undergoing a major abdominal procedure with a potential for major complications, even death, with no benefit to them self. The preanesthetic evaluation should be part of the selection process and explain the events and procedures to be undertaken in the perioperative period, including surgical and anesthetic risks.

A right hepatectomy for living donation is a lengthy procedure, approximately 8 to 12 hours in duration and usually involves a chevron incision with an upper midline extension or an extended right subcostal incision. The mean blood loss is reported to be 900 mL with a range of 150 to 2600 mL depending on the institution.[32] Both the surgical time and the blood loss improve with increasing experience.[25] Unless there is a known potential recipient contraindication (eg, concern for more extensive liver cancer than previously recognized), the donor surgery generally begins shortly before the recipients procedure. Frequent communication among the surgical teams is necessary to ensure donor and recipient safety.

The anesthetic management is essentially that of a major abdominal procedure with the additional concern to optimize the condition of the donated hepatic lobe by using an appropriate drug and perfusion management.[33]

Because of the risks associated with heterologous blood transfusion (eg, infection, immunosuppression, and anaphylactic reactions) most institutions require a prehospital autologous blood donation of 1 to 3 U and some will routinely give an injection of erythropoietin at that time.[34] Additional measures taken are hemodilution and retrieval of 1 to 3U of blood in the operating room and/or intraoperative cell salvage. With this management, and because donors would be expected to have normal preoperative hemoglobin levels, the majority of patients will not require banked blood products.[32] It is to be kept in mind though, that studies have shown similar postoperative infectious complications and immunosuppression in patients receiving autologous blood donated before surgery and those receiving homologous blood.[35] This is a compelling reason to avoid blood transfusions when possible.[36]

The recognition and treatment of untoward events requires anesthesia providers to seek a balance between the risks and benefits of procedures in patient assessment.[3] Aside from the American Society of Anesthesiologists (ASA) standards for monitoring, which include continuous electrocardiography, capnography, pulseoximetry, measurements of inhaled anesthetics, noninvasive blood pressure measurement, and core body temperature (esophageal), most centers use a radial arterial line and central venous access (internal jugular vein).

Additionally neuromuscular blockade and urine output are monitored and the latter is maintained at > 0.5 mL/kg/hr. The usage of fluid warmer and forced-air warming systems is necessary to prevent or treat intraoperative hypothermia, which frequently occurs. Sequential compression devices should be applied to prevent deep venous thrombosis.

Reports of brachial plexus injury,[3] ulnar nerve palsy,[16] radial neuropraxia,[19] peroneal nerve palsy,[26] and alopecia areata[27] emphasize the importance of patient positioning. Pressure points have to be adequately padded, and attention has to be paid to arm extension. The head position should be changed frequently to prevent undue pressure in one area of the scalp and hair loss.

The anesthetic management has to take into account its effect on the liver, as it might be significant because of the small residual liver volume after these surgeries.[33]

The patient is premedicated with a benzodiazepine and after positioning and application of standard monitors is preoxygenated with and $FiO_2$ of 1.0. The choice of induction agent is probably not crucial considering that the patients are healthy individuals and is supplemented by the administration of an opioid. Once under general anesthesia the patient is mask ventilated, and a neuromuscular blocking agent is administered. Cisatracurium has the advantage that it undergoes organ-independent chemodegredation and therefore is not affected by and does not affect liver function. Tracheal intubation is performed after complete muscle relaxation has been verified and general anesthesia is maintained with an inhalation anesthetic, air, and oxygen. Isoflurane dilates the hepatic artery and may protect against renal and splanchnic vasoconstriction and, although the total hepatic blood flow decreases, it preserves oxygen delivery to the liver well. In light of these attributes, and the fact that only 0.2% of Isoflurane is metabolized by the liver, it may be the preferred choice in these cases. Nitrous oxide is avoided to prevent intestinal distention and

the distention of a possible air embolus, which have been documented during hepatectomies.[36]

Invasive monitors are placed after induction.

Intraoperatively crystalloids and colloids are used as fluid replacement. Because an intraoperative increase in lactate levels has been demonstrated, it may be worth avoiding lactated containing solutions.[33] Normoglycemia should be maintained, if necessary, by using glucose-containing solutions. Hetastarch can contribute to intraoperative bleeding by affecting coagulation, although it has been used without adverse effects, by limiting its administration to less than 1 g/kg body weight. Alternatively albumin, 5%, is used as volume expander. Maintaining a low central venous pressure (CVP less than 5) is a simple way to decrease blood loss during hepatic resection. It has been shown in several nonrandomized, retrospective studies to decrease intraoperative blood loss and even decrease morbidity and hospital stay after hepatic resections.[37] It augments venous drainage, therefore reducing graft edema formation, decreases hepatic venous bleeding and allows easier control of inadvertent venous injury. However, a negative CVP can readily allow the entrance of air through unrecognized hepatic vein lacerations, which may result in significant air embolism.[38] There has been concern about evidence of renal dysfunction and renal failure associated with the maintenance of a low CVP in recipients of orthotopic liver transplants, which frequently suffer from renal dysfunction at the time of surgery. On the other hand maintaining a healthy patient in a controlled hypovolemic state for a short period of time has few risks, because intrinsic autoregulation and physiologic reserve are adequate to maintain organ perfusion.[39] Therefore, for the short period of the hepatic resection, it seems reasonable to maintain a low positive CVP in the donor by limiting fluid administration and using volatile agents. The use of diuresis is also possible, although rarely necessary. Nitroglycerin administration should probably be avoided to maintain adequate hepatic perfusion. Vasoactive drugs, although rarely needed, can be used to augment systemic blood pressure and improve hepatic perfusion. After the hepatic resection the CVP control should be liberalized, while still avoiding overhydration. Again the risks versus benefits, especially in a healthy patient, have to be weighed carefully. It has been shown that invasive monitors do not reveal more subtle changes in hemodynamic and liver functions. Nieman et al showed a significant increase in heart rate and cardiac output and a decrease in systemic vascular resistance after right lobe resections using indocyanine green to measure cardiac output and hepatic clearance. The hepatic clearance of indocyanine green was severely impaired after resection and only moderately improved after 5 days.[40]

Intraoperative measurements of arterial blood gas, hemoglobin, electrolytes, coagulation factors, and pH are useful in the management of these patients.

Assuming an uneventful surgical course without massive transfusions or overt blood loss, normal laboratory values, and the absence of hemodynamic and respiratory abnormalities, the donor should be extubated in the operating room.[3,19,33]

### Postoperative Care and Liver Regeneration

Postoperatively, the donor is admitted to the intensive care unit for 24 hr. Deep venous thrombosis (DVT) prophylaxis with either heparin[19] or low-molecular-weight heparin and sequential compression devices is routinely instituted.[24] Some centers perform ultrasound examinations to rule out a DVT before ambulation.[41] The donor usually receives stress ulcer prophylaxis with

H2 blockers and antibiotic prophylaxis for 3 days including the day of surgery. Chest physiotherapy and incentive spirometry are initiated, and early ambulation is encouraged.[19,27,33]

Adequate postoperative analgesia is very important for donor comfort and recovery. Persistent pain causes physical and psychological distress and impairs lung function, patient mobility, and the quality of life in an otherwise healthy person.[42] Thoracic epidural analgesia provides efficient pain relief, while minimizing systemic side effects, and therefore has been commonly used for postoperative pain control. The catheter is placed preoperatively at the midthoracic level. Using a continuous opoid and/or local anesthetic infusion, it can provide postoperative and may provide preemptive analgesia. It can also supplement the general anesthetic and therefore lower the anesthetic requirements.

Heparin is being used intraoperatively by some centers at the end of the dissection phase to prevent clotting in the remaining liver and in the inflow vessels of the graft following interruption of the vasculature.[33] Additionally postoperative changes in coagulation after liver resection peak in the early postoperative period (2–5 days) have been documented.[43] This raises concerns about the risk for epidural hematomas intraoperatively or on catheter removal. To avoid this risk some centers have abandoned the use of epidural catheters in conjunction with heparin use and in this patient population. Intravenous or intramuscular administration of pain medication is being used instead.[27,33] At our institution no intraoperative heparin is used, and we do place an epidural catheter at the level of T 6/7 for intraoperative and postoperative management. After establishing functionality with Lidocaine 2% with epinephrine, while the patient is still awake, Lidocaine 2% is used throughout the surgery to maintain a level and decrease anesthetic requirements. For postoperative pain control we use an infusion of 0.125% bupivacaine with 2 μg/ mL of Fentanyl at rate of 8–10 cc/hr. Depending on the institution, infusions of 0.5% bupivacaine with morphine or intraoperative loading doses of morphine have been used. Different combinations of epidural opoids and local anesthetics can be used successfully and safely depending on institutional experience. If epidural narcotics are being used, adequate communication with those treating breakthrough pain about all relevant recent sedatives or pain medications has to be ensured to prevent life-threatening respiratory depression. Additionally, metabolism in the residual liver is presumably slowed because of postoperative dysfunction, although the specific kinetic of drug distribution and metabolism in this population have not been studied. This puts the donor at an increased risk for respiratory side effects.[3]

The epidural catheter is usually removed on the second to fourth postoperative day. Following the recommendations of the American society of regional anesthesia consensus statement,[44] to minimize the risk of epidural hematomas on removal of the catheter, the INR has to be < 1.5. In patients receiving subcutaneous heparin. the catheter should be removed at the nadir of the heparin half life. Ideally for patient receiving heparin twice daily this would be 2 to 3 hours prior to the next heparin dose. For low-molecular-weight heparin the catheter should be removed at least 10 to 12 hours after the last dosing. The next administration of either heparin or low-molecular-weight heparin has to be postponed to at least 2 hours after removal of the catheter. In either case the patient has to be monitored for motor or sensory deficits for 24 hr postremoval.

Additionally to incisional pain some patients suffer postoperatively from right shoulder pain. This is most likely secondary to the retractor pulling on the chest wall to gain adequate surgical exposure. The pain is generally short-lived and easily treated with oral pain medication and physical therapy.

The patients are closely monitored for liver dysfunction and complications as well as for liver regeneration. Doppler ultrasound is used to monitor venous outflow and portal inflow of the residual liver. Daily laboratory tests, wound inspections, and evaluations of drainage fluids are performed.[19,24]

### *Any Electrolyte Abnormality is Treated Appropriately*

The occurrence of hypophosphatemia in the postoperative period is of special concern, because it can be associated with significant patient morbidity. Hypophosphatemia (and low intracellular adenosine triphophate [ATP]) can cause cerebral dysfunction, anorexia, bone pain, hemolysis, platelet dysfunction, renal tubular defects, myocardial suppression, muscular weakness, rhabdomyolysis, and respiratory depression. It usually does not become clinically apparent because of the efficient buffering system and large phosphorus reserve. Nevertheless, if phosphate levels drop below 1 mg/dL, it can develop into a life-threatening event.[45] Buell et al have demonstrated increased postoperative complications in hypophophatemic patients.[46] Some degree of hypophosphatemia seems to be a common occurrence after major hepatic surgery and is usually transient and most apparent on postoperative day 1 to 4. The cause is not entirely clear, but it was postulated to result from flux of phosphate into the regenerating liver as well as a complex interplay among hormonal and endocrinologic interactions. Other contributing factors may include blood loss, prolonged glucose infusions, which leads to increased excretion by the renal tubules, the liver volume resected, surgical technique, and patient selection.[45] Because of the risk of postoperative complications it was suggested to place all donors on a hyperalimentation to assure that the patient will receive supratherapeutic levels of phosphorus.[47] Tan et al on the other hand did not find profound hypophophatemia to be prevalent in their donors. Although some of their patients did experience transient hypophophatemia, there was no increased morbidity, when it was aggressively treated with intravenous or oral phosphates. In their Institution the time to oral intake is bridged by intravenous glucose containing electrolyte solutions, and so far none of their patients required hyperalimentation for metabolic derangements or prolonged inability to take oral feedings.

Hyperalimentation itself is associated with a potential morbidity, including the need for central venous access and the possibility of subsequent line infections and catheter related complications. The advantages and disadvantages of both ways to bridge the time to adequate oral intake have to be carefully considered for the benefit of patient safety.

In general oral intake is encouraged as soon as bowel activity has returned.

All donors show elevated liver enzymes postoperative in secondary to the liver injury and coagulation parameters peak early in the postoperative period. Most of these parameters normalize within the first weeks postoperatively, although some of them may remain elevated for months after the resection, as seen with the gamma-glytamyl transferase and alkaline phophatase in a Belgium study.[33] The laboratory profiles seem to follow a predictable pattern, and deviation from this pattern or failure to return to baseline requires further evaluation.[48]

The average hospital stay reported by most transplant centers is 10 to 13 days, ranging from 7 to 60 days. All donors have scheduled follow up appointments to detect possible liver dysfunctions and monitor liver regeneration (CT or MRI).[24] Most of the regeneration process takes place in the first week after hepatectomy[48] to approximately 70% of its original volume. Within a month it will reach approximately 80% of its original volume, but it may not have fully returned to a predonation level by 1 year.[19,49] Nadalin showed that the liver volume reached only 83% of its original volume by 1 year. He also showed that liver biochemistries, international normalized ratio (INR), and bilirubin returned to normal within 10 days, whereas cholinesterase and albumin recovered over 90 days. Although the full functional recovery is the norm, it occurs much slower than the recovery of volume and biochemistries, and it can take a year until it is reached. Interestingly hepatic functional recovery corresponds with the time of full psychophysical recovery.[50]

## CONCLUSIONS

LDLT has undoubtedly several advantages including a decrease in waiting time and transplantation of a healthy organ under optimal conditions. Nevertheless, a healthy person is subjected to an extensive abdominal surgery with its potential for significant morbidity and mortality.

The safety of the donor always has to be the main concern.

But it also has been shown that the risks to the donor can be minimized, if an experienced transplant team that carefully considers all aspects of the transplantation process performs the surgery. Performance of the donor surgery under optimal conditions starts with the careful selection of appropriate candidates, avoiding unnecessary risks, and ends with a thorough postoperative and long-term follow up.

The establishment of a living donor liver transplantation databank and the introduction of a standardized classification of complications will aid in ongoing evaluation and research and lead to further improvement of living donor liver transplantation.

## References

1. Organ Procurement and Transplant Network. OPTN/SRTR Annual Report 2004. Available at http://www.optn.org. Accessed May 6, 2005.
2. Strong RW, Lynch SV, Ong TH, et al. Successful liver transplantation from a living donor to her son. *N Engl J Med* 1990;322:1505–1507.
3. Merrit WT. Living donor surgery: overview of surgical and anesthesia issues. *Anesthesiology Clin N Am* 2004;22:633–650.
4. Yamaoka Y, Washida M, Honda K, et al. Liver transplantation using a right lobe graft from a living donor. *Transplantation* 1994;57:1127–1130.
5. Wachs ME, Bak TE, Karrer FM, et al. Adult living donor liver transplantation. 1998;66:1313–1316.
6. Trotter JF, Wachs M, Everson GT, et al. Adult-to-adult transplantation of the right hepatic lobe from a living donor. *N Engl J Med* 2002;346:1074–1082.
7. Brown RS, Russo MW, Lai ML, et al. A survey of liver transplantation from adult donors in the United States. *N Engl J Med* 2003;348:818–825.
8. Jassem W, Koo DDH, Cerundolo L, et al. Cadaveric versus living-donor livers: Differences in inflammatory markers after transplantation. *Transplantation* 2003;76:1599–1603.
9. New York State Committee on quality Improvement in Living Liver Donation. A report to: New York State Transplant Council and New York State Department of Health, December 2002.
10. Anderson-Shaw L, Schmidt ML, Elkin J, et al. Evolution of a Living Donor Liver Transplantation Advocacy Program. *J Clin Ethics* 2005;16(1);46–57.
11. Broelsch CF, Frilling A, Testa G, et al. Living donor transplantation in adults. *Eur J Gastroentero Hepatol* 2003;15:3–6.
12. Live Organ Donor Consensus Group. Consensus statement on the live organ donor. *JAMA* 2002;284:2919–2926.
13. Lo CM, Fan ST. Living donor liver transplantation: donor selection, evaluation, and surgical complications. *Curr Opin Organ Transplantn* 2001;6:120–25, 2001.
14. Florman S, Miller C. Living donor liver transplantation in adults. *Transplantation* 2003;8:131–138.
15. Papachristu C, Walter M, Dietrich K, Danzer G, et al. Motivation for Living-Donor Liver Transplantation from the Donor's Perspective: An In-Depth Qualitative Research Study. *Transplantation* 2004;78:1506–1514.
16. Chisuwa H, Hashikura Y, Mita A, et al. Living liver donation: preoperative assessment, anatomic considerations, and long-term outcome. *Transplantation* 2003;75:1670–1676.
17. Crowley-Matoka M, Switzer G. Nondirected Living Donation: a Survey of Current Trends and Practices. *Transplantation* 2005;79:515–519.
18. Price D. The texture and content of living donor transplant laws and policies. *Transplant Proc* 1996;28:378–379.
19. Pomfret EA, Pomposelli JJ, Lewis WD, et al. Live Donor Adult Liver Transplantation Using Right Lobe Grafts: Donor Evaluation and Surgical Outcome. *Arch Surg* 2001;136:425–433.
20. Rinella ME, Alonso E, Rao S, et al. Body mass index as a predictor of hepatic steatosis in living liver donors. *Liver Transplant* 2001;7:409–414.
21. Williams RS, Alisa A, John B, et al. Adult-to-adult living donor liver transplant: UK experience. *Eur J Gastroenterol Hepatol* 2003;15:7–14.
22. Marcos A. Right-lobe living donor liver transplantation: a review. *Liver Transplant* 2000;6:3–20.
23. Brandhagen D, Fidler J, Rosen C. Evaluation of the donor liver for living donor liver transplantation. *Liver Transplant* 2003;9:S16–28.
24. Malago M, Testa G, Frilling A, et al. Right living donor liver transplantation: An option for adult patients: single institution experience with 74 patients. *Ann Surg* 2003;238:853–863.
25. Lo CM, Fan ST, et al. Lessons learned from one hundred right lobe living donor liver transplants. *Transplantation* 2004;240:151–158.
26. Lui CL, Fan ST, et al. Right live donor liver transplantation improves survival of patients with acute liver failure. *Brit J Surg* 2002;89:317–322.
27. Soejima Y, Harada N, et al. Perioperative management and complications in donors related to living-donor liver transplantation. *Surgery* 2002;131:S195–99.
28. Hata S, Sugawara Y, et al. Volume regeneration after right lobe donation. *Liver Transplant* 2004;10:65–70.
29. Kapoor V, et al. Intrahepatic biliary anatomy of living adult liver donors: correlation of mangafodipir trisodium-enhanced MR cholangiography and intraoperative cholangiography. *AJR* 2002;179:1281–1286.
30. Goyen M, et al. Right-lobe living related liver transplantation: Evaluation of a comprehensive magnetic resonance imaging protocol for assessing potential donors. *Liver Transplant* 2002;8:241–250.
31. Akabayashi A, Slingsby B, Fujita M. The first donor death after living-related liver transplantation in Japan. *Transplantation* 2004;77:634.
32. Lutz JT, Valentin-Gamazo C, et al. Blood Transfusion requirements and blood salvage in donors undergoing right hepatectomy for living related liver transplant. *Anesth Analg* 2003;96:351–355.
33. Cammu G, Troisi R, et al. Anesthetic Management and Outcome in right-lobe living donor liver transplantation. *Eur J Anaesthesiol* 2002;19:93–98.
34. Morgan GR, Diflo T, et al. Selection and imaging of the living liver donor. *Curr Op Organ Transpl* 2001;6:350–354.
35. Nielsen HJ. Detrimental effects of perioperative blood transfusion. *Br J Surg* 1995;82:582.
36. Hatano Y, Murakwa M, et al. Venous air embolism during hepatic resection. *Anesthesiology* 1990;73:1282–1285.
37. Jones RM, Moulton CE, Hardy KJ. Central venous pressure and its effect on blood loss during liver resection. *Br J Surg* 1998;85:1058–1060.
38. Chen C-L, Chen Y-S, et al. Minimal blood loss Living Donor Hepatectomy. *Transplantation* 2000;69:2580–2586.
39. Schroeder R, Collins BH, Tuttle-Newhall E, et al. Intraoperative fluid management during orthotopic liver transplant. *J Cardiothorac Vasc Anesth* 2004;18:438–441.

40. Nieman CU, Roberts JP, Ascher NL, et al. Intraoperative hemodynamics and liver function in adult-to-adult living liver donors. *Liver Transplant* 2002;8:1126–1132.

41. Broering DC, Wilms C, Bok P, et al. Evolution of donor morbidity in living related liver transplantation: A single-center analysis of 165 cases. *Ann Surg* 2004;24:1013–1026.

42. Cywinski JB, Parker BM, Xu MMS, et al. A comparison of postoperative pain control in patients after right donor hepatectomy and major hepatic resection for tumor. *Anesth Analg* 2004;99:174–1752.

43. Borromeo CL, Stix MS, et al. Epidural catheter and increased prothrombin time after right lobe hepatectomy for living donor liver transplantation. *Anesth Analg* 2000;91:1139–1141.

44. Second Consensus Conference on Neuroaxial Anesthesia and Anticoagulation April 25-28 2002. http://www.asra.com/consensus_conferences/consensus_statements.html. Accessed June 27, 2005.

45. Tan H, Madep R, et al. hypophosphatemia after 95 right-lobe living-donor hepatectomies for liver transplantation is not a significant source of morbidity. *Transplantation* 2003;76:1085–1088.

46. Buell JF, Berger AC, et al. The clinical implications of hypophophatemia following major hepatic resection. *Arch Surg* 1998;133:757.

47. Pomposelli JJ, Pomfret EA, Burns DL, et al. Life threatening hypophophatemia after right hepatic. Lobectomy for live donor adult liver transplantation. *Liver Transplant* 2001;7:637.

48. Marcos A, Fisher RA, Ham JM, et al. Liver regeneration and function in donor and recipient after right lobe adult to adult living donor liver transplantation. *Transplantation* 2000;69:1375–1379.

49. Olthoff KM. Hepatic regeneration in living donor liver transplantation. *Liver Transplant* 2003;9(Suppl 2)S35–41.

50. Nadalin S, Testa G, et al. Volumetric and functional recovery of the liver after richt hepatectomy for living donation. *Liver Transpl* 2004;10:1024–1029.

51. Clavien PA, Camargo CA, et al. Definition and classification of negative outcomes in solid organ transplantation. Application in liver transplantation. *Ann Surg* 1994;220:109–120.

52. Beavers KL, Sandler RS, et al. The living donor experience: donor health assessment and outcomes after living donor liver transplantation. *Liver Transplant* 2001;7:943–947.

53. Diaz GC, Renz JF, et al. Donor health assessment after living donor liver transplantation. *Ann Surg* 2002;236:120–126.

54. Otte JB: Living liver donation: Preoperative assessment, anatomic considerations, and long-term outcome. *Transplantation* 2003;75:1625–1626.

55. Neuberger J, Lucey M. The first donor death after living related liver transplantation in Japan. *Transplantation* 2004;77:489–490.

56. Karliova M, Malago M, et al. Living–related liver transplantation from the view of the donor: a 1-year follow-up survey. *Transplantation* 2002; 73:1799–1804.

57. Kim-Schluger L, Florman S, et al. Quality of life after lobectomy for adult liver transplantation. *Transplantation* 2002;73:1593–1597.

## 29.5   DONOR MORBIDITY AND MORTALITY

*Dianne LaPointe Rudow, DrNP,*
*Milan Kinkhabwala, MD,*
*Jean C Edmond, MD*

### INTRODUCTION

Living donor liver transplantation (LDLT) poses an inherent conflict between two ethical principles. On the one hand, it is accepted as care givers that we should do no harm —"Primum nil nocere"—, yet as members of the transplantation community in service of the public health, we aim to maximize the utilization of available organs and thereby save lives. In the United States the first systematic application of LDLT was preceded by a comprehensive clinical–ethical analysis of the issues involved in the introduction of a radical innovation.[1] In pediatric recipients, LDLT was ethically justified because of the unacceptably high pediatric waiting list mortality and the relatively low surgical risks of lateral segmentectomy. The parents' interest in preserving the life of their child, and the interest of society in supporting the parents in this regard, was felt to trump the small, though very real risk of morbidity. Few would now argue that pediatric LDLT has not been an unqualified success in the treatment of pediatric liver failure, preserving life while efficiently allocating scarce resources; but nonetheless there have been deaths in donors of pediatric grafts. As adult-to-adult live donor transplantation (ALDLT) becomes more commonplace, appraisal of risk of potential donors has never been more important as we seek to gain public acceptance and trust in live donor transplantation.

The aim of this chapter is to review the existing experience in living donor liver transplantation from the context of morbidity of the donor operation. Quantifying true relative risk associated with donor hepatectomy has been difficult due to a lack of definition of outcome measures and inconsistent follow up of donors. In aLDLT, data on long outcomes of liver donation are limited due to a smaller clinical experience and poorer long-term compliance with follow-up compared to left lateral segment donors. In an attempt to address the paucity of data, the National Institutes of Health commissioned a multicenter study of adult-to-adult living donor liver transplantation (A2ALL) in order to accurately determine donor risk, among other aims.[2]

Donor morbidity is influenced by a complex set of variables including center experience, extent and technique of hepatic resection, anatomic factors, and general health of the donor. A recent consensus conference held in Vancouver in September 2005 sought to address the variability in selection criteria and donor evaluation and will soon publish guidelines. It is also apparent that a uniform definition of surgical morbidity is required in order to meaningfully compare outcomes. In this regard, modifications of the Clavien scale for LDLT may ultimately gain acceptance as the standard for reporting surgical morbidity.[3] The Clavien scale (Table 29.5-1) scores morbidity from grade 1 to 4 based on likelihood of the complication requiring intervention or the possibility of long-term or irreversible injury.

Donor complications appear to be more frequent in centers performing fewer procedures,[4] and in single-center reports there is an inverse correlation between experience and donor morbidity.[3] This parallels a learning curve in recipient implantation as well, which has also been observed. How best to establish a threshold for credentialing expertise is a subject of considerable debate in the transplant community. Similar concerns regarding donor safety during a "learning curve" were also raised with laparoscopic donor nephrectomy for kidney transplantation, though ultimately no policy or consensus emerged from the debate. However, regulatory agencies charged with public safety are not likely to wait for consensus within the transplant community with respect to LDLT, which in adults has a substantially greater risk of morbidity, mortality, and a steep learning curve. For example, the New York State Department of Health exerted its responsibility as a public agency in 2002 when it issued standards of care for LDLT, which were developed in cooperation with the State's transplant centers.[5] The most important contribution of the NYS standards (now regulation) was the requirement for an independent evaluation of the donor and recipient. Though a separate pathway for donor and recipient evaluation dates back to the original kidney transplant

TABLE 29.5-1

## MODIFIED CLASSIFICATION OF MORBIDITY FOR LIVER DONORS[a]

TABLE 1    Classification of Common Complications of the Donor After LDLT

Grade I

Any complication that is not life threatening, does not result in residual disability, and does not require a therapeutic invasive intervention or the use of drugs, except analgesics, antipyretics, anti-inflammatory, or antiemetic drugs

Examples

(1)   Superficial wound infection without antibiotics

(2)   Transient bile leak treated conservatively and diminished within 1 wk (bile leak: total bilirubin in drainage 2 times higher than in serum)

(3)   Transient positioning damage

(4)   Postoperative urinary retention (without necessity of permanent catheterization)

Grade II

Any complication that is potentially life-threatening, that requires the use of drug therapy or > 1 foreign blood units, but that does not require a therapeutic invasive intervention and does not result in residual disability

Examples

(1)   Bacterial, viral, or fungal infection requiring antibiotic, antiviral, or antifungic therapy

(2)   Postoperative bleeding withour requiring relaparotomy

(3)   Local controlled deep venous thrombosis without thrombembolic complications

(4)   Intrapleural or pericardial effusion (without necessity of pleurocardialcentesis or pericardialcentesis)

Grade III

Any complication that is potentially life-threatening that requires a therapeutic invasive intervention, the use of drug therapy/blood transfusions and/or leads to readmission in the ICU but does not result in residual disability

Examples

(1)   Bile leak requiring endoscopic or surgical procedures

(2)   Postoperative bleeding requiring relaparotomy

(3)   Deep wound infections requiring relaparotomy or interventional drainage and antibiotic therapy

(4)   Complicated venous thrombosis with pulmonary embolism

(5)   Gastrointestinal bleeding treated endoscopically or surgically

Grade IV

Any complication with residual or lasting disability or that leads to death

Examples

(1)   Any disease leading to death

(2)   Progressive liver failure requiring liver transplantation

(3)   Renal failure requiring persistent hemodialysis or renal transplantation

(4)   De novo human immunodeficiency virus, hepatitis B, or hepatitis C infection

(5)   Myocardial infarction with persistence of disability (NYHA classification III–IV)

(6)   Persisting neurologic disability (positioning damage)

[a]Reprinted with permission from Lippincott Williams and Wilkins.

by Murray et al. in 1954, it was not until the NYS guidelines were issued that this concept was codified as an ethical standard in living donation. Although the composition of the donor's evaluation team, the optimal evaluation and selection process, and the role of an "independent donor advocate" are left to the center, there is little debate about the necessity of having a distinct evaluation process. At Columbia, decisions regarding candidacy are achieved by consensus at biweekly Independent Donor Advocate Team (IDAT) meetings. The IDAT also functions as the group responsible for education of staff in LDLT, publication and dissemination of educational tools, documentation and regulatory issues, and quality assurance tracking of both donor and recipient LDLT. Though not specified in the regulation, the donor advocate at Columbia is a board-certified internist who participates in donor evaluation and provides support for the transplant team in the postoperative period. There is therefore frequent contact between the recovering donor and the physicians, reducing anxiety and providing opportunities for questions and answers.

Following New York's lead, the federal department of Health and Human Services through The Advisory Council on Transplant (ACOT) issued similar guidelines. United Network for Organ Sharing (UNOS) requires data submission by centers indicating donor follow-up, and now requires credentialing of all centers performing LDLT in the United States. The credentialing criteria include experience in LDLT and hepatic resection, and infrastructure to sustain a LDLT program.

## MORTALITY AFTER LIVE DONOR HEPATECTOMY

Although deaths are never acceptable in healthy donors undergoing hepatectomy, deaths are also inevitable in any major invasive procedure such as a right hepatectomy. In addition to the generic surgical risk, donor hepatectomy involves potential damage to a major life-sustaining organ. This distinction seems to account for the nearly 10-fold increase in operative risk of right hepatectomy when compared to donor nephrectomy.[6] Based on a worldwide experience of over 3000 cases, it appears that operative mortality after donor hepatectomy is less than 1%. There have been an estimated 9 to 14 deaths following live donor hepatectomy. In addition, several donors have undergone liver transplantation or been temporarily listed for liver transplant.[4,7-9] Actual mortality figures are difficult because most of the donor deaths are not actually published but by obtained personal communication, through lay press, and so forth. Therefore additional deaths may have been unreported and unpublicized. In recent years, the Scientific Registry of Transplant Recipients (SRTR), which has been charged with monitoring outcomes of living donors as well as recipients, has performed correlation with the social security death master file to verify the center-reported outcomes in the United States.

Public analysis of the causes of death in both pediatric and adult donors has led to meaningful adjustments in clinical practice. After two deaths related to thromboembolism were reported in lateral segment donors, preoperative health of the donor has been more carefully scrutinized and preoperative intervention (weight loss, discontinuation of smoking, and oral contraception) is recognized as a means of reducing risk. Unfortunately only one right lobe donor death has been published. In this case, death was the result of late postoperative liver failure and portal hypertension caused by underlying steatohepatitis not appreciated during preoperative screening of the donor.[8] After this event, there has been more attention to standardized algorithms for evaluation of steatosis in potential donors. In a second case, unpublished in the peer-review literature, but investigated by regulatory agencies and widely discussed in the lay press, the donor death accelerated the development of minimum standards for perioperative care, evaluation, and education of donors.[5]

Potential causes of mortality are known from the experience in hepatic resection in nontransplant situations. Mortality and the steps to reduce mortality risk should be discussed with potential donors during the educational process that must accompany all donor evaluations. Operative mortality after right hepatectomy for other indications has been 2% to 5% in experienced centers, which is somewhat greater than the mortality reported for hepatectomy associated with living donation. The highly selective criteria for live donor hepatectomy is likely to account for this difference, though there have been no controlled comparative studies reported.

## MORBIDITY AFTER LIVE DONOR HEPATECTOMY

### Classification of Morbidity

A modification of the Clavien scale for surgical complications has been proposed for uniform reporting of LDLT complications.[10] The previous scale, adopted for donor hepatectomy, grades complications based on the requirement for intervention, and the potential for long-term effects.[3,11,12] A modification of this scheme has been adopted for reporting outcomes in the NIH-sponsored study of adult-to-adult LDLT (A2ALL) in the United States. Grade I complications, such as self-limited bile staining of drain fluid or a narcotic induced ileus, are usually minor and non-life-threatening. Grade II complications are potentially life threatening but are managed noninvasively and with no residual effects. Grade III complications, like postoperative intrabdominal abscess requiring a percutaneous drain and antibiotic therapy, are potentially life threatening and require invasive therapy and/or hospitalization, but no residual disability is likely. Grade IV complications are likely to result in residual disability or death. The majority of donor morbidity can be classified as Grade I and Grade II,[3,12,13] with Grade III complications less frequent but more verifiable. Because Grade I and II complications are subjective in interpretation, acceptance of standardized definitions of low morbidity complications are required to serve as a prospective tracking tool in LDLT.

## EXTENT OF RESECTION AND MORBIDITY

Morbidity after live donor hepatectomy is influenced by the extent of resection, because of the influence of functional residual hepatic reserve in postoperative recovery. Right lobe donors experience increased morbidity compared to left lobe or lateral segment donors and complications tend to be more serious.[3,12,14,15] Commonly reported morbidity is shown in Table 29.5-2. Beavers et al pooled published reports to conclude that the aggregate morbidity of right lobe donation based on 409 reported cases was 31%. Grade I and II complications like bile leaks, prolonged ileus, and wound problems were the most frequently reported complications, though interpretation of this type of pooled data is limited by the lack of standardized definitions of complications in different published reports.[13]

Serious, life-threatening complications are much less frequent. Liver failure in the absence of an early technical complication like arterial or portal venous thrombosis is likely to be caused by a small-for-size remnant liver. We described this syndrome of graft injury leading to early synthetic dysfunction and prolonged cholestasis as we transitioned from pediatric LDLT, in which the graft is ample for the recipient, to adult LDLT, in which the graft is usually smaller than the projected needs of the recipient.[16] In donor evaluation, 30% functional residual volume is a proposed minimum threshold, though some centers use calculated remnant volume in relation to donor weight. Remnant volumes less than 30% have been associated with prolonged cholestasis, portal hypertension, and normal or near enzymes and synthetic function after hepatectomy ("small-for size-syndrome"), especially in the presence of moderate steatosis.[3,17,18] Pharmacological therapies

**TABLE 29.5-2**

## DONOR MORBIDITY REPORTED IN THE LITERATURE

Death
Aborted procedure
Non autologous blood transfusion
Biliary Complications
- Leak
- Stricture

Vascular complications
- Portal vein thrombus
- Hepatic vein thrombus
- Hepatic artery thrombosis
- Pulmonary emboli
- DVT

Pulmonary complications
- Pleural effusion
- Pneumonia

Wound complications
- Infection
- Hernia

Other
- Anesthesia complications
- Line/IV complications
- Transient nerve injury
- Illeus

Psychiatric
- Chronic pain
- Depression

such as intraportal glucose and insulin infusions to accelerate regeneration in a small remnant have been reported, though in fact some data on the types of agents selected are actually conflicting.[19] Because excess portal blood flow may contribute to injury of the small graft, Roberts has proposed Octreotide therapy to decrease portal pressure after LDLT (personal communication). Outcome data for small for size syndrome in donors are sparse, though any donor with a small calculated remnant is at theoretic risk for small-for-size syndrome and liver failure, especially if there is underlying steatosis. Furthermore, small-for-size remnants tolerate additive complications poorly. The presence of a concomitant complication like bile leak, infection, or bleeding may exacerbate the poor recovery in a small-for-size liver. Caution and full disclosure to the potential donor is therefore advised when the calculated remnant volume is thought to be less than ideal. Surprisingly, however, in our recent analysis of recipient outcomes in 385 LDLT in the A2ALL study, graft size was not a predictor of graft loss in a multivariate analysis.[20]

More recently extended right hepatic grafts incorporating the middle hepatic vein (MHV) have been reported with good donor and recipient results. The rationale behind inclusion of the MHV with the graft is the consistency of graft venous outflow in the anterior sectors obtained when the MHV is always procured. Advocates of procurement of the MHV argue that donor risk is not increased, but outcomes are more predictable in the recipient, especially when the graft size is at the margins (below a graft to body weight ratio of 0.8). Advocates of preservation of the MHV with the donor's remnant argue that any enhancement of potential donor risk is unacceptable, given the numerous options available for venous reconstruction of large anterior sector veins.[21] Regeneration of the remnant left lobe may be impaired in the absence of a middle vein, though the functional long-term consequence of this finding is not clear. The Toronto group recently reported no clinical difference in donor morbidity based on the fate of the MHV.[22] At this point the question is unanswered and will have to await a larger experience. In our center an individualized approach is taken, in which the transection plane is decided in the operating room by the donor surgeon based on sonographic characteristics of the venous circulation in the context of graft and remnant size in addition to other considerations.[21]

## HOSPITAL RESOURCE UTILIZATION

Hospital resource utilization has been poorly documented in live donation. Patients are typically hospitalized for 5 to 7 days with 1 to 2 days in a monitored care setting.[23] Resolution of postoperative ileus is the most common cause for prolonged hospitalization, followed by bile leakage and fever. There are no national standards for nursing care in the postoperative period, but New York State does mandate a nursing ratio of 4:1 for all recovering live liver donors for the duration of their hospital stay.[5] Most early complications occur within the initial hospitalization, less commonly after discharge. Readmission rates after discharge are 5% at Columbia, and the most common cause of readmission is pain.

## RECOVERY OF LIVER FUNCTION AFTER LIVE DONOR HEPATECTOMY

Early aminotransferase elevation is common after donor hepatectomy. Liver enzymes peak early, in the first 48 hours, whereas bilirubin tends to peak later in the postoperative course, ap-

**TABLE 29.5-3**

## RESOLUTION OF DONOR LABORATORY VALUES

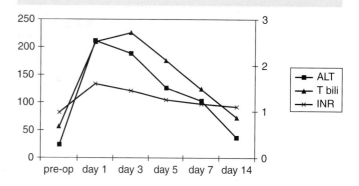

proximately postoperative day 3 (Table 29.5-3) Unusual clinical patterns of liver function are generally investigated with initial duplex sonography and possibly cross-sectional imaging (multiphase computed tomography [CT]), which is especially useful in investigating differential areas of perfusion in the liver or segmental biliary obstruction. Exaggerated enzyme leak in the absence of synthetic dysfunction suggests focal ischemia, which can occur for example with a devascularized segment 4 following lateral segmentectomy.

Prolonged or exaggerated cholestasis in the absence of a biliary complication suggests ischemia or a small residual volume. Treatment of small-for-size syndrome is supportive care and avoidance of further injury to the remnant. The natural history of small-for-size syndrome after hepatectomy is poorly documented but can be associated with significant morbidity and even mortality, most commonly as a result of infection and complications of portal hypertension. Cholestatic, small-for-size livers are susceptible to further injury and can even develop acute on chronic failure with minor infections or manipulation. Invasive diagnostic procedures like "exploratory" reoperations, endoscopic retrograde cholangiopancreatography (ERCP), or percutaneous cholangiography should therefore be approached with extreme caution and circumspection, despite the natural tendency to want to be "aggressive" when faced with a poorly functioning liver in a donor.

Encephalopathy and acidosis, when present, are ominous findings and suggest acute liver failure. Early postoperative acute liver failure suggests a vascular event like portal vein or arterial thrombosis, or acute outflow obstruction. Although acute vascular events can be reversible with immediate intervention (usually surgical), the patient should be listed for transplantation because survival in acute liver failure is directly related to the timing of liver replacement before the development of multiorgan failure or neurologic injury. Pharmacologic interventions like n-acetylcysteine or prostaglandin E1 infusion are of unproven value when there is insufficient hepatic mass resulting in cholestasis or frank liver failure. Currently there is at least one documented case of a right lobe donor requiring liver replacement as a result of acute liver failure.[4]

## HEMORRHAGE

Bleeding is inevitable during hepatic resection and is influenced by the extent of parenchymal transection. Transfusion requirements have, if anything, been lower in live donor hepatectomy than in hepatic resection for other indications, despite the fact that live donor hepatectomy is generally performed with no inflow occlusion. Experienced centers report a very low incidence of heterologous transfusion.[25] Expected blood loss in donor hepatectomy is difficult to accurately ascertain from published reports, given differences in reporting and measurement of blood loss, but estimates range from 300 {ts} cc to 800 {ts} cc for uncomplicated cases, with less blood loss in lateral segment resections.[26,27] Many techniques for parenchymal transection have been described, and new technologies are routinely applied to facilitating transection, but no controlled trials have indicated superiority of one technique over another. The most important factor is the experience of the surgical team in performing hepatic resection.

Most centers have well-established systems for blood conservation in live donor surgery, including the use of autologous banked blood, routine use of a cell saver, and in some cases isovolumetric hemodilution. An anesthesiology team that is experienced in hepatic resection and has a good working relationship with the surgical team is essential. Limitation of crystalloid resuscitation during transection in order to maintain a low central venous pressure, for example, is an important means of controlling blood loss and must be carefully orchestrated between surgeon and anesthesiologist intraoperatively.

The incidence of postoperative bleeding requiring transfusion is low, less than 5%,[4,12,213,18,25] but because a postoperative bleeding event can be unpredictable and life threatening, surveillance for bleeding in the initial postoperative period is a routine feature of care and includes frequent clinical examinations and serial hemoglobin assessments. Drains are commonly employed in hepatic surgery, though without controlled data. While drains are useful for early diagnosis of bile leaks, they are less effective in diagnosis of acute hemorrhage because of their tendency to become obstructed by clot. The absence of bloody drainage should not therefore exclude the diagnosis of hemorrhage when other signs are present, including tachycardia, hypotension, or abdominal distension. In such cases immediate intervention by an experienced clinician is the best strategy for prevention of mortality or serious morbidity. It should also be recognized by the care team that late hemorrhage can also occur, for example, hemorrhage related to removal of an abdominal drain, when the drain dislodged a clip that was securing a diaphragmatic vessel. Ultimately vigilance and an integrated care system incorporating motivated, empowered nurses is the best strategy to reduce poor outcomes related to unexpected complications.[27,28]

## VASCULAR COMPLICATIONS

Vascular complications of donor hepatectomy are fortunately rare,[4,15,25,27] but potentially catastrophic, and require immediate attention. Complex anatomy, such as portal vein trifurcation, may increase the potential for vascular compromise of the remnant by increasing the technical challenge of removing the graft. In this anatomic variant, the right anterior and the right posterior branches of the portal vein join the left portal vein separately. This means that the left portal vein is shorter and prone to being injured or narrowed as the right veins are removed with the graft. We have observed an increase in morbidity in donors with portal trifurcation anatomy, though we do not exclude donors on the basis of this anatomy alone. This vascular anomaly may also increase the difficulty of biliary reconstruction in the recipient because the right anterior and posterior bile ducts are also separated in this variation. During donor hepatectomy, when a stenosis or appearance of kinking is suspected or observed, the problem should be

corrected before leaving the operating room, with venous reconstruction or venoplasty if necessary. In most cases we now use silk ties for ligation and transection of the portal vein rather than vascular clamps and suture lines, which may increase the possibility of a stenosis. The silk ligatures can be bolstered with a clip, but it is difficult to impinge on the remnant portal vein with a well-placed tie several millimeters off the main venous bifurcation.

Postoperative diagnosis of portal vein occlusion or stenosis is based on suspicious clinical findings confirmed by sonography or cross-sectional imaging. Some centers perform routine day 1 baseline sonography for this reason. Clinical findings may be subtle, such as increased ascitic drainage suggestive of portal hypertension or mild encephalopathy. Overt signs include evidence of liver ischemia with rising enzymes, synthetic dysfunction, and progressive encephalopathy. Acute liver insufficiency in the early postoperative period is almost always technical in nature, and management is almost always surgical. At reoperation, the surgeon should be prepared to procure venous conduits for venoplasty or as interposition grafts and to use anticoagulation. Although data on success of surgical correction of postoperative portal vein thrombosis are very limited because of the rarity of these events, success is likely to be based on timely intervention before propagation of thrombus or development of liver injury related to ischemia.[18,25,27]

Arterial thrombosis of the remnant is not reported after live donor hepatectomy, though there may be occult or unreported events. Because inflow occlusion is generally not used in live donor operations and dissection is limited to the arterial circulation feeding the graft, the remnant arterial inflow is generally well protected from inadvertent surgical injury. Late portal vein thrombosis or stenosis, however, is a known complication of donor hepatectomy and can be completely asymptomatic. A problem may be suspected only on the basis of subtle signs of portal hypertension such as splenomegaly or moderate thrombocytopenia and has been reported.[25] Intervention in asymptomatic late portal complications may not be required, other than increased surveillance with physical, laboratory, and imaging examination. The true incidence of late portal complications is unknown, but because routine 1-year surveillance imaging has been adopted as a standard component of follow up care, additional data are likely to become available as worldwide experience grows.

## BILIARY COMPLICATIONS

Biliary complications are the most commonly reported Grade II or greater postoperative event in living donors. Leaks are more common than stricture. Leaks in left lateral segment donation range from 5% to 10%,[9] with a somewhat higher rate (up to 13%) in right hepatectomy.[18,29] Routine intraoperative or preoperative cholangiography is employed by some centers during donor hepatectomy, but it is not clear that routine fluoroscopic cholangiography reduces the incidence of biliary complications in the donor. Most leaks are diagnosed in the early postoperative period during the initial hospitalization, though late leaks (diagnosed after discharge) are also reported.[18] Grade I leaks are classified are those diagnosed by simple assessment of postoperative drain fluid and persisting for at least 7 days without need for further intervention, whereas Grade II and III leaks require an interventional radiology procedure, endoscopic biliary, or reoperation.[25] There is some inconsistency in the grading system because of reporting differences and differential management strategies of bile leaks at various centers. Early ERCP and stenting with any bile leakage is routine practice at some centers, whereas simple observation of the otherwise asymptomatic patient is the norm at others.

Irrespective of management most bile leaks are classified as Grade I, suggesting that simple external drainage through a Jackson Pratt or similar drain will be sufficient to avoid sepsis until the leak spontaneously resolves.[18,25] The source of leaks are typically the cut surface, though Ito et al reported that 10 of 26 leaks were confirmed to have their origin at the stump of the right hepatic stump, and no difference was found in the incidence of leaks with single biliary stumps verses multiple ducts.[18]

Strictures are reported less commonly than leaks, with an incidence under 5% but will more likely require invasive intervention for management.[13,15,18,25,29,30] Due to a paucity of long-term follow up data in liver donors, the risk of long-term biliary stricture is unknown. There may be some overlap between leaks and strictures, as stump leak may predispose to later stricture.[18] At least one right hepatic donor (unpublished data) is thought to have developed late biliary cirrhosis in the context of a postoperative stricture, which highlights the necessity of lifelong follow-up of donors.

## PULMONARY COMPLICATIONS

Pulmonary complications are common following upper abdominal surgery, especially in hepatic resection where there may be diaphragmatic dissection and elevation of the costal margins with mechanical retraction, resulting in splinting and atelectasis. Because donors are a carefully screened group, serious pulmonary complications are rare in live donor hepatic surgery. Aseptic atelectasis is the most common cause of early postoperative fever, which can progress to pneumonia requiring treatment in some cases. Right pleural effusion is almost always present following major hepatectomy, especially right hepatectomy, possibly related to diaphragmatic irritation. Drainage is not necessary in the majority of cases, but when significant (greater than 50% of the hemithorax), associated with respiratory embarrassment, or when associated with fever despite simple chest physiotherapy, placement of a pleural catheter is preferred.[13,18,25,27,29] In nonurgent situations, we have preferred percutaneous pigtail catheters for drainage of simple pleural effusions, though for complex effusions or in urgent conditions a chest tube is used.

Pulmonary embolism has been described in both left and right lobe donors and is a potential cause of significant morbidity and even mortality. Risk factors for pulmonary embolism are well known in the surgical literature and include obesity, smoking, and oral contraception. Because live donor transplantation is generally an elective procedure, interventions to reduce risk are possible prior to hepatectomy in potential donors with known risk factors. Intraoperative compression devices during general anesthesia are now standard of care in most hospitals. Some centers view any major hepatic resection as a high-risk procedure and utilize subcutaneous heparin in addition to venous compression devices. Subcutaneous heparin has not been shown to increase the risk of bleeding complications. Low-molecular-weight heparin is not superior to subcutaneous unfractionated heparin for prophlyaxis during surgery. Although many centers routinely perform preoperative screening for potential coagulation abnormalities like Factor V Leiden, antiphospholipid antibodies, and protein C and S levels, there is no evidence-based recommendations in the surgical literature to support routine screening in the absence of a prior history of clotting abnormality or thrombosis, other than standard prothrombin time-INR, partial thromboplastin time, and platelet count.

## WOUND COMPLICATIONS

Wound complications are among the most common events following hepatic resection and can be a significant sourced of disability even if they are generally not life threatening. Typical risk factors for wound complications are usually not present in live donors, who are excluded if they are diabetic, exhibit nutritional or systemic constitutional signs, or are taking steroids. Nevertheless, hernia is the most common reason for reoperation following live donor hepatectomy[25] so that even in a carefully screened population wound complications can occur and seem to occur more frequently in the presence of obesity (body mass index over 30), which is not an absolute exclusion for donation.[31] Potential donors who are dependent on physical activity for livelihood or those who are overweight should be counseled preoperatively about the possibility of prolonged recovery related to wound complications and the impact of such complications on return to work, and be encouraged to lose weight preoperatively. A single dose of preoperative antibiotic is supported by the evidence-based recommendations for infection prophylaxis in surgery, but routine additional doses of antibiotics have not been shown to reduce the rate of wound events in general surgery.

## UNKNOWN RISKS AND MORBIDITY

Numerous isolated events have been reported in the surgical literature and are potential sources of morbidity following donor hepatectomy. Although sporadic, some of these events can be significant, such as anaphylaxis or transfusion reactions. All donors should be counseled about known and unknown complications related to hospitalization, anesthesia, and abdominal surgery. Iatrogenic complications are an important cause of potential morbidity and are largely avoidable with carefully designed care systems. This requires broader attention to overall hospital infrastructure and administration, areas which may not be best managed by transplant surgeons in isolation.[4,5,28] However, the live donor team charged with protection of the donor's well-being (IDAT) is in an excellent position to audit the systems in place at the center, such as floor-based nursing protocols, education of staff in signs and symptoms, nursing ratios, anesthesia and monitoring practices, and medication ordering controls; and to partner with hospital administration in development of corrective plans before LDLT programs are even initiated. Ultimately a multidisciplinary proactive approach is the key to avoidance of donor morbidity.

## FINANCIAL AND PSYCHOSOCIAL MORBIDITY

Known or occult psychological illness such as depression and anxiety are risk factors for morbidity after donation. All donors are therefore evaluated by a psychiatrist, social worker, and financial counselor to assess the available level of support for the potential donor.[28,332,33] Most donors will underestimate the potential emotional and financial impact of donation. For donors of modest means, out-of-pocket expenses such as travel costs to the center, hotel stay if travel is from a long distance, parking, cost of prescription drugs, and unpaid leave from work are all significant potential factors in postoperative financial stress. More subtle effects of donation on well-being have yet to be studied. It is not clear at this point, for example, whether the act of donation will influence future insurability of the donor, especially if there is a complication. This is a greater issue in the United States, where there is no guarantee of universal health coverage, as compared to nations like Canada where donors will always have access to care irrespective of economic status. A recent survey of several insurance carriers in the United States suggested that there might well be a negative impact of donation on the access and/or cost of future insurance for the donor.[34]

Not all centers require active health insurance in potential donors, as the initial hospitalization costs are reimbursed through the recipient's insurance in the United States. However, the areas of greatest concern for donors are the complications requiring health resource utilization after discharge from the hospital. In these cases, it is not clear who has primary responsibility for payment of services: the recipient, the donor, or the transplant center. Most recipient insurance carriers will have specific policies for coverage of the donor, which are generally restricted to coverage of the hospitalization itself and possibly 90 days of perioperative coverage of treatment-related complications, though even this cannot be assumed, and there are generally no provisions for prescription medications. Donors with limited economic means may find it impossible to pay for prescriptions for even pain medication or acid suppression therapy upon discharge. Centers are generally unwilling to ask the donor or the donor insurance to be responsible for care related to the donation in the immediate postoperative period. Most centers will therefore provide perioperative services without charge for a specified period of time when the services are provided for complications of the donation at our center for up to 1 year. It is crucial for the center to have a clear written policy that is acceptable to hospital administration, and that the donor be educated about the center's policies regarding financial responsibility for postoperative care.

### Psychiatric Complications of LDLT

Psychiatric complications of LDLT have not been well studied, though it is our impression that they are a potentially serious and underreported risk of the procedure. The issues surrounding donation are superimposed on the enormously stressful scenario of a family coping with life-threatening illness. Nearly half of the donors in our series have required counseling in the year after donations. A smaller number have required medical therapy of depression. Trotter recently reported suicide in two patients as a late complication of donation in the 390 donors in the A2ALL series.[35] Two other patients died, one in a train accident and the other due to surgical complications. Eleven patients (2.8%) were reported as have experienced severe psychiatric complications. This important preliminary survey suggests that there is much work to be done in the assessment of psychiatric risk of living donation.

### Long-Term Morbidity

The lack of standardization for donor follow-up in the transplant community limits full accounting of long-term complications of living donation, and the current literature only superficially examines the true donor experience. The literature examining morbidity of hepatectomy for nontransplant indications is also sparse in describing long-term risks. Currently we cannot provide donors with accurate long-term assessments of risk, and there are likely subtle findings that will emerge with increased long-term scrutiny of donors undergoing hepatectomy. For example, at Columbia we have observed a 22% incidence of persistent thrombocytopenia.[25] A clearly operative factor was identified in

only one donor with thrombocytopenia; in the remaining four no technical complication could be identified, suggesting that right hepatectomy alone can result in this laboratory finding, the functional significance of which is not clear. Ongoing prospective studies such as the NIH-sponsored A2ALL study may better define the scope of long-term complications, but for know it is important to disclose to potential donors the possibility of unknown long-term complication

## RISK ASSESSMENT AND INTERVENTION TO REDUCE MORBIDITY

Although center-specific protocols for donor selection vary, the evaluation process is conducted for two main purposes: first, to assess the medical and psychosocial fitness of the donor to undergo donor hepatectomy, and second, to determine suitability of the proposed graft in restoring the health of the recipient. Because fitness and suitability are highly subjective terms that may change even within the center between different donor–recipient pairs, it is the responsibility of the evaluating team to educate the donor and his or her family and to incorporate them into the risk assessment/decision-making process even when they may be reluctant to absorb or acknowledge the information. For example, a father donating to a son may have a very different risk threshold than a cousin, and these varying thresholds should be included in the final calculation rather than rely on fixed criteria. Accurate assessment of risk is therefore crucial to both donor selection and disclosure. Allthough there are no quantitative risk scores that have been developed specifically for stratification of potential live donor/recipient pairs, most centers have developed algorithms that include the common absolute and relative risks. Absolute contraindications may include the presence of underlying liver disease, other end organ disease (renal, cardiac, pulmonary), transmissible infections, malignancy that is not considered cured, diabetes mellitus, and donor incapacity in comprehension and decision making. Relative contraindications include age, body mass index, and psychiatric history or personality disorders. (Table 29.5-4)

### Age

It is generally accepted that nonemancipated minors under the age of 18 are not candidates for donation because they are not able to freely consent to surgery. Some centers consider emancipated minors as candidates for their children who require transplantation, but not for adult-to-adult transplantation. Whether 18-year-olds have developed the maturity to consent to right hepatic donation is debatable; our center's minimum age of consent for adult-to-adult LDLT is 21.[28,33] Younger patients

**TABLE 29.5-4**

## DONOR FACTORS AFFECTING MORBIDITY

Age

BMS >30

Medical co-morbidities

Psychological co-morbidities

Hepatic mass

Liver anatomy

between the ages of 18 and 21 may be more susceptible to even subtle family coercion, especially when donating to a parent or younger sibling.

At the other end of the spectrum, older donors have been shown to have a higher peak aspartate aminotransferase (AST) and alanine aminotransferase (ALT) on the first postoperative day compared to younger donors. Donors over 50 years of age were found to have an elevated gamma-glutamyltranspeptidase (GGTP) for longer than 1 month, though the significance of this finding remains unclear.[18] Older age may also influence regeneration, and the functional reserve of the remnant liver after hepatectomy.[36] Although there is a perception that older age is associated with longer recovery after major abdominal surgery, there have been no data that implicate donor age as an independent factor in morbidity, likely due to the careful screening that excludes individuals with underlying risk factors for surgery. Many centers have arbitrarily established a relative (not absolute) center-specific upper age of 60 years because of the concern that the older donor may have more difficulty with functional rehabilitation and recovery after surgery, but final decisions are individualized.

## Body Mass Index

Obesity defined as a body mass index (BMI) >28[13] is prevalent in the United States. Obesity is associated with diabetes, hyperlipidemia, and hypertension, all of which increase surgical risk. Increased BMI is also associated with hepatic steatosis and its most pathogenic form, steatohepatitis.[33] Steatosis may reduce the functional hepatic mass of the graft, whereas steatohepatitis may have significant risk for postoperative remnant liver dysfunction, which was the etiology of donor death in one reported case.[8] Unrecognized steatosis may also increase the possibility of an aborted procedure if significant steatosis is found at the time of operation, especially if screening algorithms are not in place during the evaluation phase.[3] Although obesity without steatosis has not been associated with increased overall morbidity, there are specific complications that are more common in the obese population, mostly wound related. In addition, the obese patient poses an increased technical challenge for the donor surgeon and may therefore increase the operative time and risk of bleeding compared to nonobese individuals.[4,18,31,37]

The impact of steatosis in live donor graft function is uncertain, though significant steatosis (> 25%) has been associated with poor graft function in deceased donor liver transplantation in numerous reports. The mechanism of steatosis-associated injury is not clear but may involve an increase in postreperfusion oxygen-free radical injury arising from lipid peroxidation. The relatively short cold ischemia times in live donor liver transplantation may mitigate some of the reperfusion effects of steatosis, but Marcos and others have proposed that the functional hepatic mass is reduced by the proportion of liver cells replaced with macrosteatosis, so that in planning graft size for the purposes of estimating residual volume in the donor and graft to body weight in the recipient, the donor planning team needs to incorporate the degree of steatosis into the calculation.[38] The implication for the donor is that in general a preoperative biopsy will add considerable value in the evaluation of potential donors who have risk factors for steatosis or who have evidence of steatosis on imaging studies, and also serve to exclude steatohepatitis. Biopsy will help to quantify steatosis, which will aid in a proper formulation of risk for the donor in proceeding with hepatectomy. Although steatosis alone without inflamma-

tion has been associated with impairment in liver regeneration in animal models, no clinical studies have confirmed this observation. The practical debate, which remains unresolved, is the issue of whether every potential donor should undergo liver biopsy. This issue was debated extensively at the consensus conference on the liver donor in Vancouver. Some centers biopsy every donor candidate, whereas others (including our own) selectively biopsy those who have evidence of steatosis on serum tests or imaging studies.

Obesity is a relative but not absolute contraindication to donor hepatectomy in our center. Obese donors are required to initiate a weight loss program prior to final approval. Ultrasonography is performed for all donors with BMI > 30, with biopsy quantification of steatosis if the liver parenchyma exhibits sonographic echogenicity. The presence of abnormal liver enzymes and obesity also requires biopsy, irrespective of sonography, in order to exclude steatohepatitis. Steatohepatitis, unlike steatosis in the absence of inflammation, is a chronic liver disease that has been associated with progression to cirrhosis and hepatocellular carcinoma and is an absolute contraindication to donor hepatectomy at our center. This view is not necessarily shared by all worldwide centers performing LDLT: donor exclusion criteria must always be placed in the context of the availability of nonliving sources of organs. In Asian centers without access to deceased donor organs, for example, exclusion criteria for both donor and recipient LDLT are markedly different than in the west.[36]

## Medical and Psychological Factors

Because risk thresholds vary according to differences in worldwide access to donor organs, absolute criteria for medical contraindications in donor hepatectomy are impossible. Controlled mild to moderate hypertension may not be a reason for exclusion at some centers or for some donor/recipient pairs, but may be for others. Like other factors in assessment, the medical condition of the donor, family history, and asymptomatic findings on screening tests become part of a larger calculation. The assessment of cardiac risk for surgery is beyond the scope of this chapter; however, it is well established that cardiovascular or chronic pulmonary disease may increase perioperative surgical risk and these are therefore relative contraindications when[2] the disease is controlled and[3] the functional impairment would not preclude general anesthesia and elective hepatic resection. Significant impairment in ventricular function, symptomatic cardiovascular disease, or significant chronic obstructive pulmonary disease are all absolute contraindications to donor hepatectomy at Columbia. Because of the association between oral contraception, smoking, and venous thromboembolism, prospective donors are must discontinue both several weeks prior to surgery. Donors with risk factors for cardiovascular disease undergo cardiac stress screening and echocardiography.

## SUMMARY

Donor hepatectomy carries substantial risk that is managed by careful patient selection, meticulous operative technique, and highly attentive postoperative care. Experience of the team has been shown to be important in recipient outcomes,[39] and is likely to impact donor results. For this reason, UNOS has developed rigorous guidelines for team expertise which will be used to certify centers for LDLT.

Mortality and morbidity of right donor hepatectomy are approximately 0.2% and 45%, respectively, based on available information.[4] Mortality and morbidity of left lateral segmentectomy are approximately 0.1% and 40 %, respectivly.[9] Common causes of morbidity after donor hepatectomy are wound infection, ileus, bile leak, and pulmonary complications (atelectasis, effusion, and pneumonia). Causes of mortality have included liver failure, pulmonary thromboembolism, and cerebrovascular event, though details of the majority of donor deaths are lacking. There is lack of international standards in reporting, which limits the analysis of donor morbidity. The modified Clavien scale has been proposed as a standard mechanism for reporting after Liver donor hepatectomy. Long-term morbidity is even less well studied than perioperative morbidity, but it is clear that some donors may suffer long-lasting effects related to their surgery, both physical and psychosocial in nature.

Because of the importance of donor safety, and the devastating public consequences of donor harm, centers performing LDLT must have structured algorithms and support for live donor evaluation. In addition to surgical expertise, the organization of the postoperative care and the long-term follow-up must be rigorous and distinct from the posttransplant care team which is devoted to the recipients.

# References

1. Singer PA, Siegler M, Lantos JD, et al. CE: Ethics of liver transplantation with living donors. *N Engl J Med* 1989;321:620–621.
2. www.nih-a2all.org. Accessed May 27,2005.
3. Broering DC, Wilms C, Bok P, et al. Evolution of donor morbidity in living related liver transplantation: a single-center analysis of 165 cases. *Ann Surg* 2004;240(6):1013–1024.
4. Brown RS, Russo MW, Lai M, et al. A survey of liver transplantation from living adult donors in the United States. *N Engl J Med* 2003;348(9):818–825.
5. New York State Committee on Quality Improvement in Living Liver Donation. A report to New York State Transplant Council and New York State Department of Health. Available at: http://www.health.state.ny.us. Accessed April 21, 2004.
6. Najarian JS, Chavers BM, McHugh LE, et al. 20 years or more of follow-up of living kidney donors. *Lancet* 1992;340:807–810.
7. Wiederkehr JC, Pereira JC, Ekermann M, et al. Results of 132 Hepatectomies for Living Donor Liver Transplantation: Report of One Death. *Transplant Proc* 2005;37:1079–1080.
8. Akabbayashi A, Slingsby BT, Fujita M. The first donor death after living related liver transplantation in Japan. *Transplantation* 2004;77(4): 634–639.
9. Busuttil Ronald W, ed. *Transplantation of the Liver.* Elsevier Saunders, Chapter 47;
10. Clavien PA, Camargo CA Jr, Croxford R, et al. Definition and classification of negative outcomes in solid organ transplantation: application in liver transplantation. *Ann Surg* 1994;220:109–120.
11. Broelsch CE, Frilling A, Testa G, et al. Living donor liver transplantation in adults. *Eur J Gastroenterol Hepatol* 2003;15:3–6.
12. Salvalaggio PRO, Baker TB, Koffron AJ. Comparative analysis of live liver donation risk using a comprehensive grading system for severity. *Transplantation* 2004;77(11):1765–1767.
13. Beavers KL, Sandler RS, Shrestha R: Donor morbidity associated with right lobectomy for living donor liver transplantation to adult recipients: a systematic review. *Liver Transplant* 2003;8(2):110–117.
14. Umeshita K, Fujiwara K, Kiosawa K, et al. Operative Morbidity of Living Donors in Japan. *Lancet* 2003;362(9385):687–690.
15. Lo C. Complications and long-term outcomes of living liver donors: a survey 1508 cases in five Asians centers. *Transplantation* 2003;75:s12–s15.

16. Emond JC, Renz JF, Lim RC, et al. Functional characterization of liver grafts from living donors: implications for the treatment of older children and adults. *Ann Surg* 1996;224(4):544–552.
17. Fan ST, Lo, CM, Liu Chi- Leung et al: Safety of Donors in Live Donor Liver Transplantation Using Right Lobe Grafts. Arch Surg.135: 336–340, 2000.
18. Ito T, Kiuchi T, Egawa H, et al. Surgery-related morbidity in living donors of right-lobe liver grafts: lesions from the first 200 cases. *Transplantation* 2003;76(1):158–163.
19. Moon DB, Lee SG. Adult-to-adult living donor liver transplantation at the Asian Medical Center. Yonsei Med J 2004;45(6):1162–1168.
20. Olthoff KM, Merion RM, Ghobrial RM. A2ALL Study Group. Outcomes of 385 adult-to-adult living donor liver transplant recipients: a report from the A2ALL Consortium. Ann Surg. 2005;Sep;242(3): 314–323.
21. Kinkhabwala MM, Guarrera JV, Leno R, Brown RS, et al. Outflow reconstruction in right hepatic live donor liver transplantation. *Surgery* 2003;133(3):243–250.
22. Shah SA, Grant DR, Greig PD, et al. Analysis and outcome of right lobe hepatectomy in 101 consecutive living donors. *Am J Transplant* 2005;5:2764–2769.
23. LaPointe Rudow D, Charlton M, Sanchez C, et al. Kidney and liver living donors: a comparison of experiences. *Progr Transplant* 2005;15(2): 185–191.
24. Russo MW, LaPointe Rudow D, Teixeira A, et al: Interpretation of Liver Chemistries in Adult Donors after Living Donor Liver Transplantation. *J Clin Gastroenterol* 2004;38(9): 810–814.
25. LaPointe Rudow D, Brown RS, Emond JC, et al: One- Year morbidity after donor right hepatectomy. *Liver Transplant* 2004;10(11): 1428–1431.
26. Kiuchi T, Tanaka K. Liver transplantation from living donors: current status in Japan and safety/ long term results in the donor. *Transplant Proc* 2003;35:1172–1173.
27. Pomfret EA, Pomposelli JJ, Gordon FD, et al. Liver regeneration and surgical outcome in donors of right-lobe liver grafts. *Transplantation* 2003;76 (1):5–10.
28. LaPointe Rudow D, Brown RS, JR. Evaluation of living liver donors. *Progr Transplant* 2003;13(2):110–116.
29. Shiffman ML, Brown RS, Olthoff KM, et l: Living donor liver transplantation: summary of a conference at the national institutes of health. *Liver Transplant* 2002;8:174–188.
30. Renz JF, Roberts JP. Long term complications of living donor liver transplantation. *Liver Transplant* 2000;6(2):s73–s76.
31. Moss, LaPointe Rudow D, Renz JF, et al. Select Utilization of Obese Donors in Living Donor Liver Transplantation: Implications for the Donor Pool. *Am J Transplant* 2005;5:2974–2981.
32. Kita Y, Fukunishi I, Harihara M, et al. Psychiatric disorders in living related liver transplantation. *Transplant Proc* 2001;33:1350–1352.
33. Troter JF. Selection of donors for living donor liver transplantation. *Liver Transplant* 2003;9(10,2):S2–S7.
34. Nissing MH, Hayashi PH. Right Hepatic Lobe Donation Adversely Affects Donor Life Insurability Up to One Year After Donation. *Liver Transplant* 2005;11(7):843–847.
35. Trotter JF, Hill-Callahan M, Gillespie BW, et al. Deaths due to psychiatric complications in right hepatic lobe donors for adult to adult living donor liver transplantation. *Hepatology* 2005;42:suppl 1:451A.
36. Makuuchi M, Miller CM, Olthoff K, et al. Adult-adult living donor liver transplantation. *J Gastrointest Surg* 2004;8(3):303–312.
37. Allison DB, Saunders SE. Obesity in North America. *Med Clin North Am* 2000;84:305–332.
38. Marcos A, Fisher R, Ham JM, et al. Selection and outcome of living donors for adult to adult right lobe transplantation. *Transplantation* 2000;69(11):2410–2415.
39. Olthoff KM, Merion RM, Ghobrial RM, et al. A2ALL Study Group. Outcomes of 385 adult-to-adult living donor liver transplant recipients: a report from the A2ALL Consortium. *Ann Surg* 2005;Sep; 242(3): 314–23.

# 29.6   LONG-TERM DONOR OUTCOMES

*James F. Trotter, MD, Jeff Campsen, MD, Igal Kam, MD*

## LDLT LONG-TERM DONOR OUTCOME

In the United States, adult-to-adult right hepatic lobe living donor liver transplantation (LDLT) became popularized as a therapy for selected patients with end-stage liver disease in the late 1990s. The number of cases peaked in 2001 at 512 operations or about 10% of all liver transplantations.[1] Thereafter, the volume of LDLTs has declined to about 350 cases per year, which is due in part to concerns over donor outcomes and safety. In fact, the long-term outcome of living liver donors is one of the most important factors limiting the widespread application of this procedure in the United States. This chapter describes the medical, surgical, and psychological outcomes in right hepatic lobe donors following the donor surgery. Almost all of the findings are related to right hepatic lobe donation (unless otherwise specified) because this is the most commonly utilized lobe for this procedure. It is important to recognize the limitations of the current data. There are no large, controlled studies with sufficient follow-up to provide an accurate assessment of donor complications. The current data are based on either single-center reports or survey data. The single-center reports have the advantage of complete data collection on donor complications, but include small numbers of patients. As a result, uncommon complications may be missed or underappreciated. In addition, the findings in these reports may be skewed by the "learning curve" which is characterized by a higher incidence of complications early in the center experience. Surveys of LDLT centers include more patients, but have the disadvantages of retrospective data collection, absence of consensus definitions of complications between centers, and in some cases inadequate donor follow-up.

## SURGICAL COMPLICATIONS

### Mortality

The most important outcome for donors is survival. Currently, the exact risk of death following a right hepatic lobe donor surgery is not known, because throughout the world the precise number of donor deaths after living liver donation is unknown. Therefore, estimates of donor mortality are derived from single-center reports and surveys of LDLT centers. Table 29.6-1 shows the total worldwide number of living liver donor deaths that can be documented through published references, through which we were able to confirm 13 living liver donor deaths. Two of these deaths occurred long after the donor surgery and are likely to be unrelated to complications of surgery. The Western experience with the longest follow-up is derived from the National Institutes of Health (NIH) Adult-to-Adult Living Donor Liver Transplantation Study (A2ALL) which includes all LDLT cases from nine participating U.S. centers and comprises 390 donors.[2] In this cohort, there have been 4 donor deaths: one from surgical complications, 1 from self-inflicted gunshot wound, 1 from drug overdose, and 1 from an occupational train versus pedestrian accident. The results of this study are strengthened by independent verification of each patient's status (dead vs alive) through the Social Security Death Index. A survey report of all U.S. centers included 449 donors and reported only 1 donor death.[3] Because this study did not have independent verification of donor status, the risk of donor death may have been underestimated. A large Asian experience was published by Lo, representing 1508 cases five Asian centers where 561 right lobes or right lateral segments grafts were removed.[4] There were no perioperative deaths reported, although 1 donor died 3 years after surgery of unknown causes. However, long-term follow-up (> 3 months) was available in only 15% of donors leading to the possibility of underreporting donor deaths. Umeshita et al reported outcomes in 1853 donors from Japan including 443 right hepatic lobes.[5] (Two of the centers in the Lo paper also contributed cases to the Umeshita report.) There were no deaths reported in the 1853 donor operations. However, after publication of this report, the first donor death in Japan was published and reportedly caused by progressive liver failure.[6] The European Liver Transplant Registry has reported outcomes in 806 living liver donors with over half donating to pediatric recipients at 46 centers between 1991 and 2001.[7] Four deaths were registered due to the following causes: cardiac failure (1 patient), sepsis (2 patients) and pulmonary embolus (1 patient). Additional deaths have been reported, as noted in Table 29.6-1.[8–10] In summary, the U.S. experience reflects a risk of approximately 1 operative death in 390 cases (0.25 %) (and 3 other deaths whose attribution to the surgical procedure is unknown). In Asia there has been 1 death in approximately

**TABLE 29.6-1**

## LIVING LIVER DONOR DEATHS REPORTED IN THE MEDICAL LITERATURE

| Author | Year | n | Location | Cause |
|---|---|---|---|---|
| Trotter[2] | 2005 | 4 | United States | Drug overdose/suicide – 2, operative – 1, Other – 1 |
| Lo[4] | 2003 | 1 | Asia | Unknown, 3 y post-op |
| Akabayashi[6] | 2004 | 1 | Japan | Liver failure |
| Adam[7] | 2003 | 4 | Europe | Sepsis – 2, cardiopulmonary – 2 |
| Miller[8] | 2002 | 1 | New York | Sepsis |
| Wiederkehr[9] | 2005 | 1 | Brazil | Intracerebral hemorrhage |
| Soin[10] | 2003 | 1 | India | Unknown |

500 right hepatic lobe donor operations (0.2%; and an additional death whose attribution to surgery is unknown), and in Europe there have been 4 deaths out of 806 operations (0.5%). It is very likely that there have been other donor deaths that have occurred worldwide that have yet to be reported in the medical literature.

## Nonfatal Surgical Complications

There are several large series reporting the spectrum and incidence of donor complications. The results from these studies are summarized in Table 29.6-2. The largest is by Umeshita et al, which reports outcomes of donors for 1852 LDLTs with 1853 donors who were registered in the database of the Japanese Liver Transplantation Society, including 463 right hepatic lobe donors. Donors were identified in the database, and questionnaires were then retrospectively sent to the respective transplant centers regarding donor complications. This survey reported no donor deaths (although, as noted above, 1 death has been reported subsequently in Japan). Two hundred twenty-eight donors (12%) experienced 244 complications, the most common of which was a biliary leak (4%) followed by gastric stasis (2%) and infection (1%). Reoperation was reported in 1% of donors. Compared to left hepatic lobe (or one of its segments) donors, right lobe donors experienced significantly more biliary leaks and longer duration of hospitalization. Although this study included a large number of patients, limitations in the data include retrospective data collection, absence of clear definitions of complications, and absence of outside verification of complications, all of which could lead to underreporting of complications. Brown et al reported the largest U.S. experience in a retrospective survey study of donor complications at 84 U.S. LDLT centers, which included 449 donors.[3] The survey was conducted by sending questionnaires to 122 U.S. LDLT programs of which 84 (69%) returned the survey. Sixty-five of the 449 donors (14.5%) had one or more complications and one patient (0.2%) died. Biliary leak was the most common complications (6%), followed by nonautologous blood transfusion (4.9%) and reoperation (4.3%). Although this report acquired data retrospectively, the outcomes at eight centers performing 147 LDLTs were audited, and no discrepancies in data reporting were noted. Although this study represents a large experience, 31% of the U.S. LDLT centers did not respond to the survey and therefore did not contribute data, which could lead to underestimating actual complications. Another large report was published by Lo describing donor complications from 1508 LDLTs from the Asian experience (Taiwan, Hong Kong, Seoul, Tokyo, and Kyoto).[4] Some of these cases were reported in the combined Japanese experienced described above.[5] Five hundred and sixty-one of the LDLTs utilized a right hepatic lobe graft. The reported complication rate was 15.8% or 238 patients. The most commonly reported problem was bile leak (75 patients), wound infection (45 patients), and hyperbilirubinemia (43 patients). The complication rate in right hepatic lobe donors (28 %) was higher than that in the left lobe (7.5%) or left lateral segment (9%). In addition, 5 patients had chronic biliary problems and 1 patient developed renal failure from the nephrotoxic effects of contrast dye. Of note, only 15% of the donors had follow-up beyond 3 months which could lead to underreporting of long-term complications. The findings in a large number of single-center reports largely reflect the data from the survey publications noted above.[11-29] However, in general, the reported incidence of complications is slightly higher in the single-center reports which may reflect a bias toward underreporting complications in the large survey studies. Based on all of these studies we can conclude the following about surgical donor complications: first, the risk of death is small and probably about 1 in 300. Second, the nonfatal complication rate is about 15% in each of the large survey series. Third, the most commonly reported donor complication is postoperative biliary leak. Finally, the currently reported estimates of donor complications are likely to be lower than the actual risk due to the inherent problems of retrospective data collection in large survey studies.

The most effective means of preventing postoperative complications is careful surgical technique and the appropriate selection of patients. From a technical standpoint, the most important test in this evaluation is cross-sectional imaging to define the hepatic parenchymal, vascular, and biliary anatomy. The specific type of cross-sectional imaging utilized varies from center to center depending on local preference and expertise. However, all donors must have either a computed tomographic (CT) or magnetic resonance abdominal imaging study. A review of the

**TABLE 29.6–2**
## DONOR COMPLICATIONS

| Author | Year | n | n right lobe donors | Complications |
|--------|------|---|---------------------|---------------|
| Umeshita | 2003 | 1853 | 463 | 12.5%<br>Biliary leak 4%<br>Gastric stasis 2%<br>Infection 1%<br>Reoperation 1% |
| Brown | 2003 | 449 | 449 | 14.5%<br>Biliary leak 6%<br>Blood transfusion 5%<br>Reoperation 4% |
| Lo | 2003 | 1508 | 561 | 15.8%<br>Biliary leak 5%<br>Wound infection 3%<br>Hyperbilirubinemia 3% |

experience at our center demonstrated that biliary abnormalities discovered during cross-sectional imaging are an uncommon indication for rejection of a potential donor. Cross-sectional imaging also allows identification of the donor's vascular anatomy, which is important in planning the operative dissection. At our center, the intraoperative cholangiogram can be correlated with the findings of cross-sectional imaging and provides an important guide for the operation. Finally, if the surgeon identifies unexpected anatomical variations that could compromise donor safety, then he or she should consider termination of the donor operation. One of the most important considerations is to preserve the anatomy of the donor's remnant left lobe. The donor's left hepatic lobe should never be invaded during the right lobectomy.

Following the removal of the right hepatic donor lobe, the remnant liver undergoes intense regeneration. However, several studies have documented that hepatic regeneration is incomplete in living donors. Three months after donor hepatectomy, Humar et al. found that the remnant liver regenerated to only 78% of the ideal liver volume.[30] Hata et al. reported restoration to only 75% to 80% of preoperative liver volume in right hepatic lobe donors 3 months after surgery. In another similar study, the remnant liver increased to 87% of preoperative volume by 1month in 30 male right hepatic lobe donors.[14] Although standard liver function tests normalize in almost all right hepatic lobe donors shortly after surgery, there are very little data on quantitative liver function. Nadalin et al. performed serial hepatic volumetric measurements and galactose elimination capacity (GEC) in 27 right hepatic lobe donors preoperatively and then at days 10, 90, 180, and 360 postoperatively.[32] They showed regeneration of the remnant hepatic lobe to 83% of preoperative volume 1 year after surgery. Quantitative liver function, as measured by GEC, decreased to 57% of preoperative values by postoperative day 10 and then increased to 87%, 93%, and 97% of baseline by days 90, 180, and 360, respectively. Measurements of GEC per volume of liver showed a reduction to 75% of baseline at day 10 and subsequently increases to 115%, 124%, and 100% of baseline by days 90, 180 and 360, respectively. Serum cholinesterase values largely mirrored those of GEC. In summary, most studies shows that following the right donor hepatectomy that the donor's remnant left lobe regenerates to a mean volume of approximately 80% of total hepatic preoperative volume. Although quantitative liver function data are limited in right hepatic lobe donors, there does not appear to be a significant reduction in hepatic function as measured by standard liver function tests, GEC, and cholinesterase. Whether incomplete hepatic regeneration has any impact on donor health is unknown, because the follow-up intervals in the published studies are relatively short and the number of donors is small. Further studies will focus on subsequent changes in liver volume and function over time as well as differences in hepatic regeneration based on specific patient characteristics (size of donor graft, donor age, donor gender, and preoperative quantitative liver function).

## MEDICAL COMPLICATIONS

The most serious complications following donor surgery are surgical problems. However, there are numerous medical complications that have been reported following the right hepatic lobe donor operation. Many of these are common complications of a major abdominal surgery including (but not limited to): neuropraxia, ileus, urinary infection, pressure sores, pleural effusion, pneumonia, atelectasis, and pneumothorax. Several complications have been somewhat unexpected and deserve special consideration. Although hypophosphatemia has been previously noted following major hepatic resection in patients with hepatic tumors, there are conflicting data regarding hypophosphatemia in right hepatic lobe donors for LDLT.[33,34] The cause of hypophosphatemia after hepatectomy is not clear. The presumed mechanism is that intracellular phosphorous requirements are increased with the creation of new hepatocytes during hepatic regeneration. However, recent data suggest that renal excretion of phosphorous may be the most important factor.[35] Pomposelli et al first described "life-threatening hypophosphatemia" in 70% of donors in whom serum phosphorous levels dropped below 1.0 mg/dL in the immediate postoperative period.[36] Of note, all of the donors received total parenteral nutrition (TPN) which may have contributed to the low phosphorous levels. With increased phosphorous repletion in the TPN solution the incidence of severe hypophosphatemia (< 1.0 mg/dL) was reduced to only 8% of patients. Tan et al analyzed phosphorous levels in 95 right hepatic lobe donors and reported that none of these patients had phosphorous levels below 1.3 mg/dL.[37] None of these patients received TPN, which suggests that TPN itself may have contributed to the hypophosphatemia noted in the Pomposelli study. Finally, Burak et al reported hypophosphatemia (< 1.0 mg/dL) in 2 of 9 living donors during the first postoperative week and hypophosphatemia in 56% of all donors, none of whom received TPN.[38] In summary, hypophosphatemia has been reported in some but not all reports. There is currently no evidence that hypophosphatemia has any detrimental effect on the donor, but physicians should be aware of this potential problem. At our center, we have never recognized a clinical problem related to hypophosphatemia in over 100 LDLT cases.

Several centers have reported changes in liver function tests in living hepatic lobe donors. In the immediate perioperative period virtually all donors have transient increases in aspartate aminotransferase (AST), alanine aminotransferase (ALT), alkaline phosphatase (AP), total bilirubin (TB), and international normalized ratio (INR). These values return to normal or near-normal after 7 to 10 days.[25,27,39–41] However, there are very little long–term data recording changes in liver function tests in living liver donors, perhaps because less than 40% of LDLT centers mandate laboratory tests in their donors at 6 and 12 months.[42] One recent study reported long-term follow-up of liver function tests in 22 of 70 right hepatic lobe donors and found that 97% had normal values.[43]

Thrombocytopenia may occur in a small fraction of living liver donors. The platelet count drops in most donors in the immediate postoperative period.[11,44] Rudow et al. found that at 1 year after donor surgery, 5 of 22 donors (23%) had thrombocytopenia and 1 donor was found to have an asymptomatic portal vein thrombosis.[45] The cause of thrombocytopenia in liver donors may be due to postoperative splenomegaly in the donor, because the spleen has been shown to increase in size by 34% within 10 days of surgery.[46] The cause of the splenomegaly is not known, but could be due to a slight increase in portal pressure following the right hepatectomy. The long-term problems related to thrombocytopenia, if any, are unknown, because there is no long-term follow-up of a sufficient number of living donors to make this determination.

Deep venous thrombosis (DVT) and pulmonary embolus (PE) are a special concern, because the consequences can be devastating. Numerous donors have developed DVT and/or PE[5,28–30] and at least one donor has died as a result of this complication.[46]

As a result, most LDLT centers will reject potential donors with a history of deep venous thrombosis, hypercoaguable state or prior pulmonary embolus. In addition, most centers exclude patients with risk factors for DVT such as obesity and ongoing oral contraceptive use. Other centers utilize a comprehensive coagulation evaluation in all donor candidates, that is, protein C, protein S, antithrombin III, etc.[46] However, at our center, we have found that virtually all patients will have one or more minor abnormalities in these comprehensive coagulation screens (either in absolute level or in function). The risk of thrombosis attributed to these minor abnormalities has been, in our experience, sufficiently unclear that we no longer obtain these tests in our donor evaluation. In summary, screening donor candidates for hypercoaguable states varies from center to center, because the utility of these tests in this special population is unclear.

The most comprehensive picture of donor complications will include a record of problems attributed to invasive procedures (liver biopsy, endoscopic retrograde cholangiography, and angiogram) or diagnostic imaging tests (allergic reaction or renal dysfunction from intravenous contrast dye) performed during the evaluation process. It is important to remember that these complications may occur in some donor candidates who are rejected for donation. The most commonly utilized test during the donor evaluation with the greatest risk is the liver biopsy. Centers, which perform a mandatory liver biopsy on all donor candidates, may have a higher rate of complications in their donor candidates. Future studies will need to assess the risk and benefit of each test used in the donor evaluation to determine the most appropriate donor evaluation process.

## PSYCHOLOGICAL COMPLICATIONS

Psychological outcomes are important to assess in living liver donors. All of the data in this area are derived from single-center reports, almost all of which are from retrospective data collection. At our center, we reported results in 65 of 75 surveyed LDLT donors with a mean/median postdonation follow-up interval of 3.0 and 2.8 years, respectively. The donation experience was positive for almost all donors: 83% described a complete recovery, mean time to return to work was 2.5 months, 87% felt that they had benefited from the donation, and 95% would donate again. There were three categories of negative findings: 48% reported abdominal discomfort/scar numbness, gastrointestinal symptoms were present in 26% (dyspepsia 15% and diarrhea 11%) and 31% had self-reported depression. SF-36 surveys were completed before and after surgery in one third of donors. Compared to preoperative results, we found that postoperative scores were significantly lower in seven of eight domains. However, compared to the general population, SF-36 scores were the same or higher in all domains before and after surgery. Other centers have reported similar findings. Karliova et al reported outcomes in 24 right hepatic lobe donors who donated to 3 pediatric and 21 adult recipients.[47] The response rate to the quality-of-life survey was 22/24 (92%), and the mean follow-up interval was 10.4 months. Ninety-one percent would donate again if given the opportunity. The mean time to return to work was 9 weeks and one half reported "adverse financial affects" of the donation. The donors scored higher on the SF-36 "general health" axis compared to the normative population. The group from Mt. Sinai published their findings in 48 donors (of either right or left hepatic lobe) for adult recipients.[48] The donor response rate for the survey was 30/48 (63%) at a mean follow-up interval of 280 days. Fifty-seven percent reported on-

going "medical symptoms," although 83% reported that they felt that the donation had not negatively impacted their health. The mean time to return to work was 8.8 weeks. Fifty-three percent reported postoperative pain that was greater than expected. One donor (2%) reported that the donation was a "severe financial burden" and 9 (30%) felt the donation was a "moderate financial burden." The donors scored higher than the general population in seven of the eight domains of the SF-36. Beavers et al reported findings in 27 donors of either a right or left hepatic lobe.[21] All donors (100%) completed the donor survey, although 3 donors were excluded (2 patients with aborted donations and 1 donor death). Mean follow-up interval was 20 months. Thirty-three percent reported experiencing more pain than expected and 80% returned to their previous level of physical and social activity. Ninety-two percent returned to their predonation employment. There was no difference in the mean SF-12 scores for the donors compared to the general U.S. population. Complete recovery time for the right hepatic lobe donors was 18 weeks, and 100% would donate again. In summary, the reported psychological outcomes have been favorable. The vast majority of donors have been pleased with their decision to donate and have returned to their predonation job in a relatively short interval following surgery.

The inherent problems with the single-center reports on psychological outcomes include, incomplete donor participation, short follow-up intervals, and reporting bias toward favorable outcomes on the part of the patients and physicians. A complete understanding of the psychological complications in living donors awaits studies, which will include comprehensive, prospective preoperative, and postoperative analysis with comparisons to donor control subjects. These studies will likely report less favorable results than the retrospective studies noted above. In fact, a preliminary report from the retrospective portion of the NIH A2ALL study found that severe psychiatric reactions were reported in some donors including suicide and a fatal drug overdose. These results may have been unexpected by some physicians given the generally favorable reports from the retrospective single-center studies.

## SUMMARY

We have summarized the long-term complications in living liver donors. However, as noted above, the current data are inadequate to provide an accurate description of the incidence and spectrum of postoperative problems. Two recent efforts will help to rectify this situation. The United Network for Organ Sharing (UNOS) has initiated a nationwide reporting system for all living liver donors who are taken to the operating room for the purpose of donation. Over time, this dataset will likely provide the most complete appraisal of donor mortality because a large number of donors will be tracked, and follow-up through use of the Social Security Death Index will likely provide a definitive assessment regarding short-term and long-term donor mortality. However, this database will not likely be able to track other donor complications due to the inherent problems of a large multicenter database (limited donor follow-up and absence of clear definitions of complications from center to center). The National Institutes of Health Living Donor Cohort Study (A2ALL) has begun prospective enrollment of all living donors (and recipients) at nine U.S centers and will prospectively follow donors (and recipients) for at least 4 years relative to complications. This cohort will have the distinct advantages of (1) comparing outcomes to donor controls (patients evaluated for donation, but rejected for nonmedical indications), (2) clear definitions of donor complications, and (3) comprehensive reporting of donor complications by dedicated research coordinators whose primary job is to prospectively track donor and recipient outcomes. The A2ALL dataset will likely provide the most comprehensive information about the long-term outcomes of living liver donors.

## References

1. Trotter JF, Wachs M, Everson GT, Kam I. Adult-to-adult right hepatic lobe living donor liver transplantation. Medical Progress Review. *New Engl J Med* 2002;346:1074–1082.

2. Trotter JF, Hill-Callahan MM, Gillespie BW and the A2ALL Study Group. Severe psychiatric problems in right hepatic lobe donors for living donor liver transplantation. *Transplantation* 2007; 83: 1506–1508.

3. Brown RS Jr, Russo MW, Lai M, et al. A survey of liver transplantation from living adult donors in the United States. *N Engl J Med* 2003; 348:818–825.

4. Lo CM. Complications and long-term outcome of living liver donors: a survey of 1,508 cases in five Asian centers. *Transplantation* 2003;75: S12–S15.

5. Umeshita K, Fujiwara K, Kiyosawa K, et al. Operative morbidity of living liver donors in Japan. *Lancet* 2003;30;362:687–690.

6. Akabayashi A, Slingsby BT, Fujita M. The first donor death after living-related liver transplantation in Japan. *Transplantation* 2004; 77(4):634.

7. Adam R, McMaster P, O'Grady JG, et al. Evolution of liver transplantation in Europe: report of the European Liver Transplant Registry. *Liver Transplant* 2003;9:1231–1243.

8. Miller C, Florman S, Kim-Schluger L, et al. Fulminant and fatal gas gangrene of the stomach in a healthy live liver donor. *Liver Transplant* 2003;9:1231–1243.

9. Wiederkehr JC, Pereira JC, Ekermann M, et al. Results of 132 hepatectomies for living donor liver transplantation: report of one death. *Transplant Proc* 2005;37(2):1079–1080.

10. Soin AS. Ethical dilemmas in living donor liver transplantation. *Ind J Med Ethics* 2003;11(4).

11. Liu CL, Fan ST, Lo CM, et al. Safety of donor right hepatectomy without abdominal drainage: a prospective evaluation in 100 consecutive liver donors. *Liver Transplant* 2005;11:314–319.

12. Broering DC, Wilms C. Bok P. et al. Evolution of donor morbidity in living related liver transplantation: a single-center analysis of 165 cases. *Ann Surg* 2004;240:1013–1026.

13. Rudow DL, Brown RS Jr, Emond JC, et al. One-year morbidity after donor right hepatectomy. *Liver Transplant* 2004;10:1428–1431.

14. Kwon KH, Kim YW, Kim SI, et al. Postoperative liver regeneration and complication in live liver donor after partial hepatectomy for living donor liver transplantation. *Yonsei Med J* 2003;Dec 30;44(6): 1069–1077.

15. Pomfret EA. Early and late complications in the right-lobe adult living donor. *Liver Transplant* 2003;9:S45–S49.

16. Ito T, Kiuchi T, Egawa H, et al. Surgery-related morbidity in living donors of right-lobe liver graft: lessons from the first 200 cases. *Transplantation* 2003;76:158–163.

17. Chisuwa H, Hashikura Y, Mita A, et al. Living liver donation: preoperative assessment, anatomic considerations, and long-term outcome. *Transplantation* 2003;75:1670–1676.

18. Shoji M, Ohkohchi N, Fujimori K, et al. The safety of the donor operation in living-donor liver transplantation: an analysis of 45 donors. *Transpl Int* 2003;16:461–464.

19. Ghobrial RM, Saab S, Lassman C, et al Donor and recipient outcomes in right lobe adult living donor liver transplantation. *Liver Transpl* 2002;8:901–909.

20. Pascher A, Sauer IM, Walter M, et al. Donor evaluation, donor risks, donor outcome, and donor quality of life in adult-to-adult living donor liver transplantation. *Liver Transplant* 2002;8:829–837.

21. Beavers KL, Sandler RS, Shrestha R. Donor morbidity associated with right lobectomy for living donor liver transplantation to adult recipients: a systematic review. *Liver Transplant* 2002;8:110–117.

22. Sugawara Y, Makuuchi M, Takayama T, et al. Safe donor hepatectomy for living related liver transplantation. *Liver Transplant* 2002;8:58–62.

23. Beavers KL, Sandler RS, Fair JH, Johnson MW, Shrestha R. The living donor experience: donor health assessment and outcomes after living donor liver transplantation. *Liver Transplant* 2001;7:943–947.

24. Miller CM, Gondolesi GE, Florman S, et al. One hundred nine living donor liver transplants in adults and children: a single-center experience. *Ann Surg* 2001;234:301–312.

25. Bak T, Wachs M, Trotter J, et al. Adult-to-adult living donor liver transplantation using right-lobe grafts: results and lessons learned from a single-center experience. *Liver Transplant* 2001;7:680–686.

26. Pomfret EA, Pomposelli JJ, Lewis WD, et al. Live donor adult liver transplantation using right lobe grafts: donor evaluation and surgical outcome. *Arch Surg* 2001;136:425–433.

27. Marcos A, Fisher RA, Ham JM, et al. Selection and outcome of living donors for adult to adult right lobe transplantation. *Transplantation* 2000;69:2410–2415.

28. Malago M, Testa G, Frilling A, et al. Right living donor liver transplantation: an option for adult patients. *Ann Surg* 2003;238:853–863.

29. Broering DC, Wilms C, Bok P, et al. Evolution of donor morbidity in living related liver transplantation. *Ann Surg* 2004;240:1013–1026.

30. Humar A, Kosari K, Sielaff TD, et al. Liver regeneration after adult living donor and deceased donor split-liver transplants. *Liver Transplant* 2004;Mar;10(3):374–378.

31. Hata S, Sugawara Y, Kishi Y, et al. Volume regeneration after right liver donation. *Liver Transplant* 2004;10:65–70.

32. Nadalin S, Testa G, Malago M, et al. Volumetric and functional recovery of the liver after right hepatectomy for living donation. *Liver Transplant* 2004;10:1024–1029.

33. George R, Shiu MH. Hypophosphatemia after major hepatic resection. *Surgery* 1992;111:281–286.

34. Buell JF, Berger AC, Plotkin JS, Kuo PC, Johnson LB. The clinical implications of hypophosphatemia following major hepatic resection or cryosurgery. *Arch Surg* 1998;133:757–761.

35. Salem RR, Tray K. Hepatic resection-related hypophosphatemia is of renal origin as manifested by isolated hyperphosphaturia. *Ann Surg* 2005;241:343–348.

36. Pomposelli JJ, Pomfret EA, Burns DL, Lally A, Sorcini A, Gordon FD, Lewis WD, Jenkins R. Life-threatening hypophosphatemia after right hepatic lobectomy for live donor adult liver transplantation. *Liver Transplant* 2001;7:637–642.

37. Tan HP, Madeb R, Kovach SJ, et al. Hypophosphatemia after 95 right-lobe living-donor hepatectomies for liver transplantation is not a significant source of morbidity. *Transplantation* 2003;76: 1085–1088.

38. Burak KW, Rosen CB, Fidler JL, et al. Hypophosphatemia after right hepatectomy for living donor liver transplantation. *Can J Gastroenterol* 2004;18:729–733.

39. Marcos A, Fisher RA, Ham JM, et al. Liver regeneration and function in donor and recipient after right lobe adult to adult living donor liver transplantation. *Transplantation* 2000;69:1375–1379.

40. Russo MW, LaPointe-Rudow D, Teixeira A, et al. Interpretation of liver chemistries in adult donors after living donor liver transplantation. *J Clin Gastroenterol* 2004 Oct;38(9):810–814.

41. Pszenny C, Krawczyk M, Paluszkiewicz R, et al. Biochemical function of the donor liver in living related liver transplantation. *Transplant Proc* 2002;34:621–622.

42. Beavers KL, Cassara JE, Shrestha R. Practice patterns for long-term follow-up of adult-to-adult right lobectomy donors at US transplantation centers. *Liver Transplant* 2003;9:645–648.

43. Rudow DL, Brown RS Jr, Emond JC, et al. One-year morbidity after donor right hepatectomy. *Liver Transplant* 2004;10:1428–1431.

44. Siniscalchi A, Begliomini B, De Pietri L, et al. Increased prothrombin time and platelet counts in living donor right hepatectomy: implications for epidural anesthesia. *Liver Transplant* 2004;10:1144–1149.

45. Kamel IR, Erbay N, Warmbrand G, et al. Liver regeneration after living adult right lobe transplantation. *Abdom Imag* 2003;28:53–57.

46. Durand F, Ettorre GM, Douard R, et al. Donor safety in living related liver transplantation: underestimation of the risks for deep vein thrombosis and pulmonary embolism. *Liver Transplant* 2002;8:118–120.

47. Karliova M, Malago M, Valentin-Gamazo C, et al. Living-related liver transplantation from the view of the donor: a 1-year follow-up survey. *Transplantation* 2002;73:1799–1804.

48. Kim-Schluger L, Florman SS, Schiano T, et al. Quality of life after lobectomy for adult liver transplantation. *Transplantation* 2002;73: 1593–1597.

# 29.7 PSYCHOLOGICAL ASPECTS

*Roshan Shrestha, MD*

Since the first successful living donor liver transplant in a pediatric patient in 1988, this procedure has been considered the standard of care for children with end-stage liver disease (ESLD).[1] Since 1993, this procedure has been expanded to adult recipients. Thanks to its early success and the continued critical shortage of deceased donor (DD) livers, many transplant centers around the world are now using this procedure to prevent death while transplant candidates wait on the list. More than 50% of the transplant centers in the United States are either already performing or soon will be performing adult-to-adult living donor (LD) liver transplants.[2]

## PSYCHOLOGICAL ASSESSMENT OF RECIPIENTS

Almost all liver transplant candidates undergo routine psychological assessment as part of their comprehensive evaluation to determine their candidacy for a DD liver transplant. Most transplant centers would not consider anyone for a LD transplant if not (already) approved for a DD transplant. LD transplant candidates must be fully aware of potential complications for their donors as well as for themselves given the unique nature of the donor surgery and the implantation of only a partial graft into recipients. It is critical to ensure that LD transplant candidates are psychologically prepared to proceed. In our center, a formal family meeting with the prospective donor and recipient, their immediate family members, and the transplant team is routine in order to outline all aspects of the actual surgery beforehand.

## PSYCHOLOGICAL ASSESSMENT OF PROSPECTIVE DONORS

Prospective LDs—for both pediatric and adult recipients—must be in excellent medical and psychological condition. The most important goals of their evaluation are as follows (1) to evaluate their psychological, emotional, and social stability; (2) to establish their competency to give informed consent; and (3) to confirm that their decision to donate is entirely voluntary and free of undue pressure or coercion. These 10 factors must be carefully assessed:

1. Ambivalence
2. Guilt
3. Depression
4. Substance abuse
5. Vulnerability to psychological pressure or coercion
6. Relationship with the recipient
7. Potential benefits of donation
8. Potential medical risks and urgency of donation
9. Potential economic risks of donation
10. Potential hardships (for donor and family) of donation

A trained transplant psychiatrist, psychologist, clinical social worker, and psychiatric nurse should perform this psychological assessment.[3]

In general, biological parents are the most likely potential donors for children in need of a liver transplant. It is natural for parents to want to donate a portion of their liver to their ailing young child. However, in adult-to-adult (LD) liver transplants, the adult donor's personal relationship with the adult recipient—a relationship potentially colored by psychosocial conflicts—takes on new significance. For obvious reasons, most LD liver transplants involve a donor and a recipient who are members of the same family. If the potential donor is not from the same family, he or she must have a demonstrable, long-term, significant emotional relationship with the recipient. So, potential donors not only include first-degree relatives (parents or adult children) but also spouses, second-degree relatives (adult cousins, grandparents, or adult grandchildren), long-term friends, coworkers, and step-relatives. In addition, at least three "Good Samaritans," unrelated either genetically or emotionally, have donated part of their liver for adult-to-adult (LD) liver transplant recipients.[2]

Becoming an LD may have both positive and negative psychological effects. Goldman[4] noted a great willingness on the part of parents to donate a partial liver to their sick children. Doing so can enhance one's individual sense of self-worth. LDs of a kidney reported improved self-esteem after donation.[5] Similarly, Beavers, Trotter, and Diaz found that LDs of a partial liver were satisfied with their decision; a high percentage had a better relationship with their recipient after donation.[6–8]

Potential negative psychological aspects of donation must also be considered during the assessment, including indirect costs (such as transportation to the transplant center for evaluation, for the surgery, and for postsurgical care; lodging; and lost wages). Trotter et al.[6] found that LDs incurred mean out-of-pocket expenses of $3660.

The recipient's insurance carrier covers medical expenses for the actual evaluation, surgery, and immediate postoperative care. However, there is no guarantee that any long-term medical problems related to donation will be reimbursable. In addition, stresses on the donor (and family), any change in body image, and the inability to work for 1 to 3 months after donation could all have significant psychological effects. Short- and long-term disability might affect employment status, interpersonal relationships, and future issuance of health and life insurance.

The issue of Good Samaritan donors was first raised in the field of kidney transplantation.[9] Such donors have no previous, long-term significant relationship with the recipient. Their motives are apparently altruistic, although some have questioned the true underlying motivation.[10] Good Samaritan donors have less chance of being subjected to coercion or psychological pressure—which could be a danger for long-term emotionally related donors in particular. Given questions about LD morbidity and mortality, most transplant centers in the United States do not consider evaluating Good Samaritans as potential LDs of a partial liver.

Donor selection is the rate-limiting step in LD liver transplants. Most transplant centers consider psychological assessment as important as medical, surgical, and anatomic assessment in making decisions about prospective LDs of a partial liver. The nonacceptance rates for psychological reasons are as high as 20% to 36%.[11–13] Renz at al[11] evaluated the frequency of acceptance of LDs for pediatric liver transplants: they found that, of 75 prospective LDs, only 10 (13%) were found to be acceptable for donation. Psychological assessment (20%) was among the leading causes of nonacceptance. Psychological issues that resulted in nonacceptance included substance abuse, current incarceration, psychiatric illness under treatment, emotional lability, and single parenthood without substantial extended family support.

Similarly, Sterneck et al[12] found that of 73 prospective LDs, 24 (33%) were not accepted for pediatric liver transplants. Of these 24 donors, 6 (20%) were turned down because of psychological issues. Beavers et al[13] found that, of 161 prospective LDs for both pediatric and adult liver transplants, 57 (35%) were turned down. One of the leading reasons was psychosocial issues (36%). Such issues include ambivalence (45%), lack of adequate social support (35%), significant stress (15%), and history of a suicide attempt (5%). Valentine-Gamazo et al[14] found that, of 700 prospective LDs for adult-to-adult (LD) liver transplants, about 10% of those who underwent formal evaluation were turned down after psychological assessment. Persistent ambivalence was the leading psychological reason for exclusion. In contrast, none of the prospective LDs for pediatric liver transplants were turned down for psychological reasons.[14]

No strict guidelines exist for psychological assessment of prospective LDs of a partial liver. However, most transplant centers have adopted formal psychological assessment as an integral part of their donor evaluation.[13–18] The professional(s) responsible for psychological assessment should be part of the transplant team and must be experienced in the assessment of liver transplant recipients, so that they understand the particular context and unique psychological demands of liver transplants. Any experience in evaluating prospective LDs of other organs (eg, a kidney) would help provide the necessary expertise to evaluate whether the decision to donate is voluntary and free of coercion. Psychological evaluators (transplant psychiatrist, psychologist, clinical social worker, and psychiatric nurse) should not be involved in the care of the recipient.

Psychological assessment should be done early in the formal evaluation process. It is very important to inform prospective LDs that they can back out anytime before the actual surgery. If the donor is not accepted, the reasons must be kept confidential from the recipient. Most transplant centers will inform the recipient that the donor was not a suitable candidate on medical grounds, even when the actual reason may be different. This is done to protect the donor and to avoid any deterioration in the relationship with the recipient. In addition, to avoid conflict of interest, many centers use independent, separate evaluators for the medical vs. psychological assessment. The U.S. Department of Health and Human Services Advisory Committee on Organ Transplantation (ACOT) recommended that an independent donor advocate team evaluate the potential donor.[19] Similarly, the state of New York formed a Committee on Quality Improvement in Living Liver Donation that also recommends an independent donor advocate team to determine suitability of potential donors for donation.[20]

Various tools are available for psychological assessment of prospective LDs (Table 29.7-1). Walter et al[21] performed preoperative psychometric evaluation of 40 prospective LDs of a partial

**TABLE 29.7-1**

**COMMON INSTRUMENTS USED FOR PSYCHOSOCIAL EVALUATION OF PROSPECTIVE LIVING DONORS (LDs) OF A PARTIAL LIVER**

Symptom Checklist-90-Revised (SCL-90-R)
Minnesota Multiphasic Personality Inventory (MMPI-2)
Beck Depression Inventory (BDI)
Short Form-36 Health Survey Trail (SF-36)
Hopkins Symptom Checklist
Anamnestic Comparative Self-Assessment Scale (ACSA)
Berlin Mood Questionnaire (BSF)
Giessen Complaint Questionnaire (GBB)
Questionnaire on Self-efficacy, Optimism, and Pessimism (SWOP)

liver. All were assessed for motivation, ambivalence, and anxiety. Of these 40 individuals, 33 were found to be suitable LDs; 7, unsuitable. Suitable donors had superior scores on global quality of life, physical complaints, mood and self-efficacy, optimism, and pessimism. Most had a high level of willingness to donate, yet a few were subjected to very clear psychological pressure.

Currently, we lack criteria for an adequate psychometric evaluation as part of psychological assessment and selection of prospective LDs. A well-defined qualitative approach might provide a better understanding of the specific situation of individual prospective LDs and might improve our ability to identify those who are exposed to pronounced psychological pressure and are forced to develop defenses against the perceived danger to them.

## PSYCHOLOGICAL OUTCOME AFTER DONATION

The overall attitude toward living liver donation has been positive.[6–8] Trotter et al[6] found that, of 24 LDs for adult-to-adult LD liver transplants, 96% benefited from the donor experience, and all would donate again if necessary. Beavers et al[7] found that, of 27 LDs for both pediatric and adult liver transplants, 100% would donate again—regardless of the recipient's outcome. Similarly, Diaz et al[8] found that, of 41 LDs for pediatric liver transplants, 100% overwhelmingly endorsed living donation, regardless of the recipient's outcome; 89% advocated "increased" application of living donation beyond "emergency situations"; 0% responded that living donation should be abandoned or that he or she felt "forced" to donate. Simpson et al[22] found that, of 47 LDs for adult-to-adult LD liver transplants, 67% reported an improved spousal relationship and 98% said they would donate again; they were studied at 1 week and then 1, 3, 6, and 12 months after donation.

Walter et al[23] conducted a pilot study to evaluate the psychological outcome of LDs of livers. A total of 23 donors underwent psychological assessment before, and 6 months after, donation. The main objective of the study was to investigate the relationship between psychological findings and postoperative complications. Most (65%) donors showed an improved quality of life after donation, as compared with preoperative findings. Only 26% of donors had higher rates of symptoms of tiredness, fatigue, and limb pain after donation. The postoperative complications had no influence on the psychological outcome.

Short- and long-term psychological assessment of LDs after adult-to-adult LD liver transplants has not yet been well established. Beavers et al[24] evaluated practice patterns for long-term follow-up

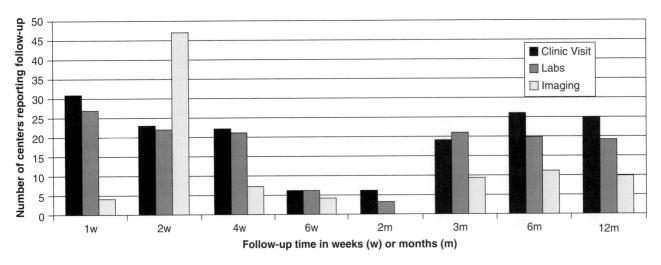

**FIGURE 29.7-1**

Living donor (LD) follow-up after right lobe liver donation for adult-to-adult transplants (N=51). Percentage of transplant centers reporting clinic visits, laboratory data, and imaging studies at specific intervals after initial hospital discharge.

of right lobectomy donors after adult-to-adult liver LD transplants at U.S. transplant centers. Of 97 centers, 90 (92.8%) responded to the survey. A total of 51 (56.7%) have performed right lobectomies. Personal psychological support services after donation were unusual, but included regular phone calls from the coordinator (5), administration of quality of life instruments (3), routine follow-up with a psychologist (1), and administration of a satisfaction survey (1). Long-term care of donors varies significantly. Formal psychological support and assessment after donation are rare (Figure 29.7-1).

Kidney donation has been shown to have psychological effects on LDs. The most common diagnoses after donation were obsession (25%), depression (17.5%), and anxiety (17.5%). Some authors have suggested that LDs need reassurance, education, support, empathy, and assistance in developing coping mechanisms and accepting the consequences of surgery.[25] In comparison, psychological assessment of LDs of a partial liver after donation is very limited. Fukunishi et al[26] found that 10% of LDs of a partial liver developed psychiatric complications 1 month after donation, and Kita et al[27] reported that 7.1% had major depression diagnosed within 1 year after donation. Similarly, Goldman[4] found psychological problems after donation in 15%. Lam et al[28] reported maladjustment in 5 of 8 LDs who had donated a partial liver to their spouse. Results from a survey sent to all liver donors in Japan through 2003 was presented at the International Conference on the Care of the Live Organ Donor (held in Vancouver, Canada, September 15–16, 2005) by the Japanese Liver Transplantation Society. Of the 2 667 live liver donors, 62% completed the survey with only half of the donors reporting complete recovery by 4 months postoperatively. Another 45% of donors reported near complete recovery with 90% of those individuals back to work or school. This means that 10% of the donors were not successfully reintegrated into society. Although only 3% of donors considered their recovery to be poor, about 40% expressed anxiety regarding their future health. Of note, this anxiety was independent of the extent of liver resection, since left lateral segment donors were equally concerned when compared with the right lobe donors. The participants of the Vancouver Forum agreed that the

Transplantation Committee must continue to monitor the health (including the psychological health issues) and long-term outcome of the live liver donor.[29]

LDs of a partial liver are currently not formally followed after donation for the development of psychological problems. Given the frequency of psychological problems after kidney donation, similar complications are likely to occur after liver donation.

In summary, LD liver transplants represent an alternative lifesaving procedure for patients with ESLD. Psychological assessment is critical, not only during donor selection but also after donation. After donation, although most liver transplant centers do evaluate the medical health and physical well-being of LDs, formal psychological support is rare. The development of standardized strict guidelines for long-term psychological follow-up after living liver donation should be considered. Such guidelines might become available in the near future, once results become available from the adult-to-adult LD liver transplant cohort study (A2ALL) sponsored by the National Institutes of Health (NIH), the American Society of Transplant Surgeons (ASTS), and the Health Resources and Services Administration (HRSA).

## References

1. Raia S, Nery JR, Mies S. Letters to the Editor: Liver transplantation from live donors. *The Lancet* 1989;497.
2. Brown RS, Jr., Russo MW, Lai M, et al. A survey of liver transplantation from living adult donors in the United States. *N Engl J Med* 2003;348:818–825.
3. Abecassis M, Adams M, Adams P, et al. Consensus statement on the live organ donor. *JAMA* 2000;284:2919–2926.
4. Goldman LS. Liver transplantation using living donors. Preliminary donor psychiatric outcomes. *Psychosomatics* 1993;34:235–240.
5. Karrfelt HM, Berg UB, Lindblad FI, et al. To be or not to be a living donor: questionnaire to parents of children who have undergone renal transplantation. *Transplantation* 1998;65:915–918.
6. Trotter JF, Talamantes M, McClure M, et al. Right hepatic lobe donation for living donor liver transplantation: impact on Donor Quality of Life. *Liver Transpl* 2001;7:485–493.

7. Beavers KL, Sandler RS, Fair JH, et al. The living donor experience: donor health assessment and outcomes following living donor liver transplantation. *Liver Transpl* 2001;7:943–947.

8. Diaz GC, Renz JF, Mudge C, et al. Donor health assessment after living-donor liver transplantation. *Ann Surg* 2002;236:120–126.

9. Matas AJ, Garvey CA, Jacobs CL, et al. Nondirected donation of kidneys from living donors. *N Engl J Med* 2000;343:433–436.

10. Levinsky NG. Organ donation by unrelated donors. *N Engl J Med* 2000;343:430–432.

11. Renz JF, Mudge CL, Heyman MB, et al. Donor selection limits use of living-related liver transplantation. *Hepatology* 1995;22:1122–1126.

12. Sterneck MR, Fischer L, Nischwitz U, et al. Selection of the living liver donor. *Transplantation* 1995;60:667–671.

13. Beavers KL, Fried MW, Zacks SL, et al. Evaluation of potential living donors for living donor liver transplantation. *Am J Transplant* 2001;1:318.

14. Valentine-Gamazo C, Malago M, Karliova M, et al. Experience after the evaluation of 700 potential donors for living donor liver transplantation in a single center. *Liver Transpl* 2004;10:1087–1096

15. Trotter JF. Selection of donors and recipients for living donor liver transplantation. *Liver Transpl* 2000;6:S52–S58.

16. Marcos A, Fisher RA, Ham JM, et al. Selection and outcome of living donors for adult to adult right lobe transplantation. *Transplantation* 2000;69:2410–2415.

17. Chen YS, Cheng YF, De Villa VH, et al. Evaluation of living liver donors. *Transplantation* 2003;75:S16–S19.

18. Samstein B, Emond J. Liver transplants from living related donors. *Annu Rev Med* 2001; 52:147–160.
http://www.organdonor.gov/acot.html.
http://www.health.state.ny.us/nysdoh/liver_donation/pdf/liver_donor_report_web.pdf.

19. Walter M, Bronner E, Steinmuller T, et al. Psychosocial data of potential living donors before living donor liver transplantation. *Clin Transplant* 2002;16:55–59.

20. Simpson MA, Richman E, Chang H, et al. Donor quality of life (QOL) after living donor adult liver transplantation (LDALT). *Am J Transplant* 2005;5:207.

21. Walter M, Bronner E, Pascher A, et al. Psychosocial outcome of living donors after living donor liver transplantation: a pilot study. *Clin Transplant* 2002;16:339–344.

22. Beavers KL, Cassara JE, Shrestha R. Practice patterns for long-term follow-up of adult-to-adult right lobectomy donors at US transplantation centers. *Liver Transpl* 2003;9:645–8.

23. Taghavi R, Mahdavi R, Toufani H. The psychological effects of kidney donation on living kidney donors (related and unrelated). *Transplant Proc* 2001;33:2636–2637.

24. Fukunishi I, Sugawara Y, Takayama T, et al. Psychiatric disorders before and after living-related transplantation. *Psychosomatics* 2001;42:337–343.

25. Kita Y, Fukunishi I, Harihara Y, et al. Psychiatric disorders in living-related liver transplantation. *Transplant Proc* 2001;33:1350–1351.

26. Lam BK, Lo CM, Fung AS, et al. Marital adjustment after interspouse living donor liver transplantation. *Transplantation Proc* 2000;32:2095–2096.

27. A Report of the Vancouver Forum On the Care of the Live Organ Donor: Lung, Liver, Pancreas and Intestine: Data and Medical Guidelines. *Am J Transplant* (in press) 2006.

# CHAPTER 30

# LIVER TRANSPLANTATION: THE RECIPIENT

## 30.1 SELECTION AND WORKUP

*Henkie P. Tan, MD, PhD, Thomas Shaw-Stiffel, MD, Kusum Tom, MD, Amadeo Marcos, MD*

### INTRODUCTION

Two major reasons for transplantation in the patient with end-stage liver disease (ESLD) are (1) to prolong survival and (2) to improve the quality of life. Therefore, transplantation should be considered in any potential recipients in whom transplantation would extend life expectancy beyond what the natural history of the underlying liver disease would predict or in whom the quality of life is likely to improve.

The most common indications of orthotopic liver transplantation (OLT) in adults are ESLD from chronic hepatititis C (HCV), alcoholic liver disease, chronic hepatitis B (HBV), cholestatic diseases (including primary biliary cirrhosis [PBC] and primary sclerosing cholangitis [PSC]), and autoimmune hepatitis. The most common indications of OLT in pediatrics are extrahepatic biliary atresia and alpha-1-antitrysin deficiency. In general, the diseases are generally not the indications of OLT; rather, it is the complications of these diseases that create the indications for OLT. Most patients undergoing OLT have complications related to (1) presence of portal hypertension (eg, gastrointestinal bleed), and/or (2) a reflection of impaired/reduced liver mass (eg, coagulopathy).

The evaluation of patients for OLT involves a multidisciplinary team approach, which includes transplant surgeons, hepatologists, psychologists/psychiatrists, social workers, nurse coordinators, and other consultants. All potential living donor liver transplantation (LDLT) recipients must first be listed with the United Network for Organ Sharing (UNOS). The indications for LDLT are the same as those for deceased donor liver transplantation (DDLT). The initial steps include the comprehensive assessment of the recipients. This chapter focuses on key issues related to the selection and evaluation of potential recipients for adult-to-adult LDLT.

### THE MELD SCORE AND IMPACT ON SELECTION OF RECIPIENTS FOR LDLT

The new liver allocation system in the United States based on the Model End-Stage Liver Disease (MELD) score (see Figure 30.1-1) was implemented on February 27, 2002. This new system was developed using an evidence-derived model that provided a much more objective measure of short-term liver disease-related mortality. In development of this new policy, the MELD score was validated against several different cohorts of patients, with and without inclusion of the subjective clinical variables, and proved to be consistent and highly predictive of 3-month mortality.[1] However, not all appropriate liver transplant candidates have a high risk of death even though they may have an increased urgency for transplantation. This exception includes early-stage hepatocellular carcinoma (HCC). Because of this, an alternative pathway for prioritization was developed utilizing a regional peer-review process through regional review boards.[2] An initial summary report of a national conference on liver allocation in the MELD era concluded that MELD has had a successful initial implementation, meeting the goal of providing a system of allocation that emphasizes the urgency of the candidate while diminishing the reliance on waiting time, and that it has proven to be a powerful tool for auditing the liver allocation system.[3,4] The MELD score, however, does not provide a highly accurate measure of the patient's chance for survival after liver transplantation.

The Scientific Registry for Transplant Recipients (SRTR) has recently analyzed the benefit of transplant in terms of life-years gained with a transplant compared with waiting on the list.[5] For patients with MELD score below 17, the risk of the transplant surgery appears to outweigh the risk of death from the liver disease. For all other MELD score ranges, liver transplantation results in an increase in life-years compared with waiting.

The MELD score is calculated using the following formula:

* MELD score = $10\{0.957 \text{Ln(Scr)} + 0.378 \text{Ln(Tbil)} + 1.12 \text{Ln(INR)} + 0.643\}$

where, Ln = $\log_e$

Scr = serum creatinine (mg/dL); Tbil-total bilirubin (mg/dL); INR = international normalized ratio; Alb = albumin (g/dL)

* MELD score ≥ 30 = 2a listing status

       24 – 29 = 2b listing status

       < 24 = 3 listing status

**FIGURE 30.1-1**

The MELD score.

Therefore, it is suggested that a score of 18 may be a reasonably good cutoff level above which LDLT is indicated, because a patient with a MELD score above 18 has a greater than 10% risk of 90-day mortality without transplantation; this exceeds the 1-year mortality after LDLT (10%). As a result, all patients with a MELD score higher than 18 should be considered potential candidates for LDLT. However, some of the patients with a low MELD score (below 18) including those with cholestatic disorders such as PBC and PSC may have other medically compelling reasons (eg, severe pruritus, recurrent infections, or recurrent encephalopathy) that prompt the transplant team to consider early transplantation with LDLT. For these sick patients with complications but a low MELD score (< 18), the odds of imminent DDLT are low at most transplant centers. According to the proponents of this approach, recipient candidates with low MELD scores (and some of the longest waiting times) will benefit from a partial liver graft earlier in the natural history of their disease and especially before transplantation becomes no longer feasible (eg, PSC complicated by cholangiocarcinoma). In fact, a substantial number of LDLT recipients have stable liver disease at the time of transplantation. Nevertheless, the potential risk of complications and death in the living donor should always be considered paramount when contemplating LDLT in stable patients with chronic ESLD.

As a result, LDLT recipients tend to have a lower MELD score at the time of transplantation than those with DDLT. Freeman et al.[6] reported that the mean MELD score for candidates receiving deceased donor grafts was 23.5 compared to 14.8 for candidates receiving living donor grafts. With a MELD < 20, a greater proportion of LDLT recipients (71%) than recipients of DDLT (48%) received liver transplants. A recent report by Sugarawa et al.[7] suggests that left-lobe grafts can be used safely in adult recipients if their MELD < 15. These results suggest the MELD score is not only a highly predictive measure of mortality risk but also a reasonable measure of functional hepatic reserve. Freeman et al suggest the ideal recipients for LDLT have a MELD scores between 14 and 25 would appear to derive the most lifetime benefit, yet face the lowest odds of posttransplantation mortality.[6] This is derived from minimal lifetime benefit for the recipients with MELD < 10, perhaps < 14. The relative risk for posttransplantation mortality starts to increase for candidates with MELD > 25.

Interestingly, preliminary results from the University of Colorado Health Sciences Center (UCHSC) in 62 LDLT recipients with greater than 6 months of follow-up, reported that MELD scores did not predict post-LDLT patient or graft survival at 1 year.[8] Higher MELD scores (> 18), however, were associated with more hospital days during the 3-month post-LDLT period. Hence, evolving data from DDLT studies may not be applicable to LDLT. Two major limitations to UCHSC's recipients were that none of their patients evaluated and treated were under the current MELD system, and there were relatively few LDLT recipients with MELD > 30. At the University of Pittsburgh Medical Center Starzl Transplantation Institute (UPMC STI), we would generally not recommend recipients with MELD scores < 10 (except selected complicated PBC and PSC) to undergo LDLT. These patients generally have compensated cirrhosis and have a low mortality without transplantation.

Whether there is an upper limit for the MELD score above which LDLT may not be a viable option due to the need for a whole liver graft rather than a partial graft is unclear. The UCHSC data found recipients with MELD > 18 spent twice as much time in the hospital during the first 3 months than did those with

MELD ≤ 18 (8). In addition, the following factors were found to predict a poor outcome after LDLT independent of the MELD score: the need for mechanical ventilation or hemodialysis and a very low Karnofsky (functional) score. Poorly decompensated patients have a comparatively poor prognosis and may not tolerate right-lobe LDLT very well.[9] The long-term mortality rate following LDLT (57%) versus DD (18%) transplantation is threefold higher for recipients with chronic liver disease and severe decompensation (former UNOS status 2A).[10] Therefore, some transplantation center and the New York State Health Department has recommended that LDLT should not be offered to patients with Model for Endstage Liver Disease (MELD) score > 25.[11] It is thought that smaller grafts are unable to meet the needs of patients experiencing severe and prolonged illness. It is important that the recipients understand and accept that the donation will put the donor at significant risk. UPMC STI propose that all recipients should be assessed for LDLT regardless of the presence of a medical urgency for transplantation (precluding any contraindications), but potential recipients with MELD <14, but >25 should be evaluated on a case-by-case basis.

## RECIPIENT EVALUATION AND SELECTION

The first step in the evaluation of a recipient for LDLT is to list the patient for DDLT according to UNOS criteria; this not only ensures that the recipient is an appropriate candidate for OLT to begin with but also more importantly avoids LDLT potentially being done in futile situations (eg, inoperable HCC). This listing for DDLT is also important for the following important reasons. Should there be any post-LDLT complications including poor- or nongraft function, the recipient can be immediately upgraded as a UNOS status 1 to obtain a whole liver via DDLT; the retransplantation rate for LDLT recipients can be as high as 10%. Additionally, all third-party payers require listing of recipient for DDLT before evaluating and approving a patient for LDLT. On the other hand, some of the patients listed for DDLT are not suitable for LDLT. DDLT candidates may qualify for LDLT, if they are deemed medically eligible and surgically suitable for the procedure.

Although the pretransplant workup varies with transplant centers, most programs require a basic battery of laboratory tests and thorough evaluation of the patient's general medical condition and fitness for major surgery[12] (see Table 30.1-1 for general pretransplant evaluation). The evaluation of potential recipients for LDLT involves a multidisciplinary team approach which includes transplant surgeons, hepatologists, psychologists/psychiatrists, social workers, nurse coordinators, financial counselors, and other consultants (anesthesiologist, cardiologist, pulmonologist, infectious disease, neurologist, gastrointestinal, gynecologist, nutritionist, dentist, etc).

A thorough psychosocial assessment is very important. Addictive behavior and compliance with medications can adversely affect the outcome of LDLT. Over 40% of candidates for OLT have at least one psychiatric disorder.[12]

At UPMC STI, the absolute and relative contraindications for recipients undergoing LDLT are similar to DDLT (see Table 30.1-2). Common relative contraindications that preclude LDLT include morbid obesity, advanced age, adverse psychosocial factors, and HIV at UPMC STI. Of the 25% listed potential recipients who are considered medically eligible for LDLT, at the UCHSC, only about half (12.5% of all recipient candidates) are found to be surgically suitable and are able to accept volunteers

**TABLE 30.1-1**

## AN OVERVIEW OF PRETRANSPLANT MEDICAL EVALUATION

**Laboratory tests**
CBC, electrolytes,
Liver function tests
Viral hepatitis
Coagulation panel
Serology (including RPR, HIV, CMV, EBV, etc)
ABO blood typing
BUN, creatinine, urinalysis
Miscellaneous (PPD, α-1 antitrypsin, ferritin, iron, transferring, ceruloplasmin, ANA, hypercoagulable state, toxicology, etc.)

**Radiographic studies**
CXR
Ultrasound: assess patency of portal and hepatic vasculature, presence of ascites, liver size, and exclude mass/lesions
CT/MRI: to exclude HCC (with increase AFP), and for clarification of abnormalities seen in ultrasound

**12 lead-EKG/cardiac stress test**
If abnormal EKG, proceed to cardiac stress test, and if positive, proceed to coronary angiogram

**Endoscopy**
EGD: Evaluate/treat esophageal/gastric varices, evaluate for presence of Barrett metaplasia
Colonoscopy

**PPD skin test**
**Female patients**
Mammography, Pap and pregnancy tests

**Selected patients**
Pulmonary function tests, arterial blood gas
Dental and dermatology clearance
Cardiac echocardiogram (bubble to exclude intrapulmonary shunting)
Carotid duplex, bone scan, bone density, MRI/MRA, AFP
Liver biopsy, ERCP
Hepatic angiogram

**TABLE 30.1-2**

## CONTRAINDICATIONS TO RECIPIENT LISTING FOR LDLT

**Absolute**
- Not a candidate for DDLT
- Multisystem organ failure/severe and uncontrolled sepsis
- Irreversible brain damage
- Extrahepatic malignancy
- Advanced cardiac or pulmonary disease
- Active substance abuse
- Medical noncompliance

**Relative**
- HIV infection
- Primary hepatobiliary malignancy
- Adverse psychosocial factors
- Age > 65 years
- Morbidly obese (BMI > 40)

will therefore always remain. This risk must be offset by beneficence to the recipient, and the continued use of these organs can only be justified if the outcome is consistently good for both the healthy donor and sick recipient.

## SPECIFIC LDLT RECIPIENT CONSIDERATIONS

The advantages of LDLT are (1) it is frequently performed electively, (2) recipient condition pre-transplant can be and should be optimized, (3) liver allograft cold ischemic time is shorter, and (4) pretransplant cross-match can be performed.

Contraindications to DD transplantation also apply to living donation. LD mortality rate is estimated to be about 0.2%. Total major and minor morbidities in donors are currently reduced to 10% to 15%. Donor biliary complications are < 5% in our experience; the majority were managed nonoperatively or resolved spontaneously. One-year graft and recipient survival after LDLT has improved to at least 80% and 86%, respectively.[15–17] Hepatic artery thrombosis occurs in about 5%,[18] and biliary complications has improved to less than 20%[15,17,19] but can be as high as 40%.[16]

There are two specific groups of patients who are ideally suited for LDLT. The first group of patients with HCC could benefit substantially from rapid LDLT transplantation prior to metastasize even with increased UNOS priority. Patients with tumors smaller than 5 cm, fewer than three tumors, and no evidence of concurrent malignant disease can be considered for LDLT, which is probably the best option for the growing number of patients with cirrhosis and small tumors. Data from Japan demonstrate that LDLT for hepatocellular carcinoma (HCC) is feasible with satisfactory results, even when liver function is markedly impaired, or HCC is uncontrolled by conventional antitumor treatments.[20] With 316 LDLT recipients, 1- and 3-year patient survivals were 78% and 69%, respectively. One- and 3-year recurrence-free survivals were 73% and 65%, respectively. LDLT recipients are generally younger and tend to have lower MELD scores.[21] LDLT results in a better outcome for patients with HCC and a lower risk of death (relative risk 0.35). Furthermore, every transplantation with a liver obtained from a living donor potentially frees up a deceased donor liver for transplantation into another recipient. A reduced waiting period for a living donor organ may decrease the risk for decompensation or death before transplantation and thus improve the chance for

for evaluation for donor surgery.[8] Overall, it appears that about a third of adult patients on the waiting list for OLT may have a potential donor and half will undergo the procedure, thus indicating that LDLT may be applicable in up to 15% of patients on the waiting list.[13] At UPMC STI, about 30% are medically eligible and 20% are surgically suitable, possibly because a larger number and wider spectrum of potential LDLT recipients are assessed. For the year 2005, out of the 279 liver transplants performed, 41 were LDLT and 188 were liver only transplants. Trotter et al. estimate the expected annual number of LDLT performed at a transplant center will probably not exceed 5% of the number of patients listed for transplantation.[14]

Once the recipient is considered medically eligible for LDLT, the recipient is then considered to be surgically suitable by the surgical team. Recipients with portal vein thrombosis and Budd-Chiari syndrome are not absolute surgical contraindications and are successfully transplanted at UPMC STI. These potential recipients are evaluated on a case-by-case basis. Poor recipient outcomes that cannot be blamed on underlying medical conditions can often be traced to intraoperative donor events, suggesting that most of the risk to healthy donors can be controlled and minimized. Even with refinement of donor surgical technique, risk will never be eliminated completely and an ethical dilemma success. Data have shown shorter waiting times and improved survival on the waiting list for patients with potential donors for LDLT, with mortality being half that of those listed for DDLT.[22,23]

Another group of potential recipients are patients whose severity of illness that is not accurately reflected by their MELD score.[24] These include patients with symptomatic benign hepatic masses (eg, hemangioma, hemangioendothelioma, polycystic liver diseases), metabolic disorders (eg, familial amyloidosis, hyperoxaluria, tyrosinemia, glycogen storage disease), complicated cholestatic liver disease or patients with ascites, uncontrolled encephalopathy and/or severe cachexia. PSC patients who have recurrent cholangitis and frequent endoscopic/percutaneous procedures that significantly impair the quality of life may have low MELD scores. PBC patients may also have a significant impairment of their quality of life with intractable pruritus, xanthomatous neuropathy, and severe metabolic bone disease. Because of their low MELD score, these patients usually have little to no chance for imminent DDLT and are, therefore, good candidates of LDLT.

Because hepatitis C viral infection (HCV) is the most common indication for liver transplantation in the United States, the issue of recurrent HCV in LDLT is of paramount importance. Although some early reports have shown earlier and more severe recurrence of HCV following LDLT compared to DD recipients,[25] this issue is still highly controversial.[26] Recent data have shown that this may not be true.[27–29] Given the current decrease in waiting list mortality with LDLT, we strongly feel that HCV cirrhosis potential recipients should be treated like any other potential recipients on the waiting list for LDLT.

Emergency LDLT for fulminant hepatic failure should be perform only on a case-by-case basis as the donor is placed in a very compromised medical and emotional/psychological position with ethical, medical, logistic and economic concerns.[30] A national survey of U.S. transplant centers reported acute liver failure as the indication for LDLT in only 2.2% of recipients.[31]

The University of Southern California has developed strategies for transfusion-free LDLT in Jehovah witnesses.[32] The use of preoperative blood augmentation with erythropoietin of selected recipients (eg, without appreciable portal hypertension), intraoperative cell salvage and acute normovolemic hemodilution, have resulted in transfusion-free LDLT.

The ideal candidate is one who is sick enough to derive a benefit from transplantation but not so sick that a potentially high posttransplant mortality risk is incurred; that is, the ideal LDLT candidate is a patient in whom transplantation would be performed today if organs were unlimited. The ideal LDLT recipient profile is listed in Table 30.1-3.[33]

To assess the efficacy of LDLT, the National Institutes of Health has funded the LDLT A2ALL Cohort Study to measure the outcomes of LDLT recipients in comparison to recipients of DDLT. Preliminary results of 385 adult-to-adult LDLT recipients at nine centers were studied with analysis of over 35 donor, recipient, intraoperative, and postoperative variables.[34] One-year recipient survival was 89% with 9.6% undergoing retransplantation. One-year graft survival was 81% with 13.2% of grafts failed in the first 90 days. The most common causes of graft failure were vascular thrombosis, primary nonfunction, and sepsis. Biliary complications were common (30% early, 11% late). Older recipients age and length of cold ischemia were significant predictors of graft failure. Center experience greater than 20 LDLT was associated with a significantly lower risk of graft failure and outcomes improve with increasing center experience. Recipient MELD score and graft size were not significant predictors.

**TABLE 30.1-3**

## THE IDEAL LDLT RECIPIENT PROFILE

| Parameters | Ideal Criteria |
| --- | --- |
| Listing | Must first be listed with UNOS |
| MELD score | $\geq 14$ but $\leq 25$, except specific recipient subgroups listed below to maximize transplant benefit[6,11] |
| Recipient risk factors | No thrombosis of multiple visceral veins, multiple medical problems, multiple significant abdominal surgeries; advanced age[24] |
| Specific recipient subgroups | |
| • HCC | Benefit substantially from rapid LDLT since DDLT may allow for metastasize[20] |
| • Severity of illness not accurately MELD score | Complicated cholestatic liver disease, reflected by patients with ascites, uncontrolled encephalopathy and/or severe cachexia[24] |

## CONCLUSIONS

Due to the ongoing shortage of deceased donors, adult-to-adult right lobe LDLT is a safe and viable option, but only in a select group of recipients and donors who meet specific criteria. MELD can help identify candidates for LDLT who are not likely to benefit because they are either too sick or too well to undergo transplantation. The ideal LDLT recipients should potentially have maximum posttransplant lifetime benefits and the least posttransplant mortality, be listed on the deceased donor list with UNOS, have MELD $\geq 14$ but $\leq 25$, or if MELD is low benefit substantially from rapid LDLT (eg, HCC, complicated PSC and PBC).

**TABLE 30.1-4**

## KEY POINTS IN RECIPIENT SELECTION FOR LDLT

1. Selection of the ideal recipients for LDLT requires assessment of recipient risk of death without a transplant, risk of death with a transplant, and donor risk. The donor risk is guided by 2 key principals: (1) donor safety with minimal acceptable morbidity and no mortality, and (2) identifying optimal donor partial hepatic allograft with resultant graft and recipient survival at least equivalent to that of DDLT. Thus, donor mortality rate should be < 0.2%. Total major and minor donor morbidities are estimated to be < 10% to 15%. Donor biliary complications are less than 5% in our experiences; the majority were managed nonoperatively and resolved spontaneously.

2. Contraindications to transplantation are becoming fewer. LDLT should optimally be performed to maximize transplant benefit and the ultimate decision to perform LDLT on a specific patient rests with the expertise of the transplant center. We prefer right lobe to left lobe donation in adult LDLT. An ideal GRBW of 0.8, corrected for degree of steatosis, is a safe lower limit with maximal 60% resection of the donor liver volume.

3. Less than 20% of recipients on the DDLT waiting list will have donors, and < 5% of the number of patients listed will undergo LDLT.

4. One-year graft and recipient survival after LDLT has improved to at least 81% and 89%, respectively. Hepatic artery thrombosis occurs in about 5% and biliary complications have improved to less than 20%.

5. HCV recurrence post LDLT is still highly controversial.

6. With improvement of surgical techniques, organs from living donors may give superior results with decrease vascular and biliary complications, and improved graft and recipient survival.

With continued improvement of surgical techniques, organs from living donors might give superior results with decreased vascular and biliary complications, and improved graft and recipient survival.[17] Table 30.1-4 lists the key points in LDLT. We implore the ASTS to continue to take the leadership and initiative in establishing an immediate long-term national registry to track the outcome of all living donors and recipients.

## References

1. Tan HP, Marcos A, Shapiro R, Eds. Living Donor Transplantation. Informa Healthcare, New York, May 2007.
2. Wiesner RH, Edwards EB, Freeman RB, et al. Model for end stage liver disease (MELD) and allocation of donor livers. *Gastroenterology* 2003;124:91–96.
3. Freeman RB. Overview of the MELD/PELD system of liver allocation. Indications for liver transplantation in the MELD era: evidence-based patient selection. *Liver Transpl* 2004;10(Suppl 2):S2–S3.
4. Olthoff KM, Brown RS, Delmonico FL, et al. Summary report of a national conference: evolving concepts in liver allocation in the MELD and PELD era. *Liver Transpl* 2004;10(Suppl 2):A6–A22.
5. Freeman RB, Harper A, Edwards EB. Liver transplantation outcomes under the model for end-stage liver disease and pediatric end-stage liver disease. *Curr Opin Organ Transplant* 2005;10:90–94.
6. Merion RM, Schaubel DE, Dykstra DM, et al. The survival benefit of liver transplantation. *Am J Transplant* 2005;5:307–313.
7. Freeman RB. The impact of the model for end-stage liver disease on recipient selection for adult living liver donation. *Liver Transpl* 2003;9(Suppl 2):S54–S59.
8. Sugarawa Y, Makuuchi M, Kaneko J, et al. MELD score for selection of patients to receive left liver graft. *Transplantation* 2003;75:573–574.
9. Hayashi PH, Forman L, Steinberg T, et al. Model for end-stage liver disease score does not predict patient or graft survival in living donor liver transplant recipients. *Liver Transpl* 2003;9:737–740.
10. Marcos A, Ham J, Fisher R, et al. Single-center analysis of the first forty living donor transplants using the right lobe. *Liver Transpl* 2000;6:296–301.
11. Testa G, Malago M, Nadalin S, et al. Right-liver living donor transplantation for decompensated end-stage liver disease. *Liver Transpl* 2002;8:340–346.
12. New York State Health Department. New York State Committee on quality improvement in living liver donation 2002.
13. Fink SA, Brown RS. Current Indications, contraindications, delisting criteria, and timing for liver transplantation. In: Busuttil RW, Klintmalm GB, eds. *Transplantation of the Liver.* Philadelphia: Elsevier; 2005: 95–114.
14. Rudow DL, Russo MW, Hafliger S, et al. Clinical and ethnic differences in candidates listed for liver transplantation with and without potential living donors. *Liver Transpl* 2003;9:254–259.
15. Trotter JF, Hayashi PH, Kam I. Donor and recipient evaluation and selection for adult-to-adult right hepatic lobe liver transplantation. In: Busuttil RW, Klintmalm GB, eds. *Transplantation of the Liver.* Philadelphia: Elsevier; 2005:655–674.
16. Marcos A, Ham JM, Fisher RA, et al. Surgical management of anatomical variations of the right lobe in living donor liver transplantation. *Ann Surg* 2000;231:824–831.
17. Gondolesi GE, Varotti G, Florman S, et al. Biliary complications in 96 consecutive right lobe living donor transplant recipients. *Transplantation* 2004;77:1842–1848.
18. Lo CM, Fan ST, Liu CL, et al. Lessons learned from one hundred right lobe living donor liver transplants. *Ann Surg* 2004;240:151–158.
19. Marcos A, Killackey M, Orloff MS, et al. Hepatic arterial reconstruction in 95 adult right lobe living donor liver transplants: evolution of anastomotic technique. *Liver Transpl* 2003;9:570–574.
20. Brown RS Jr, Russo MW, Lai M, et al. A survey of liver transplantation from living adult donors in the United States. *N Engl J Med* 2003;348:818–825.
21. Todo S, Furukawa H: Japanese study group on organ transplantation. Living donor liver transplantation for adult patients with hepatocellular carcinoma: experience in Japan. *Ann Surg* 2004;240:451–459.
22. Lo CM, Fan S, Liu C, et al. The role and limitation of living donor liver transplantation for hepatocellular carcinoma. *Liver Transpl* 2004;10:440–447.
23. Liu CL, Lam B, Lo CM. Impact of right-lobe live donor liver transplantation on patients waiting for liver transplantation. *Liver Transpl* 2003;9:863–869.
24. Russo MW, LaPointe-Rudow D, Kinkhabwala M, et al. Impact of adult living donor liver transplantation on waiting time survival in candidates listed for liver transplantation. *Am J Transplant* 2004;4:427–431.
25. Trotter JF. Living donor liver transplantation: is the hype over? J Hepatol 2005; 42:20–25.
26. Garcia-Retortillo M, Forns X, Llovet JM, et al. Hepatitis C recurrence is more severe after living donor compared to cadaveric liver transplantation. *Hepatology* 2004; 40:699–707.
27. Sugawara Y, Makuuchi M. Should living donor liver transplantation be offered to patients with hepatitis C virus cirrhosis? J Hepatol 2005; 42:472–475.
28. Shiffman ML, Stravitz RT, Cantos MJ, et al. Histologic recurrence of chronic hepatitis C virus in patients after living donor and deceased donor liver transplantation. *Liver Transpl* 2004; 10:1248–1255.
29. Russo MW, Shrestha R. Is severe recurrent hepatitis C more common after living donor liver transplantation? *Hepatology* 2004;40:524–526.
30. Bozorgzadeh A, Jain A, Ryan C, et al. Impact of hepatitis C viral infection in primary cadaveric liver allograft versus primary living-donor allograft in 100 consecutive liver transplant recipients receiving tacrolimus. *Transplantation* 2004;77:1066–1070.
31. Marcos A, Ham JM, Fisher RA, et al. Emergency adult-to-adult living donor liver transplantation for fulminant hepatic failure. *Transplantation* 2000;69:2202–2205.
32. Beavers KL, Cassara JE, Shrestha R. Practice patterns for long-term follow-up of adult-to-adult right lobectomy donors at US transplantation centers. *Liver Transpl* 2003;9:645–648.
33. Jabbour N, Gagandeep S, Mateo R, et al. Live donor liver transplantation without blood products: strategies developed for Jehovah's Witnesses offer broad application. *Ann Surg* 2004;240:350–357.
34. Tan HP, Patel-Tom K, Marcos A. Adult living donor liver transplantation: who is the ideal donor and recipient. *J Hepatol* 2005;43:13–17.
35. Olthoff KM, Merion RM, Ghobrial RM, et al. Outcomes of 385 adult-to-adult living donor liver transplant recipients: A report from the A2ALL consortium. *Ann Surg* 2005;242:314–325.

# 30.2 ANESTHESIOLOGIC CONSIDERATIONS

*Susanne Shamsolkottabi, MD,*
*Kumar G. Belani, MBBS, MS*

## INTRODUCTION

Between January 1989 and June 30, 2005, 2 802 living donor liver transplants (LDLTs) were performed in the United States (based on Organ Procurement and Transplantation Network [OPTN]-United Network for Organ Sharing [UNOS] data accessed September 11, 2005). Of these, 983 were performed in children; and 1 815, in adults. The youngest surviving living related liver transplant recipient was transplanted at 45 days of age; another transplanted from a living related liver donor at age 1 year is currently 13 years old and doing well (based on OPTN UNOS data accessed September 11, 2005).

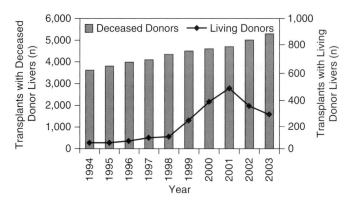

**FIGURE 30.2-1**

Liver transplant recipients from deceased and living donors, 1994–2003 (data from 2004 OPTN/SRTR Annual Report)

Living donor liver recipients may receive a reduced liver (either a lobe or a segment) from either a living related or an unrelated donor. The 1-year adjusted graft survival is approximately 80%, and the 5-year survival is approximately 63% (Source: OPTN/SRTR Data as of May 3, 2004). Figure 30.2-1 compares numbers of liver transplants from living versus deceased donors performed in the United States on a yearly basis between 1994 and 2003. LDLTs may be done in adults and pediatric recipients with end-stage liver disease (ELSD) from a variety of causes.[1,2] These may be congenital (eg, biliary atresia), metabolic (eg, Wilson's disease), infective (eg, hepatitis C cirrhosis), drug induced (eg, acetaminophen hepatic failure), alcoholic (eg, alcoholic cirrhosis), or immunological (eg, primary sclerosing cholangitis and other causes (eg, localized hepatic malignancies). In a recent review,[3] it appears that cholestatic disease as a reason for ESLD constitutes a higher frequency as eti-

ology for liver failure in the living donor liver recipients (LDLRs). Liver transplantation should not be done in patients with extrahepatic malignancy, cholangiocarcinoma, active untreated sepsis, advanced cardiopulmonary disease, patients with active alcoholism and substance abuse, and when significant surgical anatomic abnormalities are present in the recipient.[3] When performing living donor liver transplantation, the anesthesia care of both the donor and recipient occurs in the same center. Anesthesia induction and surgery usually start in the donor, followed by anesthesia induction and surgery in the recipient. This coordination is necessary to minimize ischemic time of the donated liver segment or lobe.

## ANESTHESIA CARE OF LIVING DONOR LIVER RECIPIENTS (LDLR)

The living donor liver recipient (LDLR) may be an adult or a pediatric patient with end-stage liver disease (ESLD) and will need to be assessed preoperatively. ESLD involves multiple systems as summarized in Figure 30.2-2. In most instances, since the donor is identified electively, the recipient can be prepared and optimized prior to the planned transplantation procedure.[1–2] However, this is not always the case, and emergency living donor liver transplantation has been reported.[4] In addition to performing a routine review of systems, the etiology of ESLD is noted as is the extent of other organ involvement including the current status of the recipient that will be dependent on the medical care he or she has received. Table 30.2-1 lists the problems and severity assessment that needs to be evaluated preoperatively.

Following the evaluation of items listed in Table 30.2-1, secondary consultation must be obtained when required to clarify and optimize pre-existing comorbidities if any are present.[12–16] This is done in conjunction with the hepatologist, and the surgical and critical care teams. Patients with pulmonary hypertension

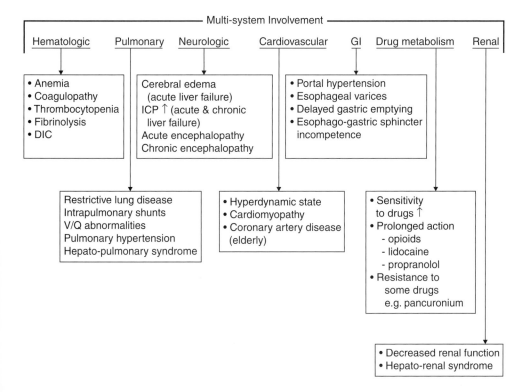

**FIGURE 30.2-2**

Summary of multisystem involvement in adults and pediatric patients with end-stage liver disease (ESLD). Each system needs to be evaluated during preoperative assessment of the living related liver donor recipient.

**TABLE 30.2-1**

## PREOPERATIVE EVALUATION OF LIVING LIVER DONOR RECIPIENTS (LDLR)

| Item | Clinical Implication |
|---|---|
| • End-stage liver disease | Note etiology: congenital, metabolic, drug induced, immunological, infective, alcoholic, or other cause. Duration of disease and functional status of liver needs to be verified. |
| • Review of systems | Rule out or confirm extent of: hepatopulmonary syndrome, hepatorenal syndrome, esophageal varices, severity of portal hypertension and effects (note if ascites is mild, moderate, or severe). Assess for esophagogastric sphincter incompetence, if any, including predisposition to regurgitation on induction. Assess if patient is preencephalopathic or has recovered from recent encephalopathic episode. Assess for cardiomyopathy secondary to chronic liver failure/cirrhosis. Review for status of esophageal varices (active esophageal varices will preclude the use of intraoperative transesophageal echo monitoring that may be used for monitoring) |
| • Coagulation status | Severity of liver disease will suggest more critical coagulopathy. Spleen enlargement may be associated with thrombocytopenia. Note if recipient is easily bruisable. |
| • Serum albumin level | Very low serum albumin levels will decrease protein binding of anesthetic agents |
| • Metabolic and intravascular fluid volume status | Recipients are typically on diuretics and may be glucose dependent. Assess electrolytes and need for glucose replacement |
| • Vascular access sites | Note for patency of jugular and subclavian veins and available peripheral veins. Assess radial artery availability for arterial line placement. Pediatric patients with chronic ESLD may be a challenge |
| • Perform routine assessments | Note allergies, upper airway & intubation feasibility, medications list, other problems if any |
| • Laboratory tests | Hgb level, platelet count, PT (including INR), aPTT, Fibrinogen level, serum electrolyte battery including blood glucose, creatinine, magnesium levels |
| • Radiological and cardiac assessment | CXR, 12-lead ECG, cardiac echo (note cardiac function, right sided enlargement if any and an estimate of pulmonary artery pressure); other tests as indicated. |

and those with severe hepatopulmonary syndrome and significant hypoxemia are high-risk candidates[17] and may require additional intervention preoperatively,[25] intraoperatively,[18] and postoperatively.[19-22] Although controversial,[19,23] patients with pulmonary hypertension may benefit from the use of nitric oxide intraoperatively[24] or preoperative preparation with epoprostenol.[25] Those with severe hypoxemia from hepatopulmonary syndrome[26] may

require a prolonged postoperative intensive care unit sojourn.[20] This needs to be discussed with the transplant team including the patient and family. If they have hepatorenal syndrome, then the intraoperative fluid care plan will have to be modified. Intraoperative hemofiltration has been described for these patients.[27] Preexisting coagulopathy must be corrected, especially in children. This may require the need for exchange transfusion.

## Preinduction Planning

Once assessment has been completed, an anesthesia care plan needs to be generated. The patient is informed about anesthesia care issues, and in addition to routine preparation, several decisions need to be made as listed in Table 30.2-2. The decision to use aprotinin and antithrombin III is usually done intraoperatively. When bleeding is nonsurgical and fibrinolysis appears to be the problem, aprotinin is instituted. Similarly, the decision to start an infusion of antithrombin III is made by the surgeon during hepatic artery and portal vein anastomosis. This is particularly important in young infants in whom the risk of newly anastomosed

**TABLE 30.2-2**

## PREPARATION OF THE LIVING LIVER DONOR RECIPIENTS (LDLR)

| | |
|---|---|
| Routine preparation measures | • Patient needs to be NPO; routine medications may be taken on day of surgery with a sip of water, eg, diuretics, antihypertensives, gut antiseptics (decrease bowel ammonia production), systemic preoperative antibiotic prophylaxis, IV immunosuppression initiation. |
| Plan for vascular access and invasive monitoring | • 2 large peripheral IVs, large-size double-lumen Hickman catheter for infants and children (serves for CVP monitoring, infusion of fluids, blood sampling, drug infusion), large bore 15F heparin-coated right internal jugular cannula for adults (portal-vein and inferior vena cava bypass), left-sided jugular or subclavian pulmonary artery catheter in adults (for intracardiac pressure monitoring, blood sampling and drug infusion), right femoral venous cannula for inferior vena cava (IVC) pressure monitoring. Radial artery catheter for blood pressure monitoring and arterial blood gases. Transesophageal echo[a] |
| Plan and set up for special infusions/drugs | • Dopamine (support renal circulation), aprotinin (to promote coagulation), anti-thrombin III (in infants and young children; dosing in consultation with hematology/surgical team), inhaled nitric oxide (in consultation with pulmonary medicine for pulmonary hypertension), inhaled or IV epoprostenol (in consultation with pulmonary medicine for pulmonary hypertension) |
| Hypothermia prevention | • Upper and lower body forced air-warming devices; fluid warmers; humidivent for inhaled gas humidification and warming. |
| Blood product availability | • Packed red cells, fresh frozen plasma, platelets, cryoprecipitate (need based on preoperative patient status and institutional practice)—notify blood bank. |
| Venovenous bypass and blood salvage set up | • Notify cardiopulmonary perfusionists (in adults) |

vessel thrombosis is quite high.[28] Because LDLRs are usually done electively and are in optimal condition, bleeding and the need for factor and platelet replacement may be predicted to be less than cadaveric transplants but this is not always true.[29] In fact, massive hemorrhage has been reported during living donor liver transplantation.[30] Blood clotting factor and platelet therapy is guided by intraoperative need and an inspection of the surgical field. For instance, platelets are infused when there is increased oozing and the count is below 50,000/μL and the international normalized ration (INR) is not increased. Thromboelastography is used in some institutions to guide factor and platelet therapy and to detect and treat fibrinolysis.[31]

## ANESTHESIA INDUCTION AND MAINTENANCE

Even though LDLRs are usually done electively and may be NPO, one should ascertain the need to do a rapid sequence induction to decrease the likelihood of aspiration. This should be determined during preoperative assessment. Successful inhalation induction with the application of cricoid pressure has been described in children receiving living related donor livers.[1] Because of the possibility of preexisting pulmonary shunting and the presence of ascites, functional residual capacity may be decreased in patients with ESLD,[34–37] and it may take longer to denitrogenate with oxygen. In children, sevoflurane may be used for induction because of better patient acceptance,[38] but because of its metabolism,[39] it should be replaced following induction with either desflurane or isoflurane. The latter two agents have been used in adults and children for many years at our institution for liver transplantation.[40,41] The choice of agent for intravenous induction will depend on the preoperative status of the patient. In most instances, propofol or thiopental are well tolerated. Succinylcholine may be used for rapid sequence induction. The same may be achieved with nondepolarizing drugs using a priming technique. Both cisatracurium and rocuronium have been used as satisfactory nondepolarizing muscle relaxants during the surgical procedure. Nitrous oxide is not recommended because of its bowel distending properties.[1] Fentanyl used either as an infusion or intermittently is the opioid of choice at our institution. Following successful induction and endotracheal intubation, controlled ventilation is instituted and the patient prepared with vascular access as illustrated in Figure 26.2-3. During placement of invasive and monitoring cannulae a sterile technique using a surgical drape and gown and glove is employed (see Figure 30.2-4).

## INTRAOPERATIVE CARE

Soon after induction and placement of invasive and vascular access cannulae, the patient is prepped and surgery begins with the dissection phase to allow the completion of native hepatectomy. This is followed by donor graft anastomosis that occurs during the anhepatic phase. After this, the donor graft is reperfused (reperfusion phase). The surgical team then completes the procedure by performing a biliary drainage procedure and then closing the abdomen. At our institution, the cardiopulmonary perfusionists are responsible for setting up the rapid infusion device system that is piggybacked into the venovenous bypass system as illustrated in Figure 30.2-3. The same system also has available a Cell-Saver® (Hemonetics Laboratories, Boston, MA) that allows for washing of both bank and salvaged blood for rapid infusion when needed. Listed in Table 30.2-3 are details about intraoperative care. During surgery arterial blood gases, electrolytes (Na$^+$, K$^+$, and ionized Ca$^{2+}$), glucose, hemoglobin,

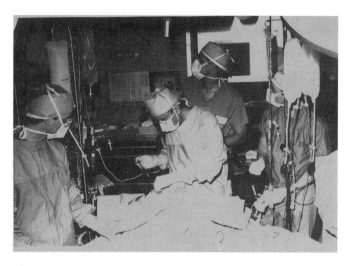

**FIGURE 30.2-4**

A sterile technique using surgical preparation, gown and glove are used for placement of invasive and vascular access cannulae during the preparation of liver recipients.

and lactate should be monitored at least hourly. Coagulation parameters such as INR, PT, PTT, fibrinogen, and platelet count or thromboelastography should be utilized as needed to guide correction of coagulopathy.

## EMERGENCY AND POSTOPERATIVE CONSIDERATIONS

At our institution, postoperatively, patients are transferred directly to the intensive care unit (ICU). This is done after removal of the large right-sided internal jugular and femoral vein catheter. Many of the LDLRs can be extubated within a few hours. This is dependent on their preoperative status and intraoperative course. Criteria for early extubation have been described and include good donor liver function, < 10 U packed red blood cells administered, hemodynamic stability, and alveolar-arterial oxygen gradient < 200 mm Hg.[42] In a prospective, randomized, double-blind, placebo-controlled clinical trial, Ponnudurai et al found that the use of an adjuvant vasopressor, together with controlled fluid administration, to maintain a stable hemodynamic status reduces the need for endotracheal reintubation and its associated morbidities in the postoperative period.[43] Postoperative pulmonary hypertension may occur; however, interestingly moderate postoperative pulmonary hypertension is not associated with increased morbidity.[44] Major postoperative problems include graft vessel thrombosis, bile leak, sepsis, and rarely graft dysfunction.[28] Graft vessel thrombosis is more likely following living versus cadaveric whole liver donor transplantation because of smaller vessels.[45] This may require percutaneous removal and placement of an expandable metallic stent.[45] Another problem that can arise is small-for-size graft syndrome.[46] This is a dreaded complication generally associated with a ratio of graft to recipient body weight of less than 0.8% which manifests as a progressive increase in intracellular cholestasis, coagulopathy, and ascites.[46] Patients with small-for-size syndrome are at risk for developing acute hepatic insufficiency and are predisposed to infectious complications with a mortality rate near 50% at 4 to 6 weeks secondary to sepsis.[46] A graft-to-recipient body weight of 1.5% to 2% has been suggested as ideal for right lobe graft recipients.[46] Vessel thrombosis is more likely in smaller infants that are less than 9 kg.[28] Portal

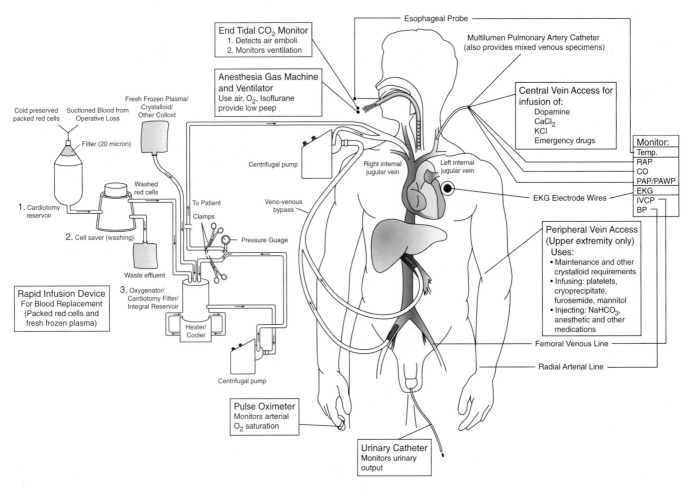

**FIGURE 30.2-3**

Diagram showing preparation of the adult living donor liver recipient. The right internal jugular canula serves as a port for rapid fluid infusion and also for venovenous and portovenous bypass. The femoral venous catheter serves to monitor inferior vena cava pressure (IVCP) and helps monitor renal perfusion pressure (mean BP less IVCP). Because venovenous and portovenous bypass is not used in children, the large right-sided internal jugular canula is not used. Instead a tunneled large double-lumen central venous catheter (Hickman) is placed either via the internal jugular or via the subclavian vein. This allows for rapid fluid replacement, measurement of CVP and blood sampling. (Reprinted from Fig. 2. Sketch of a typical patient undergoing liver transplantation in Anesthetic Principles for Organ Transplantation with permission from Raven Press, Ltd, New York)

**TABLE 30.2-3**

## SUMMARY OF INTRAOPERATIVE CARE DURING LIVER TRANSPLANTATION

| | |
|---|---|
| Dissection phase | This phase involves dissection and mobilization of the liver beginning with surgical incision and ending with cross clamping of the portal vein, supra and infrahepatic inferior vena cava, and the hepatic artery. Observe and treat hypotension during ascites drainage with colloid (FFP if coagulopathy present). Prior surgery in right upper quadrant may prolong this phase and increase bleeding. Glucose supplementation may be necessary in pediatric patients, patients with inborn errors of metabolism, and some patients with culminant hepatic failure. |
| Anhepatic phase | Begins with cross-clamping of vascular inflow to the liver and ends with reperfusion of the new liver graft. Suprahepatic and infrahepatic vena cava cross-clamping decreases venous return significantly and can lead to severe hemodynamic instability. A reduction in cardiac output of greater than 50% is associated with increased morbidity and mortality. At most centers, hemodynamic instability following test clamping of the inferior vena cava is the most common indication for initiating venovenous bypass. Advantages of using venovenous bypass include maintenance of intraoperative renal function, reduced hemodynamic instability, and possibly reduction of blood loss and facilitation of surgery. There is also a theoretical advantage in patients with pulmonary hypertension and cardiomyopathy who might tolerate the anhepatic stage poorly and in patients with acute fulminant failure by maintaining cerebral perfusion pressure by avoiding rapid swings in blood pressure. Disadvantages include possible air embolism, clot formation and thromboembolization, and inadvertent decannulation. |

Considerable variability exists between transplant centers with regards to utilization of venovenous bypass. Alternatively, use of the "piggyback" technique, with inferior vena cava preservation or cavaplasty technique combined with surgical experience and shorter surgery duration has decreased the need for venovenous bypass. Cardiac output and mean systolic pressure decline significantly without venous bypass, but cardiac output is usually still adequate as patients usually have a hyperdynamic circulation with a higher than normal cardiac output. Attempting to return cardiac output to preclamping levels with fluid boluses is not recommended and can lead to fluid overload and subsequent venous congestion of the new liver graft. Adjuvant use of vasopressor with moderate fluid boluses to maintain stable hemodynamics at greater than eighty percent of preoperative values decreases the need for postoperative endotracheal reintubation.

Coagulopathy may worsen during this phase due to continued blood loss from adhesions and collateral vessels, continued blood replacement, absence of hepatic clotting factor production. Fibrinolysis can occur due to increased intravascular release or decreased hepatic clearance of tissue-type plasminogen activator, and absence of liver-synthesized plasminogen activator inhibitor. Antifibrinolytic use varies significantly among centers.

Several metabolic changes occur during the anhepatic phase. Metabolic acidosis, which often contributes to myocardial depression, occurs as a result of accumulation of lactic acid and other endogenous organic acids normally metabolized to carbon dioxide and water by the liver. Plasma potassium levels frequently elevate as a result of anemia, reduced urine output, and potassium load from blood products. Citrate present in blood products chelates calcium and reduces ionized calcium levels. Magnesium levels also decline. Blood glucose may decline secondary to absence of liver gluconeogenesis and glucose supplementation may be necessary particularly in pediatric patients.

**Reperfusion neohepatic phase**

The neohepatic stage begins with reperfusion of the new liver graft after preservative solution is removed by flushing. The liver may be flushed with blood, colloid, or crystalloid.[a] A variety of techniques exist to accomplish flushing of the new graft. Millis and colleagues, in a randomized controlled study concluded portal vein flush without vena caval venting provided a lower incidence of postreperfusion syndrome, and vena caval venting decreased the release of potassium into the circulation.

Reperfusion is associated with an increase in preload, decreased systemic vascular resistance and blood pressure, and an increase in potassium and hydrogen ion concentrations. Preemptive administration of calcium to correct hypocalcemia; sodium bicarbonate, tris-hydroxymethyl aminomethane (THAM), or dichloroacetate to modify pH; and inotropes or vasopressor to optimize circulation should be considered. Hyperkalemia may be severe and even life threatening; EKG changes require immediate treatment with calcium chloride and sodium bicarbonate, and as time permits insulin and albuterol. Intraoperative dialysis may need to be performed in select situations and should be available intraoperatively if needed. Supraventricular or ventricular arrhythmias including ventricular tachycardia and ventricular fibrillation may occur and require prompt cardioversion (at our institution we routinely place R2 pads before surgical incision). Elevated pulmonary artery pressures and even right heart failure can occur. Rarely, pulmonary embolization of air or thrombus can further cause difficulties with patient management.

A Roux-en-Y biliary anastomosis is usually performed because of limited ductal structures available.

---

[a]Ring et al. recently report using histidine-tryptophan-ketoglutarate (HTK) solution in living related liver transplantation citing potential advantages of HTK in comparison to other preservative solutions to be low potassium concentration, low viscosity, no particles, in situ perfusion, no need to flush before perfusion, improved biliary protection, better recovery of microcirculatory changes, ready to use, and lower costs.

---

vein thrombosis is a late complication of liver transplantation which occurs at a higher rate in pediatric patients.[47]

## SUMMARY AND CONCLUSIONS

Anesthesia care for living donor liver transplant recipients requires a thorough assessment of the patient. The co-morbid conditions of the living donor liver recipients should be optimized when possible. Careful planning and coordination between the anesthesia, medical, and surgical teams preoperatively, intraoperatively, and postoperatively is essential to a good outcome for both the recipient and donor.

## ACKNOWLEDGMENTS

This work was supported in part by Health Resources and Services Administration Contract 231-00-0015. The content is the responsibility of the authors alone and does not necessarily reflect the views or policies of the Department of Health and Human Services, nor does mention of trade names, commercial products, or organizations imply endorsement by the U.S. Government.

## References

1. Djurberg H, et al. Anesthesia care for living-related liver transplantation for infants and children with end-stage liver disease: report of our initial experience. *J Clin Anesth* 2002;14(8): 564–570.

2. Niemann CU, et al. Intraoperative fluid management of living donor versus cadaveric liver transplant recipients. *Transplant Proc,* 2004;36(5): 1466–1468.

3. Steadman R H. Anesthesia for liver transplant surgery. *Anesthesiol Clin North Am* 2004; 22(4): 687–711.

4. Marcos A, et al. Emergency adult to adult living donor liver transplantation for fulminant hepatic failure. *Transplantation* 2000;69(10): 2202–2205.

5. Liu H, Lee SS. Cardiopulmonary dysfunction in cirrhosis. *J Gastroenterol Hepatol,* 1999;14(6): 600–608.

6. de la Morena G, et al. Ventricular function during liver reperfusion in hepatic transplantation. A transesophageal echocardiographic study. *Transplantation* 1994;58(3): 306–310.

7. Lim YC, et al. Intraoperative transesophageal echocardiography in orthotopic liver transplantation in a patient with hypertrophic cardiomyopathy. *J Clin Anesth* 1995;7(3): 245–249.

8. Steltzer H, et al. Two-dimensional transesophageal echocardiography in early diagnosis and treatment of hemodynamic disturbances during liver transplantation. *Transplant Proc* 1991;23(3): 1957–1958.

9. Suriani RJ, et al. Intraoperative transesophageal echocardiography during liver transplantation. *J Cardiothorac Vasc Anesth* 1996;10(6): 699–707.

10. Hofer CK, et al. Therapeutic impact of intra-operative transoesophageal echocardiography during noncardiac surgery. *Anaesthesia* 2004; 59(1):3–9.

11. Sharma A, Pagel PS, Bhatia A. Intraoperative iatrogenic acute pericardial tamponade: use of rescue transesophageal echocardiography in a patient undergoing orthotopic liver transplantation. *J Cardiothorac Vasc Anesth* 2005;19(3): 364–366.

12. Cywinski JB, et al. Dynamic left ventricular outflow tract obstruction in an orthotopic liver transplant recipient. *Liver Transpl*, 2005;11(6):692–695.

13. Neelakanta G, Mahajan A, Antin C. Systemic vasodilation is a predominant cause of hypotension in a patient with familial amyloid polyneuropathy during liver transplantation. *J Clin Anesth* 2005;17(3): 202–204.

14. Prediletto R , et al. Role of the chest radiograph in the preoperative assessment of the pulmonary function in patients with cirrhosis candidates to liver transplant. *Radiol Med (Torino)* 2004;108(4): 320–334.

15. Starkel P, et al. Outcome of liver transplantation for patients with pulmonary hypertension. *Liver Transpl* 2002;8(4): 382–388.

16. McGilvray ID, Greig PD. Critical care of the liver transplant patient: an update. *Curr Opin Crit Care* 2002;8(2): 178–182.

17. Lamps LW, et al. Pulmonary vascular morphological changes in cirrhotic patients undergoing liver transplantation. *Liver Transpl Surg* 1999;5(1): 57–64.

18. Gillies BS, Perkins JD, Cheney FW. Abdominal aortic compression to treat circulatory collapse caused by severe pulmonary hypertension during liver transplantation. *Anesthesiology* 1996;85(2): 420–422.

19. Ramsay MA, et al. Nitric oxide does not reverse pulmonary hypertension associated with end-stage liver disease: a preliminary report. *Hepatology* 1997;25(3): 24–27.

20. Kaspar MD, et al. Severe pulmonary hypertension and amelioration of hepatopulmonary syndrome after liver transplantation. *Liver Transpl Surg* 1998;4(2): 77–79.

21. Csete M.: Intraoperative management of liver transplant patients with pulmonary hypertension. *Liver Transpl Surg* 1997;3(4): 454–455.

22. Akinci SB, et al. Cardiac tamponade in an orthotopic liver recipient with pulmonary hypertension. *Crit Care Med* 2002;30(3): 699–701.

23. De Wolf AM, et al. Hemodynamic effects of inhaled nitric oxide in four patients with severe liver disease and pulmonary hypertension. *Liver Transpl Surg* 1997;3(6): 594–597.

24. Mandell MS, Duke J. Nitric oxide reduces pulmonary hypertension during hepatic transplantation. *Anesthesiology* 1994;81(6): 1538–1542.

25. Plotkin JS, et al. Successful use of chronic epoprostenol as a bridge to liver transplantation in severe portopulmonary hypertension. *Transplantation* 1998;65(4):457–459.

26. Swanson KL, Krowka MJ. Arterial oxygenation associated with portopulmonary hypertension. *Chest* 2002;121(6): 1869–1875.

27. Tuman KJ, et al. Effects of continuous arteriovenous hemofiltration on cardiopulmonary abnormalities during anesthesia for orthotopic liver transplantation. *Anesth Analg* 1988; 67(4): 363–369.

28. Wagner C, et al. Living related liver transplantation in infants and children: report of anesthetic care and early postoperative morbidity and mortality. *J Clin Anesth* 2000;12(6): 454–459.

29. Ulukaya S, Acar L, Ayanoglu HO. Transfusion requirements during cadaveric and living donor pediatric liver transplantation. *Pediatr Transplant* 2005;9(3): 332–337.

30. Kaku R, et al. [Massive bleeding due to hyperfibrinolysis during living-related liver transplantation for terminal liver cirrhosis; report of two cases]. *Masui* 2003;52(11): 1195–1199.

31. Whitten CW, Greilich PE. Thromboelastography: past, present, and future. *Anesthesiology* 2000;92(5): 223–225.

32. Emre S, et al. Selective decontamination of the digestive tract helps prevent bacterial infections in the early postoperative period after liver transplant. *Mt Sinai J Med* 1999; 66(5–6): 310–313.

33. Muller CM, et al. Forced-air warming maintains normothermia during orthotopic liver transplantation. *Anaesthesia* 1995;50(3):229–232.

34. Greenough A, et al. Functional residual capacity related to hepatic disease. *Arch Dis Child* 1988;63(7):850–852.

35. Hourani JM, et al. Pulmonary dysfunction in advanced liver disease: frequent occurrence of an abnormal diffusing capacity. *Am J Med* 1991;90(6):693–700.

36. Krowka MJ, et al. Primary biliary cirrhosis: relation between hepatic function and pulmonary function in patients who never smoked. *Hepatology* 1991;13(6):1095–1100.

37. Mohamed R, et al. Pulmonary gas exchange abnormalities in liver transplant candidates. *Liver Transpl* 2002;8(9):802–808.

38. Green DW, Ashley EM. The choice of inhalation anaesthetic for major abdominal surgery in children with liver disease. *Paediatr Anaesth* 2002;12(8):665–673.

39. Van Obbergh LJ, et al. Extrahepatic metabolism of sevoflurane in children undergoing orthotopic liver transplantation. *Anesthesiology* 2000;92(3):683–686.

40. Zaleski L, Abello D, Gold MI. Desflurane versus isoflurane in patients with chronic hepatic and renal disease. *Anesth Analg* 1993;76(2): 353–356.

41. Weiskopf RB, et al. Desflurane does not produce hepatic or renal injury in human volunteers. *Anesth Analg*, 1992. 74(4): p. 570–4.

42. Cammu G, et al. Criteria for immediate postoperative extubation in adult recipients following living-related liver transplantation with total intravenous anesthesia. *J Clin Anesth* 2003;15(7): 515–519.

43. Ponnudurai RN, et al. Vasopressor administration during liver transplant surgery and its effect on endotracheal reintubation rate in the postoperative period: a prospective, randomized, double-blind, placebo-controlled trial. *Clin Ther* 2005;27(2): 92–98.

44. Veloso CA, et al. Retrospective analysis of patients who developed pulmonary hypertension during the early postoperative period after liver transplantation. *Transplant Proc* 2004;36(4): 938–940.

45. Yamagiwa K, et al. Intrahepatic hepatic vein stenosis after living-related liver transplantation treated by insertion of an expandable metallic stent. *Am J Transplant* 2004;4(6): 1006–1009.

46. Heaton N: Small-for-size liver syndrome after auxiliary and split liver transplantation: donor selection. *Liver Transpl* 2003;9(9):S26–S28.

47. Ueda M, et al. Portal vein complications in the long-term course after pediatric living donor liver transplantation. *Transplant Proc* 2005;37(2):1138–1140.

48. Veroli P, el Hage C, Ecoffey C. Does adult liver transplantation without venovenous bypass result in renal failure? *Anesth Analg* 1992;75(4): 489–494.

49. Grande L, et al. Effect of venovenous bypass on perioperative renal function in liver transplantation: results of a randomized, controlled trial. *Hepatology* 1996;23(6):1418–1428.

50. Chari RS, et al. Venovenous bypass in adult orthotopic liver transplantation: routine or selective use? *J Am Coll Surg* 1998;186(6): 683–690.

51. Shaw BW Jr, et al. Venous bypass in clinical liver transplantation. *Ann Surg* 1984;200(4): 524–534.

52. Reddy K, Mallett S, Peachey T. Venovenous bypass in orthotopic liver transplantation: Time for a rethink? *Liver Transpl* 2005;11(7):741–749.

53. Schumann R. Intraoperative resource utilization in anesthesia for liver transplantation in the United States: a survey. *Anesth Analg* 2003; 97(1): 21–28, table of contents.

54. Tzakis A, Todo S, Starzl TE. Orthotopic liver transplantation with preservation of the inferior vena cava. *Ann Surg* 1989;210(5): 649–652.

55. Wu YM, et al. Suprahepatic venacavaplasty (cavaplasty) with retrohepatic cava extension in liver transplantation: experience with first 115 cases. *Transplantation* 2001;72(8): 1389–1394.

56. Jovine E, et al. Piggy-back versus conventional technique in liver transplantation: report of a randomized trial. *Transpl Int* 1997;10(2): 109–112.

57. Wu Y, et al. Vasopressor agents without volume expansion as a safe alternative to venovenous bypass during cavaplasty liver transplantation. *Transplantation* 2003;76(12): 1724–1728.

58. Estrin JA, et al. Hemodynamic changes on clamping and unclamping of major vessels during liver transplantation. *Transplant Proc* 1989;21(2):3500–3505.

59. Dzik WH, et al. Fibrinolysis during liver transplantation in humans: role of tissue-type plasminogen activator. *Blood* 1988;71(4):1090–1095.

60. Bakker CM, et al. Increased fibrinolysis in orthotopic but not in heterotopic liver transplantation: the role of the anhepatic phase. *Transpl Int* 1992;5(Suppl 1): S173–S174.

61. Millis JM, et al. Randomized controlled trial to evaluate flush and reperfusion techniques in liver transplantation. *Transplantation* 1997;63(3):397–403.

62. Ringe B, et al. Safety and efficacy of living donor liver preservation with HTK solution. *Transplant Proc* 2005;37(1):316–319.

# 30.3 SURGICAL PROCEDURES

## 30.3.1a  Right Lobe Liver Transplant

*Rainer W.G. Gruessner, MD*

### INTRODUCTION

Refinements in the surgical techniques of liver resections and the evolution of reduced-size and split-liver transplants from deceased donors (DDs) have made the development of living donor (LD) liver transplantation possible[1–4] (Color Plates, Figure LI-1). The first LD liver transplant, using the left lateral segments (Couinaud segments 2 and 3) from an adult to a child, was reported in 1989;[5] the ethical justification and the technical success of this procedure resulted in its widespread application worldwide.[6–8] Subsequently, LD grafts were also used for adult recipients. The first LD liver transplant of the left lobe from an adult to an adult was reported in 1994.[9]

Because of concern about the magnitude of the donor operation (leaving only about 40% of liver tissue behind), removal of a full right lobe from an LD was initially not considered. In fact, the first successful transplant of an LD right lobe, reported in 1994,[10] was accidentally done—based on the intraoperative decision not to use the left lateral segments because of the presence of 2 separate, small segmental donor arteries. The recipient was a 9-year-old child. That accidental transplant of an LD right lobe demonstrated its technical feasibility with good donor and recipient outcome.

The first right-lobe liver transplant from an adult to an adult was not reported until 1997.[11] Of note, the use of the left lobe and the right lobe from an LD was first pioneered by Asian transplant centers. The initial lack of legalization of, and (ongoing) public reluctance to embrace, the brain death concept was the stimulus for liver transplant centers in Kyoto and Hong Kong to aggressively pursue the option of LD left-lobe and right-lobe grafts. The first LD right-lobe liver transplant in the United States was reported in 1998.[12]

Although the number of LD liver transplants in the United States initially increased to 500 per year, a widely publicized donor death in 2001 led to a decrease and to subsequent stabilization at about 300 LD liver transplants per year;[13–14] the donor's right lobe is now most commonly used for LD liver transplants.

The LD partial hepatectomy and the recipient operation are technically advanced procedures that require extensive experience in both hepatobiliary surgery and whole-liver transplants. To minimize donor morbidity and mortality, in the United States, the United Network for Organ Sharing (UNOS) has established minimum criteria for surgeons (20 major hepatic resections including seven live donor procedures within a 5-year period) to be qualified to perform such procedures (Attachment 1 to Appendix B of UNOS Bylaws[13]).

Transplanting the right lobe is now considered preferable over the left lobe by most liver transplant centers because of the right lobe's greater graft volume and, therefore, the reduced risk of small-for-size syndrome in the recipient. The generally accepted safe graft-to-recipient weight ratio (GRWR) is ≥ 0.8% or at least 45% of the recipient's liver volume, which has been estimated by several formulas.[15–16] Although successful LD liver transplants have been reported with significantly lower GRWR and ideal liver volume, the risk of developing small-for-size syndrome (characterized by allograft dysfunction, cholestasis, coagulopathy, and renal dysfunction) increases significantly with a GRWR < 0.8%.

As with DD liver transplants, optimal perioperative care of adult LD liver transplant recipients is crucial to achieve the best possible outcome. As mentioned in Chapter 30.2, the surgeon and the anesthesiologist should discuss, before the beginning of the transplant operation, strategies to minimize, and adequately substitute for, blood loss during the recipient hepatectomy. Adult recipients of an LD (vs DD) liver graft in the United States are generally not as critically ill (as evidenced by a lower average Model for End-Stage Liver Disease [MELD] score).[13] Nonetheless, the degree of portal hypertension is a crucial intraoperative risk factor for adult LD liver recipients. Consideration must also be given to optimal treatment of preexisting renal dysfunction (eg, perioperative dialysis) and pulmonary dysfunction (eg, perioperative treatment for pulmonary hypertension): either condition is associated with increased mortality. A good understanding of the essential teamwork between anesthesia and surgery staff provides a solid basis for successful outcomes in these challenging cases.

An important factor in LD liver transplants is the timing of the donor procedure in relation to the recipient procedure. Recipients with noncancerous disorders of the liver are usually brought to the operating room after the anatomy in the donor has been assessed and found to be suitable for donation. Liver recipients with cancerous lesions (in particular, patients with tumor stage ≥ T2) should undergo exploratory hepatectomy before the incision in the donor is made.[17] The recipient's abdomen should be explored through a relatively small right subcostal incision (without extension beyond the midline); specifically, the porta hepatis, the superior margin of the head of the pancreas, and the tissues adjacent to the suprarenal cava and aorta should be palpated for any suspicious lymph nodes. If enlarged lymph nodes are found, biopsies should be sent for frozen section. If metastatic spread is noted, the transplant must be aborted before the donor is anesthetized and an incision is made. If extrahepatic metastatic disease is excluded, the incision should be extended (see below) and the recipient operation should proceed.

In contrast to DD liver transplants, the technique of choice for the recipient hepatectomy in LD liver transplants is the piggyback (not the orthotopic) technique, as originally described by Calne[18] and later popularized by Tzakis.[19] The piggyback technique is necessary to preserve the continuity of the recipient's suprarenal abdominal vena cava (although the native cava can be replaced by DD cava/iliac vein). Also in contrast to DD liver transplants, the hilar structures of the LD liver recipient (in particular, the recipient bile ducts and hepatic arteries) should be individually ligated as high as possible; any accessory and replaced arteries should also be left as long as possible. Doing so usually allows for a variety of different reconstruction options because of the numerous variations in liver anatomy. Many centers prefer the use of portal bypass during the recipient procedure, or at least use it in selected recipients, to preserve hemodynamic stability and to prevent intestinal and pancreatic edema. The transplant procedure itself requires technical flexibility to accommodate the numerous anatomic variations of hepatic and portal veins, arteries, and bile ducts (Color Plates, Figures LI-2-5). To avoid the development of nonanatomic small-for-size graft syndrome, portal overflow and hepatic vein outflow obstruction must be prevented by surgical and/or pharmacologic means.

## OPERATIVE PROCEDURE

### Recipient Hepatectomy

The day before surgery, the recipient should undergo some form of bowel decontamination and cleaning. The function of the cirrhotic liver should be assessed by both the surgeon and the anesthesiologist, in order to optimize the peritransplant care of the recipient.

On the day of surgery, the recipient is placed on the operating table in a supine position. After induction of general endotracheal anesthesia, appropriate lines are placed by the anesthesia team (see Chapter 30.2); they usually include a central vein or Swan-Ganz catheter, infrarenal caval line, arterial line, large-bore central line for rapid transfusion (during flushing of the donor graft), Foley catheter, and nasogastric tube. Antibiotics are given prophylactically (and repeated every 4 hours during the course of the procedure). Sequential compression devices and a warming blanket are used. Blood products and coagulation-modifying drugs are administered as needed throughout the procedure. The anesthesiologic team usually requires 60 to 90 minutes of preparation before the incision is made.

The abdomen is prepped and draped in standard fashion. A bilateral subcostal incision, with less extension to the left than to the right side and with a midline extension toward the xiphoid, is made. Electrocautery is used to divide the subcutaneous tissue and to extend the incision through the fascia. Already at this point, the degree of portal hypertension and bleeding can be appreciated: the recipient may need to be started on platelet transfusions, fresh frozen plasma (FFP), cryoprecipitate, and/or aprotinin. The abdomen is entered by ligating and dividing the falciform and teres ligaments; most commonly, ascites is suctioned first. The incision is then completed and the abdomen explored for any other nonhepatic pathologies. Adhesions (quite common after a previous cholecystectomy or other types of upper abdominal surgery) are taken down between the liver and the stomach, colon, and duodenum.

The falciform ligament is taken down to the level of the hepatic veins. The retractors are then placed to provide optimal exposure of the liver. The ribcages are retracted in a cephalad direction; the stomach, duodenum, and transverse colon, in a caudad direction. Doing so facilitates complete exposure of the liver (Figures 30.3.1a-1, 30.3.1a-2). The left triangular ligament is divided using electrocautery to mobilize the left lobe of the liver; likewise, the right triangular ligament and the peritoneal attachments on the right lobe of the liver are divided (Color Plates, Figure LI-9). Thus, both lobes are dissected off the diaphragm, and prominent diaphragmatic veins are ligated and divided. The hepatic veins are identified. Overlying attachments with the diaphragm are taken down.

The gastrohepatic ligament is opened toward the left hepatic vein and the porta hepatis. If an accessory or replaced left hepatic artery is found, the vessel is ligated and divided close to the liver (leaving it as long as possible, so that it can be used for arterial reconstruction, if necessary).

The porta hepatis is addressed next. The right and left hepatic arteries are identified high in the hilum (Figure 30.3.1a-3). Dissection between the right hepatic artery and the bile duct(s) is kept to a minimum, in order to decrease the risk of distal bile duct ischemia. The left and right hepatic arteries are separately ligated with 2-0 or 3-0 nonabsorbable sutures and, as mentioned, ligated and divided as high in the hilum as possible (Color Plates, Figure LI-8A). The hepatic arteries are then freed, back to the

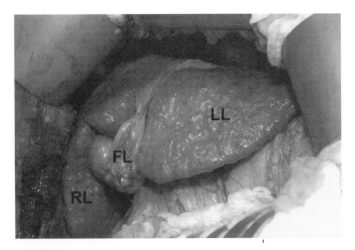

**FIGURE 30.3.1a-1**

The native, cirrhotic liver is exposed; the falciform ligament (FL) is divided (RL, right lobe; LL, Left lobe).

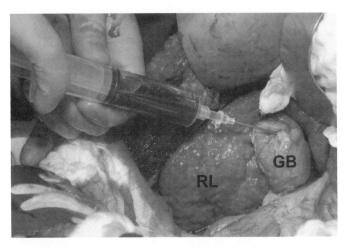

**FIGURE 30.3.1a-2**

The gallbladder (GB) is decompressed to facilitate the hilar dissection (RL, right lobe).

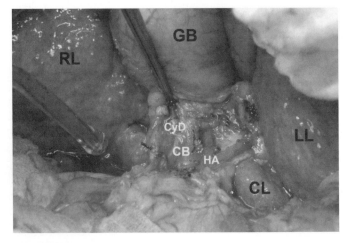

**FIGURE 30.3.1a-3**

The common bile duct (CD) is exposed, the cystic duct (CyD) is ligated and divided; the proper hepatic artery (HA) with its bifurcation is dissected free (RL, right lobe; LL, left lobe; CL, caudate lobe; GB, gallbladder).

bifurcation of the proper hepatic artery (after ligating and dividing the cystic artery off the right hepatic artery). The left and right hepatic arteries as well as the proper hepatic artery are then circumferentially dissected free from the surrounding tissues, but dissection close to the bile duct(s) is avoided. Vascular dissection may continue, following down to the takeoff of the gastroduodenal artery. During this dissection, the right gastric artery can also be identified, ligated, and divided. Overlying nerval and lymphatic tissues, as well as lymph nodes adjacent to the arteries, are ligated and divided, which frequently results in exposure of the medial aspect of the portal vein.

The cystic duct is then identified, ligated, and divided close to the neck of the gallbladder (the purpose being to preserve as much length as possible in case it will be needed for biliary reconstruction). The common bile duct is now in view. It is traced high up in the hilum, if possible, above the bifurcation of the right and left hepatic bile ducts in the hilar plate (Color Plates, Figure LI-10A). During dissection of the bile duct(s), it is important to preserve the periductal connective tissue encompassing the axial periductal microcirculation. The axial blood supply of the common bile duct is provided mainly by branches of the superior posterior pancreaticoduodenal artery (a branch of the gastroduodenal artery) and the right hepatic artery;[19-25] these branches ascend along the lateral and medial margins (at 3 and 9 o'clock) and the posterior wall (6 o'clock) of the common bile duct. Obviously, minimal dissection of the bile ducts avoids skeletonization and impaired blood supply. Several groups have described techniques that preserve the entire hilar plate with as many proximal biliary duct bifurcations as possible (at least all second-order branches to maximize the anastomotic options).[20,21] This type of dissection is started at the top of the hilar plate and leaves the common bile duct and the main hepatic ducts untouched, thus resulting in optimal preservation of the axial blood supply. Moreover, a dissection between the common bile duct and the right hepatic artery is avoided.[21] To preserve the blood supply to the bile ducts, only sharp dissection (and no electrocautery) is used; the viability of the bile duct after transection can be confirmed by the presence of pulsatile arterial bleeding from the cut ends.[21]

Lee et al. described a Glissonian dissection technique, at the high hilar level, called high hilar dissection (HHD). It involves total occlusion of the hepatoduodenal ligament with a tourniquet and blunt high hilar plate dissection with a scissors or suction tip. The Glissonian pedicles are cut intrahepatically at the third level of pedicles or beyond.[22] After removal of the liver, the portal vein and the hepatic artery are isolated from the hepatoduodenal ligament and transected separately with vascular clamps. After adequate bile ducts for anastomosis are selected, bleeding vessels and unnecessary bile ducts at the end of the hilar plate are sutured continuously with 5-0 nonabsorbable sutures.

The hilar plexus, which consists of collateral vessels that bridge the left and right hepatic arteries, is found on the inferior aspect of the hilar plate; blood supply to the right hepatic duct and right sectoral ducts arises from both the right hepatic artery and the hilar plexus.[22-26] For that reason, Lee et al. prefer the left (over the right) hepatic artery for arterial anastomosis, in order to fully preserve the right hepatic artery's blood supply into the hilar plate.[26] One potential concern of the HHD technique is that dissection deep in the hilar plate might miss tiny caudate lobe branch openings and account for early bile leakage.

If the proximal bile ducts cannot be individually transected in the hilar plate (or should not be used for anastomosis, for example, in patients with sclerosing cholangitis), the common

bile duct is circumferentially dissected free from surrounding tissues and distally ligated with one 0-nonabsorbable sutures and divided (Figure 30.3.1a-3 and Color Plates, Figure LI-10B). The (venous) blood vessels next to the common bile duct (usually at 3 and 9 o'clock) are ligated with 5-0 absorbable sutures.

The last structure in the hilum to be identified is the portal vein. All surrounding tissues, including lymph nodes, are ligated and divided. The portal vein is then circumferentially mobilized and, if possible, traced toward and beyond the takeoff of the right and left portal vein branches; posterior and lateral branches to the caudate lobe may need to be ligated and divided for complete mobilization. If the HHD technique is used, second-order branches, such as the right anterior and posterior portal vein branches, can also be preserved and, thus, increase the variability of anastomotic options if more than one portal vein anastomosis needs to be constructed. Regardless of the extent of the proximal dissection, the portal vein is fully mobilized all the way down to the superior margin of the head of the pancreas. If an accessory or replaced right hepatic artery laterally to the portal vein is noted at this point, it should be ligated and divided close to the liver to leave it as long as possible (so that it can be used, if necessary, for the arterial reconstruction).

The recipient can now be placed on portal bypass (if this option is chosen for the remainder of the hepatectomy). Alternatively, the recipient infra- and suprahepatic vena cava is isolated and encircled with vessel loops and the retrohepatic veins are ligated and divided (Color Plates, Figure LI-9) in the presence of portal flow to the liver (thus avoiding portal bypass). If portal bypass is used, the distal portal vein is clamped with a Bainbridge vascular clamp (Teleflex Medical, Pilling Weck Division, Research Triangle Park, NC; Figure 30.3.1a-4). Nonabsorbable 0-silk sutures are used either to ligate the main trunk of the portal vein close to the liver or, preferentially, to separately ligate the right and left portal vein branches (or second-order branches if dissection was carried out more proximally). The portal vein, or the left and right branches, is then divided below the ligated sutures.

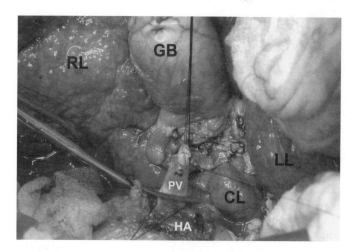

**FIGURE 30.3.1a-4**

The distal portal vein (PV) is suture ligated, the anterior wall close to the portal vein bifurcation is opened, and two 4-0 Prolene stay sutures are placed (the posterior wall will be transected next). A Bainbridge clamp is placed on the proximal portal vein at the level of the superior margin of the pancreas, and an 0-silk tie is placed around the proximal portal vein to hold the portal vein cannula in position (RL, right lobe; LL, left lobe; CL, caudate lobe; GB, gallbladder; HA, hepatic artery).

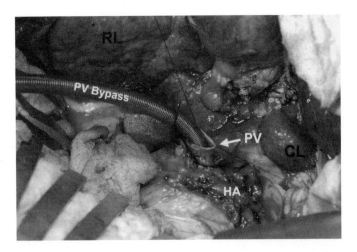

**FIGURE 30.3.1a-5**

A cannula is placed in the proximal portal vein (PV) and secured with a silk tie. The two 4-0 Prolene stay stitches are kept in place for traction (RL, right lobe; CL, caudate lobe).

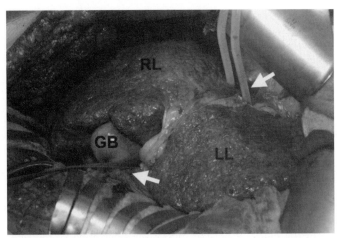

**FIGURE 30.3.1a-6**

The infra- and suprahepatic portions of the vena cava are encircled and looped (white arrows) as a safety measure before ligating and dividing the main hepatic and retrohepatic veins (piggyback technique) (RL, right lobe; LL, left lobe; GB, gallbladder).

The portal vein stump above the Bainbridge clamp (3 to 5 cm in length) is flushed with heparinized saline. Two 4-0 nonabsorbable stay sutures are used for traction on the transected portal vein stump(s) (at 3 and 9 o'clock) to facilitate placement of the cannula into the portal vein. Before the Bainbridge vascular clamp is removed, one 0-nonabsorbable suture is placed below it, and the Bainbridge clamp is removed. Usually a 24-French cannula is then placed in the portal vein and secured with the 0-nonabsorbable suture. After successful cannulation, the recipient goes on portal bypass (Figure 30.3.1a-5). A flow rate between 750 and 1,500 mL/min can easily be achieved; if the portal vein pressure is not determined, the bypass flow rate allows assessment of portal inflow. To decrease portal or mesenteric flow, octreotide, a somatostatin analog, may be started at this point.

The retractors below the liver are now repositioned: the stomach, duodenum, transverse colon, and ligated hilar structures are pulled in a caudad direction. Doing so opens up the space that is needed for mobilizing the infrahepatic vena cava. The peritoneum overlying the anterior surface of the vena cava is incised with electrocautery. The infrahepatic, suprarenal vena cava is then circumferentially freed up by blunt and sharp dissection; a vessel loop is placed around it for vascular control. After encircling the cava, the peritoneal attachments on the medial edge of the vena cava are divided, using the cautery along the caudate lobe all the way up to the origin of the left hepatic vein. In a similar fashion, the lateral peritoneal attachments overlying the vena cava are taken down, and the right adrenal vein is ligated and divided. Mobilization of the medial and lateral aspects of the vena cava usually results in circumferential mobilization of the full length of the retrohepatic cava, providing infra- and suprahepatic control in case of bleeding (Figure 30.3.1a-6).

Next, the right (or, if technically easier, the left) lobe of the liver is peeled off the cava by ligating and dividing all retrohepatic veins entering the vena cava (Color Plates, Figure LI-11). This dissection can be tedious (Figures 30.3.1a-7 and 30.3.1a-8). If brisk bleeding occurs, the infrarenal (and/or suprarenal) cava may need to be clamped, in order to control the bleeding source with suture ligation. Once all retrohepatic veins are divided, the liver is attached only by the hepatic vein pedicles. Depending on the anatomy, the hepatic veins are then individually mobilized

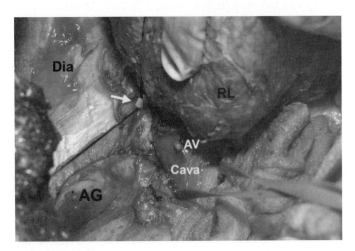

**FIGURE 30.3.1a-7**

The right lobe (RL) is retracted medially and cranially and the retrohepatic veins on the right side of the vena cava are individually ligated and divided, as is the right adrenal vein (AV). The infrahepatic/suprarenal vena cava is looped. The right hepatic vein is not yet exposed (Dia, diaphragm; AG, adrenal gland).

and stapled across with the endovascular stapler (Endopath®; ETS/FLEX/Endoscopic articulating linear cutter; Ethicon Endo-Surgery Inc., Cincinnati, OH; Figure 30.3.1a-9). Three loads of staples are used if all 3 veins need to be transected separately; two loads, if the middle and left vein are on a common trunk. At the completion of the hepatic vein division, the liver is free and passed out of the field. The piggyback technique leaves the inferior vena cava intact and hemostasis is obtained (Color Plates, Figure LI-12; Figure 30.3.1a-10).

I personally prefer the use of portal bypass. I usually do not use systemic bypass, because the piggyback technique allows partial clamping of the vena cava with a side-biting clamp; thus, little change in infrarenal vena cava pressure is observed. A partial bypass diminishes some of the complications seen with both portal and

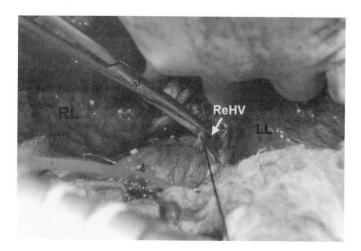

**FIGURE 30.3.1a-8**

The left lobe (LL) of the liver is retracted laterally and cranially. Retrohepatic veins (ReHV) from the left (LL) and caudate lobes (CL) are individually ligated and divided. The infrahepatic vena cava is looped.

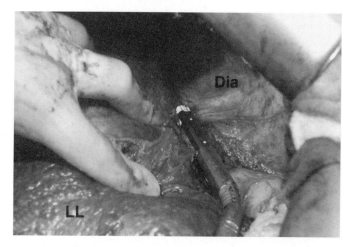

**FIGURE 30.3.1a-9**

The left and middle hepatic veins are stapled across with an endovascular 35-mm GIA stapler. The liver is pushed distally to open the space between the liver and the suprahepatic cava (Dia, diaphragm; LL, left lobe).

systemic bypass, such as pulmonary air embolism, hemolysis, fibrinolysis, and platelet trapping.[17,27,28] Most recipients tolerate portal clamping without hemodynamic instability, and construction of hepatic and portal vein anastomoses requires less than 60 minutes; therefore, portal bypass is used by many centers only in selected recipients. If portal bypass is not used, the hepatectomy is performed in a way that maintains portal flow as long as possible, in order to decrease portal clamp time and, thus, intestinal and pancreatic edema. Doing so requires full mobilization of the liver until only the portal vein and one of the hepatic veins are left intact.

Shortly before the native liver is passed out of the field, word is given to the donor team to proceed with removal of the donor graft. Communication with the donor team is important throughout the recipient procedure. If the middle hepatic vein is not retained with the graft, large segment 5 or segment 8 vein(s) may require separate implantation into the recipient cava. In those circumstances, while the recipient team is waiting to receive the

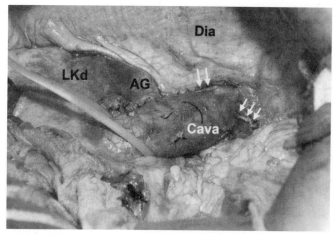

**FIGURE 30.3.1a.10**

Completion of the piggyback technique with removal of the native liver. The white arrows depict the staple line of the right as well as the left and middle hepatic veins. All retrohepatic veins are ligated. A vessel loop is placed around the cava (Dia, diaphragm; AG, adrenal gland; LKd, left kidney).

donor graft, an autologous vessel graft (eg, saphenous vein, inferior mesenteric vein, internal iliac artery) can be retrieved. If a saphenous vein graft is used, a groin incision in the recipient is made (most commonly on the left side, because the right side is usually used for placement of the infrarenal vena cava catheter). The incision is carried down to the saphenous vein. Once the vessel is identified, it is dissected for about 8 to 12 cm distal to the saphenofemoral junction. A clamp is placed at the saphenofemoral junction and distally on the saphenous vein. The vein is divided proximally and distally. The segment of saphenous vein is stored in heparinized saline. The saphenofemoral junction is oversewn using 5-0 nonabsorbable sutures. Care is taken not to cause any narrowing of the common femoral vein. The distal stump of the saphenous vein is ligated. A segment of saphenous vein can also be retrieved by one surgeon while the other surgeon is starting the bench work. As mentioned above, another important aspect during the recipient hepatectomy is ongoing assessment of the splanchnic flow, specifically at the beginning of the recipient hepatectomy, at the time of initiating portal bypass flow, and during the anhepatic phase. Assessment includes monitoring cardiac index and portal flow through the bypass machine. If the recipient is not placed on portal bypass, placing a cannula via the inferior mesenteric vein into the portal vein can help the surgeon assess the portal blood pressure. The need for surgical or pharmacologic inflow modifications can, therefore, be assessed before the graft is implanted.

## Bench Work on the Back Table

Once the donor graft is removed, it is weighed to determine the true GRWR. It is then brought to the back table (preferably in the recipient room) for flushing with University of Wisconsin (UW) (Via Span, Duramed Pharmaceuticals, Inc., subsidiary of Barr Pharmaceuticals, Inc., Pomona, NY) or histidine-tryptophane-ketoglutarate (HTK; Custodial, Odyssey Pharmaceuticals, Inc., East Hanover, NJ) preservation solution (4°C). A basin is partly filled with ice. An open bag filled with chilled preservation solution is placed in the basin so that the graft is submerged. The right lobe is flushed through the stump of the right portal veins(s) with 500 to 800 mL of preservation solution, until the effluent from the right hepatic vein is clear. The right hepatic artery is carefully dilated with a small clamp and flushed with 20 to 50 mL mL of preservation solution, until clear effluent emerges from the right hepatic or portal vein. The remaining preservation solution can be used to flush the bile duct(s) clean.

In preparation for graft implantation, vascular reconstruction may be required. Tributaries of the donor middle hepatic vein may require extension(s) with an autologous (saphenous) vein graft(s); the right hepatic vein may require a venoplasty using an autologous (portal) vein graft. If two right hepatic veins are present, and if they are not too far apart, they can be sewn together in the middle (see below; Color Plates, Figure LI-18B). If two portal vein orifices are present (right anterior and posterior branches), and if they are not too far apart, they can be sewn together in the middle; alternatively, a venous Y-graft (of autologous portal vein branches from the recipient's resected native liver) can be used. Likewise, if two arteries are present, arterial reconstruction (eg, extension or Y-graft) can be performed using auto- or allograft(s) (see below).

The liver's cut surface is inspected. Leaks that were identified during flushing are individually oversewn. The orifices of the bile duct(s), if they are not too far apart, can be sewn together in the middle; they can also be incised to create a larger anastomosis. If the graft is not immediately transplanted, it is submerged in the preservation solution and packed on ice. Once the recipient hepatectomy is completed, the donor graft is brought onto the table for implantation.

## Graft Implantation (Color Plates, Figures LI- 13 and 14)

### Caval Anastomosis

Optimal venous outflow is critical for the success of an LD liver transplant. A great deal of consideration must be given to correctly aligning the right-lobe graft, so that the right hepatic vein is orthotopically oriented. A side-biting clamp is placed on the anterolateral wall of the recipient vena cava, encompassing the stapled end of the native right hepatic vein (which usually runs in an oblique or vertical direction), and about 3 cm of anterolateral cava distal to the end of the staple line (Figure 30.3.1a-11).

For construction of the hepatocaval anastomosis, the staple line can be removed and the venotomy enlarged horizontally (Color Plates, Figure LI-17 and LI-18A). Alternatively, a venotomy can be made along the anterolateral wall of the cava, midway and medial to the stapled end of the right hepatic vein with distal extension (Figure 30.3.1a-11). Personally, I prefer creating a new venotomy using the orifice of the native right hepatic vein. The orifice frequently does not represent the optimal location (too cranial and too lateral); it may lead to subsequent obstruction, because liver regeneration causes the right lobe to axially rotate from right to left.[17] Whatever location is chosen, the venotomy should optimally accommodate the final lay of the donor right lobe, and the venous anastomosis must be in orthotopic position, in order to diminish the risk of outflow obstruction. Also, to assure proper positioning, the caval groove located posteriorly and inferiorly along the medial aspect of the right lobe can be used for optimal alignment.[17] The donor right hepatic vein should be short to avoid twisting or torsion, which could compromise venous outflow.

The most anterocranial point of the donor right hepatic vein is usually marked during the donor operation with a felt-tip pen

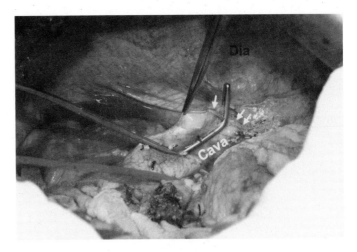

**FIGURE 30.3.1a-11**

A side-biting clamp is placed on the anterolateral wall of the vena cava for partial occlusion. Arrows depict the staple lines of the right hepatic vein, as well as of the stump of the right and middle hepatic vein trunk. An incision is made just distal to the recipient right hepatic vein stump; the cavotomy is made in anterolateral position. Holding stitches are placed (Dia, diaphragm).

or a suture, thereby facilitating proper alignment at the time of the hepatocaval anastomosis. Two 5-0 nonabsorbable sutures are placed at the proximal and distal corners of the venotomy. Two stitches are placed halfway between the two corner stitches on the anterior aspects of the venotomy edges, on both the donor and recipient side. The proximal corner suture is tied down, and the donor graft is lowered into the field. The posterior wall is usually sewn from the inside (from the proximal to the distal corner stitch, using one 5-0 nonabsorbable suture in running fashion). The suture is then brought outside and tied to the distal corner stitch (Figure 30.3.1a-12). In a similar fashion, the distal corner stitch is run toward the proximal corner stitch, but not yet tied, in order to allow venting of the liver on reperfusion.

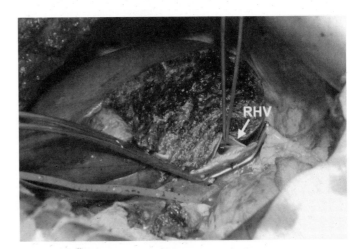

**FIGURE 30.3.1a-12**

The right donor lobe with its cut surface is shown. The posterior wall of the end-to-side anastomosis between the donor right hepatic vein (RHV) and the recipient cava is completed. The lumen of the donor right hepatic vein is shown. The anterior wall will be completed next, but will not yet be tied until after liver reperfusion and venting.

Controversy exists regarding whether to include the middle hepatic vein (MHV) with the right-lobe graft (see Chapters 29.3.1a and b; Color Plates, Figure LI-14). The main reason to include the MHV with the graft is optimal drainage of the anterior sector (Couinaud segments 5 and 8), thus avoiding venous congestion. Signs of poor venous outflow are usually evident immediately after reperfusion: segments 5 and 8 typically become swollen, turgid, and dusky-blue; even rupture has been described.[29,30] Poor venous outflow has been associated with increased sinusoidal pressure, disruption of sinusoidal epithelium, hepatic artery thrombosis, impaired liver regeneration, and dismal outcome.[29–33] Typically, restoration of the hepatic artery flow clears the dusky-blue discoloration, but such clearance cannot be interpreted as disappearance of congestion; rather, it represents adequate drainage of arterial blood via the right anterior portal vein.[34]

Because the MHV lies in the midplane of the liver, it drains not only segments 5 and 8 (the anterior sector of the right lobe) but also segment 4, where it typically originates. However, in about 30% of livers, the MHV originates in segment 5, indicating that segment 5 is the major portion of the right lobe.[34] Flow measurements by Cattral et al. demonstrated that the MHV can account for 25% to 30% of the total venous outflow of the graft.[29]

The MHV controversy has been addressed surgically in four different ways: (1) including the MHV with the right-lobe graft, (2) including the distal portion of the MHV (leaving the proximal remnant in the donor), (3) excluding the MHV, with separate caval anastomosis of the segmental vein(s), and (4) excluding the MHV, without separate caval anastomosis of the segmental vein(s).

Including the MHV in its entire length always poses the question of undue risk in the LD. Contraindications to including the MHV are a small predicted residual liver volume (< 30%) in the LD or anatomic circumstances that may increase the risk of injury to the left hepatic vein.[29] Obviously, if venous drainage from segments 5 and 8 is predominately via the right hepatic vein, including the MHV with the right-lobe graft is unnecessary. Proponents of including the entire MHV have also argued that ligating segment 4a and 4b tributaries has few consequences, with no adverse impact on early liver function test results or on long-term outcome in LDs, with sufficient residual liver volume.[29] Initially, preserving the MHV with the right-lobe graft was called the *extended right-lobe graft technique*—with the transection line about 1 cm to the left of the MHV, in order to provide adequate functional mass in case the LD was much smaller than the recipient. Subsequently, the name changed to *the right-lobe graft with MHV technique*, because the amount of segment 4 tissue included in the graft was insignificant.[34,35]

Procurement of the distal half of the MHV (draining segment 5) was proposed by Marcos et al.; the disadvantage of this technique is that segment 8 remains insufficiently drained.[34,36] The technique described by Cattral et al. preserves large segment 4a venous tributaries into the MHV in its most proximal portion; the MHV is divided at least 1 cm above its termination, avoiding risk of compromising the left hepatic vein. Revascularization of these foreshortened MHVs in the recipient usually requires an interposition graft.[29] Thus, determining the level of transection has become the center of discussion for proponents of preserving the MHV with the donor graft.

Either way, retaining the distal portion of the MHV with the graft and the proximal portion with the donor causes some degree of venous congestion in both. Removing the proximal MHV with the graft may compromise regeneration of segment 4; retaining the distal portion of the MHV in the donor may result in

some degree of small-for-size graft injury of the right posterior sector.[29,34] The small-for-size graft injury may also be due to the small size of venous collaterals, which do not fully open up within the first 7 posttransplant days.

Proponents of using a portion of the MHV (instead of reconstructing its lesser tributaries) argue that doing so is simpler and more straightforward, decreasing the risk of thrombosis as well as improving regeneration of the anterior sector.[38] Others have suggested that the lack of anterior sector regeneration is resolved by compensatory regeneration of the posterior sector and that graft congestion in the anterior segment does not affect overall graft regeneration, particularly if the GRWR is sufficient.[33,39]

If neither the entire MHV nor a portion is retained with the graft, an alternative is to restore drainage of the right anterior sector by venous jump grafts (Color Plates, Figure LI-13). Prominent segment 5 and 8 veins are anastomosed into the inferior vena cava.[34,40] However, anastomosing only the most prominent branch may not guarantee uniform drainage of the right anterior sector,[34] and composite or multiple reconstructions may be needed. Thus, an unresolved issue is which hepatic venous tributaries from segments 5 and 8 should be anastomosed, that is, when such anastomoses are mandatory as opposed to optional.[29,41–44] Doppler waveform characteristics may identify tributaries that could benefit from separate anastomosis[29,42,45]—reversed flow in the MHV tributaries may indicate that reconstruction is not required.[58] Reconstructing MHV tributaries according to diameter (> 5 mm[29] or > 8 mm[47]) has also been recommended.

Reconstructing segment 5 and 8 veins has been accomplished with LD inferior mesenteric vein, DD iliac vein (stored at 4°C), cryopreserved DD iliac vein, cryopreserved DD iliac artery, LD ovarian vein, recipient saphenous vein, recipient umbilical vein, recipient left portal vein, and recipient left hepatic vein.[40,44,46,49–52] In addition, recipient superficial femoral vein, LD external iliac vein, and recipient internal jugular vein have been used.[47,48,51] If the most commonly used vascular graft, the recipient saphenous vein, is too small in diameter, two sheets of greater saphenous vein can be used.[44,47] Reconstruction of interposition grafts is, preferably, done on the back table; it can also be done after restoration of portal flow, in order to first assess the degree of venous congestion. Either way, reconstruction of these branches with interposition grafts results in a more complex operation, longer operating time, and longer warm ischemia time. Also, a relatively long segment of interposition graft makes it more prone to thrombosis, and long-term patency is not assured.[31,38] In fact, radiologic studies have shown that reconstruction of tributaries from the anterior segment produces only suboptimal results. Improved volume regeneration of the right anterior sector has been demonstrated, but reconstruction does not completely substitute for an entirely preserved MHV with its surrounding communication.[53,54]

In contrast to venous tributaries of segments 5 and 8, tributaries of segment 6 are usually best anastomosed directly to recipient vena cava, given their posterior and inferior position.

If the functional mass of the right-lobe graft is adequate without the MHV (high GRWR), some degree of congestion may be tolerated early posttransplant, until the graft has regenerated or the anterior sector drainage is rerouted.[15,38,55] In this setting, graft congestion is short-lived, and the redirection of intrahepatic venous flow occurs rapidly. Moreover, obliterated tributaries of the MHV recanalize in a retrograde direction, eventually draining into the right hepatic vein through intrahepatic channels.[37,38] In such cases, a simple right hepatic vein anastomosis is sufficient to assure good graft function.[56–58]

One study compared the regeneration rate of right-lobe liver grafts according to three techniques (1) without MHV trunk preservation or MHV reconstruction, (2) without MHV trunk preservation but with MHV reconstruction, and (3) with MHV trunk preservation. As one would expect, the regeneration rate of the right anterior sector was lowest in right-lobe grafts without MHV trunk preservation or MHV reconstruction. The factors that significantly correlated with the regeneration rate were preoperative graft volume and graft type.[50] That study showed that, if the trunk is not preserved, MHV reconstruction should be performed in selected recipients.

Villa et al. proposed an algorithm to address the issue of preserving the MHV with the right-lobe graft and the need to reconstruct MHV tributaries. If the donor-to-recipient body weight (DRBW) ratio is > 1, then the MHV does not need to be retained with the graft; if it is ≤ 1, and the right lobe-to-recipient standard liver volume (RLRSLV) estimate is < 50, then the MHV should be retained with the graft. If the RLRSLV is > 50%, the decision should be based on the anatomy of the graft's hepatic and portal veins. In general, in the experience of Villa et al. LDs who weighed at least 10% more than the recipient will likely have a right lobe that can provide sufficient liver mass without the MHV.[38] An algorithm based on right versus MHV dominance, GRWR, and remnant liver volume has also been proposed.[39]

### Portal Vein Anastomosis

In most cases, a single anastomosis is typically performed between the donor right portal vein and either the recipient main portal vein or the recipient right portal vein branch. The portal vein anastomosis must be constructed without undue tension, redundancy, or twisting.

If portal bypass is used, the recipient is taken off of it on completion of the caval anastomosis. The recipient portal vein is occluded with a Bainbridge vascular clamp at the superior margin of the pancreas. The donor and recipient portal veins are fashioned to an appropriate length, in order to avoid any kinking after completion of the anastomosis. The anastomosis is done using 5-0 or 6-0 nonabsorbable sutures in running fashion: two sutures are anchored at the corresponding medial and lateral aspects of the recipient and donor portal veins, but only the suture on the medial side is tied; two additional running stitches are placed midway on the anterior portal vein edges (one each on the recipient and donor side), in order to improve exposure when the back wall anastomosis is sewn from the inside (Figure 30.3.1a-13). The anastomosis is completed by running the suture on the anterior wall from the medial to the lateral aspects of the recipient and donor portal veins. The suture is tied at the lateral side with incorporation of a "growth factor." Creation of a growth factor prevents portal vein narrowing at the anastomotic site itself.[59] On completion of the portal vein anastomosis, the anesthesiologist and the surgeon reassess the recipient's clinical status in preparation for reperfusion. Frequently, the recipient is given calcium, bicarbonate, and vasopressors (see Chapter 30.2).

The Bainbridge vascular clamp is removed from the recipient portal vein and the liver is reperfused. About 500 to 1,000 mL of blood are vented through the (untied) medial aspect of the vena cava anastomosis (Figure 30.3.1a-14). The blood is recirculated via the cell saver. After flushing is completed, the portal vein is clamped again, and the running suture of the medial aspect of the caval anastomosis is tied to the corner stitch. The clamps on the vena cava and the portal vein are now removed, and the liver graft is reperfused.

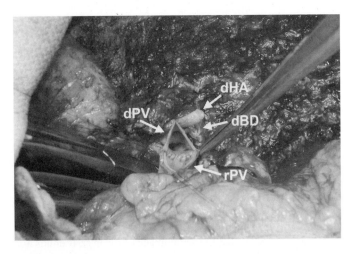

**FIGURE 30.3.1a-13**

The posterior wall between the donor portal vein (dPV) and the recipient portal vein (rPV) is completed. Holding stitches are placed and the anterior wall will be completed next (dHA, donor hepatic artery; dBD, donor bile duct).

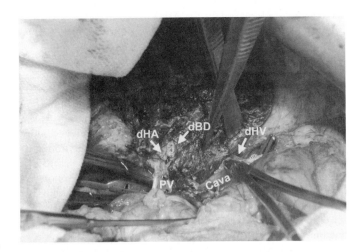

**FIGURE 30.3.1a-14**

The portal vein (PV) anastomosis is completed. The sutured (but not tied) anterior wall of the hepatic vein anastomosis (dHV) is spread open with a clamp to remove the potassium-rich venous effluent. The liver is usually flushed with 500 to 1,000 mL of standard preservation solution (dHA, donor hepatic artery; dBD, donor bile duct).

In the absence of major bleeding from the anastomoses, the anesthesiologist establishes hemodynamic stability and corrects the immediate consequences of graft ischemia and reperfusion injury; the central venous pressure (CVP) should be on the lower side (5 to 9 mm Hg), in order to prevent generalized graft swelling. The surgeon assesses the quality of liver perfusion and stops any significant bleeding with suture ligation. Usually, the liver pinks up immediately; if the MHV was not included in the graft or if venous tributaries were not reconstructed, the medial aspects of segments 5 and 8 (right anterior or paramedian segments) may be dusky-blue and are frequently swollen (see caval anastomosis). The cut surface is assessed for bleeding and hemostasis is obtained; bile leaks are identified and oversewn. Doppler ultrasound is recommended to assess triphasic flow in the hepatic vein(s) and flow velocities in the portal vein.

If the right lobe has separate right anterior and posterior portal vein branches that could not be joined as part of the bench work reconstruction and that require separate anastomoses, the recipient right and left portal vein branches can be used. Or, the donor anterior and posterior portal vein branches can be separately anastomosed to the recipient main portal vein or to the recipient right portal vein (the left portal vein usually results in an anatomically less favorable alignment). If, during the recipient hepatectomy, the second-order branches were preserved, the donor right anterior and posterior portal vein branches can be anastomosed end-to-end to their recipient counterparts. Another option is to resect the recipient portal vein bifurcation (during or after the hepatectomy) and attach this Y-graft to the donor anterior and posterior portal vein branches on the back table (see back table preparation): the Y-graft can then be anastomosed to the recipient main right portal vein at the most suitable location and angle. If the portal Y-graft is not available, a DD iliac Y-graft can also be used for reconstruction (Color Plates, Figure LI-12).

In recipients with portal vein thrombosis who cannot undergo a thrombectomy, mesenteric interposition grafts are necessary (using recipient saphenous vein grafts or DD iliac vein grafts). In addition, caval transposition and arterialization techniques have been described[60] but may be associated with higher morbidity and mortality.

Poor graft function may be the result not only of compromised venous outflow, as described above (see caval anastomosis), but also of portal hypertension and venous overperfusion. Venous overperfusion can cause excessive shear stress (ie, mechanical force against sinusoidal cells) followed by poorly understood liver injury. Such injury has been linked to sinusoidal congestion, mitochondrial swelling, disruption of the sinusoidal lining cells, and collapse of the space of Disse with impaired bile secretion and severe cholestasis.[61–63] With a GRWR < 0.8%, small-for-size syndrome (hyperbilirubinemia, portal cholestasis, delayed synthetic function, and intractable ascites) is more common than with a GRWR ≥ 0.8% (nonanatomical small-for-size syndrome). The association of portal hypertension and small-for-size syndrome may be due to intragraft upregulation of endothelin-1, reduction of plasma nitric oxide levels, and downregulation of heme oxygenase-1 and heat shock protein 70.[33]

A significant increase in portal vein flow after reperfusion is usually noted in the recipient, as compared with the LD's hemodynamic features;[64,65] surgical or pharmacologic intervention may be required if the recipient's portal flow is increased more than three- to fourfold over the LD's values[61,64] (Chapter 30.6).

Several procedures to attenuate portal venous overperfusion (and to protect the small-for-size graft) have been proposed (1) creating a portosystemic shunt; (2) intraportally infusing hepatoprotective drugs; (3) ligating the splenic artery and/or performing a splenectomy; (4) implanting auxiliary or dual-liver grafts; and (5) preventing outflow obstruction by including the MHV or reconstructing its tributaries (see caval anastomosis).

A number of different portosystemic shunts have been described. Boillot et al. reported creating a mesocaval shunt with downstream ligation of the superior mesenteric vein; the shunt completely diverted the superior mesenteric venous flow in a DD left-lobe recipient with a GRWR of 0.6%.[66] That graft then received venous blood only from the gastroduodenal and splenopancreatic veins; the graft increased twofold in volume within a week.

Troisi et al. and Takada et al.[61,67] reported portal inflow modulation by constructing a hemiportacaval shunt. During, or at the end of, the recipient hepatectomy, they created a permanent shunt between the left portal branch and the suprarenal vena cava. The right portal branch was anastomosed to the donor right portal vein.[61] The indication for creating a hemiportacaval shunt was portal vein flow at reperfusion that exceeded the one recorded in the donor by 3 to 4 times. The combination of portal hypertension and low GRWR appears to favor construction of a hemiportacaval shunt; persistent reduction of more than 50% of portal inflow has been reported. Another technique for reducing excessive shear stress due to portal hypertension involves construction of a shunt between the inferior mesenteric vein and the left renal vein, significantly reducing portal pressure.[68]

But, potential drawbacks of portosystemic shunts must be considered (1) portal blood flow competition between the shunt and the graft, resulting in hepatofugal flow and ensuing graft dysfunction (which can be prevented by shunt banding) and (2) development of hyperammonemia (which can be corrected by shunt closure, once regeneration of the graft is completed).[67] Perioperative hemodynamic monitoring (with precise flow measurements) is essential to calibrate the shunt and to avoid graft hyperperfusion.[61] If and when the shunt should be removed remains a controversial and poorly studied question.

Pharmacologic options to prevent portal overflow and small-for-size syndrome have also been suggested. Most commonly, octreotide has been used to decrease mesenteric flow and, thus, reduce portal flow.[17] Intraportally infusing hepatotrophic substances has also been recommended to improve small-for-size graft function. If the graft weight-to-recipient standard liver volume ratio (GV/SLV) is < 50%, one study recommended intraportally infusing (via a 16-G double-lumen catheter) prostaglandin $E_1$ (vasodilator and hepatoprotective effect; 500 μg/d), thromboxane $A_2$ synthetase inhibitor (vasodilator and anticoagulant; 160 mg/d), and nafamostat mesilate (protease inhibitor; 200 mg/d), in an effort to improve microcirculation, protect the hepatocytes, and inhibit platelet aggregation. The incidence of small-for-size graft syndrome was reduced, but a prospective study is warranted.[69]

Other surgical techniques to reduce portal hypertension are splenic artery ligation and splenectomy. Splenic artery ligation was initially reported in patients with hepatocellular cancer who underwent a major hepatectomy because of a cirrhotic liver. Splenic arterial ligation resulted in decompression of surplus portal hypertension (lower portal vein pressure), so this concept was successfully adopted for LD liver transplant recipients with elevated portal vein pressure early posttransplant (days 0 to 4) and small-for-size grafts (GRWR < 0.8%).[63,70] Splenectomy has also been suggested to reduce excessive portal hypertension, but this operation is rarely performed given its magnitude (in coagulopathic patients) and the risk of serious postsplenectomy infections.[61]

Other surgical options to reduce excessive portal inflow, such as auxiliary or dual-liver graft transplants and optimization of venous outflow, are reported below and in Chapters 30.3.1d and 30.4).

## Arterial Anastomosis

The arterial anastomosis can be performed either before or after reperfusion of the liver. Because of its small size, the arterial anastomosis is usually tedious and requires great attention to detail; for that reason, I prefer to perform the arterial anastomosis after reperfusion of the liver. The donor artery is usually only 2 to 5 mm in diameter and relatively short. Some degree of caliber discrepancy between the donor and recipient arteries should be anticipated (Color Plates, Figure LI-17). The smaller vessel should be gently dilated or its end should be cut obliquely to enlarge the diameter. Most of the time, the donor hepatic artery is the smaller vessel. The donor cystic artery stump (if preserved with the graft) can be used as a branch patch when creating the anastomosis.[71]

If only one donor artery is present, an end-to-end anastomosis to the recipient right hepatic artery is preferable. The recipient right hepatic artery is usually a good size-match for the donor right hepatic artery. The anastomosis must be created without any tension, usually by removing the retractors that pull the recipient hilum in a caudad direction. If the recipient right hepatic artery cannot be used, the proper hepatic artery at its bifurcation into the right and left hepatic arteries, or a recipient right aberrant or accessory artery, can be used. Use of the recipient left hepatic artery frequently results in imperfect alignment, although its standard use has been reported by groups that propagate the HHD technique (see above).[22]

The arterial anastomosis is usually performed end-to-end with 7-0 or 8-0 nonabsorbable sutures in interrupted fashion and the use of surgical loop magnification (Figures 30.3.1a-15 and 30.3.1a-16). Alternatively, an operating microscope can be used. In many Japanese centers, a separate microsurgical team performs the arterial anastomosis. The use of an operating microscope can pose technical challenges (1) the recipient artery is located deep in the abdominal cavity and the operating field is limited[72] and (2) interference from cardiac and respiratory movements is constant (making it difficult to achieve stability of the relatively small operative field).[73] To avoid instability, handling of the microforceps or needle holders should be adjusted to the biphasic ventilation movements. Respiration can be withheld temporarily during suture placement. The large amplitude movement caused passively by heart movement is occasionally problematic. Quick insertion and release of the needle into the arterial wall is necessary, so that the arterial wall is not injured by the needle.[72]

In case of multiple donor arteries, controversy remains regarding how many require reconstruction.[74–77] With good (or even pulsatile) back bleeding from the smaller artery (or arteries)

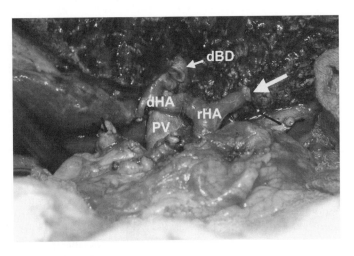

**FIGURE 30.3.1a-16**

The hepatic artery anastomosis (dHA, rHA) is completed. The recipient left hepatic artery (arrow) is shown. The completed portal vein anastomosis (PV) is located underneath the hepatic artery anastomosis (dBD, donor bile duct).

after anastomosing the main donor hepatic artery, assuming no patchy discoloration of the donor liver, ligating the smaller artery or arteries is recommended.[76] Retrograde backflow bleeding through the smaller artery may indicate some form of hilar or intrahepatic collateralization: these collaterals are usually not demonstrable on angiography (hepatic arteries are considered to be end arteries), unless they actively function as collaterals.[17,78] It remains somewhat unclear what impact a smaller ligated artery (in the presence of good pulsatile backflow) has on the arterial blood supply to segmental bile ducts.[74] On completion of the main hepatic artery anastomosis (in the presence of a smaller pulsatile, nonanastomosed artery), arterial signals in each segment should be examined by intraoperative color Doppler ultrasonography, in order to confirm sufficient arterial circulation in all segments of the graft.

If no backflow bleeding can be demonstrated from the smaller artery after the main artery has been anastomosed, an attempt should be made to anastomose the smaller artery as well. A number of different options have been described, most commonly anastomosis to another recipient hepatic artery branch, usually the right and left hepatic artery.[79] Alternatively, the recipient proper hepatic artery with the bifurcation into the left and right hepatic arteries can be divided (during or after the hepatectomy); then, a Y-graft can be reconstructed on the back table under optimal conditions. Doing so requires only one (technically less demanding) anastomosis in the recipient, with either the native proper or common hepatic artery. The disadvantage of this technique is that removing the recipient proper hepatic artery may (partly or fully) devascularize the proximal bile duct(s), requiring creation of a Roux-en-Y limb for biliary reconstruction. If the recipient cystic artery is of adequate length and diameter, it may also be used for arterial anastomosis.

On completion of all arterial anastomoses, intraoperative Doppler ultrasonography should confirm good arterial flow pattern to all segments of the donor graft.

If the recipient right hepatic artery or the proper hepatic artery cannot be used for reconstruction (eg, extended intimal dissection), the common hepatic artery can be dissected out and freed up. Ligating and dividing the gastroduodenal artery may be

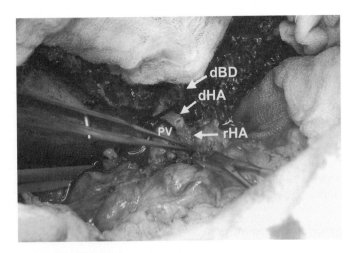

**FIGURE 30.3.1a-15**

The posterior wall between donor hepatic artery (dHA) and recipient right hepatic artery (rHA) is completed. The portal vein (PV) anastomosis is depicted right beneath the hepatic artery anastomosis. The donor bile duct (dBD) is also shown.

needed to release the hepatic artery, providing additional length to reach the hilum for the arterial reconstruction.[17] Various interposition grafts (eg, saphenous vein, inferior mesenteric vein, inferior epigastric artery, splenic artery, right gastroepiploic artery, left gastric artery, gastroduodenal artery, internal iliac artery) as well as DD artery and vein grafts have been used to provide adequate length or to perform multiple arterial reconstructions.[73–85] Even a mesenteric artery of a Roux-en-Y limb has been successfully used for hepatic arterial reconstruction.[86]

If the recipient hepatic artery is thrombosed (in extreme cases, all the way to the origin of the celiac axis), an interposition graft to the infrarenal aorta may be required. A variety of vascular grafts have been used, including saphenous vein, inferior epigastric artery, radial artery, and DD iliac artery.[83,84] The need for an interpositional vascular graft between the donor hepatic artery and the recipient infrarenal aorta can also be the result of previous interventional studies involving the proper and common hepatic artery, such as intraarterial chemotherapy or chemoembolization.[84] Arterial conduits may be preferable over saphenous vein grafts, because saphenous vein grafts tend to develop pseudoaneurysms and have an unsatisfactory long-term patency rate.[84]

### Biliary Anastomosis

Biliary reconstruction of LD (vs. DD) liver grafts is technically more demanding (1) even if only 1 duct needs to be reanastomosed, its diameter is only about half that of a common bile duct and it is shorter; (2) more frequently, multiple small ducts (only 2 to 4 mm in diameter) that were cut flush in the donor's hilar plate are present; and (3) the biliary tree of the right-lobe graft has many anatomic variations that do not correlate well with portal venous and hepatic arterial branching patterns.[87] As a consequence, the incidence of technical complications, such as leaks and strictures, is significantly higher with LD (vs. DD) liver grafts. In larger series, the incidence of biliary complications for adult LD liver transplants ranges from 8% to 67% (vs. 5% to 35% for adult DD liver transplants).[20,21,88,89] To decrease the rate of biliary complications, some suggest that biliary reconstruction should be done by microsurgeons (rather than by fatigued transplant surgeons at the end of a long and demanding procedure).[17] In practice, most biliary anastomoses are performed with loop magnification rather than with a microscope.

The two key requirements for a low biliary complication rate are (1) constructing a tension-free anastomosis and (2) preserving periductal connective tissue to maintain the bile ducts' ascending axial vascular circulation (which originates from the right hepatic artery and the superior posterior pancreaticoduodenal artery).[23,100]

Initially, the standard biliary reconstruction of LD grafts, irrespective of the number of ducts, involved the creation of a Roux-en-Y loop. The steps are as follows: in preparation, the ligament of Treitz is identified and the proximal jejunum is divided about 40 cm below the ligament of Treitz. The distal stump is oversewn using 4-0 nonabsorbable sutures. This end is then brought up to the liver graft, preferably in a retrocolic (vs. antecolic) fashion. The Roux limb is fashioned, an opening in the mesocolon of the transverse colon is made, and the Roux limb is pulled through in a cranial direction. The Roux limb needs to be of appropriate length and mobility, so that the biliary anastomosis can be created without any tension. Before the biliary reconstruction begins, the proximal end of the divided jejunum is anastomosed about 40 cm distal to the Roux limb (ie, the divided distal end of the jejunum). I usually prefer a two-layer, handsewn, end-to-side or side-to-side anastomosis.

The outer layer is created with 4-0 nonabsorbable sutures in either a running or an interrupted fashion, and the inner full-thickness layer is created with 4-0 absorbable sutures in a running fashion. The mesenteric defect of the jejunum is closed, as is the transverse colonic defect, in order to prevent internal herniation.

In preparation for the hepaticojejunostomy, dissection of the bile duct(s) is kept to a minimum, because the periductal tissue that carries the blood supply is critical to avoid anastomotic complications. Bleeding at the cut surface of the bile duct(s) should be stopped with fine suture ligations. Use of the electrocautery should be avoided. If only one donor bile duct needs to be anastomosed, a small stab incision (equal in size to the diameter of the donor bile duct) is made. If a serosa-splitting technique is used, the mucosa is tacked to the serosa with fine, absorbable sutures.[17] Full-thickness bites should be taken about 5 mm away from the bile duct edge, in order to decrease the risk of stenosis. The stitches should also not be placed too close together, in order to reduce the risk of ischemia and subsequent stricture.

On completion of the posterior wall, I prefer to place an internal stent (ie, a radiopaque 4- or 5-French pediatric feeding tube with several side holes) across the anastomosis into the Roux limb. The anterior wall of the anastomosis is then created in a similar fashion. One absorbable suture attaches the stent and keeps it in position, until the suture dissolves and the stent can pass through the gastrointestinal tract. I prefer internal (over external) stents, because they eliminate the long waiting periods until external stents can be removed safely and prevent leaks at the insertion site; in addition, symptoms related to tube removal (eg, fever, abdominal pain, infection) do not occur, and extended drainage in the presence of posttransplant ascites is not necessary.

If an external stent or T tube is used, a Witzel tunnel is created. The Roux-en-Y loop at the distal end of the Witzel tunnel is secured with several interrupted 4-0 nonabsorbable sutures to the peritoneum (to ensure easy access for interventional procedures) at a location where the stent or T tube is brought out through the abdominal wall.

If several donor bile ducts are present, options are as follows: (1) if the ducts are in close proximity or share a common wall, they can be joined together ("syndactylized") and only 1 anastomosis needs to be done; (2) if the donor bile ducts are close to each other (< 0.5 cm), but cannot be syndactylized, only one enterotomy needs to be made, and the anastomosis is created in the same way as described above (individual stents should be placed in each bile duct); and (3) if the distance between the two bile ducts is > 1 cm, two enterotomies may need to be made (separate anastomoses and separate stents).

With increasing surgical experience and improved surgical techniques, direct duct-to-duct anastomosis is now increasingly performed.[26,31,89,91,94–96] It was first described by Wachs et al.;[12] however, in that case, a biliary stricture developed 3 weeks later and the anastomosis was subsequently revised to a Roux-en-Y hepaticojejunostomy.[12] In general, a duct-to-duct anastomosis is advantageous because it (1) reduces operative time; (2) represents a simpler biliary anastomosis, by preserving physiologic bilioenteric and bowel continuity; (3) preserves the physiologic sphincter mechanism with a decreased risk of ascending or reflux cholangitis; (4) eliminates the need for bowel manipulation, with a decreased risk of intraabdominal contamination and of postoperative ileus; (5) results in earlier return of gastrointestinal function; and (6) allows easy radiologic access to the biliary tract.[20,94,103] Despite these advantages, several studies indicate better long-term outcome for Roux-en-Y hepaticojejunostomy (vs. duct-to-duct anastomosis).[20,21,89,90,94,102] The most common contraindications for direct duct-to-duct anastomosis are primary sclerosing cholangitis, previous radiologic intervention (eg, transarterial chemoembolization), and injury during the recipient hepatectomy.

Before constructing the duct-to-duct anastomosis, the viability of the donor and recipient bile ducts should be confirmed by the presence of pulsatile arterial bleeding from the cut ends.[21] If a single donor duct is present, the end-to-end anastomosis is typically created by using interrupted 6-0 or 7-0 absorbable sutures. (But, running sutures may be associated with a lower incidence of biliary complications, especially strictures.)[89] After the posterior wall of the anastomosis is completed, an internal stent is placed across the anastomosis and secured with a single 6-0 absorbable suture (Figures 30.3.1a-17 and 30.3.1a-18). The distal end of the stent is placed across the ampulla of Vater and is endoscopically removed about 4 weeks posttransplant. If an external stent or a T tube is used, the exit site of the stent or T tube is distal to the anastomosis in the recipient common bile duct.[20]

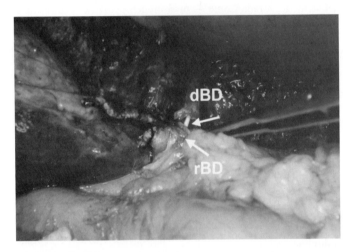

**FIGURE 30.3.1a-17**

The posterior wall between the donor right bile duct (dBD) and the recipient bile duct (rBD) is completed in interrupted fashion; then, a stent is placed internally across the anastomosis.

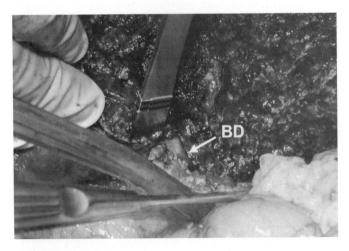

**FIGURE 30.3.1a-18**

The bile duct anastomosis (BD) is completed; the liver cut surface shows good hemostasis.

If several donor ducts are present (Color Plates, Figure LI-12), depending on the number of recipient bile ducts in the preserved hilar plate, several duct-to-duct anastomoses can be created (using the techniques as described above). If the recipient hilar plate with second- or even third-order ductal branches is preserved, multiple and widely separated graft bile ducts can be directly anastomosed to the corresponding orifices in the recipient hilar plate.[21]

If more than one duct-to-duct anastomosis is required, the recipient cystic duct has also been used successfully.[104,105] Some recommend externally stenting any anastomosis involving the cystic duct, in order to keep the lumen open (particularly when dealing with a spiral duct) and to avoid obstruction from fibrous tissue replacing the anastomotic site.[98,102,105,106] Before construction of the cystic duct anastomosis, others suggest straightening the spiral form of the cystic duct, by gently prodding it with a metal probe until it is dilated and entirely passable.[104]

If only one recipient bile duct is available for anastomosis, the remaining ducts require construction of a Roux-en-Y loop. Thus, both duct-to-duct and Roux-en-Y reconstructions can be used in the same recipient.[88] The risk of complications increases with multiple biliary reconstructions.[88,102,103]

In contrast to internal stents, T tubes (brought out through the recipient bile duct) or external stents (brought out through the Roux-en-Y loop) allow monitoring of bile juice production and radiologic study by cholangiography (eg, completion cholangiogram during the transplant, with the first posttransplant study 7 to 10 days later). When a T tube or externalized stent is placed, a completion cholangiogram should be obtained. Leaks are usually best identified and corrected at the time of the transplant. The external stents and T tubes remain in place for at least 3 months; cholangiography is routinely performed before tube removal.[20]

External and internal stents and T tubes are believed to decrease the intrahepatic biliary pressure secondary to edema and technical manipulation and to decrease the incidence of partial obstruction of the anastomosis. But, several groups have advocated nonsplinted biliary reconstruction and avoidance of external stents or T tubes and of internal stents altogether, because of implant-related complications such as leaks and dislocation.[20,26,89,91,102,107,108] If the anastomosis is created without stent placement, routine intraoperative cholangiography is recommended.[20] Supporters of a nonsplinted bilary anastomosis point to a randomized controlled trial of biliary reconstruction in DD liver transplant recipients, which showed an increase in the biliary complication rate in the T-tube group.[109] Liu et al. reported that the incidence of biliary complications after duct-to-duct biliary reconstruction with versus without biliary drainage was 31% in the experience of the Kyoto group versus 24% in the experience of the Hong Kong group, with similar follow-up duration.[89,94]

Avoiding bile duct complications is crucial, because they adversely affect the recipient's quality of life and can occasionally even cause graft loss and death.[94] For those reasons, Calne et al. termed bile duct anastomosis the Achilles' heel of liver transplantation some 30 years ago.[110]

### Closure

Once all anastomoses are completed with satisfactory results, hemostasis is assured and the cut surface is reassessed. Two drains are brought through separate stab incisions and secured to the skin. One drain is located along the diaphragm and the lateral edge of the right lobe toward the hepatic vein-to-cava anastomosis. The second drain is placed along the cut surface of the liver toward the hilum and the biliary anastomosis. The abdomen is copiously irrigated and the fascia is closed with #2 nonabsorbable sutures in a running fashion (occasional interrupted sutures can be placed for reinforcement). The skin is closed with staples. The recipient is usually transferred directly to the surgical intensive care unit.

## OPERATIVE VARIANTS

Despite its frequent anatomic variations, the right lobe is now considered the standard graft for adult liver transplants at most centers. Only a few operative variants have been described.

### Right Lateral Sector Graft

The surgical technique for removing a right lateral segment graft (Couinaud segments 6 and 7) was first described by Sugawara et al. in 2002.[111] A right lateral segment graft is used if its estimated volume is greater than that of the left-lobe graft, and if removing the right-lobe graft is deemed unsafe (due to the small volume of the remaining left lobe). Donors of right-lobe grafts suffer the greatest loss of hepatic function, with the highest postoperative serum bilirubin levels and international normalized ratios (INRs). After procurement of a right lateral segment graft, the remnant liver in the donor is larger, so the procedure is less invasive for donors.[112]

The Kyoto group has recommended not using a right-lobe graft when the potential volume of a non-right-lobe graft (eg, a right lateral sector graft, a left lobe with or without the caudate lobe) is greater than the minimal volume requirement for the recipient,[112] which has been set at 40% of the recipient's standard liver volume.[15,113] A right lateral sector graft, then, is a good alternative to a full right-lobe graft; it is larger in volume than the left lobe.[112]

In preparation for removing the right lateral sector graft, the left and right paramedian branches of the portal veins and hepatic arteries are occluded, revealing the demarcation line of the liver surface. The dissection plane is about 5 mm to the left of the right portal fissure. Liver transection under occlusion of the right paramedian branches of the portal veins and hepatic arteries is recommended.[111]

Alternatively, a Pringle maneuver (10 min preconditioning, 5 min reperfusion, and several cycles of 5 min of clamping and 5 min of release) can be applied during the parenchymal transection; an ultrasound dissector with electrocautery has been used for the parenchymal dissection.[112] The right lateral bile duct is identified using intraoperative cholangiography before the parenchymal transection.

Technically, procurement of a right lateral sector graft is the most demanding; it requires the longest ischemic time for parenchymal dissection and also the longest time for hilar dissection.[112]

In the recipient operation, Sugawara et al. recommend routine hepatic venoplasty to obtain a wider anastomotic orifice and a longer vascular pedicle. The anterior wall of the right hepatic vein is incised for about 1.5 cm. A V-shaped venous patch is obtained from the recipient left native portal vein and sutured to the incised right hepatic vein. The recipient hepatic vein with its patch plasty is then anastomosed end-to-end to the donor right hepatic vein, using 6-0 nonabsorbable sutures. The portal vein, hepatic artery, and bile duct anastomoses are as described above. Because of the large transection surface, bile leaks of up to 50% have been reported, so meticulous ligation of the bile ducts during the parenchymal transection is mandatory.[111,112]

### Domino Liver Transplants

As discussed in detail in Chapter 30.13, domino liver transplants were developed to expand the donor pool: the domino grafts are obtained from patients with familial amyloid polyneuropathy (FAP). In the first recipient (who undergoes an LD right-lobe or left-lobe liver transplant), the FAP-diseased native liver (hereafter called the FAP liver) is removed, as described above except that hepatic inflow via the portal vein and hepatic artery is preserved as long as possible, in order to minimize graft ischemia time. The resected FAP liver usually has vessels of insufficient length and multiple vascular and biliary orifices,[114] making the domino transplant technically complex. Transplants of a whole FAP liver, a right FAP lobe, a left FAP lobe, and a split FAP whole liver have all been described. The choice of procedure depends on (1) the FAP graft size and (2) the recipient size. The use of vascular auto- or allografts for vessel extension and patch plasty is frequent. In general, from a technical perspective, a whole liver is a less ideal domino graft than a lobe graft because of the complexity of multiple vascular and biliary anastomoses.

If only the left or the right lobe of the FAP recipient is removed (and not the whole FAP liver), an auxiliary partial orthotopic LD liver transplant can be performed. More commonly, in the FAP recipient, the left lobe is removed and an LD left lobe is transplanted orthotopically.[114] The advantage of an LD left-lobe transplant is avoidance of venous congestion and of portal bypass, because the right portal vein of the FAP recipient remains patent and acts as a temporary portosystemic shunt. Once the LD left lobe is revascularized, the right lobe (with vessels and bile ducts of sufficient length) is removed for the domino transplant. Likewise, the FAP left-lobe liver graft can be used for another domino recipient (split domino liver transplant).[114]

If the recipient of the domino liver has an underlying noncirrhotic liver disease and if the left lobe of the FAP liver is used, the right hepatic lobe of the recipient may not have to be removed. In these circumstances, Yazaki et al. recommend ligating and transecting the right anterior portal vein, leaving the right posterior portal vein patent. This procedure causes hypertrophy of the left liver graft as well as atrophy of the recipient's right anterior segment.[115] Thus, if a small-for-size graft (in the case by Yazaki et al. just mentioned, 26% of the recipient's standard liver volume) is used, the combination of a domino transplant and an auxiliary partial orthotopic liver transplant (APOLT) is indicated.[115]

LD domino liver transplants have also been performed in the presence of complex vascular abnormalities in the recipient. In 1 recipient with congenital absence of the portal vein, the LD domino transplant used the whole liver of a FAP patient. The recipient portal vein, which had drained directly into the inferior vena cava, was transected together with a cuff of the wall of the inferior vena cava, then anastomosed with the graft liver portal vein in an end-to-end fashion.[116]

In Asian countries, DD organs are scarce. LD domino liver transplants increase the overall number of liver transplants. According to Takeichi et al., by the end of 2003, 25 domino liver transplants had been done in Japan, a number equal to the total number of DD liver transplants since legalization of brain death there in 1997.[116]

### Auxiliary Partial Orthotopic LD Transplants

Auxiliary partial orthotopic liver transplants (APOLTs) were initially performed in recipients (1) with reversible fulminant hepatic failure and (2) with noncirrhotic metabolic liver disease, in order to correct for enzyme deficiency. For those with reversible fulminant hepatic failure, the concept is to support the remnant native liver during regeneration and to withdraw immunosuppressive therapy once the native liver has fully recovered. For those with noncirrhotic metabolic liver disease, immunosuppressive therapy must continue indefinitely, but only a relatively small graft is usually required to correct the enzyme deficiency.

The Kyoto group expanded the indication of APOLTs to treat patients with a GRWR < 0.8%. The rationale of APOLTs for small-for-size grafts is that the remnant native liver is expected to support the function of the implanted graft during the early posttransplant period. After the liver graft has grown sufficiently, it usually meets the hepatic functional demands of the recipient.[117]

Yet another indication for APOLTs is ABO incompatibility. In Asian countries, transplants of ABO-incompatible grafts are often unavoidable (given the limited number of suitable donors), but a high incidence of allograft failure due to a high rate of biliary and vascular complications has been reported.[117,118] When the anticipated graft failure occurs after an ABO-incompatible transplant, the remnant native liver can sustain the recipient's life.

Most auxiliary liver grafts are either the left lateral segments or the left lobe. The Kyoto group also reported use of the right lobe in auxiliary grafts in 3 recipients. In most APOLT recipients, the Kyoto group has recommended diverting the native portal vein to prevent functional portal vein competition between the native liver and the graft, i.e., interrupting portal flow to the native liver, with all portal flow going through the graft.[117,119,120] However, sufficient portal blood flow might be essential for the native liver's recovery and subsequent regeneration. Hepatic artery construction is usually performed without vascular grafts, using microvascular techniques or loop magnification.

The results of APOLTs in recipients with fulminant hepatic failure have been disappointing: withdrawal of immunosuppressive therapy is rarely achieved. So, APOLTs are now primarily recommended for toxic injuries, such as acetaminophen-induced toxicity, where recovery of the native liver is more likely, as compared with idiopathic viral fulminant hepatic failure.[117,121] For recipients with noncirrhotic metabolic liver disease, APOLTs have provided satisfactory outcomes, with a liver graft survival rate > 80%. For recipients who underwent APOLTs for small-for-size grafts, the Kyoto experience reported a high surgical complication rate and a low patient survival rate. After an initial experience with APOLTs using left-lobe grafts, which partially relieved the problems of small-for-size grafts, the Kyoto group eventually introduced systemic use of right-lobe LD liver transplants. The 1-year graft survival rates for right-lobe LD recipients were significantly higher, as compared with recipients of APOLTs for small-for-size grafts. APOLTs of the right-lobe graft for small-for-size grafts remain an option if donor safety is jeopardized by removing an extended right lobe with the MHV.[117]

The application of APOLTs for ABO-incompatible transplants remains less favorable, and has been abandoned by some groups.[117] The best indication for APOLTs appears to be noncirrhotic metabolic liver disease.

Of note, the high incidence of rejection in APOLT recipients has been explained by an increased expression of class II MHC-antigens on hepatocytes after auxiliary liver transplants. Experimental studies showed that auxiliary liver grafts are more susceptible to rejection than non-auxiliary grafts.[117,122,123] The incidence of biliary complications may also be higher, with a greater need for retransplants in APOLT recipients.[117]

Heterotopic auxiliary partial liver transplants (HAPLTs), at the time of this writing, have been described only for 1 left-lobe LD recipient. A small-for-size graft (only 24% of the recipient's standard liver volume) was heterotopically transplanted in a recipient with fulminant liver failure, given the possibility of regeneration of the native liver posttransplant.[124] Technical difficulties associated with HAPLTs are lack of space, atrophy of the graft due to inadequate portal blood inflow, and outflow congestion.

### Transplants for Situs Inversus

Situs inversus totalis (of both thoracic and abdominal viscera) is rare: the incidence is about 0.0075%.[125,126] Associated malformations are common. Biliary atresia has been reported in 10% to 20% of patients with a situs inversus.[125,127] LD liver transplants in pediatric patients with situs inversus and biliary atresia have been reported,[126,128,129] all using left lateral LD liver segments. Haimbach et al. reported transplanting an LD right-lobe graft in an adult recipient with situs inversus. The donor right lobe was positioned in the midline. The recipient left hepatic vein was anastomosed with the donor right hepatic vein. The donor right portal vein was anastomosed with the recipient main portal vein. The arterial anastomosis was performed between the donor right hepatic artery and the recipient right hepatic artery stump. The final position of the liver was in the midline, directly over the vena cava.[125]

In patients with situs inversus, use of a left-lobe liver graft is ideal if the graft provides sufficient liver mass. If the left lobe is a small-for-size graft, then the right lobe is the better choice.[125]

### Transplants with Concurrent Pancreatoduodenectomy

Varotti et al. described a patient with primary sclerosing cholangitis and simultaneous distal bile duct tumor who was treated with a combined LD right-lobe liver transplant and pancreatoduodenectomy.[130] Vascular liver graft implantation was as described above. Gastrointestinal continuity was established with a Roux-en-Y hepaticojejunostomy, followed by a pancreaticojejunostomy and gastrojejunostomy. In future cases, if a pylorus-sparing Whipple procedure is performed, the gastrojejunostomy should be replaced by a duodenojejunostomy.

### "Orphan" Graft Transplants

Siegler et al. raised the question of what to do with a graft if the intended recipient dies after the donor graft has been procured but before it has been transplanted. They offered the following recommendations for handling an orphan liver graft: (1) before donation, informed consent should be obtained from all donors indicating what the donor would want to have done with the orphan graft; (2) premature removal of the donor graft should be avoided until the recipient hepatectomy is completed and survival is likely; and (3) the orphan graft should be allocated according to preestablished institutional guidelines.[131]

### References

1. Bismuth H, Houssin D. Reduced-sized orthotopic liver graft in hepatic transplantation in children. *Surgery* 1984;95: 367–370.
2. Pichlmayr R, Ringe B, Gubernatis G, Hauss J, Buzendahl H. Transplantation einer Spenderleber auf zwei Empfänger (Splitting-Transplantation):Eine neue Methode in der Weiterentwicklung der Lebersegmenttransplantation. *Langenbecks Arch Chir* 1988;373: 127–130.

3. Bismuth H, Morino M, Castaing D, et al. Emergency orthotopic liver transplantation in two patients using one donor liver. *Br J Surg* 1989; 76: 722–724.

4. Rogiers X, Malagó M, Gawad K, et al. *In situ* splitting of cadaveric livers: the ultimate expansion of a limited donor pool. *Ann Surg* 1996;224: 331–341.

5. Raia S, Nery JR, Mies S. Liver transplantation from live donors. *Lancet* 1989;2: 497.

6. Strong RW, Lynch SV, Ong TH, et al. Successful liver transplantation from a living donor to her son. *N Engl J Med* 1990;322:1505–1507.

7. Broelsch CE, Emond JC, Whittington PF, et al. Application of reduced-size liver transplants as split grafts, auxiliary orthotopic grafts, and living related segmental transplants. *Ann Surg* 1990;212:368–375.

8. Ozawa K, Uemoto S, Tanaka K, et al. An appraisal of pediatric liver transplantation from living relatives. *Ann Surg* 216:547–553.

9. Hashikura Y, Makuuchi M, Kawasaki S, et al. Successful living-related partial liver transplantation to an adult patient. *Lancet* 1994;343: 1233–1234.

10. Yamaoka Y, Washida M, Honda K, et al. Liver transplantation using a right lobe graft from a living related donor. *Transplantation* 1994;57: 1127–1130.

11. Lo C-M, Fan S-T, Liu C-L, et al. Extending the limit on the size of adult recipient in living donor liver transplantation using extended right lobe graft. *Transplantation* 1997;63: 1524–1528.

12. Wachs ME, Bak TE, Karrer FM, et al. Adult living donor liver transplantation using a right hepatic lobe. Transplantation 1998;66: 1313–1316.

13. United Network for Organ Sharing (UNOS): http://www.unos.org (accessed March 2006).

14. Gorman C. The ultimate sacrifice. *Time Magazine.* January 28, 2002; 41.

15. Urata K, Kawasaki S, Matsunami H, et al. Calculation of child and adult standard liver volume for liver transplantation. *Hepatology* 1995;21: 1317–1321.

16. Gondolesi GE, Yoshizumi T, Bodian C, et al. Accurate method for clinical assessment of right lobe liver weight in adult living-related liver transplant. *Transplant Proc* 2004;36:1429–1433.

17. Florman SS, Miller CM. Adult living donor hepatectomy and recipient operation. Chapter 45. In: Busuttil RW, Klintmalm G (eds.), *Transplantation of the Liver*, second edition, Elsevier Saunders; 2005: 675–702.

18. Calne, RY, Williams R. Liver transplantation in man. I. Observations on technique and organization in five cases. *Br Med J* 1968;4:535–540.

19. Tzakis A, Todo S, Starzl TE. Orthotopic liver transplantation with preservation of the inferior vena cava. *Ann Surg* 1989;210:649–652.

20. Yi N-J, Suh K-S, Cho JY, et al. In adult-to-adult living donor liver transplantation hepaticojejunostomy shows a better long-term outcome than duct-to-duct anastomosis. *Transplant Int* 2005;18:1240–1247.

21. Dulundu E, Sugawara Y, Sano K, et al. Duct-to-duct biliary reconstruction in adult living-donor liver transplantation. *Transplantation* 2004;78:574–579.

22. Lee K-W, Joh JW, Kim SJ, et al. High hilar dissection: new technique to reduce biliary complication in living donor liver transplantation. *Liver Transpl* 2004;10:1158–1162.

23. Northover J, Terblanche J. Bile duct blood supply. *Transplantation* 1978;26:67–69.

24. Stapleton GN, Hickman R, Terblanche J. Blood supply of the right and left hepatic ducts. *Br J Surg* 1998;85:202–207.

25. Rath AM, Zhang J, Bourdelat D, et al. Arterial vascularization of the extrahepatic tract. *Surg Radiolol Anat* 1993;15:105.

26. Shokouh-Amiri MH, Grewal HP, Vera SR, et al. Duct-to-duct biliary reconstruction in right lobe adult living donor liver transplantation. *J Am Coll Surg* 2001;192:798–803.

27. Neelakanta G, Colquhoun S, Csete M, et al. Efficacy and safety of heat exchanger added to venovenous bypass circuit during orthotopic liver transplantation. *Liver Transpl Surg* 1998;4:506–509.

28. Arcari M, Phillips SD, Gibbs P, Rela SM, Heaton ND. An investigation into the risk of air embolus during veno-venous bypass in orthotopic liver transplantation. *Transplantation* 1999;68:150–152.

29. Cattral MS, Molinari M, Vollmer CM Jr, et al. Living-donor right hepatectomy with or without inclusion of middle hepatic vein: comparison of morbidity and outcome in 56 patients. *Am J Transpl* 2004;4: 751–757.

30. Marcos A, Fisher RA, Ham JM, et al. Emergency portacaval shunt for control of hemorrhage from a parenchymal fracture after adult-to-adult living donor liver transplantation. *Transplantation* 2000; 69:2218–2221.

31. Miller CM, Gondolesi GE, Florman S, et al. One hundred nine living donor liver transplants in adults and children: a single-center experience. *Ann Surg* 2001;234:301–312.

32. Man K, Fan S-T, Lo C-M, et al. Graft injury in relation to graft size in right lobe live donor liver transplantation: a study of hepatic sinusoidal injury in correlation with portal hemodynamics and intragraft gene expression. *Ann Surg* 2003;237:256–264.

33. Maetani Y, Itoh K, Egawa H, et al. Factors influencing liver regeneration following living-donor liver transplantation of the right hepatic lobe. *Transplantation* 2003;75:97–102.

34. Fan S-T, Lo C-M, Liu C-L, Wang W-X, Wong J. Safety and necessity of including the middle hepatic vein in the right lobe graft in adult-to-adult live donor liver transplantation. *Ann Surg* 2003;238: 137–148.

35. Lo C-M, Fan S-T, Liu C-L, et al. Adult-to-adult living donor liver transplantation using extended right lobe grafts. *Ann Surg* 1997;226: 261–270.

36. Marcos A, Orloff M, Mieles L, et al. Functional venous anatomy for right-lobe grafting and techniques to optimize outflow. *Liver Transpl* 2001;7:845–852.

37. Kaneko T, Kaneko K, Sugimoto H, et al. Intrahepatic anastomosis formation between the hepatic veins in the graft liver of the living related liver transplantation: observation by Doppler ultrasonography. *Transplantation* 2000;70:982–985.

38. de Villa VH, Chen C-L, Chen Y-S, et al. Right lobe living donor liver transplantation—addressing the middle hepatic vein controversy. *Ann Surg* 2003;238:275–282.

39. Kasahara M, Takada Y, Fujimoto Y, et al. Impact of right lobe with middle hepatic vein graft in living-donor liver transplantation. *Am J Transpl* 2005;5:1339–1346.

40. Cattral MS, Greig PD, Muradali D, Grant D. Reconstruction of middle hepatic vein of a living-donor right lobe liver graft with recipient left portal vein. *Transplantation* 2001;71:1864–1866.

41. Kinkhabwala MM, Guarrera JV, Leno R, et al. Outflow reconstruction in right hepatic live donor liver transplantation. *Surgery* 2003;133: 243–250.

42. Sugawara Y, Makuuchi M, Sano K, et al. Vein reconstruction in modified right liver graft for living donor liver transplantation. *Ann Surg* 2003;237:180–185.

43. Fan S-T, Lo C-M, Liu C-L. Technical refinement in adult-to-adult living donor liver transplantation using right-lobe graft. *Ann Surg* 2000;231:126–131.

44. Lee SG, Park KM, Hwang S, et al. Modified right liver graft from a living donor to prevent congestion. *Transplantation* 2002;74: 54–59.

45. Sano K, Makuuchi M, Miki K, et al. Evaluation of hepatic venous congestion: proposed indication criteria for hepatic vein reconstruction. *Ann Surg* 2002;236:241–247.

46. Lee KW, Lee DS, Lee HHJW, et al. Interposition vein graft in living donor liver transplantation. *Transpl Proc* 2004;36:2261–2262.

47. Sato K, Sekiguchi S, Fukumori T, et al. Experience with recipient's superficial femoral vein as conduit for middle hepatic vein reconstruction in a right-lobe living donor liver transplant procedure. *Transpl Proc* 2005;37:4343–4346.

48. Moreno Elola-Olaso A, Moreno Gonzalez E, Meneu Diaz JC, et al. Hepatic vein reconstruction in living donor liver transplantation. *Transpl Proc* 2005;37:3891–3892.

49. Ghobrial RM, Hsieh C-B, Lerner JS, et al. Technical challenges of hepatic venous outflow reconstruction in right lobe adult living donor liver transplantation. *Liver Transpl* 2001;7:551–555.

50. Akamatsu N, Sugawara Y, Kaneko J, et al. Effects of middle hepatic vein reconstruction on right liver graft regeneration. *Transplantation* 2003; 76:832–837.

51. Kornberg A, Heyne J, Schotte U, Hommann M, Scheele J. Hepatic venous outflow reconstruction in right lobe living-donor liver graft using recipient's superficial femoral vein. *Am J Transpl* 2003;3:1444–1447.

52. Sugawara Y, Makuuchi M, Akamatsu N, et al. Refinement of venous reconstruction using cryopreserved veins in right liver grafts. *Liver Transpl* 2004;10:541–547.

53. Ito T, Kiuchi T, Yamamoto H, et al. Efficacy of anterior segment drainage reconstruction in right-lobe liver grafts from living donors. *Transplantation* 2004;77:865–868.

54. Morioka D, Sekido H, Matsuo K, et al. Middle hepatic vein tributary reconstruction could not act as a complete substitute for an entirely preserved middle hepatic vein. *Hepato-Gastroenterology* 2005;52: 208–211.

55. Nishizaki T, Ikegami T, HirosHige S, et al. Small graft for living donor liver transplantation. *Ann Surg* 2001;233:575–580.

56. Bogetti D, Panaro F, Jarzembowski T, et al. Hepatic venous outflow reconstruction in adult living donor liver transplants without portal hypertension. *Clin Transplant* 2004;18:222–226.

57. Cescon M, Sugawara Y, Sano K, et al. Right liver graft without middle hepatic vein reconstruction from a living donor. *Transplantation* 2002;73:1164–1166.

58. Maema A, Imamura H, Takayama T, et al. Impaired volume regeneration of split livers with partial venous disruption: a latent problem in partial liver transplantation. *Transplantation* 2002;73:765–769.

59. Starzl TE, Iwatsuki S, Shaw BW Jr. A growth factor in fine vascular anastomoses. *Surg Gynecol Obstet* 1984;159:164–165.

60. Miyamoto A, Kato T, Dono K, et al. Living-related liver transplantation with reniportal anastomosis for a patient with large spontaneous splenorenal collateral. *Transplantation* 2003;79:1596–1598.

61. Troisi R, Ricciardi S, Smeets P, et al. Effects of hemi-portacaval shunts for inflow modulation on the outcome of small-for-size grafts in living donor liver transplantation. *Am J Transpl* 2005;5:1397–1404.

62. Man K, Lo C-M, Ng IO-L Ng et al. Liver transplantation in rats using small-for-size grafts. *Arch Surg* 2005;136:280–285.

63. Sato Y, Kobayashi T, Nakatsuka H, et al. Splenic arterial ligation prevents liver injury after a major hepatectomy by a reduction of surplus portal hypertension in hepatocellular carcinoma patients with cirrhosis. *Hepato-Gastroenterology* 2001;48:831–835.

64. Troisi R, Cammu G, Militerno G, et al. Modulation of portal graft inflow: a necessity in adult living-donor liver transplantation? *Ann Surg* 2003;237:429–436.

65. Marcos A, Olzinski AT, Ham JM, Fisher RA, Posner MP. The interrelationship between portal and arterial blood flow after adult to adult living donor liver transplantation. *Transplantation* 2000;70:1697–1703.

66. Boillot O, Delafosse B, Méchet I, Boucaud C, Pouyet M. Small-for-size partial liver graft in an adult recipient; a new transplant technique. *Lancet* 2002;359:406–407.

67. Takada Y, Ueda M, Ishikawa Y, et al. End-to-side portacaval shunting for a small-for-size graft in living donor liver transplantation. *Liver Transpl* 2004;10:807–810.

68. Sato Y, Yamamoto S, Takeishi T, et al. Inferior mesenteric venous left renal vein shunting for decompression of excessive portal hypertension in adult living related transplantation. *Transpl Proc* 2004;36:2234–2236.

69. Suehiro T, Shimada M, Kishikawa K, et al. Effect of intraportal infusion to improve small for size graft injury in living donor adult liver transplantation. *Transpl Int* 2005;18:923–928.

70. Ito T, Kiuchi T, Yamamoto H, et al. Changes in portal venous pressure in the early phase after living-donor liver transplantation: pathogenesis and clinical implications. *Transplantation* 2003;75:1313–1317.

71. Di Benedetto F, Lauro A, Masetti M, et al. Use of a branch patch with the cystic artery in living-related liver transplantation. *Clin Transplant* 2004;18:480–483.

72. Okazaki M, Asato H, Takushima A, et al. Hepatic artery reconstruction with double-needle microsuture in living-donor liver transplantation. *Liver Transpl* 2006;12:46–50.

73. Alper M, Gundogan H, Tokat C, Ozek C. Microsurgical reconstruction of hepatic artery during living donor liver transplantation. *Microsurgery* 2005;25:378–384.

74. Suehiro T, Ninomiya M, Shiotani S, et al. Hepatic artery reconstruction and biliary stricture formation after living donor adult liver transplantation using the left lobe. *Liver Transpl* 2002;8:495–499.

75. Tanaka K, Uemoto S, Tokunaga Y, et al. Surgical techniques and innovations in living-related liver transplantation. *Ann Surg* 1993;217:82–91.

76. Ikegami T, Kawasaki S, Matsunami H, et al. Should all hepatic arterial branches be reconstructed in living-related liver transplantation? *Surgery* 1996;119:431–436.

77. Sakamoto Y, Takayama T, Nakatsuka T, et al. Advantage in using living donors with aberrant hepatic artery for partial liver graft arterialization. *Transplantation* 2002;74:518–521.

78. Redman HC, Reuter SR. Arterial collaterals in the liver hilus. *Radiology* 1970;94:575–579.

79. Marcos A, Killackey M, Orloff MS, et al. Hepatic arterial reconstruction in 95 adult right lobe living donor liver transplants: evolution of anastomotic technique. *Liver Transpl* 2003;9:570–574.

80. Katz E, Fukuzawa K, Schwartz M, Mor E, Miller C. The splenic artery as the inflow in arterial revascularization of the liver graft in clinical liver transplantation. *Transplantation* 1992;53:1373–1374.

81. Cherqui D, Riff Y, Rotman N, Julien M, Fagniez PL. The recipient splenic artery for arterialization in orthotopic liver transplantation. *Am J Surg* 1994;167:327–330.

82. Ikegami T, Kawasaki S, Hashikura Y, et al. An alternative method of arterial reconstruction after hepatic arterial thrombosis following living-related liver transplantation. *Transplantation* 2000;69:1953–1955.

83. Nakatsuka T, Takushima A, Harihara Y, et al. Versatility of the inferior epigastric artery as an interpositional vascular graft in living-related liver transplantation. *Transplantation* 1999;67:1490–1492.

84. Mizuno S, Yokoi H, Isaji S, et al. Using a radial artery as an interpositional vascular graft in a living-donor liver transplantation for hepatocellular carcinoma. *Transplant Int* 2005;18:408–411.

85. Itabashi Y, Hakamada K, Narumi S, et al. A case of living-related partial liver transplantation using the right gastroepiploic artery for hepatic artery reconstruction. *Hepato-Gastroenterology* 2000;47:512–513.

86. Kasahara M, Sakamoto S, Ogawa K, et al. The use of a mesenteric artery of Roux-en-Y limb for hepatic arterial reconstruction after living-donor liver transplantation. *Transplantation* 2005;80:538.

87. Macdonald DB, Haider MA, Khalili K, et al. Relationship between vascular and biliary anatomy in living liver donors. *AJR* 2005;185:247–252.

88. Testa G, Malagó M, Valentin-Gamazo C, Lindell G, Broelsch CE. Biliary anastomosis in living related liver transplantation using the right liver lobe: techniques and complications. *Liver Transpl* 2000;6:710–714.

89. Ishiko T, Egawa H, Kasahara M, et al. Duct-to-duct biliary reconstruction in living donor liver transplantation utilizing right lobe graft. *Ann Surg* 2002;236:235–240.

90. Kawachi S, Shimazu M, Wakabayashi G, et al. Biliary complications in adult living donor liver transplantation with duct-to-duct hepaticocholedochostomy or Roux-en-Y hepaticojejunostomy biliary reconstruction. *Surgery* 2002;132:48–56.

91. Sugawara Y, Makuuchi M, Santo K, Ohkubo T, et al. Duct-to-duct biliary reconstruction in living-related liver transplantation. *Transplantation* 2002;73:1348–1350.

92. Icoz G, Kilic M, Zeytunlu M, et al. Biliary reconstructions and complications encountered in 50 consecutive right-lobe living donor liver transplantations. *Liver Transpl* 2003;9:575–580.

93. Settmacher U, Steinmüller TH, Schmidt SC, et al. Technique of bile duct reconstruction and management of biliary complications in right lobe living donor liver transplantation. *Clin Transplant* 2003;17:37–42.

94. Liu C-L, Lo C-M, Chan S-C, Fan S-T. Safety of duct-to-duct biliary reconstruction in right-lobe live-donor liver transplantation without biliary drainage. *Transplantation* 2004;77:726–732.

95. Grewal HP, Shokouh-Amiri MH, Vera S, et al. Surgical technique for right lobe adult living donor liver transplantation without venovenous bypass or portacaval shunting and with duct-to-duct biliary reconstruction. *Ann Surg* 2001;233:502–508.

96. Malagó M, Testa G, Hertl M, et al. Biliary reconstruction following right adult living donor liver transplantation end-to-end or end-to-side duct-to-duct anastomosis. *Langenbeck's Arch Surg* 2002;387:37–44.

97. Dalgic A, Moray G, Emiroglu R, et al. Duct-to-duct biliary anastomosis with a "corner-saving suture" technique in living-related liver transplantation. *Transpl Proc* 2005;37:3137–3140.

98. Kadry Z, Cintorino D, Scotti Foglieni C, Fung J. The pitfall of the cystic duct biliary anastomosis in right lobe living donor liver transplantation. *Liver Transpl* 2004;10:1549–1550.

99. Egawa H, Inomata Y, Uemoto S, et al. Biliary anastomotic complications in 400 living related liver transplantations. *World J Surg* 2001;25:1300–1307.

100. Terblanche J, Allison HF, Northover JMA. An ischemic basis for biliary strictures. *Surgery* 1983;94:52–57.

101. Suh K-S, Choi SH, Yi N-J, Kwon CH, Lee KU: Biliary reconstruction using the cystic duct in right lobe living donor liver transplantation. *J Am Coll Surg* 199:661–664.

102. Gondolesi GE, Varotti G, Florman SS, et al. Biliary complications in 96 consecutive right lobe living donor transplant recipients. *Transplantation* 2004;77:1842–1848.

103. Fan S-T, Lo C-M, Liu C-L, Tso W-K, Wong J. Biliary reconstruction and complications of right lobe live donor liver transplantation. *Ann Surg* 2002;236:676–683.

104. Asonuma K, Okajima H, Ueno M, et al. Feasibility of using the cystic duct for biliary reconstruction in right-lobe living donor liver transplantation. *Liver Transpl* 2005;11:1431–1434.

105. Suh KS, Choi SH, Yi NJ, Kwon CH, Lee KU. Biliary reconstruction using the cystic duct in right lobe living donor liver transplantation. *J Am Coll Surg* 2004;199:661–664.

106. Foerster EC, Matek W, Domschke W. Endoscopic retrograde cannulation of the gallbladder: direct dissolution of gallstones. *Gastrointest Endosc* 1990;36:444–450.

107. Azoulay D, Marin-Hargreaves G, Castaing D, Adam R, Bismuth H. Duct-to-duct biliary anastomosis in living related liver transplantation: The Paul Brousse technique. *Arch Surg* 2001;136:1197–1200.

108. Soejima Y, Shimada M, Suehiro T, et al. Feasibility of duct-to-duct biliary reconstruction in left-lobe adult-living-donor liver transplantation. *Transplantation* 2003;75:557–559.

109. Scatton O, Meunier B, Cherqui D, et al. Randomized trial of choledochocholedochostomy with or without a T tube in orthotopic liver transplantation. *Ann Surg* 2001;233:432–437.

110. Calne RY, A new technique for biliary drainage in orthotopic liver transplantation utilizing the gall bladder as a pedicle graft conduit between the donor and recipient common bile ducts. *Ann Surg* 1976;184: 605–609.

111. Sugawara Y, Makuuchi M, Takayama T, Imamura H, Kaneko J. Right lateral sector graft in adult living-related liver transplantation. *Transplantation* 2002;73:111–114.

112. Kokudo N, Sugawara Y, Imamura H, Sano K, Makuuchi M. Tailoring the type of donor hepatectomy for adult living donor liver transplantation. *Am J Transplant* 2005;5:1694–1703.

113. Sugawara Y, Makuuchi M, Kaneko J, et al. Living-donor liver transplantation in adults: Tokyo University experience. *J Hepatobiliary Pancreat Surg* 2003;10:1–4.

114. Hashikura Y, Ikegami T, Nakazawa Y, et al. Domino liver transplantation in living donors. *Transpl Proc* 2005;37:1076–1078.

115. Yazaki M, Hashikura Y, Takei Y-I, et al. Feasibility of auxiliary partial orthotopic liver transplantation from living donors for patients with adult-onset type II citrullinemia. *Liver Transpl* 2004;10:550–554.

116. Takeichi T, Okajima H, Suda H, et al. Living domino liver transplantation in an adult with congenital absence of portal vein. *Liver Transpl* 2005;11:1285–1288.

117. Kasahara M, Takada Y, Egawa H, et al. Auxiliary partial orthotopic living donor liver transplantation: Kyoto University experience. *Am J Transpl* 2005;5:558–565.

118. Demetris AJ, Jaffe R, Tzakis A, et al. Antibody-mediated rejection of human orthotopic liver allografts. A study of liver transplantation across ABO blood group barriers. *Am J Pathol* 1996;132:489–502.

119. Inomata Y, Kiuchi T, Kim ID, et al. Auxiliary partial orthotopic living donor liver transplantation as an aid for small-for-size grafts in larger recipients. *Transplantation* 1999;67:1314–1319.

120. Kasahara M, Takada Y, Kozaki K, et al. Functional portal flow competition after auxiliary partial orthotopic living donor liver transplantation in noncirrhotic metabolic liver disease. *J Pediatr Surg* 2004;39:1138–1141.

121. Devlin J, Wendon J, Heaton N, Tan K-C, Williams R: Pretransplantation clinical status and outcome of emergency transplantation for acute liver failure. *Hepatology* 1995;21:1018–1024.

122. Icard P, Sawyer GJ, Houssin D, Fabre JW. Marked differences between orthotopic and heterotopic auxiliary liver allografts in the induction of class II MHC antigens on hepatocytes. *Transplantation* 1990;49:1005–1007.

123. Astarcioglu I, Gugenheim J. Gigou M, et al. Immunosuppressive properties of auxiliary liver allografts into sensitized rats. *Transplantation* 1990;49:1186–1188.

124. Sato Y, Yamamoto S, Takeishi T, et al. Living related heterotopic auxiliary partial liver transplantation for extremely small-for-size graft in fulminant liver failure. *Hepato-Gastroenterology* 2003;50: 1220–1222.

125. Heimbach, JK, Narayanan Menon KV, Ishitani MB, et al. Living donor liver transplantation using a right lobe graft in an adult with situs inversus. *Liver Transpl* 2005;11:111–113.

126. Sugawara Y, Makuuchi M, Takayama, T, et al. Liver transplantation from situs inversus to situs inversus. *Liver Transpl* 2001;7:829–830.

127. Karrer FM, Hall RJ, Lilly JR, Biliary atresia and the polysplenia syndrome. *J Pediatr Surg* 1991;26: 524–527.

128. Hasegawa JT, Kimura T, Sasaki T, Okada A. Living-related liver transplantation for biliary atresia associated with polysplenia syndrome. *Pediatr Transplant* 2002;6:78–81.

129. Bak T, Wachs M, Trotter J, et al. Adult-to-adult living donor liver transplantation using right-lobe grafts: results and lessons learned from a single-center experience. *Liver Transpl* 2001;7:680–686.

130. Varotti G, Gondolesi GE, Roayaie S, et al. Combined adult-to-adult living donor right lobe liver transplantation and pancreatoduodenectomy for distal bile duct adenocarcinoma in a patient with primary sclerosing cholangitis. *J Am Coll Surg* 2003;197:765–769.

131. Siegler J, Siegler M, Cronin DC, II. Recipient death during a live donor liver transplantation: who gets the "orphan" graft? *Transplantation* 2004;78:1241–1244.

## 30.3.1b    Extended Right Lobe Transplant

*See Ching Chan, MD, MS,*
*Chung Mau Lo, MD, MS*

## INTRODUCTION

Soon after deceased donor liver transplantation (DDLT) became a practical treatment for patients with end-stage liver disease (ESLD), the supply of deceased donor liver grafts was outstripped. In order to overcome the rarity of deceased child donor liver grafts, reduced-size liver transplantation was developed.[1] Split-liver transplantation further allowed transplantation for one child and one adult recipients[2] and later, two adult recipients using one liver graft.[3] *In-situ* splitting further shortened the cold-ischemic time and lessened the inevitable graft rewarming of various degree during back-table procedure.[4] These technical innovations paved the way for living donor liver transplantation (LDLT), an idea first promulgated by Smith as early as 1969 after transplanting animals with partial liver grafts.[5] With extensive experience in liver resection for tumors, reduced-size and split-liver transplantation, Strong performed the first successful LDLT in 1989 for a 17-month-old Japanese boy using the left lateral segment graft of his mother. This recipient from Japan was not eligible to deceased donor graft allocation in Australia but to resort to his mother for the donor organ. Concerns over donor safety were already alluded to in this seminal publication on LDLT[6] and in subsequent articles by Strong himself.[7,8]

In a background of practically no deceased donor organs, LDLT using the left liver for children[9,10] and adults[11] bloomed in Japan. The left lobe often small-for-size for the adult recipient, had poor results.[12] Resistance to the use of the right liver was anecdotally broken by the Kyoto group for a 9-year-old recipient. Confirmed at laparotomy, the branching of the hepatic arteries to segments 2 and 3 had separate origins from the proper hepatic artery. These branches were considered too small for anastomosis using a surgical loupe. The group thus improvised donor right hepatectomy on table. The possibility of using the right lobe graft in the case of a relatively large child or an adult recipient was raised by the authors.[13] On May 9, 1996, the right lobe graft including the middle hepatic vein (MHV) was first transplanted to an adult who had a body weight of 90 kg with acute liver failure from Wilson's disease. Prior to anastomosis of the MHV with the inferior vena cava (IVC) the graft was congested.[14] Many centers gradually started using the right lobe for adult recipients.[15–17]

## SMALL-FOR-SIZE SYNDROME

In ALDLT, when the graft volume is less than 50%[18] of the standard liver volume,[19] or the graft weight to recipient body weight ratio less than 1%,[12] graft survival is compromised. Graft survival also worsens incrementally as this ratio decreases.[12,20] The graft size requirement also becomes higher in the presence of portal hypertension of the recipient.[21] The mode of failure for small-for-size grafts often manifested as small-for-size syndrome and is exemplified as coagulopathy, cholestasis, ascites, sepsis, encephalopathy, and eventually graft failure.[18] With maturation of surgical techniques and perioperative care, this ratio has decreased from 40%[22] to 36% in our center.[23]

Portal hyperperfusion[24] and portal hypertension[25] are currently conceived as possible mechanisms conducive to the damage of the small-for-size graft. Techniques for alleviation of portal inflow were described. These include mesocaval shunt,[26] hemiportocaval shunting,[27] and inflow modulation by splenic artery ligation.[28,29] It has been conceptualized that a bearable inflow, unimpeded outflow and adequate graft size are factors intercalated to achieve recipient success.[30] Given the common scenario of preexisting portal hypertension in the recipient and limited choice of donors to provide a large right liver graft, a reliable graft venous outflow becomes crucial. The inclusion of the MHV could only be justified with unimpeded venous outflow capacity of the graft. This is achieved by converting the right hepatic vein (RHV) and MHV to a single triangular cuff by venoplasty[31] (Color Plates, Figures LI-18B and LI-18C). This will match the triangular venotomy made on the IVC. Exploiting the resilient of the liver parenchyma between the MHV and RHV and the stretchability of the right and middle hepatic veins, the single cuff is kept widely open.[32] The single cuff-to-cuff anastomosis reliably maintains patency regardless of size of the graft and the subphrenic space. Triphasic Doppler pulsatility of the MHV and RHM after perfusion testifies satisfactory outflow capacity of the graft.[32] Being a single cuff, warm ischemic time is also shortened by expediting the suturing *in-vivo*.[33]

## RECIPIENT WORKUP

The potential recipient evaluations for DDLT and LDLT are similar. Attitude toward ALDLT as a treatment option is carefully assessed by the surgeon and the clinical psychologist. Nevertheless, recipients with multiple operations before render recipient hepatectomy difficult and sometimes impossible. Portal vein thrombosis extended into the superior mesenteric vein often present with multiple collaterals which can bleed profusely. It is important that the liver transplantation is indicated and does not risk the donor unnecessarily.

Vascular invasion by tumor is the single most important factor in treatment failure of hepatocellular carcinoma by resection[34] and liver transplantation.[35] Major vascular invasions, though apparent for larger tumors, may not be so for the small ones. The Milan Criteria[36] and the University College of San Francisco Criteria,[37] based on preoperative imaging and explant histopathology respectively, use tumor size and number as surrogate parameters for likelihood of vascular invasion. It has now been shown that tumor grade[38] and tumor diameter[39] are predicators of vascular invasion. Tumor diameter itself is also a predictor of high tumor grade.[39] Standard indications may be extended modestly for unresectable hepatocellular carcinoma with no gross vascular involvements.[40–42]

Although ALDLT is not the preferred procedure for high-urgency situation in Europe and the United States,[43–45] it was the impetus of development of ALDLT in Hong Kong. All seven recipients of our first series reported were of high urgency with hepatic encephalopathy.[46] Right lobe ALDLT is advantageous to patients waiting for DDLT. The waiting time is much shortened, and the transplant rate and survival rate are both improved.[47,48] In a series of 86 patients (fulminant hepatic failure = 17, acute-on-chronic liver failure = 69), those who were able to undergo right lobe ALDLT (31/86, 36%) had a survival of 93.5% (29/31).[48] Nevertheless, surgeons know implicitly that under such circumstances, it is associated with more a treacherous course of recovery and perhaps higher mortality. This only calls for an efficacious graft from a live donor.

## RECIPIENT HEPATECTOMY

In the presence of vascular adhesions from previous surgery, spontaneous bacterial peritonitis, and substantial portal hypertension, recipient hepatectomy could be the most difficult part of the recipient operation. Technical misadventure here can compromise recipient surgical outcome.[49] For adequate access, a generous bilateral subcostal incision and upward midline extension are made. The subcostal incisions are made more caudal for recipients with gross ascites. The incision starts from the lateral border of the left rectus to the right anterior axillary line to provide adequate access to the IVC. The xiphoid process with the fat in the upper midline that often contains vascular collaterals is excised completely to facilitate access to the suprahepatic IVC and minimize blood loss. A Bookwalter retractor is used with three retractors blades lifting up and widening the subcostal angle. The ligamentum teres which often includes a recannulated umbilical vein is ligated and divided. The falciform ligament is then divided till the suprahepatic IVC is exposed (Color Plates, Figure LI-9). Inadvertent damage to the major vessels is avoided if the electrocautery only divides the adventitia overlying that could be picked up by the DeBakey forceps.

Hilar dissection starts with opening up of the peritoneum just to the right of the common bile duct. The cystic artery and cystic ducts are then ligated and divided (Color Plates, Figure LI-10A). Peritoneum along the superior border of the hilum is further opened. Lymphatics and small vessels within the heptoduodenal ligament are cauterized if small or divided between ligatures if larger than 2 mm. The duodenum is retracted by the second assistant in the caudal direction gently to facilitate the dissection.

After careful bimanual palpation, the right and left hepatic arteries are identified, isolated, and slung with fine vessel loops. Dissection around the common hepatic duct is kept to a minimal to preserve its blood supply.[50] After defining the most cephalic portion of the common hepatic duct, a Lahey clamp is applied to the proximal end. The common hepatic duct is severed by sharp dissection and the proximal portion plicated. The 3 and 9 o'clock feeding arteries on the borders of the severed common hepatic duct are plicated with 6/0 Prolene. Care is taken not to detach it from the right hepatic artery usually in juxtaposition of it posteriorly. Although enough length for the subsequent duct-to-duct anastomosis is necessary, a very long recipient bile duct is particularly prone to ischemic stricture formation. The division of the hepatic artery is preceded by control of the proximal end by a suitable size microvascular clamp to minimize trauma to the arterial stump. This is followed by ligation of the distal portions. The main, the proximal right and left portal veins are isolated. A pancreaticoduodenal branch of the portal vein usually present anteriorly and inferiorly is ligated and divided only if it is necessary to gain enough length for application of the clamp on the main portal vein. Portal vein anastomotic stricture is usually a result of kinking due to excessive length of the portal vein. Experience from segmental resection of the portal vein of up to 4 cm testifies to the feasibility of portal vein anastomosis even when lengths of the two portions appear deficient.

The right and left triangular ligaments are detached and the short hepatic veins are divided between ligatures from the IVC. In contrast to DDLT, the recipient IVC is preserved in ALDLT. Nevertheless, circumferential control of the IVC is still necessary during hepatic vein anastomosis. Early mobilization of the retrohepatic IVC by dividing the lumbar veins between ligatures allows lifting up of the liver for dividing the short hepatic veins (Color Plates, Figure LI-11). This is further facilitated after dividing the portal vein when the donor liver graft is ready for delivery. Then, the main portal vein is controlled with a Blalock 18 mm pulmonary vascular clamp and the right and left portal veins divided close to the liver hilum. The right hepatic vein is clamped and divided. The middle and left hepatic veins are cross-clamped by Satinsky vascular clamp and divided, thus allowing delivery of the native liver out of the abdominal cavity. In the case of hepatocellular carcinoma, an Endo GIA vascular stapler (ATW 35, Ethicon Endo-Surgery, Inc. Cincinnati, OH) could be used to prevent spillage of cancer cells from the native liver. Several lumbar and phrenic veins have to be ligated and divided before the IVC is completely mobilized from the diaphragm down to the level of the right adrenal vein. Presence of the inferior right hepatic vein of over 5 mm in the graft calls for freeing of the IVC more inferiorly for vascular anastomosis.

After hemostasis of the retroperitoneum, the IVC is occluded by a Rommel tourniquet of cotton tape on the caudal side and an Ulrich-Swiss Clamp on the cephalad side. The clamp controlling the right hepatic veins is removed. The hepatic vein stump is slit open and cut into the anterior wall of the IVC to fashion a triangular venotomy opening that matches in size and shape with the hepatic vein opening of the liver graft (Figure 30.3.1b-1; Color Plates, Figure LI-18A). The height of this triangular opening with the base on the right side and apex on the left should not be longer than half the circumference of the IVC to prevent stricture of the latter.

## RIGHT LIVER GRAFT IMPLANTATION
(Color Plates, Figure LI-14 and LI-17)

### Hepatic Vein to IVC Anastomosis

The implantation starts with the hepatic vein anastomosis performed in a triangular fashion using 10 Prolene. Running sutures are applied to the posterior wall or the base of the triangle (Figure 30.3.1b-2). This is followed by the cephalic and then the caudal side. A suspensory suture applied to the apex helps in the alignment of these two walls during the suturing. A laparotomy pad helps the approximation of the vein wall for small-for-size grafts. After the hepatic vein anastomosis is completed, the portal vein of the liver graft is inspected for correct orientation and clamped by a bulldog vascular clamp. The vascular clamp and tape controlling the IVC are then released to allow restoration of the IVC blood flow. At this time, the liver graft is partially perfused in a retrograde manner by blood regurgitating from the hepatic veins. Gradual re-warming of the graft will take place while the portal vein anastomosis is completed.

HTK solution with much lower potassium content allows restoration of graft circulation without prior flushing.[52] By applying a vascular clamp onto the graft portal vein, circulation through the IVC could be restored before portal vein anastomosis.[53] Sooner restoration of inferior vena caval circulation has the advantage

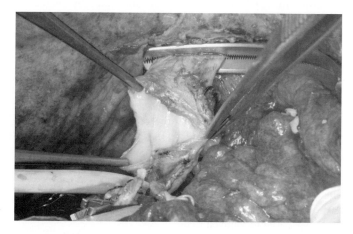

**FIGURE 30.3.1b-1**

A triangular venotomy is prepared in the inferior vena cava.

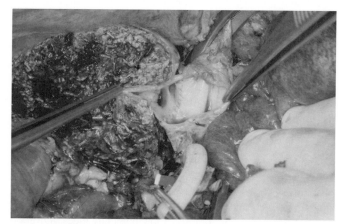

**FIGURE 30.3.1b-2**

Suturing of the posterior wall of the hepatic vein to the inferior vena cava.

of hemodynamic stability even without venovenous bypass. The latter has been shown in our series to be associated with worse outcomes, related to hypothermia and bleeding diathesis.[54] The slightly shorter preservation of HTK solution compared with UW solution is probably irrelevant in LDLT.

Venovenous bypass allows decompression of the splanchnic and retroperitoneal circulations, and prevents major hemodynamic changes during the anhepatic phase. It also provides more time for venous anastomoses by younger surgeons. Our experience, however, showed that the recipients had significantly more blood, fresh frozen plasma, and platelet infusion, and had a lower body temperature. The liver and renal functions of the first postoperative weeks were worse, and hospital mortality was also higher. By multivariate analysis, the lower body temperature was the significant factor that determined hospital death.[54]

## Portal Vein Anastomosis

When the Blalock clamp is applied to the proximal portion of the main portal vein, the blades are inline with the bifurcation of the portal vein, corresponding to its largest dimension. Recipient portal vein is divided just proximal to the bifurcation for adequate size and length. To avoid redundancy, the length of the graft portal vein and recipient portal vein is adjusted and the ends trimmed if necessary. Portal vein anastomosis is performed with 6/0 Prolene by running sutures. The graft right portal vein is often thin and liable to damage by the needle if it does not follow a smooth path of insertion and withdrawal. Bringing the vein wall with the DeBakey forceps to the needle minimizes needle movement. The graft is also raised with a gauze pack to approximate the portal veins. Just before completion of the suture, stagnant portal venous blood is released by loosening of the Blalock clamp applied to the recipient main portal vein. A Satinsky vascular clamp replacing the Balock clamp can facilitate this step. Following the suturing, the knot is placed away from the vessel walls to incorporate a growth factor about the diameter,[55] or two thirds the transverse dimension of the portal vein. Clamp on the graft side is released before the recipient side. Minor bleeding from the needle holes is expected to stop spontaneously.

## Hepatic Artery Anastomosis

In view of the high incidence of hepatic artery thrombosis employing magnifying loupes, the Kyoto group initiated hepatic artery anastomosis under high magnification with operating microscope (Wild M650; Leica, Heerbrugg, Switzerland) at a magnification of x 10 to x 15.[56] A paired Acland microvascular clamp (S&T, Neuhausen, Switzerland) is applied to both vessel ends to relieve the tension and maintain proper alignment of the two vessels. Our 10-year experience of hepatic artery anastomosis under the operating microscope showed a complication rate of 2%.[57] Multiple interrupted stitches with 9-0 nonabsorbable nylon monofilament sutures are used. Adequate lengths of both the recipient and the graft hepatic arteries are necessary to allow rotating the vessels for placement of sutures on the posterior wall. Long microvascular surgical instruments are often required to operate in the depth of the operating field. Doppler ultrasonography is performed immediately after anastomosis and after closure of the abdominal wound to ensure patency of the anastomosis. A low pulsatility index and good diastolic flow indicate satisfactory anastomosis. Hepatic artery flow is adversely affected by high portal inflow.[58] The selection of recipient hepatic artery for anastomosis is based on length, caliber, and

orientation. If the left hepatic artery satisfies the above criteria, it is preferable as rotation of the right liver graft to the left for hemostasis of the right subphrenic structures does not stretch the arterial anastomosis. Patients who had undergone transarterial oily chemoembolization may sustain damage to the hepatic artery. The gastroduodenal artery may be an alternative for anastomosis. A note is made of the course of the hepatic artery in relation to the bile ducts in case biliary reconstruction is necessary for biliary stricture at a later date.

## Biliary Reconstruction

Duct-to-duct anastomosis is our preferred technique for ALDLT except in the case of sclerosing cholangitis or choledochal cyst with extrahepatic involvement. The advantages include shorter operation time and avoidance of contamination of the operation field by bowel contents from enterotomy prior to anastomosis with the Roux loop. The sphincter of Oddi as a defense against enteric reflex and ascending infection is preserved. The risk of internal herniation is also eliminated.[59] In case of bile leakage from the anastomosis, the contamination to the peritoneal cavity is also less catastrophic. It also allows access to the biliary anastomosis by endoscopic retrograde cholangiopancreatography. The biliary complication rate for duct-to-duct anastomosis (n = 41) and the historic control of hepaticojejunostomy (n = 71) were 24% and 31%, respectively ($P = 0.457$).[60] A very low stricture rate for hepaticojejunostomy (5.3%) had been demonstrated by one series.[61] Comparison of results among centers is difficult as anastomotic techniques vary, so do the graft and recipient factors. A high Model for End-Stage Liver Disease score[60] and probably small-for-size grafts leading to poor artery perfusion[58] increase biliary complication rates.

Prior to ductal anastomosis, absence of common bile duct stones of the recipient is confirmed by choledochoscopy. Duct-to-duct anastomosis is performed between the graft right hepatic duct and the recipient common hepatic duct. We use 6-0 PDS sutures that are resorbable. The posterior wall is approximated with continuous sutures and the anterior wall by interrupted ones, with stitches not closer than 1 mm to avoid ischemia. Knots are tied after placement of all the sutures. In the case of double graft right hepatic duct, approximation of the adjacent ductal orifices to form a single cuff is done after hepatic artery anastomosis.[62] Insertion and withdrawal of needles to the graft bile duct should follow the curve of the needle to avoid creating a hole in the bile duct larger than the suture. Gentle retractor of the duodenum by the second assistant providing just enough exposure and not creating undue traction to the bile ducts is also important. We believe that microleakage through needle holes is conducive to formation of biliary anastomotic stricture. A 3.5-Fr Argyl cannula could be useful in guiding placement of sutures on the anterior wall. The catheter is removed prior to tying of the knots.

The issue of stenting of the biliary anastomosis is controversial. Currently, we do not insert T-tube or stent in either duct-to-duct anastomosis or hepatico-jejunostomy and have observed no deleterious effect. In case when the graft hepatic duct orifice is tiny and hepaticojejunostomy is made, some surgeons advocate insertion of an external biliary stent to prevent partial occlusion of the anastomosis by swollen mucosa and subsequent cholangitis. However, the value of such approach has not been documented by prospective randomized trials.

Doppler ultrasonography is mandatory before and after wound closure to check the patency and pulsatility of the graft blood vessels. We no longer place abdominal drains. We have shown in our series that abdominal drains are associated with a higher wound infection rate in liver resection of cirrhotic livers.[63] Conventionally abdominal drains placed in the proximity of the liver transection surface serve to detect and contain bile leakage. By meticulous liver transection with ligation and clipping of vasculobiliary channels, bile leakage could be avoided. Abdominal drains also allow release of ascitic fluid. However, the drain as a foreign body which transgresses the body barrier invites infection. Coupled with this policy is the reliable biliary anastomosis and unimpeded venous outflow.

## CONCLUSIONS

To justify ALDLT, donor voluntarism, acceptable donor morbidity, and good recipient outcomes are the least that could be expected. The Live Organ Donor Consensus Group has largely supported this viewpoint.[64] Given the often limited "choice" of living donors, the graft size could hardly be improved for a recipient. In the face of recipient portal hypertension the full potential of the partial liver graft has to be utilized. By including the MHV and coupled with a venoplasty with the right hepatic vein the maximal functional liver parenchyma of the graft is transplanted to the recipient.

Although a single technique of right liver ALDLT is described in this chapter, the choice of grafts should be individualized which includes using the left liver graft with the caudate lobe. The choice of the grafts should not compromise recipient surgical outcome. Thus, the judicious use of the right lobe grafts in the appropriate recipient is to be practiced. Shortage of deceased donor liver grafts will probably remain refractory. Although xenografts and stem cell transplantation are to date clinically not applicable, our immediate task is to improve donor safety and recipient success through technical innovations, careful operations and meticulous perioperative care.

## References

1. Bismuth H, Houssin D. Reduced-sized orthotopic liver graft in hepatic transplantation in children. *Surgery* 1984;95:367.
2. Pichlmayr R, Ringe B, Gubernatis G, et al. [Transplantation of a donor liver to 2 recipients (splitting transplantation)—a new method in the further development of segmental liver transplantation]. *Langenbecks Arch Chir* 1988;373:127.
3. Bismuth H, Morino M, Castaing D, et al. Emergency orthotopic liver transplantation in two patients using one donor liver. *Br J Surg* 1989;76:722.
4. Strong R, Ong TH, Pillay P, et al. A new method of segmental orthotopic liver transplantation in children. *Surgery* 1988;104:104.
5. Smith B. Segmental liver transplantation from a living donor. *J Pediatr Surg* 1969;4:126.
6. Strong RW, Lynch SV, Ong TH, et al. Successful liver transplantation from a living donor to her son. *N Engl J Med* 1990;322:1505.
7. Strong RW. Whither living donor liver transplantation? *Liver Transpl Surg* 1999;5:536.
8. Strong RW, Fawcett J, Lynch SV. Living-donor and split-liver transplantation in adults: right versus left-sided grafts. *J Hepatobiliary Pancreat Surg* 2003;10:5.
9. Ozawa K, Uemoto S, Tanaka K, et al. An appraisal of pediatric liver transplantation from living relatives. Initial clinical experiences in 20 pediatric liver transplantations from living relatives as donors. *Ann Surg* 1992;216:547.
10. Makuuchi M, Kawasaki S, Noguchi T, et al. Donor hepatectomy for living related partial liver transplantation. *Surgery* 1993;113:395.
11. Hashikura Y, Makuuchi M, Kawasaki S, et al. Successful living-related partial liver transplantation to an adult patient. *Lancet* 1994;343:1233.

12. Kiuchi T, Kasahara M, Uryuhara K, et al. Impact of graft size mismatching on graft prognosis in liver transplantation from living donors. *Transplantation* 1999;67:321.
13. Yamaoka Y, Washida M, Honda K, et al. Liver transplantation using a right lobe graft from a living related donor. *Transplantation* 1994;57:1127.
14. Lo CM, Fan ST, Liu CL, et al. Extending the limit on the size of adult recipient in living donor liver transplantation using extended right lobe graft. *Transplantation* 1997;63:1524.
15. Kiuchi T, Inomata Y, Uemoto S, et al. Evolution of living donor liver transplantation in adults: a single center experience. *Transpl Int* 2000;13 (Suppl 1):S134.
16. Marcos A, Ham JM, Fisher RA, et al: Single-center analysis of the first 40 adult-to-adult living donor liver transplants using the right lobe. *Liver Transpl* 2000;6:296.
17. Malago M, Testa G, Frilling A, et al. Right living donor liver transplantation: an option for adult patients: single institution experience with 74 patients. *Ann Surg* 2003;238:853.
18. Emond JC, Renz JF, Ferrell LD, et al. Functional analysis of grafts from living donors. Implications for the treatment of older recipients. *Ann Surg* 1996;224:544.
19. Urata K, Kawasaki S, Matsunami H, et al. Calculation of child and adult standard liver volume for liver transplantation. *Hepatology* 1995;21:1317.
20. Sugawara Y, Makuuchi M, Takayama T, et al. Small-for-size grafts in living-related liver transplantation. *J Am Coll Surg* 2001;192:510.
21. Ben-Haim M, Emre S, Fishbein TM, et al: Critical graft size in adult-to-adult living donor liver transplantation: impact of the recipient's disease. *Liver Transpl* 7:948, 2001.
22. Lo CM, Fan ST, Liu CL, et al. Minimum graft size for successful living donor liver transplantation. *Transplantation* 1999;68:1112.
23. Fan ST, Lo CM, Liu CL, et al. Determinants of hospital mortality of adult recipients of right lobe live donor liver transplantation. *Ann Surg* 2003;238:864.
24. Man K, Lo CM, Ng IO, et al. Liver transplantation in rats using small-for-size grafts: a study of hemodynamic and morphological changes. *Arch Surg* 2001;136:280.
25. Man K, Fan ST, Lo CM, et al. Graft injury in relation to graft size in right lobe live donor liver transplantation: a study of hepatic sinusoidal injury in correlation with portal hemodynamics and intragraft gene expression. *Ann Surg* 237:256, 2003.
26. Boillot O, Delafosse B, Mechet I, et al. Small-for-size partial liver graft in an adult recipient; a new transplant technique. *Lancet* 2002;359:406.
27. Troisi R, Ricciardi S, Smeets P, et al. Effects of hemi-portocaval shunts for inflow modulation on the outcome of small-for-size grafts in living donor liver transplantation. *Am J Transplant* 2005;5:1397.
28. Lo CM, Liu CL, Fan ST. Portal hyperperfusion injury as the cause of primary nonfunction in a small-for-size liver graft-successful treatment with splenic artery ligation. *Liver Transpl* 2003;9:626.
29. Troisi R, Cammu G, Militerno G, et al. Modulation of portal graft inflow: a necessity in adult living-donor liver transplantation? *Ann Surg* 2003;237:429.
30. Marcos A, Orloff M, Mieles L, et al. Functional venous anatomy for right-lobe grafting and techniques to optimize outflow. *Liver Transpl* 2001;7:845.
31. Lo CM, Fan ST, Liu CL, et al. Hepatic venoplasty in living-donor liver transplantation using right lobe graft with middle hepatic vein. *Transplantation* 2003;75:358.
32. Chan SC, Lo CM, Liu CL, et al. Versatility and viability of hepatic venoplasty in live donor liver transplantation using the right lobe with the middle hepatic vein. *Hepatobiliary Pancreat Dis Int* 2005;4:618.
33. Liu CL, Zhao Y, Lo CM, et al. Hepatic venoplasty in right lobe live donor liver transplantation. *Liver Transpl* 2003;9:1265.
34. Vauthey JN, Lauwers GY, Esnaola NF, et al. Simplified staging for hepatocellular carcinoma. *J Clin Oncol* 2002;20:1527.
35. Shetty K, Timmins K, Brensinger C, et al. Liver transplantation for hepatocellular carcinoma validation of present selection criteria in predicting outcome. *Liver Transpl* 2004;10:911.
36. Mazzaferro V, Regalia E, Doci R, et al. Liver transplantation for the treatment of small hepatocellular carcinomas in patients with cirrhosis. *N Engl J Med* 1996;334:693.

37. Yao FY, Ferrell L, Bass NM, et al. Liver transplantation for hepatocellular carcinoma: expansion of the tumor size limits does not adversely impact survival. *Hepatology* 2001;33:1394.

38. Esnaola NF, Lauwers GY, Mirza NQ, et al. Predictors of microvascular invasion in patients with hepatocellular carcinoma who are candidates for orthotopic liver transplantation. *J Gastrointest Surg* 2002;6:224.

39. Schwartz M: Liver transplantation for hepatocellular carcinoma. *Gastroenterology* 2004;127(5 Suppl 1):S268.

40. Kaihara S, Kiuchi T, Ueda M, et al. Living-donor liver transplantation for hepatocellular carcinoma. *Transplantation* 2003;75(3 Suppl):S37.

41. Todo S, Furukawa H. Living donor liver transplantation for adult patients with hepatocellular carcinoma: experience in Japan. *Ann Surg* 2004;240:451.

42. Broelsch CE, Frilling A, Malago M. Should we expand the criteria for liver transplantation for hepatocellular carcinoma—yes, of course! *J Hepatol* 2005;43:569.

43. Abt PL, Mange KC, Olthoff KM, et al. Allograft Survival Following Adult-to-Adult Living Donor Liver Transplantation. *Am J Transplant* 2004;4:1302.

44. Thuluvath PJ, Yoo HY: Graft and patient survival after adult live donor liver transplantation compared to a matched cohort who received a deceased donor transplantation. *Liver Transpl* 2004;10:1263.

45. Neuhaus P: Live donor/split liver grafts for adult recipients: When should we use them? *Liver Transpl* 2005;11(11 Suppl 2):S6.

46. Lo CM, Fan ST, Liu CL, et al. Adult-to-adult living donor liver transplantation using extended right lobe grafts. *Ann Surg* 1997;226:261.

47. Liu CL, Lam B, Lo CM, et al: Impact of right-lobe live donor liver transplantation on patients waiting for liver transplantation. *Liver Transpl* 2003;9:863.

48. Liu CL, Fan ST, Lo CM, et al: Living-donor liver transplantation for high-urgency situations. *Transplantation* 2003;75(3 Suppl):S33.

49. Eghtesad B, Kadry Z, Fung J. Technical considerations in liver transplantation: what a hepatologist needs to know (and every surgeon should practice). *Liver Transpl* 2005;11:861.

50. Vellar ID. Preliminary study of the anatomy of the venous drainage of the intrahepatic and extrahepatic bile ducts and its relevance to the practice of hepatobiliary surgery. *ANZ J Surg* 2001;71:418.

51. Poon RT, Fan ST, Lo CM, et al. Pancreaticoduodenectomy with en bloc portal vein resection for pancreatic carcinoma with suspected portal vein involvement. *World J Surg* 2004;28:602.

52. Testa G, Malago M, Nadalin S, et al. Histidine-tryptophan-ketoglutarate versus University of Wisconsin solution in living donor liver transplantation: results of a prospective study. *Liver Transpl* 2003;9:822.

53. Chan SC, Liu CL, Lo CM, et al. Applicability of histidine-tryptophan-ketoglutarate solution in right lobe adult-to-adult live donor liver transplantation. *Liver Transpl* 2004;10:1415.

54. Fan ST, Yong BH, Lo CM, et al. Right lobe living donor liver transplantation with or without venovenous bypass. *Br J Surg* 2003;90:48.

55. Starzl TE, Iwatsuki S, Shaw BW Jr. A growth factor in fine vascular anastomoses. *Surg Gynecol Obstet* 1984;159:164.

56. Mori K, Nagata I, Yamagata S, et al. The introduction of microvascular surgery to hepatic artery reconstruction in living-donor liver transplantation—its surgical advantages compared with conventional procedures. *Transplantation* 1992;54:263.

57. Wei WI, Lam LK, Ng RW, et al. Microvascular reconstruction of the hepatic artery in live donor liver transplantation: experience across a decade. *Arch Surg* 2004;139:304.

58. Marcos A, Olzinski AT, Ham JM, et al. The interrelationship between portal and arterial blood flow after adult to adult living donor liver transplantation. *Transplantation* 2000;70:1697.

59. Liu CL, Lo CM, Chan SC, et al. Internal hernia of the small bowel after right-lobe live donor liver transplantation. *Clin Transplant* 2004;18:211.

60. Liu CL, Lo CM, Chan SC, et al: Safety of duct-to-duct biliary reconstruction in right-lobe live-donor liver transplantation without biliary drainage. *Transplantation* 2004;77:726.

61. Yi NJ, Suh KS, Cho JY, et al. In adult-to-adult living donor liver transplantation hepaticojejunostomy shows a better long-term outcome than duct-to-duct anastomosis. *Transpl Int* 2005;18:1240.

62. Fan ST, Lo CM, Liu CL, et al. Biliary reconstruction and complications of right lobe live donor liver transplantation. *Ann Surg* 2002;236:676.

63. Liu CL, Fan ST, Lo CM, et al. Abdominal drainage after hepatic resection is contraindicated in patients with chronic liver diseases. *Ann Surg* 2004;239:194.

64. Abecassis M, Adams M, Adams P, et al. Consensus statement on the live organ donor. *JAMA* 2000;284:2919.

## 30.3.1c  Left Lobe Transplant With and Without the Caudate Lobe

*Yasuhiko Sugawara, MD, M. Makuuchi, MD*

### INTRODUCTION

In early adult-to-adult living donor (LD) liver transplants, left liver grafts were routinely used,[1] and satisfactory results were reported.[2] Some transplant surgeons, however, suggested that the unsatisfactory results in adults might be due to undersized grafts that did not meet the metabolic demands of the patient.[3] Accordingly, recent reports indicate that left liver grafts for adult patients have been almost abandoned. Right liver grafts are almost always used in the Western world.[4] The minimal graft volume for success, however, depends on the pretransplant condition[5] and disease of the recipient.[6]

In our institution, left liver plus caudate lobe grafts[7] are now used. The caudate lobe is a small part of the whole liver, but its volume is not negligible in the partial liver graft, providing an 8% to 12% gain in left graft weight.[8] For maximum use of the caudate lobe, reconstruction of the major short hepatic vein draining the caudate lobe should be performed.

### INDICATIONS

We have contended that left liver grafts are feasible for good-risk adult recipients. Previously, we reported successful results of left liver transplants for adult recipients.[3] The basic principles are as follows (1) graft size should be over 40% (35% for good-risk recipients) of the recipient's standard liver volume; (2) the parenchymal resection percentage should be under 70% (under 65% with extended right liver grafts, Fig. 30.3.1c-1). The minimum graft size for good-risk recipients who have a Model for End-Stage Liver Disease (MELD) score of less than 15 can be 35% of the recipient's standard liver volume.[9] Grafts that are over 30% of the recipient's standard liver volume may be acceptable for patients with metabolic disorders, such as citrullinemia or familial amyloid polyneuropathy.

### RECIPIENT OPERATION (Color Plates, Figures LI-15, LI-16, and LI-17)

#### Total Hepatectomy

The operative technique for recipients is based on the technique of whole-liver resection with preservation of the inferior vena cava, as used for orthotopic liver transplants.[10] A J-shape incision is made to open the abdominal space, as for a right hepatectomy. An argon beam coagulator is useful to stop bleeding from the hepatic surface. Each step of this operation requires meticulous technique and great care, in order to achieve an uneventful resection of the whole liver, while avoiding injury to other visceral organs. It is important to make a large and long opening along the sides of the hepatic veins, as well as to maintain satisfactory portal, biliary, and hepatic arterial sources for reconstruction. The right

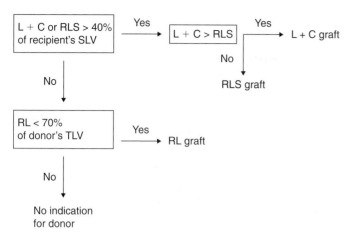

**FIGURE 30.3.1c-1**

Diagram for graft selection. The graft size should be over 40% of the recipient's SLV. The parenchymal resection percentage should be under 70%. Abbreviations used: L+C, left liver plus caudate lobe; RL, right liver; RLS, right lateral sector, SLV: standard liver volume, TLV: total liver volume.

and left hepatic arteries should be dissected out as distally as possible (Color Plates, Figure LI-10A); the left portal vein should be dissected up to the umbilical portion, which is just distal to the point of origin of the branch to segment 2; and the right portal vein should be dissected up to its bifurcation into the paramedian and lateral branches.

In recipients with little portosystemic collateral circulation, preventing portal congestion is necessary during the anhepatic phase. A temporary shunt between the portal vein and the inferior vena cava should be made.[11] Briefly, the portal vein branch, which will not be used for reconstruction, is anastomosed end-to-side or connected by a tube to the inferior vena cava. Blood flow through this shunt is maintained until portal venous reperfusion to the graft is achieved by portal vein anastomosis.

To ensure adequate hepatic venous flow, it is necessary to obtain a wide ostium and sufficient length for anastomosis of the hepatic veins.[12] Adequate hepatic venous flow should be ensured by venoplasty of the hepatic veins of the graft and of the recipient. For left liver transplants, the left and middle hepatic veins in the recipient are used for venoplasty. When the orifice of the combined left and middle hepatic veins is smaller than the graft hepatic vein, a wide orifice is created by venoplasty of three hepatic veins. Afterward, the approximation is checked with another clamp placed at the distal end.

## HEPATIC VEIN ANASTOMOSIS

In the initial LD liver transplants,[13] the drainage vein of the caudate lobe was not reconstructed. Complete revascularization of the caudate lobe should contribute to full graft regeneration.[14] Reconstruction of the caudate vein, however, is technically demanding. The hepatic vein of the caudate lobe can be resected with a cuff of the vena cava, which resembles a Carrel patch (Figure 30.3.1c-2). In the recipient operation, the caudate hepatic vein is constructed; then the trunks of the left and middle hepatic veins of the recipient and of the graft are anastomosed (Figure 30.3.1c-3). When the orifice of the short hepatic vein is located near those of the left and middle hepatic veins, the caudate vein with a cuff of the inferior vena cava can be sutured to the common orifice of the

left hepatic vein and middle hepatic vein. Thereafter, end-to-end anastomoses are made between the recipient and graft common trunks of the middle-left hepatic veins.

A new venoplasty technique has recently been applied to decrease warm ischemic time during venous reconstruction. A conduit vein graft and a patch vein graft are used to make a wide single orifice, with a large cuff consisting of the left and middle hepatic veins and the short hepatic vein. One side of a conduit vein graft is cut longitudinally to widen the orifice, which is anastomosed to the orifice of the short hepatic vein. The other side is first cut longitudinally and then horizontally. The opened edge is sutured to the posterior cuff of the left and middle hepatic veins (the lumen of a conduit vein graft cannot be narrowed). The right side of the middle hepatic vein cuff and the left side of the superficial branch of the left hepatic vein are cut longitudinally, and a rectangular-shaped vein patch is attached to the cuff for venoplasty. A circular cuff vein patch is used when the vein cuff of the liver graft is not sufficient for anastomosis. Thus, the liver graft is connected to the recipient inferior vena cava by a single and wide anastomotic site.

## PORTAL VEIN ANASTOMOSIS

When there is no stenosis or vein thrombosis leading to reduced portal vein flow, direct anastomosis is performed without a vein graft, using 6-0 monofilament.[15] When the recipient portal vein is stenotic, the vein graft is mounted over the recipient portal vein, which is incised longitudinally. When the portal vein trunk is judged inappropriate to function as a conduit (because of a narrow diameter or damaged intima), it is sacrificed; the portal conduit is anastomosed to the proximal portal vein of the recipient, near the confluence of the splenic and superior mesenteric veins. Thrombectomy is the first choice for recipients with portal vein

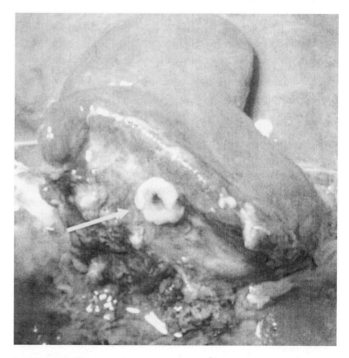

**FIGURE 30.3.1c-2**

The hepatic vein of the caudate lobe can be resected with a cuff of the vena cava. Arrow indicates the short hepatic vein.

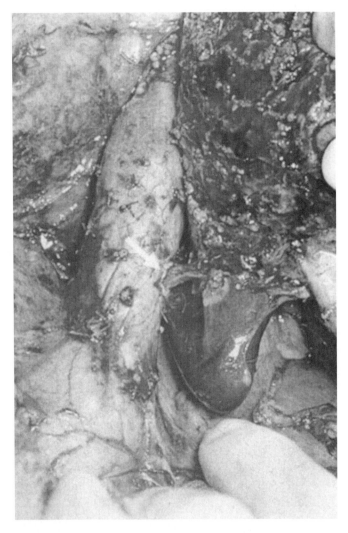

**FIGURE 30.3.1c-3**

Reconstruction of the caudate hepatic vein. Arrow indicates the anastomotic site.

thrombosis. However, a venous jump graft is indicated for recipients with complete portal vein and proximal superior mesenteric vein thrombosis.[15]

A previous study[17] reveals that 13% of recipients have an isolated caudate portal vein originating from the left sidewall of the portal branches of the Spiegelian lobe. For full graft function of the caudate lobe, the isolated caudate portal vein should be reconstructed.[18]

## HEPATIC ARTERY ANASTOMOSIS

### Use of a Microscope

Hepatic arterial reconstruction in LD liver recipients is technically difficult, given the existence of the short and thin hepatic arteries on a liver graft. A significant association has been noted between hepatic arterial thrombosis and the presence of hepatic arteries under 3 mm in diameter.[19] In LD liver recipients, the median diameter of the arterial branch is under 3 mm,[20] so microsurgery is inevitable and indispensable.[21] The information provided

by preoperative angiography is essential for surgical planning,[22] because hepatic arteries are subject to many variations.

When it is difficult to turn over the graft artery, a 9-0 monofilament nylon microsuture with double needles (W10V43-9N, Keisei Medical Industrial, Tokyo, Japan) is used for anastomosis.[23] The first suture is placed at the most difficult point (usually at the middle of the posterior wall) in the artery to be visualized through the microscope. Each suture is always placed from the inner side of the arterial wall to the outer side. The posterior suture is tied, pulling toward the back. The subsequent sutures are advanced anteriorly on either side adjacent to the previous suture. When there is a discrepancy in the diameter between the graft and the recipient artery, each suture is placed to gradually compensate for the discrepancy.

## NO NEED TO RECONSTRUCT ALL BRANCHES

In our previous series, the frequency of multiple arterial orifices was 48% in left liver grafts.[24] A double arterial supply to the liver graft was thought to be unsuitable for LD liver transplants.[25] The Kyoto group[21] reconstructed all the hepatic arteries of a liver graft.

Accessory hepatic arteries usually communicate with the original lobar arteries in the hepatic hilum.[26] Reconstruction of all hepatic arterial branches is usually unnecessary.[27] The existence of aberrant hepatic arteries is convenient for reconstruction: they are thick and can be harvested long. In arterial reconstruction of grafts with multiple arterial orifices, an adequate arterial flow to the nonanastomosed arterial branches should be confirmed.[28]

First, during the completion of the donor hepatectomy, before smaller branches of the hepatic artery are cut, they are clamped and arterial flow is examined by Doppler ultrasonography. When smaller branches of the hepatic artery are cut, pulsatile back bleeding is observed. Second, on the bench, when perfusion fluid is flushed though the largest artery, it should be observed to flow out from the smaller arterial branches. Third, arterial flow can be confirmed during the recipient operation, after reconstruction of the largest hepatic artery, by the presence of pulsatile back bleeding from the stump of the other graft's arteries. Finally, the hepatic arterial signal can be checked by Doppler ultrasonography of each segment of the liver graft.

## BILE DUCT ANASTOMOSIS

In the initial series, bile duct reconstruction was performed with a Roux-en-Y bile duct-jejunostomy. The main left hepatic ducts were reconstructed in a standard manner. Small bile ducts of the caudate lobe were anastomosed to the intestine without mucosa-to-mucosa alignment, with an external biliary drainage tube, positioned transanastomotically.[29]

Since 2000, duct-to-duct biliary reconstruction has been used instead.[30] This procedure may preserve physiologic bilioenteric and bowel continuity, thus preventing a delayed bowel movement. Duct-to-duct reconstruction allows for easy endoscopic access to the biliary tree for diagnostic and therapeutic instrumentation and management; it also prevents ascending cholangitis.

In the recipient, the hilar plate is dissected at the second-order branch of the bile ducts. Anastomosis is performed using interrupted sutures with an external stent tube. When the left bile duct and that of the caudate lobe are closely approximated, they are joined into one.[31] If they are widely separated, they are anastomosed independently. A stent tube is not fixed at the anastomotic site, but at the opposite orifice of the hilar plate. The anastomosis is begun at the posterior wall. The needle is inserted into the bile duct of the graft from the outside to the inside, then to the orifice of the hilar plate from the inside to the outside. The knots are always outside of the bile duct. The anastomotic site can be turned around for better access.

## SUMMARY

A left liver with or without a caudate lobe graft can be an alternative to a right liver graft. Secure hepatic vein reconstruction is crucial. If the caudate lobe is included with the liver graft, short hepatic vein reconstruction should result in proportional regeneration of the caudate lobe with the left liver.

## References

1. Hashikura Y, Makuuchi M, Kawasaki S, et al. Successful living-related partial liver transplantation to an adult patient. *Lancet* 1994;343:1233.
2. Kawasaki S, Makuuchi M, Matsunami H, et al. Living related liver transplantation in adults. *Ann Surg* 11998;227:269.
3. Sugawara Y, Makuuchi M, Takayama T, et al. Small-for-size grafts in living-related liver transplantation. *J Am Coll Surg* 2001;192:510.
4. Marcos A, Fisher RA, Ham JM, et al. Right lobe living donor liver transplantation. *Transplantation* 1999;68:798.
5. Lo CM, Fan ST, Liu CL, et al. Minimum graft size for successful living donor liver transplantation. *Transplantation* 1999;68:1112.
6. Ben-Haim M, Emre S, Fishbein TM, et al. Critical graft size in adult-to-adult living donor liver transplantation: impact of the recipient's disease. *Liver Transpl* 2001;7:948.
7. Takayama T, Makuuchi M, Kubota K, et al. Living-relatedtransplantation of left liver plus caudate lobe. *J Am Coll Surg* 2000;190:635.
8. Akamatsu N, Sugawara Y, Tamura S, et al. Regeneration and function of hemiliver graft: right versus left. *Surgery* 2006;139:765.
9. Sugawara Y, Makuuchi M, Kaneko J, et al. Living-donor liver transplantation in adults: Tokyo University experience. *J Hepatobiliary Pancreat Surg* 2003;10:1.
10. Tzakis A, Todo S, Starzl TE. Orthotopic liver transplantation with preservation of the inferior vena cava. *Ann Surg* 1989;210:649.
11. Kawasaki S, Hashikura Y, Matsunami H, et al. Temporary shunt between right portal vein and vena cava in living related liver transplantation. *J Am Coll Surg* 1996;183:74.
12. Makuuchi M, Sugawara Y. Living-donor liver transplantation using the left liver, with special reference to vein reconstruction. *Transplantation* 2003;75:S23.
13. Miyagawa S, Hashikura Y, Miwa S, et al. Concomitant caudate lobe resection as an option for donor hepatectomy in adult living related liver transplantation. *Transplantation* 1998;66:661.
14. Sugawara Y, Makuuchi M, Takayama T. Left liver plus caudate lobe graft with complete revascularization. *Surgery* 2002;132:904.
15. Sugawara Y, Makuuchi M, Tamura S, et al. Portal vein reconstruction in adult living donor liver transplantation using cryopreserved vein grafts. *Liver Transpl* (in press)2006.
16. Yerdel MA, Gunson B, Mirza D, et al. Portal vein thrombosis in adults undergoing liver transplantation: risk factors, screening, management, and outcome. *Transplantation* 2000;69:1873.
17. Kokudo N, Sugawara Y, Kaneko J, et al. Reconstruction of isolated caudate portal vein in left liver graft. *Liver Transpl* 2004;10:1163.
18. Yamazaki S, Takayama T, Inoue K, et al. Interposition of autologous portal vein graft in left liver transplantation. *Liver Transpl* 2005;11:1615.
19. Mazzaferro V, Esquivel CO, Makowka L, et al. Hepatic artery thrombosis after pediatric liver transplantation: a medical or surgical event? *Transplantation* 1989;47:971.
20. Sakamoto Y, Takayama T, Nakatsuka T, et al. Advantage in using living donors with aberrant hepatic artery for partial liver graft arterialization. *Transplantation* 2002;74:518.
21. Mori K, Nagata I, Yamagata S, et al. The introduction of microvascular surgery to hepatic artery reconstruction in living-donor liver transplantation: its surgical advantages compared with conventional procedures. *Transplantation* 1992;54:263.
22. Sugawara Y, Kaneko J, Akamatsu N, et al. Arterial anatomy unsuitable for a right liver donation. *Liver Transpl* 2003;9:1116.
23. Okazaki M, Asato H, Takushima A, et al. Hepatic artery reconstruction with double-needle microsuture in living-donor liver transplantation. *Liver Transpl* 2006;12:46.
24. Kishi Y, Sugawara Y, Kaneko J, et al. Hepatic arterial anatomy for right liver procurement from living donors. *Liver Transpl* 2004; 10:129.
25. Broelsch CE, Whitington PF, Emond JC, et al. Liver transplantation in children from living-related donors:surgical techniques and results. *Ann Surg* 1991;214:428.
26. Redman HC, Reuter SR. Arterial collaterals in the liver hilus. *Radiology* 1970;94:575.
27. Ikegami T, Kawasaki S, Matsunami H, et al. Should all hepatic arterial branches be reconstructed in living-related liver transplantation? *Surgery* 1996;119:431.
28. Kubota K, Makuuchi M, Takayama T, et al. Simple test on the back table for justifying single hepatic-arterial reconstruction in living related liver transplantation. *Transplantation* 2000;70:696.
29. Kubota K, Takayama T, Sano K, et al. Small bile duct reconstruction of the caudate lobe in living-related liver transplantation. *Ann Surg* 2002;235:174.
30. Sugawara Y, Sano K, Kaneko J, et al. Duct-to-duct biliary reconstruction for living donor liver transplantation: experience of 92 cases. *Transplant Proc* 2003;35:2981.
31. Dulundu E, Sugawara Y, Sano K, et al. Duct-to-duct biliary reconstruction in adult living-donor liver transplantation. *Transplantation* 2004;78:574.

## 30.3.1d   Double Liver Transplant

*SungGyu Lee, MD, PhD*

The major limitation of adult-to-adult living donor (LD) liver transplant is the insufficiency of graft size. More than 40% of the recipient's standard liver volume (SLV) is the minimum required graft volume for an adequate functioning hepatic mass. A left-lobe graft from a relatively small donor will not meet the metabolic demands of a larger recipient or of a critically ill recipient with portal hypertension. With increasing experience in left-lobe adult-to-adult liver transplants, a statistically significant negative impact of small-for-size grafts was realized. To overcome the barrier of left-lobe size mismatching, use of right-lobe grafts that increase the extent of liver resection in the donor was introduced[1] and rapidly spread to most centers.

Right-lobe procurement, however, accounts for 60% to 70% of the LD's total liver volume and is not always safe, depending on the remaining left lobe's volume and quality, particularly the grade of fatty degeneration. The LD's safety is an utmost concern. Even in nontransplant liver resectional surgery, a clear relationship between mortality and the extent of resection has been demonstrated.[2] Thus, an LD with a smaller remaining liver volume (less than 30% of his or her total liver volume) will have a higher risk of morbidity and mortality. If the LD has a sufficiently large right lobe (> 70% of total liver volume) adequate as a graft for an adult recipient, the remaining left lobe will be small (< 30% of total liver volume) and thus will threaten donor safety. This variety is found in 25% of all potential donors.[3] Such donors cannot be allowed to donate either side of their liver for adult recipients because donor safety will be endangered after a right hepatectomy and small-for-size graft syndrome may develop in the recipient after a left-lobe transplant.

In Asian countries, where decreased donor (DD) organ allocation remains below 5 per million population per year, the opportunity for a full-size DD liver transplant is very limited, even in high-urgency recipients. An alternative is to simultaneously transplant two small liver grafts (left lobe or left lateral segment) from two different LDs; that is, a double- or dual-graft transplant, to solve graft-size insufficiency and provide donor safety. Furthermore, if the large-size recipient requires more liver graft volume than the volume of two left-lobe grafts, and if a right hepatic lobectomy in one of two potential LDs seems to be safe, then one right-lobe and one left-lobe graft from two different LDs can be simultaneously transplanted into the recipient to avoid small-for-size graft syndrome.

## INDICATIONS

A dual left-lobe or lateral segment transplant requires two concurrent situations. First, the donor's left lobe must be too small and thus unable to meet the recipient's metabolic demand. Second, the proportion of the donor's right lobe (as compared with the left lobe) must be unusually high (greater than 70% of total liver volume; Figure 30.3.1d-1), so that right lobectomy would be too risky to the donor in the immediate postoperative period.

## OPERATIVE PROCEDURE

The recipient and two donor operations are started simultaneously.[3] The first graft is orthotopically positioned in the original left position. The second graft is heterotopically positioned to the right-upper-quadrant fossa, rotating it 180°, so that the graft's hilar structures are at the same level as the recipient's right hilar structures. This procedure requires two technical modifications when implanting the heterotopic right-sided second liver graft. Rotation of the heterotopic second liver graft through 180° of sagittal orientation brings the hilar structures into a reversed

position. That is, the bile duct comes to lie behind portal vein and hepatic artery. Hepaticojejunostomy of the second graft will be difficult in such a limited area, once the portal vein anastomosis is performed. Thus, the first technical modification is that the bile duct is reconstructed by duct-to-duct anastomosis, then followed by a ventrally lying portal vein anastomosis (Figure 30.3.1d-2).

The left-lobe graft is always too small to replace the space of the right lobe of the recipient's resected liver. Thus, the second technical modification is that a tissue expander filled with saline solution (from 200 to 450 mL) is inserted underneath the graft to relieve undue tension on the hilar anastomoses (Figure 30.3.1d-2).

In the recipient operation, both the right and the left branch of the portal vein and the hepatic artery are dissected free from the surrounding tissue, as peripherally as possible, to obtain the maximal length for future bilateral vascular anastomoses. The bile duct is similarly dissected to the level of the hilum. The total hepatectomy is performed after the suprahepatic and the retrohepatic vena cava (below the insertion of the right hepatic vein) are clamped. Venovenous bypass is necessary if a test clamp of the vena cava suggests unstable hemodynamics.

The first left-lobe graft is orthotopically placed and its hepatic vein anastomosis performed. The second 180° rotated left-lobe graft is heterotopically placed, and its hepatic vein anastomosis to the recipient's right hepatic vein is completed. Then, the portal vein anastomosis of the first orthotopic graft is performed to the recipient's left portal vein. A vascular clamp is applied to the recipient's right hepatic vein to prevent regurgitation of caval flow into the second graft after the vena caval clamps are released. The portal vascular clamp is applied to the right branch of the recipient's portal vein. Then vascular clamps to the vena cava and main portal vein are removed together, and the first (orthotopic) graft is reperfused.

Next, the bile duct of the second (heterotopic) graft is anastomosed to the recipient's bile duct in a duct-to-duct fashion. The portal vein anastomosis between the second graft and the recipient's right portal branch follows. Then, the vascular clamps on the recipient's right hepatic vein and right portal vein are released, and reperfusion of the second (heterotopic) graft is allowed. Hepatic artery anastomoses to both grafts are performed under a microscope. Finally, a Roux-en-Y hepaticojejunstomy to the first (orthotopic) liver graft is performed.

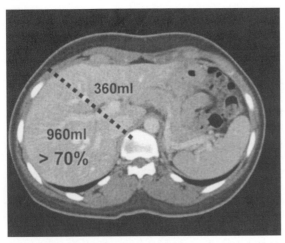

Potential Donor 1

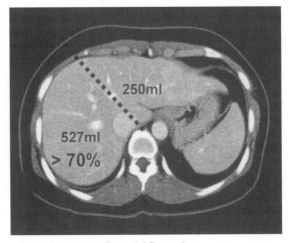

Potential Donor 2

**FIGURE 30.3.1d-1**

Two potential donors demonstrating a large right-lobe and a small left-lobe by preoperative volumetric CT.

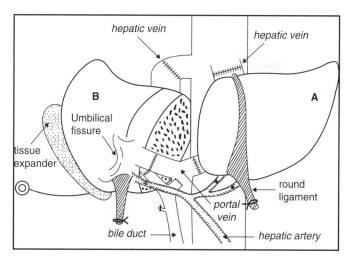

**FIGURE 30.3.1d-2**

Living donor liver transplant using dual left lobe grafts.

The number of right-lobe LD liver transplants has recently increased in many institutions, in an attempt to overcome the limitation of small-for-size grafts. However, because the donor's safety takes precedence over the recipient's outcome, the donor's remaining liver volume should not be less than 30% of his or her total liver volume. If the donor has a relatively large right lobe that is suitable as a graft for an adult recipient but the remaining left lobe is too small, then this donor cannot be accepted for a larger-size recipient. Dual left-lobe transplants using two LDs can expand application of adult-to-adult LD liver transplants—despite the limitation of the left lobe being the available largest graft. The mean graft–recipient weight ratio (GRWR) with dual left-lobe LD

transplants (median, 0.95%; range, 0.59% to 1.25%) approaches that of right-lobe LD transplants (median, 0.98%; range, 0.64% to 1.29%).

Dual-graft LD transplants raise the following questions

- Does donor morbidity increase twofold because two LDs undergo operations?

- Do recipient complications develop more frequently, since vascular and biliary anastomoses are performed twice?

- Does competitive liver regeneration between the two grafts develop?

The donor risk increases in parallel with the extent of the donor hepatectomy.[5,6] An analysis of morbidity of 1,000 LDs at our institution revealed that major donor complications requiring a prolonged hospital stay and specific interventions were more common in right-lobe LDs than in left-lobe donors.[7] Of 343 LDs who donated to 172 dual-graft recipients (note: one lateral segment was obtained from a DD) (Figure 30.3.1d-3), one LD underwent reexploration for a persistent cut-surface bile leak after lateral segmentectomy. The prevalence and the severity of donor complications were lower in the left-lobe subgroup.

The most common complications in dual-graft recipients were biliary strictures (28%) and hepatic venous outflow obstruction of the heterotopic right-sided left-lobe graft (15%). Hepatic venous outflow obstruction occurred neither to the orthotopic left-sided left-lobe graft nor to the right-sided right-lobe graft which is orthotopically positioned in its original location if a dual right-lobe and left-lobe transplant is performed. Rather, the mechanism of outflow obstruction was related to the progressive compression of the hepatic vein anastomosis by the regenerating second liver graft, which is heterotopically positioned and initially suspended on tissue expander until the 15th day posttransplant. The unrecognized

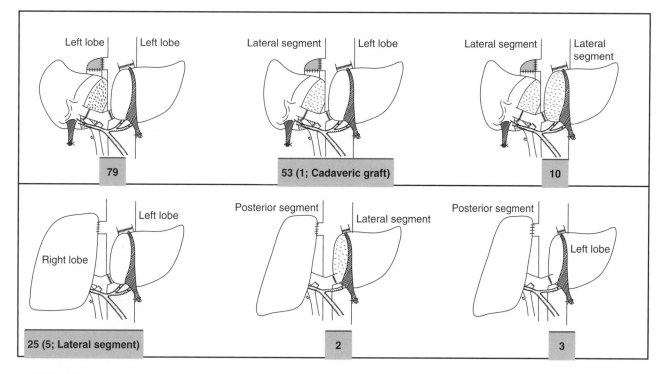

**FIGURE 30.3.1d-3**

Various kinds of 172 living donor dual liver transplants (of 938 adult living donor liver transplants) from February 1997 to September 2005 at the Asan Medical Center.

Pre-OP ➔ Post-transplant on 7th day ➔ Post-transplant 3 weeks after two left-lobe dual LDLT

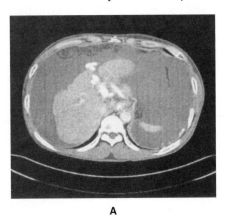
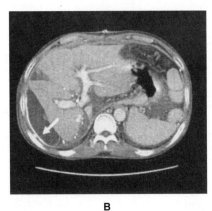
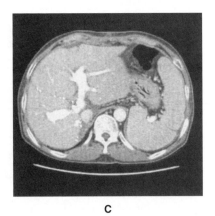

A                                    B                                    C

**FIGURE 30.3.1d-4**

Regeneration of two left-lobe liver grafts. (A) Preoperative. CT scan of the recipient showed large amounts of ascites and shrunken liver. (B) CT scan on the 7th day after transplant showed well-functioning two left-lobe liver grafts. The right-sided left lobe graft was not fully regenerated and needed tissue expander support from the behind. (C) CT scan taken 3 weeks after transplant showed that two regenerated left-lobe liver graft looked like triangular shape of normal liver.

outflow obstruction led to congestion and atrophy of the liver graft. Thus, if the recipient's liver function deteriorates, Doppler ultrasonography should be immediately done, especially to investigate outflow disturbance. Hepatic venography can confirm outflow obstruction which can then be properly managed by hepatic vein stenting.

Unlike with auxiliary partial orthotopic liver transplants (APOLTs), competition between the two liver grafts in dual-graft transplants does not develop during the regeneration period: instead, the two grafts regenerate simultaneously (Figure 30.3.1d-4).

## ASAN MEDICAL CENTER EXPERIENCE

After our first successful pediatric LD liver transplant in December 1994 and the first successful adult-to-adult LD transplant in February 1997, 938 adult-to-adult LD transplants were performed at our institution through September 2005. Of these 938 recipients, 172 underwent dual-graft transplants from March 2000 on. Indications were the same as for right-lobe LD and full-size DD liver transplants. Urgent dual-graft transplants were performed for fulminant hepatic failure (4.6%) and acute-on-chronic liver failure (19.3%). All these procedures were approved by the ethics committee of our institution and the Korean Network for Organ Sharing under the Ministry of Health. Recipient age ranged from 15 to 69 years; donor age, from 18 to 64 years.

The incidence of biopsy-proven acute rejection in dual-graft transplants is similar to that in single-graft LD recipients (17%). Three fourths of the time, in our 172 dual-graft recipients, acute rejection developed simultaneously in both of the grafts. Our in-hospital mortality rate was 5.3%—comparable to that for single-graft LD recipients—and the 1-year graft survival rate was 89.0%. The incidence and the severity of long-term complications in dual-graft and single-graft LD recipients were similar. Infrequently, unilateral graft atrophy developed in recipients of two left lobes, but it did not affect their liver function and survival.

LD transplants of dual left-lobe grafts are technically complex and elaborate, but this procedure can help solve problems related to small-for-size grafts and can help expand the indications for LD transplants and for split-liver transplants in adult recipients.

## References

1. Lo CM, Fan ST, Liu CL, et al. Adult-to-adult living donor liver transplantation using extended right lobe grafts. *Ann Surg* 1997;226:261–270.
2. Iwatsuki S, Sheahan DG, Starzl TE. The changing face of hepatic resection. *Curr Probl Surg* 1989;26:281–379.
3. Leelaudomlipi S, Sugawara Y, Kaneko J, et al. Volumetric analysis of liver segment in 155 living donors. *Liver Transpl* 2002;8:612–614.
4. Lee SG, Hwang S, Park KM, et al. An adult-to-adult living donor liver Transplant using dual left lobe grafts. *Surgery* 2001;129:647–650.
5. Dondero F, Taille C, Mal H, et al. Respiratory complications: a major concern after right hepatectomy in living liver donor. *Transplantation* 2006;81:181–186.
6. Russo MW, Brown RS Jr. Ethical issues in living donor liver transplantation. *Curr Gastroenterol Rep* 2003;5:26–30.
7. Hwang S, Lee SG, Lee YJ, et al. Lessons learned from 1,000 living donor liver transplantations in a single center: how to make living donations safe? *Liver Transpl* 2006; 12:920–927.

## 30.3.2   The Pediatric Recipient

*David C. Cronin II, MD, PhD,*
*Julian Losanoff, MD, J. Michael Millis, MD*

## BACKGROUND

Pediatric liver transplantation began with Starzl's early work in Denver, which continued in Pittsburgh.[1–3] Through these experiences the indications for pediatric liver transplantation were being established.[4] However, as the demand for grafts increased and the size discrepancy between the majority of pediatric recipients and the organ supply; technical advances were needed to reduce the pretransplant mortality. The technical advances necessary to allow successful living donor liver transplantation began with split and reduced deceased donor pediatric transplantation in several centers in Europe and the University of Chicago in the mid 1980s.[5,6] The success of these procedures allowed for the same technical concepts to be applied to the recipient living donor operation.

The first living donor liver transplants occurred in Australia and Brazil, both technically successful, although neither patient experienced long-term survival.[7,8] Broelsch, while at the University of Chicago, completed the first prospective controlled trial of living donor liver transplantation.[9] The success of this trial was pivotal in the development and refinement of the surgical techniques for both recipient and donor, defining the ethical and safety requirements for donor selection and use, and established justification for dissemination of the technique throughout the world as a standard-of-care in pediatric liver transplantation.

## INDICATIONS

The indications for living donor pediatric liver transplantation are the same as those for standard full-size, reduced-size, or split deceased donor liver transplantation and are listed in Table 30.3.2-1. The major advantage of living donor liver transplantation over deceased donor liver transplantation is the ability to prospectively determine the timing of the transplant. Thus, availability and use of the living donor has dramatically decreased the pretransplant [waiting list] mortality among children.[10]

Application of living donor liver transplantation varies dramatically around the world due to many cultural, religious, and societal differences. For example, in many Asian countries, living donors are the major source of grafts, while in the North America and Europe living donation accounts for a approximately 10% of the pediatric transplants.[11] Despite its relatively small contribution in terms of numbers, the importance of this organ source cannot be overstated, as the ability to provide living donor transplantation for the pediatric population has become the standard-of-care throughout the world.

With respect to the recipient operation living donor liver transplantation does not present specific contraindications that differ from standard deceased donor pediatric liver transplantation. However, consideration of the utility of the transplant must be more cautiously contemplated when a living donor serves as the source. First discussed, by the Chicago group prior to the initiation of the living donor trial, the concept of avoiding the use a living donor in futile situations was established.[12] Experience with both living donor grafts, split and reduced deceased donor grafts, has demonstrated that use of segmental grafts should be avoided when the organ is being placed in a hostile local environment in which the risk of intra-abdominal infection is high such as in retransplantation[13] or when the metabolic demands can be anticipated to exceed the hepatic mass being provided.

## RECIPIENT EVALUATION

Pediatric liver transplantation can be practically and technically viewed to encompass three classes of patients: infants (<10 kg), toddlers (10–20 kg), and adolescents. Alternative classification systems have described newborns [< 1 year of age], infants, and children older than 5 years of age.[14–16] These classifications represent unique technical challenges and graft requirements specific for each group.[17]

In general the recipient evaluation for living donor and deceased donor transplantation is the same and is described in Table 30.3.2-2. Additional considerations when using segmental grafts from deceased or living donors includes an evaluation of the hepatic mass required. Greater than 50% of pediatric transplant candidates present with ESLD secondary to biliary atresia within the first 2 years of life. This is also the pediatric group in which living donor liver transplantation is commonly performed. Consequently, the mass of the left lateral segment of the adult donor supplies more than an adequate hepatic mass. In fact, occasionally, the left lateral segment is too large and monosegment transplantation should be considered. Hepatic mass is also an issue in the teenage candidate when greater mass may be required. Care should be taken to avoid situations in which the graft-to-recipient weight ratio (GRWR) is less than 0.8.[18–22] In such cases, a full left or right lobe from the donor may be necessary. At the other extreme, the neonate who needs a transplant may not have enough intra-abdominal space to accommodate an adult left lateral segment, and monosegmental living donor grafts may be necessary.[23,24]

**TABLE 30.3.2-2**

## EVALUATION OF LIVING-RELATED LIVER TRANSPLANT CANDIDATE

**Laboratory Exam List**
    CBC with differential & platelets
**ABO blood type**
    PT/INR
    Electrolytes, BUN, Creatinine
    Hepatic Function Panel
    Hepatitis A IgG & IgM,
    Hepatitis B Surf Ab & Ag,
    Hepatitis C serology
    EBV serology
    CMV serology
    HIV serology
    Varicella titer
    Measles titer
    Alpha-fetoprotein
    ANA
    SMA
    Vitamin A,D, & E levels
**Radiology Examination**
    Abdominal ultrasound

**TABLE 30.3.2-1**

## INDICATIONS AND CONTRAINDICATION FOR LIVING RELATED PEDIATRIC LIVER TRANSPLANTATION

Indication

    Progressive acute or chronic Liver Disease +
        Hyperbilirubinemia
        Encephalopathy
        "Falling off " growth curve
        Deceased synthetic function
        Cholangitis
        Portal Hypertension with hemorrhage
        Wilson's disease

    Metabolic Diseases that do not cause intrinsic liver disease, but liver transplantation improves outcomes
        Glycogen Storage Disease (I, II and IV)
        Urea Cycle Diseases
    Oxalosis type 1

    Primary Hepatic Malignancy

ContraIndications (all relative)
    Non-Hepatic Organ failure that precludes successful transplantation
    Major Systemic Infection
    Extra-hepatic malignancy

## OPERATIVE PROCEDURE

### Room Preparation

Participation of a skilled and experienced anesthesia team is an absolute requirement for a safe and successful pediatric liver transplant program. Ideally, the donor and recipient operations are conducted in two adjoining rooms in order to minimize the cold ischemic storage time of the liver segment and facilitate communication and timing between the surgical teams. To highlight two often overlooked but critical components of the recipient room preparation, the operating room should be adequately heated prior to the patient's arrival and blood products should be available in the room or in close proximity, and checked and verified before the patient arrives in the room. Due to the increased surface area-to-body-weight ratio, even the smallest exposure for seemingly short periods of time can result in significant heat loss from the patient and hypothermia.[25] A drop in core body temperature at this stage of the case imposes significant physiology stress and sets up a series of potential complications (coagulopathy, arrhythmias, infection). Efforts to avoid hypothermia include increasing the ambient room temperature, application of active warming devices (forced-air warming, radiant heaters, heating mattress), use of fluid warmers for intravenous crystalloid and blood products, and heated ventilator circuit. All irrigation fluids used during the transplant (except during the anhepatic phase) should be in a temperature-controlled bath.

### Patient Positioning

Recipients less than 20 kg are positioned in the supine position close to the top of the table with the arms positioned on either side of the head, elbows at 90 degrees. This allows easy and direct access by the anesthesia team to the airway and intravenous lines. The lower extremities are protected from pressure injury by use of foam padding under and on top of the legs. Once the lower surgical drapes are in place and the equipment is in position, the lower extremities are often inaccessible. Foley catheter is placed, and in small infants a feeding tube may be needed as the catheter.

Once the patient is appropriately positioned, lined, and padded, the pediatric forced-air warmer is placed in such a fashion to cover the lower extremities, which are subsequently wrapped in plastic along with the head.

### Surgical Sequence

#### Vascular Access

Once the patient is prepped and draped, the operative procedure begins with an internal jugular vein cut down. The right side is preferred; if the left internal jugular vein is utilized care should be taken to avoid injury to the thoracic duct, which is in close proximity. Once the vein is localized the distal branch is ligated with silk or a purse-string suture on 5.0 polypropylene is placed. A venotomy is made and a tunneled double-lumen 10-French catheter is advanced into the central circulation. Injury to the vein should be avoided and the venotomy made as close to the thoracic inlet as possible preserving the distal segment of vein for use as a venous conduit, if needed. The incision is closed in multiple layers and a sterile bio-occlusive dressing is applied. The catheter is sutured securely at the exit site, and the lure-lock ends of the catheter are passed under the drape to the anesthesiologist to be used for vascular access during the transplant.

### Abdominal Incision

Often an adequate abdominal incision in the pediatric population can be accomplished with a sigmoid type bilateral subcostal incision. The key to exposure is to allow sufficient visualization of the suprahepatic vena cava. Access to this area should provide direct vertical visualization along the undersurface of the diaphragm.

On entry into the abdomen, a brief inspection should be made to identify anomalies (preduodenal portal vein, interrupted inferior vena cava, poly splenia, situs inversus, malrotation, Ladd's bands, etc) and assess the degree and location of adhesions if previous intra-abdominal procedures have been undertaken (Kasai procedure). If the transplant is being undertaken for hepatoblastoma, inspection for extrahepatic disease is critical to determine if transplant should be performed (Figure 30.3.2-1).

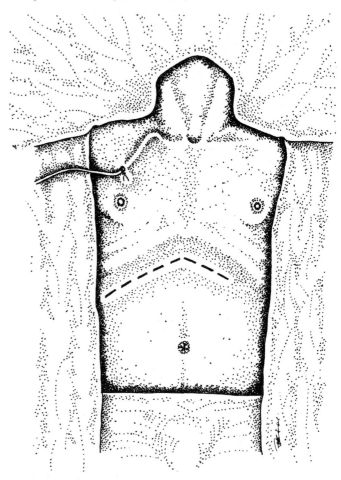

**FIGURE 30.3.2-1**

Patient positioned, access established, and abdominal incision marked.

### Recipient Hepatectomy

*Mobilization of the liver and Hilar Dissection.* Dissection is begun with division of the left triangular ligament. This is easily accomplished with the electrocautery. With the left lateral segment freed, access to the gastrohepatic ligament is obvious. Division of the gastrohepatic ligament is undertaken with the electrocautery. During this dissection, care is taken to incise the ligament close to the liver avoiding the lesser curvature of the stomach. This technique avoids many small vagal branches, which traverse this ligament to innervate the pylorus, stomach, and duodenum.

In addition, a search for and identification of the presence of accessory or replaced left hepatic artery contained in this ligament must be undertaken. In children, this artery is often of insufficient size to provide arterial inflow to the graft, but identification and purposeful division and ligation avoid inadvertent division and bleeding.

Attention is next directed to the hilum. This area of the hepatectomy should proceed with caution, patience, and skill. If there has been a prior surgical procedure in this area (hepaticojejunostomy or portoenterostomy) adhesions can be quiet dense. Vascular injury should be avoided. If there has been previously hilar dissection, postponement of this dissection until the liver is fully mobilized may be appropriate. This strategy allows the surgeon to cross-clamp the hilar structure and remove the liver quickly if significant bleeding complicates the hilar dissection.

If there has been a previous portoenterostomy, identification of the Roux limb is accomplished first in the hilar dissection. We find it easier to dissect along the antimesenteric boarder of this limb proximally toward the retrocolic tunnel in the mesentery. After mobilization we divide the jejunal limb just proximal to the portoenterostomy with a GIA, preserving the limb for subsequent use as biliary drainage from the graft. The stapled end is over sewn with a 5.0 polypropylene suture.

Once the Roux limb has been transected, or in cases without prior biliary drainage procedures, the dissection continues to identify the left hepatic artery first. Once identified, the investing tissue is carefully dissected away from the artery to allow passage of silk ties. The artery is ligated and divided. Care must be taken to avoid distraction or stretch of the vessel. Inadvertent distraction of the vessel can result in an intimal dissection. The dissection is often not appreciated at this point because flow through the vessel has been interrupted. However, the dissection can be readily apparent at the time of preparation for the arterial anastomosis, after arterial reconstruction, or delayed in presentation only to result in hepatic artery thrombosis. With the left hepatic artery divided, the proximal stump is dissected back to its confluence with the right hepatic artery and the proper hepatic artery. Dissection across the hilum continues laterally with division of lymphatic nerve, and connective tissue. The next structure to identify is the bile duct (if present). This structure is ligated and divided. Once divided the right hepatic artery is identified, ligated as far distal from the bifurcation as easily possible, and divided. Once again, it cannot be stressed enough to perform the arterial isolation without distraction. With isolation of the right hepatic artery, both arteries are dissected back to the origin of the gastroduodenal artery.

The remaining hilar structure is the portal vein. Dissection of the portal vein is performed to enable ligation of right and left branches independently. This structure is left intact until the liver has been fully mobilized and is ready for removal. This delayed ligation and division of the portal vein helps to lessen the degree of mesenteric edema and swelling that occurs during the anhepatic phase. The portal vein must be inspected, as sclerosis is not an uncommon consequence of the prior surgery and or the inflammatory changes associated with biliary atresia. If the portal vein is found to be sclerotic (usually as it emerges from under the pancreas) a venous graft (from recipient internal jugular vein or donor saphenous vein, ovarian vein or inferior mesenteric vein) should be prepared to provide satisfactory inflow and avoid portal vein thrombosis.

The right lobe of the liver is fully mobilized by division of the right triangular ligament with electrocautery. This is facilitated by identification and isolation of the infrahepatic vena cava. The right lobe is retracted in an anterior medial fashion, as the retroperitoneal attachments are divided avoiding injury to the right adrenal vein. This dissection is carried superior to the suprahepatic vena cava and identification of the right hepatic vein, medially to the lateral border of the retrohepatic vena cava. Short hepatic veins maybe isolated and ligated at this point or addressed after hepatectomy.

### Vena Cava Preservation and Preparation

Liver transplantation in the pediatric (infant and child) recipient almost always requires use of a reduced-size graft (left lateral segment from a living donor or left lateral segment from a spilt deceased donor or other segmental graft), and therefore the native vena cava must be preserved and used for venous outflow from the graft. Consequently, we have found the following technique to allow for an efficient and quick hepatectomy. With adequate mobilization, the native liver is attached only to the vena cava and portal vein. During the dissection of the right lobe of the liver several short hepatic veins may be identified, controlled, ligated, and divided. As the dissection of the vena cava proceeds toward the major hepatic veins, the portal vein is ligated and divided above the level of the bifurcation. A vascular clamp is applied to the infrahepatic cava and another to the suprahepatic cava as close to the diaphragm as possible (in small children and infants the right branch of the phrenic nerve runs close to the vena cava hiatus and can be injured with application of the suprahepatic vena cava vascular clamp. Postoperatively this presents with paralysis of the right diaphragm). Next the liver is sharply cut away from the vena cava in the following fashion: the liver is retracted inferiorly, and a curved Mayo scissors is used to transect the hepatic veins. The dissection is carried along the front of the retrohepatic vena cava by continued reflection of the liver inferiorly and anteriorly off the cava. Any short veins that were not ligated and divided previously are transected until the liver is freed and removed from the field. The vena cava is inspected and 5.0 polypropylene sutures are used to close all transected short hepatic veins. The left, middle, and right hepatic veins are cleaned of remnant liver. If the recipient is to receive a left lateral segment graft, the right hepatic vein is oversewn while the middle and left vein are opened to create a common orifice. At this point a vascular clamp can be applied to the left and middle common vein confluence and the infrahepatic and suprahepatic vascular clamps are removed. This reestablishes continuity of the vena cava and provides drainage of the lower extremities.

Bleeding from the retrohepatic space is controlled with the use of the argon beam coagulator. If space is not an issue (appropriate size graft for the abdominal space), the retrohepatic area is oversewn with running 4-0 polypropylene sutures by approximating the reflections of the right triangular ligament. This maneuver provides additional hemostasis. If adequate intra-abdominal space is likely to be a problem after re-perfusion, this area is not oversewn (Figure 30.3.2-2).

### Portal Vein Assessment and Preparation

During the hepatectomy the portal vein was ligated and divided above the bifurcation. Prior to removing the graft from iced storage, the portal vein should be assessed for caliber and quality. If the ligated left and right branches of the portal vein have dilated behind the portal pressure then it is likely that the portal flow and vein will be adequate. If the portal vein branches have not dilated and the entire portal vein continues to be small and not engorged, then the portal vein is likely sclerotic and modification will be necessary.

There are two primary methods of reconstructing a sclerotic portal vein. Both require procurement of a vein segment. Our preferred veins are the saphenous vein from the donor for the first technique

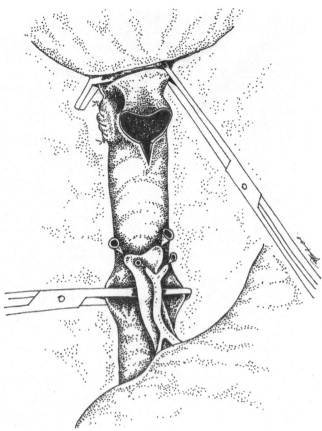

**FIGURE 30.3.2-2**

Anhepatic phase with caval preservation.

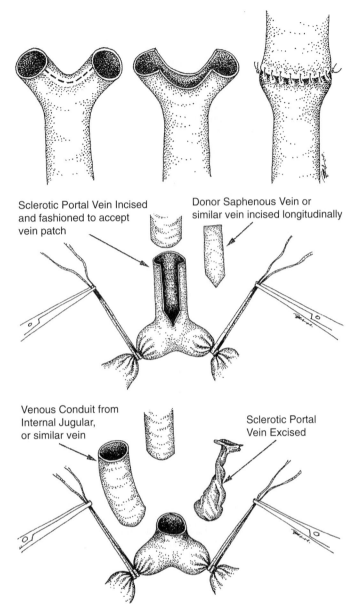

**FIGURE 30.3.2-3**

Portal Vein reconstruction methods. A. Standard branch patch method. B. Vein patch venoplasty. C. Venous conduit with sclerotic vein excision.

and the internal jugular vein from the recipient for the second method. The first method is to dissect the portal vein proximally, exposing the confluence of the splenic vein and the superior mesenteric vein. The vein at this point [confluence] is usually not sclerotic. The splenic and superior mesenteric branches are temporarily occluded with vessel–loops or similar device. The anterior leaf of the portal vein is then incised. Using a segment of saphenous vein, stripped of its valves and incised longitudinally, the sclerotic portal vein is patched. This allows for an enlarged portal vein segment tracing toward the graft. The second method utilizes a segment of internal jugular vein as a conduit from the confluence of the superior mesenteric vein and splenic vein or from the superior mesenteric vein below the pancreas. The splenic and superior mesenteric venous confluence is isolated, and each vein is controlled separately. The sclerotic segment of portal vein is excised and the internal jugular vein used as an end-to-end conduit. Alternatively, the superior mesenteric vein can be isolated below the pancreas, and then an end-to-end anastomosis between the internal jugular vein conduit and thesuperior mesenteric vein is created. The conduit is passed in a retropancreatic fashion to the right upper quadrant. Either of these latter two methods entirely eliminates the sclerotic segment of portal vein (Figure 30.3.2-3).

## GRAFT PREPARATION AND IMPLANTATION

### Graft Preparation

After the graft is removed from the donor, back-table inspection and preparation of the graft is the responsibility of the recipient surgeon. The graft is immediately submerged in ice-cold preservation solution ViaSpan (Barr Pharmaceuticals, Pomona, NY) solution or Histidine–tryptophan–ketoglutarate (HTK) solution (Human BioSystems, Palo Alto, CA). The graft is then flushed through the artery stump with a small angiocath under gravity feed system. This flush continues until the hepatic vein effluent is a clear, light-red quality. Next the portal vein is flushed with approximately 500 mL of solution. Finally the bile duct(s) are flushed with a size-appropriate angiocath connected to a 10-mL syringe. Care is taken to inspect the graft for damage or unequal perfusion during the exsanguination/flush procedure. With completion of the preservation phase, the anatomy is inspected and the graft is prepared for implantation.

First the hepatic vein is inspected to ensure there are no inadvertent injuries to the vein. If there is more than one vein (unusual in left lateral segment grafts) the veins should be joined together creating a common orifice (Figure 30.3.2-4). Assuming

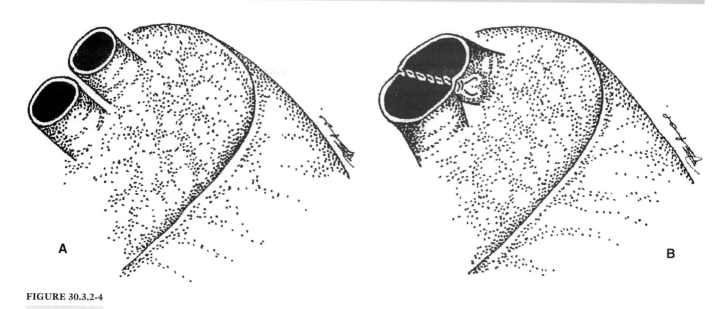

**FIGURE 30.3.2-4**

Back table hepatic vein re-construction. **A.** Two hepatic veins from Left Lateral Segment. **B.** Reconstruction of veins into a common orifice for implantation.

the graft is a left lateral segment the left hepatic vein is incised on its posterior leaflet to correspond to the incised portion of the anterior surface of the recipient's vena cava. The portal vein is then dissected to allow length and mobility for the anastomosis. A few small branches may need to be sacrificed in order to accomplish this. The bile duct or ducts are inspected next. The duct is probed to ensure that both segment 2 and segment 3 duct branches are in continuity. If more than one duct is present, the segment 2 and 3 ducts may be able to be joined into one orifice or will need to be anastomosed independently in the recipient. Finally the hepatic artery is inspected to ensure that there are no intimal injuries, and it is freed of surrounding connective tissue to ensure an adequate length for anastomosis. We do not insert any probes or dilators into the artery thereby avoiding the risk of creating an intrahepatic arterial intimal dissection. The graft is placed back in cold storage solution surrounded by ice if there will be a significant amount of time before it is to be implanted.

## Graft Implantation

The graft is now delivered from its hypothermic storage. As first described by Broelsch, pediatric living donor transplanation utilized the recipient's right hepatic vein.[9] The graft rotation associated with this position mandated the use of cryopreserved venous and donor-derived saphenous vein conduits for portal vein and arterial reconstruction. The long-term complication rate reached 50% in some groups.[26] Moving the outflow to a confluence of the middle and left hepatic vein eliminated the graft rotation; thus the routine need for conduits. Cryopreserved veins should be utilized only when there is absolutely no other alternative.[27] Implantation is started with the suprahepatic cava anastomosis. In the typical clinical scenerio, the graft is placed as a "piggyback," and the graft and hepatic veins and vena cava are prepared as noted above and below, respectively. At this point, vascular clamps are reapplied to stop blood flow through the cava. A vascular clamp is applied inferior and a Satinsky clamp is applied in the supraheaptic position. The left-middle common orifice is then extended inferior along the anterior surface of the vena cava creating a triangle.[28] This allows for the anastomosis of the hepatic

vein of the graft to the recipient vena cava and is performed in a triangular fashion. The base of the triangle is the opened left and middle hepatic vein of the recipient and the width of the left hepatic vein of the graft; the apex of the triangle is the incised portion of the recipient's vena cava and the incised portion of the left hepatic vein on the graft. The anastomosis is performed with a 4-0 polypropylene, polydioxanone, or polyglyconate suture. The use of an absorbable suture is advocated by some who feel the anastomosis can enlarge as the child grows. We have not identified any difference. The anterior portion of the anastomosis (or base of the triangle) may be left untied if a blood flush is to be used to flush out the preservation solution. This is a required step if ViaSpan is used; this step is not necessary if HTK is utilized. We find it beneficial to utilize a blood flush regardless of the preservation solution used, as it provides an indication of the robustness of portal flow.

In situations of an interrupted vena cava, there is no cava to piggyback on to; in those situations the graft cava is not incised on its posterior leaflet and the graft is anastomosed end-to-end into the cloaca of hepatic veins from the recipient's liver.

Following completion of the hepatic venous anastomosis, attention is directed to the portal vein. With prior preparation [creation of conduit if needed] during the anhepatic phase the portal anastomosis is straightforward. If the portal vein demonstrated typical distension, then a Blalock clamp (Figure 30.3.2-5) is placed on the portal vein just above the pancreas, and the left and right portal vein branches are cut just proximal to the ligatures. A branch patch is then fashioned from the right and left portal vein. Care should be taken at this point to ensure proper orientation of the portal vein (or portal venous conduit) and the graft. It is this step in which the Blalock clamp is particularly helpful. The Blalock clamp allows for precise determination of the recipient's portal vein orientation, as the jaws of the clamp are not encumbered by long laterally placed handles. The portal vein anastomosis is performed with a 6-0 suture (polypropylene, polydioxanone, or polyglyconate). A growth factor of approximately 50% of the diameter of the anastomosis is provided. If the anterior row [base of the triangle] of the suprahepatic cava anastomosis was tied then the suprahepatic clamp is removed, the anastomosis is inspected for bleeding, and if no major bleeding is noted, the liver

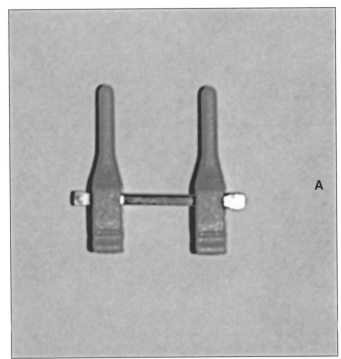

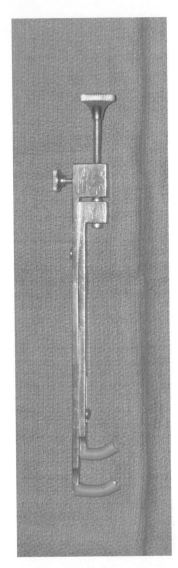

**FIGURE 30.3.2-5**

Blalock Clamp.

**FIGURE 30.3.2-6**

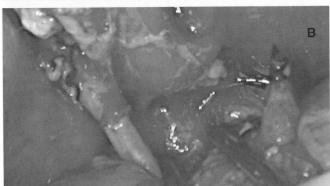

**A.** Micro-vascular arterial clamps. **B.** Completed Anastomosis.

is reperfused through the portal vein. If the anterior row was not tied in anticipation of a blood flush, then the portal vein is temporarily opened, the graft is perfused, and shed blood is collected in the cell saver. With an adequate flush, the portal vein is occluded, the anterior portion of the suprahepatic caval anastomosis is tied, the vena cava clamp is removed, the suprahepatic caval anastomosis is inspected for hemorrhage, and if none noted, the portal vein is reopened. After reperfusion, the cut edge is inspected for bleeding. Significant bleeding is rarely encountered at this point, as any major bleeding is addressed during the donor operation.

Following reperfusion and rewarming of the graft and assessment and control of hemorrhage, attention is directed to the hepatic artery. While there is still discussion regarding the optimal technique for hepatic artery reconstruction,[29,30] the best-published results are obtained with the routine use of microvascular techniques. The rate of thrombosis utilizing the operating microscope and microvascular techniques ranges from 0% to 2%.[27,31] We routinely utilize both the operating microscope and the microvascular techniques to reconstruct the artery. Under the microscope both the recipient and the donor artery are cleared of the surrounding connective tissue, and the artery is cut to a point where the artery intima and media are adherent. Microsurgical vascular clamps are placed, and vessel approximation is facilitated using the microsurgical vascular clamps attached to a microvascular metal platform (Figure 30.3.2-6). The

artery anastomosis is performed with interrupted 8–0 polypropylene. The clamps are removed, and the anastomosis is assessed for bleeding and the artery is assessed for adequate flow.

Following arterial reconstruction, biliary drainage is established, most commonly with utilization of the Roux limb from the previous portoenterostomy. Inspection of the graft on the back table would have disclosed the need to perform more than one biliary enteric anastomosis. Data from the 2006 Studies of Pediatric Liver Transplantation (SPLIT) annual report indicate that internal stents are utilized just as frequently as no stents overall in pediatric liver transplantation (42% and 44%, respectively).[32] These percentages are likely similar in pediatric living donor liver transplantation. We favor utilizing an internal stent secured by one of the posterior interrupted stitches, but their use is not routine (Figure 30.3.2-7).

Following completion of the biliary anastomosis, the surgical field is inspected once again for hemorrhage and vascular patency. The final critical step in the operation is placement of the implantable Doppler probe (Cook Medical, Blooming, IN). We have found this device to be of particular value to assessing both the hepatic artery and the portal vein in the postoperative period[33] (Figure 30.3.2-8). Drains are placed prior to the placement of

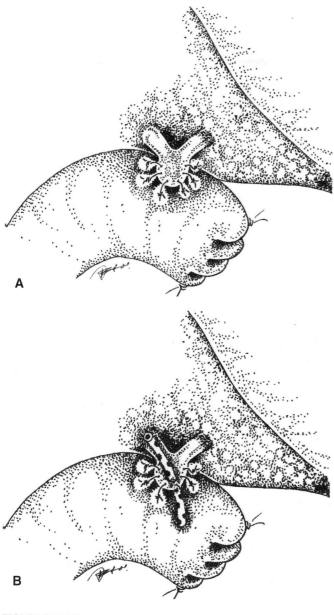

**A**

**B**

**FIGURE 30.3.2-7**

Biliary – Enteric Anastomosis. **A.** Biliary – Enteric Anastomosis without stent. **B.** Biliary- Enteric Anastomosis with Stent.

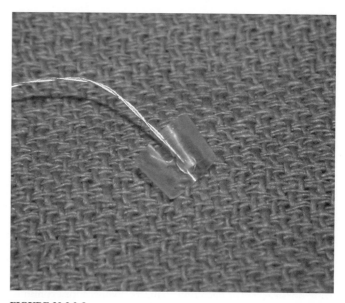

**FIGURE 30.3.2-8**

Implantable Doppler.

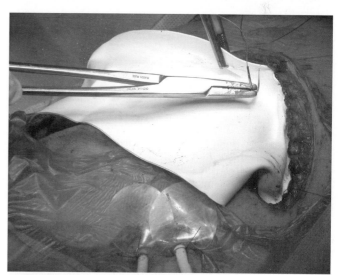

**FIGURE 30.3.2-9**

Gore-tex closure of Abdomen.

## POSTOPERATIVE MANAGEMENT

Standard postoperative pediatric liver transplant management is maintained. Immunosuppression and fluid management is similar to that in standard deceased donor transplantation. Given the higher incidence of vascular complications associated with living donor liver transplantation, a duplex Doppler ultrasound examination is performed on the first postoperative day. The critical factors to examine during this examination are hepatic venous outflow, portal vein flow, and intrahepatic arterial flow. If these parameters are adequate and signals can still be obtained from the implantable Doppler, no additional "routine" Doppler ultrasound studies need be performed. Obviously if there is clinical suspicion of a change, repeat ultrasound should be obtained especially if the implantable Doppler signal has changed or the probes have been removed. We request the nurse to interrogate the implantable Doppler every 2 hours. We leave the probes in place for the

the flow probe, and the probes are secured in place by the use of fibrin glue or similar product.

Closure of the abdomen is occasionally difficult. If the patient has required significant quantities of fluids resulting in edema in the soft tissues and intestine, or the graft size exceeds the abdominal compartment, primary closure can result in an increase in intra-abdominal pressure which can compromise ventilation as well as flow in either the portal vein or the hepatic artery. If there is concern for increased intra-abdominal pressure on closure, a Gore-tex (W.L. Gore, Flagstaff, AZ) patch can be used for temporary closure. This technique allows time for resolution of edema while providing protection of the internal visera and limiting insensible losses of heat and fluid from the recipient. Abdominal closure can be carried out by sequential patch removal or in one procedure depending on the recipient's response (Figure 30.3.2-9).

first 5 postoperative days. It has been our experience that the probe provides valuable information for at least the first 5 days. We routinely place the patient on a heparin infusion and attempt to achieve a goal partial thromboplastin time of 55 to 60 seconds for the first 5 postoperative days. We initiate the heparin infusion once the INR drops below 2.0. If bleeding ensues, modification or elimination of the heparin is required.

## OUTCOMES

Single centers report 1-year patient survival ranges from 84% to 94%. Graft survival in several experienced centers is nearly equivalent to patient survival at 94% to 92%.[27,34,35] The near-equivalent patient and graft survival is a result of the inherent superior quality of living donor grafts and the technical modifications developed at these centers. This is contrasted with registry type data indicating an increased risk (RR 1.3 vs whole) of graft loss with living donor grafts.[36] These differences between single center and registry data are likely due to the significant learning curve associated with the living donor recipient operation.[27] Biliary complications continue to be the most common postoperative complications occurring in 14% to 35% of patients.[34,37-40] Most biliary compications can be managed with aggressive interventional radiology techniques.[41]

## References

1. Starzl TE, Esquivel C, Gordon R, Todo S. Pediatric liver transplantation. *Transplantation Proceedings* 1987;19(4):3230–3235.
2. Starzl TE, Koep LJ, Schroter GP, Halgrimson CG, Porter KA, Weil R, 3rd. Liver replacement for pediatric patients. *Pediatrics* 1979; 63(6):825–829.
3. Weil R, 3rd, Putnam CW, Porter KA, Starzl TE. Transplantation in children. *Surgical Clin North Am* 1976;56(2):467–476.
4. Malatack JJ, Schaid DJ, Urbach AH, et al. Choosing a pediatric recipient for orthotopic liver transplantation. *J Pediatr.* 1987;111(4):479–489.
5. Bismuth H, Houssin D. Reduced-sized orthotopic liver graft in hepatic transplantation in children. *Surgery* March 1984;95:367–370.
6. Broelsch CE, Emond JC, Whitington PF, et al. Application of reduced-size liver transplants as split grafts, auxiliary orthotopic grafts, and living related segmental transplants. *Ann Surg* Sep 1990;212(3): 368–375; discussion 375–367.
7. Raia S, Nery JR, Mies S. Liver transplantation from live donors. *Lancet* Aug 26, 1989 1989(0140–6736 (Print)):497.
8. Strong RW, Lynch SV, Ong TH, Matsunami H, Koido Y, Balderson GA. Successful liver transplantation from a living donor to her son. *N Eng J Med* May 24, 1990 1990;322(21):1505–1507.
9. Broelsch CE, Whitington PF, Emond JC, et al. Liver transplantation in children from living related donors. Surgical techniques and results. *Ann Surg* Oct 1991;214(4):428–437; discussion 437–429.
10. Lloyd-Still JD. Impact of orthotopic liver transplantation on mortality from pediatric liver disease. *J Pediatr Gastroenterol Nutr* Apr 1991; 12(3):305–309.
11. UNOS. Annual Report. http://www.ustransplant.org/annual_reports/ current/904b_age_li.htm. Accessed November 28, 2006.
12. Singer PA, Siegler M, Whitington PF, et al. Ethics of liver transplantation with living donors. *N Engl J Med* Aug 31 1989;321(9):620–622.
13. Newell KA, Millis JM, Bruce DS, et al. An analysis of hepatic retransplantation in children. *Transplantation* May 15 1998;65(9):1172–1178.
14. Colombani PM, Cigarroa FG, Schwarz K, et al. Liver transplantation in infants younger than 1 year of age. *Ann Surg* Jun 1996;223(6):658–662; discussion 662–654.
15. Grabhorn E, Schulz A, Helmke K, et al. Short- and long-term results of liver transplantation in infants aged less than 6 months. *Transplantation* Jul 27 2004;78(2):235–241.
16. Woodle ES, Millis JM, So SK, et al. Liver transplantation in the first three months of life. *Transplantation* Sep 15 1998;66(5):606–609.
17. Feng S, Si M, Taranto SE, et al. Trends over a decade of pediatric liver transplantation in the United States. *Liver Transpl* Apr 2006;12(4):578–584.
18. Lee DS, Gil WH, Lee HH, et al. Factors affecting graft survival after living donor liver transplantation. *Transplant Proc* Oct 2004;36(8):2255–2256.
19. Lee HH, Joh JW, Lee KW, et al. Small-for-size graft in adult living-donor liver transplantation. *Transplant Proc* Oct 2004;36(8):2274–2276.
20. Man K, Fan ST, Lo CM, et al. Graft injury in relation to graft size in right lobe live donor liver transplantation: a study of hepatic sinusoidal injury in correlation with portal hemodynamics and intragraft gene expression. *Ann Surg* Feb 2003;237(2):256–264.
21. Sugawara Y, Makuuchi M, Takayama T, et al. Small-for-size grafts in living-related liver transplantation. *J Am Coll Surg* Apr 2001;192(4):510–513.
22. Tucker ON, Heaton N. The 'small for size' liver syndrome. *Curr Opin Crit Care* Apr 2005;11(2):150–155.
23. Enne M, Pacheco-Moreira L, Balbi E, et al. Liver transplantation with monosegments. Technical aspects and outcome: a meta-analysis. *Liver Transpl* May 2005;11(5):564–569.
24. Kasahara M, Kaihara S, Oike F, et al. Living-donor liver transplantation with monosegments. *Transplantation* Aug 27 2003;76(4):694-696.
25. Huang CJ, Chen CL, Tseng CC, et al. Maintenance of normothermia at operation room temperature of 24 degrees C in adult and pediatric patients undergoing liver transplantation. *Transpl Int* Apr 2005;18(4):396–400.
26. Millis JM, Seaman DS, Piper JB, et al. Portal vein thrombosis and stenosis in pediatric liver transplantation. *Transplantation* Sep 27 1996;62(6):748–754.
27. Millis JM, Cronin DC, Brady LM, et al. Primary living-donor liver transplantation at the University of Chicago: technical aspects of the first 104 recipients. *Ann Surg* Jul 2000;232(1):104–111.
28. Emond JC, Heffron TG, Whitington PF, Broelsch CE. Reconstruction of the hepatic vein in reduced size hepatic transplantation. *Surg Gynecol Obstet* Jan 1993;176(1):11–17.
29. Guarrera JV, Sinha P, Lobritto SJ, Brown RS Jr, Kinkhabwala M, Emond JC. Microvascular hepatic artery anastomosis in pediatric segmental liver transplantation: microscope vs loupe. *Transpl Int* Nov 2004;17(10):585–588.
30. Heffron TG, Welch D, Pillen T, et al. Low incidence of hepatic artery thrombosis after pediatric liver transplantation without the use of intraoperative microscope or parenteral anticoagulation. *Pediatr Transplant* Aug 2005;9(4):486–490.
31. Inomoto T, Nishizawa F, Sasaki H, et al. Experiences of 120 microsurgical reconstructions of hepatic artery in living related liver transplantation. *Surgery* Jan 1996;119(1):20–26.
32. (SPLIT) SoPLT. 2006 Annual Report. In: 3-5 T, ed; 2006:Biliary Reconstruction by Use and Type of Biliary Stent: Patient's First Transplant.
33. Cronin DC, 2nd, Schechter L, Lohman RF, et al. Advances in pediatric liver transplantation: continuous monitoring of portal venous and hepatic artery flow with an implantable Doppler probe. *Transplantation* 2002;74(6):887–890.
34. Darwish AA, Bourdeaux C, Kader HA, et al. Pediatric liver transplantation using left hepatic segments from living related donors: surgical experience in 100 recipients at Saint-Luc University Clinics. *Pediatr Transplant* May 2006;10(3):345–353.
35. Ueda M, Oike F, Ogura Y, et al. Long-term outcomes of 600 living donor liver transplants for pediatric patients at a single center. *Liver Transpl.* Sep 2006;12(9):1326–1336.
36. Diamond IR, Fecteau A, Millis JM, et al. Impact of graft type on outcome in pediatric liver transplantation: A report from Studies of Pediatric Liver Transplantation (SPLIT). *Ann Surg* (In Press)
37. Cronin DC, 2nd, Alonso EM, Piper JB, et al. Biliary complications in living donor liver transplantation. *Transplant Proc* Feb-Mar 1997;29 (1-2):419–420.
38. Soejima Y, Taketomi A, Yoshizumi T, et al. Biliary strictures in living donor liver transplantation: incidence, management, and technical evolution. *Liver Transpl* Jun 2006;12(6):979–986.

39. Karakayali H, Boyvat F, Sevmis S, et al. Biliary complications and their management in pediatric liver transplantations: one center's experience. *Transplant Proc* Sep 2005;37(7):3174–3176.

40. Kling K, Lau H, Colombani P. Biliary complications of living related pediatric liver transplant patients. *Pediatr Transplant* Apr 2004;8(2):178–184.

41. Lorenz JM, Denison G, Funaki B, et al. Balloon dilatation of biliary-enteric strictures in children. *AJR Am J Roentgenol* Jan 2005;184(1):151–155.

42. Diamond IR, Fecteau A, Millis JM, et al. Impact of graft type on outcome in pediatric liver transplantation: A report from Studies of Pediatric Liver Transplantation (SPLIT). *Ann Surg* (In Press)

# 30.4   OPTIMIZED VENOUS OUTFLOW

*Giuliano Testa, MD,*
*Enrico Benedetti, MD*

## INTRODUCTION

The construction of an optimal venous outflow is one of the technical points that determine the good outcome of a segmental liver transplantation.

Already in the era of left lateral liver transplantation, the importance of a wide anastomosis between the left hepatic vein of the graft and the vena cava of the recipient was recognized.

Although reconstruction of the graft venous outflow when more than one hepatic vein is present had been described in left lateral and extended left lateral grafts, the importance of complete venous outflow in graft function and survival became manifested with the routine use of right liver grafts.[2]

The first right liver living donor transplant was performed in 1994. The venous outflow was based only on the right hepatic vein, and no mention of congestion of the graft was reported.[3] In 1997 Lo et al. published the first series of right liver living donor transplants and immediately addressed the importance of the middle hepatic vein in the venous drainage of the anterior sector of the liver corresponding to segments 5 and 8.[4,5] In the same series the direct anastomosis to the vena cava of a large accessory inferior hepatic vein is reported.[5] In the coming years several transplant centers around the world will start performing right liver living donor transplants. The routine anastomosis of the accessory inferior hepatic veins with a diameter larger than 0.5 cm was accepted from the beginning as part of the recipient operation by almost all centers.[6,7] On the other hand, although graft congestion was a recognized phenomenon, the importance of adequate drainage of the anterior sector became the topic of intense study only when greater cumulative experience was achieved.[8–10]

The reasons to modify the venous outflow lay in the universal recognition of the role of the middle hepatic vein, in draining the anterior sector of the right liver, and at times of catastrophic consequences of graft congestion.[11]

The anatomy of venous outflow of the liver has been known for decades, but only in the early 1980s, the concept of adequate venous drainage began to be applied to liver surgery.[12,13] Observations like the nature of communication between hepatic veins, the early response of reversal of portal blood flow in case of abrupt cessation of venous outflow in the same territory, the late response of intrahepatic collateral formation, the importance of residual mass, and intact arterial inflow in the tolerability of congestion became at a later date the physiologic basis of promoting different surgical techniques in venous outflow construction of the segmental graft. Many surgeons experienced cases of graft congestion and subse-

quent failure.[14–16] Moreover, the observation of Cheng in 1998 that the absence of proper venous outflow in the left liver graft causes lack of regeneration in the territories that are not drained was confirmed by other groups.[17–19] The reversal of flow in the portal branch serving that territory was recognized as the compensatory mechanism and as the cause of lack of regeneration because of failed delivery of growth factors.[18,20] Moreover as pointed out by Lee the presence of severe portal hypertension may play an additional negative role by impeding the reversal of flow in the congested parenchyma thus precipitating graft failure.[21] Sophisticated studies with the use of the near-infrared spectrometry aimed at detecting oxygen saturation and hemoglobin concentration in the outflow-challenged territories were performed by the Japanese groups showing controversial results in terms of congestion of the anterior sector of the liver.[22–24] These studies further demonstrated, if necessary, that a right hepatectomy keeping the plan of transection to the right of the middle hepatic vein causes an impairment to the venous outflow of the anterior sector of the right liver and that the technical approach to the right hepatectomy for living donation could not be the mimic of a standard right hepatectomy for tumor. The fact that the middle hepatic vein drains the anterior sector of the liver including in all or partial segments 5 and 8 could not be ignored and became widely accepted what had been addressed by Lo in his initial experience: the optimal outcome of the right grafts lies as much on the venous outflow as on the inflow.[5,7,11,25] By modification of the venous outflow, taking in account the drainage of the anterior sector by tributaries of the middle hepatic vein, a general improvement of liver function recovery and overall outcome was documented.

All surgeons involved in the development of right living donor liver transplantation have changed the technique used to construct the venous outflow.

Two major changes have occurred: a wider outflow for the right hepatic vein anastomosis and the development of surgical strategies to allow better drainage of the anterior sector (Color Plates, Figures L1-12 and L1-18 A-D).

The first reports of right living donor liver transplant described a straight end-to-end anastomosis between the ostium of the right hepatic vein and its correspondent on the recipient with or without a slit on the wall of the vena cava.[9,10] The benefit of a better right hepatic vein outflow is recognized in subsequent reports. Marcos proposed a larger cavotomy of 1.5 to 2 times the size of the right hepatic vein of the graft and oriented caudally with a 45-degree angle with the longitudinal axis of the vena cava.[27] Kinkhabwala adds to a wider cavotomy a resection of the anterior wall of the ostium of the graft right hepatic vein to create a functional side-to-side anastomosis.[28] Nakamura describes a cavotomy very similar to the one proposed by Marcos.[29] (Sugawara proposes an elongation technique with the aim of avoiding the compression of the outflow due to the rotation of the graft that occurs during its regenerative growth. The technique is based on the use of cryopreserved veins that are cut in a diamond shape and anastomosed to the anterior wall of the right hepatic vein of the graft and to the enlarged ostium of the right hepatic vein of the recipient.[30]

Overall, besides the more complicated anastomosis proposed by Sugawara, the general practice is to create a larger cavotomy than the diameter of the right hepatic vein of the graft, with or without the inclusion of the ostium of the middle hepatic vein of the recipient. The cavotomy is almost in all cases brought toward the anterocaudal wall of the vena cava with the aim of avoiding kinking or compression of the anastomosis as the graft grows.

The reconstruction of the venous outflow of the anterior sector pertinent to the middle hepatic vein is a more complicated issue.

From an anatomical point of view the middle hepatic vein is responsible for the drainage of the anterior sector of the right liver in the great majority of the cases. When the middle hepatic vein is not taken with the graft or the largest tributaries from segments 5 and 8 are ligated, a variable portion of the anterior sector of the right liver remains congested.[31] The relief of the congestion may occur either through intraparenchymal capillary communication between the venous outflow of the anterior sector and the posterior sector drained by the right hepatic vein or by reversal of flow in the anterior branch of the portal vein into the posterior branch.

The volume percentage of the congested parenchyma in relation to the overall volume of the graft, the ratio between graft and recipient weight, the degree of portal hypertension, and the compliance of the liver are all factors that determine the magnitude of graft malfunction after transplantation. The malfunction may be insignificant in the presence of a dominant right hepatic vein, small anterior sector tributaries, and high graft/recipient weight ratio; or significant in the presence of large tributaries to the middle hepatic vein draining a high volume percentage of the graft and of a low graft–recipient weight ratio.

To accomplish anterior sector venous drainage and avoid graft malfunction either the middle hepatic vein, in toto or partially, or its tributaries must be drained in the vena cava.

The Hong Kong group is from the beginning the proponent of complete middle hepatic vein harvest. Their technique has evolved in time. In their early experience the middle hepatic vein was anastomosed end to end to the ostium of the middle hepatic vein or left hepatic vein of the recipient.[5] The finding that medial rotation of the graft after reperfusion or later during regenerative growth could in certain cases cause a compression of the middle vein brought a change in the technique. The new technique consists in the construction of a common orifice of the right and middle hepatic vein of the graft similar to what Kubota had described for joining two left graft hepatic veins.[32] The anastomosis is performed directly to the cava where the cavotomy is shaped in a triangular fashion on the anterior wall (Color Plates, Figures L1-18 A and B). The distance between the ostia of the right and the middle hepatic vein of the graft can be eliminated by dissection of the interposed parenchyma, and horizontal suturing of the vertical incision can be performed on both adjacent walls.[33]

The grafts transplanted with this outflow technique have had no problem with kinking or stretching of the anastomosis and demonstrated an improvement in functional recovery, although there was no significant difference in overall outcome in comparison with the grafts transplanted with the former technique.[34]

The complete harvest of the middle hepatic vein guarantees the most complete drainage of the anterior sector of the right graft. The critics of this technique state that in the presence of less than 30% of donor residual liver volume the harvest of the middle hepatic vein may pose the donor at a higher risk of postoperative complications also because the regeneration of segment 4 is stunned by the lack of adequate venous drainage.[19,21,25,30] From a pure technical point of view the greater risk of this procedure is an injury to the left hepatic vein that in the great majority of the cases forms a common trunk with the middle hepatic vein.[35,36]

In a review of their first 100 right liver living donor transplants Lo did not report any significant complications in the donors and stressed again the safety of complete harvest of the middle hepatic vein and the excellent results in the recipients.

The other technique that has been widely accepted is the one of anastomosing the major tributaries draining the anterior sector of the right liver into the middle hepatic vein to the vena cava leaving the middle hepatic vein with the donor rest liver.

In this technique the plane of parenchymal transection is kept to the right of the middle hepatic vein. The tributaries from segments 5 and 8 are anastomosed on the back table to venous conduits of various origins that serve as jump grafts (Color Plates, Figures L1-13 and L1-14).

Lee has been a strong proponent of the routine reconstruction of the tributaries from segments 5 and 8 with jump grafts in name of less parenchymal resection, increased safety in the donor and data demonstrating the inconsistency of intraparenchymal communication between tributary veins of the middle hepatic vein and the right hepatic vein. A hydrostatically dilated recipient saphenous vein is used as favorite conduit that is anastomosed to the stump of the recipient middle or left hepatic vein.[21] The vein stumps instead of the retrohepatic cava are chosen to facilitate venous outflow because of the exposure to a stronger negative intrathoracic pressure. The patency of these jump grafts is confirmed even at long-term follow-up. Other surgeons, including Lee, have described jump grafts constructed with left portal vein of the recipient. Superficial femoral vein, cryopreserved iliac vein and vena cava, cadaveric iliac veins and vena cava.[14,29,38–39]

Modifications to the straight jump graft technique by Lee have been proposed by several surgeons.

The approach to selective and not routine reconstruction of the venous outflow of the anterior sector is proposed by the Tokyo group and echoed by others.[24,42] The rationale is that not all right grafts present with congestion after reperfusion, and simple right hepatic vein anastomosis is sufficient in selected cases. With the donor middle hepatic vein clamped and reversal of flow in the anterior branch of the portal vein detected by Doppler, the temporary occlusion of the right hepatic artery will determine the portion of right liver affected by congestion. When the volume of the graft without the congested parenchyma is less than 40% of the calculated liver standard volume of the recipient, the tributaries must be anastomosed.[24] A selective approach based on donor/recipient weight ratio, greater or less than 1; graft/recipient standard liver, greater or less than 50%; and size of the middle hepatic vein tributaries, greater or less than 5 mm in diameter; is used by the Chen group to decide whether the graft will be harvested with or without the middle hepatic vein.[42]

The Tokyo group proposes also the use of cryopreserved iliac veins that are anastomosed to the segments 5 and 8 tributary veins and then to the wall of the right hepatic vein to form a single conduit. This conduit is the anastomosed to a cryopreserved vena cava. A side-to-side anastomosis between the cava of the graft and the cava of the recipient forms a wide outflow. This technique, named double cava technique (Color Plates, Figure L1-18D), in the experience of the authors, maintains optimal venous flow when the graft grows and rotates.[43]

A similar concept is present in the techniques described by Malago and Testa. The venous conduits utilized are not cryopreserved but simply stored cadaveric vessels that are anastomosed to the outflow veins of the graft on the back table (Color Plates, Figure L1-18C). The anastomosis is constructed between the venous conduit fully open in a patchlike fashion or with a long slit on its anterior wall and an ample cavotomy on the anterior wall of the recipient cava.[14,41]

The single-conduit technique albeit may slightly prolong the back-table reconstruction has the advantage of making the implantation of the graft very simple and by creating an anastomosis as wide as the one normally done in the piggyback for cadaveric livers practically eliminates any outflow problem. Moreover by not routinely harvesting the middle hepatic vein any potential injury to the outflow of the rest of the liver and any risk of decreased regeneration are eliminated.

The technique described by Marcos is based on the observation that the tributaries to the middle hepatic vein, and especially the one draining segment 5, have intrahepatic communication with the right hepatic vein. The lateral branch of the middle hepatic vein mainly draining segment 5 is harvested with the graft, proximal to the confluence with the branch draining segment 4A. The plan of parenchymal transection is then kept to the right of the middle hepatic vein. The portion of middle hepatic vein harvested with the graft is not anastomosed to the cava of the recipient. Likewise, very seldom the tributary vein draining segment 8 is anastomosed either directly or with a jump graft to the cava of the recipient. This operation that Marcos calls an "anterior extended right lobe resection" has the advantage of leaving almost intact the outflow from segment 4 and avoiding any dissection close to the confluence between middle hepatic vein and left hepatic vein.[27]

The same technical solution has been reported by the Colorado group.[26] Marcos has reported excellent results with this approach that seems to simplify back-table reconstruction and graft implantation and minimize outflow impairment in the donor.

The recognition of the importance of venous outflow in the postoperative function and survival of the right living donor graft has decreased to the minimum the incidence of early graft failure and delayed function. Independently, from the technique chosen, there is general agreement that adequate venous outflow reconstruction is together with the inflow a determinant factor of good outcome. Whether one technical approach is sounder than the other is probably not possible to decide. What appears clear is that graft weight and ratio with recipient and donor weight and especially each liver individual venous anatomy must be considered and carefully evaluated when a technical approach is chosen. Certain versatility in all the surgical approaches described above is possibly the best guarantee for a good donor and recipient outcome.

## References

1. Emond JC, Heffron TG, Whitington PF, et al. Reconstruction of the hepatic vein in reduced size hepatic transplantation. *Surg Gynecol Obstet* 176(1):11–17, 1993.
2. Kubota K, Makuuchi M, Takayama T, et al.: Successful hepatic vein reconstruction in 42 consecutive living related liver transplantations. *Surgery* 2000;128(1):48–53.
3. Yamaoka Y, Washida M, Honda K, et al. Liver transplantation using a right lobe graft from a living related donor. *Transplantation* 1994;57(7):1127–1130.
4. Lo CM, Fan ST, Liu CL, et al. Extending the limit on the size of adult recipient in living donor liver transplantation using extended right lobe graft. *Transplantation* 1999;63(10):1524–1528.
5. Lo CM, Fan ST, Liu CL, et al. Adult-to-adult living donor liver transplantation using extended right lobe grafts. *Ann Surg* 1997;226(3):261–270.
6. Nakamura T, Tanaka K, Kiuchi T, et al. Anatomical variations and surgical strategies in right lobe living donor liver transplantation: Lessons from 120 cases. *Transplantation* 2002;73(12):1896–1903.
7. Miller CM, Gondolesi GE, Florman S, et al. One hundred nine living donor liver transplants in adult and children: A single-center experience. *Ann Surg* 2001;234(3):301–312.
8. Wachs M, Bak TE, Karrer FM, et al. Adult living donor lover transplantation using a right hepatic lobe. *Transplantation* 1998;66(10):1313–1316.
9. Testa G, Malago M, Broelsch CE, Living-donor liver transplantation in adults. *Langenbeck's Arch Surg* 1999;384:536–534.
10. Marcos A, Fisher RA, Ham JM, et al. Right lobe living donor liver transplantation. *Transplantation* 1999;68:798–803.
11. Lee SG, Park KM, Hwang S, et al. Congestion of right liver graft in living donor liver transplantation. *Transplantation* 20001;71(6):812–817.
12. Nakamura S, Tsuzuki T. Surgical anatomy of the hepatic veins and the inferior vena cava. *Surg Gynecol Obstet* 1981152:43–50.
13. Ou QJ, Hermann RE.The role of hepatic veins in liver operations. *Surgery* 198495(4):381–391.
14. Malago M, Testa G, Frilling A, et al. Right living donor liver transplantation: An option for adult patients. Single institution experience with 74 patients. *Ann of Surg* 2003;238(6):853–863.
15. Marcos A, Olzinski AT, Ham JM, et al. The interrelationship between portal and arterial blood flow after adult to adult living donor liver transplantation. *Transplantation* 2000;70(12):1697–1703.
16. Lee SG, Park KM, Hwang S, et al. Modified right liver graft from a living donor to prevent congestion. *Transplantation* 2002;74(1):54–59.
17. Cheng YF, Chao LC, Tung LH, et al. Post-transplant changes of segment 4 after living related liver transplantation. *Clin Transplant* 1998;12:476–481.
18. Maema A, Imamura H, Takayama T, et al. Impaired volume regeneration of split livers with partial venous disruption: A latent problem in partial liver transplantation. *Transplantation* 2002;73(5):765–769.
19. Kido M, Ku Y, Takumi F, et al. Significant role of middle hepatic vein in remnant liver regeneration of right-lobe living donors. *Transplantation* 2003;75(9):1598–1600.
20. Starzl TE, Francavilla A, Halgrimson CG, et al. The origin, hormonal nature, and action of hepatotrophic substances in portal venous blood. *Surg Gynecol Obstet* 1973;137(2):179–199.
21. Lee SG, Park KM, Hwang S, et al. Anterior segment congestion of a right liver lobe graft in living-donor liver transplantation and strategy to prevent congestion. *J Hepato Pancreat Surg* 2003;10:16–25.
22. Ciu D, Kiuchi T, Egawa H, et al. Microcirculatory changes in right lobe grafts in living-donor liver transplantation: A near-infrared spectrometry study. *Transplantation* 2001;72(2):291–295.
23. Ohdan H, Kazuyuki M, Tashiro H, et al. Intraoperative near-infrared spectroscopy for evaluating hepatic venous outflow in living-donor right lobe liver. *Transplantation* 2003;76(5):791–797.
24. Sano K, Makuuchi M, Miki K, et al. Evaluation of hepatic venous congestion: Proposed indication criteria for hepatic vein reconstruction. *Ann Surgery* 2002;236(2):241–247.
25. Marcos A, Orloff M, Mieles L, et al. Functional venous anatomy for right-lobe grafting and techniques to optimize outflow. *Liver Transplant* 2001;7(10):845–852.
26. Bak T, Wachs M, Trotter J, et al. Adult-t-adult living donor liver transplantation using right-lobe grafts: Results and lessons learned from a single-center experience. *Liver Transplant* 20011;7(8):680–686.
27. Marcos A, Orloff M, Mieles L, et al. Functional venous anatomy for right-lobe grafting and techniques to optimize outflow. *Liver Transplant* 2001;7(10):845–852.
28. Kinkhabwala MM, Guarrera JV, Leno R, et al. Outflow reconstruction in right hepatic live donor liver transplantation. *Surgery* 2003;133:243–250.
29. Nakamura T, Tanaka K, Kiuchi T, et al. Anatomical variations and surgical strategies in right lobe living donor liver transplantation: Lessons from 120 cases. *Transplantation* 2002;73(12):1896–1903.
30. Sugawara Y, Makuuchi M, Akamatsu N, et al. Refinement of venous reconstruction using cryopreserved veins in right liver grafts. *Liver Transplant* 2004;10(4):541–547.
31. Yamamoto H, Maetani Y, Kiuchi T, et al. Background and clinical impact of tissue congestion in right-lobe living-donor liver grafts: A magnetic resonance imaging study. *Transplantation* 2003;76(1):164–169.
32. Kubota K, Makuuchi M, Takayama T, et al. Successful hepatic vein reconstruction in 42 consecutive living related liver transplantations. *Surgery* 2000;128(1):48–53.

33. Lo CM, Fan ST, Liu CL, et al. Hepatic venoplasty in living-donor liver transplantation using righ lobe graft with middle hepatic vein. *Transplantation* 2003;75(3):358–360.

34. Liu CL, Lo CM, Fan ST. Hepatic venoplasty in right lobe live donor lover transplantation. *Liver Transplant* 9(12):1265–1272, 2003.

35. Fan ST, Lo CM, Liu CL, et al. Safety of donors in live donor liver transplantation using right lobe grafts. *Arch Surg* 2000;135:336–340.

36. Wind P, Douard R, Cugnenc PH, et al. Anatomy of the common trunk of the middle and left hepatic veins: application to liver transplantation. *Surg Radiol Anat* 1999;21:17–21.

37. Lo CM, Fan ST, Liu CL, et al. Lessons learned from one hundred right lobe living donor liver transplants. Ann Surg 2004;240(1):1511–1518.

38. Cattral MS, Greig PD, Muradali D, et al. Reconstruction of middle hepatic vein of a living-donor right lobe liver graft with recipient left portal vein. *Transplantation* 2001;71(12):1864–1866.

39. Kornberg A, Heyne J, Schotte U, et al. Hepatic venous outflow reconstruction in right lobe living-donor liver graft using recipient's superficial femoral vein. *Am J Transplant* 2003;3:144–1447.

40. Sugawara Y, Makuuchi M, Imamura H, et al. Outflow reconstruction in extended right liver grafts from living donors. *Liver Transplant* 2003;9(3):306–309.

41. Dong G, Sankary HN, Malago M, et al. Cadaver iliac vein outflow reconstruction in living donor right lobe liver transplantation. *J Am Coll Surg* 2004;199(3):504–507.

42. de Villa VH, Chen CL, Chen YS, et al. Right lobe living donor liver transplantation-Addressing the middle hepatic vein controversy. *Ann Surg* 2003;228(2):275–282.

43. Hata S, Sugawara Y, Kishi Y, et al. Volume regeneration after right liver donation. *Liver Transpl* 2004;10(1):65–70.

# 30.5   ISCHEMIA AND REPERFUSION INJURY

*Sei-ichiro Tsuchihashi, MD, PhD, Fady Kaldas, MD, Ronald W. Busuttil, MD, PhD, Jerzy W. Kupiec-Weglinski, MD, PhD*

## INTRODUCTION

Ischemia and reperfusion injury (IRI) to the liver, an antigen-independent process, is an unavoidable consequence of liver transplantation (LT) and surgical manipulation. It causes up to 10% of early organ failure, and can lead to a higher incidence of both acute and chronic rejection.[1,2] Moreover, IRI contributes to the shortage of livers available for transplantation because of the higher susceptibility of marginal livers to the ischemic insult. Indeed, minimizing the impact of IRI could significantly increase the number of patients successfully undergoing LT. Living donor LT results in fewer episodes of graft dysfunction and acute rejection compared with cadaveric transplants.[3] These superior outcomes are due to the fact that livers from living donors are retrieved from healthy individuals under elective conditions and with minimal cold ischemia times (CIT). Prolonged cold ischemia can cause alterations in cytoskeleton and organelle structures of cells and disrupt the membrane electrical potential gradient, resulting in ion redistribution. After cold ischemia and reperfusion, reactive oxygen species are generated, causing activation of endothelial cells (EC) and increased expression of adhesion molecules.[4] Subsequently, Kupffer cells become activated and produce a variety of proinflammatory molecules, such as cytokines and chemokines that contribute to the inflammatory process and facilitate leukocyte infiltration into the parenchyma.[5]

Here, we address the mechanisms of IRI and therapeutic interventions aimed at reducing its severity in LT.

## PATHOPHYSIOLOGY OF HEPATIC IRI

### Preservation Injury

The mechanism of the injury caused by ischemia is due to the depletion of adenosine triphosphate (ATP) and the lack of oxygen, leading to anaerobic metabolism and the accumulation of lactate and hypoxanthine resulting in intracellular acidosis.[6] Under ischemic conditions, xanthine dehydrogenase is converted into xanthine oxidase, which on reperfusion converts hypoxanthine to xanthine and urate accompanied by the release of oxygen-free radicals (OFR).[7] This process causes lipid peroxidation, a potent cause of graft dysfunction. Concomitantly, there is activation of Kupffer cells with release of OFR, nitric oxide, and proinflammatory cytokines.[8,9] Cold preservation causes morphological changes in sinusoidal endothelial cells (SEC). They become rounded, detached, and slough into the sinusoidal lumen. The degree of SEC detachment correlates with the duration of cold ischemia and has been associated with sinusoidal cell damage and hypercoaguability.[4] Indeed, grafts with more than 14 hours of cold ischemia have been associated with a twofold increase in preservation damage resulting in prolonged postoperative courses, biliary structures, and decreased graft survival.[10] Therefore, it is very likely that cadaveric LT with extended CIT increases the intensity of oxidative stress, which leads to a severe inflammatory response at reperfusion.

### Inflammatory Responses After Reperfusion

The process of IRI to the liver combines many interrelated factors that produce a cascade of events ultimately leading to hepatic failure (Figure 30.5-1). OFR produced after ischemia/reperfusion (I/R) can directly damage cell membranes or cause tissue damage indirectly through the initiation of an inflammatory response. The production of cytokines, such as TNF-α and IL-1, by Kupffer cells after I/R has been thought to be the primary initiating event leading to propagation of the hepatic inflammatory response. Both cytokines induce chemokine synthesis and up-regulate the expression of adhesion molecules giving rise to increased leukocyte-SEC interaction, which results in further cytokine and chemokine production at the site of injury.[14–16] Although a characteristic feature of IRI is the rapid accumulation of leukocytes in hepatic sinusoids, a multistep series of adhesive and signaling events are responsible for regulating the recruitment of these leukocytes.

The selectin family of adhesion molecules, L-, E-, and P-selectin, and their ligands, are considered the primary mediators of leukocyte tethering and rolling on the surface of EC.[17] L-selectin is expressed on most leukocytes. E- and P-selectin are expressed on activated EC, and P-selectin is also expressed on activated platelets. The three selectins have a high affinity for, and bind a variety of, carbohydrate ligands. One such glycoprotein expressed on the surface of leukocytes is P-selectin glycoprotein ligand-1 (PSGL-1), which can bind all three selectins.[18] Subsequent activation of leukocytes and EC leads to firmer adhesion mediated through integrin adhesion molecules (CD11/CD18) and their receptors (ICAM-1, VCAM-1).[17] Leukocyte transmigration finally occurs between EC. Guided by a concentration gradient of cytokines and chemokines, leukocytes then travel through the extracellular matrix to the site of injury and contribute to the ensuing inflammatory response.[19]

In the setting of brain death, the release of inflammatory mediators before ischemia is a pertinent contributor to the inflammatory response after I/R. Animal studies have shown that after brain death there is a release of proinflammatory mediators including cytokines and chemokines, such as TNF-α, IL-1β, and

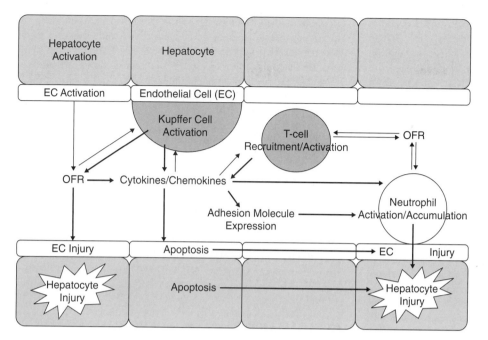

**FIGURE 30.5-1**

Mechanistic cascade of cellular events in liver IRI. OFR produced during the acute phase of IRI initiate the inflammatory cascade that gives rise to the subacute phase response, characterized inflammation, and activation of neutrophils in the liver shortly after reperfusion. Activation of Kupffer cells and T cells produces proinflammatory cytokines/chemokines and promotes neutrophils recruitment, assisted by up-regulated adhesion molecules.

macrophage inflammatory protein (MIP)-1α.[20] In addition, livers from brain-dead rats have increased expression of ICAM-1 and VCAM-1 with significant leukocyte infiltration and increased liver enzymes.[21] The effects of donor brain death have been shown to have a synergistic adverse effect with long cold preservation times, resulting in an increased susceptibility to reperfusion injury and a significant reduction in survival after LT.[22] In clinical transplantation, evidence of inflammatory events associated with brain death and intensive care management has been demonstrated through elevated levels of ICAM-1 and leukocyte infiltration in cadaveric donor livers.[23] Living donor liver allografts with shorter CIT have minimal levels of neutrophils after reperfusion. In contrast, cadaveric livers with prolonged cold storage showed neutrophil infiltration with increased levels of P-selectin.[24]

## Apoptotic Change After Reperfusion

Apoptosis is an important event after reperfusion of liver grafts, the severity of which correlates with the degree of hepatic injury. Apoptotic machinery becomes activated during the early phase of reperfusion after liver ischemia and transplantation. Induction of apoptosis can be initiated by way of various interactions and stimuli. Two major pathways activate effector caspases, which lead to apoptotic cell death after reperfusion.[25] The first pathway is mediated by OFR, which leads to disruption of mitochondrial membrane integrity, resulting in the release of proapoptotic factors. In the second pathway, TNF-α or Fas ligand activate receptors (TNF-receptor type-1 or Fas) resulting in the formation of a death complex, which leads to the activation of caspase-8. Blocking the early pathway of apoptosis can prevent hepatic injury and improve animal survival after reperfusion. In fact, inhibition of caspase-3 and -7 improves survival and reduces early graft injury after I/R in rat LT.[26] Furthermore, apoptosis is controlled through the expression of specific genes. Among these, the Bcl-2 gene family is the most important. The protein encoded by the Bcl-2 gene has been implicated in prolongation of cell survival by blocking apoptosis and preventing hepatic IRI.[27–28]

The increased apoptotic change within the cadaveric liver graft may accelerate IRI after transplantation. In the brain-dead animal,

a significant increase in the number of apoptotic cells and caspase-3 activity has been observed in the liver graft compared with controls.[29] In human livers, the percentage of Fas ligand positive cells, a potent factor in apoptosis, is significantly higher in biopsies obtained from cadaveric livers compared with living donor livers.[24]

## PREVENTIVE AND THERAPEUTIC STRATEGIES OF HEPATIC IRI

Recently, several novel molecules have been studied to reduce IRI. These include molecules interfering with OFR, proinflammatory cytokines/chemokines, adhesion molecules, and apoptosis.

Kupffer cells and activated neutrophils lead to the production of OFR during I/R. Antioxidant therapy reduces OFR and attenuates hepatic IRI. The radical scavenging properties of N-acetylcysteine (NAC) have shown a beneficial effect against hepatic IRI. In animal models, the use of NAC caused an improvement in hepatic macro- and microcirculation after reperfusion following cold and warm liver ischemia.[30] In a steatotic rat liver model of cold IRI, NAC given before 24 h of cold ischemia exhibited diminished sinusoidal microcirculatory injury and lower enzyme release after reperfusion.[31] In human LT, NAC treatment after reperfusion decreased leukocyte adherence and improved microhemodymamics.[32]

The Th2 cytokines, IL-4, IL-10, and IL-13, are known to modulate inflammatory responses in part by down-regulating the production of proinflammatory cytokines and chemokines. IL-13 gene transfer in rat LT increased IL-4 and IL-13 expression and reduced I/R-induced expression of TNF-α and MIP-2, critical mediators for the hepatic neutrophil recruitment.[33] Exogenous administration of IL-4 or IL-13 at reperfusion reduced serum TNF-α, liver neutrophil accumulation, and hepatocellular injury in a mouse hepatic warm I/R model. Donor pigs given recombinant IL-10 markedly decreased transaminase release after transplantation preceeded by 5 hr of cold ischemia.[35]

Soluble forms of adhesion molecule receptor blockers prevent leukocytes and platelets from adhering to the EC surface. The expression of proinflammatory cytokines and adhesion molecules increases in brain-dead compared with living donor transplantation.

In a series of *ex-vivo* liver perfusions of steatotic liver grafts and in a group of LTs utilizing steatotic Zucker livers into lean Zuker rats, blockade of selectins by recombinant PSGL-1 immune globulin (rPSGL1-Ig) significantly improved liver function over control animals. *Ex-vivo* livers perfused with rPSGL1-Ig had lower transaminase release, increased portal venous flow, and increased bile production compared with controls. Histologic liver architecture after reperfusion showed minimal changes in the rPSGL1-Ig treated grafts versus severe centrilobular disruption, dropout, and necrosis in controls. Survival of lean rats transplanted with steatotic livers was only 40% compared with 90% in the same model treated with PSGL1-Ig at time of harvest and before reperfusion.[36]

A number of antiapoptotic strategies have been shown to confer a high degree of protection, including improved animal survival following prolonged ischemic insult. Gene-therapy-induced Bag-1, which exerts powerful antiapoptotic effects by binding and stabilizing Bcl-2 and interacting with the TNF receptor-type I-induced death signal, prevented cold IRI in rat livers.[37] Adenovirus-mediated gene transfer of Bcl-2 into mouse livers resulted in increased resistance to IRI with dramatically reduced transaminase release, decreased hepatocyte apoptosis, and significantly prolonged animal survival as compared with controls.[27] Overexpression of Bcl-2 in transgenic mice inhibited caspase-3 activation and apoptosis after I/R, significantly reduced liver injury and increased survival.[28]

Among the many potential therapies, the heme oxygenase (HO) system is the most critical of the cytoprotective mechanisms activated during cellular stress, exerting antioxidant, anti-inflammatory, and anti-apoptotic functions (Figure 30.5-2). Heme oxygenase-1 (HO-1) belongs to a family of enzymes involved in the catabolism of heme into biliverdin/bilirubin, free iron, and carbon monoxide (CO).[38–40] HO-1 induction in normal or even in steatotic ("marginal") livers by pharmacological means (eg, cobalt protoporphyrin, hemin) or genetic engineering maintains tissue architecture, preserves organ function, and leads to prolonged graft survival after LT.[41–43] Moreover, HO-1 overexpression has been shown to reduce macrophage infiltration into liver grafts.[43] The heme degradation step by HO-1 and HO-1 byproducts (biliverdin/bilirubin and CO) have anti-inflammatory and antiapoptotic functions. Biliverdin/bilirubin exerts prominent antioxidant function against OFR during hepatic IRI. A simple

supplementation of bilirubin to the pretransplant graft rinse reduced hepatocellular damage and improved graft function in rat cold hepatic IRI[44]. *Ex-vivo* livers perfused with biliverdin demonstrated significantly increased portal venous flow, bile production, and decreased hepatocyte damage after cold preservation.[45] Biliverdin treatment, after LT inhibited liver leukocyte infiltration through the inhibition of cellular adhesion molecules (P-selectin, ICAM-1), decreased the expression of proinflammatory cytokines (TNF-α, IL-1β), and promoted an increased expression of antiapoptotic genes (Bcl-2/Bag-1) resulting in marked cytoprotection against IRI.[46] The modulation of the p38 MAPK signaling pathway by CO mediates anti-inflammatory and antiapoptotic effects in IRI.[47] CO exposure inhibited an early up-regulation of proinflammatory cytokines (TNF-α, IL-1β, IL-6), chemokines, and up-regulated Bcl-2 and reduced caspase-3 during cold IRI[48]. Ad-HO-1 gene transfer-induced CO selectivelydepressed expression of Th1 cytokines (IL-2, IFN-α), increased expression of the anti-inflammatory cytokines (IL-4, IL-10) and prevented CD95/Fas ligand-mediated apoptosis after LT.[49]

## CONCLUSIONS

The I/R induced insult, an antigen-independent component of procurement injury, has a complex pathophysiology with a number of contributing factors and represents an important problem affecting organ transplantation outcomes. Cadaveric donor livers incur inflammatory damage before explantation that may contribute to subsequent IRI and increase the susceptibility of the organ to further immune responses. Minimizing the adverse effects of IRI would significantly increase the number of patients successfully undergoing organ transplantation and reduce wait-list times.

### References

1. Yu YY, Ji J, Zhou GW, et al. Liver biopsy in evaluation of complications following liver transplantation. *World J Gastroenterol* 2004;10: 1678–1681.
2. Fellstrom B, Akuyrek LM, Backman U, et al. Postischemic reperfusion injury and allograft arteriosclerosis. *Transplant Proc* 1998;30: 4278–4280.

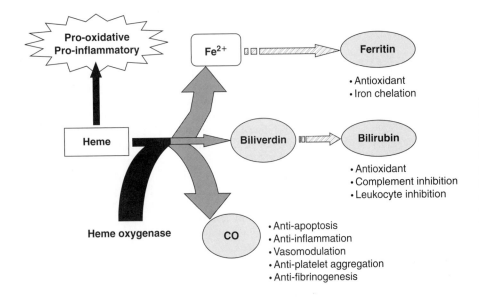

**FIGURE 30.5-2**

Mechanistic scheme of HO-1 cytoprotective role in liver IRI. HO-1 enzyme activity degrades heme to biliverdin, CO, and $Fe^{2+}$. Biliverdin is rapidly reduced to bilirubin. Biliverdin and bilirubin scavenge OFR and inhibit complement activation and leukocyte infiltration. CO not only provides anti-inflammatory and antiapoptotic effects but also modulates the vascular tone, which leads to diminished platelet aggregation and depressed fibrinogenesis. Increased $Fe^{2+}$ is channeled toward ferritin production. Ferritin prevents cell injury by antioxidant action and iron chelation.

3. Farmer DG, Yersiz H, Ghobrial RM, et al. Early graft function after pediatric liver transplantation: comparison between in situ split liver grafts and living-related liver grafts. *Transplantation* 2001;72:1795–1802.

4. Clavien PA. Sinusoidal endothelial cell injury during hepatic preservation and reperfusion. *Hepatology* 1998;28:281–285.

5. Koo DD, Welsh KI, Roake JA, et al. Ischemia/reperfusion injury in human kidney transplantation: an immunohistochemical analysis of changes after reperfusion. *Am J Pathol* 1998;153:557–566.

6. Bronk SF, Gores GJ: Acidosis protects against lethal oxidative injury of liver sinusoidal endothelial cells. *Hepatology* 1991;14:150–157.

7. Peralta C, Bulbena O, Xaus C, et al. Ischemic preconditioning: a defense mechanism against the reactive oxygen species generated after hepatic ischemia reperfusion. *Transplantation* 2002;73:1203–1211.

8. Taniai H, Hines IN, Bharwani S, et al. Susceptibility of murine periportal hepatocytes to hypoxia-reoxygenation: role for NO and Kupffer cell-derived oxidants. *Hepatology* 2004;39:1544–1552.

9. Kojima Y, Suzuki S, Tsuchiya Y, et al. Regulation of pro-inflammatory and anti-inflammatory cytokine responses by Kupffer cells in endotoxin-enhanced reperfusion injury after total hepatic ischemia. *Transpl Int* 2003;16:231–240.

10 Briceno J, Marchal T, Padillo J, et al. Influence of marginal donors on liver preservation injury. *Transplantation* 2002;74:522–526.

11. Fan C, Zwacka RM, Engelhardt JF. Therapeutic approaches for ischemia/reperfusion injury in the liver. *J Mol Med* 1999;77:577–592.

12. Okaya T, Lentsch AB. Cytokine cascades and the hepatic inflammatory response to ischemia and reperfusion. *J Invest Surg* 2003;16:141–147.

13. Jaeschke H: Molecular mechanisms of hepatic ischemia-reperfusion injury and preconditioning. *Am J Physiol Gastrointest Liver Physiol* 2003;284:G15–26.

14. Colletti LM, Kunkel SL, Walz A, et al. The role of cytokine networks in the local liver injury following hepatic ischemia/reperfusion in the rat. *Hepatology* 1996;23:506–514.

15. Thornton AJ, Strieter RM, Lindley I, et al. Cytokine-induced gene expression of a neutrophil chemotactic factor/IL-8 in human hepatocytes. *J Immunol* 1990;144:2609–2613.

16. Collins T, Read MA, Neish AS, et al. Transcriptional regulation of endothelial cell adhesion molecules: NF-kappa B and cytokine-inducible enhancers. *Faseb J* 1995;9:899–909.

17. Chamoun F, Burne M, O'Donnell M, et al. Pathophysiologic role of selectins and their ligands in ischemia reperfusion injury. *Front Biosci* 2000;5:E103–109.

18. Constantin G: PSGL-1 as a novel therapeutic target. *Drug News Perspect* 2004;17:579–586.

19. Lentsch AB, Kato A, Yoshidome H, et al. Inflammatory mechanisms and therapeutic strategies for warm hepatic ischemia/reperfusion injury. *Hepatology* 2000;32:169–173.

20. Skrabal CA, Thompson LO, Potapov EV, et al. Organ-specific regulation of pro-inflammatory molecules in heart, lung, and kidney following brain death. *J Surg Res* 2005;123:118–125.

21. van der Hoeven JA, Ter Horst GJ, Molema G, et al. Effects of brain death and hemodynamic status on function and immunologic activation of the potential donor liver in the rat. *Ann Surg* 2000;232:804–813.

22. van der Hoeven JA, Lindell S, van Schilfgaarde R, et al. Donor brain death reduces survival after transplantation in rat livers preserved for 20 hr. *Transplantation* 2001;72:1632–1636.

23. Koo DD, Welsh KI, McLaren AJ, et al. Cadaver versus living donor kidneys: impact of donor factors on antigen induction before transplantation. *Kidney Int* 1999;56:1551–1559.

24. Jassem W, Koo DD, Cerundolo L, et al. Leukocyte infiltration and inflammatory antigen expression in cadaveric and living-donor livers before transplant. *Transplantation* 2003;75:2001–2007.

25. Rudiger HA, Graf R, Clavien PA. Liver ischemia: apoptosis as a central mechanism of injury. *J Invest Surg* 2003;16:149–159.

26. Mueller TH, Kienle K, Beham A, et al. Caspase 3 inhibition improves survival and reduces early graft injury after ischemia and reperfusion in rat liver transplantation. *Transplantation* 2004;78:1267–1273.

27. Bilbao G, Contreras JL, Eckhoff DE, et al. Reduction of ischemia-reperfusion injury of the liver by in vivo adenovirus-mediated gene transfer of the antiapoptotic Bcl-2 gene. *Ann Surg* 1999;230:185–193.

28. Selzner M, Rudiger HA, Selzner N, et al. Transgenic mice overexpressing human Bcl-2 are resistant to hepatic ischemia and reperfusion. *J Hepatol* 2002;36:218–225.

29. van der Hoeven JA, Moshage H, Schuurs T, et al. Brain death induces apoptosis in donor liver of the rat. *Transplantation* 2003;76:1150–1154.

30. Glantzounis GK, Yang W, Koti RS, et al. Continuous infusion of N-acetylcysteine reduces liver warm ischaemia-reperfusion injury. *Br J Surg* 2004;91:1330–1339.

31. Nakano H, Nagasaki H, Barama A, et al. The effects of N-acetylcysteine and anti-intercellular adhesion molecule-1 monoclonal antibody against ischemia-reperfusion injury of the rat steatotic liver produced by a choline-methionine-deficient diet. *Hepatology* 1997;26:670–678.

32. Taut FJ, Schmidt H, Zapletal CM, et al. N-acetylcysteine induces shedding of selectins from liver and intestine during orthotopic liver transplantation. *Clin Exp Immunol* 2001;124:337–341.

33. Ke B, Shen XD, Lassman CR, et al. Interleukin-13 gene transfer protects rat livers from antigen-independent injury induced by ischemia and reperfusion. *Transplantation* 2003;75:1118–1123.

34. Kato A, Yoshidome H, Edwards MJ, et al. Regulation of liver inflammatory injury by signal transducer and activator of transcription-6. *Am J Pathol* 2000;157:297–302.

35. Donckier V, Loi P, Closset J, et al. Preconditioning of donors with interleukin-10 reduces hepatic ischemia-reperfusion injury after liver transplantation in pigs. *Transplantation* 2003;75:902–904.

36. Amersi F, Farmer DG, Shaw GD, et al. P-selectin glycoprotein ligand-1 (rPSGL-Ig)-mediated blockade of CD62 selectin molecules protects rat steatotic liver grafts from ischemia/reperfusion injury. *Am J Transplant* 2002;2:600–608.

37. Sawitzki B, Amersi F, Ritter T, et al. Upregulation of Bag-1 by ex vivo gene transfer protects rat livers from ischemia/reperfusion injury. *Hum Gene Ther* 2002;13:1495–1504.

38. Katori M, Anselmo DM, Busuttil RW, et al. A novel strategy against ischemia and reperfusion injury: cytoprotection with heme oxygenase system. *Transpl Immunol* 2002;9:227–233.

39. Katori M, Busuttil RW, Kupiec-Weglinski JW. Heme oxygenase-1 system in organ transplantation. *Transplantation* 2002;74:905–912.

40. Tsuchihashi S, Fondevila C, Kupiec-Weglinski JW. Heme oxygenase system in ischemia and reperfusion injury. *Ann Transplant* 2004;9:84–87.

41. Amersi F, Buelow R, Kato H, et al. Upregulation of heme oxygenase-1 protects genetically fat Zucker rat livers from ischemia/reperfusion injury. *J Clin Invest* 1999;104:1631–1639.

42. Kato H, Amersi F, Buelow R, et al. Heme oxygenase-1 overexpression protects rat livers from ischemia/reperfusion injury with extended cold preservation. *Am J Transplant* 2001;1:121–128.

43. Coito AJ, Buelow R, Shen XD, et al. Heme oxygenase-1 gene transfer inhibits inducible nitric oxide synthase expression and protects genetically fat Zucker rat livers from ischemia-reperfusion injury. *Transplantation* 2002;74:96–102.

44. Kato Y, Shimazu M, Kondo M, et al. Bilirubin rinse: A simple protectant against the rat liver graft injury mimicking heme oxygenase-1 preconditioning. *Hepatology* 2003;38:364–373.

45. Fondevila C, Katori M, Lassman C, et al. Biliverdin protects rat livers from ischemia/reperfusion injury. *Transplant Proc* 2003;35:1798–1799.

46. Fondevila C, Shen XD, Tsuchiyashi S, et al. Biliverdin therapy protects rat livers from ischemia and reperfusion injury. *Hepatology* 2004;40:1333–1341.

47. Amersi F, Shen XD, Anselmo D, et al. Ex vivo exposure to carbon monoxide prevents hepatic ischemia/reperfusion injury through p38 MAP kinase pathway. *Hepatology* 2002;35:815–823.

48. Nakao A, Kimizuka K, Stolz DB, et al. Carbon monoxide inhalation protects rat intestinal grafts from ischemia/reperfusion injury. *Am J Pathol* 2003;163:1587–1598.

49. Ke B, Buelow R, Shen XD, et al. Heme oxygenase 1 gene transfer prevents CD95/Fas ligand-mediated apoptosis and improves liver allograft survival via carbon monoxide signaling pathway. *Hum Gene Ther* 2002;13:1189–1199.

# 30.6    SMALL-FOR-SIZE GRAFTS

*Roberto Troisi, MD, PhD, Marleen Praet, MD, PhD,*
*Bernard de Hemptinne MD, PhD*

## INTRODUCTION

Adult-to-adult living donor (LD) liver transplants have become an established procedure worldwide. They are considered a good, or even the best, alternative for recipients with limited or delayed access to a deceased donor (DD) graft. Their application is principally motivated by the chronic organ shortage.[1] The procedure is continuously evolving over time; improved results are principally due to refined surgical techniques.[2–7] New 3-D reconstructive imaging of the liver, with precise anatomic reconstruction and more accurate calculation of the LD's remnant liver mass, has made donor selection more reliable and the operation safer.[8] Strategies for operational tolerance (combined stem cell or bone marrow transplants) currently under investigation could open unexpected frontiers and give a new boost to adult-to-adult LD liver transplants.[9–12]

Although the number of such transplants rapidly grew from 1997 through 2001 in Western countries, the anticipated exponential growth after that has not occurred. Today, the procedure accounts for only 5% of all liver transplants in the United States and for 3% in Europe.[13,14] In fact, the number of such transplants decreased in the United States from 408 in 2001 to 273 in 2004 and in Europe from 216 in 2002 to 140 in 2004.[13–17] The negative trend we are facing in Western countries is partly due to the application of the Model for End-Stage Liver Disease (MELD) score to select liver transplant candidates. This score system provides an expeditious transplant for patients with rapid decompensation for which an adult-to-adult LD transplant was an elegant solution in the past.[13] Another reason for the decrease in such transplants is their high complication rate for recipients, combined with concerns about donor morbidity. The relative risk of graft loss posttransplant is indeed higher than that after DD liver transplants, because of the higher vascular and biliary complication rates. The average 1-year graft survival rate is between 73% and 75%.[14,16,17] The complication rate for recipients is between 34% and 63%.[18–24]

The precise causes of graft dysfunction and loss and of recipient mortality have not been analyzed in detail in national registries. The incidence of primary nonfunction (PNF) and technical complications reported to the European Liver Transplantation Registry (ELTR) as the reason for graft failure is significantly higher after adult-to-adult LD transplants (13%, PNF; 26%, technical complications) than after DD transplants (10%, PNF; 15%, technical complications).[14] With adult-to-adult LD transplants, the cold ischemic time remains very short, and the quality of a LD graft should, by definition, be optimal. Thus, we can presume that PNF is of a quite different nature, as compared with DD transplants. What is being reported as PNF is probably a form of a functional small-for-size syndrome causing severe early graft dysfunction, often complicated by vascular thrombosis and biliary ischemia. Moreover, we have insufficient data on possible outflow insufficiency, which could also contributive to the reported technical problems.[22]

## MECHANISMS OF SMALL GRAFT INJURY

Most of the time, a partial liver graft transplanted into an adult recipient is, by definition, a small-for-size graft. Such a graft is, however, well tolerated when it is not under a critical size. It is generally admitted that the graft-weight-to-recipient body-weight (GRBW) ratio should be higher than 0.8, to ensure a proper balance between liver regeneration and liver function after graft reperfusion. But under this GRBW limit, the risk of progressive irreversible liver damage is generally too high to still proceed.

Small-for-size syndrome is characterized by a combination of early postoperative progressive cholestasis, persistent portal hypertension, ascites production associated with kidney failure, and coagulopathy. Microscopic features include cholestasis with hepatocyte ballooning, vacuolar degeneration, sinusoidal disruption, and mitochondrial swelling.[25,26] Graft dysfunction reduces the graft survival rate and increases the mortality rate. Recipients die of septic complications or, in some cases, of gastrointestinal hemorrhages or perforations.[25,27] The first mention of this clinical picture was made in 1993 by Adam et al., who transplanted pediatric donor livers into adults. They observed a complicated course posttransplant for recipients the smallest grafts, that is, those with a GRBW ratio less than 0.5% (< 600 g); the vascular thrombosis and retransplant rates were high.[28] The pathogenesis of the syndrome is primarily tied to graft volume, but three other factors have been proved to contribute to its occurrence: *functional liver mass* (volume, donor age, steatosis), *recipient status* (United Network for Organ Sharing [UNOS] status, MELD score); and *graft perfusion* (immune-mediated cellular infiltration, portal hyperperfusion, impaired venous outflow.

Evidence has emerged documenting the importance of preoperative evaluation of functional liver mass. Although the minimum graft mass capable of meeting the recipient's metabolic demand has not yet been determined, very small graft size and poor outcome are clearly related. Grafts with a GRBW ratio of less than 0.8 (graft volume less than 45% of the standard liver weight) have a reported 1-year actuarial survival of 40% to 58%.[29,30] The transplanted liver volume is often overestimated by standard imaging techniques and does not always reflect functional graft mass.[31] In older LDs and those with steatotic liver disease, liver volume measurements alone can be misleading.

Grafts from older donors are more susceptible to cold preservation injury and have a reduced capacity for protein synthesis and regeneration.[32] Steatosis exceeding 30% is known to be responsible for a higher incidence of PNF or graft dysfunction in DD liver recipients. Both could very well contribute in some cases to small-for-size syndrome. Because ischemic time can be kept very short in adult-to-adult LD liver transplants, either older donor age alone or steatosis alone is not an important risk factor, as long as they do not coexist and as long as occult liver disease is not present. Acceptance of LDs with macrovesicular steatosis is controversial: mild and moderate fatty infiltration (less than 50%) may provide good recipient and graft outcome, but only as long as the cold ischemic time is kept short. Still, steatosis does increase donor morbidity and mortality after partial liver resection, so caution is advisable.[33–37] Occult donor liver disease (congenital lipodystrophy combined with steatosis) has led to severe liver insufficiency and donor death.[38] Some groups now systematically perform histologic assessments of potential LD liver.

*Recipient status* and the severity of hepatic disease at the time of the transplant clearly affect posttransplant outcome. Hepatorenal syndrome, the need for pretransplant intensive care unit (ICU) hospitalization, and high MELD or Child-Pugh scores are known indicators of poor posttransplant outcome. Exclusion of such candidates has even been advocated for.[39–42] Recipient selection is thus of paramount importance to avoid small-for-size syndrome and to improve overall results. Ideally, adult-to-adult LD liver transplants should be preferentially proposed to candidates with a low MELD score. On the whole, it is generally accepted that such transplants should be denied to UNOS status 2A candidates.[13,39,40,43] Patients whose illness severity is not accurately reflected by their MELD score (ie, those with pronounced cholestatic liver disease, severe encephalopathy, or cachexia) or patients with hepatocellular carcinoma should be evaluated on a case-by-case basis.

The third group of factors responsible for severe graft injury relate to graft *perfusion*. If cellular infiltration (as seen in acute cellular rejection) has an impact on liver resistance and parenchymal perfusion, the most important factors influencing liver perfusion depend on the outflow and inflow conditions. Indeed, recipients of a graft volume of less than 35% of the standard liver weight, in which middle hepatic vein (MHV) drainage is not patent or liver segments do not optimally drain, have a statistically significantly higher risk of in-hospital mortality.[29–31,44] The reason is that splanchnic venous drainage after reperfusion is forced through the graft, whatever its volume. The smaller the graft, the higher the portal flow per gram of liver and the higher the risk of postoperative complications leading to graft dysfunction and failure.[45,46] Thus, posttransplant parenchymal graft perfusion is inversely proportional to the GRBW.[45,47–49]

Segmental congestion can further precipitate a small-for-size syndrome with a small but sufficient graft, if the right posterior sector accommodates all portal and arterial blood when venous drainage through the MHV is absent. This scenario has a direct impact on the sinusoidal pressure and shear stress.[20,50,51] High portal vein flow (PVF) causes compression of Disse's spaces, activation of Kupffer cells, and production of cytokines.[49,52–54] Experimental animal models have shown that portal hypertension is, on its own, a risk factor predisposing to graft failure, at least in part through increased microvascular injury. PVF and portal vein pressure (PVP) increase in an inverse proportion to graft size, despite decreased arterial flow.[28,55–58] Enhanced PVF induces shear stress and endothelial injury with progressive alterations of hepatic microcirculation.[27] Shear stress is responsible for up-and-down regulation of vasoregulatory genes, alteration of tissue repair mechanisms, and imbalance of intracellular homeostasis. Endothelin-1 (ET-1) and early growth response (Egr-1) are up-regulated, whereas heme-oxygenase-1 (HO-1) and heat shock protein 70 (Hsp-70) are down-regulated.

The loss of a small-for-size graft is primarily attributed to release of cytokines and to the upregulation of adhesion molecules and vascular endothelial growth factor (VEGF). Activated macrophages infiltrate the graft, resulting in sinusoidal inflammation and apoptotic cell death.[58–61] In rare cases, it exacerbates acute rejection.[62]

## STRATEGIES

To overcome the occurrence of the small-for-size syndrome, different strategies have been proposed. Some of these are currently under evaluation. A *pharmacologic approach* would aim to reduce portal pressure. The first evidence, to date, that a pharmacologic decrease of portal hypertension can have a protective effect on microcirculation was recently found in a rat model by infusing nitric oxide and a vasodilator, FK 409, in small-for-size graft donors.[63] Beta-blockers, efficient in the treatment of massive ascites production, could be beneficial.[64] However, caution must be recommended, as very efficient splanchnic vasoconstrictors like terlipressin can cause acute graft ischemia.[65] Intraportal infusion of nafamostat mesilate, prostraglandin E$_1$, and thromboxane A$_2$ have been shown to reduce perfusion injury in

SFSG.[66] Somatostatin and ET-1 antagonists have also been used in attempts to attenuate portal hypertension posttransplant.[67,68]

*Ischemic preconditioning* of the liver protects the parenchyma against prolonged ischemic periods (69,70). In an experimental reduced-size liver transplant model in rats, such preconditioning clearly decreased oxidative stress, enhancing liver regeneration.[71] In human LD surgery, preconditioning decreased bleeding and was beneficial to the quality of the graft.[72] However, in our prospective study of preconditioning in adult-to-adult LD liver transplants, with liver volume ranging from 0.63 to 1 GRBW, we found no beneficial effects on donor bleeding or on caspase activity, apoptosis, or postoperative cytolysis (Figure 30.6-1).[73]

*Extracorporeal liver support*, given its ability to remove hepatotoxins, could improve hepatic functional recovery and regeneration in the initial phase of small-for-size syndrome. The molecular adsorbent recycling system (MARS) may help treat posttransplant graft dysfunction by removing toxins through its membrane separation system and by lowering intracellular cholestasis. We were able to reverse small-for-size syndrome in two out of four transplant recipients.[74] Ongoing trials are needed to assess the effectiveness of MARS.

Numerous surgical refinements to optimize outflow reconstruction have been recently reported in right-lobe transplants.[4–7] No consensus has so far been reached on the precise indications of selective reconstruction of liver venous drainage. Clearly, dominant MHV-draining segments V and VIII, as seen on 3-D computed tomography, should be reconstructed better or kept with the right liver graft. Including the MHV in the procured graft is an easy way to obtain optimal outflow, but increases donor risk. However, whether optimal venous outflow helps avoid small-for-size syndrome remains an unsettled issue.[51,75,76]

Optimizing *graft inflow* is another option. Several surgical techniques to control high PVF and PVP after graft reperfusion have been proposed. Graft inflow modulation by splenic artery ligation has been advocated to improve postreperfusion hepatic arterial flow.[77] The beneficial effect of splenic artery ligation was erroneously attributed to correction of splenic artery steal syndrome.[78] Splenectomy has been principally used in left-lobe transplants to decrease portal graft hypertension in cirrhotic recipients, but without analyzing any specific effect on small-for-size syndrome.[79] Splenic artery ligation was first clearly shown to be very useful with small grafts by decreasing total portal perfusion.[3,30] Its effects on graft inflow modulation have been shown by measuring PVF and PVP.[81] According to Poiseuille's law, flow equals pressure on resistance; thus, portal pressure alone does not integrate the liver resistance parameter; splanchnic venous measurements alone are insufficient to estimate precisely the quantity of liver flow. When spontaneous portosystemic shunts are present, excessive liver resistance can lead to hepatofugal flow.

Shear stress can be reduced even without changes in PVP, as shown by the flow and pressure parameters before and after splenic artery ligation in small-for-size liver recipients. Despite stable general hemodynamic parameters in such recipients, ligation of the splenic artery can be followed by a 25% reduction of the splenic return, whereas the hepatic artery gains 50% flow (Figure 30.6-2).

Thus, a temporary significant portal and arterial flow modification can be expected even in the absence of changes in portal pressure. Splenic artery ligation corrects excessive portal flow and is sufficient to prevent small-for-size syndrome when postreperfusion portal flow per gram liver does not exceed three to four times the physiologic flow of that lobe in the donor

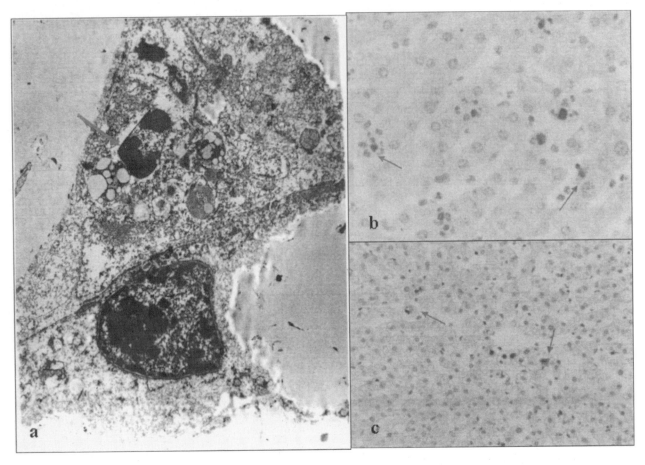

**FIGURE 30.6-1**

Effects of ischemic preconditioning in small-for-size grafts: (a) per electronmicroscopy, a single apoptotic hepatocyte (arrow); (b): TUNEL staining of postreperfusion features in without ischemic preconditioning; and (c): with ischemic preconditioning. Rare apoptotic hepatocytes appear in both stains. (Troisi R, 2005, unpublished data).

Abbreviations used: TUNEL, terminal deoxynucleotidl transferase biotin-dUTP Nick End Labeling.

(equivalent to what is expected after a partial hepatectomy of 60% to 80%).

In case of PVF more than fourfold of the physiologic values, more drastic modulations are required.[3] Portal vein banding and partial portocaval or mesocaval shunts can be lifesaving. Mesentericoportal disconnection has also been successfully described in five left-lobe grafts.[2,82] We described how a calibrated partial side-to-side portocaval shunt (hemiportocaval shunt) improved outcome of recipients of small grafts and avoiding small-for-size syndrome.[64] Recipients transplanted with a GRBW ratio of 0.8 or less had a significantly better outcome and higher survival rates with partial portal blood shunting, as compared with recipients without graft inflow modulation. In recipients with shunted grafts, PVF was, as expected, significantly lower, as compared with recipients without hemiportocaval shunts (with shunts, $190 \pm 70$ mL/min/100 g of liver versus without shunts, $401 \pm 225$ mL/min; p = 0.002). Subsequently, hepatic arterial flow significantly increased in recipients with shunted grafts. Surprisingly, liver regeneration was not affected by the shunt; hepatocytes as well as nonsinusoidal lining cells were well-preserved (Figures 30.6-3, 30.6-4, 30.6-5).

## POTENTIAL ADVANTAGES

The preference for using a right-lobe liver graft for adult recipients appears to be appropriate, because adults require a bigger liver mass than children. However, frequent vascular and biliary anatomic variations, as well as the necessity to maximize outflow reconstruction, often make the right-lobe graft implantation technique more complex. The presumed reduction in donor morbidity with left-lobe grafts also argues in their favor if problems related to size could be overcome.[83,84]

Initial experience with left-lobe grafts, in the United States and in Europe (as opposed to the Asian experience), has been disappointing, with a high incidence of complications and poor graft survival rates. However, the number of left-lobe recipients is still low, and the learning curve must be taken into account (Figure 30.6-6). Nonetheless, the ELTR reported 1-year overall graft survival rates of only 47% for left-lobe (n = 46) versus 76% for right-lobe (n = 735) recipients. The evidence that left-lobe donation may be safer for LDs (ie, fewer biliary complications and reduced liver insufficiency), as shown by the Asian survey, has not yet been confirmed in Western countries.[14,83,84]

According to published international surveys, overall, living LD morbidity rates range from 14% to 16%, with a mortality rate of 0.25%. By individually analyzing the results of these surveys, donor morbidity appears to be significantly lower for left-lobe LDs (n = 1 384, 9%), as compared with right-lobe LDs (n = 1 395, 21%); the donor mortality rate is also lower for left-lobe LDs (0.3%), as compared with right-lobe LDs (0.07%).[14,23,24] The

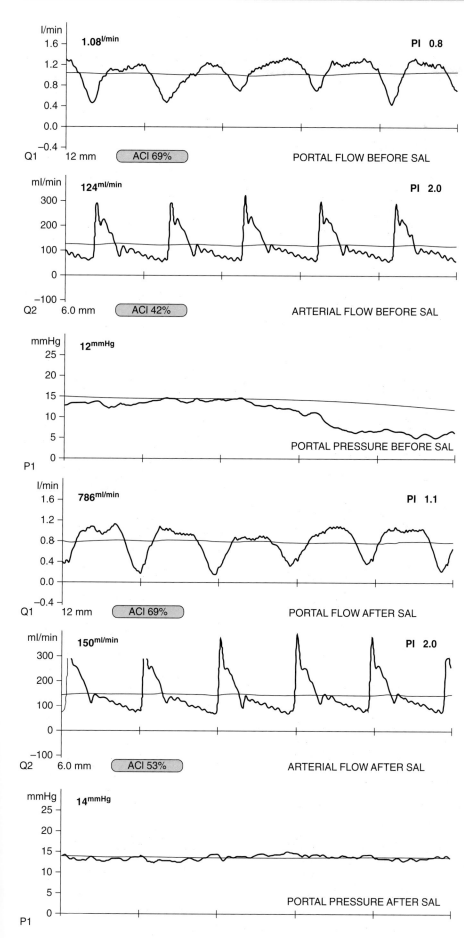

**FIGURE 30.6-2**

(A) Relationships between portal pressures and transit time flow measurements: left lobe weighing 409 g with a GRBW ratio of 0.61. Systemic hemodynamics: cardiac index of 4.2 L/m2/min, cardiac output of 8 L/min, central venous pressure of 5 mm Hg GRBW: graft weight to recipient body weight. SAL, splenic artery ligation. (B) Hemodynamic effects on graft inflow after ligature of the splenic artery: unreliability of the portal pressures to determine whether or not to proceed with inflow modulation. SAL, splenic artery ligation.

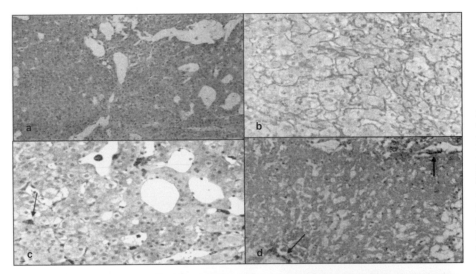

**FIGURE 30.6-3**

Routine liver biopsies of a deceased donor liver 1 to 4 weeks posttransplant: (a): normal liver parenchymal, absence of centrolobular cholestasis (hematoxylin-eosin staining x 400); (b): reticulin staining showing sinusoidal integrity (x 400); (c): CD 68 antibody staining, showing few Kupffer cells surrounded by normal parenchyma (x 400); and (d): smooth muscle actin staining showing absence of myofibroblasts (x 400).

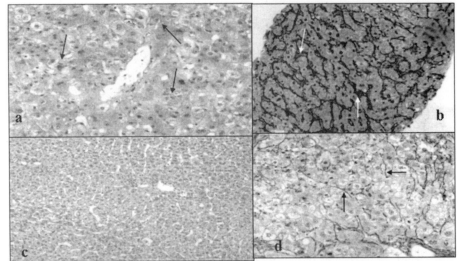

**FIGURE 30.6-4**

Liver biopsies from recipients of small-for-size grafts without (a, b) and with hemi-portocaval shunts (c, d): (a): strong cholestasis and well-preserved lobular architecture (hematoxylin-eosin staining x 400); (b): increased amount of reticulin along sinusoids with network disruption (x 400); (c): less or no cholestasis and cholangitis (x 100); and (d): less pronounced reticulin fiber stains, due to better preservation of the network (x 400).

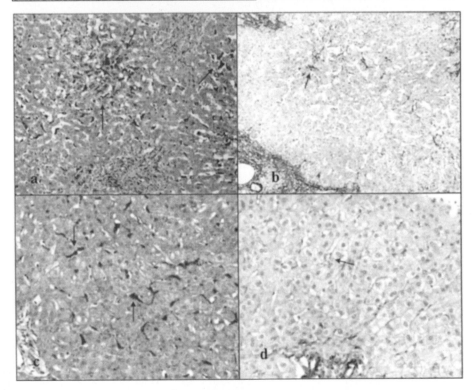

**FIGURE 30.6-5**

Liver biopsies from recipients of small-for-size grafts without (a,b) and with hemi-portocaval shunts (c, d): (a): increased staining for activated histiocytes (Kupffer cells) loaded by bile pigments (CD 68 staining x 200); (b): enhanced smooth muscle actin staining showing activation of stellate cells into myofibroblasts (SMA staining x 200); (c): less Kupffer cell activation (CD 68 staining x 200); and (d): inconspicuous stellate cells without deposition of positive staining membranes along the sinusoids (SMA staining x 200). SMA: superior mesenteric artery.

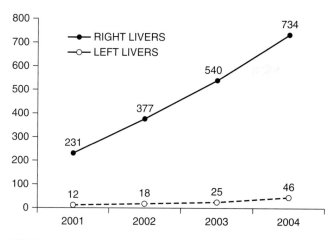

**FIGURE 30.6-6**

Type of graft used for adult-to-adult living donor liver transplants (Data from European Liver Transplant Registry, update June 2004).

left-lobe LD mortality rate is thus closer to that for kidney LDs (0.03%).[85] This lower LD mortality rate could be an argument to preferentially advocate the use of left lobes, if the problems related to small-for-size syndrome in recipients can be safely overcome.

## CONCLUSIONS

Transplant centers that perform adult-to-adult LD liver transplants are faced with the new clinical entity of small-for-size syndrome, responsible for higher morbidity and mortality rates. Its occurrence is multifactorial, but it is primarily observed when small grafts are transplanted into adult recipients. Its pathophysiology is basically related to sinusoidal shear stress, which is directly dependent on portal flow and pressure. Small grafts may be successfully transplanted into selected recipients with well-compensated cirrhosis, minimal or absent portal hypertension, and low MELD scores whose splanchnic flow is not dramatically increased. Proper venous drainage is an absolute prerequisite for implantation, and is even more important with partial liver grafts, where reversed segmental flow can adversely affect an already fragile balance. Intraoperative flow measurements are essential to estimate the extent of changes in the graft's parameters posttransplant. Inflow modulation may significantly improve overall results. However, better understanding of the mechanism involved is needed to establish precise indications for the type and extent of inflow modulation, according to graft size and recipient status. Such an understanding will certainly help us to more successfully manage postoperative liver insufficiency after major liver resections. The evidence that left-lobe donation reduces LD morbidity and mortality should encourage us to further improve posttransplant results with small grafts.

## References

1. Trotter JF, Wachs M, Everson GT, Kam I. Adult-to-adult transplantation of the right hepatic lobe from a living donor. *N Engl J Med* 2002;346:212–218.
2. Boillot O, Delafosse B, Méchet I, Boucaud C, Pouyet M. Small-for-size partial liver graft in an adult recipient: a new transplant technique. *Lancet* 2002;359:406–407.
3. Troisi R, Cammu G, Militerno G, et al. Modulation of portal graft inflow: a necessity in adult living donor liver transplantation? *Ann Surg* 2003;237:429–436.
4. Liu CL, Zhao Y, Lo CM, Fan ST. Hepatic venoplasty in right lobe live donor liver transplantation. *Liver Transplant* 2003;9:1265–1272.
5. Sugawara Y, Makuuchi M, Akamatsu N. Refinement of venous reconstruction using cryopreserved veins in right liver grafts. *Liver Transplant* 2004;10:541–547.
6. Takemura N, Sugawara Y, Hashimoto T, et al. New hepatic vein reconstruction in left liver graft. *Liver Transplantat* 2005;11:356–360.
7. Malago M, Molmenti EP, Paul A, et al. Hepatic venous outflow reconstruction in right live donor liver transplantation. *Liver Transplant* 2005;11:364–365.
8. Frericks BB, Caldarone FC, Nashan B, et al. 3D CT modeling of hepatic vessel architecture and volume calculation in living donated liver transplantation. *Eur Radiol* 2004;14:326–333.
9. Donckier V, Troisi R, Toungouz M, et al. Donor stem cell infusion after non-myelo-ablative conditioning for tolerance induction to HLA mismatched adult living-donor liver graft. *Transplant Immunol* 2004;13:139–146.
10. Kadry Z, Mullhaupt B, Renner EL, et al. Living donor liver transplantation and tolerance: a potential strategy in cholangiocarcinoma. *Transplantation* 2003;76:1003–1006.
11. Li Y, Koshiba T, Yoshizawa A, Yonekawa Y, et al. Analyses of peripheral blood mononuclear cells in operational tolerance after pediatric living donor liver transplantation. *Am J Transplant* 2004;4:2118–25.
12. Mellgren K, Fasth A, Saalman R, Olausson M, Abrahamsson J. Liver transplantation after stem cell transplantation with the same living donor in a monozygotic twin with acute myeloid leukemia. *Ann Hematol* 2005;Jul 7, 2005[Epub ahead of print].
13. Trotter JF. Living donor liver transplantation: is the hype over? *Liver Transplant* 2005;43:20–25.
14. ELTR registry: LRLT, update June 2004.
15. Ghobrial RM, Busuttil RW. Future of adult living donor liver transplantation. *Liver Transplant* 2003;9:S73–S79.
16. UNOS data: www.opt.org/latestData/rptData.asp. Accessed July 15th, 2005.
17. Abt PL, Mange KC, Olthoff KM, et al. Allograft survival following adult-to-adult living donor liver transplantation. *Am J Transpl* 2005;4: 1302–1307.
18. Wachs ME, Bak TE, Karrer FM, et al. Adult living donor liver transplantation using a right hepatic lobe. *Transplantation* 1998;66:1313–1316.
19. Marcos A, Ham J, Fisher R, Olzinski AT, Posner MC. Single center analysis of the first 40 adult-to-adult living donor liver transplants using the right lobe. *Liver Transplant* 2000;6:296–301.
20. Miller CM, Gondolesi GE, Florman S, et al.One-hundred nine liver donor transplants in adults and children; A single-center experience. *Ann Surg* 2001;234:301–312.
21. Ghobrial RM, Saab S, Lassman C, et al. *Liver Transplant* 2002;8:901–909.
22. Broelsch CE, Frilling A, Testa G, et al. Early and late complications in the recipient of an adult living donor liver. *Liver Transplant* 2003;9:S50–S53.
23. Brown RS, Russo MW, Lai M, et al. A survey of liver transplantation from living adult donors in the United States. *New Engl J Med* 2003;348:818–825.
24. Lo CM, Fan ST, Liu CL, et al. Lessons learned from one hundred right lobe living donor liver transplants. *Ann Surg* 2004;240:151–158.
25. Emond J, Renz JF, Ferrel LD, et al. Functional analysis of grafts from living donors. Implications for the treatment of older recipients. *Ann Surg* 1996;224:544–554.
26. Sugawara Y, Makuuchi M, Takayama T, et al. Small-for-size grafts in living-related liver transplantation. *J Am Coll Surg* 2001;192:510–513.
27. Man K, Lo CM, Ng IOL, et al. Liver transplantation in rats using small-for-size grafts. *Arch Surg* 2001;136:280–285.
28. Adam R, Castaing D, Bismuth H. Transplantation of small donor liver in adult recipients. *Transplant Proc* 1993;l25:1105–1106.
29. Kiuchi T, Kasahara M, Uryuhara K, et al. Impact of graft size mismatching on graft prognosis in liver transplantation from living donors. *Transplantation* 1999;67:321–327.

30. Lo CM, Fan S-T, Liu CL, et al. Minimum graft size for successful living donor liver transplantation. *Transplantation* 1999;68:1112–1116.

31. Sakamoto S, Uemoto S, Uryuhara K, et al. Graft size assessment and analysis of donors for living donor liver transplantation using right lobe. *Transplantation* 2001;71:1407–1413.

32. Ikegami T, Nishizaki T, Yanaga K, et al. The impact of donor age on living donor liver transplantation. *Transplantation* 2000;70:1703–1707.

33. Strasberg SM, Howard TK, Molmenti EP, Hertl M. Selecting the donor liver: risk factors for poor function after orthotopic liver transplantation. *Hepatology* 1994;20:829–838.

34. Todo S, Demetris AJ, Makowka L, et al. Primary nonfunction of hepatic allografts with preexisting fatty infiltration. *Transplantation* 1989;47:903–905.

35. Marsman WA, Wiesner RH, Rodriguez L, et al. Use of fatty donor liver is associated with diminished early patient and graft survival. *Transplantation* 1996;62:1246–1251.

36. Soejima Y, Shimada M, Suehiro T, et al. Use of steatotic graft in living-donor liver transplantation. *Transplantation* 2003;76:344–348.

37. Behrns KE, Tsiotos GG, DeSouza NF. Hepatic steatosis as a potential risk factor for major hepatic resection. *J Gastrointest Surg* 1998;2:292–298.

38. Malago M, Testa G, Frilling A, et al. Right living donor liver transplantation: an option for adult patients. Single institution experience with 74 patients. *Ann Surg* 2003;238:853–863.

39. Ben-Haim M, Emre S, Fishbein TM, et al. Critical graft size in adult-to-adult living donor liver transplantation: impact of the recipient's disease. *Liver Transplant* 2001;7:948–953.

40. Testa G, Malago M, Nadalin S, et al. Right-liver living donor transplantation for decompensated end-stage liver disease. *Liver Transplant* 2002;8:340–346.

41. Goldstein MJ, Salame E, Kapur S, et al. Analysis of graft failure in living donor liver transplantation: differential outcomes in children and adults. *World J Surg* 2003;27:356–364.

42. Lo CM, Fan ST, Liu CL, et al. Lessons learned from one hundred right lobe living donor liver transplants. *Ann Surg* 2004;240:151–158.

43. Tan HP, Patel-Tom K, Marcos A. Adult living donor liver transplantation: who is the ideal donor and recipient? *J Hepatol* 2005;43:13–37.

44. Fan S-T, Lo CM, Liu CL, Yong BH, Wong J. Determinants of hospital mortality of adult recipients of right lobe live donor liver transplantation. *Ann Surg* 2003;238:864–870.

45. Marcos A, Olzinski AT, Ham JM, Fisher RA, Posner MP. The interrelationship between portal and arterial blood flow after adult to adult living donor liver transplantation. *Transplantation* 2000;70:1697–1703.

46. Shimamura T, Taniguchi M, Jin MB, et al. Excessive portal venous inflow as a cause of allograft dysfunction in small-for-size living donor liver transplantation. *Transplant Proc* 2001;33:1331.

47. Hadengue A, Lebrec D, Moreau R, et al. Persistence of systemic and splanchnic hyperkinetic circulation in liver transplant patients. *Hepatology* 1993;17:175–178.

48. Henderson JM, Gilmore GT, Mackay GJ, et al. Hemodynamics during liver transplantation: the interactions between cardiac output and portal venous and hepatic arterial flows. *Hepatology* 1992;16:715–718.

49. Kanematsu T, Takenaka K, Furuta T, et al. Acute portal hypertension associated with liver resection. Analysis of early postoperative death. *Arch Surg* 1985;120:1303–1305.

50. Lee S, Park K, Hwang S, Lee Y, et al. Congestion of a right liver graft in living donor liver transplantation. *Transplantation* 2001;71:812–814.

51. Fan ST, De Villa VH, Kiuchi T, Lee SG, Makuuchi M. Right anterior sector drainage in right-lobe live-donor liver transplantation. *Transplantation* 2003;75:S25–S27.

52. Lee SS, Hadengue A, Girod C, Braillon A, Lebrec D. Reduction of intrahepatic vascular space in the pathogenesis of portal hypertension. In vitro and in vivo studies in the rat. *Gastroenterology* 1987;93:157–161.

53. Gertsch P, Stipa F, Ho J, et al. Changes in hepatic portal resistance and in liver morphology during regeneration: in vitro study in rats. *Eur J Surg* 1997;163:297–304.

54. Panis Y, McMullan DM, Emond JC. Progressive necrosis after hepatectomy and the pathophysiology of liver failure after massive resection. *Surgery* 1997;121:142–149.

55. Ku J, Fukumoto T, Nishida T, et al. Evidence that portal vein decompression improves survival of canine quarter orthotopic liver transplantation. *Transplantation* 1995;59:1388–1392.

56. Smyrniotis V, Kostopanagiotou G, Kondi A, et al. Hemodynamic interaction between portal vein and hepatic artery flow in small-for-size split liver transplantation. *Transpl Int* 2002;15:355–360.

57. Boillot O, Mechet I, Le Derf Y, et al. Portomesenteric disconnection for small-for-size grafts in liver transplantation: Preclinical studies in pigs. *Liver Transplant* 2003;9:S42–46.

58. Man K, Fan ST, Lo CM, et al. Graft injury in relation to graft size in right lobe live donor liver transplantation. *Ann Surg* 2003;237:256–264.

59. Liang TB, Man K, Lee TKW, et al. Distinct intragraft response pattern in relation to graft size in liver transplantation. *Transplantation* 2003;75:673–678.

60. Kobayashi T, Sato Y, Yamamoto S, et al. Augmentation of heme oxygenase-1 expression in graft immediately after implantation in adult living-donor liver transplantation. *Transplantation* 2005;79:977–980.

61. Yang ZF, Poon RT, Cheung CK, et al. Up-regulation of vascular endothelial growth factor (VEGF) in small-for-size liver grafts enhances macrophage activities through VEGF receptor 2-dependent pathway. *J Immunol* 2004;173:2507–2515.

62. Yang ZF, Ho DWY, Chu ACY, Wang YQ, Fan ST. Linking inflammation to acute rejection in small-for-size liver allografts: the potential role of early macrophage activation. *Am J Transpl* 2003;4:169–209.

63. Man K, Lee TK, Liang TB, et al. FK 409 ameliorates small-for-size liver graft injury by attenuation of portal hypertension and down-regulation of Egr-1 pathway. *Ann Surg* 2005;240:159–168.

64. Troisi R, Ricciardi S, Smeets P, et al. Effects of hemi-portocaval shunts for inflow modulation on the outcome of small-for-size grafts in living donor liver transplantation. *Am J Transpl* 2005;5:1–8.

65. Bernall W. Small-for-size syndrome; ICU supporting care. *Liver Transplant* 9:S15–S17.

66. Suheiro T, Shimada M, Kishikawa K, et al. Effect of intraportal infusion to improve small for size graft injury in living donor adult liver transplantation. *Transpl Int* 2005;18:923–928.

67. Reynaert H, Vaeyens F, Qin H, et al. Somatostatin suppresses endothelin-1-induced rat hepatic stellate cell contraction via somatostatin receptor subtype 1. *Gastroenterology* 2001;121:915–930.

68. Ricciardi R, Schaffer BK, Shah SA, et al. Bosentan, an endothelin antagonist, augments hepatic graft function by reducing graft circulatory impairment following ischemia/reperfusion injury. *J Gastrointest Surg* 2001;3:322–329.

69. Clavien PA, Yadav S, Sindram D, Bentley RC. Protective effects of ischemic preconditioning for liver resection performed under inflow occlusion in humans. *Ann Surg* 2000;232:163–165.

70. Clavien PA, Selzner M, Rudiger HA, et al. A prospective randomized study in 100 consecutive patients undergoing major liver resection with versus without ischemic preconditioning. *Ann Surg* 2003;238:843–850.

71. Franco-Gou R, Peralta C, Massip-Salcedo M, et al. Protection of reduced-size liver for transplantation. *Am J Transpl* 2004;4:1408–1420.

72. Imamura H, Takayama T, Sugawara Y, et al. Pringle's manoeuvre in living donors. *Lancet* 360:2049–2050.

73. Troisi R, 2005 (unpublished data).

74. Hoste E. Artificial liver support after living donor liver transplantation. Personal communication at the *"2nd Meeting on the small-for-size in liver surgery."* Ghent, March 11, 2005. www.smallforsize.be.

75. Cattral MS, Molinari M, Vollmer CM Living donor right hepatectomy with or without inclusion of middle hepatic vein: comparison of morbidity and outcome in 56 patients. *Am J Transpl* 2004;4:751–757.

76. Fan ST. Outflow reconstruction in live liver donor transplantation. Personal communication at the *"2nd Meeting on the small-for-size in liver surgery."* Ghent, March 11, 2005. www.smallforsize.be.

77. Troisi R, Hoste E, Van Langenhove P, et al. Modulation of liver graft hemodynamics by partial ablation of the splenic circuit: a way to increase hepatic artery flow? *Transplant Proc* 2001;33:1445–1446.

78. Settmacher U, Haase R, Heise M, Bechstein WO, Neuhaus P. Variations of surgical reconstruction in liver transplantation depending on vasculature. *Langenbeck's Arch Surg* 1999;384:378–383.

79. Soejima Y, Shimada M, Suehiro T, et al. Outcome analysis in adult-to-adult donor liver transplantation using the left lobe. *Liver Transplant* 2003;9:581–586.

80. Troisi R, de Hemptinne B. Clinical relevance of adapting portal vein flow in living donor liver transplantation in adult patients. *Liver Transpl* 2003;9:S36–41.

81. Ito T, Kiuchi T, Yamamoto H, et al. Changes in portal venous pressure in the early phase after living-donor liver transplantation: pathogenesis and clinical implications. *Transplantation* 2003;75:1313–1317.

82. Boillot O, Adam M, Sagnard P. Porto-mesenterical disconnection in liver transplantation: a new technique for small-for-size grafts in adult recipients. *Liver Transplant* 2003;6:539(333).

83. Shimada M, Shiotani S, Ninomiya M, et al. Characteristics of liver grafts in living-donor adult liver transplantation: Comparison between right and left-lobe grafts. *Arch Surg* 2002;137:1174–1179.

84. Lo CM. Complications and long-term outcome of living liver donors: a survey of 1508 cases in five asian centers. *Transplantation* 2003;75:S12–S15.

85. Najarian JS, Chavers BM, McHugh LE, Matas AJ. Twenty-years or more of follow-up of living kidney donors. *Lancet* 1992;340:807–810.

# 30.7   PERIOPERATIVE CARE OF THE LIVER RECIPIENT

*Mark L. Sturdevant, MD, Ty Dunn, MD,*
*Rainer W.G. Gruessner, MD*

## INTRODUCTION

Live donor liver transplantation (LDLT) will soon be entering its second decade of existence in a continuing effort to reach those patients who may otherwise be subjected to years of progressive debilitation potentially ending in death. While now accepted as ethical and useful in expanding the donor pool, LDLT remains the most high-profile of all surgical enterprises and demands technical expertise coupled with thoughtful, precise postoperative care. This chapter will concentrate on the array of perioperative surgical and medical issues the recipient experiences and, in particular, the subtle differences seen in live donor recipients when compared to deceased donor, whole liver recipients. Physiologic derangements universally occur after a major surgical procedure is performed in the setting of end-stage liver disease (ESLD); it is the manner in which the clinician identifies and manages these abnormalities along with the frequent graft-specific complications that will greatly influence the ultimate outcome.

## IMMEDIATE POSTOPERATIVE CARE

### Hemodynamic Monitoring

Regardless of the sometimes fit nature of the live donor recipient and smoothness of the elective transplant procedure, most recipients leave the operating room with the aid of mechanical ventilation destined for the intensive care unit (ICU). Universal monitoring of the electrocardiogram (ECG), arterial blood pressure, oxygen saturation, hourly urine output, pulmonary dynamics, and pulmonary artery catheter (PAC) parameters allow for constant reassessment of the intravascular volume and cardiopulmonary function and their combined effect on global perfusion. For the first 24 hours, a hemogram, electrolytes, renal function panel, coagulation profile, lactate, and liver function tests (LFTs) should be evaluated every 4 to 8 hours to monitor for bleeding, electrolyte derangements, and graft function, respectively.

## Cardiovascular Care

In general, although live donor recipients typically have a hyperdynamic circulation they are not afflicted by the profound cardiac dysfunction and pulmonary hypertension seen in those with much higher Model of End-Stage Liver Disease (MELD) scores. Insightful interpretation of the PAC parameters (eg, central venous pressure [CVP], pulmonary artery wedge pressure [PAWP], and systemic vascular resistance index [SVRI]) allows the clinician to optimize preload and judiciously add inotropic and peripheral vasoactive therapy in the appropriate settings. Mediators from the liver or intestine may lead to a reperfusion syndrome after the graft is revascularized. Common manifestations include hypotension from peripheral vasodilation, bradycardia, hyperkalemia, and pulmonary hypertension (PH) which may lead to cardiac arrest if not managed expeditiously. Precise fluid resuscitation along with inhaled nitric oxide,[1] prostacyclin infusion therapy,[2] or methylene blue infusion[3] may reduce PH and reverse the hemodynamic collapse. These therapeutic maneuvers are initiated in the operating room but often will continue into the early postoperative time period.

The gross appearance of the liver graft with varying CVP, blood pressure, and PAWP should be observed before closing the abdomen; this will aid in postoperative, goal-directed resuscitation and maintenance fluid management. Optimizing arterial blood pressure and preload will allow for ideal graft perfusion which when coupled with patent outflow should result in excellent initial graft function.

## Pulmonary Care

Positive-pressure ventilation and the use of positive end-expiratory pressure (PEEP) may lead to decreased graft oxygenation due to altered flow in the splanchnic region and congestion of the inferior vena cava (IVC) and hepatic vein drainage areas.[4] Early tracheal extubation after deceased donor liver transplantation (DDLT) has been found to be advantageous and safe especially in those recipients with minimal intraoperative blood transfusions who are absent of renal insufficiency and pulmonary edema.[5] Most live donor recipients meet these criteria and an aggressive approach to posttransplant extubation (ie, within 3–8 hours) is reasonable. In the Adult-to-Adult Living Donor Liver Transplant Consortium Study (A2ALL),[6] pulmonary complications were common in the first 90 postoperative days but a rare source of mortality: pleural effusions occurred in 18% of the recipients and pulmonary edema in 10%. Frequent monitoring with CXR and daily weights in addition to the more invasive hemodynamic monitoring should guide precise fluid management, thus minimizing these potential complications.

## Renal Issues

Only 2% of the recipients in the A2ALL study were receiving dialytic therapy at the time of transplant, and posttransplant acute renal failure (ARF) is rare after LDLT compared to a 10% incidence in the DDLT population. Common etiologies of posttransplant oligoanuria or azotemia include hypovolemic renal hypoperfusion leading to acute tubular necrosis (ATN), liver graft dysfunction, and medication toxicity (eg, calcineurin inhibitors [CNI] such as tacrolimus, aminoglycosides). If needed, renal replacement therapy may be better tolerated via the continuous venovenous hemodialysis approach.

## Infectious Disease Management and Prophylaxis

Almost 50% of the deaths following LDLT at 90 days and 1 year are attributable to infection and sepsis; it is by far the most common source of mortality and one-third of LDLT recipients experience at least one infectious complication in the first 90 days.[6] In the early postoperative period (ie, first 30 days posttransplant), more than 90% of the infections are bacterial or fungal in etiology and originate from the usual postsurgical sources: intravascular access lines, lung (eg, pneumonia), urinary tract (UTI), surgical wound, and the biliary system.[7] In the DDLT population, Winston et al noted a greater than 50% incidence of posttransplant bacterial infection, 80% of which occurred within 8 weeks; these included intraabdominal and surgical site infection, pneumonia, and UTI.[8] Intravascular access line infections account for greater than 50% of bacteremias with coagulase-negative staphylococcus and *Staphylococcus aureus* as the most common culprits.[9] Gram-negative (GN) infections (eg, enterobacter, pseudomonas) often originate from an intraabdominal source such as the liver (bile ducts) or bowel. Risk factors for GN infection posttransplant include bile leak, hepatic artery thrombosis with subsequent liver necrosis, biliary stricture, and the use of hepaticojejunostomy drainage.[10] All of these factors occur more often in LDLT when compared to DDLT. Accordingly, any GN infection in a live donor recipient mandates a thorough evaluation to rule out these posttransplant surgical complications as the septic source.

In the A2ALL study, an almost 10% incidence of fungal infection was noted in the first 90 days.[6] In the DDLT population, 80% of fungal infections are caused by invasive candidiasis. Historically, amphotericin B was the drug of choice for fungemia; however, the echinocandin, Caspofungin, appears to have equal efficacy with less toxicity (eg, nephrotoxicity),[11] and the azoles (eg, fluconazole) are an option for susceptible species. Aspergillus accounts for 15% of fungemias and carries with it an ominous mortality rate of at least 75%; 75% of all invasive Aspergillus infections occur in the first 90 days.[12]

Herpes simplex virus (HSV)-seropositive patients will have a 25% incidence of a clinically significant reactivation in the first posttransplant month if no prophylaxis is provided at the time of transplant.[13] Acyclovir is an effective prophylactic in this setting and should be offered in seropositive recipients. The remainder of the clinically active viral infections (eg, cytomegalovirus [CMV], Epstein-Barr virus [EBV], and adenovirus) occur after the first posttransplant month, and their evaluation and management are beyond the scope of this chapter. Likewise, most parasitic and protozoan infections occur several months posttransplant and will not be reviewed here.

Prophylaxis for posttransplant bacterial and fungal infections is center specific due to the lack of conclusive data; for the live donor recipient who is free of active infection a reasonable regimen consists of (1) 2 to 3 days of systemic antibacterial antibiotics with a beta-lactam penicillin or a third-generation cephalosporin + aminoglycoside and (2) fluconazole 400 mg/day for up to 10 weeks.[14] Long-term prophylactic antimicrobials are initiated immediately posttransplant. Daily administration of sulfamethoxazole-trimethoprim (SMX-TMP) is standard prophylaxis for *Pneumocystis carinii* pneumonia, as well as *Listeria monocytogenes* and Nocardia infections; by starting it postoperatively it also serves to minimize the incidence of urinary tract infections. Success has been achieved in preventing CMV infection with prophylactic 9-(1,3-dihydroxy-2-propoxymethyl) guanine (DHPG) in parenteral (ganciclovir) or enteral (valganciclovir) forms. The efficacy of oral DHPG (valganciclovir) was found to be equivalent to that of oral ganciclovir in preventing CMV disease in high-risk recipients.[15] Clotrimazole troches are used to prophylax against oropharyngeal candidiasis.

## Neuropsychiatric Care

Central nervous system (CNS) complications posttransplant occur in up to 26% of DDLT recipients.[16] Diffuse encephalopathies, seizures, and intracranial infarct/hemorrhages were noted in 11%, 6%, and 3% of recipients, respectively. The exact etiology of posttransplant diffuse encephalopathy is unknown; however, anoxic-ischemic changes in the brain are the most common findings on postmortem examinations.[17] Likewise, the pathophysiology of seizures posttransplant has not been fully elucidated; however, seizure thresholds are reduced with CNI and high-dose steroid use and during electrolyte derangements (eg, hypomagnesemia, hyponatremia). Judicious use of narcotics and benzodiazepines is also important to minimize iatrogenic causes of mental status deterioration; meperidine should be of last resort for analgesia due to its neurotoxic biometabolite, normeperidine. LDLT recipients have a lower incidence of preoperative encephalopathy, metabolic and electrolyte derangements, and coagulopathy when compared to their DDLT counterparts; these factors may lead one to believe that neurologic complications are less frequent in this population; however, very little data regarding this issue has been published in the initial LDLT outcomes.

## Fluid and Electrolyte Management

Chronic hyperaldosteronism in ESLD leads to overall increases in total body water and sodium; the result typically is a pretransplant mild-to-moderate hyponatremia with general fluid overload. Immediately posttransplant, the live donor recipient is most often euvolemic or possibly hypervolemic if blood loss is countered with excessive blood transfusion. As stated previously, goal intravascular volume parameters (eg, CVP and PAWP) are initially estimated by the gross appearance of the liver graft at the time of closure; adequate global perfusion of the recipient is equally important, and if suboptimal, additional fluid resuscitation may be needed. Maintenance crystalloid infusions are minimized in the perioperative period, and the recipient generally is kept in a euvolemic or slightly hypovolemic state to optimize graft function and avoid pulmonary edema. If needed, D5 0.45% NS is used unless the serum sodium is less than 130 mEq/L. D5 0.9% NS can be used in that case, but the excessive sodium load is undesirable in these patients; packed red cell and albumin transfusions are the preferred resuscitation fluid when volume expansion is required. If the patient is hypervolemic and hyponatremic, a gentle diuresis with a loop diuretic will be beneficial in both decreasing the intravascular volume and correcting hyponatremia. With a functioning graft and intact renal function the serum sodium will normalize in several days. The dextrose is especially valuable in the recipient with a dysfunctional graft, as hypoglycemia may occur. Hyponatremia should be corrected slowly to avoid central pontine myelinolysis.

Derangements in serum potassium are quite common posttransplant. Intraoperatively, the potassium level is minimized in preparation for a possible potassium egress from the graft postreperfusion. This may continue into the immediate postoperative period and should be cautiously treated as mild-to-moderate hypokalemia is well tolerated. Hyperkalemia, especially in the recipient with pretransplant renal impairment, is a more formidable problem, and the renal dysfunction may be exacerbated by ATN from intraoperative hypoperfusion. Medications (eg, CNI, SMX-TMP) may play some minor role in hyperkalemia as well. Standard hyperkalemia monitoring and management is usually effective but renal replacement therapy must be readily available in the ICU.

Hypomagnesemia is common in the ESLD population and may be exacerbated posttransplant by excessive blood loss and medications. In particular, the CNIs (eg, tacrolimus, cyclosporine A), loop diuretics, and amphotericin B cause magnesium wasting. Low serum magnesium levels may manifest with cardiac arrhythmias, myopathies, or impaired mentation; replacement in the form of magnesium sulfate (parenteral) or magnesium oxide (enteral) is available. Hypermagnesemia is rarely an issue unless excessive magnesium-containing antacids are given to a recipient with renal insufficiency.

Ionized serum calcium levels should be followed as total calcium levels depend on the albumin concentration which may fluctuate widely in the early posttransplant period. Hypercalcemia is typically iatrogenic in nature. Pretransplant hypocalcemia in the cirrhotic patient is attributed to malnutrition and vitamin D dysfunction primarily; this state may be exacerbated early posttransplant by citrate chelation (occurs with high blood transfusion requirement), gastrointestinal malabsorption, and hepatocyte injury resulting in an intracellular shift of calcium. Intravenous calcium chloride (200–1,000 mg) or calcium gluconate (10%) will correct this common deficiency.

Recipients with renal dysfunction may have pretransplant hyperphosphatemia which can be controlled with enteral phosphate binders. Posttransplant liver regeneration may lead to hypophosphatemia which can be corrected with parenteral phosphate (eg, sodium phosphate, potassium phosphate) or enteral potassium phosphate.

### Endocrine Management

Posttransplant hyperglycemia is prevalent due to intraoperative high-dose steroids, calcineurin inhibitors, and surgical stress. Landmark studies in postsurgical (nontransplant) and critically ill populations now provide guidance to direct the intensity of glycemic control. Golden et al reported significant decreases in surgical site infections without increases in hypoglycemic episodes in patients undergoing coronary bypass operations when glucose levels are kept below 150 mg/dL.[18] An actual decrease in mortality was noted by Van den Berghe et al when critically ill patients entering the ICU were managed with a goal blood glucose level of 80 to110 mg/dL.[19] Considering the recipient carries the additional infectious risk factor of immunosuppression and septic complications are the most common cause of death after LDLT, tight glycemic control seems prudent.

## GRAFT-SPECIFIC MANAGEMENT

### Graft Function Monitoring

Frequent evaluation of graft function is crucial and begins with the intraoperative findings by the surgical team in regards to (1) the gross appearance of the graft and vascular anastomoses, (2) biliary production and flow, and (3) improvement in hemodynamic stability and clearance of acidosis after reperfusion. In the intensive care unit, a recipient who awakens readily, remains

normoglycemic without therapeutic maneuvers and has a normal acid–base profile most likely has a functioning graft. Serial examinations of LFTs (eg, AST, ALT, total and direct bilirubin, alkaline phosphatase, GGT), coagulation parameters, and Doppler sonography (US) are mandatory and the most sensitive way to follow graft function at the hepatocellular, biliary, and vascular levels.

Normalization of the INR over the first 72 hours is an excellent sign of good engraftment and function, whereas a persistent or worsening coagulopathy may suggest primary nonfunction. Liver transaminases in the live donor recipient behave in a similar manner to that of the deceased donor recipient; that is, the AST and ALT typically peak within the first 48 to 72 hours at levels two- to fourfold normal, and then precipitously fall to near normal levels after the first posttransplant week. Of all the LFTs, AST has the initial and most marked decrease in serum levels with a functioning graft. The bilirubin level often will remain elevated or can have a dramatic drop immediately posttransplant (eg, in chronic cholestatic diseases) followed by a mild increase as tissue bilirubin is mobilized; often live donor recipients will have protracted decline in bilirubin levels before a normal range is entered.

Liver transplant Doppler ultrasonography studies play a vital role in graft monitoring and identification of surgical complications in the early posttransplant course. It has sensitivity and specificity > 90% in evaluating for one of the most ominous posttransplant complications: hepatic artery thrombosis (HAT). In addition it investigates the portal vein, hepatic veins, IVC, and the bile duct for signs of thrombosis or stenosis; extrahepatic fluid collections can easily be measured, serially followed, or percutaneously drained with the aid of US. Recommendations on the frequency of postoperative sonography range widely from two studies over the first several posttransplant days after adult-to-adult LDLT to TID evaluations for 7 days followed by a second week of BID sonograms after pediatric LDLT. A hepatic artery resistive index (RI) < 0.6 in any study should prompt additional monitoring or even angiography to further evaluate for a progressing stenosis.[18]

### Immunosuppression

No significant changes in immunosuppression are necessary for the live donor recipients compared to their deceased donor counterparts. The genetic similarities of the recipient and a related donor in LDLT has been a double-edged sword for several recipients: two sets of identical twins underwent LDLT without requiring any immunosuppression,[37] whereas a second case-series described four cases of graft-versus-host disease after LDLT when HLA-homozygous donors were used.[38] A thorough discussion regarding immunosuppression in liver transplantation is beyond the scope of this chapter (see Chapter 30.10).

### Vascular Thrombosis Prophylaxis

In the A2ALL study, HAT and portal vein thrombosis (PVT) occurred at a 6% and 2% incidence, respectively, and over half of those grafts were lost.[6] There are as many vascular thrombosis prophylaxis regimens as there are centers performing LDLT; none of these protocols have been proven to be superior in reducing the incidence of thrombosis or stenosis. Meticulous microsurgical techniques are paramount to keeping this incidence in the low single digits, especially in pediatric LDLT. Almost all regimens include some form of antiplatelet agent, most commonly a simple daily aspirin (81 mg); however, although this appears to be safe, it has not had significant success.[19] Early postoperative heparin infusions or daily subcutaneous low-molecular-weight-heparin (eg, enoxaparin) injections are also used at many centers especially in children, adults with small arteries, or in recipients with hypercoagulable states. Still others promote dextran infusions, dipyridamole, and clopidogrel. A large multicenter study is lacking in this area, and therefore no one regimen can be recommended.

## GRAFT DYSFUNCTION EVALUATION

Graft function monitoring as previously outlined is a highly sensitive way to identify graft dysfunction in the immediate and early posttransplant period. Typically, the dysfunction manifests as subtle, yet progressive increases in the transaminases or cholestatic enzymes. The exact laboratory abnormality coupled with the timing of the dysfunction allow the clinician to formulate a relatively short differential diagnosis list as to the etiology of the graft dysfunction (Table 30.7-1). Regardless of the chronology, the evaluation is initiated with US, which should exclude vascular thrombosis as a possibility. If a bile leak is likely based on clinical impressions and a perihepatic fluid collection is identified, the next step is to proceed with percutaneous drainage, which will confirm the diagnosis and control the biloma. Biliary scintigraphy

**TABLE 30.7-1**

## ALLOGRAFT DYSFUNCTION IN THE PERIOPERATIVE PERIOD

**Immediate Dysfunction ( 1–7 days)**
  Hepatocellular abnormality
    Primary nonfunction
    Primary slow function
    Small-for-size syndrome
    Drug hepatotoxicity
  Vascular thrombosis
    Hepatic artery thrombosis
    Portal vein thrombosis
    Outflow obstruction (IVC or hepatic veins)
    Bile leak or fistula

**Early Dysfunction (1–3 weeks)**
  Hepatocellular abnormality
  Acute cellular rejection
  Small-for-size syndrome
  Drug hepatotoxicity
  Vascular thrombosis
  Hepatic artery thrombosis
  Portal vein thrombosis
  Outflow obstruction (IVC or hepatic veins)
  Biliary leak or fistula
  Sepsis

**Late Dysfunction ( > 3 weeks)**
  Hepatocellular abnormality
    Acute cellular rejection
    Recurrent viral hepatitis (Hepatitis B, C, or D)
    Drug or TPN hepatotoxicity
  Vascular thrombosis
    Delayed hepatic artery thrombosis
  Biliary tract abnormality
    Bile leak or fistula
    Biliary stricture
**Sepsis**
  Primary graft infection
    Liver graft abscess
    Opportunistic (eg, CMV, EBV, adenovirus)

(eg, HIDA scan) can noninvasively demonstrate an active leak. Any additional concern regarding the bilary anastomosis would be best evaluated with magnetic resonance cholangiography (MRC) or endoscopic retrograde cholangiography (ERC).

Typically, a normal or equivocal US is followed by percutaneous liver graft biopsy to evaluate for hepatocellular abnormalities. It is crucial that the clinical team review the histopathology with the liver pathologist; differentiating cellular rejection and recurrent viral hepatitis is difficult and serial biopsies over time may be necessary. The pathologist can also be quite helpful in identifying opportunistic infection or drug toxicity based on pathognomonic histologic findings.

This straightforward algorithm (Figure 30.7-1) will lead to a diagnosis for the graft dysfunction in the vast majority of recipients. A rapid, systematic approach to graft dysfunction in the perioperative period will increase the likelihood of graft salvage by initiating appropriate therapy. The management of these complications is reviewed here; more comprehensive reviews of each complication are found elsewhere in the text.

## LDLT COMPLICATIONS LEADING TO GRAFT DYSFUNCTION

### Primary Nonfunction (PNF)

In LDLT, ischemia times are minimal and donor quality typically excellent; therefore, PNF is uncommon with a 3% incidence in the A2ALL study as compared to 5% to 10% rates in DDLT.[6] It is more likely if the live donor is older than 50 years or graft macrosteatosis (> 30%) is noted; postoperative suspicion should be high if the graft is firm and produces scant bile intraoperatively. Posttransplant, the recipient will be in acute liver failure (eg, encephalopathic, coagulopathic, acidotic) and typically a marked transaminitis (eg, AST > 2,500 IU/L) develops. Once vascular thrombosis is excluded a confirmatory percutaneous biopsy should be performed. Urgent retransplantation is prudent.

### Vascular Thrombosis

*Hepatic artery thrombosis* (HAT) occurs in 2% to 8% of LDLT recipients;[6,21,22] a recent LDLT series comparing adult-to-pediatric recipients did not show a significant difference in the incidence of HAT.[23] HAT may present in a variety of ways ranging from an insidious rise in LFTs to profound hepatic failure, frank bile leak, or recurrent episodes of bacteremia. This exemplifies the need for aggressive and liberal use of doppler US or more invasive studies (eg, magnetic resonance or CT angiography, conventional angiography)[24,25] after LDLT when graft dysfunction is evident. The timing and presentation of HAT will dictate the most efficacious therapeutic route; options include microsurgical reconstruction, angiography plus or minus thrombolytics and stenting, expectant management, or retransplantation.[26]

Graft dysfunction accompanied by signs of worsening portal hypertension (eg, ascites, variceal hemorrhage) suggests *portal vein thrombosis* which occurred in 2% of the A2ALL recipients.[6] This can be imaged with Doppler US, dual-phase CT, or magnetic resonance venography (MRV). Again, therapy depends on the timing and clinical manifestations of the thrombosis; surgical reconstruction,[27] surgical shunt placement[28] or retransplantation are typically reserved for the early thrombosis causing marked graft dysfunction whereas percutaneous transhepatic portal venoplasty plus or minus anticoagulation/stenting[29] is used for delayed thrombosis.

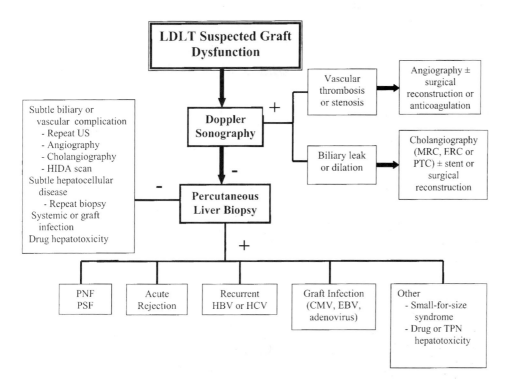

**FIGURE 30.7-1**

If graft dysfunction is suspected (eg, abnormal LFTs), a rapid evaluation with Doppler US and possibly a liver graft biopsy is performed. Repeat US and biopsy along with more invasive studies may be warranted if the diagnosis is allusive. PNF, primary nonfunction; PSF, primary slow function; MRC, magnetic resonance cholangiography; ERC, endoscopic retrograde cholangiography; HIDA, hepatobiliary iminodiacetic acid scan; CMV, cytomegalovirus; EBV, Epstein-Barr virus; HBV, hepatitis B virus; HCV, hepatitis C virus; CTA, computed tomographic angiography; MRA, magnetic resonance angiography

## Biliary Complications

The nemesis of DDLT, namely, the *bile leak*, is even more troublesome in LDLT; a 30% incidence of early bile leak was noted in the A2ALL study.[6,30,31] The presentation is variable and may be as subtle as an isolated mild hyperbilirubinemia. Large, early leaks may cause significant abdominal pain and tenderness, fever, and leukocytosis; examination of the wound and surgical drains may show gross bile. Noninvasive studies such as US with percutaneous drainage of perihepatic fluid or biliary scintigraphy (eg, HIDA) will confirm the leak and its activity but will not localize it. Cholangiography (eg, PTC, ERC) is confirmatory, can localize the leak to the anastomosis or cut liver surface, and can allow for endoscopic stenting of small leaks. Recipients with early, large leaks are best served with a biliary reconstruction possibly with a Roux-en-Y hepaticojejunostomy. Late leaks are often due to HAT and are formidable problems in that they are often accompanied by infected bilomas or cholangitis. These recipients must receive a biliary drainage procedure, adequate antibacterial and antifungal coverage, and a thorough vascular evaluation; retransplantation may be the only long-term solution for a recipient with HAT and a necrotic biliary system.

Late graft dysfunction heralded by an isolated increase in cholestatic enzymes may be secondary to a *biliary stricture*. These are typically ischemic in nature, may be multiple in numbers, and are usually found on the donor side of the anastomosis. Doppler US not only is vital as a screening tool to evaluate for biliary dilation but also to survey the vascular inflow, as HAT or stenosis may be the inciting event. Once confirmed with cholangiography (eg, PTC or ERC), most of these strictures are initially managed with endoscopic ballooning and stenting.[32] Isolated, recalcitrant strictures may be amenable to surgical reconstruction; however, a recipient with multiple, diffuse stricturing may require retransplantation for adequate long-term graft survival.

## Recurrent Viral Hepatitis

Early studies suggested that HCV recurrence was more common and virulent after LDLT compared to those undergoing DDLT.[33]

However, studies in both the United States and Japan concluded that graft and patient survival was equivalent between the groups and that recurrent HCV did not appear to be a more significant problem in LDLT.[34,35] Recurrent HCV typically presents primarily as an asymptomatic increase in LFTs; HCV-RNA PCR levels should be obtained weekly to follow the viral load. Ribavarin and interferon therapy should be considered in any recipient with graft dysfunction secondary to recurrent HCV; a complete discussion of this topic is beyond the scope of this chapter.

Hepatitis B immune globulin in conjunction with lamivudine is used as prophylactic agents in recipients with HBV.[34] Active recurrence in the recipient is confirmed with positive serologic tests for HBsAg, HBeAg, and an increase in HBV-DNA PCR levels compared to pretransplant.

In both recurrent HCV and HBV, a liver biopsy is important to obtain in order to exclude rejection and monitor the severity of the acute hepatitis.

## Rejection

With modern immunosuppression protocols, the incidence of acute cellular rejection after DDLT is approximately 20% to 30% with most episodes occurring early posttransplant.[6] Most rejection episodes are heralded by asymptomatic increases in the LFTs and is readily diagnosed via liver graft biopsy. Rejection resolution is expected after treatment with high-dose steroids plus or minus an increase in the dosage of oral immunosuppressive agents. Antilymphocyte therapy is rarely required.

## Small-for-Size Syndrome

Live donor recipients may have a posttransplant course complicated by small-for-size syndrome, which is manifested by profound cholestasis and signs of portal hypertension. This typically afflicts those recipients with relatively severe liver disease and significant portal hypertension who receive a graft with a graft-to-recipient weight ratio less than 0.8%. The exact pathophysiology is unclear and the appropriate treatment is evolving. An entire chapter is devoted to this posttransplant complication (Chapter 30.6).

## Drug Hepatotoxicity

A recipient with ongoing graft dysfunction who has normal sonographic findings and an equivocal liver biopsy may have drug toxicity as the sole offending agent. The list of medications known to cause hepatotoxicity is exhaustive; however, several drugs are introduced in the peritransplant period that are known to cause liver toxicity. Both cyclosporine and tacrolimus can cause mild cholestasis, whereas yet a third immunosuppressive agent, azathioprine, leads to a mixed picture of cholestasis and hepatocellular injury. Most recipients are started on SMX-TMP, which can lead to profound and idiosyncratic hepatocellular injury; there are several case reports of fulminant hepatic failure from SMX-TMP. Other antimicrobials, such as fluconazole and ampicillin, can also be hepatotoxic but usually present as an asymptomatic increase in LFTs. The transplant pharmacist will be helpful when trying to exclude drug toxicity as a potential source for graft dysfunction.

## Infection

Systemic sepsis can have deleterious effects on the liver graft especially if it progresses to multiorgan system failure. Any bacteremia, in particular one of the gram-negative variety, should prompt a thorough investigation of the abdomen (eg, CT) and biliary system (eg, US, cholangiography) in order to locate an infectious source.

Tissue-invasive viral infections emerge no earlier than 1-month posttransplant. CMV, EBV, and adenovirus have all been noted to cause infectious hepatitis. Serologic testing is performed, but a liver biopsy is vital in this evaluation, as it will provide histological evidence of viral infection via standard microscopy and specific immunohistochemical staining. The liver graft tissue should also be cultured to confirm the correct diagnosis.

If an opportunistic infection is confirmed, antivirals (eg, ganciclovir, acyclovir) are initiated and the immunosuppression intensity lowered. In refractory CMV hepatitis, CMVIgG should be considered.

## SUMMARY

Based on the most recent data from the largest series to date, it is safe to estimate an approximately 30% to 40% complication rate in the peritransplant period after LDLT. Biliary, vascular, and infectious issues are still present in LDLT and may be more common and severe in nature than in deceased donor transplantation. In addition, new problems such as small-for-size syndrome have been introduced, and our understanding and experience with it are insufficient at this time. Despite these realities, thorough and thoughtful posttransplant care can guide many of these recipients through this labyrinth of potential complications to a state of health and wellbeing which will allow them to go home soon after transplant.

## References

1. DeWolf A, Scott V, Bjerke R et al. Hemodynamic effects of inhaled nitric oxide in four patients with severe liver disease and pulmonary hypertension. *Liver Transplant Surg* 1997;3:594–597.
2. Kuo PC, Johnson LB, Plotkin JS et al. Continuous infusion of epoprostenol for the treatment of portopulmonary hypertension. *Transplantation* 1997;63:604–606.
3. Koelzow H, Gedney JA, Baumann J et al. The effect of methylene blue on the hemodynamic changes during ischemia reperfusion injury in orthotopic liver transplantation. *Anesth Analg* 2002;94(4):824–829.
4. Dorinsky PM, Hamlin RL, Gadek JE. Alteration in regional blood flow during positive end-expiratory pressure ventilation. *Crit Care Med* 1987;15:106–112.
5. Biancofiore G, Romanelli AM, Bindi ML et al. Very early tracheal extubation without predetermined criteria in a liver transplant recipient population *Liver Transplantation* 2001;7(9):777–778.
6. Olthoff KM, Merion RM, Ghobrial RM et al. Outcomes of 385 adult-to-adult living donor liver transplant recipients. *Ann Surg* 2005;242 (3):314–325.
7. Fishman J, Rubin R: Infection in organ-transplant recipients. *N Engl J Med* 2005;338:24.
8. Winston DJ, Emmanouilides C, Busuttil RW. Infections in liver transplant recipients. *Clin Infect Dis* 1995;21:1077.
9. Wade JJ, Rolando N, Hayllar K et al. Bacterial and fungal infections after liver transplantation: An analysis of 284 patients. *Hepatology* 21:1328, 1995.
10. Patel R, Paya CV. Infections in solid organ transplant recipients. *Clin Microbiol Rev* 1997;10:86.
11. Mora-Duarte J, Betts R, Rotstein C, et al. Comparison of caspofungin and amphotericin B for invasive candidiasis *N Engl J Med* 2002;347: 2020–2029.
12. Paya CV. Fungal infections in solid organ transplantation. *Clin Infect Dis* 1993;16:677.
13. Dummer JS, Ho M. Infections in solid organ transplant Recipients. In: Mandell GL, Bennett JE, Dolin R, eds. *Principles and Practice of Infectious Diseases.* Philadelphia; Churchill Livingstone; 2000:3148–3158.
14. Winston DJ, Pakrasi A, Busutill RW, et al. Prophylactic fluconazole in liver transplant recipients: A randomized, double blind, placebo-controlled trial. *Ann Intern Med* 1999;131:729.
15. Paya C, Humar A, Dominguez E, et al. Efficacy and safety of valganciclovir vs. oral ganciclovir for prevention of cytomegalovirus disease in solid organ transplant recipients. *Am J Transplantat* 2004;4:611–662.
16. Lewis MB, Howdle PD. Neurologic complications of liver transplantation in adults. *Neurology* 2003;61(9):1174–1178.
17. Martinez AJ. The neuropathology of organ transplantation: comparison and contrast in 500 patients. *Pathol Res Pract* 1998;194:473–486.
18. Golden SH, Peart-Vigilance C, Kao WH, et al. Perioperative glycemic control and the risk of infectious complications in a cohort of adults with diabetes. *Diabetes Care* 1999;22:1408–1414.
19. Van den Berghe G, Wouters P, Weekers F, et al. Intensive insulin therapy in critically ill patients. *N Engl J Med* 2001;345:1359.
20. Uzochukwu LN, Bluth EI, Smetherman DH, et al. Early postoperative hepatic sonography as a predictor of vascular and biliary complications in adult orthotopic liver transplant patients. *AJR* 2005;185.
21. Wolf DC, Freni MA, Boccagni P, et al. Low-dose aspirin therapy is associated with few side effects but does not prevent hepatic artery thrombosis in liver transplant recipients. *Liver Transplant Surgery* 1997;3:598–560.
22. Marsman WA, Wiesner RH, Rodriguez L, et al. Use of fatty donor liver is associated with diminished early patient and graft survival. *Transplantation* 1996;62:1246–1251.
23. Malago M, Testa G, Broelsch CE, et al. Right living donor liver transplantation: an option for adult patients: single institution experience with 74 patients. *Ann Surg* 2003;238(6):853–862.
24. Kiuchi T, Inomata Y, Uemoto S, et al. Living-donor liver transplantation in Kyoto, 1997. Clinical Transplants 1997. Los Angeles, UCLA Tissue Typing Laboratory, 1998, 191–198.
25. Goldstein MJ, Salame E, Kapur S, et al. Analysis of failure in living donor liver transplantation: Differential outcomes in children and adults. *World J Surg* 2003;27:356–364.
26. Vit A, De Candia A, Como G, et al. Doppler evaluation of arterial complications of adult orthotopic liver transplantation. *J Clin Ultrasound* 2003;31:339–345.
27. Nishida S, Kato T, Tzakis A, et al. Effect of protocol doppler ultrasonography and urgent revascularization on early hepatic artery thrombosis after pediatric liver transplantation. *Arch Surg* 2002;137:1279–1283.

28. Sheiner PA, Varma CV, Guarrera JV, et al. Selective revascularization of hepatic artery thromboses after liver transplantation improves patient and graft survival. *Transplantation* 1997;64(9):1291–1299.

29. Scantelbury VP, Zajiko AB, Esquivel CO, et al. Successful reconstruction of late portal vein thrombosis after liver transplantation. *Arch Surg* 1989;84:503–505.

30. Rouch DA, Ring EJ, Roberts JP, et al. The successfulmanagement of portal vein thrombosis after liver transplantation with a splenorenal shunt. *Surg Gynecol Obstet* 1988;166: 924–928.

31. Olcott EW, Thistlewaite JR, Lichtosh et al. Percutaneous transhepatic portal vein and stent placement after liver transplantation: early experience. *J Vasc Interv Radiol* 1990;1:17–22.

32. Testa G, Malago M, Valentin- Gamazo C, et al. Biliary anastomosis in living related liver transplantation using the right lobe: techniques and complications. *Liver Transpl* 2000;6(6):710–714.

33. Ikegami T, Nishizaki T, Kishikawa K, et al. Biliary reconstruction in living donor liver transplantation with dye injection leakage test and without stent use. *Hepatogastroenterology* 2001;48(42):1582–1584.

34. Shah JN, Ahmad NA, Shetty K, et al. Endoscopic management of biliary complications after adult living donor liver transplantation. *Am J Gastroenterol* 2004;99(7):1291–1295.

35. Garcia- Retortillo M, Forns X, Llovet JM, et al. Hepatitis C recurrence is more severe after living donor compared to cadaveric liver transplantation. *Hepatology* 2004;40(3) 699–707.

36. Russo MW, Galanko J, Beavers K, et al. Patient and graft survival in hepatitis C recipients after adult living donor liver transplantation in the United States. *Liver Transpl* 2004;10(3): 340–346.

37. Sugawara Y, Makuuchi M, et al. Living donor liver transplantation to patients with hepatitis C cirrhosis. *World J Gastroenterol* 2006;12(28): 4461–446.

38. Markowitz JS, Martin P, Conrad AJ, et al. Prophylaxis against hepatitis B recurrence following liver transplantation using combination lamivudine and hepatitis B immune globulin. *Hepatology* 1998; 28:585–589.

39. Liu LU, Schiano TD, Min AD, et al. Syngeneic living donor liver transplantation without the use of immunosuppression. *Gastroenterology* 2002;123(4):1341–1345.

40. Soejima Y, Shimada M, Suehiro T, et al. Graft-versus- host disease following living donor liver transplantation. *Liver Transpl* 2004; 10(3):460–464.

# 30.8   POSTTRANSPLANT COMPLICATIONS

*Hiroyuki Furukawa, MD, Satoru Todo, MD*

## INTRODUCTION

Despite refinements in surgical technique and immunosuppression, postoperative complications continue to be a major source of morbidity and mortality in liver transplantation. In this chapter we present postoperative complications for living donor (LD) versus deceased donor (DD) liver transplants focused on the three categories; vascular, biliary and immunological.

LD liver transplants are technically demanding surgeries and expected to be more susceptible to surgical complications. Apparently the incidence of biliary complications is significant higher in LD liver transplants, compared to DD liver transplants. The incidence of vascular complications has become less frequent because of technical development in LD liver transplants and is not much different from that of DD liver transplants. The incidence of acute cellular rejection is lower in LD liver transplants compared to DD liver transplants, especially in adults. LD liver transplants conceivably confer an immunological advantage against rejection when the donor and recipient are genetically related. Other unique aspects of the complications in LD liver transplants such as outflow block and fatal GVHD are also presented.

## VASCULAR COMPLICATIONS

The spectrum of posttransplant complications is not different for living donor (LD) versus deceased donor (DD) liver transplants. However, the incidence of surgical complications is significantly higher for LD liver transplants and requires a detailed analysis.

### Hepatic Artery Thrombosis in Deceased Donor (DD) Liver Recipients

Hepatic artery thrombosis (HAT) in DD liver recipients is a devastating complication with high morbidity and mortality. In DD liver recipients, the incidence of HAT now ranges from 3 % to 9%,[1] which is significantly improved as compared with the relatively high rates reported in the early 1980s.[2–4] Early HAT (ie, occurring within 1 month posttransplant) may present with acute hepatic failure, biliary sepsis, liver abscess, or biliary complications such as bile leak[1,2,5–7] The presentation of delayed HAT (ie, occurring after 1 month) is much more variable; patients may exhibit features of cholangitis, bile leak, biliary strictures, or liver abscess, or they may even be asymptomatic, with abnormal liver function tests.[8–13] Early HAT is more likely than late HAT to be associated with a high rate of graft loss and patient mortality.[8]

The diagnosis of HAT can be suggested by duplex ultrasonography[14,15] and confirmed by angiography,[16] exploratory laparotomy, and autopsy. Early diagnosis of HAT permits immediate thrombectomy and revascularization before the patient deteriorates. Urgent revascularization can sometimes be an effective means either to avoid a retransplant or to provide a bridge until a suitable donor becomes available.[17–19] Despite attempts at graft salvage, however, 25% to 80% of recipients with HAT eventually require a retransplant, which is associated with considerable morbidity and with mortality rates ranging from 10% to 55%.[1]

Identification of risk factors for HAT is crucial both to reducing its incidence and to managing this dreadful complication. Among the postulated major variables are certain donor and recipient characteristics, surgical techniques, and perioperative care (see Table 30.8-1).[2,5–7,13,20–27]

### Hepatic Artery Thrombosis in LD Liver Recipients

In early experiences with LD liver transplants in the 1990s, the incidence of HAT was approximately 22% to 23%.[4,28] Per more recent reports on a total of 1,128 recipients at 11 liver transplant centers, the incidence of HAT after LD liver transplants now ranges from 0% to 10.0% (mean 2.8%): 1.7% to 10% in pediatric recipients and 0% to 6.8% in adult recipients (Table 30.8-2).[29–39] The mean HAT rate of 2.8% after LD liver transplants is relatively lower than the mean of 4.7% in DD recipients.[1] This finding is not surprising, however, given the better quality and shorter preservation times of hepatic grafts in LD recipients as compared with DD recipients.

Key to reducing the incidence of HAT has been the development of advanced microsurgical techniques, which have made it possible to overcome such obstacles as small-caliber hepatic arteries and multiple anastomoses.[30,39,40] At least 9 of the 11 centers (82%) whose experience is reported in Table 30.8-2 now use microsurgical techniques for hepatic artery anastomosis, either in all LD recipients or in selected recipients, such as pediatric LD recipients. Since the introduction of microsurgical techniques in Kyoto, the incidence of HAT there has been minimal: in one series, it developed in only 4 children and 2 adults out of 365 recipients, despite the fact that 3 of those 4 pediatric transplants were ABO incompatible.[30]

**TABLE 30.8-1**

## RISK FACTORS FOR HEPATIC ARTERY THROMBOSIS (DDLT)

**Donor and recipient characteristics**
  Donor weight (<15 kg)
  Donor age (>60)
  Donor cause of death
  Infant or child recipient
  Recipient body weight (<15 kg)
  Recipient cigarette smoking
  Donor and recipient CMV status (positive to negative)
  Donor and recipient gender (female donor/male recipient)
  Recipient/donor BW ratio>1.25

**Surgical technique**
  Size of hepatic artery
  Times of anastomoses
  Aberrant hepatic artery (backtable reconstruction)
  Use of an aortic or iliac graft conduit
  Biliary reconstruction (C-J>D-D)
  Retransplantation
  Cold ischemia time

**Perioperative management**
  Transfusion of FFP or packed RBC
  Anticoagulants

**Postoperative factors**
  HA flow <400 mL/min
  Acute rejection<1 week after transplant
  CMV Infection

At least 7 of the 11 centers (64%) employ routine Doppler ultrasonography screening to detect HAT. Doppler ultrasonography has high a sensitivity for the diagnosis of HAT,[41–43] and it is noninvasive, portable, repeatable, and readily available.[44] By performing serial examinations at frequent intervals during the first 1 to 2 weeks posttransplant, HAT can be detected before it becomes clinically obvious. Early diagnosis of HAT permits immediate thrombectomy and revascularization before the patient deteriorates, and ultimately may help protect patients with HAT from the need for a retransplant and from late complications, such as biliary strictures.[18,44]

ABO incompatibility and intraoperative transfusion of fresh frozen plasma (FFP) have been identified as risk factors for HAT in LD recipients[30]; data from studies to evaluate other potential risk factors are not yet available. Of 32 LD recipients with HAT (Table 30.8-2), 15 underwent revascularization; and 11, a retransplant. Currently, the mortality among LD recipients who develop HAT is as low as 25%, a decrease that appears to be attributable to early diagnosis and revascularization.

### Hepatic Artery Stenosis

Hepatic artery stenosis, although usually asymptomatic, will eventually progress to HAT in 30% to 65% of recipients if not promptly recognized and treated.[3,45] The incidence is 4% to 13% in DD recipients[46–48] and 1% to 16% in LD recipients.[31,33,49] The early clinical presentation may or may not include elevated liver function test results. Frequently, patients have biliary strictures and bile leaks, which have a significant impact on graft and patient survival rates.[47,50]

Obviously, it is critical to identify and treat hepatic artery stenosis before it progresses to biliary complications and complete occlusion. Routine Doppler ultrasonography is a sensitive method for diagnosis.[51] Stenosis should be suspected when the resistance index (RI) is less than 0.5 or the systolic ascending time (SAT) is greater than 10 msec. If Doppler values are abnormal, angiography is performed to confirm the diagnosis.

Although conventional treatment is either surgical repair or a retransplant,[47] percutaneous transluminal angioplasty (PTA) or stent placement is becoming predominant.[45,49] The success rate of PTA is 90% to 95%, but in some recipients, it must be repeated 4 to 5 times.[49] Complications related to PTA, including intimal dissection or rupture of the hepatic artery, occur in 5% to 12% of recipients.[45,49] Some centers prefer to use coronary stents instead of simple PTA.[48] The restenosis rate after stent placement is 31% at 1 year, and the complication rate is 8%. Surgical revision is reserved for recipients whose hepatic artery is inaccessible (eg, due to kinking).[45]

### Portal Vein Complications in DD Recipients

Portal vein thrombosis (PVT) is a rare complication in DD recipients, with the incidence ranging from 1% to 2%.[52,53] PVT usually occurs

**TABLE 30.8-2**

## HEPATIC ARTERY THROMBOSIS IN LDLT

| No | Author | Place | Year | Total | Pediatrics | Adults | HAT | RV | ReTX | Mortality |
|----|--------|-------|------|-------|------------|--------|-----|-----|------|-----------|
| 1 | Otte | Brussels, Belgium | 1996 | 30 | 30 | | 1 (3.3%) | 1 | 0 | 0 (0%) |
| 2 | Hatano | Kyoto, Japan | 1997 | 242 | 234 | 8 | 4 (1.7%) | 4 | 0 | 2 (50%) |
| 3 | Miller | Mount Sinai, USA | 2001 | 109 | 50 | 59 | 6 (5.5%) | 3 | 3 | 3 (33%) |
| 4 | Bak | Denver, USA | 2001 | 41 | | 41 | 1 (2.4%) | 0 | 1 | 0 (0%) |
| 5 | Lee | Seoul, Korea | 2001 | 156 | | 156 | 0 (0%) | 0 | 0 | 0 (0%) |
| 6 | Nakamura | Kyoto, Japan | 2002 | 120 | | 120 | 2 (1.7%) | 0 | 0 | 0 (0%) |
| 7 | Sugawara | Tokyo, Japan | 2002 | 82 | | 82 | 1 (1.2%) | 0 | 0 | 0 (0%) |
| 8 | Uchiyama | Fukuoka, Japan | 2002 | 52 | — | — | 2 (3.8%) | 0 | 2 | 1 (50%) |
| 9 | Malago | Essen, Germany | 2003 | 74 | | 74 | 5 (6.8%) | 0 | 5 | 1 (20%) |
| 10 | Kaneko | Tokyo, Japan | 2004 | 70 | 70 | | 7 (10.0%) | 7 | 0 | 1 (14%) |
| 11 | Wei | Hong Kong, China | 2004 | 152 | 28 | 124 | 3 (2.0%) | 0 | 0 | 0 (0%) |
| Total | | | | 1128 | 412 | 508 | 32 (2.8%) | 15 | 11 | 8 (25%) |

HAT: hepatic artery thrombosis

RV: revascularization

ReTX: retransplantation.

at the anastomotic site in the early postoperative period. Risk factors include technical complications, small diameter of the portal vein, history of pretransplant PVT, portosystemic shunt placement pretransplant, and splenectomy.[52] In addition to acute graft failure from early occurrence of PVT, the associated portal venous hypertension can produce serious complications, such as bleeding from esophageal varices, massive ascites, splenomegaly, and hypersplenism.

In the past, the only therapeutic options for PVT involved surgery, including thrombectomy, portosystemic shunt placement, and a retransplant.[52–55] More recently, many nonsurgical treatment modalities have been reported, such as percutaneous portal vein thrombolysis, angioplasty, and endovascular stent placement.[56,57] Successful recanalization of late PVT using low-dose recombinant tissue plasminogen activator has also been reported.[58]

Portal vein stenosis (PVS) is also rare. PVS can be detected by routine surveillance with Doppler ultrasonography. It should be suspected in recipients with symptoms of portal venous hypertension similar to PVT. Routine screening for portal vein patency has several advantages. By detecting and alleviating portal vein stenosis in an early stage, symptoms of portal hypertension as well as progression to complete portal vein occlusion can potentially be averted. PVS can also be treated with venoplasty and stent placement,[59,60] but the long-term patency and complication rates of these approaches have yet to be established. In the longest available follow-up study (mean, 46 months; range, 5 to 61 months), 4 children who underwent successful venoplasty, and 12 children who underwent stent placement have required no further intervention.[61]

## Portal Vein Complications in LD Recipients

The reported incidence of portal vein complications in LD recipients ranges from 1.7% to 8%, with rates of PVT ranging from 1.7% to 6.1% and PVS from 0% to 3.3% (Table 30.8-3)[29,31,33–35,37,62] Of 33 recipients with PVT in 7 transplant centers, 7 (21%) underwent successful surgical thrombectomy and revascularization.[29,31,33–35,37,62] Radiologic intervention with thrombolysis or venoplasty was done in 19 recipients (58%), but was successful in only 10. Of 3 recipients who required a retransplant, 1 died of sepsis. Another recipient died after simultaneous PVT and HAT immediately posttransplant; still another, after liver failure. Early diagnosis of PVT with Doppler ultrasonography and early treatment with radiologic intervention appear to have reduced the graft loss rate to 9% and the mortality rate to 12%.

A particular technical challenge in LD recipients is the limited length of portal vein that can be obtained from the donor. In some recipients, a direct anastomosis between the donor and the recipient portal veins results in tension on the anastomosis, because of the orientation of the graft in the recipient. Such recipients experience a high incidence of PVT immediately posttransplant.[63] Millis et al. started using interposition venous grafts to alleviate tension on the anastomosis and to decrease the incidence of early PVT in pediatric LD recipients. With use of cryopreserved iliac vein instead of reconstructed vein from the donor, they were able to eliminate early PVT, but the late incidence of PVT increased.[64] Ultimately, they recommended avoiding the venous conduit, but, if it was absolutely necessary, using cryopreserved femoral vein. In contrast, Marwan et al. have used ovarian or inferior mesenteric veins from the donor, either for interposition grafts or as patches to reconstructed portal veins, without significant complications.[65]

A high graft-weight-to-recipient body weight ratio is also a risk factor for portal vein complications, as shown in a large study in pediatric LD recipients.[62] Long-term follow-up in that study showed that, of 11 recipients with persistent PVT, 3 developed biliary cirrhosis 2 to 9 years after PVT; 2, moderate liver fibrosis at 25 and 40 months. Another 3 had no fibrosis. In the remaining 3, fibrosis was not histologically confirmed. Of the 3 recipients with biliary cirrhosis, 2 required a retransplant (1 died) and 1 developed severe portopulmonary hypertension. Interestingly, 1 of the 3 recipients with biliary cirrhosis developed severe portopulmonary hypertension, 1 of the 2 with moderate fibrosis has hepatopulmonary syndrome; presumably, both of these complications were secondary to portosystemic shunt.

## Hepatic Venous Outflow Block

In the early experience with DD liver transplants, hepatic venous outflow block (HVOB) occurred in 1% to 2% of recipients as a result of obstruction of a conventional suprahepatic caval anastomosis.[66,67] After adoption of the piggyback technique for standard reconstruction of the outflow, the incidence of HVOB ranged from 0.8% to 9% due to torsion, compression, or thrombus of the hepatic vein or inferior vena cava (IVC).[26,68] A relatively rare complication after whole-organ DD liver transplants, HVOB developed in up to 16% of pediatric recipients in early series of reduced-size liver transplants, mostly due to the small orifice or to kinking of the anastomosis.[69,70] Most transplant centers that perform LD liver transplants have been faced with this devastating complication. The recent incidence of HVOB is 0.8% to 10.5% in LD recipients (Table 30.8-4).[32,34,71–78]

**TABLE 30.8-3**
## PORTAL VEIN COMPLICATIONS IN LDLT

| No | Author | Place | Year | Total | Pediatrics | Adults | PVT | PVS |
|---|---|---|---|---|---|---|---|---|
| 1 | Otte | Brussels, Belgium | 1996 | 30 | 30 | | 1 (3.3%) | — |
| 2 | Miller | Mount Sinai, USA | 2001 | 109 | 50 | 59 | 3 (2.8%) | — |
| 3 | Lee | Seoul, Korea | 2001 | 156 | | 156 | 3 (1.9%) | 3 (1.9%) |
| 4 | Nakamura | Kyoto, Japan | 2002 | 120 | | 120 | 2 (1.7%) | 0 (0.0%) |
| 5 | Sugawara | Tokyo, Japan | 2002 | 82 | | 82 | 5 (6.1%) | — |
| 6 | Malago | Essen, Germany | 2003 | 74 | | 74 | 2 (2.7%) | — |
| 7 | Ueda | Kyoto, Germany | 2005 | 479 | 479 | | 17 (3.5%) | 16 (3.3%) |
| Total | | | | 1050 | 559 | 491 | 33 (3.1%) | 19 (1.8%) |

PVT: portal vein thrombosis

PVS: portal vein stenosis

**TABLE 30.8-4**

## HEPATIC VENOUS OUTFLOW BLOCK IN LDLT

| No | Author | Place | Year | Total | Age Pediatrics | Age Adults | Graft Rt* | Graft Lt# | HV OB | Treatment Surgery | Treatment IVR |
|----|--------|-------|------|-------|----------------|------------|-----------|-----------|-------|-------------------|---------------|
| 1 | Egawa | Kyoto, Japan | 1997 | 150 | 150 | | 1 | 151 | 8 (5.3%) | 2 (25%) | 6 (75%) |
| 2 | de Villa | Kaohsiung, Taiwan | 2000 | 38 | 37 | 1 | | 38 | 4 (10.5%) | 2 (50%) | 2 (50%) |
| 3 | Bak | Denver, USA | 2001 | 41 | | 41 | 41 | | 2 (4.9%) | — | — |
| 4 | Marcos | Rochester, USA | 2001 | 48 | | 48 | 48 | | 2 (4.2%) | 2 (100%) | — |
| 5 | Nakamura | Kyoto, Japan | 2002 | 120 | | 120 | 120 | | 1 (0.8%) | — | — |
| 6 | Buell | Chicago, USA | 2002 | 118 | 118 | | | 118 | 2 (1.7%) | — | — |
| 7 | Ko | Soul, Korea | 2002 | 313 | — | — | — | — | 27 (8.6%) | NA | 27 (100%) |
| 8 | Kinkhabwala | NYPH, USA | 2003 | 48 | | 48 | 48 | | 1 (2.0%) | — | 1 (100%) |
| 9 | Akamatsu | Tokyo, Japan | 2004 | 223 | 70 | 153 | 88 | 135 | 5 (2.2%) | 3 (60%) | 2 (40%) |
| 10 | Tannuri | Sao Paulo, Brazil | 2005 | 54 | 54 | | | 54 | 5 (9.3%) | — | 5 (100%) |
| Total | | | | 1151 | 429 | 411 | 346 | 496 | 57 (5.0%) | | |

NYPH: New York Presbyterian Hospital

HVOB: hepatic venous outflow block

IVR: interventional radiology

*Rt includes right lobe and right lateral sector grafts

#Lt includes left lobe, extended left lobe, and left lateral segment grafts

HVOB is occasionally diagnosed during transplant surgery on the basis of swelling and congestion of the graft.[37,73] The diagnosis is confirmed if intraoperative ultrasonography detects a flat waveform in the hepatic vein.[79] HVOB detected intraoperatively can usually be relieved by keeping the graft in its original position.[71] The Kyoto group employed a tissue expander in the right subphrenic fossa for this purpose.[80] Acute graft dysfunction early posttransplant may be a sign of HVOB secondary to graft dislocation. Immediate exploration to reposition the graft is necessary.[37,71] Postoperatively, the clinical presentation of HVOB can include ascites, elevated liver function test results, splenomegaly, variceal bleeding, lower-extremity edema, and kidney dysfunction.[71,74] A persistent monophasic wave pattern from the hepatic vein on Doppler ultrasonography suggests substantial stenosis.[81,82] Subsequent angiography with direct contrast can confirm the diagnosis; the pressure gradient across the stenosis is typically > 3 to 10 mm Hg.[75] In severe cases, HVOB may cause graft dysfunction or failure, requiring a retransplant.[32,37]

To prevent HVOB, wide-open anastomosis of the hepatic vein is advocated by many transplant centers. In right-lobe grafts, the right hepatic vein is enlarged by making a caudal extension to the IVC to create an oval or elliptical orifice larger than the donor hepatic vein.[32,34,73,76] In left-lobe or left lateral segment grafts, the anastomotic orifices are enlarged by extending the confluence with the middle hepatic vein and left hepatic vein in a right caudal direction onto the IVC,[71] by making a triangular orifice by dividing the bridge of tissue between the 3 hepatic veins with an anterior longitudinal extension caudally,[69,74,78] or by performing venoplasty in the recipient with the middle or left (or the right) hepatic vein.[83,84] Venoplasty in the donor has been performed to obtain a wide-open outflow orifice between the right and the middle hepatic vein in extended right-lobe grafts,[85] or between the middle and left hepatic vein in left-lobe grafts if those two veins are separated.[72] Some centers prefer enlarging the hepatic vein orifice in the donor with a longitudinal incision onto the posterior surface of the vein.[69,74]

Except in the surgical case of acute HVOB early posttransplant, the first-line treatment is angioplasty. Reported success rates of balloon angioplasty and stent placement range from 40% to 100%.[34,71–78] Especially in pediatric recipients, balloon angioplasty is preferred as an initial treatment, because stents can cause stenosis as children grow.[75] In several series, 17% to 80% of pediatric recippients with HVOB eventually required stent placement or surgical repair.[71,75,78] Recent developments in the surgical evolution of hepatic vein anastomosis and in the early diagnosis and treatment of HVOB have reduced the rates of graft failure and death to minimal levels.

### Outflow Block of Middle Hepatic Vein Tributaries

In right-lobe LD recipients, the management of middle hepatic vein tributaries is extremely controversial.[86–88] Transplantation of the right lobe with the middle hepatic vein ensures adequate venous drainage of the graft.[86] Conversely, transplantation without the middle hepatic vein can cause congestion of the right anterior sector (Couinaud segments 5 and 8)— leading to poor regeneration in the right anterior sector, as compared with the posterior lateral sector,[89,90] or, in extreme cases, to fatal graft dysfunction.[91] Inclusion of the middle hepatic vein with the graft, however, can lead to congestion of Couinaud segment 4 in the donor,[86] increasing the donor's risk for impaired regeneration in Couinaud segment 4.[92]

For safety reasons, when the right lobe is taken without the middle hepatic vein, large tributaries that drain the right anterior sector are commonly reconstructed.[76,91,93] Still unresolved, however, is the question of whether reconstruction of these tributaries is always necessary when a right-lobe graft does not include the middle hepatic vein. Sano et al. recommend venous reconstruction if the venocongestive area, as assessed by temporary arterial occlusion and intraoperative Doppler ultrasonography, is so large that the graft volume outside this area is insufficient to meet postoperative metabolic demands. Given the importance of optimal venous drainage, reconstruction of tributaries greater than 5 mm is recommended by most centers.[76,91,93] No center, however, has verified that routine reconstruction of tributaries greater than 5 mm is necessary.

Preoperative 3-dimentional computed tomographic (CT) studies in which the images are reconstructed by perspective volume-rendering software can provide information on the donor's liver volume and hepatic vascular anatomy.[94–96] This type of software delineates not only the number and size of tributaries but also the area and volume drained by them. This technique can allow a surgeon to plan preoperatively for reconstruction of tributaries. Tributaries should be reconstructed in the recipient if the volume of the right-lobe graft without the area drained by the tributaries is less than a graft volume/recipient standard volume (GV/SV) ratio of 40%.[95,96]

When reconstruction of the tributaries is indicated, the great saphenous vein, external iliac vein, ovarian vein, umbilical vein, inferior mesenteric vein, and portal vein have been used as autologous interposition grafts.[97] Though easily available, these vessels are often of inadequate caliber and length. Cryopreserved grafts have been used for venous reconstruction, but experience with them in liver transplants is limited. High complication rates have been reported in association with cryopreserved grafts (eg, vascular stenosis or thrombosis),[64,98] yet recent series from Tokyo have shown no complications using cryopreserved veins for reconstruction.[99,100]

Adverse events after reconstruction of middle hepatic vein tributaries include occlusion or stenosis of the interposition grafts secondary to vessel size mismatching, kinking of the grafts due to a long course, or venous twisting or compression from displacement of the regenerated liver graft. With interposition grafts, 1 to 2 weeks of patency is sufficient for development of collaterals and good graft function.[87] Complications that occur within the first 2 weeks can cause life-threatening deterioration of liver function. Early diagnosis and treatment is therefore essential. To treat interposition graft stenosis or occlusion, Shin et al. advocate primary stent placement instead of balloon angioplasty, because angioplasty can disrupt the anastomosis, cannot treat kinking of the redundant interposition grafts or extrinsic compression, and can require repeated interventional treatment.[101] In the series by Shin et al., the immediate technical and clinical success rates were quite high: 91% (technical) and 82% (clinical).

## BILIARY COMPLICATIONS

Biliary complications remain the most common cause of postoperative morbidity and among the most challenging complications in LD liver recipients, significantly affecting quality of life and occasionally causing graft loss and death. The incidence of biliary complications has decreased over time in DD recipients; still, the current rate of biliary complications in LD recipients is almost comparable to the incidence in the early era of DD liver transplants.

### Evolution of Biliary Reconstruction

In DD recipients, the most widely used techniques for biliary reconstruction are duct-to-duct anastomosis and choledochojejunostomy

to a Roux-en-Y limb. In adults, in the absence of contraindications, duct-to-duct anastomosis is preferred if the recipient bile duct is available, because it is less time-consuming, preserves the sphincter of Oddi, permits observation of the quality and quantity of the bile, allows easy access for cholangiography, and promises less lethal biliary complications. Currently, with either technique, the incidence of complications is less than 10%.

In the late 1980s, LD liver transplants were initiated with the left lateral segment, in order to save children who were dying on the DD waiting list. The Roux-en-Y reconstruction was the gold standard. Since the mid-1990s, LD liver transplants have been offered to adults, for whom a right hemiliver is generally a preferable choice. Initially, the hepaticojejunostomy was employed for biliary reconstruction in most adults[102–104]; Since the late 1990s, duct-to-duct anastomosis has been used, with the hope of achieving benefits similar to those obtained in DD liver transplants. The first adult LD experience with duct-to-duct anastomosis portended a difficult future; however, that recipient developed an anastomotic stricture 4 weeks later and subsequently required conversion to a hepaticojejunostomy.[32]

### Incidence and Risk Factors

#### Pediatric Recipients

In each of two early pediatric LD series, the biliary complication rate was 38%.[105,106] In more recent experience, the biliary complication rate has ranged from 4.6% to 34%[107–111] (Table 30.8-5)—comparable to that for split-liver transplants (5.7% to 25.5%),[105,111–113] but higher than that for whole-organ liver transplants (2.3%-14%).[108,114,115]

Risk factors for biliary complications in children are summarized in Table 30.8-5.[109,116]

#### Adult Recipients

The incidence of biliary complications in adult LD liver recipients is 14% to 46%[32,34,117–125]—significantly higher than that for adult DD liver recipients (9% to 15%)[114,126–128] (Table 30.8-6). Most centers use right hemilivers with duct-to-duct anastomoses, but some Asian centers use the left hemiliver. Of 836 LD recipients in 11 centers (Table 30.8-6), the incidence of biliary leaks (4.2% to 32.0%; mean, 16.0%) and biliary strictures (7.3% to 26.0%; mean, 15.7%) were similar. About 50% of those biliary leaks arose from the cut surface.

Risk factors for biliary complications in adult LD recipients are summarized in Table 30.8-7. HAT,[126] cytomegalovirus (CMV) infection,[129] and rejection—once major risk factors for biliary complications in DD recipients—are not significant risk factors in LD recipients, but this finding may be due to the relatively small population of LD recipients studied.[34,119, 122,123,125]

**TABLE 30.8-5**

## BILIARY COMPLICATIONS IN PEDIATRIC LDLT

| No | Author | Place | Year | LDLT | Biliary Complications | Leak | Stricture |
|----|--------|-------|------|------|-----------------------|------|-----------|
| 1 | Reichert | UCSF, USA | 1998 | 32 | 8 (25%) | 6 (19%) | 2 (6%) |
| 2 | Reding | Brussels, Belgium | 1999 | 41 | 14 (34%) | 10 (24%) | 3 (7%) |
| 3 | Egawa | Kyoto, Japan | 2001 | 391 | 71 (18%) | 45 (12%) | 35 (9%) |
| 4 | Kling | John Hopkins, USA | 2004 | 48 | 16 (33%) | 10 (20%) | 8 (17%) |
| 5 | Broering | Hamburg, Germany | 2004 | 44 | 2 (4.6%) | — | — |
| Total | | | | 556 | 111 (20.0%) | | |

**TABLE 30.8-6**
## BILIARY COMPLICATION IN ADULT LDLT

| No | Author | Center | Year | LDLT | Right Lobe | DD | Biliary Complications | Leak | Stricture |
|----|--------|--------|------|------|------------|-----|----------------------|------|-----------|
| 1 | Bak | Denver, USA | 2001 | 41 | all | 13 (32%) | 14 (34%) | 12 (29%) | 3 (7%) |
| 2 | Nakamura | Kyoto, Japan | 2002 | 52 | all | all | 17 (33%) | 5 (10%) | 12 (23%) |
| 3 | Settmacher | Berlin, Germany | 2003 | 50 | all | 38 (76%) | 7 (14%) | 5 (10%) | 2 (4%) |
| 4 | Soejima | Fukuoka, Japan | 2003 | 46 | all left lobe | 7 (15%) | 21 (46%) | 9 (20%) | 12 (26%) |
| 5 | Icoz | Izmir, Turkey | 2003 | 50 | all | 36 (72%) | 15 (30%) | 7 (14%) | 8 (16%) |
| 6 | Malago | Essen, Germany | 2003 | 74 | all | NA | 17 (30%) | 12 (16%) | 5 (7%) |
| 7 | Sugawara | Tokyo, Japan | 2003 | 92 | 59% | all | 28 (30%) | 11 (12%) | 9 (10%) |
| 8 | Liu | Hong Kong, China | 2004 | 41 | all | all | 10 (24%) | 3 (7%) | 10 (24%) |
| 9 | Gondoleski | Mount Sinai, USA | 2004 | 96 | all | 39 (41%) | 39 (41%) | 21 (22%) | 22 (23%) |
| 10 | Maluf | Richmond, USA | 2005 | 69 | all | NA | 18 (26%) | NA | NA |
| 11 | Hwang | Seoul, Korea | 2006 | 259 | 87% | 160 (62%) | 54 (21%) | 12 (4%) | 42 (16%) |
| Total | | | | 836 | | | 329 (30%) | 97 (14%) | 125 (16%) |

**TABLE 30.8-7**
## RISK FACTORS FOR BILIARY COMPLICATIONS IN LDLT

**Pediatrics**
   All biliary complications
      hepatic artery thrombosis, intrapulmonary shunt, CMV disease
   Bile leak;
      stent usage, intrapulmonary shunt, female gender
   Biliary stricture
      anastomotic leak, CMV disease, HAT, female gender

**Adults**
   All biliary complications
      right lobe graft, small bile duct < 4 mm, multiple bile ducts, MELD>35
   Biliary stricture
      internal stent or no stent, hepatico-jejunostomy

## Prevention of Biliary Complications in LD Recipients

### Anatomic Considerations

Constructing of perfect biliary anastomosis requires an understanding of the biliary and vascular anatomy in both the donor and recipient. The arterial flow to the supraduodenal duct is mainly supplied by the axial periductal arteries from above (38%) and below (60%).[130] The downward supply originates from the right hepatic, cystic, and left hepatic arteries, but the upward arterial supply originates from the posterior–superior pancreaticoduodenal, retroportal, and gastroduodenal arteries. The remaining 2% flows transversally from the proper hepatic artery. A fine arterial plexus is formed by the axial periductal arteries at the hepatic hilum and nourishes the common bile duct.[131] The axial periductal arteries nourish the confluence and both hepatic ducts via the hilar plexus at the inferior aspect of the hilar plate. Thus, interruption of blood supply to the hilar plate during donor hepatectomy and to the supraduodenal segment during recipient hepatectomy should be avoided.[123,132,133] In other words, the dissection between hilar plates and hepatic arteries must be minimal in both the donor and the recipient. Injury to the duct blood supply may lead to bile duct ischemia, resulting in anastomotic leaks, stricture, or even necrosis of the bile duct.

Anatomic variations in the vascular supply may contribute to biliary complications. In two LD recipients, for example, when the donor's left hepatic artery provided a significant portion of the blood supply to the right duct, they developed bile leaks secondary to ischemia of the bile duct.[123]

### Technical Considerations

For successful biliary reconstruction, especially with duct-to-duct anastomosis, it is imperative to preserve the arterial supply to the bile duct with careful and meticulous dissection in both the donor and the recipient operations. In the donor, to preserve the blood supply to the right hepatic duct, dissection should be avoided between the right hepatic artery and the right hepatic duct. The division of the right hepatic duct should be precisely localized by intraoperative cholangiography to avoid two or three duct openings. The hepatic parenchyma overlying the right hepatic duct should be preserved, to preserve the blood supply and venous drainage.[133]

In the recipient, to produce a tension-free, well-vascularized anastomosis, the common hepatic duct and right hepatic artery should be divided as close as possible to the parenchyma of the liver. Both structures should then be mobilized caudad as a single unit. Preserving the gastroduodenal artery is equally important, to supply the supraduodenal portion of the bile duct.[132] Recently, the intrahepatic Glissonian approach (ie, high hilar dissection), during the recipient hepatectomy has been proposed.[134] With this approach, the hepatoduodenal ligament is totally occluded. The Glissonian pedicles are divided at the third level of pedicles or beyond, allowing unused bile duct for anastomosis, tension-free duct-to-duct anastomosis, and preservation of good arterial flow.

Preservation solution may be an etiologic factor in biliary complications secondary to bile duct ischemia. According to this theory, the relatively high viscosity of University of Wisconsin solution may result in relatively poor flushing of the periductal capillary system, causing biliary complications.[135,136]

## Management of Biliary Complications

### Bile Leaks

Bile leaks may originate from the anastomosis, the cut surface, or the exit site of a T tube (or other types of external stents). Virtually all bile leaks are technical. Anastomotic leaks are caused either by ischemic necrosis of the end of the bile duct or by a technically unsatisfactory anastomosis. Leaks can manifest as sudden onset of biliary drainage from the abdominal drain, or they may be diagnosed by routine T-tube cholangiography. Biloma can be detected by ultrasonography or CT scan before the recipient becomes symptomatic. Biloma formation is the usual consequence of a biliary leak in the absence of abdominal drains. The enlarged or infected biloma causes fever, nausea, vomiting, abdominal discomfort or pain, and sometimes an elevation of canalicular enzymes (ALP or GGTP).

Bile leaks from any source may be serious, but those from the anastomosis are the most hazardous. Leaks from the cut surface or T tube can usually be managed by percutaneous drainage, with or without endoscopic retrograde biliary drainage (ERBD) or sphincterotomy.[137–139] Accumulated experience demonstrates that, in most recipients, nonsurgical care is effective, especially for leaks related to T tubes. Evidence of infection in bilomas requires antibiotic therapy in addition to drainage. Leaks from the anastomosis also can be successfully managed with nonsurgical treatment if they are small and localized. Stenting with percutaneous transhepatic cholangiography (PTC) or endoscopic retrograde cholangiopancreatography (ERCP) at the anastomotic site can resolve minor leaks. If the anastomosis is seriously disrupted, however, surgical revision is the safest approach. A retransplant may be required.

### Biliary Strictures

Early strictures (ie, during the first several posttransplant months) are usually at an anastomotic site, secondary to local ischemia at the anastomosis or to a suturing technique that produced excessive narrowing. Strictures can present with cholestasis with elevated liver function test results, especially elevated canalicular enzyme levels. An episode of cholangitis may occur. Direct contrast study by T-tube cholangiogram, PTC, or ERC is required to confirm the diagnosis. Early strictures are often amenable to endoscopic or transhepatic intervention with good long-term results.[137–139] Stricture recurrence is preventable if the initial or second dilatation procedure is followed by stent placement for several months. Even longer term (up to 1 year) stenting by ERC may be possible if the stents are kept inside the bile duct without sphincterotomy.[138] This method also allows multiple stenting for the multiple strictures, which often occur in LD recipients.

Late strictures are more likely to be complex. Causes of late strictures include hepatic artery complications, preservation injury, rejection, and recurrent disease. Care is largely influenced by the nature and extent of strictures. Surgical revision or a retransplant may be required for definitive treatment. Nonsurgical management of more complex hilar and intrahepatic strictures is less successful.

## IMMUNOLOGIC COMPLICATIONS

### Acute Cellular Rejection

Despite advances in immunosuppressive therapy for DD recipients, acute cellular rejection (ACR) continues to occur, particularly during the first 6 weeks posttransplant, with rates of 50% to 70% during the first year in recipients on double therapy (a calcineurin inhibitor and steroids) and 30% to 40% when mycophenolate mofetil is added.[140–143] Recipient risk factors for ACR appear to be older age, greater severity of illness (as measured by pretransplant liver and kidney function), and certain causes of the underlying liver disease (in particular, autoimmune liver diseases). Donor risk factors include HLA (DR) mismatches, sex mismatches, older donor age, and preservation injury of the graft.[142,144–146] Although ACR can usually be treated, the enhanced levels of immunosuppression may predispose to infection, recurrent hepatitis C, and malignancy.

### Pediatric LD Recipients

LD transplants conceivably confer an immunologic advantage against rejection when the donor and recipient are genetically related with a better quality graft and shorter preservation time. Kidney transplant recipients with a living related donor have survival and immunologic advantages over DD recipients.[147,148] However, the incidence and degree of rejection in liver (vs kidney) transplant recipients with a living related donor appear to be quite different, especially in children.

Comparative studies between LD and DD in pediatric recipients have shown an incidence of ACR ranging from 29% to 74% (LD) and 24% to 78% (DD)[108,149–153] (Table 30.8-8). In one series of several hundred pediatric LD recipients, the incidence was 36%.[154] Evidence suggests that LD recipients are less likely than DD recipients to develop steroid-resistant or chronic rejection.

**TABLE 30.8-8**

## ACUTE CELLULAR REJECTION IN PEDIATRIC AND ADULT LDLT

| | Author | Place | Year | Cases | | ACR | | | Steroid Resistant ACR | | |
|---|---|---|---|---|---|---|---|---|---|---|---|
| | | | | DDLT | LDLT | DDLT | LDLT | P | DDLT | LDLT | P |
| Pediatric | | | | | | | | | | | |
| 1 | Katz | Houston, USA | 1994 | 30 | 9 | 53% | 56% | NS | 25% | 20% | NS |
| 2 | Alonso | Chicago, USA | 1996 | 54 | 38 | 78% | 74% | NS | 43% | 13% | <0.01 |
| 3 | Drews | Hamburg, Germany | 1997 | 49 | 51 | 64% | 72% | NA | 24% | 20% | NA |
| 4 | Reding | Brussels, Belgium | 1999 | 68 | 42 | 24% | 29% | NS | — | — | |
| 5 | Eid | Lyon, France | 2000 | 29 | 11 | 41% | 54% | NS | — | — | |
| 6 | Toyoki | San Francisco, USA | 2002 | 51 | 37 | 78% | 68% | NS | 22% | 8% | NS |
| Adult | | | | | | | | | | | |
| 1 | Maluf | Richmond, USA | 2004 | 202 | 69 | 24% | 12% | 0.03 | — | — | |
| 2 | Liu | Mount Sinai, USA | 2005 | 64 | 64 | 73% | 32% | sig | 58% | 55% | |

ACR: acute cellular rejection

sig: significant

For example, Alsono et al. reported that the overall incidence of rejection in their pediatric living related and DD groups was similar, but that the rates of steroid-resistant rejection and chronic rejection were significantly lower in the living related group.[150] Toyoki et al also found that overall rejection rates were similar between pediatric LD and DD groups; in their study, however, late rejection episodes (greater than 1 year posttransplant) developed in 22% of DD recipients, but in none of the LD recipients).[153]

Since most LDs for pediatric recipients are parents, they are generally a 1-haplotype major histocompatibility match and should therefore confer a definite immunologic advantage. Why then do the data seem to suggest that pediatric LD liver recipients have less of an immunologic advantage than LD kidney recipients? A part of the answer might be the use of protocol liver biopsies. Although the diagnosis of ACR is usually made by liver biopsy when clinically indicated, some centers use protocol liver biopsies. In the first few weeks after liver transplant, protocol liver biopsies sometimes display histologic features of ACR, even in the absence of significant biochemical dysfunction. Barlett et al reviewed 1,566 recipients who underwent protocol liver biopsies: 1,048 (67%) had histologic evidence of ACR, but 331 (32%) had no associated biochemical graft dysfunction.[155] Without treatment, only 14% of those 331 recipients subsequently developed biochemical graft dysfunction requiring adjuvant immunosuppression.

Further investigation is necessary to determine why pediatric living related liver transplants do not confer an immunologic advantage, as compared with pediatric DD liver transplants. The answers may hold the key to other as-yet-unsolved mysteries, such as why and how tolerance to liver grafts is acquired. In studies by Kamada et al.,[156,157] rats that acquired tolerance after liver transplants had mononuclear cell infiltrates in the portal area similar to that seen in ACR. Thus, if protocol biopsies show mononuclear cell infiltrates without clinical or biochemical manifestations, they might be related to tolerance rather than rejection.

### Adult LD Recipients

The reported incidence of ACR for adult LD liver recipients ranges from 12% to 32%, considerably less than the 24% to 73% reported for adult DD recipients[124,158] (Table 30.8-8). Liu et al. matched 64 adult LD recipients with 64 DD recipients and analyzed the occurrence of ACR.[158] Interestingly, ACR rates in LD recipients and their DD matches did not differ significantly when the LDs were unrelated, but did differ for the nonsibling but related (p = 0.03) and the sibling (p = 0.03) LD subgroups. The results were similar when comparing rates of high-degree ACR for unrelated, for nonsibling but related, and for sibling pairs. Liu et al. concluded that the decreased rate of ACR for related LD recipients (vs unrelated LD or matched DD recipients) appears to have a genetic basis, as ACR rates are lower in recipient–donor pairs with increasing genetic similarity. Although theirs was a retrospective study, it nevertheless suggests the possibility of an immunologic advantage in related LD transplants.

### Human Leucocyte Antigen (HLA) Matching

The precise roles of HLA matching and lymphocytotoxic crossmatching in liver transplants are still controversial. Studies of HLA matching in DD recipients have produced contradictory results that do not justify its clinical use.[159–163] In contrast, the detrimental effects of positive lymphocytotoxic crossmatching on graft survival or on the incidence of rejection have been well described.[161,162,164–167] In the vast majority of recipients, liver transplants across a positive T-cell-

lymphocytotoxic crossmatch do not result in hyperacute rejection, yet events compatible with a diagnosis of hyperacute rejection have been reported. In DD recipients, time constraints make it impractical to select suitable donor–recipient combinations according to the results of HLA matching or lymphocytotoxic crossmatching. In LD recipients, however, the role of HLA matching and lymphocytotoxic crossmatching deserves further study.

Even in LD recipients, data on the role of HLA matching in preventing or reducing rejection are conflicting. In pediatric LD recipients, one center found that grafts from HLA-A 0-mismatch donors might be advantageous for reducing early acute rejection,[168] but another center was unable to show any beneficial effect of HLA matching.[169] Takekura et al reported that pretransplant positive T-cell flow cytometry crossmatching was closely related to ACR and to refractory ACR in a predominantly pediatric population.[170]

In adult LD recipients, a graft from an HLA-DR 0-mismatch or negative T-lymphocytotoxic crossmatch might be advantageous for decreasing episodes of acute rejection, although it would not affect patient and graft outcomes.[171] As previously reported in DD recipients, the graft failure rates were higher with positive crossmatching; such recipients might therefore require stronger immunosuppression.[172]

### Chronic Rejection

Chronic rejection of liver grafts is characterized by the histologic findings of ductopenia and a decreased number of arteries in portal tracts in the presence of obliterative arteriopathy. It still a significant cause of late graft dysfunction and failure.[173,174] In DD recipients, the incidence of chronic rejection at 5 years posttransplant has steadily decreased from 15% to 20% in the 1980s to a current expected incidence of 3% to 5%.[173–176] This decrease is likely attributable to the unique immunologic properties of liver allografts and to better recognition and control of acute rejection and of the early phase of chronic rejection with tacrolimus.[177,178] Tacrolimus-based immunosuppression has permitted the avoidance of chronic rejection in pediatric recipients.

As discussed in the section on ACR, adult-related LD recipients are thought to have an immunologic advantage. Experience with LD (vs DD) kidney recipients has shown a reduced incidence of chronic rejection, a lower frequency of graft loss, and a survival advantage.[179–181] A comparative pediatric study showed a significantly lower chronic rejection rate in related LD (vs DD) recipients: 4% (vs 16%).[182] Similar trends were seen in two other studies.[150–152] Not much information is available on chronic rejection in adult LD recipients, but the rate seems to be 1.0% to 2.0%,[154] similar to that for DD recipients.[124]

Risk factors for chronic rejection include a higher number and greater severity of acute rejection episodes,[146,183–185] younger recipient age,[183,186] older donor age (> 40 years),[186], a male-to-female sex mismatch[146], a primary diagnosis of autoimmune hepatitis or biliary disease,[186] baseline immunosuppression,[141,146] and nonwhite recipient race.[183,187] The role of histocompatibility differences is still controversial,[183] as is the effect of cytomegalovirus infection.[142,146,183,188,189] Similar risk factors have been identified in a large series of pediatric LD recipients.[182]

### Graft-Versus-Host Disease (GVHD)

Graft-versus-host disease (GVHD) after liver transplants is an uncommon but devastating complication. GVHD results from the engraftment of T lymphocytes associated with the graft. It is characterized by fever, skin rash, diarrhea, or pancytopenia, usually occurring 2 to 6 weeks posttransplant. The incidence of GVHD after liver transplants is 1% to 2%.[190,191] Its symptoms may initially be difficult to differentiate from CMV infection or drug-induced skin rash and pancytopenia. The diagnosis is confirmed by demonstrating large numbers of donor lymphocytes in the recipient's tissue or circulation. Treatment has consisted of either increasing or withdrawing immunosuppression. Either course is often ineffective, and the mortality rate is greater than 75%.[190,192,193] Death is due to infection, bleeding, or severe metabolic disorders resulting from desquamation and severe diarrhea.

Use of HLA homozygous donors leading to one-way HLA matching has been shown to significantly increase the risk of GVHD after LD transplants.[194] Recently, fatal GVHD occurred in 8 LD recipients in Japan after donor-dominant one-way HLA matching in the three loci of HLA-A, -B, and –DR (per either serologic or DNA typing).[195-197] Those LDs were a son (n = 4), a mother (n = 3), and a sister (n = 1). All recipients, at 14 to 114 days (median, 40 days) posttransplant, had a skin rash, with or without fever. They died at a median of 130 days posttransplant (range, 36 to 540 days) with a Gluckberg clinical grade of 3 to 4. In contrast, no GVHD occurred after donor-dominant one-way HLA matching in two loci or or locus. Thus, donor-dominant one-way HLA matching in the three loci appears to be a significant risk factor for fatal GVHD in LD recipients.

## References

1. Stange BJ, Glanemann M, Nuessler NC, et al. Hepatic artery thrombosis after adult liver transplantation. *Liver Transpl* 2003;9(6):612–620.
2. Tzakis AG, Gordon RD, Shaw BW Jr, et al. Clinical presentation of hepatic artery thrombosis after liver transplantation in the cyclosporine era. *Transplantation* 1985;40(6):667–671.
3. Wozney P, Zajko AB, Bron KM, et al. Vascular complications after liver transplantation: a 5-year experience. *AJR Am J Roentgenol* 1986;147(4):657–663.
4. Stevens LH, Emond JC, Piper JB, et al. Hepatic artery thrombosis in infants. A comparison of whole livers, reduced-size grafts, and grafts from living-related donors. *Transplantation* 1992;53(2):396–399.
5. Oh CK, Pelletier SJ, Sawyer RG, et al. Uni- and multi-variate analysis of risk factors for early and late hepatic artery thrombosis after liver transplantation. Transplantation 2001;71(6):767–772.
6. Silva MA, Jambulingam PS, Gunson BK, et al. Hepatic artery thrombosis following orthotopic liver transplantation: a 10-year experience from a single centre in the United Kingdom. *Liver Transpl* 2006;12(1):146–151.
7. Vivarelli M, Cucchetti A, La Barba G, et al. Ischemic arterial complications after liver transplantation in the adult: multivariate analysis of risk factors. Arch Surg 2004; 139(10):1069–1074.
8. Valente JF, Alonso MH, Weber FL, Hanto DW. Late hepatic artery thrombosis in liver allograft recipients is associated with intrahepatic biliary necrosis. *Transplantation* 1996;61(1):61–65.
9. Parera A, Salcedo M, Vaquero J, et al. [Arterial complications after liver transplantation: early and late forms]. *Gastroenterol Hepatol* 1999;22(8):381–385.
10. Drazan K, Shaked A, Olthoff KM, et al. Etiology and management of symptomatic adult hepatic artery thrombosis after orthotopic liver transplantation (OLT). Am Surg 1996;62(3):237–240.
11. Rabkin JM, Orloff SL, Corless CL, et al. Hepatic allograft abscess with hepatic arterial thrombosis. Am J Surg 1998;175(5):354–359.
12. Hidalgo E, Cantarell C, Charco R, et al. Risk factors for late hepatic artery thrombosis in adult liver transplantation. *Transplant Proc* 1999;31(6):2416–2467.
13. Gunsar F, Rolando N, Pastacaldi S, et al. Late hepatic artery thrombosis after orthotopic liver transplantation. *Liver Transpl* 2003;9(6):605–611.
14. Segel MC, Zajko AB, Bowen A, et al. Hepatic artery thrombosis after liver transplantation: radiologic evaluation. *AJR Am J Roentgenol* 1986;146(1):137–141.
15. Wellings RM, Olliff SP, Olliff JF, et al. Duplex Doppler detection of hepatic artery thrombosis following liver transplantation. *Clin Radiol* 1993;47(3):180–182.
16. Zajko AB, Bron KM, Starzl TE, et al. Angiography of liver transplantation patients. *Radiology* 1985;157(2):305–311.
17. Kwon KH, Kim YW, Kim SI, et al. Postoperative liver regeneration and complication in live liver donor after partial hepatectomy for living donor liver transplantation. *Yonsei Med J* 2003;44(6):1069–1077.
18. Pinna AD, Smith CV, Furukawa H, et al. Urgent revascularization of liver allografts after early hepatic artery thrombosis. *Transplantation* 1996;62(11):1584–1157.
19. Sheiner PA, Varma CV, Guarrera JV, et al. Selective revascularization of hepatic artery thromboses after liver transplantation improves patient and graft survival. *Transplantation* 1997;64(9):1295–1299.
20. Tan KC, Yandza T, de Hemptinne B, et al. Hepatic artery thrombosis in pediatric liver transplantation. *J Pediatr Surg* 1988;23(10):927–930.
21. Todo S, Makowka L, Tzakis AG, et al. Hepatic artery in liver transplantation. *Transplant Proc* 1987; 19(1 Pt 3):2406–2411.
22. Pungpapong S, Manzarbeitia C, Ortiz J, et al. Cigarette smoking is associated with an increased incidence of vascular complications after liver transplantation. *Liver Transpl* 2002;8(7):582–587.
23. Madalosso C, de Souza NF, Jr., Ilstrup DM, et al. Cytomegalovirus and its association with hepatic artery thrombosis after liver transplantation. *Transplantation* 1998;66(3):294–297.
24. Mazzaferro V, Esquivel CO, Makowka L, et al. Hepatic artery thrombosis after pediatric liver transplantation--a medical or surgical event? *Transplantation* 1989;47(6):971–977.
25. Todo S, Nery J, Yanaga K, et al. Extended preservation of human liver grafts with UW solution. *JAMA* 1989;261(5):711–714.
26. Sieders E, Peeters PM, TenVergert EM, et al. Early vascular complications after pediatric liver transplantation. *Liver Transpl* 2000;6(3):326–332.
27. Abbasoglu O, Levy MF, Testa G, et al. Does intraoperative hepatic artery flow predict arterial complications after liver transplantation? *Transplantation* 1998;66(5):598–601.
28. Jurim O, Shackleton CR, McDiarmid SV, et al. Living-donor liver transplantation at UCLA. *Am J Surg* 1995;169(5):529–532.
29. Otte JB, de Ville de Goyet J, Reding R, et al. Living related donor liver transplantation in children: the Brussels experience. *Transplant Proc* 1996; 28(4):2378–2379.
30. Hatano E, Terajima H, Yabe S, et al. Hepatic artery thrombosis in living related liver transplantation. *Transplantation* 1997;64(10):1443–1446.
31. Miller CM, Gondolesi GE, Florman S, et al. One hundred nine living donor liver transplants in adults and children: a single-center experience. *Ann Surg* 2001;234(3):301-311; discussion 311–312.
32. Bak T, Wachs M, Trotter J, et al. Adult-to-adult living donor liver transplantation using right-lobe grafts: results and lessons learned from a single-center experience. *Liver Transpl* 2001;7(8):680–686.
33. Lee SG, Park KM, Lee YJ, et al. 157 adult-to-adult living donor liver transplantation. *Transplant Proc* 2001;33(1–2):1323–1325.
34. Nakamura T, Tanaka K, Kiuchi T, et al. Anatomical variations and surgical strategies in right lobe living donor liver transplantation: lessons from 120 cases. *Transplantation* 2002;73(12):1896–1903.
35. Sugawara Y, Makuuchi M, Kaneko J, et al. Living-donor liver transplantation in adults: Tokyo University experience. *J Hepatobiliary Pancreat Surg* 2003;10(1):1–4.
36. Uchiyama H, Hashimoto K, Hiroshige S, et al. Hepatic artery reconstruction in living-donor liver transplantation: a review of its techniques and complications. *Surgery* 2002;131(1 Suppl):S200–S204.
37. Malago M, Testa G, Frilling A, et al. Right living donor liver transplantation: an option for adult patients: single institution experience with 74 patients. *Ann Surg* 2003;238(6):853–62; discussion 862–863.
38. Kaneko J, Sugawara Y, Akamatsu N, et al. Prediction of hepatic artery thrombosis by protocol Doppler ultrasonography in pediatric living donor liver transplantation. *Abdom Imaging* 2004;29(5):603–605.

39. Wei WI, Lam LK, Ng RW, et al. Microvascular reconstruction of the hepatic artery in live donor liver transplantation: experience across a decade. *Arch Surg* 2004;139(3):304–307.

40. Mori K, Nagata I, Yamagata S, et al. The introduction of microvascular surgery to hepatic artery reconstruction in living-donor liver transplantation—its surgical advantages compared with conventional procedures. *Transplantation* 1992;54(2):263–268.

41. Flint EW, Sumkin JH, Zajko AB, Bowen A. Duplex sonography of hepatic artery thrombosis after liver transplantation. *AJR Am J Roentgenol* 1988;151(3):481–483.

42. De Gaetano AM, Cotroneo AR, Maresca G, et al. Color Doppler sonography in the diagnosis and monitoring of arterial complications after liver transplantation. *J Clin Ultrasound* 2000;28(8):373–380.

43. Maceneaney PM, Malone DE, Skehan SJ, et al. The role of hepatic arterial Doppler ultrasound after liver transplantation: an 'audit cycle' evaluation. *Clin Radiol* 2000;55(7):517–524.

44. Nishida S, Kato T, Levi D, et al. Effect of protocol Doppler ultrasonography and urgent revascularization on early hepatic artery thrombosis after pediatric liver transplantation. *Arch Surg* 2002;137(11):1279–1283.

45. Saad WE, Davies MG, Sahler L, et al. Hepatic artery stenosis in liver transplant recipients: primary treatment with percutaneous transluminal angioplasty. *J Vasc Interv Radiol* 2005;16(6):795–805.

46. Mondragon RS, Karani JB, Heaton ND, et al. The use of percutaneous transluminal angioplasty in hepatic artery stenosis after transplantation. *Transplantation* 1994; 57(2):228–231.

47. Abbasoglu O, Levy MF, Vodapally MS, et al. Hepatic artery stenosis after liver transplantation--incidence, presentation, treatment, and long term outcome. *Transplantation* 1997; 63(2):250–255.

48. Denys AL, Qanadli SD, Durand F, et al. Feasibility and effectiveness of using coronary stents in the treatment of hepatic artery stenoses after orthotopic liver transplantation: preliminary report. *AJR Am J Roentgenol* 2002;178(5):1175–1179.

49. Kodama Y, Sakuhara Y, Abo D, et al. Percutaneous transluminal angioplasty for hepatic artery stenosis after living donor liver transplantation. *Liver Transpl* 2006;12(3):465–469.

50. Orons PD, Sheng R, Zajko AB. Hepatic artery stenosis in liver transplant recipients: prevalence and cholangiographic appearance of associated biliary complications. AJR *Am J Roentgenol* 1995;165(5):1145–1149.

51. Dodd GD, 3rd, Memel DS, Zajko AB, et al. Hepatic artery stenosis and thrombosis in transplant recipients: Doppler diagnosis with resistive index and systolic acceleration time. *Radiology* 1994;192(3):657–661.

52. Lerut J, Tzakis AG, Bron K, et al. Complications of venous reconstruction in human orthotopic liver transplantation. *Ann Surg* 1987;205(4):404–414.

53. Langnas AN, Marujo W, Stratta RJ, et al. Vascular complications after orthotopic liver transplantation. *Am J Surg* 1991;161(1):76-82; discussion 82–83.

54. Rouch DA, Emond JC, Ferrari M, et al. The successful management of portal vein thrombosis after hepatic transplantation with a splenorenal shunt. *Surg Gynecol Obstet* 1988;166(4):311–316.

55. Marino IR, Esquivel CO, Zajko AB, et al. Distal splenorenal shunt for portal vein thrombosis after liver transplantation. *Am J Gastroenterol* 1989;84(1):67–70.

56. Bhattacharjya T, Olliff SP, Bhattacharjya S, et al. Percutaneous portal vein thrombolysis and endovascular stent for management of posttransplant portal venous conduit thrombosis. *Transplantation* 2000;69(10):2195–2198.

57. Cherukuri R, Haskal ZJ, Naji A, Shaked A. Percutaneous thrombolysis and stent placement for the treatment of portal vein thrombosis after liver transplantation: long-term follow-up. *Transplantation* 1998;65(8):1124–1126.

58. Guckelberger O, Bechstein WO, Langrehr JM, et al. Successful recanalization of late portal vein thrombosis after liver transplantation using systemic low-dose recombinant tissue plasminogen activator. *Transpl Int* 1999;12(4):273–277.

59. Funaki B, Rosenblum JD, Leef JA, et al. Portal vein stenosis in children with segmental liver transplants: treatment with percutaneous transhepatic venoplasty. *AJR Am J Roentgenol* 1995;165(1):161–165.

60. Funaki B, Rosenblum JD, Leef JA, et al. Angioplasty treatment of portal vein stenosis in children with segmental liver transplants: midterm results. *AJR Am J Roentgenol* 1997;169(2):551–554.

61. Funaki B, Rosenblum JD, Leef JA, et al. Percutaneous treatment of portal venous stenosis in children and adolescents with segmental hepatic transplants: long-term results. *Radiology* 2000;215(1):147–151.

62. Ueda M, Egawa H, Ogawa K, et al. Portal vein complications in the long-term course after pediatric living donor liver transplantation. *Transplant Proc* 2005;37(2):1138–1140.

63. Broelsch CE, Whitington PF, Emond JC, et al. Liver transplantation in children from living related donors. Surgical techniques and results. *Ann Surg* 1991;214(4):428–437; discussion 437–439.

64. Millis JM, Seaman DS, Piper JB, et al. Portal vein thrombosis and stenosis in pediatric liver transplantation. *Transplantation* 1996;62(6):748–754.

65. Marwan IK, Fawzy AT, Egawa H, et al. Innovative techniques for and results of portal vein reconstruction in living-related liver transplantation. *Surgery* 1999;125(3):265–270.

66. Zajko AB, Claus D, Clapuyt P, et al. Obstruction to hepatic venous drainage after liver transplantation: treatment with balloon angioplasty. *Radiology* 1989;170(3 Pt 1):763–765.

67. Althaus SJ, Perkins JD, Soltes G, Glickerman D. Use of a Wallstent in successful treatment of IVC obstruction following liver transplantation. *Transplantation* 1996;61(4):669–672.

68. Sze DY, Semba CP, Razavi MK, et al. Endovascular treatment of hepatic venous outflow obstruction after piggyback technique liver transplantation. *Transplantation* 1999;68(3):446–449.

69. Emond JC, Heffron TG, Whitington PF, Broelsch CE. Reconstruction of the hepatic vein in reduced size hepatic transplantation. *Surg Gynecol Obstet* 1993;176(1):11–17.

70. Broelsch CE, Lloyd DM. Living related donors for liver transplants. *Adv Surg* 1993;26:209–231.

71. Egawa H, Inomata Y, Uemoto S, et al. Hepatic vein reconstruction in 152 living-related donor liver transplantation patients. *Surgery* 1997;121(3):250–257.

72. de Villa VH, Chen CL, Chen YS, et al. Outflow tract reconstruction in living donor liver transplantation. *Transplantation* 2000;70(11):1604–1608.

73. Marcos A, Orloff M, Mieles L, et al. Functional venous anatomy for right-lobe grafting and techniques to optimize outflow. *Liver Transpl* 2001;7(10):845–852.

74. Buell JF, Funaki B, Cronin DC, et al. Long-term venous complications after full-size and segmental pediatric liver transplantation. *Ann Surg* 2002;236(5):658–666.

75. Ko GY, Sung KB, Yoon HK, et al. Endovascular treatment of hepatic venous outflow obstruction after living-donor liver transplantation. *J Vasc Interv Radiol* 2002;13(6):591–599.

76. Kinkhabwala MM, Guarrera JV, Leno R, et al. Outflow reconstruction in right hepatic live donor liver transplantation. *Surgery* 2003;133(3):243–250.

77. Akamatsu N, Sugawara Y, Kaneko J, et al. Surgical repair for late-onset hepatic venous outflow block after living-donor liver transplantation. *Transplantation* 2004;77(11):1768–1770.

78. Tannuri U, Mello ES, Carnevale FC, et al. Hepatic venous reconstruction in pediatric living-related donor liver transplantation—experience of a single center. *Pediatr Transplant* 2005;9(3):293–298.

79. Kasai H, Makuuchi M, Kawasaki S, et al. Intraoperative color Doppler ultrasonography for partial-liver transplantation from the living donor in pediatric patients. *Transplantation* 1992;54(1):173–175.

80. Inomata Y, Tanaka K, Egawa H, et al. Application of a tissue expander for stabilizing graft position in living-related liver transplantation. *Clin Transplant* 1997;11(1):56–59.

81. Someda H, Moriyasu F, Fujimoto M, et al. Vascular complications in living related liver transplantation detected with intraoperative and postoperative Doppler US. *J Hepatol* 1995;22(6):623–632.

82. Ko EY, Kim TK, Kim PN, et al. Hepatic vein stenosis after living donor liver transplantation: evaluation with Doppler US. *Radiology* 2003;229(3):806–810.

83. Matsunami H, Makuuchi M, Kawasaki S, et al. Venous reconstruction using three recipient hepatic veins in living related liver transplantation. *Transplantation* 1995; 59(6):917–919.

84. Takemura N, Sugawara Y, Hashimoto T, et al. New hepatic vein reconstruction in left liver graft. *Liver Transpl* 2005;11(3):356–360.

85. Liu CL, Zhao Y, Lo CM, Fan ST. Hepatic venoplasty in right lobe live donor liver transplantation. *Liver Transpl* 2003;9(12):1265–1272.

86. Fan ST, Lo CM, Liu CL, et al. Safety and necessity of including the middle hepatic vein in the right lobe graft in adult-to-adult live donor liver transplantation. *Ann Surg* 2003;238(1):137–148.

87. Kaneko T, Kaneko K, Sugimoto H, et al. Intrahepatic anastomosis formation between the hepatic veins in the graft liver of the living related liver transplantation: observation by Doppler ultrasonography. *Transplantation* 2000;70(6):982–985.

88. de Villa VH, Chen CL, Chen YS, et al. Right lobe living donor liver transplantation-addressing the middle hepatic vein controversy. *Ann Surg* 2003;238(2):275–282.

89. Akamatsu N, Sugawara Y, Kaneko J, et al. Effects of middle hepatic vein reconstruction on right liver graft regeneration. *Transplantation* 2003;76(5):832–837.

90. Maetani Y, Itoh K, Egawa H, et al. Factors influencing liver regeneration following living-donor liver transplantation of the right hepatic lobe. *Transplantation* 2003;75(1):97–102.

91. Lee S, Park K, Hwang S, et al. Anterior segment congestion of a right liver lobe graft in living-donor liver transplantation and strategy to prevent congestion. *J Hepatobiliary Pancreat Surg* 2003;10(1):16–25.

92. Kido M, Ku Y, Fukumoto T, et al. Significant role of middle hepatic vein in remnant liver regeneration of right-lobe living donors. *Transplantation* 2003;75(9):1598–600.

93. Sugawara Y, Makuuchi M, Sano K, et al. Vein reconstruction in modified right liver graft for living donor liver transplantation. *Ann Surg* 2003;237(2):180–185.

94. Kamel IR, Lawler LP, Fishman EK. Variations in anatomy of the middle hepatic vein and their impact on formal right hepatectomy. *Abdom Imaging* 2003; 28(5):668–74.

95. Yonemura Y, Taketomi A, Soejima Y, et al. Validity of preoperative volumetric analysis of congestion volume in living donor liver transplantation using three-dimensional computed tomography. *Liver Transpl* 2005;11(12):1556–1562.

96. Taniguchi M, Furukawa H, Shimamura T, et al. Hepatic venous reconstruction of anterior sector using three-dimensional helical computed tomography in living donor liver transplantation. *Transplantation* 2006;81(5):797–799.

97. Gyu Lee S, Min Park K, Hwang S, et al. Modified right liver graft from a living donor to prevent congestion. *Transplantation* 2002;74(1):54–59.

98. Kuang AA, Renz JF, Ferrell LD, et al. Failure patterns of cryopreserved vein grafts in liver transplantation. *Transplantation* 1996;62(6):742–747.

99. Sugawara Y, Makuuchi M, Akamatsu N, et al. Refinement of venous reconstruction using cryopreserved veins in right liver grafts. *Liver Transpl* 2004;10(4):541–547.

100. Hashimoto T, Sugawara Y, Kishi Y, et al. Superior vena cava graft for right liver and right lateral sector transplantation. *Transplantation* 2005;79(8):920–925.

101. Shin JH, Sung KB, Yoon HK, et al. Endovascular stent placement for interposed middle hepatic vein graft occlusion after living-donor liver transplantation using right-lobe graft. *Liver Transpl* 2006;12(2):269–276.

102. Hashikura Y, Makuuchi M, Kawasaki S, et al. Successful living-related partial liver transplantation to an adult patient. *Lancet* 1994;343(8907):1233–1234.

103. Lo CM, Fan ST, Liu CL, et al. Adult-to-adult living donor liver transplantation using extended right lobe grafts. *Ann Surg* 1997;226(3):261–269; discussion 269–270.

104. Marcos A, Fisher RA, Ham JM, et al. Right lobe living donor liver transplantation. *Transplantation* 1999;68(6):798–803.

105. Heffron TG, Emond JC, Whitington PF, et al. Biliary complications in pediatric liver transplantation. A comparison of reduced-size and whole grafts. *Transplantation* 1992;53(2):391–395.

106. Cronin DC, 2nd, Alonso EM, Piper JB, et al. Biliary complications in living donor liver transplantation. *Transplant Proc* 1997;29(1-2):419–420.

107. Reichert PR, Renz JF, Rosenthal P, et al. Biliary complications of reduced-organ liver transplantation. *Liver Transpl Surg* 1998;4(5):343–349.

108. Reding R, de Goyet Jde V, Delbeke I, et al. Pediatric liver transplantation with cadaveric or living related donors: comparative results in 90 elective recipients of primary grafts. *J Pediatr* 1999;134(3):280–286.

109. Egawa H, Inomata Y, Uemoto S, et al. Biliary anastomotic complications in 400 living related liver transplantations. *World J Surg* 2001;25(10):1300–1307.

110. Kling K, Lau H, Colombani P. Biliary complications of living related pediatric liver transplant patients. Pediatr Transplant 2004;8(2):178–184.

111. Broering DC, Kim JS, Mueller T, et al. One hundred thirty-two consecutive pediatric liver transplants without hospital mortality: lessons learned and outlook for the future. *Ann Surg* 2004;240(6):1002–1012; discussion 1012.

112. de Ville de Goyet J. Split liver transplantation in Europe—1988 to 1993. *Transplantation* 1995;59(10):1371–376.

113. Azoulay D, Astarcioglu I, Bismuth H, et al. Split-liver transplantation. The Paul Brousse policy. *Ann Surg* 1996;224(6):737–746; discussion 746–748.

114. Greif F, Bronsther OL, Van Thiel DH, et al. The incidence, timing, and management of biliary tract complications after orthotopic liver transplantation. *Ann Surg* 1994;219(1):40–45.

115. Heffron TG, Pillen T, Welch D, et al. Biliary complications after pediatric liver transplantation revisited. *Transplant Proc* 2003;35(4):1461–1462.

116. Egawa H, Uemoto S, Inomata Y, et al. Biliary complications in pediatric living related liver transplantation. *Surgery* 1998;124(5):901–910.

117. Settmacher U, Steinmuller TH, Schmidt SC, et al. Technique of bile duct reconstruction and management of biliary complications in right lobe living donor liver transplantation. *Clin Transplant* 2003;17(1):37–42.

118. Soejima Y, Shimada M, Suehiro T, et al. Feasibility of duct-to-duct biliary reconstruction in left-lobe adult-living-donor liver transplantation. *Transplantation* 2003;75(4):557–559.

119. Icoz G, Kilic M, Zeytunlu M, et al. Biliary reconstructions and complications encountered in 50 consecutive right-lobe living donor liver transplantations. *Liver Transpl* 2003;9(6):575–580.

120. Malago M, Testa G, Hertl M, et al. Biliary reconstruction following right adult living donor liver transplantation end-to-end or end-to-side duct-to-duct anastomosis. Langenbecks *Arch Surg* 2002;387(1):37–44.

121. Sugawara Y, Sano K, Kaneko J, et al. Duct-to-duct biliary reconstruction for living donor liver transplantation: experience of 92 cases. *Transplant Proc* 2003;35(8):2981–2982.

122. Liu CL, Lo CM, Chan SC, Fan ST. Safety of duct-to-duct biliary reconstruction in right-lobe live-donor liver transplantation without biliary drainage. *Transplantation* 2004;77(5):726–732.

123. Gondolesi GE, Varotti G, Florman SS, et al. Biliary complications in 96 consecutive right lobe living donor transplant recipients. *Transplantation* 2004;77(12):1842–1848.

124. Maluf DG, Stravitz RT, Cotterell AH, et al. Adult living donor versus deceased donor liver transplantation: a 6-year single center experience. *Am J Transplant* 2005;5(1):149–156.

125. Hwang S, Lee SG, Sung KB, et al. Long-term incidence, risk factors, and management of biliary complications after adult living donor liver transplantation. *Liver Transpl* 2006.

126. Colonna JO, 2nd, Shaked A, Gomes AS, et al. Biliary strictures complicating liver transplantation. Incidence, pathogenesis, management, and outcome. *Ann Surg* 1992;216(3):344–350; discussion 350–352.

127. Neuhaus P, Blumhardt G, Bechstein WO, et al. Technique and results of biliary reconstruction using side-to-side choledochocholedochostomy in 300 orthotopic liver transplants. *Ann Surg* 1994;219(4):426–434.

128. Verran DJ, Asfar SK, Ghent CN, et al. Biliary reconstruction without T tubes or stents in liver transplantation: report of 502 consecutive cases. *Liver Transpl Surg* 1997;3(4):365–373.

129. Halme L, Hockerstedt K, Lautenschlager I. Cytomegalovirus infection and development of biliary complications after liver transplantation. *Transplantation* 2003;75(11):1853–1858.

130. Northover JM, Terblanche J. A new look at the arterial supply of the bile duct in man and its surgical implications. *Br J Surg* 1979;66(6):379–384.

131. Stapleton GN, Hickman R, Terblanche J. Blood supply of the right and left hepatic ducts. *Br J Surg* 1998;85(2):202–207.

132. Shokouh-Amiri MH, Grewal HP, Vera SR, et al. Duct-to-duct biliary reconstruction in right lobe adult living donor liver transplantation. *J Am Coll Surg* 2001;192(6):798–803.

133. Fan ST, Lo CM, Liu CL, et al. Biliary reconstruction and complications of right lobe live donor liver transplantation. *Ann Surg* 2002;236(5):676–683.

134. Lee KW, Joh JW, Kim SJ, et al. High hilar dissection: new technique to reduce biliary complication in living donor liver transplantation. *Liver Transpl* 2004;10(9):1158–1162.

135. Pirenne J, Van Gelder F, Coosemans W, et al. Type of donor aortic preservation solution and not cold ischemia time is a major determinant of biliary strictures after liver transplantation. *Liver Transpl* 2001;7(6):540–545.

136. Moench C, Moench K, Lohse AW, et al. Prevention of ischemic-type biliary lesions by arterial back-table pressure perfusion. *Liver Transpl* 2003;9(3):285–289.

137. Park JS, Kim MH, Lee SK, et al. Efficacy of endoscopic and percutaneous treatments for biliary complications after cadaveric and living donor liver transplantation. *Gastrointest Endosc* 2003;57(1):78–85.

138. Hisatsune H, Yazumi S, Egawa H, et al. Endoscopic management of biliary strictures after duct-to-duct biliary reconstruction in right-lobe living-donor liver transplantation. *Transplantation* 2003;76(5):810–815.

139. Shah JN, Ahmad NA, Shetty K, et al. Endoscopic management of biliary complications after adult living donor liver transplantation. *Am J Gastroenterol* 2004; 99(7):1291–1295.

140. A comparison of tacrolimus (FK 506) and cyclosporine for immunosuppression in liver transplantation. The U.S. Multicenter FK506 Liver Study Group. *N Engl J Med* 1994; 331(17):1110–1115.

141. Randomised trial comparing tacrolimus (FK506) and cyclosporin in prevention of liver allograft rejection. European FK506 Multicentre Liver Study Group. *Lancet* 1994;344(8920):423–428.

142. Wiesner RH, Demetris AJ, Belle SH, et al. Acute hepatic allograft rejection: incidence, risk factors, and impact on outcome. *Hepatology* 1998;28(3):638–645.

143. Wiesner R, Rabkin J, Klintmalm G, et al. A randomized double-blind comparative study of mycophenolate mofetil and azathioprine in combination with cyclosporine and corticosteroids in primary liver transplant recipients. *Liver Transpl* 2001;7(5):442–450.

144. Doran TJ, Geczy AF, Painter D, et al. A large, single center investigation of the immunogenetic factors affecting liver transplantation. *Transplantation* 2000;69(7):1491–1498.

145. Brooks BK, Levy MF, Jennings LW, et al. Influence of donor and recipient gender on the outcome of liver transplantation. *Transplantation* 1996;62(12):1784–1787.

146. Candinas D, Gunson BK, Nightingale P, et al. Sex mismatch as a risk factor for chronic rejection of liver allografts. *Lancet* 1995;346(8983):1117–1121.

147. Cecka JM. The OPTN/UNOS Renal Transplant Registry 2003. *Clin Transpl* 2003;1–12.

148. Matas AJ, Payne WD, Sutherland DE, et al. 2,500 living donor kidney transplants: a single-center experience. *Ann Surg* 2001;234(2):149–164.

149. Katz SM, Ozaki CF, Monsour HP Jr, et al. Pediatric living-related and cadaveric liver transplantation: a single center experience. *Transplant Proc* 1994;26(1):145–146.

150. Alonso EM, Piper JB, Echols G, et al. Allograft rejection in pediatric recipients of living related liver transplants. *Hepatology* 1996;23(1):40–43.

151. Drews D, Sturm E, Latta A, et al. Complications following living-related and cadaveric liver transplantation in 100 children. *Transplant Proc* 1997;29(1-2):421–423.

152. Eid B, Villard F, Stamm D, et al. Review of living related versus cadaveric donors in pediatric liver transplantation: the lyon experience. *Transplant Proc* 2000;32(2):453.

153. Toyoki Y, Renz JF, Mudge C, et al. Allograft rejection in pediatric liver transplantation: Comparison between cadaveric and living related donors. *Pediatr Transplant* 2002;6(4):301–307.

154. Minamiguchi S, Sakurai T, Fujita S, et al. Living related liver transplantation: histopathologic analysis of graft dysfunction in 304 patients. *Hum Pathol* 1999;30(12):1479–1487.

155. Bartlett AS, Ramadas R, Furness S, et al. The natural history of acute histologic rejection without biochemical graft dysfunction in orthotopic liver transplantation: a systematic review. *Liver Transpl* 2002;8(12):1147–1153.

156. Kamada N. The immunology of experimental liver transplantation in the rat. *Immunology* 1985;55(3):369–389.

157. Kamada N, Teramoto K, Baguerizo A, et al. Cellular basis of transplantation tolerance induced by liver grafting in the rat. Extent of clonal deletion among thoracic duct lymphocytes, spleen, and lymph node cells. *Transplantation* 1988;46(1):165–167.

158. Liu LU, Bodian CA, Gondolesi GE, et al. Marked Differences in acute cellular rejection rates between living-donor and deceased-donor liver transplant recipients. *Transplantation* 2005;80(8):1072–1080.

159. Donaldson PT, Alexander GJ, O'Grady J, et al. Evidence for an immune response to HLA class I antigens in the vanishing-bile-duct syndrome after liver transplantation. *Lancet* 1987;1(8539):945–951.

160. Markus BH, Duquesnoy RJ, Gordon RD, et al. Histocompatibility and liver transplant outcome. Does HLA exert a dualistic effect? *Transplantation* 1988;46(3):372–377.

161. Katz SM, Kimball PM, Ozaki C, et al. Positive pretransplant crossmatches predict early graft loss in liver allograft recipients. *Transplantation* 1994;57(4):616–620.

162. Nikaein A, Backman L, Jennings L, et al. HLA compatibility and liver transplant outcome. Improved patient survival by HLA and cross-matching. *Transplantation* 1994;58(7):786–792.

163. Poli F, Scalamogna M, Aniasi A, et al. A retrospective evaluation of HLA-A, B and -DRB1 matching in liver transplantation. *Transpl Int* 1998;11 (Suppl 1):S347–S349.

164. Takaya S, Iwaki Y, Starzl TE. Liver transplantation in positive cytotoxic crossmatch cases using FK506, high-dose steroids, and prostaglandin E1. *Transplantation* 1992;54(5):927–929.

165. Doyle HR, Marino IR, Morelli F, et al. Assessing risk in liver transplantation. Special reference to the significance of a positive cytotoxic crossmatch. *Ann Surg* 1996;224(2):168–177.

166. Bathgate AJ, McColl M, Garden OJ, et al. The effect of a positive T-lymphocytotoxic crossmatch on hepatic allograft survival and rejection. *Liver Transpl Surg* 1998;4(4):280–284.

167. Hathaway M, Gunson BK, Keogh AC, et al. A positive crossmatch in liver transplantation--no effect or inappropriate analysis? A prospective study. *Transplantation* 1997; 64(1):54–59.

168. Sugawara Y, Mizuta K, Kawarasaki H, et al. Risk factors for acute rejection in pediatric living related liver transplantation: the impact of HLA matching. *Liver Transpl* 2001;7(9):769–773.

169. Kasahara M, Kiuchi T, Uryuhara K, et al. Role of HLA compatibility in pediatric living-related liver transplantation. *Transplantation* 2002;74(8):1175–1180.

170. Takakura K, Kiuchi T, Kasahara M, et al. Clinical implications of flow cytometry crossmatch with T or B cells in living donor liver transplantation. *Clin Transplant* 2001;15(5):309–316.

171. Sugawara Y, Makuuchi M, Kaneko J, et al. Risk factors for acute rejection in living donor liver transplantation. *Clin Transplant* 2003;17(4):347–352.

172. Suehiro T, Shimada M, Kishikawa K, et al. Influence of HLA compatibility and lymphocyte cross-matching on acute cellular rejection following living donor adult liver transplantation. *Liver Int* 2005;25(6):1182–1188.

173. Demetris AJ, Murase N, Lee RG, et al. Chronic rejection. A general overview of histopathology and pathophysiology with emphasis on liver, heart and intestinal allografts. *Ann Transplant* 1997;2(2):27–44.

174. Wiesner RH, Batts KP, Krom RA. Evolving concepts in the diagnosis, pathogenesis, and treatment of chronic hepatic allograft rejection. *Liver Transpl Surg* 1999; 5(5):388–400.

175. Jain A, Demetris AJ, Kashyap R, et al. Does tacrolimus offer virtual freedom from chronic rejection after primary liver transplantation? Risk and prognostic factors in 1,048 liver transplantations with a mean follow-up of 6 years. *Liver Transpl* 2001;7(7):623–630.

176. Jain A, Mazariegos G, Pokharna R, et al. The absence of chronic rejection in pediatric primary liver transplant patients who are maintained on tacrolimus-based immunosuppression: a long-term analysis. *Transplantation* 2003;75(7):1020–1025.

177. Fung JJ, Todo S, Tzakis A, et al. Conversion of liver allograft recipients from cyclosporine to FK 506-based immunosuppression: benefits and pitfalls. *Transplant Proc* 1991;23(1 Pt 1):14–21.

178. Sher LS, Cosenza CA, Michel J, et al. Efficacy of tacrolimus as rescue therapy for chronic rejection in orthotopic liver transplantation: a report of the U.S. Multicenter Liver Study Group. *Transplantation* 1997;64(2):258–263.

179. Knight RJ, Kerman RH, Welsh M, et al. Chronic rejection in primary renal allograft recipients under cyclosporine-prednisone immunosuppressive therapy. *Transplantation* 1991; 51(2):355–359.

180. Matas AJ, Humar A, Payne WD, et al. Decreased acute rejection in kidney transplant recipients is associated with decreased chronic rejection. *Ann Surg* 1999;230(4):493–498; discussion 498–500.

181. Knight RJ, Burrows L, Bodian C. The influence of acute rejection on long-term renal allograft survival: a comparison of living and cadaveric donor transplantation. *Transplantation* 2001;72(1):69–76.

182. Gupta P, Hart J, Cronin D, et al. Risk factors for chronic rejection after pediatric liver transplantation. *Transplantation* 2001;72(6):1098–1102.

183. Freese DK, Snover DC, Sharp HL, et al. Chronic rejection after liver transplantation: a study of clinical, histopathological and immunological features. *Hepatology* 1991;13(5):882–891.

184. Farges O, Nocci Kalil A, Sebagh M, et al. Low incidence of chronic rejection in patients experiencing histological acute rejection without simultaneous impairment in liver function tests. *Transplant Proc* 1995;27(1):1142–1143.

185. Anand AC, Hubscher SG, Gunson BK, et al. Timing, significance, and prognosis of late acute liver allograft rejection. *Transplantation* 1995;60(10):1098–1103.

186. Blakolmer K, Seaberg EC, Batts K, et al. Analysis of the reversibility of chronic liver allograft rejection implications for a staging schema. *Am J Surg Pathol* 1999;23(11):1328–1339.

187. Devlin JJ, O'Grady JG, Tan KC, et al. Ethnic variations in patient and graft survival after liver transplantation. Identification of a new risk factor for chronic allograft rejection. *Transplantation* 1993;56(9):1381–1384.

188. Manez R, White LT, Linden P, et al. The influence of HLA matching on cytomegalovirus hepatitis and chronic rejection after liver transplantation. *Transplantation* 1993;55(5):1067–1071.

189. Paya CV, Wiesner RH, Hermans PE, et al. Lack of association between cytomegalovirus infection, HLA matching and the vanishing bile duct syndrome after liver transplantation. *Hepatology* 1992;16(1):66–70.

190. Smith DM, Agura E, Netto G, et al. Liver transplant-associated graft-versus-host disease. *Transplantation* 2003;75(1):118–126.

191. Taylor AL, Gibbs P, Sudhindran S, et al. Monitoring systemic donor lymphocyte macrochimerism to aid the diagnosis of graft-versus-host disease after liver transplantation. *Transplantation* 2004;77(3):441–446.

192. Cattral MS, Langnas AN, Wisecarver JL, et al. Survival of graft-versus-host disease in a liver transplant recipient. *Transplantation* 1994;57(8):1271–1274.

193. Taylor AL, Gibbs P, Bradley JA. Acute graft versus host disease following liver transplantation: the enemy within. *Am J Transplant* 2004;4(4):466–474.

194. Whitington PF, Rubin CM, Alonso EM, et al. Complete lymphoid chimerism and chronic graft-versus-host disease in an infant recipient of a hepatic allograft from an HLA-homozygous parental living donor. *Transplantation* 1996;62(10):1516–1519.

195. Nemoto T, Kubota K, Kita J, et al. Unusual onset of chronic graft-versus-host disease after adult living-related liver transplantation from a homozygous donor. *Transplantation* 2003;75(5):733–736.

196. Soejima Y, Shimada M, Suehiro T, et al. Graft-versus-host disease following living donor liver transplantation. *Liver Transpl* 2004;10(3):460–464.

197. Kamei H, Oike F, Fujimoto Y, et al. Fatal graft-versus-host disease after living donor liver transplantation: differential impact of donor-dominant one-way HLA matching. *Liver Transpl* 2006;12(1):140–145.

# 30.9 INTERVENTIONAL THERAPIES

*Erik N.K. Cressman, MD, PhD*

## INTRODUCTION

Living donor liver transplants (LDLT) are considered among the most technically demanding surgeries[1,2] performed today. Despite this and the ethical controversies[3] associated with involvement of an otherwise healthy donor,[4,5,6] supply and demand are such that application of the procedure has been increasing steadily since the first operation in 1989. In particular, although the procedure began with pediatric patients and left lateral segment transplantation, the balance has shifted in favor of right lobe transplantation in adult patients. Data from the Organ Procurement and Transplantation Network (http://www.optn.org) show that as of 5/31/05 the total number of LDLTs was 2 770 (1 789 adult, 977 pediatric). For the year to date, the total was 133 (104 adult, 28 pediatric). In the United States, adult LDLT surpassed pediatric LDLT in 1999. To put this in perspective, deceased donor liver transplants (DDLT) since 1988 were 60 147 adult and 8 325 pediatric cases. The year-to-date data show adult DDLT at 2 364 and pediatric DDLT at 218 and there are nearly 90 000 patients on the waiting list. Thus, although the percentage of LDLT is relatively small, it is increasing and some data regarding complication rates have begun to accrue. As familiarity with these procedures has increased, complication rates have declined [7,8,9] but are still considerably greater with LDLT than DDLT. This chapter focuses on the most common problems encountered in LDLT[10] and applications of interventional radiology [11,12] in treating them. Anatomic considerations are discussed followed by biliary complications, hepatic arterial complications, and finally venous complications whether portal, hepatic, or caval. Where possible, emphasis is placed on the differences in complications encountered in LDLT compared to whole organ DDLT. Interventional radiology involvement in pretransplant evaluations,[13] chemoembolization or other ablative methods for hepatocellular carcinoma as a means of delaying or preventing dropout from transplant lists, treatment of extrahepatic fluid collections, vascular access, feeding tube placement, biopsies, and surgical issues of primary nonfunction, wound infections, and wound dehiscence will not be covered. As experience with the procedure has grown and sizing the transplant has become more appropriate, the small-for-size syndrome[14,15,16] (hyperperfusion) and its counterpart, oversizing resulting in compressive hypoperfusion, have decreased in frequency and also are beyond the scope of this discussion.

## ANATOMIC AND PHYSIOLOGIC CONSIDERATIONS

### Differences in Pediatric Versus Adult LDLT

Separating procedures based on age is useful for several purposes because different anatomic and physiologic issues exist. A different spectrum of diseases is seen in pediatric patients (biliary atresia, inborn errors of metabolism, etc) with less reserve but fewer of the co-morbidities typically seen in adult patients; healing potential is greater; implications of treatment have a much longer time span in consideration; radiation doses (both whole-body and gonadal) likewise have different lifetime implications; pediatric patients may have had more temporizing surgeries such as a Kasai procedure with attendant adhesions; smaller vascular and biliary anastomoses; general anesthesia is used for procedures[17] rather than conscious sedation; a Roux-en-Y biliary-enteric anastomosis is much more likely than direct choledochocholedochostomy; and finally, pediatric LDLT is usually done using the left lateral segment,[18] which is technically somewhat less challenging than right lobe donation.

Size is an important independent risk factor. Small infants are more prone to hepatic arterial and portal venous thrombosis, which is thought to be a result of the small diameter of the vessels involved[19] in creation of the anastomoses. Although interventional radiology has served a diagnostic role with angiography, these life-threatening complications are generally treated surgically. Intra-arterial lytic therapy is not advisable due to bleeding risks in the immediate postoperative situation and the amount of time required for restoration of perfusion of an already endangered graft.

Other anatomic issues appear as well. Anastomoses of the hepatic artery, bile duct(s), portal vein, and vena cava are discussed below in more detail. In general, vascular and biliary pedicles are shorter in LDLT and therefore harder to manipulate than in conventional whole-organ transplantation. This makes them more prone to the development of stenosis. Biliary ductal variation is extremely common and it has been reported[20] that there is an association between multiple ducts and an increase in complications such as strictures. Such variability makes it imperative for the interventional radiologist to review the pertinent imaging and especially to review the operative report of the transplant procedure to know what to expect when attempting percutaneous treatment.

### Left Lateral Segment Versus Right Lobe

Four different LDLT grafts have been used. Right lobe, left lobe, extended right, and left lateral segment transplants have all been attempted, but the best results have come from right lobe transplant in adults and left lateral segment in size-matched infants and children. Right or left lobe transplantation may matter in terms of propensity for certain complications, but to date there are no data showing a significant difference in complication rates. The left lateral segment transplant involves dissection along the plane of the falciform ligament. The cut surface is considerably smaller than that in right lobe transplantation, and the attendant risk of a parenchymal bile leak or hematoma may therefore be somewhat less.

### BILIARY COMPLICATIONS AND TREATMENT

#### Leakage: Anastomotic Versus Parenchymal

Bile leaks are most likely to occur early in the postoperative course[21] leading to persistent drain outputs, biloma formation, and/or bile peritonitis. Drainage is indicated whether the leak is parenchymal (generally not an issue in whole-organ DDLT) or associated with the ductal system. Anastomotic leaks are most common and appear somewhat more likely with direct duct-to-duct anastomoses than with hepaticojejunostomies.[22] Opinions

vary regarding techniques with some authors reporting better results with T-tube placement.[23] Parenchymal leaks usually resolve in a few days to weeks with simple drainage but leakage from the biliary system generally requires biliary diversion. In the case of preserved anatomy, endoscopy[24] may be the preferred choice, but many patients will have a Roux limb precluding this option. Percutaneous transhepatic cholangiography (PTC) and percutaneous biliary drainage (PBD) then play a role. Access to a nondilated leaking system is much more difficult than conventional PTC for obstructed systems but once accomplished can allow the bile ducts to heal.[25] Tracts are usually allowed to epithelialize for 6 to 8 weeks and by this time the patient is usually ready for a clinical trial. This consists of placing a shorter tube above the leak yet preserving access. If this is successful a cholangiogram through the access is typically performed after an additional 2 weeks. The tube may then be removed provided there is no further evidence of leakage.

### Strictures: Anastomotic Versus Diffuse

Anastomotic strictures, in contrast, typically present later than leaks and often require more prolonged treatment. These are the most common complication seen in transplantion and have been referred to by many as the Achille's heel of liver transplants.[26,27,28] Differentiation of anastomotic from diffuse biliary strictures is also important as they have different etiologies, different treatments, and different prognoses. Diffuse stricturing is associated with rejection and biliary ischemia, whereas anastomotic stricturing is due to local tissue proliferation. Strictures also are more common with hepaticojejunostomies than with direct choledochocholedochostomies (Figure 30.9-1A,B). Various methods have been employed for treating these lesions (including surgical revision[29]), and there is some thought that anastomotic strictures may be more common in LDLT patients than whole-organ DDLT patients.[30] Periodic balloon cholangioplasty,[31] cutting balloons, and prolonged courses of stenting with internal/external biliary drains[32] have had the most success (Figure 30.9-2A,B). Opinions vary, but as a general rule anastomotic strictures take several months to a year of treatment to provide acceptable results. Metallic stents are rarely employed given that they severely restrict further surgical options and tend to occlude in significantly less time than the patient's life expectancy.

### Arterial Complications And Treatment

#### *Pseudoaneurysm, Stenosis*

The most devastating complication is hepatic artery thrombosis as described earlier, which is managed surgically with thrombectomy, bypass, or even retransplantation.[33] Anastomotic stenoses typically are diagnosed early on ultrasound examinations[34,35] but occasionally manifest as abnormal lab values or in extreme cases, infarction, biloma formation, and/or cholangitis (Figure 30.9-3A,B). This usually leads to either MRCP or PTC, and if there is diffuse structuring noted, an arteriogram is performed.[36] Stenosis may be treated with balloon angioplasty alone[37] or if refractory a stent may be placed.[38,39,40] Stents also have a role in the treatment of hepatic artery pseudoaneurysms in select cases but given that a stents represent foreign bodies in an immunocompromised patient, their use is rather limited. In rare cases a pseudoaneurysm has been coil embolized, but this should not be the first option in these situations.

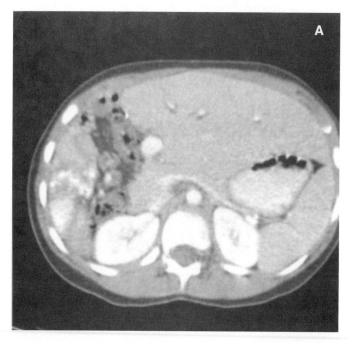
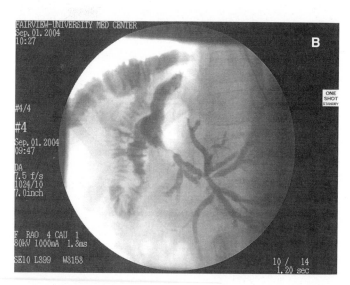

**FIGURE 30.9-1**

(A, B) Pediatric left lateral segment transplant patient demonstrating intrahepatic biliary ductal dilation on CT and pullback cholangiogram showing anastomotic stricture.

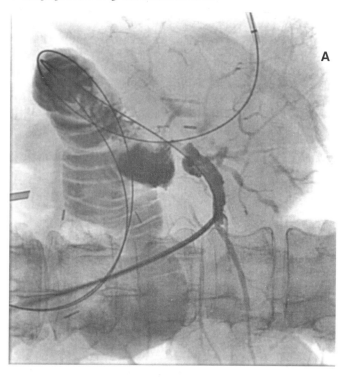
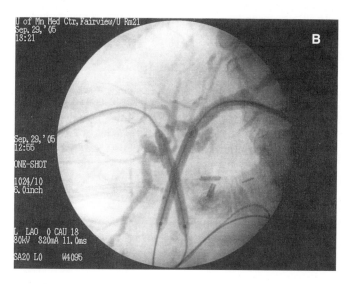

**FIGURE 30.9-2**

(A,B) Biliary-enteric stricture and treatment with balloon angioplasty.

## VENOUS COMPLICATIONS AND TREATMENT

### Portal Vein Thrombosis and Stenosis

Portal vein thrombosis is usually an early complication treated surgically for reasons similar to hepatic artery thrombosis. Late portal vein thrombosis has been treated with combined mechanical and pharmacologic thrombolysis.[41] Portal vein stenosis, on the other hand, appears later, is somewhat more common in LDLT patients than whole-organ DDLT patients, particularly pediatric patients with cryopreserved vein as a portal conduit, and is often amenable to percutaneous management.[42] Incidence of symptomatic portal vein stenosis has decreased over

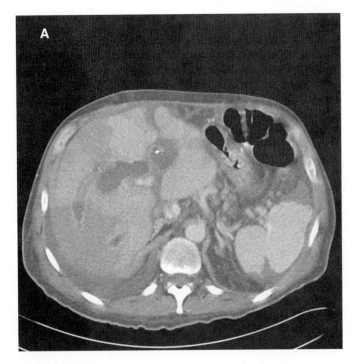
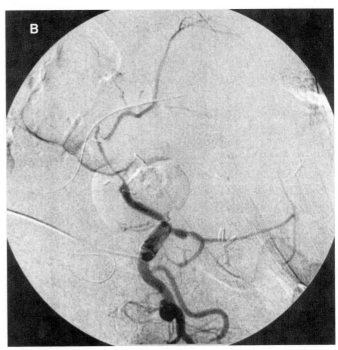

**FIGURE 30.9-3**

**(A,B)** CT scan of ischemic, failing transplant liver showing areas of hypoperfusion, infarction, and biloma formation secondary to long-segment hepatic artery stenosis demonstrated on celiac angiography.

the last decade as experience has increased.[43] Percutaneous transhepatic portography with hemodynamics may be followed where indicated by portal vein angioplasty with or without stent placement.[44] This has been successfully employed at several centers. As with all permanent devices in transplant patients, thought must be given to preserving future surgical options wherever possible.

## Hepatic Vein Thrombosis and Stenosis

Hepatic vein thrombosis occurs rarely, but is a serious complication. Provided the patient can be stabilized, a transjugular intrahepatic portosystemic shunt (TIPS) through the transplanted liver[45] may provide a means of graft salvage or, at a minimum, a bridge to retransplantation. Hepatic vein stenosis documented with hemodynamics is amenable to angioplasty and stent placement, generally from an internal jugular approach.[46,47]

## Vena Cava Thrombosis and Stenosis

Inferior vena cava stenosis is a rare complication treated by angioplasty and stent placement.[48]

## References

1. Ghobrial RM, Saab S, Lassman C, et al. *Liver Transpl* 2002;8:901.
2. Miller CM, Gondolesi GE, Florman S, et al. *Ann Surg* 2001;234:301.
3. Lee SY, Ko G-Y, Gwon DI, et al. Living donor liver transplantation: Complications in donors and interventional management. *Radiology* 2004;230:443.
4. Humar A, Carolan E, Ibrahim H, et al. A comparison of surgical outcomes and quality of life surveys in right lobe vs. left lateral segment liver donors. *Am J Transpl* 2005;5:805.
5. Renz JF, Roberts JP. Long-Term Complications of Living Donor Liver Transplantation: *Liver Transpl* 2000;6(6);(Suppl 2): S73.
6. Wiederkehr JC, Pereira JC, Ekermann M, et al. Results of 132 Hepatectomies for Living Donor Liver Transplantation: Report of One Death *Transpl Proc* 2005;37:1079.
7. Gondolesi GE, Varotti G, Florman SS, et al. Biliary Complications in 96 Consecutive Right Lobe Living Donor Transplant Recipients: *Transplantation* 2004;77(12):1842.
8. Lo C-M, Fan ST, Liu CL, et al. Lessons learned from one hundred right lobe living donor liver transplants. *Ann Surg* 2004;240(1):151.
9. Freise CE, Kam I, Pruett TL, et al. Outcomes of 385 adult-to-adult living donor liver transplant recipients: a report from the A2ALL Consortium. *Ann Surg* 2005;242(3):314.
10. Bücheler E, Nicolas V, Broelsch CE, et al. *Diagnostic and Interventional Radiology in Liver Transplantation*. New York, Springer; 2003.
11. Karani JB, Yu DFQC, Kane PA. Interventional radiology in liver transplantation. *Cardiovasc Intervent Radiol* 2005;28:271.
12. Gemmete JJ, Mueller GC, Carlos RC Liver transplantation in adults: postoperative imaging evaluation and interventional management of complications. *Sem Roentgen* 2006;41(1):36–44.
13. Rose SC, Andre MP, Roberts AC, et al. Integral role of interventional radiology in the development of a pediatric liver transplantation program. *Ped Transpl* 2001;5:331.
14. Sugimoto H, Kaneko T, Hirota M, et al. Critical progressive small-graft injury caused by intrasinusoidal pressure elevation following living donor liver transplantation. *Transpl Proc* 2004;36:2750.
15. Lee DS, Gil WH, Lee HH, et al. Factors affecting graft survival after living donor liver transplantation. *Transpl Proc* 2004;36:2255.
16. Shimada M, Ijichi H, Yonemura Y, et al. Is graft size a major risk factor in living-donor adult liver transplantation? *Transpl Int* 2004;17:310.
17. Wagner C, Beebe DS, Carr RJ, et al. Living related liver transplantation in infants and children: Report of anesthetic care and early postoperative morbidity and mortality. *J Clin Anes* 2000;12:454.
18. Broelsch CE, Frilling A, Testa G, et al. Early and late complications in the recipient of and adult living donor liver. *Liver Transpl* 2003; 9(10) Suppl 2:s50.

19. Lin C-C, Chuang F-R, Wang C-C, et al. Early postoperative complications in recipients of living donor liver transplantation. *Transpl Proc* 2004; 36:2338.

20. Salvalaggio PRO, Whitington PF, Alonso EM, et al. Presence of multiple bile ducts in the liver graft increases the incidence of biliary complications in pediatric liver transplantation. *Liver Transpl* 2005;11(2):161.

21. Humar A. Donor and recipient outcomes after adult living donor liver transplantation. *Liver Transpl* 2003;9(10);(Suppl 2):S42.

22. Egawa H, Inomata Y, Uemoto S, et al. Biliary anastomotic complications in 400 living related liver transplantations. *World J Surg* 2001;25:1300.

23. Kobayashi T, Sato Y, Yamamoto S, et al. Biliary reconstruction and complications of left lobe living donor liver transplanation. *Transpl Proc* 2005;37:1122.

24. Morelli J, Mulcahy HE, Willner IR, et al. Long-term outcomes for patients with post-liver transplant anastomotic biliary strictures treated by endoscopic stent placement *Gastrointest Endo* 2003;58(3):374.

25. Lorenz JM, Funaki B, Leef JA, et al. Percutaneous transhepatic cholangiography and biliary drainage in pediatric liver transplant patients. *AJR* 2001;176:761.

26. Pascher A, Neuhaus P. Bile duct complications after liver transplantation *Transpl Int* 2005;18:627.

27. Yazumi S, Tsutomu C. Biliary complications after right-lobe living donor liver transplantation *J Gastroenterol* 2005;40:861–865.

28. Chang JM, Lee JM, Suh KS, et al. Biliary complications in living donor liver transplantation: imaging findings and the roles of interventional procedures. *Cardiovasc & Intervent Rad* 2005;28(6):756–767.

29. Fan S-T, Lo C-M, Liu C-L, et al. Biliary reconstruction and compications of right lobe live donor liver transplantation *Ann Surg* 2002; 236(5);676.

30. Schwarzenberg SJ, Sharp HL, Payne WD, et al. Biliary stricture in living-related donor liver transplantation: Management with balloon dilation. *Ped Transpl* 2002;6:132.

31. Saad WEA, Saad NEA, Davies MG, et al. Transhepatic balloon dilation of anastomotic biliary strictures in liver transplant recipients: The significance of a patent hepatic artery. *J Vasc Intervent Rad* 2005;16(9):1221.

32. Righi D, Cesarani F, Muraro E et al: Role of Interventional Radiology in the Treatment of Biliary Strictures Following Orthotopic Liver Transplantation *Cardiovasc Intervent Radiol* 2002; 25:30.

33. Settmacher U, Stange B, Haase R et al: Arterial complications after liver transplantation. *Transplant Int* 2000; 13:372.

34. Kaneko J, Suawara Y, Togashi J et al: Simultaneous Hepatic Artery and Portal Vein Thrombosis After Living Donor Liver Transplantation *Transpl Proc* 2004; 36:3087.

35. Zanotelli ML, Vieira S, Alencastro R, et al: Management of Vascular Complications After Pediatric Liver Transplantation *Transpl Proc* 2004; 36:945.

36. Settmacher U, Stange B, Haase R, et al: Arterial complications after liver transplantation. *Transplant Int* 2000; 13:372–78.

37. Saad, WEA, Davies MG, Sahler, L, et al Hepatic Artery Stenosis in Liver Transplant Recipients: Primary Treatment with Percutaneous Transluminal Angioplasty *J Vasc Intervent Rad* 2005; 16(6): 795

38. Cotroneo AR, DiStasi C, Cina A, et al: Stent placement in four patients with hepatic artery stenosis or thrombosis after liver transplantation *J Vasc Intervent Radiol* 2002; 13:619.

39. Denys AL, Qanadli SD, Durand F, et al: Feasibility and effectiveness of using coronary stents in the treatment of hepatic artery stenoses after orthotopic liver transplantation: preliminary report *Am J Roentgenol* 2002; 178:1175.

40. Denys AL, Qanadli SD, Durand F, et al: Feasibility and effectiveness of using coronary stents in the treatment of hepatic artery stenoses after orthotopic liver transplantation: preliminary report *Am J Roentgenol* 2002; 178:1175–79.

41. Rossi C, Zambruni A, Ansaloni F, et al: Combined Mechanical and Pharmacologic Thrombolysis for Portal Vein Thrombosis in Liver-Graft Recipients and in Candidates for Liver Transplantation *Transplantation* 2004; 78(6): 938.

42. Ueda M, Egawa H, Ogawa K, et al: Portal Vein Complications in the Long-Term Course After Pediatric Living Donor Liver Transplantation *Transpl Proc* 2005; 37:1138.

43. Funaki B, Rosenblum JD, Leef J, et al: Percutaneous Treatment of Portal Venous Stenosis in Children and Adolescents with Segmental Hepatic Transplants: Long-term Results *Radiology* 2000; 215:147,

44. Buell JF, Funaki B, Cronin DC et al: Long-Term Venous Complications After Full-Size and Segmental Pediatric Liver Transplantation *Ann Surg* 2002; 236(5):658.

45. Saad, WEA, Davies, MG, Lee, DE, et al Transjugular Intrahepatic Portosystemic Shunt in a Living Donor Left Lateral Segment Liver Transplant Recipient: Technical Considerations *J Vasc Intervent Rad* 2005; 16(6): 873.

46. Narumi S, Hakamada K, Totsuka E et al: Efficacy of Cutting Balloon for Anastomotic Stricture of the Hepatic Vein *Transpl Proc* 2004; 36:3093.

47. Ko GY, Surg KB, Yoon HK, et al: Endovascular treatment of hepatic venous outflow obstruction after living-donor liver transplantation *J Vasc Intervent Rad* 2002; 13:591–99.

48. Weeksw SM, Gerber DA, Jaques PF, et al: Primary Gianturco stent placement for inferior vena cava abnormalities following liver transplantation. *J Vasc Intervent Rad* 2000; 11:177–87.

## 30.10   IMMUNOSUPPRESSIVE THERAPY

*Roberto Gedaly, MD, Hosein Shokouh-Amiri, MD, Santiago R. Vera, MD, A. Osama Gaber, MD*

Living donor liver transplantation (LDLT) was developed initially in children as a response to organ shortage and the high rates of pediatric mortality on the waiting list. Extending the application to adults was a necessity in countries without the possibility of cadaveric donation and a means to increase organ supply where the transplantation rates were inadequate to keep up with the expanding need for liver replacement. As with other transplant procedures, immunosuppression following LDLT is the key to survival of both the allograft and the patient. The availability of effective therapeutic agents allows for adequate delivery of immune suppression to even the most complex patients, and raises new challenges regarding individualization of therapy.

Immunosuppression in LDLT has evolved from protocols used in cadaveric transplant protocols. LDLT, however, has many differences from whole organ cadaveric liver transplantation that could impact the immunosuppression management. Most importantly, with LDLT there is the potential of better human leukocyte antigen (HLA) matching. Improved matching may confer to the recipient, an immunological advantage similar to that observed in living donor kidney transplantation. Traditionally, living donor kidney recipients have reduced acute and chronic rejection rates and a decreased need for potent immune therapy. Another advantage of the living donor liver procedure may be related to avoiding the activation of the inflammatory cascade seen in cadaveric livers obtained from brain dead donors,[1] which has been implicated in up-regulation of inflammatory cytokines, adhesion molecules, class II presentation and in affecting microcirculatory flow to the liver with resultant hepatocellular damage and allograft dysfunction.[2] Furthermore, with the lack of prolonged preservation living donor grafts are at low risk of primary nonfunction or initial graft dysfunction allowing rapid and early introduction of full dose immune suppressants. Because of its small size, however, the transplanted graft has to undergo compensatory hyperplasia to rebuild the liver mass. Because most of the immune suppressants, particularly the calcineurins, are hepatically metabolized, the availability and metabolism of these drugs can be altered during the post transplant regenerative phase. Other aspects related to LDLT that may impact immunosuppression protocols include the potential for development of "small-for-size" syndrome, the utilization of LDLT as first resource in cancer patients, the preferential utilization of living donor transplants in pediatric populations, the potential for accelerated hepatitis C recurrence in the regenerating liver and the use of ABO incompatible donor recipient combinations.

It should be emphasized that the field of immune suppression for living donor liver transplantation is a relatively young one with few published reports and no prospective studies. We encourage the reader to recognize the evolutionary nature of the field and to consider the opportunities available for the study of immunosuppression management in this unique population.

## TECHNICAL ASPECTS AND COMPLICATION OF LDLT

The development of LDLT has been prompted by organ shortage and restrained by practical and ethnical concern for donors. In the United States, more than 1 000 potential liver transplant candidates die each year on the waiting list.[3] In other countries such as Japan, Korea, and Egypt, LDLT provides the only source of organs for patients with advanced liver disease. Living-donation of the lateral segment of the left lobe has become highly successful in pediatric transplantation. In recent years, an increasing number of transplant centers have ventured into adult-to-adult living donor liver transplantation. Despite the high level of technical expertise in the transplant units performing LDLT, donor procedures carry significant morbidity and mortality. The morbidity of a left lateral segmentectomy, which is used primarily in pediatric LDLT, is around 10% with a small mortality of less than 1%.[4,5] The estimated mortality of the right hepatic lobectomy used in adult-to-adult LDLT is around 1.5% to 2%.[6] Concern regarding potential donor morbidity and mortality has limited the routine adoption of the procedure.

Because of the complex nature of the recipient procedure, morbidity occurs with different frequency than in whole liver cadaveric transplantation. In the pediatric population, hepatic artery thrombosis and biliary complications are most frequently encountered. The rate of hepatic artery thrombosis has been reduced from 5% to 15% to less than 2% in most recent series.[7] Modern results are typical to the results presented by Reding, who compared outcomes in children receiving LDLT to those having cadaveric transplants.[8] As expected, the living donor group (n = 68) had significantly lower waiting list mortality than cadaver recipients (n = 42). Biliary complications were, however, more common in the living donor recipients (34% vs 14%, p < .05), whereas HAT occurred more frequently in the cadaveric recipients. Importantly, 1-year patient and graft survival were similar in both groups (patient survival 87% cadaver vs 92 LDLT; graft survival 75% cadaver vs 90% LDLT).

In adult-to-adult LDLT, most series report comparable results to those seen in cadaveric liver transplantation. As with children, however, biliary complications are consistently higher in LDLT recipients (around 25%).[9] This is especially relevant in the context of immune suppression with calcineurins. Absorption of calcineurins is dependent to some extent on an intact enterohepatic circulation. The degree of cyclosporine availability is compounded in children by variations in the length and location of the Rou-en-y used in biliary drainage.[10] These considerations are less important in patients receiving Prograf or CyA microemulsion.

## IMMUNOSUPPRESSION IN LIVER TRANSPLANTATION

Immunosuppressive therapy for liver recipients in most centers is based on a calcineurin inhibitor in conjunction with an anti-proliferative agent or steroid.[11] It is now accepted that dual regimens of steroids and a calcineurin inhibitor appear as efficacious as triple therapy.[12] Long-term monotherapy with a calcineurin, double therapy with steroids and calcineurins, and complete calcineurin elimination have all been reported. The advantage of early use of triple therapy is that it may allow delaying the initiation of the calcineurin inhibitors while the post transplant changes in renal function recover. This is a lesser concern in LDLT because most of these procedures are done electively and prior to physiological deterioration of the recipient. The use of antibody therapy, particularly nondepleting anti-CD25 antibodies in the perioperative period, has been increasing during the last few years. These antibodies are usually used as part of sequential drug therapy protocols allowing a delay in the introduction of calcineurins and minimization or avoidance of steroid use.[13,14] Cyclosporin and Tacrolimus seem to be similar in terms of graft and patients survival.[15] However, Tacrolimus is associated with fewer episodes of rejection and less need for steroid use. Tacrolimus has the same degree of nephrotoxicity as cyclosporin but is associated with lower incidence of hypertension and hyperlipidemia and increased rates of diabetes and neurotoxicity.[16,17] UNOS data demonstrate that tacrolimus is being used in over 75% of liver recipient including liver donor recipients.

MMF is another immunosuppressant that is being increasingly used in liver recipients. MMF is an antiproliferative agent that blocks purine synthesis. MMF is used to allow dosage reduction or discontinuation of calcineurin inhibitors, particularly in patients experiencing significant renal dysfunction.[18,19] Sirolimus is used in kidney transplantation to allow reduction and elimination of the CNI. Sirolimus was found to be associated with higher incidence of hepatic artery thrombosis in one series.[20] This resulted in the issuance of an FDA "Black Box" warning regarding Rapamycin's utilization in the postoperative period. Subsequent studies have suggested, however, that hepatic arterial thrombosis may not be a major problem. We currently use Sirolimus in patients that develop renal dysfunction or posttransplant diabetes or in patients with neurotoxicity.

Steroid withdrawal protocols have been shown to be safe in liver transplant recipients. Recently, regimens based on complete steroid avoidance have been explored in conjunction with Tacrolimus and MMF. Results indicate that steroid avoidance is associated with similar rates of rejection compared to historical controls. In addition, steroid avoidance was associated with lower serum cholesterol, less posttransplant diabetes, and less hypertension.[21] The regenerative capacity of the liver coupled with its relative immune privileged status has stimulated interest in immune suppression withdrawal[22] or tolerance induction protocols. Tolerogenic protocols aim at eliminating the immune response to donor antigens while maintaining full reactivity to other antigens. Several different strategies have been utilized in attempts to develop tolerance to liver allografts including combined transplantation of donor bone marrow with the liver allograft. Tolerance induction was also attempted by treating with immunotherapy against antigen-presenting cells using anti-CD28-B7 and anti-CD40-CD40L given immediately posttransplant, or more recently, using anti-CD52 (Campath-1H) in conjunction with low-dose tacrolimus.[11,23] At present, complete immune suppression withdrawal has only been successful in 30% to 40% of patients.[24] Minimal success in inducing operative tolerance has been seen in the clinical experience, although some promising studies are currently ongoing.[25]

UNOS data indicate that 97% of liver recipients received CNI at hospital discharge following the transplant. At first hospital discharge, corticosteroids use was reported in more than 90% of liver transplants, mycophenolate mofetil was reported in nearly 48%, and Rapamycin was reported in 7%. Antibodies were given to 18% of recipients with the majority of antibody use being anti-IL-2 receptor antibodies.[26–28]

## SPECIAL CONSIDERATIONS IN IMMUNE SUPPRESSION IN LDLT

### Calcinuerin Doses and Levels

Trotter et al. compared 46 LDLT recipients with 66 matched concurrent cadaveric liver transplant recipients. Immunosuppression was a mix of tacrolimus and CyA in both groups. Calcineurin blood levels were recorded at weeks 1, 2, 3, and 4 and at months 2, 3, 4, 5, and 6 in both groups.[29] The ratio of level to dose was also recorded at each interval. They observed that the mean calcinuerin-level-to-dose ratio was 26% higher for those undergoing LDLT (p = 0.01), and they concluded that LDLT recipients using cyclosporine and tacrolimus achieve higher levels for a given dose compared to cadaveric recipients.[29] These findings were confirmed by Taber et al., who reported a similar decrease in tacrolimus dosing requirements in LDLT recipients compared to CAD recipients during the first 3 months Posttransplantation.[30] These variations in dose levels ratio were correlated to graft size, intestinal MDRI level, and hepatic CYP3A5*1 genotype.[31–33]

## HEPATIC REGENERATION IN THE CONTEXT OF IMMUNE SUPPRESSIVE PROTOCOLS

In response to hepatocellular damage the liver mounts inflammatory, regenerative, and repair processes with the aim of restoring the functional liver tissue mass. Liver regeneration is an orchestrated response that involves sequential changes in gene expression, growth factor production, and morphologic structure. During the regenerative process, the liver undergoes compensatory hyperplasia in order to reestablish the optimal mass set in relationship to body size. Many growth factors and cytokines, most notably HGF, EGF, TGF-alpha, IL-6, TNF-alpha, insulin, and norepinephrine, seem to play important roles in this process.[34] In the last few years several reports analyzing the pattern of regeneration in the living donor remaining liver and in the recipient liver segment have been published. An evolving consensus from these data is that the pattern of regeneration is not identical in the donor and recipient after the hepatectomy and implantation of the graft. Because several of the immune suppressants used for LDLT recipients are known to interfere with cytokine upregulation (steroids) growth factor actions (Rapamycin and calcineurins) it is possible to speculate that some of the differences could be related to immune suppression use in the recipients. Other factors known or suspected to affect the regenerative process include

portal pressure and graft size to recipient size ratio. Portal venous pressure has been studied clinically following LDLT and its impact of hepatic regeneration examined. Pressure in the portal vein of 20 mm Hg or greater was associated with rapid liver hypertrophy, and a higher peripheral blood hepatocyte growth factor level. Both these changes were associated with graft dysfunction, hyperbilirubinemia, coagulopathy, and ascites. Thus, in patients with elevated portal pressure at the time of LDLT, modifications of immune suppression such as induction with anti-CD25 antibodies with delayed introduction of the hepatically metabolized calcinuerins may be considered. Reduced graft size in relation to body size could lead to the development of small-for-size syndrome, which is later discussed in detail.

## IMMUNE SUPPRESSION IN LDLT RECIPIENTS WITH HEPATITIS C

A major advantage of living donor availability for a hepatitis C recipient is that the waiting period before transplantation can be used to render the recipient negative for HCV RNA.[35] Transplantation of HCV RNA-negative recipients is associated with low risk (40%) of posttransplant recurrence of hepatitis C infection.[36] Viral eradication and immediate transplantation using a living donor at an early stage when the patient can better tolerate the antiviral treatment could afford significant advantage to the subset of patients with successful response to antiviral therapy. Balanced immune suppression in this group of patients is crucial to keep low recurrence rates and minimize graft rejection. A major concern with LDLT for patients with persistent hepatitis C viral infections is related to the suggestion that regeneration in the transplanted graft can predispose those individuals to a more aggressive recurrence of HCV hepatitis. Two large retrospective studies, to date, have shown that the incidence and severity of HCV recurrence do not differ between cadaveric and LDLT.[37,38] However, one study has found that the incidence of fibrosing cholestatic hepatitis, a particularly virulent form of recurrence of HCV, is greater in LDLT recipients.[39] Recently a comparison of protocol biopsies from 23 LDLT and 53 deceased donor transplant recipients found no significant difference in the degree of hepatic inflammation in both groups with similar or less fibrosis in the LDLT group.[38]

Because HCV can progresses rapidly after liver transplantation the choice and extent of immunosuppression has been an area of controversy. Most studies have shown that the chance and severity of HCV recurrence are similar whether cyclosporine or tacrolimus are used.[40,41] Data with MMF are conflicting with some reports showing improved outcomes, whereas others show worse outcome. Similarly, although there are several reports indicating a negative effect of steroids on hepatitis C recurrence other reports indicate that small doses of steroids may be associated with decreased graft fibrosis. The current consensus is that it is the overall intensity of immunosuppression that affects HCV outcomes.[42] For example, high-dose or bolus steroid therapy and treatment with antilymphocyte or anti IL-2 receptor preparations is associated with rapid progression to cirrhosis, cholestatic hepatitis, and graft failure in patients with HCV.[40,42,43] Several reports have shown that treatment of rejection in this subset of patients is associated with decrease survival. Therefore, a restrained response involving increasing the CNI doses or the addition of MMF may be preferable to the use of steroids or antibodies when rejection is suspected. This is of particular relevance in the LDLT recipient where early rejection is particularly dangerous as it impacts regeneration and graft adaptation, whereas aggressive immune suppressive therapy also affects hepatic regeneration and increases HCV recurrence. Changes in the level of immunosuppression in the hepatitis C patients are most deleterious because they increase viral replication during periods intense immunosuppression, followed by allowing immune recognition and clearance of virally infected allograft cells during rapid immunosuppression withdrawal.[42] It thus seems that the best approach to LDLT recipients is to have adequate early immunosuppression to minimize the possibility of acute rejection. This is followed by a very gradual taper to avoid the need for intense treatment of rejection that could be precipitated by rapid immune suppression withdrawal.

## IMMUNE SUPPRESSION IN PATIENTS WITH SMALL-FOR-SIZE SYNDROME

Small-for-size is a clinical syndrome that occurs following segmental liver transplantation and extended hepatectomy. The syndrome is characterized by postoperative coagulopathy, liver dysfunction, poor bile production, delayed synthetic function, prolonged cholestasis, and intractable ascites leading to increased susceptibility to septic complications and mortality due to insufficient functional liver mass. Prevention is based on performing a meticulous preoperative evaluation of functional liver mass, liver quality, portal pressure, and variations in surgical technique to ensure a graft-to-recipient body-weight ratio equal or greater than 0.8% or graft-weight ratio equal or greater than 30% of standard liver volume. Other than supportive therapy during the prolonged cholestasis or retransplantation, there is no known treatment for this syndrome. Of particular importance in adult-to-adult living donor transplantation is the determination of whether the graft is a right hepatic vein dominant lobe or a middle hepatic vein dominant lobe. Tanaka et al. have proposed that in cases of small for size grafts or of middle-hepatic-vein-dominant grafts a larger right lobe graft including the middle hepatic should be utilized as long as the remnant liver volume is enough to sustain life in the donor.[44] In our center, we have resisted procuring a larger right lobe graft with the middle hepatic vein because of concern for donor safety. Our practice is to perform individual reconstruction of the veins draining segment 5 and 8 instead of taking the middle hepatic vein and to evaluate another donor if small for size graft is suspected.[45]

Management of immune suppression in patients with small-for-size syndrome is critical. Despite several hepatic dysfunctions, there is no evidence to date that the liver is less likely to undergo rejection during this period. In fact, there are unconfirmed reports that early administration of calcineurins can ameliorate hepatic injury.[46] On the other hand, because septic mortality dominates the pathophysiology of this syndrome high immune suppression levels are dangerous. Once the small-for-size syndrome occurs the trend is to decrease the overall amount of immunosuppression. Our reasoning is that a dysfunctional small graft is not as efficient as a healthy-size graft in metabolizing drugs. CNIs are excreted in the bile, and poor bile excretion during the period of cholestasis allows infrequent (once every few days) administration of very small doses based on level monitoring. One has to recognize also that other drug handling is seriously impaired in these situations such as prophylactic drugs for fungal (Diflucan) pneumocystis (Bactrim) and bacterial infections (antibiotics). Variable pharmacokinetics and interactions between the medications could complicate immune suppression management.

## IMMUNE SUPPRESSION IN PATIENTS WITH HEPATOCELLULAR CARCINOMA AND LDLT

The incidence of hepatocellular carcinoma (HCC) in North America increased from 1.4 to 3.0 cases per 100,000 persons per year, primarily because of an increase in the incidence of hepatitis C.[47] Transplantation has become one of the few curative treatment modalities for patients with HCC, especially in patients with favorable tumors.[48–50] The advent of living donor liver transplantation for adult recipients provides another major therapeutic option, in patients with HCC. Living donor transplantation may limit the transplant waiting time and, as a result, decrease the chance for progression of hepatocellular cancers. The new allocation policy of the United Network of Organ Sharing[51] gives candidates with hepatocellular carcinoma a priority MELD score beyond their degree of hepatic decompensation. This policy has led to a significant decrease in the waiting time of HCC patients from 2.28 years to 0.69 years.[51] In a recent study Sarasin et al.[52] calculated that living donor liver transplantation provides superior recipient outcomes than cadaveric liver transplantation when cadaveric transplant waiting times are longer than 7 months.

Two groups of hepatocellular cancer patients may still be candidates for LDLT. The first is patients with HCC smaller than 2 cm. These patients are not currently being allowed a status upgrade in the United States. A second group is that of patients with HCC who exceed the Milan criteria but are within the limits of expanded criteria (solitary lesions less than 6.5 cm or up to three tumors with the largest no more than 4.5 cm and the combined tumor diameter no more than 8 cm).[53] These patients do not get a status upgrade in the United States despite acceptable reported survival rates following transplantation. Immune suppression considerations in the HCC LDLT recipient are currently evolving. There is, as of yet, no formal indication of changing the immunosuppression in the HCC patient. Most HCC cases are associated with Hepatitis C or B, and this should be taken into account when the immunosuppression protocol is being tailored for individuals with HCV and HCC. Rapamycin and its derivatives are promising therapeutic agents with both immunosuppressant and antitumor properties.[54] These rapamycin actions are mediated through the specific inhibition of the mTOR protein kinase. The mTOR signaling network contains a number of tumor suppressor genes including PTEN, LKB1, TSC1, and TSC2, and a number of proto-oncogenes including PI3K, Akt, and eIF4E, and mTOR signaling is constitutively activated in many tumor types.[54] Rapamycin appears to inhibit tumor growth by halting tumor cell proliferation, inducing tumor cell apoptosis, and suppressing tumor angiogenesis. The immunosuppressant actions of Rapamycin result from inhibition of T- and B- cell proliferation through the same mTOR mechanisms that block cancer cell proliferation. It is important to note that Rapamycin should be introduced in a conversion protocol weeks after transplantation to avoid its inhibitory effect on hepatic regeneration and to avoid any possible problems with arterial flow. Up to now there are not enough clinical data to support the utilization of Rapamycin in all patients with HCC or other types of cancer and more studies to justify its systematic application are needed.

Another consideration in the immune suppression management of HCC patients following LDLT is related to the concomitant use of cancer chemotherapy in the postoperative period. Careful planning of timing, type, and degree of immune suppression should be undertaken in these situations. The timing of cancer chemotherapy should be coordinated to avoid interference with liver regeneration and to allow the graft time to achieve its maximum potential hyperplasia. It should be remembered that chemotherapeutic agents themselves impact the immune system, and most of them can interact with posttransplant immune suppression drugs leading to increased toxicities of both drug classes. It is thus prudent to consider decreasing overall immune suppression together with possible discontinuation of drugs that are likely to potentiate the side effects of the cancer chemotherapeutic used. The effects of combining chemotherapeutics and immune suppressants on coexisting hepatitis B or C should also be closely monitored.

## ABO-INCOMPATIBLE AND HLA COMPATIBILITY IN LIVING DONOR LIVER TRANSPLANTATION

The most important transplantation antigen system in solid organ transplantation is the ABO blood group system. ABO-incompatible liver transplants have been associated with a high risk of antibody-mediated rejection, poor patient and graft survival, and a high risk of vascular thrombosis and ischemic bile duct complications. In the United States, transplantation crossing the ABO barrier in solid organ transplantation is usually not done except for critically ill patient situations. Because of the difficulties in performing deceased donor liver transplantation in Asia and the lack of enough living donors transplant centers are more liberal in the utilization of LDLT from ABO incompatible donors.[55,56] Special protocols have been developed to increase utilization of ABO incompatible donors. These protocols employ a variable combination of prospective recipient treatment with Rituximab, plasma exchange, splenectomy and intra-arterial infusion of PGE1. Recently the Kyoto group published a protocol of intraarterial PGE1 infusion and rituximab with preservation of the spleen.[57] Eight patients received Rituximab at 2 to 14 days before LDLT. Methylprednisolone and PGE1 were administered via a hepatic artery catheter for 2 to 3 weeks after LDLT in addition to an immunosuppressive regimen consisting of tacrolimus and steroids. No episodes of humoral rejection were found although two patients died of causes unrelated to rejection. In 2003, Hanto et al[58] published the experience at University of Cincinnati with ABO-incompatible donors using pretransplantation and posttransplantation double-volume total plasma exchange, splenectomy, and quadruple immunosuppression (cyclophosphamide or mycophenolate mofetil, prednisone, cyclosporine or tacrolimus, and OKT3 induction) in 14 patients. Actuarial 1- and 5-year patient and graft survival rates are 71.4% and 61.2 %, and 71.4% and 61.2%, respectively, with a mean follow-up of 62.9 +/- 39.4 months. Ten acute cellular rejections occurred, and the mean time to the first episode was 62 +/- 33 days. All were steroid sensitive. No antibody-mediated rejection or vascular thromboses occurred.[58]

## HLA MATCHING AND REJECTION IN LDLT

Human leukocyte antigen (HLA) matching is, at present, not used for the allocation of cadaveric liver allografts. However, the exact role of HLA compatibility in the long-term outcome of liver transplantation is not yet clearly defined. It has been hypothesized that improved HLA matching may be associated with lower rates of rejection in LDLT, but more aggressive recurrence of viral and autoimmune liver diseases. Other reports indicated a beneficial effect of mismatching some HLA class II specificities.[59] The overall rates of rejection in LDLT are reported between 10% and 25% in

adults and 40% and 80% in children.[59,60] Kasahara et al. published in 2004 that among 324 ABO-compatible pediatric LDLT patients, the cumulative 5-year graft survivals in HLA 0-, 1-, 2- and 3-mismatch groups (A, B, and DR) were 100% (n = 10), 78.9% (n = 19), 86.2% (n = 87), and 82.9% (n = 205), respectively (P = 0.525). The overall incidence of rejection during the follow-up period (median 66 months, range 16–139 months) was 46.1%. No significant differences were found in the incidence of rejection and rejection-free survival among the four groups. Importantly, however, the trough level of tacrolimus needed for maintenance during the chronic phase tended to be lower in well-matched pairs, and a high percentage of immunosuppressant-free patients were found in the 0-mismatch group.[61] Another study from the Tokyo group demonstrated in a pediatric population that patients with HLA zero mismatching had a significantly lower chance of rejection within 6 weeks after LDLT.[62] Further confirmation of the role of HLA matching in liver rejection came from Germany where 924 cadaveric liver transplant recipients in which the donor–recipient HLA typing was retrospectively analyzed. Although the number of HLA compatibilities had no influence on graft survival, the number of acute rejections was significantly less in transplants with more HLA compatibilities (P < 0.05).[63]

The relationship between the incidence of acute rejection and lymphocytotoxic cross-matching was examined in 100 patients. Patients with HLA DR zero mismatching (p = 0.02) or negative T-lymphocytotoxic crossmatch (p = 0.04) had a significantly lower chance of rejection within 6 weeks after LDLT. However the results had no influence on the patient survival.[64] The clinical relevance of antidonor humoral immunity for living donor liver transplantation by means of flow cytometry crossmatch was examined in 58 patients. Twelve patients (20.7%) showed positive posttransplantation flow cytometry crossmatch. The incidence of acute rejection within 1 month was 100% in flow cytometry crossmatch positive patients and 17.4% in flow cytometry crossmatch negative patients (P < 0.001). This may suggest a role for donor-specific humoral immunity in acute rejection.[65] In contrast, two other reports found a similar rate of cellular rejection among pediatric patients who received a cadaveric or a living-related graft; however, in one of these reports, the rate of steroid-resistant rejection was lower in the living related group. Although the use of related donors has not yet proven to provide an immunologic benefit, larger studies with longer periods of follow-up are needed to more fully explore this issue.

## PEDIATRIC LDLT OUTCOMES AND IMMUNE SUPPRESSION

Analyzing the U.S. scientific registry of transplants evaluating recipients who received a first liver transplant from 1989 to 2000 demonstrated that in patients less than 2 years old, living donor liver transplantation was associated with significant reduction in risk of graft failure compared to deceased donor split and deceased donor full liver grafts during the first year after transplant.[66] Similar results were shown for the time period from 1996 to 1999 and for all pediatric recipients (aged <18 years).[67,68] Basic immune suppression protocols in pediatric recipients are similar to those employed in adults. In children, however, steroid withdrawal to prevent growth retardation is much more widely practiced. Surveillance of children treated by calcineurins for EBV viral infections and appropriate prophylaxis and treatment is essential to prevent the development of post transplant lymphoproliferative disorder.[69] Because differences in lymphocyte regeneration rates dosages of T-cell-active drugs have to be monitored closely in children to prevent breakthrough rejections that were noticed with the anti-CD$_3$ monoclonal OKT$_3$.

# ACKNOWLEDGMENT

This work was supported in part by a grant funded by Astellas: "Evaluation of a corticosteroid-free maintenance immunosuppression regimen in cadaveric liver transplant recipients."

# References

1. Jassem W, Koo DD, Cerundolo L, et al. Cadaveric versus living-donor livers: differences in inflammatory markers after transplantation. *Transplantation* 2003;76(11):1599–1603.
2. Golling M, Mehrabi A, Blum K, et al. Effects of hemodynamic instability on brain death-induced prepreservation liver damage. *Transplantation* 2003;75(8):1154–1159.
3. http://www.optn.org/data.
4. Grewal HP, Thistlewaite JR Jr, Loss GE, et al. Complications in 100 living-liver donors. *Ann Surg* 1998;228(2):214–219.
5. Whitington PF. Living donor liver transplantation: ethical considerations. *J Hepatol* 1996;24(5):625–627.
6. Lo CM, Fan ST, Liu CL, Wei WI, Lo RJ, Lai CL et al. Adult-to-adult living donor liver transplantation using extended right lobe grafts. *Ann Surg* 1997;226(3):261-269; discussion 269–270.
7. Inomoto T, Nishizawa F, Sasaki H, et al. Experiences of 120 microsurgical reconstructions of hepatic artery in living related liver transplantation. *Surgery* 1996;119(1):20–26.
8. Reding R, de Goyet Jde V, Delbeke I, et al. Pediatric liver transplantation with cadaveric or living related donors: comparative results in 90 elective recipients of primary grafts. *J Pediatr* 1999;134(3):280–286.
9. Inomata Y, Uemoto S, Asonuma K, Egawa H. Right lobe graft in living donor liver transplantation. *Transplantation* 2000;69(2):258–264.
10. Kehrer BH, Whitington PF, Black DD. The effect of Roux-en-Y biliary enterostomy on the absorption of cyclosporine: relevance to poor drug bioavailability in children after orthotopic liver transplantation. *Transplant Proc* 1988;20(2 Suppl 2):523–528.
11. Perry I, Neuberger J. Immunosuppression: towards a logical approach in liver transplantation. *Clin Exp Immunol* 2005;139(1):2–10.
12. Serrano J, Garcia Gonzalez M, Gomez M, et al. Tacrolimus is effective in both dual and triple regimens after liver transplantation. *Transplant Proc* 2002;34(5):1529–1530.
13. Lin CC, Chuang FR, Lee CH, et al. The renal-sparing efficacy of basiliximab in adult living donor liver transplantation. *Liver Transpl* 2005;11(10):1258–1264.
14. Schuller S, Wiederkehr JC, Coelho-Lemos IM, Avilla SG, Schultz C. Daclizumab induction therapy associated with tacrolimus-MMF has better outcome compared with tacrolimus-MMF alone in pediatric living donor liver transplantation. *Transplant Proc* 2005;37(2):1151–1152.
15. Levy G, Villamil F, Samuel D, et al. Results of lis2t, a multicenter, randomized study comparing cyclosporine microemulsion with C2 monitoring and tacrolimus with C0 monitoring in de novo liver transplantation. *Transplantation* 2004;77(11):1632–1638.
16. A comparison of tacrolimus (FK 506) and cyclosporine for immunosuppression in liver transplantation. The U.S. Multicenter FK506 Liver Study Group. *N Engl J Med* 1994;331(17):1110–1115.
17. O'Grady JG, Burroughs A, Hardy P, Elbourne D, Truesdale A. Tacrolimus versus microemulsified ciclosporin in liver transplantation: the TMC randomised controlled trial. *Lancet* 2002;360(9340):1119–1125.
18. Fisher RA, Ham JM, Marcos A, Shiffman ML, Luketic VA, Kimball PM et al. A prospective randomized trial of mycophenolate mofetil with neoral or tacrolimus after orthotopic liver transplantation. *Transplantation* 1998;66(12):1616–1621.
19. Wiesner R, Rabkin J, Klintmalm G, et al. A randomized double-blind comparative study of mycophenolate mofetil and azathioprine in combination with cyclosporine and corticosteroids in primary liver transplant recipients. *Liver Transpl* 2001;7(5):442–450.
20. Weisner R. Rapamune Liver Transplant Study Group - The safety and efficacy of sirolimus and low-dose tacrolimus versus tacrolimus in denovo orthoptic liver transplant recipients. Results for a pilot study [Abstract]. *Hepatology*;36:208A.
21. Liu CL, Fan ST, Lo CM, Chan SC, Ng IO, Lai CL et al. Interleukin-2 receptor antibody (basiliximab) for immunosuppressive induction therapy after liver transplantation: a protocol with early elimination of steroids and reduction of tacrolimus dosage. *Liver Transpl* 2004;10(6):728–733.
22. Abe M, Fuchinoue S, Koike T, Sato S, Uchida Y, Murakami T et al. Successful prednisone withdrawal after living-related liver transplantation. *Transplant Proc* 1998;30(4):1441–1442.
23. Tzakis AG, Tryphonopoulos P, Kato T, Nishida S, Levi DM, Madariaga JR et al. Preliminary experience with alemtuzumab (Campath-1H) and low-dose tacrolimus immunosuppression in adult liver transplantation. *Transplantation* 2004;77(8):1209–1214.
24. Takatsuki M, Uemoto S, Inomata Y, Egawa H, Kiuchi T, Fujita S et al. Weaning of immunosuppression in living donor liver transplant recipients. Transplantation 2001;72(3):449–454.
25. www.immunetolerance.org/research/solidorgantrials. In.
26. http://www.ustransplant.org/cgi-bin/ar?p_tables_10.htm&y 2003 Organ Procurement and Transplantation Network/Scientific Registry of Transplant Recipients Annual Report In.
27. Fung J, Kelly D, Kadry Z, Patel-Tom K, Eghtesad B. Immunosuppression in liver transplantation: beyond calcineurin inhibitors. *Liver Transpl* 2005;11(3):267–280.
28. Kaufman DB, Shapiro R, Lucey MR, Cherikh WS, R TB, Dyke DB. Immunosuppression: practice and trends. *Am J Transplant* 2004;4 Suppl 4:38–53.
29. Trotter JF, Stolpman N, Wachs M, I et al. Living donor liver transplant recipients achieve relatively higher immunosuppressant blood levels than cadaveric recipients. *Liver Transpl* 2002;8(3):212–218.
30. Taber DJ, Dupuis RE, Fann AL, et al. Tacrolimus dosing requirements and concentrations in adult living donor liver transplant recipients. *Liver Transpl* 2002;8(3):219–223.
31. Goto M, Masuda S, Kiuchi T, et al. CYP3A5*1-carrying graft liver reduces the concentration/oral dose ratio of tacrolimus in recipients of living-donor liver transplantation. *Pharmacogenetics* 2004;14(7):471–478.
32. Masuda S, Goto M, Okuda M, Ogura Y, Oike F, Kiuchi T et al. Initial dosage adjustment for oral administration of tacrolimus using the intestinal MDR1 level in living-donor liver transplant recipients. Transplant Proc 2005;37(4):1728–1729.
33. Sugawara Y, Makuuchi M, Kaneko J, Ohkubo T, Imamura H, Kawarasaki H. Correlation between optimal tacrolimus doses and the graft weight in living donor liver transplantation. Clin Transplant 2002;16(2):102–106.
34. Michalopoulos GK, DeFrances MC. Liver regeneration. *Science* 1997;276(5309):60–66.
35. Shergill AK, Khalili M, Straley S, et al. Applicability, tolerability and efficacy of preemptive antiviral therapy in hepatitis C-infected patients undergoing liver transplantation. *Am J Transplant* 2005;5(1):118–124.
36. Everson GT. Treatment of patients with hepatitis C virus on the waiting list. *Liver Transpl* 2003;9(11):S90–94.
37. Russo MW, Galanko J, Beavers K, Fried MW, Shrestha R. Patient and graft survival in hepatitis C recipients after adult living donor liver transplantation in the United States. *Liver Transpl* 2004;10(3):340–346.
38. Shiffman ML, Stravitz RT, Contos MJ, et al. Histologic recurrence of chronic hepatitis C virus in patients after living donor and deceased donor liver transplantation. *Liver Transpl* 2004;10(10):1248–1255.
39. Gaglio PJ, Malireddy S, Levitt BS, Lapointe-Rudow D, Lefkowitch J, Kinkhabwala M et al. Increased risk of cholestatic hepatitis C in recipients of grafts from living versus cadaveric liver donors. Liver Transpl 2003;9(10):1028–1035.
40. Charlton M, Seaberg E, Wiesner R, et al. Predictors of patient and graft survival following liver transplantation for hepatitis C. *Hepatology* 1998;28(3):823–830.

41. Ghobrial RM, Steadman R, Gornbein J, Lassman C, Holt CD, Chen P et al. A 10-year experience of liver transplantation for hepatitis C: analysis of factors determining outcome in over 500 patients. *Ann Surg* 2001;234(3):384-393; discussion 393–384.

42. Brown RS. Hepatitis C and liver transplantation. *Nature* 2005;436(7053): 973–978.

43. Nelson DR, Soldevila-Pico C, Reed A, et al. Anti-interleukin-2 receptor therapy in combination with mycophenolate mofetil is associated with more severe hepatitis C recurrence after liver transplantation. *Liver Transpl* 2001;7(12):1064–1070.

44. Kasahara M, Takada Y, Fujimoto Y, et al. Impact of right lobe with middle hepatic vein graft in living-donor liver transplantation. *Am J Transplant* 2005;5(6):1339–1346.

45. Shokouh-Amiri MH, Grewal HP, Vera SR, et al. Eighteen years of experience with adult and pediatric liver transplantation at the University of Tennessee, Memphis. *Clin Transpl* 2000:255–261.

46. Kato T, Sato Y, Kurasaki I, et al. FK506 may suppress liver injury during the early period following living-related liver transplantation. *Transplant Proc* 2003;35(1):79.

47. Befeler AS, Hayashi PH, Di Bisceglie AM. Liver transplantation for hepatocellular carcinoma. *Gastroenterology* 2005;128(6):1752–1764.

48. Colella G, De Carlis L, Rondinara GF, et al. Is hepatocellular carcinoma in cirrhosis an actual indication for liver transplantation? *Transplant Proc* 1997;29(1-2):492–494.

49. Jonas S, Bechstein WO, Steinmuller T, et al. Vascular invasion and histopathologic grading determine outcome after liver transplantation for hepatocellular carcinoma in cirrhosis. *Hepatology* 2001;33(5): 1080–1086.

50. Tamura S, Kato T, Berho M, et al. Impact of histological grade of hepatocellular carcinoma on the outcome of liver transplantation. *Arch Surg* 2001;136(1):25–30; discussion 31.

51. UNOS. http://www.unos.org Policy 3.6.4.4. Liver Transplant candidates with HCC.

52. Sarasin FP, Majno PE, Llovet JM, et al. Living donor liver transplantation for early hepatocellular carcinoma: A life-expectancy and cost-effectiveness perspective. *Hepatology* 2001;33(5):1073–1079.

53. Yao FY, Ferrell L, Bass NM, et al. Liver transplantation for hepatocellular carcinoma: expansion of the tumor size limits does not adversely impact survival. *Hepatology* 2001;33(6):1394–1403.

54. Law BK. Rapamycin: an anti-cancer immunosuppressant? *Crit Rev Oncol Hematol* 2005;56(1):47–60.

55. Kawagishi N, Satoh K, Enomoto Y, et al. New strategy for ABO-incompatible living donor liver transplantation with anti-CD20 antibody (rituximab) and plasma exchange. *Transplant Proc* 2005;37(2):1205–1206.

56. Kozaki K, Egawa H, Kasahara M, A et al. Therapeutic strategy and the role of apheresis therapy for ABO incompatible living donor liver transplantation. *Ther Apher Dial* 2005;9(4):285–291.

57. Yoshizawa A, Sakamoto S, Ogawa K, et al. New protocol of immunosuppression for liver transplantation across ABO barrier: the use of Rituximab, hepatic arterial infusion, and preservation of spleen. *Transplant Proc* 2005;37(4):1718–1719.

58. Hanto DW, Fecteau AH, Alonso MH, Valente JF, Whiting JF. ABO-incompatible liver transplantation with no immunological graft losses using total plasma exchange, splenectomy, and quadruple immunosuppression: evidence for accommodation. *Liver Transpl* 2003;9(1): 22–30.

59. Campos J, Quijano Y, Franco A, et al. Beneficial effects of HLA class II incompatibility in living donor liver transplantation. *Transplant Proc* 2003;35(5):1888–1891.

60. Ringe B, Moritz M, Zeldin G, Soriano H. What is the best immunosuppression in living donor liver transplantation? Transplant Proc 2005;37(5):2169–2171.

61. Kasahara M, Kiuchi T, Uryuhara K, Uemoto S, Fujimoto Y, Ogura Y et al. Role of HLA compatibility in pediatric living-related liver transplantation. *Transplantation* 2002;74(8):1175–1180.

62. Sugawara Y, Mizuta K, Kawarasaki H, et al. Risk factors for acute rejection in pediatric living related liver transplantation: the impact of HLA matching. *Liver Transpl* 2001;7(9):769–773.

63. Neumann UP, Guckelberger O, Langrehr JM, et al. Impact of human leukocyte antigen matching in liver transplantation. *Transplantation* 2003;75(1):132–137.

64. Sugawara Y, Makuuchi M, Kaneko J, et al. Risk factors for acute rejection in living donor liver transplantation. *Clin Transplant* 2003;17(4):347–352.

65. Kasahara M, Kiuchi T, Takakura K, et al. Postoperative flow cytometry crossmatch in living donor liver transplantation: clinical significance of humoral immunity in acute rejection. *Transplantation* 1999;67(4):568–575.

66. Roberts JP, Hulbert-Shearon TE, Merion RM, Wolfe RA, Port FK. Influence of graft type on outcomes after pediatric liver transplantation. *Am J Transplant* 2004;4(3):373–377.

67. Sindhi R, Rosendale J, Mundy D, et al. Impact of segmental grafts on pediatric liver transplantation—a review of the United Network for Organ Sharing Scientific Registry data (1990-1996). *J Pediatr Surg* 1999;34(1):107–110; discussion 110–101.

68. Thuluvath PJ, Yoo HY. Graft and patient survival after adult live donor liver transplantation compared to a matched cohort who received a deceased donor transplantation. *Liver Transpl* 2004;10(10):1263–1268.

69. Egawa H, Ohishi T, Arai T, et al. Application of in situ hybridization technique for quantitative assessment of ongoing symptomatic Epstein-Barr virus infection after living related liver transplantation. *Clin Transplant* 1998;12(2):116–122.

# 30.11  IMMUNOBIOLOGY

*Kenneth J. Woodside, MD,*
*John A. Daller, MD, PhD*

## INTRODUCTION

Living-related liver transplantation (LRLT) has increased in frequency over the last decade. Although adult-to-pediatric engraftments are more common, adult-to-adult transplants are also increasing. Although pediatric LRLT may have improved outcome,[1] long-term adult-to-adult LRLT data are still lacking. LRLT recipients may suffer fewer episodes of acute rejection and delayed graft function,[1–4] suggesting that the immunobiology of the LRLT may be more favorable. LRLT grafts, in contrast to deceased donor organs, are electively procured from healthy donors, with minimal ischemic time and little exposure to the multifactorial ravages of critical illness and brain death that are common in deceased donors, resulting in reduced inflammatory signal.[5] Although somewhat hypothetical, a number of factors may contribute to an improved immunological profile for LRLT recipients, including absence of prolonged ischemia time, avoidance of the physiological changes that accompany brain death and whatever mechanism caused the death of the cadaveric donor, and differing surgical techniques for procurement. In addition, while human leukocyte antigen (HLA) matching seems to have little effect on liver graft survival,[6] there may be benefit from the frequent familial relationship of the living donor. This chapter focuses on the immunological differences for the recipient of organs from living-related and cadaveric liver allografts.

## DONOR EFFECTS

Physiological changes that occur in the allograft may contribute to a more robust immunological response by the recipient following engraftment. Deceased donors have enhanced adhesion molecule expression after cold storage, as well as greater T lymphocyte and monocyte infiltration (Figures 30.11-1A and 30.11-1B).[7,8]

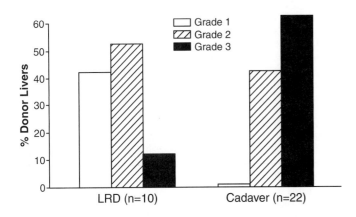

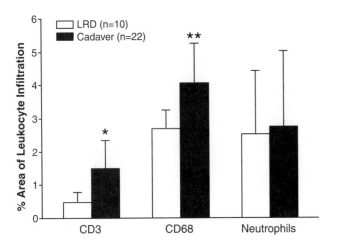

**FIGURE 30.11-1**

A. Expression of ICAM-1 on cadaveric livers and living-related livers before transplantation. Liver biopsies from cadaveric and living-related livers were stained with an anti-ICAM-1 monoclonal antibody, and the staining was assessed semiquantitatively. Cadaveric livers expressed higher levels of ICAM-1 (grade 3) compared with living-related livers (P = 0.02). (With permission from Jassem W, et al. Leukocyte infiltration and inflammatory antigen expression in cadaveric and living-donor livers before transplant. *Transplantation* 75:2001–2007, 2003, Lippincott Williams & Wilkins, Inc.) B. Leukocyte infiltration in cadaveric liver and living-related livers before transplantation. Cadaveric and living-related livers biopsies were stained with monoclonal antibodies against CD3, CD68, and neutrophil elastase; and the percentage area of positivity was calculated by morphometric point counting. Significantly higher levels of CD3+ lymphocytes (*P = 0.00004) and CD68+ Kupffer cells (**P = 0.0003) were detected in cadaveric livers compared with living-related livers. There were no significant differences in neutrophil infiltration between cadaveric and LRD livers before transplantation (P = 0.8). (With permission from Jassem W, et al. Leukocyte infiltration and inflammatory antigen expression in cadaveric and living-donor livers before transplant. *Transplantation* 75:2001–2007, 2003, Lippincott Williams & Wilkins, Inc.)

These changes may be the result of the usual critical illness of the donor,[7,9] as well as the alterations in expression of adhesion molecules and inflammatory cytokines caused by brain death.[10,11] Furthermore, brain death enhances hemodynamic instability as a result of perturbation of the normal hypothalamic–pituitary axis, further exacerbating this cascade. Inflammatory changes in the deceased donor result in hepatocyte damage and apoptosis, as well as Kupffer cell activation. These events, occurring after

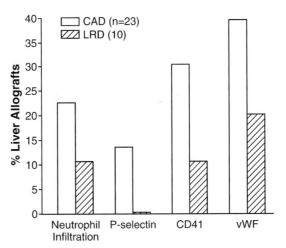

**FIGURE 30.11-2**

Percentage of cadaver (CAD) (n = 23) and living-related donor (n = 10) liver transplants with increases in P-selectin, CD41, and von Willebrand factor (vWF) expression and neutrophil infiltration after engraftment and reperfusion. (With permission from Jassem W, et al. Cadaveric versus living-donor livers: differences in inflammatory markers after transplantation. *Transplantation* 76:1599–1603, 2003, Lippincott Williams & Wilkins, Inc.)

brain death but before reperfusion, increase the susceptibility of the organ to damage following reperfusion (Figures 30.11-2 and 30.11-3).[9,11–17] Furthermore, steatosis is more likely to be present in the deceased donor liver, as such living donor candidates would likely be excluded from donating. Steatosis, amplified by the effects of brain death, can result in an increased rate of primary graft dysfunction.[18,19] In contrast, the living-donor liver is not subjected to many of these changes,[7,8,13] resulting in a much less immunologically primed organ at the time of engraftment.

## SURGICAL MANIPULATION

Manipulation of the liver *in vivo* and *ex vivo* are likewise thought to result in hypoxia, inflammation, and stress response (Figure 30.11-4).[20–24] Most centers avoid early vascular cross-clamping during the donor operation[25] to minimize warm ischemia time and the resulting ischemia-reperfusion injury initiated on revascularization in the recipient. In particular, partial hepatectomy results in increased interleukin-6 (IL-6) and C-reactive protein expression,[26] both key constituents of the acute-phase response. Interestingly, IL-6 levels are elevated to a lesser degree in LRLT donors than in patients undergoing hepatectomy for hepatocellular carcinoma. Whether this difference is the result of a blunted increase due to the underlying cirrhosis present in the hepatocellular carcinoma group or to enhanced expression due to the better health of the donor group has not been determined. In addition, a number of technical and temporal aspects of both the donor and the recipient operation can result in hepatocyte damage (eg, biliary obstruction, prolonged operative time, or transfusion requirements) and result in increased inflammation and risk of rejection.[27–29]

### Ischemia-Reperfusion Injury

Cold storage injury is initiated in the donor at the time of cross-clamping, and is amplified by ischemia-reperfusion injury following revascularization of the organ. Traditionally, the end-organ

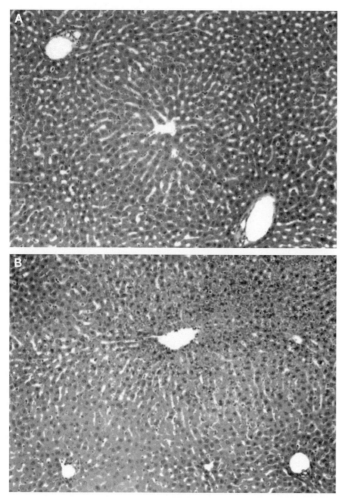

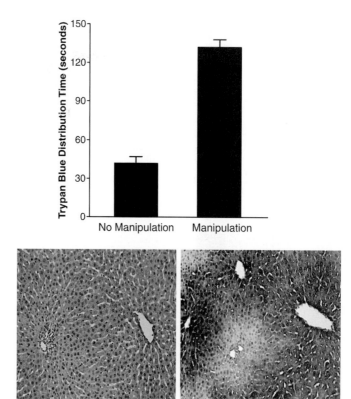

**FIGURE 30.11-3**

Biopsies of rat livers 1 h after syngeneic orthotopic transplantation. (A) Liver retrieved from a non-brain-dead donor, cold stored for 20 hr in University of Wisconsin (UW) solution before transplantation; normal histology. (B) Liver retrieved from a brain-dead donor, cold stored for 20 hours in UW solution before transplantation; vacuolization of the hepatocytes and pericentral necrosis is evident. (With permission from van der Hoeven, JA, et al. Donor brain death reduces survival after transplantation in rat livers preserved for 20 hours. *Tranplantation* 72:1632–1636, 2001, Lippincott Williams & Wilkins, Inc.)

**FIGURE 30.11-4**

Effects of surgical manipulation during harvest on microcirculation and lobular pattern of pimonidazole binding. (A) After harvest, livers were perfused with trypan blue *in situ* to index microcirculation. Values are mean ± SEM. (B) To detect hypoxia in liver tissue, pimonidazole, a hypoxia marker, was injected 5 minutes before the donor operation. At the end of experiments, livers were fixed with 10% formalin by perfusion. Immunohistochemistry was performed using antibodies to bound pimonidazole. Photomicrographs depict patterns of pimonidazole binding (dark staining) in livers after harvest. (With permission from Schemmer P, et al. New aspects on reperfusion injury to liver—impact of organ harvest. *Nephrol Dial Transplant* 19 (Suppl 4): iv26–iv35, 2004, The European Renal Association-European Dialysis and Transplant Association)

damage was thought to be superoxide respiratory burst, endothelial leak, and inflammation. However, recent studies suggest that the injury is partially mediated by apoptotic mechanisms.[30–34] Although the exact mechanism is unclear, apoptosis and adhesion molecule up-regulation is readily apparent on cold storage[7,8,16] and likely progresses after reperfusion and exposure to recipient lymphocytes.[30,35] Following reperfusion, endothelial swelling, microcirculation narrowing, and platelet deposition occur.[36] Organs procured from living related liver donors experience minimal postreperfusion changes, whereas livers from deceased donors demonstrate more neutrophil infiltration, P-selectin up-regulation, and platelet deposition[13] following reperfusion. However, the deceased organs were exposed to longer cold ischemia times in this study, and those with longer cold ischemia times had increased episodes of acute rejection. Thus, it is possible that the differences are not inherent to the donor status. However, overall hepatocellular and endothelial cell

damage is reduced for LRLT when compared to deceased liver recipients.[37]

IL-6 expression is increased in both the donor and the recipient[26,37] following operation. It serves also as a primary growth factor for hepatocytes[38] and reverses the impaired regenerative response following normothermic liver ischemia or transplantation.[39,40] Interestingly, sustained cold ischemia in a rat model of partial liver transplantation resulted in impaired IL-6 and tumor necrosis factor-α production, resulting in impaired liver regeneration (Figure 30.11-5).[41] As mentioned earlier, partial hepatectomy resulted in increased interleukin-6 (IL-6) and C-reactive protein expression,[26] although these elevated IL-6 levels were lower in LRLT donors than in patients undergoing hepatectomy for hepatocellular carcinoma. IL-6 and hepatocyte growth factor also increases after LRLT in the recipient (Figure 30.11-6),[42] suggesting an intriguing mechanism for liver regeneration following engraftment.

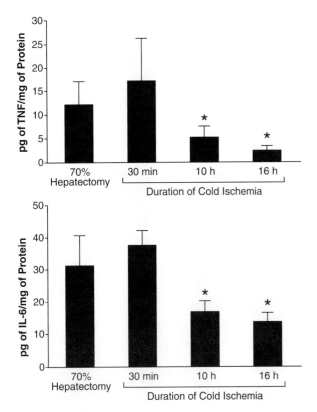

**FIGURE 30.11-5**

Effects of cold preservation on TNF-α and IL-6 levels in rat liver tissue. Tissue levels of (A) TNF-α and (B) IL-6 three hours after transplantation were significantly lower in rats with longer times of cold preservation (10 and 16 hours) compared with the respective control groups (70% liver resection alone). In contrast, short times of cold preservation (30 minutes) were associated with increased (although not statistically significant) levels compared with control (n = 5 in each group; *P ≤ .05, ANOVA). (With permission from Selzner N, et al. Cold ischemia decreases liver regeneration after partial liver transplantation in the rat: a TNF-α/IL-6-dependent mechanism. *Hepatology* 36:812–818, 2002, Wiley & Sons, Inc.)

## Hyperacute and Acute Rejection

Although the liver is thought to be relatively resistant to antibody-mediated rejection when compared to other organs, it is possible that reduced-size liver allografts may be at more risk when compared to deceased allografts.[43–45] In animal models, sensitized rats experience an increased risk of antibody-mediated rejection of reduced-size liver allografts, with histology suggestive of a hyperacute rejection pattern,[43] possibly from activation of sinusoidal endothelial cells and Kupffer cells. Larger human studies have not revealed any significant differences, however.

The perceived decrease in acute cellular rejection episodes that may be present in LRLT recipients is controversial.[5,46] It is hypothesized that closer HLA matching between the living-related donor and recipient should reduce the likelihood of rejection. However, most studies do not support a large clinical difference between these groups.[4,25,46–52] In a study of 100 pediatric primary liver transplant patients, overall rejection was observed to be similar (78% vs 68% in deceased and living-related groups, respectively). However, rejection episodes that occurred more than 1 year posttransplant were reduced in the LRLT group (22% vs 0%; Table 30.11-1).[4] Furthermore, the LRLT group was more likely to succeed in having their immunosuppression reduced. Other studies have suggested that LRLT recipients are less likely to develop steroid-resistant rejection.[47]

As in deceased donor liver transplants, the benefit of HLA matching has been difficult to demonstrate in LRLT and remains controversial.[5,6,50,53] Although some studies demonstrate limited benefit from zero mismatch pairs,[6,54] actual tangible clinical benefit seems to be limited to the need for somewhat less immunosuppression (eg, lower tacrolimus levels) or slightly lower acute rejection rates—if present at all.[6,50,54] For LRLT, it has been suggested, although not conclusively demonstrated, that increased mismatch may increase the risk of chronic rejection, however.[6]

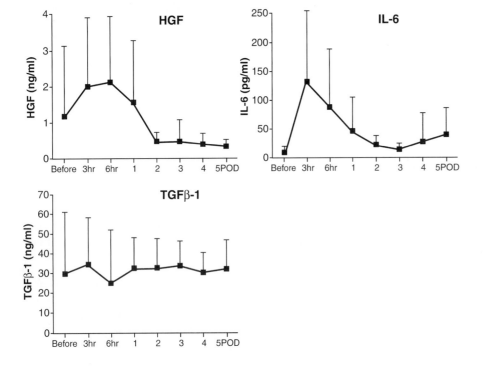

**FIGURE 30.11-6**

Changes of serum levels of HGF, IL-6, and TGF-β1 in 14 LRLT cases with no complications. Levels of HGF increased 3 hours after reperfusion and decreased to below 1 ng/mL at POD 2. Levels of IL-6 reached maximum values at 3 hours after reperfusion, and then decreased rapidly. Levels of TGF-β1 showed no significant changes. (With permission from Asakura T, et al. Changes of serum cytokines associated with hepatic regeneration after living-related liver transplantation. *Transplantation Proc* 32:2199–2203, 2000, Elsevier Science Inc.)

**TABLE 30.11-1a**

| | Cadaveric Liver Transplant (n = 51) | LRLT (n = 37) | p-value |
|---|---|---|---|
| Recipients who were diagnosed rejection | 40 | 25 | NS |
| Rejection within 1 year post-Tx | 37 | 25 | NS |
| Rejection since 1 year post-Tx | 11 | 0 | P<0.05 |
| Switch to tacrolimus-based immunosuppression | 17 | 13 | NS |
| Graft loss due to rejection | 3 | 0 | NS |

[a]With permission from Toyoki, Y, et al. Allograft rejection in pediatric liver transplantation: comparison between cadaveric and living related donors. *Pediatr Transplantation* 2002, 6:301-307, Blackwell Munksgaard.

## Chronic Rejection

Chronic rejection rates are thought to be lower in LRLT when compared to deceased donor recipients, although the risk factors are overall similar to those for any liver allograft.[47,55] In a larger study of 285 pediatric liver transplant recipients with a total of 385 grafts, recipients of living-related grafts were significantly less likely to develop chronic rejection (4% vs 16% in the cadaveric group; Figure 30.11-7).[55] However, there were a couple of significant demographic differences between the groups, including more African American patients and patients with autoimmune hepatitis. There were similar incidences of CMV, PTLD, and number and histological grade of acute rejection episodes between the groups. Furthermore, the incidence of chronic rejection is somewhat high, even for the pediatric population.

## ORGAN ACCEPTANCE

### Immunosuppression

Most transplant centers utilize similar immunosuppressive regimens for LRLT as for deceased donor liver transplantation.[4,46,48,56,57] As described previously, LRLT patients are more

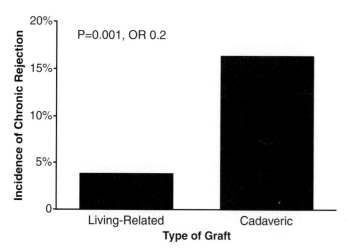

P=0.001, OR 0.2

**FIGURE 30.11-7**

Risk of chronic rejection versus type of graft. (With permission from Gupta P, et al. Risk factors for chronic rejection after pediatric liver transplantation. *Transplantation* 72:1098–1102, 2001, Lippincott Williams & Wilkins, Inc.)

likely to benefit from reduced immunosuppression—meaning that fewer patients are on triple-drug therapy.[4] As with other allografts, steroid avoidance may be beneficial.[57] Induction therapy with steroids, polyclonal antithymocyte globulin, anti-CD25 monoclonal antibody preparations, and even OKT3 has been described.[4,49,56–58] Larger studies are required to differentiate efficacy and safety between living-related and cadaveric liver transplant immunosuppressive protocols.

### Tolerance Mechanisms

Tolerance mechanisms for LRLT are likely similar to deceased donor transplants. For example, non-hepatitis-C liver transplant patients who experience an episode of early acute cellular rejection have improved long-term outcomes.[59–61] Hepatic allografts possess significant regenerative capacities when compared to other commonly transplanted organs, allowing the liver to repair damage from the rejection episode. It is likely that interleukin-2-dependent apoptosis of allospecifically activated lymphocytes occurs, thereby encouraging an acceptance reaction.[62–67] It is tempting to speculate that the decrease in late acute cellular rejection episodes seen in LRLT recipients results from this mechanism.[4,5] Similarly, mechanisms such as portal tolerance, wherein alloantigen infused via the portal vein results in allospecific tolerance, has been explored in the setting of adult living-related liver transplantation, resulting in decreased steroid and calcineurin inhibitor use in the portal infusion group.[68] Similarly, microchimerism has been described following pediatric LRLT,[69] presumably with the same immunological benefits.

## PEDIATRIC AND ADULT IMMUNE SYSTEMS

As is readily apparent from the references in this chapter, many of the immunological differences for living versus deceased liver allografts have been described in children. However, the pediatric and adult immune systems are different: pediatric and adult lymphocytes react differently, the adult thymus involutes, and so forth. Furthermore, the pediatric operation is more demanding—offering more possibilities of a technical fault that may lead to increased immunogenicity. Overall, pediatric liver recipients have higher rates of both acute and chronic rejection,[4,28,55] but the underlying systems are different. Additional studies exploring the differences of adult and pediatric LRLT are needed to better define both the technical and the immunological challenges inherent in the operation.

## References

1. Farmer DG, Yersiz H, Ghobrial RM, et al. Early graft function after pediatric liver transplantation: comparison between in situ split liver grafts and living-related liver grafts. *Transplantation* 2002;72:1795.
2. Chen CL, Fan ST, Lee SG, et al. Living-donor liver transplantation: 12 years of experience in Asia. *Transplantation* 2003;75:S6.
3. Lo CM. Complications and long-term outcome of living liver donors: a survey of 1,508 cases in five Asian centers. *Transplantation* 2003;75:S12.
4. Toyoki Y, Renz JF, Mudge C, et al. Allograft rejection in pediatric liver transplantation: Comparison between cadaveric and living related donors. *Pediatr Transplant* 2002;6:301.
5. Kelly DA, Goddard S. Is there any immunological advantage to living-related donor liver transplantation in pediatric recipients? *Pediatr Transplant* 2002;6:364.

6. Kasahara M, Kiuchi T, Uryuhara K, et al. Role of HLA compatibility in pediatric living-related liver transplantation. *Transplantation* 2002;74:1175.

7. Jassem W, Koo DD, Cerundolo L, et al. Leukocyte infiltration and inflammatory antigen expression in cadaveric and living-donor livers before transplant. *Transplantation* 2003;75:2001.

8. Jassem W, Koo DD, Muiesan P, et al. Non-heart-beating versus cadaveric and living-donor livers: differences in inflammatory markers before transplantation. *Transplantation* 2003;75:1386.

9. van der Hoeven JA, Ter Horst GJ, Molema G, et al. Effects of brain death and hemodynamic status on function and immunologic activation of the potential donor liver in the rat. *Ann Surg* 2000;232:804.

10. Toyama H, Takada M, Suzuki Y, et al. Brain death-induced expression of ICAM-1 and VCAM-1 on rat hepatocytes. *Hepatogastroenterology* 2003;50:1854.

11. van der Hoeven JA, Lindell S, van Schilfgaarde R, et al. Donor brain death reduces survival after transplantation in rat livers preserved for 20 hr. *Transplantation* 2001;72:1632.

12. Hu M, Woodside KJ, Thomas RP, et al. Altered PTHrP expression during cold storage with thymoglobulin. *Transplant Proc* 2002;34:1629.

13. Jassem W, Koo DD, Cerundolo L, et al. Cadaveric versus living-donor livers: differences in inflammatory markers after transplantation. *Transplantation* 2003;76:1599.

14. van der Hoeven JA, Moshage H, Schuurs T, et al. Brain death induces apoptosis in donor liver of the rat. *Transplantation* 2003;76:1150.

15. van der Hoeven JA, Ploeg RJ, Postema F, et al. Induction of organ dysfunction and up-regulation of inflammatory markers in the liver and kidneys of hypotensive brain dead rats: a model to study marginal organ donors. *Transplantation* 1999;68:1884.

16. Woodside KJ, Song J, Song W, et al. Immunomodulation of hepatic ischemic injury via increased Bcl-X(L) and decreased Bcl-X(S). *J Surg Res* 2003;112:59.

17. Zhang SJ, Chen S. The influence of brain death on liver in rats. *Transplant Proc* 2004;36:1925.

18. Fernandez-Merino FJ, Nuno-Garza J, Lopez-Hervas P, et al. Impact of donor, recipient, and graft features on the development of primary dysfunction in liver transplants. *Transplant Proc* 2003;35:1793.

19. Yamagami K, Hutter J, Yamamoto Y, et al. Synergistic effects of brain death and liver steatosis on the hepatic microcirculation. *Transplantation* 2005;80:500.

20. D'Alessandro AM, Stratta RJ, Southard JH, et al. Agonal hepatic arterial vasospasm. *Surg Gynecol Obstet* 1989;169:324.

21. Schemmer P, Connor HD, Arteel GE, et al. Reperfusion injury in livers due to gentle in situ organ manipulation during harvest involves hypoxia and free radicals. *J Pharmacol Exp Ther* 1999;290:235.

22. Schemmer P, Schoonhoven R, Swenberg JA, et al. Gentle in situ liver manipulation during organ harvest decreases survival after rat liver transplantation: role of Kupffer cells. *Transplantation* 1998;65:1015.

23. Schemmer P, Mehrabi A, Kraus T, et al. New aspects on reperfusion injury to liver—impact of organ harvest. *Nephrol Dial Transplant* 2004;19(Suppl 4):iv26, 2004.

24. Sollinger HW, Vernon WB, D'Alessandro AM, et al. Combined liver and pancreas procurement with Belzer-UW solution. *Surgery* 1989;106:685.

25. Lacaille F, Sokal E. Living-related liver transplantation. *J Pediatr Gastroenterol Nutr* 2001;33:431.

26. Lan AK, Luk HN, Goto S, et al. Stress response to hepatectomy in patients with a healthy or a diseased liver. *World J Surg* 2003;27:761.

27. Ghobrial RM, Amersi F, Busuttil RW. Surgical advances in liver transplantation. Living related and split donors. *Clin Liver Dis* 2000;4:553.

28. Otte JB. History of pediatric liver transplantation. Where are we coming from? Where do we stand? *Pediatr Transplant* 2002;6:378.

29. Tanaka K, Kiuchi T, Kaihara S. Living related liver donor transplantation: techniques and caution. *Surg Clin North Am* 2004;84:481.

30. Borghi-Scoazec G, Scoazec JY, Durand F, et al. Apoptosis after ischemia-reperfusion in human liver allografts. *Liver Transpl Surg* 1997;3:407.

31. Burns AT, Davies DR, McLaren AJ, et al. Apoptosis in ischemia/reperfusion injury of human renal allografts. *Transplantation* 1998;66:872.

32. Jain S, Bicknell GR, Whiting PH, et al. Rapamycin reduces expression of fibrosis-associated genes in an experimental model of renal ischaemia reperfusion injury. *Transplant Proc* 2001;33:556.

33. Jones EA, Shoskes DA. The effect of mycophenolate mofetil and polyphenolic bioflavonoids on renal ischemia reperfusion injury and repair. *J Urol* 2000;163:999.

34. Saxton NE, Barclay JL, Clouston AD, et al. Cyclosporin A pretreatment in a rat model of warm ischaemia/reperfusion injury. *J Hepatol* 2002;36:241.

35. Natori S, Selzner M, Valentino KL, et al. Apoptosis of sinusoidal endothelial cells occurs during liver preservation injury by a caspase-dependent mechanism. *Transplantation* 1999;68:89.

36. Serracino-Inglott F, Habib NA, Mathie RT. Hepatic ischemia-reperfusion injury. *Am J Surg* 2001;181:160.

37. Zhao X, Koshiba T, Fujimoto Y, et al. Proinflammatory and antiinflammatory cytokine production during ischemia-reperfusion injury in a case of identical twin living donor liver transplantation using no immunosuppression. *Transplant Proc* 2005;37:392.

38. Cressman DE, Greenbaum LE, DeAngelis RA, et al. Liver failure and defective hepatocyte regeneration in interleukin-6-deficient mice. *Science* 1996;274:1379.

39. Debonera F, Aldeguer X, Shen X, et al. Activation of interleukin-6/STAT3 and liver regeneration following transplantation. *J Surg Res* 2001;96:289.

40. Selzner M, Camargo CA, Clavien PA. Ischemia impairs liver regeneration after major tissue loss in rodents: protective effects of interleukin-6. *Hepatology* 1999;30:469.

41. Selzner N, Selzner M, Tian Y, et al. Cold ischemia decreases liver regeneration after partial liver transplantation in the rat: A TNF-alpha/IL-6-dependent mechanism. *Hepatology* 2002;36:812.

42. Asakura T, Ohkohchi N, Satomi S. Changes of serum cytokines associated with hepatic regeneration after living-related liver transplantation. *Transplant Proc* 2000;32:2199.

43. Astarcioglu I, Cursio R, Reynes M, et al. Increased risk of antibody-mediated rejection of reduced-size liver allografts. *J Surg Res* 1999;87:258.

44. Omura T, Nakagawa T, Randall HB, et al. Increased immune responses to regenerating partial liver grafts in the rat. *J Surg Res* 1997;70:34.

45. Shiraishi M, Csete ME, Yasunaga C, et al. Regeneration-induced accelerated rejection in reduced-size liver grafts. *Transplantation* 1994;57:336.

46. Encke J, Uhl W, Stremmel W, et al. Immunosuppression and modulation in liver transplantation. *Nephrol Dial Transplant* 2004;19(Suppl 4):iv22.

47. Alonso EM, Piper JB, Echols G, et al. Allograft rejection in pediatric recipients of living related liver transplants. *Hepatology* 1996;23:40.

48. Colombani PM, Lau H, Prabhakaran K, et al. Cumulative experience with pediatric living related liver transplantation. *J Pediatr Surg* 2000;35:9.

49. Evrard V, Otte JB, Sokal E, et al. Impact of surgical and immunological parameters in pediatric liver transplantation: a multivariate analysis in 500 consecutive recipients of primary grafts. *Ann Surg* 2004;239:272.

50. Reding R, de Goyet Jde V, Delbeke I, et al. Pediatric liver transplantation with cadaveric or living related donors: comparative results in 90 elective recipients of primary grafts. *J Pediatr* 1999;134:280.

51. Sebagh M, Yilmaz F, Karam V, et al. Cadaveric full-size liver transplantation and the graft alternatives in adults: A comparative study from a single centre. *J Hepatol* 2006;44:118.

52. Tanaka K, Uemoto S, Tokunaga Y, et al. Living related liver transplantation in children. *Am J Surg* 1994;168:41.

53. Francavilla R, Hadzic N, Underhill J, et al. Role of HLA compatibility in pediatric liver transplantation. *Transplantation* 1998;66:53.

54. Sugawara Y, Mizuta K, Kawarasaki H, et al. Risk factors for acute rejection in pediatric living related liver transplantation: the impact of HLA matching. *Liver Transpl* 2001;7:769.

55. Gupta P, Hart J, Cronin D, et al. Risk factors for chronic rejection after pediatric liver transplantation. *Transplantation* 2001;72:1098.

56. Janssen H, Malago M, Testa G, et al. Immunosuppression in living related and living unrelated liver transplantation. *Transplant Proc* 2002;34:1229.

57. Ringe B, Moritz M, Zeldin G, et al. What is the best immunosuppression in living donor liver transplantation? *Transplant Proc* 2005;37:2169.

58. Marino IR, Doria C, Scott VL, et al. Efficacy and safety of basiliximab with a tacrolimus-based regimen in liver transplant recipients. *Transplantation* 2004;78:886.

59. Charlton M, Seaberg E. Impact of immunosuppression and acute rejection on recurrence of hepatitis C: results of the National Institute of Diabetes and Digestive and Kidney Diseases Liver Transplantation Database. *Liver Transpl Surg* 1999;5:S107.

60. Farges O, Nocci Kalil A, Sebagh M, et al. Low incidence of chronic rejection in patients experiencing histological acute rejection without simultaneous impairment in liver function tests. *Transplant Proc* 1995;27:1142.

61. Tippner C, Nashan B, Hoshino K, et al. Clinical and subclinical acute rejection early after liver transplantation: contributing factors and relevance for the long-term course. *Transplantation* 2001;72:1122.

62. Kneitz B, Herrmann T, Yonehara S, et al. Normal clonal expansion but impaired Fas-mediated cell death and anergy induction in interleukin-2-deficient mice. *Eur J Immunol* 1995;25:2572.

63. Lenardo MJ. Interleukin-2 programs mouse alpha beta T lymphocytes for apoptosis. *Nature* 1991;353:858.

64. Li Y, Li XC, Zheng XX, et al. Blocking both signal 1 and signal 2 of T-cell activation prevents apoptosis of alloreactive T cells and induction of peripheral allograft tolerance. *Nat Med* 1999;5:1298.

65. Wells AD, Li XC, Li Y, et al. Requirement for T-cell apoptosis in the induction of peripheral transplantation tolerance. *Nat Med* 1999;5:1303.

66. Woodside KJ, Hu M, Meng T, et al. Differential effects of interleukin-2 blockade on apoptosis in naive and activated human lymphocytes. *Transplantation* 2003;75:1631.

67. Woodside KJ, Hu M, Liu Y, et al. Apoptosis of allospecifically activated human helper T cells is blocked by calcineurin inhibition. *Transplant Immunol* 2006;13:229.

68. Sato Y, Ichida T, Watanabe H, et al. Repeating intraportal donor-specific transfusion may induce tolerance following adult living-related donor liver transplantation. *Hepatogastroenterology* 2003;50:601.

69. Ueda M, Hundrieser J, Hisanaga M, et al. Development of microchimerism in pediatric patients after living-related liver transplantation. *Clin Transplant* 1997;11:193.

# 30.12   CONTROVERSIAL INDICATIONS

## 30.12.1   Hepatitis C

*John R. Lake, MD*

### INTRODUCTION

Liver disease caused by the hepatitis C virus (HCV) represents the most common indication for liver transplantation in adults throughout the world.[1] As HCV reinfection is almost universal, the recurrence of hepatitis C following liver transplantation represents the most important clinical problem facing liver transplant physicians and surgeons. Moreover, it has been suggested that recurrent hepatitis C is becoming an increasing problem posttransplant.[1] Not only is recurrence of hepatitis C becoming increasingly recognized, and the percentage of transplants being performed for hepatitis C is increasing, but there also is evidence that the disease severity may be worsening.[2] The reasons proposed for this are several including more potent immunosuppressive agents, the greater use of livers from older donors, and the increasing age of HCV–positive recipients.

The use of adult-to-adult live donor liver transplantation for the management of end-stage liver disease has been increasing throughout the world.[3,4] Although in many countries this is the only option for patients with end-stage liver disease, in North America, the use of live donor liver transplantation has been fueled by an extreme shortage of deceased donor livers. Moreover, with the conversion to the Models for End-Stage Liver Disease (MELD) allocation system in the United States, patients need to become quite ill in many parts of the country in order to qualify for receiving transplantation.[5] This extends the period of pretransplant disability and in some cases frightens patients, fueling the demand for live donor liver transplantation.

In general, the early outcomes of adult-to-adult live donor liver transplantation were somewhat less than those receiving livers from deceased donors, particularly when correcting for the fact that the donors are younger, cold ischemia time is less, and the recipients tend to be less ill at the time of transplant.[2] The use of live donor liver transplantation for HCV-positive recipients has been a particularly controversial topic, with most single-center studies suggesting no difference in outcomes, yet with some suggesting HCV-positive recipients do worse with living donor liver transplantation (LDLT) and some suggesting they do better.[6] In this chapter, I review the current outcomes of liver transplantation for cirrhosis caused by hepatitis C and compare the general results using deceased donor livers to the outcomes obtained using organs form live donors.

### OUTCOMES OF LIVER TRANSPLANTATION (OLT) FOR HEPATITIS C

In studies of OLT patients, there exists an almost universal viral recurrence and ultimately recurrence of liver disease in most HCV-positive OLT recipients. In general, the disease appears to be more aggressive posttransplantation, when compared to pretransplant with some 20% to 30% of transplant recipients with HCV developing cirrhosis in the allograft within 5 years. The enhanced disease progression is likely multifactorial in etiology and depends on the interaction among several host, donor, viral, and external factors.

Most early studies of HCV-infected recipients suggested that graft and patient survival data were similar in HCV-infected patients compared to HCV-negative recipients following OLT. While these studies did not find that graft or patient survival was significantly decreased in HCV–positive transplant recipients, in several, a trend toward decreased graft and patient survival was observed.[1,2] Moreover, most of these studies were not sufficiently powered to detect the small outcome differences that may have existed between study groups. Several recent studies have suggested that HCV infection does indeed affect patient and graft survival following OLT.

In the largest study of liver transplant recipients to date, a review of 11 036 patients from the United Network for Organ Sharing (UNOS) database indicated that survival was decreased following liver transplantation in HCV-positive patients (Figure 30.12.1-1). Kaplan-Meier survival rates were 86.4%, 77.8%, and 69.9% at 1, 3, and 5 years respectively, in HCV-positive patients, compared with 87.5%, 81.8%, and 76.6% in HCV-negative patients at the same time points (p < 0.0001). Graft survival was also affected by HCV infection and reported to be 76.9%, 66.4%, and 56.8% in HCV–positive patients at 1, 3, and 5 years, respectively, in contrast with 80.1%, 73.3%, and 67.7% in HCV-negative patients (p < 0.0001). In a prospective study of 234 OLTs in 209 HCV-positive patients,

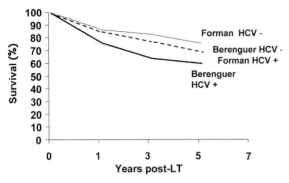

**FIGURE 30.12.1-1**

Patient survival in HCV-infected versus non-HCV-infected liver transplant recipients.

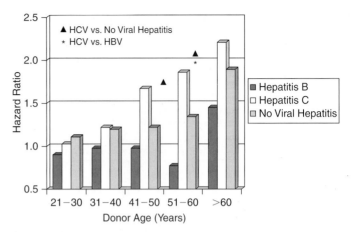

**FIGURE 30.12.1-2**

Relative risk for graft loss based on donor age.

Neumann et al. from Berlin reported that HCV recurrence was responsible for 35.9% of the reported 53 deaths in their study population in the first 10 years following OLT.

Universal viral recurrence and the early development of cirrhosis suggest that with longer follow-up, such as the 10-year study of Neumann et al., subtle survival differences will become more apparent in HCV-positive transplant recipients. In a recent publication, Terasaki et al. now demonstrate quite conclusively that the results of liver transplantation for hepatitis C have not improved over the past decade, and in fact, the outcomes of transplantation for hepatitis C were worse in the latter half of the decade of study. This observation was first made by Berenguer et al., in a multicenter study that showed the rates of fibrogenesis caused by recurrence of hepatitis C were accelerating throughout the 1990s. The present study now demonstrates that these accelerated rates of fibrogenesis translate into worse patient and graft survival. Moreover, in the Terasaki study, the authors indicate the worsening outcomes of transplantation for hepatitis C have prevented improvement in the overall results of liver transplantation. Such results are distressing and need to be a source of international concern.

Why are patient and graft survival rates decreasing for patients transplanted for hepatitis C? There are several potential reasons for this including the use of older donors, the use of more potent immunosuppressants and immunosuppressive regimens, and possibly other factors as well.

Certainly the average age of organ donors has been increasing over the past 15 years. In a study recently published, we demonstrated quite conclusively that the use of older donors for transplantation of recipients with hepatitis C is associated with worse outcomes.[1] Although there certainly is a trend toward the association of worse outcomes and donor age for other etiologies of liver disease, this association is markedly amplified in those patients transplanted with hepatitis C (Figure 30.12.1-2). In virtually every study that has looked at predictors of patient and graft survival in HCV–positive recipients, donor age has been an important factor. Unfortunately, there is little that can be done about this as the donor characteristics we have to deal with at present will be the donor characteristics that we are likely to see in the foreseeable future, and it would be untenable to suggest that livers from younger donors should be preferentially transplanted into patients with hepatitis C.

It also has been suggested that more potent immunosuppression could contribute to the worse outcomes. Certainly there is

considerable evidence that corticosteroid boluses and the use of antibody therapy to treat rejection is associated with worse outcomes. However, the data on maintenance immunosuppressive regimens or specific immunosuppressive agents on the outcomes of transplantation for hepatitis C are less convincing. One can, in fact, choose a study to support the concept that cyclosporine is better than tacrolimus or vice versa for patients with hepatitis C, or that mycophenolate mofetil (MMF) is beneficial or harmful for these recipients.

## PRETRANSPLANT ANTIVIRAL TREATMENT

Clearly the most affective way to improve the results for transplanting hepatitis C is to prevent recurrence of infection. This is what has led to substantial improvement in outcomes for transplantation for hepatitis B, which now enjoys the best outcomes (Figure 30.12.1-3), and one would expect hepatitis C (now with the worst outcomes) to have a similar benefit. However, our ability to do so is limited. There is certainly recent data from two studies that suggest that patients being treated while waiting for liver transplantation with interferon and ribavirin therapy can clear virus, and if they remain a sustained virologic responder, have ~ 80% chance of avoiding reinfection. However, it is likely that this will not benefit more than 10% to 20% of patients because of the relatively poor response and tolerability of the therapy in patients with cirrhosis. Particularly in those with a genotype 1 virus (most common in North America and Europe) one will likely not see more than 5% to 10% of patients referred for liver transplantation being able to achieve a sustained virologic response using the medications we currently have available. Thus the vast majority of recipients will continue to be plagued by HCV reinfection and disease recurrence. Moreover, in contrast to HBV, we have been thus far, unable to develop effective antibody therapy therapies to prevent reinfection at the time of transplant.

The results should cause concern for the transplant community. The current results should drive each of us to double or even triple our efforts to develop more effective therapies for hepatitis C and to assure that patients undergoing transplantation maintain good liver function as quite clearly the patients with hepatitis C seem to tolerate initial graft function, allograft rejection and

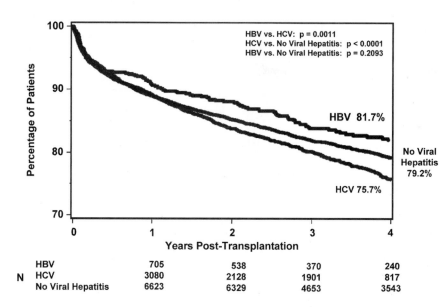

**FIGURE 30.12.1-3**

Patient survival for recipients with HBV, HCV, and no viral hepatitis.

biliary complications more poorly. If we are to expect to see an improvement in the results of liver transplants in general, this issue must be addressed.

## OUTCOMES OF LIVER TRANSPLANTATION USING LIVE DONORS FOR HCV (+) RECIPIENTS

In many ways, comparing live donor transplants to deceased donor liver transplants is like comparing "apples and oranges." First, live donors tend to be younger than deceased donors. As stated above, there is very good evidence that HCV-infected patients are disproportionately adversely affected by increasing donor age. No such relationship was found for patients transplanted for HBV-related liver disease, and although a similar relationship exists between donor age and outcomes in those with nonviral causes of liver disease, the slope of the line relating donor age to outcome was much less indicating less of an adverse effect of donor age in that population. In fact, donor age is the strongest predictor of graft loss and death in patients with HCV, starting with donors > 40 years.[1] With the age of deceased liver donors in the United States increasing, this will likely be an ever-increasing problem.

Second, quite clearly in the United States, recipients of deceased donors are more ill than those who receive live donors. In the first report of the impact on MELD on liver transplantation in the United States, the mean MELD score for deceased donor transplants was 23, whereas for LDLT it was 15. In fact, one is likely limited in the use of live donors for transplantation of the most ill patients, as the results of LDLT in those adults who were previously listed under the old U.S. allocation system as status 2A did relatively poorly. Although consensus has not yet been reached regarding above what MELD score LDLT is contraindicated, most programs use a cutoff of a calculated MELD score of > 25. In the United States, the majority of liver recipients are transplanted at a calculated MELD score < 25, and MELD score at transplant does not appear to increase the risk of patient or graft loss using livers from deceased donors until the MELD score exceeds 30.

Whether are the outcomes of liver transplantation for hepatitis C using life donors are equivalent to that using deceased donors has been an issue of some controversy.[6,7] However, by now, a large number of studies have been published supporting all dif-

fering views including that live donor liver transplantation yields worse results, equivalent results, and even better results.[8]

One of the earliest reports that suggested that the outcome of transplantation using live donors for hepatitis-C-infected individuals might yield inferior results came from the combined experience of the University of Colorado and Mt. Sinai Medical Center in New York. In this study, it was suggested that recurrence of hepatitis C occurred earlier and that graft survival might be less. However, this report, which was published in abstract form, has never to my knowledge been submitted as a full manuscript; although the Mt. Sinai program has published on their own similar results.

One of the first reports published as a manuscript suggesting that the outcome of live donor liver transplantation in hepatitis C patients may yield worse results came from Columbia University.[9] Here, they compared the results of transplantation in 45 HCV-infected adult patients who received deceased donor grafts as compared with 23 recipients who received organs from live donors. Overall, they found that the incidence of hepatitis C recurrence and time to recurrence were not different between the two groups. However, severe recurrence of hepatitis C occurred more commonly in patients receiving an organ from a live donor. Severe recurrence was defined by either the presence of cholestatic hepatitis, grade 3 or 4 inflammation, or HCV-induced graft failure requiring retransplantation. Specifically, they found that 17% of the patients transplanted using live donors developed cholestatic hepatitis C as compared to none of the patients receiving an organ from a deceased donor. Overall, however, there was no difference in patient or graft survival between the two groups.

Similarly, a report from Barcelona suggested that transplanting patients with hepatitis C using a live donor as compared to a deceased donor increased the likelihood of the recipient developing severe recurrence of hepatitis C.[10] This study compared 95 HCV–positive patients undergoing deceased transplantation to 22 HCV-positive patients undergoing transplantation using a live donor. They compared the number of patients developing a severe hepatitis C recurrence defined as biopsy-proven cirrhosis or occurrence of clinical decompensation. The 2-year probability of developing sever recurrence was significantly higher in recipients of live donor liver transplants (45%) as compared to those undergoing deceased donor transplantation (22%). When multivariate analysis was performed, the odds ratio of developing severe recurrence was 2.8-fold higher in those patients undergoing live donor liver transplantation.

A study by Thuluvath et al used the Scientific Registry of Transplant Recipients to address this issue.[11] In this study, they compared the outcome of 764 patients who received live donor liver transplantation as compared to 1,470 deceased donor liver transplant recipients who were matched for age, gender, race, diagnosis, and year of transplantation. Patient survival was similar between the two groups; however, graft survival was significantly lower in the live donor liver transplant recipients. In this study, grant survival was also lower for HCV-positive patients undergoing live donor liver transplantation, but the difference appeared no greater than that seen for the entire cohort of transplant recipients.

The majority of studies, however, have suggested the outcome is not different for HCV-positive recipients undergoing LDLT, and in one study, the outcome was reported to be better. Russo et al used the United Network for Organ Sharing liver transplant database to compare the outcomes of HCV-positive recipients receiving a liver from a live donor versus a deceased donor.[2] They found no significant differences in the outcome of those receiving an organ from a deceased donor versus a live donor. In this particular study the donor ages were comparable; however, the patients in the deceased donor group appeared to be somewhat more ill with a higher serum total bilirubin concentration and a greater INR.

Shiffman et al. from the Virginia Commonwealth University Medical Center reported results in 23 HCV–positive patients who underwent live donor liver transplantation as compared 53 HCV-positive patients who underwent deceased donor transplantation.[12] Importantly, protocol biopsies were obtained in this study. At 48 months posttransplant, the patient and graft survival rates were not different between the two groups. At 36 months, fibrosis was present in 78% of deceased donor liver transplant recipients, and the mean fibrosis score was 1.9. This compared with 59% of patients undergoing live donor transplantation who had fibrosis with a mean score of 0.9. However, these differences were not statistically significant.

A study from the University of Rochester compared 35 HCV-positive recipients of live donor transplants with 65 HCV positive recipients of deceased donor transplants.[13] In this study, the Kaplan-Meier actuarial patient survival at 39 months was 75% for deceased donor liver transplant recipients versus 89% for LDLT recipients. There were five deaths as a result of recurrent hepatitis C in recipients of deceased liver transplants versus only one in a live donor transplant recipient. Rates of recurrence, hepatitis activity indices and fibrosis scores were similar between groups. In fact, none of the differences were found to be statistically significant.

Our own data at the University of Minnesota Medical Center suggest that the outcome of liver transplantation is fact better using live donors than deceased donors in HCV–positive recipients.[14] In this study, we found that patients receiving whole livers from a deceased donor were more ill, and the livers experienced longer cold ischemia times. The most striking difference was that the age of whole liver deceased donors was 44 versus 32 years of age for the live donors and deceased donors of partial livers. When comparing the results of 32 whole liver deceased donor transplants with 12 live donor transplants, and with 7 deceased donor split transplants, we found no differences in patient or graft survival rates. The incidence o f histologic recurrence of hepatitis C was 81% in whole liver deceased donor transplants, 50% in live donor transplants, and 86% in deceased donor split transplants

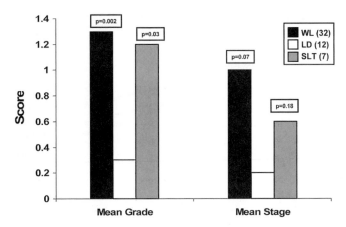

**FIGURE 30.12.1-4**

Mean grade and stage of biopsy.

(P = .06). However, the grade of inflammation on the biopsy specimens was 1.3 in whole liver deceased donor transplants, 0.33 in live donor transplants, and 1.2 in deceased donor split transplants (P = .002) (Figure 30.12.1-4). Most importantly fibrosis stage was 0.96 in whole liver deceased liver transplants, 0.22 in live donor transplants, and 066 in deceased donor split transplants (P = .07). Only one patient in each group developed cholestatic hepatitis. This suggests that, if anything, the outcomes are better in patients receiving live donor transplants.

Similarly, uncontrolled studies from Japan and Korea (reasonable given the relative lack of deceased donor activity in those countries) also have suggested good outcomes using live donors for patients with hepatitis C.[15]

## SUMMARY

It is now quite clear that the results of liver transplantation for patients with hepatitis C are similar when organs are used from live donors versus deceased donors. Previous concerns about a higher frequency of cholestatic hepatitis or more aggressive fibrogenesis with live donors have not turned out to be true. The benefits of live donor transplantation in HCV-positive patients include: younger donors, less cold ischemia time, and the possibility of successfully treating patients with antivirals prior to transplantation. The downside is potentially a higher rate of biliary complications.

At present, patients with HCV should not be denied live donor transplants. Time will tell whether improved surgical outcomes will lead to improved outcomes in this patient population.

## References

1. Lake JR, Shorr JS, Steffan BJ, et al. Differential effects of donor age in liver transplant recipients infected with hepatitis B, hepatitis C and without viral hepatitis. *Am J Transplant* 2005;(Mar);5(3):549–557.
2. Russo MW, Galanko J, Beavers K, Fried MW. Shrestha R. Patient and graft survival in hepatitis C recipients after adult living donor liver transplantation in the United States. *Liver Transplantation* 2004;10(3):340–346.
3. Barr ML, Belghiti J, Villamil FG, et al. A report of the Vancouver Forum on the care of the live organ donor: lung, liver, pancreas, and intestine data and medical guidelines. *Transplantation* 2006(May 27)81(10):1373–1385.

4. Shif fman ML, Brown RS Jr, Olthoff KM, et al. Living donor liver transplantation: summary of a conference at The National Institutes of Health. *Liver Transpl* 2002;8:174–188.

5. UNOS, Transplant Programs Appendix B, Attachment 1 (XII). Accessed 22 February 2005

6. Forman LM, Trotter JF, Emond J. Living donor liver transplantation and hepatitis C. *Liver Transplantation* 2004;10(3):347–348.

7. Tanaka K, Yamada T. Living donor liver transplantation in Japan and Kyoto University: what can we learn? *J Hepatol* 2005;42:25–28.

8. Schiano TD, Gutierrez JA, Walewski JL. Accelerated hepatitis C virus kinetics but similar survival rates in recipients of liver grafts from living versus deceased donors. *Hepatology* 2005;42(6):1420–1428.

9. Gaglio PJ, Malireddy S, Levitt BS. Increased risk of cholestatic hepatitis C in recipients of grafts from living versus cadaveric liver donors.[see comment]. [Journal Article] *Liver Transplantation* 2003;9(10): 1028–1035.

10. Garcia-Retortillo M, Forns X, Llovet JM. Hepatitis C recurrence is more severe after living donor compared to cadaveric liver transplantation. *Hepatology* 2004;40(3):699–707.

11. Thuluvath PJ, Yoo HY. Graft and patient survival after adult live donor liver transplantation compared to a matched cohort who received a deceased donor transplantation. *Liver Transplantat* 2004;10(10):1263–1268.

12. Shiffman ML, Stravitz RT, Contos MJ. Histologic recurrence of chronic hepatitis C virus in patients after living donor and deceased donor liver transplantation]. *Liver Transplantat* 2004;10(10):1248–1255.

13. Bozorgzadeh A, Jain A, Ryan C. Impact of hepatitis C viral infection in primary cadaveric liver allograft versus primary living-donor allograft in 100 consecutive liver transplant recipients receiving tacrolimus. *Transplantation* 2004;77(7):1066–1070.

14. Humar A, Horn K, Kalis A, et al. Living donor and split-liver transplants in hepatitis C recipients: does liver regeneration increase the risk for recurrence? *Am J Transplantat* 2005;(Feb)5(2):399–405.

15. Takada Y, Haga H, Ito T, et al. Clinical outcomes of living donor liver transplantation for hepatitis C virus (HCV)-positive patients. *Transplantation* 2006;81(3):350–354.

## 30.12.2 Cancer

*Greg J. McKenna, MD,*
*Goran B. Klintmalm, MD, PhD*

## INTRODUCTION

The incidence of hepatocellular carcinoma (HCC) has been steadily increasing for the past 2 decades. Although currently the 18th most common cancer in the United States,[1] it ranks sixth most common worldwide.[2,3] Between 1975 and 1996, the incidence of HCC in the United States more than doubled, from an age-adjusted rate of 1.4 cases per 100 000 to 3.0 per 100 000.[4] In 2005 we will see an estimated 18,000 new cases of HCC in the United States[5] and over 600 000 worldwide with an annual number of deaths worldwide exceeding 500 000.[2] The median survival worldwide is less than 6 months.

The rise in incidence of HCC parallels the near epidemic of the hepatitis C virus: in more than 90% of cases, HCC occurs in a setting of chronic liver disease related to hepatitis B or C virus. In hepatitis C, the HCC is a result of chronic injury from the virus over an extended period of time. This rising incidence of HCC is likely to worsen as many hepatitis C virus patients are entering the third and fourth decade of their infection, when they will become most at risk of developing HCC.

HCC originates from atypical hepatocellular hyperplasia which itself arises from adenomatous hyperplasia, and this undergoes transformation into a malignancy.[6] HCC tends to present as encapsulated and well-demarcated tumors,[7] usually in a setting of cirrhosis, and is the leading cause of death in cirrhotic patients.[8]

In those patients with HCC whose inadequate hepatic function precludes resection, transplantation represents the only treatment option for cure. Transplantation for HCC is beneficial even to those with adequate hepatic reserve, because transplantation removes the remaining preneoplastic tissue—the remaining cirrhotic liver—which limits the risk of further *de novo* HCC development. Success in treating HCC with transplantation is now widely acknowledged, but has been complicated by the supply and demand issues that affect all the other end-stage liver disease patients awaiting transplantation. In 2003 in the United States, 1,756 of the 17,853 patients with end-stage liver disease awaiting transplant died before receiving a transplant. As a solution to this imbalance between cadaveric donor graft availability and the growing number of potential recipients, living donor liver transplantation (LDLT) was developed as a way to expand the donor pool.

When LDLT was developed, it was thought that its use would be clearly indicated for HCC patients. However, in the last few years, the use of LDLT for HCC has become more controversial. Changes in organ allocation systems giving priority to specific HCC patients, and a further understanding of the outcomes and recurrence of HCC after LDLT have raised questions as to the ongoing use of LDLT as a treatment for HCC.

## HISTORICAL BASIS FOR LIVER TRANSPLANTATION FOR HCC

The role of liver transplantation as a treatment for HCC has changed significantly over the last 2 decades. The early series of studies regarding transplantation for HCC described poor outcomes, with 5-year survivals ranging from 15% to 48%.[9–13] In our early experience at Baylor University Medical Center from 1984 to 1994, of 75 patients transplanted for HCC (6% of all transplants performed) the 5-year patient survival was 34%.[14] The poor early outcomes for transplant centers even led the U.S. Department of Health and Human Services to decide in 1989 that HCC was a contraindication to transplantation. The poor results for transplantation for HCC described in these studies were due to inadequate patient selection for transplantation. In the past, liver transplantation was usually reserved for large, diffuse, multinodular tumors considered otherwise unresectable. However, in 1993, Bismuth and his group in Villejuif first proposed transplanting an "optimal" group of candidates—those with uninodular or binodular tumors < 3 cm in size, and they described an excellent 3-year survival of 83%.

Bismuth's research was followed by a landmark study by Mazzaferro and the Milan Group[15] in 1996 involving transplantation in 48 conservatively selected recipients with HCC, which established liver transplantation as a viable treatment option for HCC. They showed that by restricting transplantation to those patients with early HCC (T1 and T2 tumors as defined by the now-revised TMN staging) having 1 tumor <= 5 cm, or up to 3 tumors all <= 3 cm, survival rates equivalent to non-HCC transplants could be achieved (4-year survival of 75%). These findings were reproduced by other centers with similar outcomes,[16–18] and these selection criteria have become known as the Milan Criteria. By the end of 1990s, the ideal transplant candidates were recognized and a common agreement was that patients should be listed for liver transplant only when the probability of living 5 years after the procedure exceeded 50%.[19]

Between January 1998 and February 2002, the United Network for Organ Sharing (UNOS) implemented a system for organ allocation that assigned patients with HCC Status 2 B listing for liver transplant regardless of their Child–Turcotte–Pugh score. In February 2002, the System Model for End-Stage Liver Disease (MELD) was adopted by UNOS, and it significantly changed the allocation of organs to patients with HCC. Adopting the Milan Criteria as its standard, the MELD system assigned priority scores to HCC patients whose tumors met the guidelines. A MELD score of 24, representing a 15% pretransplantation death probability, was assigned to patients with T1 staging (1 nodule < 2.0 cm). A MELD score of 29, representing a 30% pretransplantation death probability, was assigned to patients who fit the T2 staging (1 nodule 2.0 to 5.0 cm or 2 to 3 nodules all < 3.0 cm). These priority scores had a significant impact on the number of transplants performed for HCC: in the year following the adoption of the MELD system 23% of all cadaveric liver transplants were for HCC, whereas previously HCC represented 8% of all cadaveric transplants.[20]

Since its initial adoption, the MELD system has twice been adjusted. In February 2003, it was determined that initial attempts to assign priority score gave too much advantage to HCC patients over other end-stage liver disease patients. The MELD HCC priority scores were adjusted so that a MELD score of 20, representing an 8% pretransplantation death probability, was assigned to patients with T1 staging and a MELD score of 24, representing a 15% pretransplantation death probability, was assigned to patients with T2 staging. In March 2005, these priority scores were further adjusted such that the MELD score for T2 patients was further decreased to 22. Also since less than 10% of patients with T1 lesions were dropping off the waiting list at 1 year because of tumor progression, the T1 priority score was eliminated. The subsequent impact of these two later adjustments in the MELD priority scores on transplantation rates for HCC has not yet been determined.

## LIVING DONOR LIVER TRANSPLANT FOR HCC

### Favorable Graft Size Issues

The first adult-to-adult LDLT was performed in 1998, and this procedure represented a way to address the two main issues specific to HCC patients needing transplantation: long waiting times and tumors exceeding the Milan criteria.

From an operative standpoint, the HCC patient represents an ideal LDLT recipient. Patients with advanced end-stage liver disease and significant portal hypertension are relatively poor candidates for LDLT,[21] and studies show that when a recipient's underlying liver function is severely impaired (ie, MELD > 30) the early post-op mortality after LDLT can be up to 50%. The post-op mortality risk in LDLT in HCC recipients is less, because the MELD priority points assigned to HCC patients mean they have a much lower calculated MELD score at the time of transplant.

An appropriate donor liver segment graft size is key in selecting acceptable donors and recipients for LDLT. Because hyperdynamic portal flow damages smaller grafts, the size of a donor liver required for a safe LDLT in the recipient correlates with the amount of portal hypertension. The Mount Sinai group describe a 12.5% incidence of small-for-size syndrome in LDLT recipients. In their study, however, none of the Child's Class A LDLT recipients, who would have less portal hypertension, developed small-for-size syndrome.[22] Since HCC LDLT recipients are more likely to be Child's Class A recipients they are at less risk for small-for-size syndrome.

The smaller graft size requirements for LDLT in HCC recipients may have benefits for the donor as well. Experience with LDLT suggests that in patients with significant liver failure, a donor allograft size of 40% of GV/SV or 0.8 GV/BV is required. In contrast, in patients without significant liver failure, often the case with HCC patients, a donor allograft size of only 30% of GV/SV or 0.6 GV/BW is required.[23] HCC patients generally have preserved liver function and less portal hypertension, and they are better able to tolerate implantation of a relatively undersized graft. The ability to use a smaller graft, or even the possibility of using a left lobe graft means that LDLT for HCC patients may represent less of a surgical risk to the donor and make it a more appealing option.

### Cost Effectiveness and Projected Survival Advantage

In the absence of controlled trials in clinical decision making, one can use decision analysis to assess elements and outcomes. Two studies from the pre-MELD era suggest that LDLT may be a superior strategy compared to cadaveric transplants in HCC patients in terms of gains in overall life expectancy as well as cost-effectiveness.

The group at Tufts used a Markov model, a statistical modeling technique used for decision analysis, to assess a hypothetical cohort comparing outcomes between three groups of HCC patients: those receiving a LDLT, a cadaveric transplant or no liver transplant.[24] Their hypothetical cohort assumed a 58-year-old patient with 3.5-cm tumor, Child's A cirrhosis, 82% 5-year survival, a tumor doubling time of 204 days and a waiting time typical for a UNOS stage 2B. In their analysis, LDLT offered gain in overall life expectancy of 4.5 years when compared to cadaveric transplant, making it the optimal strategy. Varying the model parameters (cirrhosis severity, age, tumor doubling time, tumor size, and rate of cirrhosis progression) did not change the dominant choice. They found that LDLT conferred a substantial survival advantage in patients with compensated cirrhosis and nonresectable early-stage HCC.

A second study from the Geneva group and the Barcelona group also used a Markov model to compare LDLT to cadaveric liver transplant.[25] The goal of the study was to integrate the various factors that affect the outcomes of LDLT and cadaveric liver transplant into practical clinical scenarios, balancing the gains and losses in life expectancy among the donors and the recipients. The analysis baseline parameters were a 5-year survival rate of 70%, a 6-month waiting time, a 4% monthly dropout rate, an 8% 3-month transplantation-related mortality and a 1% donor mortality. The study assumed equivalent outcomes for LDLT and cadaveric transplants, that all patients were less than 65 years of age and all tumors within the Milan criteria. A LDLT was defined as effective when the gain in life-years to the recipient provided from time saved on the waiting list, balanced the loss of life years due to the donor operation. In this model, LDLT for HCC becomes more beneficial compared to cadaveric transplant once the time on the waiting list exceeds 7 months. If the model is adjusted for a donor mortality of 0.5%, LDLT becomes preferred to cadaveric liver transplant after only 3.5 months on the waiting list.[25]

The same group from Geneva and Barcelona also showed that LDLT can be more cost-effective compared to cadaveric transplant by using a Markov cost-utility analysis.[25] Despite LDLT procedure itself being more expensive than a cadaveric transplant, LDLT eliminates the need for extensive neoadjuvant therapy to control tumor progression while awaiting transplant, meaning less chemoembolization, radiofrequency ablation, and surgery for a HCC recipient. Over 40% of the total expenses incurred by patients undergoing cadaveric liver transplant occur during the waiting period.[26] Additionally, LDLT eliminates the follow-up costs associated with monitoring the tumor every 3 months and also eliminates palliative care costs associated with HCC patients who drop out while awaiting a cadaveric transplant. Utilizing the standard model parameters described earlier, their analysis indicates LDLT for HCC patients becomes cost-effective compared to cadaveric transplants after 7 months on the waiting list, when improvements in life expectancy are gained as a function of waiting list time (and the situation meets a threshold of less than $50 000 per quality-adjusted life-year saved). If the model is adjusted to allow for a shorter waiting time, LDLT provides only marginal gains in cost-effectiveness, and only those settings with high dropout (> 4%) or excellent 5-year survival (> 80%) still prove to be cost-effective when the waiting list is short. Indirect costs for the donor, including time lost from work, and future liabilities such as a difficulty obtaining health insurance, are difficult to estimate and are therefore not included in these cost analyses, making the overall determination of cost-effectiveness less definitive.[27]

## Indications for Living Donor Liver Transplant

### Curbing Tumor Progression on the Waiting List

A main indication for LDLT in HCC is long waiting-list times and the resulting potential for tumor progression to an untransplantable state. The decision-making analysis models predict that LDLT for HCC has a survival advantage and is cost-effective in those settings where prolonged waitlists exist. The need for LDLT for HCC is limited in those areas where cadaveric livers are readily available; however, such an excess supply is rare. Despite the priority status for HCC patients brought in by the MELD system, prolonged waiting lists can still be common.

The Barcelona group was one of the first to report the impact of patient dropout on overall survival in HCC patients awaiting liver transplant, by utilizing an intention-to-treat analysis. They found significant reductions in overall survival in HCC patients (2-year survival of 60%), when the waiting time for transplant exceeds 6 months, and the dropout rate exceeds 20%[16]; these results have been reiterated by other centers.[28] In many programs in the United States and around the world, HCC patients can face waiting times of over 12 months, and the number of patients who become excluded while waiting for transplant equal the number who are ultimately transplanted. The group from UCSF also evaluated dropout of HCC patients from the transplant list with an intention-to-treat analysis.[28] They describe a similar 22% dropout rate from the waitlist due to tumor progression. They found that the risk of dropout generally increased with the waitlist time, and the estimated monthly dropout rates were 0% from 0 to 3 months waiting time, 1.0% from 3 to 6 months, 1.6% from 6 to 9 months and 4.9% from 9 to 12 months. Several centers have defined risk factors that are independent predictors of waiting-list dropout, and these include tumors > 3 cm in diameter, 3 tumor nodules at time of presentation, baseline AFP levels > 200 ng/mL, tumor doubling time < 6 months to be independent predictors of waiting-list dropout[28,29] (Table 30.12.2-1).

The concept of using LDLT in HCC patients to improve overall survival in a setting of prolonged waiting lists is best outlined in a retrospective study from the group at the University of

**TABLE 30.12.2-1**

## RISK FACTORS FOR WAITING-LIST DROPOUT

Risk Factors for Waiting-List Dropout
HCC > 3 cm diameter
3 tumor nodules at time of presentation
Baseline AFP levels > 200ng/mL
Tumor Doubling Time < 6 months
Des-gamma-carboxy prothrombin serum level

Hong Kong.[30] In this study of the 51 consecutive HCC patients evaluated for transplant, a potential living donor was available for almost half of the HCC patients (25/51 patients), and LDLT was performed in 21 of these 25 patients after a median waiting time of 24 days. In contrast, only 20% of the patients (6/30 patients) without a living donor and awaiting a cadaveric liver underwent transplant, after a median wait of 344 days. The majority of this group (21/30 patients) dropped off the list because of tumor progression while awaiting liver transplant. The 3-year recipient actuarial survival of those who were actually transplanted was similar for both the group with a LDLT (81%) and the group relying on cadaveric liver transplant (80%). However, the intention-to-treat analysis highlights the survival advantage of LDLT in HCC patients where there is a long waiting list. The 1- and 3-year intention-to-treat survival of the LDLT group was 88% and 66%, respectively, compared to a 1-year and 3-year intention-to-treat survival of 72% and 38% in the group relying only on cadaveric liver transplant.

According to UNOS data, prior to the introduction of the MELD system, the average waiting time in the United States for a cadaveric transplant for HCC patients was 2.28 years.[20] After the MELD system implementation, the average waiting time for transplant for HCC patients decreased to 0.69 years. Studies presented 1 year after the introduction of the MELD system showed more than 85% of all eligible HCC patients were transplanted within 90 days[20] and the 5-month dropout rate from tumor progression decreased from 16.5% to 8.5%. In a setting where there are such improvements in the waiting list time for transplant for HCC, the indication for LDLT has become less clear. However, in the years since these studies were reported, there have been two separate downward revisions of HCC tumor priority scores, and although not yet reported, an increase in dropout rate due to tumor progression is likely. These downward revisions have the potential of increasing the waiting list times for HCC patients and call into question the assumption that LDLT may not necessarily be indicated.

Despite the improvements in overall waiting list times described in these early post-MELD studies, significant variations currently exist in the waiting-list times between the various UNOS Regions themselves, making these improved outcomes only a region-specific reality.[31] According to the UNOS data for 2005, in Regions 1, 5, and 9, more than two thirds of patients transplanted had a MELD score of 25 or greater (Figure 30.12.2-1). This compares to Regions 2, 3, 6, and 10 where less than one third of patients were transplantesd with a MELD score of 25 or greater. Because the current MELD system applies a priority score of 22 points for T2 criteria, in regions such as Regions 1, 5, and 9, a wait of over 6 months is common in order to achieve a MELD score where transplantation is likely. In 2005, 78% of HCC patients in Region 9 and 41.7% of HCC patients in Region 5 were on the waiting list for greater than 1 year compared to a mean of 23.5% of patients in

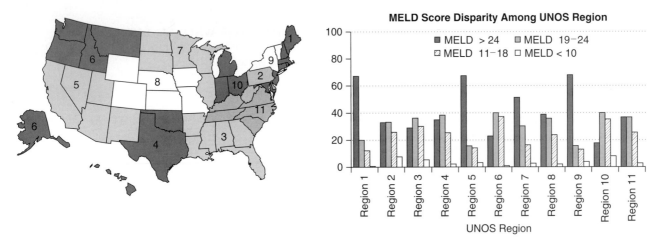

**FIGURE 30.12.2-1**

Disparity of MELD scores of recipients at the time of liver transplant across the various UNOS Regions in 2005.

the rest of the country. Also, from 1995 to 2003, only two regions experienced an increase in waitlist death rates: Region 9 (5.7% to 8.2%) and Region 5 (6.5% to 7%), whereas waitlist death rates decreased in all other regions of the United States. These data confirm that regional disparities do exist and that dropout from the waitlist due to tumor progression is still a reality in some regions of the United States despite overall improvements in organ allocation due to the MELD System.

In those regions where there is a prolonged waiting time for organs in spite of increased tumor priority points, the use of LDLT to curb tumor progression and increase survival is indicated. Even in areas where the waiting time is moderate, LDLT may still be valuable, if it can be determined that tumor progression is accelerated. The independent predictors of tumor progression described earlier may be useful to define aggressive tumors that are more sensitive to waiting list time. Thus, in those patients with large and multiple tumors, and those with doubling times < 6 months or with high AFP levels, the use of LDLT may still be indicated in those settings with short to moderate waiting time.

### HCC Exceeding the Milan Criteria

A second potential indication for LDLT in HCC patients is the presence of tumors exceeding the Milan Criteria. In patients with limited-stage HCC that fulfill the Milan Criteria, the current MELD system gives a priority for transplant. In the United States, however, since adoption of the MELD system and Milan Criteria, patients with tumors exceeding these guidelines have generally been excluded from receiving a transplant. There is evidence to suggest, however, that these criteria may be too restrictive, and that there may be patients with potentially curable tumors that go untreated because of their exclusion from a transplant. Since using a LDLT for HCC does not involve accessing the cadaveric donor pool, the possibility exists to use LDLT to transplant beyond the Milan Criteria.

The idea of using LDLT to transplant those patients with HCC exceeding the Milan Criteria requires first it be a feasible option to transplant HCC that exceed the Milan Criteria at all, and that a reasonable possibility of long-term survival exists. The idea of expanding the criteria for transplantation of HCC to something beyond the Milan Criteria has been proposed by

several centers: University of California San Francisco (UCSF), Mount Sinai, Pittsburgh, Barcelona, and Baylor University Medical Center. Despite slight differences in the proposed expansion criteria from these different centers, the common theme is that acceptable survival results can be achieved even in tumors that exceed the Milan Criteria.

The group at UCSF propose that a modest expansion of tumor size limits for transplanting HCC patients does not adversely affect survival.[32] Their proposed expansion extends to a single nodule less than 6.5 cm in diameter, or up to 3 nodules with total diameter less than 8 cm with no nodule greater than 4.5 cm. This expanded criteria was evaluated in a cohort of 70 HCC patients transplanted from 1988 to 2000,[33] and no significant difference in survival was found in those 24 patients that exceeded the Milan Criteria compared to the 46 patients who were within the criteria. For those patients transplanted with HCC using the expanded criteria, the 1-year and 5-year recurrence-free survival were 90% and 75.2%, respectively. The group at Pittsburgh corroborated the UCSF data by comparing the Milan Criteria and the expanded UCSF criteria in a large retrospective evaluation of a cohort of 403 patients who underwent transplant for HCC from 1981 to 2000. In the 248 patients of their cohort whose tumors fulfilled Milan Criteria and the 265 patients who fulfilled the expanded UCSF criteria, the 5-year patient survival was 67%.[34] There was no recurrence in half of the remaining 37% who did not fulfill Milan Criteria, and also no recurrence in 45.3% of the 32.6% of patients who did not meet UCSF criteria. A major criticism of these retrospective studies by UCSF and Pittsburgh, however, is that they are based on pathological data obtained postoperatively as opposed to pre-op imaging. Pre-op imaging is what is used in the decision-making in selecting potential recipients, bringing into question the validity of applying these studies prospectively. Since pre-op imaging has been shown to underestimate the extent of the disease in 30% of patients,[35–36] this needs to be factored into these proposed criteria based on pathological findings.

A prospective study of the issue of transplantation for HCC that exceed the Milan Criteria was done by the group at Mount Sinai, New York, instituting a protocol for transplanting patients with HCC greater than 5 cm.[37] Beyond the absence of extrahepatic disease, regional node involvement, and the presence of patent vessels, the inclusion criteria for transplant were for tumor

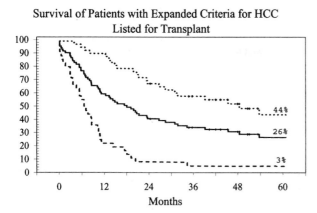

**FIGURE 30.12.2-2**

Survival of 80 patients with expanded criteria for HCC listed for transplantation. Overall intention-to-treat survival (n = 80, 5-year survival 25%, full line). Survival of patients effectively transplanted (n = 43, 5-year survival 44%, dotted line). Survival of patients dropping out from the waiting list due to tumor progression (n = 37, 5-year survival 3%, dashed line). From Roayaie S, Llovet JM. Liver transplantation for hepatocellular carcinoma: Is expansion of criteria justified. *Clin Liv Dis* 2005;9:315. With permission.

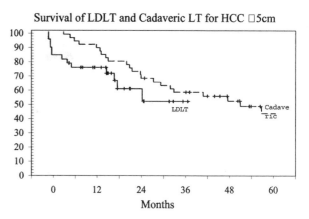

**FIGURE 30.12.2-3**

Patient survival after living donor liver transplant (solid line) for HCC compared to cadaveric liver transplant (dashed line) in patients with HCC ≥ 5 cm. From Gondolesi GE, Roayaie S, Munoz L et al. Adult living donor liver transplantation for patients with hepatocellular carcinoma: extending UNOS priority criteria. *Ann Surg* 2004;239:142. With permission.

involvement of less than 75% of the total liver volume. Multicentricity was acceptable, but if there was bilobar disease, the tumor burden in the lobe with less involvement had to be less than 5 cm. This study only included patients who exceeded the Milan Criteria (Figure 30.12.2-2), and a total of 80 patients were prospectively evaluated using this protocol, with 43 proceeding to transplant with a mean waiting time of 142 days. A total of 37 patients were ultimately excluded because of progression of disease and the dropout rate was 46%. The overall intention-to-treat 2-year and 5-year survival was 43% and 26%, respectively, because of the large dropout rate. For those HCC patients actually transplanted, the 2-year and 5-year survival was 73% and 44%, respectively. A subgroup analysis of this group exceeding the Milan Criteria, looking only at those patients who had tumors between 5 and 7 cm, showed a 55% 5-year survival.

Recently our group at the Baylor University Medical Center, Dallas, reported an analysis of the International Registry of Hepatic Tumors in Liver Transplantation (ITR).[38] The Registry consists of 1,242 HCC patients transplanted from 1992 to 2005 and represents data accumulated from 57 transplant centers on 4 continents. The analysis found those patients with tumors less than or equal to 3 cm had the best survival. There was, however, no difference in recurrence-free survival for tumors ranging between 3.1–5.0 cm and 5.1–6.0 cm. The Registry data suggest that an expansion of tumor size criteria is acceptable. Looking at the number of nodules, those patients with two to four lesions less than 5 cm did equally as well as those with two to four lesions less than 3 cm with 5-year recurrence-free survivals of 56.3% versus 63.7%, respectively, furthering the idea of a safe expansion of the Milan Criteria to include up to even four nodules.

In addition to these above-described studies that suggest a role for transplantation for HCC exceeding the Milan Criteria, there are three major studies that specifically address the use of LDLT in patients exceeding the Milan Criteria. The first of these studies is from the group at Mount Sinai, who in 2002 initially described their experience of 27 HCC patients trans-

planted with LDLT,[21] showing a 1-year patient survival of 81% and 1-year recurrence-free survival of 83%. The group expanded on these results in their 2004 follow-up study of 36 HCC patients transplanted by LDLT, and presented a longer follow-up, that stratified results based on whether the HCC exceeded the Milan Criteria[39] (Figure 30.12.2-3). For all HCC patients, those transplanted with LDLT had a 1-year and 2-year patient survival of 75% and 60%, respectively, compared to 81% and 70%, respectively, for cadaveric transplants. For patients with tumors exceeding 5 cm in diameter, the 1-year and 2-year patient survival in LDLT patients was 75% and 46%, respectively, versus 82% and 62%, respectively, for cadaveric transplants.

A retrospective study of LDLT for HCC from the group at Kyoto University describes 122 patients referred for LDLT from 1999 to 2002.[11] A total of 56 of the 122 referred were subsequently transplanted using liberal selection criteria. There was no limitation on HCC size or number of nodules, and the only exclusion criteria for transplant was extrahepatic metastasis or vascular invasion. For all patients, the overall 1-year and 3-year patient survival was 73.1% and 54.6%, respectively. There were 25 patients (44.6%) transplanted whose tumors exceeded the Milan Criteria. A subgroup analysis on this group of 25 who exceeded Milan Criteria showed a 3-year patient survival of 55%.

A recent report out of Sapporo, Japan, for the Japanese Study Group on Organ Transplantation presented data regarding LDLT for HCC accumulated from 49 centers in Japan. In these centers, about one third of the programs adopted the Milan Criteria as strict guidelines for transplant. However, the other two thirds examined those patients with HCC that exceeded Milan Criteria, on a case-by-case basis. LDLT was offered to those patients with either severely impaired liver function, or to those with failure to control the tumor by medical, radiologic, or surgical means. For all HCC patients transplanted by LDLT, the 1-year and 3-year patient survivals were 78.1% and 69.0%, respectively, and the 1-year and 3-year recurrence-free survivals were 72.7% and 64.7%, respectively. Of the 316 patients described in the study, 54.1% did not meet Milan Criteria, and the 1-year and 3-year patient survivals were 75.0% and 60.4%, respectively, compared to 81.6% and 79.1%, respectively, for those that did meet criteria.

The studies from the five centers suggest that transplanting HCC patients using criteria that exceed the Milan Criteria may be acceptable. The current restrictive MELD system of organ allocation with its priority scores for HCC based on the Milan Criteria mean that there are patients who might benefit from transplantation who are not being transplanted. The three studies that specifically address LDLT in patients with HCC exceeding Milan Criteria demonstrate acceptable survival rates in these patients, with 3-year patient survivals of 55% to 60%. However, these studies are retrospective studies that use subgroup analysis to make their conclusions limiting their applicability, and large prospective investigations are needed to assess the real outcome for LDLT for tumors that exceed the Milan Criteria. The Barcelona group has proposed such a prospective study, based in part on the results of the subgroup analysis from the Mount Sinai study, by evaluating the role of LDLT in patients with tumors from 5 to 7 cm.[37] Their proposed inclusion criteria for transplantation of HCC with single nodules <= 7cm and multiple nodules (three or fewer nodules <=5cm or five or fewer <=3cm) without macroscopic vascular invasion, or the down-staging of any tumor for greater than 6 months in order to meet the Milan Criteria. The results of this prospective study are pending and these data may be key to resolving the controversy of the role of LDLT in HCC patients who exceed the Milan Criteria.

## Impact of Living Donor Liver Transplant on HCC Recurrence

Some centers have noted an increase in the recurrence of HCC when examined on a stage-for-stage basis in those patients who have had their transplant waiting time shortened by using expanded donor options (LDLT, split liver transplants, domino liver transplants).[41] In contrast, other centers have described no difference in recurrence rates between LDLT and cadaveric transplant for HCC.[39,42]

The group from Sapporo Japan reports a 3-year recurrence-free survival of 75% in HCC patients who received a LDLT.[42] This recurrence-free survival is similar to the rates reported in the literature for cadaveric transplants, indicating a similar recurrence pattern between cadaveric and LDLT. Reports from the Mount Sinai group also describe no significant difference in 3-year overall HCC recurrence-free survival when LDLT is compared to cadaveric transplant (74% vs 83%).[39]

The results from Japan and Mount Sinai stand in contrast to results from the group at Northwestern that describe an increase in HCC recurrence in those patients who were "fast-tracked" to transplant with either a LDLT, split liver, domino liver, or MELD upgrade.[41] The rate of recurrence in the group who were "fast-tracked" was 15% compared to a rate of 0% in the "non fast-tracked" group. Although the numbers in the Northwestern study were small, they suggest that accelerating transplant for HCC with one of the many "fast-track" options such as LDLT lead to an increased rate of recurrence.

One explanation offered by the groups that report a higher rate of recurrence of HCC with LDLT is that the recurrence is related to hepatic regeneration in LDLT and the tumor-promoting effects from growth factors and cytokines that are released with regeneration. This theory, however, requires that there be a microscopic presence of extrahepatic tumor at the time of transplantation to be stimulated by the cytokines and factors that are specific to LDLT. The hepatectomy techniques used in LDLT are similar to the piggyback hepatectomy techniques used in cadaveric transplants, and these cadaveric transplants do not demonstrate

any increase in HCC recurrence.[41] Thus, the regeneration from the donor segment per se is unlikely to explain any differences in HCC recurrence that may have been observed.

Another explanation for an increased HCC recurrence when LDLT is used for HCC patients is related to the biological aggressiveness of the tumor. Time is often a substitute for tumor aggressiveness as a prolonged wait time allows a tumor to declare its biological aggressiveness and define itself as likely to metastasize. Using LDLT to shorten the time on the waiting list is done in the hope of curbing tumor progression while waiting for transplant. However, shortening the time on the waiting list may result in transplanting very aggressive tumors that have already metastasized on a microscopic level but are not yet apparent. The group at Mount Sinai showed that a tumor doubling time of less than 6 months is a bad prognostic indicator of dropout from the waiting list,[29] possibly identifying an aggressive tumor. A short waitlist time may prevent identification of these aggressive tumors with short doubling time, so that LDLT may result in transplanting those patients that will not benefit from transplantation and are likely to have recurrent HCC.

The groups at Kyushu University and University of Tokyo in Japan have investigated the role of des-gamma-carboxy prothrombin (DCP) levels in HCC recurrence and shown that high levels are strong predictors of tumor aggressiveness and vascular invasion.[43,44] In patients who received LDLT for HCC that exceeded the Milan Criteria, the 2-year recurrence-free survival was significantly better in those patients with DCP levels less than 300 mAU/mL compared to those with levels greater than 300 mAU/mL (2-year survival 80% vs 38%, respectively).[45] Using preoperative DCP levels as a marker of tumor aggressiveness may be helpful in identifying those patients who have a high chance of recurrence post-LDLT.

The group from Pittsburgh[46] has proposed analyzing the pretransplant HCC by microdissection genotyping using a panel of tumor suppressor gene markers of allelic loss. Their study examined 103 HCC specimens for tumor suppressor gene loss using PCR amplification of microdissected tissue. These results were then evaluated using an artificial neural network model designed by the group, allowing them to create a highly discriminatory model for predicting HCC recurrence after liver transplantation. The technique allows for a very accurate prediction of tumor recurrence.

Because it is debatable whether LDLT might increase tumor recurrence or may "fast-track" a tumor that has already metastasized, a better strategy would be one that first identifies a tumor with a high recurrence potential. This would prevent an LDLT being performed when no benefit from the transplantation exists.

Using such techniques as preoperative microdissection genotyping of the HCC, with measurements of DCP levels, may identify HCC with a high certainty of recurrence and allow judicious use of LDLT minimizing recurrence attributed to "fast-tracking."

## ETHICAL CONSIDERATIONS

Although ethical issues in LDLT are examined elsewhere, there are ethical issues related to LDLT specific to HCC patients that are addressed here. The main ethical issues of LDLT are related to the fact that the donor faces potential risks and complications. Because donor safety is the paramount concern, it is important to consider this issue in regards to the nature of HCC.

HCC is a potentially recurrent disease. Unlike pediatric recipients, who are essentially cured of their liver disease by a LDLT, there is potential for recurrence of tumor in HCC patients that can limit the lifetime of the graft. For a LDLT for HCC to be considered, there needs to be a minimum expected graft survival. However, when justifying LDLT based on survival outcomes, some argue that survival outcomes for LDLT for HCC should be compared to nonsurgical/no-treatment outcomes rather than compared to outcomes from transplanting non-HCC patients. The potential risks and complications to the donor mean that this is unethical, and the LDLT should only take place when there is an acceptable survival, regardless of the other potential nontransplant outcomes. The Markov models used by researchers evaluate the donor and recipient gains and losses as if they are equal; however, the donor is more important, and the death of a donor cannot be compared to recurrence of disease.

Looking at the two major indications for LDLT for HCC, LDLT is ethically justified in those cases where waiting time is disproportionately long and the prolonged waitlist increases the risk of the HCC progression to a nontransplantable state. The risk to the donor can be justified because acceptable survival results can be expected in these patients and performing the LDLT stands to improve the outcome. When LDLT is performed for HCC that exceed the Milan Criteria it is ethically less clear, because the LDLT is being done due the recipient's exclusion from a possible cadaveric transplant. It is difficult to justify the potential risks to the donor in such a situation where society prohibits a transplant because it is unlikely to be of benefit. There is accumulating evidence, however, that slightly exceeding the Milan Criteria can still yield acceptable survival and for this situation LDLT may be ethically acceptable. Beyond this, there is poor survival, and it is not acceptable to expose the donor to the risks in this situation.

There is a higher incidence of PNF and graft complications with LDLT. Normally if a graft acutely fails, it requires an urgent retransplant. If a LDLT were used in a situation where a cadaveric donor is contraindicated, such as exceeding the Milan Criteria, the urgent retransplant would require a cadaveric organ, even though the patient was originally contraindicated. In these situations, the patient should not be retransplanted.

## CONCLUSIONS

Transplantation remains the best option for cure in a majority of patients with HCC. The role for LDLT has changed as our understanding of the tumor biology has grown and organ allocation systems have been modified. From an overall patient survival, cost-effectiveness and ethical point of view, LDLT for HCC is best suited in those situations where prolonged waiting times exist. Changes in organ allocation systems have attempted to improve this waiting-time issue and if successful may render this indication for LDLT as moot. The use of LDLT for HCC that exceed the Milan Criteria is a less clear indication. There is evidence that LDLT may be useful in a subset of patients that exceed the Milan Criteria by an incremental amount, and it is this subset that may be indicated from a patient survival and ethical point of view. It is not clear whether LDLT increases the risk of tumor recurrence. Regardless, efforts to identify those HCC likely to recur represent the best way to minimize tumor recurrence and prevent unnecessary LDLT with its concomitant donor risks. Any risks to the donor must always be considered in cases with risk of tumor recurrence and poor recipient outcomes. The role for LDLT in treating HCC continues to change, and ongoing evaluation of this role is needed as the field of transplantation and the various treatment options available for HCC change.

## References

1. Ferlay J, Bray F, Pisani P et al. GLOBOCAN 2002 Cancer Incidence, Mortality and Prevalence Worldwide. IARC CancerBase. No. 5 Version 2.0 Lyon, France, IARC Press, 2004.
2. Parkin DM, Fray F, Ferlay J et al. Estimating the world cancer burden: GLOBOCAN 2000. *Int J Cancer* 2001;94:153.
3. El-Serag HB, Davila JA, Petersen NJ, et al. The continuing increase in the incidence of hepatocellular carcinoma in the United States: An Update. *Ann Intern Med* 2003;139:817.
4. El-Serag HB. Epidemiology of hepatocellular carcinoma. *Clin Liver Dis* 2001;5:87.
5. Schafer DF, Sorrell MF. Hepatocellular carcinoma. *Lancet* 1999;353:1253.
6. Molmenti EP, Klintmalm GB. Cancer and liver transplantation. *Transplant Rev* 2000;14:183.
7. Fattovich G, Giustina G, Degos F, et al. Morbidity and mortality in compensated in cirrhosis type C: A retrospective follow-up study of 384 patients. *Gastroenterology* 1997;112:463.
8. Iwatsuki S, Starzl TE, Sheahan DG, et al. Hepatic resection versus transplantation for hepatocellular carcinoma. *Ann Surg* 1991;214:221.
9. Moreno P, Jaurrieta E, Figueras J, et al. Orthotopic liver transplantation: treatment of choice in cirrhotic patients with hepatocellular carcinoma? *Transplant Proc* 1995;27:2296.
10. Ringe B, Pichmayr R, Wittekind C, et al. Surgical treatment of hepatocellular carcinoma: experience with liver resection and transplantation in 198 patients. *World J Surg* 1991;15:270.
11. Bismuth H, Chiche L, Adam R, et al. Liver resection versus transplantation for hepatocellular carcinoma in cirrhotic patients. *Ann Surg* 1993;218:145.
12. Penn I. Hepatic transplantation for primary and metastatic cancers of the liver. *Surgery* 1991;110:726.
13. McKenna GJ, Sanchez EQ, Chinnakotla S, et al. The Baylor Regional Transplant Institute: Review of a Twenty-Year Experience. *Clin Transplants* 2004;221.
14. Mazzaferro V, Regalia E, Doci R, et al. Liver transplantation for the treatment of small hepatocellular carcinomas in patients with cirrhosis. *N Engl J Med* 1996;334:693.
15. Llovet JM, Fuster J, Bruix J. Intention-to-treat analysis of surgical treatment for early hepatocellular carcinoma: resection versus transplantation. *Hepatology* 1999;30:1434.
16. Bismuth H, Majno PE, Adam R, et al. Liver transplantation for hepatocellular carcinoma. *Semin Liver Dis* 1999;19:311.
17. Klintmalm GB. Liver transplantation for hepatocellular carcinoma: a registry report of the impact of tumor characteristics on outcome. *Ann Surg* 1998;228:479.
18. Bruix J, Llovet JM. Prognostic prediction and treatment strategy in hepatocellular carcinoma. *Hepatology* 2002;35:519.
19. Sharma P, Balan V, Hernandez JL, et al. Liver transplantation for hepatocellular carcinoma: the MELD impact. *Liver Transpl* 2004;10:36.
20. Gondolesi G, Munoz L, Matsumoto, et al. Hepatocellular carcinoma: a prime indication for living donor liver transplantation. *J Gastrointest Surg* 2002;6:102.
21. Ben-Haim, Emre S, Fishbein TF, et al. Critical graft size in adult-to-adult living donor living transplantation: Impact of the recipient's disease. *Liver Transpl* 2001;7:948.
22. Lo CM, Fan ST, Liu CL, et al. Minimum graft size for successful living donor transplantation. *Transplantation* 1999;68:1112.
23. Cheng SJ, Pratt DS, Freeman RB Jr. Living-donor versus cadaveric liver transplantation for non-resectable small hepatocellular carcinoma and compensated cirrhosis: a decision analysis. *Transplantation* 2001;72:861.

24. Sarasin FP, Majno PE, Llovet JM, et al. Living donor liver transplantation for early hepatocellular carcinoma: a life expectancy and cost-effectiveness perspective. *Hepatology* 2001;33:1072.

25. Brand DA, Viola D, Rampersaud P, et al. Waiting for a liver—Hidden costs of the organ shortage. *Liver Transpl* 2004;10:1001.

26. Russo MW, Brown Jr RS. Financial impact of adult living donation. *Liver Transpl* 2003;9:S12.

27. Yao FY, Bass NM, Nikolai B, et al. A follow-up analysis of the pattern and predictors of drop-out from the waiting list for liver transplantation in patients with hepatocellular carcioma: implications for the current organ allocation policy. *Liver Transpl* 2003;9:684.

28. Roayaie S, Ben-Haim M, Fishbein TM, et al. Comparison of surgical outcomes for hepatocelllular carcinoma in patients with hepatitis B versus hepatitis C: a western experience. *Ann Surg Oncol* 2000;7:764.

29. Lo CM, Fan ST, Liu CL, et al. The role and limitation of living donor liver transplantation for hepatocellular carcinoma. *Liver Transpl* 2004;10:440.

30. Schaffer III RL, Kulkarni S, Harper A, et al. The sickest first ? Disparities with model for end-stage liver disease-based organ allocation: one region's experience. *Liver Transpl* 2003;9:1211.

31. Yao FY, Ferrer L, Bass NM, et al. Liver transplantation for hepatocellular carcinoma: Expansion of the tumor size limits does not adversely impact survival. *Hepatology* 2001;33:1394.

32. Yao FY, Ferrer L, Bass NM, et al. Liver transplantation for hepatocellular carcinoma: comparison of the proposed UCSF criteria with the Milan criteria and the Pittsburgh modified TMN criteria. *Liver Transpl* 2002;8:765.

33. Marsh JW, Dvorchik I. Liver organ allocation for hepatocellular carcinoma: are we sure ? *Liver Transpl* 2003;9:693.

34. Rizzi PM, Kane PA, Ryder SD, et al. Accuracy of radiology in detection of hepatocellular carcinoma before liver transplantation. *Gastroenterology* 1994;107:1425.

35. Burrel M, Llovet JM, Ayuso C, et al. MRI angiography is superior to helical CT for detection prior to liver transplantation: an explant correlation. *Hepatology* 2003;38:1034.

36. Roayaie S, Frischer JS, Emre SH, et al. Long-term results with multimodal adjuvant therapy and liver transplantation for the treatment of hepatocellular carcinomas larger than 5 centimenters. *Ann Surg* 2002;235:533.

37. Onaca N, Davis GL, Goldstein RM, et al. Expanded criteria for liver transplantation in patients with hepatocellular carcinoma: a report from the International Registry of Hepatic Tumors *Liver Transpl* 2007; 13: 391.

38. Gondolesi GE, Roayaie S, Munoz L, et al. Adult living donor liver transplantation for patients with hepatocellular carcinoma: extending UNOS priority criteria. *Ann Surg* 2004;239:142.

39. Kaihara S, Kiuchi T, Ueda M, et al. Living-donor liver transplantation for hepatocellular carcinoma. *Transplantation* 2003;75:S37.

40. Kulik L, Abecassis M. Living donor liver transplantation for hepatocellular carcinoma. *Gastroenterology* 2004;127:S277.

41. Todo S, Furukawa H. Living donor liver transplantation for adult patients with hepatocellulaar carcinoma. *Ann Surg* 2004;240:451.

42. Koike Y, Shiratori Y, Sato S, et al. Des-gamma-carboxy prothrombin as a useful predisposing factor for the development of portal venous invasion in patients with hepatocellular carcinoma: A prospective analysis of 227 patients. *Cancer* 2001;91:561.

43. Shimada M, Takenaka K, Fujiwara Y, et al. Des-gamma-carboxy prothrombin and alpha-fetoprotein positive status as a new prognostic indicator after hepatic resection for hepatocellular carcinoma. *Cancer* 1996;78:2094.

44. Shimada M, Yonemura Y, Ijichi I, et al. Living donor liver transplantation for hepatocellular carcioma: A special reference to a preoperative des-gamma-carboxy prothrombin value. *Transplant Proc* 2005;37:1177.

45. Marsh JW, Finkelstein SD, Demetris A, et al. Genotyping of hepatocellular carcinoma in liver transplant recipients adds predictive power for determining recurrence-free survival. *Liver Transpl* 2003;9:664.

## 30.12.3   Alcohol Abuse

*Bashar A. Aqel, MD*

### INTRODUCTION

Alcohol-related liver disease is the major cause of alcohol-related morbidity and mortality in the United States and in the world. Alcoholic liver disease encompasses a clinicohistologic spectrum of disease including fatty liver, alcoholic hepatitis, and alcoholic liver cirrhosis. Alcoholic liver cirrhosis affects 20% of patients who abuse alcohol. It is responsible for 100,000 to 150,000 hospitalizations, 10,000 deaths, and 1,500 transplants per year in the United States alone.

Alcoholic hepatitis is another distinct clinical entity that is associated with high rates of mortality. Treatment options for alcoholic hepatitis are limited and lack efficacy. Despite treatment and abstinence, recovery is not guaranteed and many patients die. Patients whose discriminant function (4.6 (Prothrombin time-control time) + bilirubin (mg/dL)) exceeds 32 have 35% to 46% risk of short-term mortality.[1]

Despite the fact that survival after liver transplantation in cases of alcoholic liver disease (ALD) is similar to that observed after transplantation for other causes, the selection of candidates with ALD for liver transplantation raises ethical and social issues and continues to be controversial. Data on liver transplantation in patients with acute alcoholic hepatitis or the utilization of living related donor are limited.

### ALCOHOLIC LIVER DISEASE: NATURAL HISTORY

Alcohol consumption was identified as a risk factor for liver disease long time ago when Laennec documented high prevalence of cirrhosis among heavy drinkers. Modern epidemiological data confirm a strong correlation between death attributable to cirrhosis and per capita consumption of alcohol.[2]

In the United States alone, data show that > 70% of Americans drink some alcohol with approximately 10 million Americans fulfilling the definition of "alcoholics" (3%). Approximately 20% to 25% of alcoholics develop cirrhosis. Alcoholic liver cirrhosis is one of the leading indications for liver transplantation worldwide.[3]

ALD is believed to progress through histological stages. Hepatic steatosis is the earliest histological abnormality associated with alcohol consumption. It develops in 80% of heavy drinkers. Synthetic liver functions are usually normal and are completely reversible with abstinence. Acute alcoholic hepatitis is another distinct clinical entity. It is characterized by significant systemic manifestations including hepatomegaly, fever, jaundice, and ascites. Treatment can be considered in severe cases with steroids or Pentoxifylline. Still this entity is associated with high rates of mortality (50% 1-month mortality). The last stage of the spectrum of ALD is alcoholic liver cirrhosis. It develops in 20% to 25% of alcoholic patients. It is responsible for 150,000 hospitalizations, 10,000 deaths, and 1,500 liver transplants annually.[4]

### ALD: INVESTIGATIONS OF PATIENTS FOR LIVER TRANSPLANTATION

Patients with ALD are at an additional risk of other organs dysfunction and require multisystem approach to determine candidacy for liver transplantation. Alcohol not only affects the liver but also other organs including heart, central and peripheral nervous system, bone marrow, and pancreas. It is usually difficult to differentiate the consequences of cirrhosis from those related to alcohol-induced organ damage. Unfortunately, the literature lacks until now any data regarding the prevalence and outcome of significant extrahepatic alcohol-related organ damage in patients evaluated for liver transplantation.

All transplant centers are satisfied with echocardiography, electrocardiogram, and stress test for cardiac evaluation. Cardiomyopathy reflected by left ventricular dysfunction is considered a contraindication for liver transplantation. The limits of left ejection fraction vary between different centers and range between 20% and 45%.

Patients with ALD should undergo a thorough neurological evaluation. Evidence of irreversible brain damage is considered a contraindication for liver transplantation. Peripheral neuropathy has no impact on the outcome and thus should not preclude patients from being considered for liver transplantation.

All patients with ALD being considered for liver transplantation should have a formal psychosocial assessment and should be monitored for alcohol drinking once listed. It is essential for these patients to have stable social support without any evidence of other substance abuse or psychiatric disability.

Recent studies showed patients transplanted for ALD are at increased incidence of some malignancies post liver transplantation, especially of the upper airway and upper gastrointestinal tract. This ahs resulted in a lower than expected long-term survival in those patients.[5–7]

## ALD: LIVER TRANSPLANTATION

Liver transplantation was first performed in 1963 by Starzl et al. The procedure was later recognized in 1983 by the National Institutes of Health (NIH) as an appropriate treatment for advanced liver disease including ALD National Institutes of Health (NIH) as an appropriate treatment for advanced liver disease including ALD later recognized the procedure in 1983. The NIH conference assumed that a minority of patient with ALD would meet the strict medical and psychosocial criteria required to be candidates for transplantation. At that time, only 5% of liver transplants were performed in patients with ALD and survival rates were very low at 20%.

In 1988, Starzl et al. published their experience at the University of Pittsburgh and showed that the outcome of liver transplantation in patients with ALD was similar to those transplanted for other indications. In addition they showed that a minority of patients (6%) returned to drinking post transplant.[8] Over the following 10 years, data from multiple transplant centers compiled by the United Network of Organ Sharing (UNOS) confirmed that posttransplant survival of patients with alcoholic liver cirrhosis were indeed comparable to those transplanted for other causes. The same data showed that alcohol relapse rates averaged 15% with few patients returning to trouble drinking.[9]

This encouraging data resulted in the collaboration of transplant hepatologists and surgeons with psychiatrists to define psychosocial predictors of long-term sobriety and compliance after liver transplantation. This collaboration led most transplant centers to adopt a minimal 6 months of sobriety which evolved as a reasonable, easily identified, and objective requirement for candidacy for liver transplantation (allow adequate time for liver functions to recover in some patients, identify those who are likely to relapse and allow adequate time for rehabilitation).[10–11]

However, the need for a set period of abstinence has been questioned on the basis of number of observations. First, the 6-months rule is based on clinical practice and not on prospectively collected data. Second, some patients including those with acute alcoholic hepatitis may die before the abstinence period is completed, thus precluding some who are good candidates for liver transplantation. Third, the length of the wait time for liver transplant in most centers recently exceeds 6 months and should be used to follow these patients and offer them the appropriate support and treatment. Fourth, pretransplant abstinence does not predict posttransplant abstinence or compliance.[12–14] Fifth, despite the fact that some patient return to some form of alcohol drinking, very few will have excessive and trouble drinking and data showed minimal impact on graft and patient survival.[15,16] Sixth, some centers (15% of the U.S. transplant centers) do not follow the 6-month rule, and their data support a multidisciplinary approach with attention to the psychosocial parameters.[17]

Thus, although most guidelines suggest that there should be a fixed period of abstinence, I think that there should be some flexibility in selected patients. A reasonable approach is to have the patient fully evaluated by a multidisciplinary team to ensure adequate social support and minimal risk of relapse, and to ensure that with abstinence the patient will not improve to an extent where liver transplantation is no longer needed.[18] Patients with acute alcoholic hepatitis should be also evaluated if failed medical therapy and, with appropriate social assessment, should be considered for liver transplantation in selected cases.

## ALD: OUTCOME AFTER LIVER TRANSPLANTATION

Rates of graft and patient survival after liver transplantation for ALD are excellent and are similar to those for other chronic liver disease.[19] It stands lower than rates for patients with cholestatic liver disease but higher than rates observed in patients with viral hepatitis. These data led to a substantial increase in the relative percentage of transplants performed for ALD over past 20 years and currently stands at 25% to 30% of all transplants currently performed in the United States.

Data from the UNOS registry in 1997 showed a 7-year patient survival of 60% in patients with ALD compared to 76% in those with primary biliary cirrhosis. Similar data were published by different centers in Europe.[20,21] However, some recent studies showed a trend of lower long-term survival in patients with ALD. Jain et al. in a long-term follow-up study from Pittsburgh showed a significantly lower survival rate after 5 years in the patients transplanted for ALD.[6] This was mainly contributed to the development of extrahepatic malignancies post-liver-transplant which was more common in the patients with ALD. A similar increase in cancer risk posttransplantation was reported in an abstract form by a French Multicenter study.[7]

The risk of recidivism of alcohol use post transplant has been one of the most important reasons for the reluctance to accept patients with ALD for liver transplantation. Even the careful selection of patients, 20% to 50% of patients acknowledge some alcohol use after transplantation. The rates of recidivism are approximately 30% to 34% as been published by various groups in Europe and the United States. However, the overall impact on patient and graft survival was low in all these studies. Alcohol drinking was minimal in most patients, and rates of significant drinking were low at 5% to 8%. Most studies showed lack of predictor factors for recidivism including the so-called 6-months abstinence rule, but confirmed that a structured management of patients with ALD by a dedicated group of specialists in alcohol and addiction medicine, a social worker, and a transplant coordinator might be the most important factor in reducing the rates of recidivism post liver transplantation.[18,22]

## ALD: TRANSPLANTATION FOR ACUTE ALCOHOLIC HEPATITIS

Acute alcoholic hepatitis is a clinical syndrome that was first described in 1961 by Beckett, Livingstone, and Hill. The syndrome is characterized by abdominal pain, fever, jaundice, high levels of transaminases, anorexia and leukocytosis. It occurs in patients after sustained consumption of alcohol. Histologically, syndrome characterized by acute lobular hepatitis, Mallory's hyaline, and hepatocyte regeneration and necrosis. Studies in humans showed that syndrome is accompanied by increased oxidative stress and increased expression of proinflammatory cytokines such as tumor necrosis factor-alpha (TNF-$\alpha$). This syndrome is associated with high rates of mortality. Patients with severe disease (Maddrey score > 32) have a short-term mortality of 35% to 46%, and if patient requires dialysis, mortality is 90% to 100%.

Treatment options for patients with acute alcoholic hepatitis are limited currently to corticosteroids and Pentoxifylline. Data regarding the efficacy of steroids are controversial. A recent meta-analysis, which included data from the French and American randomized controlled trials to study the efficacy of corticosteroids in severe alcoholic hepatitis, showed that survival at 1 month was significantly better in patients receiving corticosteroids than those in the placebo group (84.6% vs 65.1%).[23] In another study, Akriviadis et al. showed that Pentoxifylline resulted in the reduction of short-term mortality from 46% among patients who received placebo to 24.5% among patients who received Pentoxifylline.[24]

Such high mortality in patients with acute alcoholic hepatitis even among abstinent patients and those treated with corticosteroids raised the question regarding the efficacy of liver transplantation in these patients. Because most programs in North America and Europe require a period of abstinence (6-month rule) to be considered for liver transplantation, acute alcoholic hepatitis is considered an inappropriate indication for liver transplantation, as patients with this syndrome by definition have been drinking in excess in the recent past, and thus have been excluded.

Few observations are relevant in the discussion of liver transplantation for alcoholic liver disease and acute alcoholic hepatitis. These observations are helpful in determining patients who are suitable for liver transplantation.[25] First, mortality rates in patients treated medically is very high. Second, a significant number (50%–70%) of patients with acute alcoholic hepatitis will recover with abstinence and medical treatment. Third, continued alcohol use is an important contributor to mortality in the period after the initial hospital admission. Predictive factors for mortality include continued alcohol consumption, hyponatremia, and renal failure. In the study done by Veldt et al., they found that clinical signs of recovery from liver injury tend to occur within 3 months of initiation of abstinence. They found that few patients will come to liver transplant because they will either die first, return to alcohol consumption, or recover their liver functions with abstinence.[25] Patients who do not recover after 1 to 3 months of abstinence have high mortality rates and should be considered more frequently for liver transplantation.

Data on transplantation among patients with acute alcoholic hepatitis are scanty, as most centers exclude these patients from consideration. Shakil et al. conducted a retrospective study of patients who received liver transplants at University of Pittsburgh Medical Center with primary diagnosis of ALD. Seventeen patients (3.6%) had hepatic explants with histological features of acute alcoholic hepatitis; however, only 9 (1.9%) met the clinical criteria of acute alcoholic hepatitis with a Maddrey score (Discriminant function) > 32.[26] Among patients transplanted for alcoholic cirrhosis, 1-year survival was 80% and 3-year survival was 71%. In patients with acute alcoholic hepatitis and discriminant function > 32, 1- and 3-year survival was as good at 78%. Rates of recidivism were low with minimal impact on patient and graft survival, and there was no increased risk of noncompliance with immunosuppressive regimen. Bonet et al. reported similar experience in 45 patients with ALD who were transplanted and were found to have alcoholic hepatitis on the explant.[27] The study confirmed that superimposed acute alcoholic hepatitis has no impact on patient survival. Tome et al. studied the influence of acute alcoholic hepatitis seen on the explant on the outcome of liver transplantation.[28] The study included 68 consecutive patients transplanted for ALD. All had minimum of 3 months of abstinence before transplant. Superimposed acute alcoholic hepatitis was seen in 36 patients. This was characterized using the Maddrey score as severe in 10 patients and mild in 26 patients. Survival rates for patients with ALD was good and similar to those transplanted for non-alcohol-related liver diseases (Figure 30.12.3-1). The presence of acute alcoholic hepatitis on the explant had no impact on patient or graft survival (Figure 30.12.3-2). Furthermore, there was no difference in survival between those with severe and those with mild acute alcoholic hepatitis (Figure 30.12.3-3). Finally, the presence of acute alcoholic hepatitis on biopsy was not associated with increased frequency of alcoholic relapse after transplantation.

In a different study from University of Chicago, Conjeevaram et al. retrospectively reviewed 68 patients who had liver transplantation for ALD (15% with coexisting viral hepatitis).[29] Alcoholic hepatitis was seen in 8 patients on the explanted liver, and in those patients the rates of recidivism were high at 50 %, and 3 out of 8 patients died with fatal alcoholic hepatitis posttransplant.

All the above-mentioned studies were retrospective, and alcoholic hepatitis was diagnosed based on histological features in the

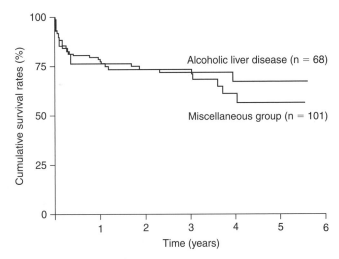

**FIGURE 30.12.3-1**

Survival rates for patients with ALD and patients with miscellaneous causes of liver disease undergoing liver transplantation. There is no significant difference among groups

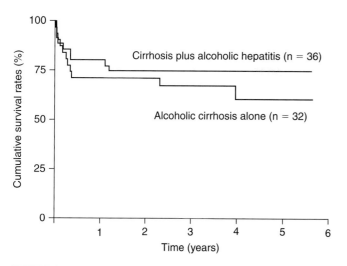

**FIGURE 30.12.3-2**

Survival rates for patients with alcoholic cirrhosis and patients with cirrhosis plus alcoholic hepatitis undergoing liver transplantation. There is no significant difference between the two groups

explanted liver. It may be reasonable for now to assume that data can be applied to patients with clinical syndrome of acute alcoholic hepatitis. All these studies except for one showed no impact of superimposed acute alcoholic hepatitis (defined histologically) on patient survival or rates of recidivism. It will be reasonable to assume that liver transplantation can have a potential role in the management of patients with acute alcoholic hepatitis. The data available are scanty but still justify the initiation of a randomized controlled prospective study. A reasonable approach will be a randomized trial of liver transplantation compared to medical management in patients with severe acute alcoholic hepatitis (MELD > 15 or Maddrey score > 32) who failed medical therapy and have been abstinent for at least 3 months (allow recovery where possible). Patients with concomitant renal failure should be considered early for liver transplant, as most studies showed short-term mortality of 90% to 100%. These patients underwent

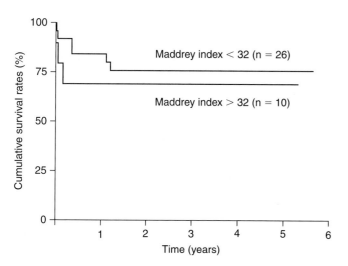

**FIGURE 30.12.3-3**

Survival rates for patients with alcoholic hepatitis according to Maddrey discriminant function (lower or higher than 32). There is no significant difference between the two groups.

extensive psychosocial evaluation to determine candidacy for liver transplant, and a support system should be maintained post liver transplantation to avoid risk of recidivism.

## LIVER TRANSPLANT FOR ALD: ETHICAL ISSUES

The shortage of donor organs, despite the greater use of marginal donors, split livers transplant and adult living donor transplantation, forces the implementation of rational criteria for selecting appropriate transplant candidates. Liver transplantation for patients with ALD is considered a medical dilemma. Clearly, the outcome of patients transplanted with ALD has been shown to be as good if not better as those transplanted for other indications, but the question of justice continues to be raised. The public, who is the main provider of donor livers and the resources for transplantation, believes that precious organs should not used to save the lives of people who have abused themselves. However, over the past few years, substantial evidence has emerged that points to successful outcome and low rates of recidivism in appropriately selected patients transplanted for ALD; thus all transplant centers in the United States and Europe accept patients with end-stage ALD for liver transplantation.

Unfortunately, most transplant centers place a lot of emphasis on the 6-months sobriety rule despite the evidence that showed poor correlation between this and risk of recidivism post liver transplant (discussed above), limiting the option of liver transplantation for patients who are too sick to wait and those with severe acute alcoholic hepatitis. Some of these patients, who are considered to be good candidates for liver transplant based on a thorough psychosocial assessment and adequate support system, may benefit from expanding the donor pool and using adult living donor liver transplantation

## ALD: ADULT LIVING DONOR LIVER TRANSPLANTATION (ALDLT)

The shortage of cadaveric liver organs has significantly inhibited further expansion of liver transplantation. With fewer than 5,000 cadaveric livers available annually, and more than 10,000 patients added to the United Network for Organ Sharing (UNOS) annually, a significant supply and demand disparity became obvious and has exponentially led to increased waiting times and increased waiting-list deaths (approximately 2,000 deaths in 2001). Although the number of registration on the UNOS liver transplant list has decreased because the implementation of the Model for End-Stage Liver Disease Score (MELD) for allocation of donor livers, the number of sick patients remained the same and waiting-list mortality for adults has increased to 10%. Because of the first report of ALDLT by Wachs et al. in the United States, the technique has gained widespread application.[30] By 2002, more than 1,000 ALDLT were performed in the United States alone, and 10% of all pediatric and adult liver transplants were done using living donors. There was a sharp decline in the number of ALDLT in 2002 due to the concern about donor mortality but the procedure continues to gain popularity.[31]

Liver transplantation is the best therapeutic option for patients with end-stage ALD. ALDLT can play an important role in those patients, and it can be utilized in both the standard and the extended indications. Clearly, the waiting-list mortality and increased waiting time are affecting patients with end stage ALD who are listed for transplant. The presence of a living donor will help a significant percentage of these patients. The main theoretical advantage is the very quick availability of an organ with optimal quality allowing these patients to have shorter waiting times, thus reducing the waiting0list mortality. In this group of patients, the outcome of ALDLT should be as good as that for cadaveric liver transplant. The use of ALDL in this group of patients should not represent any ethical dilemma.

The main ethical dilemma comes in using ALDLT for extended indications in patients with end-stage ALD. The two main indications in that category will be severe acute alcoholic hepatitis in a patient who fails to respond to medical treatment, and patients with a good psychosocial evaluation and a good support system, who otherwise are not able to wait for the minimal 6 months of sobriety due to advanced liver disease at the time of initial presentation. Although the data are scanty, there is enough evidence to suggest some benefit for liver transplant in patients with acute alcoholic hepatitis. In view that most centers are not listing these patients for liver transplants, and until we see more data in these patients using cadaveric donors, it is reasonable to avoid using ALDLT in this group. The outcome of ALDLT in those critically ill patients may be suboptimal, and the potential risk imposed on the donor may outweigh the recipient's minimal gains to be achieved with ALDLT. On the other hand, ALDLT can be utilized with caution in patients with end-stage ALD, who are too sick at their initial presentation or are not expected to be able to wait for the 6-month sobriety period due to advanced liver disease. These patients should go though an extensive medical and psychosocial evaluation. If they were found suitable candidates by the transplant team, in presence of a good social support system, ALDLT should be an option for those patients. The timely transplant and donor availability may help to improve the outcome of liver transplantation. Multiple studies showed poor correlation between the 6-months sobriety rule and alcohol relapse or patients' compliance posttransplantation; thus the outcome of ALDLT should be good and acceptable.

In conclusion, end-stage ALD is an acceptable indication for liver transplantation. ALDLT may benefit patients on the transplant list by minimizing waiting-list mortality and should be considered and encouraged in patients with suitable living donor. Until more data are available regarding the outcome of ALDLT in critically ill patients and the outcome of cadaveric liver transplant in severe acute alcoholic hepatitis, ALDLT should not be used in those patients. Long-term organized data collection and accurate results reported by multiple centers to define variables that influence recipient, graft, and donor outcomes are crucial to define the role of ALDLT in patients with ALD. The NIH-sponsored consortium of nine transplant centers in which ALDLT is performed for data collection and critical analysis will shed some light and allow safe implementation of ALDLT for end-stage liver cirrhosis in general and ALD in particular.

## References

1. Maddrey WC, Boitnott JK, Bedine MS, et al. Corticosteroid therapy of alcoholic hepatitis. *Gastroenterology* Aug 1978;75(2):193–199.
2. Mann RE, Smart RG, Govoni R. The epidemiology of alcoholic liver disease. *Alcohol Res Health* 2003;27(3):209–219.
3. Hoofnagle JH, Kresina T, Fuller RK, et al. Liver transplantation for alcoholic liver disease: executive statement and recommendations. Summary of a National Institutes of Health workshop held December 6–7, 1996, Bethesda, Maryland. *Liver Transpl Surg* May 1997;3(3):347–350.
4. Diehl AM. Alcoholic liver disease: natural history. *Liver Transpl Surg* May 1997;3(3):206–211.
5. Bellamy CO, DiMartini AM, Ruppert K, et al. Liver transplantation for alcoholic cirrhosis: long term follow-up and impact of disease recurrence. *Transplantation* Aug 27 2001;72(4):619–626.
6. Jain A, DiMartini A, Kashyap R, Youk A, Rohal S, Fung J. Long-term follow-up after liver transplantation for alcoholic liver disease under tacrolimus. *Transplantation* Nov 15 2000;70(9):1335–1342.
7. Miguet JP, Vanlemmens C, Messner M, Minello A, Duvoux C, Mondor H. Impact of Liver Transplantation on Survival in Pugh B Alcoholic Cirrhotic Patients. *Hepatology* 2003;38(Suppl 1):424.
8. Starzl TE, Van Thiel D, Tzakis AG, et al. Orthotopic liver transplantation for alcoholic cirrhosis. *Jama*. Nov 4 1988;260(17):2542–2544.
9. DiMartini A, Jain A, Irish W, Fitzgerald MG, Fung J. Outcome of liver transplantation in critically ill patients with alcoholic cirrhosis: survival according to medical variables and sobriety. *Transplantation* Aug 15 1998;66(3):298–302.
10. Foster PF, Fabrega F, Karademir S, et al. Prediction of abstinence from ethanol in alcoholic recipients following liver transplantation. *Hepatology* Jun 1997;25(6):1469–1477.
11. Gerhardt TC, Goldstein RM, Urschel HC, et al. Alcohol use following liver transplantation for alcoholic cirrhosis. *Transplantation* Oct 27 1996;62(8):1060–1063.
12. Berlakovich GA, Steininger R, Herbst F, et al. Efficacy of liver transplantation for alcoholic cirrhosis with respect to recidivism and compliance. *Transplantation* Sep 15 1994;58(5):560–565.
13. Osorio RW, Ascher NL, Avery M, et al. Predicting recidivism after orthotopic liver transplantation for alcoholic liver disease. *Hepatology* Jul 1994;20(1 Pt 1):105–110.
14. Neuberger J, Tang H. Relapse after transplantation: European studies. *Liver Transpl Surg*. May 1997;3(3):275–279.
15. Lucey MR, Carr K, Beresford TP, et al. Alcohol use after liver transplantation in alcoholics: a clinical cohort follow-up study. *Hepatology*. May 1997;25(5):1223–1227.
16. Pageaux GP, Michel J, Coste V, et al. Alcoholic cirrhosis is a good indication for liver transplantation, even for cases of recidivism. *Gut* Sep 1999;45(3):421–426.
17. Lucey MR, Beresford TP. Alcoholic liver disease: to transplant or not to transplant? *Alcohol Alcohol* Mar 1992;27(2):103–108.
18. Bjornsson E, Olsson J, Rydell A, et al. Long-term follow-up of patients with alcoholic liver disease after liver transplantation in Sweden: impact of structured management on recidivism. *Scand J Gastroenterol* Feb 2005;40(2):206–216.
19. Poynard T, Barthelemy P, Fratte S, et al. Evaluation of efficacy of liver transplantation in alcoholic cirrhosis by a case-control study and simulated controls. *Lancet* Aug 20 1994;344(8921):502–507.
20. Poynard T, Naveau S, Doffoel M, et al. Evaluation of efficacy of liver transplantation in alcoholic cirrhosis using matched and simulated controls: 5-year survival. Multi-centre group. *J Hepatol* Jun 1999;30(6):1130–1137.
21. Neuberger J. Transplantation for alcoholic liver disease: a perspective from Europe. *Liver Transpl Surg* Sep 1998;4(5 Suppl 1):S51–57.
22. Miguet M, Monnet E, Vanlemmens C, et al. Predictive factors of alcohol relapse after orthotopic liver transplantation for alcoholic liver disease. *Gastroenterol Clin Biol* Oct 2004;28(10 Pt 1):845–851.
23. Mathurin P, Mendenhall CL, Carithers RL Jr, et al. Corticosteroids improve short-term survival in patients with severe alcoholic hepatitis (AH): individual data analysis of the last three randomized placebo controlled double blind trials of corticosteroids in severe AH. *J Hepatol* Apr 2002;36(4):480–487.
24. Akriviadis E, Botla R, Briggs W, et al. Pentoxifylline improves short-term survival in severe acute alcoholic hepatitis: a double-blind, placebo-controlled trial. *Gastroenterology* Dec 2000;119(6):1637–1648.
25. Veldt BJ, Laine F, Guillygomarc'h A, et al. Indication of liver transplantation in severe alcoholic liver cirrhosis: quantitative evaluation and optimal timing. *J Hepatol* Jan 2002;36(1):93–98.
26. Shakil AO, Pinna A, Demetris J, et al. Survival and quality of life after liver transplantation for acute alcoholic hepatitis. *Liver Transpl Surg* May 1997;3(3):240–244.

27. Bonet H, Manez R, Kramer D, et al. Survival of patients transplanted with alcoholic hepatitis plus cirrhosis as compared with those with cirrhosis alone. *Transplant Proc* Feb 1993;25(1 Pt 2):1126–1127.

28. Tome S, Martinez-Rey C, Gonzalez-Quintela A, et al. Influence of superimposed alcoholic hepatitis on the outcome of liver transplantation for end-stage alcoholic liver disease. J Hepatol. Jun 2002;36(6):793-798.

29. Conjeevaram HS, Hart J, Lissoos TW, et al. Rapidly progressive liver injury and fatal alcoholic hepatitis occurring after liver transplantation in alcoholic patients. *Transplantation* Jun 27 1999;67(12):1562–1568.

30. Wachs ME, Bak TE, Karrer FM, et al. Adult living donor liver transplantation using a right hepatic lobe. *Transplantation* Nov 27 1998; 66(10):1313–1316.

31. Brandhagen D, Fidler J, Rosen C. Evaluation of the donor liver for living donor liver transplantation. *Liver Transpl* Oct 2003;9(10 Suppl 2):S16–28.

## 30.12.4  Acute Liver Failure

*Bijan Eghtesad, MD, Charles Winans, MD,*
*John J. Fung, MD, PhD*

A liver transplant is the only effective treatment for patients with irreversible acute or chronic liver failure. However, the growing number of patients on the waiting list and the relatively constant number of available deceased donor (DD) livers have resulted in an increasing number of deaths on the waiting list—particularly in children, given the limited availability of smaller grafts. Recent innovations such as reduced-size grafts and split-liver transplants have enhanced opportunities for children.[1,2] The use of living donors (LDs) has also helped (an option originally conceived to address the shortage of liver allografts in the pediatric population with end-stage liver disease).[3,4] Furthermore, the success of left lateral segment liver transplants then encouraged transplant surgeons to use full left lobe, and later right lobe, grafts to help more adults and to decrease mortality on the waiting list.[5,6]

Liver transplants are an established life-saving therapy for patients with fulminant hepatic failure (FHF) with survival rates of 60% to 90%.[7–9] FHF is classically described as severe impairment of liver function, with the development of encephalopathy within 8 weeks after the initial symptoms, in patients without a previous history of liver disease.[10] The prognosis of advanced FHF is extremely poor. The mortality rate of such patients, if untreated, can be as high as 80%. The timely availability of an allograft may be the ultimate determinant of survival. However, because of the shortage of DD livers even in high-volume Western transplant centers, mortality on the waiting list is still high—50% at some centers. This situation is even more dire in transplant programs in Asia, where DD livers are less available.

In many Asian programs, LDs were first used for pediatric patients with chronic disease; then, the use of LDs expanded to more emergent diseases such as FHF (in both children and adults).[11–13] Still, the use of LDs for patients with FHF is a matter of controversy and raises significant ethical issues.

## CHILDREN WITH FULMINANT HEPATIC FAILURE

The recent advances in reduced-size, split-liver, and LD transplants have dramatically reduced mortality on the waiting list for the pediatric population, particularly in Western transplant programs where DD livers are more available. However, in Asian

transplant centers where the supply of DD livers is scarce or nonexistent, LD liver transplants are often the only lifesaving procedure possible for children (or adults) with FHF.

The first successful LD liver transplant for a child with FHF was described in 1992.[14] Shortly thereafter, the Kyoto group reported their experience with LD liver transplants (left lobes) in 3 pediatric patients with FHF. In a subsequent report, the Kyoto group reported 11 LD liver transplants for FHF, with a patient survival rate of 73% during a 28-month follow-up. In two other reports, LD liver transplants were also used for pediatric patients with FHF: 10 in Japan (long-term patient survival rate, 90%) and 8 in Hong Kong (62%).[12,13]

In the United States, experience with LD liver transplants for pediatric patients with FHF has been limited to two series, plus a cumulative series by the Studies of Pediatric Liver Transplantation (SPLIT) Research Group. Emre et al. reported a 67% patient survival rate in 6 patients with FHF who received LD left lateral segments (mean follow-up, 27 months).[16] Mack et al described 19 pediatric patients with FHF: 8 received LD livers; 11, DD. The two groups were quite similar in disease severity. The patient survival rate at 30 days and 6 months posttransplant was 88% and 63% for the LD group versus 45% and 27% for the DD group. This marked difference was attributed to the LD groups shorter pretransplant waiting time (mean, 3.5 days, LD group, vs 6.5 days, DD group) and shorter cold ischemia time (mean 3.8 hours, LD group vs 7.9 hours, DD group).[17] The SPLIT data included 1092 primary liver transplants in children from 1995 through 2002, 141 (12.9%) of whom had FHF. Of these 141 children with FHF, 20 (14.2%) received LD livers; the rest, DD livers (whole organs, split livers, or reduced-size livers). The SPLIT Research Group found no significant differences in posttransplant survival for donor type or donor age.[18]

In all of these reported series (both Western and Asian), the overall patient survival rate after LD transplants for FHF in the pediatric age group ranged from about 60% to 75%. These survival rates are generally lower than in adults, possibly due to differences in the cause of FHF, to faster deterioration in children, or to longer waiting times in children, all of which could lead to more serious postoperative complications. Uemoto et al. suggested that rejection episodes were more severe in children with FHF, resulting in a higher rate of graft loss and a higher rate of patient death; however, this finding has not been confirmed by others.[19]

In a report on 500 primary DD liver pediatric recipients in Brussels from 1984 through 2000, the overall patient survival rate for 29 children who underwent a transplant for FHF was 72% at 5 years—significantly lower than for biliary atresia (83%) or familial intrahepatic cholestatic disease (97%) (p < 0.05).[20]

The crucial concern for children with FHF is the timely availability of a suitable liver before irreversible brain damage or death ensues. In Europe and the United States, transplant programs are now giving priority for DD livers to patients with FHF and more extensively using split-liver grafts for pediatric patients, thus allocating DD livers to children with FHF as quickly as possible.[21] In EuroTransplant, improved allocation of livers to patients with emergent diseases allowed 8 out of 11 children with FHF who were on the highly urgent liver transplant waiting list to receive DD livers within a mean waiting time of 3.1 days (of the other 3, 1 died within 2 days after being listed, and 2 recovered without a transplant).[22]

## LIVING DONOR FOR ADULTS WITH FULMINANT HEPATIC FAILURE

The results of LD liver transplants in adults with advanced chronic liver failure and acute or chronic liver disease, including FHF, have been poor. Blame has been placed on the "small-for-size syndrome" of the LD graft (typically, the left lobe) used in such situations. But with increased expertise in the use of the larger right lobe, better outcomes have been reported by transplant programs. Nonetheless, the operation itself carried a high risk of complications and mortality for LDs.

The use of LDs for adults with FHF has been reported extensively in Asia (where, again, there is not much chance of obtaining a timely DD liver in emergency situations). Lo et al, in their 1999 report, had success with LD transplants in emergency situations: of 25 patients who did not have LDs, only 2 received a DD liver; the other 23 died. However, of 13 patients who did have LDs, 11 survived.[23]

Nishizaki et al. in 2002, described left lobe transplants for FHF. A total of 15 adults (age, 22 to 59 years) with FHF received the left lobe from LDs, including the middle hepatic vein; liver volumes ranged from 260 to 570 mL, corresponding to 23% to 54% of the recipient's standard liver volume. The patient survival rate was 80% (follow-up, 3 to 43 months), with no LD mortality.[24]

Liu et al. used the right lobe from LDs in 16 adults with FHF. Within 24 hours after the recipients were listed, the evaluation process of the LD was completed. The grafts weighed 430 to 950 g (median, 615) and represented 39% to 89% (median, 48%) of the recipient's estimated standard liver mass. Of the 16 recipients, 14 survived (follow-up, 6 to 33 months) with no neurologic consequences; 1 patient died of biliary complications and 1 died of necrotizing pancreatitis.[25]

In another report from Korea, Moon and Lee reported a 90% survival rate in 19 patients with FHF who underwent adult-to-adult LD liver transplants.[26]

In the United States, the first report on the use of LDs for FHF was from the Miami group. The recipient was a pregnant woman, in her second trimester, with acute liver failure. She received the left lateral segment from her brother and had a good outcome.[27] The use of the right lobe for FHF in the United States was first reported by Marcos et al. The recipient was a 28-year-old man with FHF secondary to hepatitis B. His condition rapidly deteriorated. The lack of a DD liver prompted the transplant team to use the right lobe from one of his siblings, with a good outcome.[28] Despite the popularity of LD liver transplants for patients with end-stage liver disease in the United States, this operation has not been well accepted for patients with FHF. The reason is probably the fact that such patients are listed as high urgency and thus have an excellent chance to receive a DD liver in a short time without increased risk. According to United Network for Organ Sharing (UNOS) statistics from July 2001 through 2002, of 476 LD liver recipients, only 26 (5.5%) had been listed as "status 1." FHF constitutes about 7% of all indications for liver transplants in the United States.[29]

## ETHICAL CONSIDERATIONS

Despite the growing number of worldwide reports on the use of LD livers in adults, including those with FHF, the benefit of the operation—especially the use of the right lobe—must be weighed against the risk to the LD of a major hepatectomy. The emergency nature of FHF potentially could preclude the potential LD from making a careful decision about donation.[30] Questions about the safety of the operation and the possibility of coercion, especially in the setting of FHF, have not been answered. Patients with FHF rarely recover spontaneously, and there is a limited interval between the onset of this disease and irreversible complications and death. A

liver transplant is the only available effective treatment for this group of patients. Timely access to an organ is paramount, in order to prevent neurologic injury and to ensure irreversibility of the condition.

Many recent reports suggest that risks to the LD have been quite low. Complication rates range from 20% to 67% in different reports; mortality is estimated at between 0.13% to 0.2%.[31,32] In elective situations, the prospective LD is able to follow a predetermined, stepwise process, with enough time to assess the risks and benefits of donation and to undergo a psychological evaluation by the transplant team. However, in urgent situations such as with FHF, this process must be expedited. It is possible to finish the anatomic and biochemical workup of LDs in less than 12 hours, but that might not allow enough time for them to understand and consider the risks.

When access to DD organs is limited or nonexistent, the ethical issues of donation become radically different: potential LDs, usually parents or close family members, face only two options, namely, to let their loved one die by not agreeing to donate, or let their loved one live by accepting the risk of donor surgery. In an emergency situation, the process of informed consent by LDs could be influenced by coercion from family members or from the medical team. Autocoercion is also a strong possibility. According to a study by Crowely-Matoka et al, a significant number of LDs believe that living donation is coercive by its very nature, whether elective or emergency.[33] In this respect, and especially in the context of extending elective LD liver transplants to the more urgent situation of FHF, transplant programs must pay special attention to the autonomy of the potential LD and must ensure truly informed consent.

## CONCLUSIONS

In countries where DD transplants are limited, the use of LD livers is the only chance to rescue patients suffering from highly urgent conditions like FHF, with satisfactory overall patient and graft survival rates. Even programs with better access to DD organs should keep the LD option viable in emergency situations, when any wait increases the risk to the potential recipient. The LD morbidity rate is acceptably low. Yet, the possibly increased coercive nature of the donation process, especially when faced with a child with FHF, is a concern. Physicians are ethically required to fully inform the parents and family members about all the available therapeutic options.

## References

1. Broelsch CE, Edmond JC, Whitington PF, et al. Application of reduced-size liver transplants as split grafts, auxiliary orthotopic grafts, and living related segmental grafts. *Ann Surg* 1990;212:368.
2. Busuttil RW, Goss JA. Split liver transplantation. *Ann Surg* 1999;229:313.
3. Strong RW, Lynch SV, On TH, et al. Successful liver transplantation from a living donor to her son. *N Engl J Med* 1990;322:1505.
4. Broelcsh CE, Whitington PF, Edmond JC, et al. Liver transplantation in children from living related donors: surgical techniques and results. *Ann Surg* 1991;214:428.
5. Yamaoka Y, Washid M, Honda K, et al. Liver transplantation using a right lobe graft from a living related donor. *Transplantation* 1994;57:1127.
6. Wachs ME, Bak TE, Karrer FM, et al. Adult liver transplantation using a right hepatic lobe. *Transplantation* 1998;66:1313.
7. Bismuth H, Samuel D, Castaing D, et al. Orthotopic liver transplantation in fulminant and subfulminant hepatitis. The Paul Brousse experience. *Ann Surg* 1995;222:109.

8. Iwatsuki S, Stieber AC, Marsh JW, et al. Liver transplantation for fulminant hepatic failure. *Transplant Proc* 1989;21:2431.

9. Corbally MT, Rela M, Heaton ND, et al. Orthotopic liver transplantation for acute liver failure in children. *Transpl Int* 1994;7:S104.

10. Trey C, Davidson CS. The management of fulminant hepatic failure. *Prog Liver Dis* 1970;3:282.

11. Tanaka K, Uetomo S, Inomata Y, et al. Living related liver transplantation for fulminant hepatic failure in children. *Transpl Int* 1994; 7:S108.

12. Miwa S, Kashikura Y, Mita A, et al. Living-related liver transplantation for patients with fulminant and subfulminant hepatic failure. *Hepatology* 1999;30:1521.

13. Liu CL, Fan ST, Lo CM, et al. Live donor liver transplantation for fulminant hepatic failure in children. *Liver Transpl* 2003;9:1185.

14. Matsunami H, Makuuchi M, Kawasaki S, et al. Living-related liver transplantation in fulminant hepatic failure. *Lancet* 1992;343:1233.

15. Hattori H, Higuchi Y, Tsuji M, et al. Living-related liver transplantation and neurological outcome in children with fulminant hepatic failure. *Transplantation* 1998;65:686.

16. Emre S, Schwartz ME, Shneider B, et al. Living related liver transplantation for acute liver failure in children. *Liver Transpl Surg* 1999;5:161.

17. Mack CL, Ferrario M, Abecassis M, et al. Living donor liver transplantation for children with fulminant hepatic failure and concurrent multiple organ system failure. *Liver Transpl* 2001;7:890.

18. Baliga P, Alvarez S, Lindblad A, et al. Posttransplant survival in pediatric fulminant hepatic failure: the SPLIT experience. *Liver Transpl* 2004;10:1364.

19. Uemoto S, Inomata Y, Sakurai T, et al. Living donor liver transplantation for fulminant hepatic failure. *Transplantation* 2000;70:152.

20. Evrard V, Otte JB, Sokal E, et al. Impact of surgical and immunological parameters in pediatric liver transplantation. A multivariate analysis in 500 consecutive recipients of primary grafts. *Ann Surg* 2004;239:272.

21. Broering DC, Mueller L, Ganschow R, et al. Is there still a need for living-related liver transplantation in children? *Ann Surg* 2001;234:713.

22. Reding R. Is it right to promote living donor liver transplantation for fulminant hepatic failure in pediatric recipients? *Am J Transpl* 2005; 5:1587.

23. Lo CM, Fan ST, Liu CL, et al. Applicability of living donor liver transplantation to high-urgency patients. *Transplantation* 1999;67:73.

24. Nishizaki T, Hiroshige S, Ikegami T, et al. Living donor liver transplantation for fulminant hepatic failure in adult patients with a left-lobe graft. *Surgery* 2002;131: S182.

25. Liu CL, Fan ST, Lo CM, et al. Right-lobe live donor liver transplantation improves survival of patients with acute liver failure. *Br J Surg* 2002;89:317.

26. Moon DB, Lee SG. Adult-to-adult living donor liver transplantation at the Asan Medical Center. *Yonsei Med J* 2004;45:1162.

27. Kato T, Nery JR, Morcos JJ, et al. Successful living related liver transplantation in an adult with fulminant hepatic failure. *Transplantation* 1997;64:415.

28. Marcos A, Ham J, Fisher R, et al. Emergency adult to adult living donor liver transplantation for fulminant hepatic failure. *Transplantation* 2000; 69:2202.

29. United Network for Organ Sharing. Annual Report of the Scientific Registry of Transplant Recipients and the Organ Procurement and Transplantation Network: Transplant data 2003.

30. Abouna GJ. Emergency adult to adult living donor liver transplantation for fulminant hepatic failure—Is it justifiable? *Transplantation* 2001;71:1498.

31. Renz JF, Roberts JP. Long-term complications of living donor liver transplantation. *Liver Transpl* 2000;6:S73.

32. Beavers KL, Sandler RS, Shrestha R. Donor morbidity associated with right lobectomy for living donor liver transplantation to adult recipients. A systematic review. *Liver Transpl* 2002;8:110.

33. Crowely-Matoka M, Siegler M, Cronin D. Long-term quality of life issues among adult–to-pediatric living liver donors: a qualitative exploration. *Am J Transpl* 2004;4:744.

# 30.13   DOMINO LIVER TRANSPLANTATION

## 30.13.1   Technical Aspects

*Andreas G. Tzakis, MD, PhD, Seigo Nishida, MD, PhD, David M. Levi, MD*

Domino liver transplantation (DLTx) refers to the specific scenario whereby the recipient of a liver allograft contemporaneously donates their liver to another recipient. The first reported case of DLTx was performed in Portugal in 1955.[1] In this sentinel case, the "domino donor" had familial amyloidotic polyneuropathy (FAP). Although still relatively rare, the history of this procedure has been recorded by the Familial Amyloidotic Polyneuropathy World Transplant Registry (FAPWTR) and the Domino Liver Transplant Registry (DLTR).[2] At least 56 centers in 16 countries have performed the procedure for a total of some 700 cases to date.[2]

In principle, the DLTx procedure requires an appropriate domino donor (DD) and domino recipient (DR). A DD must be noncirrhotic with normal liver function except for a single metabolic defect. Most have FAP and consequently possess livers that produce an abnormal form of the protein transthyretin.[3] The abnormal accumulation and deposition of this protein is key to the pathogenesis of this disease. Liver transplantation with a normal liver may halt the progression of this debilitating and often lethal disease.[3] Because these are otherwise normal livers and because the natural history of FAP is measured in decades, there is a population of potential DRs that can benefit from transplantation using these grafts. The typical DR is an elderly patient with cirrhosis and limited hepatocellular carcinoma or any so-called "marginal" patient for whom the mortality risk of waiting for another graft is greater than the risk of acquiring the disease of the donor.[4]

Ironically, domino livers are usually of excellent quality and are procured under optimum conditions. Although the logistics of coordinating multiple transplants simultaneously can be resource intensive, the reward is a high-quality graft, procured from a stable DD, with minimal ischemic injury.[5]

DLTx requires careful planning and coordination. DD and DR pairs should be selected well before the procedure based on size, blood type, and anatomy. Proper informed consent must be obtained from both patients. Appropriate surgical teams are required for the cadaveric donor, DD, and DR. Excellent communication between the teams is essential. One successful demonstration of the logistics involved in these transplants was described by Azoulay in France.[6] In this report, the authors reported that a DD's native FAP liver was split *in vivo* for two DR adults. The DD received a cadaveric liver. In short, one available cadaveric liver had the domino effect of three transplants.

Although most DLTx procedures involve a DD with FAP, there have been notable exceptions reported. In one case, a neonate with fulminant liver received a metabolically abnormal liver as a "bridge" from a child (DD) with primary oxalosis.[7] The DD received a partial liver graft from his mother. In another case, the native liver of a recipient of a multivisceral graft (DD) was salvaged for a patient with advanced, decompensated cirrhosis.[8]

The DD hepatectomy is in essence of a live donor total hepatectomy.[9–11] Sufficient length of vital vascular and biliary structures must be preserved for the DD while ensuring that the graft is transplantable. The hepatic artery is divided between the splenic and gastroduodenal (GDA) arteries after ligating and dividing the latter. Some length of the GDA should be preserved with the graft especially if there is a replaced right hepatic artery. This replaced artery can be reconstructed to the GDA at the back table. If there exists an accessory left hepatic artery arising from the left gastric artery and it is small and/or there is adequate back bleeding, it may be ligated. If arterial flow to the left lobe is dependent on the accessory vessel, it should be preserved and reconstructed in the DR. The portal vein should be divided closer to its bifurcation than in the usual cadaveric donor hepatectomy. The DD with FAP may not have significant portal hypertension making it likely that venovenous bypass will be required to minimize bowel edema. Enough portal vein length should be preserved for the DD to accommodate a portal vein cannula and accomplish implantation of the new graft. The inferior mesenteric vein may be an alternative access site to the portal venous system for bypass. The common bile duct should be divided relatively close to the liver. If the retrohepatic cava is kept with the graft, the lower cava should be divided close to the liver.[12] The retrohepatic cava can be preserved for the DD if the suprahepatic veins of the graft can reconstructed at the back table.[13,14]

The hepatectomy for the DR should also be performed with attention given to preserving the length of the vascular structures and bile duct. Hepatectomy with preservation of the retrohepatic cava is preferred but not essential.[15] Venovenous bypass or a temporary portocaval shunt may be used if there is a longer than expected anhepatic phase.

The Achille's heel of the DLTx from a technical standpoint involves the hepatic veins and suprahepatic cava of the DD.[16,17] Without taking precaution, the suprahepatic cava may abe too short to be simply divided equally for both the DD and the DR. Short anastomotic cuffs for either patient may lead to poor control during implantation, prolonged warm ischemia time, or compromised hepatic venous outflow for the DD, DR, or both. This problem has been addressed with four specific technical solutions each with its own merits and disadvantages:

1.  Thorough mobilization of the suprahepatic cava maximizes the length available for both the DD and DR.[4,6] Ligation and division of the phrenic veins and freeing the cava circumferentially from the diaphragm and opening the pericardium permit exposure of the cava from the hepatic veins to the coronary sinus. Tedious dissection of the cava and opening the pericardium may increase the risk of a technical error in the DD.

2.  Liberal use of vein grafts for reconstruction of the hepatic outflow tract in the DD and/or the DR.[13,14] A variety of reconstruction techniques have been described which could be performed on the patient or on the liver graft at the back table. If the liver from the DD is removed with the cava, an extension can be added to the suprahepatic cava of the graft at the back table (Figure 30.13.1-1). If the piggyback technique is used, vein grafts can be used to unite and reconstruct the main suprahepatic veins. The caveat of the use of these extensions is that if too long they may kink restricting the venous outflow.

3.  Venoplasties between hepatic veins or between the hepatic veins and the vena cava may be performed (Figure 30.13.1-2).[12] These can be combined with venous extensions as needed. Although they simplify the construction of the venous anastomoses, they do not solve the fundamental problem of the short cuffs for anastomosis.

4.  The use of the infrahepatic cavocavostomy or "reverse-piggyback" technique avoids the problems related to the short suprahepatic cava of the domino liver (Figure 30.13.1-3).[15] The cava is preserved in the DR and the upper cava of the graft is closed with a vein patch. The infrahepatic cava of the graft is then anastomosed to the anterior wall of the preserved cava of the DR. Consequently, free drainage of the suprahepatic veins of the graft is achieved by reverse flow through the retrohepatic cava. A limitation of this technique is that it requires preservation of the cava in the DR.

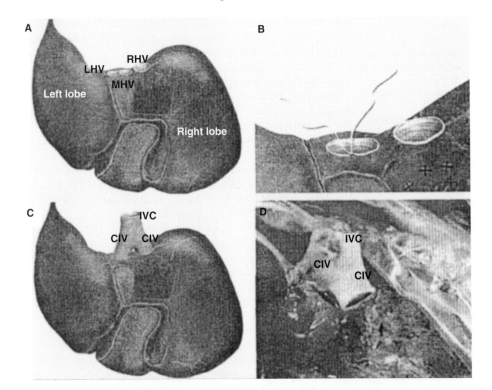

**FIGURE 30.13.1-1**

Venous conduit from the diseased donor for reconstruction of the FAP venous out flow. Abbreviations used: RHV, right hepatic vein; MHV, middle hepatic vein;LHV, left hepatic vein; IVC, inferior vena cava. Reprinted from "A new technical options for domino liver transplantation." *Liver Transplant* 2003;6:632–633; Figure 1, copyright (2003) with permission of Wiley-Liss, Inc., a subsidiary of John Wiley & Sons, Inc.

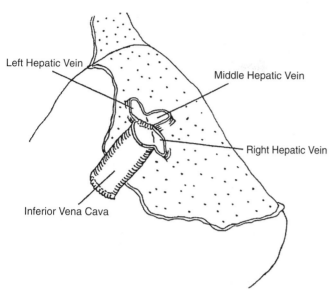

**FIGURE 30.13.1-2**

Venoplasty between the hepatic vein and inferior vena cava of the FAP liver. *Abbreviations used:* RHV, right hepatic vein; MHV, middle hepatic vein; LHV, left hepatic vein; IVC, inferior vena cava. Reprinted from Cadaveric domino liver transplant." *J Hepatobiliary Pancreat Surg* 2004;11:445–448. Figure 1, copyright (2004) with kind permission of Springer Science and Business Media.

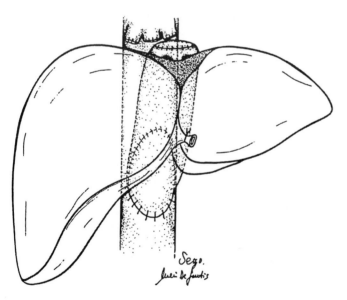

**FIGURE 30.13.1-3**

Infrahepatic cavocavostomy between the infrahepatic inferior vena cava of the FAP liver and the inferior vena cava of second recipient. Reprinted from "Domino liver transplantation with end to side infrahepatic vena cavo-cavostomy." *J Am Coll Surg* 2001;192:237–240. Figure 1, copyright (2001) with permission from American College of Surgeons.

In summary, the shortage of livers available for transplantation in conjunction with a better understanding of the etiology and pathogenesis of FAP has facilitated the use of domino liver transplantation to expand the donor pool. Hepatic venous outflow is the most important technical issue for domino liver transplantation. It can be addressed with an array of innovative surgical techniques.

## References

1. Futado A, Tomé L, Oliveira FJ, et al. Sequential liver transplantation. *Transplant Proc* 1997;29:467–468.
2. Ericzon BG, Larsson M, Herlenius G, Wilczek HE. Familial Amyloidotic Polyneuropathy World Transplant Registry (FAPWTR) and the Domino Liver Transplant Registry (DLTR). *Amyloid* 2003; Aug; 10 Suppl 1:67–76.
3. Holmgren G, Steen L, Ekstedt J, et al: Biochemical effect of liver transplantation in two Swedish patients with familial amyloidotic polyneuropathy (FAP-met 30). *Clin Genet* 1991;40:242–246.
4. Azoulay D, Samuel D, Castaing D, et al. Domino liver transplants for metabolic disorder: Experience with familial amyloidotic polyneuropathy. *J Am Coll Surg* 1999;189:584–593.
5. Inomata Y, Nakamura T, Uemoto S, et al. Domino split-liver transplantation from a living donor: Case reports of in situ and ex situ splitting. *Liver Transpl* 2001;7:150–153.
6. Azoulay D, Castaing D, Adam R, Mimoz O, Bismuth H. Transplantation of three adult patients with one cadaveric graft: wait or innovate. *Liver Transpl* 2006;6:239–2400.
7. Casas-Melley AT, Thomas PG, Krueger LJ, et al. Domino as a bridge to definitive liver transplantation in a neonate. *Pediatr Transpl* 2002; 6:249–254.
8. Tzakis AG, Nery JR, Raskin JB, "Domino" liver transplantation combined with multivisceral transplantation. *Arch Surg* 1997 Oct; 132(10): 1145–1147.
9. Hashikura Y, Ikegami T, Nakazawa Y, Domino liver transplantation in living donors. *Transplant Proc* 2005;37:1076–1078.
10. Nishizaki T, Kishikawa K, Yoshizumi T, Domino liver transplantation from a living related donor. *Transplantation* 2000;70:1236–1239.
11. Malagó M, Hertl M, jTesta G, et al. Split-liver transplantation: Future use of scarce donor organs. *Wold J Surg* 2002;26:275–282.
12. Wakayama K, Jin MB, Furukawa H, et al. Cadaveric domino liver transplantation: The first case in Japan. *J Hepatobiliary Pancreat Surg* 2004;11:445–448.
13. Pacheco-Moreira LF, De Oliveira ME, Balbi E, et al. A new technical option for domino liver transplantation. *Liver Transpl* 2003;9:632–633.
14. Pena JR, Barroso E, Martins A, Andrade JR, Pereira JP. Sequential whole liver transplant resected as piggy-back from FAP patients [Abstract]. *Liver Transpl* 2002; 8:C-24.
15. Nishida S, Pinna A, Verzaro R, et al. Domino liver transplantation with end-to-side infrahepatic vena cavo-cavostomy. *J Am Coll Surg* 2001;192:237–240.
16. Nicoluzzi JE, Massault PP, Matmar M, et al. Pitfalls of domino transplant. *Transplantation* 2001 Aug 27;72(4):751.
17. Nishida S, Tzakis AG. Pitfalls of domino transplant. *Transplantation* 2002 Mar 27;73(6):1009–1010.

## 30.13.2  Report from the Domino Liver Transplant Registry

*Henryk F. Wilczek, MD, PhD, Marie Larsson, BSc, Bo-Göran Ericzon, MD*

## BACKGROUND TO THE DOMINO PROCEDURE AND THE DOMINO LIVER TRANSPLANT REGISTRY

The continued success of liver organ transplantation is hampered by continuous shortage of suitable organs and progressively longer waiting lists. Many patients die while waiting for a transplant.[1,2] Efforts to change this have focused on, among other things, the use of living liver donors.[3–5] One group of potential living liver donors, are those individuals who are liver-recipient candidates themselves, but where their own removed liver in turn could be considered for transplantation into another patient. Familial amyloidotic polyneuropathy (FAP) is an autosomal, dominant, debilitating, and fatal condition caused by a point mutation in transthyretin (TTR), one of the prealbumins. As the liver is the main source of the circulating mutant form of TTR,[6] orthotopic liver transplantation was introduced in 1990 as a radical and hopefully curative treatment for FAP.[7] Early follow-up data were promising, showing patient improvement and that the disease progression appeared to be halted,[8] which spread the procedure worldwide. Some years later the idea came up to use these livers for transplantation, and this gave birth to the interesting therapeutic concept of the so-called sequential or domino liver transplantation procedure (DLT). The procedure was first performed in Portugal in 1995,[9] when a removed FAP-liver was transplanted into another patient in need of a liver transplantation. In order to gather as much information as possible on the DLT procedure an international register, the Domino Liver Transplant Registry (DLTR), was created in 1999 as an extension of the already existing Familial Amyloidotic Polyneuropathy World Transplant Registry (FAPWTR). This report presents our experience since the start of the DLTR 7 years ago and 11 years after the performance of the first domino liver transplantation procedure.

## THE DOMINO LIVER TRANSPLANTATION PROGRAM

The domino approach can be considered in several genetic or biochemical disorders that are nowadays treated by liver transplantation. The crucial aspect is that such livers ultimately cause severe systemic disease but do not affect other functions of the liver. The first and main indication thus far has been familial amyloidotic polyneuropathy.[10,11]

### Description of FAP—The Main Domino Donor Candidate Disease

FAP is a heritable, fatal condition in which the protein transthyretin misevolves, leading to the formation of amyloid fibrils and proteinaceous deposits that interfere with nerve and muscle function. The cause in the most common form leading to transplantation is a point mutation of methionine substituting valine at position 30. More than 80 amyloidogenic TTR variants have been described.[12,13] The mechanism for the conformational change of transthyretin and for its toxicity is largely unknown. The amyloid aggregates as insoluble fibers that are deposited in the extracellular matrix of various organ systems creating a diverse clinical picture.[14] Typically, the initial symptom is a painful sensorimotor polyneuropathy beginning in the lower extremities and progressing in an ascending fashion. In the later stages of the disease, the peripheral nerves, gastrointestinal tract, heart, kidneys, and autonomic nervous system are affected. Autonomic nervous system dysfunction may be present early in the disease, causing severe orthostatic hypotension and impotence. In the final stages of the disease, the patients are severely incapacitated, malnourished, and suffering from urinary incontinence and disturbed bowel function. The eyes are also affected with impaired vision in about 20% of the patients. The most prevalent transthyretin mutations are TTR Val30Met and TTR Val122Ile, which is carried by approximately 3.9% of Afro-Americans. Geographically, major foci of FAP occur in Portugal, Japan, and Sweden, but cases have also been found in other parts of the world mainly in Brazil, France, Spain, United Kingdom, and the United States. Although phenotypic expression varies greatly among geographical and ethnic foci, the outcome is slowly but invariably progressive and fatal within 10 to 15 years.[12,15–17] In FAP livers there are no other abnormalities than the production of the variant protein.[18]

## Rationale for the Use of FAP Livers for Transplantation

The reasons to use FAP livers for transplantation in other patients are multiple:

- The procedure expands the donor pool and makes more liver grafts available.

- The anatomy of the FAP liver is normal.

- The livers show no abnormal functionalities other than the production of the mutant form of TTR.

- The lean body habitus and the absence of portal hypertension in the FAP patients anticipate a relatively easy hepatectomy.

- The domino donor is a relatively young, stable individual, which in combination with a short cold ischemia time allows excellent conditions for the liver to be used as a graft.

- The disorder normally requires minimum 15 years to develop disease symptoms in genetically affected individuals. However, only a small proportion of all patients with the variant TTR mutation will develop clinical disease. It has been assumed that the TTR Val30Met producing liver grafts given to genetically nonaffected patients will need the same time to develop symptoms or, at best, the disease may never manifest itself.

## Other Hepatic Metabolic Disorders Used for Domino Donor Transplantation

In time, patients with other hepatic metabolic disorders have been considered as domino liver donors. Conditions that can be considered are, for example, primary hyperoxaluria, protein C deficiency, and some urea cycle disorders like citrullinemia. Until now reports on domino transplantation with livers from a patient with primary hyperoxaluria[19] and a patient with homozygous familial hypercholesterolemia[20] have been published. The rationale for using these patients as domino liver donors is essentially the same as in FAP patients. However, the issue is different regarding the recipient and requires strict assessment of the benefit–risk ratio, because the onset of manifest symptoms appears to occur much faster than in domino recipients of FAP livers. The risks for each metabolic disorder have to be assessed in the context of the clinical status and prognosis for each recipient of these grafts.

## Domino-Recipient Selection Criteria

The domino procedure, using livers from patients with hepatic metabolic disorders is justified for patients, whose condition precludes a long time on the waiting list; for example, some elderly patients and patients for whom palliative treatment rather than long-term cure remains the only option. The proportion of patients being subjected to DLT for nonmalignant disease has been increasing, and most of these patients are being transplanted for HBV- and HCV-induced cirrhosis, as well as sporadic cases with metabolic and fulminant disease. The hepatic tumors reported are primary liver tumors such as HCC and hepatoblastoma but also metastatic tumors from colonic cancer, carcinoid, and neuroendocrine tumors.

## DOMINO TRANSPLANTATION—ISSUES TO CONSIDER

### General Aspects

- Criteria for the acceptance as a domino liver recipient vary from country to country. In several centers DLT candidates are patients who otherwise would not have been considered for conventional liver transplantation because of poor prognosis and have an expected short life span,[9,11,21–26] whereas in some other centers[27,28] and at our center it is required that a DLT candidate must previously have been accepted for a conventional liver transplantation. Detailed information about the procedure and potential hazards and benefits must be given both to the donor and to the recipient. This means information not only of the operative risk but also of the possible future risk of acquiring the hepatic metabolic disease.

- Informed consent from both the domino donor and the domino recipient must be obtained well in advance of surgery.

- A thorough clinical and hepatic workup of the domino liver donor comprising liver tests, ultrasound examination of the liver, and sometimes also liver biopsy, magnetic resonance imaging, and celiac arteriography.

### Risks Associated With the Domino Liver Transplant Procedure

From a technical point of view, the domino donor and the recipient of the domino graft have to share a short segment of the suprahepatic caval vein, which is normally used for the construction of the venous outflow in both the donor and the recipient of the domino graft. This constitutes a potential risk and deserves particular attention, because it may lead to severe postoperative complications.[29,30] Several suggestions on how to handle this problem have been proposed.[9,22,31–33] At our institution we prefer to leave the longer caval segment in the domino donor, and we accept a somewhat short and sometimes somewhat "defective" cava on the explanted liver. So far, we have always managed to repair the cava and make it usable for grafting the liver into the recipient. This problem is more extensively discussed in Chapter 30.13.1.

The evident disadvantage by using livers with functional abnormalities as grafts, is the risk of transmitting the donor disease to the recipient. This risk can be made ethically justifiable by restricting the use of such livers to selected patient categories, in whom the likelihood that the domino recipient over the lifetime will develop disease symptoms caused by the hepatic metabolic disorder is estimated to be enough small. Examples of such patient categories are recipients older than 60 years and some recipients who have a malignancy such as hepatocellular carcinoma. In these patients, the life expectancy is estimated to be less than the risk of disease recurrence by the domino procedure. Other potential candidates that can be considered are certain patients with hepatitis C, in whom the risk of developing FAP symptoms can be assumed to be smaller than the risk of recurrent hepatitis in the graft. The recipient's underlying diagnosis, previous history, clinical status, and immunosuppressive treatment are all factors of importance for the course after transplantation and may modulate the hepatic disorder and disease evolution.

### Ethical Consideration—The Domino Donor

A domino liver transplant program raises new ethical issues both for the donor and for the recipient. The main priority must be guided by the clinical necessity in the domino donor, and the potential domino liver candidate must come second. In the donor, the issue is technical consideration and choosing the correct time of transplantation. The technique to remove the liver from the domino donor calls for particular attention, because it is not exactly the same as when removing a diseased liver in a conventional recipient, and the removal procedure cannot be permitted to carry a too great additional risk. The donor explantation procedure must permit a subsequent safe liver transplantation in both the domino donor and the domino recipient.

### Ethical Consideration—The Domino Recipient

In the domino liver transplant candidate, the ethical problem concerns the risk of transferring the hepatic metabolic disease with the graft. However, considering the desolate condition and expected short life span in the domino recipient, such a risk can be ethically justified if it is expected that the hepatic disorder will need many years to manifest itself as a symptomatic disease. The recipient has to be informed that the mandatory, lifelong immunosuppressive treatment after the domino liver transplantation may alter the natural course of the underlying disorder, and cause disease symptoms to manifest themselves earlier than anticipated. At present, our experience is not long enough to permit a definitive assessment of these risks. In some centers a retransplantation with a liver from a normal cadaveric donor is considered, if the recipient of a metabolically dysfunctional domino liver survives for more than 5 years.[11,22]

## MATERIALS AND METHODS

Centers are to report patients at the time of transplantation, retransplantation, patient death, or lost to follow-up; the register also requests annual follow-up data on transplanted patients. Information regarding patient demographics and clinical manifestations of peripheral and autonomic neuropathy are recorded. Each center is free to use its preferred method when evaluating the development of the neurological features after transplantation.

Patient weight, height, and serum albumin are also recorded for calculation of the modified body mass index (mBMI). This index has been reported to correlate well with the prognosis after transplantation[34] in FAP patients, but it is less clear with regard to DLT recipients. The mBMI is calculated by multiplying the BMI of the patient by the level of serum albumin, thus compensating for the presence of oedema present in a malnourished patient, which may yield falsely high BMI.

Some of the basic data from the register are displayed on the Registry's home page, www.fapwtr.org, from which it is also possible to download patient report forms. Separate forms are used for the domino liver transplantations. In the present analysis, patients reported to the DLTR until December 2005 are included.

## STATISTICAL ANALYSIS

For the difference between normally distributed means, the student's t test was used. Actuarial patient survival was calculated by the Kaplan–Meier product limit estimator. The log–rank test (Mantel-Cox) was used to test the equality of survival curves. All statistical tests were conducted at 0.05 significance level, 2-sided. Data are given as mean ± SD.

## RESULTS

Forty-six centers in 16 countries have been reporting recipients of domino liver grafts to the Domino Liver Transplant Registry (Table 30.13.2-1). With time, the annual global number of DLTs performed have increased (Figure 30.13.2-1) and presently 60 to 65 domino liver transplantations are performed. The male:female domino recipient ratio is approximately 3:1, and the mean recipient age at the time of transplantation is 54.5 ± 9.7 years (range 17–74 years).

The survival in FAP patients who became liver donors themselves did not differ from those FAP patients who did not donate a liver (Figure 30.13.2-2). Altogether, 513 patients were

**TABLE 30.13.2-1**
## NUMBER OF DOMINO TRANSPLANTATIONS PERFORMED BY DEC. 31, 2005

| Country | City | Hospital | No. of Tx | No. of Tx/ Country |
|---|---|---|---|---|
| Portugal | Porto | Hospital de Sto Antonio | 91 | 221 |
| | Coimbra | Coimbra University Hospital | 73 | |
| | Lisbon | Hospital Curry Cabral | 57 | |
| France | Villejuif | Hospital Paul Brousse/Kremlin Bicêtre | 79 | 82 |
| | Clichy | Hospital Beaujon | 3 | |
| Sweden | Stockholm | Huddinge University Hospital | 28 | 35 |
| | Gothenburg | Sahlgrenska University Hospital | 7 | |
| Brazil | São Paulo | University Hospital | 28 | 33 |
| | Rio de Janeiro | Federal University of Rio de Janeiro | 5 | |
| Germany | Mainz | Der Johannes Gutenberg Universität | 16 | 32 |
| | Hannover | Medizinische Hochschule | 10 | |
| | Heidelberg | Klinikum der Universität | 4 | |
| | Münster | Universitätsklinikum | 1 | |
| | Tübingen | Klinikum der Universität | 1 | |
| USA | Burlington | Lahey Clinic Medical Center | 8 | 28 |
| | San Francisco | UCSF Medical Center | 8 | |
| | Miami | University of Miami | 5 | |
| | Philadelphia | The Penn Transplant Center | 2 | |
| | Chapel Hill | UNC Comprehensive Transplant Center | 1 | |
| | Pittsburgh | Thomas E Starzl Transplantation Institute | 1 | |
| | Phoenix | Mayo Clinic | 1 | |
| | Rochester | Mayo Clinic | 1 | |
| | Baltimore | University of Maryland | 1 | |
| Japan | Kyoto | Kyoto University | 8 | 27 |
| | Matsumoto | Shinshu University Hospital | 7 | |
| | Kumamoto | Kumamoto University Hospital | 7 | |
| | Niigata | Niigata University Hospital | 2 | |
| | Sapporo | Hokkaido University Hospital | 1 | |
| | Fukuoka | Kyushu University | 1 | |
| | Tokyo | Tokyo University Hospital | 1 | |
| Spain | Barcelona | Hospital de Bellvitge | 27 | 27 |
| UK | London | King´s College | 11 | 12 |
| | Birmingham | Queen Elizabeth Hospital | 1 | |
| Belgium | Brussels | UCL St Luc | 4 | 8 |
| | Gent | University Hospital | 3 | |
| | Liège | University of Liège | 1 | |
| Canada | London | London Health Science Center | 4 | 7 |
| | Toronto | Toronto General Hospital | 3 | |
| Switzerland | Geneve | Hôpital Cantonal | 3 | 4 |
| | Bern | Inselspital | 1 | |
| Netherlands | Rotterdam | University Medical Center | 2 | 3 |
| | Groningen | University Hospital | 1 | |
| Italy | Milan | National Cancer Institute | 1 | 2 |
| | Milan | Ospedale Maggiore Policlinico | 1 | |
| Argentina | Buenos Aires | Hospital C Argerich | 1 | 1 |
| Australia | Sydney | Royal Prince Alfred Hospital | 1 | 1 |

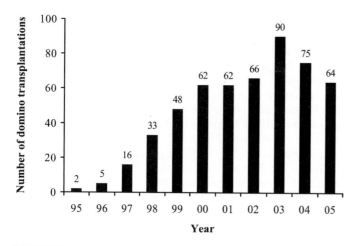

**FIGURE 30.13.2-1**

Number of domino liver transplantations per year since the start in 1995.

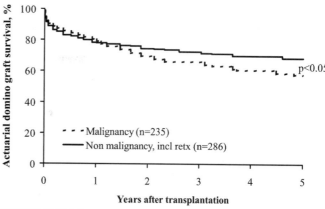

**FIGURE 30.13.2-3**

Actuarial graft survival in domino liver recipients transplanted because of malignancy and compared to domino recipients transplanted because of nonmalignant disease.

subjected to a total of 523 domino liver transplantations. The overall 1-year and 5-year graft survival in DLT recipients was 79.2% and 63.7%, respectively. Domino recipients transplanted because of malignancy had inferior survival figures compared to nonmalignant recipients (Figure 30.13.2-3). The majority (n = 513) of the DLT livers came from FAP patients, but two livers from patients with oxalosis have also been reported to the DLT registry. One of these livers was given to a patient with hepatocellular carcinoma, and this patient died 3.5 years after the transplantation because of *de novo* solid organ tumor. The other oxalosis liver was given to a patient with hepatocellular carcinoma and hepatitis B, and this patient was reported to be on dialysis 2.5 years after the transplantation because of progressive renal failure caused by oxalate renal deposition and cyclosporin medication. In eight cases the domino liver was used as a split; that is, the domino liver was divided and used for transplantation into two patients. Table 30.13.2-2 presents the indications among recipients of domino liver grafts. A total of 207 (40%) of the used FAP grafts were given to patients with a primary hepatic malignancy, of whom 113 (55%) patients also had viral hepatitis. In 86 of the 113 patients (76%) hepatitis C was diagnosed, whereas 27 (24%) patients had hepatitis B. FAP livers were used in 28 cases of retransplantation. Cirrhosis due to hepatitis C (n = 87) and

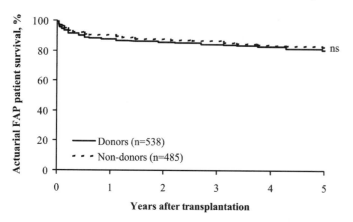

**FIGURE 30.13.2-2**

Actuarial survival in FAP patients with regard to whether they became domino liver donors or not.

**TABLE 30.13.2-2**

## INDICATIONS FOR DOMINO LIVER TRANSPLANTATION REPORTED TO THE DLTR

|  | No. of Cases |
|---|---|
| • **Primary hepatic malignancy** | **216** |
| • Hepatocellular cancer | 207 |
| • Hemangioendothelioma | 5 |
| • Cholangiocarcinoma | 3 |
| • Hepatoblastoma | 1 |
| • **Metastatic hepatic malignancy** | **19** |
| • Unspecified neuroendocrine tumor | 11 |
| • Carcinoid tumor hepatic metastases | 5 |
| • Colorectal hepatic metastases | 2 |
| • Hepatic metastase from a primary tumor of non-gastrointestinal origin | 1 |
| • **Retransplantation** | **28** |
| • **Cirrhosis secondary to hepatitis B and C** | **113** |
| • **Other miscellaneous diagnoses** | **145** |
| • Alcoholic cirrhosis | 81 |
| • Primary biliary cirrhosis | 16 |
| • Primary sclerosing cholangitis | 12 |
| • Cryptogenic cirrhosis | 4 |
| • Wilson's disease | 4 |
| • High age | 3 |
| • Autoimmune cirrhosis | 2 |
| • Virus BC related cirrhosis | 2 |
| • Virus BD related cirrhosis | 2 |
| • Secondary biliary cirrhosis | 2 |
| • Biliary artresia | 2 |
| • Fulminant Virus B hepatitis | 2 |
| • NASH | 2 |
| • Hemochromatosis | 1 |
| • Primary hyperoxaluria | 1 |
| • Polycystic disease | 1 |
| • Budd Chiari | 1 |
| • Hemangioma | 1 |
| • Citrullinemia | 1 |
| • Congenital agenesis of portal vein | 1 |
| • Liver failure after right lobe living donation | 1 |
| • Antitrypsin deficiency | 1 |
| • Rendu Osler | 1 |
| • Fulminant hepatitis, not specified | 1 |
| • **Diagnosis not specified** | **2** |

B (n = 26) as the sole indication for domino liver transplantation was reported in 22% of the patients. With time, the number of domino recipients with cirrhosis caused by excessive alcohol intake has markedly increased to become the third largest indication for the domino liver procedure (n = 81) only superseded by hepatocellular carcinoma and hepatitis C. Other, rare, miscellaneous underlying diagnoses are hemochromatosis, Wilson´s disease, primary biliary cirrhosis, and primary sclerosing cholangitis. Noteworthy, 160 (31%) of the 523 domino graft recipients were older than 60 years of age. In 63 cases, a domino graft was sent from one transplant center to another within the same country and from one European country to another in nine cases. One hundred and sixty-two out of 513 DLT recipients died. Tumor recurrence and septicemia accounted for 39% of the deaths. The remaining patients died from a variety of causes, such as peroperative death (7%), cardiac-related death (7%), and end-stage liver disease secondary to recurrence of hepatitis B and C in the graft.

## DISCUSSION

Domino liver transplantation is a procedure in which one patient receives a new liver, while that patient's functionally defective liver is removed and then used for transplantation into another patient. The main candidates to become domino donors are patients with FAP, because the onset of extrahepatic complications in FAP is in adulthood.[35] Using livers for transplantation from patients with hepatic metabolic disorders has proved to be a good alternative method to expand the donor pool. The procedure offers the chance of a cure to patients who benefit significantly by a short waiting time, or to patients who most probably otherwise would never have become transplanted. Some conditions must be fulfilled when considering the domino liver procedure

1. Apart from the metabolic disorder, the liver must be fully functional.

2. The genetic defect in the host should not be expected to recur within a too short latency time-period.

3. A close lifelong monitoring of the domino liver transplant recipient is mandatory. Such a monitoring should include clinical, laboratory, and metabolic tests, and in recipients of FAP livers also neurological follow-up.

Since the first domino liver transplantation was performed in 1995,[9] the practice of reusing FAP-livers in a domino manner has become routine in many transplant centers around the world.[11,27,36] With time, many centers have widened their indications regarding acceptance of domino liver recipients to also include patients with nonmalignant liver diseases such as viral hepatitis and elderly recipients. FAP-livers have also been used to retransplant patients in whom a primary liver disease recurred after a previous liver transplantation. DLTR data also indicate that domino liver grafts have been used in some desperate and urgent clinical situations, such as primary nonfunctioning grafts. Furthermore, it appears that domino liver transplantation is sometimes performed in patients, who otherwise in a clinical nondomino situation would be considered extremely controversial, for example, metastatic and recurrent hepatic malignancies in previously transplanted patients. It is noteworthy that domino liver grafts have been used for retransplantation in operatively high-risk scenarios, as evidenced by the fact that 2 of the 28 patients that were retransplanted with domino grafts had received two previous cadaveric grafts.

The domino liver procedure has without doubt evolved to a tool making it possible to increase the number of livers available for transplantation. The main concern with the domino transplantation strategy is the safety of the donor. The harvesting should not impose on the donor any additional risk that he or she would not encounter under conventional transplantation procedures. The Registry data do not indicate that the domino donor faces any increased risk as illustrated by the Registry survival curves presented in Figure 30.13.2-2, a finding in agreement with several single-center reports.[9,11,21,22,26] At present the DLT registry does not collect data to answer the question whether the procedure has shortened the time on the waiting list for domino liver recipients. A very important issue to be resolved in the future is the risk of inducing *de novo* hepatic metabolic manifest diseases in the recipients of domino grafts; for example, amyloidotic polyneuropathy in recipients of FAP liver grafts and renal insufficiency due to hyperoxalemia/hyperoxaluria in recipients of livers from donors with primary hyperoxaluria. Such a risk is real and cannot be disregarded as indicated by the development of renal insufficiency in one of the oxalosis cases reported to us, and, as also supported by two recent publications.[19,37] This illuminates the predicament and the necessity of thoroughly defining the risk–benefit situation in the domino situation. In this context, another related important issue is how the necessary immunosuppressive treatment after transplantation influences the course of the hepatic metabolic disorder in the domino liver transplant recipient. Defining the impact of immunosuppression on the underlying initiating biological mechanisms as well as on the course of the manifest symptoms needs to be clarified by further studies.

## SUMMARY

To summarize, liver transplantation is presently the only hope for patients afflicted with certain disabling and fatal hepatic metabolic disorders. These patients can themselves, in carefully selected cases, serve as liver organ donors. Transplanting such livers into strict selected recipients appears to be ethically justified, since it creates opportunities to transplant patients who otherwise have no access to therapy or who cannot support a long waiting time. Performed by experienced surgeons the liver explantation procedure is safe, whereas at the same time permitting a subsequent safe transplantation in the domino donor. The immediate and short-term hepatic function in the domino recipients of FAP livers is excellent, and survival during the first years of follow-up is also good, especially when considering the recipients poor prognosis without transplantation. As expected, the survival among the domino recipients transplanted because of malignancy is inferior compared to those without malignancy. Nonetheless, a much longer follow-up period is required to definitely evaluate all laboratory and clinical consequences by the use of such livers, something which is clearly illustrated by the recent report of a case developing systemic TTR amyloidosis 8 years after a FAP domino liver transplantation.[37] Thus, continuous close monitoring and more long-term follow-up studies are needed. One way of monitoring these patients and evaluating the potential risk-benefit ratio of this interesting treatment modality is through a viable international collaborative Registry.

## ACKNOWLEDGMENTS

We would like to thank all reporting centers for their excellent work in reporting to the FAPWTR. Astellas Pharma Inc., Karolinska University Hospital, Huddinge, and the Karolinska

Institutet, Stockholm, Sweden, sponsor the FAPWTR. The funding sources had no involvement in the collection, analysis, and interpretation of data or in the writing of this report.

## References

1. *2001 Annual Report of the U.S. Organ Procurement and Transplantation Network and the Scientific Registry for Transplant Recipients: Transplant Data 1991-2000:* Rockville, MD: Dept of Health and Human Services, Health Resources and Services Administration, Office of Special Programs, Division of Transplantation; Richmond, Va: United Network for Organ Sharing; and Ann Arbor, Mich: University Renal Research and Education Association; 2001.
2. Wiesner RH, Rakela J, Ishitani MB, et al. Recent advances in liver transplantation. *Mayo Clinic Proc* 2003;78(2):197–210.
3. Marcos A. Right-lobe living donor liver transplantation. *Liver Transplant* 6(6 (suppl 2)):S59–S63, 2000.
4. Strong RW, Lynch SV, Ong TH, et al. Successful liver transplantation from a living donor to her son. *New Engl J Med* 1990;322:1505–1507.
5. Wachs ME, Bak TE, Karrer FM, et al. Adult living donor liver transplantation using a right hepatic lobe. *Transplantation* 1998;66(1313–1316).
6. Soprano DR, Herbert J, Soprano K, et al. Demonstration of transthyretin mRNA in the brain and other extrahepatic tissues. *J Biological Chem* 1985;260:11793–11798.
7. Holmgren G, Steen L, Ekstedt J, et al. Biochemical effect of liver transplantation in two Swedish patients with familial amyloidotic polyneuropathy (FAP-met30). *Clin Genet* 1991;40(3):242–246.
8. Holmgren G, Ericzon BG, Groth CG, et al. Clinical improvement and amyloid regression after liver transplantation in hereditary transthyretin amyloidosis. *Lancet* 1993;341(8853):1113–1116.
9. Furtado A, Tome L, Oliveira FJ, et al. Sequential liver transplantation. *Transplant Proc* 1997;29(1-2):467–468.
10. Duvoux C. La transplantation hépatique a l'heure de la pénurie d'organes. *Gastroenterol Clin Biol* 2001;25:73–76.
11. Azoulay D, Samuel D, Castaing D, et al. Domino liver transplants for metabolic disorders: experience with familial amyloidotic polyneuropathy. *J Am Coll Surg* 1999;189(6):584–593.
12. Benson MD, Uemichi T. Transthyretin amyloidosis. *Amyloid: Int J Exp Clin Invest* 1996;3:44–56.
13. Reilly MM, King RH. Familial amyloid polyneuropathy. *Brain Pathol* 1993;3(2):165–176.
14. Glenner GG. Amyloid deposits and amyloidosis. The beta-fibrilloses (second of two parts). *N Engl J Med* 1980;302(23):1333–1343.
15. Coutinho P, Martins da Silva A, Lopes-Lima J, et al. *Forty Years of Experience with Type I Amyloid Polyneuropathy. Review of 483 Cases.* Amsterdam: Excerpta Medica; 1980.
16. Holmgren G, Haettner E, Nordenson I, et al. Homozygosity for the transthyretin-met30-gene in two Swedish sibs with familial amyloidotic polyneuropathy. *Clin Genet* 1988;34(5):333–338.
17. Saraiva MJM, Birken S, Costa PP, et al. Amyloid fibril protein in familial amyloid polyneuropathy, Portuguese type: definition of molecular abnormality in transthyretin (prealbumin). *J Clin Invest* 1984;74:104–109.
18. Hawkins PN, Rydh A, Persey MR. SAP scintigraphy in 43 patients with TTR associated FAP. *Neuromusc Dis* 1996;6:23.
19. Donckier V, El Nakadi I, Closset J, et al. Domino hepatic transplantation using the liver from a patient with primary hyperoxaluria. *Transplantation* 2001;71(9):1346–1348.
20. Popescu I, Simionescu M, Tulbure D, et al. Homozygous familial hypercholesterolemia: specific indication for domino liver transplantation. *Transplantation* 2003;76(9):1345–1350.
21. Figueras J, Pares D, Munar-Ques M, et al. Experience with domino or sequential liver transplantation in familial patients with amyloid polyneuropathy. *Transplant Proc* 2002;34(1):307–308.
22. Hemming AW, Cattral MS, Chari RS, et al. Domino liver transplantation for familial amyloid polyneuropathy. *Liver Transplant Surg* 1998;4(3):236–238.
23. Nishizaki T, Kishikawa K, Yoshizumi T, et al. Domino liver transplantation from a living related donor. *Transplantation* 2000;70(8):1236–1239.
24. Stangou AJ, Heaton ND, Rela M, et al. Domino hepatic transplantation using the liver from a patient with familial amyloid polyneuropathy. *Transplantation* 1998;65(11):1496–1498.
25. Suehiro T, Terashi T, Shiotani S, et al. Liver transplantation for hepatocellular carcinoma. *Surgery* 2002;131(1 Suppl).
26. Tome L, Ferrao J, Furtado E, et al. Sequential liver transplantation: 27 cases in 25 patients. *Transplant Proc* 2001;33(1-2):1430–1432.
27. Schmidt HH, Nashan B, Propsting MJ, et al. Familial Amyloidotic Polyneuropathy: domino liver transplantation. *J Hepatol* 1999;30(2):293–298.
28. Tzakis AG. Let's play dominos. *Liver Transplant* 2000;6(4):506–508.
29. Seigo N, Tzakis AG. Pitfalls of domino transplant: Letter to the editor. *Transplantation* 2002;73(6):1009–1010.
30. Nicoluzzi JE, Massault PP, Matmar M, et al. Pitfalls of domino transplant. *Transplantation* 2001;72(4):27.
31. Hesse UJ, Troisi R, Mortier E, et al. Sequential orthotopic liver transplantation—domino transplantation. *Chirurg* 1997;68(10):1011–1013.
32. Nishida S, Pinna A, Verzaro R, et al. Domino liver transplantation with end-to-side infrahepatic vena cavocavostomy. *J Am Coll Surg* 2001; 192(2):237–240.
33. Pacheco-Moreira LF, de Oliveira ME, Balbi E, et al. A new technical option for domino liver transplantation. *Liver Transplant* 2003;9(6):632–633.
34. Suhr O, Danielsson A, Holmgren G, et al. Malnutrition and gastrointestinal dysfunction as prognostic factors for survival in familial amyloidotic polyneuropathy. *J Int Med* 1994;235(5):479–485.
35. Pomfret EA, Lewis WD, Jenkins RL, et al. Effect of orthotopic liver transplantation on the progression of familial amyloidotic polyneuropathy. *Transplantation* 1998;65:918–925.
36. Furtado L, Oliveira F, Furtado E, et al. Maximum sharing of cadaver liver grafts composite split and domino liver transplants. *Liver Transplant Surg* 1999;5(2):157–158.
37. Stangou AJ, Heaton ND, Hawkins PN. Transmission of systemic transthyretin amyloidosis by means of domino liver transplantation. *N Engl J Med* 2005;352(22):2.

# 30.14   LIVER RETRANSPLANTATION

## 30.14.1   Adult Recipient

*SungGyu Lee, MD, PhD, Shin Hwang, MD, PhD*

Adult-to-adult living donor (LD) liver transplants have been established as a successful alternative to help solve the serious shortage of deceased donor (DD) grafts. However, in spite of a large number of adult-to-adult LD liver transplants (about 5,000 worldwide to date), LD retransplants have been uncommon. According to the registry maintained by the Japanese Liver Transplantation Society, 2,249 liver transplants had been performed in 49 institutions throughout Japan through 2002: 2,226 LD transplants in 2,164 recipients and 23 deceased donor (DD) transplants.[1] These data indicate that the retransplant rate after LD transplants was about 2.8%, most of them again using LDs.

Of 1,000 adult LD recipients at the Asan Medical Center (AMC) from February 1997 to January 2006, 19 underwent LD retransplants. Of those 19 recipients, 4 (1 heterotopic auxiliary) underwent LD retransplants; 15, DD retransplants.[2] In addition, 1 recipient underwent an LD retransplant due to primary nonfunction of the DD graft. This series showed 1.9% rate of retransplants in our adult LD liver transplant recipients. In contrast, the reported rate of retransplants from large-volume DD liver transplant programs has varied from 7% to 23%.[3] In the University of California,

Los Angeles, a series of 3,200 liver transplants (including 65 LD transplants) were performed; retransplants were performed, sometimes more than once, in 538 (20.2%) of 2,662 patients.[4]

The basic reasons that adult LD retransplants have such a low incidence (vs DD transplants) are as follows (1) The incidence of primary nonfunction is very low after LD transplants.[5,6,10] Primary nonfunction has been the most common cause of retransplants after DD transplants. A North American multicenter study group reported that 11 (2.9%) LD liver grafts failed because of primary nonfunction in 385 recipients; 37 of them underwent retransplants within the first year posttransplant, mainly because of vascular thrombosis or primary nonfunction.[5] In that study, only DD retransplants were performed. The detailed clinical sequences of primary nonfunction after LD transplants are not fully understood, although 1 case of a DD retransplant made it clear that primary nonfunction was caused by a steatotic LD liver graft.[6]

(2) The second reason for the low incidence of LD retransplants is related to the progressive decrease in graft failures from technical causes, by virtue of the advancement of surgical techniques and the improvement of imaging studies both donor and recipient hepatic vascular anatomy evaluation.[7] Various innovative techniques have decreased the incidence of refractory surgical complications after LD transplants significantly; hence, the need for retransplants has proportionately decreased.[8]

(3) The third reason is the definite shortage of available DD or LD livers for retransplants. In North America and Europe where DD liver transplants are the main types of liver transplants, a DD liver graft could probably be available after a relatively short waiting time if an urgent retransplant is required.[5] LDs are primarily used for a first liver transplant to cope with the relative shortage of DD livers. The probability of using LD grafts for retransplants is very low. Furthermore, the cumulative number of LD transplants in North America and Europe is much smaller than that in Asian countries.

However, in Asian countries where DD livers are scarce, the probability of retransplants (with either DD or LD livers) is very low because of the lack of donors. Thus, serious posttransplant complications often lead directly to death, with no chance of a retransplant. According to the AMC experience, the major causes of early graft failure in adult LD recipients were fatal technical complications, such as thrombosis or pseudoaneurysm of the hepatic artery, portal flow steal syndrome, and hepatic outflow obstruction. Massive hemorrhagic necrosis or refractory acute rejection of the liver graft seldom contributed to early graft failure as an immunologic complication.

## RETRANSPLANTS ACCORDING TO DONOR TYPE

LD retransplants can be classified into three types according to the sequences of the grafts used: LD-to-LD, LD-to-DD, and DD-to-LD. The surgical techniques in the retransplant differ according to these three different sequences. The timing of the retransplant can be either early or late.

An *early* (< 1 month) LD-to-DD retransplant is the simplest type of retransplant, because all structures belonging to the first liver graft are removed before adhesions form and the new graft can be easily anastomosed to the recipient's native structures. A *late* (> 3 months) LD-to-LD or DD-to-LD retransplant is typically the worst situation, because severe adhesions, distorted structures, and newly developed collateral veins make the recipient operation very difficult or not feasible (particularly in the absence of DD vascular grafts).

According to the AMC experience with 20 adult LD retransplants, the 1-year patient survival rate is about 60%—much lower than the 91% rate after primary LD transplants in 1,000 adult recipients.[9] Any cause of early graft failure is a possible indication for an early LD-to-DD retransplant, such as primary nonfunction, early severe dysfunction, or major surgical complications confined to the liver graft. Incidence of primary nonfunction after adult LDLT in our experience was 0.1%. Severe initial dysfunction of LD grafts has often been associated with small-for-size grafts, excessive venous congestion of right-lobe grafts from hepatic outflow obstruction, or portal flow steal syndrome (see Chapter 30.3.1a). Hepatic artery-related complications, including hepatic artery thrombosis or pseudoaneurysm, occurred in 2% to 5% of recipients at large-volume LD programs and became a leading cause of early graft failure.[11–13] Intractable biliary complications also can be an indication for retransplant, because its clinical course could be refractory and it occasionally induces life-threatening sepsis.[14,15] If recipients with intrahepatic sepsis can endure a retransplant operation itself, there might be no absolute contraindications.

For an early LD-to-LD retransplant, the eligibility criteria might be similar to those for an early LD-to-DD retransplant. Technical feasibility should be considered first. The most important concern is the availability of a hepatic arterial inflow source. A reliable source, besides the reuse of proper hepatic artery branches, is the right gastroepiploic artery because it can be easily mobilized toward the hepatic hilum after detachment from the greater curvature of the stomach and can be promptly enlarged in case of a size mismatch after splenic artery ligation. The clinical significance of this artery has been proven in LD transplants.[11,16] If it is not possible to use this artery in the retransplant, the interposition artery graft from the autogenous inferior mesenteric artery or sigmoidal artery can be used, or a fresh arterial DD graft should be procured.

For an early DD-to-LD retransplant, the indications are exactly the same as an early LD-to-LD retransplant, unless extensive hepatic artery thrombosis occurred. Hilar dissection of the failed whole-liver graft is comparable to that during the initial LD transplant. If hepatic arterial thrombosis was the cause of graft failure, an alternative arterial inflow source with mobilization of the right gastroepiploic artery or splenic artery can be used with excellent results.

For a late LD-to-DD retransplant, the indications are the same as for a typical late DD-to-DD retransplant, such as recurrence of primary liver disease or chronic rejection. This type of retransplant is considered to carry an increased risk comparable to a repeated DD retransplant.[17–20] No shortcut exists to dissect heavy adhesions and collaterals surrounding the failed primary liver graft, so the proper and harmonic timing of DD liver procurement and the recipient operation must be adjusted to minimize cold preservation time of liver graft.[21–22]

## OPERATIVE TECHNIQUES

The difficulty of recipient operation depends mainly on the timing of retransplant. An early urgent retransplant within the first 2 weeks posttransplant does not entail a difficult dissection process, because the primary liver graft has few adhesions around it. With a retransplant from 1 to 3 months after the primary transplant, some degree of adhesion will be encountered. Minute collateral vasculatures usually develop along with adhesions. Meticulous sharp dissection is mandatory to reduce blood loss.

With a late retransplant (3 months or more after the primary transplant), for progression of recurred primary liver disease (such as viral hepatitis-associated cirrhosis or chronic rejection), heavy adhesions and new portosystemic venous collaterals will be encountered. Every adhesion should be dissected sharply, and every bleeding point meticulously controlled from the beginning of the procedure. Blunt dissection for adhesiolysis is better to be avoided, because it can induce massive uncontrollable bleeding from the widely dissected surface in the presence of portal hypertension. If necessary, active venovenous bypass through inferior mesenteric vein may reduce the portal pressure and bleeding. One of the most early important steps in isolating hepatic artery, portal vein, and bile duct individually is to identify and loop the hepatoduodenal ligament from the severely adhered hepatic hilum. The foramen of Winslow should first be identified by continuing the sharp dissection downward, close to the ventral liver surface, or by completely mobilizing the right lobe of the liver graft and finding the way between the vena cava and the portal vein. Unlike an early retransplant, a late retransplant requires longer operative time (vs the primary transplant). Hence, donor and recipient operations must be scheduled so that cold preservation time of the liver graft and the LD operative time are minimized.[21,22]

## Early LD-to-DD Retransplants

After the previous incision for the initial LD transplant is opened, gentle blunt dissection with fingers may be permissible to separate the gelatinous or mild adhesions from the liver graft. The retrohepatic vena cava should be mobilized more extensively than during the primary DD transplant, thus further, cephalad to enable deep secure clamping of the suprahepatic vena cava over the diaphragm, given the necessity of new vena caval cuff construction. After sufficiently dividing the inferior vena cava down to the insertion of the right hepatic vein, the recipient's right, middle, and left hepatic vein openings are united. Doing so creates a wide new caval opening, incising septums and suturing them to make a trumpet-shaped long common cuff (Figure 30.14.1-1).

If the common hepatic artery is not healthy enough for an arterial anastomosis, an arterial interposition graft should be used as an infrarenal aortic jump graft.

After the liver graft and the inferior vena cava are completely dissected, the retransplant operation proceeds as for a DD-to-DD retransplant. The piggyback technique with side-to-side

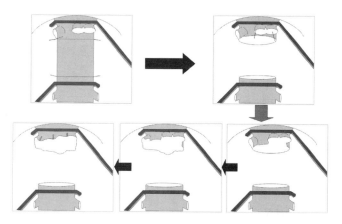

**FIGURE 30.14.1-1**

New vena caval orifice formation. After dividing the vena cava down to the insertion of the right hepatic vein, the openings of the right, middle, and left hepatic veins are united to create a wide new caval opening, incising septums and suturing them to make a trumpet-shaped long cuff.

or end-to-side cavocaval reconstruction is not recommended, because it seems to have no advantage over the standard technique.[23–25] LD transplants have often used duct-to-duct anastomosis, but if a sufficient length of bile duct from a DD liver graft is available and the recipient's healthy duct is easily isolated, a duct-to-duct anastomosis can often be redone. Otherwise, Roux-en-Y choledochojejunostomy is performed.[26,27]

## Early LD-to-LD Retransplants

For this type of retransplant, the volume and quality of the second liver graft and the hepatic arterial inflow source should be considered prudently. This type of retransplant is often performed in a highly morbid situation, so the suboptimal donor graft (such as a graft smaller than 40% of the recipient's standard liver volume, an older LD liver, or a steatotic liver) should not be used.[28–30] Donor livers with a variant anatomy, such as a variant portal vein or hepatic artery, should be cautiously used.[11,13,31,32] If a right-lobe graft is used, hepatic venous congestion should be minimized by reconstructing or concurrently procuring the middle hepatic vein.[33–36]

Arterial inflow source is another important issue to be considered in this type of retransplant. It is frequently not feasible to use proper hepatic artery branches again in recipients with hepatic artery thrombosis. The splenic artery is often not suitable for arterial reconstruction, due to its limited length, to its diameter discrepancy, and to the difficulty of mobilizing it in the presence of portal hypertension. Cryopreserved interposition vessel grafts should not be used for arterial reconstruction, because of a high risk of arterial thrombosis or of pseudoaeurysm formation, although successful outcomes have been sporadically reported.[37–39] Instead, fresh arterial interposition grafts from a DD can be used for recipients with a thrombosed hepatic artery. For such a purpose, it is reasonable to interpose a superior mesenteric artery graft from a DD, because it has many small branches that can be matched to the right or left hepatic artery of the partial liver graft. As alternatives, autogenous inferior mesenteric or sigmoidal artery interposition grafts can be used, but the available length of artery may not be sufficient.

Another reliable source of hepatic arterial inflow is the recipient's right gastroepiploic artery. In a situation requiring an arterial inflow source other than innate hepatic arteries, the right gastroepiploic artery is preferred for LD recipients because of its invariable anatomic location, its size, and its sufficient length. This artery often looks too small at a glance, but it can be rapidly dilated after clamping for a short time. Because it is fed from the arterial arcades at the pancreatic head and from the gastroduodenal artery, hepatic artery thrombosis (HAT) without extension to the celiac axis usually does not have a negative influence on the right gastroepiploic artery's blood flow. Interposition arterial grafts require two anastomoses, but the right gastroepiploic artery requires one anastomosis with less incidence of HAT. These merits of the right gastroepiploic artery as a substitute for hepatic arterial inflow have led to its use for multiple or redo arterial reconstructions in LD recipients.[11] Preoperative selective arteriography or 3-dimensional reconstruction of computed tomographic (CT) angiography can be used to evaluate it.[40]

If the use of a partial liver graft of a different type is anticipated, for example, if a left-lobe graft replaces a right-lobe graft, the suprahepatic vena cava clamping over the diaphragm should be done as for a DD retransplant, to facilitate hepatic vein anastomosis in a better surgical field. If prolonged vena cava clamping is often required, active venovenous bypass is beneficial.

After the primary liver graft and the inferior vena cava are completely dissected, the retransplant operation proceeds as for a primary LD transplant. The portal vein should be cut close to the primary liver graft across the anastomotic line, leaving a long cuff. A similar principle should be applied to the hepatic vein orifice. After vena cava clamping, the liver parenchyma should be cut to leave some hepatic tissue at the hepatic vein orifice, to preserve the edge of the hepatic vein orifice intact.

Technically, the use of a partial graft of the same type is an advantage for intra-abdominal space occupation and hepatic vein reconstruction. The same stump of portal vein can be used for portal vein reconstruction. The hepatic vein stump can be used as for a primary LD transplant, but a sufficient outflow orifice should be made. When using the right gastroepiploic artery as an alternative hepatic arterial inflow source, straightening the anastomosis site is helpful to avoid a kinking deformity. To prevent accidental excessive tension at the arterial anastomosis site, it is often necessary to transfix the periarterial omental tissue to the surrounding structures, such as gastric antrum or duodenum. Because its viability is not fully guaranteed, the recipient bile duct used for biliary reconstruction is not usually acceptable for redoing the duct-to-duct anastomosis.

### Early DD-to-LD Retransplants

This type of retransplant has been usually used for recipients with primary nonfunction of the first DD liver graft. Thus, all vascular structures remain intact. In contrast, if the cause of the graft failure is a vascular complication (such as HAT, portal vein stenosis, or vena cava stenosis), such recipients will require technical modifications. Hilar vascular structures and the retrohepatic vena cava of the failed liver graft should be dissected as for primary LD transplants. The vena cava and the portal vein of the failed liver graft should be left as interposition grafts (Figure 30.14.1-2). The hepatic artery of the failed liver graft can be used as an interposition graft (Figure 30.14.1-2), or an alternative source of arterial

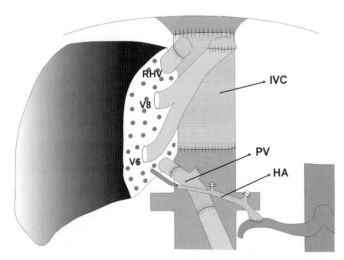

**FIGURE 30.14.1-2**

Preservation of the retrohepatic vena cava, portal vein, and hepatic artery (dotted area) of the first liver graft for use as interposition grafts for retransplants. In this retransplant, the modified right-lobe graft was implanted. Abbreviations used: RHV, right hepatic vein; V8, segment 8 hepatic venous tributary; V5, segment 5 hepatic venous tributary; IVC, inferior vena cava; PV, portal vein; HA, hepatic artery.

inflow (such as the right gastroepiploic artery) can be used. Both supra- and infrahepatic caval anastomotic lines are carefully protected when the right hepatic vein and multiple short right hepatic vein anastomoses are reconstructed. The portal vein of the failed liver graft should be dissected further distally, but this process is not difficult because the failed liver has nearly normal anatomy and hilar structures have been already dissected. Duct-to-duct anastomosis is not usually feasible, because the proximal portion of the recipient's bile duct has already been removed and the recipient's own duct cannot reach the LD graft's duct without undue tension.

### Late LD-to-DD Retransplants

Heavy adhesions and prominent venous collaterals are frequently encountered during the recipient operation. The piggyback technique is not recommended, given the heavy adhesions around the retrohepatic vena cava. Although the dissection of the hepato-duodenal ligament is difficult and heavy blood loss has to be anticipated, such a dissection can be successfully performed in most instances. The DD liver graft usually has a sufficient length of portal venous and hepatic arterial conduit to reach the near junction of the superior mesenteric vein and splenic vein as well as to reach the infrarenal aorta.

### Late DD-to-LD Retransplants

This type of retransplant is also very technically demanding. Hilar isolation of the intact portal vein and hepatic artery is difficult. The LD partial liver graft usually affords the short length of the portal vein and the hepatic artery. Surgical techniques are similar to those for early DD-to-LD retransplants, but the difficulty of hilar dissection varies depending on the associated portal hypertension and perihepatic collateral development.

### Late LD-to-LD Retransplants

This type of retransplant is almost impractical by any ordinary reconstruction method, because heavy adhesions and distorted structures of the hepatoduodenal ligament do not allow safe and sufficient isolation of healthy hilar portal vein and hepatic artery. The hilar portions of the recipient's hepatic artery and portal vein are easily injured during dissection of the hepatoduodenal ligament. With LD liver grafts, the hepatic artery and portal vein are not long enough to reach the recipient's common hepatic artery and proximal portal trunk. Alternatively, an interposition vein graft obtained from the recipient's left renal vein, 3 cm long, can bridge the gap between the liver graft's portal vein and the trunk of the recipient's portal vein (Figure 30.14.1-3). The left renal vein has many collaterals, such as the gonadal vein and the renal-azygous branch. Therefore, when the left renal vein is resected for a vein graft or ligated for preventing portal flow steal in partial LD transplants, these collateral branches must to be preserved, in order to maintain function of the left kidney.[42] Arterial lnflow is obtained from the right gastroepiploic artery by performing a microvascular anastomosis (Figure 30.14.1-3). If the vena cava wall for construction of the right hepatic vein anastomosis is injured and thin, a new right hepatic vein orifice can be created by making a circular fence to the side wall of the vena cava (Figure 30.14.1-3). The best material for the circular fence in the absence of cryopreserved DD vessels can be obtained from the autogenous great saphenous vein at the time of the retransplant.

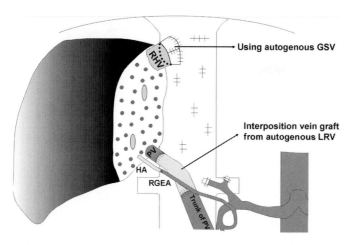

**FIGURE 30.14.1-3**

Vascular reconstruction in a *late* LD-to-LD or a late DD-to-LD retransplant. An interposition vein graft from the recipient's renal vein can bridge the gap between the liver graft's portal vein and the trunk of the recipient's portal vein. Arterial inflow is obtained from the right gastroepiploic artery. If the vena cava wall (for the right hepatic vein anastomosis) is injured and thin, the new orifice is created by making a circular fence to the side wall of the vena cava.

Abbreviations used: RHV, right hepatic vein; GSV, great saphenous vein; RGEA, right gastroepiploic artery; LRV, left renal vein; PV, portal vein; HA, hepatic artery.

## SUMMARY

Because LD retransplants have been performed in only a small number of recipients worldwide, their outcome cannot be assessed statistically (unlike with DD retransplants). Certainly, several technical limitations exists. Procurement of LD vascular grafts is not allowed. An alternative method of vascular reconstruction is often required, with increasing technical difficulty. Furthermore, the timing of a retransplant is seldom optimal, given the shortage of DD and LD grafts and the urgency involved with a failing first graft. Generally DD retransplant recipients have a higher morbidity and lower survival rate (vs primary DD recipients); nonetheless, the 1-year survival rate in adult DD retransplant recipients has recently improved to 70%.[17,41] Despite technical refinements, LD retransplants still carry an overall higher morbidity and mortality (vs DD retransplants). The 60% 1-year survival rate for LD retransplant recipients in the AMC series is comparable to that for DD retransplant recipients. Fundamental requirements for improving retransplant results include expanding the donor pool and the proper timing of retransplants.

## References

1. Tanaka K, Yamada T. Living donor liver transplantation in Japan and Kyoto University: what can we learn? *J Hepatol* 2005;42:25.
2. Hwang S, Lee SG, Lee YJ, et al. Lessons Learned from 1000 Living Donor Liver Transplantations in a Single Center: How to Make Living Donations Safe. *Liver Transpl* 2006;12:920-927.
3. Lerner SM, Markmann J, Jurim O, et al. Retransplantation. In: Busuttil RW, Klintmalm GB, eds. *Transplantation of the Liver*, 2nd ed. Philadelphia: WB Saunders; 2005:767.
4. Busuttil RW, Farmer DG, Yersiz H, et al. Analysis of long-term outcomes of 3200 liver transplantations over two decades: a single-center experience. *Ann Surg* 2005;241:905.
5. Olthoff KM, Merion RM, Ghobrial RM, et al. Outcomes of 385 adult-to-adult living donor liver transplant recipients: a report from the A2ALL Consortium. *Ann Surg* 2005;242:314.
6. Hwang S, Lee SG, Lee YJ, et al. A case of primary non-function following adult-to-adult living donor liver transplantation. *Hepatogastroenterology* 2002;49:1412.
7. Sugawara Y, Makuuchi M. Advances in adult living donor liver transplantation: a review based on reports from the 10th anniversary of the adult-to-adult living donor liver transplantation meeting in Tokyo. *Liver Transpl* 2004;10:715.
8. Moon DB, Lee SG. Adult-to-adult living donor liver transplantation at the Asan Medical Center. *Yonsei Med J* 2004;45:1162.
9. Colombani PM, Lau H, Prabhakaran K, et al. Cumulative experience with pediatric living related liver transplantation. *J Pediatr Surg* 2000; 35:9–12.
10. Ahn CS, Lee SG, Hwang S, et al. Anatomic variation of the right hepatic artery and its reconstruction for living donor liver transplantation using right lobe graft. *Transplant Proc* 2005;37:1067.
11. Wei WI, Lam LK, Ng RW, et al. Microvascular reconstruction of the hepatic artery in live donor liver transplantation: experience across a decade. *Arch Surg* 2004;139:304.
12. Marcos A, Killackey M, Orloff MS, et al. Hepatic arterial reconstruction in 95 adult right lobe living donor liver transplants: evolution of anastomotic technique. *Liver Transpl* 2003;9:570.
13. Hwang S, Lee SG, Sung KB, et al. Long-term incidence, risk factors and management of biliary complications after adult living donor liver transplantation. *Liver Transpl* 2006;12:831-838.
14. Fan ST, Lo CM, Liu CL, et al. Biliary reconstruction and complications of right lobe live donor liver transplantation. *Ann Surg* 2002; 236:676.
15. Itabashi Y, Hakamada K, Narumi S, et al. A case of living-related partial liver transplantation using the right gastroepiploic artery for hepatic artery reconstruction. *Hepatogastroenterology* 2000;47:512.
16. Yao FY, Saab S, Bass NM, et al. Prediction of survival after liver retransplantation for late graft failure based on preoperative prognostic scores. *Hepatology* 2004;39:230.
17. Burton JR Jr, Sonnenberg A, Rosen HR. Retransplantation for recurrent hepatitis C in the MELD era: maximizing utility. *Liver Transpl* 2004;10:S59.
18. Burton JR Jr, Rosen HR. Liver retransplantation for hepatitis C virus recurrence: a survey of liver transplant programs in the United States. *Clin Gastroenterol Hepatol* 2005;3:700.
19. Zimmerman MA, Ghobrial RM. When shouldn't we retransplant? *Liver Transpl* 2005;11:S14.
20. Schnitzler MA, Woodward RS, Brennan DC, et al. The economic impact of preservation time in cadaveric liver transplantation. *Am J Transplant* 2001;1:360.
21. Totsuka E, Fung JJ, Lee MC, et al. Influence of cold ischemia time and graft transport distance on postoperative outcome in human liver transplantation. *Surg Today* 2002;32:792.
22. Cescon M, Grazi GL, Varotti G, et al. Venous outflow reconstructions with the piggyback technique in liver transplantation: a single-center experience of 431 cases. *Transpl Int* 2005;18:318.
23. Navarro F, Le Moine MC, Fabre JM, et al. Specific vascular complications of orthotopic liver transplantation with preservation of the retrohepatic vena cava: review of 1361 cases. *Transplantation* 1999;68:646.
24. Miyamoto S, Polak WG, Geuken E, et al. Liver transplantation with preservation of the inferior vena cava. A comparison of conventional and piggyback techniques in adults. *Clin Transplant* 2004;18:686.
25. Nakamura N, Nishida S, Neff GR, et al. Intrahepatic biliary strictures without hepatic artery thrombosis after liver transplantation: an analysis of 1,113 liver transplantations at a single center. *Transplantation* 2005;79:427.
26. Schlitt HJ, Meier PN, Nashan B, et al. Reconstructive surgery for ischemic-type lesions at the bile duct bifurcation after liver transplantation. *Ann Surg* 1999;229:137.
27. Shimada M, Ijichi H, Yonemura Y, et al. Is graft size a major risk factor in living-donor adult liver transplantation? *Transpl Int* 2004;17:310.

28. Kiuchi T, Tanaka K, Ito T, et al. Small-for-size graft in living donor liver transplantation: how far should we go? *Liver Transpl* 2003;9:S29.

29. Ito T, Kiuchi T, Yamamoto H, et al. Changes in portal venous pressure in the early phase after living donor liver transplantation: pathogenesis and clinical implications. *Transplantation* 2003;75:1313.

30. Marcos A, Orloff M, Mieles L, et al. Reconstruction of double hepatic arterial and portal venous branches for right-lobe living donor liver transplantation. *Liver Transpl* 2001;7:673.

31. Lee SG, Hwang S, Kim KH, et al. Approach to anatomic variations of the graft portal vein in right lobe living-donor liver transplantation. *Transplantation* 2003;75:S28.

32. Lee SG, Park KM, Hwang S, et al. Modified right liver graft from a living donor to prevent congestion. *Transplantation* 2002;74:54.

33. Chan SC, Lo CM, Liu CL, et al. Tailoring donor hepatectomy per segment 4 venous drainage in right lobe live donor liver transplantation. *Liver Transpl* 2004;10:755.

34. Hwang S, Lee SG, Choi ST, et al. Hepatic vein anatomy of the medial segment for living donor liver transplantation using extended right lobe graft. *Liver Transpl* 2005;11:449.

35. Vivarelli M, Cavallari A, Buzzi M, et al. Successful arterial revascularization in liver transplantation using a cryopreserved arterial allograft. *Transplantation* 2004;77:792.

36. Kuang AA, Renz JF, Ferrell LD, et al. Failure patterns of cryopreserved vein grafts in liver transplantation. *Transplantation* 1996;62:742.

37. Settmacher U, Steinmuller T, Luck W, et al. Complex vascular reconstructions in living donor liver transplantation. *Transpl Int* 2003; 16:742.

38. Lee SS, Kim TK, Byun JH, et al. Hepatic arteries in potential donors for living related liver transplantation: evaluation with multi-detector row CT angiography. *Radiology* 2003;227:391.

39. Postma R, Haagsma EB, Peeters PM, et al. Retransplantation of the liver in adults: outcome and predictive factors for survival. *Transpl Int* 2004;17:234.

40. Moon DB, Lee SG, Hwang S, et al. Ligation of left renal vein for splenorenal collateral shunt to prevent portal flow steal in adult living donor liver transplantation. *J Korean Soc Transplant* 2005;19:182–191.

## 30.14.2   Pediatric Recipent

*Yasuhiro Ogura, MD, PhD, Koichi Tanaka, MD*

### INTRODUCTION

The only therapeutic option for patients with a failing hepatic allograft is a liver retransplant.[1,2] After the first successful living donor liver transplant (LDLT) in 1989, LDLTs are currently accepted worldwide as one of the treatment options for patients with end-stage liver disease.[3,5] Although the advantages and disadvantages of LDLTs have been discussed,[6–9] the issues surrounding retransplants, especially using LDs (Re-LDLTs), have rarely been reported. Problems that underlie Re-LDLTs are different from those that underlie deceased donor (DD) liver transplants.

Despite technical and immunologic progress, about 5% to 10% of pediatric liver transplant patients require a second liver transplant.[10,11] In the current era of the critical shortage of organs, the demand for liver allografts far exceeds the currently available supply. In many countries, LDLTs have been adopted, in order to increase the chance of a liver transplant or to expand the donor pool. In DD liver transplants, the outcome of retransplants and organ allocation are important concerns. In Re-LDLTs, ethical problems and the timing of the retransplant are more controversial. Furthermore, availability of LD and DD livers for retransplants differs in each country or region. Some

studies have been published regarding pediatric liver retransplants, but most were on DD retransplants.[12–14] Because reports on Re-LDLTs are limited,[11] we will mainly describe the pediatric Re-LDLT experience at Kyoto University Hospital, Japan. Several technical considerations in retransplants differ from primary LDLTs. Procurement of vascular grafts is particularly important in liver retransplants; prevention of infection, we believe, is another key to success.

### PEDIATRIC RE-LDLTS

From June 1990 to October 2003, a total of 590 pediatric LDLTs were performed (in recipients younger than 18 years of age) at Kyoto University Hospital. Over the same study period, a total of 32 pediatric Re-LDLTs (5.4%) were performed in 27 recipients (2 of them twice). Donor selection for Re-LDLTs is difficult if the LD must be selected from close family members. LD selection for a retransplant is sometimes even more difficult because of the blood-type combinations between a recipient and a second LD. Given the limited number of LD candidates, the proportion of incompatible blood type combinations increases for Re-LDLTs (Figure 30.14.2-1).

The vast majority (96.7%) of LDs for primary pediatric LDLTs were their parents, but other family members, such as grandparents and aunts, were LDs for Re-LDLTs or Re-Re-LDLTs (Table 30.14.2-1). With LDLTs, performance of more than one retransplant is extremely uncommon, mainly because of the limited availability of LDs among family members.

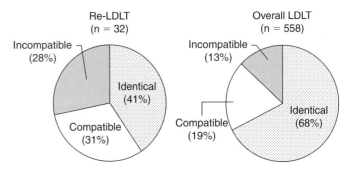

**FIGURE 30.14.2-1**

Donor-recipient blood type combinations in Re-LDLT settings (n=32) and overall LDLT settings (n=558) at Kyoto University Hospital.

**TABLE 30.14.2-1**

### THE LIVING DONOR SELECTION FOR PRIMARY LDLT, RE-LDLT, AND RE-RE-LDLT IN KYOTO LDLT SERIES

|  | Primary LDLT (n=30) | Re-LDLT (n=30) | Re-Re-LDLT (n = 2) |
|---|---|---|---|
| Father or Mother | 29 (96.7%) | 25 (83.3%) | — |
| Grandfather or Grandmother | 1 (3.3%) | 4 (13.3%) | — |
| Aunt | — | 1 (3.3%) | 2 (100%) |

## RE-LDLT TIMING AND CAUSE OF GRAFT LOSS

Posttransplant care has improved, yet many of our patients lost their liver allograft for various reasons. In DD liver transplants, primary nonfiction (PNF), hepatic artery thrombosis (HAT), and chronic rejection are the three most common causes of graft loss.[14] In contrast, in our LDLT series, the three most common causes of graft loss were chronic rejection (34.4%), chronic cholangitis (25.0%), and vascular complications (21.9%). In our entire series, we have not yet experienced PNF, a major cause of retransplants after DD liver transplants.[15] Furthermore, in our series, the interval between the previous LDLT and the Re-LDLT was relatively longer than in most DD series, a finding probably related to the cause of the graft loss. For example, pediatric Re-LDLTs as a result of chronic cholangitis were performed 5.9±1.3 years, after the primary LDLT operation; as a result of chronic rejection, 0.9±0.3 years; and as a result of vascular complications, 1.9±1.0 years (Figure 30.14.2-2).

## OUTCOME

The patient survival rate after pediatric Re-LDLTs is less satisfactory than after primary LDLTs. In our series, the 1-, 3-, and 5-year survival rate after pediatric Re-LDLTs was 48.2%, as compared with 84.7%, 84.1%, and 82.5% after our primary pediatric LDLTs (Figure 30.14.2-3A). Along with the improvement in general LDLT outcomes, we noted a comparable trend in our Re-LDLT results. As compared with our first 16 pediatric Re-LDLT cases (until May 2000), our most recent 16 cases (after May 2000) demonstrated better results (Figure 30.14.2-3B). According to recent reports in the literature, the 1-year survival rate after pediatric liver retransplants (mainly DD transplants) ranges from 63.0% to 71.7%,[12–14] results that are similar to our recent Re-LDLT cases.

The preoperative condition of the patient and the elective or emergent nature of the retransplant have an important impact on outcomes. Emergent Re-LDLTs and Re-LDLTs for patients confined to the intensive care unit (ICU) preoperatively carry higher morbidity and mortality, so patient selection and the timing of the retransplant must be considered carefully (Figure 30.14.2-3C).

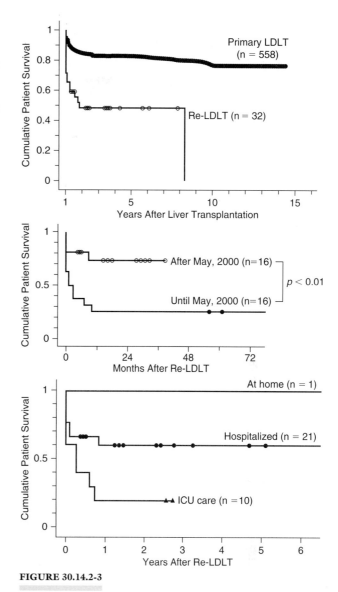

**FIGURE 30.14.2-3**

**A.** Kaplan-Meier survival curve showing the difference between primary LDLT and Re-LDLT. **B.** Improved survival of the last 16 Re-LDLT (after May 2000) recipients, as compared with our first 16 recipients (until May 2000). **C.** Kaplan-Meier survival curve showing the difference in survival after Re-LDLT by the patient's preoperative condition (at home, hospitalized, ICU-bound).

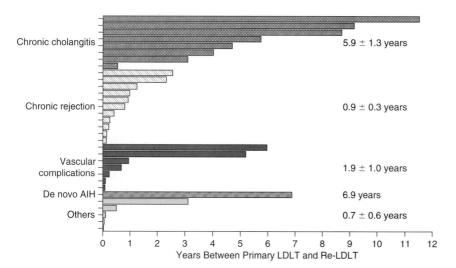

**FIGURE 30.14.2-2**

Intervals between primary LDLT and Re-LDLT, by cause of graft loss.

## CAUSE OF DEATH

The major causes of deaths after liver retransplants are sepsis and multiple organ failure. Sieders et al. reported that sepsis was the most important complication and cause of death after retransplants.[13] Of 32 pediatric Re-LDLT recipients in our series, 17 died. Of note the most common cause of death (52.9%) was infection, followed by bleeding (35.3%) and acute or chronic rejection (23.5%). Therefore, it is particularly important to control infection. High cumulative doses of immunosuppression can lead to infections, and technical difficulty during Re-LDLT procedures can also cause surgical site infections. Surgical technique modification for pediatric Re-LDLTs can reduce surgical infections, as mentioned later in this chapter.

## RE-LDLT OPERATION

The recipient Re-LDLT operation is made more difficult by the relatively long interval after the previous LDLT, an interval that gives rise to dense and fibrous adhesion. Surgeons frequently encounter this difficulty in dissecting surrounding tissues and identifying the important vessels. Moreover, due to the relatively small size and short length of vessels in LD liver grafts, the dissection and preparation of vessels should be extended as far as possible in the recipient operation. One of the most difficult dissections involves the preservation of hepatic arteries. When hepatic arteries are sacrificed or damaged, and when they are too short for reconstruction, other arteries must be selected, such as the gastroduodenal artery, the left gastric artery, or the splenic artery.

Outcome after pediatric Re-LDLTs is highly influenced by the presence of infection. To avoid surgical infection, pediatric Re-LDLTs must be performed with the highest caution. Optional technique may sometimes decrease the risk of severe infection. Since biliary anastomosis in pediatric Re-LDLTs has a higher risk of leakage (as compared with primary pediatric LDLTs), exteriorization of the distal part of the Roux-en Y limb is useful. Doing so prevents reflux of the conduit. Such exteriorization gave us many satisfactory results in our recent cases (Figure 30.14.2-4).

## SUMMARY

Pediatric Re-LDLTs are the only alternative for children with failing liver allografts. In DD liver transplants, the most common causes of graft loss are PNF, HAT, and chronic rejection. However, in our LDLT series, the most causes were chronic cholangitis, chronic rejection, and vascular complications.

Outcome after liver retransplants is less favorable than after primary liver transplants. Avoiding the need for retransplants, through optimal surgical technique and thorough postoperative care in primary liver transplants, is extremely important. In pediatric liver transplants, hepatic artery reconstruction is a key to success. Technical refinements, such as the introduction of the microscope for hepatic artery reconstruction,[16] can help prevent HAT, which leads to emergent retransplants. Furthermore, the development of more effective immunosuppressive and antirejection protocols may reduce acute and chronic rejection, which often leads to graft loss.

Outcome after pediatric Re-LDLTs can be improved by earlier identification of candidates for retransplants—before preoperative ICU care becomes necessary. Elective Re-LDLTs are much preferable to emergent situations.

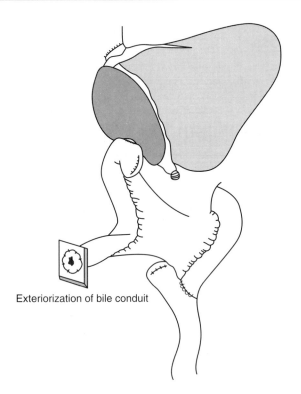

Exteriorization of bile conduit

**FIGURE 30.14.2-4**

Exteriorization of the bile conduit of the Roux-en-Y limb.

Pediatric Re-LDLTs can save patients with a failing hepatic allograft just as a DD retransplant can. To achieve more favorable results after pediatric Re-LDLTs, we need to more fully understand the factors leading to poor outcome.

## References

1. Mora NP, Klintmalm GB, Cofer JB, et al. Results after liver retransplantation (RETx): a comparative study between "elective" vs "nonelective" RETx. *Transplant Proc.* 1990;22(4):1509–1511.
2. D'Alessandro AM, Ploeg RJ, Knechtle SJ, et al. Retransplantation of the liver—a seven-year experience. *Transplantation.* 1993;55(5):1083–1087.
3. Piper JB, Whitington PF, Woodle ES, et al. Pediatric liver transplantation at the University of Chicago Hospitals. *Clin Transpl.* 1992:179–189.
4. Brolsch CE, Stevens LH, Whitington PF. The use of reduced-size liver transplants in children, including split livers and living related liver transplants. *Eur J Pediatr Surg.* 1991;1(3):166–171.
5. Broelsch CE, Emond JC, Whitington PF, et al. Application of reduced-size liver transplants as split grafts, auxiliary orthotopic grafts, and living related segmental transplants. *Ann Surg.* 1990;212(3):368–375; discussion 375–367.
6. Tanaka K, Kiuchi T. Living-donor liver transplantation in the new decade: perspective from the twentieth to the twenty-first century. *J Hepatobiliary Pancreat Surg.* 2002;9(2):218–222.
7. Malago M, Testa G, Marcos A, et al. Ethical considerations and rationale of adult-to-adult living donor liver transplantation. *Liver Transpl.* 2001;7(10):921–927.
8. Strong RW, Lynch SV. Ethical issues in living related donor liver transplantation. *Transplant Proc.* 1996;28(4):2366–2369.
9. Shiffman ML, Brown RS, Jr., Olthoff KM, et al. Living donor liver transplantation: summary of a conference at The National Institutes of Health. *Liver Transpl.* 2002;8(2):174–188.
10. Kim JS, Groteluschen R, Mueller T, et al. Pediatric transplantation: the Hamburg experience. *Transplantation.* May 15 2005;79(9):1206–1209.

11. Ogura Y, Kaihara S, Haga H, et al. Outcomes for pediatric liver retransplantation from living donors. *Transplantation.* Sep 27 2003;76(6):943–948.
12. Deshpande RR, Rela M, Girlanda R, et al. Long-term outcome of liver retransplantation in children. *Transplantation.* Oct 27 2002;74(8): 1124–1130.
13. Sieders E, Peeters PM, TenVergert EM, et al. Retransplantation of the liver in children. *Transplantation.* Jan 15 2001;71(1):90–95.
14. Achilleos OA, Mirza DF, Talbot D, et al. Outcome of liver retransplantation in children. *Liver Transpl Surg.* 1999;5(5):401–406.
15. Biggins SW, Beldecos A, Rabkin JM, Rosen HR. Retransplantation for hepatic allograft failure: prognostic modeling and ethical considerations. *Liver Transpl.* 2002;8(4):313–322.
16. Tanaka K, Uemoto S, Tokunaga Y, et al. Surgical techniques and innovations in living related liver transplantation. *Ann Surg.* 1993;217(1):82–91.

# 30.15   LONG-TERM OUTCOME

## 30.15.1   Adult Recipients

*Silvio Nadalin MD, Massimo Malagò, MD*

On November 2, 1993, the Shinshu group performed the first successful adult-to-adult living donor liver transplant (ALDLT).[1] Subsequently, the Hong Kong group (Queen Mary Hospital) performed the first series of right living donor liver transplants (RLDLTs) [2]. In the United States. The first ALDLT was reported by the Denver group in 1998. In Europe, unsuccessful ALDLTs were performed by our team in Hamburg in 1991, using a left lateral graft, and by the Madrid group in 1997, using a left graft. The first successful ALDLT using a right graft was performed in Europe by Broelsch et al in 1998.[4]

This surgical strategy evolved rapidly worldwide. By December 2005, a total of 979 ALDLTs were recorded in the European Liver Transplantation Registry (ELTR Report 2004, http://www. eltr.org). In 2005, the use of a graft from an adult living donor (LD) to an adult recipient was reported in over 385 patients in 94 centers across the United States.[5] According to the Japanese Liver Transplantation Society, 1,063 living donor liver transplants (LDLTs) were performed in Japan by the end of 2002.[6] A total of 766 ALDLTs have been performed in five Asian centers over the 12-year period from January 1990 to December 2001.[7] Considering the recent history of ALDLTs, the main data regarding long-term results are based mainly on follow-up of 2 to 5 years. The relatively short history of ALDLTs, the technical challenges, and the fact that, overall, few transplant centers have specialized in the procedure make the analysis of long-term ADLDT results more complicated than DD whole-liver transplants (DDLTs).

The main factors that have a significant impact on long-term ALDLT outcome are the country and transplant center, the operative technique preferred by the surgeons and the type of living graft chosen, the indications for the transplant and clinical status of the recipient, and the impact of technical and other complications.

## OUTCOME BY COUNTRY

### Asia

LDLTs are quite popular in Asian countries because DDs are scarce or not available at all. Improvements in results due to technical refinements and an extended range of indications have widely diffused ALDLTs (similar to that in the West).

Chen et al. reported on ALDLTs in 766 patients in five leading Asian centers (Kyoto and Tokyo in Japan, Hong Kong in China, Seoul in South Korea, and Kaoshiung in Taiwan).[7] At the time of their survey, there were 43 liver transplant centers in Japan and 25 in South Korea, less than half of which perform more than 10 transplants per year.

In the five leading liver transplant centers, the 1-year actuarial patient survival rate ranged from 78.7% to 97.8%; 5-year actuarial patient survival, from 76.1% to 97.8%. The 1-year actuarial graft survival rate ranged from 76.6% to 97.8%; 5-year actuarial graft survival, 72.4% to 97.8%.[7]

Biliary complications were more frequent in adults (7.3%, bile leakage; 10.5%, biliary stricture) than in children, probably because of the higher incidence of multiple bile ducts in right-lobe grafts. Vascular problems were more common in children (1.8%, hepatic artery thrombosis; 1.8%, portal vein thrombosis; 0.9%, outflow obstruction) than in adults. The mortality rate because of technical problems and recurrent disease was, in general, low. Infections, in the form of intraabdominal abscesses, opportunistic infections, and sepsis, remained a major complication and cause of death. Infectious complications occurred in more than 10% of adults. Sepsis was the cause of death in more than 2.5% of adults. The retransplant rate of the five centers ranged from 1% to 4.9%.

### United States

The Adult-to-Adult Living Donor Liver Transplantation (LDLT) Cohort Study (A2ALL) (National Institute of Health, www. niha2all.org) was organized by a consortium of nine North American LD liver transplant centers. This retrospective cohort study included over 700 donors and recipients treated between 1998 and 2003.[5] It analyzed in detail recipient outcomes of a large U.S. multicenter experience of 385 right-lobe ALDLT grafts. Outcomes were categorized as early (first 90 days), or late (91 to 365 days). There were 42 recipient deaths in the first year posttransplant. Kaplan–Meier estimates of patient survival were 94% at 90 days and 89% at 1 year. The largest number of deaths was due to infection and sepsis (43%), followed by multiorgan failure, graft failure, and cardiopulmonary causes. The survival rate with the original functioning graft was 87% at 90 days and 81% at 1 year. There were 72 graft failures in the first year, 71% in the first 90 days. The major causes of graft failure were hepatic artery or portal vein thromboses (n = 19) and primary nonfunction (n = 12). A total of 21 patients died with a functioning graft; 37 patients underwent retransplants, 86% in the first 90 days. Of the retransplant recipients, 7 died within a short time. The most common late complications (after the first 90 days) were biliary strictures (10%), infections (8%), and hernias (5%).[5]

### Europe

According to the last report of ELTR 2004 (http://www.eltr.org), from January 1991 to December 2004, a total of 1,709 LDLTs were performed in 63 (out of 135) liver transplant institutions in 23 European countries. ALDLTs are performed in countries with relatively poor (Germany) and excellent (Spain) donation rates, but predominantly in Western Europe. The vast majority of adults (91%) received right grafts (ELTR Report 2004, http://www. eltr.org). Globally, 979 ALDLTs were carried out all over Europe, with a patient survival rate of 81% at 1 year, 76% at 2 years, 72% at 3 years, and 69% at 5 years posttransplant; and a graft survival rate of 75% at 1 year, 71% at 2 years, 66% at 3 years, and 60% at

5 years. Interestingly, only 7 of these 63 centers performed ≥ 10 ALDTs per year, and only 4 published their own single-center experience.[8–11]

## OUTCOME BY OPERATIVE TRANSPLANT TECHNIQUE AND GRAFT TYPE

In ALDLTs, graft size is an independent predictor of mortality in adult recipients.[12] Still, ALDLTs can be performed successfully using a smaller graft in good-risk recipients.[6,7,13] Therefore, the strategy for graft selection should be influenced by the patient's preoperative condition: patients with advanced liver disease require a larger liver mass. Different techniques have been used in different centers: 11 types of grafts have been developed over the years, reflecting the versatility of surgeons in liver resection with consequently different results.[14]

The choice of the LD grafts, either the right or left liver, is dictated by surgeon preference and beliefs. Proponents of the left liver cite advantages for the donor and less risk.[6,15] Opponents of the left liver point to disadvantages for the recipient and a graft too small for the recipient's size. The same arguments, but reversed, apply to the proponents and opponents of right liver ALDLTs.[16,17] In general, right liver grafts have definitely been favored in the Western Hemisphere, because the size of recipients is normally too big to safely accommodate the smaller left graft.

Additionally, as with every evolving surgical procedure and more so with ALDLTs, the results are strongly influenced by the learning curve. In fact, analyses of the results of several major transplant centers showed a significant difference when early and late experiences were compared. The longer and greater the experience, the better the results—making the overall outcome of ALDLTs comparable to, or even better than, the outcome of DDLTs.[5–7,10,13,14,16,18–24,25]

### Left Liver Graft

In the initial adult LDLT procedures, only a left liver graft was used. By January 2004, the Shinshu group had performed 95 ALDLTs using left liver grafts.[6,15] At 5 years, the graft survival rates was 81%; patient, 82%. Their data indicate that the left liver graft provides satisfactory results for appropriately selected recipients. In the University of Tokyo program, 56% of the patients received a left liver or left liver with caudate lobe graft; at 5 years, the patient survival rates were 82%; graft, 84%.[13]

### Right Liver Graft

In 1998, the University of Colorado group[3] introduced the use of the right liver graft without reconstruction of the middle hepatic vein (MHV) trunk in ALDLTs. From January 1997 to July 2003, the group performed 80 ALDLTs. In the first 10 cases, in which the MHV branches of the graft were not preserved, 3 grafts were lost. Based on the group's preliminary experience, the resection line of the graft in the donor was moved to the left, in order to preserve the MHV branches and their connections with the right hepatic vein (RHV).[26]

Of 979 ALDLTs performed in Europe from January 1998 to December 2004, 91% used right-lobe grafts (mainly without the MHV). In right ALDLTs, the patient survival rate was 81% at 1 year and 76% at 3 years; graft, 72% at 1 year and 68% at 3 years. In left ALDLTs, the patient survival rate was 76% at 1 year and 67% at 3 years; graft, 74% at 1 year and 66% at 3 years (ELTR 2004, http://www.eltr.org).

### Right Liver Graft With MHV

The Hong Kong group was the first to transplant a right liver graft including the MHV in 1996.[2] Outcome for the initial eight donors and recipients was quite complicated: one recipient died, and the recipients as well as the donors experienced high morbidity. The next 92 patients subsequently received extended right liver grafts with the following innovations: elimination of venovenous bypass from the routine protocol, preservation of segment IV venous drainage in the donor, venoplasty of the MHV and right hepatic vein into a single orifice for better venous return, and easy vein reconstruction in the recipients.[27] Over time, the mortality rate of the recipients decreased from 16% in the initial 50 cases to 0% in 50 more recent patients. A similar experience was observed by our group. Since 2001, we performed 122 right ALDLTs—41 of them with the MHV and maximized outflow.[28] After the introduction of this new technique, we also observed an increase in the 1-year patient (87%) and graft (81%) survival rate (personal data), as compared with 79% and 75% in the earlier period.[10]

Overall, it appears that when the liver graft size is appropriately matched to the recipient's size, outcome is comparable, no matter which graft type is selected.

## OUTCOME BY INDICATIONS

The cause of liver disease continues to be an important variable affecting long-term outcomes of ALDLT recipients.[6,22,29] As with DDLTs, the best results are in patients with cholestatic liver disease, autoimmune hepatitis, and hepatitis B. The worst results are in patients with fulminant hepatic failure, advanced hepatocellular carcinoma (HCC), and hepatitis C.[6,26] Additionally, the stage of liver disease pretransplant plays a fundamental role in determining short- and long-term outcomes. For example, in patients formerly categoried as UNOS 2A, a 1-year survival rate of only 43% was observed.[30] Therefore, ALDLTs in the United States are now mostly confined to relatively well-compensated patients (former UNOS status 3);[31] recipients with Model End-Stage Liver Disease MELD scores higher than 20 represent only 17.3% of the total.[5] Note that the MELD score seems not to predict long-term outcome after ALDLTs in the same way as for 3-month mortality.[32]

### Primary Biliary Cirrhosis (PBC)

The prognosis of patients with primary biliary cirrhosis (PBC) has improved since the introduction of LTs. However, the experience with LDLTs for PBC has been limited. The Tokyo group reported about 50 LDLTs for patients with PBC.[33] Within 2 months, four died (mortality rate, 8%); three died later. At a median follow-up of 35 months (range, 4 to 84 months), the overall survival rate was 90% at 1 year, 88% at 3 years, and 80% at 5 years. No recurrence of PBC was confirmed at 3 years: LDLTs seem to provide satisfactory long-term survival for PBC patients.

### Hepatitis B Virus Cirrhosis

Outcome posttransplant for hepatitis B virus (HBV) cirrhosis patients has improved significantly in the last 2 decades, mainly as a direct consequence of the therapeutic innovations introduced to control the virus load before and after the transplant. Over the last few years, outcome after DDLTs for HBV patients, adjusting for other variables, is comparable with, if not slightly better than, outcomes for patients with other diagnoses.[34] Long-term experience with LDLTs for patients with HBV infection is still limited. Because LDLTs can be performed electively, they can provide an appropriate length of time to reduce HBV DNA levels pretransplant. Perioperative use of lamivudine and indefinite postoperative administration of hepatitis B immunoglobulin might be a rational strategy for preventing HBV reinfection after LDLTs.[35]

## Hepatitis C Virus Cirrhosis

Data indicate that the progression of hepatitis C seems to be accelerated posttransplant, as compared with nontransplanted individuals.[36]

Risk factors for posttransplant recurrence of hepatitis C virus (HCV) can be divided into those related to the virus itself, that is, pretransplant high viral loads and certain viral genotypes;[37] those related to the donor, that is, donor age and graft steatosis;[38,39] and those related to the recipient, that is, the incidence of acute cellular rejection and the amount and type of immunosuppression.[40]

In contrast to whole-organ deceased donor liver tansplants (DDLTs), survival and effects of recurrence after ALDLTs for HCV patients are not yet defined. The issue of recurrent HCV has been studied in split DD liver grafts: partial liver grafts may be associated with an increased risk for HCV recurrence.[41]

Humar et al. observed that LD recipients do not seem to be at higher risk for HCV recurrence than their DD counterparts (either full-size or split), according to exact assessment of several different markers of recurrence, including transaminase levels, viral loads, clinical course, and histologic scoring of biopsy specimens.[42] The biopsy findings for LD recipients demonstrated significantly lower grades of inflammation and less fibrosis in their grafts, as compared with DD recipients. This histologic trend was noted at 6 months and was even more prominent by 12 months. Similar results have been reported in two other cohort studies.[24,43]

Moreover, Maluf et al.[44] did not find any statistical difference comparing the patient and graft survival rates of 97 adult DDLT versus 29 ALDLT recipients with hepatitis C. Histologic recurrence of within 1 year was observed in 73% of ADDLT and 84% of ALDLT recipients. However, the patient and graft survival rates of ALDLT recipients who were HCV+ at 1 and 3 years were 12% to 15% lower, as compared with DDLT recipients.

On the contrary, Garcia-Retortillo et al.[45] in a prospective study of 117 patients with hepatitis C who underwent LTs (95 DDLTs and 22 ALDLTs) observed that, after a median follow-up of 22 months, 26 (22%) recipients developed severe recurrence of HCV (decompensation in 12)—18% of the 95 DDLT recipients, and 41% of the 22 ALDLT recipients.

The mechanisms that might explain the more aggressive course of HCV recurrence after LDLTs are unknown. Theoretically, variables are specifically linked to LDLTs that might prevent severe HCV disease recurrence, such as young donor age, the lack of significant steatosis of the graft, and the short ischemia time during surgery.[38,39,46] But other variables might negatively affect HCV disease recurrence, such as increased HLA donor–recipient matching, the type of immunosuppression, a high incidence of biliary complications posttransplant, and liver regeneration.[45,47]

The expected decrease in the graft or even the patient survival rate might make LDLTs a non-cost-effective approach for HCV-infected patients. Possible alternatives are to restrict LDLTs to patients with very long waiting times, to high waiting-list dropout rate settings, and to non-HCV-infected patients (at least during the learning curve). Or, HCV infections can be treated before

LDLTs.[48,49] If such strategies become successful, LDLTs may have an advantage over DDLTs.

## Hepatocellular Carcinoma (HCC)

Liver transplants are now acknowledged as the best therapeutic option for patients with early, nonresectable HCC. But LDLTs for HCC[50–52] patients are controversial, discussed with animosity in the literature.[53–56]

Until the beginning of the 1990s, the results of DDLTs were very poor, because the main indication for a transplant was advanced HCC. As a result, HCC became a contraindication to DDLTs until the introduction of the Milan Crieria (MC) by Mazzaferro in 1996. Applying the MC, a 4-year survival rate of 83% and a 4-year disease-free survival rate of 75% were reached.[57] Similar results were observed in LDLTs in different centers. Unfortunately, the preoperative tumor screening and tumors staging results are not always reliable: sometimes the HCC is overstaged in the preoperative workup, with consequent exclusion from transplants of a high number of patients who could benefit.[58] Additionally, the probability of dropping out from the waiting list because of HCC progression ranges from 40% to 50% at 2 years after diagnosis. To escape the dilemma of limited organ availability, LDLTs are a good alternative, offering a short waiting time with fewer dropouts and deaths on the waiting list.

Interestingly, more than 50% of patients in a published series of LDLTs for HCC were beyond the MC. The opinion of some surgeons that ALDLTs are particularly indicated for patients with HCC not strictly within the MC criteria has been voiced by Yao et al, who proposed expanding the MC in case of LDLTs. Their proposal is to expand the HCC criteria to a single nodule ≤ 6.5 cm or to ≤ 3 nodules ≤ 4.5 cm. Applying these expanded criteria, they reported a survival rate of 90% at 1 year and 75% at 5 years.[59]

Some studies showed that the number of tumor nodules represents a less important prognostic factor than diameter, presence of vascular infiltration, histologic type, and grade of malignancy.[60] Lee et al. suggested further extending the MC in selected patients with a higher number of small tumor nodules without macrovascular invasion.[60] Gondolesi et al reported good results with LDLTs for patients with large tumors.[53] Overall, in patients with tumors > 5 cm (n = 12), they found no statistically significant differences in survival or in freedom from recurrence between LD and DD recipients.

In Europe, from January 1991 to December 2004, a total of 277 ALDLTs for patients with HCC have been performed, with a patient survival rate of 84% at 1 year and 74% at 3 years, and a graft survival rate of 78% at 1 year and 70% at 3 years (ELTR Report 2004, http://www.eltr.org). These results were slightly better than for DDLT recipients.

In our center between 1998 and 2003, 34 patients with HCC (12 of them exceeding the Milan Criteria) underwent LDLTs. At a mean follow-up of 41 months, we observed an postoperative overall patient survival rate of 68% at 1 year and 62% at 3 years.[61] The recurrence-free survival rate (excluding patients who died within the first 3 months posttransplant) was 88% at 1 year and 75% at 3 years.[61]

Although complicated factors such as donor voluntarism and selection criteria limit the role of LDLTs for HCC patients, LDLTs allow more patients to undergo an early transplant, which results in a better outcome, even for patients beyond the MC.

## Long-Term Complications

The majority of complications occur, generally, within the first 90 days posttransplant: early infections, bile leaks, and hepatic artery thrombosis associated with poor function or primary nonfunction.

In a blinded survey (sponsored by the American Society of Transplant Surgeons) of 30 North American liver transplant centers that had performed a total of 208 ALDLTs within the United States and Canada, the overall incidence of complications was 30%.[62] The three most frequent complications were biliary (18%), vascular (6% allograft loss), and primary allograft nonfunction (4% allograft loss). A later survey by Brown et al.[63] of 84 U.S. transplant programs reported on 433 ALDLTs. The patient and graft survival rates were not reported, but the incidence of biliary complications was 23%; of vascular complications, 8%.

As in DDLTs, biliary complications represent the main cause of late morbidity after LDLTs—the Achilles heel of the procedure.[5,64-66] They include anastomotic leakage and stenosis, problems related to T or stent tubes, and rarely, nonanastomotic strictures or intrahepatic bilomas. These complications can lead to cholangitis, sepsis, and, eventually, a retransplant or death. The incidence of biliary complications in right ALDLT recipients ranges from 24% to 50%,[10,67-69] depending on the technique used. Hepaticojejunostomy (HJ) is mainly associated with early complications (ie, bile leaks); duct-to-duct anastomosis (DDA), mainly with late ones (ie, biliary strictures).[67,69-71] In our prospective randomized study of 80 right ALDLT recipients, we compared the results of HJ (n = 40) versus DDA (n = 40). In the HJ group, we noted more bile leaks (30% HJ, vs 4.2%, DDA; p = 0.035). In the DD group, the rate of biliary strictures was higher (33.3%, DD, vs 15%, HJ; p = 0.162). Bile leaks were often present within 30 days posttransplant; biliary strictures appeared 29 days to 12 months posttransplant, and most of them could be managed endoscopically (personal data).

Thus, in the long term, DDA is better for right ALDLT recipients whenever possible. However, HJ can always be used for recipient with complicated biliary anatomy and remains the method of choice for conversion from DDA.

The real long-term impact on graft survival of biliary complications is still difficult to assess. In fact, the literature related to ALDLTs lacks reports on the incidence of retransplants of ALDLT grafts because of biliary complications. The general opinion among transplant surgeons is that biliary complications are the single most important technical complication leading to long-term graft loss.

## CONCLUSION

One of the main principles of living liver donation recently established at the Vancouver Forum (Vancouver Forum on the Care of the Live Organ Donor, Vancouver, Canada, September 15–16, 2005) as well by the American Society of Transplant Surgeons' position paper on adult-to-adult LDLTs is that the risk to the donor should be weighed against the realistic estimate of a successful outcome in the recipient.[72] Therefore, ALDLTs should offer results similar to, or even better than, DDLTs.[29] We and other centers reported 5-year graft and patient survival rates after ALDLTs of 72% to 97%—results at least as good as after DDLTs.[10,66,73] But other centers have not demonstrated a clear advantage of ALDLTs over ADDLTs, in contrast to the excellent outcomes reported in pediatric LDLTs.[5,44,4,75]

LDLT recipients receive significantly younger donor grafts, have significantly shorter cold ischemia time and better ABO matching, and are less sick than their contemporaneous DDLT counterparts, yet they achieve the same 2-year patient survival rate of 80%.[76,77] Thuluvat et al,[75] using UNOS data, showed that LDLT recipients have similar survival rates, as compared with a matched population of DDLT recipients. However, the 1-year graft survival rate was significantly lower (≈15%) for the LDLT recipients.

The recent Organ Procurement and Transplantation Network/Scientific Registry of Transplant Recipients (SRTR) analysis showed that the unadjusted LD recipient graft survival rate is slightly lower at 1 to 3 years, as compared with DD recipient graft survival, only to become 15% greater at 5 years.[44,77]

Sugawara and Thuluvath observed that LDLT recipients with poor risk factors, like their DDLT counterparts, had a worse outcome, as compared with those with "good" risk factors.[78,79]

A statistical model to optimize the results of LDLTs was proposed by Durand et al.[80] They tried (1) to create statistical models for predicting each of the events after being listed for a transplant on the basis of variables available at the time of listing; (2) to elaborate a multistate model involving all these individual models for both DDLTs and LDLTs; (3) to use this global model to simulate different strategies of selection for LDLTs; and (4) to determine which strategy is optimal in terms of survival after listing. Interestingly, they found that the sickest patients derive the highest benefit from LDLTs. But their results are not directly applicable to countries such as the United States, where the allocation system is patient-oriented with priority given to the sickest patients according to MELD score. Their results are not even applicable to Asian countries, where DDLTs are limited or even absent.

Despite technical challenges and their relatively recent advent (as compared with DDLTs), ALDLTs have been successful and have had a tremendous impact on the lives of thousands of patients. Clearly, we should continue to strive to improve outcomes and availability of ALDLTs (whose outcomes should become better than DDLT outcomes). A multidisciplinary team approach, with objective criteria for donor and recipient selection, is imperative for ALDLTs.

## References

1. Hashikura Y, Makuuchi M, Kawasaki S, et al. Successful living-related partial liver transplantation to an adult patient. *Lancet* 1994;343(8907): 1233–1234.
2. Lo CM, Fan ST, Liu CL, et al. Adult-to-adult living donor liver transplantation using extended right lobe grafts. *Ann Surg* 1997;226(3): 261–269; discussion 269–270.
3. Wachs ME, Bak TE, Karrer FM, et al. Adult living donor liver transplantation using a right hepatic lobe. *Transplantation* 1998;66(10): 1313–1316.
4. Broelsch CE, Malago M, Testa G, et al. Living donor liver transplantation in adults: outcome in Europe. *Liver Transpl* 2000;6(6 Suppl 2): S64–S65.
5. Olthoff KM, Merion RM, Ghobrial RM, et al. Outcomes of 385 adult-to-adult living donor liver transplant recipients: a report from the A2ALL Consortium. *Ann Surg* 2005;242(3): 314–323, discussion 323–325.
6. Sugawara Y, Makuuchi M. Advances in adult living donor liver transplantation: a review based on reports from the 10th anniversary of the adult-to-adult living donor liver transplantation meeting in Tokyo. *Liver Transpl* 2004;10(6):715–720.

7. Chen CL, Fan ST, Lee SG, et al. Living-donor liver transplantation: 12 years of experience in Asia. *Transplantation* 2003;75(3 Suppl): S6–S11.

8. Garcia-Valdecasas JC, Fuster J, Charco R, et al. [Adult living donor liver transplantation. Analysis of the first 30 cases]. *Gastroenterol Hepatol* 2003;26(9): 525–530.

9. Dazzi A, Lauro A, Di Benedetto F, et al. Living donor liver transplantation in adult patients: our experience. *Transplant Proc* 2005;37(6): 2595–2596.

10. Malago M, Testa G, Frilling A, et al, Right living donor liver transplantation: an option for adult patients: single institution experience with 74 patients. *Ann Surg* 2003;238(6):853–862; discussion 862–863.

11. Williams RS,. Alisa AA, Karani JB, et al. Adult-to-adult living donor liver transplant: UK experience. *Eur J Gastroenterol Hepatol* 2003;15(1): 7–14.

12. Lo CM, Fan ST, Liu CL, et al. Minimum graft size for successful living donor liver transplantation. *Transplantation* 1999;68(8): 1112–1126.

13. Sugawara Y, Makuuchi M, Kaneko J, et al. Living-donor liver transplantation in adults: Tokyo University experience. *J Hepatobiliary Pancreat Surg* 2003;10(1):1–4.

14. Lee SG, Park KM, Hwang S, et al. Adult-to-adult living donor liver transplantation at the Asan Medical Center, Korea. *Asian J Surg* 2002;25(4):277–284.

15. Kawasaki S, Makuuchi M, MatsunamiM, et al. Living related liver transplantation in adults. *Ann Surg* 1998;227(2):269–274.

16. Miller CM, Gondolesi GE, Florman S, et al. One hundred nine living donor liver transplants in adults and children: a single-center experience. *Ann Surg* 2001;234(3):301–311; discussion 311–312.

17. Marcos A. Right lobe living donor liver transplantation: a review. *Liver Transpl* 2000;6(1):3–20.

18. Adam R, McMaster P, O'Grady JG, et al. Evolution of liver transplantation in Europe: report of the European Liver Transplant Registry. *Liver Transpl* 2003;9(12): 1231–1243.

19. Fan ST, Lo CM, Liu CL, et al. Determinants of hospital mortality of adult recipients of right lobe live donor liver transplantation. *Ann Surg* 2003;238(6):864–869; discussion 869–870.

20. Ghobrial RM, Saab S, Lassman C, et al. Donor and recipient outcomes in right lobe adult living donor liver transplantation. *Liver Transpl* 2002;8(10): 901–909.

21. Lo CM, Fan ST, Liu CL, et al. Lessons learned from one hundred right lobe living donor liver transplants. *Ann Surg* 2004;240(1):151–158.

22. Roberts MS, Angus DC, Bryce CL, et al. Survival after liver transplantation in the United States: a disease-specific analysis of the UNOS database. *Liver Transpl* 2004;10(7):886–897.

23. Tanaka K, Yamada T. Living donor liver transplantation in Japan and Kyoto University: what can we learn? *J Hepatol* 2005;42(1): 25–28.

24. Russo MW, Galanko J, Beavers K, et al. Patient and graft survival in hepatitis C recipients after adult living donor liver transplantation in the United States. *Liver Transpl* 2004;10(3):340–346.

25. Pomposelli JJ, Verbesey J, Simpson MA, et al. Improved Survival After Live Donor Adult Liver Transplantation (LDALT) Using Right Lobe Grafts: Program Experience and Lessons Learned. *Am J Transplant* 2006;6(3):589–598.

26. Bak T, Wachs M, Trotter J, et al. Adult-to-adult living donor liver transplantation using right-lobe grafts: results and lessons learned from a single-center experience. *Liver Transpl* 2001;7(8):680–686.

27. Lo CM, Fan ST, Liu CL, et al. Hepatic venoplasty in living-donor liver transplantation using right lobe graft with middle hepatic vein. *Transplantation* 2003;75(3):358–360.

28. Malago M, Molmenti EP, Paul A, et al. Hepatic venous outflow reconstruction in right live donor liver transplantation. *Liver Transpl* 2005;11(3): 364–365.

29. Busuttil RW, Farmer DG, Yersiz H, et al. Analysis of long-term outcomes of 3200 liver transplantations over two decades: a single-center experience. *Ann Surg* 2005;241(6): 905–916; discussion 916–918.

30. Testa G, Malago M, Nadalin S, et al. Right-liver living donor transplantation for decompensated end-stage liver disease. *Liver Transpl* 200;8(4): 340–346.

31. Russo MW, Brown RS Jr. Adult living donor liver transplantation. *Am J Transplant* 2004;4(4):458–465.

32. Hayashi PH, Forman L, Steinberg T, et al. Model for End-Stage Liver Disease score does not predict patient or graft survival in living donor liver transplant recipients. *Liver Transpl* 2003;9(7):737–740.

33. Hasegawa K, Sugawara Y, Imamura H, et al. Living donor liver transplantation for primary biliary cirrhosis: retrospective analysis of 50 patients in a single center. *Transpl Int* 2005;18(7):794–799.

34. Kim WR, Poterucha JJ, Kremers WK, et al. Outcome of liver transplantation for hepatitis B in the United States. *Liver Transpl* 2004;10(8): 968–974.

35. Sugawara Y, Makuuch M, Kaneko J, et al. Living donor liver transplantation for hepatitis B cirrhosis. *Liver Transpl* 2003;9(11):1181–1184.

36. Berenguer, M. Natural history of recurrent hepatitis C. *Liver Transpl* 2002;8(10 Suppl 1):S14–S18.

37. Sugo H, Balderson GA, Crawford DH, et al. The influence of viral genotypes and rejection episodes on the recurrence of hepatitis C after liver transplantation. *Surg Today* 2003;33(6):421–425.

38. Berenguer M, Prieto M, San Juan F, et al. Contribution of donor age to the recent decrease in patient survival among HCV-infected liver transplant recipients. *Hepatology*, 2002;36(1):202–210.

39. Ortiz V, Berenguer M, Rayon JM, et al. Contribution of obesity to hepatitis C-related fibrosis progression. *Am J Gastroenterol* 2002;97(9): 2408–2414.

40. Eghtesad B, Fung JJ, Demetris AJ, et al. Immunosuppression for liver transplantation in HCV-infected patients: mechanism-based principles. *Liver Transpl* 2005;11(11):1343–1352.

41. Everson GT, Trotter J. Role of adult living donor liver transplantation in patients with hepatitis C. *Liver Transpl* 2003;9(10 Suppl 2):S64–S68.

42. Humar A, Horn K, Kalis A, et al. Living donor and split-liver transplants in hepatitis C recipients: does liver regeneration increase the risk for recurrence? *Am J Transplant* 2005;5(2): 399–405.

43. Shiffman ML, Stravitz RT, Contos MJ, et al. Histologic recurrence of chronic hepatitis C virus in patients after living donor and deceased donor liver transplantation. *Liver Transpl* 2004;10(10):1248–1255.

44. Maluf DG, Stravitz RT, Cotterell AH, et al. Adult living donor versus deceased donor liver transplantation: a 6-year single center experience. *Am J Transplant* 2005;5(1):149–156.

45. Garcia-Retortillo M, Forns X, Llovet JM, et al. Hepatitis C recurrence is more severe after living donor compared to cadaveric liver transplantation. *Hepatology* 2004;40(3):699–707.

46. Berenguer M, Crippin J, Gish R, et al. A model to predict severe HCV-related disease following liver transplantation. *Hepatology* 2003;38(1): 34–41.

47. Gaglio PJ, Malireddy S, Levitt BS, et al. Increased risk of cholestatic hepatitis C in recipients of grafts from living versus cadaveric liver donors. *Liver Transpl* 2003;9(10):1028–1035.

48. Forns X, Garcia-Retortillo M, Serrano T, et al. Antiviral therapy of patients with decompensated cirrhosis to prevent recurrence of hepatitis C after liver transplantation. *J Hepatol* 2003;39(3): 389–396.

49. Brown RS. Hepatitis C and liver transplantation. *Nature* 2005;436(7053): 973–978.

50. Bigourdan JM, Jaeck D, Meyer N, et al. Small hepatocellular carcinoma in Child A cirrhotic patients: hepatic resection versus transplantation. *Liver Transpl* 2003;9(5):513–520.

52. Figueras J, Jaurrieta E, Valls C, et al. Resection or transplantation for hepatocellular carcinoma in cirrhotic patients: outcomes based on indicated treatment strategy. *J Am Coll Surg*, 2000. 190(5): p. 580–7.

53. Hemming AW, Nelson DR, Reed AI. Liver transplantation for hepatocellular carcinoma. *Minerva Chir*, 2002; 57(5): 575–85.

54. Gondolesi GE, Roayaie S, Munoz L, et al. Adult living donor liver transplantation for patients with hepatocellular carcinoma: extending UNOS priority criteria. *Ann Surg* 2004;239(2):142–149.

55. Kaihara S, Kiuchi T, Ueda M, et al. Living-donor liver transplantation for hepatocellular carcinoma. *Transplantation* 2003;75(3 Suppl):S37–S40.

56. Todo S, Furukawa H. Living donor liver transplantation for adult patients with hepatocellular carcinoma: experience in Japan. *Ann Surg* 2004;240(3):451–459; discussion 459–461.

57. Lo CM, Fan ST, Liu CL, et al. The role and limitation of living donor liver transplantation for hepatocellular carcinoma. *Liver Transpl* 2004;10(3):440–447.

58. Mazzaferro V, Regalia E, Doci R, et al. Liver transplantation for the treatment of small hepatocellular carcinomas in patients with cirrhosis. *N Engl J Med* 1996;334(11):693–699.

59. Sotiropoulos GC, Malago M, Molmenti E, et al. Liver transplantation for hepatocellular carcinoma in cirrhosis: is clinical tumor classification before transplantation realistic? *Transplantation* 2005;79(4): 483–487.

60. Yao FY, Ferrell L, Bass NM, et al. Liver transplantation for hepatocellular carcinoma: expansion of the tumor size limits does not adversely impact survival. *Hepatology* 2001;33(6): 1394–1403.

61. Lee KW, Park JW, Joh JW, et al. Can we expand the Milan criteria for hepatocellular carcinoma in living donor liver transplantation? *Transplant Proc* 2004;36(8):2289–2290.

62. Malago M, Sotiropouolos GC, Nadalin S. Living donor liver transplantation for hepatocellular carcinoma: a single-center preliminary report. *Liver Transpl* 2006.

63. Renz JF, Busuttil RW. Adult-to-adult living-donor liver transplantation: a critical analysis. *Semin Liver Dis* 2000;20(4):411–424.

64. Brown RS Jr,. Russo MW, Lai M, et al. A survey of liver transplantation from living adult donors in the United States. *N Engl J Med* 2003;348(9):818–825.

65. Testa G, Malago M, Valentin-Gamazo C, et al. Biliary anastomosis in living related liver transplantation using the right liver lobe: techniques and complications. *Liver Transpl* 2000;6(6):710–714.

66. Egawa H, Inomata S, Uemoto Y et al. Biliary anastomotic complications in 400 living related liver transplantations. *World J Surg* 2001;25(10):1300–1307.

67. Lo CM. Complications and long-term outcome of living liver donors: a survey of 1,508 cases in five Asian centers. *Transplantation* 2003;75(3 Suppl):S12–S15.

68. Gondolesi GE, Varotti G, Florman SS, et al. Biliary complications in 96 consecutive right lobe living donor transplant recipients. *Transplantation* 2004;77(12):1842–1848.

69. Icoz G, Kilic M, Zeytunlu M, et al. Biliary reconstructions and complications encountered in 50 consecutive right-lobe living donor liver transplantations. *Liver Transpl* 2003;9(6):575–580.

70. Yazumi S, Chiba T. Biliary complications after a right-lobe living donor liver transplantation. *J Gastroenterol* 2005;40(9):861–865.

71. Kawachi S, Shimazu M, Wakabayashi G, et al. Biliary complications in adult living donor liver transplantation with duct-to-duct hepaticocholedochostomy or Roux-en-Y hepaticojejunostomy biliary reconstruction. *Surgery* 2002;132(1):48–56.

72. Fan ST, Lo CM, Liu CL, et al. Biliary reconstruction and complications of right lobe live donor liver transplantation. *Ann Surg* 2002;236(5): 676–683.

73. American Society of Transplant Surgeons' position paper on adult-to-adult living donor liver transplantation. *Liver Transpl* 2000;6(6):815–817.

74. Marcos A, Ham JM, Fisher RA, et al. Single-center analysis of the first 40 adult-to-adult living donor liver transplants using the right lobe. *Liver Transpl* 2000;6(3):296–301.

75. Abt PL, Mange KC, Olthoff KM, et al. Allograft survival following adult-to-adult living donor liver transplantation. *Am J Transplant* 2004;4(8):1302–1307.

76. Thuluvath PJ, Yoo HY. Graft and patient survival after adult live donor liver transplantation compared to a matched cohort who received a deceased donor transplantation. *Liver Transpl* 2004;10(10): 1263–1268.

77. Freeman RB. The impact of the model for end-stage liver disease on recipient selection for adult living liver donation. *Liver Transpl* 2003;9 (10 Suppl 2):S54–S59.

78. Brown RS, Rush SH, Rosen HR, et al. Liver and intestine transplantation. *Am J Transplant* 2004;4(Suppl 9):81–92.

79. Sugawara Y, Makuuchi M, Imamura H, et al. Living donor liver transplantation in adults: recent advances and results. *Surgery* 2002. 132(2): 348–52.

80. Thuluvath PJ, Yoo HY, Thompson RE. A model to predict survival at one month, one year, and five years after liver transplantation based on pretransplant clinical characteristics. *Liver Transpl* 2003;9(5):527–532.

81. Durand F, Belghiti J, Troisi R, et al. Living donor liver transplantation in high-risk vs. low-risk patients: Optimization using statistical models. *Liver Transpl* 2006;12(2):231–239.

## 30.15.2   Pediatric Recipient

*Rohit Kohli, MBBS, Estella M. Alonso, MD,*
*Peter F. Whitington, MD*

### INTRODUCTION

The decision to move forward with liver transplantation in a child with end-stage liver disease (ESLD) requires careful consideration of risks and benefits. This decision, once made, initiates a series of events that provide limited opportunities for choice on the part of either the treating physician or the patient's guardian. The elective choice to perform a living donor liver transplant (LDLT) is an important exception to this general trend. Most pediatric liver transplant centers offer the living donor option to families early in the evaluation process to allow them the opportunity to take an active part in determining timing of the transplant procedure.

ESLD in children, and subsequently the need for liver transplantation, has a bimodal age distribution as evidenced by mortality rates in the pretransplant era. The first peak of mortality related to liver disease occurs in children less than 2 years of age and the second peak in those above ten years.[1] The primary indication for liver transplantation in children is biliary atresia (41%) with the majority of these children requiring transplant before 5 years of age.[2] In larger pediatric series, the median age at transplant is between 1 and 2 years of age. This age distribution contrasts with that of pediatric organs donors, very few who are less than 5 years of age. In the initial years of pediatric liver transplant experience, this recipient/donor mismatch resulted in excessive waiting-list mortality for smaller children.[3] Reduced-size liver transplantation was an important first step to address this need. However, waiting times for children remained unacceptably high. LDLT was first introduced in 1989[4,5] in response to this ongoing need and after an open and public ethical debate,[6] the first prospective and systematic serial application of LDLT was published in 1991.[7] This report was followed by a more widespread use of LDLT and by the year 2000 approximately 1000 pediatric living donor donations had been performed in the United States, Japan, and Europe.[8–10]

The goal of these innovative surgical techniques, including LDLT was to expand the organ pool for younger recipients, thus providing much needed relief to the subpopulation of children requiring smaller-size organs. This strategy was clearly successful as exemplified by a reduction in pretransplant waiting list mortality from 25% in 1989 to 5% in 1993, and reports of nearly 0% by the year 2001.[7,10–12] A comparative analysis of the waiting-list mortality rates from Belgium also showed that the patients who ultimately received LDLT had a significantly lower 2% waiting list mortality compared to the 14.5% on cadaveric lists.[8]

### RATIONALE FOR LDLT IN PEDIATRICS

The success of pediatric LDLT was made possible by surgical innovations such as reduced-size and split-liver transplantation[3,13,14] on the backdrop of a growing unmet need for pediatric-size grafts.[15] The conceptual framework of LDLT included the primary advantage of minimizing waiting time prior to transplantation, but it also provided the benefit of securing grafts independent of many of the problems inherent to cadaveric organ donation. The final theorized advantage was the likelihood of improved graft tolerance for children receiving haploidentical grafts from their parents. However, these advantages for the recipients were to be balanced against the risks undertaken by the donor; thus a lively ethical debate was an important component of the evolution of the LDLT process. The expectation was not only that LDLT would reduce waiting list mortality without significant risk to the donor but also that it would improve short- and long-term patient and graft survival.

## LONG-TERM LDLT OUTCOMES

Almost 15 years after the publication of the first prospective series of LDLT from the University of Chicago Hospitals there exist today multiple centers across the globe with technical expertise and long-term experience in performing LDLT. The cumulative world experience today was estimated in an editorial in 2003 to exceed 2000 cases.[16]

Compared to children receiving a cadaveric graft, posttransplant patient survival is consistently equal to or slightly better for children receiving a LDLT graft, with 1-year actuarial patient survival reported between 83% and 94%.[17,18] Graft survival has also been observed in large series of patients to be comparable or better for LDLT pediatric recipients, with 1-year graft survival being between 86% and 94%.[18,19] Similar survival rates have been observed at 2 years posttransplant, with these reports including infants less than 1 year of age for whom the LDLT procedure is most useful.[8] Data reported from the University of California at Los Angeles (UCLA) also found no statistically significant differences in patient survival as a function of the type of graft used for the initial transplant, with 1-year graft survival rates of 87% for living donor grafts.[20] We have summarized patient and graft actuarial survival rates from various centers in Table 30.15.2-1.

In Japan, cultural beliefs have precluded cadaveric organ donation; thus a large experience with LDLT has accumulated in this country. Experience reported from Japanese centers has been an important foundation in our understanding of patient and graft survival following LDLT. At Kyoto University, one of the larger transplant centers in Japan, a total of 547 LDLTs were performed on 519 children between 1990 and 2002. The median age for this cohort was 2.3 years while the range was from 1 month to 17.8 years. The overall patient survival rates for LDLT at this center at 1 and 5 years have been reported as 84% and 81%, respectively. This group also published their experience with using LDLT as a means of retransplantation and though their 1-year patient survival was significantly less (47%) than primary LDLT recipients, it does speak to their experience and success with using living donor transplantation in difficult cases.[17] The Studies of Pediatric Liver Transplant (SPLIT) registry in North America, which has been collecting data since 1996 and presently pools data from 39 centers, provides another large database available for review. As of June 2003, 2,139 patients were enrolled in the registry, 1,491 of whom have received a liver transplant. Of these, 226 (15.2%) were living related and 14 were living unrelated grafts. The majority of children receiving a LDLT (87.1%) were less than 4 years of age, and 28% were less than a year of age. More than 35% of all living donors were female and children of white or Asian race were more likely to receive a graft from a living donor. The percentage of transplanted patients receiving living

**TABLE 30.15.2-1**

## LONG-TERM PEDIATRIC LDLT PATIENT AND GRAFT SURVIVAL

| Institution | | 1-Year Survival | | 5-Year Survival | |
| --- | --- | --- | --- | --- | --- |
| | N | Patient | Graft | Patient | Graft |
| Brussels, Belgium[40] | 41 | 92% | 90% | 92% | 89% |
| Chicago, USA[18] | | | | | |
| 1989–1994 | 78 | 87% | 74% | NA | NA |
| 1996–1999 | 20 | 94% | 94% | NA | NA |
| Hamburg, Germany[26] | 44 | 100%[a] | 96%[a] | NA | NA |
| Kyoto, Japan[17] | 547 | 84% | NA | 81% | 79% |
| Matsumoto, Japan[41] | 160 | 88% | 88% | 85% | 85% |
| New York, USA [19] | 50 | 90% | 86% | 81% | 78% |

[a]6-month data.

related grafts has been constant over the time period SPLIT has been collecting data. The outcome of whole cadaveric transplants compared with living donor transplants in children is comparable, with relative risk calculations showing nonsignificant differences between groups.[21]

Reding et al. from Belgium published a report in 1999 that highlighted the multiple advantages of LDLT over cadaveric liver transplantation. The report included outcomes for 41 patients transplanted by LDLT and 49 patients who received cadaveric grafts between 1993 and 1997. They observed patient survival at 1 year was 92% in LDLT recipients compared to 87% for cadaveric transplants done during the same time period. Similar differences were seen in the 1-year graft actuarial survival statistics, which were 90% for the LDLT group and 75% for the cadaveric group. Although these data revealed a trend towards better outcomes in the LDLT group, the differences did not reach statistical significance. An important advantage highlighted in this report was the reduction in pretransplant mortality observed in patients awaiting LDLT as compared to those awaiting a cadaveric graft. Pretransplant mortality occurred in 10 patients (15%) on the cadaveric waiting list, whereas only 1 patient (2%) assessed to receive a LDLT died prior to transplant.[22]

Patient and graft survival following LDLT appear to be improving over time. Millis et al. reported the experience at the University of Chicago with 104 pediatric LDLTs completed by 2000.[18] Assessment of outcomes was divided into two eras. Analysis of transplants performed prior to 1994 revealed 1-year graft and patient survival rates of 74% and 87%, respectively. Both these rates improved significantly to 94% after 1994 following significant changes in surgical technique. One important determinant of this improvement was the elimination of the use of cryopreserved venous conduits for portal vein reconstruction.

### Long-Term Graft Complications

One of the expectations of LDLT that was realized was a significant reduction in primary nonfunction (PNF) rate with living donor organs. The elective nature of the surgery significantly decreased (61.7% shorter) "cold ischemia" time and improved graft preservation dropping the incidence of PNF which was 4% for cadaveric organs to less than 1%[10]

A somewhat unexpected impact of LDLT was an increased incidence of vascular complications. Dissection of the vascular structures in the living donor frequently results in shorter vascular structures compared to reduced size grafts. Complex reconstruction of these vessels is frequently required. High rates of thrombosis of the hepatic artery or portal vein reduced rates of graft survival in the early experience with LDLT.[18] However, with refinement of surgical techniques there has been steady reduction in these complications with an improvement in short and long-term graft survival. Likewise, advances in the management of immunosuppressive therapy have improved graft and patient survival, especially in long-term follow-up.

## HEPATIC ARTERIAL THROMBOSIS

Vascular complications as reported in the 2003 SPLIT annual report were the second most common post-operative complication with 15.5% of the group having at least one vascular complication.[21] The most common complication was hepatic arterial thrombosis (HAT) with 65 (9.2%) of the children who received a deceased donor graft developing an HAT versus 6.5% of those that received living donor grafts. However, the timing of these events was not categorized as early versus late. Experience from other reports has revealed that the majority of these events are early, diagnosed within the first 30 postoperative days. Risk factors that lead to late HAT which include chronic rejection, CMV infection and atherosclerosis are likely to be experienced equally by deceased donor and living donor recipients.

## PORTAL VEIN THROMBOSIS

Late portal vein stenosis and thrombosis was recognized as an important long-term problem in LDLT recipients in the mid-1990s. The University of Chicago reported a series of patients of whom 27% (32/118) developed narrowing or occlusion of the portal vein. This compared with stenosis/thrombosis rates,

which had historically been 1% for deceased donor grafts. When examined by era, there was a significant decrease in late portal vein stenosis in patients transplanted before and after 1994 (33/265 [12.5%] versus 6/335 [1.8%]). This decrease coincided with the recognition that cryopreserved venous extension grafts, used primarily in LDLT recipients, were a strong risk factor for late portal vein thrombosis.[18,23] Late-onset stenosis of the portal vein can be successfully treated with balloon venoplasty and in refractory cases with placement of an endovascular stent (see Figure 30.15.2-1). A recent report also advocates the use of thrombolytic agents with subsequent venoplasty for vessels with late thrombosis. However, in most patients with complete occlusion of the vein, shunt procedures or retransplantation is necessary to avoid life-threatening complications of advanced portal hypertension.

## HEPATIC VEIN THROMBOSIS

Hepatic venous stenosis and thrombosis can be difficult to recognize. A relatively common early postoperative complication in the initial LDLT series, it is now primarily observed as a late phenomenon.[24] Overall, stenosis has been reported to occur with an increased frequency in LDLT grafts (2%) in comparison to whole organ grafts (1%), but less commonly than in reduced-size or split grafts (4%).[23] The clinical hallmarks of this problem include unexplained hypoalbuminemia, likely secondary to protein losing enteropathy, intermittent ascites, unexplained prolonged prothrombin time, and in advanced cases, hypersplenism and varices. A high index of suspicion must be maintained to diagnose HVT since screening Doppler ultrasound is far less sensitive for abnormalities in the hepatic outflow tract than in the portal venous system.

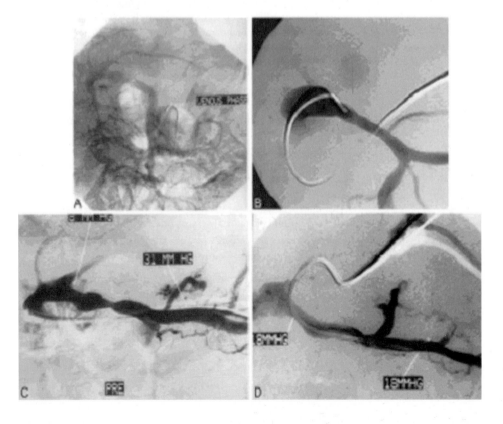

**FIGURE 30.15.2-1**

**(A)** Portal venous stenosis demonstrated by venogram obtained with contrast injection into the extrahepatic portal vein after percutaneous puncture.
**(B)** Fluoroscopic image demonstrating venoplasty of stenotic segment.
**(C)** Site of recurrent stenosis requiring stenting.
**(D)** Placement of endovascular stent at stenotic point.

## BILIARY COMPLICATIONS

Biliary strictures are the Achilles heel of living donor transplantation. Accepted risk factors for stricture formation include history of hepatic arterial thrombosis, even with successful early revascularization, and chronic rejection. In the SPLIT cohort biliary complications were observed in 20% of patients receiving technical variant grafts in the first 30 days posttransplant, compared to only 8.3% for whole organ recipients.[2] Egawa et al. reported a biliary complication rate of 14% in their series of 208 pediatric living donor transplants. Logistic regression identified HAT, CMV infection, and intrapulmonary shunting as significant risk factors for development of these complications (Egawa H. *Surgery* 1998;124:901–910). Living donor grafts do appear to be at increased risk for these complications as compared to other technical variant grafts, especially as observed in early reports. Heffron et al. reported a rate of biliary complications of 12% for reduced-size grafts compared to 38% for LDLT grafts in 1992 while at the University of Chicago. This analysis included only 13 living donor grafts, preformed during the initial surgical experience. A later publication, which included 91 LDLT recipients at the University of Chicago, described anastomotic strictures in 22 (24%).[25] The majority of these strictures were successfully treated with balloon dilatation. The University of Chicago experience would suggest that even with accumulated surgical experience, the biliary complication rate is relatively high. However, in a recent series from Germany, the rate of biliary complications for all grafts (6%) after 132 liver transplants was similar to those after split (5.7%) and LDLT grafts (4.6%) which were significantly lower than what has been previously reported.[26] The question as to whether the incidence of these complications is decreasing is still open to debate. Many of the reports do not specifically state the interval of follow-up achieved for patients, which is an important consideration since strictures may present for the first time many years after the transplant procedure.

The use of interventional radiology to perform balloon dilation of strictures has proven successful in many cases avoiding the need for surgical reoperation and decreasing the occurrence of graft loss due to biliary complications.[27,28] This technique is most successful in treating isolated strictures at the biliary–enteric anastomosis. Recurrence of stricture formation may occur months to years after radiological treatment with recurrence being more common in the setting of intrahepatic stricture formation.

## INCIDENCE OF REJECTION

At the outset of LDLT it had been hypothesized that one of the inherent benefits of a graft donated by a close relative of the recipient would be immunologic and HLA compatibility. When the donor is either a parent or a close relative it was probable that there will be greater HLA homology between the donor and the recipient as compared to the donor-to-recipient match with a cadaveric graft. It was envisioned that this homology would provide an immunologic advantage resulting in lower rates of acute and chronic rejection, and lower requirements for immunosuppression.[7]

These hypotheses were also encouraged by data showing the beneficial effect of HLA compatibility in kidney transplantation.[29] HLA-matched sibling living donation for pediatric kidney transplantation was reported to give the best outcomes both for survival of graft, and the least frequency of rejection episodes.

Living-related-adult-to-pediatric-kidney donation was also shown to have better outcomes than size-matched pediatric cadaveric donor kidneys. This was especially true for the under-5 age group where graft survival was reported to be 30% lower than when related adult kidneys (ASK) were transplanted.[30]

To test this hypothesis the incidence of rejection in LDLT recipients at the University of Chicago was retrospectively reviewed. This analysis included LDLTs performed in 38 patients between 1990 and 1993. Though the acute rejection rate (74%) was found to be comparable to that of cadaveric transplants (78%), the incidence of steroid resistant acute rejection was found to be less in LDLT recipients (13%) as compared to cadaveric recipients (43%; p < 0.1). The incidence of chronic rejection was similar in both groups in this report.[31] However, this observation regarding steroid-resistant rejection was made in patients receiving primary immunosuppression with cyclosporin (CSA) may not be generalizable to patients treated with tacrolimus.

When data from the SPLIT registry were analyzed in 2003, the overall rate of steroid-resistant acute rejection in all types of grafts was 13%.[2] This analysis showed a trend toward a decreasing incidence of acute rejection over time possibly related to the increasing use of tacrolimus. In a report by Reding et al acute rejection and steroid resistant acute ejection-free graft survival rates at 1 year were similar for the LDLT and CLT group.[22] The group from University of California at San Francisco also reported in 2002 that the overall incidence of rejection and graft survival rate were comparable in CLT (n = 51) and LDLT (n = 37); however, rejection episodes in LDLT recipients diagnosed greater than 1 year posttransplant were significantly fewer than CLT recipients (p < 0.05; see Table 30.15.2-2).[32]

All the above clinical data from single-center and registry sources led to the understanding that there may not be a strong benefit in graft tolerance for LDLT recipients. HLA matching was performed at Kyoto University, Japan, in a cohort of approximately 600 LDLT donor/recipient pairs to further investigate this issue. Complete HLA data on 321 pairs were collected and analyzed. The cumulative 5-year graft survivals in HLA 0-, 1-, 2-, and 3-mismatch groups (A, B, and DR) were 100% (n = 10), 78.9% (n = 19), 86.2% (n = 87), and 82.9% (n = 205), respectively (p = 0.525). The overall rejection and rejection-free survival rates were no different amongst these four groups. Duration of steroid use posttransplant was also found to be no different amongst the groups. However, the trough level of tacrolimus needed for

**TABLE 30.15.2-2**

## RECIPIENTS OUTCOME COMPARED BETWEEN CLT AND LDLT

|  | CLT (n551) | LDLT (n=537) | p-value |
|---|---|---|---|
| Recipients who were diagnosed rejection | 40 | 25 | NS |
| Graft loss due to rejection | 3 | 0 | NS |
| Rejection within 1 year Post-Tx | 37 | 25 | NS |
| Rejection since 1 year Post-Tx | 11 | 0 | P<0.05 |
| Switch to tacrolimus-based immunosuppression | 17 | 13 | NS |

maintenance of an acceptable liver function during the chronic phase tended to be lower in well-matched pairs, and a high percentage of immunosuppressant-free patients were found in the 0-mismatch group, but again no significant difference was found.[33] Thus, overall HLA compatibility by itself has not been found to improve graft or patient outcomes.

## Qualitative Outcomes

The true test of the long-term benefit of LDLT is the examination of qualitative outcomes for these children. Achieving normal growth and development is an important and sometimes elusive goal. Measurement of quality of life has been limited in all pediatric liver transplant recipients, and physicians struggle with how to set future expectations for these children and their families. Qualitative outcomes have not been systematically compared between pediatric deceased donor and living donor recipients. Likewise, analysis of risk factors for delayed growth and development and lower qualitative outcomes is ongoing.

## Growth and HRQOL

Few studies have focused specifically on the growth of children post-LDLT. Ohkohchi et al recruited 31 children (15 males and 16 females) who had undergone LDLT at their center from 1991 to 2001. After liver transplantation, approximately 70% of patients displayed growth restoration both in body weight and in height by 2 years posttransplant. Patients who received liver transplantation at less than 5 years of age showed significantly greater catch-up growth compared with those over 5 years of age.[34] These findings are similar to observations in series of predominantly cadaveric recipients where growth acceleration was seen between 2 and 4 years posttransplant, with younger infants showing the most pronounced catch-up growth.[35,36]

Health-related quality of life (HRQOL) for children after liver transplantation has been measured in several studies using generic instruments. At present, disease-specific instruments to measure HRQOL in transplant recipients are not available. In two single-center studies HRQOL was measured using a generic tool, the Child Health Questionnaire. These studies were a cross-sectional analysis of liver transplant recipients older than age 5. Scores for children who had received liver transplantation were compared to a normative population.[37,38] In both studies, transplant recipients had significantly lower subscale scores for general health perceptions, emotional impact on parents and disruption of family activities. In these analyses, donor source did not significantly influence subscale scores. In the report by Bucuvalas et al., children were assessed with a second generic tool, the PedsQL. PedsQL scores showed that LT recipients scored lower than normal children in all domains, with scores that were similar to those seen for children with other chronic diseases[37,38] (see Table 30.15.2-3). These findings suggest that older children and their families may not be enjoying the same level of HRQOL of life as their healthy peers, with the most significant differences in general health, physical function, and parental stress.

Cole et al. surveyed younger LT recipients below the age of 5 years, enrolling 45 patients with a mean age at transplantation of 1.4 (+/− 1.2) years. Parents completed an infant/toddler version of the CHQ (ITCHQ), which was in development. Scores on this survey improved steadily over the course of study with the largest increases seen at 6 months posttransplant. ITCHQ subscales were similar for patients who received LDLT compared with those who

**TABLE 30.15.2-3**

## PEDSQL COMPARED TO GENERAL POPULATION & CHILDREN WITH CHRONIC ILLNESS[38, 42]

| Subscale | Study Population | General Population | *P* Value | Chronic Illness | *P* Value |
|---|---|---|---|---|---|
| Physical health | 77.8 +/− 20.3 | 89.3 +/− 16.3 | <.01 | 73.2 +/− 27.0 | NS |
| Emotional Functioning | 73.2 +/− 19.0 | 82.6 +/− 17.5 | <.01 | 73.1 =/− 23.8 | NS |
| Social Functioning | 75.5 +/− 17.9 | 91.6 +/− 14.2 | <.01 | 79.8 +/− 21.9 | NS |
| School functioning | 64.4 +/− 20.7 | 85.5 +/− 17.6 | <.01 | 71.1 +/− 24.0 | <.01 |
| Psychosocial health | 71.0 +/− 15.6 | 86.6 +/− 12.8 | <.01 | 74.8 +/− 18.2 | <.05 |

received cadaver grafts at baseline and at 1 year after transplant. The study suggests that HRQOL improves after transplantation in young children irrespective of the donor type.[39]

## SUMMARY

LDLT has become a reasonable and popular method to increase organ availability for children with ESLD. It is most commonly used for young infants with biliary atresia, and multiple reports suggest reduced waiting-list mortality and a small posttransplant patient and graft survival advantage associated with LDLT used in this setting. Postoperative surgical complications may be higher in the LDLT group, but long-term graft survival is similar to that observed in cadaveric recipients. Initial expectations that living-donor recipients would have improved graft tolerance as compared to cadaveric recipients have not been validated. Qualitative outcomes for children who receive LDLT appear to be the same as those who receive cadaveric grafts, but systematic analysis of these outcomes in still forthcoming.

## References

1. Hyattsville M. Vital Statistics of the U.S. 1982. Vol 2. *Mortality* 1986;186.
2. McDiarmid SV. Current status of liver transplantation in children. *Pediatr Clin North Am* Dec 2003;50(6):1335–1374.
3. Emond JC, Whitington PF, Thistlethwaite JR, Alonso EM, Broelsch CE. Reduced-size orthotopic liver transplantation: use in the management of children with chronic liver disease. *Hepatology* Nov 1989;10(5):867–872.
4. Raia S, Nery JR, Mies S. Liver transplantation from live donors. *Lancet* Aug 26 1989;2(8661):497.
5. Strong RW, Lynch SV, Ong TH, Matsunami H, Koido Y, Balderson GA. Successful liver transplantation from a living donor to her son. *N Engl J Med.* May 24 1990;322(21):1505–1507.
6. Singer PA, Siegler M, Whitington PF, et al. Ethics of liver transplantation with living donors. *N Engl J Med* Aug 31 1989;321(9):620–622.
7. Broelsch CE, Whitington PF, Emond JC, et al. Liver transplantation in children from living related donors. Surgical techniques and results. *Ann Surg* Oct 1991;214(4):428–437; discussion 437–429.
8. Otte JB, de Ville de Goyet J, Reding R, et al. Pediatric liver transplantation: from the full-size liver graft to reduced, split, and living related liver transplantation. *Pediatr Surg Int* July 1998;13(5–6):308–318.

9. Tanaka K, Yol S. Incidence and management of biliary strictures in living-related donor graft. *Pediatr Transplant* Dec 2002;6(6):452–455.

10. Broering DC, Mueller L, Ganschow R, et al. Is there still a need for living-related liver transplantation in children? *Ann Surg* Dec 2001;234(6): 713–721; discussion 721–712.

11. de Ville de Goyet J, Hausleithner V, Reding JR, et al. Impact of innovative techniques on the waiting list and results in pediatric liver transplantation. *Transplantation* Nov 1993;56(5):1130–1136.

12. Lopez Santamaria M, Vazquez J, Gamez M, et al. Impact of liver reduction techniques on waiting list mortality in pediatric patients. *Transplant Proc* Aug 1995;27(4):2292.

13. Bismuth H, Houssin D. Reduced-sized orthotopic liver graft in hepatic transplantation in children. *Surgery* Mar 1984;95(3):367–370.

14. Broelsch CE, Emond JC, Thistlethwaite JR, et al. Liver transplantation, including the concept of reduced-size liver transplants in children. *Ann Surg* Oct 1988;208(4):410–420.

15. Malatack JJ, Schaid DJ, Urbach AH, et al. Choosing a pediatric recipient for orthotopic liver transplantation. *J Pediatr* Oct 1987;111(4): 479–489.

16. Chisuwa H, Hashikura Y, Mita A, et al. Living liver donation: preoperative assessment, anatomic considerations, and long-term outcome. *Transplantation* May 27 2003;75(10):1670–1676.

17. Ogura Y, Kaihara S, Haga H, et al. Outcomes for pediatric liver retransplantation from living donors. *Transplantation* Sep 27 2003;76(6): 943–948.

18. Millis JM, Cronin DC, Brady LM, et al. Primary living-donor liver transplantation at the University of Chicago: technical aspects of the first 104 recipients. *Ann Surg* July 2000;232(1):104–111.

19. Miller CM, Gondolesi GE, Florman S, et al. One hundred nine living donor liver transplants in adults and children: a single-center experience. *Ann Surg* Sep 2001;234(3):301–311; discussion 311–312.

20. Goss JA, Shackleton CR, McDiarmid SV, et al. Long-term results of pediatric liver transplantation: an analysis of 569 transplants. *Ann Surg* Sep 1998;228(3):411–420.

21. McDiarmid SV, Anand R. Studies of Pediatric Liver Transplantatioan (SPLIT): a summary of the 2003 Annual Report. *Clin Transpl* 2003: 119–130.

22. Reding R, de Goyet Jde V, Delbeke I, et al. Pediatric liver transplantation with cadaveric or living related donors: comparative results in 90 elective recipients of primary grafts. *J Pediatr* Mar 1999;134(3):280–286.

23. Buell JF, Funaki B, Cronin DC, et al. Long-term venous complications after full-size and segmental pediatric liver transplantation. *Ann Surg.* Nov 2002;236(5):658–666.

24. Millis JM, Seaman DS, Piper JB, et al. Portal vein thrombosis and stenosis in pediatric liver transplantation. *Transplantation.* Sep 27 1996;62(6):748–754.

25. Cronin DC, 2nd, Alonso EM, Piper JB, et al. Biliary complications in living donor liver transplantation. *Transplant Proc.* Feb-Mar 1997;29(1–2): 419–420.

26. Broering DC, Kim JS, Mueller T, et al. One hundred thirty-two consecutive pediatric liver transplants without hospital mortality: lessons learned and outlook for the future. *Ann Surg* Dec 2004;240(6):1002–1012; discussion 1012.

27. Lorenz JM, Denison G, Funaki B, et al. Balloon dilatation of biliary-enteric strictures in children. *AJR Am J Roentgenol* Jan 2005;184(1): 151–155.

28. Sung RS, Campbell DA, Jr., Rudich SM, et al. Long-term follow-up of percutaneous transhepatic balloon cholangioplasty in the management of biliary strictures after liver transplantation. *Transplantation* Jan 15 2004;77(1):110–115.

29. Thorogood J, van Houwelingen JC, van Rood JJ, et al. Factors contributing to long-term kidney graft survival in Eurotransplant. *Transplantation* Jul 1992;54(1):152–158.

30. Sarwal MM, Cecka JM, Millan MT, Salvatierra O Jr. Adult-size kidneys without acute tubular necrosis provide exceedingly superior long-term graft outcomes for infants and small children: a single center and UNOS analysis. United Network for Organ Sharing. *Transplantation* Dec 27 2000;70(12):1728–1736.

31. Alonso EM, Piper JB, Echols G, Thistlethwaite JR, Whitington PF. Allograft rejection in pediatric recipients of living related liver transplants. *Hepatology* Jan 1996;23(1):40–43.

32. Toyoki Y, Renz JF, Mudge JC, et al. Allograft rejection in pediatric liver transplantation: Comparison between cadaveric and living related donors. Pediatr *Transplant* Aug 2002;6(4):301–307.

33. Kasahara M, Kiuchi T, Uryuhara K, et al. Role of HLA compatibility in pediatric living-related liver transplantation. *Transplantation* Oct 27 2002;74(8):1175–1180.

34. Ohkohehi N, Orii JT, Kawagishi N, Satomi S. Quality of life of pediatric patients receiving living donor liver transplantation in long-term follow-up period. *Transplant Proc* Nov–Dec 2001;33(7-8): 3610–3613.

35. Bartosh SM, Thomas SE, Sutton MM, Brady LM, Whitington PF. Linear growth after pediatric live transplantation. *J Pediatr* Nov 1999; 135(5):624–631.

36. McDiarmid SV, Gornbein JA, DeSilva PJ, et al. Factors affecting growth after pediatric livre transplantation. *Transplantation* Feb 15 1999; 67(3):404–411.

37. Alonso EM, Neighbors K, Mattson C, et al. Functional outcomes of pediatric liver transplantation. *J Pediatr Gastroenterol Nutr* Aug 2003; 37(2):155–160.

38. Bucuvalas JC, Britto M, Krug S, et al. Health-related quality of life in pediatric liver transplant recipients: A single-center study. *Liver Transpl* Jan 2003;9(1):62–71.

39. Cole CR, Bucuvalas JC, Hornung JRW, et al. Impact of liver transplantation on HRQOL in children less than 5 years old. *Pediatr Transplant* Jun 2004;83(3):222–227.

40. de Ville de Goyer J, Reding R, Lerut J, et al. Paediatric orthotopic liver transplantation: lessons from a 532 transplant single centre experience with 532 transplants in 446 children. *Acta Gastroenterol Belg* Jul–Sep 1999;62(3):290–294.

41. Hashikura Y, Kawasaki S, Terada M, et al. Long-term results of living-related donor liver graft transplantation: a single-center analysis of 110 transplants. *Transplantation* Jul 15 2001;72(1):95–99.

42. Bucuvalas JC, Ryckman FC, Atheroton H, et al. Predictos of cost of liver tansplantation in children: a single center study. *J Pediatr* Jul 2001;139(1):66–74.

# 30.16 STRATEGIES TO MAXIMIZE THE DONOR POOL

## 30.16.1 ABO Incompatibility

*Giuliano Testa, MD, Enrico Benedetti, MD, Phillip J. DeChristopher, MD, PhD*

From the beginning of liver transplantation, each report dealing with liver transplantation across the blood barrier has the intrinsic premise of having to justify such a practice before the eyes of the reader. Before the era of living donor liver transplantation, the justification was the scarcity of grafts in emergent situations or in pediatric recipients. With the advent of living donation, the justification has become the lack of compatible donors in a system where cadaveric donors are not available. The hesitancy to perform incompatible liver transplantations has been dictated by the evidence that in general these transplants have poorer outcomes than identical and compatible transplants. The main reason for this outcome has been identified in the humoral response of the recipients against AB antigens expressed on the endothelial and epithelial cells of the donor graft. Although a preliminary report by Starzl excluded the possibility that the liver could be the object of a hyperacute rejection like the kidney,[1] later studies have clearly shown that an incompatible liver graft can be lost, if not immediately after reperfusion, then surely in a few days after the transplantation.[2–4] It has also been documented that even in the event that the graft does not show any signs of acute failure, a chronic damage, which significantly diminishes its life span, might occur.[5–7] In fact, the average short-term graft and patient survival of incompatible liver transplants reported in the late 1980s and early 1990s does not surpass 40%.[4,6,8–10] The acute and chronic histologic damage suffered by these grafts has been clearly documented. In 1990, Gugenheim described hemorrhagic infiltration of the portal tract and lobules, intense deposit of IgM, fibrinogen on the sinusoidal cells, and arterial and venous endothelium, confirming the findings already documented by Gordon in 1986.[4,8] In the same report, Gugenheim describes what at a later date was confirmed by Sanchez-Urdazpal in a study of 18 ABO incompatible liver grafts[6] the chronic damage to the biliary tree leading to progressive cholestasis. Both authors point out that the cause of the graft damage and shorter survival is the recipient's humoral response to AB antigens expressed on the vascular endothelium and biliary epithelium of the donor's liver. Despite these findings and outcomes, the use of incompatible liver grafts would not be fully discouraged by either authors or many others, but would rather limit their use to patients in acute failure.

Attempts at successfully transplanting cadaveric livers across the blood barrier continued by adopting strategies that had already been proven efficacious in incompatible kidney transplantation.[11–14] In particular, perioperative lowering of the preformed AB antibodies, splenectomy, and more aggressive immunosuppression were introduced. The results reported in the literature are based on a small series with short-term follow-up.[15–18] The practice of incompatible liver transplantation is a rare event limited to few centers due to both the reluctance to routinely accept incompatible liver grafts and the actual limitation dictated by the cadaveric liver allocation system. Consequently, the impact of the therapeutic strategies implemented to improve short- and long-term outcome in liver transplantation performed across the blood barrier is very hard to determine. The scenario has been completely changed by the worldwide acceptance of living donor liver transplantation both in pediatric and adult patients. Performing incompatible living donor liver transplantation, although in just a few centers, is increasing, and the data obtained contribute to a more precise analysis of its value and place in modern liver transplantation. Starting in the mid-1990s, a renewed interest in the use of grafts from blood-incompatible donors has come mainly from Japan where living donor transplantation is practically the sole source of grafts. The first reports were based on pediatric recipients, whereas lately the practice of incompatible living liver transplantation has been extended to adult patients as well.

## PLASMAPHERESIS/THERAPEUTIC PLASMA EXCHANGE

### Background

The well-recognized barrier of major ABO incompatibility to solid organ transplantation is beginning to fall. Factors contributing to high probabilities of humoral rejection are the widespread expression of A and B antigens on transplanted tissues, the ubiquitous presence of naturally occurring, preformed antibodies (isoagglutinins) directed against the A or B antigens in the recipient, and the high propensity of ABO isoagglutinins to bind complement. Serial plasmapheresis or therapeutic plasma exchange (TPE), in

proportion to recipient body size, has become accepted practice as an important modality in the immunomodulation of incompatible liver recipients. Plasmapheresis is the selective removal of large quantities of anticoagulated plasma using automated blood cell separators; technically, TPE is the same process using the same medical devices, but uses plasma, usually as fresh frozen plasma, as the isovolemic replacement fluid in the procedure. The purpose of TPE in this setting is to rapidly, albeit temporarily, drop the level of circulating the blood group isoagglutinins (anti-A, anti-B, and/or anti-A,B). Compared to cadaveric transplantation, the fact that most living donor liver transplants are elective creates a great advantage for the role of TPE. In this setting, it is possible to perform even multiple TPE treatments, in concert with various systemic immunosuppressive regimens, to abate the levels of AB isoagglutinins as much as possible.

### Serologic Determination of Isoagglutinin Levels

ABO antibody levels (titers) are determined at baseline and before (pre-) and after (post-) each TPE procedure. The standard methods used for ABO isoagglutinin determinations use the tube method, in a normal saline diluent (not albumin or other serologic potentiators), and doubling dilutions. Patient's raw serum and serial dilutions are admixed and incubated with reagent Group A or Group B red blood cells (rbc). To estimate the level of IgM, the admixture is performed at room temperature/immediate spin, incubated for 30 minutes at room temperature, then read. For IgG determination, the admixture is incubated for 30 minutes at 37°C; then antihuman globulin serum (Coombs' serum) is added and read. The *titer* of the antibody, a relative measure of the concentration of the analyte, is the reciprocal of the dilution at which physical agglutination is visually observed *in vitro*. [So, agglutination at a dilution of up to 1:16 is reported as a titer of 16.] Another important adjunct to ABO titering is to perform standard red blood cell antibody screens periodically. Because solid organ transplant recipients are frequently transfused, they can make RBC alloantibodies that could interfere with the determination of isoagglutinins, unless the antigen specificity is accounted for in the selection of rbc's used to perform the titer.

### Therapeutic Plasma Exchange Protocols

Optimal peritransplant protocols for TPE in this setting have not been established. Typically the volume removed/replaced with each procedure, the total number of procedures, their frequency, and when to resume them, if stopped, are individualized to each patient. Variables include the estimated plasma volume of the patient, the starting titer(s) of isoagglutinin(s), the relative effectiveness of concomitant immunosuppressive drugs, the degree to which titers will *rebound* (a humoral immune effect which is always expected), and the kinetics of titer rebound. These variables and the patient's coagulation status require close monitoring during TPE. In principle, it is easier to drop circulating IgM titers because approximately 80% of IgMs are distributed in the intravascular space. IgG titers are more challenging to maintain because, at any one moment in time, TPE treats only the intravascular space and only approximately 45% of IgG resides there. Usually, TPE procedures are scheduled on alternate days both in the ambulatory (pre- or posttransplant) and hospitalized settings. Also, 1 plasma volume is removed per procedure; in a typical 70-kg person, this amounts to 3,000–3,500 mL. The usual replacement fluids can be 5% human albumin and 0.9% saline (in a 2:1 vol:vol ratio). In the setting of end-stage liver disease in patients who are already coagulopathic, an important management caveat is that even alternate-day TPE can make coagulation parameters worsen. Certainly, when daily TPEs are required by high baseline ABO titers or by rapidly rising titers, the exchange fluid of choice is fresh frozen plasma to correct any acquired hemostatic deficiencies. The total number of TPE procedures is variable, with the need for 2 to 4 pre-transplant, and 4 to 6 after transplant, out to about postoperative day 10.

## Preliminary Results Correlating ABO Antibody Titers to Outcome

In a small series published on children transplanted with cadaveric-incompatible liver grafts, it was noted that keeping the titers lower than between 8 and 32 could be an important factor in improving outcome and reducing rejection.[15,16] The first report from Tanaka, based on 3 children receiving living donor grafts, proposed a titer of < 64 prior to and after the transplant. No splenectomy was performed, and the immunosuppressive regimen was based on OKT3, low-dose steroids and Tacrolimus.[19] In a subsequent publication from the same group, the estimated 1-year survival for 13 children transplanted with an incompatible graft was 77%.[20] Four years later, in 1998, Egawa reported on 28 children receiving an incompatible living donor liver graft who suffered an increased incidence of intrahepatic biliary complications compared to children receiving compatible or identical grafts. More importantly, the correlation among high ABO antibody IgM titers prior to the transplant, persistent higher titers afterwards, and biliary complications was drawn. More detailed analyses from the same group suggested that patients with high IgM titers prior to transplant have an increased incidence of biliary complications, and patients with increased titers of both IgM and IgG posttransplant have an increased incidence of hepatic necrosis.[21] Based on their experience, the Tanaka group adopted a perioperative target for ABO antibody titers of < 8. Nevertheless, in practice, it is not always possible to reach and to maintain this target. Of 12 patients who suffered intrahepatic biliary complications, all but 1 had a titer of IgM equal to or higher than 128.[22] The analysis of liver tissue obtained with a percutaneous biopsy, performed when a rise in the transaminases and AB titers occurred, allowed a precise definition of the early and late damage created by humoral rejection. In fact, prior to the series published by the Tanaka group, the description of the histologic changes associated with humoral rejection in incompatible liver transplantation was obtained in grafts with already advanced damage or during postmortem evaluation. The pathognomic injury of humoral rejection is the presence of portal edema and necrosis that might extend into the periportal areas.[22,23] One of the important findings of these studies is the correlation among recipient ages, incidence of biliary complications, poorer graft survival, and level of antibody titers. In the analysis by Egawa, it was noted that no child younger than 1 year of age developed hepatic necrosis or intrahepatic biliary damage. In these younger children, the peak perioperative antibody titers remained significantly lower than in older age groups. [This is to be expected because infants do not produce anti-A and anti-B iso-agglutinins until about 3 to 6 months of age, with typical median titers being between 16 and 32 at 1 year of age.] In the analysis made by Egawa, the overall 5-year survival was significantly higher and similar to compatible or identical liver transplant recipients; in recipients younger than 1 year of age, 76%, and when compared to recipients older than 16 years, 22%.[22] The observation of very

low or undetectable AB antibodies was already made by Yandza in 5 children younger than 1 year of age undergoing incompatible cadaveric liver transplantation and may partially explain the good results reported by Caciarelli in a series of children with a mean age of 2.2 years undergoing incompatible liver transplant without perioperative plasmapheresis.[17,24] By comparison, Hanto presented a series of 14 adult patients undergoing incompatible cadaveric liver transplant supported by TPE with a target antibody titer of < 8 who have survivals comparable to recipients of identical or compatible liver grafts.[25]

It remains unclear how long AB titers should be kept low after transplant. Although no specific study on this issue has been reported, it appears from the published literature that an arbitrary period of 1 month should suffice. After this period, a rise in antibody titer does not seem to be associated with an increased incidence of rejection or intrahepatic biliary complications.[17,22,23] The explanation for this phenomenon, that has been named *accommodation* and was first observed in incompatible kidney transplantation, is unclear and might be related to a modification of either graft antigen expression or of the antibody response.[26]

## HEPATIC ARTERY THROMBOSIS

A statistically significant increase of hepatic artery thromboses in recipients of incompatible grafts has been reported both in cadaveric and living donor transplants. Sanchez-Urdzapal had reported an incidence of hepatic artery thrombosis of 24% versus 0% in a study of 18 incompatible cadaveric liver recipients.[22] In his analysis of 66 incompatible living donors liver recipients, he noted an incidence of hepatic artery thrombosis of 15% versus 0.6% for recipients of compatible or identical grafts.[6,7,22] It appears that the triggering factor for the increased incidence of hepatic artery thrombosis is due to the binding of antibodies on the antigens expressed on the endothelium of the vessels and sinusoids and the subsequent activation of the complement cascade.[23] According to Egawa this endothelial injury leading to impaired arterial circulation could also be the cause of the intrahepatic biliary damage. In order to control the consequences of this immunoflammatory reaction that has been described as "single organ DIC," a strategy of intraportal or intra-arterial infusion has been proposed.[27,28]

The infusion using PGE1 alone or combined with steroids and Gabexate mesilate in the case of intraportal infusion is started at graft reperfusion and continued for 2 weeks afterwards. The number of reported cases performed using this approach is still very limited to assess whether this strategy to avoid thrombotic angiopathy will really improve the outcome of incompatible liver transplantation.

## SPLENECTOMY

The necessity of splenectomy in patients undergoing incompatible liver transplant is debatable. In 1989, Redding presented a rat model designed to assess the influence of splenectomy in antibody resynthesis after depletion with plasma exchange. The conclusion was that resynthesis is not influenced by splenectomy.[29] Several authors presented acceptable outcomes in children transplanted with cadaveric incompatible grafts and no splenectomy.[16,17,24] The main reason to avoid splenectomy was based on the potential increased incidence of infectious complications in the children.[16,30] Nonetheless, splenectomy is still routinely performed in all recipients older than 6 months in the largest series of incompatible living donor liver transplants published to date.[22]

## IMMUNOSUPPRESSION

Immunosuppressive therapy in recipients of an incompatible liver graft does not differ substantially from the one given to recipients of identical or compatible grafts. Most of the published series base their regimen on induction therapy with OKT3, ALG, or basiliximab followed by a calcineurin inhibitor, azathioprine or mycophenolate mofetil, cyclophosphamide, and steroids. In early reports, an increased incidence of acute cellular rejection was noticed in incompatible liver transplant recipients. In his latest analysis based on 66 patients, Egawa reports an incidence of acute cellular rejection of 46%, not dissimilar from 43% and 41% in identical and compatible liver transplant recipients.[22] The latest addition to the immunosuppressive armamentarium in incompatible liver transplants is Rituximab.[31,32] Because Rituximab is effective in depleting B cells for up to 4 weeks after a single dosing, it should guarantee a better control of humoral rejection and theoretically make splenectomy potentially unnecessary.

The overall review of the data reported above makes it possible to draw some conclusions and future directions. When drawing these conclusions one must keep in mind that the great majority of the data presented have been obtained from small series, with a limited follow-up, often analyzing recipients of very different clinical characteristics and undergoing various immunosuppressive regimens. Also important is the fact that, under the present allocation system for cadaveric livers in the Western world, the practice of incompatible liver transplantation will always be very limited and have a negligible impact on the patients awaiting liver transplant. On the other hand, there is a chance that incompatible liver transplantation will have a somewhat greater application in candidates of living donor liver transplantation. In this latter setting, it is not uncommon that the only suitable donor for a given recipient is of a different blood group. In addition, living donation offers an elective setting that allows a more standardized preparation of the recipient. The best long-term results have been obtained in children. Varela–Fascinetto reported an actuarial 10-year patient and graft survival of 70% and 67% in 28 children undergoing incompatible cadaveric liver transplant. Significantly better outcomes were noticed in children younger than 3 years of age.[33] Good outcomes have also been reported in 14 children with a mean age of 2.2 years transplanted with cadaveric grafts, who had an actuarial 3-year patient and graft survival of 79% and 71%, respectively.[24] Interestingly, the patients in these series did not undergo routine treatments to lower perioperatively the AB antibody titers. Egawa reported on 21 children younger than 1 year of age undergoing incompatible living donor liver transplant where actuarial 5-year patient, and graft survivals were as high as 59%.[22] In adult recipients of incompatible liver transplants, the outcomes have definitely been worse than in recipients of identical or compatible liver transplants. The best results presented in the literature are in 14 patients undergoing cadaveric liver transplant with an actuarial 5-year patient and survival of 71% and 61%, respectively.[25] No other series matches these outcomes. In 43 patients undergoing emergency cadaveric liver transplantation reported by Farges, the 5-year patient survival was 50%, but the graft survival only 20%.[7] In 9 patients older than 16 years of age undergoing living donor liver transplant reported by Egawa, the 5-year actuarial patient and graft survival was only 22%.

It is difficult from the data reported in the literature on incompatible liver transplant in adults to determine whether the clinical status of the recipients at the time of the transplant, the perioperative level of the AB antibody titers, or the different immunosuppressive regimens played a role in the great difference in outcome. There is evidence that incompatible liver transplantation can be performed in pediatric patients less than 5 years of age with outcomes similar to identical and compatible liver transplants. It appears that these young patients do not suffer an increased incidence of biliary complications neither short- nor long-term compared to their peers undergoing identical or compatible liver transplant. All data considered, the most important factor in achieving good long-term survival is the somewhat diminished humoral response and possibly the immature immune systems of these children. The other important factor is that many of these children may undergo transplantation with an incompatible graft utilizing the same immunosuppressive protocols used for identical or compatible liver transplantation. Very young children starting with low or nearly absent AB antibody titers did very well without routine perioperative treatments to decrease AB titers and without splenectomy. In practical terms, the transplantation of incompatible liver grafts in young children is possible with costs and efforts similar to identical and compatible grafts. The only question that has not been completely answered is whether, in these children and in the presence of negligible AB antibody titers, long-term graft failure due to chronic biliary damage will occur. In fact, none of the studies reported in the literature have sufficient data and follow-up to prove that such a chronic damage will definitely not occur at longer periods after the transplant.

In conclusion, the analysis of the data presently reported indicates that it is justifiable to transplant a child of less than 1 year of age with a graft of incompatible blood type. The same conclusion cannot be drawn for adult patients or for that matter for any patient older than 5 years of age. There is, in fact, only one study published with enough follow-up that shows outcomes comparable to the ones obtained in patients transplanted with identical or compatible grafts. In general, adult patients receiving an incompatible liver have a poor immediate outcome, and graft survival is affected by chronic biliary damage. The experience in the adult patients undergoing incompatible liver transplant is also limited in living donor liver transplantation. The largest series includes only 9 patients older than 16 years of age, and a 1-year patient and graft survival does not surpass 25%. In our Institution, 5 adult patients have received an incompatible living donor liver graft. The patients had a mean age at the time of the transplant of 59 years, range 50 to 74 years. At a mean follow-up of 14 months, range 4 to 27 months, 4 patients are alive with normal transaminases and bilirubin. Preoperatively all patients underwent plasmapheresis to lower AB antibody titers below 4. A target titer level of <16 was kept for the first 8 weeks after the transplant. All patients underwent splenectomy. The immunosuppression was based on pretransplant Rituximab, thymoglobulin induction, and postoperative maintenance with either Prograf or Neoral and Cellcept.[32] Even if these results are encouraging, more experience and longer follow-up are needed to determine whether this strategy can be proposed to a larger number of candidates.

At the present time with the experience and knowledge gathered, it can be said that incompatible living donor liver transplant can be offered to very young children when no other identical or compatible graft is available. In these cases, a survival similar to children receiving identical or compatible liver transplant should be expected. In adult patients undergoing incompatible liver transplant, outcomes similar to identical or compatible transplant cannot be expected. Too many factors regarding the humoral response of adult patient to blood incompatible tissue, the type of immunosuppressive regimen, and the chronic damage to the biliary tree are unknown or inadequately studied. Patients undergoing such transplants should be carefully selected avoiding the ones where a low preoperative AB antibody titer cannot be achieved or have already an extremely poor predicted survival due to other co-morbidities. The patients should be warned that the present results are possibly inferior to the results obtained transplanting very marginal cadaveric livers. Nevertheless, incompatible liver transplantation in adults should continue to be performed within strictly controlled protocols in institutions willing to dedicate a tremendous amount of technical and human resources. The ultimate goal of improving overall patient and graft survival should be achieved by a strong research effort in understanding the various factors responsible for current poor results.

## References

1. Starzl TE, Ishikawa M, Putnam CW, et al. Progress in and deterrents to orthotopic liver transplantation, with special reference to survival, resistance to hyperacute rejection and biliary duct reconstruction. *Transplant Proc* 1974;6:129.
2. Demetris AJ, Jaffe R, Tzakis A, et al. Antibody-mediated rejection of human orthotopic liver allografts. A study of liver transplantation across ABO blood group barriers. *Am J Path* 1988;132:489.
3. Knechtle S, Kolbeck P, Tsuchimoto S, et al. Hepatic transplantation into sensitized recipients. *Transplantation* 1987;43(1):8.
4. Gugenheim J, Samuel D, Reynes M, et al. Liver transplantation across ABO blood group barriers. *Lancet* 1990;336:519.
5. Sanchez-Urdazpal L, Sterioff S, Janes C, et al. Increased bile duct complications in ABO incompatible liver transplant recipients. *Transplant Proc* 1991;23(1):1440.
6. Sanchez-Urdazpal L, Batts K, Gores G, et al. Increased bile duct complications in liver transplantation across the ABO barrier. *Ann Surg* 1993;218(2):152.
7. Farges O, Nocci Kalil A, Samuel D, et al.: Long-term results of ABO-incompatible liver transplantation. *Transplant Proc* 27(2):1701, 1995.
8. Gordon R, Fung J, Markus B, et al. The antibody crossmatch liver transplantation. *Surgery* 1986;100(4):705.
9. Lo CM, Shaked A, Busuttil RW. Risk factors for liver transplantation across the ABO barrier. *Transplantation* 1994;58:543.
10. Busson M, Romano P, Hors J. Importance of ABO blood group matching in liver transplantation. *Transplant Proc* 1995;27:1157.
11. Slapak M, Evans P, Trickett L, et al. Can ABO-incompatible donors be used in renal transplantation? *Transplant Proc* 1984;16:75.
12. Slapak M, Digard N, Ahmed N, et al. Renal transplantation across the ABO-barrier–A 9-year experience. *Transplant Proc* 1990;22:1425.
13. Alexandre GPJ, Squifflet JP, De Bruyere M, et al. Splenectomy as a prerequisite for successful human ABO-incompatible renal transplantation. *Transplant Proc* 1985;17:138.
14. Alexandre GPJ, Squifflet JP, De Bruyere M, et al. Present experiences in a series of 26 ABO-incompatible living donor renal allografts. *Transplant Proc* 1987;19:4538.
15. Fishel RJ, Ascher NL, Payne WD, et al. Pediatric liver transplantation across ABO blood group barriers. Transplant Proc 1989;21(1):2221.
16. Renard TH, Andrews WS. An approach to ABO-incompatible liver transplantation in children. *Transplantation* 1992;53:116.
17. Yandza T, Lamert T, Alvarez F, et al. Outcome of ABO-incompatible liver transplantation in children with no specific alloantibodies at the time of transplantation. *Transplantation* 1994;58(1):46.
18. Mor E, Skerrett D, Manzarbeitia C, et al. Successful use of an enhanced immunosuppressive protocol with plasmapheresis for ABO-incompatible mismatched grafts in liver transplant recipients. *Transplantation* 1995;59(7):986.
19. Tokunaga Y, Tanaka K, Fujita S, et al. Living related liver transplantation across ABO blood groups with FK506 and OKT3. *Transplant Int* 1993;6:313.
20. Tanaka A, Tanaka K, Kitai T, et al. Living related liver transplantation across ABO blood groups. *Transplantation* 1994;58(5):548.
21. Kozaki K, Kasahara M, Oike F, et al. Apheresis therapy for living-donor liver transplantation. Experience of apheresis use for living-donor liver transplantation at Kyoto University. *Therapeutic Apheresis* 2002;6(6):478.
22. Egawa H, Oike F, Buhler L, et al. Impact of recipient age on outcome of ABO-incompatible living-donor liver transplantation. *Transplantation* 2004;77(3):403.
23. Haga H, Egawa H, Shirase T, et al. Periportal edema and necrosis as diagnostic histological features of early humoral rejection in ABO-incompatible liver transplantation. *Liver Transplant* 2004;10(1):16.
24. Cacciarelli T, So S, Lim J, Concepcion W, et al. A reassessment of ABO incompatibility in pediatric liver transplantation. *Transplantation* 1995;60(7):757.
25. Hanto D, Fecteau A, Alonso M, et al. ABO-incompatible liver transplantation with no immunological graft losses using total plasma exchange, splenectomy, and quadruple immunosuppression: Evidence for accommodation. *Liver Transplant* 2003;9(1):22.
26. Platt JL. Immunobiology of Graft Rejection: Antibodies in graft rejection. In: Bach FH, Auchincloss H, eds. *Transplantation Immunology.* New York; 1995:113.
27. Tanabe M, Shimazu M, Wakabayashi G, et al. Intraportal infusion therapy as a novel approach to adult ABO-incompatible liver transplantation. *Transplantation* 2002;73(12):1959.
28. Nakamura Y, Matsuno N, Iwamoto T, et al. Successful case of adult ABO-incompatible liver transplantation: Beneficial effects of intrahepatic artery infusion therapy: A case report. *Transplant Proc* 2004;36:2269.
29. Redding R, White D, Davies H, et al. Effect of splenectomy on antibody rebound after plasma exchange. *Transplantation* 1989;48(1):145.
30. Alexander JW, First MR, Majeski JA, et al. The late adverse effect of splenectomy on patient survival following cadaveric renal transplantation. *Transplantation* 1984;37:467.
31. Monteiro I, McLoughlin L, Fisher A, et al. Rituximab with plasmapheresis and splenectomy in ABO-incompatible liver transplantation. *Transplantation* 2003;76(11):1648.
32. Testa G, Marinov M, Schena S, et al. Successful protocol for living-related liver transplantation across blood barrier. *Clin Transpl* 2004;19 (Suppl 13):34.
33. Varela-Fascinetto G, Treacy SJ, Lillehein CW, et al. Long-term results in pediatric ABO-incompatible liver transplantation. *Transplant Proc* 1999;31:467.

## 30.16.2  Hepatitis-Positive Donors

*Chung Mau Lo, MD, MS,*
*Sheung Tat Fan, MS, MD, PhD*

### INTRODUCTION

The success of liver transplantation and the accelerating shortage of organs have stimulated the use of extended criteria or marginal donors. A graft from a marginal deceased donor is one which is associated with an unfavorable outcome in the recipient because of a greater risk for primary nonfunction or disease transmission. The risk is balanced against the benefit of increasing the donor pool and an early transplant particularly for recipients with high medical urgency. In living donor liver transplantation (LDLT), however, a marginal donor may have a more widely variable definition and implications for the risk of either the recipient or the donor, or both. A living donor may be considered marginal because of an increased risk for the recipient alone, as in the use of an ABO-incompatible liver graft, or for the donor alone, as in an older donor or one with co-morbidity. Occasionally, a marginal graft such as a small-for-size left-lobe graft may increase the risk of the recipient and yet protect the donor's safety. Because the safety of a living donor is always the primary concern, marginal living donors with added operative risks are generally not recommended.

A hepatitis-positive donor provides a key example of a marginal donor in the application of LDLT in which not only the risk of the recipient but also that of the donor may be increased. The presence of antibody to hepatitis B core antigen (anti-HBc) in the absence of hepatitis B surface antigen (HBsAg) signifies past exposure to hepatitis B virus (HBV) and may represent a state of resolved infection with immunity or recent clearance of HBsAg and yet persistent low-grade hepatitis activity. Apart from the risk of transmission of HBV infection to HBsAg-negative recipients,[1] there is concern that anti-HBc-positive donors are at an extra risk, and controversy exists as to whether seropositivity for anti-HBc should be regarded as a contraindication for living liver donation.[2] In this chapter, we reviewed the evidence available in the literature regarding the risk of both the recipient and the donor in the context of a marginal living liver donor who is seropositive for anti-HBc.

## LIMITATION OF ANTI-HBc AS AN INDICATION OF OCCULT HBV INFECTION

The presence of a positive serology for anti-HBc is usually taken as the marker for previous exposure to HBV and hence possible occult infection. The enzyme-linked immunoassay for anti-HBc, however, has a significant false-positive rate that may account for the variable rate of HBV reactivation reported in recipients who received an anti-HBc-positive liver graft. A false-positive result may lead to inappropriate exclusion of donors or unnecessary and costly prophylaxis against reactivation in the recipients. The development of more sensitive assays for viral antigens and the introduction of HBV DNA detection tests have delineated the molecular basis and led to the development of a different definition of occult infections.[3,4] Persistence of HBV DNA has been demonstrated in the liver or serum of HBsAg-negative patients with various forms of acute infection, chronic hepatitis, and hepatocellular carcinoma who test positive for anti-HBc with or without anti-HBs.[3-5] Viral DNA persistence has also been detected even in subjects with normal liver parameters including in particular blood and organ donors.[5-9] These highly sensitive HBV DNA assays, however, are mainly confined to research programs. Optimization of the sensitivity, adoption of appropriate negative controls, and standardization of techniques and type of tissue used are some of the concerns that need to be resolved before its role in clinical practice can be determined. From a clinical point of view, the information available in the literature only allows for an evaluation of a hepatitis-positive donor based on a positive serology for anti-HBc.

## RISK FOR HBV REACTIVATION IN THE RECIPIENT

Transplantation of a liver graft from an anti-HBc-positive donor to a HBsAg-negative recipient results in HBV infection after transplantation at a rate of 25% to 95%.[1] A variety of terms such as *de novo* hepatitis B, recurrent hepatitis B, transmission of hepatitis B, or reactivation of hepatitis B have been used to describe HBV infection in this setting. Because episomal form of HBV accompanied by ongoing viral replication has been identified in the majority of healthy individuals positive for anti-HBc,[7] and the genetic identity of HBV in recipients who developed infection

after transplantation is identical to that of the HBV found in the donor's liver tissue,[10] the HBV infection should be regarded as reactivation of latent infection in the liver graft.[1]

Experience with the use of anti-HBc-positive livers from deceased donors indicated that the risk of HBV reactivation varies with the recipient's HBV serology status. The presence of anti-HBs in the recipient has been reported to protect against reactivation.[11-14] The recipient's anti-HBc seropositivity has also been shown to be associated with a lower risk of HBV reactivation.[11-14] On the other hand, the concomitant presence of anti-HBs in the donor's serum does not offer any protective effect. Other factors such as the Child-Pugh score[12] and the type of immunosuppressive therapy,[12,15] have also been suggested to affect the rate of HBV reactivation through its effect on the host immune response. As a result of the small number of patients with HBV reactivation and the heterogeneity of data in most series, however, a definite conclusion based on a meaningful statistical analysis was not possible.

There are few reports on the risk of HBV reactivation when an anti-HBc-positive graft is transplanted from a living donor without prophylaxis. Uemoto et al.[10] reported that in the absence of prophylaxis, 15 of 16 (94%) recipients who were primarily anti-HBs-negative developed HBV reactivation after receiving anti-HBc-positive liver grafts from living donors. In a series of 24 LDLTs using anti-HBc-positive liver grafts from Taiwan,[14] HBV reactivation developed in 3 of 8 (37.5%) recipients without prophylaxis, including 1 recipient who was positive for anti-HBs before transplantation. In a follow-up study on the expanded experience from the same center,[16] 7 of 16 (44%) recipients developed reactivation in such circumstances. Hence, the overall risk appears to be at least as high as that of an anti-HBc-positive deceased donor graft and other risk factors are assumed to be similar. It is not certain whether the regeneration of a small-for-size graft which is common in LDLT may stimulate and increase the rate of reactivation of the latent infection. Nonetheless, with the recognition of the problem of reactivation and widespread use of various prophylactic measures, it may be difficult to find an answer to this question by elucidating the natural course of reactivation.

## STRATEGIES FOR THE USE OF ANTI-HBc-POSITIVE GRAFTS

### Matching

Matching is the most logical and cost-effective way to optimize the use of an anti-HBc-positive liver graft from a deceased donor.[1] Such a graft is usually allocated first to HBsAg-positive recipients who would in any case need prophylaxis against recurrence. Because the prevalence of anti-HBc seropositivity in a geographic region is closely related to that of chronic HBV infection, the number of suitable recipients on the list should match the supply. If an HBsAg-positive recipient is not available, the graft will be offered to an HBsAg-negative recipient who usually has a high medical urgency and should be fully informed of the risk of HBV reactivation. Although recipients with anti-HBc have a lower risk of HBV reactivation, particularly if anti-HBs is positive, the chance of HBV reactivation exists and all recipients of anti-HBc-positive livers should be placed on long-term prophylaxis as discussed later.

Unfortunately, a matching policy is not appealing and has little role in the practice of LDLT. A living donor is evaluated for the possibility of donation to a specific recipient and the graft is a dedicated gift that cannot be allocated to an alternative recipient for matching purpose. Frequently, there may be no more than one voluntary donor, and the only decision that needs to be made is whether to accept the risk of HBV reactivation and the need for long-term prophylaxis.

## Prophylaxis Against HBV Reactivation

Recipients of liver grafts from anti-HBc-positive donors should receive prophylaxis to minimize the risk of HBV reactivation. Even if the risk may be lower for recipients who test positive for anti-HBc and/or anti-HBs, prophylaxis needs to be considered. The most cost-effective regimen, however, remains to be defined. The various strategies to prevent recurrent hepatitis B in HBsAg-positive recipients have been explored, including hepatitis-B-immune globulin (HBIG) and lamivudine, either alone or in combination. HBIG alone is not always effective and is associated with a small but definite risk of HBV reactivation.[11,18] In prophylaxis against HBV recurrence, HBIG works by binding circulating HBV and preventing entry of the virus into the liver cells. Because the source of the infecting virus responsible for HBV reactivation is not in the recipient's circulation but already in the donor's liver cells, it is conceivable that the HBIG monoprophylaxis may fail.

Adding lamivudine to HBIG has been shown to completely protect against HBV reactivation. High-dose HBIG similar to the regimen used for the prevention of recurrence in HBsAg-positive recipients has been used,[17] but the regimen is prohibitively expensive and carries all the adverse effects and inconvenience of high-dose HBIG therapy. Regimens with lower doses and a shorter course of HBIG have been shown to have similar effectiveness. Finally, the success of lamivudine monoprophylaxis in preventing reactivation suggests that HBIG may not be necessary at all.[14,15] The number of study patients, however, was small, and the duration of follow-up was short. The major concern is the emergence of lamivudine-resistant viral mutants particularly with long-term administration. Nonetheless, unlike patients with chronic hepatitis B infection, the viral load in anti-HBc-positive donors with occult HBV infection is very low,[2] and the risk of emergence of viral mutants with drug resistance is expected to be low. Loss et al.[19] studied the presence of HBV DNA by polymerase chain reaction (PCR) in liver grafts of patients receiving lamivudine prophylaxis against HBV reactivation. Of the eight patients with HBV DNA-positive donor livers, seven became PCR-negative for liver HBV DNA at 1 to 20 months after transplantation, suggesting that the viral load in the liver continued to decrease and the risk of selecting out viral mutant was small. So far, there has not been any report of breakthrough infection due to HBV mutant with drug resistance in HBsAg-negative patients receiving lamivudine prophylaxis against HBV reactivation.

While awaiting results of larger studies on the durability of lamivudine monoprophylaxis, a study from Taiwan reported the induction of active immunity through pretransplant vaccination in addition to lamivudine prophylaxis in 16 patients receiving anti-HBc-positive grafts from living donors.[14] Fifteen patients seroconverted before transplant and none developed reactivation at a mean follow-up of 25 months. Nonetheless, the posttransplant anti-HBs status was not reported, and the role of the additional protection provided by the vaccine-induced immunity is unknown, as reactivation in vaccinated anti-HBs-positive recipients has been reported.[20] The efficacy of this approach would clearly

be limited by the low response rate of patients with chronic liver disease to vaccination.

A selective prophylaxis protocol based on serum and liver HBV DNA status has been proposed. Fabrega et al.[21] reported seven recipients of anti-HBc-positive grafts who received combination prophylaxis until HBV DNA results from the donor were available. All seven were PCR-negative in serum and liver samples, and the prophylaxis was stopped. None of the patients developed reactivation after a follow-up of 9 to 36 months. Nery et al.[22] performed PCR assay for detection of HBV DNA in serum and liver samples of both donors and recipients. If the donor or recipient was positive for HBV DNA, combination of HBIG and lamivudine would be administered. Otherwise, only anti-HBs-negative recipients were given lamivudine monoprophylaxis, whereas anti-HBs-positive recipients received no prophylaxis. At a median follow-up of 23.5 months, HBV reactivation developed in 2 of 45 patients, and was attributed to noncompliance with medications in both cases. In a survey on the use of anti-HBc positive donors in the United States,[23] two thirds of the respondents supported the idea that additional information on the HBV DNA status of the donor might guide the prophylaxis protocol. If HBV DNA were to be used routinely, it appears that liver tissue rather than serum, should be tested, because serum HBV DNA has little value in predicting HBV reactivation.[10–12] Nonetheless, detection of HBV DNA in liver tissue remains controversial, and numerous technical limitations need to be resolved. There is a need for more clinical studies before any conclusion can be drawn on this selective prophylactic approach.

## DONOR'S RISK

In the United States, 50% of the programs would transplant an anti-HBc-positive liver from a deceased donor into a HBV naïve recipient, and an additional 7% would do that for selective high-risk recipients such as the desperately ill or those with hepatocellular carcinoma.[23] Yet, exclusion of anti-HBc-positive living donors has been generally advocated.[2,24,25] Although the risk of HBV reactivation in a recipient may be balanced by its benefit and may be prevented by effective prophylaxis, objection to its use in LDLT is based primarily on the assumption of the extra risks for the donor. Theoretically the underlying hepatitis infection may delay the recovery and regeneration of the liver remnant and the surgical risk will be increased. There may be a risk of reactivation of integrated HBV virus in the postoperative period, and these risks are likely to be more significant if an extensive resection such as a right hepatectomy is to be performed. In the longer term, the occult hepatitis infection may progress to chronic liver disease or liver malignancy[26–28] and the previous hepatic resection for liver donation may compromise the prospects for appropriate treatment.

These potential problems in anti-HBc-positive donors, however, are theoretical, and the assumption of the extra risks has never been supported by clinical data. Because most programs in Western countries advocate exclusion of anti-HBc-positive living donors, these data would only come from Asian countries where HBV infection is endemic. Hwang et al.[29] retrospectively studied 86 right-lobe and 34 left-lobe living liver donors in the Asan Medical Center in Korea. Fifty (39%) donors were positive for anti-HBc but the anti-HBs status was not reported. The anti-HBc seropositivity had no significant effect on the short-term outcome in terms of blood loss, recovery of liver function, and morbidity in either right-lobe or left-lobe donors. The liver remnant regeneration rate at 1 week and 2 months was also comparable in right-lobe donors.

A report from The University of Hong Kong at Queen Mary Hospital in Hong Kong[30] specifically addressed this issue in right-lobe liver transplant. Twenty-nine (54%) of 54 right-lobe donors were anti-HBc-positive, and of these, 24 (83%) had anti-HBs as well. All donors were negative for HBV DNA in serum by PCR, but the liver HBV DNA status was not available. Anti-HBc seropositivity was associated with older age and the proportion of anti-HBc-positive donors increased with age from 18% below 30 years of age to 100% after the age of 50. There was no significant difference in graft size or histologic findings of fatty change or fibrosis, but interestingly, there was a higher operative blood loss and postoperative bilirubin level in anti-HBc-positive donors. Three donors developed significant postoperative cholestasis and all were positive for anti-HBc, older than 45 years, and had mild fatty change. It remains unclear whether the higher blood loss and cholestasis might be related to the subtle difference in the consistency and function of the liver attributed to increasing age, fatty change, or anti-HBc seropositivity. Older donors are at a greater risk for cholestasis after right lobe donation,[31] and steatosis is also associated with increased intraoperative blood loss and cholestasis.[32,33] Whether anti-HBc seropositivity has an independent effect on these short-term outcome measures remains to be determined by larger studies.

Although these two studies indicated that the overall short-term surgical risk of liver resection is not significantly increased in selected Asian donors seropositive for anti-HBc, there is concern, though unproven, that difference in the prevalence of steatosis and other factors may affect the recovery of these living donors in Western countries.[2] More importantly, there may be long-term issues such as the risk for the development of cirrhosis or hepatocellular carcinoma.[26–28] In the study from Hong Kong[30] with a follow-up that ranged from 21 to 72 months, all anti-HBc-positive donors had normal liver function, and none experienced any episode of hepatitis or other liver diseases. Nonetheless, the possibility of reactivation and progressive development of cirrhosis remains, particularly if immunosuppression is required for other diseases in future.[34,35] Past exposure to HBV infection has also been shown to increase the risk of the development of hepatocellular carcinoma in patients with chronic liver disease,[27] but whether the risk is significant in patients with biochemically and histologically normal liver is controversial. Transplant centers that accept living donors positive for anti-HBc are obliged to continue lifelong follow-up of these donors in order to assess these potential long-term sequels.

## PREVALENCE OF ANTI-HBc SEROPOSITIVITY AND IMPLICATION FOR A RECOMMENDED STRATEGY

The prevalence of serum anti-HBc parallels the overall rate of HBV infection in the general population. It varies widely in different geographical areas, ranging from about 5% in low-prevalence areas such as the United States[36] to 12% in moderately prevalent areas such as Spain,[12] and over 25% in endemic areas that include a large part of Asia.[14,29,30,37] In the endemic areas, HBV-related liver disease is a common indication for liver transplantation.[38,39] Because HBV infection tends to cluster within families, the prevalence of anti-HBc in potential living donors for HBsAg-positive recipient is even higher than that in the general population.[30] Reports from Taiwan, Korea, and Hong Kong where the prevalence of HBsAg positivity is 10% to 20% show that 39% to 57% of living

**TABLE 30.16.2-1**

**INCIDENCE OF ANTI-HBc SEROPOSITIVITY IN LIVING LIVER DONORS**

| Author (ref) | Geographic Area | Year | No. of Donors | No. of Anti-HBc-Positive Donors |
|---|---|---|---|---|
| Uemoto et al.[10] | Japan | 1998 | 171 | 16 (9%) |
| Chen et al.[14] | Taiwan | 2002 | 42 | 24 (57%) |
| Hwang et al.[29] | Korea | 2003 | 127 | 50 (39%) |
| Lo et al.[30] | Hong Kong | 2003 | 54 | 29 (54%) |
| Lee et al.[37] | Korea | 2004 | 128 | 58 (45%) |

donors are positive for anti-HBc (Table 30.16.2-1). Regarding a positive serology as a contraindication for living liver donation would result in exclusion of nearly 50% of the living donors. More importantly, many of these HBV-endemic areas in Asia coincidentally also have a very low organ donation rate,[38] and LDLT may account for over 50% of all liver transplants.

The considerations are very different in Western countries with low prevalence of HBV infection. In the United States, for example, less than 5% of the deceased donor liver grafts transplanted were anti-HBc positive, and the proportion of anti-HBc-positive living donor was even lower.[40] In addition, LDLT accounts for only 6.3% of all liver transplants performed in 2003. Acceptance of a positive serology for anti-HBc in living donor will have a minor effect (< 5%) in maximizing LDLT and an even more infinitesimal impact (about 0.3%) on the overall practice of liver transplantation.

While awaiting results of large studies particularly on the long-term risk for anti-HBc-positive donors, it appears reasonable for individual transplant programs to consider the prevalence of anti-HBc as well as the role of LDLT in the local population regarding a policy on anti-HBc-positive living donors. When anti-HBc seropositivity is uncommon and LDLT accounts for a small proportion of all liver transplants, as in most Western countries, exclusion of all anti-HBc-positive living donors may be the simplest and easiest answer. For many HBV endemic areas in Asia, where living donors provide the major source of liver grafts, the recipient's risk of HBV reactivation and the donor's unproven extra risk are probably superseded by the benefit of accepting an anti-HBc-positive donor in order to maximize LDLT.

## RECOMMENDATION FOR ANTI-HBc-POSITIVE LIVING DONORS

For liver transplant centers that decide to accept living donors positive for anti-HBc, detailed preoperative assessment and postoperative follow-up are mandatory for both the donor and the recipient. Donors with ongoing chronic hepatitis and viremia as indicated by abnormal liver biochemistry and positive serum HBV DNA should be excluded. A routine preoperative percutaneous liver biopsy[41] seems justified to assess the degree of steatosis and to exclude any degree of occult hepatitis or fibrosis, but the clinical role of HBV DNA assay in liver tissue remains unclear. The elective nature of LDLT allows donors seronegative for anti-HBs to receive HBV vaccination to protect against the risk of future HBV reactivation. The possibility of adoptive immunity transfer may also potentially enhance the recipient's immune response to HBV and prevent reactivation or recurrence.[42]

For the HBsAg-positive recipients, there is no need for any adjustment to the appropriate prophylaxis against HBV recurrence. All HBsAg-negative recipients should receive active immunization if possible before transplantation and prophylactic treatment with lamivudine alone or in combination with HBIG after transplantation. Both the donor and the recipient should receive regular and lifelong follow-up with close serological and virological monitoring, and an episode of liver dysfunction should be investigated thoroughly for HBV reactivation.

## CONCLUSION

The development of LDLT has generated more controversies and distinctly different issues with the use of a marginal anti-HBc-positive graft as compared to deceased donor liver transplant. The ethical consideration is complicated by the additional concern with the safety of a healthy living donor. Instead of the justice of the organ allocation system, we have to reflect the worthiness of a dedicated donation. Matching a recipient from a long waiting list for a better outcome is not possible, as there is only a limited choice of donors, if any, for a particular recipient. On the other hand, the possibility of a more thorough preoperative assessment of the living donor provides the unique opportunity for decisions to be based on the results of investigations such as HBV DNA in serum and liver tissue of the donor before transplantation. It would also allow pretransplant intervention by immunologic manipulation of the donor's HBV immunity status. Finally, living donors provide the novel model to study the effect of liver resection on latent HBV in individuals with resolved infection and a normal liver. With the information available at present, transplant centers may decide to accept these marginal donors based on their rate of anti-HBc-seropositivity and the need for LDLT. Nonetheless, it is imperative that protocols are developed for prospective collection of data and tissue samples in order to clarify the scientific basis for this approach.

## References

1. Munoz SJ. Use of hepatitis B core antibody-positive donors for liver transplantation. *Liver Transpl* 2002;8:S82–S87.
2. Fontana RJ, Merion RM. Are we ready for marginal hepatitis B core antibody-positive living liver donors? *Liver Transpl* 2003;9:833–836.
3. Brechot C, Thiers V, Kremsdorf D, et al. Persistent hepatitis B virus infection in subjects without hepatitis B surface antigen: clinically significant or purely "occult"? *Hepatology* 2001;34:194–203.
4. Hu KQ. Occult hepatitis B virus infection and its clinical implications. *J Viral Hepatitis* 2002;9:243–257.
5. Marrero JA, Lok AS. Occult hepatitis B virus infection in patients with hepatocellular carcinoma: Innocent bystander, cofactor, or culprit? *Gastroenterology* 2004;126:347–350.
6. Hui CK, Sun J, Au WY, et al. Occult hepatitis B virus infection in hematopoietic stem cell donors in a hepatitis B virus endemic area. *J Hepatol* 2003; 42:813–819.
7. Marusawa H, Uemoto S, Hijikata M, et al. Letent hepatitis B virus infection in healthy individuals with antibodies to hepatitis B core antigen. *Hepatology* 2000; 31:488–495.
8. Kleinman SH, Kuhns MC, Todd DS, et al. Frequency of HBV DNA detection in US blood donors testing positive for the presence of anti-HBc: implications for transfusion transmission and donor screening. *Transfusion* 2003;43:696–704.
9. Dreier J, Kroger M, Diekmann J, et al. Low-level viraemia of hepatitis B virus in an anti-HBc- and anti-HBs-positive blood donor. *Transfus Med* 2004;14:97–103.
10. Uemoto S, Sugiyama K, Marusawa H, et al. Transmission of hepatitis B virus from hepatitis B core antibody-positive donors in living related liver transplants. *Transplantation* 1998;65:494–499.
11. Roque-Afonso AM, Feray C, Samual D, et al. Antibodies to hepatitis B surface antigen prevent viral reactivation in recipients of liver grafts from anti-HBC positive donors. *Gut* 2002;50:95–99.
12. Prieto M, Gomez MD, Berenguer M, et al. De novo hepatitis B after liver transplantation from hepatitis B core antibody-positive donors in an area with high prevalence of anti-HBc positivity in the donor population. *Liver Transpl* 2001;7:51–58.
13. Manzarbeitia C, Reich DJ, Ortiz JA, et al. Safe use of livers from donors with positive hepatitis B core antibody. *Liver Transpl* 2002;8:556–561.
14. Chen YS, Wang CC, de Villa VH, et al. Prevention of de novo hepatitis B virus infection in living donor liver transplantation using hepatitis B core antibody positive donors. Clin *Transplant* 2002;16:405–409.
15. Yu AS, Vierling JM, Colquhoun SD, et al. Transmission of hepatitis B infection from hepatitis B core antibody-positive liver allografts is prevented by lamivudine therapy. *Liver Transpl* 2001;7:513–517.
16. de Villa VH, Chen YS, Chen CL. Hepatitis B core antibody-positive grafts: recipient's risk. *Transplantation* 2003;75:S49–S53.
17. Dodson SF, Bonham CA, Geller DA, et al. Prevention of de novo hepatitis B infection in recipients of hepatic allografts from anti-HBc positive donors. *Transplantation* 1999;68:1058–1061.
18. Holt D, Thomas R, Van Thiel D, et al. Use of hepatitis B core antibody-positive donors in orthotopic liver transplantation. *Arch Surg* 2002;137:572–576.
19. Loss GE Jr, Mason AL, Nair S, et al. Does lamivudine prophylaxis eradicate persistent HBV DNA from allografts derived from anti-HBc-positive donors? *Liver Transpl* 2003;9:1258–1264.
20. Lee KW, Lee DS, Lee HH, et al. Prevention of de novo hepatitis B infection from HbcAb-positive donors in living donor liver transplantation. *Transplant Proc* 2004;36:2311–2312.
21. Fabrega E, Garcia-Suarez C, Guerra A, et al. Liver transplantation with allografts from hepatitis B core antibody-positive donors: a new approach. *Liver Transpl* 2003;9:916–920.
22. Nery JR, Nery-Avila C, Reddy KR, et al. Use of liver grafts from donors positive for antihepatitis B-core antibody (Anti-HBc) in the era of prophylaxis with prophylaxis-B immunoglobulin and lamivudine. *Transplantation* 2003;75:1179–1186.
23. Burton JR Jr, Shaw-Stiffel TA. Use of hepatitis B core antibody-positive donors in recipients without evidence of hepatitis B infection: A survey of current practice in the United States. *Liver Transpl* 2003; 9:837–842.
24. Brown RS Jr, Russo MW, Lai M, et al. A survey of liver transplantation from living adult donors in the United States. *N Engl J Med* 2003;348:818–825.
25. Trotter JF, Wachs M, Everson GT, et al. Adult-to-adult transplantation of the right hepatic lobe from a living donor. *N Engl J Med* 2002;346:1074–1082.
26. Tanaka H, Iwasaki Y, Nouso K, et al. Possible contribution of prior hepatitis B virus infection to the development of hepatocellular carcinoma. *J Gastroenterol Hepatol* 2005;20:850–856.
27. Okada S, Sato T, Okusaka T, et al. Past exposure to hepatitis B virus as a risk factor for hepatocellular carcinoma in patients with chronic liver disease. *Br J Cancer* 1998;77:2028–2031.
28. Yano Y, Yamashita F, Sumie S, et al. Clinical features of hepatocellular carcinoma seronegative for both HBsAg and anti-HCV antibody but positive for anti-HBc antibody in Japan. *Am J Gastroenterol* 2002;97:156–161.
29. Hwang S, Moon DB, Lee SG, et al. Safety of anti-hepatitis B core antibody-positive donors for living-donor liver transplantation. *Transplantation* 2003;75:S45–S48.
30. Lo CM, Fan ST, Liu CL, et al. Safety and outcome of hepatitis B core antibody-positive donors in right-lobe living donor liver transplantation. *Liver Transpl* 2003;9:827–832.
31. Sakamoto S, Uemoto S, Uryuhara K, et al. Graft size assessment and analysis of donors for living donor liver transplantation using right lobe. *Transplantation* 2001;71:1407–1413.
32. Fan ST, Lo CM, Liu CL, et al. Safety of donors in live donor liver transplantation using right lobe grafts. *Arch Surg* 2000;135:336-340.

33. Behrns KE, Tsiotos GG, DeSouza NF, et al. Hepatic steatosis as a potential risk factor for major hepatic resection. *J Gastrointest Surg* 1998;2:292–298.

34. Law JK, Ho JK, Hoskins PJ, et al. Fatal reactivation of hepatitis B post-chemotherapy for lymphoma in a hepatitis B surface antigen-negative, hepatitis B core antibody-positive patient: Potential implications for future prophylaxis recommendations. *Leuk Lymphoma* 2005;46:1085–1089.

35. Knoll A, Pietrzyk M, Loss M, et al. Solid-organ transplantation in HBsAg-negative patients with antibodies to HBV core antigen: low risk of HBV reactivation. *Transplantation* 2005;79:1631–1633.

36. McQuillan GM, Coleman PJ, Kruszon-Moran D, et al. Prevalence of hepatitis B virus infection in the United States: the National Health and Nutrition Examination Surveys, 1976 through 1994. *Am J Public Health* 1999;89:14–18.

37. Lee KH, Wai CT, Lim SG, et al. Risk for de novo hepatitis B from antibody to hepatitis B core antigen-positive donors in liver transplantation in Singapore. *Liver Transpl* 2001;7:469–470.

38. Chen CL, Fan ST, Lee SG, et al. Living-donor liver transplantation: 12 years of experience in Asia. *Transplantation* 2003;75:S6–S11.

39. Lo CM, Fan ST, Liu CL, et al. Prophylaxis and treatment of recurrent hepatitis B after liver transplantation. *Transplantation* 2003;75:S41–S44.

40. University Renal Research and Education Association. United Network for Organ Sharing Annual 2002 Report of the US Organ Procurement and Transplantation Network and the Scientific Registry of Transplant Recipients: Transplant Data 1992-2003. Available at: http://www.ustransplant.org/annual.html.Accessed June 30, 2005.

41. Ryan CK, Johnson LA, Germin BI, et al. One hundred consecutive hepatic biopsies in the workup of living donors for right lobe liver transplantation. *Liver Transpl* 2002;8:1114–1122.

42. Lo CM, Fung JT, Lau GK, et al. Development of antibody to hepatitis B surface antigen after liver transplantation for chronic hepatitis B. *Hepatology* 2003;37:36–43.

# LIVER TRANSPLANTATION: COST ANALYSIS

*Mark W. Russo, MD, MPH, Robert S. Brown, MD, MPH*

## INTRODUCTION

The financial aspects of health care and economic forces have made costs of treating patients with end-stage liver disease an important issue. Declining reimbursement, more advanced and costly procedures and medications, managed care, and increased regulation have made a drive toward cost-effectiveness essential. For liver diseases, liver transplantation, which is perhaps the most costly of interventions used in patients with end-stage liver disease, is at the forefront of these efforts to understand and control costs. The initial barriers to liver transplantation were to document success in terms of patient and graft survival. Now that liver transplantation is a well-accepted therapy for end-stage liver disease, strategies to provide this life-saving technique in the broadest and most cost-effective manner have emerged as central issues.

With the development and success of living donor liver transplantation (LDLT) there is the opportunity to improve the access, effectiveness, and cost of a life-saving treatment. By increasing the number of patients who can undergo transplantation as well as by performing the procedure in an elective manner, it is possible to improve costs without compromising quality or outcomes. There is the potential to select patients who are less ill at the time of transplant, which could potentially reduce the cost of transplantation as well as the cost of managing complications of end-stage liver disease. The focus of this chapter is on the financial aspects of liver transplantation, with comparison between deceased donor liver transplantation (DDLT) and adult-to-adult living donor liver transplantation (LDLT).

## COST OF DECEASED DONOR LIVER TRANSPLANTATION

A discussion on costs of medical care and liver transplantation warrants making the distinction between costs and charges. Cost is the economic value of both labor and resources required to provide a service or perform a procedure, excluding markup. Charges are the amount billed to a patient or third-party payer by a health-care organization. Charges typically include costs as well as profit. Costs should be less variable than charges and it is the preferred data for economic analyses. Obtaining the cost of a procedure is more difficult than obtaining its associated charges. Results in economic analyses can report total costs, but more commonly studies of cost-effectiveness of an intervention are reported. Cost-effectiveness reflects what is obtained (ie, the benefits) for any given cost. Terms used in cost analyses are defined in Table 31-1.

**TABLE 31-1**

**TERMS USED IN COST ANALYSES**

| Term | Definition |
|------|------------|
| Cost | Economic value of labor and resources to provide a service or procedure |
| Charge | Value a patient or payer is billed by a health-care provider including markup |
| Discounting | An estimate that incorporates the concept that a year of life or quantity of money currently is worth more now than at a time point in the future |
| Utility measure | An estimate that is used to quantitate quality of life. Range is typically for 0 to 1 with 0 death and 1 complete health |
| Incremental cost-effectiveness ratio | The additional cost of a more effective intervention for each additional year of life saved compared to a less effective, less costly intervention |
| Sensitivity analysis | An analysis that uses a range of assumptions for variables used in the model to determine the effect of changes in that variable on the outcome. |

Cost-effectiveness studies are economic analyses that incorporate the ratio of the change in effectiveness between two or more interventions and their relative costs. Typically, the cost for the improvement in survival for the more effective intervention is reported as dollars per life-years saved, and is termed *incremental cost-effectiveness* for the intervention of interest compared to the reference intervention. In addition, a measure of quality of life or utility can be incorporated into economic analyses. When quality of life is incorporated the results are reported as quality adjusted life year saved (QALYS). Cost-effectiveness analyses may use data for costs and outcomes obtained from the literature. If values for costs or outcomes are estimates then sensitivity analyses can be performed. Sensitivity analyses are conducted to determine how variability in the inputs used for cost or outcome would affect the results of the analysis.

There are published guidelines for criteria that should be used in cost-effectiveness analyses.[1] The purpose of the guidelines is to provide a uniform approach to these types of studies so the results are generalizeable and reproducible. Cost-effectiveness analyses can be performed from the perspective of society, payer, or patient. Analyses from the perspective of society are the most complete analyses, but are difficult to conduct because indirect costs are hard to obtain. Examples of indirect costs include costs associated with time away from work, rent, and electricity. Many cost-effectiveness analyses are from the perspective of the payer and include direct costs only. Professional fees are usually not included in cost-effectiveness analyses because of the wide variability in fees across geographic regions.

## Total Cost of Deceased Donor Liver Transplantation

Economic analyses of liver transplantation may report actual dollar (or other types of currency) amounts for interventions or they may elect to report results in arbitrary cost units. Arbitrary units may be used because costs and charges are considered proprietary information by many institutions. Results from studies using arbitrary units are useful for making comparisons between two or more interventions in a single study, but these types of studies do not provide a true understanding of the absolute costs involved or allow comparisons to other time periods or institutions.

The cost of liver transplantation is typically determined from the time of transplant to the time of discharge or through the first post-transplant year (Table 31-2). LDLT candidates may have less advanced liver disease at the time of transplantation and therefore have a more rapid posttransplant recovery. In addition, determining costs starting at the time of transplant may not capture potential benefits from living donor liver transplantation. Liver transplant candidates who undergo LDLT may be less likely to be hospitalized prior to transplantation from complications of portal hypertension compared to candidates awaiting deceased donor liver transplantation. These potential cost benefits should be balanced against the potential for greater complications after LDLT compared to DDLT and the costs associated with evaluating potential living donors.

Costs associated with liver transplantation include the cost of organ procurement; cost of the procedure itself, including professional fees, hospital fees, procedural fees, postoperative care, pharmacy costs; and the cost of treating complications (Figure 31-1). Studies on "cost" of liver transplantation have typically reported charges; these results have ranged from $150,000 to $300,000.[2-7] Average billed charges for liver transplantation and the first year after liver transplantation are shown in Table 31-2. Hospital charges are the largest component of total charges accounting for 60% of total charges. Professional fees account for 13.5% of total charges of transplantation. If pretransplant care is included average physicians charges caring for liver

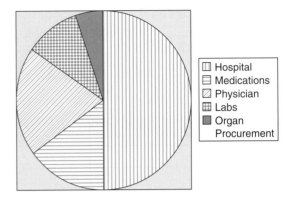

**FIGURE 31-1**

Cost centers as a proportion of total cost of liver transplantation.

transplant candidates may be $72,269. The nonphysician costs of pretransplant care is even greater and associated hospital charges may be more than $3 million for patients with end-stage liver disease.[8] Thus the economic benefit of shortening waiting time is likely quite significant.

## FACTORS ASSOCIATED WITH COST OF DDLT

Severity of illness at the time of transplantation has a substantial effect on the cost of transplantation.[9-11] Costs will be higher at centers that transplant patients with more advanced liver disease. Similarly, patients with more advanced liver disease may be hospitalized more frequently compared to patients with less advanced disease. Greater resources may be needed to treat patients with decompensated cirrhosis.[12] The increase in resource utilization is associated with an exponential increase in pretransplant cost. Furthermore, transplant candidates who are sicker at the time of transplant have a longer recovery time increasing both direct and indirect costs posttransplant.

### Pretransplant Factors

Studies have demonstrated increased posttransplant costs are associated with pretransplant factors that also increase pretransplant resource utilization, such as etiology of liver disease, renal function, severity of illness, and mechanical ventilation.[3,6,14] (Table 31-3). Patients with alcoholic liver disease incurred higher resource use compared to patients with other etiologies of liver disease.[3] The previous UNOS status 2A, decompensated ICU-bound, patients

**TABLE 31-2**

### CHARGES ASSOCIATED WITH LIVER TRANSPLANTATION TO FIRST YEAR AFTER TRANSPLANT[a]

|  | Average Charge ($) |
|---|---|
| Evaluation | 11,000 |
| Candidacy (per month) | 10,600 |
| Procurement | 24,700 |
| Hospital (to discharge) | 188,900 |
| Physician fees | 42,600 |
| Follow-up | 26,400 |
| Immunosuppressants | 10,300 |
| Total | 314,500 |

[a]From Milliman and Robertson, Inc., R. Hauboldt, 1996. Accessed at: http://www.gao.gov/special.pubs/organ/chapter7.pdf#search='gao%20and%20costs%20and%20organ%20transplant'.

**TABLE 31-3**

### FACTORS ASSOCIATED WITH INCREASED COST OF LIVER TRANSPLANTATION

Dialysis
Cytomegalovirus infection
Mechanical ventilation
Recipient age
Alcoholic cirrhosis
Preservation time
Advanced liver disease
Retransplantation
Biliary complications

Compiled from references 3, 6, 7, 9, 10, 11, 13, 14, 15, 16, 18 incurred more than $50,000 compared to less ill patients.[6] The cost of liver transplantation for patients with fulminant hepatic failure is 58% higher compared to patients with chronic liver disease.[6] Recipients 60 years of age and older have higher costs compared to younger recipients.[3] Renal insufficiency with or without dialysis is the factor most consistently associated with increased costs.[6,9,11,14] Thus these factors have a profound impact on total cost, and transplantation prior to the development of these complications can reduce both pre- and posttransplant costs.

## Peritransplant Factors

Transplant factors that affect cost are length of hospital stay, donor age, blood transfusion, and preservation time.[3,6,16] Donor age greater than 60 years old is associated with increased resource utilization and length of stay.[3] Increased costs have been associated with greater use of intraoperative blood transfusions and increased preservation time.[6,16] A 1-hour increase in preservation time was associated with a 1.4% increase in standardized resource utilization.[16] Donor serum sodium and AST have not consistently been shown to be associated with increased costs.[11]

## Posttransplant Factors

Posttransplant factors associated with increased costs include length of stay, infection, requiring mechanical ventilation, and surgical complications.[6,7,10,11,17] Dialysis posttransplant is associated with excess cost of approximately $100,000.[6] Biliary complications and CMV infection are also associated with increased posttransplantation costs.[6,15] CMV infection can increase hospital charges by 49%, independent of other factors, compared to recipients who do not develop CMV infection.[15] Surgical complications requiring a return to the operating room can increase cost significantly and are unpredictable; in one study the impact was to increase mean charges from $146,000 to $442,000 and median length of stay in the ICU from 11 to 46 days.[18] Retransplantation may cost $300,000 more compared to first deceased donor liver transplant.[3,18]

## Cost-Effectiveness of Deceased Donor Liver Transplantation

Cost-effectiveness analysis typically compares an intervention that is more effective, but more expensive to a less effective and less costly intervention. One purpose of the analysis is to determine if the increase in cost is worth the increase in effectiveness, usually from a payer perspective. In the case of deceased donor liver transplantation there has not been an effective alternative intervention until living donor liver transplantation. There have been no randomized controlled trials comparing the efficacy of liver transplantation to supportive care in patients with end-stage liver disease. Therefore, cost-effectiveness analysis would need to compare liver transplantation to the natural history of a patient with end-stage liver disease. Because there are natural history data on survival in patients with end-stage liver disease, such as those with alcoholic liver disease or primary biliary cirrhosis, cost-effectiveness can be performed using data from these studies.

Liver transplantation for chronic liver failure has been shown to be cost-effective.[20,21] The incremental cost for liver transplantation for patients with end stage liver disease from alcohol, primary sclerosing cholangitis, or primary biliary cirrhosis

ranges from 12,000 to 25,000 British pounds per quality adjusted life-year saved.[21] Costs are increased in patients with alcohol-related liver disease because some patients may undergo evaluation and may not be candidates compared to patients with cholestatic liver disease. Costs for the care of patients with primary sclerosing cholangitis may be lower after liver transplantation because of decreased rates of hospitalization and lower resource utilization compared to rates before transplantation. The estimates for the cost-effectiveness of deceased donor liver transplantation fall within the range of other accepted medical procedures, such as screening mammography, considered affordable by society. However, given that survival after transplantation is so dramatically improved compared to survival without transplantation in patients with end-stage liver disease, the cost-effectiveness of liver transplantation compared to supportive care is not very clinically meaningful. However, these early studies did reveal the significant costs of managing ESLD without transplantation; decreasing these costs is the potential cost saving of LDLT.

## Costs of Medical Therapy Posttransplant

### Immunosuppression

Medical treatment after liver transplantation is expensive. The cost for immunosuppression alone can be more than $10,000 per year. Average retail prices for commonly used immunosuppressants are shown in Table 31-4. Tacrolimus may be more cost-effective than cyclosporine because it is associated with lower rates of severe rejection.[22] Hospitalization for rejection and antibody preparations for induction or the treatment of steroid-refractory rejection are the costs most amenable to modification at the current time, thus decreasing rejection rates is likely cost saving. However, the cost-effectiveness of immunosuppressive drugs has not been compared prospectively; thus the optimal method of immunosuppression remains conjectural.

### Hepatitis B

The recurrence rate of hepatitis B with subsequent graft loss is high without prophylaxis against reinfection of the graft with hepatitis B. Therefore, long-term prophylaxis against hepatitis B is required indefinitely after transplantation. Prophylactic regimens include hepatitis B immune globulin (HBIg) with or without an oral antiviral agent.[23] Lamivudine is currently the most commonly added to the prophylactic regimen at a daily dose of 100 mg/day.

Hepatitis-B-immune globulin can be administered intravenously or intramuscularly. The cost of intramuscular HBIg exceed

**TABLE 31-4**

## CHARGES FOR COMMONLY USED POSTTRANSPLANTATION DRUGS[a]

|  | Cost ($) |
| --- | --- |
| Cyclosporine 100 mg bid | $400 for 30 day supply |
| Tacrolimus 5 mg bid | $690 for 30 day supply |
| Ganciclovir | $9,500 for 21 days |
| Valacyclovir | $900–$1 500/ month |
| Hepatitis B Immune globulin (IV) | $10,000 per infusion |

[a]Charges obtained from retail pharmacies or www.drugstore.com, in 2005 dollars. Charge for HBIG was obtained from reference 26.

$750 per injection and the cost of intravenous HBIg are up to $10,000 per infusion.[24] However, if a recipient develops, graft failure from hepatitis B costs of retransplantation can exceed $400,000.[18] Treatment with HBIg is cost-effective.[23–25] Intramuscular administration of HBIg when administered with lamivudine is effective in preventing recurrent disease.[26] Adequate titers of anti-HBS can be achieved with intramuscular administration. The combination of intramuscular HBIg and lamivudine results in 60% lower costs compared to intravenous HBIg.[23,24] Another approach that results in costs savings without comprising efficacy is on-demand administration of intravenous HBIg only when titers drop below a specified level (usually 100–500 IU/mL) instead of fixed monthly dosing. A 50% reduction of costs of prophylactic therapy can be achieved with on-demand dosing.[25]

The concurrent administration of oral agents that inhibit hepatitis B replication could potentially reduce the frequency of HBIg administration and result in lower costs. Treatment with lamivudine monotherapy after the first year posttransplantation may lead to substantial cost savings, but concerns about emergence of recurrence with lamivudine resistant HBV has led to slow adoption. With the development of better oral agents that are associated with lower rates of resistance compared to lamivudine there may be associated reductions in cost of prophylactic therapy. Adefovir dipivoxil and entecavir are approved by the FDA for the treatment of chronic hepatitis B in nontransplant patients. The role of these agents in posttransplantation prophylaxis has not been determined. Adefovir has been shown to be effective for recurrence with lamivudine resistant Hepatitis B posttransplant and is the treatment of choice in that scenario.[27] Entecavir has not yet been studied in posttransplant patients.

Combination therapy with oral agents may be associated with lower rates of resistance. If combination therapy results in sustained inhibition of hepatitis B viral replication then target anti-HBS levels could be lowered or HBIg could potentially be discontinued, which would result in cost savings that would outweigh the costs on the antivirals.

### Prophylaxis Against Cytomegalovirus (CMV) Infection

CMV infection occurs in 5% of liver transplant recipients during the first year after transplantation. The highest rate of CMV infection is during the first 3 months after liver transplant, and drug therapy for prevention against CMV is typically restricted to this time period. Prophylactic regimens against CMV infection have evolved from prolonged intravenous ganciclovir to short-course intravenous ganciclovir followed by acyclovir, oral ganciclovir, or oral valganciclovir. The approach to CMV prophylaxis varies among centers. Some centers tailor therapy based on donor and recipient CMV status. Other centers use a universal, standardized approach for all recipients.

The efficacy of oral valacyclovir is similar to intravenous ganciclovir for prophylaxis against CMV infection in renal transplant recipients, including high-risk groups.[28] Studies with oral valganciclovir in renal transplant recipients demonstrate similar efficacy compared to IV ganciclovir, but these studies are smaller than the studies with valacyclovir.[29,30] The efficacy of valacyclovir for CMV prophylaxis has not been studied in a randomized trial in liver and other solid organ transplant recipients. Oral valganciclovir showed similar rates of CMV disease to oral ganciclovir in high-risk liver transplant recipients.[52] The costs for intravenous ganciclovir are higher than for valganciclovir. The cost for CMV prophylaxis with ganciclovir is approximately $500 per day assuming treatment with 5 mg/kg/day for a 70 kg recipient. Treatment

with valganciclovir is $25 to $50 per day for a 450 mg to 900 mg daily dose. Therefore oral valganciclovir is a much more attractive alternative from a cost perspective.

CMV prophylaxis in liver transplant recipients is cost-effective.[31] Median hospital charges for a recipient who develops CMV disease are $148,300 compared to median charges of $114,000 for recipients who do not develop CMV.[15] Prophylaxis with ganciclovir is associated with a $40,000 reduction in charges compared to prophylaxis with acyclovir. Restricting prophylaxis to high-risk groups or extending prophylaxis beyond 3 months is not cost-effective.[31] Valacyclovir may be more cost-effective compared to intravenous ganciclovir under certain circumstances in renal transplant recipients.[32] The comparison has not been made to oral valganciclovir or in liver transplant recipients.

## COSTS OF LIVING DONOR LIVER TRANSPLANTATION

Before the advent of adult-to-adult living donor liver transplantation there was no therapeutic alternative to compare to deceased donor liver transplantation. Because there is the potential to perform living donor liver transplantation (LDLT) electively in candidates who are less ill at the time of transplant, it can potentially reduce the cost of transplantation as well as the cost of managing complications of end-stage liver disease. However, the costs of LDLT are not well studied. Furthermore, any cost-savings seen with LDLT will need to be balanced against the health care costs of the donor, including direct costs of medical care, indirect costs of work lost, and potential future liabilities, such as inability to obtain insurance.

### Cost-Effectiveness of LDLT

Because a randomized trial of LDLT compared to deceased donor transplantation cannot be done, economic analyses using modeling of costs and outcomes must be used. A weakness of economic modeling is that they by their nature must incorporate assumptions, and if these estimates are inaccurate, then the results from the analysis may not reflect actual practice.

Typically, studies on cost of liver transplantation incorporate costs starting from the time of transplantation. However, because transplantation is a treatment for end-stage liver disease, the costs associated while patients are waiting for liver transplantation should be captured. In the era of LDLT this is particularly true, because a major benefit of LDLT is shortened waiting time and potentially reduced pretransplant complications and costs. End-stage liver disease is resource intensive because of morbidity associated with complications from portal hypertension. The total direct health-care costs for the management of hepatitis C alone is estimated to have exceeded $1 billion.[33] Hospitalizations from complications associated with portal hypertension are associated with substantial costs. Patients may be hospitalized for variceal bleeding, ascites, spontaneous bacterial peritonitis, or encephalopathy. The cost of transjugular intrahepatic portosystemic shunting (TIPS) for treatment of complications of portal hypertension may be in the order of $15,000.[34]

As patients become more debilitated with progressive liver failure, complications from portal hypertension may increase in frequency leading to increased hospitalizations. Pretransplant costs while waiting for transplantation may account for 41% of total costs from listing through discharge from the transplant admission.[35] Additionally, patients with cirrhosis awaiting liver transplantation may incur substantial personal financial losses with high indirect costs. Patients with end-stage liver disease may not be able to work because of their disease. This typically leads to reduced income and financial pressures. Because many transplant recipients are of working age the economic impact is substantial, but this has not been well quantified.

Cost-effectiveness analyses have not demonstrated a cost benefit of LDLT compared to DDLT[36-38](Table 31-4). A model comparing deceased donor liver transplant, deceased donor transplant with living donor transplant offered, or conservative therapy demonstrated that the cost-effectiveness of deceased donor and living donor liver transplantation were similar when compared to conservative therapy, that is, the natural history of end-stage liver disease.[36] A second analysis, which incorporated donor costs including donors evaluated and rejected, compared 24 recipients of living donor transplant to 43 deceased donor recipients.[37] The costs were lower in deceased donor recipients, but the difference was not statistically significant. Much of the cost in the living donor group is a result of the evaluation of donors, some who were rejected. In addition, even though patients who undergo LDLT are transplanted with less severe liver disease, which should lower costs, postoperative complications may occur more frequently after LDLT. LDLT recipients have higher rates of biliary complications compared to DDLT recipients, which increases resource utilization.[39] In pediatric living donor liver transplantation LDLT is more expensive compared to DDLT partly due to higher rates of biliary complications.[41]

Any benefits seen with LDLT in reducing pre-transplant resource utilization by avoiding complications from portal hypertension may be offset by increased posttransplant complications compared to DDLT. Although it seems that LDLT should be more cost-effective than DDLT because it is performed in patients with less advanced liver disease and associated with fewer complications from portal hypertension due to shorter waiting times, results from studies that use actual cost data have not yet demonstrated that LDLT is more cost-effective compared to DDLT (Table 31-5). As experience with LDLT increases, donor selection and technical advances should improve, which would lower complications rates and reduce costs of LDLT.

Comparison of LDLT to DDLT should incorporate costs associated with retransplantation. Initially, graft failure and retransplantation rates were higher with LDLT. In recent years graft survival and retransplantation rates for LDLT approach those seen with DDLT. Cost of retransplantation can be double costs associated with the first transplant, especially if the retransplant occurs early on. Much of the increase in cost is due to increase in length of stay and intensive unit care.

## LDLT for Hepatocellular Carcinoma

Liver transplantation can cure patients with hepatocellular carcinoma who meet certain restricted size criteria. Increased tumor size and number of lesions are associated with higher rates of tumor recurrence after liver transplantation. Therefore, once a diagnosis of early hepatocellular carcinoma is confirmed, patients would likely benefit from earlier transplantation prior to tumor progression. However, with the shortage of deceased donor organs, even with increased priority given to patients with hepatocellular carcinoma under the MELD system in the United States, prompt transplantation is usually not feasible.

Patients with hepatocellular carcinoma may derive an additional benefit from LDLT compared to patients with other

**TABLE 31-5**

**COST STUDIES OF LIVING DONOR AND DECEASED DONOR LIVER TRANSPLANTATION**

| Reference | Design | Findings |
|---|---|---|
| Sagameister et al.[36] | Markov Model | Offering DDLT plus LDLT is cost-effective 23,530 Euros per quality adjusted life year saved |
| Sarasin et al.[43] | Markov Model, LDLT for HCC | LDLT cost-effective for HCC if waiting time exceeds 3.5 months |
| Trotter et al.[37] | Retrospective | LDLT 21% higher costs compared to DDLT. Costs of evaluating living donor 1% higher than organ acquisition costs for DD |
| Cole et al.[41] | Retrospective, pediatric | Mean costs for first year in pediatric LDLT 60% higher than DDLT |
| Oostenbrink, Kok, Verheul | Retrospective | Total costs for: Cadaveric kidney transplant: 70,723 Euros Living donor kidney transplant: 76,577 Euros Deceased donor liver transplant: 141,510 Euros Heart transplant: 171,828 Euros |
| Ouwens et al.[51] | Retrospective | Cost per life year saved for: Lung transplant = $77,000 Liver transplant = $26,000 Heart transplant = $38,000 |

etiologies of liver disease. In addition to having end-stage liver disease, patients with HCC have a tumor that may grow beyond the criteria accepted for transplantation. There is always the concern of developing a tumor associated portal vein thrombosis or extrahepatic metastatic disease that would preclude transplant. Thus, LDLT could potentially offer a survival and cost benefit. LDLT also allows the planning of pretransplant locoregional ablative therapy (eg, chemoembolization, radiofrequency ablation) with a scheduled transplant and without the concern about potential decompensation without a subsequent deceased donor graft being available in a timely manner.

Liver transplantation is cost-effective for cirrhotic patients with hepatocellular carcinoma.[42] Modeling supports a survival benefit with LDLT compared to DDLT in patients with hepatocellular carcinoma if waiting time exceeds 3.5 months.[43] Because waiting time exceeds 6 months in many areas, LDLT may be the best option for patients with HCC if a suitable donor has volunteered. In this model, the cost per quality adjusted life-year for LDLT is less than $50,000 per quality adjusted life year saved under a wide range of assumptions.[42]

## Donor Costs

Donor safety of LDLT is of paramount importance and has been a major focus of interest. Though donor morbidity and mortality associated with right hepatectomy are important issues, costs are a reality and need to be discussed with the donor and incorporated in formal economic analyses. The evaluation of the donor varies among centers, including variable use of invasive diagnostic testing such as angiography and liver biopsy.[44] These costs are usually covered by the recipient's insurance so the short-term financial burden on the donor should not be substantial. The surgical procedure and postoperative care are also typically covered by the recipient's insurance.

Medical costs that the living donor patient may be responsible for, depending on the timing and the philosophy of the program, are those incurred after hospital discharge, including potential late complications of the procedure, such as incisional hernia. These costs incurred later may be substantial and potential living donors need to be made aware of these costs. A financial counselor may review with the potential donor costs that the recipient's health insurance will cover. In one study, mean out-of-pocket expenses for the donor were $3,660.[45] Early complications occur in 31% of donors and donors should be aware that they may be responsible for costs that are not covered by the recipient's insurance, even if it is related to a complication.[39] Additionally travel, lodging, parking, and incidental costs are usually not reimbursed, and, though unusual, can even be viewed as financial remuneration and thus illegal by some programs.

Right hepatectomy donors can anticipate not returning to work for at least 2 to 3 months, which can result in significant income loss depending on the leave policy of their employer. Despite increased use of Family Medical Leave Act or federal government or some state governments, Organ Donor Leave Acts, many donors may have inadequate benefits for the convalescence period. All donors should assess whether their household can support this period of time off and if their employer will allow it. Finally, the impact on future insurance premiums for liver donors is unknown. Higher rates for life and health insurance have not been reported for kidney donors, though these concerns persist.[46] One study reported that some life insurance companies would not offer the lowest "preferred" rate to an otherwise healthy person who had undergone an uncomplicated right liver lobe donation procedure in the past.[47] The overall burden of these costs must be incorporated into economic analyses and will partially offset any potential cost savings of LDLT.

## LDLT Compared to Living Donor Kidney and Other Solid Organ Transplantation

LDLT in adults had been performed for a relatively short period of time; however, living donor kidney transplantation has been performed for over 50 years. Although there are obvious differences between the two procedures, there are also similarities, such as the potential to reduce pre-transplant morbidity and costs. Over $11 billion is spent on end stage renal disease each year and these costs may be reduced after kidney transplantation.[48] The average charge of kidney transplantation of $84 000 is less than that for liver transplantation, but some of the same principals of cost that apply to kidney transplantation also apply to liver transplantation.[48,49] Patients with end-stage kidney disease who undergo living donor kidney transplantation do not absorb the costs of continuing on dialysis as do their counterparts awaiting cadaveric kidney transplantation. An analogous argument can be made for liver transplant recipients from living donors who may experience fewer complications of portal hypertension, and thus less economic burden, compared to deceased-donor recipients. Indeed, an analysis of 42,868 cadaveric kidney transplant recipients and 13,754 living donor kidney transplants demonstrated significantly lower costs in the living donor group.[49] The largest

source of difference in payments was from inpatient hospitalizations. Thus, cost analyses comparing deceased and living donor organ transplantation should incorporate pretransplant morbidity and its associated costs.

Liver transplantation may be more expensive than heart transplantation, but because posttransplant survival is longer it may be more cost-effective. Studies conducted in the Netherlands demonstrate that the costs associated with liver transplantation are more than those associated with heart and kidney transplantation.[51,59] However, liver transplantation was the most cost-effective as the cost per life year gained for lung, heart, and liver transplantation were $77,000, $38,000 and $26,000, respectively. These results may not be generalizeable to the United States because of differences in health-care systems.

## SUMMARY AND CONCLUSIONS

Liver transplantation is effective in improving survival in patients with end-stage liver disease, and is also cost-effective compared to conservative medical management. The costs of living donor liver transplantation are similar to deceased donor liver transplantation. LDLT has the potential to reduce pretransplant morbidity and associated costs, although this has not yet been demonstrated in cost-effectiveness studies. Candidates with hepatocellular carcinoma may have the most to gain in terms increased life expectancy and cost-effectiveness compared to DDLT. Long-term data on costs incurred by the living donor will need to be captured in economic analyses to adequately assess the cost-effectiveness of LDLT. With progressively longer waiting times for DDLT and increased experience and lower complication rates with LDLT, LDLT may prove to be more cost-effective than DDLT.

## References

1. Weinstein MC, Siegel JE, Gold MR, Kamlet MS, Russell LB. Recommendations of the panel on cost-effectiveness in health and medicine. *JAMA* 1996;276:1253–1258.
2. Gilbert JR, Pascual M, Schoenfeld DA, et al. Evolving trends in liver transplantation: an outcome and charge analysis. *Transplantation* 1999;67:246–53.
3. Showstack J, Katz P, Lake JR, et al. Resource utilization in liver transplantation. Effects of patient characteristics and clinical practice. *JAMA* 1999;281:1381–1386.
4. van Agthoven M, Metselaar HJ, Tilanus HW, et al. A comparison of the costs and effects of liver transplantation. *Transpl Int* 2001;14:87–94.
5. Best JH, Veenstra DL, Geppert J. Trends in expenditures for Medicare liver transplant recipients. *Liver Transpl* 2001;7:858–862.
6. Whitting JF, Martin J, Zavala E, Hanto D. The influence of clinical variables on hospital costs after orthotopic liver transplantation. *Surgery* 1999;125:217–222.
7. Taylor MC, Greig PD, Detsky AS, et al. Factors associated with the high cost of liver transplantation adults. *Canad J Surg* 2002;45:425–434.
8. Cohen SM, Gundlapalli S, Shah AR, et al. The downstream financial effect of hepatotogy. *Hepatology* 2005;41:968–975.
9. Markmann JF, Markmann JW, Markmann DA, et al. Preoperative factors associated with outcome and their impact on resource use in 1148 consecutive primary liver transplants. *Transplantation* 2001;72:1113–1122.
10. Rufat P, Fourquet F, Conti F, e al. Costs and outcomes of liver transplantation in adults: a prospective, 1-year, follow-up study. *Transplantation* 1999;68:76–83.
11. Filipponi F, Pisati R, Cavicchini G, et al. Cost and outcome analysis and cost determinants of liver transplantation in a European National Health Service Hospital. *Transplantation* 2003;75:1731–1736.

12. Brown Jr. RS, Kumar KS, Russo MW, et al. Model for end stage liver disease and Child-Turcotte-Pugh score as predictors of pretransplant disease severity, post-transplant outcome and resource utilization in UNOS status 2A patients. *Liver Transpl* 2002;8:278–284.

13. Brown RS Jr, Lake JR, Ascher NL, Emond JC, Roberts JP. Predictors of the cost of liver transplantation. *Liver Transpl Surg* 1998;4:170–176.

14. Brown RS Jr, Lombardero M, Lake JR. Outcome of patients with renal insufficiency undergoing liver or liver-kidney transplantation. *Transplantation* 1996;62:1788–1993.

15. Kim WR, Badle AD, Wiesner RH, et al. The economic impact of cytomegalovirus infection after liver transplantation. *Transplantation* 2000;69:357–361.

16. Schnitzler MA, Woodward RS, Brennan DC, et al. The economic impact of preservation time in cadaveric liver transplantation. *Am J Transpl* 2001;1:360–365.

17. Brown RS Jr, Ascher NL, Lake JR, et al. The impact of surgical complications after liver transplantation on resource utilization. *Arch Surg* 1997;132:1098–1103.

18. Reed A, Howard RJ, Fujita S, et al. Liver retransplantation: a single-center outcome and financial analysis. *Transpl Proc* 2005;37;1161–1163.

19. Azoulay D, Linhares MM, Huguet E, et al. Decision for retransplantation of the liver: an experience-and cost-based analysis. *Ann Surg* 2002;236:713–721.

20. Bambha K, Kim WR. Liver transplantation is effective, but is it cost-effective? *Liver Transpl* 2003;9:1308–1311.

21. Longworth L, Young T, Buxton MJ, et al. Midterm cost-effectiveness of the liver transplantation program of England and Wales for three disease groups. *Liver Transpl* 2003;9:1295–1307.

22. Lake JR, Gorman KJ, Esquivel CO, et al. The impact of immunosuppressive regimens on the cost of liver transplantation-results from the U.S. FK506 multicenter trial. *Transplantation* 1995;60:1089–1095.

23. Buti M, Mas A, Preito, M, et al. A randomized study comparing lamivudine monotherapy after a short course of hepatitis B immune globulin (HBIg) and lamivudine with long-term lamivudine plus HBIg in the prevention of hepatitis B virus recurrence after liver transplantation. *J Hepatol* 2003;38:711–717.

24. Faust D, Rabenau HF, Allwinn R, Caspary WF, Zeuzem S. Cost-effective and safe ambulatory long-term immunoprophylaxis with intramuscular instead of intravenous hepatitis B immunoglobulin to prevent reinfection after orthotopic liver transplantation. *Clin Transplant* 2003;17:254–258.

25. Di Paolo D, Tisone G, Piccolo P, et al. Low-dose hepatitis B immunoglobulin given 'on-demand' in combination with lamivudine: a highly cost-effective approach to prevent recurrent hepatitis B virus infection in the long-term follow-up after liver transplantation. *Transplantation* 2004;77:1203–1208.

26. Han SH, Martin P, Edelstein M. Conversion form intravenous to intramuscular hepatitis B immune globulin in combination with lamivudine is safe and cost-effective in patients receiving long-term prophylaxis to prevent hepatitis B recurrence after liver transplantation. *Liver Transpl* 2003;9:182–187.

27. Schiff ER, Lai CL, Hadziyannis S, et al. Adefovir dipivoxil therapy for lamivudine-resistant hepatitis B in pre- and post-liver transplantation patients. *Hepatology* 2003;38;1419–1427.

28. Lowance D, Neumayer HH, Legendre CM, et al. Valacyclovir for the prevention of cytomegalovirus disease after renal transplantation. International Valacyclovir Cytomegalovirus Prophylaxis Transplantation Study Group. *N Engl J Med* 1999;341:921.

29. Akalin E, Sehgal V, Ames S, Hossain S, et al. Cytomegalovirus disease in high-risk transplant recipients despite ganciclovir or valganciclovir prophylaxis. *Am J Transplant* 2003;3:731–735.

30. Babel N, Gabdrakhmanova L, Juergensen JS, et al. Treatment of cytomegalovirus disease with valganciclovir in renal transplant recipients: a single center experience. *Transplantation* 2004;78:283–285.

31. Das A. Cost-effectiveness of different strategies of cytomegalovirus prophylaxis in orthotopic liver transplant recipients. *Hepatology* 2000;31: 311–317.

32. Mauskopf JA, Richter A, Annemans L, Maclaine G. Cost-effectiveness model of cytomegalovirus management strategies in renal transplantation. Comparing valacyclovir prophylaxis with current practice. *Pharmacoeconomics* 2000;18:239–251.

33. Kim WR. The burden of hepatitis C in the United States. *Hepatology* 2002;36:(5 Suppl) 1:S30–S34.

34. Russo MW, Zacks SL, Sandler, RS, Brown Jr RS. Cost-effectiveness analysis of transjugular intrahepatic portosystemic shunt versus endoscopic therapy for the prevention of esophageal variceal bleeding. *Hepatology* 2000;31:358–363.

35. Brand DA, Viola D, Rampersaud P, et al. Waiting for a liver-Hidden costs of the organ shortage. *Liver Transpl* 2004;10;1001–1010.

36. Sagmeister M, Mullhaupt B, Kadry Z, et al. Cost-effectiveness of cadaveric and living-donor liver transplantation. *Transplantation* 2002;73: 616–622.

37. Trotter JF, Mackenzie S, Wachs M, et al. Comprehensive cost comparison of adult-adult right hepatic lobe living-donor liver transplantation with cadaveric transplantation. *Transplantation* 2003;75:473–476.

38. Sagmeister M, Mullhaupt B. Is living donor liver transplantation cost-effective? *J Hepatol* 2005;43:27–32.

39. Russo MW, Brown Jr. RS. Adult Living Donor Liver Transplantation. *Am J Transpl* 2004;4:458–465.

40. Russo MW, Brown Jr, RS. Financial Impact of Adult Living Donation. *Liver Transpl* 2003;9 (Suppl 2):S12–S15, 2003.

41. Cole CR, Bucuvalas JC, Hornung R, et al. Outcome after pediatric liver transplantation impact of living donor transplantation on cost. *J Pediatr* 2004;144:729–735.

42. Llovet JM, Fuster J, Bruix J. Intention-to-treat analysis of surgical treatment for early hepatocellular carcinoma: resection versus transplantation. *Hepatology* 2001;33:1073–1079.

43. Sarasin FP, Majno PE, Llovet JM, et al. Living donor liver transplantation for early hepatocellular carcinoma: A life-expectancy and cost-effectiveness perspective. *Hepatology* 2001;33;1073–1079.

44. Brown RS Jr., Russo MW, Lai M, Shiffman ML, Richardson MC, Everhart JE, Hoofnagle JH. A survey of liver transplantation from living adult donors in the United States. *N Engl J Med* 2003;348:818–825.

45. Trotter JF, Talamantes M, McClure M, et al. Right hepatic lobe donation for living donor liver transplantation: impact on donor quality of life. *Liver Transpl* 2001;7:485–493.

46. Spital A, Jacobs C. Life insurance for kidney donors:another update. *Transplantation* 2002;74:972–973.

47. Nissing MH, Hayahsi PH. Right hepatic lobe donation adversely affects donor life insurability up to one year after donation. *Liver Transpl* 2005;11:843–847.

48. Evans RW, Kitzmann DJ. An economic analysis of kidney transplantation. *Surgical Clinics of North America* 1998;78:149-174Spital A, Jacobs C. Life insurance for kidney donors: another update. *Transplantation* 2002;74:972–973.

49. Smith CR, Woodward RS, Cohen DS, et al. Cadaveric versus living donor kidney transplantation: A Medicare payment analysis. *Transplantation* 2000;69:311–314.

50. Oostenbrink JB, Kok ET, Verheul RM. A comparative study of resource use and costs of renal, liver, and heart transplantation. *Transpl Int* 2005;18;437–443.

51. Ouwens JP, van Enckevort PJ, TenVergert EM, et al. The cost effectiveness of lung transplantation compared with that of heart and liver transplantation in the Netherlands 2003;16:123–127.

52. Paya C, Humar A, Dominguez E, et al. Efficacy and safety of valganciclovir vs. oral ganciclovir for prevention of cytomegalovirus disease in solid organ transplant recipients. *Am J Transplant* 2004;4:611–620.

# CHAPTER 32

# HISTORY OF LIVING DONOR INTESTINAL TRANSPLANTATION

*Rainer W.G. Gruessner, MD*

Intestinal transplantation is a treatment option for patients with short bowel syndrome or short bowel dysfunction and life-threatening complications of total parenteral nutrition (TPN). *Short bowel syndrome* is defined as the presence of < 80% of an individual's expected bowel length. *Short bowel dysfunction* is defined as a condition that does not afford normal growth and development of enteral feedings despite the presence of normal bowel length. Despite their different etiologies, both conditions result in inadequate absorption of solids derived from the product of digested food, causing diarrhea, steatorrhea, malnutrition, and fluid and electrolyte losses. As a consequence, patients with irreversible intestinal failure require special nutritional consideration by depending on TPN. The incidence of shortbowel syndrome in Western countries is estimated at 2 to 3 individuals per million.[1]

In adults, short bowel syndrome may develop after extensive resection of the intestine for vascular compromise of the mesenteric vessels (eg, embolic or thrombotic occlusion of the superior mesenteric artery or vein, herniation of the intestine), primary intestinal compromise (eg, Crohn's disease, desmoid tumor, familial polyposis), and trauma. In children, the most common causes of short bowel syndrome are congenital malformations (eg, intestinal atresia, gastroschisis, malrotation, midgut volvulus), infections (eg, necrotizing enterocolitis, inflammatory bowel diseases), and trauma. Short bowel dysfunction—associated with normal bowel length, but impaired bowel motility and absorption—is more common in children than adults: neuroendocrine abnormalities (eg. Hirschsprung's disease, intestinal pseudo-obstruction) are the leading causes in children; radiation enteritis and refractory sprue, in adults.[2]

Several surgical nontransplant procedures have been devised for patients with short bowel syndrome, including interposition of antiperistaltic segments, valve replacement procedures, and bowel lengthening procedures.[3–8] But, by and large, the results of these surgical procedures have been disappointing.

Experimental models of intestinal transplantation were developed in the late 1950s and early 1960s before the introduction of TPN.[9–11] At that time, patients with short bowel syndrome were doomed to die within a short time. However, the early experience with intestinal transplants in the precyclosporine era was dismal.[12] With the introduction of TPN in the late 1960s, survival rates of patients with short bowel syndrome markedly improved. For that reason, interest in intestinal transplantation waned, only to revive in the 1980s after the side effects and limitations of TPN became apparent and cyclosporine was successfully used for other solid organ transplants. But, a real improvement in outcome was not seen until tacrolimus was introduced and patient and graft survival

rates markedly improved in the 1990s.[12] Less than 5% of intestinal transplants have been from living donors, mainly because of concern of the potential consequences of the donor operation and the initial lack of standardized surgical techniques for the donor and recipient procedures.

## PRECYCLOSPORINE ERA

The first documented and independently reported intestinal transplant from a deceased donor (DD) was performed by Richard Lillehei in 1967 at the University of Minnesota.[13] However, this was not the first clinical intestinal transplant: at the 11th Annual Meeting of the Society for Surgery of the Alimentary Tract in Chicago, Illinois, in 1970, on the occasion of what was believed to be the first intestinal transplant from a living donor (LD), Ralph Deterling reported during the ensuing discussion that he had already performed in 1964 such a transplant (Table 32-1). Deterling's case was not only the first intestinal transplant but also the first extrarenal LD solid organ transplant.[14] Deterling reported that, for an infant recipient "a segment of the mother's ileum was used, but the child's condition was so poor that in about 12 hours, the child died of medical conditions. The transplant appeared to be in fine condition and did not show any signs of rejection. The vasculature was open . . . The transplantation of the vessels was into the aorta and vena cava."[14] Although this LD transplant preceded Lillehei's DD intestinal transplant by 3 years, it was never formally reported to the literature. Thus, Richard Lillehei's transplant in 1967 remains the first reported intestinal transplant (although the technical feasibility of the procedure was demonstrated, Lillehei's recipient died 12 hours after the procedure).[13]

The first documented and independently reported case of an intestinal transplant from an LD was reported by Fikri Alican from the University of Mississippi, Jackson, at the above mentioned 11th Annual Meeting of the Society for Surgery of the Alimentary Tract in 1970 (Figure 32-1). The proceedings, including the ensuing discussion with Deterling's comments were published in the *American Journal of Surgery* in 1971.[14] Alican et al reported the case of an 8-year-old boy whose "entire small bowel from the ligament of Treitz to the ileocecal valve was gangrenous, secondary to strangulation, . . . and was resected."[15] Because of recurrent line infections and sepsis and the then "extremely poor" results of the very few clinical intestinal transplants from DDs, the idea of an LD transplant was pondered. "If a living adult donor with high histocompatibility would be willing to sacrifice a small portion (about 3 feet) of his small intestine, this length would mean considerable absorptive surface for this small patient."

**TABLE 32-1**

## LD INTESTINAL TRANSPLANTS IN THE PRECYCLOSPORINE AND CYCLOSPORINE ERAS

| Year | Author | Disease | Donor–Recipient Relationship | Type of Graft | Graft Length | Immuno-suppression | Outcome |
|---|---|---|---|---|---|---|---|
| **Precyclosporine Era** | | | | | | | |
| 1964 | Deterling[14] | Mesenteric Thrombosis | Mother-to-Infant | Ileum | NA | NA | Died < 12 hr |
| 1969 | Alican et al.[15] | Mesenteric Band | Mother-to-Child (11 years) | Ileum | 95 cm | ALG, AZA, P | Graft removed after 9 days; died after 32 days |
| 1970 | Fortner et al.[16] | Gardner's Syndrome | Sister-to-Sister HLA-Id (37 years) | Jejunoileum | 170 cm | ALG, AZA, P | Died after 76 days |
| **Cyclosporine Era** | | | | | | | |
| 1987 | Deltz[19] | Volvulus | Mother-to Child (5 years) | Jejunoileum | 60 cm | CSA, P | Graft removed after 12 days |
| 1988 | Deltz[19] | Mesenteric Thrombosis | Sister-to-Sister (41 years)(0-Ag MM) | Jejunoileum | 60 cm | ALG, CSA, P | TPN independence > 2 years |

ALG, antilymphocyte globulin; AZA, azathioprine; CSA, cyclosporine; P, prednisone

The experimental nature of the procedure and the ethical issues were also addressed by Alican and his associates: "the full Committee on Human Investigation met and it was agreed unanimously that a small bowel transplant would be in order in this case... The parents were fully aware of the risks to the child (very definite) and to the mother (negligible) and of the limited promise of long-term success of the transplant."

On September 9, 1969, the transplant was performed. The donor (who did not undergo a preoperative angiogram) at laparotomy had

> ... the continuation of the superior mesenteric artery with its accompanying vein beyond their ileocolic branch ... isolated. These vessels supplied about 3 feet of ileum ... this ileal segment ... was divided at both ends and the mother's ileum was reanastomosed end to end. The excluded ileal segment to be used as the allograft was allowed to remain on its intact vascular pedicle until the child had been prepared in an adjacent operating room. When the recipient was ready, the graft was removed, perfused with cold lactated Ringer's solution and transplanted.

The recipient procedure was complicated by the finding of "thrombosis of the vena cava (extending) almost up to the level at which the renal veins entered the vena cava... we decided to expose the left renal vein where it crossed the aorta and anastomosed the vein of the graft to this, and the artery of the graft to the aorta of the recipient ... We brought both ends of the allograft through the right upper quadrant." Posttransplant, the patient was placed on antilymphocyte globulin, azathioprine, and prednisone.

> Unfortunately, (on the 9th posttransplant day) it was noted that the stomas ... appeared necrotic and ... the patient ... returned to the operating room ... The allograft was still perfused, though it did not appear really healthy ... We re-

luctantly decided to remove the allograft ... Microscopic examination of the excised allograft revealed patchy necrosis of the submucosa and muscularis of the entire segment of the allograft ... The pathologists did not find evidence of an advanced state of allograft rejection.

Alican et al. believed "that limited arterial perfusion may have contributed substantially to the atrophic changes observed," and, in fact, during the transplant procedure, the allograft, although initially pinking up after revascularization became cyanotic for over an hour: "Administration of Rheomacrodex® and heparin in addition to moderate selective hypothermia of the allograft gradually improved its appearance." In retrospect, it appears that technical problems contributed to allograft failure. The recipient died 3 weeks later.[15]

The third attempt at an LD intestinal transplant in the precyclosporine era was reported by Fortner et al from the Transplantation Service at the Sloan-Kettering Institute and published in 1972[16] (Figure 32-1). Fortner et al reported the case of a 37-year-old female with Gardner's syndrome who had

> ... previously had the entire jejunum, ileum, and right to mid-transverse colon resected for recurrent desmoid tumor ... On November 16, 1970, an allograft of 170 cm of lower jejunum and upper ileum was obtained from her (HLA-identical) sister. The graft was vascularized by anastomosing the terminal portion of donor superior mesenteric artery and vein, respectively, to the recipient's internal iliac artery and common iliac vein ... Intestinal continuity was established by taking down the original duodeno-colonic

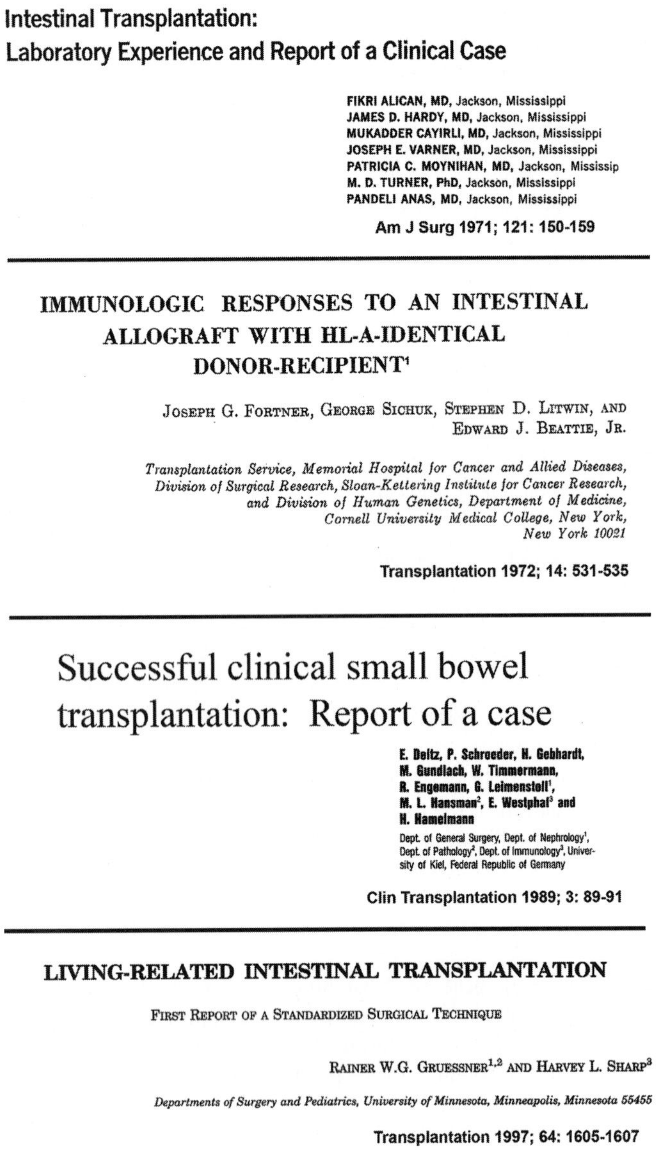

**Intestinal Transplantation:**
**Laboratory Experience and Report of a Clinical Case**

FIKRI ALICAN, MD, Jackson, Mississippi
JAMES D. HARDY, MD, Jackson, Mississippi
MUKADDER CAYIRLI, MD, Jackson, Mississippi
JOSEPH E. VARNER, MD, Jackson, Mississippi
PATRICIA C. MOYNIHAN, MD, Jackson, Mississip
M. D. TURNER, PhD, Jackson, Mississippi
PANDELI ANAS, MD, Jackson, Mississippi

Am J Surg 1971; 121: 150-159

## IMMUNOLOGIC RESPONSES TO AN INTESTINAL ALLOGRAFT WITH HL-A-IDENTICAL DONOR-RECIPIENT[1]

Joseph G. Fortner, George Sichuk, Stephen D. Litwin, and Edward J. Beattie, Jr.

*Transplantation Service, Memorial Hospital for Cancer and Allied Diseases, Division of Surgical Research, Sloan-Kettering Institute for Cancer Research, and Division of Human Genetics, Department of Medicine, Cornell University Medical College, New York, New York 10021*

Transplantation 1972; 14: 531-535

## Successful clinical small bowel transplantation: Report of a case

E. Deltz, P. Schroeder, H. Gebhardt, M. Gundlach, W. Timmermann, R. Engemann, G. Leimenstoll[1], M. L. Hansman[2], E. Westphal[3] and H. Hamelmann

Dept. of General Surgery, Dept. of Nephrology[1], Dept. of Pathology[2], Dept. of Immunology[3], University of Kiel, Federal Republic of Germany

Clin Transplantation 1989; 3: 89-91

## LIVING-RELATED INTESTINAL TRANSPLANTATION

FIRST REPORT OF A STANDARDIZED SURGICAL TECHNIQUE

Rainer W.G. Gruessner[1,2] and Harvey L. Sharp[3]

*Departments of Surgery and Pediatrics, University of Minnesota, Minneapolis, Minnesota 55455*

Transplantation 1997; 64: 1605-1607

**FIGURE 32-1**

Pivotal publications on LD intestinal transplantation: Alican et al (1971): first independently reported LD intestinal transplant. Fortner et al (1972): first technically successful LD intestinal transplant, lost secondary to graft rejection. Deltz et al (1989): first LD intestinal transplant in the cyclosporine era with long-term graft and patient survival. Gruessner et al (1997): first standardized technique for LD intestinal transplants.

anastomosis and inserting the graft between the 2 cut ends in an isoperistaltic fashion ... An auxiliary jejunal pouch was constructed... from the uppermost portion of the graft. The opening of the pouch was sutured to the skin and the innermost portion was closed; this permitted sequential biopsies so that the histological status of the graft could be evaluated.

A rejection episode "developed by the 17th posttransplant day. It was reversed." However, the patient continued to have various infections and liver dysfunction and "died with E. coli sepsis and ... symptoms of consumption coagulopathy 76 days

after transplantation... At necropsy, the graft wall was atrophic but intact; epithelial crypts were present. All vascular anastomoses were normal and there° was no evidence of vascular compromise." The authors concluded that "current methods of immunotherapy seem unlikely to permit long-term survival of any intestinal allograft without the occurrence of some degree of rejection."[16]

For immunosuppressive therapy, equine antilymphocyte globulin, steroids, and azathioprine were used: "Oral intake was started on the 21st posttransplant day and the recipient progressed to a soft diet, although supplemental i.v. hyperalimentation was continued." This graft allowed oral food intake and showed that intestinal transplantation can be successful if the immunologic barrier is overcome.

## CYCLOSPORINE ERA

The introduction of cyclosporine markedly improved outcome for solid organ transplants. The first successful combined small bowel and liver transplant from a DD (using cyclosporine-based immunosuppression) was reported by David Grant in 1990.[17] However, by the late 1980s, it had become apparent that the use of cyclosporine was not as beneficial for intestinal as for most other solid organ transplants. Until June 1995, only a total of 49 intestinal transplants were performed with cyclosporine-based immunosuppression: 1-year graft survival rates were only 17% for solitary intestinal transplants and 41% for intestinal and liver or multivisceral transplants.[18]

In the cyclosporine era, only two intestinal transplants from living donors were reported by Deltz et al.[19] (Figure 32-1). The first recipient was a 4-year-old boy with volvulus who received 60 cm of jejunoileum from his mother in November 1987. However, the graft had to be removed on the 12th postoperative day following an intractable rejection episode.

The second recipient was a 42-year-old woman with a history of "subtotal small bowel resection after thrombotic occlusion of mesenteric veins induced by strangulation." The recipient received a 0-antigen-mismatched graft from her sister on August 9, 1988. In the donor, "the graft of 60 cm length was taken from the lower part of jejunum and upper ileum. A vascular pedicle was prepared by separating one mesenteric artery and vein respectively from the mesenterium. The vessels as well as the lumen of the excised graft were perfused with 4° C Collins solution." In the recipient, "mesenteric vessels of the graft were anastomosed to the common iliac vein and artery of the recipient ... The graft was placed to the left abdominal cavity and both its ends were exteriorized as stomas." Posttransplant immunosuppressive therapy consisted of cyclosporine, steroids, and antithymocyte globulin. On posttransplant day 6, the patient was treated for rejection with steroid boluses. About 6 weeks posttransplant, "in the second operative step, the oral end of the graft was anastomosed to the distal portion of the duodenum and the aboral end was connected in an end-to-end fashion to the sigmoid stump." Two weeks later, the patient was on full oral intake.[19] Her course was rocky: "Over the years, the patient developed several acute rejection episodes that were reversed with steroid boluses. She remained off parenteral nutrition until mid 1990, when graft function was lost because of chronic rejection. The patient became diabetic, developed renal failure, and died in September, 1993."[20] This case was the first successful LD intestinal transplant with long-term function because the patient remained off TPN for over 3 years.

Thus, all five LD intestinal transplants in the precyclosporine and cyclosporine eras (Table 32-1) were not successful in the long term because they all lacked standardized surgical donor and recipient techniques as well as potent immunosuppressive and antimicrobial therapy.

## TACROLIMUS ERA

With the introduction of tacrolimus in the 1990s, a new chapter in intestinal transplantation began (Table 32-2). Just as cyclosporine in the 1980s had significantly increased the survival rates of kidney, liver, pancreas, and heart transplants, tacrolimus propelled intestinal (and lung) transplantation to clinical acceptance. Initial work at the University of Pittsburgh demonstrated that tacrolimus significantly decreased the incidence of rejection and increased graft and patient survival rates after intestinal transplantation.[21,22] Although tacrolimus-based immunosuppression markedly increased the number of intestinal transplants from DDs, the role and the technical aspects of intestinal transplants from LDs remained unclear in the early tacrolimus era.

The first LD intestinal transplant in the tacrolimus era was reported by Morris et al. in 1995.[23] A 31-year-old man with a desmoid tumor underwent excision of the tumor, and in the same session, a small bowel transplant from his monozygotic twin. The twin donor underwent resection of the distal ileum, ileocecal valve, and portion of the cecum (110 cm of bowel); the intestinal graft was on a vascular pedicle comprising the ileocolic vessels with subsequent anastomosis between the ileum and the ascending colon. The vascular anastomoses in the recipient were between the donor ileocolic artery and vein and the recipient SMA and SMV (portal drainage); bowel continuity was restored by duodenoileostomy and cecocolostomy. However, by removing the

donor's terminal ileum, the donor became dependent on monthly vitamin $B_{12}$ injections.[23] This and other potential donor complications (eg, bacterial overgrowth) hindered this technique from gaining more widespread acceptance. Shortly thereafter, Pollard et al.[24] reported an LD intestinal transplant between a 27-year-old female with short bowel syndrome secondary to familial adenomatosis and her mother: 180 cm of donor ileum on a pedicle of distal SMA and SMV was transplanted, the vascular pedicle of the graft was anastomosed to the inferior aorta and vena cava, the bowel continuity was restored with a duodenoileostomy, and the distal end was brought out as a terminal stoma. Posttransplant immunosuppression was tacrolimus-based; three rejection episodes early posttransplant were successfully reversed.

Also in the mid-1990s, Tesi and Jaffe reported two LD intestinal transplants, one in a patient with Gardner's syndrome, the other in a patient with pseudo-obstruction.[25,26] The adult recipients received 200 and 180 cm of proximal donor bowel. Because the jejunum was used, the vascular anatomy was not favorable; the vascular pedicle in one patient contained two arteries and two veins; the other, four arteries and three veins. Despite induction therapy with OKT3 and maintenance therapy with tacrolimus, both patients had several rejection episodes and both went back on TPN about 6 months posttransplant.

At the University of Minnesota, preparations for LD intestinal transplantation started in the early 1990s. Many of the transplant fellows involved at the time have subsequently advanced the field of intestinal transplantation in their own right (Enrico Benedetti, Jacques Pirenne, Jon Fryer, and others).[27–32] The technical aspects of LD intestinal transplantation were studied in a pig model; the results of this experimental work became the basis of the first

TABLE 32-2

## LD INTESTINAL TRANSPLANTS IN THE EARLY TACROLIMUS ERA (1995–1998)

Tacrolimus Era

| Year | Author | Disease | Donor–Recipient Relationship | Type of Graft | Graft Length | Ostomy | Vascular Anastomosis | Immuno-suppression |
|---|---|---|---|---|---|---|---|---|
| 1995 | Morris et al.[23] | Desmoid | Twin brothers (31 years) | Ileum + Cecum | 100 cm | — | SMA, SMV | — |
| 1996 | Pollard et al.[24] | FAP Desmoid | Mother-to-daughter (27 years) | Ileum | 180 cm | TI | Aorta, Cava | TAC,AZA,P |
| 1996/ 1977 | Gruessner et al.[33] | Trauma, Crohn's | Father-to-son (16 years), Mother-to-son (39 years) | Ileum<br>Ileum | 200 cm<br>200 cm | TI<br>TI | Aorta, Cava<br>Aorta, Cava | OKT3,TAC, MMF,P<br>OKT3,TAC, P |
| 1997 | Tesi et al.[25]<br>Jaffe et al.[26] | Gardner's Pseudo-Obstruction. | Mother-to-daughter (26 years), Mother-to-son (29 years) | Jejunum<br>Jejunum | 200 cm<br>180 cm | TI<br>— | Aorta, Cava<br>SMA, SMV | OKT3, TAC, MMF,P NA |
| 1997 | Calne et al.[35] | Mesenteric Thrombosis | Twin brothers (40 years) | Ileum | 150 cm | BK | Aorta, Cava (jump grafts) | — |
| 1998 | Uemoto et al.[37]<br>Fujimoto et al.[40] | Volvulus, Gastroschisis | Mother-to-child (2 years)<br>Mother-to-child (4 years) | Ileum<br>Ileum | 100 cm<br>120 cm | BK<br>LI | Aorta, Cava<br>IMA, IMV | TAC,AZA,P<br>OKT3,TAC, CP,P |
| 1998 | Morel et al.[36] | Volvulus | Twin brothers (13 years) | Ileum | 160 cm | — | Aorta, Cava (jump grafts) | — |

TI, terminal ileostomy; BK, Bishop–Koop ileostomy; LI, loop ileostomy; TAC, tacrolimus; MMF, mycophenolate mofetil; P, prednisone; CP, cyclophosphamide

LD intestinal transplant at the University of Minnesota.[33] The following conclusions were drawn from this bench-to-bedside approach (1) the ileum was preferable to the jejunum because of its greater absorptive capacity of bile acids, vitamins, fat, water, and solutes, and its greater adaptation potential (despite the fact that the jejunum may have an immunologic advantage because of a lower rejection risk)[34]; (2) the terminal ileum (most distal 30 cm), the ileocecal valve, and the cecum should remain in the donor to minimize short- and long-term morbidity; (3) a vascular pedicle should be used, consisting of only one artery and vein (either the ileocolic artery and vein, comprising the distal branches of the SMA and SMV with a few ileal tributaries, or only the terminal branches of the SMA and SMV; the right colic artery with its descending branch has to remain in the donor to guarantee adequate blood supply to the terminal ileum, ileocecal valve, and cecum); (4) and bowel continuity should be restored with a proximal bowel anastomosis and creation of a distal ileostomy (to allow easy access for graft biopsy); ileostomy takedown should occur about 6 months posttransplant or 6 months after treatment of the last rejection episode. After the University of Minnesota's first two technically successful LD intestinal transplants, our group published these guidelines for a standarized technique for intestinal transplants in 1997[33] (Figure 32-1).

Since then, at least 25 more LD intestinal transplants have been performed worldwide (see Chapter 34.5). Calne et al reported an intestinal transplant between two of identical triplets in 1997.[35] The recipient had short bowel syndrome secondary to SMV thrombosis and underwent transplantation of 150 cm of the donor's distal ileum on a vascular pedicle comprising the distal SMA and SMV. Vascular reconstruction included the use of recipient saphenous vein jump grafts between the donor distal SMA and SMV and the recipient infrarenal aorta and cava. Bowel continuity was accomplished via a duodenoileostomy and creation of a "chimney" spout ileostomy. In contrast to the intestinal transplant reported by Morris et al., Calne et al used no immunosuppression. Another identical twin intestinal transplant was performed in 1998 in Geneva; the difference between this and the other two twin cases (by Morris et al and Calne et al.) was that both donor and recipient were minors, requiring permission of the institution's ethics committee.[36] Both the Calne and the Geneva identical twin transplants are basically isografts, making it "possible to study the physiology of the grafted bowel ... in the absence of an immune reaction."[35]

Initially, LD intestinal transplants were performed in North America and Europe. Over time, LD intestinal transplants have also been reported in Asian countries, such as Japan, China, and Korea.[37–39] The first Japanese case was performed in Kyoto in a 2-year 6-month-old boy who received 100 cm of distal donor ileum.[37] Despite tacrolimus-based immunosuppression, four rejection episodes occurred and the patient died 16 months later from *Pneumocystis carinii* pneumonia. In a second Kyoto case of a 4-year 5-month-old girl, 120 cm was transplanted; the donor vein was anastomosed to the recipient's inferior mesenteric vein, utilizing portal drainage.[40]

As shown in Chapter 34.5, 41 LD intestinal transplants have been reported worldwide between January 1985 and March 2005. Of note, with the exception of the identical twin transplants, there appears to be no significant (graft and patient) survival advantage 95 compared with the results of DD intestinal transplants—this finding has been critically acknowledged in the literature and has stirred a debate about whether the use of LDs for segmental intestinal transplants is justified.[41,42] However, what is frequently overlooked is that short bowel syndrome is not a static process and that serious TPN-associated complications, such as liver failure, lack of vascular access, and recurrent infections, continue to progress and become life-threatening. According to United Network for Organ Sharing (UNOS) data, between January 1, 2003, and December 31, 2005, a total of 68 patients were listed initially for an intestinal transplant alone, but, 7 or more days later, were listed for an additional liver transplant. Of those, 36 (53%) received a transplant (26, intestine and liver; 10, intestine alone [only 2 needed a subsequent liver]) and 8 (12%) remained on the waiting list. However, 24 (35%) patients died or had to be removed from the waiting list (12 died; 3 were removed or too sick to be transplanted; 9 were removed for other reasons including LD transplants) (personal communication, Sarah Taranto, BA, UNOS Data Specialist, June 2006). These figures clearly demonstrate that LD intestinal grafts are life-saving if DD grafts do not become available in time or if the recipient progresses to end-stage liver disease and then requires an additional (scarce) liver graft.

One of the most disturbing facts of TPN dependence and associated liver failure (specifically in children) is, in fact, the high mortality on the DD waiting list.[43] For that reason, LD intestinal and liver transplants have been considered since 1998,[34] but not successfully performed before 2004.[44] The first sequential intestinal and liver transplant from the same donor was performed at the University of Illinois; two previous attempts in Japan failed long-term.[45] Testa et al. reported a case of a 2-year-old boy with short bowel syndrome secondary to gastroschisis who underwent an LD small bowel transplant (150 cm of terminal ileum from his grandmother). However, 4 months posttransplant, the graft had to be removed because of posttransplant lymphoproliferative disease (PTLD). As the patient's liver function deteriorated (progression to cirrhosis on biopsy), he was initially listed for a combined DD small bowel and liver transplant, but a suitable DD did not become available. After approval by the institution's ethics committee, the patient underwent LD liver transplantation first to eliminate preformed antibodies. A week after the LD liver transplant, the recipient underwent transplantation of 150 cm of terminal ileum from the mother, using the above described standard technique.

Since this initial case of sequential LD liver and bowel transplantation, the University of Illinois group has performed two successful combined liver and intestinal transplants in pediatric recipients.[46] At the University of Minnesota, the first combined LD intestinal and liver transplant was performed in November 2005. It appears that combined LD liver and small bowel transplants may become a viable option when a suitable DD donor is not available (Color Plates, Figure IN-6).

At the University of Minnesota, since 1996, a total of five isolated LD intestinal transplants and one combined LD liver and intestinal transplant have been performed. The first patient in 1996 underwent the aforementioned and now generally accepted standardized surgical technique; the 16-year-old recipient had been involved in a car accident that left him paraplegic and with short bowel syndrome after undergoing extensive bowel resection for massive mesenteric bleeding. He received a 4-antigen-matched ileal graft of 200 cm on a vascular pedicle comprising the ileocolic artery and vein from his father.[33] The patient was completely off TPN at the time of discharge (3 weeks posttransplant), he gained about 20 kg within the first posttransplant year, and showed no evidence of rejection, graft-versus-host disease (GVHD), or infection. About 4 years posttransplant, he developed cytomegalovirus (CMV) enteropathy with complete mucosal denudation. About 5 years posttransplant, he was diagnosed with chronic rejection; the graft was removed 5½ years posttransplant. The second transplant was performed in a 39-year-old man with a longstanding history of Crohn's disease and immunosuppression. He received 200 cm of ileal graft from his 3-antigen-matched mother despite a positive B-cell crossmatch. About 2 weeks after surgery he developed severe rejection, requiring treatment with OKT3; he developed pulmonary aspergillosis and died of sepsis about 3 months posttransplant. The third patient was a 1-year-old child who had lost most of her bowel from midgut volvulus. Because of recurrent catheter infections, lack of vascular access, and incipient liver dysfunction, she received a 4-antigen-matched bowel graft from her father. She was initially TPN-independent, but developed adenoviral enteropathy with mucosal denudation 6 months posttransplant, followed by two severe rejection episodes. One year posttransplant, the graft had to be removed because of PTLD. The fourth patient was a 32-year-old woman who had lost most of her small bowel due to a volvulus about 1 year after undergoing a gastric bypass procedure (with a weight decrease from 130 to 50 kg). She had developed liver dysfunction with bilirubin levels in the 20 mg/dL range and biopsy-proven liver fibrosis, grade 3. She received an HLA-identical graft from her brother and has been TPN-independent since, without evidence of rejection, PTLD, or infection. The fifth patient also received an HLA-identical graft from his brother. He developed short bowel syndrome secondary to thrombosis of his SMA secondary to an underlying coagulopathy. The transplant was initially successful; however, despite systemic anticoagulation, he lost the graft on posttransplant day 9 from graft thrombosis. The sixth patient was a 9-month-old infant with short bowel syndrome secondary to gastroschisis and midgut volvulus. He developed progressive liver failure (cirrhosis on biopsy) and a DD donor did not become available in time. Thus, he received a combined LD intestinal and liver graft from his mother but developed hepatic artery thrombosis on the first posttransplant day. Four weeks later he underwent a liver retransplant when a size-matched DD organ became available.

In light of the historical development and the overall results of LD intestinal transplantation, the question is where to go from here.

As with all other solid organ transplants, an LD must only be placed at risk when the chance of a successful outcome in the recipient is high, and a comparable result unlikely to be achieved by other approaches.[47] This requirement is fulfilled particularly in patients with irreversible intestinal failure and documented, but still reversible, liver disease and in whom a solitary intestinal graft from a DD may not become available in time. Thus, the primary rationale for performing LD intestinal transplants is not only to improve posttransplant outcome and to reduce the waiting time but also to decrease the mortality on the waiting list: solitary LD intestinal transplants in patients with TPN-associated incipient liver dysfunction can prevent the progression to end-stage liver disease and eliminate the need for a simultaneous or sequential liver transplant. There are other advantages aside from the just-mentioned justification for the core requirement for LD intestinal transplants. Elective surgery such as an LD intestinal transplant allows optimal preparation of the donor and recipient, reducing the risk of perioperative complications. LD intestinal transplants are also associated with shorter preservation times and possibly lower rates of rejection due to better HLA matching. LD intestinal transplants may also facilitate the application of immunomodulatory peritransplant strategies.[48,49]

But, irrespective of what the advantages for the recipient are, the ethical issues regarding the use of an LD remain. Therefore, as for all other solid organ transplants that use LDs, the risks and benefits need to be analyzed for each individual intestinal donor and recipient pair. The overall risk for an intestinal donor is small (similar to the risk of general anesthesia, approximately 0.03%),[50] but the donor must also be informed about long-term risks such as small-bowel obstruction or vitamin $B_{12}$ deficiency. If donor outcome data were to be reported to an LD registry, surgeons and physicians would be able to accurately inform donors about the postoperative risks and not rely on anecdotal or incomplete information.[47]

At an International Consensus Conference on the Care of Live Organ Donors in Vancouver, Canada, in September 2005, LD intestinal transplants were not considered experimental, but the recommendation was to regard this procedure as innovative evolving technology. Because of the evolving nature of the procedure, the Vancouver forum participants recommended that centers performing LD intestinal transplants should submit their proposals for ethical review and report outcomes to an international registry.[50]

Looking beyond donor safety, LD intestinal transplants warrant systematic analysis regarding quality of life for both donors and recipients and critical assessment of new developments such as nondirected donation and commercialization.

## References

1. Van Gossum A, Espen-Han Group. Home parenteral nutrition (NPN) in adults: a multicentre survey in Europe in 1933. *Clin Nutr* 1996;15:53–58.
2. Buchman AL. Etiology and initial management of short bowel syndrome. *Gastroenterology* 2006;130:55–S15.
3. Panis Y, Messing B, Rivet P, et al. Segmental reversal of the small bowel as an alternative to intestinal transplantation in patients with short bowel syndrome. *Ann Surg* 1994;225:401–407.
4. Glick PL, de Lorimier AA, Adzick NS, et al. Colon interposition: an adjuvant operation for short-gut syndrome. *J Pediatr Surg* 1984;19:719–725.
5. Waddell WR, Kern Jr. F, Halgrimson CG, Woodbury JJ. A simple jejunocolic "valve". For relief of rapid transit and the short bowel syndrome. *Arch Surg* 1970; 100:438–444.
6. Grieco GA, Reyes HM, Ostrovsky E. The role of a modified intussusception jejunocolic valve in short-bowel syndrome. *J Pediatr Surg* 1983;18: 354–358.
7. Bianchi A. Intestinal loop lengthening – a technique for increasing small intestinallength. *J Pediatr Surg* 1980;15:145–151.
8. Kim HB, Fauza D, Garza J, et al. Serial transverse enteroplasty (STEP): a novel bowel lengthening procedure. *J Pediatr Surg* 2003;38:425–429.
9. Lillehei RC, Goott B, Miller FA. The physiological response of the small bowel of the dog to ischemia including prolonged in vitro preservation of the bowel with successful replacement and survival. *Ann Surg* 1959;150:543–560.
10. Lillehei RC, Goott B, Miller FA. Homografts of the small bowel. *Surg Forum* 1959; 10:197–199.
11. Starzl TE, Kaupp HA, Brock DR, Butz GW, Linman JW. Homotransplantation of multiple visceral organs. *Am J Surg* 1962;103:219–229.
12. McAlister VC, Grant DR. Clinical small bowel transplantation. In: Grant DR, Wood RMW, eds. *Small Bowel Transplantation*. London: Edward Arnold Publ.; 1994. Chapter 12:121–132.
13. Lillehei RC, Idezuki Y, Feemster JA, et al. Transplantation of stomach, intestine, and pancreas: experimental and clinical observations. *Surgery* 1967;62:721–741.
14. Deterling R. Comment on living donor intestinal transplantation. In: Alican F, Hardy JD, Cayirli M, et al. eds. Intestinal transplantation:

Laboratory experience and report of a clinical case. *Am J Surg* 1971;121:150–159.

15. Alican F, Hardy JD, Cayirli M, et al. Intestinal transplantation: laboratory experience and report of a clinical case. *Am J Surg* 1971;121:150–159.

16. Fortner JG, Sichuk G, Litwin SD, Beattie EJ, Jr. Immunological responses to an intestinal allograft within HL-A-identical donor-recipient. *Transplantation* 1972;14: 531–535.

17. Grant D, Wall W, Mimeault R, et al. Successful small-bowel/liver transplantation. *Lancet* 1990;335:181–184.

18. Grant D, Current results of intestinal transplantation. *Lancet* 1996;347: 1801–1803.

19. Deltz E, Schroeder P, Gebhardt H, et al. Successful clinical small bowel transplantation: report of a case. *Clin Transpl* 1989;3:89–91.

20. Margreiter R. Living-donor pancreas and small-bowel transplantation. *Langenbeck's Arch Surg* 1999;384:544–549.

21. Todo S, Tzakis AG, Abu-Elmagd K, et al. Cadaveric small bowel and small bowel-liver transplantation in humans. *Transplantation* 1992;53: 369–376.

22. Todo S, Reyes J, Furukawa H, et al. Outcome analysis of 71 clinical intestinal transplantations. *Ann Surg* 1995;222:270–282.

23. Morris JA, Johnson DL, Rimmer JA, et al. Identical-twin small-bowel transplant for desmoid tumour. *Lancet* 1995;Jun 17;345:1577–1578.

24. Pollard SG, Lodge P, Selvakumar S, et al. Living related small bowel transplantation: The first United Kingdom case. *Transplant Proc* 1996; 28:2733.

25. Tesi R, Bech R, Lambiase L, et al. Living-related small-bowel transplantation: donor evaluation and outcome. *Transplant Proc* 1997;29:686–687.

26. Jaffe BM, Beck R, Flint L, et al. Living-related small bowel transplantation in adults: a report of two patients. *Transplant Proc* 1997;29:1851–1852.

27. Benedetti E, Pirenne J, Moon-Chul S, et al. Simultaneous en bloc transplantation of liver, small bowel, and large bowel in pigs. *Tanspl Proc* 1995; 27:341–343.

28. Benedetti E, Testa G, Sankary H, et al. Successful treatment of trauma-induced short bowel syndrome with early living related bowel transplantation. *J Trauma* 2004;57:164–170.

29. Fryer JP, Kim S, Wells CL, et al. Bacterial translocation in a large animal model of small bowel transplantation: portal vs systemic venous drainage and effect of FK 506 immunosuppression. *Arch Surg* 1996;131: 77–84.

30. Fryer JP. Intestinal transplantation: an update. *Curr Opin Gastroenterol* 2005;21:162–168.

31. Pirenne J, Gruessner A, Benedetti E, et al. Donor-specific unmodified bone marrow transfusion does not facilitate intestinal engraftment after bowel transplantation in a porcine model. *Surgery* 1997;121:79–88.

32. Pirenne J, Koshiba T, Geboes K, et al. Complete freedom from rejection after intestinal transplantation using a new tolerogenic protocol combined with low immunosuppression. *Transplantation* 2002;73:966–968.

33. Gruessner RWG, Sharp HL. Living-related intestinal transplantation. *Transplantation* 1997;64:1605–1607.

34. Nakkleh RE, Gruessner AC, Pirenne J, et al. Colon versus small bowel rejection after total bowel transplantation in a pig model. *Transpl Int* 1996;9:S269–S274.

35. Calne RY, Friend PK, Middleton S, et al. Intestinal transplant between two of identical tripleits. *Lancet* 1997;350:1077–1078.

36. Morel P, Kadry Z, Charbonnet P, Bednarkiewicz, M, Faidutti B. Paediatric living related intestinal-transplantation between two monozygotic twins: a 1-year follow-up. *Lancet* 2000;355:723–724.

37. Uemoto S, Fujimoto Y, Inomata Y, et al. Living-related small bowel transplantation: the first case in Japan. *Pediatr Transpl* 1998;2:40–44.

38. Wu GS, Wang WZ, Song WL, Lin R, Duraj FF. The living-related small bowel transplant: the first case in China. *Transpl Proc* 2000;32:1218.

39. Lee MD, Kim DG, Ahn ST, et al. Isolated small bowel transplantation from a living-related donor at the Catholic University of Korea–a case report of rejection–Free Course. *yonsei Med J* 2004;45:1198–1202.

40. Fujimoto Y, Uemoto S, Inomata Y, et al. Small bowel transplantation using grafts from living-related donors. Two case reports. *Transpl Int* 2000;13 [Suppl 1]:S179–S184.

41. Tzakis AG, Gruessner RWG, Future of living-related small bowel transplantation in children. *Pediatr Transpl* 1998;2:1–2.

42. Fryer J, Angelos P. Is there a role for living donor intestine transplants? *Progr Transpl* 2004;14:321–329.

43. Fryer J, Pellar S, Ormond D, Koffron A, Abecassis M. Mortality in candidates waiting for combined liver-intestine transplants exceeds that for other candidates waiting for liver transplants. *Liver Transpl* 2003;9:748–753.

44. Testa G, Holterman M, John E, et al. Combined living donor liver/small bowel transplantation. *Transplantation* 2005;79:1401–1404.

45. Tanaka K. Personal communication. July 2004.

46. Benedetti E. Personal communication. January 2006.

47. Gaston RS, Eckhoff DE. Whither living donors? *Am J Transpl* 2004;4: 203.

48. Gruessner RWG, Nakhleh RE, Harmon JV, Dunning M, Gruessner AC. Donor-specific portal blood transfusion in intestinal transplantation: a prospective, preclinical large animal study. *Transplantation* 1998;66:164–169.

49. Gruessner RWG, Levay-Young BK, Nahkleh RE, et al. Portal donor-specific blood transfusion and mycophenolate mofetil allow steroid avoidance and tacrolimus dose reduction with sustained levels of chimerism in a pig model of intestinal transplantation. *Transplantation* 2004;77:1500–1506.

50. Barr ML, Belghiti J, Villamil FG, et al. A report of the Vancouver Forum on the care of the live organ donor: lung, liver, pancreas, and intestine data and medical guidelines. *Transplantation* 2006; 81: 1373-1385.

# INTESTINAL TRANSPLANTATION – THE DONOR

## 33.1  SELECTION AND WORKUP

*Enrico Benedetti, MD, Mark J. Holterman, MD, PhD, Giuliano Testa, MD*

### OVERVIEW

The early results from the largest reported cohort of small bowel donors indicates that in terms of donor safety, living donor intestinal transplantation (LDITx) can be proposed as a valid solution for patients affected by irreversible intestinal failure (IF). In comparison to liver, kidney, lung, and pancreas living donor operations, the resection of the terminal ileum is technically less challenging and presents fewer immediate and long-term risks for the donor.[1]

Although the number of LDITx donors is still relatively small, there have not been any reports of patient mortality and the only short-term morbidity is characterized by increased number of bowel movements per day and fecal urgency. Undesired weight loss has not been a problem. At the present time no donor has complained of persistent diarrhea, new onset of food intolerance, or has shown evidence of anemia due to vitamin $B_{12}$ deficiency or malabsorption of fat-soluble vitamins. Longer follow-up is necessary to determine the incidence of postsurgical intestinal adhesions, which could be the only potential remaining long-term complication in small bowel donors.

To optimize the success and minimize the complications of LDITx, one needs to choose the donor carefully. As a general guideline, when faced with a number of potential donors, one should choose the healthiest ABO-compatible donor with the greatest degree of human leukocyte antigen (HLA) matching.

On the other hand, sometimes there are no healthy ABO-compatible donors available and LDITx is not an option. As in most living related donors it is imperative that one chooses a donor with minimal physical problems. The initial screening involves an interview session in which the idea and process of living donor intestinal transplantation are described in detail, and the potential donors have a chance to ask any questions concerning perioperative care and short- and long-term complications. During this session it should be made clear to the patients the advantages and disadvantages of living related intestinal transplants including the available results from transplant centers with LDITx experience. It is important for patients and their families to consider cadaver ITx and be aware of the latest excellent outcomes reported by these centers.[2–4] In the case of children with IF, it is critical that families are made aware of the 30% to 40% mortality rate associated with time spent on the organ waiting list and the associated high incidence of progression to liver failure necessitating both a liver and a bowel transplant.[5] In the case of patients who have already developed advanced liver disease, the possibility of combined living donor liver and intestinal transplantation will be discussed.[6]

### OVERALL HEALTH

One aspect of the initial discussions is to rule out those family members that cannot serve as donors for medical reasons. Because donor safety is paramount, the selected donor must be able to tolerate an elective surgical procedure that results in loss of nearly one third of their small intestine. The potential donor must be free of significant cardiovascular, pulmonary, and renal problems. A donor with a history of malignancy, type 1 diabetes or other autoimmune disease would be disqualified. Any type of inflammatory bowel disease, gastrointestinal polyposis, arteriovenous malformation, malabsorption, or dysmotility syndromes would preclude the donor.[7]

At this point, all of the family members that are interested in donation and are not disqualified by immediately identifiable medical issues undergo a blood test to determine ABO compatibility and HLA type. Once these tests are back, the compatible donor(s) undergoes an extensive evaluation in search of medical, psychosocial, or ethical determinants that would disqualify them as acceptable donors (Table 33.1-1).

### DONOR SELECTION

Potential living related small bowel donor selection starts with the preliminary determination of ABO blood type and HLA.

#### ABO Compatibility

Potential donors are screened for ABO compatibility with the recipient. The standard ABO-compatibility guidelines apply with one additional caveat. With LDITx there is a significant amount of passenger lymphocytes carried along with the intestinal graft. These lymphocytes can generate an antibody response against the donor's A, B, or Rh antigens that can result in antibody-mediated hemolytic anemia.[8]

This rare complication can result in significant transient hyperbilirubinemia and is usually self-limited. This potential for complication can be avoided with appropriate donor selection whenever possible. It is important to stress that the pool of acceptable donors should not be restricted to donors with zero chance of donor

**TABLE 33-1**
## LIVING-RELATED DONOR EVALUATION FOR LDIT$_X$

- MEDICAL HISTORY SCREENING: significant medical or surgical conditions preclude donation (e.g. history of malignancy, previous intestinal surgery, etc.)

- ABO-COMPATIBILITY

- HLA-DETERMINATION

- COMPLETE HISTORY AND PHYSICAL

- CHEST RADIOGRAPH

- ELECTROCARDIOGRAM

- LABORATORY TESTS: glucose, BUN, electrolytes, creatinine, bilirubin, alkaline phosphatase, AST, ALT, GGT, albumin, ammonia, alpha-fetoprotein, prothrombin time, partial thromboplastin time, triglycerides, Vitamin A, D, E, K,

- B-12

- INFECTIOUS DISEASE ASSESSMENT: Hepatitis screen, HIV, CMV (IgG, IgM), EBV (IgG, IgM), Herpes zoster (IgA, EIA), stool culture, urine culture

- LYMPHOCYTOTOXIC CROSS-MATCH

- ETHICS CONSULTATION: An in-depth interview with a member of the institutional ethics committee to evaluate the patient's motivation for, and understanding of the risks involved in, intestinal donation.

- PSYCHOSOCIAL ASSESSMENT: Psychiatric and/or psychological consultation, social worker consultation.

- ANATOMIC ASSESSMENT: Abdominal CT-scan, selective superior mesenteric angiogram or 3-D-angio-CT-scan

- ANESTHESIOLOGY ASSESSMENT: consultation, anesthesia and surgical history, drug allergies

passenger lymphocyte-mediated hemolysis. Such a restriction precludes too many donors solely based on the possibility of a rare nonfatal complication.

## HLA Matching

Where possible, it seems most prudent to choose donors who have a close HLA match. For example, a parent-to-child donation ensures at least a three out of six HLA antigen match. Sibling to sibling donations may share even more HLA antigens. Worldwide experience is not sufficiently extensive to draw definite conclusions about the role that HLA antigen matching has on short- and long-term graft function. In addition, there may be a theoretical advantage to a mother-to-child donation, based on the child receiving a tolerogenic innoculation to maternal antigens through *in utero* exposure or via breast-feeding.

After the initial donor pool is narrowed to ABO-compatible donors with an optimal degree of HLA antigen match, the donors undergo a further workup involving a complete history and physical, laboratory tests and infectious disease assessment. These tests include screening for infectious viral agents and in the case of adult-to-child donation; the ideal donor would be EBV and CMV negative. This possibility is unusual, however, because of the high incidence of these latent viral infections in the adult population. A donor with HIV-AIDS or hepatitis B and C would be disqualified.

Additionally the immune responsiveness of the recipient to the donor cells is assessed through the performance of a lymphocytotoxic crossmatch. Recipients are also screened for preformed anti-HLA antibodies against the various donors under consideration. Potential donors who have not been disqualified by problems such as anemia or cardiac, renal, pulmonary, or liver disease then undergo a psychosocial evaluation and an in-depth consultation by a member of the institution's ethics committee. A final preoperative evaluation is undertaken by the anesthesiology team.

## Psychosocial Evaluation

Many important issues must be considered in the psychological evaluation of LDITx donors. These mainly have to deal with identifying the psychological strengths and weaknesses of each individual donor candidate. A history of mental disease and/or psychological impairment would predict that patients might not be able to cope with the stress of surgery and the postoperative care. In addition, depending on the psychological status of the patient, their ability to make a competent decision to donate a segment of their small intestine must be clearly and professionally determined. It is obvious that the intense search for a suitable donor provides the opportunity for excessive coercion to be brought to bear by well-meaning family members or members of the transplant team. This is especially problematic for potential donors with impaired coping skills or altered views of reality.

## Ethical Considerations

As discussed in detail throughout this monograph, there are important ethical considerations that pertain to volunteering for elective organ donations. It is appropriate for a member of the institution's bioethics committee to perform an in-depth independent interview of all potential donors for LDITx. It is important that the interview(s) with the ethicist occurs early on in the evaluation process and certainly before invasive procedures are performed (eg, angiography). An early disqualification on ethical grounds can also allow for the donor to resist coercion and avoid the momentum that occurs if such a disqualification occurs as the last step prior to the actual donation. The potential donor should be reminded of the risks involved in the operation and the ramifications to them and their family should a complication or fatality occur. The serious nature of this decision to donate can be underscored by asking the potential donor if they have made their own will including arrangements for the care of their other family members. The ethicist should discern the presence of donor coercion being applied by the donor/recipient family and encourage the free discussion of alternatives to donation and techniques to extricate the donor from this coercion. The ethicist must grant their approval before the donor can proceed to the final workup and surgery.[9]

Provided that all medical, psychosocial, and ethical factors have been deemed acceptable it is important to complete the final stage of the workup, which is mainly involved with determining the vascular anatomy of the donor's small intestine and evaluating the anesthetic risk for the donor. It should be noted that the size match between the donor and the recipient, critical in cadaver cases, is not important in the setting of LDITx since a segment of bowel is used. In order to evaluate anatomy and patency of the donor's superior mesenteric vessels, conventional selective

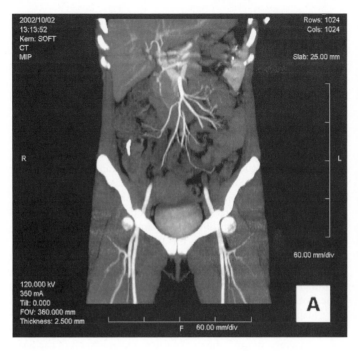
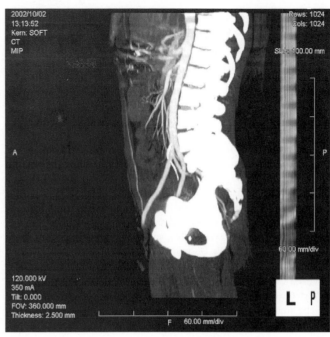

**FIGURE 33.1-1**

CT angiography followed by 3-D reconstruction can be used to evaluate the anatomy of the superior mesenteric vessels without the need for an invasive angiogram. This donor's mesenteric vasculature is appreciated from the anterior and lateral position. The arrows indicate the superior mesenteric artery and the main branch supplying the ileum that will be harvested for the transplant.

angiography is performed. Abdominal CT-scan completes the study of the donor's abdomen to rule out unknown associated pathologies. This basic CT scan can be enhanced to include a detailed study of the splanchnic vasculature with 3-D image reconstruction. This novel test can provide images that are comparable to those obtained with standard angiography, but is less invasive and can complete in a single step all the necessary imaging[10] (Figure 33.1-1).

Prior to surgery, a detailed anesthesia evaluation is performed to ensure that the patient's medical condition does not pose an unacceptable anesthetic risk. This interaction can also provide the potential donor with a valuable opportunity to allay any fears concerning surgery and anesthesiology and encourages excellent communication and trust between patient and anesthesiologist.

The final step before surgery involves a meeting between those surgeons, anesthesiologists, social workers, and ethicists who have performed evaluations on the available donors. Appropriate attention to all expressed concerns is essential for optimal donor selection and surgical outcomes.

## Postoperative Evaluation

It is important that the donors have adequate follow-up care. Their initial postoperative course usually requires 3 to 4 days in the hospital. As mentioned the most frequent complaint of the donor is a sense of fecal urgency and loose stools. This has always resolved over a course of several weeks. Undesired weight loss and/or persistent diarrhea may indicate fat absorption problems that could be treated with dietary modification or motility slowing agents. After their discharge home their eating and defecation

patterns need to be evaluated on a monthly basis initially and then on an annual basis. There currently are few short-term complications associated with segmental ileum donation for LDITx, but it is important that the donors can contact the transplant team and all involved remain vigilant for the possibility of long-term complications.

## References

1. Testa G, Panaro F, Schena S, et al. Living related small bowel transplantation: donor surgical technique. *Ann Surg* 2004;240(5):779–784.
2. Bond GJ, Mazariegos GV, Sindhi R, et al. Evolutionary experience with immunosuppression in pediatric intestinal transplantation. *J Pediatr Surg* 2005;40(1):274–279.
3. Goulet O, Sauvat F, Ruemmele F, et al. Results of the Paris: ten years of pediatric intestinal transplantation. *Transplant Proc* 2005;37(4):1667.
4. Grant D, Abu-Elmagd K, Reyes J, et al. On behalf of the Intestine Transplant Registry. 2003 report of the intestine transplant registry: a new era has dawned. *Ann Surg* 2005;241(4):607.
5. UNOS Registry. Available at: http://www.unos.org. Accessed May 2005.
6. Testa G, Holterman M, John E, et al. Combined living donor liver/small bowel transplantation. *Transplantation* 2005;79(10):1401.
7. Seda NJ, Macedo C, Jaffe R, et al. Carcinoma of donor origin after liver-intestine transplantation in a child. *Pediatr Transplant* 2005;9(2):244.
8. Panaro F, DeChristopher PJ, Rondelli D, et al. Severe hemolytic anemia due to passenger lymphocytes after living-related bowel transplant. *Clin Transplant* 2004;18(3):332.
9. Anderson-Shaw L, Schmidt ML, Elkin J, et al. Evolution of a living donor liver transplantation advocacy program. *J Clin Ethics* 2005;16(1):46.
10. Panaro F, Testa G, Balakrishnan N, et al. Living related small bowel transplantation in children: 3-dimensional computed tomography donor evaluation. *Pediatr Transplant* 2004;8(1):65.

## 33.2 SURGICAL PROCEDURES AND PERIOPERATIVE CARE

*Rainer W.G. Gruessner, MD*

### INTRODUCTION

As shown in Chapter 32, a standardized and easily reproducible procurement technique for intestinal grafts from living donors (LDs) was not reported until 1997.[1] Until then, controversy existed regarding (1) whether the donor ileum or the donor jejunum should be used, (2) what the optimal length of procured donor bowel should be (in order to free the recipient from total parenteral nutrition (TPN) and to spare the donor the development of short-bowel syndrome), and (3) what the technically least complicated vascular reconstruction in the recipient should be.[2–6]

At the University of Minnesota, we developed a technique that focused on both donor safety and recipient TPN independence.[1] We determined that the distal ileum is the most suitable portion of the small bowel to transplant because of its absorptive capacity (of bile acids, vitamins, water, electrolytes, and nutrients) and its adaptation potential. We also believed that the most distal 20 to 30 cm of ileum had to remain in the donor to provide adequate vitamin $B_{12}$ absorption and to avoid the development of macrocytic anemia (as a result of vitamin $B_{12}$ deficiency). By leaving the most distal ileum in the donor, along with the ileocecal valve and the cecum, we also eliminated such negative effects of an ileocecal resection as shortened transit time (diarrhea) and bacterial overgrowth.[5,7] We also determined that the optimal LD bowel length for an adult recipient should be about 200 cm (vs 120 to 150 cm

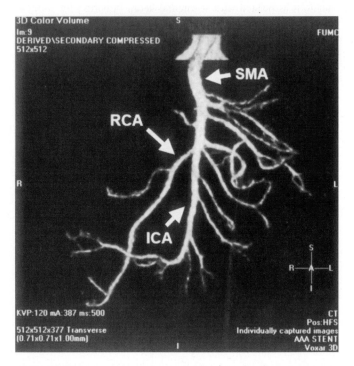

**FIGURE 33.2-1**

A 3-D postprocessed image of the donor superior mesenteric artery (SMA), the ileocolic artery (ICA), and the right colic artery (RCA).

for a pediatric recipient), leaving the donor with two-thirds or three-fifths of native small bowel.

Having determined the optimal location and length of donor small bowel, we realized another advantage of this technique: it would require anastomosis of only one donor inflow and one outflow vessel in the recipient. We chose the ileocolic artery (ICA) and vein (ICV), leaving the right colic artery (RCA) with its descending branch (supplying the cecum, ileocecal valve, and terminal ileum) in the donor (Color Plates, Figure IN-1). Other clinicians, and more recently, Testa et al in nine adult donors, described a technique that uses the terminal branch of the superior mesenteric artery (SMA), rather than the ICA.[8]

These two anatomical variants are shown in Figure IN-1 (Color Plates). The first variant depicts the ICA, which is formed by the terminal branch of the SMA and usually one to three additional distal ileal branches; the ICA ends at the takeoff of the RCA. The second variant shows the ICA as a separate branch off the SMA; in such patients, the terminal branch of the SMA is another different vessel that, independently of the ICA, supplies the distal ileum. Irrespective of the anatomical variant, the ICA is usually slightly larger in diameter than the terminal branch of the SMA, an advantage if the LD is a small person. In LDs who are of average weight, the use of the terminal branch of the SMA is sufficient (as shown by the largest series of LD intestinal transplants by the University of Illinois transplant group).[8]

### OPERATIVE PROCEDURES

#### LD Intestinal Donation

The pretransplant preparation of an LD is the same as for any patient undergoing major elective bowel surgery. In the afternoon before the day of surgery, the donor takes GoLYTELY (polyethylene glycol and electrolyte solution) orally until the rectal effluent is clear. For intestinal decontamination, 3 doses of neomycin (1 g by mouth) and metronidazole (500 mg) are given (18, 17, and 10 hours before surgery).[8] A single perioperative dose of an intravenous cephalosporin (for antibiotic prophylaxis) is also administered.

The donor is placed on the operating table in the supine position. After induction of general endotracheal anesthesia, a Foley catheter and a nasogastric tube are placed. A central venous line and an arterial line are usually not required. Sequential compression devices for thrombosis prophylaxis are used.

The donor is prepped and draped in standard fashion, and a lower midline incision is made. After general exploration of the entire abdominal cavity, the colon is retracted cephalad and the small bowel approached. First, the entire length of the small bowel, from the ligament of Treitz to the ileocecal valve, is measured along its antimesenteric border, by using an umbilical tape.

Next, the cecum is identified and the terminal ileum marked 30 cm proximal from the ileocecal junction: this point serves as the distal end of the resection. From there, 200 cm (for adult recipients, as compared with 120 to 150 cm for pediatric recipients) is measured on the distal ileum. The proximal end of the resection is also marked. The stitches that are used to mark the proximal and distal ends of the small bowel should be different in length (or in strength) to distinguish both ends after the bowel has been removed. The remainder of the bowel is measured one more time to assure that > 60% of its length is left in the donor. Of note, mobilization and manipulation of the bowel induce peristalsis, resulting in a different length every time though the same bowel segment is measured; Testa et al. recommend accepting the first measurement of the entire bowel as the final one.[8]

The transverse colon is kept in a cephalad position and the root of the mesentery with the superior mesenteric vessels is identified. With the help of the preoperative computed tomography (CT) or magnetic resonance (MR) angiogram, the takeoff of the RCA is identified, but the vessel itself is left untouched. As described previously, preservation of the RCA with its descending branch is paramount, because it provides the blood supply to the remaining cecum, ileocecal valve, and terminal ileum. Distal to the takeoff of the RCA, the ICA is typically identified as the distal extension of the SMA trunk. Usually, one to three small distal ileal side branches originate from the ICA; the most distal and longest branch of the ICA is called the terminal branch of the SMA. In contrast to the ICA, its most distal (terminal) branch has no ileal side branch(es).

Given the abundant collateralization of the small bowel's blood supply, procurement of the ICA along with one to three distal ileal side branches (and the terminal branch of the SMA) does not jeopardize the recipient's blood supply to the remaining ileum.

On occasion, the ICA is a separate branch off the main trunk of the SMA (Color Plates, Figure IN-1), and the terminal branch of the SMA is an independent vessel; in such donors, the ICA can be preserved and the terminal branch of the SMA is procured. Typically, the ICA is larger in diameter than the terminal branch of the SMA and is the preferred donor vessel if the donor is a small person. In donors who are of at least average weight, the terminal branch of the SMA can also be used.

If the ileocolic vessels are chosen for procurement, they are identified and then dissected free a few cm distal to the takeoff of the RCA. The ICA is encircled with a vessel loop, at or close to the level of transection; the vessel is dissected free and cleared from surrounding tissue over a length of 2 to 3 cm. The corresponding segment of the ICV is usually found immediately adjacent (laterally) to the ICA. Likewise, the ICV is dissected free and cleared over a length of 2 to 3 cm from the surrounding mesenteric tissue; the ICV is also encircled with a vessel loop. Segments of about 2 to 3 cm of free vessels are needed to facilitate the construction of the almost rectangular end-to-side anastomoses in the recipient and to avoid the use of extension grafts (see Chapter 34.2).

When the ICA and ICV are completely dissected free (or, alternatively, the terminal branches of the SMA and SMV), the mesentery is divided by using the transilluminating technique ("diaphanoscopy") along the distribution of the ileocolic vessels, targeting the two ends of the bowel transection. The mesentery is usually divided sequentially between clamps, and the mesentery vessels are ligated with 3-0 silk sutures and divided. The mesentery is thus divided in a "V"-shaped fashion, with the bottom of the "V" superimposing the transection line of the ileocolic vessels.[8] Once the entire mesentery is divided on both sides, the bowel is divided at the two resection points with a gastrointestinal anastomosis (GIA)-55 stapler. At this point, the entire bowel should be viable and have excellent blood flow, even at the distal ends throughout the mesenteric division.

Once word is given that the recipient operating room is ready, the donor is given 70 U/kg of heparin. Then, either vascular spoon-shaped clamps or Hendren clamps are applied to the ICA and ICV, about 2 cm distal to the takeoff of the RCA. The anterior portions of the ICA and ICV (or the terminal branches of the SMA and SMV) are marked with a pen; doing so will allow the recipient team to properly orient and align the donor vessels. The donor

vessels are divided with a knife, leaving a short stump on the clamps. The heparin is reversed with an equivalent dose of protamine. After the vessels are transected, the bowel graft is removed and the specimen is delivered to the recipient team (Color Plates, Figure IN-2).

The arterial and venous stumps of the ileocolic vessels are then oversewn with 6-0 nonabsorbable sutures in a running fashion. The clamps are released, and the oversewn stumps are checked for hemostasis. If necessary, a clip can be placed above the suture line. The mesentery is reevaluated: it should be hemostatic. The two small-bowel ends are also evaluated: they should have excellent perfusion. The stapled ends are oversewn with 4-0 absorbable sutures in a running fashion. The two ends of the ileum are anastomosed in side-to-side (functional end-to-end) fashion, by using a running handsewn two-layer technique with an inner layer of 4-0 absorbable sutures and an outer layer of 4-0 absorbable or nonabsorbable sutures; alternatively, the GIA stapler can be used to create the jejunoileostomy. On completion of the anastomosis, patency is assured. The mesenteric defect is reapproximated with 3-0 nonabsorbable sutures in a running or interrupted fashion. The abdomen is thoroughly irrigated, and any remaining bleeding is stopped. The incision is closed in standard fashion.

Although the donor team is oversewing the ileocolic vessels, the recipient team is perfusing the graft at the back table, through the ICA, with University of Wisconsin (UW) solution (100 to 300 mL at 4°C) until the graft can blanch and the perfusate is clear. The graft is now ready for implantation.

In contrast to LD kidney, pancreas, and liver grafts, LD bowel grafts have not (yet) been procured laparoscopically. In fact, the laparoscopic approach may not present a significant advantage with LD bowel grafts, because the size of the incision needed to safely extract the graft is about the same size of the incision that is made for open procurement. The only cosmetic advantage of the laparoscopic approach would be graft procurement through a Pfannenstiel incision, but even so, three to four trocar incisions (each 5 to 15 mm) are also needed. From a technical point of view, laparoscopic feasibility has already been demonstrated in a pig model with procurement of 200 cm of proximal jejunum.[9]

## LD Intestinal and Liver Donation

Combined intestinal and liver transplants have only been done for pediatric recipients, requiring procurement of liver segments 2 and 3 and the ileal graft. For adult recipients, combined procurement of a full liver lobe and the ileal graft currently does not appear safe, given the magnitude of the LD procedure (see Chapter 29.3).

If the recipient is to undergo a combined LD intestinal and liver transplant, the donor operation becomes logistically and technically more complex. Because of the recipient's advanced liver disease, the liver should be procured and transplanted first. Only if the recipient remains stable throughout the liver transplant procedure can the intestinal procurement and transplant ensue.

If the recipient is not stable throughout the transplant procedure, the donor's incision should be closed; the intestinal transplant can then be rescheduled for a later time (preferably, within the first 2 weeks after the liver transplant) when the recipient is stable. The recipient could instead undergo an intestinal transplant from a deceased donor (DD) if a graft became available shortly after the liver transplant; however, if the liver and intestinal grafts are from different donors, the grafted liver may no longer offer immunologic protection for the intestinal graft.

The technical aspects of procurement for a combined LD intestinal and liver transplant are not significantly different from those for an isolated liver transplant (Chapter 29.32) or for a bowel transplant alone. One difference, however, is that the donor undergoes an upper midline incision between the xiphoid process and umbilicus for procurement of liver segments 2 and 3; if intestinal procurement proceeds in the same session, the upper midline incision may be slightly extended a few centimeters below the umbilicus. If intestinal procurement is delayed, the upper midline incision is closed in standard fashion (using interrupted sutures for the fascia); if the donor were to undergo intestinal procurement several days later, a periumbilical incision is made, thus extending all or portions of the previous midline incision a few centimeters below the umbilicus. Although combined LD intestinal and liver procurement for a pediatric recipient is of no greater magnitude than a right donor lobectomy, anesthesia time is usually longer (because of the need to wait until the liver transplant is completed and until a decision is made about proceeding with intestinal procurement in the same session). The disadvantage of sequential liver and intestinal procurement is that the donor is exposed to operative stress twice and to the risks of non-organ-specific complications (eg, wound infections, pneumonia, thrombosis) of two major surgical procedures. Only a handful of combined LD intestinal and liver transplants have been performed (at the university hospitals of Kyoto, Illinois, and Minnesota). At the time of this writing (August 2006), only one such case has been described in the literature so far.[10]

## POSTOPERATIVE CARE

The postoperative care of an intestinal LD is not different from that of any patient undergoing a small-bowel resection for benign or malignant disease. The donor is transferred from the postanesthesia control unit (PACU) to a regular floor within 2 hours after surgery and is placed on intravenous fluid and electrolyte substitution. The nasogastric tube is usually removed within a few days, once bowel activity is noted.

When oral intake is tolerated, the donor is discharged to home, usually between postoperative day 4 and day 7. Initial diarrhea (up to five bowel movements) is uncommon, but if it occurs, usually resolves on its own within the first 2 to 8 weeks after surgery[1,11,12]; rarely is the use of Imodium indicated. The donor should undergo vitamin $B_{12}$ assays (1, 6, and 12 months postdonation) to ascertain normal vitamin $B_{12}$ absorption. Donor weight loss has not been reported in many series[1,5,6,13,14]; in others, it has been minimal (range 0–5kg).[8] Onset of new food intolerance has not been reported.[8] With the standardized procurement technique (above), postoperative complications—except for wound infections[8]—have not been reported. However, if the terminal ileum, the ileocecal valve, and the cecum were procured, vitamin $B_{12}$ injections at regular intervals are required.[5]

For combined intestinal and liver LDs, postoperative recovery is delayed. Discharge plans are usually not made until 7 to 10 days after surgery. Otherwise, their postoperative care is the same as for intestinal LDs.

## References

1. Gruessner RWG, Sharp HL. Living-related intestinal transplantation: first report of a standardized surgical technique. *Transplantation* 1997;64:1605–1607.

2. Alican F, Hardy JJD, Cayirli M, et al. Intestinal transplantation: laboratory experience and report of a clinical case. *Am J Surg* 1971;121L:150–159.

3. Fortner JG, Sichuk G, Litwin SD, Beattie EJ, Jr. Immunological responses to an intestinal allograft with HL-A-identical donor-recipient. *Transplantation* 1972;14:531–535.

4. Delta E, Schroeder P, Gebhardt H, et al. Successful clinical small bowel transplantation: report of a case. *Transplantation* 1989;3:89–91.

5. Morris JA, Johnson DL, Rimmer JAP, et al. Identical twin small bowel transplant after resection of abdominal desmoid tumor. *Trans Proc* 1996;28:2731–2732.

6. Pollard SG, Lodge P, Selvakumar S, et al. Living related small bowel transplantation: the first United Kingdom case. *Trans Proc* 1996;28:2733.

7. Pollard SG. Intestinal transplantation: living related. *Brit Med Bull* 1977;53:868–878.

8. Testa G, Panara F, Schena S, et al. Living related small bowel transplantation: donor surgical technique. Ann Surg 2004; 5: 779–784.

9. Kim WW, Gagner M, Fukuyama S, et al. Laparoscopic harvesting of small bowel graft for small bowel transplantation. Surg Endosc 2002; 16: 1786–1789.

10. Testa G, Holterman M, John E, et al. Combined living donor liver/small bowel transplantation. *Transplantation* 2005;79:1401–1404.

11. Lee MD, Kim DG, Ahn ST, et al. Isolated small bowel transplantation from a living-related donor at the Catholic University of Korea—a case report of rejection-free course. *Yonsei Med J* 2004;45:1198–1202.

12. Benedetti E, Testa G, Sankary H, et al. Successful treatment of trauma-induced short bowel syndrome with early living related bowel transplantation. *J Trauma* 2004;57:164–170.

13. Morel P, Kadry Z, Charbonnet P, et al. Paediatric living related intestinal-transplantation between two monozygotic twins: a 1-year follow-up. *Lancet* 2004;355:723–724.

14. Fujimoto Y, Uemoto S, Inomata Y, et al. Small bowel transplantation using grafts from living-related donor. Two case reports. *Transpl Int* 2000;13(Suppl 1): S179–S184.

# 33.3  MORBIDITY, MORTALITY, LONG-TERM OUTCOME

*Giuliano Testa, MD, Fabrizio Panaro, MD, Enrico Benedetti, MD*

## INTRODUCTION

Living donation of abdominal organs is practiced in many transplant centers around the world. The necessity of using living donor organ is clear and well explained in other chapters of this book. For kidney transplantation, living donors have become the greater source of organs in the United States.[1] In Asia the great majority of renal and liver transplants are performed with living donor organs. It is evident that even if not universally accepted, living donation has become part of the modern practice of transplantation. Living donor organs work as well and better than cadaveric ones, and the primary issue remains the one of not harming, neither short nor even more importantly long term, the donor.[2,3]

Although the experience with renal and liver donation is decennial and vast, the same cannot be said for intestinal donation. Until March 2003 only 32 cases of intestinal living donor transplantation had been reported to the Intestinal Transplant Registry (ITR).[4] In the world literature, only case reports can be found, and there is one single article that specifically studies the outcome of the intestinal donors.[5,6]

Outside of the experience of the University of Illinois, which has the largest series of living donor intestinal transplantation and where a standardized technique has been used, most of the other centers have reported single cases with different surgical approaches.[7–9]

The living donor operation for intestinal transplantation has been performed by resection of part of the jejunum (literature) or part of the ileum (literature).

The short-term complications are the same as those for any major abdominal operation involving intestinal or colonic surgery. The major difference with the aforementioned surgeries is that no pathology is present in the bowel and that the donor is perfectly and electively prepared for the surgery.

Although electivity and perfect preparation do not totally eliminate the general complications of any major surgery, including infections, deep vein thrombosis, and even death, they definitely limit to the lowest possible chance their occurrence.

Peculiar to the small bowel resection are the complications of dehiscence of the intestinal anastomosis, volvulus, and prolonged ileus or small bowel obstruction due to adhesions.

None of the aforementioned complications have been reported in the University of Illinois series published in 2003[6]; neither has been seen by the authors in any of the donors operated on thereafter.

The closest possible reference to the above data could be extrapolated by a review of the literature on exploratory laparotomy for abdominal trauma or for colorectal surgery.

The incidence of early or late small bowel obstruction due to adhesions after intestinal surgery for cancer or inflammatory bowel disease has been reported to be between 6% and 9.5%.[10–12] In the trauma literature, the incidence of early small bowel obstruction after exploratory laparotomy has been reported to be between 4% and 14%.[13–15] Overall the incidence and risk of early postoperative small bowel obstruction has been reported at 0.69%.[16]

Intestinal anastomosis dehiscence is reported to occur at an incidence between 2% and 5% in patients with preexisting conditions. Factors like malnutrition, older age, cancer, and medical conditions do favor the occurrence of anastomosis dehiscence (see references 1–4 of the Behrman article). The trauma literature reports an incidence of 1.8% of dehiscence of a small bowel anastomosis in patients with an average age similar to the one of the intestinal donors and presumably in healthy conditions before the trauma. It also points out that the dehiscence is definitely more prone to occur in patients with heavy blood loss and large fluid requirements, conditions that do not occur in intestinal donors.[17]

Unplanned readmissions to the hospital within 90 days from discharge after colorectal surgery have an incidence of 9%, as published in a study in 2001.[18] The risk of ventral hernia after laparotomy ranges from 11% to 20% depending on the type of surgery, its indication, and electivity.[19]

All the above data cannot directly reflect the conditions of an intestinal resection for living donation where no other co-morbid factors may favor the development of complications. Nonetheless, because of the lack of data on intestinal donors, exploratory laparotomy for inflammatory bowel disease, cancer, and trauma appear to be the closest surgical examples from which to draw indications on the potential incidence of complications after segmental intestinal resection for living donation.

This predicted incidence compares favorably with the reported incidence of complication for living liver and kidney donation. In the kidney donor population the complication rate has been reported from 5% to 265 for the laparoscopic approach and from 3% to 38% for the open approach.[20]

For donors of the liver the complication rate varied from 28% for donors of the right lobe to 7.5% for donors of the left lateral segment in a review of 1,508 donors from five Asian countries.[21] An incidence of 14% of serious complications and a readmission incidence of 8.5% was reported in a publication reporting the result of a survey of the transplant centers performing living donor liver transplantation in the United States.[22]

In the experience of the authors of this chapter, only 1 out of 16 patients, 6.5%, suffered an early complication in the form of a wound infection. No long-term complications have been encountered at the present time. Overall it seems that even in the worst scenario the overall incidence of complications after intestinal resection for living donation should not be higher than 5% to 10%.

Almost all donors have manifested a temporary chance in bowel habits. In the donors we have personally followed, the change related to consistency and frequency of the stool has been limited at a maximum period of 2 to 3 months after the intestinal resection. The average number of bowel movements experienced by the donors was 1.5 per day. The weight loss the donors experienced was related to the postoperative decrease in food intake and not to malabsorption due to excessive diarrhea. Practically a moderate weight decreased was experienced by only three donors for an average of 2.8 kg and rapidly regained once the oral intake returned to normal.

## THE LONG-TERM COMPLICATIONS

Sixteen donors underwent intestinal resection at our program. In all cases, the ileocecal valve, in continuity with a segment of 20 cm of terminal ileum and a least 60% of small bowel, has been preserved in the donor.[6] The mean follow-up is 33 months (range 1–86 months. Eleven donors have a follow-up longer than 18 months (mean 45 months, range 18–86 months).

At the present time no patient has been readmitted to the hospital or has suffered partial or total small bowel obstruction. Since mechanical ileus due to adhesions may occur many years after the surgery, it is still possible that some patients will suffer from this complication in the future. No patients have manifested persistent changes of bowel habits and or signs of malabsorption.

Specifically we have monitored the hemoglobin level and the red cell MCV to exclude macrocytic anemia due to vitamin $B_{12}$ deficiency. None of the donors in our series have manifested macrocytic anemia, and most of the donors have had vitamin $B_{12}$ levels routinely checked and always found being within normal range. One report in the literature describes the living donor graft consisting of distal ileum, ileocecal valve, and a portion of the cecum.[7] In this case the donor suffered from prolonged diarrhea and dysvitaminosis. These complications have not occurred in our donors. In fact when the operation is performed leaving at least 20 cm of terminal ileum and the ileocecal valve in place like in the donor of our series, the risk of vitamin $B_{12}$ deficiency is eliminated and the bowel habits return to normal.

The data available to us show that distal ileum resection with preservation of 20 cm of distal ileum prior to the ileocecal valve, and at least 60% of the entire length of the small intestine is a safe operation in terms of both short- and long-term complications and donor recovery. Living donor small bowel transplantation assures an optimal equilibrium between donor discomfort, risk, and return

**TABLE 33.3-1**
## THE DONOR FOLLOW-UP

| | |
|---|---|
| N° Donor | 10 |
| M/F | 5/5 |
| Age | 31 years old (25–53 years) |
| Races | 8 Caucasian and 2 African Americans |
| Preoperative vascular analysis | 5 3D-CT-scan; 5 Angiography |
| Operative time Range (min) | 118 (95–175) |
| Length of the graft Range (cm) | 150–200 cm |
| Operative complications Need of blood transfusion (U) | 0 0 |
| Postoperative complications | 1 wound infection on POD 5, treated conservatively |
| Postoperative hospital stay Range (days) | 3–5 |
| Length of follow-up Range (months) | 6–80 |
| Bowel movement Range (n/day) | 1.5 SBM/day; range 1–3 |
| Weight decreased Range (kg) | 2.8 kg (0–5 kg). |

**TABLE 33.3-2**
## LIVING DONOR MONITORING[31,32]

- Clinical assessment: 1 week, 2 weeks, 1 month, 3 months, 6 months, 1 year
- GI x-ray: 1 month later
- Laboratory assessment (RBC, WBC, Hb, PTL, total bilirubin, Vit. B-12, MCV, Sideremy, transferrinemy, ferritinemy, fecal examination): 1 week, 1 month, 6 months, 1 year
- Psychologic and social worker assessment (quality of life, social work, and psychological change): 1 month, 6 months

to normal life and functional result in the recipient. Having proved that no functional deficiency are present after the ileal resection in the donor, the only possible long-term complication remains mechanical ileum due to postoperative adhesions (see Table 33.3-1 and Table 33.3-2).

## COMMENTS

Living donor intestinal transplantation is a relatively new procedure, and as all new operations that involve living donors, it is being carefully evaluated and closely followed.[6,7,23] Among the initial questions were (1) how much bowel graft is needed for success after transplantation? and (2) how much can be left in the donor to have a safe margin to avoid malabsorption? Two other reports of attempts at jejunum transplantation resulted in vascular complications due to complex vascular reconstruction.[6,7] In yet another report of a living intestinal transplantation, the ileum with the distal superior mesenteric artery (SMA) and vein were used, but no information was given regarding the very distal terminal ileum and blood supply to the remaining ileocecal valve and cecum.[6] It has

been just well demonstrated that intestinal grafts develop early adsorption adaptations.[5,24] On the basis of all these considerations, we decided to use 150 to 200 cm of small bowel graft resecting primarily the ileum, respecting the last 15 to 20 cm before the ileocecal valve. We found that a graft of this size is sufficient to obtain TPN independence and avoids the complications associated with the resection of the terminal ileum and ileocecal valve in the donor.

Another factor that favors the ileum over the jejunum as a graft is based on the vascular anatomy of the bowel. The vascular anatomy of the jejunum is more complicated than that of the ileum, and therefore the dissection in the donor and the reconstruction of the graft on the back table following the resection are more laborious. The donor's specific anatomic considerations also guide the resection of the distal ileum. It is important to preserve the descending branch of the right colic artery to provide adequate vascular supply to the distal terminal ileum, the ileocecal valve, and the cecum. We resect the SMA after the takeoff of the vascular branch for the cecum. This protects the donor ileocecal valve and the cecum from ischemic injury.[6]

Last but not least is the question of the real risk for the donor during and after the operation. The first problem concerns the risk of malabsorption. The preservation of the last 15 to 20 cm of the terminal ileum and ileocecal valve prevents lipid and/or vitamin $B_{12}$ malabsorption and does not accelerate intestinal transit time in the donor. Additional risks are those correlated with surgical intestinal resection (general anesthesia, bowel anastomotic obstruction or leakage, peritoneal adhesions, incisional hernias, increase of risk for the donor in future bowel resection or laparotomies; see Figure 33.3-1). In the worldwide experience, none of these potential complications have been reported to date.[4–8,24–28]

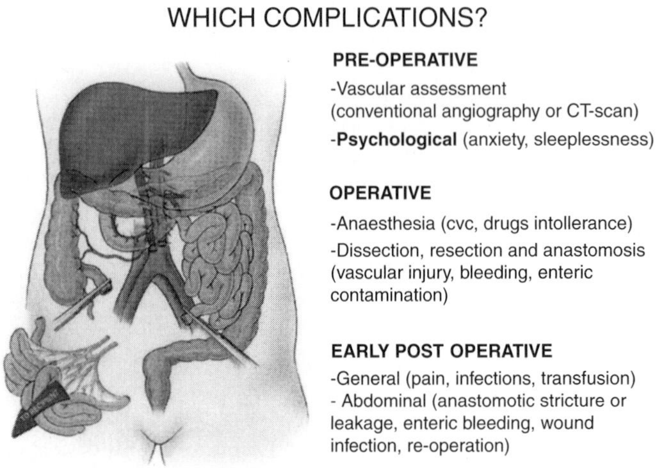

## WHICH COMPLICATIONS?

**PRE-OPERATIVE**
-Vascular assessment (conventional angiography or CT-scan)
-**Psychological** (anxiety, sleeplessness)

**OPERATIVE**
-Anaesthesia (cvc, drugs intollerance)
-Dissection, resection and anastomosis (vascular injury, bleeding, enteric contamination)

**EARLY POST OPERATIVE**
-General (pain, infections, transfusion)
- Abdominal (anastomotic stricture or leakage, enteric bleeding, wound infection, re-operation)

**FIGURE 33.3-1**

Donor's Complications

But for a better evaluation of the donor risk, a longer period of follow-up (>10 years) is clearly necessary.[4,29,30]

## References

1. United Network Organ Sharing. Available at www.unos.org. Accessed August 2005.

2. Manzer J. Transplant group to study altruism of kidney donors. *Medical Post* 2000;36(2).

3. Arlene Judith Klotzko, JD, Mphil. The Good Samaritan as Organ Donor. Medscape Transplantation.

4. The Intestinal Transplant Registry. Availableat:www.intestinaltransplant.org. Accessed January 7, 2002.

5. Jaffe B. Current indications for and prospects of living related intestinal transplantation. *Curr Opin Organ Transplant* 2000;5:290–294.

6. Testa G, Panaro F, Schena S, et al. Living related small bowel transplantation: donor surgical technique. *Ann Surg* 2004;240(5):779–784.

7. Gruessner RW, Sharp HL. Living-related intestinal transplantation: First report of a standardized surgical technique. *Transplantation* 1997;11: 271–274.

8. Pollard SG. Intestinal transplantation: living related. *Br Med Bull* 1997;53(4):868–878.

9. Wu GS, Wang WZ, Song WL, et al. Living-related small bowel transplant: the first case in China. *Transplant Proc* 2000;32(6):1218.

10. Edna TH, Bjerkeset T. Small bowel obstruction in patients previously operated on for colorectal cancer. *Eur J Surg* 1998;164(8):587–592.

11. Ellozy SH, Harris MT, Bauer JJ, et al. Early postoperative small-bowel obstruction: a prospectiove evaluation in 242 consecutive abdominal operations. *Dis Colon Rectum* 2002;45(9):1214–1217.

12. Duepree HJ, Senagore AJ, Delaney CP, et al. Does means of access affect the incidence of small bowel obstruction and ventral hernia after bowel resection? Laparoscopy versus laparotomy. *J Am Coll Surg* 2003;97(2):177–181.

13. Tortella BJ, Lavery RF, Chandrakantan A, et al. Incidence and risk factors for early small bowel obstruction after celiotomy for penetrating abdominal trauma. *Am Surg* 1995;61(11):956–958.

14. Henderson VJ, Organ CH Jr, Smith RS. Negative trauma celiotomy. *Am Surg* 1993;59(6):365–370.

15. Weigelt JA, Kingman RG. Complications of negative lapartomoy for trauma. *Am J Surg* 1988;156(6):544–547.

16. Stewart RM, Page CP, Brender J, et al. The incidence and risk of early postoperative small bowel obstruiction. A cohort study. *Am J Surg* 1987;154(6):643–647.

17. Behrman SW, Bertken KA, Stefanacci HA, et al. Breakdown of intestinal repair after lapartomy for trauma: incidence, risk factors, and strategies for prevention. *J Trauma* 1998;45(2):227–231.

18. Azimuddin K, Rosen L, Reed JF 3rd, et al. Readmissions after colorectal surgery cannot be predicted. *Dis Colon Rectum* 2001;44(7):942–946.

19. Luijendijk RW, Hop WC, van den Tol MP, et al. A comparison of suture repair with mesh repair for incisional hernia. *N Engl J Med* 2000;343(6):392–398.

20. Tooher RL, Rao MM, Scott DF, et al. A systematic review of laparoscopic live-donor nephrectomy. *Transplantation* 2004;78(3):404–414.

21. Lo CM, Fan ST, Liu CL, et al. Hepatic venoplasty in living-donor liver transplantation using right lobe graft with middle hepatic vein. *Transplantation* 2003;75(3):358–360.

22. Brown RS Jr, Russo MW, Lai M, et al. A survery of liver transplantation from living adult donors on the United States. *N Engl J Med* 2003;348(9):818–825.

23. Tzoracoleftherakis E, Cohen M, Sileri P, et al. Small bowel transplantation and staged abdominal wall reconstruction after shotgun injury. *J Trauma* 2000;53(4):770–776.

24. Benedetti E, Baum C, Cicalese L, et al. Progressive functional adaptation of segmental bowel graft from living related donor. *Transplantation* 2001;27(7):569–571.

25. Cicalese L, Rastellini C, Sileri P, et al. Segmental living related small bowel transplantation in adults. *J Gastrointest Surg* 2001;5(2): 168–173.

26. Fujimoto Y, Uemoto S, Inomata Y, et al. Small bowel transplantation using grafts from living-related donors. Two case reports. *Transpl Int* 2000 ;13(Suppl 1):S179–S184.

27. Taguchi T, Suita S. Segmental small-intestinal transplantation: a comparison of jejunal and ileal grafts. *Surgery* 2002;131(1 Suppl):S294–S300.

28. Margreiter R. Living-donor pancreas and small-bowel transplantation. *Langenbecks Arch Surg* 1999;384(6):544–549.

29. Broering DC, Wilms C, Bok P, et al. Evolution of donor morbidity in living related liver transplantation: a single-center analysis of 165 cases. *Ann Surg* 2004;240(6):1013–1024.

30. Fryer J, Angelos P. Is there a role for living donor intestine transplants? *Prog Transplant* 2004;14(4):321–329.

31. Ghobrial RM, Farmer DG, Amersi F, et al. Advances in pediatric liver and intestinal transplantation. *Am J Surg* 2000;180:328–334.

32. Dudrick SJ, Wilmore DW, Vars HM. Long term total parenteral nutrition with growth, development and positive nitrogen balance. *Surgery* 1968;169:134–142.

# INTESTINAL TRANSPLANTATION – THE RECIPIENT

## 34.1   SELECTION AND WORKUP

*Enrico Benedetti, MD, Stefano DiDomenico, MD, Giuliano Testa, MD*

## INTRODUCTION

Intestinal transplantation (ITx) is the physiological alternative to lifelong dependency on total parenteral nutrition (TPN) for patients with intestinal failure. However, mostly because of the historically suboptimal results of bowel transplantation, TPN remains the mainstay therapy for short bowel syndrome. Only patients with irreversible intestinal failure who are experiencing life-threatening complications of TPN are currently considered appropriate candidates for bowel transplantation.

The indications for living donor bowel transplantation are in general the same as cadaver bowel transplant. Registry data suggest that patient and graft survival are similar regardless of the source of the graft.[1] Using a living donor can potentially help to reduce the mortality on the waiting list, which is particularly high for candidates less than 5 years of age (up to 35%) according to United Network of Organ Sharing (UNOS) data.[2] Furthermore, the recent development of a viable technique for combined liver–bowel transplant from a living donor in children offers further hope for a growing role of living donors in the field of intestinal transplantation.[3]

In special circumstances, such as the availability of an identical twin as the donor, a living related bowel transplant can be offered before occurrence of TPN complications with a high grade of success.[4] Furthermore, intestinal transplant candidates with human leukocyte antigen (HLA)-identical potential donors should be preferentially considered for living donor bowel transplant.

The goals of the patient evaluation for intestinal transplantation are to determine the cause and extent of the intestinal failure, to evaluate any associated organ dysfunctions, and to determine that appropriate therapy, including other surgical or medical options, have been already offered to the patient. Once the candidacy to bowel transplant has been established, the patient will need to be counseled about the potential advantages and disadvantages of living donor versus cadaver intestinal transplantation, at least in centers offering both options.

## CAUSES OF INTESTINAL FAILURE

Intestinal failure (IF) can be caused by a reduced surface area or intestinal mass as a result of massive surgical resections or anatomic loss of intestine due to congenital anomalies; indeed intestinal failure may occur despite a normal length as a result of chronic mucosal dysfunction or severe motility disorders (Table 34.1-1).

## INTESTINAL FAILURE IN PEDIATRIC PATIENTS

The majority of candidates to intestinal transplantation are children. As of March 2005, according to current UNOS data, out of a total of 189 patients listed for intestinal transplant in the United States, 137 (72%) were less than 18 years of age and of those 88 were less than 5 years of age.[2] These data reflect the fact that long-term TPN is not as well tolerated in pediatric patients compared to adult patients, and the risk of life-threatening complications is increased in the pediatric population. To follow, a short profile of the most important causes of intestinal failure in pediatric patients is summarized.

Volvulus results from a mal-rotation of the bowel around a fixed point formed by congenital or adhesive bands or from abnormal motility along the mesenteric axis. Extensive bowel resection is usually needed because ischemic necrosis secondary to vascular compromise. Mal rotation with volvulus is often diagnosed within the first 2 months, but may occur at any age. Volvulus has been historically one of the leading indications to bowel transplant in children.

**TABLE 34.1-1**
## CAUSES OF INTESTINAL FAILURE

| | Pediatric | Adult |
|---|---|---|
| **Reduced Surface Area** | Gastroschisis | Crohn's disease |
| | Small bowel atresia | Trauma |
| | Midgut volvulus | Vascular accident |
| | Necrotizing enterocolitis (NEC) | Volvulus |
| | Crohn's disease | Familial polyposis |
| | Gardener's syndrome | Gardener's syndrome |
| | Vascular accident | Desmoid tumor |
| **Motility Dis.** | Hirschprung's disease | |
| | Pseudoobstruction syndrome | |
| | Megacystis microcolon syndrome | |
| **Mucosal Dis.** | Microvillus inclusion disease | Radiation enteritis |
| | Tufting enteropathy | |

Gastroschisis occurs when variable length of the intestine and occasionally part of the liver, without a peritoneal sac, herniates through an abdominal wall defect located to the right of the umbilical cord. Although surgical treatment is frequently successful in repairing the defect and preserving the intestine, occasionally extensive small bowel resection becomes necessary. The disease has a higher incidence in premature babies and may be associated with stenoses or atresias of jejunum or ileum.[5] Gastroschisis is another leading indication to bowel transplant in children.

Atresia and stenoses are congenital defects of the small intestine. Duodenal atresia results when the lumen fails to recanalize during week 8 to 10 of gestation and is associated with prematurity in 25% of the cases. Jejunoileal atresias are more common, with most cases involving complete obstruction of the distal ileum and proximal jejunum. An association with common variable immune deficiency has been reported in infants with intestinal atresia.[6]

Necrotizing enterocolitis (NEC) is an inflammatory disorder that occurs more commonly in premature infants and constitutes the most common surgical emergency in neonates. The mortality can be as high as 44% in infants of less than 1,500 g of weight. Survivors are at risk for short-gut syndrome in consequence of surgical resection and ischemia. NEC is associated with bronchopulmonary dysplasia and intraventricular hemorrhage that require careful pulmonary and neurologic evaluation during the evaluation for ITX. Patients with necrotizing enterocolitis historically have had a poor prognosis after ITx with a survival rate of less than 30% at 1-year postoperative.[7] However, more recent data from the University of Miami suggest a better outcome with 1- and 3-year patient survival rate of 60%, comparable to results obtained in other indications.[8]

Long segment Hirschprung's disease is a common indication for ITx in children. In this condition there is a congenital absence of intramural nerve plexus (agangliosis) resulting in a functional obstruction of the bowel with dilatation of the non affected gut. The length of the intestine involved in this disease varies and the resection of an extensive aganglionic portion may lead to intestine failure. It is important to assess motility of the residual bowel and stomach during the transplant evaluation since pseudo-obstruction may be present. Hirschprung's disease is associated with other anomalies including ventricular septal defect, deformities-agenesis of kidney, and hydrocephalus.[9]

Chronic intestinal pseudo-obstruction is a heterogeneous group of disorders in which ineffective intestinal contractions lead to intestinal obstructions in absence of an anatomical obstruction. It is often associated with urinary bladder neuromuscular disease and immunodeficiencies. An accurate pretransplant study of motility and length of residual intestine as well as urological evaluation to establish further organ involvement is essential.[10,11]

Megacystis microcolon intestinal hypoperistalsis syndrome is a poorly understood disease affecting the smooth muscle of the gastrointestinal and urinary tract. The lack of motility of the intestine, despite the presence of ganglionic cells, determines the inability of the patients to tolerate enteral feeding and the need for long-term TPN. The disease is almost uniformly fatal within the first year of life. Recently, multivisceral transplantation has been performed with some success in three children affected by the syndrome, with at least one patient achieving long-term survival.[12]

Microvillus inclusion disease (MID) is a rare autosomal recessive disorder of the brush border of the enterocyte that causes severe secretory diarrhea. Diagnosis must be confirmed through electron microscopy of intestinal biopsies, which reveal severe atrophy without crypt injury and absence or hypoplasia of the microvilli. Patients affected by congenital MID have an extremely reduced life expectancy with a 1-year survival rate of less than 25%, whereas patients with atypical or late-onset MID have a better prognosis. Given the good success rate of small bowel transplant in MID, it is recommended that once the diagnosis of congenital MID has been made and the child is in a eutrophic phase under TPN, ITx should be considered without delay to avoid hepatic failure. Conversely, patients with a late-onset or atypical form of MID should not be automatically scheduled for small bowel transplant. The individual course of the disease will help to decide whether an individual child is a candidate for ITx.[13,14]

Intestinal epithelial dysplasia ("tufting enteropathy") is an epithelial disorder of the intestinal mucosa involving both small intestine and colon that cause intractable diarrhea and profound mal-absorption. Several cases of intestinal epithelial dysplasia have been reported as being associated with choanal atresia, rectal and esophageal atresia.[15]

## Intestinal Failure in Adult Patients

Although TPN is better tolerated in adults, their prospects for successful weaning from parenteral nutrition are probably reduced. Adults with less than 35 cm of residual jejunum have no more than a 50% chance of being successfully weaned from TPN, even in the presence of intact colon.[16] Once an adult patient is listed for ITx, the mortality on the list remains substantial, being estimated in the order of 11% in the United States.[2] The main causes of IF in adults are briefly described in the following paragraphs.

Crohn's Disease is a chronic inflammatory disease potentially involving any location of the alimentary tract with a propensity for the distal small bowel and the proximal colon. The disease may be severe and widespread, requiring multiple bowel resections and resulting in IF. Extra intestinal manifestations of the disease are common, and the presence of amyloidosis, primary sclerosing cholangitis, autoimmune hepatitis, and renal disease and prothrombotic states must be carefully considered during the evaluation.[17–19]

Intestinal vascular insufficiency leading to massive bowel resection may occur as consequence of thromboembolic occlusion of the superior mesenteric artery. Severe intestinal ischemia may also complicate a direct injury of the mesenteric vessels due to trauma, or gastrointestinal involvement of systemic vasculitis such as Churg-Strauss syndrome.[20] Less frequently, intestinal ischemia may be due to mesenteric vein thrombosis secondary to hypercoagulable states such as factor V mutation, antiphospholipidies syndrome, protein S or C deficiencies, or antithrombin III deficiency.[21]

Gastrointestinal neoplasms can necessitate extensive gut resections leading to permanent intestinal failure. ITx is indicated only for relatively benign tumors such mesenteric desmoid tumors, Gardener's Syndrome, and other diffuse polypoid syndromes.[22]

Radiation therapy may induce mucosal damage with villous atrophy and progressive fibrosis. As a result, patients can develop bloody diarrhea and mal-absorption syndrome with protein-losing enteropathy.[23] Of course, ITx can be considered only if the primary neoplastic disease originally treated with radiation is radically cured with no evidence of recurrence for at least 5 years.

## Limits of Intestinal Adaptation

In the majority of adult and pediatric patients, IF is a consequence of extensive small bowel resections. Intestinal adaptation is a compensatory process by which the remaining functioning bowel improves its ability to absorb nutrients by structural and motility changes. Structural adaptation increases intestinal surface area by slight lengthening, but more importantly, by villous elongation and augmentation in diameter; intestinal motor activity is also modulated in this process leading to prolonged transit time.[24,25] Intestinal adaptation starts soon after resection and evolves over 1 to 2 years period before being completed. Irreversible IF will ensue if the compensatory process will prove unable to allow weaning from TPN.[26]

Several factors are important determinants in the functional adaptation process and clinical outcome: presence of the colon, presence of the ileocecal valve, length and health of remaining bowel, presence of co-morbidities, and age. Newborns and children have great adaptation potentialities. However, about 10% of the children started early in life on TPN are unable to be weaned off completely and die of complication of long term TPN. Furthermore, if a child has not been weaned off by age 3, the chance of successful discontinuation of TPN is minimal.[27] Risk factors for failure to adapt include a remaining small intestinal length of < 30 to 40 cm, absence of the ileocecal valve, resection of some colon and minimal tolerance of enteral nutrition within the fist few months following resection. Although adaptation to full enteral nutrition has been reported with as little as 10 cm of remnant intestine, infants with duodenum, or at most 10 cm of jejunum and no ileocecal valve, have virtually no chance of survival even with optimal parenteral nutrition. In the particular case of congenital intractable mucosal disorders, the IF never resolves or improves sufficiently to permit termination of TPN.[28] As previously mentioned, adults have an inferior degree of intestinal adaptation. Patients with residual bowel length >100 cm in the absence of an intact and functional colon or > 60 cm in the presence of functional colon have high probability of weaning TPN, whereas patients with a small bowel length of < 50 cm and end-enterostomy have low rate of TPN weaning and poor survival prospective with 5-year survival rates of 44% to 57%.[29]

Surgical "lengthening" procedures may improve the outcome of patients with chronic IF but can be applied only in a subset of them. Nevertheless patients referred to an intestinal transplant center must be evaluated regarding length and functionality of the remnant bowel in order to identify the best surgical approach. In the presence of established TPN-related liver disease, all the above-mentioned surgical procedures may not be indicated and referral for transplant should be immediately initiated.

## Limits of Total Parenteral Nutrition (TPN)

TPN remains the standard therapy for chronic IF with a survival rate between 85% to 90% at 5 years in patients tolerating TPN at home.

However, complications of TPN can damage the quality of life of these patients and lead to a significantly lower survival rate.[28,30] ITx is the treatment of choice for patients whose life expectancy is jeopardizing by the life-threatening complications of TPN.

Hepatic complications can present as a broad spectrum of pathologic entities, including steatosis, cholestasis, steatohepatitis, fibrosis, and cirrhosis.[31,32] About 15% of patients receiving TPN for more than 1 year develop end-stage liver disease which is associated with 100% mortality within 2 years of onset. In children the incidence of liver disease is higher, especially in patients with > 30 to 40 cm of remnant bowel developing jaundice soon after birth with no improvement by age 3 to 4 months.[33,34] Liver disease remains the leading reason to perform ITx in children. Steatosis

and cholestasis can resolve after isolated bowel transplantation, but the presence of bridging fibrosis with architectural distortion or cirrhosis mandates combined liver–bowel transplantation.[35]

Sepsis is a common complication of protracted parenteral nutrition with an average of one expected episode/year/patient.[36] The most common source of the sepsis is the central line used for TPN. A single episode of life-treating sepsis does not constitute an indication for small bowel transplantation. However, recurrent septic episodes along with the development of metastasis infectious foci, such as endocarditis, may be considered a reasonable indication to ITx.

Loss of central venous access becomes an indication for bowel transplantation when it is jeopardizing the ability to provide parenteral nutrition and the possible post transplant recovery period. In children, ITx is indicated when two of the four available standard accesses, the subclavian and jugular veins, have been lost to thrombosis. In older children, and by extension, in adult patients, ITx is indicated when three of the six available standard sites, jugular, subclavian, and femoral veins have been lost.[28] In patients referred for this particular indication, a careful hematological evaluation for the presence of defects of the fibrinolytic system is mandatory.

## Indications and Contraindications for Intestinal Transplantation

As previously stated, ITx is reserved for those patients with permanent IF with no prospects of discontinuation of TPN that are experiencing life threatening complications. Lately, early ITx regardless TPN complications has also been recommended for infants with ultrashort bowel syndrome (with only duodenum or >10 cm of jejunum) since they have virtually no chance of survival.[28]

Standard absolute contraindications, shared with any other organ transplant, include severe and irresolvable cardiac, respiratory, and neurological diseases, multiorgan failure, overwhelming sepsis, and malignancy outside of the intestine.

Relative contraindications are often center-specific and include physical debilitation, poor family support or noncompliance, advanced age, and low weight (children weighing less than 5 kg).

## Evaluation for Intestinal Transplantation

Comprehensive multidisciplinary evaluation of patients with IF is essential to assess appropriate candidacy for transplantation and provide for the best outcome for these complex patients.

The evaluation process must clarify several points:

1. The failure of TPN as well as the failure of nontransplant surgical strategies

2. The need of isolated intestine or combined liver–bowel transplantation

3. the state of remnant intestine and the patency of great vessel

4. The absence of absolute contraindications and the presence of associated diseases that may jeopardize the procedure and postoperative course

This process includes clinical history and assessment, laboratory test, diagnostic procedures focusing on the anatomy and function of GI tract, nutritional state, hepatic function, vascular patency, infection history and immunological status, abdominal compliance, psychosocial issues, and child development (Table 34.1-2).

**TABLE 34.1-2**

## EVALUATION FOR INTESTINAL TRANSPLANTATION

| Component of Evaluation | Tests and Procedures |
| --- | --- |
| Physical examination | Complete physical examination and review of systems |
| Medical and Surgical History | Neonatal history<br>Complete review of all medical and surgical problems and procedures |
| Gastroenterology Assessment | Gastroenterology consultation<br>Upper and lower GI barium studies<br>Gastric emptying study (if indicated)<br>Motility tests (if indicated)<br>Endoscopy (if indicated)<br>Absorption testing (D-xylose, fecal fat)<br>Abdominal ultrasound<br>CT / NMR (if indicated) |
| Hepatic Function Assessment | **Laboratory tests:**<br>Serum bilirubin, ALP, AST, ALT, GGT, albumin, prothrombin time, partial thromboplastin time, ammonia, AFP<br>**Procedure:**<br>Liver eco color doppler<br>Liver biopsy (if indicated) |
| Venous Access Assessment | Ultrasound of great vessels for patency<br>Number of placement of Broviac lines |
| Nutritional Assessment | **Nutritional status:**<br>Height, weight<br>Anthropometric measurements<br>Caloric intake<br>**Nutritional support:**<br>TPN<br>Enteral feeds<br>Oral intake history / aversion / behaviors<br>**Laboratory tests:**<br>Electrolytes, creatinine, bun<br>Triglycerides<br>Zinc |
| Infectious Disease Assessment | History of infection episodes<br>Immunization<br>Laboratory screen: Hepatitis, HIV, CMV, EBV, VZV, measles, mumps and rubella titers<br>Cultures of Blood, Urine, Stool |
| Pulmonary Assessment | Pulmonary consultation (if indicated)<br>Assessment for pulmonary complications:<br>Bronchopulmonary dysplasia<br>Hepatopulmonary syndrome<br>Cystic fibrosis |
| Cardiac Assessment | Cardiology consultation<br>Electrocardiogram<br>Chest X-ray<br>Echocardiogram |
| Anesthesiology Assessment | Anesthesiology consultation<br>Anesthesia history<br>Surgical procedures<br>Drug allergies |
| Developmental Assessment | Child life<br>Child development<br>Speech therapy<br>Occupational therapy |
| Psychosocial Assessment | Psychiatry / Psychology consultation<br>Social Work consultation<br>Clinical nurse specialist consultation |

The nutritional assessment comprises a meticulous feeding history, assessment of caloric intake, and measurement of growth parameters in children. Head circumference is measured in infants and young children with an evaluation of their growth curve. Infants and children should also be evaluated for oral aversion and abnormal oral or eating behaviors, excessive oral intake of water, or bulimia that can be compromise the outcome after ITx.

Caloric intake is estimated through assessment of the TPN solution and enteral and oral feedings. Nutritional state is also evaluated by laboratory tests including electrolytes, blood urea nitrogen, creatinine, calcium, magnesium, phosphorus, zinc, trace elements, cholesterol, triglycerides, and levels of vitamins A, D, E, K, and $B_{12}$.

Hepatic function is evaluated to assess patients for possible TPN-induced liver disease with particular emphasis on the identification of those with irreversible liver failure requiring combined liver–bowel transplantation. Laboratory values related to liver function are routinely obtained, including alanine- aminotransferase, aspartate-aminotransferase, gamma glutamyl transpeptidase, direct and indirect bilirubin, albumin, prothrombin time, partial thromboplastin time, alpha-fetoprotein, platelets, ammonia, and factors V and VII. An ultrasound of the liver and abdomen is obtained to assess liver size, vasculature, and evidence of portal hypertension. An upper endoscopy is obtained to assess the possible presence of varices in cirrhotic patients. A liver biopsy must be routinely performed for any patients with abnormal liver function tests.

### Anatomy and Function of Gastroenteric Tract

Upper and lower GI barium studies are done to clarify the extension and characteristics of the remnant bowel in order to detect any abnormalities that can be surgically corrected and to plan the required surgical anastomosis during ITx. In patients with functional indications for ITx, gastrointestinal motility and gastric emptying are also assessed in details. Esofagogastroduodenal endoscopy, ERCP, and colonoscopy are indicated as required for specific clinical conditions or when the previous tests are inadequate. Absorption is evaluated in patients with longer segments of residual bowel through D-xylose testing and fecal fat absorption to determine whether TPN can be weaned and enteral feedings increased to enhance or promote intestinal adaptation.

### Vascular Patency

Patients may require TPN or intravenous fluids for prolonged periods of time after ITx before being converted to full enteral support. Vascular assessment requires a complete history of the number of intravenous line placements, locations, durations, and reasons for replacement. A baseline ultrasound of the great vessels is obtained to evaluate the splanchnic venous anatomy as well as the internal jugular, subclavian, and iliac veins. However, especially in patients with a history of previous central vein thrombosis, appropriate definition of venous anatomy may require angiography, MRA, or double spiral CT.

Immunologic status: A detailed infectious history is obtained to assess the etiology and frequency of infection, pathogens, response to treatment, and resistant organisms. All potential source of infection after transplantation must be screened. Cultures of the blood, urine, stool, throat, and ascitic fluid may be obtained for bacterial, fungal, or viral pathogens. The presence of hepatitis C virus, hepatitis B virus, and HIV must also be checked as well as IgG and IgM titers for cytomegalovirus (CMV), Epstein–Barr virus (EBV), herpes zoster, varicella, measles, mumps, and rubella.

Indeed, immunologic deficiencies must be excluded with particular attention in children affected by intestinal atresia.

## Abdominal Space

The patient's abdominal cavity may be extremely small or shrunken as a result of decreased or absence of bowel mass. Furthermore, abdominal wall compliance may be compromised by previous surgical interventions or trauma. These situations must be evaluated to plan the appropriate strategy to maximize the chances of obtaining a proper closure of the abdominal cavity. Pretransplant may be appropriate preserving the native bowel to maintain adequate volume and introducing tissue expander to increase the intraabdominal capacity.

Additional consultations may be necessary to complete the evaluation: cardiology to rule out cardiac abnormalities or contraindications to surgery, pulmonology for patients with respiratory complications such as bronchopulmonary dysplasia or cystic fibrosis, urology for kidney and bladder diseases often associated with motility disorders and neonatal indications, neurology for patients with seizure disorders or neurologic impairments.

## Psychosocial Evaluation

A psychosocial evaluation is crucial to assess for the patient's and family's ability to cope with the rigors of the ITx process.

Experienced clinical psychologists or psychiatrists must complete a full psychosocial evaluation of the patient and family focusing on family functioning, physical functioning, coping skills, and family support. This evaluation must be very accurate in the case of children because some cases of Munchausen's by proxy syndrome have been reported in children referred for functional bowel disease.[37] During this evaluation, patients and families must acquire an understanding of posttransplant care requirements and recognize their ability to provide that care. Children undergoing evaluation for ITx may also be assessed from the developmental standpoint by a child development therapist, child life specialist, physical therapist, occupational therapist, and/or speech therapist.

## Specific Indications for Living Donor Intestinal Transplant

The decision to accept a patient as a transplant candidate must be taken in the setting of a multidisciplinary meeting with all the information available. Although the criteria for listing for cadaver donor are the same used for living donor candidates, we believe that some patients may be best served by the living donor option.

In adults, the reported results of living donor intestinal transplant using identical twin as donor suggest that a patient with such an ideal donor available should be transplanted without delay. The same may hold true for HLA-identical siblings as donors. Our own experience on 11 cases of living donor ITx performed using donors with at least one haplotype match has been extremely favorable, with no instances of acute rejection during the first year after transplantation. Therefore, we believe that in adult candidates with an available donor at least one haplotype match, this option should be considered as a valid alternative to cadaver ITx.

In children affected by ultrashort bowel syndrome with no potential of successful weaning of TPN and therefore very likely to die, living donor ITx should be considered early in order to prevent progression to end-stage liver failure and avoid death on the waiting list. For children suffering of TPN-related cirrhosis, the novel option of combined segmental liver–bowel transplant from an adult donor may contribute to minimize death on the waiting list, particularly common in this subpopulation.

## References

1. The Intestinal Transplantation Registry. http://www.lhsc.on.ca/itr/.
2. UNOS Registry. http://www.unos.org
3. Testa G, Holterman M, John E, et al. Combined living donor liver/small bowel transplantation. *Transplantation* 2005;79(10):1401.
4. Berney T, Genton L, Buhler LA, et al. Five-year follow-up after pediatric living related small bowel transplantation between two monozygotic twins. *Transplant Proc* 2004;36(2):316.
5. Langer JC. Abdominal wall defects. *World J Surg* 2003;27(1):117.
6. Grosfeld J. Jejunoileal atresia and stenosis. In: O'Neill JA, Rowe MI, Grosfeld JL, et al. eds. *Pediatric Surgery, 5th ed*. St. Louis, Mosby, 1998:1145.
7. Bueno J, Ohwada S, Kocoshis S, et al. Factors impacting the survival of children with intestinal failure referred for intestine transplantation. *J Pediatr Surg* 1999;34(1):27.
8. Vennarecci G, Kato T, Misiakos EP, et al. Intestinal transplantation for short gut syndrome attributable to necrotizing enterocolitis. *Pediatrics* 2000;105(2):E25.
9. Brown RA, Cywes S. Disorders and congenital malformations associated with Hirschprung's disease, in Holschneider AM, Puri P, eds. *Hirschprung's Disease and Allied Disorders*. Amsterdam, Harwood Academic Publishers, 2000:137.
10. Shuffler M, Pagon RA, Schwartz R, et al. Visceral myopathy of the gastrointestinal and genitourinary tracts in infants. *Gastroenterology* 1988;94(4):892.
11. Pulliam TJ, Schuster MM. Congenital markers for chronic intestinal pseudo obstruction. *Am J Gastroenterol* 1995;90(6):922.
12. Masetti M, Rodriguez MM, Thompson JF, et al. Multivisceral transplantation for megacystis microcolon intestinal hypoperistalsis syndrome. *Transplantation* 1999;68(2):228.
13. Phillips AD, Schmitz J. Familial microvillous atrophy: a clinicopathological survey of 23 cases. *J Pediatr Gastroenterol Nutr* 1992;14(4):380.
14. Bunn SK, Beath SV, McKeirnan PJ, et al. Treatment of microvillous inclusion disease by intestinal transplantation. *J Pediatr Gastroenterol Nutr* 2000;31(2):176.
15. Abely M, Hankard GF, Hugot JP, et al. Intractable infant diarrhea with epithelial dysplasia associated with polymalformative syndrome. *J Pediatr Gastroenterol Nutr* 1998;27(3):348.
16. Carbonnel F, Cosnes J, Chevret S, et al. The role of anatomic factors in nutritional autonomy after extensive small bowel resection. *J Parenter Enteral Nutr* 1996;20(4):275.
17. Veloso FT, Carvalho J, Magro F. Immune-related systemic manifestation of inflammatory bowel disease. A prospective study of 792 patients. *J Clin Gastroenterol* 1996;23(1):29.
18. Rasmussen HH, Fallingborg JF, Mortensen PB. Hepatobiliary dysfunction and primary sclerosing cholangitis in patients with Crohn's disease. *Scand J Gastroenterol* 1997;32(6):604.
19. Jackson LM, O'Gorman PJ, O'Connell J, et al. Thrombosis in inflammatory bowel disease: clinical setting, procoagulant profile and factor V Leiden. *QJM* 1997;90(3):183.
20. Guillevin L, Lhote F, Gallais V, et al. Gastrointestinal tract involvement in polyarterities nodosa and Churg-Strauss syndrome. *Ann Med Interne (Paris)* 1995; 146(4):260.
21. Amitrano L, Brancaccio V, Guardascione MA, et al. High prevalence of thrombophilic genotypes in patients with acute mesenteric vein thrombosis. *Am J Gastroenrerol* 2001;96(1):768.
22. Winter HS. Intestinal polyps. In: Walker WA, Durie PR, Hamilton JR, Walker-Smith JA, Watkins JB, eds. *Pediatric Gastrointestinal Disease: Pathophysiology, Diagnosis, Management 2nd ed*. 1996:891.

23. Kelijo DJ, Squires RH. Anatomy and anomalies of the small and large intestine. In: Feldman M, Scharschmidt BF, eds. *Gastrointestinal and Liver Disease: Pathophysiology, Diagnosis, Management, 6th ed.* Philadelphia: Pennsylvania, Saunders, 1998:1419.

24. Bristol JB, Williamson, RC. Nutrition, operation and intestinal adaptation. *J Parenter Nutr* 1988;12(3):299.

25. Uchiymna M, Iwafuchi M, Matsuda Y, et al. Intestinal motility after massive intestinal resection in conscious canines: comparison of acute and chronic phases. *J Pediatr Gastroenterol Nutr* 1996;23(3):217.

26. Messing B, Crenn P, Beau P, et al. Long term survival and parenteral nutrition dependence in adult patients with short bowel syndrome. *Gastroenterology* 1999;117:1043.

27. Sondheimer JM, Cadnapaphornchai M, Sontag M, et al. Predicting the duration of dependence on parenteral nutrition after neonatal intestinal resection. *J Pediatr* 1998;132(1):80.

28. Kaufman SS, Atkinson JB, Bianchi A, et al. Indications for pediatric intestinal transplantation: a position paper of the American Society of Transplantation. *Pediatr Transplantation* 2001;5(2):80.

29. Messing B, Crenn P, Beau P, et al. Long term survival and parenteral nutrition dependence in adult patients with short bowel syndrome. *Gastroenterology* 1999;117(5):1043.

30. Scolapio JS, Fleming CR, Kelly DG, et al. Survival of home parenteral nutrition treated patients: 20 years of experience at the Mayo Clinic. *Mayo Clin Proc* 1999;74(3):217.

31. Chan S, McCowen KC, Bistrian BR, et al. Incidence, prognosis, and etiology of end stage liver disease in patients receiving home total parenteral nutrition. *Surgery* 1999;126(1):28.

32. Briones ER, Iber FL. Liver and biliary tract changes associated with total parenteral nutrition: pathogenesis and prevention. *J Am Coll Nutr* 1995;14(3):219.

33. Kelly DA. Liver complication of pediatric parenteral nutrition–epidemiology. *Nutrition* 1998;14(1):153.

34. Sondeheimer JM, Asturias E, Cadnapaphornchai M. Infection and cholestasis in neonates with intestinal resection and long term parenteral nutrition. *J Pediatr Gastroenterol Nutr* 1998;27(2):131.

35. Beath SV, Needham SJ, Kelly DA, et al.: Clinical features and prognosis of children assessed for isolated small bowel or combined small bowel and liver transplantation. *J Pediatr Surg* 1997;32(3):459.

36. Bakker H, Bozzetti F, Staun M, et al. Home parenteral nutrition in adults: a European multicentre survey in 1997. *Clin Nutr* 1999;18(3):135.

37. Kosmach B, Tarbell S, Reyes J, et al. "Munchausen by proxy" syndrome in a small bowel transplant recipient. *Transplant Proc* 1996;28(5):2790.

## 34.2  SURGICAL PROCEDURES AND PERIOPERATIVE CARE

*Rainer W.G. Gruessner, MD*

## INTRODUCTION

The first documented (though not described independently in a published article) extrarenal organ transplant was the small bowel[1] (see Chapter 32). But today, the total number of living donor (LD) intestinal transplants trails the total number not only of LD kidney and liver transplants but also of LD pancreas transplants. According to the international Intestinal Transplant Registry (ITR; see Chapter 34.5), only 41 LD intestinal transplants have been performed in the last 2 decades (1985 to 2005). Two reasons help explain this relatively low number of LD intestinal transplants: (1) deceased donor (DD) intestinal grafts are not in short supply, and, unless the prospective recipient has end-stage liver disease as a result of total parenteral nutrition (TPN), the mortality rate on the waiting list for solitary intestinal transplants is relatively low, and (2) unlike the kidney,

the intestine is not a paired (nor a sterile) organ, so restoration of intestinal continuity after graft removal from an LD requires surgical reconstruction (ie, creation of an enteroenterostomy) with its own intrinsic risk.

What is frequently overlooked, however, is that the magnitude of the LD procedure is less for the small bowel than for the kidney, liver, or pancreas: only 25% to 40% of the LD's small bowel is removed. Thus, the percentage of resected functioning organ mass is significantly higher for kidney (50%), pancreas (> 50%), and liver (> 55% in case of right lobectomy) LDs.

The results of intestinal transplants are still poorer than the results of other solid-organ transplants,[2] specifically because of a higher incidence of rejection, infection, and posttransplant lymphoproliferative disease (PTLD). Accordingly, LD intestinal transplants provide the best results if the donor and the recipient are HLA-identical. And even in the non-HLA-identical setting, the use of LD intestinal grafts may be advantageous if the recipient has life-threatening complications from TPN (ie, liver dysfunction with fibrosis, lack of vascular access, or recurrent episodes of septicemia) and a DD graft is not available, or if the recipient has high panel-reactive antibody (PRA) levels (> 80%) and the prospective LD is crossmatch-negative. Such indications are mainly responsible for the moderate increase in LD intestinal transplants in the last 10 years (1996 to 2005), as shown in the ITR analysis in Chapter 34.5.

Overall, the intestinal transplant literature is scant, but it appears that 180 to 200 cm of donor graft length for an adult recipient and about 120 to 150 cm for a pediatric recipient is sufficient to provide TPN independence.[3] Long-term studies on absorption and weight grain are not available, nor are comparisons with full-length DD small-bowel grafts. Short-term results, however, indicate that, if the distal donor ileum is used, absorption is sufficient; a lack of trace elements (including vitamins such as $B_{12}$) has not been observed.[4]

With regard to the vascular reconstruction, systemic vein drainage via the infrarenal cava is preferable (over portal vein drainage) because of its technical simplicity. Systemic vein drainage offers these advantages: direct (end-to-side) anastomosis between the donor ileocolic vein and the recipient vena cava; drainage from a low-flow to a high-flow system; and avoidance of extension grafts. All of these advantages may decrease the risk of graft thrombosis. Conversely, portal vein drainage (via the recipient superior or inferior mesenteric vein, or via the splenic vein) is technically more challenging and may require the use of venous extension graft(s); moreover, drainage into the recipient's low-flow portal system may increase the risk of graft thrombosis. Studies both in animals[5,6] and in humans[7,8] have not shown significant disadvantages to bypassing the liver and using venous drainage into the systemic circulation. Long-term studies are not available, but are certainly warranted.

To restore bowel continuity, the distal native bowel of the recipient (usually duodenum or jejunum) is anastomosed to the proximal end of the donor graft, usually in a side-to-side (functionally end-to-end) fashion.[3] Whether a terminal (Brooke) ileostomy, a "chimney" (Bishop-Coop) ileostomy, or a loop-ileostomy should be created is controversial. A terminal (Brooke) ileostomy has this advantage: a second, distal anastomosis (between the distal donor graft and the remaining recipient colon) is not required during the transplant procedure, thus reducing the risk of technical complications from an anastomotic leak. But the disadvantage is that a second laparotomy is required for distal bowel reanastomosis. The distinct advantage of the loop-ileostomy is that closure can be accomplished without a standard laparotomy and with a relatively short recovery time.

Also unclear is the optimal timing for ileostomy takedown. In my experience, takedown should be done about 6 months post-transplant or, if rejection has occurred, 6 months after the last rejection episode.

Clearly, LD intestinal transplantation is an evolving, underused option. If it becomes more popular, insight into immunologic and absorptive issues could eventually be deepened.

## OPERATIVE PROCEDURES

### Solitary LD Intestinal Transplants

The day before surgery, the recipient is given GoLYTELY (polyethylene glycol electrolyte solution; either orally or via a gastric [G-] tube) until the stomal effluent is clear. Decontamination of the remaining small bowel is normally not required, but neomycin (1 g) and metronidazole (500 mg) can be given about 12 hours before surgery. In addition, the recipient is given enemas from below (in case the intraoperative decision is made to perform an ileocolostomy). Also, the day before surgery, the optimal ostomy site (and one alternative site) should be selected.

The recipient is placed on the operating table in a supine position. After induction of general endotracheal anesthesia, a central venous catheter, an arterial line for constant blood pressure monitoring, a Foley catheter for bladder drainage, nasogastric suction, prophylactic antibiotics (repeated every 4 hours during the course of the procedure), and sequential compression devices for thrombosis prophylaxis are all used. The existing duodenostomy/jejunostomy is oversewn; existing G or jejunal (J)tubes are prepped out of the field. The abdomen is prepped and draped in the standard surgical fashion.

A midline incision is made; frequently, in case of previous laparotomies, the skin and scar tissues are excised. The incision is carried through all layers of the abdomen with the electrocautery device. In some recipients, the peritoneal cavity can easily be entered: the only remaining bowel is the duodenum (with or without a segment of proximal jejunum), a portion of the colon (of variable length), and the remaining small bowel mesentery. But in other recipients, tense adhesive bands throughout the abdomen (despite the absence of bowel loops) need to be sharply and bluntly taken down, in order to isolate the distal portion of the remaining duodenum/jejunum. The ostomy is taken down, and the most distal portion with the ostomy is resected using the gastrointestinal anastomosis (GIA) stapler. The stapled stump is then oversewn with 4-0 as per 30.3.1a nonabsorbable sutures; the nasogastric tube or the previously placed G as per 30.3.1a or J tubes are put on suction. The fascia at the ostomy site is closed with #2 nonabsorbable sutures in a running fashion.

The liver is inspected. A liver biopsy may be obtained at this time to assess the extent of histopathologic changes before the bowel transplant. A decision is also made whether or not to perform a cholecystectomy (eg, in case of multiple gallstones as a result of longstanding TPN dependence).

After the remaining small bowel is mobilized, the infrarenal aorta and cava are identified and dissected free from the takeoff of the renal vessels to their iliac bifurcations. The lumbar vessels are carefully dissected out and looped around for vascular control. Once the vascular dissection in the recipient is completed, the donor team is given word to remove the donor small bowel. Although the donor small bowel is flushed and prepared (eg, patching and

spatulating the donor artery and vein to an appropriate length) on the back table, the recipient is given heparin intravenously (40 to 70 U/kg body weight, depending on the amount of bleeding). Once the back-table work is finished, the recipient infrarenal aorta and cava are clamped proximally and distally (with separate control of the lumbar vessels), or side-biting clamps are placed (which do not require separate control of the lumbar vessels).

The arterial anastomosis is done first (Color Plates, Figure IN-3): it is technically more challenging than the venous anastomosis because of the donor artery's small diameter. The position of the arterial anastomosis is distal to the venous anastomosis. The arteriotomy is made somewhere between the origins of the inferior mesenteric artery and the renal arteries. The arteriotomy can be enlarged and optimally size-fashioned with an aortic punch. The aorta is flushed with heparinized solution. The graft is removed from the back-table basin (containing preservation solution); a wet lap is used to cover the bowel loops, in order to keep them out of the field during the vascular reconstruction. The vascular pedicle of the graft is inspected and the correct orientation is assessed. As described in Chapter 33.2, the ileocolic artery and vein (or alternatively, the terminal branches of the superior mesenteric artery [SMA] and superior mesenteric vein [SMV]), are marked anteriorly, either with fine stitches or with a felt pen. For construction of the arterial anastomosis, 6-0 or 7-0 nonabsorbable sutures are used. Given the small size of the ileocolic artery (about 5 mm), the end-to-side ileocolic artery-to-infrarenal aorta anastomosis is constructed in an interrupted fashion. If the recipient abdomen is deep, the anastomosis can be accomplished with the parachuting technique. The 6-0 or 7-0 nonabsorbable sutures are tied as the intestinal graft is lowered into the operative field.

If the ileocolic artery is of good size, the arterial anastomosis can be constructed with the quadrangulation technique. Four double-armed 6-0 nonabsorbable sutures are placed at the corners and sides of the arteriotomy. The sutures are taken to their respective points on the donor ileocolic artery and tied. The arterial anastomosis is completed by running the 6-0 nonabsorbable corner sutures continuously, from one end to the other end, and tying them at the corners.

An appropriate site on the cava is chosen for the venotomy (usually 2 to 3 cm proximal to the arterial anastomosis). The venotomy is made, and the site is flushed with heparinized solution. The venous anastomosis is done with the quadrangulation technique. Four double-armed 6-0 or 7-0 nonabsorbable sutures are placed at the corners and sides of the venotomy. The sutures are taken to their respective points on the donor ileocolic vein. The end-to-side ileocolic vein-to-infrarenal cava anastomosis is completed by running the 6-0 or 7-0 nonabsorbable corner sutures continuously, from one end to the other, and tying them at the corners (Color Plates, Figure IN-3).

At the beginning of the venous anastomosis, mannitol (0.5 to 1.0 g/kg body weight) is given to the recipient to diminish the extent of bowel edema as a result of the reperfusion injury. On completion of the vascular anastomoses, all vascular clamps on the intrarenal aorta and cava are removed. Any bleeding sites, specifically on the anastomotic site or on the cut surface of the mesentery, are identified and carefully controlled with fine-suture ligation techniques. If good arterial inflow and venous outflow is achieved, the graft immediately pinks up and shows some peristalsis.

Next, the proximal end of the intestinal graft is identified (different marking sutures were placed during the donor operation to distinguish the proximal and distal bowel end). A decision is made as to whether the anastomosis to the remaining recipient duodenum/

jejunum should be made in an end-to-end, end-to-side, or side-to-side fashion. I prefer a handsewn, two-layer side-to-side anastomosis (which is basically a functional end-to-end anastomosis); to that effect, the proximal stapled end of the donor small bowel is oversewn with a running 4-0 nonabsorbable suture. The handsewn technique decreases the risk of intraluminal anastomotic bleeding (as compared with a stapled anastomosis). The posterior outer layer of the anastomosis is constructed first, with a 4-0 nonabsorbable suture in running or interrupted fashion. Enterostomies are made on the corresponding recipient and donor (antimesenteric) bowel sites. An inner full-thickness layer between the remaining recipient duodenum/jejunum and the donor graft is constructed circumferentially with running 4-0 absorbable sutures. An outer posterior layer of interrupted 4-0 nonabsorbable sutures completes the anastomosis (Color Plates, Figure IN-4).

The nasogastric tube is advanced and placed across the anastomosis into the intestinal graft and placed on intermittent suction. If the recipient only had a previous G tube, it is replaced with a G/J or a J tube, and the J limb is placed across the anastomosis. If a new J tube is placed, a stab enterotomy is made in the remaining recipient duodenum/jejunum, and the tube is advanced across the anastomosis; the tube is secured in the bowel wall with a purse string suture at the enterotomy site and further secured along the bowel wall with the Witzel technique.

Except with identical twins, the distal end of the donor graft should be brought out as a stoma to allow easy access for endoscopy and biopsy. The stoma can be created three ways (Color Plates, Figure IN-5) (1) an end-ileostomy, without construction of a distal anastomosis at the time of the transplant (thus avoiding a second bowel anastomosis); (2) a loop-ileostomy, with the distal end of the intestinal graft anastomosed to the remaining recipient colon (again, I prefer a handsewn side-to-side [functional end-to-end] two-layer anastomosis) and with the diverting loop-ileostomy created about 15 cm from the distal anastomosis; or (3) a distal anastomosis (ileocolostomy), in a side-to-side or side-to-end fashion, with the distal end of the graft brought out as a "chimney" spout ileostomy (Bishop-Koop ileostomy).

The site of the ostomy is now chosen at the most ideal location, as identified the day before surgery (see above). A quarter-size skin hole is opened down to the fascia, and 2 finger widths of fascia are opened. The distal end of the bowel graft (Brooke ileostomy), the "chimney" (Bishop-Koop) ileostomy, or the distal loop (loop-ileostomy) is brought out through the stoma site. The intestinal graft is then secured to the peritoneum with several interrupted 4-0 nonabsorbable sutures.

The mesenteric defects are now closed with 4-0 nonabsorbable sutures in an interrupted or continuous fashion. The abdomen is thoroughly irrigated with antibiotic- and antifungal-containing solutions. After hemostasis is again confirmed, the abdomen is closed in the standard fashion. The skin is stapled closed, and a sterile dressing is applied. Finally, the ostomy is opened and matured with 4-0 absorbable sutures; a stoma bag is applied.

This technique for solitary LD small bowel transplants is identical for adult and pediatric recipients; the only difference is that the donor bowel length for pediatric recipients is shorter, ranging from 120 to 150 cm; a length of > 100 cm may not be sufficient to guarantee TPN independence, as suggested by the Kyoto group.[9]

## Technical Variations

Variations of the vascular anastomoses are common. Several different recipient vessels can be used as alternatives. Recipients with an underlying clotting disorder may have a thrombosed infrahepatic cava; an end-to-side anastomosis to the renal vein[10] or to the iliac vein can be considered. Both iliac vessels (artery and vein), as alternatives to the infrarenal aorta and cava, have been used for vascular anastomoses.[11,12] Calne et al. described the use of autologous saphenous vein grafts to bridge the gap between the donor ICA/ICV and the recipient infrarenal aorta/cava, because the bulk of the specimen and fat in the mesentery obstructed the view[13]; the recipient superficial femoral artery has also been used as an interposition arterial graft.[14] However, in my opinion, extension grafts can usually be avoided by clearing the most proximal 2 to 3 cm of the donor ileocolic vessels from surrounding tissues.

Another technically more demanding alternative to systemic venous drainage is portal venous drainage. Initially, the ileocolic vessels were considered to be too short for portal vein drainage.[15] However, two Asian groups have shown that the ileocolic vein can be successfully anastomosed to the recipient inferior mesenteric vein. The Kyoto group in 2000 reported that portal vein drainage is feasible.[9] The Seoul group in 2004 reported that the donor ileocolic vessels (both artery and vein) can successfully be anastomosed to the recipient inferior mesenteric vessels; the artery required reconstruction under the microscope with 10-0 nonabsorbable sutures.[16]

Not infrequently, the abdominal wall cannot be closed primarily after an LD intestinal transplant because of the recipient's limited intraabdominal space: previous bowel resection(s) can result in contraction or obliteration of the peritoneal cavity.[15] In general, the longer the time interval between the initial extensive bowel resection and the subsequent intestinal transplant, the greater the likelihood of an abdominal wall defect. This complication is more commonly observed in pediatric recipients, because they receive (despite their small size) up to three-fourths of the donor small bowel that adult recipients do. To prevent closure of the abdomen with undue tension, the University of Illinois group has recommended the use of a double-layered polyglycolic mesh, sewn circumferentially to the fascial edges. This defect can subsequently be closed primarily, or a split-thickness skin graft can be applied over the granulation tissue on the mesh.[17,18]

## Combined LD Liver and Intestinal Transplants

Patients with short bowel syndrome and TPN-induced liver failure may also undergo sequential or combined LD liver and intestinal transplants (Color Plates, Figure IN-6). This option was first mentioned by the Kyoto group in 2000.[9] It appears to be an alternative if a DD donor is not available in time and if the recipient's liver function continues to deteriorate (see Chapter 32). The decision as to whether to proceed with a simultaneous or a sequential liver and intestinal transplant should be made intraoperatively: if the recipient is stable throughout the LD liver transplant, the LD intestinal transplant can ensue in the same session; if the recipient is not stable during the LD liver transplant, the recipient should be stabilized first in the intensive care unit and, once stable, undergo a subsequent LD intestinal transplant about 1 week later. Thus far, only a handful of combined liver and intestinal transplants have been performed worldwide (at the university hospitals in Kyoto, Illinois, and Minnesota), all in pediatric recipients.

Recipients should undergo the LD liver transplant first to correct the existing coagulopathy and replace the cirrhotic native liver (Figures 34.2-1–34.2-3). A bicostal incision, with midline extension to the xiphoid, is made in the standard fashion; transplantation of the LD segments 2 and 3 then proceeds as described in Chapter 30.3.3. After the vascular anastomoses are

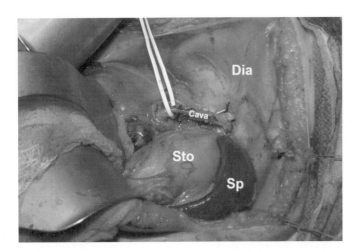

**FIGURE 34.2-1**

The operating field in the recipient after removal of the liver; preservation of the native cava (Dia, diaphragm; Sto, stomach; Sp, spleen).

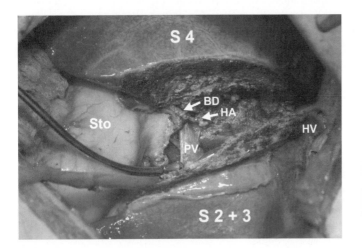

**FIGURE 34.2-2**

Donor lateral segmentectomy. The liver parenchyma has been transected just to the right of the falciform ligament. The portal vein (PV) and hepatic vein (HV) are dissected free and still intact, the hepatic artery (HA) has been cut, as has the bile duct (BD); the BD is already oversewn on the donor side (white arrow) (S2 + 3, segments 2 and 3; S4, segment 4; Sto, stomach).

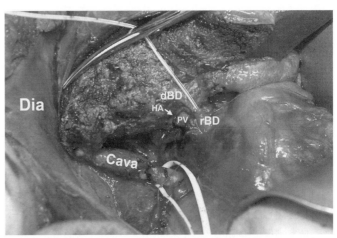

**FIGURE 34.2-3**

Recipient liver transplant procedure: implantation of liver segments 2 and 3. The recipient hepatic veins with the caval cuff have been anastomosed to the donor left hepatic vein in standard triangular fashion. The suprarenal cava is encircled. The portal vein (PV) and hepatic artery (HA) anastomoses are completed in end-to-end fashion. The posterior wall of the recipient common bile duct (rBD)-to-donor left bile duct (dBD) anastomosis is completed. A small feeding tube is used for internal stenting. The anterior wall of the bile duct anastomosis still needs to be completed (Dia, diaphragm).

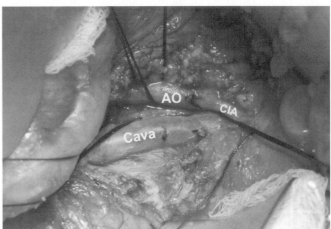

**FIGURE 34.2-4**

The recipient infrarenal aorta (AO) and cava are dissected free and mobilized in preparation for intestinal graft implantation. The aortic bifurcation with the right common iliac artery (CIA) is shown. Lumbar arteries and veins coming off of the infrarenal aorta and cava are looped with 2-0 ties for inflow and outflow control.

completed and blood supply to the liver is restored, the incision should be closed if the recipient is not hemodynamically stable. The bile ducts of the transplanted liver can be anastomosed to either the recipient's Proper hepatic duct or to the native duodenum, or the ducts can be stented and brought out through the skin.[19] If the recipient is hemodynamically stable throughout the LD liver transplant, the midline extension should be extended toward the pubic bone. The cruciate incision in the recipient provides excellent exposure, but the anesthesia team must pay great attention to maintaining normal body temperature and to avoiding hypothermia (which can result in impaired synthetic function of the grafted liver).

The intestinal transplant is performed as described above (Figures 34.2-4–34.2-7). The proximal end of the donor graft is anastomosed to the donor bile duct(s). Given the significantly shorter length of an LD (vs a DD) intestinal graft, the Roux-en-Y limb can only be 10 to 20 cm in length.[19] The duodenoileostomy is constructed in a side-to-side fashion, with the same two-layer technique as described above. The cruciate incision should only be closed primarily in the absence of tension (Figure 34.2-8). If the abdomen cannot be closed primarily, attempts should be made to approximate the bicostal incision and to close the midline incision with absorbable (polyglycolic) mesh, which subsequently can be covered with a skin graft.[19]

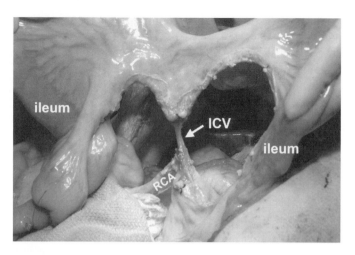

**FIGURE 34.2-5**

Procurement of the donor ileum. The ileocolic vessel (ICV) is shown; the mesentery has been divided between ligatures. The donor ileum is shown on both sides of the vascular pedicle. The ileocolic vessels will be transected just distal to the takeoff of the right colic artery (RCA).

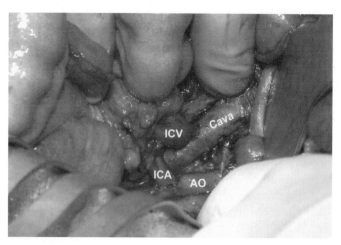

**FIGURE 34.2-7**

Completion of the donor ileocolic artery (ICA)-to-recipient aorta (A) and ileocolic vein (ICV)-to-recipient cava anastomoses.

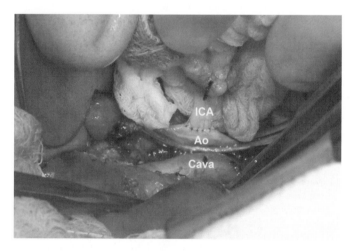

**FIGURE 34.2-6**

Recipient intestinal transplant procedure. The ileocolic artery (ICA) has been anastomosed end-to-side to the recipient infrarenal aorta (Ao). The recipient infrarenal cava is shown, and the venous anastomosis between the donor ileocolic vein and the recipient cava will be constructed proximal to the arterial anastomosis.

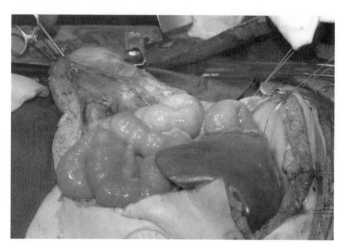

**FIGURE 34.2-8**

The recipient abdomen after combined LD intestinal and liver transplant. In this case, the abdomen was closed primarily; if this is not possible, absorbable mesh can be used and subsequently covered with a skin graft.

## POSTOPERATIVE CARE

Postoperative care is different for recipients of a solitary LD intestinal transplant versus a combined LD intestinal and liver transplant.

### Solitary LD Transplants

Recipients of a solitary LD intestinal transplant, after closure of the abdomen, are brought to the postanesthesia care unit (PACU) or directly to the intensive care unit (ICU). As with any surgical procedure, hemodynamic and ventilatory assessment is essential during recovery. The endotracheal tube is usually removed in the operating room. However, if the abdomen is closed with undue tension, extubation may not be possible immediately posttransplant. On transfer from the operating room,  recipients

rontinely undergo blood tests, chest x-ray, and EKG are routinely obtained. Blood pressure, pulse rate, and urine output are monitored. Initially, a complete blood count, complete chemistry, and coagulation profile are also obtained in the PACU or ICU.

The first 24 to 48 hours posttransplant are most crucial: the recipient undergoes the physiologic response to surgical trauma; the transplanted organ is in a varying degree of ischemia or reperfusion injury; and immunosuppression begins (see Chapter 34.3). Initially, vital signs, color of the ostomy, and laboratory parameters (specifically hemoglobin and partial thromboplastin time (PTT) are monitored every 4 hours. For electrolyte management, recipients are usually placed on ½ NS and D5W. Intravenous fluids are initially infused at an In = Out ratio until hemodynamic stability is obtained. After the first 12 to 24 hours, the recipient goes back on (glutamine-enriched) TPN at a straight rate.

The crucial element immediately posttransplant is systemic anticoagulation: the ileocolic vessels of the LD are significantly smaller than the vessels procured from a DD (SMA with aortic cuff, SMV/portal vein) and are thus more prone to vascular thrombosis. In the operating room, before closure of the abdominal incision, LD recipients are started on a heparin drip (about 200 U/hour). The target PTT within the first 24 hours is 40 to 50; thereafter, 40 to 60. Over the next 5 to 7 days, recipients are weaned off heparin and usually started on daily baby aspirin (81.5 mg) on posttransplant day 5. Recipients who lost their native small bowel secondary to thrombotic or embolic events remain on systemic anticoagulation for the first 6 months, or even indefinitely (depending on the underlying coagulopathy).

Dressing and ostomy care are per the standard routine if the abdomen was closed primarily. If a mesh graft was used, saline-moistened gauzes should be changed several times per day. The ileostomy is initially visualized every 3 hours to determine its viability. On posttransplant day 7, a small bowel follow-through barium study is performed to confirm intactness of the anastomosis(es). The following day, the recipients undergo the first graft biopsy. Endoscopy with graft biopsy is initially performed two to three times per week; as with DD intestinal transplant recipients, zoom endoscopy has also been recommended for LD recipients.[20] Within the first few months posttransplant, a marked increase in the length of intestinal villi can be noted, resulting in a marked increase in absorptive surface.[17]

After an anastomotic leak is radiologically ruled out, recipients begin clear liquids. Alternatively, enteral nutrition via the J tube placed beyond the proximal anastomosis can slowly be started within the first 48 hours posttransplant. Once oral or tube feeding is tolerated, bilirubin levels in recipients with liver dysfunction start to decrease. Of note, oral intake may be prolonged in recipients with delayed gastric emptying[21,22], a finding that is not uncommon with small bowel syndrome or dysfunction.

If the stomal output is high immediately posttransplant (in the absence of rejection or infection), supplemental intravenous hydration may become necessary; usually the high stomal output decreases within a few weeks, and then intravenous fluids are no longer required.[4] To assess the absorptive capacity of the intestinal graft, Beneditti et al have suggested checking fat-soluble vitamin and albumin levels, performing the Schilling test (for vitamin $B_{12}$ absorption), quantifying fecal fat excretion, and performing D-xylose absorption tests at 1, 6, and 12 months posttransplant.[4] Normal results are expected within 3 to 6 months.

Antimicrobial prophylaxis, usually initiated perioperatively, consists of antibacterial, antifungal, and antiviral medications. Blood, urine, stool, and sputum are collected routinely for microbiologic assessment. Broad-spectrum antibiotics are given intraoperatively, every 4 hours, and for the first 3 days posttransplant. Antifungal medication (eg, fluconazole) is administered for 7 days. Antiviral medications, specifically cytomegalovirus (CMV) prophylaxis, are first given intravenously, immediately posttransplant, and then orally when the patient tolerates a diet. Depending on the recipient and donor CMV status, anti-CMV prophylaxis continues for up to 6 months posttransplant. In addition, sulfamethoxazole/trimethoprim is given as long-term prophylaxis against *Pneumocystis carinii* and *Nocardia* infections.

## Combined LD Intestinal and Liver Transplants

For recipients of a combined LD intestinal and liver transplant, postoperative care is more complex. It is initially dictated by liver graft function. Once liver function has stabilized (usually within the first few days posttransplant), attention then shifts toward monitoring the intestinal graft.

## References

1. Deterling R. Discussion on living donor intestinal transplantation. In: Alican F, Hardy JD, Cayirli M, et al. Intestinal transplantation: laboratory experience and report of a clinical case. *Am J Surg* 1971;121:159.
2. Grant D, Abu-Elmagd K, Reyes J, et al. 2003 report of the intestinal transplant registry: a new era has dawned. *Ann Surg* 2005;241:607–613.
3. Gruessner RWG, Sharp HL. Living-related intestinal transplantation. *Transplantation* 1997;64:1605–1607.
4. Benedetti E, Baum C, Cicalese L, et al. Progressive functional adaptation of segmental bowel graft from living related donor. *Transplantation* 2001;71:569–571.
5. Kaneko H, Fischman MA, Buckley TM, Buckley TM. A comparison of portal versus systemic vernous drainage in the pig small-bowel allograft recipient. *Surgery* 1991;109:663–670.
6. Fryer JP, Kim S, Wells CL, et al. Bacterial translocation in a large-animal model of small-bowel transplantation: portal vs systemic venous drainage and the effect of tacrolimus immunosuppression. *Arch Surg* 1996;131:77–84.
7. Todo S, Tzakis A, Reyes J, et al. Small intestinal transplantation in humans with or without the colon. *Transplantation* 1994;57:840–848.
8. Berney T, Kato T, Nishida S, et al. Systemic versus portal venous drainage of small bowel grafts: similar long-term outcome in spite of increased bacterial translocation. *Transplant Proc* 2002;34:961–962.
9. Fujimoto Y, Uemoto S, Inomata Y, et al. Small bowel transplantation using grafts from living-related donors. Two case reports. *Transpl Int* 2000;13[Suppl 1]:S179–S184.
10. Alican F, Hardy JD, Cayirli M, et al. Intestinal transplantation: laboratory experience and report of a clinical case. *Am J Surg* 1971;121:150–159.
11. Fortner JG, Sichuk G, Litwin SD, Beattie EJ, Jr. Immunological responses to an intestinal allograft within HL-A-identical donor-recipient. *Transplantation* 1972;14:531–535.
12. Deltz E, Schroeder P, Gebhardt H, et al. Successful clinical small bowel transplantation: report of a case. *Clin Transplantation* 1989;3:89–91.
13. Calne RY, Friend PJ, Middleton S, et al. Intestinal transplant between two of identical triplets. *Lancet* 1997;350:1077–1078.
14. Morel P, Kadry Z, Charbonnet P, et al. Paediatric living related intestinal-transplantation between two monozygotic twins: a 1-year follow-up. *Lancet* 2000;355:723–724.
15. Pollard SG. Intestinal transplantation: living related. *Brit Med Bull* 1997;53:868–878.
16. Lee MD, Kim DG, Ahn ST, et al. Isolated small bowel transplantation from a living-related donor at the Catholic University of Korea—A case report of rejection-free course. *Yonsei Med J* 2004;45:1198–1201.
17. Benedetti E, Testa G, Sankary H, et al. Successful treatment of trauma-induced short bowel syndrome with early living related bowel transplantation. *J Trauma* 2004;56:164–170.
18. Holterman MJ, Holterman AL, Carrol, R, et al. Living-related bowel transplantation to treat short bowel syndrome in a four-year-old child: A case report. *J Ped Surg* 2003;38:1763–1765.
19. Testa G, Holterman M, John E, et al. Combined living donor liver/small bowel transplantation. *Transplantation* 2005;79:1401–1404.
20. Sasaki, T, Hasegawa T, Nakai H, et al. Zoom endoscopic evaluation of rejection in living-related small bowel transplantation. *Transplantation* 2002;73:560–564.
21. Cicalese L, Rastellini C, Sileri P, et al. Segmental living related small bowel transplantation in adults. *J Gastrointest Surg* 2001;5:168–173.
22. Pollard SG, Lodge P, Selvakumar S, et al. Living related small bowel transplantation: The first United Kingdom case. *Transplant Proc* 1996; 28:2733–2732.

## 34.3   IMMUNOSUPPRESSIVE THERAPY AND POSTOPERATIVE COMPLICATIONS

*Enrico Benedetti, MD, Antonio Gangemi, MD, Giuliano Testa, MD*

Several factors are involved in conferring to the intestinal graft an immunologic peculiarity in respect to other solid organ transplants. First of all, the rejection after intestinal transplantation (IT) interplays with infectious complications. In fact rejection alters the mucosal barrier of the bowel allowing endotoxines to translocate.[1–3] On the other hand endotoxines are a powerful immune adjuvant that can aggravate the antigraft alloimmune response.[4,5] The ability of enteric-derived cells to function as facultative antigens presenting cells (APC) represents an additional factor. The transplant event itself produces a favorable microenvironment by switching cells of enteric origin in direction of APC line.[6,7] Specific stimulatory factors are the inflammation deriving from the ischemia-reperfusion injury, rejection-associated inflammatory changes, or viral infection.[6,7]

In addition intestinal grafts combine high immunogenicity with the ability to mount a graft versus host disease (GVHD).[8] It has been already demonstrated in experimental models that GVHD can mitigate rejection in a canine animal model. Short intestinal segments were quickly rejected, whereas recipients of full-length intestinal grafts died at least in part due to GVHD and with no signs of rejection.[9]

These immunologic considerations originally induced most centers to use heavy immunosuppression, initially based on high-dose cyclosporine A (CsA).[10,11] The price of this strategy has been paid in terms of increased rate of infections determining high mortality. On the other hand, attempts of using lower doses of CsA resulted in loss of a considerable number of grafts due to acute and chronic rejection. As final result, IT under CsA immunosuppression resulted in overall poor outcome.[12–15]

The introduction of tacrolimus (TAC) signed a critical step in the improvement of the outcomes after IT.[10,11] Currently, all the protocols for clinical IT are based on tacrolimus. The better therapeutic efficacy of TAC in respect to CsA allows a reduced rate of rejection and lower rate of complications related to the immunosuppressive therapy.

Nevertheless IT is still threatened by a wide range of complications. The recent introduction of living related small bowel transplantation (LR-SBTx) may contribute in making the IT a more successful procedure.

Intestinal grafts are extremely sensitive to preservation injury, which is minimized in the setting of LR-SBTx. Further potential advantages of LR-SBTx include the optimal donor–recipient human leukocyte antigen (HLA) matching, the reduced waiting-list time, the better donor bowel preparation associated with the elective context of the operation, the total absence of hemodynamic instability and of preharvesting bowel hypoperfusion. According to these considerations in 1998, we have initiated, in our institution, an IT program using segmental bowel grafts obtained from living related donors. Of note, the worldwide experience in LD-SBTx is limited to only 32 cases including 7 children (15 cases performed at University of Illinois at Chicago).[16–19]

Because of the small number of cases in LR-SBTx most of the data presented in this chapter are derived from the cadaver SBTx experience.

## REJECTION AND IMMUNOSUPPRESSIVE THERAPY

Despite the advancement in immunosuppressive therapy, rejection represents still the most challenging postoperative complication and the main obstacle to the widespread use of intestinal transplantation.[20]

In a large published series, the incidence of rejection severe enough to be treated in children and adults was 93%![20] The overall incidence of acute allograft rejection is reported at 78% or greater. Rejection is seen most frequently and is most severe in isolated IT (88%) as compared to combined liver–intestine–grafts (66%) and multivisceral grafts.[21–22] Rejection is liable to result in graft loss and can also precipitate opportunistic infections and contribute to the patient death from other complications.[23]

The lack of reliable markers of rejection is a significant problem since clinical manifestations such as abdominal distension, abdominal pain, diarrhea, and fever are late and unreliable signs and symptoms of rejection. In fact the patient may be totally asymptomatic. The most common symptom is a change in the bowel habits usually with significant increase in ileostomy output or worsening diarrhea. Severe rejection can result in graft paralytic ileus and bleeding from mucosal sloughing.

The most effective mean of diagnosing rejection in the intestinal allograft is intensive serial surveillance by videoendoscopy and biopsy. The creation of an ileostomy at the time of the transplant is critical for performing endoscopies and for obtaining biopsy specimens (Figure 34.3-1). General endoscopic signs of rejection include mucosal edema, erythema, friability, and focal ulcerations. Signs of severe rejection are a granular mucosal pattern with diffuse ulcerations, mucosal sloughing, and absence of peristalsis.

The primary goal of current immunosuppressive protocols is to maximize efficacy while minimizing the morbidity of immunosuppressive agents. The recent evidence that both high doses of steroids and calcineurin inhibitors can prevent induction of tolerance represents a logical rationale to move in direction of low immunosuppressive regimens.[24,25] It has been hypothesized that some mechanism of tolerance induction (ie, development of regulatory cells) may depend on a normal signaling by Th1 cytokines (IL-2 and IFNγ) potentially limited by high immunosuppressive regimens.[26–29]

Virtually all the currently available immunosuppressive agents have been used in different combination in clinical IT.[11,20,30,31–36]

The use of induction agents in IT is becoming more popular.[11,20,32,34,37] Recently, enthusiasm for the use of interleukin-2 receptor antagonists has increased.[37–39] Daclizumab has been associated with a significant reduction in the incidence of rejection compared with rejection rates under historic immunosuppressive protocols that did not include induction agents.[40]

However, recent data suggest that thymoglobulin may be the best induction therapy in the setting of IT.[41] Reyes et al. treated 36 IT pediatric recipients (age 5 months-20 years) with 2 doses of rabbit antithymocyte globulin just before (3 mg/kg) and early post transplant (2 mg/kg). Tacrolimus PO was begun within 24 hours after graft reperfusion with aggressive reduction of dose after 3 months; no steroids were given. Methyloprednisolone or other agents were used to treat breakthrough rejection. At 8 to 28 months follow-up 1- and 2-year patient and graft survival was 100% and 94%, respectively. There was a low incidence of immunosuppression-related complications.[30] The same group has successfully applied this strategy to adult recipients.[41]

The University of Pittsburg group previously attempted a radically different approach based on the hypothesis that the

WEEK 1                    WEEK 2                    WEEK 3

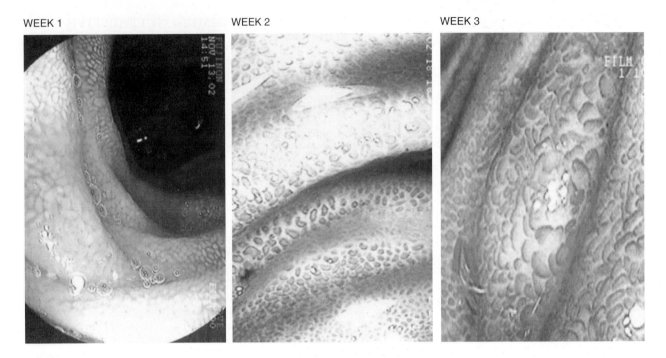

**FIGURE 34.3-1**

Magnified video endoscopy.

persistence of donor-derived hematopoietic cells correlate with better outcome in solid organ transplant recipients.[42–45]

Donor-specific bone marrow transfusion (DSBMT) has been used to increase this natural phenomenon. The results of IT under this protocol have not been superior to standard immunosuppression. In a bowel transplant large animal model, addition of DSBMT resulted in increased risk of acute rejection, GVHD, and infection.[46] Chimerism may be an important mechanism in tolerance development but does not represent an absolute requirement as it has been already proven.[47]

Tzakis et al. have used Campath 1-H, a monoclonal depleting antibody against the CD52 receptor, for induction therapy in IT, after previous reports of its effectiveness in kidney transplantation.[48,49] Early experience with this depleting antibody has led to acceptable early survival rates in adults. Longer follow-up will be required to determine the impact of Campath on long-term graft and patient survival.

Protocols based on a combination of low immunosuppression and strategies for induction of operational tolerance have been also attempted. Pirenne has proposed a new tolerogenic strategy that combines the administration of donor-specific blood transfusion in the portal vein the day of transplantation, the avoidance of bolus of steroids, and the administration of low-dose calcineurin inhibitors.[50]

Mycophenolate mofetil (MMF) and rapamycin have been associated occasionally to tacrolimus for maintenance immunosuppression after IT.[51] Fishbein et al. have recently used rapamycin in 12 patients concomitantly with tacrolimus, steroids and Basiliximab obtaining a decreased incidence of early rejection and a significantly increased 1 year graft survival in comparison to a control group without rapamycin (16.7% vs 73.7% and 91.7% vs 73.7%, respectively).[52]

In our living donor bowel transplant program we originally used a regimen consisting of short thymoglobulin induction,

steroids, and tacrolimus maintenance. For the last five cases we have weaned adult and pediatric patients off steroids within 6 days after transplant. For the patients treated with early steroids withdrawal, MMF at standard doses is added to the immunosuppressive regimen; MMF is discontinued at 6 months if the patient has had no rejection episodes. Thymoglobulin (1.5 mg/kg) is given for 1 dose perioperatively and then for 1 to 3 doses postoperatively until therapeutic levels of tacrolimus are reached. We aim to tacrolimus level of ~15 ng/mL for the first month, 10 to 15 ng/mL for the second and third months, and 5 to 10 ng/mL thereafter. In our series, during the first year after transplant, only one patient who received a totally mismatched graft out of 11 cases experienced one episode of rejection (8%).[16] The role of HLA matching and short ischemia time in this setting is still under investigation.

## Treatment of Acute Rejection

Acute rejection is initially treated with a corticosteroid bolus and taper. Rejection of the intestinal graft can alter TAC absorption and levels, and doses may need to be altered in this setting. Because rejections in IT are often steroid-resistant, monoclonal and polyclonal antibodies are widely used at standard doses.

Pascher et al. treated successfully two patients, who were diagnosed with steroid-resistant and OK73 refractory severe acute cellular rejection, with Infliximab, a monoclonal antibody against TNF-alpha (at a dose of 3 mg/kg).[53] Fishbein et al. more recently obtained similar results using Infliximab in four patients diagnosed with late-ulcerating rejection.[54] One patient was refractory to treatment with thymoglobulin, whereas the other three had relative contraindications to depleting antibody therapy. All patients presented with mucosal ulcerations and met standard histological criteria for moderate or severe rejection; all had full resolution of the process after Infliximab therapy.

## OTHER POSTOPERATIVE COMPLICATIONS

According to the Intestinal Transplantation Registry (ITR), there is no significant difference in terms of graft and patient survival between the LR-SBTx and the cadaver bowel transplantation.[55] Table 34.3-1 summarizes the causes of mortality and graft loss in living donor versus cadaver intestinal transplant recipients according to registry data. Our discussion focuses on common complications highly associated with graft loss and mortality.

### Infectious Complications in Intestinal Transplant Recipient

Infectious complications represent a major challenge in IT recipients and remain the leading cause of death after IT. Intestinal grafts, unlike other transplanted abdominal organs, are directly exposed to bacteria and viral agents from outside the body. Furthermore, since the intestine has an essential role as a barrier against intraluminal microorganisms, any insult to the allograft, whatever ischemic or immunologic, can lead to bacteriemia and sepsis.

General predisposing factors to bacteria translocation are shock, trauma, bowel obstruction, immunosuppression, TPN, and antibiotic therapy.[56–58] Additional mechanisms predisposing to bacterial translocation specific to the setting of IT include graft ischemia, preservation–reperfusion injury, lymphatic disruption, alteration in venous drainage, and rejection. The duration of cold ischemia time strongly influences the rate of bacterial translocation after IT. As previously published a preservation time of less than 7 hours was associated with BT in 14% of patients, whereas prolongation of 9 hours or longer was associated with BT in 76% of patients. Prolonged preservation of the small bowel graft should be avoided to minimize early infectious complications.[59] The minimization of cold ischemia time easily obtainable in the setting of LDBTx may potentially contribute to the reduction of bacterial translocation and septic complications.

#### Bacterial Infections

Bacterial infection represents the most common cause of sepsis after IT, accounting for 73% of the infectious complications.[60] Although the origin of bacteremia cannot be determined in a significant number of cases, the most common sources are, in order of frequency, central venous catheters, intra-abdominal, respiratory, and wound related. *Staphylococci, Enterococci, Pseudomonas,* and different genders of *Enterobacteriaceae* are the most frequent agents isolated from the involved sites.[61]

A rare but frequently fatal bacterial complication recently reported is necrotizing fasciitis after IT.[62] This is a rapidly spreading subcutaneous infection characterized by necrosis of subcutaneous tissue with fulminant course associated with high mortality (24% to 58%).[63,64] In the setting of IT, it can develop even after many years posttransplant, in presence of minimal immunosuppression.

#### Viral Infections

The most relevant viral infections after IT are those caused by cytomegalovirus (CMV) and Epstein–Barr virus (EBV), although recently other important sources of viral enteritis have been identified.

CMV can manifest as severe enteritis leading to graft loss. The main risk factor is the combination of a CMV-positive donor and CMV-negative recipients, which is often the case in children. Some centers routinely rule out potential donors otherwise suitable based on CMV positivity. The clinical manifestations of CMV enteritis are not unlike those of rejection with fever, increased stoma output and gastrointestinal symptoms. Only careful review of properly stained intestinal biopsies may reveal tissue-invasive CMV and allow appropriate differential diagnosis. The prophylaxis and treatment of CMV disease after IT are based on gancyclovir and high titer anti-CMV immunoglobulin, as in other solid organ transplant. However, there is a clear trend for more intensive prophylaxis and monitoring in IT recipients. In a large published series by Farmer et al. prophylactic therapy with gancyclovir administered for 100 days after IT (5 mg/kg) intravenously (IV) BID for 14 days, followed by 6 mg/kg IV QD and then by oral acyclovir (40 mg/kg per day) until 2 years after IT, lead to excellent control of CMV and EBV.[65] Monitoring was performed weekly during hospitalization, monthly during the first outpatient year, and every 4 months thereafter. Monitoring was accomplished using either a quantitative or a qualitative PCR assay of peripheral blood to detect virus-specific DNA. Persistent viremia or intolerance to therapy was treated with CMV IV immunoglobulin: 150 mg/kg IV load followed by 100 mg/kg IV QOD X 2 doses, then 100 mg/kg IV Q week thereafter. More than 50% of patients did not have evidence of CMV and EBV viremia or disease after IT. Frequent monitoring with virus-specific PCR demonstrated viremia in 46% of IT recipients. However, CMV and EBV disease occurred in only 15.4% and 7.7% of recipients, respectively.

In our center, we extend routinely the prophylaxis in LDBTx recipients with valgancyclovir for at least 1 year posttransplant.

An acute EBV infection may be associated with severe malaise and fever and flulike symptoms; however, the majority of the EBV infection is clinically silent. The most dreaded complication of EBV infection is posttransplant lymphoproliferative disorder (PTLD), which is discussed in a specific section.

Adenovirus historically has been thought of as having a secondary importance in the context of viral infection in IT when compared to CMV and EBV infections. Adenovirus has a wide range of clinical manifestations ranging from a self-limited fever to gastroenteritis, hepatitis, or pneumonia. Recent evidence seems to suggest that the role of this virus in IT has been underestimated. In a recently published series, all the 14 IT recipients studied had evidence of adenoviral infection (intestinal graft 13; liver graft 1).[66] Eight of 14 developed tissue-invasive disease with identifiable adenoviral intranuclear inclusions. Intensive corticosteroid therapy was recognized as a risk factor for tissue-invasive disease. Adenovirus had its onset in the large majority of the recipients (64.2%) within the first month after the IT. There are no proven antiviral agents of certain efficacy against adenovirus; cidofovir may have a role, although its activity is based on anecdotal evidence only.[67]

The occurrence of human Calicivirus enteritis in five pediatric recipients of IT been recently reported.[68] Three of the five infants developed severe diarrhea and necessitated intravenous fluid therapy for 40 days or more. Human Caliciviruses, both Norwalk-like (Noroviruses) and Sapporo viruses, commonly cause epidemic or endemic viral gastroenteritis of short duration in healthy individuals.

Similarly to what is seen with CMV infection, the differentiation of calicivirus enteritis from allograft rejection has been difficult in this case too, both being disorders associated with increased enterocyte apoptosis and inflammation. Intensification of immunosuppressive therapy because of suspected rejection appeared to prolong the duration of symptoms.

### *Fungal Infections*

The incidence of fungal infection in IT recipients has been estimated at 59%.[69] Candida albicans represents the most common fungal infection after solid organ transplantation.[70] Common sites of involvement are oropharynx, esophagus, and genitalia. The clinical presentation is usually in the form of white plaques or nodules at the level of the gastrointestinal tract or in the form of vaginitis for the genitalia localization. The invasive infection is characterized by fever, superficial nodules, rash, and sepsis. CT scan and echocardiogram, in order to rule out abscess/fungal pockets or cardiac vegetations, respectively, are mandatory in this circumstance.

While *C. albicans* species can be usually treated successfully with fluconazole, others (such as *C. parapsilosis, C. tropicalis, T. glabrata*, etc) tend to be resistant to this drug. In the past amphotericin B IV for 28 days, or liposome amphotericin in case of renal insufficiency was the obligate alternative. However, a new generation of antifungal agents such as voraconazole and caspifungin is now an excellent alternative for sensitive species because of the lack of nephrotoxicity.

Aspergillus infection represents the second most common fungal infection in transplant recipients. Lungs and sinuses are the most common sites involved by the primary infection.[71] The CNS is almost invariably involved in the secondary infection followed by liver and kidneys.[72] The onset is usually within 6 months after transplantation. The mortality rate is >90%.[73] Many factors have been characterized to increase the risk of infection like prolonged OR time (>12 hr), "second-look" surgery, prolonged use of broad spectrum antibiotics and of course heavy immunosuppression.[74] Although amphotericin was the only therapeutic option in the past, both caspifungin and voraconazole have demonstrated good activity against the fungus.[75–77]

## INFECTIOUS COMPLICATIONS IN LIVING DONOR RECIPIENTS

Published information regarding infectious complications in recipient of LR-SBTx is scarce. In a paper published by our group the rate of infectious complications was low compared with reports from other centers using cadaver LR-SBTx.[78] The bowel decontamination protocol we used consisted of donor bowel mechanical preparation and preoperative cefoxitin administration (2 g intravenously). Recipients received perioperative antibiotic prophylaxis with vancomycin (1 g IV before surgery) and piperacillin (3 g IV six or eight times per day, depending on renal function, for 3 days). In addition, to evaluate the efficacy of the donor bowel preparation we evaluated BT in two of the donors. Mesenteric lymph nodes and peritoneal swabs were obtained at the time of surgery, immediately before the bowel was harvested, and were sent for microbiologic evaluation.

We did not witness any bacterial infection. Furthermore, we did not encounter a single episode of rejection that could also be associated with BT.

Mesenteric lymph nodes and peritoneal swabs, considered initial stations of BT, were sterile in these patients. Optimal HLA matching and the consequent lower levels of immunosuppression used, a short cold ischemia time (<10 minutes), minimization of preservation injury, optimal donor condition, and hemodynamic stability have been considered in this circumstance. Most likely the low rate of infections associated with LR-SBTx in our experience is the consequence of the association of these factors with our graft preparation protocol.

## SURGICAL COMPLICATIONS IN THE INTESTINAL TRANSPLANTATION RECIPIENT

Surgical complications can cause graft loss and usually decrease in frequency with the learning curve. The most common are postoperative hemorrhage, vascular thrombosis, and biliary leaks or obstructions. Intestinal perforation, wound dehiscence, intra-abdominal abscesses, and chylous ascites have also been reported.[21,79–81] The experience of the surgical team is fundamental to reduce and appropriately manage these complications. Theoretically the elective context of living donor transplantation may represent an important factor in decreasing the incidence of technical complications in comparison with emergent cadaver intestinal transplant. The living donor graft is exposed to a minimal cold and warm ischemia time. In our series the cold ischemia time was only 5 minutes average, whereas the warm ischemia time was about 30 minutes. We did not encounter any technical complications, either from the intestinal anastomosis or from the vascular anastomosis in our 15 cases of LR-SBTx. In general, the reported rate of technical complications in the ITR in LR-SBTx compares favorably with the rates reported for cadaver IT.[55]

### Graft-Versus-Host Disease (GVHD)

IT is a high-risk procedure for the development of GVHD because of small bowel is a major lymphoid organ laden with both mesenteric lymph nodes (MLN) and gut-associated lymphoid tissue (GALT) in the form of Peyer's patches, as well as lamina propria and intraepithelial lymphocytes. The reported incidence of GVHD in intestinal transplant recipients is 5% to 14%.[82] Many symptoms of GVHD are not specific and may be confused with others disorders such as CMV infection, drug toxicity, and allergic manifestations. Skin rashes, ulceration of oral mucosa, diarrhea, lymphadenopathy, and native liver dysfunction have all been reported.[83] The diagnosis must always be confirmed by tissue biopsy and demonstration of donor-type chimerism on peripheral blood cells or recipient tissue after transplant. GVHD may be identified histologically even though typical clinical manifestations are not observed.[84] Reported histopathological criteria include keratinocyte necrosis, epithelial apoptosis of the native gastrointestinal tract, and epithelial cell necrosis of oral mucosa and donor-cell tissue infiltration.[83] The management of GFHD is often based on control of the symptoms like fever, diarrhea, and skin lesions; and on transfusion and careful use of immunosuppressive agents. The removal of the graft is at times the only option associated with positive results. However, some cases have been successfully treated with steroid administration and optimization of tacrolimus immunosuppression.[83] The increasing use of thymoglobulin as induction therapy in IT may potentially decrease the rate of GVHD, according to bone marrow literature.[85]

### Posttransplant Lymphoproliferative Disorders (PTLD)

The term *PTLD* encompasses a wide spectrum of lymphoproliferative processes in transplanted patients. Chronic EBV infection of seronegative naïve B cells may result in B-cell transformation and mono- or policlonal expansion. Although PTLD can occur in previously EBV-seropositive recipients, seronegativity remains the main risk factor for PTLD.[86] Because pediatric patients are usually EBV negative, they are at increased risk of PTLD compared to adults. The clinical manifestations of PTLD range from mild benign hyperplasia, usually policlonal, to severe monoclonal disease histologically indistinguishable from Hodgkin's lymphoma. Currently, the disease is classified according a system developed by Harris et al. in 1997.[87] Bowel transplant recipients have the highest incidence of PTLD in solid organ transplant.[88] The aggressive immunosuppressive regimens commonly used in IT represent the main factor responsible for this trend. Invasive monitoring of the intestine graft for PTLD as well as serial assessment of serological EBV status are warranted in these high-risk patients in order to institute timely treatment. Long-term prophylactic treatment is commonly used and is based on oral gancyclovir. The optimal management of PTLD remains controversial.[89] Reduction of immune suppression has been used routinely as first-line management. Additional treatments include antiviral therapy, monoclonal B-cell antibodies (Rituximab), chemotherapy, and cytotoxic T-lymphocyte infusion. The mortality related to PTLD is considerable. In a recent paper, we proposed to proceed with immediate removal of the intestinal graft and discontinuation of immunosuppression in the face of an aggressive monomorphic PTLD limited to the bowel graft. Because the bowel graft is not a life-supporting organ, this modality leaves open the opportunity of eradicating the disease and retransplanting the patient, as described in our clinical case.[18] The current practice of using less aggressive immunosuppressive protocols may contribute to the decrease of this serious complication in the future.

## CONCLUSIONS

The results of intestinal transplant have been steadily improving in the last decade. The procedure is still high risk for immunological, infectious, and technical complications. The development of less aggressive immunosuppressive regimens and strategies for tolerance induction are the keys to future growing success. LR-SBTx has potential advantages that may lead to a decrease in immunological and infectious complications after IT. Further study and a larger clinical experience will be necessary to determine if these potential advantages will translate in real benefit for IT recipients.

## References

1. Browne BJ, Johnson CP, Roza AM, et al. Endotoxemia after small bowel transplantation. *Transplant Proc* 1992;24(3):1107.
2. Price BA, Cumberland NS, Ingham Clark CL, et al. Changes in small intestinal microflora following small bowel transplantation in the rat and bacterial translocation in rejection and graft-versus-host disease. *Transplant Proc* 1992;24(3):1194.
3. Grant D, Hurlbut D, Zhong R, et al. Intestinal permeability and bacterial translocation following small bowel transplantation. *Transplantation* 1001;52(2):221–224.
4. Gifford GE, Lohmann-Matthes ML. Gamma interferon priming of mouse and human macrophages for induction of tumor necrosis factor production by bacterial lipopolysaccaride. *JNCI* 1987;78(1):121–124.
5. Waage A. Production and clearance of tumor necrosis factor in rats exposed to endotoxin and dexamethasone. *Clin Immunol Immunopathol* 1987;45:348–355.
6. Li XC, Zhong R, Zhu L, et al. Donor specific cytotoxicity induced by allogeneic intestinal epithelial cells in a sponge matrix model. *Transplant Int* 1995;8:13–19.
7. Bland P: MHC class II expression by the gut epithelium. *Immunol Today* 1988;9(6):174–188.
8. Johnsson C, Gannedahl G, Scheynius A, et al. Simultaneous occurrence of rejection and graft-versus-host reaction after allogeneic small bowel transplantation. *Transplantation* 1995;59(11):1524–1529.
9. Cohen Z, MacGregor AB, Moore KTH, et al. Canine small bowel transplantation. *Arch Surg* 1976;111:248–253.
10. Goulet O, Michel JL, Jobert A, et al. Small bowel transplantation alone or with the liver in children: changes by using FK506. *Transplant Proc* 1998;30:1569–1570.
11. Todo S, Tzakis AG, Abu-Elgmagd K, et al. Intestinal transplantation in composite visceral grafts or alone. *Ann Surg* 1992;216:112–123.
12. Reyes J, Bueno J, Kocoshis S, et al. Current status of intestinal transplantation in children. *J Pediatr Surg* 1998;33:243-254.
13. Kusne S, Manez R, Bonet H, et al. Infectious complications after small bowel transplantation in adults. *Transplant Proc* 1994;26:1682.
14. Todo S, Reyes J, Furukawa H, et al. Outcome analysis of 71 clinical intestinal transplantations. *Ann Surg* 1995;l222:270.
15. Abu Elgmad K, Todo S, Tzakis A, et al. Three years clinical experience with intestinal transplantation. *J Am Coll Surg* 1994;179:385.
16. Benedetti E, Marinov M, Porubsky M, et al. Living related segmental small bowel transplantation: from experimental to standardized procedure. *American Journ of Transpl* 2005; 5(11):429.
17. Benedetti E, Testa G, Holterman M, et al. Application of living-donor bowel transplantation to pediatric patients. *Clinical Transplant* 2004;18(S13):INV-134.
18. Talisetti A, Testa G, Holterman M, et al. Successful treatment of post-transplant lymphoproliferative disorder with removal of small bowel graft and subsequent second bowel transplant. *J Pediatric Gastroenterol Nutr* 2005;41(3):354–356.
19. Benedetti E, Testa G, Sankary H, et al. Successful treatment of trauma-induced short bowel syndrome with early living related bowel transplantation. *J Trauma* 2004;57:164–170.
20. Abu-Elgmad K, Reyes J, Todo S, et al. Clinical intestinal transplantation: new perspectives and immunologic considerations. *J Am Coll Surg* 1998;186:512–527.
21. Reyes J, Bueno J, Kocoshis S, et al. Current status of intestinal transplantation in children. *J Pediatr Surg* 1998;33:243–254.
22. Lee RG, Nakamura K, Tsamandas AC, et al. Pathology of human intestine transplantation. *Gastroenterology* 1996;110:1820–1834.
23. Sigurdsson L, Kocoshis S, Todo S, et al. Severe exfoliative rejection after intestinal transplantation in children. *Transplant Proc* 1996;28:2783–2784.
24. Koshiba T, Kitade H, Waer M, et al. Break of tolerance via donor-specific blood transfusion by high doses of steroids: a differential effect after intestinal transplantation and heart transplantation. *Transplant Proc* 2003;35(8):3153–3155.
25. Lan F, Hayamizu K, Strober S. Cyclosporine facilitates chimeric and inhibits nonchimeric tolerance after posttransplant total lymphoid irradiation. *Transplantation* 2000;69(4):649–655.
26. Pirenne J, D'Silva M, Jacquet N, et al. The use of spleen transplantation and cyclosporine. A treatment to ameliorate survival after small bowel transplantation. *Transplant Proc* 1993;25:1206.
27. Qian S, Lu L, Fu F, et al. Apoptosis within spontaneously accepted mouse allografts. Evidence for deletion of cytotoxic T cells and implications for tolerance induction. *J Immunol* 1997;158:4654–4661.
28. Sharland A, Yan Y, Wang C, et al. Evidence that apoptosis of activated T cells occurs in spontaneous tolerance of liver allografts and is blocked by manipulations which break tolerance. *Transplantation* 1999;68(11):1736–1745.
29. Furtado GC, Curotto de Lafaille MA, Kutchukhidze N, et al. Interleukin 2 signaling is required for CD4+ regulatory T cell function. *J Exp Med* 2002;196(6):851–857.
30. Reyes J, Bueno J, Kocoshis S, et al. Current status of intestinal transplantation in children. *J Pediatr Surg* 1998;33:243.
31. Langnas AN, Sudan DL, Kaufman S, et al. Intestinal transplantation: a single center experience. *Transplant Proc* 2000;32:1228.
32. Pinna AD, Weppler D, Nery J, et al. Intestinal transplantation at the University of Miami-five years of experience. *Transplant Proc* 2000;32:1226–1227.
33. Vennarecci G, Kato T, Misiakos EP, et al. Intestinal transplantation for short gut syndrome attributable to necrotizing enterocolitis. *Pediatrics* 2000;105:E25.

34. Jan D, Michel JL, Goulet O, et al. Up-to-date evolution of small bowel transplantation in children with intestinal failure. *J Pediatr Surg* 1999;34:841–844.

35. Beath SV, Protheroe SP, Brook GA, et al. Early experience of pediatric intestinal transplantation in the United Kingdom, 1993 to 1999. *Transplant Proc* 2000;32:1225.

36. Abu-Elgmagd K, Todo S, Tzakis AG, et al. Three years clinical experience with intestinal transplantation. *J Am Coll Surg* 1994;179(4):385–400.

37. Farmer DG, McDiarmid SV, Yersiz H, et al. Improved outcome after intestinal transplantation: an 8-year, single-center experience. *Transplant Proc* 2000;32:1233–1234.

38. Kato T. New techniques for prevention and treatment of rejection in intestinal transplantation. Current Opin Organ Transplant 2000;5:284–289.

39. Abu-Elmagd K, Fung J, McGhee W, et al. The efficacy of daclizumab for intestinal transplantation: preliminary report. *Transplant Proc* 2000;32:1195–1196.

40. Demetris AJ, Nalesnik MA. Transplant Pathology Internet Services. Available at http://www.tpis.upmc.edu. Accessed June 2005.

41. Starzl TE, Murase N, Abu-Elmagd K, et al. Tolerogenic immunosuppresion for organ transplantation. *Lancet* 2003;361:1502–1510.

42. Starzl TE, Murase N, Thomson A, et al. Liver transplants contribute to their own success. *Nat Med* 1996;2(20):163–165.

43. Starzl TE, Demetris AJ, Rao AS, et al. Spontaneous and iatrogenically augmented leukocite chimerism in organ transplant recipients. *Transplant Proc* 1994;26(5):3071–3076.

44. Starzl TE, Demetris AJ, Murase N, et al. Cell migration, chimerism, and graft acceptance. *Lancet* 1992 ;339:1579–1582.

45. Iwaki Y, Starzl TE, Yagihashi A, et al. Replacement of donor lymphoid tissue in small bowel transplants. *Lancet* 1991;337:818–819.

46 Pirenne J, Gruessner AC, Benedetti E, et al. Donor-specific unmodified bone marrow transfusion does not facilitate intestinal engraftment after bowel transplantation in a porcine model. *Surgery* 1997;121:79–88.

47. Bushell A, Pearson TC, Morris PJ, et al. Donor-recipient microchimerism is not required for tolerance induction following recipient pretreatment with donor-specific transfusion and anti-CD4 antibody: evidence of a clear role for short-term antigen persistence. *Transplantation* 1995;59:1367–1371.

48. Calne R, Friend P, Moffatt S, et al. Tolerance, perioperative campath 1H, and low-dose cyclosporin monotherapy in renal allograft recipients. *Lancet* 1991;6:351(9117):1701.

49. Tzakis AG, Kato T, Nishida S, et al. Preliminary experience with campath 1H (C1H) in intestinal and liver transplantation. *Transplantation* 2003;75(8):1227.

50. Pirenne J, Koshiba T, Geboes K, et al. Complete freedom from rejection after intestinal transplantation using a new tolerogenic protocol combined with low immunosuppression. *Transplantation* 2002;73(6):966–968.

51. Gruessner RW, Levay-Young BK, Nakhleh RE, et al. Portal donor-specific blood transfusion and mycophenolate mofetil allow steroid avoidance and tacrolimus dose reduction with sustained levels of chimerism in a pig model of intestinal transplantation. *Transplantation* 2004;77(10):1500–1506.

52. Fishbein TM, Florman S, Gondolesi G, et al. Intestinal transplantation before and after the introduction of sirolimus. *Transplantation* 2002;73(10):1538–1542.

53. Pascher A, Radke C, Dignass A, et al. Successful infliximab treatment of steroid and OK73 refractory acute cellular rejection in two patients after intestinal transplantation. Transplantation 2003;76(3):615–618.

54. Fishbein TM: The Current State of Intestinal *Transplantation. Transplantation* 2004;78(2):175–178.

55. The Intestinal Transplantation Registry. Available at: htpp://www.lhsc.on.ca/itr/. Accessed July 21, 2005.

56. Wang ZT, Yao YM, Xiao GX, et al. Risk factors of development of gut-derived bacterial translocation in thermally injured rats. *World J Gastroenterol* 2004;10(11):1619–1624.

57. Kane TD, Johnson SR, Alexander JW, et al. Bacterial translocation in organ donors: clinical observations and potential risk factors. *Clin Transplant* 1997;11(4):271–274.

58. Sedman PC, Macfie J, Sagar P, et al. The prevalence of gut translocation in humans. *Gastroenterology* 1994;107(3):643–649.

59. Cicalese L, Sileri, P, Green M, et al. Bacterial translocation in clinical intestinal transplantation. *Transplantation* 2001;71(10):1414–1417.

60. Roberts CA, Markin RS, Radio SJ, et al. Histopatologic evaluation of primary intestinal transplant recipients at autopsy: a single center experience. IV International Small Bowel Symposium (Syllabus), 6-9 October 1999, Omaha, NB.

61. Loinaza C, Katoa T, Nishidaa S, et al. Bacterial infections after intestine and multivisceral transplantation. *Transplant Proc* 2003;35(5):1929–1930.

62. Kobayashi S, Kato T, Nishida S, et al. Necrotizing fasciitis following liver and small intestine transplantation. *Pediatr Transplant* 2002;6:344–347.

63. Wall DB, De Virgilio C, Black S, et al. Objective criteria may assist in distinguishing necrotizing fasciitis from nonnecrotizing soft tissue infection. *Am J Surg* 2000;179:17–21.

64. Hsieh T, Samson LM, Jabbour M, et al. Necrotizing fasciitis in children in eastern Ontario: A case-control study. *CMAJ* 2000;163:393.

65. Farmer DG, McDiarmidb SV, Winstonc D, et al. Effectiveness of aggressive prophylatic and preemptive therapies targeted against cytomegaloviral and Epstein–Barr viral disease after human intestinal transplantation. *Transplant Proc* 2002;34(3):948–949.

66. Pinchoff RJ, Kaufman SS, Magid MS, et al. Adenovirus infection in pediatric small bowel transplantation recipients. *Transplantation* 2003;76(1):183–189.

67. Cundy KC, Bidgood AM, Lynch G, et al. Pharmacokinetics, bioavailability, metabolism, and tissue distribution of cidofovir (HPMPC) and cyclic HPMPC in rats. *Drug Metab Dispos* 1996;24(7):745–752.

68. Kaufman SS, Chatterjee NK, Fuschino ME, et al. Characteristic of human calicivirus enteritis in intestinal transplant recipients. *J Pediatr Gastroenterol Nutr* 2005;40(3):328–333.

69. Kusne S, Furukawa H, Abu-Elgmad K, et al. Infectious complications after small bowel transplantation in adults: an update. *Transplant Proc* 1996;28:2761.

70. Green M, Michaels MG, Weber SA, et al. The management of Epstein-Barr virus associated post-transplant lymphoproliferative disorders in pediatric solid organ transplant recipients. *Pediatr Transplant* 1999;3(4):271–281.

71. Torre-Cisneros J, Manez R, Kusne S, et al. The spectrum of aspergillosis in liver transplant patients: comparison of FK506 and cyclosporine immnunosuppression. *Transplant Proc* 23(6):3040–3041.

72 Henwick S, Hetherington SV. "Aspergillosis" Infections in immunocompromised infants and children. Patrick CC, ed. New York: Churchill Livingstone; 1992:557–572.

73. Lin SJ, Schranz J, Teutsch SM. Aspergillosis case-fatality rate: systematic review of the literature. Comprehensive, systematic review describing significant mortality related to aspergillus despite advances in diagnosis and treatment. *Clin Infect Dis* 2001;32:358–366.

74. Gavalda J, Len O, San Juan R, et al. RESITRA (Spanish Network for Research on Infection in Transplantation). Risk factors for invasive aspergillosis in solid-organ transplant recipients: a case-control study. *Clin Infect Dis* 2005;41(1):52–59.

75. Dinser R, Grgic A, Kim YJ, et al. Successful treatment of disseminated aspergillosis with the combination of voriconazole, caspofungin, granulocyte transfusions, and surgery followed by allogeneic blood stem cell transplantation in a patient with primary failure of an autologous stem cell graft. *Eur J Haematol* 2005;74(5):438.

76. Schuster F, Moelter C, Schmid I, et al. Successful antifungal combination therapy with voriconazole and caspofungin. *Pediatr Blood Cancer* 2005;44(7):682–685.

77. Kartsonis NA, Saah AJ, Joy Lipka C, et al. Salvage therapy with caspofungin for invasive aspergillosis: results from the caspofungin compassionate use study. *J Infect* 2005;50(3):196–205.

78. Cicalese L, Sileri P, Coady N, et al. Proposed protocol to reduce bacterial infectious complications in livig related small bowel transplant recipients. *Transplant Proc* 2002;34(3):950.

79. Reyes J, Selby R, Abu-Elmagd K, et al. Intestinal and multiple organ transplantation. In: Shoemaker WC, Ayers SM, Grenvik NA, Holbrook PR, eds. *Textbook of Critical Care*, 4th ed. Philadelphia: W.B. Saunders Company;1999:1678–1687.

80. Abu-Elgmagd KM, Reyes J, Fung JJ, et al. Clinical intestine transplantation in 1998: Pittsburgh experience. *Acta Gastro-Enterologica Belgica* 1999;62:244–247.

81. Mousa H, Bueno J, Griffiths J, et al. Intestinal motility after small bowel transplantation. *Transplant Proc* 1998;30:2535–2536.

82. Pirenne J, Benedetti E, et al. Graft versus host response: clinical and biological relevance after transplantation of solid organs. *Transplant Rev* 1996;10(1):46–48.

83. Mazariegos GV, Abu-Elmagd K, Jaffe R, et al. Graft versus host disease in intestinal transplantation. *Am J Transplant* 2004;4(9):1459–1465.

84. Langrehr JM, Hoffman RA, et al. Induction of graft versus host disease and rejection by sensitized small bowel allograft. *Transplantation* 1991;52:399.

85. Basara N, Baurmann H, Kolbe K, et al. Antithymocyte globulin for the prevention of graft-versus-host disease after unrelated hematopoietic stem cell transplantation for acute myeloid leukemia: results from the multicenter German cooperative study group. *Bone Marrow Transplt* 2005;35(10):1011–1018.

86. Ho M, Miller G, Atchison RW, et al. Epstein-Barr virus infections and DNA hybridization studies in post transplant lymphoma and lymphoproliferative lesions. *J Infect Dis* 1985;152:876–881.

87. Harris NL, Ferry JA, Swerdlow SH. Post-transplant lymphoproliferative disorders. Summary of Society for Hematopathology Workshop. *Semion Diagn Pathol* 1997;14:8–15.

88. Sudan DL, Kaufman SS, Shaw BW Jr, et al. Isolated intestinal transplantation for intestinal failure. *Am J Gastroenterol* 2000;(6):1506–1515.

89. Green M, Michaels MG. Infectious complications of solid-organ transplantation in children. *Adv Pediatr Infect Dis* 1992;7:181–204.

# 34.4 PATHOLOGY OF SMALL BOWEL TRANSPLANTATION

*Jose Jessurun, MD, Stefan Pambuccian, MD*

Although the outcome of patients who have undergone small-bowel transplantation has been steadily improving, numerous challenges remain. The clinical management of these patients is strongly influenced by the information derived from the microscopic examination of biopsy specimens obtained from the transplanted organ. In this chapter we present a brief summary of the pathology associated with small-bowel transplants based on published information and our experience at the University of Minnesota Medical Center, Fairview.

## HISTORICAL VIGNETTE

Intestinal transplantation was first envisioned by Alexis Carrel as a therapeutic option that would become available once the techniques for vascular anastomosis became feasible. Preclinical studies in dogs were performed by Richard Lillihei at the University of Minnesota in 1959 which were followed 5 years latter by the first human intestinal transplant which was carried out by Ralph Deterlin in Boston.[1] This and other attempts were discouraging and most patients died within few days as a result of sepsis, allograft rejection, and technical complications. This situation persisted during the next 20 years until surgical techniques improved and cyclosporine became available. The first successful small-bowel transplants were performed in France and Germany. Further refinement of the surgical techniques, analysis of outcomes and basic science research has made small-bowel transplantation a reasonable therapeutic modality for the management of intestinal insufficiency.[2,3] Today there are over 40 centers in North America and over 60 worldwide that perform this type of surgery.[4] Over the years the number of cases has increased from 11 in 1990 to a rate of 140 per year in 2003. Of all transplants, 75.5% were performed in the United States.[5] At present most organs continue to be obtained from cadaveric donors. Recently, transplants from living related donors have been carried out to overcome the critical shortage of organs.[6]

## PATIENT CHARACTERISTICS

According to the 2003 report on the intestine transplant registry, slightly more than half of transplants were performed in adults. However, proportionally more combined intestinal and liver transplants occurred in children. Thirty-two grafts were obtained from living donors. In children, intestinal failure was more frequently the result of gastroschisis, volvulus, necrotizing enterocolitis, pseudo-obstruction, and Hirshsprung's disease; whereas in adults ischemia, Crohn's disease, trauma, and other disorders associated with short gut were the main indications.[5]

Graft survival has considerably improved over time. The two factors most significantly associated with increased graft survival were transplants performed in patients waiting at home versus at the hospital and antibody induction immune suppression with monoclonal IL-alpha 2 receptor blockers or polyclonal antilymphocyte agents. Of the 919 recipients reported to the registry since 1985, 47.6% have died. The most common causes of death were sepsis and rejection. After 1998, the 1-year graft/patient survival rate were 65%/77% for intestinal grafts, 59%/60% for small-bowel and liver grafts, and 61%/66% for multivisceral grafts. The 1-year overall graft/patient survival rates for patients receiving living donor grafts were slightly (but not significantly) better than for those whose with cadaveric grafts.[5]

## PRESERVATION INJURY

Despite the high number and diversity of cells present in the small bowel that may release toxic mediators on reperfusion such as reactive oxygen and nitrogen intermediates and various proteases and cytokines, preservation and reperfusion injury have not been a major problem in small-bowel transplantation. The extraordinary regenerative capacity of the intestinal mucosa may explain this fortunate event. The molecular events that participate in intestinal regeneration have recently begun to be deciphered.[7] In experimental animal modes, when the different segments of the small intestine are compared, the ileum appears to withstand ischemic injury better than the jejunum and, despite the abundance of lymphoid tissue in the latter segment, the frequency and severity of acute rejection is not encountered more often than in jejunal grafts.

Preimplantation specimens frequently show surface epithelial detachment from the underlying edematous lamina propria. After reperfusion focal epithelial denudation may be present. Shortly thereafter, numerous mitotic figures appear within the crypts indicating vigorous regeneration. Mild neutrophilic infiltrates on the superficial lamina propria and surface epithelium may be occasionally present. Follow-up biopsies takes as early as 2 days may either be normal or show minimal changes; by 10 days posttransplant, the majority of the biopsy specimens show a normal mucosa. Due to the rapid repopulation of enterocytes, bacterial translocation does not appear to be problem at this stage.[8]

# REJECTION

Clinical signs of rejection are nonspecific and include abdominal pain, fever, ileus, stomal bloody output from stoma, nausea, and vomiting. The same clinical manifestation may be caused by a variety of infections or other complications such as ischemia. Histologic examination of mucosal biopsy specimens is the gold-standard test for the diagnosis of rejection and, in conjunction with cultures, for the identification of infections.

## ACUTE REJECTION

Most patients experience one or multiple episodes of acute rejection, which generally occurs between posttransplant days 5 and 60. However, acute rejection occurring several months after transplantation is not uncommon. Endoscopic examination of the mucosa reveals a variety of lesions ranging from edema and hyperemia in mild cases to granularity, loss of the vascular pattern, and ulcers. It is important to keep in mild that the areas showing rejection may have a multifocal or patchy distribution. For this reason it is recommended to take a minimum of three biopsies from the affected areas. If the lesions are ulcerated, in addition to biopsies from the ulcer, the mucosa at the periphery of the ulcer and in between ulcers should be sampled since it is at these sites where the diagnostic lesions are going to be found. If possible, biopsies of the native bowel should be included and submitted separately since comparative evaluation of these specimens are extremely helpful in the differential diagnosis of rejection.

As in other organs, small-bowel allografts may be affected by cellular and humoral rejection. The histologic diagnosis of cellular acute rejection requires the presence of inflammatory infiltrates in the lamina propria, evidence of epithelial cell injury, and the identification of apoptotic cells.[9] (Figure 34.4-1)

The inflammatory infiltrate is composed of a mixture of lymphocytes, eosinophils, neutrophils, plasma cells, and histiocytes. In the majority of cases, lymphocytes are the predominant cells;

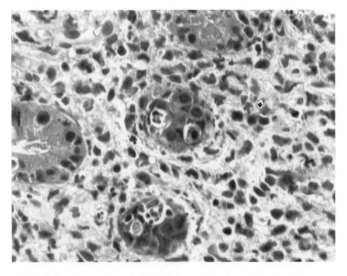

**FIGURE 34.4-1**

Small-bowel transplant biopsy specimen showing acute rejection. The lamina propria contains numerous inflammatory cells including activated lymphocytes. Several apoptotic lesions are present within the crypts.

however, occasionally eosinophils may be quite abundant. Within the infiltrating lymphoid population several cell types are universally present: in addition to typical small lymphocytes with round hyperchromatic nuclei there are larger lymphoid cells with dispersed chromatin and small nucleoli which have been called blastic or activated lymphocytes.

Epithelial cell injury is identified by shortening of the epithelial cells, mucin depletion, and nuclear hyperchromatia. Focal or diffuse infiltration of crypts by lymphocytes, eosinophils, and neutrophils is generally present.

Apoptotic cells are identified as clear spaces within crypts containing fragmented (karryorhectic) nuclei. Most of the apoptotic bodies are located toward the base of the crypts.[8,9] When evaluating these lesions, several important considerations should be kept in mind

1. Occasional apoptotic bodies (usually no more than 2 per 10 crypts) are found in the normal intestinal mucosa.

2. In addition to rejection, apoptotic bodies are part of the constellation of changes present in infectious enteritis of viral etiology.

3. Apoptotic enteric cells should be differentiated from degenerating infiltrating inflammatory cells.

Apoptotic cells may predominate over lamina propria inflammation and crypt degeneration in acute rejection that occurs several months after transplantation, mimicking the changes seen in graft-versus-host disease.

A grading schema has been proposed to evaluate the severity of acute rejection. Grading, coupled with the clinical findings and endoscopic observations, may influence therapeutic decisions.[10] Mild acute rejection may require an increase in basal immunosuppressive drug treatment, whereas a more aggressive therapy may be indicated for moderate and severe rejection. The following five grades have been proposed

| No evidence of acute cellular rejection | Normal histology |
|---|---|
| Indeterminate for ACR | Minimal inflammation and epithelial cell injury. Few apoptotic cells (<6/10 crypts). |
| Mild ACR | Localized inflammation, epithelial cell injury. Frequent apoptosis; no ulcers. |
| Moderate ACR | Abundant dispersed infiltrates; diffuse epithelial cell injury, confluent apoptosis, mild to moderate intimal arteritis; no ulcers. |
| Severe ACR | Similar features plus ulcers; possible severe intimal or transmural arteritis. |

Endoscopic biopsies taken 4 to 5 days after successful treatment show evidence of epithelial regeneration. Actively proliferating mucin-depleted enterocytes derived from the adjacent viable mucosa cover the luminal surface of the lamina propria. This is followed by penetration into the lamina propria and differentiation toward the different cellular components of the crypts and formation of villi. In addition, there is a decrease in the amount of inflammation and number of apoptotic lesions. In our experience, biopsies taken less than 3 days after the initiation of treatment do not provide clinically relevant information, because few if any changes are present when compared to the pretreatment biopsy specimens.

In addition to T-cell-mediated cellular rejection, humoral mechanism may play a role in acute bowel allograft rejection. According to a recent study, humoral-mediated injury to the microvasculature develops in a considerable proportion of cases during the first 30 days after transplantation and seldom after more than 3 months. On light microscopy vascular congestion and erythrocyte extravasation appear to be the main findings.[11] Of interest, no capillary leukocyte margination and/or thrombosis, as seen in the acute humoral rejection of the kidney, was identified. We recommend caution in using these criteria for humoral rejection, because congestion and microhemorrhages in the lamina propria are relatively nonspecific and may be due to trauma from the biopsy procedure. Credible evidence of humoral rejection relies on the demonstration of C4d and immunoglobulin deposition on small vessels. According to the aforementioned study graft survival is significantly lower in patients with early vascular humoral rejection.[10]

## Chronic Rejection

Progressive graft failure clinically manifested as persistent diarrhea and nonhealing mucosal ulcers characterize chronic rejection. The hallmark lesion is obliterative arteriopathy. However vessels of the size affected by this process are not present in endoscopic biopsy specimens. When histologic evidence of chronic ischemic injury is present, the diagnosis of chronic rejection is entertained along with other causes of persistent ischemia. Early changes consist of patchy fibrosis of the lamina propria, focal crypt loss and shortening. Late changes include loss of villous architecture and crypts, chronic ulcers, pyloric gland metaplasia and mucosal fibrosis[12] (Figure 34.4-2).

The events that increase the likelihood for the development of chronic graft failure include acute rejection within the first month, multiple rejection episodes, high grade rejection, isolated small

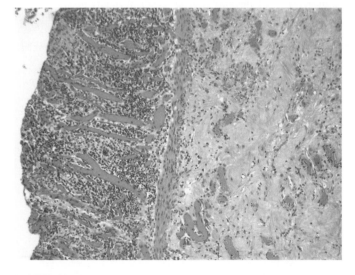

**FIGURE 34.4-2**

Small-bowel transplant resection specimen. This patient developed chronic rejection. The lamina propria is devoid of crypts and villi; the underlying submucosa is fibrotic.

bowel grafts rather than combined bowel-liver grafts, older recipient age, non-Caucasian race and Caucasian to non-Caucasian transplant.[12]

## INFECTIONS AFTER INTESTINAL TRANSPLANTATION

An essential differential diagnosis that has to be considered when analyzing biopsy specimen from small-bowel transplant patients is infectious enteritis versus rejection because selection of the wrong therapy may exacerbate either problem. Achieving an adequate level of immunosuppression that does not translate into a facilitation of infections is an extraordinarily complex task. The transgression to the mucosal barrier caused either by rejection or infections, in addition to bowel dysfunction, leads to translocation of infectious organisms and sepsis, which is the leading cause of death after intestinal transplantation. However, the differentiation of these conditions by histopathologic analysis alone may be extremely difficult because the cells responsible for infectious (and immunologic) surveillance, which constitute the inflammatory infiltrates, are derived form the recipient. These cells are of a different HLA type than the surrounding stromal and antigen-presenting cells. Thus, a similar inflammatory response would be expected irrespective of whether the cells are responding to viral epitopes presented by foreign HLA antigens or to the foreign HLA antigen epitopes themselves. To further complicate this diagnostic dilemma several viral infections do not produce easily recognizable cytopathic changes. For this reason, it is essential to submit adequate cultures at the time when the endoscopic biopsies are obtained. For viruses, the use of shell vial assays with probes directed against specific viral antigens or PCR-based techniques to detect viral genome sequences are excellent options that provide results within 48 hours.[13]

The prevalence of viral infections in small bowel transplant recipients is very high and account for a substantial number of graft loss. These infections tend to be more common in male children than in females and adults. Adenovirus and rotavirus account for the majority of the infections. Rotavirus produces a self-limited disease, which is treated by supportive care. Adenovirus infection is a more serious condition. Mortality rates among children who have undergone liver transplantation are as high as 10%. The histopathologic inflammatory pattern associated with adenovirus infection of small intestinal mucosa includes crypt cell apoptosis and nuclear disarray, Eosinophilic nuclear inclusions, the so-called "smudge cells" with enlarged basophilic nuclei, and an inflammatory infiltrate with abundant plasma cells[14] (Figure 34.4-3). As has been mentioned before, in some cases the nonspecific inflammatory pattern and the absence of clear-cut viral cytopathic changes make histopathologic analysis unreliable because the inflammatory pattern overlaps with that of rejection. Immunohistochemical reactions are now available that aid in the identification of infected cells.

The use of prophylactic therapies directed against cytomegalovirus (CMV) and Epstein–Barr virus (EBV) have lowered the incidence of these infections. In immunosuppressed patients, CMV infection is almost always associated with cytopathic changes that can be easily identified on hematoxylin- and eosin-stained slides and by immunohistochemistry. In the past CMV and EBV infections were problematic with disease rates as high as 40%.[15] Another virus that has been recently identified as a cause of prolonged diarrheal illness in pediatric recipients of small intestinal transplant is calicivirus. Norwal-like virus and Sapporuo virus are the two subgroups of calicivirus pathogenic

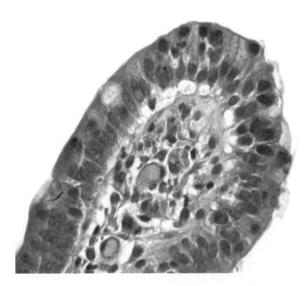

**FIGURE 34.4-3**

Small-bowel transplant biopsy specimen showing adenovirus infection. Several cells at the tip of this villus contain ill-defined intranuclear inclusions giving the nuclear chromatin a smudged appearance.

in humans. The pathologic changes associated with this infection include mononuclear infiltrates in the lamina propria, villous blunting, disarray of surface epithelial cells, increased apoptosis in the surface epithelium, and superficial lamina propria. The diagnosis can be confirmed by the use of reverse-transcription polymerase chain reaction to detect viral RNA polymerase genes in stool and tissues.[16]

Due to antimicrobial therapy, bacterial infections do not appear to be a major problem. However, for the same reason, infections by *Clostridium difficile* have been reported.[13]

Infection by *Cryptosporidium* and *Giardia lamblia* has also been reported, with inconsistent response to therapy. Patients should be advised to avoid untreated tap and well water to avoid these infections.[17,18]

## POSTTRANSPLANT LYMPHOPROLIFERATIVE DISORDERS (PTLDS)

A serious complication of chronic immunosuppression is the development of life-threatening lymphoproliferations. In most instances, infection by EBV is etiologically related to the development of these complications. PTLDs have been extensively characterized on morphologic, phenotypic, and molecular bases.

The incidence of PTLDs is higher with intestinal transplant recipients especially in the pediatric population where absence of EBV exposure is more common. PTLDs develop in as many as 11.1% of pediatric small–bowel-only transplants, in 10.4% of those with combined liver–intestine transplants and in 18.6% of those with multivisceral transplants in the pediatric population compared to 3.4%, 2.9%, and 6.0%, respectively, in the adult population. PTLDs involve native and allograft organs. Morphologically, the proliferative lesions range from those that have a polymorphic appearance resembling other reactive conditions to frank lymphomas. The diagnosis of EBV infection can be confirmed in the biopsy material by in situ hybridization studies for EBV early RNA (EBER).[19]

## References

1. Lillehei R, Groott B, Miller FA. The physiological responses of the small bowel of the dog to ischemia including prolonged in vitro preservation of the small bowel with successful replacement and survival. *Ann Surg* 1959;150:543–560.
2. McAllister VC, Grant DR. Clinical small bowel transplantation. In: Grant DR, Woods RFM, eds. *Small Bowel Transplantion*. Great Britain: Edward Arnold; 1994;121–132.
3. Fryer JP. Intestinal transplantion: an update. Curr Opin Gastroenterol 2005;21:162–168.
4. Intestinal transplant registry: www.intestinaltransplantregistry.com
5. Grant D, Abu-Elmagd K, Reyes J, et al. 2003 Report of the Intestine Transplant Registry. A New Era Has Dawned. *Ann Surg* 2005;241:607–613.
6. Gruessner RW, Sharp HL. Living-related intestinal transplantation: first report of a standardized surgical techniques. *Transplantation* 1997;64:1605–1607.
7. Abraham C, Cho HC. Inducing Intestinal Growth. *N Engl J Med* 2005;353:2297–2299.
8. Lee RG, Nakamura K, Tsamandas AC, et al. *Gastroenterology* 1996;110:1820–1834.
9. Ruiz P, Bagni A, Brown R, et al. Histological Criteria for the Identification of Acute Cellular Rejection in Human Small Bowel Allografts: Results of the Pathology Workshop at the VIII International Samll Bowel Transplant Symposium. *Transplant Proc* 2004;36:335–337.
10. Wu T, Abu-Elmagd K, Bond G, et al. A schema for Histologic Grading of Small Intestine Allograft Acute Rejection. *Transplantation* 2003;75:1241–1248.
11. Ruiz P, Garcia M, Pappas P, et al. Mucosal Vascular Alterations in Isolated Small-Bowel Allografts: Relationship to Humoral Sensitization. *Am J Transpl* 2003;3:43–49.
12. Parizhskaya M, Redondo C, Demetris A, et al. Chronic Rejection of Small Bowel Grafts: Pediatric and Adult Study of Risk Factors and Morphologic Progression. *Pediatr Dev Pathol* 2003;6:240–260.
13. Ziring D, Tran R, Edelstein S, et al. Infectious Enteritis After Intestinal Transplantation: Incidence, Timing and Outcome. *Transplantation* 2005;79:702–709.
14. Pinchoff RJ, Kaufman SS, Magid MS, et al. Adenovirus infection in pediatric small bowel transplantation recipients. *Transplantation* 2003;76:183–189.
15. Pascher A, Klupp J, Schulz RJ, et al. CMV, EBV, HHV6 and HHV7 Infections After Intestinal Transplantation Without Specific Antiviral Prophylaxis. *Transplant Proc* 2004;36:381–382.
16. Morotti RA, Kaufman SS, Fishbein TM, et al. Calicivirus Infection in Pediatric Small Intestine Transplant Recipients : Pathological Considerations. *Hum Pathol* 2004;35:1236–1240.
17. Delis SG, Tector J, Kato T, et al. Diagnosis and treatment of Cryptosporidium infection in intestinal transplant recipients. *Transplant Proc* 2002;34:951–952.
18. Chen XM, Keithly JS, Paya CV, et al. Current concepts: cryptosporidiosis. *N Engl J Med* 2002;346:1723–1731.
19. Finn L, Reyes J, Bueno J, Yunis E. Epstein-Barr Virus Infections in Children Alter Transplantation of the Sami Intestine. *Am J Surg Pathol* 1998;22:299–309.

## 34.5  REGISTRY REPORT AND LONG-TERM OUTCOME

*Shimul A. Shah, MD,*
*David R. Grant, MD*

Living donor intestine transplantation has become a valid alternative to deceased donor intestine transplantation. Potential advantages include reduced waiting times with attendant reductions in morbidity and mortality, better organ preservation, and less rejection. This chapter reviews (1) Registry data on the current status of deceased donor intestine grafting, (2) pre-Registry data on live donation and evolution of techniques, (3) current outcomes of live donor intestine transplantation, and (4) future directions.

## CURRENT STATUS OF DECEASED DONOR INTESTINE TRANSPLANTATION

Intestinal transplantation has become the treatment of choice for patients with end-stage gut failure and life-threatening complications on parenteral nutrition. As the results improve, this procedure is poised to become the preferred option for treatment of intestine failure, much as kidney transplantation is preferred to dialysis for the treatment of end-stage renal disease.

Over the last 20 years, there has been a remarkable improvement in short-term graft- and patient survival rates after intestine transplantation and a resulting growth in the application of this procedure (Figures 34.5.1 and 34.5.2). Over 1,292 transplants have been performed in 1,210 patients in 65 centers from 12 countries. Children are more susceptible than adults to liver injury from parenteral nutrition. Thus, isolated intestine grafts are more commonly performed in adults, whereas combined liver and intestine grafts or multivisceral grafts are more commonly performed in infants. Factors contributing to improved outcomes in recent years include center experience, transplantation of a higher ratio of patients who are waiting at home, and the use of induction therapy to prevent exfoliative rejection. One-year patient survival rates of more than 80% are now being achieved. More than 90% of survivors stop parenteral nutrition, resume oral intake, and return to normal daily activities.[1,2] Quality of life in intestinal recipients is excellent and successful intestine grafting is cost-saving compared with maintenance parenteral nutrition.[3–5]

Two factors currently limit deceased donor intestine grafting from more widespread application (1) a shortage of deceased

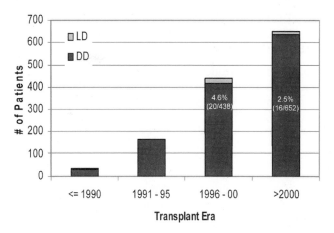

**FIGURE 34.5-2**

Ratio of living donor intestine transplants to deceased donor intestinal transplants (all types).

donor organs, which is associated with a high mortality rate on the waiting list for intestine transplants[6]; and (2) high rates of late graft and patient loss due to rejection and infection.[1,7,8] Living donor intestine transplantation offers theoretical advantages which could help to address these problems.

Patients awaiting intestine transplants in the United States have the highest mortality of any group on the waiting list based on the United Network of Organ Sharing (UNOS) registry (available at http://www.unos.org). Although there are a small number of patients on the waiting list for intestine transplantation, the waiting time is long, averaging 220 days. The mortality on the waiting list for a deceased donor graft is up to 25% for adult recipients and 60% for pediatric recipients.[6,7] Early referral and living donor intestinal transplantation can reduce waiting time, thus decreasing mortality and preventing progression of the complications caused by total parenteral nutrition (TPN).[6,9] UNOS has recently allocated more points to patients waiting for intestine and liver grafts; whether this change in practice will significantly improve mortality rates remains to be seen.

Currently, the 5-year patient survival rates for all types of intestine transplants are approximately 50%. In contrast to the dramatic improvement in short-term survival after intestine grafting, the longer-term survival of grafts in patients who have lived for more than 1 year after intestine transplantation has failed to improve (2005 Intestine Registry Report, www.Intestinetransplant.org). Graft rejection and/or infection are still the most common causes of early and late deaths. The use of living donors has the theoretical potential to reduce the risk of rejection and sepsis after transplantation, although these advantages are as yet unproven. Potential factors that may reduce the risk of rejection using live donor grafts include: better donor bowel decontamination; improved tissue antigen matching, reduced cold ischemic injury; and optimization of recipient medical status.[10,11] If live donation permits the use of reduced immune suppression, this would also help to reduce the infection rates.

The potential benefits of live donation must be weighed against the potential disadvantages of living donor intestinal transplantation which include: risk to the donor, poorer function because a smaller segment of bowel is transplanted, and limited experience to date, largely confined to adolescents and identical twins.[4,7]

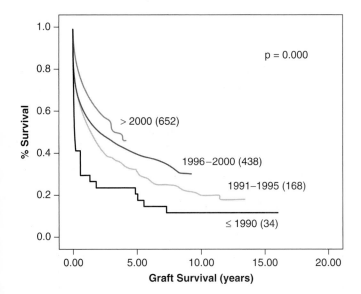

**FIGURE 34.5-1**

Comparison of graft survival of all intestine transplants by era.

## PRE-REGISTRY DATA ON LIVE DONOR INTESTINE TRANSPLANTATION AND EVOLUTION OF TECHNIQUES

The potential for live donation to reduce the risk of intestine graft rejection was demonstrated in the infancy of this procedure, but it took many years before reliable surgery techniques were worked out.

The surgical techniques for intestine grafting were first established in dogs.[12–14] Early experiments in rodent, dog, and pig models of intestine grafting demonstrated a survival advantage with matching of histocompatibility antigens.[15–17] These advantages were subsequently confirmed in mice also.[15,18,19]

Seven attempts were made to transplant the intestine in the 1960s and early 1970s in the precyclosporine era with limited success. Most failed because of technical complications. It is noteworthy, however, that the longest survivor received an HLA-identical ileal segment from her sister, surviving for 76 days after transplantation.[20]

Many of the early clinical cases of living donor intestine transplantation were plagued by poor function. In one case, only 60 cm of distal jejunum and proximal ileum was removed and this graft never functioned well.[21] In another case, the ileocecal valve was removed along with the terminal ileum resulting in diarrhea due to increased transit times and a vitamin $B_{12}$ deficiency.[22] Two other early cases of proximal small bowel transplantation failed because of vascular complications. In both of these cases, procurement of the jejunum necessitated a complex vascular reconstruction of several small jejunal vessels to create only one arterial and venous anastomosis with the recipient vessel leading to anastomotic vascular stenosis and graft failure.[23] Based on this experience, most centers currently now prefer to procure a jejunal graft which has a single vascular pedicle that can be easily anastomosed to recipient vessels.

Gruessner has described the surgical technique for live donation of isolated intestine grafts which is most commonly used today. The graft consists of a 100- to 200-cm segment of donor terminal ileum (no more than one third of the donor small bowel) with preservation of the ileocecal valve in the donor. Arterial inflow is provided by the ileocolic branch of the superior mesenteric artery; venous outflow is via the ileocolic branch of the superior mesenteric vein.[9]

Benedetti has described a technique for simultaneous procurement segments of the intestine and the liver from a single live donor.[24] This combined graft consists of a left lateral segment of liver, which is implanted first in a standard piggyback fashion. Despite the complete absence of intestine, the flow in the portal vein appears to be sufficient for perfusion of the liver. One week later, both the donor and the pediatric recipient are brought back to the operating room for harvest and implantation of 150 cm of terminal ileum.[24] To date, Benedetti et al. have performed four simultaneous living donor liver and intestine transplants with excellent results (Benedetti, manuscript in preparation).

The intestine grafts are transplanted using an arterial anastomosis to the native superior mesenteric artery stump or more commonly the infrarenal aorta. The vein is usually anastomosed end-to-side to the vena cava. Intestine continuity is restored with proximal and distal anastomoses to the native gut; a loop ileostomy or chimney stoma is exteriorized to provide access to the graft for biopsies. The stoma is closed approximately 3 months after the transplanted, provided the patient is doing well.

Intestinal grafts show evidence of adaptation, characterized by increased length and size of the villi.[25] Thus, it is possible for ileal grafts measuring 150 to 200 cm of terminal ileum without the ileocecal valve to provide sufficient nutrient absorption to achieve independence from parenteral nutrition.

## CURRENT OUTCOMES

### Single-Center Reports

Living donor intestinal transplant is not routinely performed and therefore few reports of short- and long-term outcomes exist. The largest series, reported by Benedetti at the University of Illinois at Chicago, included nine patients who underwent transplantation of 150 to 200 cm resection of terminal ileum proximal to the ileocecal valve. The 1- and 3-year actuarial patient and graft survival rates were 78% and 67%, respectively.[6] In Benedetti's series, six or seven living donor intestinal transplants HLA matching achieved long-term function and survival. No rejection has been documented in these grafts during the first year posttransplant at their institution (Benedetti, personal communication). Benedetti's team believes that their low rate of acute rejection is due to the use of live donor grafts. However, to balance this perspective, it must be pointed out that other centers have reported rates with graft rejection comparable to deceased donor organs[10] and very low rates of intestine graft rejection have also been reported with deceased donor grafts (A. Langnas, Omaha, personal communication).

Four identical twin intestinal transplants of 150 to 200 cm small bowel have enjoyed complete recovery with no adverse long-term side affects.

Case reports of living donor intestinal transplants at other centers have described similar outcomes to the larger programs.[9,23,26,27] None of the reports of live donor intestine transplants have described any serious, long-term adverse effects in the donor, and no donor deaths have been reported.

### 2005 Registry Report on Live Donor Intestine Transplantation

The International Registry report was established to evaluate results of intestinal transplantation and long-term outcomes. There has been a 100% participation rate in the Registry; to the best of our knowledge the Registry captures more than 99% of all intestine transplants performed worldwide between January 1985 and March 2005. Of 1,292 intestinal transplants performed to date, 41 grafts (3.2%) were obtained from living donors at 16 centers (Table 34.5-1) in 7 different countries (Figure 34.5-2).

Living related intestinal transplants were performed more commonly in males (male 63%; female 57%) and in the pediatric population (< 18 years; Figure 34.5-3). The causes of intestinal failure requiring living donor intestinal transplant are shown in Figure 34.5-4. Volvulus, followed by intestinal ischemia, is the most common indication, which reflects the procedure being done more commonly in children.

Intestinal graft survival has steadily improved over time. Close to half of the patients who have undergone living donor intestinal transplantation are currently alive today (21/41; 51%). Causes of death included sepsis (n = 12; 29%), liver failure (n = 2; 4.9%), rejection (n = 2; 4.9%), and other causes (n = 4; 9.8%). Only one patient lost their intestinal graft due to vascular thrombosis (2.5%). This suggests that the small vascular pedicle in living donor intestinal transplant is not a significant risk factor for graft loss when compared to deceased donor grafts as technical results

**TABLE 34.5-1**

## LIVING DONOR INTESTINE TRANSPLANT CENTERS

| Transplant Centers | Country |
|---|---|
| **Asia** | |
| KJinling Hospital, Nanjing | China |
| Tianjin University Medical Hospital, Tianjin | China |
| Kyoto University, Kyoto | Japan |
| Osaka University Medical School, Osaka | Japan |
| Tohoku University Hospital, Sendai | Japan |
| Shahid Beheshti Medical University, Tehran | Iran |
| **Europe** | |
| Hospitaux Universitaires de Geneve, Geneva | Switzerland |
| University Hospital, Innsbruck | Austria |
| Friedrich-Ebert Hospital, Neumunster | Germany |
| Addenbrooke's Hospital, Cambridge | UK |
| St. James University Hospital, Leeds | UK |
| **North America** | |
| University of Illinois at Chicago, Chicago | USA |
| Northwestern Memorial Hospital, Chicago | USA |
| University of Minnesota, Minneapolis | USA |
| Stanford University Medical Center, Palo Alto | USA |
| Tulane Univ. School of Medicine, New Orleans | USA |

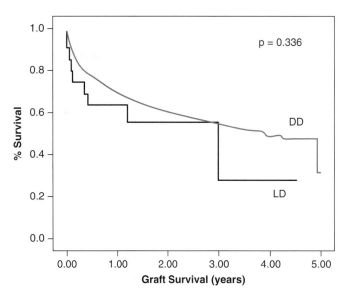

**FIGURE 34.5-5**

Graft survival comparing deceased and living donor intestinal transplants.

are at least comparable to deceased donors (2.5% vs 15%–20% graft loss, respectively).

Center volume had no effect on graft survival, but this may reflect the small number of procedures performed worldwide. There was no difference in graft survival (Figure 34.5-5) or patient survival (Figure 34.5-6) when comparing living donor and deceased donor intestinal transplantation.

## FUTURE DIRECTIONS

Living donor intestine transplantation has become a life-saving procedure for selected patients with end-stage intestinal failure. The outcomes of living donor intestine transplant are at least comparable to deceased donor transplantation. More data are needed to (1) document donor safety and (2) determine if potential theoretical benefits such as decreased waiting times and reduced graft rejection rates can be achieved in clinical practice.

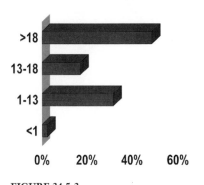

**FIGURE 34.5-3**

Age distribution of living donor intestine transplants.

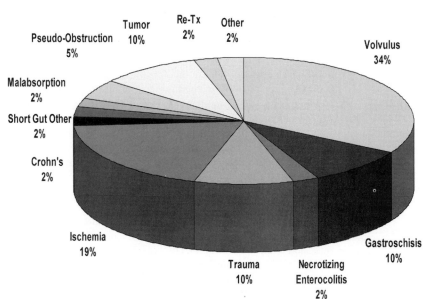

**FIGURE 34.5-4**

Causes of intestinal failure in living donor intestinal transplant recipients.

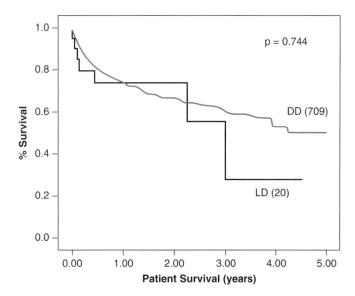

**FIGURE 34.5-6**

Patient survival comparing deceased and living donor intestine transplants.

## References

1. Grant D, Abu-Elmagd K, Reyes J, et al. 2003 report of the intestine transplant registry: a new era has dawned. *Ann Surg* 2005;241(4):607–613.
2. Grant D. Intestinal transplantation: 1997 report of the international registry. Intestinal Transplant Registry. *Transplantation* 1999;67(7):1061–1064.
3. Abu-Elmagd K, Reyes J, Bond G, et al. Clinical intestinal transplantation: a decade of experience at a single center. *Ann Surg* 2001;234(3):404–416.
4. Cicalese L, Sileri P, Gonzales O, et al. Cost-effectiveness of early living related segmental bowel transplantation as therapy for trauma-induced irreversible intestinal failure. *Transplant Proc* 2001;33(7-8):3581–3582.
5. Rovera GM, Sileri P, Rastellini C, et al. Quality of life after living related small bowel transplantation. *Transplant Proc* 2002;34(3):967–968.
6. Testa G, Panaro F, Schena S, et al. Living related small bowel transplantation: donor surgical technique. *Ann Surg* 2004;240(5):779–784.
7. Fishbein TM. The current state of intestinal transplantation. *Transplantation* 2004;78(2):175–178.
8. Fishbein TM, Schiano T, LeLeiko N, et al. An integrated approach to intestinal failure: results of a new program with total parenteral nutrition, bowel rehabilitation, and transplantation. *J Gastrointest Surg* 2002;6(4):554–562.
9. Gruessner RW, Sharp HL. Living-related intestinal transplantation: first report of a standardized surgical technique. *Transplantation* 1997;64(11):1605–1607.
10. Cicalese L, Rastellini C, Sileri P, Abcarian H, Benedetti E. Segmental living related small bowel transplantation in adults. *J Gastrointest Surg* 2001;5(2):168–172.
11. Cicalese L, Baum C, Brown M, et al. Segmental small bowel transplant from adult living-related donors. *Transplant Proc* 2001;33(1–2):1553.
12. Sarr MG, Duenes JA. Early and long term effects of a model of intestinal autotransplantation on intestinal motor patterns. *Surg Gynecol Obstet* 1990;170(4):338–346.
13. Libsch KD, Zyromski NJ, Tanaka T, et al. Role of extrinsic innervation in jejunal absorptive adaptation to subtotal small bowel resection: a model of segmental small bowel transplantation. *J Gastrointest Surg* 2002;6(2):240–247.
14. Tsiotos GG, Kendrick ML, Libsch K, et al. Ileal absorptive adaptation to jejunal resection and extrinsic denervation: implications for living-related small bowel transplantation. *J Gastrointest Surg* 2001;5(5):517–524.
15. Koltun WA, Madara JL, Smith RJ, Kirkman RL. Metabolic aspects of small bowel transplantation in inbred rats. *J Surg Res* 1987;42(4):341–347.
16. Tanaka T, Zyromski NJ, Libsch KD, Kendrick ML, Sarr MG. Canine ileal motor activity after a model of jejunoileal autotransplantation. *Ann Surg* 2003;237(2):192–200.
17. Murr MM, Miller VM, Sarr MG. Contractile properties of enteric smooth muscle after small bowel transplantation in rats. *Am J Surg* 1996;171(1):212–217.
18. Kirkman RL, Lear PA, Madara JL, Tilney NL. Small intestine transplantation in the rat--immunology and function. *Surgery* 1984;96(2):280–287.
19. Kirkman RL. Small bowel transplantation. *Transplantation* 1984;37(5):429–433.
20. Fortner JG, Sichuk G, Litwin SD, Beattie EJ Jr. Immunological responses to an intestinal allograft with HL-A-identical donor-recipient. *Transplantation* 1972;14(5):531–535.
21. Deltz E, Schroeder P, Gebhardt H, et al. [First successful clinical small intestine transplantation. Tactics and surgical technic]. *Chirurg* 1989;60(4):235–239.
22. Morris JA, Johnson DL, Rimmer JA, et al. Identical-twin small-bowel transplant for desmoid tumour. *Lancet* 1995;345(8964):1577–1578.
23. Jaffe BM, Beck R, Flint L, et al. Living-related small bowel transplantation in adults: a report of two patients. *Transplant Proc* 1997;29(3):1851–1852.
24. Testa G, Holterman M, John E, et al. Combined living donor liver/small bowel transplantation. *Transplantation* 2005;79(10):1401–1404.
25. Benedetti E, Baum C, Cicalese L, et al. Progressive functional adaptation of segmental bowel graft from living related donor. *Transplantation* 2001;71(4):569–571.
26. Pollard SG. Intestinal transplantation: living related. Br Med Bull 1997; 53(4):868–878.
27. Benedetti E, Baum C, Raofi V, et al. Living related small bowel transplantation: progressive functional adaptation of the graft. *Transplant Proc* 2000;32(6):1209.

## 34.6  INTESTINAL TRANSPLANTATION: COST ANALYSIS

*Giuliano Testa, MD, Aaron J. Simon, MHA, CHE, Enrico Benedetti, MD*

This chapter evaluates the cost analysis of living related intestinal transplantation.

The economical factor, although crude when one compares the chance of cure given by transplantation to palliative therapy like total parenteral nutrition (TPN), is of importance especially when the cost of treatment is so elevated, and only specialized centers can deliver it. In a group report of the Second World Congress of Pediatric Gastroenterology, Hepatology, and Nutrition, the problem of the high cost of intestinal failure therapies is recognized as one of the factors that need intervention in order to improve the outcome of the affected patients.[1]

The information on the cost of living donor intestinal transplantation are limited, at the present time, by the fact that only few centers have performed the procedure and even fewer have cumulated enough cases to allow a meaningful analysis and a comparison with the costs of cadaver intestinal transplantation and TPN.

On the other hand, cost analyses for cadaver intestinal transplantation have already been done, both in the United States and in Europe, and comparison with the costs of TPN have been drawn.

In 1999, a cost analysis of cadaver intestinal transplantation was made at the University of Pittsburgh. It was noticed that, when the period 1990 to 1994 was compared to the period 1994 to 1998, a significant reduction of the costs had been achieved for both isolated and combined liver–intestine transplantations. Most importantly, the reduction in costs was associated to a significant improvement in survival. The principal conclusion of the study was that intestinal transplantation became cost-effective therapy in comparison to TPN by the second year after transplantation.[2] A subsequent cost analysis done at the University of Nebraska looked at the gross billed hospital charges for a cadaver intestinal transplant. The result was an average of $234,858 (range $112,000–$667,000) based on an average stay of 53.4 days (range 18–119 days). This figure included the organ recovery fees but not the preoperative evaluation that was calculated at an average of $10,000. Finally the average charges related to posttransplant care were calculated at $25,000/year beginning with the first anniversary of the transplant. The actual average cost of intestinal transplantation has been reported with a wide range between $150,000 and $500,000.[3]

In a publication analyzing economics in short bowel syndrome, Schalamon, from the University of Graz, in Austria estimated the cost of isolated intestinal transplantation at $35,000 and of combined liver–intestine at $45,000, with an hospital stay set at 30 days.[4]

Data from 1998 estimated the annual cost for TPN ranging between $60,000 and $250,000 in the United States and around $100,000 in the UK.[5-7] A more recent publication from the University of Graz reports an approximate annual cost of $205,000 for in hospital TPN and $90,000 for home TPN.[4]

At the present time, it is estimated that the annual cost of home TPN in the United States is approximately $150,000.[7] This cost does not include all the other additional expenses that are part of the routine care of the patients on TPN. In fact, the cumulative cost for a patient on TPN, considering frequent hospital admissions, medical equipment, and nursing care can rise to a sum between $300,000 and $500,000 per year.[8] This number is likely to rise as the cost of hospital and home-care increases.

Just by taking in consideration the average costs reported above it appears that, cadaver intestinal transplantation not only has the advantage of offering a cure to intestinal failure but also is also economically competitive in comparison to TPN.

The nature of the disease and the clinical conditions of the patients make it normal that a wide range in the reported costs of a cadaver intestinal transplant is found. It appears that the final sum varies from as low as $100,000 up to $500,000, including the organ procurement fees. The wide range of cost is directly attributed to the variability of the length of stay and/or complications associated with the operation. Additionally, patients who received an intestinal transplantation may have received an isolated intestine, combined liver–intestine transplantation, or a multivisceral procedure, thus adding to the variation of cost. It is important to point out that many of the candidates to intestinal transplantation are patients who have exhausted any form of medical treatments and are referred to the transplant surgeons as a last resort. Consequently, the clinical conditions of these patients are often very poor making a prolonged, more costly recovery the norm and can explain hospital length of stay longer than 3 months.

Fourteen patients underwent 15 living donor intestinal transplants at the University of Illinois Medical Center at Chicago from 1998 to 2004. The average charges for the living related donor workup and hospitalization was calculated at $20,000 ± $5,000 (based on an average length of stay of 5.75 days). No donor has required any additional care related to the donor surgery and these costs can be regarded as accurate. The local procurement

organization charges about $21,000 for a cadaver intestinal graft to which an additional 10% is added if the donor is out of state.

The average charges for the recipient of a living donor intestinal transplant have been calculated at around $294,000, based on an average length of stay of 41 days (range 12–111 days). To this sum, an average of $14,000 per year for the immunosuppression therapy and another $4,000 for follow-up care must be added. Thus, at this institution the total average charges for a living donor intestinal transplant for the first year is approximately $332,000 (see Table 34.6-1).

The only other reference for comparison of costs for a living donor transplant can be found in a publication of the University of Graz, although no precise source of the data is given. The cost of donor workup and hospitalization is reported at $16,000; the average cost for the recipient, at $113,000; and the follow-up care, at $3,900 per year.[4]

Based on the data available it appears that in terms of crude charges cadaveric intestinal transplantation has an economical advantage on the living donor procedure.

This conclusion would be in reality unfounded because the comparison of the economical aspect of the two procedures is faulted by two important facts. The data are extrapolated by different institutions, and then affected by regional variation. The data do not take in account the fact that by eliminating waiting time living donor transplantation decreases the overall cost of the treatment of intestinal failure. Specifically the latter can significantly alter the economics of intestinal transplantation in favor of the living donor procedure. United Network for Organ Sharing (UNOS) reports that the average waiting time for a small bowel graft is between 370 and 540 days for a child age < 1 to 5 years of age.[9]

Living donor intestinal transplantation is not yet a widely performed operation, like kidney and liver living donor transplants. A comparative cost analysis between living donor and cadaveric transplantation is possible with kidney transplant were the variables are less and the experience is vast. Smith et al. in 2000 analyzed the Medicare payments for living donor versus cadaveric donor kidney transplant.[10] He concluded that the payments were considerably lower for living donor kidney transplants and the single largest cost saving comes from inpatient hospital services.[10] A very accurate analysis performed by Oostenbrink in the Netherlands similarly demonstrated that the mean direct cost of patient care are almost the same for cadaver versus living donor kidney transplant and that although the costs for living donor are higher

**TABLE 34.6-1**

### AVERAGE CHARGES FOR A LIVING RELATED INTESTINAL TRANSPLANTATION AND TOTAL PARENTERAL NUTRITION[a]

|  | Average | Range |
| --- | --- | --- |
| Donor workup and hospitalization | $20,000 | $15,000–$25,000 |
| Recipient | $294,000 | $100,000–$500,000 |
| Follow-up evaluation | $4,000 |  |
| Immunosuppression Therapy | $14,000 |  |
| **TOTAL** | $332,000 |  |
| TPN (yearly cost) | $150,000 | $60,000–$250,000 |
| **TOTAL** | $150,000 |  |

[a]Ranges, where noted, are provided and explain the wide variability reported by different transplant centers

because of the surgery they are largely offset by the reduction in costs of inpatient days.[11] In living donor liver transplantation, the great variability in recipient conditions, the potential for complications and a learning curve that still in many centers has not been exhausted make a precise comparison more difficult. Nonetheless, a review from Russo points out that also in end-stage liver disease pretransplant hospital care is the responsible for a large part of the economical burden. A more accurate cost analysis comparing cadaveric and living donor liver transplant should consequently take in account that the decrease in waiting time for the living donor candidates means a decrease in the number of complications and an overall reduction of the treatment costs.[12]

The same case holds true for living donor intestinal transplantation. Moreover, few other factors in favor of living donor over cadaveric intestinal transplantation should be considered. Although the number of intestinal donors is small, no readmissions or treatment of postoperative complications has increased the overall cost.

Regarding the recipients the preliminary experience shows that the incidence of technical complications is minimal, and so is the incidence of acute cellular rejection. These factors and the practical elimination of the waiting time should with increasing experience show a definite economical advantage of living donor over cadaver intestinal transplantation.

If based on the presented data, living related intestinal transplantation becomes cost-effective from the second to third year posttransplant when compared to TPN, it is possible to conclude that in the near future, the economical advantages over cadaver intestinal transplantation will become clearer and that living donor intestinal transplantation will become cost effective within a year in comparison to TPN.

# References

1. Kocoshis SA, BEath SV, Booth IW, et al. Intestinal failure and small bowel transplantation, including clinical nutrition: Working Group report of the second World Congress of Pediatric Gastroenterology, Hepatology, and Nutrition. *J Pediatr Gastroenterol Nutr* 2004;39(Suppl 2):S655–S661.
2. Abu-Elmagd KM, Reyes J, Fung JJ, et al. Evolution of clinical intestinal transplantation: improved outcome and cost effectiveness. *Transplant Proc* 1999;31(1–2):582–584.
3. Chaney M. Financial considerations insurance and coverage issues in intestinal transplantation. *Prog Transplant* 2004;14(4):312–320.
4. Schalamon J, Mayr JM, Hollwarth ME. Mortality and economics in short syndrome. *Best Pract Res Clin Gastroenterol* 2003;17(6):931–942.
5. Puntis JW. The economics of home parenteral nutrition. *Nutrititon* 1998;14(10):809–812.
6. Reddy P, Malone M. Cost and outcome analysis of home parenteral and enteral nutrition. *J Parenter Enteral Nutr* 1998;22(5):302–310.
7. Colomb V. Economic aspects of paediatric home parenteral nutrition. *Curr Opin Clin Nutr Metab Care* 2000;3(3):237–239.
8. Benedetti E, Testa G, Sankary H, et al. Successful treatment of trauma-induced short bowel syndrome with early living related bowel transplantation. *J Trauma* 2004;57:164–170.
9. United Network Organ Sharing. Available at www.unos.org. Accessed on July 2005.
10. Smith CR, Woodward RS, Cohen DS, et al. Cadaveric versus living donor kidney transplantation: a Medicare payment analysis. *Transplantation* 2000;69(2):311–314.
11. Oostenbrink JB, Kok ET, Verheul RM. A comparative study of resource use and costs of renal, liver and heart transplantation. *Transpl Int* 2005;18(4):437–443.
12. Russo MW, Brown RS Jr. Financial impact of adult living donation. *Liver Transpl* 2003;9(10Suppl2):S12–S15.

# PART IV

# FUTURE DEVELOPMENTS AND ALTERNATIVES TO LIVING DONOR TRANSPLANTATION

CHAPTER 35

# DUAL-ORGAN DONATION

*Rainer W.G. Gruessner, MD*

As shown in previous chapters, donation of one organ alone can be associated with considerable morbidity and mortality. For that reason, donation of two organs from one living donor (LD) has rarely been done. The vast majority of such procurements were performed over the last decade. As of December 1, 2006, dual-organ procurements have been performed in at least 97 LDs.

Dual-organ procurements from 1 LD can be performed either sequentially or simultaneously. For the LD, the advantage of undergoing sequential procurements is the reduced magnitude of the procedure. Sequential procurements also offer the option to postpone or cancel the second procurement, if the LD or recipient endured any complications from the first procurement. The disadvantage of sequential procurements is that the LD (and the recipient) must undergo surgery and anesthesia twice.

Given concern over the magnitude of simultaneous procurement of two organs in one procedure, the first successful dual-organ transplant from one LD was performed sequentially.[1] As of December 1, 2006, either sequential or simultaneous procurements from one LD has been described for the kidney and (distal) pancreas (n > 78); the kidney and liver (lateral segments or a full lobe; n > 12); and (a portion of) the small bowel and liver segments 2 and 3 (n > 7). Of the 12 sequential or simultaneous liver and kidney procurements, 9 involved the lateral liver segments[2,3]; 3 involved a full liver lobe. The first type of dual-organ procurement was that of a kidney and (distal) pancreas; the most recent type of dual-organ procurement was that of (a portion of) the small bowel and liver segments 2 and 3.

The first successful segmental pancreas procurement after the LD had undergone a previous (donor) nephrectomy was performed on June 20, 1979, at the University of Minnesota.[1] At the same institution, subsequently, a total of 24 segmental pancreas after kidney (PAK) procurements (ie, sequential transplants) was performed from the same LDs.[2] One donor–recipient pair was concerned about the prospect of undergoing surgery and anesthesia twice, so that LD underwent the first technically successful simultaneous segmental pancreas and kidney procurement on March 10, 1994, also at the University of Minnesota.[3] An earlier attempt at Jackson Memorial Hospital, Miami, on November 12, 1980, was not successful because the recipient died—though with functioning organs—5 weeks posttransplant[4] (J. Miller, personal communication, December 1, 2006).

As of December 1, 2006, according to the International Pancreas Transplant Registry (IPTR), at least 54 simultaneous and 24 sequential segmental pancreas and kidney procurements from one LD have been reported from four countries: the United States (four institutions), Japan, South Korea, and Norway.[4] To date, the LD mortality rate of simultaneous or sequential segmental pancreas and kidney procurements is 0%.[4] The morbidity of simultaneous segmental pancreas and kidney procurement appears

to be no different than that for single-organ procurement,[5] but the exact risk still needs to be determined.

According to United Network for Organ Sharing (UNOS) data, from October 1, 1987, to December 1, 2006, in the United States, four LDs underwent sequential procurement of a kidney and liver segments 2 and 3.[6] Those four sequential procurements occurred 16 days, 7 weeks, 5 months, and 8 months apart. In three of the four sequential transplants, lateral liver segments 2 and 3 were transplanted first; in one of them, the kidney was transplanted first. At the time of this writing (December 1, 2006), a simultaneous kidney and full liver lobe procurement from the same LD has not been done in the United States.

Of note, according to UNOS data, in the United States, an additional 15 transplants involved sequential or simultaneous kidney and liver procurements from different LDs. Of these 15 recipients, 5 underwent simultaneous transplants (all adults, from 21 to 61 years of age) from different LDs; 10, sequential transplants (7 adults, 3 pediatric recipients) (Sarah Taranto, B.A., UNOS Research Department).

Outside the United States, at least eight simultaneous or sequential kidney and liver procurements have been performed. The first simultaneous kidney and liver (lateral segments) procurement was performed in Turkey in May 1992; however, the 23-year-old recipient died 15 days posttransplant of cerebral hemorrhage.[7] Also in Turkey, in November 2001, a 20-year-old woman simultaneously donated her right kidney and the left lobe of her liver (segments 2 to 4) to her 9-year-old brother to treat primary hyperoxaluria type I.[8] The first simultaneous LD kidney and right-lobe liver transplant (a father donating to his son) was performed by Marujo et al. in Brazil and reported in 1999.[9] Another report from Brazil described a sequential LD kidney and right lobe liver transplant, with a 20-year interval, between two brothers.[10] In Japan, three transplants in pediatric recipients (< 3 years old) were reported after sequential kidney and liver (segments 2 and 3) procurements.[11] In Sweden, a simultaneous LD procurement of a kidney and auxiliary liver segments 2 and 3 was done in a highly sensitized recipient; the auxiliary liver graft was done first to protect the kidney from (hyperacute) rejection (see Chapter 16.16.3c).[12] However, in the absence of a worldwide donor registry, the exact number of simultaneous or sequential kidney and liver procurements from the same LD is unknown (see Chapter 1).

A few sequential or simultaneous procurements of liver segments 2 and 3 and a portion of the small bowel from one LD have been performed to treat short bowel syndrome and liver failure associated with total parenteral nutrition. The first successful sequential (2003) and the first successful simultaneous (2004) segmental liver and small-bowel procurements were performed at the University of Illinois.[13] Sequential or simultaneous segmental liver and bowel procurements have also been performed at the

University of Kyoto (n = 2)[14] and at the University of Minnesota (n = 1). Worldwide, at least seven such procedures (all in pediatric recipients) have been performed. But, in the absence of an international donor registry, the exact number remains unknown.

To date, no LD deaths after dual-organ procurements have been reported. Yet, undoubtedly, procurement even of only a portion of a second organ increases the risks of mortality and morbidity. In addition, no long-term studies have examined the long-term consequences of donating more than one organ. The introduction of laparoscopic technology has diminished, but not completely abrogated, the surgical trauma of donation (as shown for simultaneous laparoscopic procurement of the distal pancreas and kidney[15]). Laparoscopic techniques may also confer a short-term advantage (eg, shorter hospitalization, faster recovery) for simultaneous procurement of liver segments 2 and 3 and a kidney. In contrast, simultaneous procurement of liver segments 2 and 3 and a portion of the small bowel appears to be less amenable to laparoscopy because of the need for a relatively large incision to recover the graft and to restore the LD's bowel continuity.

Regarding the ideal relationship between dual-organ LDs and their recipients, we at the University of Minnesota (having performed a total of 63 dual-organ procurements) feel strongly that only directed donation should be considered. Nondirected dual-organ donation by altruistic LDs, given the lack of long-term donor outcome data, should not be encouraged at this time. It is evident that parents are willing to accept the higher morbidity and mortality risk associated with dual-organ procurement if their child's life is at stake (eg, in cases of liver and intestinal failure, or liver and kidney failure); the same motivation is often noted for other family members and emotionally related individuals.

If the prospective recipient's disease is not immediately life-threatening (eg, diabetes mellitus and end-stage renal disease), dual-organ procurements are justified from LDs who are HLA-identical siblings or twins, given the excellent recipient and graft survival rates. Dual-organ procurements are also justified in non-life-threatening situations from non-HLA-identical LDs, if the recipient has a high panel-reactive antibody (PRA) level and if the donor–recipient crossmatch result is negative. However, LDs considered for dual-organ procurement should undergo twice the medical, psychological, and social scrutiny than donors of one organ alone. Only then will this field continue to have a place in cutting-edge medicine.

## References

1. Sutherland DER, Goetz FC, Najarian JS. Pancreas transplants from related donors. *Transplantation* 1984;38 (6):625–633.
2. Gruessner RWG. Living donor pancreas transplantation. In: Gruessner RWG, Sutherland DER, eds. *Pancreas Transplantation*. New York: Springer-Verlag; 2004:423–440.
3. Gruessner RWG, Sutherland DER. Simultaneous kidney and segmental pancreas transplants from living related donors – the first two successful cases. *Transplantation* 1996;(8):1265–1268.
4. International Pancreas Transplant Registry (IPTR). Personal communication. November 30, 2006.
5. Gruessner RWG, Kendall DM, Drangstveit MB, Gruessner AC, Sutherland DER. Simultaneous pancreas-kidney transplantation from live donors. *Ann Surg* 1997;226(4):471–482.
6. United Network for Organ Sharing (UNOS) (Sarah Taranto, B.A., UNOS Research Department).
7. Haberal M, Abbasoğlu, Büyükpamukçu N, Bilgin N, et al. Combined liver-kidney transplantation from a living-related donor. *Transpl Proc* 1993;25(3):2211–2213.
8. Astarcioglu I, Karademir S, Gűlay H, Bora S, et al. Primary hyperoxaluria: simultaneous combined liver and kidney transplantation from a living related donor. Liver Transplantation 2003, 9(4):433–436.
9. Marujo WC, Barros MFA, Cury RA, Pacheco-Silva A, Sette Jr. H. Successful combined kidney-liver right lobe transplant from a living donor. *Lancet* 1999;353:641.
10. Pacheco-Moreira LF, Balbi E, Enne M, et al. One living donor and two donations: sequential kidney and liver donation with 20-year interval. *Transpl Proc* 2005;37:4337–4338.
11. Nakamura M, Fuchinoue S, Nakajima I, et al. Three cases of sequential liver–kidney transplantation from living-related donors. *Nephrol Dial Transpl* 2001;16:166–168.
12. Olausson M. Personal communication. December 1, 2006.
13. Testa G, Holterman M, John E, et al. Combined living donor liver/small bowel transplantation. *Transplantation* 2005;27(10):401–404.
14. Tanaka K. Personal communication. April 1, 2004.
15. Gruessner RWG, Kandaswamy R, Denny R. Laparoscopic simultaneous nephrectomy and distal pancreatectomy from a live donor. *J Am Coll Surg* 2001;193(3):333–337.

# CHAPTER 36

# USE OF LIVING DONORS FOR HIV-POSITIVE TRANSPLANT CANDIDATES

*Peter G. Stock, MD, PhD*

## INTRODUCTION—ETHICS OF LIVING DONOR TRANSPLANTATION IN THE HIV-POSITIVE RECIPIENT

The ethical balance of potentially harming a healthy person during a live donor operation for the life-saving benefit of another is heavily impacted by the risk/benefit ratio. For the majority of living donor kidney transplant procedures, the relative risk to the donors is minimal compared to the life-enhancing and saving qualities for the recipient. The benefit is increased even more by minimizing or eliminating the time on dialysis for the person in renal failure, particularly in light of 6- to 7-year waiting times for some blood types in certain regions of the country. Although donor morbidity is higher for the living donor liver transplant procedure, the ability to proceed with transplantation prior to progression of disease in the recipient to a transplantable Model for End-Stage Liver Disease (MELD) score outweighs the risk for the donor. However, there is an increased ethical dilemma when performing a living donor procedure for a recipient with an unknown outcome. There is an ongoing perception that morbidity and mortality following transplantation and immunosuppression in people with HIV is too high to justify the risks to a living donor. This chapter discusses the increasing need for transplantation in people with HIV, the current experience and success rates following liver and kidney transplantation in people with HIV, and the important role for living donation.

## RATIONALE FOR SOLID ORGAN TRANSPLANTATION IN THE HAART ERA

The transplant community has been slow to recognize that HIV has evolved to a chronic condition, with the majority of U.S. transplant centers still considering HIV to be a contraindication to transplantation.[1] Significant progress has been achieved in several areas, which has provided the impetus for several major transplant centers to reconsider HIV positivity as a contraindication to transplantation. The advent of highly active antiretroviral therapy (HAART) has decreased the morbidity and mortality in people with HIV, so they are no longer dying from progression of HIV to AIDS.[2,3] HAART typically involves the use of protease inhibitor or nonnucleoside reverse transcriptase inhibitor in combination with two nucleoside analogs. This combination therapy has been effective in providing virologic, immunologic, and survival benefits for patients with HIV.

The ability to suppress HIV viral replication with HAART therapy provided the initial motivation for reconsidering transplantation in people with HIV. However, further impetus for transplantation in this group of patients with an immunodeficient state has been provided by improved prophylaxis and treatment for opportunistic infections. Perhaps the best example of this is the treatment of tissue invasive cytomegalovirus (CMV) disease, which once was a fatal disease in both the immunosuppressed transplant recipient and people with HIV, but has evolved to outpatient management with an oral antiviral agent.

One of the major barriers to moving forward with transplantation in people with HIV related to the logical concerns that the immunosuppressive agents essential for successful transplantation would further weaken the compromised immunologic status of the HIV recipient. Interestingly, many of the commonly used immunosuppressive agents have antiretroviral qualities. Cyclosporine may suppress HIV replication associated with inhibition of interleukin-2-dependent T-cell proliferation.[4] Other antiretroviral qualities of cyclosporine are mediated by binding to cyclophilin A, preventing formation of the HIV gag protein/cyclophilin A complex necessary for nuclear import of the HIV-1 DNA.[5,6] Mycophenolate mofetil (MMF), one of the most efficacious and frequently used immunosuppressive agents, inhibits inosine monophosphate dehydrogenase and diminishes the pool of intracellular nucleosides. MMF therefore acts synergistically with nucleosides analogs, such as abacavir, which are integral components of HAART therapy.[7,8] Sirolimus, a more recent addition to immunosuppressive regimens, down-regulates the CCR5 receptor, the T-cell receptor for the HIV virion.[9] The surprising antiretroviral qualities of many of the currently effective immunosuppressive agents has increased the enthusiasm for transplanting people with HIV, and the immunosuppressive agents with antiretroviral qualities have been the most frequently used drugs in the initial clinical trials.

## INCREASING DEMAND FOR SOLID ORGAN TRANSPLANTS IN HIV-POSITIVE RECIPIENTS

Better control of HIV viral replication has changed HIV infection from a rapidly progressive disease to a chronic condition. As a result, people are no longer dying from progression of HIV disease to AIDS. Unfortunately, people with HIV infection are representing a rapidly increasing population of kidney and liver transplant waiting lists as a result of co-morbidities associated with HIV.

End-stage renal failure secondary to HIV nephropathy (HIVAN) is now the third most common etiology of end-stage renal disease among African Americans ages 20 to 64.[10] HIVAN is a collapsing variant of focal sclerosing glomerulonephritis (FSGS), and about 800 patients per year with this diagnosis have been reported to the United States Renal Data System (USRDS) to start dialysis.[11] The etiology of HIVAN and the reason it effects principally African American males remains unclear, but there is evidence that direct infection of renal tubular and/or mesangial cells by HIV-1 may be a significant factor.[12] Other patients at risk for the development of glomerulonephritis are patients co-infected with hepatitis B (HBV) and C (HCV). Membranous nephropathy has been observed in the HIV/HBV co-infected patient. IgA nephropathy has also been observed in people with HIV and is likely a direct result of the HIV infection.[13–15] Finally, kidney disease may be exacerbated by nephrotoxicity related to the multiple medications associated with HAART and infection prophylaxis.[16]

Liver disease is now the leading cause of death for HIV-positive patients co-infected with Hepatitis C, and a major cause of death for HIV-HBV co-infected patients.[17] The prevalence of end-stage liver disease in HIV-infected patients continues to increase as a result of HCV infection and HBV co-infection, reported at 22% to 33% and 9%, respectively.[15] There is also data to support that progression of liver disease mediated by viral hepatitis is exacerbated in people with HIV/HCV co-infection, and possibly HIV/HBV co-infection.[18,19] Adding to the difficulties, people with HIV have a great deal of difficulty tolerating interferon therapy, thus minimizing the chance for successful treatment of hepatitis C. Finally, antiretroviral therapy may further exacerbate liver insufficiency as a direct result of drug toxicity, as well as immune restoration hepatitis or the development of lamivudine-resistant HBV.[20–23] For all these reasons, the demand for liver transplantation in the co-infected patients will continue to increase, further increasing already stressed waiting lists.

## PATIENT SELECTION, DONOR ISSUES, CLINICAL MANAGEMENT, AND EARLY OUTCOMES IN SOLID ORGAN TRANSPLANTATION IN PEOPLE WITH HIV IN THE HAART ERA

### Patient Selection Criteria

In most of the prospective trials during the HAART era, HIV-positive kidney transplant recipients were required to have an undetectable HIV viral load (HIV RNA<50 copies/mL) on a stable HAART regimen and CD4 counts greater than 200 cells/mL. These CD4 requirements were based on lack of significant HIV disease progression at these CD4+ T-cell counts. For liver transplant recipients, the CD4 requirements were dropped to 100 cells/mL to accommodate a large percentage of referred patients who had lower counts in the presence of massive splenomegaly seen in HIV disease. Because many of these patients had undetectable HIV viral loads, the lower CD4 counts were attributed to splenic sequestration, and as a result the CD4 requirements were dropped to 100 cells/mL in this cohort. Another issue confronting the potential liver transplant recipients has been hepatoxicity related to HAART therapy, requiring termination of HAART therapy secondary to exacerbation of liver insufficiency. In these patients, a detectable HIV viral load was acceptable as long as control of the virus could be predicted posttransplant. Patients with HAART-resistant HIV virus were excluded. Although the a history of opportunistic infections or neoplasm was considered a relative contraindication in the early trials of solid organ transplantation in people with HIV, the lack of opportunistic infections

(OIs) or neoplasms in the pilot trials has prompted most centers to change this philosophy. Protocols have been modified to allow a history of most opportunistic infections, provided the infectious problem has been treated and cleared prior to transplantation. OIs that cannot be cleared or adequately treated, such as chronic cryptosporidiosis or progressive multifocal leukoencephalopathy (PML), remain a contraindication. Cutaneous Kaposi's sarcoma (KS) that has resolved with reconstitution of the immune system with HAART therapy is not an exclusion criterion, although transplantation in patients with a history of visceral KS remains controversial.

### Donor Issues

With expanding waiting lists and stagnant donor pools, waiting times for kidney recipients are now exceeding 6 or 7 years for some blood types in certain parts of the country. These excessive waiting times are problematic for the entire recipient pool, and there is evidence that these problems are further exacerbated in people with HIV. Early data showed the 2-year survival for patients with HIVAN was 36%, compared to 64% for all other causes of ESRD.[24] More recent data suggest these dismal early survival rates have been improved, but the exact improvement remains to be determined.[25] As a result, many centers have capitalized on the use of "high infectious risk" organs. These are organs that are from donors that have engaged in behavior that puts them at increased risk for HIV, but are serologically negative for hepatitis B, hepatitis C, and HIV. There are a surprising number of donors who fit that criteria, but previously were not utilized secondary to the unknown risk of HIV transmission. The majority of HIV patients have been willing to accept these organs, and this has been an excellent source of kidneys that have permitted the HIV patients to minimize the lengthy wait times. Interestingly, livers have not been available from these high-risk donors, secondary to their utilization in the HIV negative recipient pool. It should be emphasized that at this point in time, utilization of the "high-risk donor" applies to organs that are serologically negative for HIV. There has been some interest in the potential use of HIV positive deceased donors, but the risk of super-infection with a drug-resistant or more virulent form of HIV has precluded the use of this potential source.

The waiting times for potential HIV positive liver recipients are even more problematic, in that the MELD scores necessary for the allocation of a liver are getting higher with expanding lists. By the time the HIV-positive candidate achieves the MELD score required for allocation, their deterioration has been so severe that they no longer meet the entry criteria (CD4 counts, HIV viral load) required at most transplant centers. This problem was recently emphasized in a report demonstrating shorter pre-transplantation survival times in HIV-positive liver transplant patients compared with HIV negative recipients, despite comparable MELD scores at the time of listing.[26,27] The inability to obtain high-risk donors for liver transplantation in the HIV-positive recipients combined with a rapid deterioration on waiting lists has prompted centers to use living donor liver transplants (adult-to-adult, R lobes) to facilitate transplantation, whereas the HIV-positive recipients are healthy enough to tolerate the procedure. There is a debate as to whether HCV recurrence is exacerbated in (HIV positive or negative) the ambience of a regenerating liver. However, the opportunity to receive a living donor prior to significant deterioration on the waiting lists outweighs the unknown risks of more rapid recurrence of hepatitis C, and has prompted several centers to move forward with living donor liver transplantation in people with HIV.

Similarly, in light of the increasing length of waiting lists for kidney transplant recipients compounded by dialysis-associated mortality in the HIV-positive patient, living donation kidney transplantation is an important option. For both living donor kidney and liver transplant donors, complete informed consent should include a disclosure of the recipients HIV status. Although this could be perceived as an unfair requirement, it is important that the donor be aware of the unknown risks to transplantation in the HIV-positive recipient. This is analogous to the situation in which a living donor should be made aware of high-risk cardiac scenarios (ie, living donor kidney transplantation to the high-risk diabetic recipient), in the event of recipient morbidity or mortality following the procedure. Although disclosure of recipient HIV status to potential donors is necessary for these reasons, this disclosure should only occur after sufficient review of the donor eligibility status. The discovery of donor hypertension, diabetes, or incompatibility after a HIV recipient has disclosed serologic status to the donor can lead to unnecessary conflict between the health-care team, the potential donor, recipient, and family members.

## POSTTRANSPLANT CLINICAL MANAGEMENT

### Immunosuppression and HAART

For the HIV-positive recipient, most centers have elected to use immunosuppressive agents, which also have antiretroviral qualities. These include CSA, mycophenolate mofetil, and sirolimus. Induction agents with lymphocyte-depleting agents have been avoided due to concerns for overimmunosuppression in the HIV-positive patient, although they have been required to treat a surprisingly high incidence of moderate-severe rejection in the kidney transplant recipients (see below). The posttransplant management of the HIV-positive patients is complicated by the drug interactions between HAART and immunosuppressive regimens. The calcineurin inhibitors, sirolimus, and the antiretroviral protease inhibitors cause a significant inhibition of the cytochrome p4503A metabolism.[28–30] Maintenance immunosuppressant dosages are significantly decreased in patients receiving protease inhibitors. As an example, most patients require about 50 mg of CSA per day, and about 2 mg of sirolimus per week. The nonnucleoside reverse transcriptase inhibitors are inducers of cytochrome P4503A; thus immunosuppressant dosages must be slightly increased when used with these agents.[31] If patients are on both protease inhibitors and nonnucleoside reverse transcriptase inhibitors, the dosing of the immunosuppressant agents are similar to those used with protease inhibitors alone. The effects of other agents commonly used in transplant patients, such as antibiotics and antifungals, can have profound effects on the levels of immunosuppressive drugs. Agents such as erythromycin or flucanazole also inhibit the cytochrome P4503A system, and therefore necessitate even further reduction in the dosing of calcineurin inhibitors and sirolimus.

In light of the profound impact of the protease inhibitors on drug metabolism, some centers have switched HAART regimens to eliminate these from the drug regimens. However, the current recommendations are to continue the regimen that has been effective in terms of HIV suppression. Rather than switch regimens, close drug monitoring should be used to maintain therapeutic levels of immunosuppressive agent while continuing the HAART regimen which has been efficacious in controlling HIV.

It is important to hold all components of HAART therapy following the transplant procedure until patients can reliably take oral medications. Unless therapeutic levels of the HAART agents can be achieved, the risk of developing resistance is high.

### HBV and HCV Management

Lamivudine has been a component of HAART therapy since the 1990s, and as a consequence many HIV/HBV co-infected patients have developed HBV resistance. In HIV-negative patients, HBV resistance develops in 50% of patients following 3 years of therapy. In fact, many patients co-infected with HBV present with hepatic decompensation related to a flare from resistant HBV. Fortunately, lamivudine-resistant HBV is sensitive to other agents, including tenofovir and adefovir.[32,33] A particularly challenging time occurs during the immediate period following liver transplantation, when it is imperative to control reinfection from HBV. During this period, hepatitis B immune globulin (HBIg) remains a critical component of the treatment regimen. However, lamivudine and/or tenofovir cannot be restarted until all the components of HAART therapy can be reinitiated to avoid the development of HIV resistance. A better choice in circumstances when HAART cannot be reinitiated posttransplant is adefovir, because the development of HIV resistance associated with this agent is low. Another newer anti-HBV agent that lacks anti-HIV properties is entecavir, and is a more appropriate agent to use to prevent HBV reinfection when lamividine or tenofovir cannot be used.

The recurrence of HCV following liver transplantation in HCV/HIV co-infected patients remains a significant concern secondary to the lack of consistently effective therapy to control HCV recurrence (see results below). Similar to the strategy used in HIV-negative HCV-positive recipients, the current recommendations are that HCV treatment not be initiated preemptively posttransplant. Rather, HCV treatment should be initiated posttransplant when there is liver biopsy documentation of progressive and severe HCV infection, with an HAI score >8 and/or fibrosis stage >2.[34] The concurrent use of interferon and ribavirin therapy compounds the difficulty in managing an already challenging immunosuppressive and HAART regimen. Adjunctive therapy with antidepressants and growth factors are necessary, and managing these complex regimens requires significant oversight by a multidisciplinary team.

### HIV-Specific Opportunistic Infection Prophylaxis

HIV-positive transplant recipients require standard prophylaxis used by transplant centers for CMV, PCP, and fungal infections. There are a few HIV-specific specific additions to these standard regimens which are recommended. PCP prophylaxis should continue for life in these recipients, as most transplant centers eliminate this after the first year of transplant in the HIV negative recipient. If CD4 T-cell counts drop below 75 cells/mL, the HIV-positive recipient is at risk for disseminated mycobacterium avium complex (MAC).[31] These recipients should receive weekly azithromycin until the CD4 counts increase above 100 cells/mL for 6 months. Similarly, patients with CD4 counts below 50 cell/mL are at an increased risk for CMV retinitis, and should receive close ophthalmologic follow-up. Finally, the risk of developing tuberculosis in HIV-infected people is approximately 10% per year in those with a positive PPD, and these patients should be screened every 6 months. A positive PPD should be treated for 9 months. As with any transplant recipient, a patient who has been treated for active tuberculosis should undergo secondary prophylaxis for another 9 months posttransplant.

## HIV-Specific Neoplasms

Women with HIV are at a significantly elevated risk for the development of cervical cancers and should undergo screening every 6 to 12 months. Men and women who are at risk for human papilloma virus (HPV)-mediated anal cancers. Anal examinations and pap smears should should be performed, although the impact of immunosuppression, as well as the management of these lesions, is currently under investigation.

## EARLY OUTCOMES IN SOLID ORGAN TRANSPLANTATION IN PEOPLE WITH HIV IN THE HAART ERA

Comparisons of the historical data for patient and allograft survival rates in HIV-positive versus HIV-negative solid organ recipients are difficult to interpret, in that many of these retrospective studies were done prior to the availability of HAART therapy. Difficulties in the interpretation of these data are further complicated by unavailability of data regarding the HIV viral loads or CD4 counts in many of these studies. However, more recent reports of solid organ transplants performed in HIV-positive recipients during the HAART era have demonstrated comparable results to HIV-negative recipients in selected patients. Furthermore, there has not been a significant increase in technical complications or infections in HIV-positive patients undergoing solid organ transplantation. Both living donor kidney and liver transplants (adult-to-adult) are being performed in the HIV-positive population, and the technical results have been equivalent to the HIV-negative population. Based on the increasing waiting times and relatively poor outcomes of the HIV-positive patients on waiting lists,[27,35] the living donor option for both kidney and liver transplants in HIV-positive patients is justified and an important option.

## Results of Liver Transplantation in the HAART Era

There have been numerous reports of successful liver transplantation in people with HIV during the HAART era,[36-44] with 1-year survival rates ranging between 60% and 100%. In one report, which pooled the data from the larger centers performing liver transplantation in HIV-positive patients during the HAART era,[45] survival data were compared to a UNOS database cohort of matched HIV-negative controls. Patient and graft survival was not significantly different between the HIV co-infected patients and their HIV-negative matched cohorts at 12, 24, and 36 months posttransplant. However, poorer survival rates within the HIV-positive recipients were associated with HCV infection, intolerance of HIV medication posttransplant, and CD4 counts less than 200 cells/mL.

Progression of HIV following liver transplantation and initiation of immunosuppression has not been an issue in the vast majority of cases that have been reported during the HAART era. Similarly, results from clinical trials suggest that recurrence of hepatitis B can be prevented following transplantation in the co-infected patients, similar to the excellent results seen in the HIV-negative population. Although there was some concern with the control of hepatitis B in the high percentage of co-infected patients with lamivudine resistance, the development of further resistance to adefovir or tenofovir has not been observed. Further increases in the number of agents available to treat breakthrough hepatitis B suggest that long-term control of hepatitis B will be feasible.

Unfortunately, hepatitis C recurrence remains a significant concern in the co-infected patients. Despite earlier reports demonstrating fulminant recurrence of hepatitis C following transplantation in the co-infected patients,[38] other reports have suggested that the recurrence is not significantly different than the experience seen in the hepatitis C recipients who are HIV negative.[37] Most centers are treating with interferon and ribavirin when there is histologic evidence of hepatitis C progression, and there have been some cases of viral clearance in the co-infected recipients.

## Results of Kidney Transplantation in the HAART Era

Excellent early results from prospective pilot trials of kidney transplants in the HIV-positive patients during the HAART era suggest that this is a safe and efficacious procedure. One-year graft survival has been comparable to HIV-negative patients, and in one series was 100% at a mean follow-up of 480 days.[36] Progression of HIV disease was not an issue, and all patients remained undetectable for the HIV virus. Surprisingly, acute rejection was seen in over half of the patients, a rate double of that seen in HIV-negative patients. This may represent immune dysregulation, although it could also represent insufficient immunosuppression. Another prospective trial using more aggressive induction therapy with an anti-CD25 antibody, and maintenance with sirolimus therapy has had lower rejections rates, but a 1-year patient and graft survival of 85% and 75%, respectively.[46] In any case, progression of HIV has not been seen in any of the trials and supports the role of kidney transplantation in the HIV-positive patient.

## CONCLUSIONS

Early results from transplants performed in the HAART era dispute the convention that HIV is a contraindication to transplant. Progression of HIV or development of opportunistic infections following transplantation and immunosuppression has not been observed. Patient and graft survival rates following both kidney and liver transplantation have been similar to the general transplant population, and these procedures can no longer be denied in patients with well-controlled HIV. Drug interactions between the antiretroviral agents and immunosuppressive agents require close monitoring to prevent toxicity. Nonetheless, the HIV-positive patient clearly requires therapeutic levels of immunosuppression, as evidenced by the higher than expected rejection rates in the kidney transplant recipients. Patients undergoing liver transplantation for lamivudine-resistant HBV have done extremely well, and further resistance has not been observed with the use of HBIg and newer antivirals. As with the HIV-negative liver transplant recipients, recurrence of hepatitis C remains a variable problem. Although there have been reports of aggressive HCV recurrence in the co-infected recipients, there have also been cases where HCV has been cleared following the procedure.

Based on the increasing demand for solid organ transplants in people with HIV, as well as on the excellent early results in the HIV-positive recipient, living donation should be an option for these recipients. In light of the excessive waiting times on deceased donor kidney lists, as well as the high incidence of morbidity of HIV-positive patients on dialysis, living donation is well justified. For the HIV-positive liver transplant recipients, the situation is more problematic, in that the MELD system for liver allocation does not serve the HIV-positive patient well. By the time the MELD score becomes high enough to warrant allocation, many of the co-infected patients are no longer candidates for the transplant. Furthermore, operative morbidity associated with the HIV-positive recipients of living donor organs (kidney and R lobe liver) has been similar to that seen in the HIV-negative recipients. It is imperative that HIV clinicians, nephrologists, hepatologists, and patients are aware that transplantation is an option for HIV-infected patients, and that live donor operations are ethically justified based on the promising early results in the HAART era. Delays in referral have resulted in unnecessary morbidity and mortality in this deserving group of patients.

# References

1. Halpern SA, Stock DA, Shaked P, Blumberg A. Determinants of transplant surgeons willingness to provide organs for patients with the hepatitis B, hepatitis C, and human immunodeficiency viruses [abstract]. *Am J Transplant* 2004;4(Suppl 8):425.

2. Palella FJ Jr, et al. Declining morbidity and mortality among patients with advanced human immunodeficiency virus infection. HIV Outpatient Study Investigators. *N Engl J Med* 1998;338(13):853–860.

3. Kaplan JE, et al. Epidemiology of human immunodeficiency virus-associated opportunistic infections in the United States in the era of highly active antiretroviral therapy. *Clin Infect Dis* 2000;30 Suppl 1:S5–S14.

4. Rizzardi GP, et al. Treatment of primary HIV-1 infection with cyclosporin A coupled with highly active antiretroviral therapy. *J Clin Invest* 2002;109(5):681–688.

5. Andrieu JM, et al. Effects of cyclosporin on T-cell subsets in human immunodeficiency virus disease. *Clin Immunol Immunopathol* 1988;47(2):181–198.

6. Calabrese LH, et al. Placebo-controlled trial of cyclosporin-A in HIV-1 disease: implications for solid organ transplantation. *J Acquir Immune Defic Syndr* 2002;29(4):356–362.

7. Chapuis AG, et al. *Effects of mycophenolic acid on human immunodeficiency virus infection in vitro and in vivo. Nat Med* 2000;6(7):762–768.

8. Margolis D, et al. Abacavir and mycophenolic acid, an inhibitor of inosine monophosphate dehydrogenase, have profound and synergistic anti-HIV activity. *J Acquir Immune Defic Syndr* 1999;21(5):362–370.

9. Heredia A, et al. Rapamycin causes down-regulation of CCR5 and accumulation of anti-HIV beta-chemokines: an approach to suppress R5 strains of HIV-1. *Proc Natl Acad Sci USA* 2003;100(18):10411–10416.

10. US Renal Data System. USRDS 2004 annual data report: Atlas of end-stage renal disease in the United States. 2004, National Institute of Health, National Institute of Diabetes and Digestive and Kidney Diseases: Bethesda, MD.

11. USRDS. The United States renal data system. *Am J Kidney Dis* 2003;42:1–230.

12. Ray PE, et al. Infection of human primary renal epithelial cells with HIV-1 from children with HIV-associated nephropathy. *Kidney Int* 1998;53(5):1217–1229.

13. Nochy D, et al. Renal disease associated with HIV infection: a multicentric study of 60 patients from Paris hospitals. *Nephrol Dial Transpl* 1993;8(1):11–19.

14. D'Agati V, Appel GB. Renal pathology of human immunodeficiency virus infection. *Semin Nephrol* 1998;18(4):406–421.

15. Ockenga J, et al. Hepatitis B and C in HIV-infected patients. Prevalence and prognostic value. *J Hepatol* 1997;27(1):18–24.

16. Currier JS, Havlir DV. Complications of HIV disease and antiretroviral therapy. Highlights of the 11th Conference on Retroviruses and Opportunistic Infections, February 8-11, 2004, San Francisco, California, USA. *Top HIV Med* 2004;12(1):31–45.

17. Bica I, et al. Increasing mortality due to end-stage liver disease in patients with human immunodeficiency virus infection. *Clin Infect Dis* 2001;32(3):492–497.

18. Soto B, et al. Human immunodeficiency virus infection modifies the natural history of chronic parenterally-acquired hepatitis C with an unusually rapid progression to cirrhosis [see comments]. *J Hepatol* 1997;26(1):1–5.

19. Lesens O, et al. Hepatitis C virus is related to progressive liver disease in human immunodeficiency virus-positive hemophiliacs and should be treated as an opportunistic infection. *J Infect Dis* 1999;179(5):1254–1258.

20. Zylberberg H, et al. Rapidly evolving hepatitis C virus-related cirrhosis in a human immunodeficiency virus-infected patient receiving triple antiretroviral therapy. *Clin Infect Dis* 1998;27(5):1255–1258.

21. Vento S, et al. Enhancement of hepatitis C virus replication and liver damage in HIV-coinfected patients on antiretroviral combination therapy [letter]. *Aids* 1998;12(1): 116–117.

22. Sulkowski MS, et al. Hepatotoxicity associated with antiretroviral therapy in adults infected with human immunodeficiency virus and the role of hepatitis C or B virus infection [see comments]. *JAMA* 2000;283(1):74–80.

23. Puoti M, et al. Liver damage and kinetics of hepatitis C virus and human immunodeficiency virus replication during the early phases of combination antiretroviral treatment. *J Infect Dis* 2000;181(6):2033–2036.

24. Abbott KC, et al. Human immunodeficiency virus infection and kidney transplantation in the era of highly active antiretroviral therapy and modern immunosuppression. *J Am Soc Nephrol* 2004;15(6):1633–1639.

25. Ahuja TS, Borucki M, Grady J. Highly active antiretroviral therapy improves survival of HIV-infected hemodialysis patients. *Am J Kidney Dis* 2000;36(3):574–580.

26. Ragni M, et al. Pre-Transplant Survival is Shorter in HIV-Positive than HIV-Negative subjects with End-Stage Liver Disease. *Liver Transpl* 2005.

27. Stock PG. Rapid deterioration of HIV co-infected patients waiting for liver transplantation is not predicted by MELD. *Liver Transpl* 2005;11(11):1315–1317.

28. Jain A, et al. The interaction between anti-retroviral agents and tacrolimus in liver and kidney transplant patients. in American Transplant Congress. 2002. Washington DC.

29. Frassetto L, et al. Cyclosporine pharmacokinetics and dosing modifications in human immunodeficiency virus-infected liver and kidney transplant recipients. *Transplantation* 2005;80(1):13–17.

30. Guaraldi G, et al. Role of therapeutic drug monitoring in a patient with human immunodeficiency virus infection and end-stage liver disease undergoing orthotopic liver transplantation. *Transplant Proc* 2005;37(6):2609–2610.

31. 1999 USPHS/IDSA guidelines for the prevention of opportunistic infections in persons infected with human immunodeficiency virus. U.S. Public Health Service (USPHS) and Infectious Diseases Society of America (IDSA). *MMWR Recomm Rep* 1999;48(RR-10):1–59, 61–66.

32. Benhamou Y, et al. Safety and efficacy of adefovir dipivoxil in patients co-infected with HIV-1 and lamivudine-resistant hepatitis B virus: an open-label pilot study. *Lancet* 2001;358(9283):718–723.

33. Ying C, et al. Inhibition of the replication of the DNA polymerase M550V mutation variant of human hepatitis B virus by adefovir, tenofovir, L-FMAU, DAPD, penciclovir and lobucavir. *J Viral Hepat* 2000;7(2):161–165.

34. Ishak K, et al. Histological grading and staging of chronic hepatitis. *J Hepatol* 1995;22(6):696–699.

35. Ragni MV, et al. Pretransplant survival is shorter in HIV-positive than HIV-negative subjects with end-stage liver disease. *Liver Transpl* 2005;11(11):1425–1430.

36. Stock PG, et al, Kidney and liver transplantation in human immunodeficiency virus-infected patients: a pilot safety and efficacy study. *Transplantation* 2003;76(2):370–375.

37. Ragni MV, et al. Survival of human immunodeficiency virus-infected liver transplant recipients. *J Infect Dis* 2003;188(10):1412–1420.

38. Prachalias AA, et al. Liver transplantation in adults coinfected with HIV. Transplantation 2001;72(10):1684–1688.

39. Norris S, et al. Outcomes of liver transplantation in HIV-infected individuals: the impact of HCV and HBV infection. *Liver Transpl* 2004;10(10):1271–1278.

40. Neff GW, et al. Orthotopic liver transplantation in patients with human immunodeficiency virus and end-stage liver disease. *Liver Transpl* 2003;9(3):239–247.

41. Moreno S, et al. Liver transplantation in HIV-infected recipients. *Liver Transpl* 2005; 11(1):76–81.

42. Rafecas A, et al. Liver transplantation without steroid induction in HIV-infected patients. *Liver Transpl* 2004;10(10):1320–1323.

43. Vogel M, VE, Wasmuth JC, Brackmann H, et al. Orthotopic liver transplantation in HIV-positive patients: Outcome of 10 patients from the Bonn cohort. In: *12th Conference on Retroviruses and Opportunistic Infections*. 2005. Boston, MA.

44. Radecke K, et al. Outcome after orthotopic liver transplantation in five HIV-infected patients with virus hepatitis-induced cirrhosis. Liver Int 2005;25(1):101–108.

45. Ragni M, BS, Im K, Neff G, et al. *Survival in HIV-infected liver transplant recipients*. in *10th Conference on Retroviruses and Opportunistic Infections*. 2003. Boston, MA.

46. Kumar MS, et al. Safety and success of kidney transplantation and concomitant immunosuppression in HIV-positive patients. *Kidney Int* 2005;67(4):1622–1629.

# NEW IMMUNOSUPPRESSIVE PROTOCOLS

*Rolf N. Barth, MD, Stuart J. Knechtle, MD*

## INTRODUCTION

The challenge of any novel immunosuppressive strategy, especially with respect to living donor transplantation, is to maintain the high success rates of current strategies, while attaining longer-term benefit. The current standards for living donor renal transplants include 1- and 5-year graft survivals of 95% and 80%.[1] Results for living donor liver transplants are reported 1-year graft survival rates from 55% to 85%.[2] The aim of any new regimen should be guided by the ultimate goals of improved long-term patient and graft survival. Attempts to reach this goal have included the following (1) reduction in the morbidity of chronic exposure to steroids and calcineurin inhibitors, (2) improved therapies for humoral rejection, (3) novel immunosuppressive therapies, and (4) improved monitoring of the immunologic status of patients. These strategies must be strictly measured against the highly successful therapies currently employed in transplantation, and only those that demonstrate benefit to long-term graft and patient survival should be adopted for widespread application. Until clear evidence arises, data exist that point us down the path of improved results, clinical trials must be created, updated, and reported on to provide reliable data.

The development of new strategies may provide the ultimate answers to improved long-term results. The living donor transplant recipient may be the ideal candidate for these strategies to improve on long-term graft survival. New and wider application of induction therapies, including lymphocyte depletion and IL-2 receptor blockade, provides potential for superior longer-term graft survival. These therapies may also open the door to greater success with steroid and calcineurin minimization and withdrawal strategies. New drug development may also expand the pharmacologic arsenal to improve graft function without additional morbidity. Finally, more accurate monitoring of the immunologic status of recipients may guide more appropriate levels of immunosuppression tailored to individual recipients.

## LYMPHOCYTE DEPLETION

### Alemtuzumab (Campath-1H)

Lymphocyte depletion strategies have been used in recent years with good short-term results with regard to patient and graft survival, and with acceptable morbidity. Alemtuzumab was approved by the U.S. Food and Drug administration for treatment of lymphoid malignancies in 1999, and has been subsequently utilized in off-label clinical trials, induction therapies, and maintenance immunosuppression for kidney, kidney–pancreas, small-bowel, and liver transplantation. Alemtuzumab is a humanized monoclonal antibody directed against the CD52 epitope expressed on T and B cells, NK cells, and monocytes and macrophages. CD52 is not expressed on bone marrow cells, erythrocytes, and granulocytes. Alemtuzumab provides for profound and durable depletion of T cells within the periphery and lymph node compartments via both complement and antibody-dependent cell cytotoxicity. Development and initial studies of alemtuzumab have attempted to find the optimal treatment regimens of alemtuzumab as well as co-administered immunosuppression. Induction therapy with alemtuzumab is usually performed by the intraoperative and optional postoperative day 1 administration of 20 to 30 mg. Lymphocyte depletion exceeds 99% in peripheral blood and at 12 months recovers to only one third of pretreatment CD3 counts.[3] There has been no documentation of increased infectious or malignant complications with lymphocyte depletion provided for by standard alemtuzumab therapy.

Short-term benefits of alemtuzumab induction therapy may be greatest in high-risk patients. This has been demonstrated in recipients of renal allografts that demonstrate delayed graft function more likely associated with extended criteria donors than with living donors. Recipients of renal allografts that demonstrated delayed graft function who have received alemtuzumab induction demonstrated a 20% reduction in rejection rates during the first 6 months posttransplant as compared to patients receiving either thymoglobulin or basiliximab.[4] High-risk living donor recipients who are highly sensitized based on panel-reactive antibody titers, positive crossmatch, or ABO incompatibility may similarly benefit from a lymphocyte-depletion strategy. This could provide potent immunosuppression while clinicians await adequate renal function to tolerate additional immunosuppression most commonly including calcineurin inhibitor therapy.

Most of the initial trials with alemtuzumab induction therapy have attempted immunosuppressive withdrawal or minimization and have demonstrated success at having a high proportion of patients successfully decrease their subsequent immunosuppressive regimens. These studies have predominantly focused on low-risk deceased donor and living donor renal allografts. Data from 5-year follow-up have demonstrated comparable patient and graft survival results with alemtuzumab-treated patients and cyclosporine monotherapy as compared to standard immunosuppression without induction therapy.[5] Recipients have not demonstrated increased malignant or infectious complications at 5-year follow-up. Alemtuzumab therapy has been combined with sirolimus in an effort to avoid both steroid and calcineurin therapies. Results from this trial at 3 years have demonstrated 96% graft survival with two thirds of patients on steroid-free regimens and over half of patients remaining on monotherapy.[6]

Increased rates of humoral rejection were observed in some alemtuzumab trials that did not utilize calcineurin inhibitor or mycophenolate based therapies.[7,8] Increased rates of humoral rejection were not observed in alemtuzumab trials that utilized calcineurin inhibitors and mycophenolate therapies.[3] The reason for higher rates of humoral rejection may be related to the combination of alemtuzumab induction with novel strategies of drug monotherapy; however, this has not been conclusively demonstrated, and it is possible that humoral mechanisms may be uncovered by T-cell depletion. This could theoretically include populations of T regulatory cells that modulate antibody production.

The potential for lymphocyte depletion pretransplant to provide for the development of a posttransplant tolerant state has been investigated with alemtuzumab therapy. Transplant tolerance was defined by stable renal allograft function after alemtuzumab induction and without continued immunosuppressive therapy. This approach failed to demonstrate success as all seven recipients demonstrated evidence of rejection within the first month posttransplant.[9] Alternately, alemtuzumab maintenance therapy has been investigated as method of avoidance of both steroids and calcineurin inhibitors. In a study population of pancreas and simultaneous kidney pancreas recipients, alemtuzumab maintenance therapy was administered to maintain a lymphocyte count below 200 cells/mm$^3$ and was combined only with mycophenolate mofetil.[10] At 6 months evaluation, patients treated with alemtuzumab maintenance therapy demonstrated higher graft loss in pancreas-alone transplants and earlier rejection episodes but comparable graft survival in simultaneous kidney pancreas recipients. These early results confirm the need for additional therapies combined with lymphocyte-depletion strategies.

Experience with alemtuzumab induction therapy in children is limited, but has demonstrated efficacy in lymphocyte depletion and acceptable morbidity.[11] The obvious benefit in children might be a greater ability to proceed with steroid and calcineurin inhibitor minimization and withdrawal strategies. Ongoing trials are examining the potential of these approaches to realize long-term benefits while maintaining traditional excellent results, especially in living donor combinations.

## Antithymocyte Globulin (Thymoglobulin)

Thymoglobulin is a polyclonal antithymocyte antibody preparation that also provides for efficacious depletion of T cells. Thymoglobulin induction therapy has been used with success in steroid withdrawal protocols.[12] Patients were recipients of either living or deceased donor kidneys and had rapid discontinuation of steroids 5 days after induction therapy with thymoglobulin. Patients were maintained on calcineurin inhibitor therapy plus either mycophenolate mofetil or sirolimus. At 3 years, graft survival was 93%, and 84% of patients remained on steroid-free regimens. Updated results from this trial demonstrated 5-year graft survival of 84% with a continued high proportion of patients off steroids.[13] Statistically significant reduced rates of cataracts, diabetes, fractures, and avascular necrosis were observed in the steroid-free population.

Although no prospective randomized trial has compared thymoglobulin to alemtuzumab, some studies have suggested the superiority of alemtuzumab as compared to thymoglobulin with respect to drug minimization or withdrawal. In one study, renal transplant recipients treated with either alemtuzumab or thymoglobulin induction therapy followed by calcineurin monotherapy that was attempted to be weaned to low doses or off as tolerated. Alemtuzumab-treated patients demonstrated reduced incidence and time to rejection, and decreased rates of chronic allograft nephropathy.[14] As compared to thymoglobulin, alemtuzumab provides for a more complete and durable depletion of CD52+ T cells and thus may be viewed as a more efficacious strategy to achieve lymphocyte depletion.

## Rituximab (Rituxan)

Rituximab is a monoclonal antibody directed against the CD20 epitope expressed on mature B cells, but importantly, not on plasma cells. Rituximab is administered as an intravenous dose (375 mg/m$^2$) and accomplishes depletion of CD20+ B cells in the periphery with 24 hours.[15] It has been approved for treatment of B-cell lymphomas and has been used off-label in organ transplantation. Studies support use for treatment of rheumatoid arthritis and treatment of antibody-mediated rejection in renal allografts.[16] There is at least one ongoing trial examining a role for rituximab as an induction agent in renal transplantation to allow for calcineurin inhibitor free immunosuppression (Sollinger communication). This includes low-risk patient populations including living donor combinations. The potential of rituximab as an effective therapy to either treat or prevent B-cell-mediated graft loss may provide for another method to improve long-term graft survival.

The benefits of induction therapy in living donor transplantation are twofold: (1) in high-risk patients or sensitized patients to decrease the incidence of early rejection episodes; and (2) in low-risk patients to provide potential for greater success with drug minimization, withdrawal, or avoidance strategies. This latter point has not been clearly demonstrated, and in fact, many questions and contradictory data exist as to whether the expected benefits of steroid and calcineurin minimization or avoidance correlate with improved patient or graft survival. Nonetheless, the long-term toxicity of calcineurin inhibitors and morbidity of steroid therapy are two important topics to address improved long-term success in living donor transplant recipients who generally do very well during the first 5 to 10 years posttransplantation.

## STEROID WITHDRAWAL

Steroid minimization and withdrawal strategies have now been applied and studied for decades and might not be regarded as part of new immunosuppressive protocols. Transplant physicians have been tapering doses of steroids in patients with stable allografts since the beginning of clinical transplantation, and many transplant centers have established protocols for steroid withdrawal in HLA-identical renal transplants. Known complications of steroid therapy include diabetes, osteoporosis, cushingoid physical changes, and growth retardation in children. Patients with predicted excellent long-term potential for graft function are therefore appropriately interested in reducing the morbidity of corticosteroid therapy.

Trials aimed at withdrawing steroids from patients under contemporary immunotherapy regimens that included calcineurin inhibitors and mycophenolate mofetil have demonstrated increased rates of rejection. A meta-analysis of nine trials demonstrated increased risks of both rejection and graft loss.[17] European and U.S. trials using cyclosporine-MMF combinations with steroid withdrawal have similarly demonstrated significant increases in rejection rates.[18,19] Additional meta-analyses have confirmed higher rates of graft rejection; however, this did not always correlate with higher rates of graft loss at 5 years follow-up.[20] Additionally, follow-up of a decade has been reported in a cohort of low-risk renal transplant recipients treated without induction therapy with cyclosporine and mycophenolate mofetil and steroid withdrawal either before or after 6 months.[21] Patients demonstrated excellent 10-year graft survival of between 82% and 88% depending on the timing of steroid withdrawal. The conclusions of steroid withdrawal attempts without induction therapy are that in low-risk patients, steroid withdrawal may be achieved with possible increases in rejection and graft loss rates.

The introduction of induction therapies and/or addition of sirolimus to maintenance therapies, however, may offer even greater potential to avoid the increased rejection rates observed in earlier trials. Induction therapy regimens include previously described lymphocyte depletion strategies or IL-2-receptor monoclonal antibodies. As previously stated, studies with alemtuzumab induction and sirolimus monotherapy in living donor and low immunologic risk patients have demonstrated that two thirds of patients have been maintained on steroid-free regimens at 3 years with excellent graft survival of 96%.[6] Complementary studies with deceased donor kidneys have demonstrated comparable graft and patient survival at 5 years between patient groups treated with alemtuzumab induction and cyclosporine monotherapy and conventional triple immunotherapy.[5] Also as stated prior, thymoglobulin induction appears to be permissive toward steroid discontinuation. Five-year results have demonstrated that patients treated with five doses of thymoglobulin demonstrated excellent graft survival with over 80% maintained on steroid-free therapies.[13]

IL-2 receptor antibody-induction therapy also appears to improve success with steroid minimization and weaning protocols. Two alternate preparations of IL-2 receptor antibodies are currently available: the chimeric monoclonal basiliximab and the humanized monoclonal daclizumab. Three randomized trials are currently evaluating the ability of IL-2 receptor antibody induction to permit steroid withdrawal and avoidance. The THOMAS trial is a multicenter European study that has demonstrated similar rates of rejection, graft, and patient survival at 6 months when withdrawing steroids 3 months after daclizumab induction and maintenance therapy with tacrolimus and mycophenolate mofetil.[22] The CARMEN trial is another European multicenter study comparing standard triple therapy to daclizumab induction and steroid avoidance and has demonstrated comparable rejection rates during the first 6 months posttransplant.[23] The good results with daclizumab therapy and steroid withdrawal may not translate to basiliximab-induction strategies. The ATLAS trial compares standard triple therapy to either basiliximab induction and tacrolimus monotherapy or tacrolimus/mycophenolate mofetil therapy. The latter two groups do not utilize steroid therapy, and both revealed significantly higher rates of rejection at 1 year, with no significant difference in patient or graft survival.[24]

If long-term follow-up studies confirm the success of steroid withdrawal after induction therapy, the timing of steroid withdrawal remains to be resolved. Daclizumab-induction therapy has been demonstrated to allow weaning and steroid discontinuation after 6 months with equivalent 1-year serum creatinine levels to patients maintained on steroids, tacrolimus, and mycophenolate mofetil.[25] One prospective multicenter study comparing daclizumab induction and steroid cessation after 3 days to that of no induction and withdrawal after 4 months has demonstrated no differences in rejection rates or graft survival at 1 year.[26] These low-risk recipients of either living or deceased donor renal allografts appear to better tolerate steroid withdrawal at earlier time points after daclizumab induction therapy.

High immunologic risk patients do not appear to benefit from IL-2 receptor antibody induction alone allowing steroid withdrawal and are unlikely candidates for this approach. High-risk patients treated with daclizumab induction and triple therapy consisting of tacrolimus, sirolimus, and mycophenolate mofetil demonstrated a 60% rate of acute rejection.[27] This point may as well be applicable to calcineurin inhibitor withdrawal strategies, as well. The poor results of IL-2 receptor antibody therapy and steroid withdrawal in high-risk patients are an important distinction to make as compared to lymphocyte depletion strategies that demonstrate some benefit in high-risk groups of patients.

The benefits of steroid minimization and avoidance are predictably greater in a pediatric transplant population that would traditionally necessitate steroid therapy through the growth and development period. Increased rejection rates with withdrawal or alternate-day steroid treatment regimens have been reported with standard immunosuppressive protocols as applied to pediatric renal allograft recipients.[28] Success with steroid weaning and avoidance protocols in pediatric populations may be better realized when combined with induction and early therapy with daclizumab. The use of daclizumab induction therapy continued for 6 months postoperatively and combined with calcineurin inhibitor and mycophenolate mofetil in low-risk pediatric recipients of both living and deceased donor renal allografts demonstrated only 8% incidence of acute rejection at 1 year.[29,30] The ability to achieve complete steroid avoidance would presumably maximize benefits in terms of growth as compared to steroid minimization. Pediatric recipients of living related renal transplants may have the most to gain from induction therapy and steroid withdrawal.

## CALCINEURIN INHIBITOR MINIMIZATION AND AVOIDANCE

Although calcineurin inhibitors are credited with much of the improvement in graft survival and decreased rates of acute rejection over the last 20 years, improved long-term graft survival remains elusive. The same calcineurin inhibitors that have decreased rates of early rejection and graft loss may be contributing to chronic allograft nephropathy. The goal of minimizing long-term exposure to calcineurin inhibitors, thus, attempts to improve on the long-term graft damage that has been attributed to both tacrolimus and cyclosporine.

Similar to steroid minimization and withdrawal studies, efforts to reduce exposure to calcineurin inhibitors are dependent on induction strategies. The most aggressive strategies attempt to completely withdraw all immunosuppressive therapy. Lymphocyte-depletion strategies have been used in an attempt to completely avoid all immunosuppressive therapies with mixed results. As previously described, Kirk et al. at the NIH demonstrated that alemtuzumab-induction therapy used alone was not sufficient for stable renal graft function without additional immunosuppression even within the first month.[9] Lymphocyte depletion, however, may provide for greater success with steroid avoidance and calcineurin weaning. Spaced weaning protocols provide for the gradual reduction in immunosuppression, thus allowing clinical parameters to determine the ability to proceed with further reduction. The University of Pittsburgh has compared thymoglobulin to alemtuzumab in the ability to proceed with weaning of calcineurin monotherapy. Results at 18 months suggest that alemtuzumab induction may provide for reduced rates of acute rejection as compared to thymoglobulin, and that both strategies were at early points allowing for monotherapy and/or weaning strategies in nearly 90% of patients.[14] This study has also found that lymphocyte depletion by thymoglobulin combined with calcineurin weaning does not reduce chronic allograft nephropathy observed at timepoints up to 40 months after transplant. The alemtuzumab cohort of patients did not have sufficient follow-up to confirm this observation. The failure to see long-term benefit with respect to chronic allograft nephropathy with any induction or withdrawal strategy should be recognized as evidence that the underlying etiology for chronic graft loss remains untouched by such strategies. Nonetheless, if equivalent clinical outcomes are achieved, the benefits of reduced immunosuppressive protocols may still be important enough to pursue.

Studies investigating the ability of sirolimus therapy to reduce or withdraw renal transplant patients from calcineurin inhibitors have demonstrated mixed results. Meta-analysis of trials looking at sirolimus therapy and calcineurin withdrawal have demonstrated increased risk of acute rejection, no 1-year difference in graft or patient survival, and improved blood pressure control.[31] These studies did not use or report any induction therapy, which as mentioned previously may improve on these rejection events within the first year posttransplant. Basiliximab induction with subsequent triple therapy with either cyclosporine or sirolimus has been compared in one prospective randomized trial of renal transplant recipients.[32] At 2-year follow-up, sirolimus-treated patients (off cyclosporine) demonstrated lower serum creatinine levels, improved glomerular filtration rate, and diminished evidence of chronic allograft nephropathy based on protocol biopsies. The University of Wisconsin experience has demonstrated that alemtuzumab-induction therapy with postoperative sirolimus monotherapy in renal transplant recipients has yielded 3-year graft survival of 96% with nearly 80% of patients off calcineurin inhibitor therapy.[6]

The ultimate endpoint of improved long-term graft survival with calcineurin inhibitor minimization or avoidance has yet to be realized. Although early results from a combination of new induction therapies and new maintenance therapies are promising, the chronic allograft damage currently seen with calcineurin-based therapies may be exchanged for other forms of long-term graft damage or patient morbidity. Long-term follow-up is therefore requisite in all attempts to substitute new therapies for established successful calcineurin-based regimens. Patients should be exposed to the possibilities and risks of both improved outcomes or increased graft loss and morbidity as parts of well-designed clinical trials until these long-term outcomes have been evaluated.

## NEW AGENTS

### Belatacept (LEA-29Y)

CTLA4-Ig, a soluble recombinant immunoglobulin fusion protein was developed to inhibit T-cell activation caused by CD80 and CD86 molecules interacting with their CD28 receptor. Application of CTLA4-Ig to non-human primate models demonstrated relatively low efficacy, perhaps because of relatively low affinity for the receptors.[33-35] Belatacept (LEA-29Y) was subsequently developed in order to provide more potent immunosuppression in organ transplant models. Two amino acids were substituted on CTLA4-Ig resulting in fourfold greater binding avidity to CD86 and twofold greater avidity in CD80 binding compared

to CTLA4-Ig.[36] This translated into greater *in vitro* and *in vivo* inhibition of T-cell activation and prevention of renal transplant rejection in non-human primates.[36]

Subsequently, a phase II clinical trial was performed to evaluate safety and efficacy of belatacept versus cyclosporine in human renal transplantation. These results appear to be encouraging in that equivalence was achieved with respect to rejection rates. The renal function was significantly better in patients receiving belatacept. Cardiovascular and metabolic endpoints were also better in the belatacept cohort.[37] This phase II trial is being followed up with two phase III trials which include basiliximab induction, mycophenolate, and prednisone maintenance therapy. Unlike antibody or fusion protein therapies in the past, the design of belatacept therapy includes monthly administration of the fusion protein via a parenteral route. The response of patients to receiving an intravenous maintenance drug as part of their immunosuppressive therapy has so far been quite positive, but this has only occurred in the context of well-controlled clinical trials. Broader acceptance by patients awaits further evaluation.

### FK778

Experimental work has been reported with FK778 (Astellas), a malononitrilamide derived from leflunomide with both anti-T- and B-cell activity. FK778 inhibits pyrimidine synthesis, thus blocking proliferation of immune cells. This compound has been shown to reduce the production of various cytokines including TGFβ which are implicated in the development of allograft fibrosis. There has been some preliminary data that FK778 may have some activity against BK polyoma virus. FK778 is currently in early clinical trials to assess its utility in reducing either antibody-mediated injury or BK virus injury. Its principal side effect is dose-related anemia.

### FTY720

FTY720 (Novartis), an analog of sphingosine-1-phosphate (S1P), is currently in clinical trials in renal transplantation as a novel immunosuppressant. This agent has been shown to modify the trafficking of leukocytes in the peripheral blood and in particular to cause lymphocyte sequestration in the lymph nodes. Although its mechanism of action remains to be better elucidated, it appears to be effective when used in combination with calcineurin inhibitors to prevent rejection and allow lower doses of calcineurin inhibitors to be used. FTY720 is phosphorylated *in vivo* and interacts as an agonist with a family of G-protein-coupled receptors that recognize S1P as the endogenous ligand. Activation of S1P signal regulates multiple immunologic functions of T cells including proliferation, apoptosis, differentiation, migration, and cytokine secretion. Exposure to the drug results in receptor internalization and down-regulation on the surface of lymphocytes. This effect is thought to be the major mechanism of action. The safety and efficacy of this drug in humans is currently under investigation in clinical trials, some of which have been stopped due to concern about macular edema in diabetic patients, and due to lack of additional clinical benefit compared to mycophenolate mofetil.

## TREATMENT OF HUMORAL REJECTION

It has recently become clear that alloantibody may comprise an important component of acute rejection and less frequently occurs as an independent process without cell-mediated rejection.

Antibody-mediated rejection typically targets endothelial cells, and kidney and heart allografts have the highest incidence of documented antibody-mediated rejection. By staining for the complement component C4d, histologic evidence of antibody is indirectly demonstrated. C4d immunofluorescence or immunohistochemistry has developed as an important adjunct to the diagnosis of acute rejection and, in particular, antibody-mediated rejection. The treatment of humoral rejection is less clear, in terms of both appropriate agents and anticipated outcomes. Removal of antibody can be accomplished through plasmapheresis, although multiple serial applications of plasmapheresis are necessary. Treatment with the anti-CD20 antibody, rituximab, is being commonly used, although controlled clinical trials to address its efficacy in this setting are missing. Anti-T-cell therapy including bolus steroid therapy and thymoglobulin treatment are also frequently employed in order to treat the either presumed or confirmed role of T-cell-mediated rejection. Finally, the role of intravenous immune globulin again remains controversial, but may be helpful in arresting antibody-mediated injury.

## IMMUNOLOGIC MONITORING

With the goal of improving diagnostic accuracy following organ transplantation, various molecular and genetic tests are being developed. Generally, these assays are in the research phase rather than clinical approval. Nuclear magnetic resonance (NMR) spectroscopy is being used by Nickerson et al to perform proteomic profiling of urine in patients with renal transplants.[38] Hricik has reported on the use of ELISPOT assays of peripheral blood cells to measure IFNγ released by recipient cells in response to donor cell or donor peptide.[39] The level of IFNγ appears to correlate with the eventual outcome of the kidney as measured by serum creatinine. In other words, high IFNγ production by recipient cells portends a poor outcome for renal allograft function. The difficulty with this approach to date has been that although patients can be placed in a high-risk category based on such an assay, there is no specific treatment for a particular patient that would be guided by the assay.

Urine markers including CD3 perforin and granzyme B have been measured in urine by PCR and reported to correlate with acute cellular rejection.[40] However, IP-10 and CXCR3 may be more accurate predictors of acute cellular rejection.[40–42] Development of a protein-based assay to measure chemokines may also be more diagnostically useful than a PCR-based assay.[42]

An alternative strategy is to monitor urinary BK virus infection as a barometer of overimmunosuppression. Brennan has reported the usefulness of monitoring viruria as a means of reducing immunosuppression and effectively preventing viremia.[43] The Cylex immunoassay which measures phosphate energy stores within CD4+ T cells is being evaluated for its correlation with overimmunosuppression.[44] Again, the clinical application of these tests requires considerable further study to determine whether individual patient decisions can be made based on results.

Clearly, the field of transplantation begs for improved diagnostic tests to individualize immunosuppression, detect the rare possibility of tolerance, and detect rejection before it develops into full-blown clinical injury with elevated creatinine in kidney transplantation. Given the sensitivity of new tools such as PCR-based and proteomic-based methodologies, these possibilities seem realistic, but have not yet been reduced to a practical clinical application. Nevertheless, there are considerable research opportunities in the immunologic monitoring which have potential to change the means of monitoring transplant patients.

## References

1. Gjertson DW. Look-up survival tables for living-donor renal transplants: OPTN/UNOS data 1995-2002, in Cecka JM, Terasaki PI (eds): *Clin Transpl 2003*. Los Angeles, UCLA Immunogenetics Center; 2004:337.
2. Renz JF, Kin CJ, Saggi BH, et al. Outcomes of living donor liver transplantation, in Busuttil RW, Klintmalm GB (eds): *Transplantation of the Liver*. Philadelphia: Elsevier Saunders; 2005:713.
3. Ciancio G, Burke GW, Gaynor JJ, et al. The use of Campath-1H as induction therapy in renal transplantation: preliminary results. *Transplantation* 2004;78:426.
4. Knechtle SJ, Fernandez LA, Pirsch JD, et al. Campath-1H in renal transplantation: The University of Wisconsin experience. *Surgery* 2004;136:754.
5. Watson CJ, Bradley JA, Friend PJ, et al. Alemtuzumab (CAMPATH 1H) induction therapy in cadaveric kidney transplantation—efficacy and safety at five years. *Am J Transplant* 2005;5:1347.
6. Barth RN, Janus CA, Lillesand CA, et al. Three-year success of Campath-1H induction for renal transplantation (abstract). *Am J Transplant* 2005;5:569.
7. Knechtle SJ, Pirsch JD, Fechner JH Jr, et al. Campath-1H induction plus rapamycin monotherapy for renal transplantation: results of a pilot study. *Am J Transplant* 2003;3:722.
8. Cai J, Terasaki PI, Bloom DD, et al. Correlation between human leukocyte antigen antibody production and serum creatinine in patients receiving sirolimus monotherapy after Campath-1H induction. *Transplantation* 2004;78:919.
9. Kirk AD, Hale DA, Mannon RB, et al. Results from a human renal allograft tolerance trial evaluating the humanized CD52-specific monoclonal antibody alemtuzumab (CAMPATH-1H). *Transplantation* 2003;76:120.
10. Gruessner RW, Kandaswamy R, Humar A, et al. Calcineurin inhibitor- and steroid-free immunosuppression in pancreas-kidney and solitary pancreas transplantation. *Transplantation* 2005;79:1184.
11. Bartosh SM, Knechtle SJ, Sollinger HW. Campath-1H use in pediatric renal transplantation. *Am J Transplant* 2005;5:1569.
12. Khwaja K, Asolati M, Harmon J, et al. Outcome at 3 years with a prednisone-free maintenance regimen: a single-center experience with 349 kidney transplant recipients. *Am J Transplant* 2004;4:980.
13. Matas AJ, Kandaswamy R, Gillingham KJ, et al. Prednisone-free maintenance immunosuppression-a 5-year experience. *Am J Transplant* 2005;5:2473.
14. Shapiro R, Basu A, Tan H, et al. Kidney transplantation under minimal immunosuppression after pretransplant lymphoid depletion with Thymoglobulin or Campath. *J Am Coll Surg* 2005;200:505.
15. Schroder C, Azimzadeh AM, Wu G, et al. Anti-CD20 treatment depletes B-cells in blood and lymphatic tissue of cynomolgus monkeys. *Transpl Immunol* 2003;12:19.
16. Becker YT, Becker BN, Pirsch JD, et al. Rituximab as treatment for refractory kidney transplant rejection. *Am J Transplant* 2004;4:996.
17. Kasiske BL, Chakkera HA, Louis TA, et al. A meta-analysis of immunosuppression withdrawal trials in renal transplantation. *J Am Soc Nephrol* 2000;11:1910.
18. Vanrenterghem Y, Lebranchu Y, Hene R, et al. Double-blind comparison of two corticosteroid regimens plus mycophenolate mofetil and cyclosporine for prevention of acute renal allograft rejection. *Transplantation* 2000;70:1352.
19. Ahsan N, Hricik D, Matas A, et al. Prednisone withdrawal in kidney transplant recipients on cyclosporine and mycophenolate mofetil—a prospective randomized study. Steroid Withdrawal Study Group. *Transplantation* 1999;68:1865.
20. Pascual J, Quereda C, Zamora J, et al. for the Spanish Group for Evidence-Based Medicine in Renal Transplantation: Steroid withdrawal in renal transplant patients on triple therapy with a calcineurin inhibitor and mycophenolate mofetil: a meta-analysis of randomized, controlled trials. *Transplantation* 2004;78:1548.

21. Rama I, Cruzado JM, Gil-Vernet S, et al. Steroids can be safely withdrawn from cyclosporine and mycophenolate mofetil-treated renal allograft recipients: long-term results. *Transplantation* 2005;80:164.

22. Vanrenterghem Y, Van Hooff JP, Squifflet JP, et al. for the European Tacrolimus/MMF Renal Transplantation Study Group: Minimization of immunosuppressive therapy after renal transplantation: results of a randomized controlled trial. *Am J Transplant* 2005;5:87.

23. Rostaing L, Cantarovich D, Mourad G, et al. for the CARMEN Study Group: Corticosteroid-free immunosuppression with tacrolimus, mycophenolate mofetil, and daclizumab induction in renal transplantation. *Transplantation* 2005;79:807.

24. Kramer BK, Kruger B, Mack M, et al. Steroid withdrawal or steroid avoidance in renal transplant recipients: focus on tacrolimus-based immunosuppressive regimens. *Transplant Proc* 2005;37:1789.

25. Kuypers DR, Evenepoel P, Maes B, et al. The use of an anti-CD25 monoclonal antibody and mycophenolate mofetil enables the use of a low-dose tacrolimus and early withdrawal of steroids in renal transplant recipients. *Clin Transplant* 2003;17:234.

26. ter Meulen CG, van R, I, Hene RJ, et al. Steroid-withdrawal at 3 days after renal transplantation with anti-IL-2 receptor alpha therapy: a prospective, randomized, multicenter study. *Am J Transplant* 2004;4:803.

27. Alloway RR, Hanaway MJ, Trofe J, et al. A prospective, pilot study of early corticosteroid cessation in high-immunologic-risk patients: the Cincinnati experience. *Transplant Proc* 2005;37:802.

28. Roberti I, Reisman L, Lieberman KV, et al. Risk of steroid withdrawal in pediatric renal allograft recipients (a 5-year follow-up). *Clin Transplant* 1994;8:405.

29. Sarwal MM, Vidhun JR, Alexander SR, et al. Continued superior outcomes with modification and lengthened follow-up of a steroid-avoidance pilot with extended daclizumab induction in pediatric renal transplantation. *Transplantation* 2003;76:1331.

30. Vidhun JR, Sarwal MM. Corticosteroid avoidance in pediatric renal transplantation. *Pediatr Nephrol* 2005;20:418.

31. Mulay AV, Hussain N, Fergusson D, et al. Calcineurin inhibitor withdrawal from sirolimus-based therapy in kidney transplantation: a systematic review of randomized trials. *Am J Transplant* 2005;5:1748.

32. Flechner SM, Kurian SM, Solez K, et al. De novo kidney transplantation without use of calcineurin inhibitors preserves renal structure and function at two years. *Am J Transplant* 2004;4:1776.

33. Kirk AD, Harlan DM, Armstrong NN, et al. CTLA4-Ig and anti-CD40 ligand prevent renal allograft rejection in primates. *Proc Natl Acad Sci USA* 1997;94:8789.

34. Levisetti MG, Padrid PA, Szot GL, et al. Immunosuppressive effects of human CTLA4Ig in a non-human primate model of allogeneic pancreatic islet transplantation. *J Immunol* 1997;159:5187.

35. Greene JL, Leytze GM, Emswiler J, et al. Covalent dimerization of CD28/CTLA-4 and oligomerization of CD80/CD86 regulate T cell costimulatory interactions. *J Biol Chem* 1996;271:26762.

36. Larsen CP, Pearson TC, Adams AB, et al. Rational development of LEA29Y (belatacept), a high-affinity variant of CTLA4-Ig with potent immunosuppressive properties. *Am J Transplant* 2005;5:443.

37. Vincenti F, Larsen C, Durrbach A, et al. for the Belatacept Study Group: Costimulation blockade with belatacept in renal transplantation. *N Engl J Med* 2005;353:770.

38. Schaub S, Rush D, Wilkins J, et al. Proteomic-based detection of urine proteins associated with acute renal allograft rejection. *J Am Soc Nephrol* 2004;15:219.

39. Hricik DE, Rodriguez V, Riley J, et al. Enzyme linked immunosorbent spot (ELISPOT) assay for interferon-gamma independently predicts renal function in kidney transplant recipients. *Am J Transplant* 2003;3:878.

40. Tatapudi RR, Muthukumar T, Dadhania D, et al. Noninvasive detection of renal allograft inflammation by measurements of mRNA for IP-10 and CXCR3 in urine. *Kidney Int* 2004;65:2390.

41. Hu H, Aizenstein BD, Puchalski A, et al. Elevation of CXCR3-binding chemokines in urine indicates acute renal-allograft dysfunction. *Am J Transplant* 2004;4:432.

42. Kotsch K, Mashreghi MF, Bold G, et al. Enhanced granulysin mRNA expression in urinary sediment in early and delayed acute renal allograft rejection. *Transplantation* 2004;77:1866.

43. Brennan DC, Agha I, Bohl DL, et al. Incidence of BK with tacrolimus versus cyclosporine and impact of preemptive immunosuppression reduction. *Am J Transplant* 2005;5:582.

44. Kowalski R, Post D, Schneider MC, et al. Immune cell function testing: an adjunct to therapeutic drug monitoring in transplant patient management. *Clin Transpl* 2003;17:77.

# CHAPTER 38

# STRATEGIES TO INDUCE TOLERANCE

*Gregor Warnecke, MD, Kathryn J. Wood, DPhil*

## INTRODUCTION

Donor-specific tolerance, if achievable in the routine clinical practice of transplantation, has the potential to transform the field and is therefore often considered as the holy grail of transplantation research. Ideally, a state of immunologic tolerance or unresponsiveness would be induced in recipients of allogeneic organ transplants that would prevent rejection of the transplant without the need for lifelong pharmacologic immunosuppression with its hazardous and potentially life-threatening side effects. This state of tolerance would completely prevent destructive immune responses against the graft but would not interfere with normal immune responses against environmental pathogens and tumor cells. Thus the burden of opportunistic infections and malignancies that are today so frequent in pharmacologically immunosuppressed transplant recipients might be resolved.

The deliberate induction of transplantation tolerance was first described by Billingham et al. in 1953,[1] who translated the earlier findings of Owen and colleagues into this applied setting.[2] Owen had shown that dizygotic twin cattle that exchange blood in fetal life through anastomoses of their placental vessels maintain red cell chimerism throughout their lifetime. Billingham and Medawar could not only show that these cattle twins are fully tolerant of each other's skin grafts,[3] but also that they succeeded in injecting allogeneic lymph node cells into unborn mouse fetuses rendering these mice tolerant to donor strain skin grafts after birth.[1] In this latter experiment, the skin grafts were accepted indefinitely, whereas third-party skin grafts were promptly rejected. These findings reflect the strict criteria that are still valid, now more than 50 years later, to define experimental donor-specific tolerance. These criteria state that a "tolerant" recipient of an allograft must neither reject the graft nor a second transplant from the same (or a syngeneic) donor, and the recipient must be able to mount a "normal" immune response against a transplant from a third party donor (ie, a donor, that is MHC-mismatched to both the recipient and the original organ donor), as well as against normal environmental pathogens. The criteria for "true" transplantation tolerance are very strict and the subject of ongoing debate. They have been established in part as a result of the observation that many tolerance induction protocols that are successful in rodents are not necessarily reproducible in large animals, primates, or humans.[4,5] It is therefore argued by some that the organ or tissue transplanted should ideally be skin, because tolerance to skin grafts is considered to be more robust than tolerance toward other organs.[5] However, achieving tolerance to other types of organ and cell transplants experimentally is equally valid and relevant to the development of strategies that can be transplanted to the clinic in the future. Prolonged heart allograft survival sometimes referred to as operational tolerance in rodents, for example, is more easily accomplished in some donor–recipient combinations, using an abundance of protocols, including administration of a short course of cyclosporine[6,7] or other immunosuppressive agents, such as anti-CD4 therapy.[8] These findings are clearly not directly transferable into humans if all other forms of immunosuppression are to be withdrawn as part of the protocol. The long-term acceptance of skin allografts, however, is more challenging to achieve in large animal, as well as in rodent models.[9] Only few protocols can provide long-term skin allograft survival in immunocompetent primary recipients, and those that are effective might be considered as the protocols that have the greatest potential value once transferred into a large animal model. On the other hand, it is reasonable to ask whether meeting these strict criteria is absolutely necessary.

The answer to this question really depends on the objective of tolerance protocols in clinical transplantation. If the objective of tolerance induction is to achieve long-term graft survival in the complete absence of immunosuppressive therapy, so-called drug-free immunosuppression, then it might be necessary to adhere to this strict definition. However, if the objective is to reduce the load of immunosuppressive drug therapy required to achieve long-term graft survival, thereby reducing the unwanted side effects of nonspecific immunosuppression and improving the quality of life of transplant recipients, a less strict definition may be acceptable. In humans, a protocol providing operational tolerance, that is, tolerance that is maintained by peripheral mechanisms might be of great value for reduction of maintenance immunosuppressive drug levels or the important issue of steroid withdrawal, providing that there were no unwanted immune responses actively targeting the transplant.

Living donor organ transplantation offers several unique advantages in the setting of tolerance induction. Because it is an elective procedure that is planned well in advance of the actual surgery, tolerance induction protocols could easily make use of techniques that require manipulation of the recipient days or weeks before the transplant. In addition, as the identity of the organ donor is also known well ahead of the transplantation procedure, donor blood, leukocytes, or other necessary tissues could be processed, stored if necessary, and used for tolerance induction protocols days or weeks before transplantation. Moreover, many living donors are related to the recipient, providing superior MHC-matching, and, as the procedures are usually performed in one center, ischemic times are short. Both of these factors potentially lower the risk of rejection and therefore theoretically improve the chances for the success of a tolerance induction protocol. Clinical trials of tolerance induction have therefore been conducted preferentially in living donor kidney (or liver) transplantation recipients to date.[10–16]

## MECHANISMS OF TOLERANCE

In order to understand the underlying mechanisms of transplantation tolerance, it is important to grasp the fundamental concepts of self-tolerance in the immune system. The adaptive immune system, consisting of the T- and B-cell compartments, within an individual has the inherent ability to mount an immune response against all antigens, not only against environmental pathogens and allogeneic organs but also against antigens originating from the individual themselves, so-called self-antigens. If this response against self-antigens is left unchecked, it will lead to autoimmunity resulting in the damage or destruction of tissues within the host. Therefore, self-tolerance, that is, the failure to make a destructive immune response to self-antigens, is critical for prevention of autoimmune disease.

Naïve B cells that emerge from the bone marrow and T cells that emerge from the thymus have an extremely diverse repertoire of B-cell and T-cell receptors (BCR or Ig and TCR, respectively). These BCR and TCR molecules determine the antigen specificity of the lymphocyte. The generation of these receptors result from random rearrangements at the DNA level, of the gene segments encoding the variable domains of the BCR and TCR chains.[17] The random nature of these rearrangements results in the production a high proportion of potentially self-reactive naïve lymphocytes. Nearly 50 years ago clonal selection (or: clonal deletion) was proposed as the mechanism that the immune system used to distinguish between receptors that could recognize self and nonself.[18] Clonal selection affects self-reactive juvenile T cells that have migrated from the bone marrow into the thymus to undergo the gene rearrangements required to produce a functional TCR. During this selection process, a major proportion of juvenile T cells that have rearranged TCRs with the capacity to recognise self-antigens are deleted or eliminated, a process also termed *negative selection*. Negative selection is accomplished by specialized antigen-presenting cells (APC) that include thymic epithelial cells. These cells present self-antigens in the context of MHC class I and II molecules, and juvenile T cells with TCRs that bind to these with high affinity are recognized and physically deleted.[19] Although this very effective mechanism has been shown to be mandatory for T cell[20] and indeed for B-cell[21] self-tolerance, where a similar process resulting in the elimination of self-reactive B cells occurs in the periphery, it is known that these processes are incomplete and many self-reactive lymphocytes escape clonal deletion and arrive in the periphery as potential harmful effector cells.[22]

To prevent the self-reactive lymphocytes that emerge into the periphery from causing damage to the individual's own tissues, several mechanisms have been characterized as potentially playing a role in preventing damage. For example, the self-reactive lymphocytes may fail to be activated (ie, they ignore self-antigens) because of lower avidities of their receptors for self-antigens presented by host APC; they may be rendered functionally inactive or anergic whenever they encounter self-antigen due to the absence of the correct accessory and costimulatory molecules required for activation, whereas in other circumstances the self-reactive cells may be deleted on encounter with peripheral self-antigens in the

**TABLE 38-1**

## MECHANISMS OF TOLERANCE TO ALLOANTIGENS

| | |
|---|---|
| Deletion | 1. Central thymic deletion can be induced by donor bone marrow infusion after cytoreductive irradiation or immunotherapy. This enables donor APCs to trigger the deletion of alloreactive maturing lymphocytes in the recipient thymus.<br>2. In the periphery, deletion can be triggered by alloantigen recognition under suboptimal conditions, including costimulation blockade. |
| Anergy | Functional inactivation of the T-cell response to restimulation by alloantigen. Some forms of T-cell anergy result in the development of regulatory activity. |
| Clonal exhaustion | Chronic alloantigen stimulation or alloantigen recognition under suboptimal conditions may lead to deletion or functional inactivation of alloreactive lymphocytes. Clonal exhaustion can occur after liver transplantation, where the large number of donor-derived APCs migrating from the liver to the draining lymphoid tissues after transplantation can trigger this type of response. This may also occur after infusion of donor bone marrow or donor-specific transfusions in the context of tolerance induction in living donor transplantation. |
| Ignorance | Uncommon mechanism in the induction phase of unresponsiveness to alloantigens as it is difficult to perform any form of transplantation without alerting the immune system. Depriving the immune system of "help" at the time of alloantigen recognition will facilitate long-term graft survival, although the stability of such a state is questionable. |
| Immunoregulation | Active process, whereby one population of cells regulates the activity of another population. Both the innate and adaptive immune responses to alloantigen can be controlled by various leukocyte populations. |

periphery. However, in addition to each of these "passive" mechanisms of peripheral self-tolerance, there is a further dominant mechanism, that of active suppression or regulation that inhibits or controls the activity of self-reactive lymphocytes in the periphery. Suppressor T cells, more recently termed *regulatory T cells*, have been shown to actively downregulate the activation and expansion of self-reactive lymphocytes, thereby controlling any self-reactive lymphocytes that escape deletion.[23] Table 38-1 lists mechanisms that are known to be relevant for mediating tolerance to alloantigens.

## STRATEGIES FOR TOLERANCE INDUCTION

By taking these naturally occurring mechanisms of self-tolerance into account, two distinct approaches of tolerance induction can be defined. Approaches that harness the potential of *central tolerance* may be used to modulate the fate of naïve T cells with TCRs that recognize donor alloantigen in the thymus, resulting in the deletion of donor reactive cells. This goal may be achieved by protocols aimed at generating bone marrow chimeras and will be discussed in more detail in the section of the chapter entitled Strategies to Induce Central Tolerance. Approaches that harness the potential of *peripheral tolerance* will enable a state of so-called immune privilege of an allograft that is induced by a variety of induction protocols that inactivate donor-reactive lymphocytes in the periphery. Some of the protocols that use this strategy are covered in the section of the chapter entitled Strategies to Induce Peripheral Tolerance.

## ROLE OF REGULATORY T CELLS IN TRANSPLANTATION TOLERANCE

Early evidence for the role of regulatory T cells in the maintenance of transplantation tolerance was derived from rodent adoptive transfer models.[24] Lymphocytes isolated from an animal exhibiting operational tolerance to an allograft could transfer the tolerant state to a naïve animal leading to the acceptance of allografts matched to the original donor without any further treatment. The principle of this type of study is shown in Figure 38-1.

A variety of T-lymphocyte subsets have been shown experimentally to include populations with suppressor activity, for example, CD8+ (25), CD8+CD28− (26), T-cell-receptor (TCR)+CD4−CD8− (double-negative)[27] and natural killer T cells.[28] Moreover, each of these subsets have been described in different models as having the potential to contribute to the induction and/or maintenance of the tolerant state. In addition, CD4+ T cells have been shown to have the potential to suppress immune responses, and arguably this T-cell subset includes the single most important population of T cells with suppressor function described to date.

Unfortunately, no definitive marker for identification of CD4+ regulatory T cells has been described so far, but enriching these cells for expression of high levels of the surface marker CD25, the α-subunit of the interleukin-2 (IL-2) receptor, has been shown to be very useful in practical terms.[29]

The first demonstration that tolerance could be adoptively transferred by CD25+CD4+ T cells was obtained using a rat heart transplantation model, where recipients accepted heart allografts indefinitely after cyclosporine treatment.[30] Subsequently, CD25+CD4+ T cells were shown to have potent regulatory properties in both the induction and the maintenance phases of *in vivo* tolerance to alloantigens in mice.[31–34] Donor-derived CD25+CD4+ T cells have also been found to protect against graft-versus-host disease (GvHD) after bone marrow transplantation.[35] Importantly, it has been shown, that CD25+CD4+ regulatory T cells are not a rodent-specific phenomenon, and that cells with similar regulatory properties are present in human peripheral blood, thymus, and lymph nodes.[36–40] Regulatory T cells might thus used as a surrogate marker for tolerance in the clinical transplantation setting.[41]

With respect to phenotype and function of regulatory T cells only two of the more important molecules associated with regulatory activity, CTLA4 (CD152) and Foxp3, are discussed here. CTLA4 is expressed on naturally occurring regulatory T cells[42] and on regulatory T cells in tolerant transplant recipients in experimental models[33] at high levels intracellularly. The interaction between CTLA4 and its ligands, members of the B7 family of

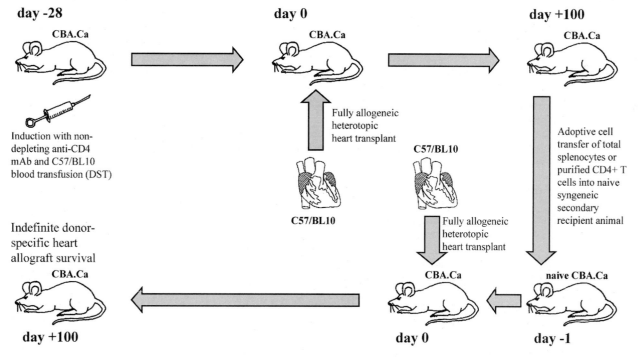

**FIGURE 38-1**

Demonstration of operational tolerance to alloantigen by regulatory T cells. This experiment utilizes two inbred mouse strains that are fully mismatched at the MHC locus. The pretreatment of CBA.Ca animals with non-depleting anti-CD4 Ab YTS177 on day −28 and with a C57/BL10 blood transfusion (donor-specific transfusion, DST) on day −27 results in indefinite heterotopic C57/BL10 heart allograft survival. Total splenocytes or purified CD4+ cells that are harvested from those long-term survivors on day +100 and are adoptively transferred into secondary CBA. Ca-recipient animals render these animals tolerant to C57/BL10 antigens. A heterotopic C57/BL10 heart allograft is accepted indefinitely in these animals without the need for further pretreatment or immunosuppressive therapy.

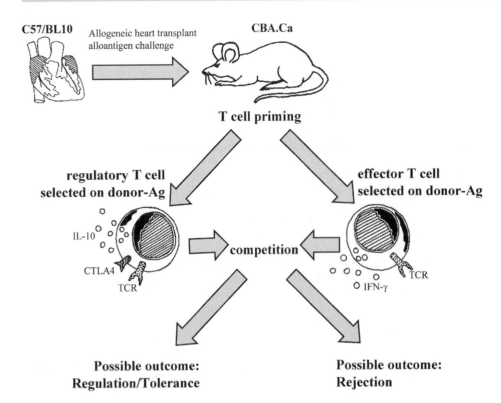

**FIGURE 38-2**

Alloantigen-driven T-cell priming. Exposure to alloantigen after an experimental heart transplant primes naïve T cells that may then mature to regulatory or effector T cells. Depending on the specific circumstances of the antigen challenge, one arm of the immune response may outcompete the other, leading to two distinct possible outcomes.

molecules[43] have been suggested to transmit a "negative" (or inhibitory) signal to the APC, that might be responsible for the regulatory activity of CD25+CD4+ T cells and consequently costimulatory blockade with CTLA4-Ig can abrogate tolerance under some circumstances. Alternative hypotheses have also been proposed and are reviewed by Chikuma and Bluestone.[44] Unfortunately, although expression of CTLA4 is associated with regulatory T cells it is not specific for this specialized population.[45]

Gene expression of *Foxp3* (forkhead box P3) is currently the most promising marker with respect to specificity and stability for regulatory T cells. *Foxp3* encodes a forkhead/winged helix transcription factor, scurfin, that is expressed by CD25+CD4+ regulatory T cells in the thymus and the periphery of normal mice and humans.[46] Expression of *Foxp3* cannot be induced in naïve T cells by activation,[47] in contrast to the expression of CTLA4. *Foxp3*-deficient mice (scurfy mice) develop autoimmune disease,[46] whereas the retroviral reintroduction of the gene into T cells renders them to a regulatory phenotype, indicating important functional properties of the gene. Analogously, in humans, the fatal autoimmune disorder "immune dysregulation, polyendocrinopathy, enteropathy, X-linked" (IPEX) has been shown to be caused by mutations in the *Foxp3* gene.[48] Stimulated by these findings, Fontenot et al. have published an exhaustive series of experiments supporting the hypothesis that *Foxp3* indeed is the lineage specification factor of regulatory T cells, irrespective of their cell surface expression of CD25.[49]

How is regulation of immune responses to alloantigens induced? It is generally accepted that the primary stimulus for activation and proliferation of both alloreactive effector and regulatory T cells is the alloantigen challenge. As a general rule, it can be assumed that in most situations both populations are actually stimulated by the same antigens and possibly even at the same time, but that one of the two responses is quicker or stronger and eventually overcomes the other. For example, after organ transplantation in humans or animals without immunosuppression,

alloreactive effector T cells are obviously the dominant arm of the immune response; rejection is the inevitable consequence of transplantation under these conditions. However, if early alloreactivity is inhibited, regulatory T cells potentially have time to expand in a donor antigen-specific manner, and eventually a controlled or regulated immune response might succeed enabling the allograft to survive (Figure 38-2). This mechanism has been shown in a variety of animal models in our own laboratory[50] and by others.

Evidence for this mechanism also comes from observations in adoptive transfer models in rodents (Figure 38-1). It is well known that the transfer of CD4+ T cells from rodent recipients with accepted, long-term surviving cardiac grafts into naïve animals could render them capable of accepting cardiac allografts without further treatment. However, adoptive transfer of CD4+ T cells from recipients of *recently rejected* cardiac allografts into naïve hosts unexpectedly also leads to long-term survival of cardiac grafts in those secondary recipients (Steger, Kingsley, Bushell, and Wood, unpublished observations). Similar findings in a rat kidney transplant model have been published by Schmidt et al.[51] Apparently, under these conditions, where donor alloantigens continue to be released from the graft after rejection, regulatory T cells enrich *in vivo* among CD4+ lymphocytes despite the fact that other populations present at the same time initially outcompeted the activity of the regulatory cells and rejected the allograft. In this situation, initially the regulatory activity was not strong enough, either quantitatively due to low numbers of regulatory cells or qualitatively due to low activity, and was therefore unable to prevent rejection in time; but generation or expansion of regulatory T cells might continue to take place over time in the presence of a persistent source of alloantigen such that regulatory activity can be demonstrated at a later time point. These data raise an important issue regarding identifying T cells with regulatory activity: highlighting the overall status of the immune system must be taken into account.

How can the knowledge of the immune system's mechanisms to control self-reactive lymphocyte clones be of use for the development of a clinically applicable tolerance induction protocol for solid organ or bone marrow transplantation? The recent discoveries in the field of $CD25^+CD4^+$ regulatory T cells have resulted in an upsurge of activity around the induction of peripheral tolerance. Protocols describing the induction of peripheral tolerance in rodents have been around for decades and have frequently been criticized because they are felt to provide only an unstable state of tolerance that might easily be broken by relatively minor immunologic challenges. If antigen-specific regulatory T cells could be generated *in vivo* or *in vitro* under controlled conditions in sufficient numbers intentionally, a therapeutic tool would be on hand that could solve the uncertainties of peripheral tolerance induction protocols. The successful experimental expansion of $CD4^+CD25^+Foxp3^+$ regulatory T cells that are capable of inducing antigen-specific immunologic tolerance has been described both *in vivo* and *in vitro* in 2004 by Nishimura.[52] Exciting new protocols for induction of tolerance will almost certainly arise from these results.

## STRATEGIES TO INDUCE CENTRAL TOLERANCE

### Bone Marrow Transplantation and Full Chimerism

Two years after Billingham's early work[1] on the intentional induction of transplantation tolerance in mouse fetuses was published, it was shown that a lethal preconditioning protocol followed by allogeneic bone marrow transplantation enables *full chimerism* of donor hematopoietic cells and transplantation tolerance in adult animals.[53] Within this approach, that resembles the classic protocol for clinical bone marrow transplantation for hematologic malignancies, the recipient's own bone marrow (including mature circulating leukocytes) is ablated by whole body irradiation and/or administration of chemotherapeutics. To rescue the then aplastic patient, allogeneic bone marrow cells are infused to reconstitute the hematopoietic system. After engraftment of the allogeneic bone marrow, 100% of the circulating leukocytes are of donor origin, thus the term *full chimerism* is used. This approach has been shown to reproducibly induce transplantation tolerance when a solid organ from the original bone marrow donor or a syngeneic donor is transplanted thereafter into the chimeric recipient in a variety of models in rodents[54,55] and large animals[56,57] and in humans.[58,59]

In clinical medicine, the vigorous treatment necessary for allogeneic bone marrow transplantation has the potential to cure patients with otherwise lethal malignancies, but it has several major drawbacks. The myeloablative conditioning regimen causes a high rate of morbidity and mortality, especially when the bone marrow transplant fails to engraft.[60] The development of acute GvHD is a frequent and severe complication and may require more aggressive pharmacologic immunosuppression. Acute GvHD can be reversed in most cases but progresses to chronic GvHD in a significant proportion of cases. Treatment strategies to resolve chronic GvHD are not known. The incidence of GvHD can be reduced by depletion of $CD3^+$ cells from the donor bone marrow before transplantation, but this T-cell depletion has a negative impact on engraftment.[61] These problems have hindered allogeneic bone marrow transplantation for many years and have restricted clinical application to transplants between carefully selected closely related individuals such as siblings with sufficient histocompatibility.[62]

In recent years techniques have been developed to derive growth-factor-mobilized $CD34^+$ hematopoietic stem cells from peripheral blood, large-scale donor registers have been established, wherein the tissue types of large numbers of potential donors are registered, and molecular genetic techniques have been developed for routine tissue typing that are far more exact than the serologic typing techniques used before. All these developments contribute to the recent success of allogeneic bone marrow transplantation, since perfectly HLA-A-, -B-, and -DR-matched allogeneic transplants have become routine clinical procedures. Although minor antigen mismatches still may cause GvHD, its incidence and severity are low enough to allow for the widespread application of this type of transplantation.

The drawback for the use of allogeneic bone marrow transplantation as an adjunct of solid organ transplantation for the induction of tolerance is that the necessary degree of HLA matching is feasible neither in cadaver organ transplantation nor in any living donor organ transplant other than between HLA-identical siblings. However, the practical value of this approach has been repeatedly proven in rare cases of bone marrow allograft recipients that developed secondary kidney failure and eventually received a living-related renal transplantation from the original bone marrow donor, as mentioned above.[58,59] These patients have been reported to be indefinitely free of pharmacologic maintenance immunosuppression with completely normal graft function. Although not reproducible on any larger scale, these rare cases have been regarded as an inspiration for further development of the bone marrow chimerism approach for induction of clinical transplantation tolerance.

### Bone Marrow Transplantation and Mixed Chimerism

The prohibitive hurdles of allogeneic bone marrow transplantation after myeloablative conditioning for tolerance induction have stimulated an extensive number of experimental studies investigating less invasive conditioning protocols for allogeneic bone marrow transplantation. The first descriptions of mixed hematopoietic chimerism after nonmyeloablative conditioning were published in the late 1980s.[63,64] Cobbold and Waldmann demonstrated in a mouse model that fully MHC-mismatched marrow engraftment and specific tolerance could be achieved by pretreating recipients with depleting doses of anti-CD4 and anti-CD8 monoclonal antibodies along with a sublethal dose (6 Gy) of whole body irradiation. Sharabi and Sachs showed that the whole body irradiation dose could be reduced further to 3 Gy, if 7 Gy of additional selective thymic irradiation were added along with the anti-CD4 and anti-CD8 antibody treatment before allogeneic bone marrow transplantation was performed.[64] This protocol resulted in sustained *mixed chimerism* as characterized by the presence of both donor- and recipient-derived mononuclear cells of all three lineages (ie, lymphocytes, granulocytes and monocytes) in the recipient's peripheral blood and lymphatic organs. Donor-specific skin grafts were accepted indefinitely by these animals, whereas third-party skin was rejected.

Several variations of this protocol have since been published by these and other authors, but the main components remain essentially the same. In a primate model, 3 Gy whole body irradiation, 7 Gy thymic irradiation, recipient splenectomy, antithymocyte globulin (ATG), and 28 days of cyclosporine treatment are required to allow for simultaneous bone marrow and kidney engraftment.[65] Using this conditioning regimen, mixed hematopoietic chimerism and kidney allograft survival could be followed up for many years. One common finding of several studies has been the absolute requirement for the higher dose thymic irradiation.[66,67] More recently, more rigorous T-cell-depleting antibody treatment protocols, utilizing multiple injections, have been developed that allow for the omission of selective thymic irradiation.[68,69]

The need to modify the thymic environment to achieve hematopoietic chimerism has been attributed to the requirement to overcome intrathymic alloresistance.[67] As a mechanism of tolerance induction through the establishment of mixed chimerism, it has been proposed that in mixed chimeras, naïve hematopoietic cells from both the recipient and the donor locate to the thymus and hence delete both host-reactive and donor-reactive T cells, resulting in a peripheral T-cell repertoire that is tolerant toward the donor and the host.[70] This form of transplantation tolerance relies on a central, that is, thymic, mechanism, and is thus believed to be especially robust. Donor-reactive T cells are subjected to central (thymic) deletion, and this physical destruction prevents them from later reactivation. However, central deletion of donor-reactive T-cell clones has been shown to rely on the continuing presence of donor cells in the thymus in the long term, resulting in potential for break of tolerance even when central deletional mechanisms are invoked initially. An advantage of mixed over full chimerism is the superior immunocompetence. The immunoincompetence after induction of full chimerism across complete MHC barriers results from the full MHC disparity between the positive selecting elements in the thymus, which are of host origin, and the APC in the periphery, which are entirely of donor origin in full chimeras. These T cells are ineffective at mounting relevant donor-restricted immune responses and lack host APC that could induce generation of host-restricted responses. In contrast, mixed chimeras have a lifelong source of host APC to allow effective generation of host-restricted immune responses.

Based on the experimental successes in both rodents and large animals, Sachs et al. initiated a clinical trial for the investigation of combined kidney and bone marrow transplantation after nonmyeloablative conditioning for multiple myeloma.[71] Only two cases have been published so far, although more transplants have been performed, and the donor-recipient pairs have been selected with a high MHC match, but both patients are off immunosuppression several years after the procedure, proving that transplantation tolerance can be intentionally induced.

Why have these tolerance induction protocols, that are so successful experimentally, not been used in clinical transplantation on any larger scale so far? This question can easily be answered. The nonmyeloablative conditioning protocols that are used in young and healthy experimental animals with satisfactory safety and success are only transferable into humans by putting the patients at some degree of risk. This risk might be acceptable in individuals with hematologic malignancies, who need cytoreductive treatment for their underlying disease. However, for recipients of solid organ transplants, without any hematologic malignancy, the risk is generally considered to be too high at present, as they might develop life-threatening infections, tumors, posttransplant lymphoproliferative disease, or GvHD even more likely during the postoperative course after nonmyeloablative conditioning than under conventional immunosuppression.

### Alternative Protocols for the Generation of Mixed Chimerism

For the reasons outlined above, various strategies to develop less invasive protocols for establishment of mixed chimerism have been investigated. For example, it has been reported that thymic irradiation can be replaced by repeated injections of depleting anti-T-cell antibodies,[67] with pretransplant cyclosporine treatment,[72] or with a costimulatory blocker[69] in a number of studies. Both thymic irradiation and T-cell-depleting antibodies can be omitted when costimulatory blockade is used[73] and when very high doses of bone marrow are used whole-body irradiation can also be omitted.[74] By combining these modifications Wekerle et al. found that all preconditioning could be eliminated by giving a high dose of fully MHC-mismatched donor marrow followed by a single injection of each of two costimulatory blockers[75] or repeated injections of anti-CD40 ligand as reported by Durham et al.[76]

The administration of very large numbers of hematopoietic cells has been described as causing a "mass effect" in terms of antigen load and that this overcomes the requirement to create space with myelosuppressive treatment to achieve bone marrow engraftment.[77] It has to be said that the administration of very large hematopoietic cell doses is only an experimental approach as it would be very difficult to harvest enough hematopoietic cells from one cadaver organ donor to provide sufficient numbers of cells. However, it might be feasible in the setting of living donor transplantation, where the donor could be pretreated with stem-cell-mobilizing growth factors, and stem cells could then be enriched from the peripheral blood in high numbers, potentially in several subsequent sessions until the necessary cell numbers are on hand. Indeed, Trivedi et al have published a clinical study applying this approach to living-related renal transplants with encouraging preliminary results.[10]

## STRATEGIES TO INDUCE PERIPHERAL TOLERANCE OR UNRESPONSIVENESS

In rodent models, a large number of protocols have been published that induce specific unresponsiveness or operational transplantation tolerance without engraftment of donor bone marrow. These strategies rely on peripheral rather on than central thymic mechanisms for both the induction and the maintenance of the tolerant state. From a practical standpoint, these protocols have major advantages over mixed chimerism protocols, because either no or only minor cytoreductive conditioning is necessary to achieve the unresponsive state. However, the stability of the tolerance induced using these approaches is believed to be inferior to that achieved using central deletional mechanisms.

### Induction of Tolerance by Donor-Specific Blood Transfusion

In the early days of clinical kidney transplantation it was observed that patients that had received frequent blood transfusions before allografting had a significantly improved 1-year graft survival compared to patients that had not received blood transfusions before transplantation (71% vs 41%, respectively).[78] Although this striking difference seemed to vanish in the cyclosporine era, and as a result the deliberate transfusion of patients waiting for kidney transplantation was discontinued by most clinical transplant centres, a more recent prospective trial on more than 400 patients still found significant differences under calcineurin-inhibitor based immunosuppressive regimens.[79] In that latter study, the 1-year graft survival in patients pretreated with three blood transfusions was 90+/–2%, as opposed by 82+/–3% in patients who did not receive any transfusions (P = 0.020). The respective 5-year figures were 79+/–3% vs. 70+/–4%, P = 0.025.

Experimentally, it was shown a number of years ago, in a rat model of donor-specific blood transfusions in our laboratory, that a population of CD4+ T cells arises *in vivo* under treatment with donor-specific transfusions that bears suppressor activity and prevents subsequent allograft rejection indefinitely.[80] These CD4+ suppressor T cells have been characterized further in an adoptive transfer mouse model more recently and shown to express high levels of CD25.[81] CD25+CD4+ T cells are now referred to as regulatory T cells and have been shown to play important roles in both transplantation tolerance[82] and the prevention of autoimmune disease,[83] as discussed earlier in this chapter. It has been concluded from these data, that exposure to foreign antigen does not invariably generate sensitization, but might in certain circumstances rather induce regulation. This regulation, despite being potentially reversible, can have an extraordinarily long-standing effect, as suggested by the significantly improved renal allograft survival after pretransplant blood transfusions in the aforementioned clinical study, indicating stable operational tolerance.

To generate regulation rather than sensitization reliably in one of the mouse models investigated in this laboratory, a single dose of nondepleting anti-CD4 antibody is to be administered preferentially a day before donor-specific[84] or random[85] blood is transfused. Cardiac grafts, transplanted 4 weeks after the blood transfusion, were then accepted indefinitely. One component of many experimental tolerance induction protocols is the adjuvant infusion of isolated donor cells (usually splenocytes)[86] or purified donor antigen (eg, MHC I or II molecules),[87–89] basically providing an alloantigen load in a more or less similar fashion as a blood transfusion. Because in living donor organ transplantation the identity of the organ donor is known before the procedure is to be performed, blood or cell infusions from the organ donor could be given to the recipient, eliminating the necessity of random (donor-non-specific) blood transfusions with their potential risk of transmission of infectious diseases.

### Induction of Tolerance by Costimulatory Blockade

Co-stimulatory blockade in itself does not lead to true tolerance in large animal transplantation models.[90,91] This conclusion is supported by data from several more recent rodent studies, among them a report from Kanaya et al.[92] using an ACI to Lewis rat hind-limb transplantation model to study the effect of combined CD28-B7 and CD154-CD40 co-stimulatory blockade by administering adenoviral vectors transfecting genes encoding for CTLA4-Ig or CD40-Ig. Allograft survival was prolonged under these conditions, but rejection eventually occurred, ruling out the induction of stable tolerance using this approach. However, blockade of the CD154-CD40 pathway can induce specific immunologic unresponsiveness and long-term cardiac allograft survival in some mouse strain combinations. In agreement with the observation, that CD154 blockade mainly affects CD4+ T cells, it was shown in our laboratory, that CD154-independent CD8+ T cells are responsible for rejecting allografts after costimulatory blockade using anti-CD154 antibody in a mouse model.[93] Thus, in this situation, controlling the activity of the CD8+ T cells is also important. CD25+CD4+ regulatory T cells could be found 100 days after cardiac transplantation when anti-CD154 treatment was used in CD8+ T-cell-depleted recipients. Upon adoptive transfer of CD25+CD4+-enriched lymphocytes from the long-term survivors to naïve animals, rejection of a cardiac allograft transplanted the day after cell transfer was prevented.[50] In this latter study, rejection was also prevented by CD25+CD4+-enriched

lymphocytes from anti-CD154-treated long-term survivors, when a TCR-transgenic model was used. In this case, rejection is solely dependent on the presence of CD8+ T cells specific for a MHC class I donor antigen. These TCR-transgenic CD8+ T cells themselves are not susceptible to anti-CD154 treatment, but their antidonor activity could be controlled by CD4+ regulatory T cells. Further experiments within that study showed as a mechanism that the regulatory cells did not delete the CD8+-effector T cells; rather they prevented their clonal or homeostatic proliferation and inhibited their switch to a memory (CD44+) phenotype.[50]

### Induction of Tolerance by T-Cell-Depleting Protocols

Thomas et al. have described a very relevant series of kidney transplants in rhesus monkeys.[94] Although only limited success was observed with a protocol utilizing antithymocyte globulin, donor bone marrow infusion and posttransplant total lymphoid irradiation,[95] its replacement with anti-CD3ε-CRM9 and 15-deoxyspergualin (DSG) in an attempt to use a clinically feasible approach to induce transplantation tolerance was more successful. Anti-CD3ε-CRM9 is a fusion molecule consisting of an anti-CD3 antibody targeted to the ε-subunit and the potent neurotoxin CRM9, functionally resulting in an immunotoxin with remarkable T-cell-depleting abilities. DSG is an immunosuppressive drug with a variety of effects on cells of the immune system, among them prevention of dendritic cell maturation, resulting in deficient antigen presentation to T cells and B cells early after transplantation,[96] partly due to the lack of expression of co-stimulatory molecules on APC. The combination of these two drugs without further conditioning, drug treatment, or donor cell infusions proved to be very effective in the induction of long-term graft acceptance and tolerance in more than 50% of the experimental animals.[97] This protocol does not comprise any measurable donor cell chimerism, thus central thymic tolerance is unlikely to be the underlying mechanism and a form of peripheral tolerance maintenance may be operational.

## POTENTIAL BARRIERS AND LIMITATIONS OF TOLERANCE INDUCTION

A major concern in tolerance induction protocols that are entirely or in part based on intrathymic clonal deletion is the fact that thymus involution occurs in adults. A dramatic reduction in thymic cellularity is seen in early adulthood, and although it might be disputed whether the process is most pronounced from puberty or occurs progressively from the postnatal period, it eventually leads to a state where the aged thymus may export fewer than 5% of the T cells produced by a young adult.[19] Although the thymus remains functional, the rate at which it exports T cells is insufficient to replace the number of naïve T cells lost daily from the periphery; thus homeostatic proliferation of peripheral T cells is triggered to prevent lymphopenia, and the memory pool expands.[98] Eventually, less than 5% of mature T cells may have passed the thymus before appearing in the periphery with the remainder being produced by homeostatic proliferation of existing memory clones.

Homeostatic proliferation has been recently described as a major barrier to tolerance induction in adults.[99] This had been observed by Adams et al, who were investigating the reasons for the differential efficacy of tolerance induction protocols using costimulatory blockade in rodents and primates.[100] These authors hypothesized that a critical distinction between specific pathogen-free mice on the one hand and nonhuman primates on the other might be their acquired immune history. In an elegant set of experiments, naïve mice were infected with several viruses, and the mice were then allowed to recover from their infection before the transplantation experiments, using costimulatory blockade protocols that would promote tolerance in naïve animals, were performed. The data they obtained showed that viral infections promoted the generation of specific CD8[+] memory T cells. Despite being specific for certain viral antigens, these memory T cells were cross-reactive with alloantigens, a condition described as heterologous immunity, and the memory populations were found to undergo homeostatic proliferation when an allotransplant was performed and consequently caused rejection. This proliferation of central memory cells was not sensitive to costimulatory blockade. These data provided an explanation for the difficulties that are encountered when a tolerance induction protocol is applied in primates or humans. Homeostatic proliferation might also be a major problem after cytoreductive induction therapy in transplantation using anti-CD3ε-CRM9, antithymocyte globulin, antilymphocyte globulin, OKT-3, or the newer Campath-1 antibodies, since extensive homeostatic T-cell proliferation can occur under conditions of lymphopenia, leading to potentially alloreactive memory cell expansion[99] not seen in naïve laboratory rodents that lack a significant acquired immune history.

Is clinical tolerance induction thus doomed by heterologous immunity and homeostatic proliferation of viral-antigen-induced alloreactive T-cell memory? Certainly careful reevaluation of tolerance-inducing strategies that have been proposed in the past is necessary in the light of the new evidence. This might be achieved by refined animal models using a more senescent immune system that already has a significant T-cell memory in recipient animals for transplantation experiments. However, some existing data support optimism for tolerance induction. The blood transfusion effect inducing significant T-cell regulation has been observed in humans that have an acquired immune history. Experimentally, it has been shown that CD25[+]CD4[+] T cells have the capacity to control homeostatic expansion of both CD4[+] and CD8[+] T-cell subsets.[101,102] Protocols are currently under investigation that can expand regulatory CD25[+]CD4[+] T cells *in vitro* and *in vivo*.[52] This could provide the transplant clinician with a powerful tool to influence alloreactivity in the recipient.

## SUMMARY

The unique advantages of living donor transplantation render it a natural candidate for the implementation of tolerance induction protocols. Both the induction of central tolerance by co-transplantation of donor bone marrow and the induction of peripheral tolerance by donor-specific transfusion-based protocols could benefit from the accessibility of donor material before transplantation in the setting of living donor transplants. We are now at the exciting time of early clinical trials, applying techniques of tolerance induction that have been developed in animal experiments over decades. Allogeneic bone marrow transplantation-based protocols with the intention to induce central tolerance as well as protocols aimed at inducing peripheral tolerance or unresponsiveness have made tremendous experimental progress recently, and feasible clinical protocols, especially in the setting of living donor transplantation, are now emerging from both. Additionally, the rapid development of knowledge related to regulatory T cells will almost certainly translate into important clinical implications within the next few years. Clinical living donor

transplantation programs should thus be encouraged to initiate or participate in further trials evaluating tolerance induction protocols, and although it may not be feasible to induce tolerance to donor alloantigens in all transplant recipients, significant advances in promoting unresponsiveness to donor antigens will undoubtedly be made, enabling immunosuppressive drug therapy to be minimised in the long term after transplantation.

## ACKNOWLEGDMENTS

Work from the authors' own laboratory described in this chapter was supported by grants from the Wellcome Trust, MRC, and the European Union.

## References

1. Billingham RE, Brent L, Medawar P. "Actively acquired tolerance" of foreign cells. *Nature* 1953;172:603–606.
2. Owen RD. Immunogenetic consequences of vascular anastomoses between bovine twins. *Science* 1945;102:400–401.
3. Anderson D, Billingham RE, Lampkin GH, Medawar PB. The use of skin grafting to distinguish between monozygotic and dizygotic twins in cattle. *Heredity* 1951;5:379.
4. Kirk AD. Crossing the bridge: large animal models in translational transplantation research. *Immunol Rev* 2003;196:176–196.
5. Wekerle T, Sykes M. Induction of tolerance. *Surgery* 2004;135:359-364.
6. Nagao T, White DJ, Calne RY. Kinetics of unresponsiveness induced by a short course of cyclosporin A. *Transplantation* 1982;33:31–35.
7. Hall BM, Gurley KE, Pearce NW, Dorsch SE. 1989. Specific unresponsiveness in rats with prolonged cardiac allograft survival after treatment with cyclosporine. II. Sequential changes in alloreactivity of T cell subsets. *Transplantation* 47:1030–1033.
8. Madsen JC, Peugh WN, Wood KJ, and Morris PJ. 1987. The effect of anti-L3T4 monoclonal antibody treatment on first-set rejection of murine cardiac allografts. *Transplantation* 1987;44:849–852.
9. Larsen CP, Elwood ET, Alexander DZ, et al. Long-term acceptance of skin and cardiac allografts after blocking CD40 and CD28 pathways. *Nature* 1996;381:434–438.
10. Trivedi HL, Shah VR, Shah PR, et al. Megadose approach to DBMC infusion-induced allograft hyporesponsiveness in living-related renal allograft recipients. *Transplant Proc* 2001;33:71–76.
11. Mathew JM, R. Garcia-Morales L, Fuller A. et al. Donor bone marrow-derived chimeric cells present in renal transplant recipients infused with donor marrow. I. Potent regulators of recipient antidonor immune responses. *Transplantation* 2000;70:1675–1682.
12. Millan MT, Shizuru JA, Hoffmann P, et al. Mixed chimerism and immunosuppressive drug withdrawal after HLA-mismatched kidney and hematopoietic progenitor transplantation. *Transplantation* 2002;73:1386–1391.
13. Sellers MT, Deierhoi MH, Curtis JJ, et al. Tolerance in renal transplantation after allogeneic bone marrow transplantation-6-year follow-up. *Transplantation* 2002;71:1681–1683.
14. Donckier V, Troisi R, Toungouz M, et al. Donor stem cell infusion after non-myeloablative conditioning for tolerance induction to HLA mismatched adult living-donor liver graft. *Transpl Immunol* 2004;13:139–146.
15. Kadry Z, Mullhaupt B, Renner EL, et al. Living donor liver transplantation and tolerance: a potential strategy in cholangiocarcinoma. *Transplantation* 2003;76:1003–1006.
16. Kirk AD, Hale DA, Mannon RB, Results from a human renal allograft tolerance trial evaluating the humanized CD52-specific monoclonal antibody alemtuzumab (CAMPATH-1H). *Transplantation* 2003;76:120–129.
17. Garcia KC, Teyton L, and Wilson IA. Structural basis of T cell recognition. *Annu Rev Immunol* 1999;17:369–397.

18. Burnet FM. 1959. The Clonal Selection Theory of Acquired Immunity. London: Cambridge Univ. Press: London; 1959.

19. Gill J, Malin M, Sutherland J. Thymic generation and regeneration. *Immunol Rev* 2003;195:28–50.

20. Kappler JW, Roehm N, Marrack P. T cell tolerance by clonal elimination in the thymus. *Cell* 1987;49:273–280.

21. Goodnow CC, Cyster JG,. Hartley SB, et al. Self-tolerance checkpoints in B lymphocyte development. *Adv Immunol* 1995;59:279–368.

22. Van Parijs L, Abbas AK. Homeostasis and self-tolerance in the immune system: turning lymphocytes off. *Science* 1998;280:243–248.

23. Sakaguchi, S. Regulatory T cells: key controllers of immunologic self-tolerance. *Cell* 2000;101:455–458.

24. Kilshaw PJ, Brent L, Pinto M. 1975. Suppressor T cells in mice made unresponsive to skin allografts. *Nature* 2000;255:489–491.

25. Gilliet M, Liu YJ. Generation of human CD8 T regulatory cells by CD40 ligand-activated plasmacytoid dendritic cells. *J Exp Med* 2002;195: 695–704.

26. Ciubotariu R, Colovai AI, Pennesi G, et al. Specific suppression of human CD4+ Th cell responses to pig MHC antigens by CD8+CD28- regulatory T cells. *J Immunol* 1998;161:5193–5202.

27. Zhang ZX, Yang L, Young KJ, DuTemple B, Zhang B. Identification of a previously unknown antigen-specific regulatory T cell and its mechanism of suppression. *Nat Med* 2000;6:782–789.

28. Seino KI, Fukao K, Muramoto K, et al. Requirement for natural killer T (NKT) cells in the induction of allograft tolerance. *Proc Natl Acad Sci USA* 2001;98:2577–2581.

29. Sakaguchi S, Sakaguchi N, Asano M, Itoh M, Toda M. Immunologic self-tolerance maintained by activated T cells expressing IL-2 receptor alpha-chains (CD25). Breakdown of a single mechanism of self-tolerance causes various autoimmune diseases. *J Immunol* 1995;155: 1151–1164.

30. Hall BM, Pearce NW, Gurley KE, Dorsch SE. Specific unresponsiveness in rats with prolonged cardiac allograft survival after treatment with cyclosporine. III. Further characterization of the CD4+ suppressor cell and its mechanisms of action. *J Exp Med* 1990;171:141–157.

31. Sakaguchi, S., N. Sakaguchi, J. Shimizu, S. Yamazaki, T. Sakihama, M. Itoh, Y. Kuniyasu T, Nomura M, Toda, Takahashi T. Immunologic tolerance maintained by CD25+ CD4+ regulatory T cells: their common role in controlling autoimmunity, tumor immunity, and transplantation tolerance. *Immunol Rev* 2001;182:18–32.

32. Hara M, Kingsley CI, Niimi M, et al. IL-10 is required for regulatory T cells to mediate tolerance to alloantigens in vivo. *J Immunol* 2001;166:3789–3796.

33. Kingsley CI, Karim M, Bushell AR, Wood KJ. CD25+CD4+ regulatory T cells prevent graft rejection: CTLA-4- and IL-10-dependent immunoregulation of alloresponses. *J Immunol* 2002;168: 1080–1086.

34. Graca L, Thompson S, Lin CY. Both CD4(+)CD25(+) and CD4(+)CD25(-) regulatory cells mediate dominant transplantation tolerance. *J Immunol* 2002;168:5558–5565.

35. Hoffmann P, Ermann J, Edinger M., Fathman CG, Strober S. Donor-type CD4(+)CD25(+) regulatory T cells suppress lethal acute graft-versus-host disease after allogeneic bone marrow transplantation. *J Exp Med* 2002;196:389–399.

36. Baecher-Allan C, Brown JA, Freeman GJ, Hafler DA. CD4+CD25high regulatory cells in human peripheral blood. *J Immunol* 2001;167: 1245–1253.

37. Ng WF, Duggan PJ, Ponchel F, et al. Human CD4(+)CD25(+) cells: a naturally occurring population of regulatory T cells. *Blood* 2001;98: 2736–2744.

38. Levings MK, Sangregorio R, Roncarolo MG. Human cd25(+)cd4(+) t regulatory cells suppress naive and memory T cell proliferation and can be expanded in vitro without loss of function. *J Exp Med* 2001;193:1295–1302.

39. Jonuleit H, Schmitt E, Stassen M. Identification and functional characterization of human CD4(+)CD25(+) T cells with regulatory properties isolated from peripheral blood. *J Exp Med* 2001;193: 1285–1294.

40. Stephens LA, Mottet C, Mason D, Powrie F. Human CD4(+) CD25(+) thymocytes and peripheral T cells have immune suppressive activity in vitro. *Eur J Immunol* 2001;31:1247–1254.

41. Meloni F, Vitulo P, Bianco AM. Regulatory CD4+CD25+ T cells in the peripheral blood of lung transplant recipients: correlation with transplant outcome. *Transplantation* 2004;77:762–766.

42. Takahashi T, Tagami T, Yamazaki S. Immunologic self-tolerance maintained by CD25(+)CD4(+) regulatory T cells constitutively expressing cytotoxic T lymphocyte-associated antigen 4. *J Exp Med* 2000;192: 303–310.

43. Greenwald RJ, Freeman GJ, Sharpe AH. 2005. The B7 family revisited. *Annu Rev Immunol* 2005;23:515–548.

44. Chikuma S, Bluestone JA. CTLA-4 and tolerance: the biochemical point of view. *Immunol Res* 2003;28:241–253.

45. Egen JG, Allison JP. 2002. Cytotoxic T lymphocyte antigen-4 accumulation in the immunological synapse is regulated by TCR signal strength. *Immunity* 2002;16:23–35.

46. Brunkow ME, Jeffery EW, Hjerrild KA. Disruption of a new forkhead/winged-helix protein, scurfin, results in the fatal lymphoproliferative disorder of the scurfy mouse. *Nat Genet* 2001;27:68–73.

47. Hori S, Nomura T, Sakaguchi S. Control of regulatory T cell development by the transcription factor Foxp3. *Science* 2003;299:1057–1061.

48. Bennett CL, Christie J, Ramsdell F, et al. The immune dysregulation, polyendocrinopathy, enteropathy, X-linked syndrome (IPEX) is caused by mutations of FOXP3. *Nat Genet* 2001;27:20–21.

49. Fontenot JD, Rasmussen JP, Williams LM, et al. Regulatory T cell lineage specification by the forkhead transcription factor foxp3. *Immunity* 2005;22:329–341.

50. van Maurik A, Herber M, Wood KJ, Jones ND. Cutting edge: CD4+CD25+ alloantigen-specific immunoregulatory cells that can prevent CD8+ T cell-mediated graft rejection: implications for anti-CD154 immunotherapy. *J Immunol* 2002;169:5401–5404.

51. Schmidt H, Filantenkov A, Reutzel-Selke A, et al. Adoptive transfer of regulatory T cells following chronic allograft rejection induces tolerance for secondary allografts. *Transplant Proc* 2002;34:2893–2894.

52. Nishimura E, Sakihama T, Setoguchi R, Tanaka K, Sakaguchi S. Induction of antigen-specific immunologic tolerance by in vivo and in vitro antigen-specific expansion of naturally arising Foxp3+CD25+CD4+ regulatory T cells. *Int Immunol* 2004;6:1189–1201.

53. Main JM, Prehn RT. Successful skin homografts after the administration of high dosage X radiation and homologous bone marrow. *J Natl Cancer Inst* 1955;15:1023.

54. Auchincloss H Jr, Sachs DH. Mechanisms of tolerance in murine radiation bone marrow chimeras. I. Nonspecific suppression of alloreactivity by spleen cells from early, but not late, chimeras. *Transplantation* 1983;36:436–441.

55. Auchincloss H Jr, Sachs DH. Mechanisms of tolerance in murine radiation bone marrow chimeras. II. Absence of nonspecific suppression in mature chimeras. *Transplantation* 1983;36:442–445.

56. Weiden PL, Storb R, Tsoi MS, et al. Infusion of donor lymphocytes into stable canine radiation chimeras: implications for mechanism of transplantation tolerance. *J Immunol* 1976;116:1212–1219.

57. Guzzetta PC, Sundt TM, Suzuki T, et al. Induction of kidney transplantation tolerance across major histocompatibility complex barriers by bone marrow transplantation in miniature swine. *Transplantation* 1991;51:862–866.

58. Sayegh MH, Fine NA, Smith JL, et al. Immunologic tolerance to renal allografts after bone marrow transplants from the same donors. *Ann Intern Med* 1991;114:954–955.

59. Jacobsen N, Taaning, E, Ladefoged J, Kristensen JK, and Pedersen FK. Tolerance to an HLA-B,DR disparate kidney allograft after bone-marrow transplantation from same donor. *Lancet* 1994;343:800.

60. Quinones RR. Hematopoietic engraftment and graft failure after bone marrow transplantation. *Am J Pediatr Hematol Oncol* 1993;15:3–17.

61. Kernan NA, Flomenberg N, Dupont B, O'Reilly R. Graft rejection in recipients of T-cell-depleted HLA-nonidentical marrow transplants for leukemia. *Transplantation* 1987;43:842.

62. Clift RA, Storb R. Histoincompatible bone marrow transplants in humans. *Ann Rev Immunol* 1987;5:43.

63. Cobbold S, Martin G, Qin S, Waldmann H. Monoclonal antibodies to promote marrow engraftment and tissue graft tolerance. *Nature* 1986;323:164.

64. Sharabi Y, Sachs DH. 1989. Mixed chimerism and permanent specific transplantation tolerance induced by a nonlethal preparative regimen. *J Exp Med* 1989;169:493–502.

65. Kawai T, Cosimi AB, Colvin, RB, et al. Mixed allogeneic chimerism and renal allograft tolerance in cynomolgus monkeys. *Transplantation* 1995;59:256–262.

66. Kimikawa M, Sachs DH, Colvin RB, et al. Modifications of the conditioning regimen for achieving mixed chimerism and donor-specific tolerance in cynomolgus monkeys. *Transplantation* 1997;64: 709–716.

67. Nikolic B, Khan A, Sykes M. Induction of tolerance by mixed chimerism with nonmyeloblative host conditioning: the importance of overcoming intrathymic alloresistance. *Biol Blood Marrow Transpl* 2001;7:144–153.

68. Tomita Y, Sachs DH, Khan A, Sykes M. Additional monoclonal antibody (mAB) injections can replace thymic irradiation to allow induction of mixed chimerism and tolerance in mice receiving bone marrow transplantation after conditioning with anti-T cell mABs and 3-Gy whole body irradiation. *Transplantation* 1996;61:469–477.

69. Wekerle T, Sayegh MH, Ito H, 1999. Anti-CD154 or CTLA4Ig obviates the need for thymic irradiation in a non-myeloablative conditioning regimen for the induction of mixed hematopoietic chimerism and tolerance. *Transplantation* 1999;68:1348–1355.

70. Tomita Y, Khan A, Sykes M. Role of intrathymic clonal deletion and peripheral anergy in transplantation tolerance induced by bone marrow transplantation in mice conditioned with a nonmyeloablative regimen. *J Immunol* 1994;153:1087–1098.

71. Buhler LH, Spitzer TR, Sykes M, et al. Induction of kidney allograft tolerance after transient lymphohematopoietic chimerism in patients with multiple myeloma and end-stage renal disease. *Transplantation* 2002;74:1405–1409.

72. Nikolic B, Zhao G, Swenson K, Sykes M. A novel application of cyclosporine A in nonmyeloablative pretransplant host conditioning for allogeneic BMT. *Blood* 2000;96:1166–1172.

73. Wekerle T, Sayegh MH, Hill J, et al. Extrathymic T cell deletion and allogeneic stem cell engraftment induced with costimulatory blockade is followed by central T cell tolerance. *J Exp Med* 1998;187: 2037–2044.

74. Sykes M, Szot GL, Swenson KA, Pearson DA. Induction of high levels of allogeneic hematopoietic reconstitution and donor-specific tolerance without myelosuppressive conditioning. *Nat Med* 1997;3:783–787.

75. Wekerle T, Kurtz J, Ito H, et al. Allogeneic bone marrow transplantation with co-stimulatory blockade induces macrochimerism and tolerance without cytoreductive host treatment. *Nat Med* 2000;6: 464–469.

76. Durham MM, Bingaman AW, Adams AB, et al. Cutting edge: administration of anti-CD40 ligand and donor bone marrow leads to hemopoietic chimerism and donor-specific tolerance without cytoreductive conditioning. *J Immunol* 2000;165:1–4.

77. Sykes M, Szot GL, Swenson K, Pearson DA, Wekerle T. Separate regulation of peripheral hematopoietic and thymic engraftment. *Exp Hematol* 1998;26:457–465.

78. Opelz G, Terasaki PI. Dominant effect of transfusions on kidney graft survival. *Transplantation* 1980;29:153–158.

79. Opelz G, Vanrenterghem Y, Kirste G, et al. Prospective evaluation of pretransplant blood transfusions in cadaver kidney recipients. *Transplantation* 1997;63:964–967.

80. Quigley RL, Wood KJ, Morris PJ. Mediation of antigen-induced suppression of renal allograft rejection by a CD4 (W3/25+) T cell. *Transplantation* 1989;47:684–688.

81. Bushell A, Karim M, Kingsley CI, Wood KJ. Pretransplant blood transfusion without additional immunotherapy generates CD25+CD4+ regulatory T cells: a potential explanation for the blood-transfusion effect. *Transplantation* 76:449–455.

82. Wood, K.J., and S. Sakaguchi. 2003. Regulatory T cells in transplantation tolerance. *Nat Rev Immunol* 3:199–210.

83. Sakaguchi, S. 2004. Naturally arising CD4+ regulatory t cells for immunologic self-tolerance and negative control of immune responses. *Annu Rev Immunol* 2003;22:531–562.

84. Saitovitch D, Bushell A, Mabbs DW, Morris PJ, Wood K.J. Kinetics of induction of transplantation tolerance with a nondepleting anti-Cd4 monoclonal antibody and donor-specific transfusion before transplantation. A critical period of time is required for development of immunological unresponsiveness. *Transplantation* 1996;61: 1642–1647.

85. Bushell A, Morris PJ, Wood KJ. Induction of operational tolerance by random blood transfusion combined with anti-CD4 antibody therapy. A protocol with significant clinical potential. *Transplantation* 1994;58:133–139.

86. Tsui TY, Jager MD, Deiwick A, Klempnauer J, Schlitt HJ. Induction of peripheral tolerance by posttransplant infusion of donor splenocytes. *Transplant Proc* 2001;33:187–188.

87. Saitovitch D, Morris PJ, Wood KJ. Recipient cells expressing single donor MHC locus products can substitute for donor-specific transfusion in the induction of transplantation tolerance when pretreatment is combined with anti-Cd4 monoclonal antibody. Evidence for a vital role of Cd4+ T cells in the induction of tolerance to class I molecules. *Transplantation* 1996;61:1532–1538.

88. Wong W, Morris PJ, Wood KJ. Pretransplant administration of a single donor class I major histocompatibility complex molecule is sufficient for the indefinite survival of fully allogeneic cardiac allografts: evidence for linked epitope suppression. *Transplantation* 1997;63:1490–1494.

89. Spriewald BM, Billing JS, Jenkins S, et al. Syngeneic bone marrow transduced with a recombinant retroviral vector to express endoplasmic reticulum signal-sequence-deleted major histocompatibility complex class-I alloantigen can induce specific immunologic unresponsiveness in vivo. *Transplantation* 2003;75:537–541.

90. Pearson TC, Trambley J, Odom K, et al. Anti-CD40 therapy extends renal allograft survival in rhesus macaques. *Transplantation* 2002;74: 933–940.

91. Adams AB, Shirasugi N, Jones TR, et al. Development of a chimeric anti-CD40 monoclonal antibody that synergizes with LEA29Y to prolong islet allograft survival. *J Immunol* 2005;174:542–550.

92. Kanaya K, Tsuchida Y, Inobe M, et al. Combined gene therapy with adenovirus vectors containing CTLA4Ig and CD40Ig prolongs survival of composite tissue allografts in rat model. *Transplantation* 2003;75:275–281.

93. Jones ND, Van Maurik A, Hara, M, et al. CD40-CD40 ligand-independent activation of CD8+ T cells can trigger allograft rejection. *J Immunol* 2000;165:1111–1118.

94. Thomas F, Ray P, Thomas JM. Immunological tolerance as an adjunct to allogeneic tissue grafting. *Microsurgery* 2000;20: 435–440.

95. Thomas J, Alqaisi M, Cunningham P, et al. The development of a posttransplant TLI treatment strategy that promotes organ allograft acceptance without chronic immunosuppression. *Transplantation* 1992; 53:247–258.

96. Thomas JM, Contreras JL, Jiang XL, et al. Peritransplant tolerance induction in macaques: early events reflecting the unique synergy between immunotoxin and deoxyspergualin. *Transplantation* 1999; 68:1660–1673.

97. Hutchings A, Wu J, Asiedu C, et al. The immune decision toward allograft tolerance in non-human primates requires early inhibition of innate immunity and induction of immune regulation. *Transpl Immunol* 2003;11:335–344.

98. Haynes BF, Markert ML, Sempowski GD, Patel DD, Hale LP. The role of the thymus in immune reconstitution in aging, bone marrow transplantation, and HIV-1 infection. *Annu Rev Immunol* 2000;18:529–560.

99. Wu Z, Bensinger SJ, Zhang J, et al. Homeostatic proliferation is a barrier to transplantation tolerance. *Nat Med* 2004;10:87–92.

100. Adams AB, Williams MA, Jones TR, et al. Heterologous immunity provides a potent barrier to transplantation tolerance. *J Clin Invest* 2003;111:1887–1895.

101. Annacker O, Pimenta-Araujo R, Burlen-Defranoux O, et al. CD25+ CD4+ T cells regulate the expansion of peripheral CD4 T cells through the production of IL-10. *J Immunol* 2001;166: 3008–3018.

102. Murakami M, Sakamoto A, Bender J, Kappler J, P. Marrack P. 2002. CD25+CD4+ T cells contribute to the control of memory CD8+ T cells. *Proc Natl Acad Sci USA* 2002;99:8832–8837.

# XENOTRANSPLANTATION

*Kazuhiko Yamada, MD, PhD, Prashanth Vallabhajosyula, MD, David H. Sachs, MD*

## INTRODUCTION

The field of xenotransplantation provides verification of the old adage "Necessity is the mother of invention." With the possible exception of kidney transplants between human leukocyte antigen (HLA)-identical siblings, the use of living donors as a source for organ transplantation has been the result of the shortage of available cadaver donor organs. As is evident in many of the other chapters of this volume, the use of living donors is not without risk to the donor and, in the case of partial organ transplants (ie, liver lung and pancreas), often provides an organ of inferior quality to an intact cadaver organ. In addition, there are organs like the heart that will never be amenable to living donation. Thus, if transplantation is to reach its full potential. There is an urgent necessity to find another source of donor organs. This necessity has led to a resurgence of interest in the clinical potential of xenotransplants over the past decade.

Xenotransplantation actually has a long history, the first attempts having been carried out long before allogeneic transplantation, as will be reviewed below. However, until recently, these attempts have all resulted in dismal failure. In the past decade, enormous progress has been made in the quest for successful xenotransplantation, but the field remains one of preclinical research, not of applicable clinical therapy. Nevertheless, it seems reasonable to include a chapter on this modality in a volume on Living Donor Organ Transplantation, because future developments in this field could potentially obviate the need for use of living human donors.

## A BRIEF HISTORY OF XENOTRANSPLANTATION

Although the anecdotal history of xenotransplantation dates back to ancient times, it was not until the 1960s, along with the advent of immunosuppressive drugs, that serious attempts at clinical xenotransplantation began. In 1963, Reemtsma transplanted a kidney from a rhesus monkey into a 43-year-old male, using available immunosuppression.[1] The patient died 63 days posttransplantation. The following year, he transplanted a chimpanzee kidney into a human, with a 9-month survival, which remains the longest known survival of a xenotransplanted organ into a human.[1] Also in 1964, Hardy performed the first heart xenotransplantation, replacing a human heart with that of a chimpanzee,[2] but the patient died 90 minutes after the transplant. Soon thereafter, Hitchcock and Starzl transplanted baboon kidneys into six human patients, with variable survival ranging from 19 to 98 days.[3] In 1969, Bertoye and Marion reported two liver

xenotransplantations, from baboon to human, one patient surviving 4 months, the other 39 hours.[4] In the early 1970s, Starzl reported liver xenotransplantation from chimpanzee to human, with survivals up to 15 days.[5,6]

For the next 15 years, interest in clinical xenotransplantation almost disappeared, as interest and activity in allogeneic transplantation intensified. However, as allogeneic transplantation became increasingly successful, the inability of supply to meet the demand became quickly apparent, and interest in xenotransplantation returned. In 1984, Bailey transplanted an ABO-incompatible baboon heart into a 12-day-old baby girl named Baby Fae.[7] There was enormous media attention to this event, but the baby's survival of only 20 days led to disappointment with the potential of this modality. It was not until 1992, with the advent of immunosuppression with FK-506, that Starzl reinitiated clinical efforts in this field, transplanting baboon livers into two human recipients, one of whom survived for 70 days and the other for 26 days after surgery. At about this time, most workers in the field concluded (see below) that pigs should be far preferable to baboons as xenograft donors and research efforts in the field were redirected toward preclinical studies of pig-to-non-human primate organ transplantation. A series of advances have been made over the subsequent years, many of which will be detailed in the remainder of this chapter. Although the studies have so far remained in the preclinical realm, these advances are sufficiently impressive that it seems likely that renewed clinical efforts will be forthcoming in the near future.

## CHOICE OF THE MOST APPROPRIATE DONOR SPECIES

A major consideration in the quest for xenografts is determination of the most appropriate donor species. From a phylogenetic viewpoint, nonhuman primates would clearly be the best choice. However, the only nonhuman primates of adequate size to provide a heart to an adult human would be chimpanzees or apes, both of which are endangered species and therefore out of consideration as potential sources of xenograft organs. The baboon, on the other hand, is relatively available and could potentially be used as donor for organs such as the liver, which regenerates, or the kidney, which has considerable excess functional capacity and could be transplanted as a pair of organs. However, the problems of potential pathogenic viruses, which are more likely to cross into humans from a closely related species than from a more distant one, as well as ethical considerations associated with the use of any nonhuman primate donor, have led most workers in the field to the conclusion that a discordant species, in particular the pig, will be the most suitable xenograft donor.

Pigs have the advantages of essentially unlimited availability, favorable breeding characteristics and similarity of many organ systems to those of humans. Partially inbred miniature swine, which have been pedigree-bred for the past 35 years in the laboratory of the authors, are a particularly attractive choice.[8] Their adult weights of up to 120 kg are similar to those of humans, in contrast to domestic swine that can reach weights over 500 kg. Their physiology is also similar to humans for many organ systems, and their breeding characteristics have permitted inbreeding and genetic manipulation.[9] There are currently three lines of inbred miniature swine, each homozygous for a different MHC haplotype (SLA$^a$, SLA$^c$, and SLA$^d$ ) and five lines bearing different intra-MHC-recombinant haplotypes (Figure 39-1). In addition, one subline of the SLA$^{dd}$ line has been maintained over the last 15 years by sequential brother–sister mating, to produce an inbred line of that now has a coefficient of inbreeding of > 94%. This high degree of consanguinity permits acceptance of skin and organ transplants among offspring within the line without immunosuppressive drugs.[9] Thus, if immunologic tolerance can be induced across xenogeneic barriers (see below), this property should make it possible to exchange an organ that might fail with another immunologically identical organ without further manipulation of the immune response.

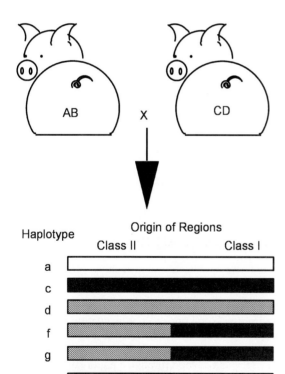

**FIGURE 39-1**

Origin of haplotypes of available partially inbred miniature swine.

## POTENTIAL ADVANTAGES OF XENO- OVER ALLO- TRANSPLANTATION

The single most compelling rationale for xenotransplantation is the severe shortage of organs and the tremendous improvement in morbidity and mortality seen with organ transplantation. However, in addition to availability, xenogeneic organs could have a number of benefits over their allogeneic counterparts. Among these are:

1. The potential to cure or alleviate diseases caused by human-specific viruses: For example, many human-tropic viruses, including viral hepatitis and HIV[10] F[11]would be incapable of infecting a pig liver.

2. Potential for gene delivery: The transplantation of tissues or organs from genetically engineered animals producing desired gene products, either constitutively or under regulation, would be uniquely possible for xenotransplants.[12,13]

3. Avoidance of risk of human disease transmission to the organ recipient and/or to health care personnel: Although the risk of infection with endogenous viruses (such as porcine endogenous retrovirus) has been the subject of considerable interest and investigation,[14] the unfortunate occurrence of transmission of occult tumors and infections with rare organisms which have been reported following allotransplantation should be completely avoidable with the use of xenografts.

4. Ease of coordination and cost-effectiveness: The administrative efforts and the multilevel coordination required to perform cadaveric organ transplantation is both time-consuming and costly. Both would be avoided for xenotransplants, as transplantation would be an elective and conveniently timed procedure. The elective nature of the procedures would avoid many of the errors that are caused by the time pressure of current cadaver donor selection and distribution.

5. Capacity for retransplantation: Given the essentially unlimited supply of organs, a recipient would be able to receive a replacement organ as needed—whether because of technical failure or because of loss of function for other reasons. Indeed, using the approach being developed in the laboratory of the authors, the donors will be inbred (ie, genetically identical) animals and tolerance induction to many of the major antigens will be part of the preparative regimen.[9,15,16] In these circumstances, replacement of a failed organ for any reason other than rejection should be possible without need for any additional immunosuppression.

## IMMUNOLOGIC BARRIERS OF XENOTRANSPLANTATION

Because the antigenic differences recognizable by the immune system of a recipient of a different species are greater than those within a species, the immunologic barriers to xenotransplantation are more powerful than those encountered for allotransplantation. Among the immunologic reactions that characterize xenograft rejection are

1. Hyperacute Rejection (HAR): By definition, hyperacute rejection occurs only between discordant (ie, distantly related) species. Concordant (closely related) species reject transplants in much the same way as they reject allotransplants,

although at an accelerated pace.[17,18] Hyperacute preformed rejection occurs within the first 24 hours and is caused by xenoreactive antibodies (predominately of the IgM subclass) circulating in large quantities in the recipient's blood, which bind to cell surface molecules on vascular endothelial cells of the graft.[19–23] This binding induces a conformational change in the antibody that exposes a binding site for complement. The complement cascade then attacks the endothelial cells, either activating or killing them. Blood cells and fluid leak out of the damaged endothelium into surrounding tissues, resulting in diffuse interstitial hemorrhage and edema. Activated endothelial cells change their shape and lose their anticoagulant functions, leading to coagulation and the formation of thrombi in small and large vessels.[24–28] The resulting graft is left black, swollen, and nonfunctional.

The predominant initiators of this HAR immune response of primates to pigs are the preformed natural antibodies (Nabs) found in all primates against the antigenic sugar moiety alpha-galactose-1,3-galactose (Gal).[29–33] It is believed that the reason for the predominance of these antibodies is the fact that during evolution, at the level of old-world primates, a frameshift mutation in the gene encoding the enzyme alpha-1,3 galactosyltransferase (GalT) rendered it inactive, that is, a "pseudogene."[31,34] Old-world primates and humans are presumably sensitized to Gal soon after birth by Gal-expressing microorganisms that colonize the gut, leading to preformed anti-Gal antibodies. In the xenotransplantation setting, these Nabs, interact with Gal expressed on the vascular endothelial cells of the pig organ and mediate the HAR response. It has been estimated that as much as 70% to 90% of human preformed IgM antibodies to pig are directed against this single sugar epitope.[35,36] The aggregate cytotoxicity of all other human anti-pig Nabs is less than one tenth that of the anti-Gal Nabs.[23]

2.  Delayed Xenograft Rejection (DXR): Hyperacute acute rejection can be avoided through the depletion of Nabs,[37,38] complement inhibition,[39–41] or the use of transgenic pig donors expressing complement down-regulatory proteins.[39,42,43] In all of these cases, a delayed form of xenograft rejection, also termed *acute humoral xenograft rejection* (AHXR), occurs. DXR begins within 3 to 10 days of transplantation and is associated with the increased deposition of anti-pig antibodies in the graft. The immunologic basis of delayed xenograft rejection is not fully understood, but is likely to involve induced antibodies to both Gal and other determinants, complement, NK cells, macrophages, and activation of coagulation.[44–46]

    Morphologically, DXR is characterized by the development of thrombotic microangiopathy with endothelial cell apoptosis and necrosis, followed by the destruction of the microvasculature and platelet aggregation.[44,46,47] NK cell and macrophage cell infiltrates may also play a role in the graft's destruction. Because the same measures that have been used to avoid HAR have also been found to postpone or eliminate DXR, it is likely that either residual Nabs or newly induced, T cell-dependent antibodies to other pig determinants are important initiators of this process.

3.  Acute T cell Rejection: Because of the intense rejection processes that are induced by antibodies against discordant transplants, until recently much greater attention has been given to humoral response to xenografts than to the cellular response. However, the cellular immune responses to xenotransplants are clearly also of great importance to their success. Extensive cellular studies of discordant xenogeneic reactions were originally conducted in mice and suggested that responder antigen presenting cells (APC) were required for T cell recognition (*indirect pathway*) of xenogeneic antigens.[48–50] However, it now appears that the mouse may be unusual in this regard, since human T cells have been demonstrated to react directly with stimulators of other species (direct pathway),[50,51] including endothelial cells of the pig. Among the reasons proposed for failure of murine T cells to respond via direct pathway are deficiencies in CD4-class II and CD8-class I MHC interactions, lower frequencies of reactive precursors, and species specificities of some cytokine-mediated or costimulatory pathways.[52–56] Once measures have been instituted to avoid humoral immunity (see below), a strong T cell-mediated cellular response of primates to porcine xenotransplants has been observed.[50,57–61]

## Chronic Rejection

One of the major obstacles to long-term survival of clinical allografts remains the development of chronic rejection,[51,62–64] a process involving gradual loss of function and characterized histologically by chronic vasculopathy and fibrosis. Although the number of factors that can cause chronic rejection is still a matter of controversy, both cellular and humoral immune responses have been implicated in the process.[65–68] Other factors, such as ischemia-reperfusion injury, acute tubular necrosis, and viral infections may also be involved.[69–72] To date, no transplanted pig organ has survived long enough in a primate to determine how much of an obstacle chronic rejection will pose to xenotransplantation. Given its prevalence in allotransplantation, however, it seems likely that chronic rejection will occur at least to the extent that it does in allotransplants.

## STRATEGIES TO PREVENT XENOGRAFT REJECTION

The numerous interconnected elements of the immune system ensure that strategies that inhibit one type of rejection often have an effect on other types as well. Here, strategies are grouped according to the type of rejection at which they were originally targeted.

### Avoiding Hyperacute Rejection (HAR)

Several approaches have been successful in avoiding HAR. Among these are

1.  Absorption of anti-Gal antibodies: Absorption of anti-Gal Nabs from primate blood prior to transplantation has been accomplished by a number of methods, all of which have been effective in preventing HAR.[73–78] These include perfusion of the recipient's blood through a pig organ, absorption of all immunoglobulins on anti-Ig columns, specific antibody absorption by plasmapheresis through immunoaffinity columns bearing Gal oligosaccharides bound covalently to an insoluble matrix, and administration of soluble Gal-containing molecules intravenously to absorb the anti-Gal antibodies *in vivo*.[37,73,75,77–82] Sequential plasmapheresis with replacement of serum proteins by albumin has also been utilized as a means of removing Nabs

nonspecifically.[83,84] All of these methods have reduced the Nab level to a sufficiently low level to avoid HAR, but none has proved capable of maintaining this depletion long term. As anti-Gal antibody production increases after each absorption, eventually the humoral response overcomes any method used to maintain depletion.

2. Inhibition of Complement: A number of agents capable of inhibiting complement activity *in vivo* have been utilized to reduce the damage caused by binding of Nabs to vascular endothelial cells. These include cobra venom factor,[85–88] soluble human complement receptor I (SCR1),[89–92] and several peptide inhibitors of serine proteases.[93] Again, all of these reagents are capable of delaying HAR, but none has provided long-term protection against antibody-mediated destruction of vascularized organ xenografts.

3. Use of transgenic donors expressing complement-inhibitory proteins: Pigs have been prepared that express one or more human complement regulatory proteins, which protect the organs from human complement. These regulatory proteins include hDAF (CD55, human decay accelerating factor), MCP (membrane cofactor protein), CD59 (inhibitor of the formation of the membrane attack complex), and hMCP (human membrane cofactor protein, CD46). Studies with hDAF pig-to-baboon kidney or heart transplantation with intensive immunosuppressive therapy have shown survivals between 1 and 2 months.[42,94] The protection against complement supplied by these transgenes seems to prevent HAR, but this protection can be overwhelmed by the humoral response, resulting in DXR.

4. Genetic engineering of donors to decrease Gal expression: Lactosamine serves as the substrate in the production of the Gal sugar in normal pigs. The Gal transferase enzyme adds a Gal terminal sugar onto lactosamine.[95–97] The production of the Gal sugar can be 90% inhibited by the expression of the gene for the enzyme alpha-1,2-fucosyltransferase which competes with GalT for the lactosamine base. Alpha-galactosidase reduces the amount of Gal expressed by cleaving Gal from its lactosamine base with 60% to 70% efficiency.[98–102] Experiments with partial knockout pigs that express about 5% of the normal quantity of Gal on their fibroblasts suggest that a 95% reduction of Gal expression may prevent HAR, but is not sufficient to prevent DXR. Xenokidneys donated in two such experiments showed uretal humoral rejection within 11 days of transplantation (Yamada et al., unpublished data).

5. Elimination of Gal expression by production of GalT knock-out animals: Complement-controlling pharmacologic agents, transient antibody-depleting strategies, and the use of transgenic animals have proven to be insufficient to prevent the eventual rejection of xenografts via a humoral mechanism. A more complete elimination of Gal from the surface of the donor pig cells was therefore deemed necessary. The technology of nuclear transfer, first publicized following the production of the sheep Dolly,[103] combined with homologous recombination, was utilized to accomplish this goal.[104–106] In 2002, two groups reported the use of nuclear transfer to produce α-1,3-galactosyltransferase knockout (GalT-KO) swine, which lack the gene responsible for adding the Gal terminal sugar onto lactosamine.[107,108] These pigs thus express no Gal. In the laboratory of the authors, the nucleus was taken

from a fibroblast cell line derived from the most highly inbred subline of miniature swine and then subjected to homologous recombination and selection to ablate expression of the GalT gene.[105,107] Initial results with organs from these GalT-KO pigs in baboons have shown the absence of hyperacute rejection without the need for inhibition of anti-Gal antibodies or of complement. Life-supporting renal grafts maintained on a protocol designed to induce tolerance led to survivals of up to 83 days,[109] with the longest survivors dying of other causes with functioning kidney grafts (Creatinine < 1.4 mg/dL). Heterotopic non-life-supporting heart xenografts maintained with chronic immunosuppression survived up to 179 days,[110] with eventual graft failure associated with thrombotic microangiopathy, induced by cellular and humoral rejection. These results are promising and hint at the possibility of transplanting vascularized tissues and organs from pigs to primates with neither the immediate nor the inexorable delayed forms of humoral rejection caused by anti-Gal NAbs in primates.

6. **Avoiding Delayed Xenograft Rejection (DXR)** Although the precise causes and mechanisms of DXR remain unclear, the fact that natural killer (NK) cells, antibodies, and macrophages have all been shown to play a role has led to several strategies aimed at silencing these immune responses:

1. Prevention of the induced antibody response: Induced high-affinity anti-Gal IgG antibodies are thought to be produced by a T cell-dependent mechanism.[111,112] The co-stimulation pathway of CD40 and CD154 (CD40L) plays a role in the activation of T cells in response to antigen and in the activation of resting B cells by CD4+ T cells.[113] Therefore, the administration of anti-CD154 mAb has been attempted as a means of preventing the induced antibody response to a transplanted pig organ in a baboon.[114–116] Although this therapy was effective in preventing induced IgG antibodies, it was insufficient to completely prevent DXR.

2. Silencing of NK cell: NK cells recognize self-class I MHC molecules through inhibitory receptors, so that if a target cell lacks self-class I it becomes susceptible to NK killing.[117–121] NK cells also express natural cytotoxicity receptors (NCR) that are activating receptors and can recognize their targets in an MHC-independent manner. Although the activating NCR on NK cells function between species, the inhibitory signals do not, making xenogeneic cells very susceptible to NK killing. The role NK cells play in xenograft rejection could therefore potentially be ameliorated by the production of a transgenic pig that expressed human class I molecules, and thus provided the inhibitory signal necessary to avoid attack by human NK cells.[122] However, while NK killing has been demonstrated clearly for target cells in suspension, it remains unclear how important inhibition of NK cells will be in avoiding rejection of solid organ xenografts.[123]

3. Avoiding Acute T Cell Rejection: The same immunosuppressive drugs that have been developed to suppress cellular immunity to allografts have also been used in xenotransplantation, but in considerably higher doses.[124–127] Even with such doses, complete inhibition of T cell-dependent antibody formation has not

been achieved. Therefore, it seems likely that the intensity of immunosuppression that will be required to avoid rejection of a xenograft will be much greater than that required for control of an allograft reaction, and possibly too immunosuppressive to be used clinically without unacceptable levels of complications, such as infections and tumors. These considerations have suggested the importance of inducing immunologic tolerance, at least to some of the most important xenogeneic antigens.[79,85,124,127–131] A tolerant recipient would regard the graft as self, thus avoiding rejection but leaving the recipient fully immunocompetent. In addition, induction of tolerance at the T Cell level would also avoid the production of T Cell-dependent antibody responses to pig antigens other than Gal (elicited antibodies).

The two approaches to induction of T Cell tolerance that have been investigated extensively in the laboratory of the authors and their colleagues at the Massachusetts General Hospital in Boston are (1) a mixed chimerism (ie, mixed lymphohematopoietic reconstitution) approach and (2) a thymic transplantation approach. Tolerance to both concordant and discordant xenografts has been achieved by both approaches in mice.[132–143] In pig-to-baboon combination, however, although there has been considerable progress, full tolerance (ie, withdrawal of all immunosuppression) has not yet been achieved.

## Tolerance Induction Strategies

1. Mixed Chimerism: Using either bone marrow (BM) or cytokine-mobilized peripheral blood progenitor cells (PBPC) as the source of hematopoietic stem cells (HSC), large doses of HSC from either miniature swine or hDAF donor pigs have been infused into immunocompromised baboons.[144–146] In the initial attempts to achieve long-term, hematopoietic chimerism, 2–3 x 10^8 pig bone marrow cells/ kg and swine recombinant growth factors (IL-3 and SCF)

were administered to immunosuppressed baboons.[145,146] Although only transient and low levels of chimerism could be detected by fluorescent sorting, porcine colony forming units (CFU) were detectable in the recipients for over 6 months by polymerase chain reaction (PCR). However, over this time, positive assays were often interspersed with negative assays, indicating that detection of pig cells by this technique was probably at very low levels, close to the threshold level of detection.

In an attempt to increase engraftment, the dose of progenitor cells administered was next raised to a "megadose" using cytokine-mobilized PBPC.[147–150] These enormous yields obtained following mobilization and pheresis permitted administration of pig PBPC to baboons at doses of 2–4 x 10^10 cells/kg. However, even these enormous doses of pig cells led to detection of pig cells in the baboon circulation for only 2 to 5 days, with the exception of one animal, in which a second appearance of pig cells was observed peripherally from days 16 to 21,[151] suggesting transient engraftment (Figure 39-2). There did appear to be an effect at the T cell level, as monitored by in vitro assays,[152] but this specific hyporesponsiveness was also transient. To explain these findings, it was reasoned that because HSC do not express Gal, the failure of these cells taken from miniature or hDAF swine to establish peripheral chimerism could be due to the appearance of Gal on progeny of these HSC and subsequent elimination by natural anti-Gal antibodies (Nab). Only a very limited number of transplants of bone marrow from the new GalT-KO swine to baboons have been possible to date, but the data obtained support this hypothesis in demonstrating higher levels and longer lasting peripheral chimerism than had been detected in previous studies.[153]

2. Thymic transplantation: Using T cell depletion and thymectomy to prepare recipient baboons, Yamada et al. have transplanted a source of vascularized porcine thymus along with a porcine organ xenograft in an attempt to induce tolerance at the T cell level.[124,154,155] Again, the initial studies were carried out using miniature swine or hDAF swine as donors. The vascularized xenografts survived for up to 30 days, with evidence of viable thymic epithelium and Hassall's corpuscles in the thymic implants, and with evidence of donor-specific hyporesponsiveness by *in vitro* assays in some of the animals even after immunosuppression had been stopped. Grafts were rejected simultaneously with the return of anti-Gal antibodies and the grafts demonstrated humoral damage without evidence of cellular infiltrates. It was concluded that the vascularized thymic grafts induced specific hyporesponsiveness a the T cell level, with avoidance of new T cell-dependent antibody responses, but that eventual rejection due to the anti-Gal antibody response could not be overcome.

3. Vascularized thymic transplantation: Transplantation of vascularized thymus in the form of a composite organ has most recently been tested as a tolerance inducing strategy in baboons using GalT-KO pig donor thymo kidneys.[109] There was a major increase in survival of renal xenografts from GalT-KO versus hDAF donors using the same protocol that had been used previously for miniature or hDAF renal xenografts, although now without the need for inhibition of anti-Gal.[109] The survival of such life-supporting kidneys was prolonged from a previous maximum of about 30 days to over 80 days using GalT-KO donors. In addition

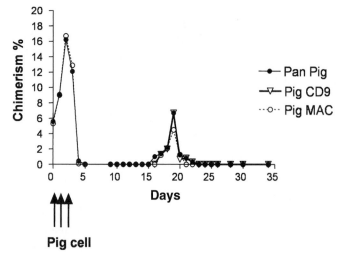

**FIGURE 39-2**

Pig cell chimerism detected by FACS in a baboon that received a "megadose" of pig peripheral blood progenitor cells.

the longest surviving kidneys were all still functioning when the animals expired for other reasons. Indeed, the longest survivor in this series died with a normal creatinine from a myocardial infarct on day 83, possibly arug-related or possibly caused by an iatrogenic embolism to the coronary artery from a misplaced carotid arterial catheter. At the time of death, its kidney appeared normal by both gross inspection and by histology. These data are early, but very encouraging, as they suggest that tolerance induction may be of great importance in achieving long-term xenograft survival.

4. Prevention of Chronic Rejection: As pointed out above, although transplanted pig organs in primates have not yet survived long enough to develop chronic rejection, it seems likely that it will become a problem once survivals approach those of allotransplants. Because the elimination of chronic rejection in clinical allotransplantation has proved elusive, one might expect the same difficulty for xenotransplants. One advantage of xenotransplantation over allotransplantation with respect to chronic rejection is the possibility of offering the patient another organ when the first is near the end of its functional life—an opportunity that is only rarely available for recipients of human organs. Such retransplantation would of course only be reasonable if the cause of the chronic rejection was predominantly nonimmunologic.

5. Preventing nonimmunologic loss of xenotransplants: As indicated above, a prominent feature of porcine Gal-KO heart grafts prolonged by chronic immunosuppression has been thrombotic microangiopathy.[156] Because these lesions were less prominent in renal xenografts prolonged by a protocol designed to induce tolerance,[157] they could, at least in part, be induced by low-level antibody responses, and therefore also be ultimately immunologic in origin. However, thrombotic reactions could also be caused by molecular incompatibilities of the coagulation pathway, of nonimmunologic origin.[158,159] In this case, even if the xenogeneic cellular and humoral responses are fully controlled, incompatible regulators of coagulation could lead to thrombotic complications and thereby constitute another barrier to long-term xenograft survival and function. Genetic engineering of donor animals to express human anticoagulant and platelet-regulatory factors could provide a means of overcoming this barrier, and experimental work in this direction is already under way.[160,161]

## PREPARING THE DONOR

### Choice of Donor Organ

As xenotransplantation is not yet being performed clinically, the decision on which organ should be transplanted first remains one of active debate. Among the most likely candidates are (1) kidney, (2) heart, (3) liver, (4) lung, and (5) pancreas; and each has its proponents and detractors. In favor of the kidney is the fact that failure of the transplant would not necessarily be fatal, as the patient could presumably be put back on dialysis. In addition, there are numerous patients on most waiting lists for kidneys who are highly sensitized to potential donors (ie, high panel reactive antibody, or PRA).[162] On the other hand, the availability of living donor transplants and the fact that renal failure is treatable by dialysis provide alternatives to xenotransplantation that argue against its use until there is a reasonable expectation of long-term success.

The heart, liver, and lungs are organs, without which life cannot be sustained, making the need for an alternative source unquestionable when a human donor cannot be obtained in time. For this reason, some workers have suggested that xenotransplanted organs might be used as a "bridge" to sustain life while the search for a human donor organ goes on. However, others argue that the use of a xenogeneic organ as a bridge does not solve the problem of organ shortage; rather it increases the number of people on the waiting list for a human organ. Nevertheless, it seems possible that one might learn enough about the potential of clinical xenotransplantation from such cases that they could provide a stepping-stone toward long-term therapy by this modality. In the case of liver, some have argued that the number of proteins (eg, enzymes, coagulation factors, complement components, etc) produced by this organ is so large that some of them will undoubtedly be unable to function properly across such a large species disparity. However, that many of the most important functions are intact is evidenced by the fact that hepatectomized baboons that have received pig liver transplants have been reported to wake up and show relatively normal cognitive and metabolic function, as well as to normalize their coagulation parameters.[163] Because one could not awaken or normalize such functions without a liver, clearly many of the vital functions of this organ must have been intact. Furthermore, even if some proteins produced by the liver do prove to be incompatible with their required function in humans, genetic engineering now opens the possibility of exchanging the genes for such proteins in the pig for their human counterparts.

Pancreas or islet xenotransplantation would most likely be carried out for treatment of type I diabetes. Because porcine insulin, which is very similar to human insulin, and until the recent advent of the recombinant human product, was used to treat diabetic patients,[164,165] it is very likely that the pig islets would support the insulin needs of a diabetic as well as an allograft. However, as for human pancreas transplantation, there is debate concerning the wisdom of subjecting a diabetic patient to the effects of immunosuppression for a condition that can be treated with exogenous insulin. Because the immunosuppressive regimen required for a xenotransplant would undoubtedly be more dangerous than that used for an allogeneic graft, this argument would be even more problematic for the xenograft. More likely, as for human pancreas transplantation, whole pancreatic xenogeneic organ transplants would be carried out in combination with transplantation of another organ (such as pancreas-kidney). Because there is a high incidence of renal failure from diabetic nephropathy in diabetic patients, the number of potential recipients for such combined transplants would undoubtedly be large. Xenograft islet transplants may likewise be offered to the same kind of patients, as they are now for either brittle diabetics or diabetics who also need a kidney transplant.[166–168]

### Microbiology

The spread of infection between species has been termed *zoonosis*[14] and involves a large number of potential pathogens that are known to infect both animals and humans.[169,170] One might expect, based on experience with human transplants and experimental transplantation in swine, that after immunosuppression, recipients would be susceptible to similar bacterial and fungal infections to those that are seen in clinical transplantation today. These would include a variety of organisms that infect both swine and primates, including Staphylococci, Streptococci, Aspergillus, Salmonella, Klebsiella, Enterococcus, and Actinomyces. Under the intensive immunosuppression required to control early rejection, infections to additional organisms, usually controlled by normal host defenses, may also occur. These would include cytomegalovirus, other herpes viruses, adenovirus, and the hepatitis viruses, as well as numerous other opportunistic infections (eg, Pneumocystis, Toxoplasma, Histoplasma, Brucella, and Leptospira), although it is not clear whether humans would be infected by the porcine equivalents of many of these pathogens.

Importantly, all of these are organisms that can be easily diagnosed by microbiologic assays should they occur, and can be treated in a recipient of a xenograft as in current recipients of allografts. Even more importantly, these are organisms that can readily be excluded from pigs raised specifically to be xenograft donors. Indeed, it would be easier to assure absence of most known pathogens—bacteria, viruses, and fungi—in xenograft donors that it currently is in human cadaver donors, for whom complete microbiologic histories are rarely available.

What cannot be excluded by screening and re-derivation are retroviruses, which are endogenous to each species and carried in the genome.[14,171] Infections due to these retroviruses are generally very species-specific. However, the uncertainty about whether such species specificity might break down in the face of the intimate exposure of the human tissues to those of the pig xenograft has led to a whole new field, sometimes called "xenozoonosis," attempting to assess the risk of new infections that might occur after a xenotransplant. The possibility that such an infection, once established, might spread to other members of the human species has led to intense activity at regulatory levels and to recommendations for how patients undergoing xenotransplantation should be handled. Despite this intense activity, there has been no evidence uncovered to date to indicate that any pig endogenous retroviruses (PERV) have ever infected a human, much less caused any disease.[172] The only cross-species transmission of PERV detected to date has been from infected porcine cells mixed in tissue culture with certain infectious human cell lines.[171] Even this level of transmission is not observed when the porcine cells are obtained from certain "nontransmitting" strains of miniature swine. Therefore, although the risk posed by the possibility of cross-species infection will be something that will engender intense regulation an scrutiny after the first clinical xenotransplants, there is little evidence at present that any new diseases will occur as a result of this process. For a full discussion of the biology of PERV and of its potential risks, the reader is referred to several excellent reviews.[173–177]

## PREPARING THE RECIPIENT

### Choosing the Recipient

Hand in hand with choice of the most appropriate organ, goes choice of the most appropriate patient to receive that organ. As mentioned above, one potential patient population may be highly allosensitized (high PRA) recipients on waiting lists for renal transplants. There are currently over 60 000 patients on waiting lists for kidney transplants in the United States, of whom approximately 20% have PRA > 80%. Due to the difficulty in finding a suitable crossmatch-negative human donor organ, this 20% of the population generally accounts for less than 5% of kidney transplants performed.

Although there have been reports of cross-reactivity of anti-HLA antibodies with swine leukocyte antigens (SLA), which

might suggest increased risk of rejection in high PRA recipients,[178,179] these studies have been difficult to interpret due to the high levels of anti-Gal antibodies in all humans, the removal of which is often problematic. The recent development of GalT-KO miniature swine has eliminated the effects of anti-Gal antibodies and thereby provided a unique opportunity to study the role that anti-non-Gal antibodies play in xenoreactivity. Recent studies from the authors' laboratory have used these GalT-KO cells to compare the xenoreactivity of sera from allosensitized and nonallosensitized patients. Patients with high PRA were found to have no increase in levels of anti-non-Gal antibodies compared to low PRA patients. Indeed, serum xenoreactivity against the GalT-KO swine cells in high PRA sera was generally much lower than alloreactivity of these sera against random human blood donors. These findings would support the possibility of recruiting high PRA patients as potential recipients of porcine renal xenografts. Some feel that the dire need of patients awaiting heart or liver transplants may make them more likely candidates for the first clinical xenografts.

### Surveillance Pre- and Postxenotransplantation

The first recipients of xenografts in a controlled clinical trial will be heavily monitored both before and after transplantation, according to guidelines formulated by an FDA panel, to which the reader is referred for details.[180] Recipients will have to have the support necessary and be sufficiently responsible to handle the required immunosuppressive regimen, the required testing, and the detailed follow-up of the patient and the patient's intimate contacts. The potential public health risk that xenotransplantation represents, no matter how small (see above), will necessitate careful monitoring of the first recipients of xenografts and of their contacts.

### Immunosuppression and/or Tolerance Induction

Immunosuppression with drugs similar to those used for allogeneic transplantation today will undoubtedly be part of all xenotransplantation protocols. The plethora of immunosuppressive agents now available for targeting T cell-immune responses have been responsible for major increases in survival rates for allografts. These include both pharmacologic and antibody reagents.[181–188] Because most antibody responses to allografts are T cell dependent, these same reagents have been effective in avoiding antibody responses as well. In most cases, these agents can be titrated to a level at which they are effective in inhibiting the response to the transplant without undue side effects. Unfortunately, for xenografts, the levels of these agents needed to fully suppress the immune response is greater than for allografts, and might be expected to lead to greater complications. In addition, antibody-mediated responses appear to be more prevalent and more robust in xenograft rejection than in allograft rejection, and even when the major response to Gal has been eliminated by use of GalT-KO donors, it appears likely that low levels of T cell-dependent antibodies may still form, possibly contributing to the thrombotic complications that are associated with xenograft rejection.[189]

It is therefore perhaps not entirely surprising that chronic immunosuppression has so far not been effective in long-term maintenance of xenografts. The authors' laboratory has recently reported the longest survival to date of a heterotopic heart transplant maintained by chronic immunosuppression.[110] This non-life-supporting transplant was from a GalT-KO donor and continued to beat for 179 days, but was then rejected, with evidence of cellular and humoral components as well as thrombotic microangiopathy.[110] The same immunosuppressive regimen maintained life-supporting GalT-KO kidney xenografts in baboons to day 3, again being rejected despite a rigorous immunosuppressive regimen.[109]

On the other hand, an approach utilizing tolerance induction, at least to some of the most important xenogeneic antigens, may be capable of avoiding such persistent immune reactivity. Initial results also from the authors' laboratory have demonstrated that when co-transplanted with donor vascularized thymic grafts, a method for inducing tolerance at the T Cell level (see Avoiding Acute T Cell Rejection), life-supporting GalT-KO renal xenografts showed no evidence of rejection for up to 83 days.[109] This animal also showed *in vitro* evidence for donor-specific unresponsiveness, suggesting that the baboon may have been on a path toward development of tolerance.

## CONCLUSIONS

As a field, xenotransplantation is still in its early stages. We have attempted here to review briefly the history of this field, to summarize where the field now stands with regard to overcoming its numerous obstacles, and to present what we consider the most likely potential donors and recipients for the first clinical attempts at xenotransplantation in the future. The most compelling reason for continuing this pursuit is the large number of patients who continue to die every year while on the waiting list for an organ transplant. There are clearly ethical questions that continue to surround xenotransplantation, especially with regard to the concerns about xenozoonoses (see under Microbiology). However, the current alternative of using normal living donors and thereby subjecting human beings to invasive and potentially life-threatening procedures that they do not need clearly raises competing and perhaps equally troubling ethical questions. The burgeoning fields of stem cell biology and tissue engineering may eventually offer solutions to this dilemma with fewer ethical and technical problems, but these solutions will require many years of further research before they can be brought to the clinic. In the meantime, xenotransplantation, despite its potential risks, remains the best hope we have to solve the organ shortage for the thousands of patients who will otherwise perish while waiting for an organ.

## References

1. Reemtsma K, McCracken BH, Schlegel JU. Renal heterotransplantation in man. *Ann Surg* 1964;160:384.
2. Hardy JD, Kurrus FD, Chavez CM, et al. Heart transplantation in man. Developmental studies and report of a case. *JAMA* 1964; 188:1132–1140.
3. Starzl TE, Marchioro TL, Peters GN. Renal heterotransplantation from baboon to man: experience with six cases. *Transplantation* 1964;2:752.
4. Bertoye A, Marion P, Mikaeloff P, Bolot JF. [Attempt at treatment of various severe acute hepatic insufficiencies by temporary heterotopic heterologous liver graft (baboon liver)]. *Lyon Med* 1969;222(33): 347–354.
5. Giles GR, Boehmig HJ, Amemiya H, Halgrimson CG, Starzl TE. Clinical heterotransplantation of the liver. *Transplant Proc* 1970;2(4): 506–512.
6. Starzl TE, Ishikawa M, Putnam CW, et al. Progress in and deterrents to orthotopic liver transplantation, with special reference to survival,

7. resistance to hyperacute rejection, and biliary duct reconstruction. *Transplant Proc* 1974;6(4 Suppl 1):129–139.
7. Bailey LL, Nehlsen-Cannarella SL, Concepcion W, Jolley WB. Baboon-to-human cardiac xenotransplantation in a neonate. *JAMA* 1985;254(23):3321–3329.
8. Sachs DH. The pig as a potential xenograft donor. *Vet Immunol Immunopathol* 1994;43:185–191.
9. Mezrich JD, Haller GW, Arn JS, et al. Histocompatible miniature swine: an inbred large-animal model. *Transplantation* 2003; 75(6):904–907.
10. Mueller NJ, Barth RN, Yamamoto S, et al. Activation of cytomegalovirus in pig-to-primate organ xenotransplantation. *J Virol* 2002;76(10): 4734–4740.
11. Starzl TE, Fung J, Tzakis A, et al. Baboon-to-human liver transplantation. *Lancet* 1993;341:65–71.
12. Lin SS, Platt JL. Genetic therapies for xenotransplantation. *J Am Coll Surg* 1998;186(4):388–396.
13. Platt JL. Xenotransplantation - New risks, new gains. Nature 2000; 407(6800):27–30.
14. Patience C, Takeuchi Y, Weiss RA. Zoonosis in xenotransplantation. *Curr Opin Immunol* 1998;10(5):539–542.
15. Utsugi R, Barth RN, Lee RS, et al. Induction of transplantation tolerance with a short course of tacrolimus (FK506): I. Rapid and stable tolerance to two-haplotype fully mhc-mismatched kidney allografts in miniature swine. *Transplantation* 2001; 71(10): 1368–1379.
16. Ierino FL, Yamada K, Hatch T, Rembert J, Sachs DH. Peripheral tolerance to class I mismatched renal allografts in miniature swine: donor antigen-activated peripheral blood lymphocytes from tolerant swine inhibit antidonor CTL reactivity. *J Immunol* 1999;162(1):550–559.
17. Lin Y, Vandeputte M, Waer M. Natural killer cell- and macrophage-mediated rejection of concordant xenografts in the absence of T and B cell responses. *J Immunol* 1997; 158:5658–5667.
18. Lin Y, Vandeputte M, Waer M. Factors involved in rejection of concordant xenografts in complement-deficient rats. *Transplantation* 1997;63:1705–1712.
19. McKenzie IFC, Xing PX, Vaughan HA, et al. Distribution of the major xenoantigen (gal (alpha 1-3)gal) for pig to human xenografts. *Transpl Immunol* 1994;2(2):81–86.
20. Sandrin MS, Vaughan HA, Dabkowski PL, McKenzie IF. Anti-pig IgM antibodies in human serum react predominantly with Gal(alpha 1-3) Gal epitopes. *Proc Natl Acad Sci USA* 1993;90:11391–11395.
21. Sandrin MS, McKenzie IF. Gal alpha (1,3)Gal, the major xenoantigen(s) recognised in pigs by human natural antibodies. *Immunol Rev* 1994; 141:169–190.
22. Oriol R, Ye Y, Koren E, Cooper DK. Carbohydrate antigens of pig tissues reacting with human natural antibodies as potential targets for hyperacute vascular rejection in pig-to-man organ xenotransplantation. *Transplantation* 1993;56:1433–1442.
23. Parker W, Bruno D, Holzknecht ZE, Platt JL. Characterization and affinity isolation of xenoreactive human natural antibodies. *J Immunol* 1994;153:3791–3803.
24. Kearns-Jonker MK, Cramer DV, Dane LA, Swensson JM, Makowka L. Human serum reactivity to porcine endothelial cells after antisense-mediated down-regulation of GpIIIa expression. *Transplantation* 1997; 63:588–593.
25. Platt JL, Dalmasso AP, Vercellotti GM, et al. Endothelial cell proteoglycans in xenotransplantation. *Transplant Proc* 1990;22:1066.
26. Platt JL, Lindman BJ, Geller RL, et al. The role of natural antibodies in the activation of xenogenic endothelial cells. *Transplantation* 1991;52:1037–1043.
27. Platt JL, Holzknecht ZE, Lindman BJ. Porcine endothelial cell antigens recognized by human natural antibodies. *Transplant Proc* 1994;26:1387.
28. Platt JL, Lindman BJ, Chen H, Spitalnik SL, Bach FH. Endothelial cell antigens recognized by xenoreactive human natural antibodies. *Transplantation* 1990;50:817–822.

29. Cooper DK, Good AH, Koren E, et al. Identification of alpha-galactosyl and other carbohydrate epitopes that are bound by human anti-pig antibodies: relevance to discordant xenografting in man. *Transpl Immunol* 1993;1:198–205.

30. Cooper DK, Koren E, Oriol R. Oligosaccharides and discordant xenotransplantation. *Immunol Rev* 1994;141:31–58.

31. Galili U. Evolution and pathophysiology of the human natural anti-alpha- galactosyl IgG (anti-Gal) antibody. Springer Semin Immunopathol 1993; 15:155–171.

32. Galili U. Interaction of the natural anti-Gal antibody with alpha-galactosyl epitopes: a major obstacle for xenotransplantation in humans. *Immunol Today* 1993;14(10):480–482.

33. Galili U, Macher BA, Buehler J, Shohet SB. Human natural anti-alpha-galactosyl IgG. II. The specific recognition of alpha (1-3)-linked galactose residues. *J Exp Med* 1985; 162:573–582.

34. Galili U, Shohet SB, Kobrin E, Stults CL, Macher BA. Man, apes, and Old World monkeys differ from other mammals in the expression of alpha-galactosyl epitopes on nucleated cells. *J Biol Chem* 1988;263:17755–17762.

35. Buonomano R, Tinguely C, Rieben R, Mohacsi PJ, Nydegger UE. Quantitation and characterization of anti-Galalpha1-3Gal antibodies in sera of 200 healthy persons. *Xenotransplant* 1999;6(3):173–180.

36. Diaz I, Veira P, Valdes F, Alonso C, Sanchez P. Quantitation and comparison of anti-Gal-alpha-1,3-Gal antibodies in sera of healthy individuals and patients waiting for kidney transplantation. *Transplant Proc* 2003;35(5):2043–2044.

37. Taniguchi S, Neethling FA, Korchagina EY, et al. In vivo immunoadsorption of antipig antibodies in baboons using a specific Gal(alpha)1-3Gal column. *Transplantation* 1996;62(10):1379–1384.

38. Cooper DKC, Koren E, Oriol R. Manipulation of the anti-aGal antibody-aGal epitope system in experimental discordant xenotransplantation. *Xenotransplant* 1996;3(1):102–111.

39. Dalmasso AP, Vercellotti GM, Platt JL, Bach FH. Inhibition of complement-mediated endothelial cell cytotoxicity by decay-accelerating factor. Potential for prevention of xenograft hyperacute rejection. *Transplantation* 1991;52:530–533.

40. Davis EA, Pruitt SK, Greene PS, et al. Inhibition of complement, evoked antibody, and cellular response prevents rejection of pig-to-primate cardiac xenografts. *Transplantation* 1996;62(7):1018–1023.

41. Pruitt SK, Bollinger RR, Collins BH, et al. Effect of continuous complement inhibition using soluble complement receptor type 1 on survival of pig-to-primate cardiac xenografts. *Transplantation* 1997;63:900–902.

42. Bhatti FN, Schmoeckel M, Zaidi A, et al. Three-month survival of HDAFF transgenic pig hearts transplanted into primates. *Transplant Proc* 1999;31(1–2):958.

43. White DJG. hDAF transgenic pig organs: are they concordant for human transplantation? *Xeno* 1996;4(3):50–54.

44. Bach FH, Winkler H, Ferran C, Hancock WW, Robson SC. Delayed xenograft rejection. *Immunol Today* 1996;17(8):379–384.

45. Chen D, Cao R, Guo H, et al. Pathogenesis and pathology of delayed xenograft rejection in pig-to-rhesus monkey cardiac transplantation. *Transplant Proc* 2004;36(8):2480–2482.

46. Ierino FL, Kozlowski T, Siegel JB, et al. Disseminated intravascular coagulation in association with the delayed rejection of pig-to-baboon renal xenografts. *Transplantation* 1998;66(11):1439–1450.

47. Candinas D, Belliveau S, Koyamada N, et al. T cell independence of macrophage and natural killer cell infiltration, cytokine production, and endothelial activation during delayed xenograft rejection. *Transplantation* 1996;62:1920–1927.

48. Dorling A, Lombardi G, Binns R, Lechler RI. Detection of primary direct and indirect human anti-porcine T cell responses using a porcine dendritic cell population. *Eur J Immunol* 1996;26(6):1378–1387.

49. Garrovillo M, Ali A, Oluwole SF. Indirect allorecognition in acquired thymic tolerance: induction of donor-specific tolerance to rat cardiac

allografts by allopeptide-pulsed host dendritic cells. *Transplantation* 1999;68(12):1827–1834.

50. Yamada K, Sachs DH, DerSimonian H. Human anti-porcine xenogeneic T cell response. Evidence for allelic specificity of MLR and for both direct and indirect pathways of recognition. *J Immunol* 1995;155(11):5249–5256.

51. Baker RJ, Hernandez-Fuentes MP, Brookes PA, et al. Loss of direct and maintenance of indirect alloresponses in renal allograft recipients: implications for the pathogenesis of chronic allograft nephropathy. *J Immunol* 2001;167(12):7199–7206.

52. Moses RD, Pierson RN, III, Winn HJ, Auchincloss H, Jr. Xenogeneic proliferation and lymphokine production are dependent on CD4$^+$ helper T cells and self antigen-presenting cells in the mouse. *J Exp Med* 1990;172:567–575.

53. Auchincloss H, Jr., Lee R, Shea S, Markowitz JS, Grusby MJ, Glimcher LH. The role of "indirect" recognition in initiating rejection of skin grafts from major histocompatibility complex class II-deficient mice. *Proc Natl Acad Sci USA* 1993;90(8):3373–3377.

54. Moses RD, Winn HJ, Auchincloss H Jr. Evidence that multiple defects in cell-surface molecule interactions across species differences are responsible for diminished xenogeneic T cell responses. *Transplantation* 1992;53:203–209.

55. Alter BJ, Bach FH. Cellular basis of the proliferative response of human T cells to mouse xenoantigens. *J Exp Med* 1990;171:333–338.

56. Dorling A, Binns R, Lechler RI. Cellular xenoresponses: Observation of significant primary indirect human T cell anti-pig xenoresponses using co-stimulator-deficient or SLA class II-negative porcine stimulators. *Xenotransplant* 1996;3:112–119.

57. Yamada K, Sachs DH, DerSimonian H. Direct and indirect recognition of pig class II antigens by human T cells. *Transplant Proc* 1995;27:258–259.

58. Chan DV, Auchincloss HJr. Human anti-pig cell-mediated cytotoxicity in vitro involves non-T as well as T cell components. *Xenotransplant* 1996;3:158–165.

59. Kumagai-Braesch M, Satake M, Korsgren O, Andersson A, Moller E. Characterization of cellular human anti-porcine xenoreactivity. *Clin Transpl* 1993;7:273–280.

60. Yamada K, Seebach JD, DerSimonian H, Sachs DH. Human anti-pig T-cell mediated cytotoxicity. *Xenotransplant* 1996;3:179–187.

61. Kirk AD, Li RA, Kinch MS, Abernethy KA, Doyle C, Bollinger RR. The human antiporcine cellular repertoire. In vitro studies of acquired and innate cellular responsiveness. Transplantation 1993; 55:924–31X.

62. Häyry P, Isoniemi H, Yilmaz S, et al. Chronic allograft rejection. *Immunological Rev* 1993;134:33–80.

63. Paul LC. Chronic renal transplant loss. Kidney Int 1995; 47:1491-1499.

64. Tullius SG, Tilney NL. Both alloantigen-dependent and -independent factors influence chronic allograft rejection. *Transplantation* 1995;59:313–318.

65. Baid S, Saidman SL, Tolkoff-Rubin N, et al. Managing the highly sensitized transplant recipient and B cell tolerance. *Curr Opin Immunol* 2001;13(5):577–581.

66. Womer KL, Stone JR, Murphy B, Chandraker A, Sayegh MH. Indirect allorecognition of donor class I and II major histocompatibility complex peptides promotes the development of transplant vasculopathy. *J Am Soc Nephrol* 2001;12(11):2500–2506.

67. Crespo M, Pascual M, Tolkoff-Rubin N, et al. Acute humoral rejection in renal allograft recipients: I. Incidence, serology and clinical characteristics. *Transplantation* 2001; 71(5):652–658.

68. Russell PS, Chase CM, Winn HJ, Colvin RB. Coronary atherosclerosis in transplanted mouse hearts. II. Importance of humoral immunity. *J Immunol* 1994;152:5135–5141.

69. Gupta P, Hart J, Cronin D, et al. Risk factors for chronic rejection after pediatric liver transplantation. *Transplantation* 2001;72(6):1098–1102.

70. Randhawa PS, Magnone M, Jordan M, et al. Renal allograft involvement by Epstein-Barr virus associated post- transplant lymphoproliferative disease. *Am J Surg Pathol* 1996; 20(5):563–571.

71. Walker RC, Paya CV, Marshall WF, et al. Pretransplantation sero-negative Epstein-Barr virus status is the primary risk factor for post-transplantation lymphoproliferative disorder in adult heart, lung, and other solid organ transplantations. *J Heart Lung Transplant* 1995;14(2):214–221.

72. Williams MA, Tan JT, Adams AB, et al. Characterization of virus-mediated inhibition of mixed chimerism and allospecific tolerance. *J Immunol* 2001;167(9):4987–4995.

73. Alwayn IPJ, Xu Y, Basker M, et al. Effects of specific anti-B and/or anti-plasma cell immunotherapy on antibody production in baboons: depletion of CD20- and CD22-positive B cells does not result in significantly decreased production of anti-alphaGal antibody. *Xenotransplant* 2001;8(3):157–171.

74. Buhler L, Yamada K, Kitamura H, et al. Pig kidney transplantation in baboons: anti-Gal(alpha)1-3Gal IgM alone is associated with acute humoral xenograft rejection and disseminated intravascular coagulation. *Transplantation* 2001;72(11):1743–1752.

75. Cooper DKC, Cairns TDH, Taube DH. Extracorporeal immunoadsorption of alphaGal antibodies. *Xeno* 1996;4(2):27–29.

76. Galili U. Anti-alpha galactosyl (anti-Gal) antibody damage beyond hyperacute rejection. In: Cooper DKC, Kemp E, Platt JL, White DJG, eds. *Xenotransplantation*. Heidelberg: Springer; 1997:95–103.

77. Kozlowski T, Ierino FL, Lambrigts D, et al. Depletion of anti-Gal(alpha)1-3 Gal antibody in baboons by specific alpha-Gal immunoaffinity columns. *Xenotransplant* 1998;5(2):122–131.

78. Xu Y, Lorf T, Sablinski T, Gianello P, Bailin M, Monroy R et al. Removal of anti-porcine natural antibodies from human and nonhuman primate plasma in vitro and in vivo by a Galalpha1-3Gbeta1-4beta-Glc-X immunoaffinity column. *Transplantation* 1998;65(2):172–179.

79. Alwayn IP, Basker M, Buhler L, Cooper DK. The problem of anti-pig antibodies in pig-to-primate xenografting: current and novel methods of depletion and/or suppression of production of anti-pig antibodies. *Xenotransplant* 1999;6(3):157–168.

80. Lambrigts D, Van Calster P, Xu Y, et al. Pharmacologic immunosuppressive therapy and extracorporeal immunoadsorption in the suppression of anti-alphaGal antibody in the baboon. *Xenotransplant* 1998;5(4):274–283.

81. Simon PM, Neethling FA, Taniguchi S, et al. Intravenous infusion of Galalpha1-3Gal oligosaccharides in baboons delays hyperacute rejection of porcine heart xenografts. *Transplantation* 1998;65(3):346–353.

82. Ye Y, Neethling FA, Niekrasz M, Koren E, Richards SV, Martin M et al. Evidence that intravenously administered alpha-galactosyl carbohydrates reduce baboon serum cytotoxicity to pig kidney cells (PK15) and transplanted pig hearts. *Transplantation* 1994;58(3):330–337.

83. Brewer RJ, Del Rio MJ, Roslin MS, et al. Depletion of preformed antibody in primates for discordant xenotransplantation by continuous donor organ plasma perfusion. *Transplant Proc* 1993;25:385–386.

84. Kroshus TJ, Dalmasso AP, Leventhal JR, et al. Antibody removal by column immunoabsorption prevents tissue injury in an ex vivo model of pig-to-human xenograft hyperacute rejection. *J Surg Res* 1995;59(1):43–50.

85. Appel JZ, III, Alwayn IP, Buhler L, et al. Modulation of platelet aggregation in baboons: implications for mixed chimerism in xenotransplantation. I. The roles of individual components of a transplantation conditioning regimen and of pig peripheral blood progenitor cells. *Transplantation* 2001;72(7):1299–1305.

86. Basker M, Alwayn IPJ, Buhler L, et al. Clearance of mobilized porcine peripheral blood progenitor cells is delayed by depletion of the phagocytic reticuloendothelial system in baboons. *Transplantation* 2001;72(7):1278–1285.

87. Kobayashi T, Taniguchi S, Neethling FA, et al. Delayed xenograft rejection of pig-to-baboon cardiac transplants after cobra venom factor therapy. *Transplantation* 1997;64:1255–1261.

88. Scheringa M, Schraa EO, Bouwman E, et al. Prolongation of survival of guinea pig heart grafts in cobra venom factor-treated rats by splenectomy. No additional effect of cyclosporine. *Transplantation* 1995;60(11):1350–1353.

89. Heckl-Östreicher B, Wosnik A, Kirschfink M. Protection of porcine endothelial cells from complement- mediated cytotoxicity by the human complement regulators CD59, C1 inhibitor, and soluble complement receptor type 1—Analysis in a pig-to-human in vitro model relevant to hyperacute xenograft rejection. *Transplantation* 1996;62:1693–1696.

90. Lam TT, Hausen B, Hook L, Lau M, et al. The effect of soluble complement receptor type 1 on acute humoral xenograft rejection in hDAF-transgenic pig-to-primate life-supporting kidney xenografts. *Xenotransplant* 2005;12(1):20–29.

91. Pruitt SK, Kirk AD, Bollinger RR, et al. The effect of soluble complement receptor type 1 on hyperacute rejection of porcine xenografts. *Transplantation* 1994;57(3):363–370.

92. Weisman HF, Bartow T, Leppo MK, et al. Soluble human complement receptor type 1: in vivo inhibitor of complement suppressing post-ischemic myocardial inflammation and necrosis. *Science* 1990;249(4965):146–151.

93. Basker M, Buhler L, Alwayn IP, Appel JZ, III, Cooper DK. Pharmacotherapeutic agents in xenotransplantation. *Expert Opin Pharmacother* 2000;1(4):757–769.

94. Buhler L, Yamada K, Alwayn I, et al. Miniature swine and hDAF pig kidney transplantation in baboons treated with a nonmyeloablative regimen and CD154 blockade. *Transplant Proc* 2001;33(1-2):716.

95. Gorelik E, Duty L, Anaraki F, Galili U. Alterations of cell surface carbohydrates and inhibition of metastatic property of murine melanomas by alpha 1,3 galactosyltransferase gene transfection. *Cancer Res* 1995; 55:4168–4173.

96. Gustafsson K, Strahan K, Preece A. Alpha 1,3galactosyltransferase: a target for in vivo genetic manipulation in xenotransplantation. *Immunol Rev* 1994;141:59–70.

97. Strahan KM, Gu F, Andersson L, Gustafsson K. Pig alpha 1, 3galactosyltransferase: sequence of a full-length cDNA clone, chromosomal localisation of the corresponding gene, and inhibition of expression in cultured pig endothelial cells. *Transplant Proc* 1995;27:245–246.

98. Sandrin MS, Fodor WL, Mouhtouris E, et al. Enzymatic remodelling of the carbohydrate surface of a xenogenic cell substantially reduces human antibody binding and complement- mediated cytolysis [see comments]. *Nat Med* 1995;1:1261–1267.

99. Chen CG, Salvaris EJ, Romanella M, et al. Transgenic expression of human a1,2-fucosyltransferase (H-transferase) prolongs mouse heart survival in an ex vivo model of xenograft rejection. *Transplantation* 1998;65(6):832–837.

100. Cowan PJ, Chen CG, Shinkel TA, et al. Knock out of a1,3-galactosyltransferase or expression of a1,2-fucosyltransferase further protects CD55- and CD59-expressing mouse hearts in an ex vivo model of xenograft rejection. *Transplantation* 1998;65(12):1599–1604.

101. Sepp A, Skacel P, Lindstedt R, Lechler RI. Expression of a-1,3-galactose and other type 2 oligosaccharide structures in a porcine endothelial cell line transfected with human a-1,2-fucosyltransferase cDNA. *J Biol Chem* 1997;272:23104–23110.

102. Sharma A, Okabe J, Birch P, et al. Reduction in the level of Gal(a1,3)Gal in transgenic mice and pigs by the expression of an a(1, 2)fucosyltransferase. *Proc Natl Acad Sci USA* 1996; 93:7190–7195.

103. Wilmut I, Schnieke AE, McWhir J, Kind AJ, Campbell KH. Viable offspring derived from fetal and adult mammalian cells. *Nature* 1997;385(6619):810–813.

104. Dai Y, Vaught TD, Boone J, et al. Targeted disruption of the alpha1,3-galactosyltransferase gene in cloned pigs. *Nat Biotechnol* 2002;20(3):251–255.

105. Dor FJ, Tseng YL, Cheng J, et al. alpha1,3-Galactosyltransferase gene-knockout miniature swine produce natural cytotoxic anti-Gal antibodies. *Transplantation* 2004;78(1):15–20.

106. Kolber-Simonds D, Lai L, Watt SR, et al. Production of {alpha}-1,3-galactosyltransferase null pigs by means of nuclear transfer with fibroblasts bearing loss of heterozygosity mutations. *Proc Natl Acad Sci USA* 2004;101(19):7335–7340.

107. Lai L, Kolber-Simonds D, Park K, et al. Production of -1,3-Galactosyltransferase Knockout Pigs by Nuclear Transfer Cloning. *Science* 2002;295(5557):1089–1092.

108. Phelps CJ, Koike C, Vaught TD, et al. Production of alpha 1,3-galactosyltransferase-deficient pigs. *Science* 2003;299(5605): 411–414.

109. Yamada K, Yazawa K, Shimizu A, et al. Marked prolongation of porcine renal xenograft survival in baboons through the use of alpha1,3-galactosyltransferase gene-knockout donors and the cotransplantation of vascularized thymic tissue. *Nat Med* 2005;11(1):32–34.

110. Kuwaki K, Tseng YL, Dor FJ, et al. Heart transplantation in baboons using alpha1,3-galactosyltransferase gene-knockout pigs as donors: initial experience. *Nat Med* 2005;11(1):29–31.

111. Minanov OP, Itescu S, Neethling FA, et al. Anti-Gal IgG antibodies in sera of newborn humans and baboons and its significance in pig xenotransplantation. *Transplantation* 1997;63(2):182–186.

112. Teranishi K, Manez R, Awwad M, Cooper DK. Anti-Galalpha1-3Gal IgM and IgG antibody levels in sera of humans and old world non-human primates. *Xenotransplant* 2002;9(2):148–154.

113. Grewal IS, Flavell RA. CD40 and CD154 in cell-mediated immunity. *Annu Rev Immunol* 1998;16:111–135.

114. Kawai T, Andrews D, Colvin RB, Sachs DH, Cosimi AB. Thromboembolic complications after treatment with monoclonal antibody against CD40 ligand [In Process Citation]. *Nat Med* 2000 Feb;6(2):114 2000;6(2):114.

115. Knosalla C, Ryan DJ, Moran K, et al. Initial experience with the human anti-human CD154 monoclonal antibody, ABI793, in pig-to-baboon xenotransplantation. *Xenotransplant* 2004;11(4):353–360.

116. Sun H, Subbotin V, Chen C, et al. Prevention of chronic rejection in mouse aortic allografts by combined treatment with CTLA4-Ig and anti-CD40 ligand monoclonal antibody. *Transplantation* 1997;64(12):1838–1843.

117. Kärre K. Express yourself or die: Peptides, MHC molecules, and NK cells. *Science* 1995; 267:978–979.

118. Lanier LL. NK cell receptors. *Annu Rev Immunol* 1998;16:359–393.

119. Ruggeri L, Capanni M, Mancusi A, et al. Natural killer cell alloreactivity in haploidentical hematopoietic stem cell transplantation. *Int J Hematol* 2005; 81(1):13–17.

120. Velardi A, Ruggeri L, Alessandro, Moretta, Moretta L. NK cells: a lesson from mismatched hematopoietic transplantation. *Trends Immunol* 2002;23(9):438–444.

121. Young NT. Immunobiology of natural killer lymphocytes in transplantation. *Transplantation* 2004;78(1):1–6.

122. Münz C, Holmes N, King A, et al. Human histocompatibility leukocyte antigen (HLA)-G molecules inhibit NKAT3 expressing natural killer cells. *J Exp Med* 1997;185:385–391.

123. Benda B, Karlsson-Parra A, Ridderstad A, Korsgren O. Xenograft rejection of porcine islet-like cell clusters in immunoglobulin- or Fc-receptor gamma-deficient mice. *Transplantation* 1996;62:1207–1211.

124. Barth RN, Yamamoto S, LaMattina JC, et al. Xenogeneic thymokidney and thymic tissue transplantation in a pig-to-baboon model: I. Evidence for pig-specific T cell unresponsiveness. *Transplantation* 2003;75(10):1615–1624.

125. Garcia B, Sun HT, Yang HJ, Chen G, Zhong R. Xenotransplantation of human decay accelerating factor transgenic porcine kidney to non-human primates: 4 years experience at a Canadian center. *Transplant Proc* 2004;36(6):1714–1716.

126. Hammer C. Immunosuppression in xenotransplantation. *Transplant Proc* 1996;28:3017–3020.

127. Kozlowski T, Shimizu A, Lambrigts D, et al. Porcine kidney and heart transplantation in baboons undergoing a tolerance induction regimen and antibody adsorption. *Transplantation* 1999;67(1):18–30.

128. Appel JZ, III, Alwayn IP, Correa LE, Cooper DK, Robson SC. Modulation of platelet aggregation in baboons: Implications for mixed chimerism in xenotransplantation. II. The effect of cyclophospamide on pig peripheral blood progenitor cell-induced aggregation. *Transplantation* 2001;72(7):1306–1310.

129. Lan P, Wang L, Diouf B, et al. Induction of human T cell tolerance to porcine xenoantigens through mixed hematopoietic chimerism. *Blood* 2004.

130. Smith RM, Mandel TE. Pancreatic islet xenotransplantation: the potential for tolerance induction. *ImmunolToday* 2000;21(1):42–48.

131. Sykes M, Sachs DH. Xenogeneic tolerance through hematopoietic cell and thymic transplantation. In: Cooper DKC, Kemp E, Platt JL, White DJG, eds. *Xenotransplantation*. New York: Springer-Verlag; 1997:496–518.

132. Arnold B, Schonrich G, Hammerling GJ. Induction of tolerance in mature peripheral T cells. *Exp Nephrol* 1993;1:72–77.

133. Bhattacharyya S, Chawla A, Smith K, et al. Multilineage engraftment with minimal graft-versus-host disease following in utero transplantation of S-59 psoralen/ultraviolet a light-treated, sensitized T cells and adult T cell-depleted bone marrow in fetal mice. *J Immunol* 2002;169(11):6133–6140.

134. Burkly LC, Lo D, Flavell RA. Tolerance in transgenic mice expressing major histocompatibility molecules extrathymically on pancreatic cells. *Science* 1990;248:1364–1368.

135. Colson YL, Wren SM, Schuchert MJ, et al. A nonlethal conditioning approach to achieve durable multilineage mixed chimerism and tolerance across major, minor, and hematopoietic histocompatibility barriers. *J Immunol* 1995;155(9):4179–4188.

136. Colson YL, Schuchert MJ, Ildstad ST. The abrogation of allosensitization following the induction of mixed allogeneic chimerism. *J Immunol* 2000;165(2):637–644.

137. Eto M, Kong YY, Uozumi J, Naito S, Nomoto K. Importance of intrathymic mixed chimerism for the maintenance of skin allograft tolerance across fully allogeneic antigens in mice. *Immunology* 1999;96(3): 440–446.

138. Hoffmann MW, Allison J, Miller JF. Tolerance induction by thymic medullary epithelium. *Proc Natl Acad Sci USA* 1992;89(7): 2526–2530.

139. Ito H, Kurtz J, Shaffer J, Sykes M. CD4 T cell-mediated alloresistance to fully MHC-mismatched allogeneic bone marrow engraftment is dependent on CD40-CD40 ligand interactions, and lasting T cell tolerance is induced by bone marrow transplantation with initial blockade of this pathway. J Immunol 2001; 166(5):2970–2981.

140. Marrack P, Lo D, Brinster R, Palmiter R, Burkly L, Flavell RH et al. The effect of thymus environment on T cell development and tolerance. *Cell* 1988;53:627–634.

141. Tomita Y, Khan A, Sykes M. Role of intrathymic clonal deletion and peripheral anergy in transplantation tolerance induced by bone marrow transplantion in mice conditioned with a non-myeloablative regimen. *J Immunol* 1994;153:1087–1098.

142. Nikolic B, Gardner JP, Scadden DT, et al. Normal development in porcine thymus grafts and specific tolerance of human T cells to porcine donor MHC. *J Immunol* 1999;162(6):3402–3407.

143. Rodriguez-Barbosa JI, Zhao Y, Zhao G, Ezquerra A, Sykes M. Murine CD4 T cells selected in a highly disparate xenogeneic porcine thymus graft do not show rapid decay in the absence of selecting MHC in the periphery. *J Immunol* 2002;169(12):6697–6710.

144. Kozlowski T, Monroy R, Xu Y, et al. Anti-a Gal antibody response to porcine bone marrow in unmodified baboons and baboons conditioned for tolerance induction. *Transplantation* 1998;66(2):176–182.

145. Kozlowski T, Monroy R, Giovino M, et al. Effect of pig-specific cytokines on mobilization of hematopoietic progenitor cells in pigs and on pig bone marrow engraftment in baboons. *Xenotransplant* 1999; 6(1):17–27.

146. Kozlowski T, Monroy R, Giovino M, et al. Effect of pig-specific cytokines on mobilization of hematopoietic progenitor cells in pigs and on pig bone marrow engraftment in baboons. *Xenotransplantation* 1999; 6(1):17–27.

147. Bachar-Lustig E, Reich-Zeliger S, Gur H, et al. Bone marrow transplantation across major genetic barriers: the role of megadose stem cells and nonalloreactive donor anti-third party CTLS. *Transplant Proc* 2001;33(3):2099–2100.

148. Handgretinger R, Klingebiel T, Lang P, Gordon P, Niethammer D. Megadose transplantation of highly purified haploidentical stem cells: current results and future prospects. *Pediatr Transplant* 2003;7(Suppl 3): 51–55.

149. Rachamim N, Gan J, Segall H, et al. Tolerance induction by "megadose" hematopoietic transplants - Donor-type human CD34 stem cells induce potent specific reduction of host anti-donor cytotoxic T lymphocyte precursors in mixed lymphocyte culture. *Transplantation* 1998;65(10):1386–1393.

150. Reisner Y, Gur H, Reich-Zeliger S, Martelli MF, Bachar-Lustig E. Hematopoietic stem cell transplantation across major genetic barriers: tolerance induction by megadose CD34 cells and other veto cells. *Ann NY Acad Sci* 2003;996:72–79.

151. Ohdan H, Swenson KG, Kitamura H, Yang YG, Sykes M. Tolerization of Gal alpha 1,3Gal-reactive B cells in pre-sensitized alpha 1,3-galactosyltransferase-deficient mice by nonmyeloablative induction of mixed chimerism. *Xenotransplant* 2001;8(4):227–238.

152. Buhler L, Awwad M, Treter S, et al. Pig hematopoietic cell chimerism in baboons conditioned with a nonmyeloablative regimen and CD154 blockade. *Transplantation* 2002;73(1):12–22.

153. Tseng YL, Dor FJ, Kuwaki K, et al. Bone marrow transplantation from alpha1,3-galactosyltransferase gene-knockout pigs in baboons. *Xenotransplant* 2004;11(4):361–370.

154. Wu A, Yamada K, Neville DM, Awwad M, Wain JC, Shimizu A et al. Xenogeneic thymus transplantation in a pig-to-baboon model. *Transplantation* 2003;75(3):282–291.

155. Kamano C, Vagefi PA, Kumagai N, et al. Vascularizecd thymic lobe transplantation in miniature swine: thymopoiesis and tolerance induction across fully MHC-mismatched barriers. Proc Natl Acad Sci U S A. 2004;101(11):3827–3832.

156. Kuwaki K, Tseng YL, Dor FJ, et al. Heart transplantation in baboons using alpha1,3-galactosyltransferase gene-knockout pigs as donors: initial experience. *Nat Med* 2005;11(1):29–31.

157. Yamada K, Yazawa K, Shimizu A, et al. Marked prolongation of porcine renal xenograft survival in baboons through the use of alpha1,3-galactosyltransferase gene-knockout donors and the cotransplantation of vascularized thymic tissue. *Nat Med* 2005;11(1):32–34.

158. Robson SC, Schulte aE, Bach FH. Factors in xenograft rejection. *Ann NY Acad Sci* 1999;875:261–276.

159. Robson SC, Cooper DK, d'Apice AJ. Disordered regulation of coagulation and platelet activation in xenotransplantation. *Xenotransplantation* 2000;7(3):166–176.

160. Somerville CA, Kyriazis AG, McKenzie A, et al. Functional expression of human CD59 in transgenic mice. *Transplantation* 1994;58: 1430–1435.

161. Chen D, Weber M, McVey JH, et al. Complete inhibition of acute humoral rejection using regulated expression of membrane-tethered anticoagulants on xenograft endothelium. *Am J Transplant* 2004;4(12): 1958–1963.

162. Duquesnoy RJ, Howe J, Takemoto S. HLAmatchmaker: a molecularly based algorithm for histocompatibility determination. IV. An alternative strategy to increase the number of compatible donors for highly sensitized patients. *Transplantation* 2003;75(6):889–897.

163. Ramirez P, Chavez R, Majado M, et al. Life-supporting human complement regulator decay accelerating factor transgenic pig liver xenograft maintains the metabolic function and coagulation in the nonhuman primate for up to 8 days. *Transplantation* 2000;70(7): 989–998.

164. Rayat GR, Rajotte RV, Korbutt GS. Potential application of neonatal porcine islets as treatment for type 1 diabetes: a review. Ann N Y Acad Sci 1999; 875:175–188.

165. Schernthaner G. Immunogenicity and allergenic potential of animal and human insulins. *Diabetes Care* 1993;16 (Suppl 3):155–165.

166. Rayat GR, Gill RG. Pancreatic islet xenotransplantation: barriers and prospects. *Curr Diab Rep* 2003;3(4):336–343.

167. Korsgren O, Buhler LH, Groth CG. Toward clinical trials of islet xenotransplantation. *Xenotransplant* 2003;10(4):289–292.

168. Matsumoto S, Okitsu T, Iwanaga Y, et al. Insulin independence after living-donor distal pancreatectomy and islet allotransplantation. *Lancet* 2005;365(9471):1642–1644.

169. Fishman JA. Miniature swine as organ donors for man: Strategies for prevention of xenotransplant-associated infections. *Xenotransplant* 1994;1:47–57.

170. Michaels MG, Simmons RL. Xenotransplant-associated zoonoses. Strategies for prevention. *Transplantation* 1994;57:1–7.

171. Patience C, Takeuchi Y, Weiss RA. Infection of human cells by an endogenous retrovirus of pigs. *Nat Med* 1997;3(3):282–286.

172. Dinsmore JH, Manhart C, Raineri R, Jacoby DB, Moore A. No evidence for infection of human cells with porcine endogenous retrovirus (PERV) after exposure to porcine fetal neuronal cells. *Transplantation* 2000;70(9):1382–1389.

173. Karlas A, Kurth R, Denner J. Inhibition of porcine endogenous retroviruses by RNA interference: increasing the safety of xenotransplantation. *Virology* 2004;325(1):18–23.

174. Le Tissier P, Stoye JP, Takeuchi Y, Patience C, Weiss RA. Two sets of human-tropic pig retrovirus. *Nature* 1997;389:681–682.

175. Martin U, Kiessig V, Blusch JH, Haverich A, Von der H, Herden T et al. Expression of pig endogenous retrovirus by primary porcine endothelial cells and infection of human cells. *Lancet* 1998;352(9129): 692–694.

176. Paradis K, Langford G, Long Z, et al. Search for cross-species transmission of porcine endogenous retrovirus in patients treated with living pig tissue. *Science* 1999;285(5431):1236–1241.

177. Takeuchi Y, Patience C, Magre S, et al. Host range and interference studies of three classes of pig endogenous retrovirus. *J Virol* 1998;72(12):9986–9991.

178. Bartholomew A, Latinne D, Sachs DH, et al. Utility of xenografts; lack of correlation between PRA and natural antibodies to swine. *Xenotransplant* 1997;4:34–39.

179. Baertschiger RM, Dor FJ, Prabharasuth D, Kuwaki K, Cooper DK. Absence of humoral and cellular alloreactivity in baboons sensitized to pig antigens. *Xenotransplant* 2004;11(1):27–32.

180. Bloom ET. New FDA xenotransplantation documents: a proposed rule and a draft guidance. *Xenotransplantation* 2001;8(3):153–154.

181. Allan JS, Slisz JK, Vesga L, et al. Enhanced efficacy of repeated anti-CD8 monoclonal antibody therapy by high-dose cyclosporine treatment. *Transplant Proc* 1998;30(8):4062–4063.

182. Bourdage JS, Hamlin DM. Comparative polyclonal antithymocyte globulin and antilymphocyte/antilymphoblast globulin anti-CD antigen analysis by flow cytometry. *Transplantation* 1995;59(8): 1194–1200.

183. Costanzo MR, Koch DM, Fisher SG, Heroux AL, Kao WG, Johnson MR. Effects of methotrexate on acute rejection and cardiac allograft vasculopathy in heart transplant recipients. *J Heart Lung Transpl* 1997;16(2):169–178.

184. Delmonico FL, Cosimi AB, Colvin R, et al. Murine OKT4A immunosuppression in cadaver donor renal allograft recipients—A cooperative clinical trial in a transplantation pilot study. *Transplantation* 1997;63:1087–1095.

185. Haug CE, Colvin RB, Delmonico FL, et al. A phase I trial of immunosuppression with anti-ICAM-1 (CD54) mAb in renal allograft recipients. *Transplantation* 1993;55:766–72; discussion.

186. Isobe M, Suzuki J, Yagita H, et al. Immunosuppression to cardiac allografts and soluble antigens by anti-vascular cellular adhesion molecule-1 and anti-very late antigen-4 monoclonal antibodies. *J Immunol* 1994;153:5810–5818.

187. Knoll GA, Bell RC. Tacrolimus versus cyclosporin for immunosuppression in renal transplantation: meta-analysis of randomised trials. *BMJ* 1999;318(7191):1104–1107.

188. Matthews JB, Ramos E, Bluestone JA. Clinical trials of transplant tolerance: slow but steady progress. *Am J Transplant* 2003;3(7): 94–803.

189. Cretin N, Bracy J, Hanson K, Iacomini J. The role of T cell help in the production of antibodies specific for Gal alpha 1-3Gal. *J Immunol* 2002;168(3):1479–1483.

# CHAPTER 40

# GENE THERAPY

*Jonathan S. Bromberg, MD, Peter Boros, MD, Nan Zhang, PhD*

## INTRODUCTION

This chapter surveys developments, issues, and challenges in the field of gene transfer and gene therapy. Although gene therapy has received much attention and interest over the last decade for the treatment of a wide variety of diseases, there are numerous challenges that have so far prevented this modality from becoming a common clinical approach. Nonetheless, with the tremendous amount of ongoing investment in the field, it is anticipated that the challenges and hurdles will eventually be solved, and that administration and manipulation of genetic material will become common approaches in many fields of medicine, including solid organ transplantation. In a general sense, gene transfer and gene therapy have often been used as interchangeable terms to describe the introduction of novel genetic sequences into recipient cells, tissues, organs, or the entire individual. With the development of many new techniques and vectors, and with the increased understanding of genetic structures and changes, gene transfer, and gene therapy have broadened to include a variety of other considerations, including regulation of endogenous genes, repair or alteration of endogenous gene structure, and various types of genetic manipulations to enable cellular therapies with autologous or allogeneic cellular transplants.

The rationales for the application of gene transfer and gene therapy to solid organ transplantation are generally twofold. The first rationale is that gene transfer vectors can be administered to an organ to produce an immunosuppressive or tolerogenic milieu. Local immunosuppression may be able to avoid the side effects and toxicities associated with conventionally administered systemic immunosuppression. Local immunosuppression may also be able to interface directly with the immune system and alloantigen, thereby not interfering with the interaction of the immune system with other antigens, particularly with microbial antigens. Anatomically restricted, immunologically nonspecific immunosuppression confined to the allograft may result in a state that is functionally equivalent to antigen specific immunosuppression, and perhaps even result in antigen-specific tolerance.

The second major rationale for the application of gene transfer and gene therapy to solid organ transplantation is that genetic transfer may be performed on the back table of the operating room in an *ex vivo* and *in vitro* fashion. The ability to perform back-table transduction avoids many of the targeting problems that plague other applications in which gene transfer must take place *in vivo*. Thus, the vector does not need to be administered systemically. With anatomic targeting to a solid organ, such as through the artery or other tubular structures like the biliary tract or the ureter, the ability to deliver concentrated solutions of targeting vectors becomes straightforward, rather than rely on complicated and expensive targeting strategies with catheters, delivery vehicles, and specialized genetic constructs. Strong promiscuous promoters, rather than weaker cell-specific promoters, may be employed because there will not be systemic administration of the vector. Localized administration of vectors diminishes the toxicity and immunogenicity of systemic in vivo delivery. The validity of these two rationales will be considered in more detail below.

The separate sections of this chapter will cover the types of vectors that are currently available, their advantages and disadvantages, and what we may look forward to in the future. Regulation of gene expression is key to all of gene therapy and will be discussed from the standpoint of solid organ transplantation. Perhaps one of the most important facets of gene therapy and gene transfer is the fact that all vectors incite both innate and adaptive immune responses. The implications of these immune responses to solid organ transplantation and the response to alloantigens will be discussed. The broadening of the field of gene transfer, along with the development of new techniques, raise the possibility of many and varied gene delivery strategies to cells, tissues and organs. A greater understanding of immune reactivity and tolerance has generated many hypotheses for the best possible approaches to immunosuppression and tolerance in gene transfer. These approaches will be considered in the context of when, where, and which immunosuppressive genes to deliver.

## VECTORS

Vector structure and vector–host interaction are two important areas of development. The choice of vector is restricted by features such as immunogenicity and the size of insert, and also by therapeutic requirements such as persistence of gene expression and the type and location of cells that are targeted for transduction. As the limitations of certain vectors have become better understood, they have been strategically targeted to specific therapies, such as adenovirus for short-term gene expression or retroviruses for long-term expression. In addition to viral vectors, plasmid DNA can also be used to deliver genes to cells, either in its naked form or complexed with carrier agents such as liposomes.

So far no "ideal" vector yet exists. New technologies including small interfering RNA (siRNA), adenoassociated virus-inverted terminal-repeat (AAV ITR)-based plasmids, novel classes of lentivirus (EIAV, FIV), lentivirus-herpesvirus hybrids, and other vectors are in development. Their efficacies in transplantation remain to be tested.

## Viral Vectors

### Adenovirus

Adenoviral vectors are versatile. Their most important feature is the ability to generate high titers (up to $10^{12}$ pfu/mL) and to infect a broad range of cell types. Thus, the greatest number of *in vitro* and *in vivo* gene therapy experiments has been carried out with adenoviruses. The major limitations of these vectors are transient gene expression and high immunogenicity. Adenoviral-mediated transduction induces the production of a number of chemokines and their respective receptors in either solid organ or cellular grafts, resulting in subsequent recruitment of inflammatory cells and impairment of engraftment. The inflammatory response is dependent at least in part on the presence of expressed sequences in the vector backbone. Several strategies have succeeded in generating "gutless" adenoviral vectors, but it has been challenging to grow these vectors to high titer without the presence of contaminating helper virus.

### Adenoassociated Virus

Adenoassociated virus (AAV) vectors were first developed 20 years ago, and AAV vector was first administered to a human subject in November 1995. AAV vectors offer advantages over adenoviral vectors. The features of this human parvovirus that make it an attractive tool for gene therapy include persistent gene expression in episomal or genomic loci, lack of nonpathogenicity, that viral genes can be completely removed from the recombinant virus, and that replication is dependent on co-infection with a lytic helper virus so that reversion to replication-competent virus is an unlikely event. The barriers to AAV as a vector include limited tropism due to cell-surface receptors, proteasome-mediated degradation of vector, inefficiency of nuclear entry and conversion to double-stranded DNA, small capacity, and inefficient stable integration of vector DNA in a form that will persist within the target cell population. Novel approaches to overcome these barriers have included the introduction of new AAV serotypes, capsid mutants, proteasome inhibitors, self-complementary AAV vectors, double-stranded AAV vectors, tyrosine phosphatase inhibitors, and AAV-Rep-mediated site-specific integration. Its small packaging capacity has led to the development of dual vectors. In this strategy, components of the transcription regulatory unit or the transgene itself are split into two parts and packaged into two independent AAV vectors that are delivered simultaneously to target cells, leading to the reconstruction of intact expression cassettes through inverted terminal repeat mediated intermolecular concatamerization. So far at least 11 different AAV vectors have now entered into clinical trials for *in vivo* delivery for different diseases.

### Retrovirus

Retroviral vectors, derived from lipid-enveloped particles containing two identical copies of a linear single-stranded RNA genome of around 711 kb, were among the earliest vectors in gene therapy models. They have been used for stable gene transfer into mammalian cells for more than 20 years. Vectors based on the Moloney murine leukemia virus (MuLV) have been pivotal in thousands of experiments and continue to constitute the best tool available for stable gene transfer into a number of cell types and applications. They easily infect replicating cells and integrate into the host genome. Actively replicating immune cells, especially T cells, while highly resistant to transfection by most other vectors, were among the first cell types to be transduced by retroviruses.

A serious concern over retroviral vector use is the risk of insertional mutagenesis, in which the ectopic chromosomal integration of viral DNA either disrupts the expression of a tumor suppressor gene or activates an oncogene, leading to the malignant transformation of cells. This is evidenced in an MuLV-based clinical trial for X-linked severe combined immunodeficiency, in which 3 of 11 treated children developed a type of T-cell leukemia, resulting in one death. The large-scale production of retroviral vectors for clinical applications also faces challenges such as high titer vector production and the generation of replication-competent particles. Improving vector designs through strategies for cell targeting, regulated and tissue-specific expression, modulating transgene expression and silencing, and controlling immune responses to the transgene products constitutes important issues that must be resolved if retroviral vectors are to be widely applied in clinical transplantation.

### Lentivirus

Lentiviruses are members of the retroviral family but can infect cells at both mitotic and postmitotic stages of the cell cycle, thus creating the possibility of targeting nondividing cells for stable gene expression. The best characterized lentiviral vector system is based on the human immunodeficiency virus type 1 (HIV-1). HIV-1-based vectors have been widely used recently in preclinical trials and for *in vitro* genetic manipulation studies. However, safety concerns preclude the use of HIV-1-derived vectors in clinical trials. Nonprimate lentiviruses, such as feline immunodeficiency virus (FIV), equine infectious anemia virus (EIAV), and Visna-Maedi virus (VMV), are currently undergoing active development. Lentiviral vectors offer low to no immunogenecity, but their target cell range is limited and the titers are significantly lower compared to adenovirus. Targeting has been improved by the incorporation of heterologous envelope proteins onto lentiviral cores, in order to combine the specific tropisms of envelope glycoproteins with the biological properties of lentiviral vectors.

### Nonviral Vectors

Non-viral-mediated gene transfer commonly refers to direct administration of naked plasmid DNA or transfection of cells by DNA in complex with various cationic polymers. Nonviral vectors are non- or low-immunogenicity and are easy to produce in large quantities amenable to rigid quality control. However, plasmid DNA-mediated gene transfer is of low efficiency. To improve DNA uptake by cells or tissue, a number of innovations has been developed including the use of electroporation, gene guns, diverse liposomal formulations, or basic proteins and polymers, such as polyethylenimine, in complex with DNA prior to gene delivery. Cationic liposomes are artificial membrane vesicles that can complex with DNA. The resulting liposome–DNA complex is thought to fuse with the negatively charged plasma membrane or become endocytosed, resulting in gene delivery to the nucleus. Cationic peptides consist either of consecutive basic amino acids, for example, polylysine, which compact DNA into spherical complexes, or of chromatin components such as histones or protamine, which compact DNA in a structured manner. Polyethylenimine is either a linear or a branched polymer that has high cationic charge to allow stable complex with DNA and contains many amino nitrogen groups that, after cell entry, attract abundant protons and cause osmotic swelling and rupture of endosome to release polyethylenimine–DNA complexes into the cytoplasm. Such complexes enter target cells by their interaction with sulfated membrane-bound proteoglycans.

Naked recombinant DNA plasmid can be generated at considerably lower cost compared to viral vectors. Newer generation plasmid vectors have been designed to have a low immunogenic profile. Additionally, polycistronic vectors are easily constructed compared to viral vectors. Nonetheless, naked DNA cannot attain stable transgene persistence in transduced cells, and high concentrations are often required along with multiple dosings. Plasmid DNA vectors and naked DNA also evoke innate immune response via triggering Toll-like receptors (TLR), although this effect may be weaker compared to viral vectors.

### Antisense and RNA Interference

An antisense oligonucleotide is a single-stranded, chemically modified DNA-like molecule that is 17 to 22 nucleotides in length and designed to be complementary to the mRNA of a selected gene, thereby specifically inhibiting expression of that gene. Several mechanisms of action have been determined for antisense oligonucleotides. These include inhibition of transcription, inhibition of splicing, inhibition of mRNA maturation by prevention of 5'-cap formation and polyadenylation, and inhibition of ribosomal readthrough. Most importantly, antisense drugs hybridized with target RNA have been shown to serve as substrates for RNase H enzymes that cleave the RNA in DNA–RNA hybrids or RNA–RNA hybrids (as in RNA interference) and decrease mRNA levels of the target gene. Major problems with antisense include nonspecific effects and inefficient delivery to target cells.

There is increasing enthusiasm for developing therapies based on RNA interference (RNAi), a posttranscriptional gene-silencing mechanism mediated by small RNA duplexes of 19 to 23 base pairs. The major mechanisms of RNAi effects involve a two-step mechanism. In the first step, double-stranded RNA is processed into 21–23-nucleotide guide sequences. The guide RNAs are incorporated into a nuclease complex, called the RNA-induced silencing complex (RISC), which acts in the second effector step to destroy mRNAs that are recognized by the guide RNAs through base-pairing interactions. The mechanism of RNAi can be manipulated for inducing gene-specific silencing through administration of short interfering RNA (siRNA) and microRNA (miRNA). siRNA are short RNA duplexes that direct the degradation of homologous mRNA through the RNAi pathway. miRNA in contrast, are single-stranded RNAs that bind to partially complementary (50%–85%) 3' untranslated regions of mRNA leading to translational repression without target degradation. Both siRNA and miRNA are produced from longer double-stranded precursor RNA by the multidomain ribonuclease III enzyme Dicer. Dicer cleaves long dsRNAs approximately every 22, nucleotides yielding small duplexes containing 2 to 3 nucleotide overhangs, 5' phosphates, and free 3' hydroxyl-termini. Applying RNAi to mammalian systems, some vectors have been engineered to express short hairpin RNA (shRNA) that is processed into 21 nucleotide long siRNA-like molecules to trigger RNAi following transcription in target cells. The ability to stably express siRNA/shRNA in human cells using viral vectors raises the possibility of using RNAi to selectively inhibit the expression of disease-specific genes.

Many features of siRNA remain to be further defined, including metabolic stability, delivery approach, nonspecific or off-target effects, and immune stimulation through TLR signaling. Many approaches have been designed to increase stability and improve cellular delivery of siRNA, including complexes with atelocollagen, polyethyleneimine containing nanoparticles, lipid complexes, and covalent linkage to cholesterol.

### Regulation of Gene Expression

In the context of gene therapy, the persistent expression and imprecise regulation of the delivered gene could be harmful to the host. It is exceedingly important to tightly control the expression of transgenes in target cells. Such agents should be externally delivered drugs, natural compounds or, most preferably, factors that are indicative of the need for the gene product. In the context of transplantation, this could be inflammation or organ specific factors. The development of inducible expression systems in recent years has conferred the ability to control the timing and level of transgene expression and to minimize the systemic effects of the gene expression profile on the host. Existing gene expression regulatory systems comprise three components. One is an inducible promoter, which should ideally exhibit minimal transcription in potential target cells. A second component is a modulator-controlled transactivator, comprised of three domains: a DNA-binding domain that recognizes and binds unique cis elements in the inducible promoter, a transcription activation domain, and a site for the modulator to bind to. The final component is a modulator, which interacts with the transactivator to alter the ability of the latter to bind and activate the inducible promoter. The modulators are usually small molecules including antibiotics, hormone analogs, and metal ions.

A number of artificial regulation systems have been reported for the control of transgene expression, including tetracycline and its derivative doxycycline, the insect hormone ecdysone, the progesterone antagonist mifepristone, and rapamycin. The tetracycline-regulated transcription system has been the most studied for tight regulation of transgene expression for gene therapy applications. The rapamycin system has been engineered into AAV and successfully used in muscle and liver in preclinical trials.

## IMMUNE RESPONSES TO VECTORS

Immune responses against gene transfer vectors, a major challenge with all vector types, may eliminate the vector and the transfected cells, decreasing both the intensity and the duration of transgene expression. Furthermore, the immune response to vectors involves the production of proinflammatory cytokines and chemokines that may have harmful effects on the graft or recipient. The first immune response occurring after vector transfer emerges from the innate immune system. TLRs play a pivotal role in this innate response, recognizing pathogenic epitopes in the viral capsids or nucleic acids, leading to the production of proinflammatory cytokines and chemokines, nonspecific stimulation of the immune system, and an influx of nonspecific inflammatory cells (macrophages, NK cells, neutrophils) to the transduced tissues. Such responses are exuberant with adenovirus, but relatively minor with AAV. It is noteworthy that plasmid DNA vectors and siRNA also stimulate innate immunity via TLRs. Adaptive immunity is stimulated days or weeks later and includes humoral responses of B cells producing specific antibodies that neutralize vectors or transgene products and cell-mediated responses involving CD4 and CD8 T cells attacking transduced target cells. Adaptive immunity also results in a memory response that hinders further efforts to use the same vector or transgene. Some gene delivery parameters such as route of administration, dose, or promoter type are all critical factors influencing immunity to the vector.

## Innate Immunity

The innate immune system represents the first line of defense against invading pathogens. Vectors derived from viruses or bacterial plasmids carry many of the microbial features, which mammalian hosts consider as foreign, such as unusual nucleic acids, lipids, carbohydrates, and proteins. One of the principal functions of the innate immune system is pathogen recognition through the TLR family. TLR are mammalian homologs of Drosophila Toll receptors, expressed on the cell surface or in intracellular compartments. Distinct TLRs are key molecules in the selective recognition of different vector components. For example, viral envelope glycoproteins trigger TLR2 and TLR4, and CpG motifs, a characteristic feature of bacterial nucleic acids, are detected by TLR9. dsRNA stimulates TLR3, and ssRNA stimulates TLR7 and TLR8. TLR3, TLR7, and TLR8 are located in the endosomal compartment, which place them in an ideal position to recognize intracellular genetic invasion. Synthetic siRNAs formulated in nonviral delivery vehicles can be potent inducers of interferons and inflammatory cytokines, both *in vivo* in mice and *in vitro* in human blood. The immunostimulatory activity of formulated siRNAs and the associated toxicities are dependent on the nucleotide sequence.

The recognition of pathogen-associated molecular patterns by innate receptors triggers a series of events that serves to limit and eradicate infection or vectors. The intracellular signal transduction pathways of TLR3 and TLR9 promote transcription of genes regulated by NF-kB and mitogen-activated protein kinases (MAPKs), such as extracellular signal-regulated kinase (ERK) and p38 MAPK, resulting in the transcription of host proinflammatory cytokine and chemokine genes. These proinflammatory molecules play a direct role in clearing pathogens or vectors and recruiting effector leukocytes.

## Adaptive Immunity

### Cell-Mediated Immune Response

Adaptive immunity to viral vectors is induced by capsid proteins or by transgene products, inhibiting the intended therapeutic effect, and in the context of transplantation potentially causing damage to the target tissues. For example, expression of viral genes by first-generation adenoviral vectors results in an immune response specifically directed against the products of these genes. Gutless adenoviral vectors, which are devoid of viral genes, induce a weaker T-cell response. However, even in the absence of viral transcription, adenoviruses can induce a cytotoxic T-cell response as well as infiltration by CD4 and CD8 T cells. This response is due to the immunogenicity of adenoviral capsid proteins, which may result in elimination of the transduced cells that express the antigen. Immune mechanisms involve internalization by dendritic cells (DC) of capsid antigens which are then presented by class II MHC antigens, followed by priming and activation of CD4 T cells which in turn help CD8 T cell and B-cell responses. All viral vectors and many novel transgene products have the capacity to induce cell-mediated responses.

Viral vector tropisms to antigen-presenting cells (APC) are central to the induction of innate and adaptive immune responses. One of the major reasons adenovirus-induced immune responses are so prominent is the ability of these vectors to infect APCs such as DC and macrophages and inducing cytokines such as IL-6, IL-12, or TNF. Activated APCs then present viral antigens to CD4 and CD8 T cells, generating responses that clear the vector

and preclude its readministration. Adaptive cell-mediated immunity is weaker with AAV or other vectors because these vectors have markedly lower ability to efficiently infect APCs.

### Humoral Response

Administration of vectors, such as adenoviral or AAV, leads to presentation of the viral capsid antigens to CD4 T cells and B cells within lymph nodes, inducing differentiation of B cells to plasma cells. Neutralizing antibodies specific to viral capsid proteins can prevent infection by the vectors during subsequent gene therapy attempts. In humans, the problem is compounded by preexisting immunity against wild-type adenovirus or AAV, because hosts are frequently exposed to natural infections.

When creating new vectors and developing gene therapy strategies for transplantation, the consequences of antivector immunity must be kept in mind. Manipulation of the immune system to induce tolerance to the vector may deserve consideration, although the most satisfying approach will consist of developing vectors with little or no potential to induce an immune response.

## GENE THERAPY IN SOLID ORGAN TRANSPLANTATION

The introduction of potent immunosuppressive agents has reduced significantly the incidence of acute rejection and improved 1-year allograft survival rates to the current levels of 80% to 95% for kidney, heart, or liver transplants. Despite these positive developments, however, significant challenges remain in clinical transplantation. The lifelong treatment with nonspecific and toxic immunosuppressive medications is associated with serious complications including malignancy, infections, hyperlipidemia, and diabetes. Long-term allograft function may be compromised by both nonimmune mechanisms (eg, ischemia/reperfusion injury or drug toxicity) as well as immune-mediated events such as chronic allograft rejection. By allowing cell-specific manipulation and alteration of the graft's local milieu, gene therapy provides an opportunity to intercede at the molecular level, and address some of these existing challenges in transplantation.

A unique opportunity in transplantation compared to other fields of medicine is that genetic modification can be performed *ex vivo*, resulting in localized expression of the gene of interest, while minimizing systemic hazards. Preclinical transplant models support the idea that gene therapy can improve allograft function and survival. Some of these strategies are aimed to mitigate inflammation, while most are primarily designed to achieve immunosuppression. Immunosuppression can be attained by altering the immunogeneic properties of the graft, by interfering with antigen recognition pathways, or by targeting antibody production and complement. The long-term function of allografts may also be improved by genetic modifications (Table 40-1).

## Reducing Ischemia/Reperfusion Injury

Reducing ischemia/reperfusion injury to allografts has multiple beneficial effects in clinical transplantation. Successful treatment would increase the number of organs available for transplantation, and improve early graft function. The process of reperfusion triggers an inflammatory process characterized by endothelial activation, complement deposition, cytokine release, and infiltration of inflammatory cells. The depletion of available adenosine triphosphate energy sources within the graft generates membrane

**TABLE 40-1**

## STRATEGIES FOR GENE THERAPY IN ORGAN TRANSPLANTATION

1. Reducing ischemia/reperfusion injury

2. Immunosuppressive strategies

   i. Altering alloantigens of the graft

      Hematopoietic chimerism

      Soluble MHC

      Induction of regulatory T cells

   ii. Blockade of antigen recognition

      Co-stimulatory pathways

      Dendritic cell maturation

      Death ligands

      Chemokines and chemokine receptors

   iii. Alloantibodies and complement as targets for gene therapy

3. Genetic approaches to improve long-term graft performance

potential alterations that cause cell swelling and damage. The production of oxygen-free radicals initiates intracellular signaling that can cause apoptotic cell death and reduced availability of nitric oxide. Ischemia/reperfusion stimulates the innate immune response, and complement has been shown to play an important role in the inflammatory response.

The complex cascade of mediators associated with ischemia/reperfusion injury offers multiple targets for gene therapy. Overexpression of antiapoptotic genes and free radical scavengers have protective effects as pretreatment of liver grafts with antiapoptotic Bcl-2 adenoviral vectors significantly decreased organ injury and apoptosis. Similarly, genetic modification of endothelial cells to express caspase-resistant Bcl-2 resulted in increased resistance to apoptosis and cytotoxic T-cell-mediated lysis. Expression of antiapoptotic proteins such as Bcl-xL and A20 may also have long-term effects as they prevented antibody-induced transplant atherosclerosis in cardiac allograft models. Genetic transfer of superoxide dismutase and heme oxygenase-1 results in the blockade of free radical production. Overexpression of heme oxygenase-1 or adenoviral-mediated expression of copper-zinc superoxide dismutase protects rat livers from ischemia/reperfusion-induced tissue damage and apoptosis. Increased manganese superoxide dismutase production via *ex vivo* adenoviral transfection has been shown to protect cardiac allografts from ischemia/reperfusion injury. Inhibition of complement activation during ischemia/reperfusion via genetic deletion of C3 or C4 complement components causes a significant reduction in skeletal muscle injury.

Genetic engineering strategies accomplishing the blockade of leukocyte adhesion have also been beneficial in reducing ischemia/reperfusion injury. Blockade of intercellular adhesion molecule (ICAM)-1, with the use of antisense oligonucleotides, leads to a reduction in rat cardiac allograft reperfusion injury. Increased gene expression of anti-inflammatory cytokines has also been shown to ameliorate the effects of ischemic reperfusion injury. Intratracheal adenoviral administration of IL-10-reduced lung ischemia/reperfusion injury and IL-13 adenoviral gene expression resulted in an increase in liver graft survival rates. Intramuscular

application of TGF-$\beta$1 adenoviral vector resulted in enhanced oxygenation and improved function of lung allografts.

## Immunosuppressive Strategies

The initiation of the immune response in transplant rejection is dependent on the recognition of alloantigens by T cells of the recipient, making alloantigens and the recognition process primary targets for gene therapy. MHC class I molecules are present on all nucleated cells, whereas MHC class II antigens are limited to B cells, activated T cells, monocytes, macrophages, Langerhans cells, DC, and endothelial and epithelial cells. The recipient T cells recognize donor alloantigens via two main pathways: direct and indirect. The direct pathway involves recognition by recipient CD4 and CD8 T cells of the donor MHC on donor APC. In the indirect pathway, the recipient APC present donor-derived MHC class I or II peptides in the context of self-MHC. In addition, for T cells to become fully activated and acquire effector function, such as the ability to produce cytokines, they must also receive signals from the interaction of co-stimulatory molecules expressed on their surface with ligands expressed on APC. Co-stimulatory molecule interactions can result in T-cell activation or inhibition. Modification of MHC allorecognition via gene therapy may lead to transplant tolerance.

## Altering Alloantigens of the Graft

Mixed host–donor hematopoietic cellular chimerism, induced by allogeneic bone marrow transplantation, is known to result in long-term stable donor-specific tolerance. Molecular chimerism involving the transfer of genes encoding allogeneic donor-type MHC proteins into autologous hematopoietic stem cells may also result in tolerance, without the complications associated with allogeneic bone marrow transplants. Modification of MHC gene expression by gene therapy allows for tolerance induction via molecular chimerism. Retroviral transduction of MHC class I antigens to autologous murine bone marrow cells results in a permanent state of molecular chimerism, which is specific for the transduced MHC, and has been associated with long-term acceptance of skin allografts. Hyporesponsiveness to allogeneic renal transplants has also been induced in pigs following induction of molecular chimerism. The mechanism by which induction of molecular chimerism induces CD8 T-cell tolerance has been recently elucidated using a T-cell receptor (TCR) transgenic mouse model. In this system, $H$-$2K^b$-specific TCR transgenic CD8 T cells underwent negative selection in the thymus after encountering bone-marrow-derived cells expressing the transduced MHC class I gene. Because central deletion of alloreactive T cells is the most stable form of tolerance, the proof that deletion occurs in molecular chimeras suggests that gene therapy can be used to permanently change the T-cell repertoire.

Soluble MHC antigens have immunosuppressive properties, and elevated levels of donor-specific soluble MHC are found in the circulation of recipients of spontaneously accepted liver allografts. Genetic modification of recipient lymphocytes to overexpress class I antigens has been shown to suppress the immune response in rat recipients, and elevated levels of donor-specific soluble MHC have been shown to inhibit anti-donor-immune responses in sensitized rats.

Subpopulations of CD4 T cells can suppress allograft rejection. These regulatory cells can be induced using a variety of approaches including administration of nondepleting anti-CD4 antibodies and exposure to a tolerizing antigen in the form of donor-specific transfusions. Treatment of immunocompetent mice with nondepleting anti-T-cell antibodies together with syngeneic bone marrow infected with adenoviruses carrying an allogeneic MHC class I gene can lead to the acceptance of fully allogeneic cardiac transplants. These experiments suggest that the use of gene transfer-modified bone marrow may be capable of inducing regulatory T cells that can inhibit the responses to the transduced gene product.

## Blockade of Antigen Recognition

The ability of naïve T cells to initiate an immune response is dependent on their interaction with APC, and DC are the most efficient APC. Following antigen capture, maturation of the DC occurs with presentation of the MHC-peptide complex. MHC–peptide complexes cluster with costimulatory molecules CD80, CD86, and CD40 and are thought to be critical in initiating TCR activation. Engagement of the TCR without additional co-stimulatory signaling leads to induction of T-cell anergy. Co-stimulatory blockade also enhances DC ability to induce T-cell apoptosis. Blockade of T-cell activation and the subsequent inflammatory process is critical to the prevention of allograft rejection.

Genetic modification of either DC or the graft to inhibit the engagement of the co-stimulatory molecules can potentially eliminate the need for immunosuppression. Various animal models based on antibody-mediated co-stimulatory blockade against CD28, CD80, CD154, CD40, and CTLA4 have led to varying degrees of donor-specific hyporesponsiveness. Combination of an anti-CD154 monoclonal antibody with donor-specific transfusion resulted in prolonged murine islet and cardiac allograft survival. Combinations of antibodies directed at multiple cell-surface costimulatory proteins prolong allograft survival more effectively than the blockade of a single molecule. The necessity of repeated doses to maintain the immunosuppressive effects, however, makes antibody-mediated blockade difficult; and thromboembolic complications in both humans and primates have been reported in association with the use of anti-CD154 antibody.

Blocking the interaction of CD28 with CD80 and CD86 using an immunoglobulin fusion protein containing the extracellular portion of CTLA-4 (CTLA-4Ig) can result in immunosuppression *in vivo* and prevent transplant rejection. Permanent acceptance, however, was associated with nonspecific inhibition of T-cell responses to unrelated third-party antigens. It appears, that transduction of CTLA-4Ig can result in systemic immunosuppression, and it may be detrimental to host immunity. To overcome this long-term immunosuppressive effect, adenovirus vectors carrying the gene-encoding CTLA-4Ig flanked by two *loxP* sequences were developed. Administration of this CTLA-4Ig gene construct in combination with adenoviruses carrying the gene-encoding Cre recombinase permitted excision of the CTLA-4Ig gene, terminating expression *in vivo* and *in vitro*. Pancreatic islets transplanted into the liver of mice receiving *loxP*-flanked adenovirus-encoded CTLA-4Ig remained functional 40 days after serum CTLA-4Ig was no longer detectable following Cre-mediated excision of the CTLA-4Ig gene. Cre-mediated deletion of CTLA-4Ig was associated with the restoration of responses to adenovirus, permitting control of the duration of immunosuppression.

Using the principal of costimulatory blockade, alternative approaches to antibody treatment were also developed. Bone marrow-derived DC can be modified to express CTLA4-Ig and impair allogeneic T-cell proliferation, and thus

induce alloantigen-specific hyporesponsiveness. *Ex vivo* treatment of rat islets with AdCTLA4-Ig protected the islets from alloimmune destruction in spontaneously diabetic BB rats.

Adenoviral-mediated transfer of the gene encoding CD40-Ig into rat livers resulted in long-term survival following transplantation into allogeneic recipients. Expression of CD40-Ig in rat cardiac transplants has also been shown to delay acute rejection. At early time points after transplantation there was nonspecific immunosuppression, but response to third-party alloantigens returned later along with donor-specific T-cell activity and chronic rejection. The development of chronic rejection suggests the need for additional therapeutic interventions.

T-cell activation can also be inhibited by preventing DC maturation as immature DC are poor stimulators of naïve T cells, and may induce alloantigen-specific hyporesponsiveness. IL-10, vitamin D, *ex vivo* expansion of cells in low-dose granulocyte-macrophage colony-stimulating factor (GM-CSF) medium, and TGF-β1 are known inhibitors of DC maturation. Genetic engineering that leads to increased TGF-β1 expression can maintain DC in an immature state. Transduction of rhesus monkey monocyte-derived DC with active rhesus TGF-β1 resulted in inhibition of in vitro CD4 and CD8 cellular proliferation. In rodents, genetic modification of donor-derived DC with Ad TGF-β1 has been reported to prolong cardiac allograft survival. The results obtained with cytokine-gene-transduced DC were similar to those obtained with transduced organs. Both result in modest increases in transplant survival.

Recently, rat DC were transfected with an adenoviral vector encoding a kinase-defective dominant negative form of IKK2 (dnIKK2) to block NF-kB activation. Since NF-kB is central to DC maturation, dnIKK2-DC acquired potent regulatory properties, inhibiting naïve T-cell proliferation toward allogeneic stimuli. Pretransplant infusion of allogeneic donor dnIKK2-DC prolonged the survival of a kidney allograft from the same allogeneic donor, without the need for immunosuppressive therapy.

Engagement of Fas (CD95) on the surface of T cells by Fas ligand (CD95L) leads to the induction of apoptosis in activated T cells. This process plays a role in the establishment of immunoprivileged sites, and may also be involved in the killing of CD4 T cells. DC genetically engineered to express CD95L on their surface are able to inhibit alloreactive T-cell proliferation *in vitro*, and a slight prolongation of cardiac graft survival following *in vivo* administration has also been demonstrated in rodents.

Chemokines and chemokine receptors may also be relevant targets for gene therapy. Chemokines are divided into four subfamilies (C, CC, CXC, and CX3C) based on the presence and positioning of their conserved cysteine residues. These small proteins are involved in the recruitment of hematopoietic cells to sites of inflammation, and as signaling mediators, regulate cell trafficking to maintain tissue homeostasis. The actions of chemokines are mediated through a large family of seven-transmembrane-spanning G-protein–coupled receptors. Cell-surface expression of these receptors varies from cell to cell, and cells may express multiple chemokine receptors. Many of these receptors tend to have promiscuous ligand binding specificity. In the early posttransplant period, chemokine production is triggered by tissue injury inflicted by the surgical procedure and ischemia/reperfusion. This leads to recruitment of macrophages and neutrophils, which is shortly followed by increased levels of chemokines directed at increasing trafficking of alloantigen-activated T cells into the graft. In transplantation, the use of gene therapy to alter the chemokine-signaling response is limited by the redundancy within the chemokine signaling system. Targeted deletions of chemokine receptors have been shown to delay allograft rejection. Viral proteins vMIP-II and MC148 with antagonistic properties against multiple CC and CXC chemokine receptors prevent acute allograft rejection. vMIP-II is a human herpes virus product that prevents chemokine receptor activation by blocking calcium signaling, whereas MC148 is a chemotaxis inhibitor. Injection of plasmid DNA encoding for these viral proteins prolonged cardiac graft survival.

## Targeting Alloantibodies and Complement Products

Formation of alloantibodies most frequently occurs in patients sensitized by prior transplants, transfusions, or pregnancies but can also develop in the nonsensitized transplant recipient by mechanisms not yet well understood. In patients with prior sensitization, the initial exposure to alloantigen leads to the development of alloreactive B cells that present donor-specific allopeptides on their MHC II complexes. Alloantibodies initiate complement-mediated destruction of the graft. Donor-specific antibodies trigger polymerization of C5–C9 complement molecules with formation of the cell membrane attack complex. Antibody-mediated cell toxicity can also occur by Fc receptor signaling of NK cells. Preformed antibodies and complement activation also play a role in the rejection of xenotransplants. Complement activation is the primary component of hyperacute rejection of xenogeneic organ transplants. Gene therapy strategies that reduce complement-mediated rejection include the use of soluble inhibitory complement receptors, such as sCR1 (a potent regulator of C3 and C5 activation), which has been shown to be beneficial in pig lung allotransplantation. Engineering of xenografts to express human membrane-associated proteins can also prevent complement-mediated rejection. Transfection of porcine endothelial cells with human CD59 protected the cells from complement-mediated destruction. Baboons transplanted with hearts derived from CD55-transgenic pigs were protected from hyperacute rejection.

## Genetic Approaches to Improve Long-Term Graft Performance

Chronic allograft dysfunction is a progressive decline of allograft function leading ultimately to allograft loss. In addition to persistent low-grade alloimmune responses, other nonimmune factors, such as ischemia/reperfusion injury, age, infection, and drug toxicity may contribute to the progressive deterioration of allografts. The deterioration and pattern of graft loss varies from organ to organ, in the kidney as tubular atrophy and fibrosis, in the lungs as bronchiolitis obliterans, in the liver as obliteration of the bile ducts, and in the heart as coronary artery arteriosclerosis. Vasculopathy and interstitial fibrosis are the most common and prominent histological features associated with graft failure. Injury to the vascular endothelial cells results in the release of various cytokines and growth factors (eg, FGF, VEGF, HGF and TGF-$\beta$1) that stimulate smooth muscle cell proliferation. Various gene therapy approaches have been used to prevent chronic allograft dysfunction. Costimulatory blockade has been shown to be beneficial, rats treated with AdCTLA4-Ig displayed a significant reduction in lung fibrosis and obstruction. Adenoviral-mediated expression of the immunosuppressive cytokine IL-10 also reduced the development of bronchiolitis obliterans, whereas inhibition of ICAM-1 by antisense oligonucleotides reduced intimal hyperplasia and vascular occlusion of rat cardiac

allografts. Up-regulation of inducible nitric oxide synthase by adenoviral vectors protects aortic allografts from the development of arteriosclerosis.

## GENE THERAPY IN TISSUE AND CELL TRANSPLANTATION

### Islet Transplantation

Type 1 diabetes results from insulin deficiency caused by autoimmune destruction of insulin-producing pancreatic cells. Islet transplantation, $\beta$-cell regeneration, and insulin gene therapy have been explored in attempts to cure type 1 diabetes. Significant improvements in islet isolation technology and less toxic immunosuppressive drug regimes are critical for success. The limited availability of human islets from cadaveric organs can be addressed by using islet growth factors to increase -cell replication, to improve -cell function, and to enhance -cell survival. Transgenic mice overexpressing hepatocyte growth factor (HGF) in the pancreatic -cell display increased -cell proliferation, function, and survival. Their islets markedly improve transplant performance in severe combined immunodeficiency (SCID) mice and reduce the number of islets necessary for successful islet transplantation. Adenoviral-mediated gene transfer of HGF into normal rodent islets also has been shown to be beneficial in different marginal mass islet transplant models. Human vascular endothelial growth factor (hVEGF) gene delivery has the potential to improve islet survival by promoting revascularization. Transfection of hVEGF to murine islet grafts resulted in increased insulin release in response to glucose. Immunohistochemical staining of transplanted islets suggested that the islets were functional, and there was new blood vessel formation.

The persisting hostile $\beta$-cell-specific autoimmune response remains a major clinical challenge. Insulin gene therapy might be helpful with respect to vulnerability to autoimmune attack. This method replaces the function of cells by introducing various components of the insulin synthetic and secretory machinery into non-cells, which are less likely to be targets of -cell-specific autoimmune responses. Additionally, gene transfer of immunoregulatory molecules such as soluble type 1 tumor necrosis factor receptor (TNFR) immunoglobulin-Fc fusion transgene (TNFR-Ig) may protect islets from cytokine-induced apoptosis. TNFR-Ig transgenic islets were protected from cytokine-induced apoptosis in culture, and diabetic mice transplanted with islets expressing TNFR-Ig returned to and maintained normoglycemia significantly longer than untransduced islet recipients. Although there is no perfect solution for the cure of type 1 diabetes at the present time, research on a variety of potential strategies may offer a multilayered approach to the cure of type 1 diabetes.

### Stem Cells

Stem cells are defined by their capacity for limitless self-renewal and multilineage differentiation. These unique characteristics may allow their use to treat a broad spectrum of human diseases. Hematopoietic stem cells (HSC) can reconstitute the entire blood system, and bone marrow transplantation (BMT) has long been used in the clinic to treat various diseases. The transplantation of other tissue specific stem cells, such as those isolated from epithelial and neural tissues, could replace damaged epithelial and neural cells. An alternative to tissue-specific stem cell therapy takes advantage of embryonic stem (ES) cells, which are capable of differentiating into any tissue type. Nuclear transfer, the transfer of a postmitotic somatic cell nucleus into an enucleated oocyte, creates a limitless source of autologous cells that are similar to ES cells and when combined with gene therapy can serve as a powerful therapeutic tool.

## Adult Stem Cells

The presence of HSC in the bone marrow of humans led to the use of BMT to treat patients afflicted with cancer and inherited diseases including immune deficiencies, metabolic diseases, and hemoglobinopathies. HSCs are isolated to 85% to 95% purity using cell-surface markers, ensuring proper dosage. The transplantation regimen must eradicate abnormal cells, suppress the immune response of the recipient to prevent donor cell rejection, and create space for the newly transplanted cells. Chemotherapy and/or radiation eradicate abnormal cells and suppress the immune system. The donor marrow degree of matching to the recipient affects both the chance of graft rejection and graft-versus-host disease (GVHD).

HSC are excellent targets for gene therapy because of their capacity for self-renewal and multilineage differentiation. The first example of a gene therapy trial in humans was performed in SCID disease. CD34 cells were infected *ex vivo* with a retrovirus containing the gene for the γ-chain of the common cytokine receptor complex and transplanted into SCID patients. This created a functional immune system with detectable functional B and T cells 8 months after transplantation. A major risk associated with retrovirus-mediated gene transfer is caused by the insertion of the retrovirus into proto-oncogenes resulting in acute lymphocytic leukemia in some patients. The leukemic cells contained a viral insertion near the LMO2 site on chromosome 11, which is a known oncogene activated by translocations. From these results has come the realization that each gene transfer attempt must be closely monitored for insertional mutagenesis. A recent report further demonstrates that there were two separate insertions in the tumor cells, one near LMO2 and one near the γ-c gene, which acted as collaborating oncogenes. Therefore, the leukemias were probably caused by a double hit, and this vector may be prone to insertional mutagenesis at oncogenes.

A novel approach to treat HIV infection is the introduction of antiviral genes in HSC stem cells, and thereby control of HIV replication and the progression to AIDS. These antiviral genes could create a host cell population that is specifically resistant to HIV infection. Current gene therapy clinical trials have established the safety of gene therapy of HIV-1 infection. Several issues remain to be resolved, including increasing the efficiency of HSC transduction as well as better understanding of the high turnover of CD4 cells in HIV-infected patients.

Epidermal stem cells can be easily harvested and expanded and may provide a more efficient therapy in a broad array of diseases and injuries. Skin epithelial stem cells have already proven useful in the clinical practice as they have been removed from patients, cultured to form epithelial sheets, and then reapplied to burns, wounds, and ulcers. Purification is difficult, as their characterization is limited to the expression of cell-adhesion molecules.

Epithelial stem cells could treat genetic diseases affecting the skin. Cultured epithelial stem cells from individuals suffering from recessive dystrophic epidermolysis bullosa, a disease caused by mutations in the collagen VII (COL7A1) gene, were corrected by genomic integration and transplanted into immunodeficient mice. The transplanted cells maintained the corrected gene expression

suggesting that skin disorders caused by genetic lesions may be corrected by *ex vivo* strategies through nonviral and lentiviral approaches.

Neural stem (NS) cells have been isolated from both central and peripheral adult nervous systems, and these populations can generate neurons and glia. Transplantation of enriched neural populations has shown clinical utility in neurological disorders including Parkinson's disease. Ventral midbrain tissue containing dopaminergic neurons extracted from 7- to 8-week-old human embryos is capable of establishing functional synapses, and increased the number of surviving dopaminergic neurons, often resulting in alleviation of symptoms. In a double-blind study, most patients showed long-term survival of dopaminergic neurons, although the clinical benefit was questionable.

Genetic modification of NS cells recently has attracted interest in terms of their therapeutic potential in neurological diseases and tumors. C17.2, an immortalized mouse NS cell line was transduced with two enzymes (tyrosine hydroxylase [TH] and GTP cyclohydrolase 1 [GTPCH1]) involved in dopamine biosynthesis. Implantation of the transduced C17.2 cells into the striata of parkinsonian rats lead to an improvement in amphetamine-induced turning behavior compared with controls, indicating that genetically modified NS cells grafted into the brain are capable of survival, migration, and neuronal differentiation. The ability of genetically engineered NS to migrate toward a tumor mass can be used for the treatment of gliomas. NS cells transduced with the herpes simplex virus-thymidine kinase (HSVtk) gene (NStk) were intracranially co-implanted in athymic nude mice and rats along with C6 rat glioma cells. A potent bystander effect was observed as animals treated with ganciclovir (GCV) following co-implantation survived more than 100 days, whereas those treated with saline died of tumor progression. NStk cells were also injected into the preexisting C6 tumors, and treatment with GCV resulted in significant tumor regression.

Although the pancreas exhibits limited cell turnover, an endogenous source of stem cells able to regenerate pancreatic insulin-secreting cells has been suggested. The insulin-secreting islets that modulate glucose levels in humans are destroyed by autoimmune attack in type I diabetes. The replenishment of pancreatic β-cell populations is accompanied by endogenous insulin secretion; therefore, the isolation of stem cells in the pancreas that can produce new β-cells could lead to a cure for type I diabetes. Genetic strategies for manipulation of these cells would be similar to those used for mature islets as noted above.

## Embryonic Stem Cells

The problems associated with transplantation of tissue-specific stem cells, including isolation, limited quantities, and the questionable existence of tissue-specific stem cells for some adult organs, may be circumvented by the use of ES cells. These cells have the potential to differentiate down specific lineages used for cell-replacement therapy. ES cells can be directed to differentiate into hematopoietic precursors capable of long-term reconstitution in irradiated mice. ES cells transplanted into patients, however, carry the risk of tumor formation, reinforcing the need for directed differentiation strategies. Normal expansion of ES cells into HSC can be achieved by introducing the homeobox gene *HoxB4*, and animals engrafted with *HoxB4*-expressing cells showed long-term reconstitution of HSC.

ES-cell-derived HSC may be of greater clinical use than BMT. The generation of ES cell lines ensures a standardized stock of cells, whereas bone marrow, despite marrow banks, may be in short supply. Bone-marrow-derived HSC may also accumulate defects as a result of aging, leading to decreased long-term survival. The advantages of deriving HSC from ES support the development of methods to manipulate ES cells to differentiate into HSC and other tissue specific stem cells.

Nurr1 is a transcription factor critical for the development of midbrain dopaminergic (DA) neurons. Mouse ES can be engineered to constitutively express Nurr1 under the elongation factor-1 alpha promoter, leading to up-regulation of DA neuronal markers, and a four- to fivefold increase in the proportion of DA neurons. These neurons represent a midbrain neuronal phenotype, demonstrating that genetic manipulation of ES cells with key transcription factor facilitates differentiation to midbrain DA neurons.

Gene therapy has led to reconsideration of standard therapies for cardiac disease such as the cardiac pacemaker, which has been used in both high-degree heart block and sinoatrial node dysfunction. Gene therapy has been used to explore the overexpression of β2-adrenergic receptors, the down-regulation of inward rectifier current, and the overexpression of pacemaker current as potential sources of biological pacemakers.

ES-derived cells also offer a strategy for overcoming immunological barriers and the need for lifelong immunosuppression. Co-transplantation of HSC along with the tissue of choice can induce lifelong tolerance to grafts in mouse models.

## FUTURE DIRECTIONS AND CHALLENGES

The discussion has highlighted many exciting possibilities and challenges for gene transfer and gene therapy, not only for solid organ transplantation but also for virtually all other applications of these modalities. The first challenge is the search for the right vector. This vector must be high capacity, high transduction or transfection efficiency, low immunogenicity, low inflammatory potential, regulatable, persistent, nononcogenic, and nonmutagenic. The genetic material delivered must be long lasting, specific to the needs of the disease entity, and have no adverse consequences with regard to specific integration sites and replicative potential, whether it is genomic or remains episomal. The second major challenge is to understand what constitutes the innate immune response to transfer vectors and how this innate response may be regulated, prevented, or channeled in a direction appropriate for gene expression, while ensuring organ function and survival, without stimulation of the adaptive immune response. It has only recently become widely recognized that innate immunity is perhaps the greatest barrier to all applications of gene therapy, because all cells possess a variety of molecular mechanisms that degrade, subvert, or otherwise prevent incorporation and expression of exogenous nucleic sequences. A third major challenge is to devise the appropriate immunosuppressive strategy to achieve localized immunosuppression and/or tolerance. Our knowledge and understanding of immunity and tolerance suggest that simple blockade of T-cell receptors or co-stimulatory receptors, or the inhibition of a few major cytokines or chemokines will not ensure prolonged graft survival or tolerance. Other than strategies that promote bone marrow chimerism, it is not yet clear how effective immunosuppression or tolerance will yet be achieved with gene transfer and gene therapy. Indeed, this challenge questions our assumption that local immunosuppression by the transfer of one or a few immunosuppressive genes will be adequate for solid organ transplantation. We must question our assumptions and determine if regional immunosuppression, or perhaps even a brief period of systemic immunosuppression, is required for tolerization. As is outlined in other chapters in this section of the book, the development of tissue engineering, therapeutic cloning, and embryonic stem cells will present alternative opportunities for genetic therapy and manipulation that may prove more tractable from an immunologic standpoint, particularly if these cells and tissues are autologous and syngeneic.

## References

1. Carter BJ. Adeno-associated virus vectors in clinical trials. *Hum Gene Ther* 2005;16:541–550.
2. Ryther RCC, Flynt AS, Phillips JA III, et al. siRNA therapeutics: big potential from small RNAs. *Gene Ther* 2005;12: 5–11.
3. Kafri T. Air-conditioning for regulated transgene expression. *Gene Ther* 2005;12:383–385.
4. Bessis N, GarciaCozar FJ, Boissier MC. Immune responses to gene therapy vectors: influence on vector function and effector mechanisms. *Gene Ther* 2004;11:S10–S17.
5. Judge AD, Sood V, Shaw JR, et al. Sequence-dependent stimulation of the mammalian innate immune response by synthetic siRNA. *Nat Biotech* 2005;23:457–462.
6. Bagley J, Iacomini J. Gene therapy progress and prospects: gene therapy in organ transplantation. *Gene Ther* 2003;10:605.
7. Prockop DJ, Gregory CA, Spees JL. One strategy for cell and gene therapy: harnessing the power of adult stem cells to repair tissues. *Proc Natl Acad Sci USA* 2003;100;1917.
8. Wong W, Wood KJ. Transplantation tolerance by donor MHC gene transfer. *Curr Gene Ther* 2004;4:329.
9. Imai E, Takabatake Y, Mizui M, et al: Gene therapy in renal diseases. *Kidney Int.* 65:1551, 2004.
10. Tian C, Bagley J, Cretin N, et al. Prevention of type 1 diabetes by gene therapy. *J Clin Invest.* 2004;114:969.
11. Bottino R, Lemarchand P, Trucco M, et al. Gene- and cell-based therapeutics for type I diabetes mellitus. *Gene Ther* 2003;10:875.

# CHAPTER 41

# ORGANOGENESIS AND CLONING

*Marilia Cascalho, MD, PhD, Brenda M. Ogle, PhD, Jeffrey L. Platt, MD*

## INTRODUCTION

No advance in medicine and surgery has sparked more excitement and offered more promise than organ transplantation. The first attempts at organ transplantation in the early years of the 20th century were greeted with extraordinary celebration. Although these transplants functioned only for periods of days to weeks, Alexis Carrell was awarded the Nobel Prize in 1912 for the "successful" transplantation of the kidney.[1] But true and enduring success in transplantation and clinical application had to await the discovery of drugs that would suppress the immune response of the recipient against the graft. Today, with increasingly effective immunosuppressive therapy, transplantation of the heart, liver, lung, or kidney (and some would add the pancreas) is considered the preferred therapy for organ failure. Indeed, transplantation not only corrects devastating pathophysiology but also potentially reverses disability and prolongs life.

Yet, for all of the excitement and promise it generates, organ transplantation has had only a fraction of the impact on human health that might seem possible. What limits the success and the impact of organ transplantation are first the limited availability of organs for transplantation and second the need to suppress the function of the immune system of the recipient to prevent rejection of the graft. In this chapter we discuss how certain new technologies, organogenesis and cloning, might be exploited to overcome the limitations of organ transplantation and thus to allow organ replacement to achieve the full potential envisioned during the past century.

## THE NEED FOR ORGAN REPLACEMENT

Before we consider how new technologies might be applied for the replacement of organ function, it is fitting to consider whether the need for organ replacement might change in one direction or another over time. One might imagine that rapid advances in biomedical knowledge, engineering, and technologies eventuate the cure or even the prevention of some of the diseases that today call for organ transplantation as the last resort. For example, the development of a vaccine or immunotherapy for the prevention or treatment of insulin-dependent diabetes would abolish much of the demand for pancreas transplantation and some demand for kidney transplantation. Development of an effective vaccine for hepatitis C might potentially eradicate the major indication for liver transplantation. If these examples were to be extended, one might be forgiven for questioning whether organ transplantation will occupy such an important place in the treatment of diseases in the future.

Despite these considerations, we think the demand for organ replacement may very well increase over time.[2,3] Advances in therapeutics will probably lead to progressive improvements in longevity, and these improvements will increase the prevalence of type 2 diabetes and of failure of the kidney and heart, all of which increase with age. Furthermore, some of the advances will allow early diagnosis of diseases such as cancer, renal, cardiac, or pulmonary failure that might be treated preemptively by removing and replacing the affected organ with a transplanted healthy one. However, preemptive indications for transplantation will be eclipsed by the imperative to treat organ failure, except for organs obtained from living donors. Finally, new indications for transplantation may emerge or become apparent. Thus, unforeseen epidemics, environmental catastrophes, and use of transplantation to address metabolic disorders could extend the indications and demand for transplantation well beyond current use.[2,3]

To meet what may be new indications for transplantation and to provide effective preemptive therapy, the ideal transplant must function at a normal level (not simply at a level that is better than the failed organ), and it must be deliverable without ongoing immunosuppression. Neither of these objectives can be achieved by organ allotransplantation as currently practiced. Perhaps the ideal transplant is most likely to be provided by continued improvements in immunosuppression or development of approaches to inducing immunologic tolerance and/or by treatments that would improve graft function. We shall consider, however, an alternative if more remote scenario that the ideal approach to organ replacement can be achieved by application of cloning and organogenesis.

## CLONING

The word "clone" derives from a Greek word, *klon*, meaning twig. Clone was originally used to refer to the offspring of plants, derived by asexual reproduction. As used in biology and medicine, clone refers to a genetically identical cell or cells derived from one parental cell or from one individual (or identical gene sequences derived from one sequence). Lower vertebrates have been cloned by parthenogenesis; however, until recently, higher animals, particularly mammals, were thought to derive exclusively from sexual reproduction. As we shall presently discuss, cloning generates pluripotential stem cells and potentially solves several of the challenges of transplantation—the derivation of cells that are genetically identical to and thus histocompatible with a parental cell and the generation of stem cells capable of proliferation and differentiation.

The concept of cloning can be traced over 100 years. In the early 20th century, Hans Spemann showed that one primitive cell type could direct the development of more mature tissues. Later Spemann performed the first nuclear cloning by transferring the nucleus from a cell of the salamander embryo to a cell in which the cytoplasm had been isolated by literally constricting the non-nuclear part of the cell. In the early 1980s, nuclear transfer was used by others to show that the nucleus of an embryonic cell could direct the development of an enucleated egg, zygote, or early-stage embryo. Since then, cloning has been approached by transferring the nucleus of the cell or individual to be cloned to a primitive recipient cell. In 1997, Wilmut et al. produced Dolly, the first mammal cloned from a cell from a mature individual.

## Cloning in Current Practice

Cloning is generally carried out by removing the nucleus from cells of the individual to be cloned and injecting the nucleus into an enucleated immature cell from another individual. Among the immature cells used in cloning are eggs, zygotes and cells from early stage embryos.[4] Once inside an immature cell, the nucleus is "reprogrammed," which is to say modifications that limit the potential of the nucleus are removed and the newly generated cell begins to proliferate.[2,5] Complete reprogramming of the nucleus probably occurs during the course of several cell divisions so that the cluster of proliferating cells has the potential to become any cell in the body, which is to say it is pluripotential.[6]

The generation of cloned mammals demonstrated that the nuclei of relatively mature cells have not undergone irreversible changes with differentiation. This point was ultimately proved when Hochedlinger and Jaenisch showed that the nucleus of a lymphocyte with rearranged receptor DNA can generate a living animal.[7]

Cloning accomplishes several important objectives that could contribute to a solution to the replacement of organs. First, cloning allows the chromosomal DNA of a given individual to be used to generate new cells. For example, if the cells of a patient were used as the source of nuclei for cloning, the resulting cells would have the same genes of the major histocompatibility locus, and most minor loci as the patient. Second, the reprogrammed cells behave like embryonic stem cells, which is to say they are capable of extensive proliferation and have the capacity to form any cell in the body. In fact the generation and breeding of Dolly proved that the stem cells formed by nuclear transfer could become any cell including germ cells that thus could potentially generate a line of related individuals.

The feasibility of obtaining pluripotential stem cells by nuclear cloning was demonstrated by recent successes in cloning large animals[8] (reproductive cloning). Cloning was carried out by transfer of the nucleus from a somatic cell to a recipient enucleated cell capable of reverting the epigenetic modifications of chromatin characteristic of the differentiated state. The molecular basis for reprogramming of chromatin to allow de-differentiation and subsequent re-differentiation has only now begun to be understood. A provocative report suggests that faulty imprinting of such genes as Igf2, Igf2r, and H19 in the extra-embryonic tissue rather than in the embryo may underlie low efficiency in cloning.[9]

Cloning is sometimes referred to as "reproductive" or "therapeutic," depending on the use made of the cloned cells. If the cloned cells are used to generate intact animals, the cloning is reproductive cloning; if the cloned cells are grown in culture to generate a specific type of tissue, the cloning is called "therapeutic"

(implying that the cells grown in this way might be of some clinical benefit, which is yet to be proved). Despite the different uses made of cloned cells, the techniques for reproductive and therapeutic cloning are generally the same.

Recent studies have suggested that efficiency in generating blastocysts by nuclear transfer may be inversely related to the state of differentiation of the donor nucleus source.[9] Successful therapeutic cloning for functional tissue engineering does not require the orchestration of gene expression needed for development of the body plan, and faulty reprogramming and accumulation of mutations may not preclude use of nuclear transfer to generate new tissues. One critical advantage of therapeutic cloning is that tissues or cells so derived are genetically similar to the source of the nuclei.

Although reproductive cloning and therapeutic cloning are carried out in the same way, they have profoundly different ethical and biological implications. From an ethical perspective, many would oppose the use of cloning for reproduction of people (the cloned offspring would be identical or nearly so to the nucleus donor); fewer oppose use for generation of stem cells. Some oppose both types of cloning because both involve the generation and destruction of an early stage embryo (ie, the proliferating cells generated by nuclear transfer). From a biological perspective, reproductive cloning is an imperfect and inefficient way to generate new individuals—cloned animals are found to have various defects that compromise well-being and survival.[4] On the other hand, tissues generated from cloned cells are not known to be less functional than tissues generated with embryonic stem cells. Probably, the errors from DNA replication and possibly acquired defects limit the ability of the cloned cells for generating all tissues and organs much more than one given tissue or organ.

## The Limitations of Cloning

Cloning is not applied today for clinical therapeutics, much less for human reproduction. Besides the ethical problems mentioned above and the possibility that a whole organism produced by cloning would suffer defects, there are several important limitations. Reproductive cloning is intrinsically inefficient. In mice, only 0.5% to 2% of implanted blastocysts lead to newborn animals.[10] Part of the reason for loss of efficiency is that creation of a new individual requires recapitulation of early embryogenesis and, thus, reprogramming of the chromatin to revert the epigenetic alterations of differentiation: (1) silencing of differentiated transcripts, (2) activation of early genes, (3) reactivation of both X chromosomes in female nuclei, (4) maintenance of imprinting of the maternal and paternal chromosomes, and (5) the reversal of shortened telomeres. While these events may occur, allowing development to adulthood,[10] reprogramming, as such, is often faulty. In addition, the nuclei used to generate embryos may have accumulated mutations that preclude normal development. Another limitation of cloning and a limitation pertinent to therapeutic cloning is that the enucleated egg, zygote, or early embryonic cell used for reprogramming comes from an individual other than the patient to be treated, and it will have mitochondria and hence mitochondrial DNA foreign to that patient. Hence the reconstructed cells will not be fully identical genetically with the patient. Because mitochondrial DNA encodes several minor histocompatibility antigens, the tissues or organs generated from those cells may be immunogenic. The extent to which such tissues are immunogenic has not been thoroughly explored. Preliminary studies in a large animal system have failed to reveal immune responses,[11] but whether that system can predict no response in humans is uncertain.

Other limitations of cloning are that it is inefficient, as already mentioned, and expensive. Cloning has been conducted for experimental applications and it can be used to generate lines of animals of value for research or commercial purposes. However, widespread application of nuclear transfer would require development of new facilities, training of personnel, and the carrying out of additional labor-intensive procedures for each person to be treated.

The most difficult limitation of cloning stems from the question of how the cells would be used. If one wants to replace the function of complex organs, one must focus on technologies that can provide whole organs, not just tissues. A tissue such as lung or kidney tissue might make a nice illustration, but it would hardly help support the physiology of a person. Later we shall consider how stem cells might be used to generate intact organs, but for the moment we should point out that no technology available today could begin to produce a whole organ from stems cells without producing an intact organism, that is, without having to perform reproductive cloning to generate fetal cells.

## The Future of Cloning

While the barriers to application of cloning may seem to be considerable, some of these barriers may soon be overcome. Hansis et al[6] recently reported that extracts prepared from frog eggs and early-stage frog embryos can partially reprogram mature human cells. Particularly important for inducing reprogramming was BRG1, an ATPase involved in remodeling of chromatin. These preliminary findings suggest to us that a set of cloning factors might be identified, which when applied to mature cells will drive reprogramming of the cells. Were such factors to be identified, some of the more challenging problems associated with cloning might be overcome. First, by using cloning factors (or extracts), one does not transmit mitochondrial DNA and hence the expression of minor antigens encoded by mitochondrial DNA is avoided. Second, the use of factors or extracts avoids nuclear transfer, the most difficult and expensive step in cloning, and thus might allow the procedure to be applied much more widely than possible to this point. Finally, because the reprogrammed cells still lack the full potential of embryos generated by nuclear transfer, the cells probably lack the ability to become a whole, intact organism and hence bypass the ethical problems associated with nuclear cloning. However, the problem of how to generate whole organs remains to be solved. As we shall, see this problem might succumb to organogenesis.

## ORGANOGENESIS

Organogenesis refers to the stage or period in fetal development when organs form. In humans this period spans weeks 9 through 20 of fetal life; in the mouse this period spans days 11 through 16. Because some organs continue to develop during the later period of fetal life and even after birth, these periods really represent the times during which organ development begins.

Tissues removed from a fetus at a suitable point in development can mature spontaneously in culture or can be driven to mature by a suitable inducing stimulus. For example, Grobstein[12] reported more than 50 years ago that nephrogenic mesenchyme from the genital ridge of a chick can be induced by tubular epithelium to undergo nephrogenesis. Similar systems were used to study the lung, liver, and pancreas.[13] Tissues that can develop spontaneously are being removed from the fetus are said to be "specified." Once specified, a tissue might in principle be grown to generate an organ. Human embryonic stem cells have been coaxed to form organotypic tissues, such as kidney.[14]

Two factors limit this approach to organogenesis. First the size of tissues (or organs) that can be grown in culture is quite small. Although one might imagine using matrices to grow a large mass of cells such as hepatocytes that would provide a metabolic function, the three-dimensional structure of the kidney, heart, and lungs would preclude achieving a physiological size at least with existing technologies. Second, tissues grown in culture lack blood vessels.[15] Thus, methods of cell culture do not allow the formation of physiologically relevant organs.

Some of the limitations of *in vitro* organogenesis might be circumvented if organogenesis could be carried out *in vivo*. Indeed, fetal tissues of various types have been found to mature after implantation into adult animals.[16–21] Organs grown in this way might achieve physiologic size (although to date they have not) because the organs are vascularized by in-growth of blood vessels of the "recipient."

If organogenesis is to be applied for the treatment of disease in people, the major question that must be addressed is the source of cells to be used. Human fetal cells probably will not be used because of ethical concerns. Even if those concerns were addressed, the cells would be allogeneic with respect to the person to be treated. Later we discuss the possibility of using cloned cells to address this problem.

## Limitations of Organogenesis

Besides identifying a suitable source of cells that could be used to grow an organ, the main challenge of organogenesis is identifying the conditions in which an organ can be grown. Growing an organ *de novo* in an individual with severe disease might be difficult because the organ would draw on the metabolism and oxygen supply of the treated individual. Although diverting nutrients and oxygen to a growing organ and generating more waste might not challenge the well-being of a normal individual, it might be difficult for those with organ failure. Furthermore, the normal development of some organs, such as the lung, requires the microenvironment of the fetus.

## The Future of Organogenesis

We have proposed that some of the limitations of organogenesis could be overcome if organogenesis were carried out using an animal as a temporary recipient for the human cells.[22] Thus, human stem cells could be introduced into fetal animals in which the local microenvironment supports and directs the development of the organ of interest. One limitation to applying this approach is that the temporary graft of human cells might be subject to immune-mediated injury.[23] This problem could be overcome by using immunodeficient animals as temporary hosts. The use of a temporary host for organogenesis does, however, engender another problem: the blood vessels in the organ derive from the animal host[16] and on transfer to a human, these blood vessels would be subject to vascular rejection.[24] Unless vascular rejection is avoided, for example, by genetic engineering,[25] or unless human blood vessels can be induced to grow,[26] this problem may limit application of organogenesis as it has organ xenotransplantation. However, as we discuss next, those organs such as the kidney and pancreas that can potentially be grown from isolated cells to treat conditions (renal failure and diabetes) for which alternative therapies can compensate for some metabolic stress might be induced in a foreign host and then grown in the patient.

## Fusion of Technologies for the Replacement of Organ Function

For some time we have thought that no one technology—cloning, stem cells, tissue engineering, building of devices or xenotransplantation—can provide the ideal approach to replacing organ function.[2,27,29] Instead, we think the solution is likely to come from the combining of two or more strategies to address the limitations and hurdles of each strategy. In this chapter, we have considered how cloning and organogenesis might be applied some day for the replacing of organ function. In this closing section we consider how the two technologies might be optimally combined.

As one future approach to organ replacement, we envision the following steps might be undertaken. First, somatic cells from the patient would be cloned, preferably by treating those cells with cloning factors. Cloning will reprogram the nuclei of the treated cells so the cells can proliferate and differentiate into many different tissues.

Second, the cloned cells might be introduced into fetal animals in which induction and cell–cell and matrix interactions would generate fetal organs. We have recently found that human bone marrow cells after administration to a fetus can develop as part of fetal organs and contribute to mature tissues.[30]

Third, the "human" fetal organs grown in animals would be harvested and the induced human cells would be isolated and transferred back into the person from whose cells the cloned cells derived. Kidney, pancreas, and liver might then be allowed to grow in the patient. This strategy will not suffice for the lung because, as explained above, the development of normal lung outside the thorax of the fetus has not been achieved. Replacement of the lung will thus require other technologies. One potential approach that might be pursued would involve the use of vascular precursor cells grown from the cloned cells to populate the lung with human blood vessels. Also uncertain is whether and how this approach could be used to replace the heart. At present, one can envision growing cardiac muscle cells and cardiac tissue in a foreign host (or in the patient), but growing of an intact heart remains to be accomplished.

## ACKNOWLEDGMENT

Work in the authors' laboratories is supported by grants from the National Institutes of Health.

## References

1. Carrel A. Transplantation in mass of the kidneys. *J Exp Med* 1980; 10:98–140.

2. Cascalho M, Platt J. New technologies for organ replacement and augmentation. *Mayo Clin Proc* 2005;80:370–378.

3. Cascalho M, Ogle BM, Platt JL. Emerging strategies in kidney transplantation. In: Pereira BJG, Sayegh MH, Blake P, eds. *Chronic Kidney Disease, Dialysis, and Transplantation* Elsevier: Philadelphia, 2005: 750–758.

4. Hochedlinger K, Jaenisch R. Nuclear transplantation, embryonic stem cells, and the potential for cell therapy. *New Engl J Med* 2003;349: 275–286.

5. Pomerantz J, Blau HM. Nuclear reprogramming: a key to stem cell function in regenerative medicine. *Nat Cell Biol* 2004;6:810–816.

6. Hansis C, Barreto G, Maltry N, et al. Nuclear reprogramming of human somatic cells by xenopus egg extract requires BRG1. *Curr Biol* 2004;14:1475–1480.

7. Rossant J. A monoclonal mouse? *Nature* 2002;415:967–969.

8. Wilmut I, Schnieke AE, McWhir J, et al. Viable offspring derived from fetal and adult mammalian cells. *Nature* 1997;385:810–813.

9. Humpherys D, Eggan K, Akutsu H, et al. Abnormal gene expression in cloned mice derived from embryonic stem cell and cumulus cell nuclei. *Proc Natl Acad Sci USA* 2002;99:12889–12894.

10. Rideout III WM, Eggan K, Jaenisch R. Nuclear cloning and epigenetic reprogramming of the genome. *Science* 2001;293:1093–1098.

11. Lanza RP, Chung HY, Yoo JJ, et al. Generation of histocompatible tissues using nuclear transplantation. *Nat Biotechnol* 2002;20:689–696.

12. Grobstein C. Inductive epithelio-mesenchymal interaction in cultured organ rudiments of the mouse. *Science* 1953;118:52–55.

13. Bernfield M, Banerjee SD, Koda JE, et al. Remodelling of the basement membrane: morphogenesis and maturation. *CIBA Found Symp* 1984;108:179–197.

14. Thomson JA, Itskovitz-Eldor J, Shapiro SS, et al. Embryonic stem cell lines derived from human blastocysts. *Science* 1998;282:1145–1147.

15. Ekblom P. Formation of basement membranes in the embryonic kidney: an immunohistological study. *J. Cell Biol* 1981;91:1–10.

16. Sariola H. Interspecies Chimeras: An experimental approach for studies on embryonic angiogenesis. *Med Biol* 1985;63:43–65.

17. Dekel B, Burakova T, Ben-Hur H, et al. Engraftment of human kidney tissue in rat radiation chimera: II. Human fetal kidneys display reduced immunogenicity to adoptively transferred human peripheral blood mononuclear cells and exhibit rapid growth and development. *Transplantation* 1997;64:1550–1558.

18. Rogers SA, Lowell JA, Hammerman NA, et al. Transplantation of developing metanephroi into adult rats. *Kidney Int* 1998;54:27–37.

19. Rogers SA, Hammerman MR. Transplantation of rat metanephroi into mice. *Am J Physiol* 2001;280:R1865–R1869.

20. Hammerman MR. Transplantation of embryonic organs. *Am J Transplant* 2004;4(Suppl 6):14–24.

21. Dekel B, Burakova T, Arditti FD, et al. Human and porcine early kidney precursors as a new source for transplantation. *Nat Med* 2003;9: 53–60.

22. Cascalho M, Platt JL. Xenotransplantation and other means of organ replacement. *Nat. Rev Immunol* 2001;1:154–160.

23. Dekel B, Marcus H, Herzel BH, et al. In vivo modulation of the allogeneic immune response by human fetal kidneys: the role of cytokines, chemokines, and cytolytic effector molecules. *Transplantation* 2000;69:1470–1478.

24. Cascalho M, Platt JL. The immunological barrier to xenotransplantation. *Immunity* 2001;14:437–446.

25. Ogle BM, Platt JL: Genetic therapies and xenotransplantation. *Expert Opin Biol Ther* 2002;2:299–310.

26. Kocher AA, Schuster MD, Szabolcs MJ, et al. Neovascularization of ischemic myocardium by human bone-marrow-derived angioblasts prevents cardiomyocyte apoptosis reduces remodeling and improves cardiac function. *Nat Med* 2001; 7:430–436.

27. Cascalho M, Ogle BM, Platt JL. New approaches to replacing failing organs. *Transplant Proc* 2004;36:1629.

28. Ogle BM, Cascalho M, Platt JL. Fusion of approaches to the treatment of organ failure. *Am J Transplant* 4(Suppl 6):74–77.

29. Cascalho M, Ogle BM, Platt JL. Xenotransplantation and the future of renal replacement. *J Am Soc Nephrol* 2004;15:1106–1112.

30. Ogle BM, Butters KB, Plummer TB, et al. Spontaneous fusion of cells between species yields transdifferentiation and retroviral in vivo. *FASEB J* 2004;18:548–550.

# INDEX

Page numbers followed by f indicate figures; numbers followed by t indicate tables.
LD, living donor.